BRADY

INTERMEDIATE EMERGENCY CARE PRINCIPLES & PRACTICE

BRYAN E. BLEDSOE, D.O., F.A.C.E.P., EMT-P

Clinical Associate Professor of Emergency Medicine
University of North Texas Health Sciences Center
Fort Worth, Texas

ROBERT S. PORTER, M.A., NREMT-P

Senior Advanced Life Support Educator
Madison County Emergency Medical Services
Canastota, New York
and
Flight Paramedic
AirOne, Onondaga County Sheriff's Department
Syracuse, New York

RICHARD A. CHERRY, M.S., NREMT-P

Clinical Assistant Professor of Emergency Medicine
Assistant Residency Director
SUNY Upstate Medical University
Syracuse, New York

D0164832

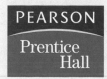

PEARSON

Prentice
Hall

Upper Saddle River, New Jersey 07458

Library of Congress Cataloging-in-Publication Data

Bledsoe, Bryan E. (date).
   Intermediate emergency care: principles & practice / Bryan E. Bledsoe, Robert S. Porter,
Richard A. Cherry.
      p. ; cm.
   Includes bibliographical references and index.
   ISBN 0-13-113607-0 (pbk.)
     1. Emergency medicine. 2. Medical emergencies. 3. Emergency medical personnel. I.
Porter, Robert S. (date). II. Cherry, Richard A. III. Title.
   [DNLM: 1. Emergencies. 2. Emergency Medical Services—methods. 3. Emergency
Medical Technicians—education. WX 105 B646b 2004]
RC86.7.B5945 2004
616.02'5—dc22

                                                        2003056537

Publisher: Julie Levin Alexander
Executive Assistant and Supervisor: Regina Bruno
Executive Editor: Marlene McHugh Pratt
Assistant Editor: Monica Silva
Managing Development Editor: Lois Berlowitz
Development Editors: Josephine Cepeda, Sandra Breuer
Senior Marketing Manager: Katrin Beacom
Product Information Manager: Rachele Triano
Director of Manufacturing and Production: Bruce Johnson
Managing Production Editor: Patrick Walsh
Production Liaison: Jeanne Molenaar
Production Editor: Trish Finley, Carlisle Communications, Ltd.
Manufacturing Manager: Ilene Sanford
Manufacturing Buyer: Pat Brown
Design Director: Cheryl Asherman
Design Coordinator: Christopher Weigand
Interior Design: Jill Yutkowitz
Cover Design: Blair Brown
Cover Photography: Eddie Sperling
Managing Photography Manager: Michal Heron
Interior Photographers: Michal Heron, Richard Logan,
   George Dodson, © Scott Metcalfe Photography
Printer/Binder: Banta Book Group
Cover Printer: Lehigh Press
Composition: Carlisle Communications, Ltd.

Pearson Education LTD.
Pearson Education Australia PTY, Limited
Pearson Education Singapore, Pte. Ltd
Pearson Education North Asia Ltd
Pearson Education Canada, Ltd
Pearson Educación de Mexico, S.A. de C.V.
Pearson Education—Japan
Pearson Education Malaysia, Pte. Ltd
Pearson Education Upper Saddle River, NJ

Studentaid.ed.gov, the U.S. Department of Education's website on
college planning assistance, is a valuable tool for anyone thinking
of pursuing higher education. A guide to the financial process, it is
designed to help students at all stages of schooling, including
international students, returning students, and parents. The
website presents information on applying to and attending college
as well as on funding your education and repaying loans. It also
provides links to useful resources, such as state education agency
contact information, assistance in filling out financial aid forms,
and an introduction to various forms of student aid.

Art Acknowledgments
Rolin Graphics, Plymouth, Minnesota
Algorithms created by Joseph J. Mistovich, M.Ed., NREMT-P,
and rendered by Precision Graphics.

Photo Acknowledgments
All photographs not credited adjacent to the photograph were
photographed on assignment for Brady/Prentice Hall Pearson
Education.

Organizations: We wish to thank the following organizations
for their valuable assistance in creating the photo program for
this edition:

Rockland Paramedic Services, Orangeburg, New York
Ovilla Fire Department, Ovilla, Texas

Technical Advisors: Acknowledgment for providing technical
support during the photo shoots to:

Rockland Paramedic Services, Orangeburg, New York
Michael Murphy, RN, EMT-P, Assistant Chief of Operations;
Richard Greer, EMT-P; Christopher Westbrook, EMT-P;
William Oliver, EMT-P; Jennifer Legge, EMT-P; Gregory
Pekera, EMT-P; Tara Florida, EMT; Craig Sherman, EMT

Ovilla Fire Department, Ovilla, Texas
Donnie Pickard, Fire Chief; Joni Sidler; Tom Leverentz;
Phillip Brancato

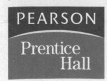

PEARSON
Prentice
Hall

10 9 8 7 6 5 4 3 2
ISBN 0-13-113607-0

NATIONAL EMS MEMORIAL

The National EMS Memorial is the federally designated memorial to honor emergency medical services personnel who have died in the line of duty. The memorial, located at the To the Rescue Museum in Roanoke, Virginia, serves to ensure that all are recognized for the ultimate sacrifice they made for fellow human beings. The names of those who have been honored are permanently engraved on bronze oak leaves as a part of a "Tree of Life." The oak leaf is universally accepted as a symbol of strength, valor, and solid character. A memorial book contains each honoree's biography and photograph.

The National EMS Memorial Service is held in Roanoke, Virginia, on the Saturday prior to Memorial Day. The service began in 1993 and is held annually. Various events occur on that weekend whereby the inductees and their families are honored. The service is a reverent and emotional tribute to those who gave their lives so others may live. During the service, a family member or agency representative is presented with a U.S. flag denoting the honoree's service to our country, a white rose representing undying love, and an engraved medallion signifying eternal memory.

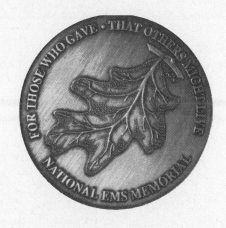

Content Overview

Detailed Contents

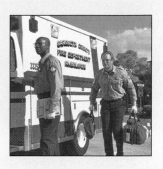
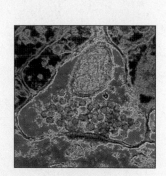

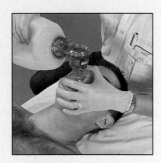

DIVISION 2   PATIENT ASSESSMENT

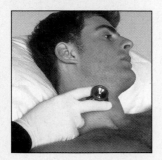

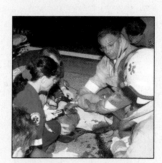

DIVISION 3   TRAUMA EMERGENCIES

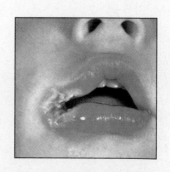

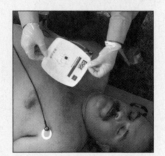

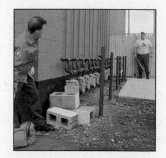

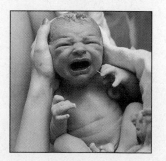

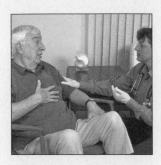
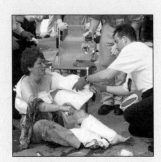

Preface

Congratulations on your decision to further your EMS career by undertaking the course of education required for certification as an Emergency Medical Technician-Intermediate! The world of emergency care is one that you will find both challenging and rewarding. Whether you will be working as a volunteer or paid professional, you will find the field of advanced prehospital care very interesting.

This book is based on the 1999 United States Department of Transportation *EMT-Intermediate: National Standard Curriculum* and is organized into five divisions. The first division, entitled *Preparatory Information,* addresses the fundamentals of Intermediate-level practice, including pathophysiology, pharmacology, medication administration and advanced airway management. The second division, *Patient Assessment,* builds on assessment skills with special emphasis on advanced patient assessment at the scene. *Trauma Emergencies,* the third division of the text, discusses advanced prehospital care from the mechanism of injury analysis to shock/trauma resuscitation. The fourth division of the book, *Medical Emergencies,* is the most extensive and addresses Intermediate-level care of medical emergencies. Particular emphasis is placed on the most common medical problems as well as serious emergencies, such as respiratory and cardiovascular emergencies. The last division addresses *Special Considerations,* including neonatal, pediatric, and geriatric emergencies as well as a new chapter on responding to terrorist acts.

SKILLS

The psychomotor skills of fluid and medication administration, advanced airway care, ECG monitoring and defibrillation, and advanced medical and trauma patient care are best learned in the classroom, skills laboratory, and then the clinical and field setting. Common advanced prehospital skills are discussed in the text as well as outlined in the accompanying procedure sheets. Review these before and while practicing the skill. It is important to point out that this or any other text cannot teach skills. Care skills are only learned under the watchful eye of an instructor and perfected during your clinical and field internship.

HOW TO USE THIS TEXTBOOK

Intermediate Emergency Care: Principles & Practice is designed to accompany an education program that includes ample classroom, practical laboratory, in-hospital clinical, and prehospital field experience. These educational experiences must be guided by instructors and preceptors with special training and experience in their areas of participation in your program.

It is intended that your program coordinator will assign reading from the text in preparation for each classroom lecture and discussion section. The knowledge gained from reading this text will form the foundation of the information you will need in order to function effectively in your EMS system. Your instructors will build upon this information to strengthen your knowledge and understanding of advanced prehospital care so that you may apply it in your practice. The in-hospital clinical and prehospital field experiences will further refine your knowledge and skills under the watchful eyes of your preceptors.

The workbook that accompanies this text can also assist in improving classroom performance. It contains information, sample test questions, and exercises designed to assist learning. Its use can be very helpful in identifying the important elements of Intermediate-level education, in exercising the knowledge of prehospital care, and in helping you self-test your knowledge.

Intermediate Emergency Care: Principles & Practice presents the knowledge of emergency care in as accurate, standardized, and clear a manner as is possible. However, each EMS system is uniquely different, and it is beyond the scope of this text to address all differences. You must count heavily on your instructors, the program coordinator, and ultimately the program medical director to identify how specific emergency care procedures are applied in your system.

Acknowledgments

CONTRIBUTORS

We wish to acknowledge the remarkable talents and efforts of the following people who contributed to the development of *Intermediate Emergency Care: Principles & Practice*. Individually, they worked with extraordinary commitment on this new program. Together, they form a team of highly dedicated professionals who have upheld the highest standard of EMS instruction.

B.E.B., R.S.P., R.A.C.

Beth Lothrop Adams, M.A.; R.N.; NREMT-P; ALS Coordinator, EHS Programs, Adjunct Assistant Professor, Emergency Medicine, The George Washington University, Fairfax, Virginia.

J. Nile Barnes, B.S.; NREMT-P; Associate Professor of EMS Professions, Austin Community College, Austin, Texas and Paramedic, Williamson County (Texas) EMS Department.

Brenda Beasley, R.N., B.S., EMT-P; EMS Program Director, Calhoun College, Decatur, Alabama.

Lawrence C. Brilliant, M.D.; F.A.C.E.P.; Clinical Assistant Professor, Department of Primary Care Education and Community Services, Hahnemann University; Emergency Physician, Doylestown Hospital, Doylestown, Pennsylvania.

Eric C. Chaney, M.S.; NREMT-P; Administrator, Office of the State EMS Medical Director, Maryland Institute for Emergency Medical Services Systems, Baltimore, Maryland.

Elizabeth Coolidge-Stolz, M.D.; Medical Writer; Health Educator; North Reading, Massachusetts.

Robert A. De Lorenzo, M.D.; F.A.C.E.P.; Lieut. Colonel, Medical Corps, US Army, Brooke Army Medical Center.

Kate Dernocoeur, B.S., EMT-P, Lowell, Michigan.

James W. Drake, M.S.; NREMT-P; EMS Coordinator, Jameson Memorial Hospital, New Castle, Pennsylvania.

Robert Feinberg, EMT-P, PA-C, Emergency Medicine, Wayne, Pennsylvania.

Joseph P. Funk, M.D., F.A.C.E.P., Peachtree Emergency Associates, Piedmont Hospital, Atlanta, Georgia.

Kathleen G. Funk, M.D., F.A.C.E.P., Emergency Medicine Physician, Atlanta, Georgia.

William E. (Gene) Gandy, J.D., LP, Hill-Gandy Associates, Albany, Texas.

Eric W. Heckerson, R.N., M.A., NREMT-P, EMS Coordinator, Mesa Fire Department, Mesa, Arizona.

Sandra Hultz, B.S.; NREMT-P; EMS Instructor, University of Mississippi Medical Center, Jackson, Mississippi.

Jeffrey L. Jarvis, M.S.; EMT-P; Medical Student, University of Texas Medical Branch, Galveston, Texas.

Deborah Kufs, R.N.; B.S.; C.C.R.N.; C.E.N.; NREMT-P; Clinical Instructor, Hudson Valley Community College, Institute for Prehospital Emergency Medicine, Troy, New York.

Daniel Limmer, A.S.; EMT-P; Instructor/Clinical Coordinator, Southern Maine Community College, South Portland, ME; Paramedic, Kennebunk Fire Rescue, Kennebunk, Maine.

William Marx, D.O.; Associate Professor of Surgery and Critical Care; Director, Surgical Critical Care SUNY Upstate Medical University, Syracuse, New York.

Michael O'Keefe, NREMT-P; EMS Training Coordinator; Vermont Department of Health.

John M. Saad, M.D.; Medical Director of Emergency Services, Navarro Regional Hospital, Corsicana, Texas; Medical Director of Emergency Services, Medical Center at Terrell, Terrell, Texas.

John S. Saito, M.P.H.; EMT-P; Director, EMS/Paramedic Education; Assistant Professor, Oregon Health Sciences University, School of Medicine, Department of Emergency Medicine, Portland, Oregon.

Jo Anne Schultz, B.A.; NREMT-P; Paramedic, Lifestar Ambulance Inc., Salisbury, Maryland; Level II Emergency Medical Services Instructor, Maryland Fire and Rescue Institute, University of Maryland; Paramedic Instructor, Maryland Institute of Emergency Medical Services Systems, University of Maryland; ACLS, BTLS, and PALS instructor.

Craig A. Soltis, M.D.; F.A.C.E.P.; Assistant Professor of Clinical Emergency Medicine, Northeastern Ohio Universities College of Medicine; Chairman, Department of Emergency Medicine, Forum Health, Youngstown, Ohio.

Marian D. Streger, R.N.; B.S.N.; C.E.N., Cleveland, Ohio.

Emily Vacher, Esq.; M.P.A.; EMT-CC; Associate Director of Judicial Affairs, Syracuse University, Syracuse, New York.

Kevin Waddington, EMT-P, MedStar, Fort Worth, Texas.

Gail Weinstein, M.A., EMT-P, Director of Paramedic Training, State University of New York Upstate Medical University, Syracuse, New York.

Howard A. Werman, M.D.; F.A.C.E.P.; Associate Professor of Clinical Emergency Medicine, The Ohio State University College of Medicine and Public Health, Columbus, Ohio; Medical Director, MedFlight of Ohio.

Matthew S. Zavarella, B.S., A.S.; NREMT-P; CCTEMT-P; Director Prehospital Education, Medical College of Ohio, Toledo, Ohio.

DEVELOPMENT AND PRODUCTION

The task of writing, editing, reviewing, and producing a textbook the size of *Intermediate Emergency Care: Principles & Practice* is complex. Many talented people have been involved in developing and producing this new program.

First, the authors would like to acknowledge the support of Julie Alexander, Marlene Pratt, and Lois Berlowitz. Their belief in us and support of EMS has allowed us to ensure that *Intermediate Emergency Care: Principles & Practice* is at the forefront of Intermediate-level education. Special thanks go to Josephine Cepeda, who served as project coordinator for our new text. Jo exhibits the finest in editorial talent and brought special dedication to developing this program. We also thank Sandy Breuer, with whom we have worked for many years, for the research, analysis, and support she provided in initially moving the project forward. The extraordinary efforts of these exceptional editors are deeply appreciated.

The challenges of production were in the very capable hands of Patrick Walsh and Jeanne Molenaar of Prentice Hall and Trish Finley at Carlisle Publishers Services, who skillfully supervised all production stages to create the final product you now hold. In developing our art and photo program we were fortunate to work with yet additional talent, leaders within their professions. Most of the staged photographs are by Michal Heron of New York City, whose commitment to excellence never falters. The new art was drafted by Rolin Graphics of Plymouth, Minnesota; algorithms were prepared by Precision Graphics.

MEDICAL REVIEW BOARD

Our special thanks to the following physicians for their review of material in this program. Their reviews were carefully prepared, and we appreciate the thoughtful advice and keen insight each shared with us.

Dr. Robert De Lorenzo, Lieutenant Colonel, Medical Corps, U.S. Army; Associate Clinical Professor of Military and Emergency Medicine, Uniformed Services University of Health Sciences.

Dr. Edward T. Dickinson, Assistant Professor and Director of EMS Field Operations in the Department of Emergency Medicine, University of Pennsylvania School of Medicine in Philadephia.

Dr. Howard A. Werman, Associate Professor, Department of Emergency Medicine, The Ohio State University College of Medicine and Public Health, Columbus, Ohio.

INSTRUCTOR REVIEWERS

The reviewers of *Intermediate Emergency Care: Principles & Practice* have provided many excellent suggestions and ideas for improving the text. The quality of the reviews has been outstanding, and the reviews have been a major aid in the preparation and revision of the manuscript. The assistance provided by these EMS experts is deeply appreciated.

Mary E. Alston, RN, BSN, CEN
Montana State University
Extended Studies
Bozeman, MT

P. A. Ambrose, NREMT-P, CCEMT-P
EMS/Continuing Education
    Coordinator
St. Vincent/Medical College of Ohio
Life Flight
Toledo, OH

Brenda M. Beasley, RN, BS, EMT-
    Paramedic
Calhoun Community College
Department Chair, Allied Health
EMS Program Director
Decatur, AL

Rhonda J. Beck, NREMT-P
Paramedic Instructor
Houston County EMS
Georgia

John L. Beckman, FF/EMT-P
Fire Fighter/Paramedic
EMS Instructor
Lincolnwood Fire Dept
Affiliated with Addison Fire Protection
    District
Lincolnwood, IL

Christopher Black, Director
Department of EMS
Eastern Arizona College

Harvey Conner, AS, NREMT-P
Professor of EMS
Oklahoma City Community College
Oklahoma City, OK

Tony Crystal
Director, Emergency Medical Services
Lake Land College
Mattoon, IL

Cathey Eide
EMS Program Coordinator
University of Illinois
Fire Service Institute
Champaign, IL

Bruce Evans, MPA
Henderson Fire Dept
Henderson, NV

Joseph W. Ferrell
Iowa Dept of Public Health
Bureau of EMS
Des Moines, IA

Stephen L. Garrison, RN, NREMT-P
EMS Coordinator
Memorial Hospital
South Bend, IN

David Gurchiek, M.S., NREMT-P
Paramedic Program Director
Montana State University-Billings
Billings, MT

Nicholas Klimenko, BS, NREMT-P
Nicholas Klimenko & Assoc Inc
Williamsburg, VA

William S. Krost, NREMT-P
Program Manager
Emergency Medicine Special
    Operations Institute
University of Cincinnati Dept of
    Emergency Medicine
Cincinnati, OH

William R. Montrie, EMT-P
EMT Certification Coordinator
Perrysburg, OH

Randell Pitts LP, NREMT-P
Critical Care Paramedic II
Scott & White Hospital
Prehospital Services
Temple, TX

Liam Proctor, NREMT-P, CCEMT-P,
    EMS-I
Advisory Committee
School of EMS
Clinic Health Systems
Ohio

Michael W. Robinson, MA, NREMT-P
Fire Rescue Academy
Baltimore County Fire Dept
Sparrows Point, MD

Notices

It is the intent of the authors and publishers that this textbook be used as part of a formal EMS education program taught by a qualified instructor and supervised by a licensed physician. The care procedures presented here represent accepted practices in the United States. They are not offered as a standard of care. Intermediate-level emergency care is to be performed only under the authority and guidance of a licensed physician. It is the reader's responsibility to know and follow local care protocols as provided by medical advisors directing the system to which he or she belongs. Also, it is the reader's responsibility to stay informed of emergency care procedure changes.

NOTICE ON DRUGS AND DRUG DOSAGES

Every effort has been made to ensure that the drug dosages presented in this textbook are in accordance with nationally accepted standards. When applicable, the dosages and routes are taken from the American Heart Association's Advanced Cardiac Life Support Guidelines. The American Medical Association's publication *Drug Evaluations,* the *Physician's Desk Reference,* and the *Prentice Hall Health Professionals Drug Guide 2004* are followed with regard to drug dosages not covered by the American Heart Association's guidelines. It is the responsibility of the reader to be familiar with the drugs used in his or her system, as well as the dosages specified by the medical director. The drugs presented in this book should only be administered by direct order, whether verbally or through accepted standing orders, of a licensed physician.

NOTICE ON GENDER USAGE

The English language has historically given preference to the male gender. Among many words, the pronouns "he" and "his" are commonly used to describe both genders. Society evolves faster than language and the male pronouns still predominate in our speech. The authors have made great effort to treat the two genders equally, recognizing that a significant percentage of EMS professionals and patients are female. However, in some instances, male pronouns may be used to describe both male and female EMTs and patients solely for the purpose of brevity. This is not intended to offend any readers of the female gender.

NOTICE ON PHOTOGRAPHS

Please note that many of the photographs contained in this book are taken of actual emergency situations. As such, it is possible that they may not accurately depict current, appropriate, or advisable practices of emergency medical care. They have been included for the sole purpose of giving general insight into real-life emergency settings.

Precautions on Bloodborne Pathogens and Infectious Diseases

Prehospital emergency personnel, like all health care workers, are at risk for exposure to bloodborne pathogens and infectious diseases. In emergency situations it is often difficult to take or enforce proper infection control measures. However, as an EMT-Intermediate, you must recognize your high-risk status.

Infection control is designed to protect emergency personnel, their families, and their patients from unnecessary exposure to communicable diseases.

Laws, regulations, and standards regarding infection control include:

* *Centers for Disease Control (CDC) Guidelines.* The CDC has published extensive guidelines regarding infection control. Proper equipment and techniques that should be used by emergency response personnel to prevent or minimize risk of exposure are defined.
* *The Ryan White Act.* The Ryan White Act of 1990 allows emergency personnel to find out if they were exposed to an infectious disease while rendering patient care. Employers are required to name a "designated officer" to coordinate communications with the treating hospital.
* *Americans with Disabilities Act.* This act prohibits discrimination against individuals with disabilities including those with contagious diseases. It guarantees equal employment opportunities and job protection if the infected individual can perform essential job functions and does not pose a threat to the safety and health of patients and coworkers.
* *Occupational Safety and Health Administration (OSHA) Regulations.* OSHA recently enacted a regulation entitled Occupational Exposure to Bloodborne Pathogens that classifies emergency response personnel as being at the greatest risk of occupational exposure to communicable diseases. This regulation requires employers to provide hepatitis B (HBV) vaccinations free of charge, maintain a written exposure control plan, and provide personal protective equipment (PPE). These requirements primarily apply to private employers. Applicability to local and state governmental employees varies by locality. Many states have developed their own OSHA plans.

* *National Fire Protection Association (NFPA) Guidelines.* This is a national organization that has established specific guidelines and requirements regarding infection control for emergency response agencies, particularly fire departments and EMS services.

BODY SUBSTANCE ISOLATION PRECAUTIONS AND PERSONAL PROTECTIVE EQUIPMENT

Emergency response personnel should practice *Body Substance Isolation (BSI)*, a strategy that considers ALL body substances potentially infectious. To achieve this, all emergency personnel should utilize *Personal Protective Equipment (PPE)*. Appropriate PPE should be available on every emergency vehicle. The minimum recommended PPE includes the following:

* *Gloves.* Disposable gloves should be donned by all emergency response personnel BEFORE initiating any emergency care. When an emergency incident involves more than one patient, you should attempt to change gloves between patients. When gloves have been contaminated, they should be removed as soon as possible. To remove gloves, first hook the gloved fingers of one hand under the cuff of the other glove. Then pull that glove off without letting your gloved fingers come in contact with bare skin. Then slide the fingers of the ungloved hand under the remaining glove's cuff. Push that glove off, being careful not to touch the glove's exterior with your bare hand. Always wash hands after gloves are removed, even when the gloves appear intact.
* *Masks and Protective Eyewear.* Masks and protective equipment should be present on all emergency vehicles and used in accordance with the level of exposure encountered. Proper eyewear and masks prevent a patient's blood and body fluids from spraying into your eyes, nose, and mouth. Masks and protective eyewear should be worn together whenever blood spatter is likely to occur, such as arterial bleeding, childbirth, endotracheal intubation, invasive procedures, oral suctioning, and clean-up

of equipment that requires heavy scrubbing or brushing. Both you and the patient should wear masks whenever the potential for airborne transmission of disease exists.

* *HEPA Respirators.* Due to the resurgence of tuberculosis (TB), prehospital personnel should protect themselves from TB infection through use of a high-efficiency particulate air (HEPA) respirator, a design approved by the National Institute of Occupational Safety and Health (NIOSH). It should fit snugly and be capable of filtering out the tuberculosis bacillus. The HEPA respirator should be worn when caring for patients with confirmed or suspected TB. This is especially true when performing "high hazard" procedures such as administration of nebulized medications, endotracheal intubation, or suctioning on such a patient.

* *Gowns.* Gowns protect clothing from blood splashes. If large splashes of blood are expected, such as with childbirth, wear impervious gowns.

* *Resuscitation Equipment.* Disposable resuscitation equipment should be the primary means of artificial ventilation in emergency care. Such items should be used once, then disposed of.

Remember, the proper use of personal protective equipment ensures effective infection control and minimizes risk. Use ALL protective equipment recommended for any particular situation to ensure maximum protection.

Consider ALL body substances potentially infectious and ALWAYS practice body substance isolation.

HANDLING CONTAMINATED MATERIAL

Many of the materials associated with the emergency response become contaminated with possibly infectious body fluids and substances. These include soiled linen, patient clothing, and dressings, and used care equipment, including intravenous needles. It is important that you collect these materials at the scene and dispose of them appropriately to assure your safety as well as that of your patients, their family members, bystanders, and fellow caregivers. Properly dispose of any contaminated materials according to the recommendations outlined below.

* Handle contaminated materials only while wearing the appropriate personal protective equipment.

* Place all blood- or body-fluid-contaminated clothing, linen, dressings and patient care equipment and supplies in properly marked biohazard bags and assure they are disposed of properly.

* Ensure all used needles, scalpels and other contaminated objects that have the potential to puncture the skin are properly secured in a puncture-resistant and clearly-marked sharps container.

* Do not recap a needle after use, stick it into a seat cushion or other object, or leave it lying on the ground. This increases the risk of an accidental needle stick.

* Always scan the scene before leaving to assure all equipment has been retrieved and all potentially infectious material has been bagged and removed.

* Should you be exposed to an infectious disease, have contact with body substances with a route for system entry (such as an open wound on your hand when a glove tears while moving a soiled patient), or receive a needle stick with a used needle, alert the receiving hospital and contact your service's infection control officer immediately.

Following these recommendations will help protect you and the people you care for from the dangers of disease transmission.

Welcome to Intermediate Emergency Care

ONE LAKE STREET
UPPER SADDLE RIVER, NJ 07458

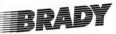

Dear Instructor:

Brady, your partner in education, is pleased to present *Intermediate Emergency Care: Principles & Practice*. This new textbook was developed specifically to meet the 1999 U.S. DOT National Standard Curriculum for EMT-Intermediates.

Intermediate Emergency Care: Principles & Practice is the result of more than two years of research in the form of focus groups, surveys, interviews, content reviews, and everyday contact with customers. We learned how and why the Intermediate curriculum was built and examined how it was used across the country. Based on our findings, we determined that a comprehensive approach was needed—that it is important students understand both the theory and practice of Intermediate care, not just be taught to perform the skills themselves. We asked Bryan Bledsoe, Robert Porter, and Dick Cherry to approach Intermediate care with the same student-friendly, easy-to-understand style that has been so successful in their Paramedic series.

In addition to the tried-and-true features of Chapter Objectives, Content Review, Key Terms, Key Points, Scans, Documentation, Medical Calculations, and Summaries, we added some new features—*Patho Pearls*, explaining the pathology students will encounter in the field; *Legal Notes*, presenting instances in which legal or ethical considerations should be evaluated for both provider and patient protection; and *Cultural Considerations*, providing insight into the different cultures encountered in the field and awareness of specific beliefs or actions that would affect patient care. We also added a chapter on *EMS Response to Weapons of Mass Destruction*, a topic whose inclusion is critical for the world in which EMS operates today.

Our package also includes comprehensive support for both students and instructors. The following pages provide a complete walkthrough of the text and its features, as well as information about our Instructor's Resource Manual, Test Program, PowerPoint Slides, Student Workbook, and Companion Website.

Intermediate Emergency Care: Principles & Practice offers you the high-quality content you've come to know and trust. We continue in our tradition of bringing the best to EMS education with the highest standards of writing, development, and production that our customers deserve.

Welcome to the next generation of EMS education.

Sincerely,

Julie Levin Alexander
Publisher

Katrin Beacom
Senior Marketing Manager

Marlene McHugh Pratt
Executive Editor

Thomas Kennally
District Manager, Brady Sales

BRADY
Your Partner in Education

Chapter Objectives with Page References

Each chapter begins with clearly stated **Objectives** that follow the U.S. DOT EMT-I curriculum. Students can refer to these objectives while studying to make sure they understand the material fully. Page references after each objective indicate where relevant content is covered in the chapter.

CHAPTER 4

Venous Access and Medication Administration

Objectives

Part 1: Principles and Routes of Medication Administration
(begins on page 274)

After reading Part 1 of this chapter, you should be able to:

1. Review the specific anatomy and physiology pertinent to medication administration. (pp. 274–303)
2. Discuss the legal aspects of medication administration, including the "six rights" of drug administration. (pp. 274–276)
3. Discuss medical asepsis, the differences between clean and sterile techniques, the use of antiseptics and disinfectants. (pp. 275–276)
4. Describe how body substance isolation (BSI) precautions relate to medication administration. (p. 275)
5. Describe the indications, equipment, techniques, precautions, and general principles of administering medications by the inhalation route. (pp. 280–283)
6. Differentiate among the different dosage forms of oral medications, and describe the

equipment and general principles of their administration. (pp. 284–288)
7. Describe the indications, equipment, techniques, precautions, and general principles of rectal medication administration. (pp. 288–298)
8. Describe the equipment, techniques, complications, and general principles for the preparation and administration of parenteral medications. (pp. 289–303)
9. Describe proper disposal of contaminated items and sharps. (p. 276)
10. Synthesize a pharmacological management plan including medication administration. (pp. 273–275)
11. Integrate pathophysiological principles of medication administration with patient management. (pp. 273–275)

Continued

Key Points

Key Points in the margins help students identify and learn the fundamental principles of EMT-I practice.

Content Review

Content Review summarizes important content and gives students a format for quick review.

Key Terms

Reinforcement of **Key Terms** helps students master new terminology.

Treat all blood and body fluids as potentially infectious.

Content Review

NEEDLE HANDLING PRECAUTIONS
- Minimize tasks in a moving ambulance.
- Properly dispose of all sharps.
- Recap needles only as a last resort.

sharps container rigid, puncture resistant container clearly marked as a biohazard.

Content Review

ROUTES OF DRUG ADMINISTRATION
- Percutaneous
- Pulmonary
- Enteral
- Parenteral

topical medications material applied to and absorbed through the skin or mucous membranes.

DISPOSAL OF CONTAMINATED EQUIPMENT AND SHARPS

Blood and body fluid can harbor infectious material that endangers the health-care provider, family, bystanders, or the patient himself. Many times, the patient is infected with pathogenic organisms long before signs and symptoms appear. Therefore, you must treat all blood and body fluids as potentially infectious.

Drug administration commonly involves needles in direct contact with the patient's blood and body fluid. Once used, a needle presents a significant risk. Inadvertent needle sticks, the most common accident in health care as a whole, can transmit diseases between the patient and the EMT-I. Properly handling needles and other sharps before and after patient use can prevent many of these accidental needle sticks. To minimize or eliminate the risk of an accidental needle stick, take these precautions:

- *Minimize the tasks you perform in a moving ambulance.* Use needles as sparingly as possible in the back of a moving ambulance. When appropriate, perform all interventions involving needles on scene. If en route, it may be occasionally necessary to have the driver pull the ambulance to the side of the road and stop briefly. Most EMT-Is become quite proficient at completing these procedures in a moving ambulance.
- *Immediately dispose of used sharps in a sharps container.* A **sharps container** is a rigid, puncture-resistant container clearly marked as biohazardous. You can deposit whole needles and prefilled syringes in it, thus eliminating the need for bending or cutting. Some sharps containers have adapters that permit the easy removal of needles from blood-draw equipment and syringes. You should also dispose of items such as used ampules in the sharps container. Avoid dropping sharps onto the floor for later disposal. In the heat of the moment, you may forget the sharp or mentally misplace it.
- *Recap needles only as a last resort.* If you absolutely must recap a needle, never use two hands to do so. Place the sharp on a stationary surface, and replace the cap with one hand. Although the one-hand method is still hazardous, it at least reduces the chance for an accidental needle stick.

By law, every medical organization must have a biological hazard exposure plan. Be familiar with yours. If you are exposed to blood or other body substances, follow the plan and immediately notify the appropriate resources. Remember that prevention is the best medicine.

MEDICATION ADMINISTRATION AND DOCUMENTATION

When administering medications, proper and thorough documentation is extremely important. You must record all information concerning the patient and the medication, including:

- Indication for drug administration
- Dosage and route delivered
- Patient response to the medication—both positive and negative

You must also document the patient's condition and vital signs before medication administration, as well as after. In addition to communicating all information to those to whom you transfer care, you must record it on a copy of the patient care report.

In emergent and nonemergent situations alike, you will administer a variety of medications through a variety of delivery routes. The routes of drug administration fall into four basic categories: percutaneous, pulmonary, enteral, and parenteral. Technically, drug deliveries through the rectum and pulmonary system are **topical** applications; however, accepted practice classifies these routes separately. Which route you use will depend on the drug you are administering and your patient's status.

Table 7-4	NORMAL BREATH SOUNDS		
Sound	Description	Location	Duration
Tracheal	Very loud, harsh	Over the trachea	Nearly equal inspiratory and expiratory phases
Bronchial	Loud, high pitch, hollow	Over the manubrium	Prolonged expiratory phase
Bronchovesicular	Soft, breezy, lower pitch	Between the scapulae/ 2nd–3rd ICS lateral to the sternum	Approximately equal inspiratory and expiratory phases
Vesicular	Soft, swishy, lowest pitch	Lung periphery	Prolonged inspiratory phase

Tables and Illustrations

Tables and **illustrations** offer visual support to enhance students' understanding of EMT-I principles and practice.

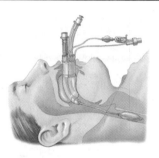

FIGURE 5-31 Pharyngo-tracheal lumen airway.

- Does not require direct visualization of the larynx and, thus, does not require the use of a laryngoscope or additional specialized equipment.
- Can be used in trauma patients, since the neck can remain in neutral position during insertion and use.
- Helps protect the trachea from upper airway bleeding and secretions.

Disadvantages of the Pharyngo-Tracheal Lumen Airway

Disadvantages of the PtL airway include the following:

- It does not isolate and completely protect the trachea from aspiration.
- The oropharyngeal balloon can migrate out of the mouth anteriorly, partially dislodging the airway.
- Intubation around the PtL is extremely difficult, even with the oropharyngeal balloon deflated.
- It cannot be used in conscious patients or those with a gag reflex.
- It cannot be used in pediatric patients.
- It can only be passed orally.

Inserting the Pharyngo-Tracheal Lumen Airway

Do the following to insert the PtL airway:

1. Complete basic manual and adjunctive maneuvers and provide supplemental oxygen and ventilatory support with a BVM and hyperventilation.
2. Place the patient supine and kneel at the top of his head.
3. Prepare and check the equipment.
4. Place the patient's head in the appropriate position. Hyperextend the neck if there is no risk of cervical spine injury. Maintain neutral position with stabilization of the cervical spine if cervical spine injury is possible.
5. Insert the PtL gently, using the tongue-jaw-lift maneuver.
6. Inflate the distal cuffs on both PtL tubes simultaneously with a sustained breath into the inflation valve.

394 CHAPTER 5 *Airway Management and Ventilation*

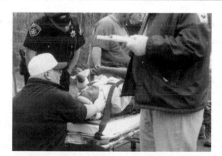

FIGURE 15-14 Emotional support for the seriously injured trauma patient is an important part of shock patient care.

as dopamine, and the other cardiac drugs are indicated (see Chapter 20, "Cardiovascular Emergencies"). For spinal and obstructive shock, consider IV fluids such as normal saline and lactated Ringer's solution. For distributive shock, consider IV fluids, dopamine, and use of the PASG.

The patient who has experienced trauma sufficient to induce hemorrhage and hypovolemia will be anxious and bewildered. As the care provider at the patient's side, it is your responsibility to be calm and reassuring, thus counteracting the natural "fight-or-flight" response (Figure 15-14). By acting in this manner, you not only help your patient deal with the event's emotional trauma but also combat some of the negative effects of sympathetic stimulation.

UMMARY

Significant hemorrhage and its serious consequence, shock, are genuine threats to the trauma patient's life. The signs of these threats are often subtle or hidden, especially if bleeding is internal. Only through careful analysis of the mechanism of injury during the scene size-up and careful evaluation of the patient during the assessment process can you recognize and then treat these life-threatening problems. Treatment often involves rapidly bringing the patient to the services of a trauma center and, while doing so, providing aggressive care—supplemental oxygen, positive pressure ventilations, fluid resuscitation, and use of a PASG as necessary—aimed at maintaining vital signs, not necessarily improving them. With this approach, you afford your patient the best chance for survival.

ON THE WEB

For additional practice and review, go to the companion website at www.prenhall.com/bledsoe and click on *Intermediate Emergency Care: Principles & Practice.*

670 CHAPTER 15 *Hemorrhage and Shock*

End-of-Chapter Summary

Each end-of-chapter **Summary** reviews the main topics covered.

EMPHASIZING PRACTICE

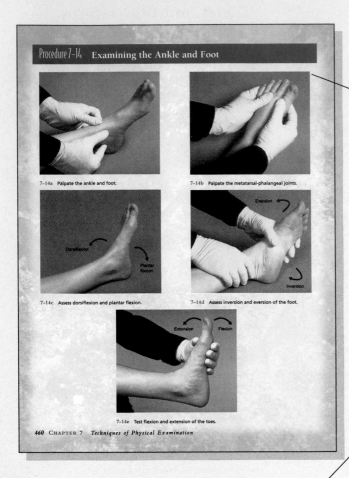

Procedure 7-14 Examining the Ankle and Foot

7-14a Palpate the ankle and foot.

7-14b Palpate the metatarsal-phalangeal joints.

7-14c Assess dorsiflexion and plantar flexion.

7-14d Assess inversion and eversion of the foot.

7-14e Test flexion and extension of the toes.

460 CHAPTER 7 *Techniques of Physical Examination*

Procedure Scans

Specially photographed **Procedure Scans** provide step-by-step visual support on how to perform skills included in the DOT curriculum.

Patho Pearls

Almost since the inception of advanced prehospital care, aggressive fluid resuscitation has always been a major component of trauma treatment. However, several recent studies have questioned the role of aggressive fluid resuscitation. Research has shown that fewer than 10% of trauma patients (blunt and penetrating) present with hypotension. Many of these are hypotensive for reasons other than blood loss (i.e., pneumothorax, gastric distension).

It has been demonstrated that the body has natural compensatory mechanisms that are activated when the blood pressure falls to between 70 and 85 torr. Even at this lowered blood pressure, cerebral and renal perfusion is maintained. Elevation of the blood pressure to pre-injury levels, through aggressive fluid resuscitation and PASG, can result in progressive re-bleeding at the injury site. In addition, as blood is lost, it is replaced with crystalloid solutions that do not contain any hemoglobin or clotting factors. Thus, over time, with aggressive fluid resuscitation, the blood becomes more dilute and its capacities to transport oxygen and initiate clotting are diminished.

Many trauma experts are now calling for trauma patients to be maintained in a region of "permissive hypotension," where fluids are judiciously given to maintain the systolic blood pressure between 70 and 85 torr. Like many issues in EMS, practices should only change when there is overwhelming scientific data. Soon, however, "permissive hypotension" may be the standard of care for trauma patients.

Legal Notes

Burn patients require highly specialized care in a facility specifically designed for burn injuries. Burn centers offer a multi-disciplinary approach to burn care utilizing plastic surgeons, general surgeons, orthopedic surgeons, rehabilitation specialists, pain management specialists, and others. In addition, burn centers provide nutritional counseling (very important to burn healing), pastoral care, and psychological care. Burn care facilities are expensive to operate and patients tend to remain in them for prolonged periods of time. The American Burn Association (ABA) has published guidelines for determining which patients might benefit from treatment in a burn center.

Most burn centers are regional facilities, and frequently patients must be transported some distance to them. Personnel who routinely transport burn patients should be familiar with burn care including dressings, fluid therapy, and escharotomy (if required). In addition, continued adequate analgesia should be provided according to local protocols and interhospital transfer orders. Burn care should be addressed in any trauma system plan.

Cultural Considerations

Many religions and cultures have specific beliefs about blood loss and transfusions. Because of these, it is important for EMS personnel to understand and respect these beliefs. For example, large numbers of Hmong immigrated to the United States and Canada after the Vietnam conflict. The Hmong are among the oldest group of people in Asia and are often referred to as the "Hill People." They put great faith in folk medicine and sometimes will trust a shaman more than a Western medical practitioner. Many Hmong believe that the body has a limited amount of blood, and any blood loss can cause permanent problems. Furthermore, many Hmong believe that any injuries or surgical procedures sustained in life will remain with them when they enter the spirit world. Thus, many Western practices, such as surgery and autopsy, may be forbidden by members of this culture.

The Jehovah's Witnesses are a religious group that has specifically forbidden blood transfusions. This belief comes from their interpretation of a Bible verse (Acts 15:29) that states, "That ye abstain from meats offered to idols, and from blood, and from things strangled, and from fornication: from which if ye keep yourselves, ye shall do well. Fare ye well." Although some have interpreted this verse to mean the literal "eating of blood," the Jehovah's Witnesses have interpreted it to include the transfusion of blood. The beliefs will vary from individual to individual. Some Jehovah's Witnesses will allow the administration of crystalloid fluids, while others will allow the actual administration of some blood components (plasma, globulins, and platelets). However, many will refuse all blood or similar products (including IV fluids). Regardless, the EMT-I must respect this wish and change treatment plans accordingly.

Special Features

Patho Pearls offer a snapshot of pathological considerations students will encounter in the field.

Legal Notes present instances in which legal or ethical considerations should be evaluated.

Cultural Considerations provide an awareness of beliefs that might affect patient care.

USES FOR DOCUMENTATION

Your PCR is a valuable resource for a variety of people. They include medical professionals, EMS administrators, researchers, and occasionally, lawyers.

MEDICAL

Hospital staff (nurses and physicians) may need more information from you than they can get before you have to take another call. For example, they may want a chronological account of your patient's mental status from the time you arrived on the scene. Your PCR can tell the emergency department staff of your patient's condition before he arrived at the hospital. It serves as a baseline for comparing assessment findings and detecting trends that indicate improvement or deterioration. The surgical staff will want to know the mechanism of injury and other pertinent findings during your initial assessment of your patient and the scene.

Your PCR is an important document that helps ensure your patient's continuity of care.

If your patient is admitted to the hospital, the floor or intensive care unit staff may need more information about his original condition than he can remember. In addition, your PCR provides them with information from people at the scene to whom they might not have access—family, bystanders, first responders, or other witnesses. Knowing about the circumstances that led to the event or the mechanism of injury may also help rehabilitation specialists to provide better therapy. Your PCR becomes an important document that helps ensure your patient's continuous effective care (Figure 11-1).

ADMINISTRATIVE

response time time elapsed from when a unit is alerted until it arrives on scene.

EMS administrators must gather information for quality improvement and system management. Information regarding **response times**, call location, the use of lights and siren, date and time is vital to evaluating your system's readiness to respond to life-threatening emergencies. It also is essential to providing information of community needs. The quality improvement or quality assurance committee use PCRs to identify problems with individual EMT-Is or with the EMS system. In some agencies, the billing department needs to determine which services are billable. Insurance carriers may need to know more about the illness or injury to process the claim. Some states use your PCR data to allocate funding for regional systems.

RESEARCH

Your PCR provides the basis for continuously improving patient care in your EMS system.

Your PCR may give researchers useful data about many aspects of the EMS call. For example, they may analyze your recorded data to determine the efficacy of certain medical devices or interventions such as drugs and invasive procedures. They also may use the data to cut costs, alter staffing, and shorten response times. Some systems use computerized or electronic

Prehospital Care Report

Agency Name	ARLINGTON RESCUE	MILEAGE		USE MILITARY TIMES
Dispatch Information	CARDIAC	END 2 4 4 9 6	CALL REC'D	0 7 0 5
Call Location	124 CYPRUS ST 2nd FLOOR	BEGIN 2 4 4 7 6	ENROUTE	0 7 0 7
		TOTAL 0 0 0 2 0	ARRIVED AT SCENE	0 7 1 9
CHECK ONE ☑ Residence ☐ Other Work Loc. ☐ Health Facility ☐ Farm ☐ Roadway ☐ Recreational ☐ Indus. Facility ☐ Other	LOCATION CODE 0 1 2 1 4	FROM SCENE	0 7 3 8
CALL TYPE AS REC'D	MECHANISM OF INJURY	AT DESTIN	0 7 5 4
☑ Emergency	☐ MVA (✓ seat belt used __) ☐ Knife	IN SERVICE	0 8 1 0
☐ Non-Emergency	☐ Fall of ___ feet N/A ☐ Machinery	IN QUARTERS	0 8 3 2
☐ Stand-by	☐ Unarmed assault ☐ GSW		

FIGURE 11–1 Run data in a prehospital care report is vital to your agency's efforts to improve patient care.

Documentation

Covered thoroughly throughout the text, **proper documentation techniques** are critical to ensuring provider protection on the job as well as patient safety during the transition of care.

To use this formula, you must express all weight and volume measurements with the same metric prefix. For example, if the desired dose is expressed in *milli*grams, the dosage on hand must also be expressed in *milli*grams, volume on hand in *milli*liters.

CALCULATING DOSAGES FOR ORAL MEDICATIONS

The following example illustrates how to calculate the volume of a specific drug dosage:

Example 1: A physician orders you to administer 90 mg of acetaminophen to a pediatric patient. The liquid acetaminophen is packaged as a concentration of 500 mg in 8 mL of solution. How much of the medication will you administer?

Because you cannot see the 90 mg of acetaminophen, you must convert this weight to a volume. To do so you need these facts:

$$\text{desired dose} = 90 \text{ mg}$$
$$\text{dosage on hand} = 500 \text{ mg}$$
$$\text{volume on hand} = 8 \text{ mL}$$

Use the formula to calculate the dosage's volume:

$$\text{volume to be administered} = \frac{\text{volume on hand } (8 \text{ mL}) \times \text{desired dose } (90 \text{ mg})}{\text{dosage on hand } (500 \text{ mg})}$$

$$\text{volume to be administered} = (8 \times 90)/500$$
$$\text{volume to be administered} = 720/500$$
$$\text{volume to be administered} = 1.44$$

Administer 1.44 mL of solution to deliver 90 mg of acetaminophen.

Another way to calculate drug dosages is the ratio (fraction) and proportion method. A ratio (fraction) illustrates a relationship between two numbers. A proportion is the comparison of two numerically equivalent ratios. Using the variable x, the above problem can be stated:

$$8 \text{ mL}/500 \text{ mg} = x \text{ mL}/90 \text{ mg}$$

To solve the problem, cross multiply the numerals:

$$8/500 = x/90$$
$$720/500 = x$$
$$1.44 = x$$
$$x = 1.44 \text{ mL}$$

CONVERTING PREFIXES

The following example shows how to calculate the volume to be administered when the desired dose, the dosage on hand, and the volume on hand are not all expressed in metric units with the same prefix.

Example 2: A physician orders you to give 250 mg of a drug via IV bolus. The multidose vial contains 2 grams of the drug in 10 mL of solution. How much of the medication should you administer?

Because the desired dose is expressed as *milli*grams, the dosage on hand must be converted from grams to milligrams. In the metric system, 2 grams equal 2,000 milligrams. You now know:

$$\text{desired dose} = 250 \text{ mg}$$
$$\text{dosage on hand} = 2,000 \text{ mg}$$
$$\text{volume on hand} = 10 \text{ mL}$$

Medical Calculations

Mathematical examples are provided to give students practice in medical calculations, a critical skill in prehospital care.

Teaching & Learning Package

For the Instructor

Instructor's Resource Manual (ISBN 0-13-1136321)

The Instructor's Resource Manual contains everything needed to teach the 1999 U.S. DOT National Standard Curriculum for EMT-Intermediates. It fully covers the DOT curriculum with:

- lecture outlines
- innovative teaching strategies
- suggestions for additional resources
- student activities handouts for reinforcement and evaluation
- a transition guide from competing product

The manual is also available on CD-ROM so instructors can customize resources to their individual needs.

PowerPoint® Presentations on CD-ROM (ISBN 0-13-1136348)

This CD-ROM offers a comprehensive PowerPoint® presentation that contains more than 2,700 word slides and images. The entire presentation can be tailored to your course needs.

TestGen (ISBN 0-13-113633X)

The TestGen test software contains more than 1,700 textbook-based questions in a format that enables instructors to select questions based on topic area and degree of difficulty.

For the Student

Student Workbook (ISBN 0-13-1136399)

A student workbook with review and practice activities accompanies *Intermediate Emergency Care: Principles & Practice.* The workbook includes a review of chapter objectives, multiple-choice questions, labeling exercises, case studies, and special projects, along with an answer key with text page references.

Online Resources

Companion Website: www.prenhall.com/bledsoe

This free site, tied chapter-by-chapter to the text, reinforces student learning through interactive online study guides, key terms, quizzes based on the new curriculum, and links to important EMS-related Internet resources. The Companion Website also allows instructors to create a customized syllabus.

For information on additional media to support the series, please contact your Brady representative: 1-800-638-0220

CHAPTER 1

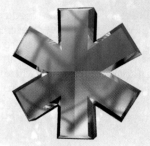

Foundations of the EMT-Intermediate

Objectives

Part 1: Introduction to Advanced Prehospital Care (begins on p. 5)

After reading Part 1 of this chapter, you should be able to:

1. Describe the relationship between the EMT-Intermediate and other members of the allied health professions. (pp. 5–7)
2. Identify the attributes and characteristics of an EMT-Intermediate. (pp. 6–7)

3. Explain the elements of EMT-Intermediate education and practice that support its stature as a profession. (pp. 6–7)

Part 2: EMS Systems (begins on p. 7)

After reading Part 2 of this chapter, you should be able to:

1. Describe key historical events that influenced the national development of Emergency Medical Services (EMS) systems. (pp. 7–10)
2. Define the following terms: EMS systems (p. 7), licensure (p. 14), certification (p. 14), reciprocity (p. 14), registration (p. 14), profession (p. 15), professionalism (p. 15), health-care professional (p. 15), ethics (p. 19), peer review (p. 19), medical direction (p. 11), protocols (p. 11).
3. Identify national groups important to the development, education, and implementation

of EMS as well as the role of national associations, the National Registry of EMTs, and the roles of various EMS standard-setting agencies. (pp. 15–16)
4. Identify the standards (components) of an EMS system as defined by the National Highway Traffic Safety Administration. (pp. 9–10)
5. Differentiate among EMS provider levels: First Responder, EMT-Basic, EMT-Intermediate, and EMT-Paramedic. (pp. 14–15)
6. Describe what is meant by "citizen involvement in the EMS system." (p. 12)

Continued

7. Discuss the role of the EMS physician in providing medical direction, prehospital and out-of-hospital care as an extension of the physician, the benefits of on-line and off-line medical direction, and the process for the development of local policies and protocols. (pp. 10–11)

8. Describe the relationship among a physician on the scene, the EMT-Intermediate on the scene, and the EMS physician providing on-line medical direction. (pp. 11–12)

9. Describe the components of continuous quality improvement and analyze its contribution to system improvement, continuing medical education, and research. (pp. 18–19)

10. Describe the importance, basic principles, process of evaluating and interpreting, and benefits of research. (pp. 19–20)

Part 3: Roles and Responsibilities of the EMT-Intermediate (begins on p. 21)

After reading Part 3 of this chapter, you should be able to:

1. Describe the attributes of an EMT-Intermediate as a health-care professional. (pp. 24–28)

2. Describe the benefits of EMT-Intermediate continuing education and the importance of maintaining an EMT-Intermediate license/certification. (p. 28)

3. List the primary and additional responsibilities of EMT-Intermediates. (pp. 21–28)

4. Define the role of the EMT-Intermediate relative to the safety of the crew, the patient, and bystanders. (pp. 21–23)

5. Describe the role of the EMT-Intermediate in health education activities related to illness and injury prevention. (p. 24)

6. Describe examples of professional behaviors in the following areas: integrity, empathy, self-motivation, appearance and personal hygiene, self-confidence, communications, time management, teamwork and diplomacy, respect, patient advocacy, and careful delivery of service. (pp. 25–28)

7. Identify the benefits of EMT-Intermediates teaching in their community. (p. 24)

8. Analyze how the EMT-Intermediate can benefit the health-care system by supporting primary care for patients in the out-of-hospital setting. (p. 23)

9. Describe how professionalism applies to the EMT-Intermediate while on and off duty. (pp. 24–25)

Part 4: Well-Being of the EMT-Intermediate (begins on p. 28)

After reading Part 4 of this chapter, you should be able to:

1. Discuss the concept of wellness and its benefits, components of wellness, and role of the EMT-Intermediate in promoting wellness. (p. 28)

2. Discuss how cardiovascular endurance, weight control, muscle strength, and flexibility contribute to physical fitness. (pp. 28–32)

3. Describe the impact of shift work on circadian rhythms. (p. 41)

4. Discuss the contributions that periodic risk assessments and warning-sign recognition make to cancer and cardiovascular disease prevention. (p. 30)

5. Differentiate proper from improper body mechanics for lifting and moving patients in emergency and non-emergency situations. (pp. 30, 32)

6. Describe the problems that an EMT-Intermediate might encounter in a hostile situation and the techniques used to manage the situation. (pp. 44–45)

7. Describe the considerations that should be given to using escorts, dealing with adverse environmental conditions, using lights and siren, proceeding through intersections, and parking at an emergency scene. (pp. 44–45)

8. Discuss the concept of "due regard for the safety of all others" while operating an emergency vehicle. (p. 45)

9. Describe the equipment available in a variety of adverse situations for self-protection, including body substance isolation steps for protection from airborne and bloodborne pathogens. (pp. 33–35, 44–45)

10. Given a scenario where equipment and supplies have been exposed to body substances, plan for the proper cleaning, disinfection, and disposal of the items. (p. 35)

11. Describe the benefits and methods of smoking cessation. (p. 30)
12. Identify and describe the three phases of the stress response, factors that trigger the stress response, and causes of stress in EMS. (p. 40)
13. Differentiate between normal/healthy and detrimental physiological and psychological reactions to anxiety and stress. (pp. 39–40)
14. Describe behavior that is a manifestation of stress in patients and those close to them, and describe how that behavior relates to EMT-Intermediate stress. (pp. 39–44)
15. Identify and describe the defense mechanisms and management techniques commonly used to deal with stress and the role of a personal support system in dealing with EMS stress. (pp. 41–44)
16. Given a scenario involving a stressful situation, formulate a strategy to help adapt to the stress. (pp. 39–44)
17. Describe the stages of the grieving process (Kübler-Ross) and the unique challenges for EMT-Intermediates in dealing with themselves, adults, children, and other special populations related to their understanding or experience of death and dying. (pp. 36–37)
18. Given photos of various motor-vehicle collisions, assess scene safety and propose ways to make the scene safer. (pp. 44–45)

Part 5: Illness and Injury Prevention (begins on p. 45)

After reading Part 5 of this chapter, you should be able to:

1. Describe the incidence, morbidity and mortality, and the human, environmental, and socioeconomic impact of unintentional and alleged unintentional injuries. (pp. 45–46)
2. Identify health hazards and potential crime areas within the community. (pp. 49–50)
3. Identify local municipal and community resources available for physical, socioeconomic crises. (pp. 47–48, 50–52)
4. List the general and specific environmental parameters that should be inspected to assess a patient's need for preventive information and direction. (pp. 49–52)
5. Identify the role of EMS in local municipal and community prevention programs. (pp. 50–52)
6. Identify the injury and illness prevention programs that promote safety for all age populations. (pp. 49–52)
7. Identify patient situations where the EMT-Intermediate can intervene in a preventive manner. (pp. 49–52)
8. Document primary and secondary injury prevention data. (pp. 50–52)

Part 6: Medical–Legal Considerations in Prehospital Care (begins on p. 52)

After reading Part 6 of this chapter, you should be able to:

1. Differentiate legal, ethical, and moral responsibilities. (p. 52)
2. Describe the basic structure of the legal system and differentiate civil and criminal law. (pp. 52-53)
3. Differentiate licensure and certification. (p. 55)
4. List reportable problems or conditions and to whom the reports are to be made. (p. 55)
5. Define: abandonment (p. 64), advance directives (p. 66), assault (p. 65), battery (p. 65), breach of duty (p. 57), confidentiality (p. 59), consent (expressed, implied, informed, involuntary) (pp. 61–62), do not resuscitate orders (p. 66), duty to act (p. 56), emancipated minor (p. 62), false imprisonment (p. 65), immunity (p. 55), liability (p. 52), libel (p. 61), minor (p. 62), negligence (p. 56), proximate cause (p. 57), scope of practice (p. 54), slander (p. 61), standard of care (p. 57), tort (p. 53).
6. Discuss the legal implications of medical direction. (pp. 54, 59
7. Describe the four elements necessary to prove negligence. (p. 56)
8. Explain liability as it applies to emergency medical services. (pp. 52, 56–59)
9. Discuss immunity, including Good Samaritan statutes, as it applies to the EMT-Intermediate. (pp. 55–56)
10. Explain the necessity and standards for maintaining patient confidentiality that apply to the EMT-Intermediate. (pp. 59–61)

Continued

11. Differentiate expressed, informed, implied, and involuntary consent and describe the process used to obtain informed or implied consent. (pp. 61–62)
12. Discuss appropriate patient interaction and documentation techniques regarding refusal of care. (pp. 62–64)
13. Identify legal issues involved in the decision not to transport a patient or to reduce the level of care. (pp. 64–65)
14. Describe the criteria and the role of the EMT-Intermediate in selecting hospitals to receive patients. (pp. 65–66)
15. Differentiate assault and battery. (p. 65)
16. Describe the conditions under which the use of force, including restraint, is acceptable. (p. 65)
17. Explain advance directives and how they impact patient care. (pp. 66–67)
18. Discuss the EMT-Intermediate's responsibilities relative to resuscitation efforts for patients who are potential organ donors. (p. 67)
19. Describe how an EMT-Intermediate may preserve evidence at a crime or injury scene. (pp. 67–68)
20. Describe the importance of providing accurate documentation of an EMS response. (pp. 68–69)
21. Describe what is required to make a patient care report an effective legal document. (pp. 68–69)

Part 7: Ethics in Advanced Prehospital Care (begins on p. 69)

After reading Part 7 of this chapter, you should be able to:

1. Define ethics and morals and distinguish between ethical and moral decisions in EMS. (pp. 69–71)
2. Identify the premise that should underlie the EMT-Intermediate's ethical decisions in out-of-hospital care. (pp. 70–71)
3. Analyze the relationship between the law and ethics in EMS. (p. 69)
4. Compare and contrast the criteria used in allocating scarce EMS resources. (pp. 76–77)
5. Identify issues surrounding advance directives in making a prehospital resuscitation decision and describe the criteria necessary to honor an advance directive in your state. (pp. 73–74)

CASE STUDY

It is a beautiful Fourth of July. You and your family are traveling down the interstate on your way to a concert and fireworks show. Just an hour from your destination, a tire blows out on the vehicle ahead of you. It skids into the median and crashes into some pine trees. You pull onto the shoulder. As an experienced EMT-Intermediate, you ensure scene safety before approaching the mangled car. You see no movement inside the passenger compartment.

Your daughter grabs the cell phone and calls 9-1-1. The dispatcher asks for the location of the crash and transfers the call to the 9-1-1 center for that area. The emergency medical dispatcher gathers the appropriate information and dispatches the local volunteer fire service and an advanced life support (ALS) ambulance. While you attempt to gain access to the patients, your daughter continues to provide the dispatcher with information that he, in turn, relays to the responding units.

The local volunteer fire and rescue team arrives on scene in about 7 minutes. You provide a verbal report to the arriving rescuers. They do their own scene safety check, approach the car, and determine that there are four patients. Two are priority-1 patients (one of these is a 2-year-old child), and two are priority-3 patients. Based on the initial assessment, Rescue Lt. C. J. Greenlee requests a medical helicopter and a second ALS unit. Approximately 2 minutes later, a fire truck crew arrives. They reroute traffic and establish a landing zone.

When all EMS personnel summoned are on scene, they decide that the 2-year-old patient will be flown to Children's Hospital, a pediatric specialty center. The other priority-1 patient will be transported by ground to the closest level-one trauma center. The priority-3 patients will be taken to the local hospital by ground transport.

Working as a team, the fire and ambulance personnel extricate the patients and package them for transport.

Approximately 22 minutes after the arrival of the first ALS unit, all patients are extricated and en route to a receiving facility capable of providing the level of care they need. Within 15 minutes of arrival at the pediatric trauma center and just 31 minutes after the crash, the 2-year-old is moved to surgery for the repair of a ruptured liver and spleen. The other patients are being treated at their destinations as well.

INTRODUCTION

Congratulations on your decision to become an Emergency Medical Technician-Intermediate (EMT-Intermediate or EMT-I). Before you begin this rewarding endeavor, it is important to understand what the job of an EMT-I in the twenty-first century entails. Emergency Medical Services (EMS) has made significant advances over the last 30 years. Not that long ago, the ambulance was simply a vehicle that provided rapid, horizontal transportation to the hospital. Today, equipped with the latest in equipment and technology, the ambulance is truly a mobile emergency room. The EMT-I of the twenty-first century is a highly trained health-care professional.

Part 1: Introduction to Advanced Prehospital Care

The EMT-I is the second-highest level of prehospital care provider and an important member of the prehospital care team (Figure 1-1). As a member of the **allied health professions,** the EMT-I is highly regarded by society.

allied health professions
ancillary health care professions, apart from physicians and nurses.

DESCRIPTION OF THE PROFESSION

The primary task of the EMT-I is to provide emergency medical care in an out-of-hospital setting, extending the care of the emergency physician to the patient in the field. To function as an EMT-I you must have fulfilled the prescribed requirements of the appropriate licensing or credentialing body. The EMT-I may only function under the direction and license

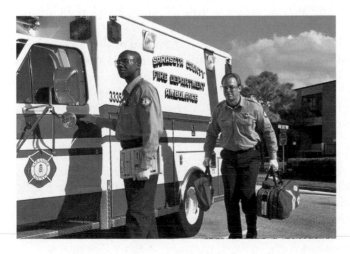

FIGURE 1-1   The EMT-Intermediate is an important member of the prehospital care team.

of the EMS system's medical director. Because of this, the EMT-I must also be approved by the system's medical director before being permitted to practice.

There are many different types of EMS system designs and operations. As an EMT-I, you may work for a fire department, private ambulance service, third city service, hospital, police department, or other operation. Regardless of the type of service, you will be an essential component in the continuum of care and will often serve as a link between various health resources. Although the EMT-I of the twenty-first century will continue to fill the well-defined and traditional role of 9-1-1 response, he will also encounter a wide variety of additional responsibilities. The emerging roles and responsibilities of the EMT-I include public education, health promotion, and participation in injury and illness prevention programs. As a consequence of the need to cut costs, you may be charged with ensuring that your patient gets to the appropriate health-care facility, which may be a facility other than the hospital emergency department. Thus, the EMT-I may begin to function as a facilitator of access to care as well as an individual treatment provider.

An EMT-I must always strive toward maintaining high quality health care at a reasonable cost. Nevertheless, you must always be an advocate for your patient and make sure he receives the best possible care—without regard to his ability to pay or insurance status.

An EMT-I is responsible and accountable to the system medical director, his employer, the public, and peers. Although this may seem like a difficult standard to meet, if you always act in the best interest of the patient, you will seldom run into problems.

> *You must always be an advocate for your patient and make sure that the patient receives the best possible care.*
>
>

> *EMT-Is are accountable to their medical director, their employer, the public, and peers.*
>
>

EMT-INTERMEDIATE CHARACTERISTICS

As an EMT-I, you must be a confident leader who can accept the challenge and responsibility of the position. You must have excellent judgment and be able to prioritize decisions so as to act quickly in the best interest of the patient. You must be able to develop rapport with a wide variety of patients so that, for example, you can safely interview hostile patients and communicate with members of diverse cultural groups and the various ages within those groups. Overall, you must be able to function independently at an optimum level in a nonstructured, constantly changing environment. The job is never easy and always challenging.

> *You must be able to function independently at an optimum level in a nonstructured, constantly changing environment.*

EMT-INTERMEDIATE: A TRUE HEALTH PROFESSIONAL

Despite its relative youth as a profession, the field of emergency medical services is now recognized as an important part of the health-care system. As an EMT-I, you must never take this status for granted. Instead, you must always strive to earn your acceptance as a health-care professional. Consider the completion of your initial EMT-I course to be the beginning of your professional education, not the end. Participate in continuing education programs. Frequently review and practice skills, especially those used less frequently. Participate in routine peer-evaluation and assume an active role in professional and community organizations.

A major step toward the development of EMS as a true health-care profession has been to raise the standards of education for prehospital personnel. A significant advance was the U.S. Department of Transportation's 1998 publication of the revised *EMT-Intermediate: National Standard Curriculum,* which has taken EMT-I's education to a much higher level. The course now requires a far more extensive foundation of medical knowledge to underlie the required skills. DOT's EMT-I curriculum is the guideline for this textbook.

As an EMT-I, you must actively participate in the design, development, evaluation, and publication of research on topics relevant to your profession. For years, EMT-I practice was based on anecdotal data and tradition. Only during the 1990s did EMS truly begin applying the scientific method to various aspects of prehospital practice. Surprisingly, there was little or no scientific data to support many prehospital practices. As a result of research, many traditional EMS treatments have been abandoned or refined. There are still unanswered questions about EMT-I practice, and these can only be answered by sound, ongoing scientific research.

Another essential aspect of a health professional is acceptance and adherence to a code of professional ethics and etiquette. The public must feel confident that, for the EMT-I, the patient's and public's interests are always placed above personal, corporate, or financial interests. You must never forget that the patient is your primary concern.

An essential aspect of a health professional is acceptance and adherence to a code of professional ethics and etiquette.

Part 2: EMS Systems

An **emergency medical services (EMS) system** is a comprehensive network of personnel, equipment, and resources established to deliver aid and emergency medical care to the community. An EMS system is comprised of both out-of-hospital and in-hospital components. The out-of-hospital component includes:

- Members of the community who are trained in first aid and cardiopulmonary resuscitation (CPR)
- A communications system that allows public access to emergency services dispatch and allows EMS providers to communicate with each other
- EMS providers, including EMT-Intermediates
- Fire/rescue and hazardous-materials services
- Public utilities, such as power and gas companies
- Resource centers, such as regional poison control centers

The in-hospital component includes:

- Emergency nurses
- Emergency physicians and specialty physicians
- Ancillary services, such as radiology and respiratory therapy
- Specialty physicians, such as trauma surgeons and cardiologists
- Rehabilitation services

emergency medical services (EMS) system a comprehensive network of personnel, equipment, and resources established for the purpose of delivering aid and emergency medical care to the community.

A typical EMS operation begins with citizen activation when someone contacts a 9-1-1 dispatch center. EMS dispatch collects essential information and sends out the closest appropriately staffed and equipped unit. In many EMS systems, the dispatcher also provides pre-arrival instructions to caller.

The first EMS provider at the scene may be a police officer, firefighter, lifeguard, teacher, or other community member who has been trained as a First Responder. The First Responder's role is to stabilize the patient until more advanced personnel arrive. The next EMS provider likely to arrive depends on the type of EMS system. In most areas, the dispatcher will send either a **basic life support (BLS)** or an **advanced life support (ALS)** ambulance. Other EMS systems use a "tiered response," sending multiple levels of emergency care personnel to the same incident. In still other areas, ALS personnel respond to every incident regardless of the level of care needed.

basic life support (BLS) refers to basic life-saving procedures such as artificial ventilation and cardiopulmonary resuscitation (CPR).

advanced life support (ALS) refers to advanced life-saving procedures such as intravenous therapy, drug therapy, and intubation.

Once care has been initiated, EMS providers must quickly decide on the medical facility to which the patient should be transported—based on the type of care needed, transport time, and local protocols. Where specialty centers have been designated (such as pediatric, trauma, and burn centers), it may be necessary to transport the patient to a facility other than the closest hospital. At the receiving medical facility, an emergency nurse or physician assumes responsibility, and the patient is assigned a priority of care. If needed, a surgeon or other specialist will be summoned.

HISTORY OF EMS

Evidence suggests that emergency medicine has a very long history, beginning as far back as biblical times.

ANCIENT TIMES

Emergency medicine may be traced to biblical times when it was recorded that a "good Samaritan" provided care to a wounded traveler by the side of a road. In fact, about 4,000 to 5,000 years ago, Sumerians inscribed clay tablets with some of the earliest medical records. Similar to EMS protocols today, the tablets provided step-by-step instructions for care based on the patient's description of symptoms as well as instructions on how to create and administer medications. The most striking difference between these first "protocols" and EMS today is the absence of a physical exam.

In 1862, the Egyptologist Edwin Smith purchased a papyrus scroll dating to about 1500 B.C.E. It contained forty-eight medical case histories with data arranged in head-to-toe order and in order of severity, an arrangement very similar to today's patient assessment. One section, the "Book of Wounds," explains the treatment of injuries such as fractures and dislocations.

At about the same time as that scroll was written, King Hammurabi of Babylon created a code of laws known today as the "Code of Hammurabi." A section of the code regulated medical fees and penalties based on the social class of the patient. For example, if a surgeon operated successfully on a commoner, he would be paid only half of what his fee would be if he had operated on a rich man. If a surgeon caused the death of a rich man, the surgeon's hand would be cut off, but if a slave died under his care, he only had to replace the slave.

EIGHTEENTH AND NINETEENTH CENTURIES

During the Napoleonic Wars of the early nineteenth century, one of Napoleon's chief surgeons, Jean Larrey, formed the *ambulance volante,* or "flying ambulance," which focused efforts on providing emergency surgery as close to the battlefield as possible. Though the *ambulance volante* was little more than a covered horse-drawn cart, Larrey is credited with the development of the first prehospital system that used **triage** and transport.

triage a method of sorting patients by the severity of their injuries.

Between 1861 and 1865, during the U.S. Civil War, a nurse named Clara Barton coordinated care for the sick and injured. Defying army leaders, she persisted in going to the front where wounded men suffered and often died from lack of the simplest medical attention. She organized the triage and transport of injured soldiers to improvised hospitals in nearby houses, barns, and churches away from the battlefield.

The first civilian ambulance service was formed about the same time (1865) in Cincinnati, Ohio. Four years later in 1869 the New York City Health Department Ambulance Service began operating out of Bellevue Hospital. The ambulances of both services were specially designed horse-drawn carts, which were staffed with physician interns from the various hospital wards.

TWENTIETH CENTURY

During World War I, a high mortality rate of soldiers was associated with an average evacuation time of 18 hours. As a result, in World War II a system was created in which battlefield ambulance corps transported wounded soldiers from the front lines to higher echelons (levels) of care. However, many of the echelons were so far from the battlefield and each other that there were huge delays in patient care. In many cases, it was often days from the injury itself to definitive surgery.

During the Korean and Vietnam conflicts, there were great advances in the patient care delivery system. The wounded soldier was treated on the battlefield when the injury occurred and evacuated by helicopter to a field hospital to receive definitive surgery. In Vietnam, in many cases, this occurred within 10 to 20 minutes. Once stabilized and able to be moved (generally within 24 to 48 hours), the patient would be transported by jet to Clark Air Force Base in the Philippines for further treatment. The decrease in the amount of time to definitive care plus the advances in medical procedures significantly reduced mortality rates.

trauma a physical injury or wound caused by external force or violence.

Throughout history, significant advances in **trauma** care occurred during wartime. However, until the late 1960s, few areas of the United States provided adequate civilian prehospital emergency care. Medical care began in the hospital emergency department. Rescue techniques were crude, ambulance attendants poorly educated, and equipment minimal.

Police, fire, and EMS personnel had no radio communication. Proper medical direction was not available, and the only interaction between physicians and EMS personnel was at the receiving facility.

Eventually, as costs and demand for additional services forced many rural mortician-operated ambulances to withdraw, local police and fire departments found that they had to provide the ambulance service. In many areas, volunteer ambulance services made up of local, independent EMS provider agencies proliferated. In the urban setting, the increased demand on hospital-based EMS systems resulted in the development of municipal services at city, county, or regional levels. However, because they could not communicate with each other, it was impossible to coordinate a response to any but the simplest local calls.

In 1966 the publication of *Accidental Death and Disability: The Neglected Disease of Modern Society* by the National Academy of Sciences, National Resource Council, focused attention on the problem. "The White Paper," as the report was called, spelled out the deficiencies in prehospital emergency care. It suggested guidelines for the development of EMS systems, the training of prehospital emergency medical providers, and the upgrading of ambulances and their equipment. This landmark publication set off a series of federal and private initiatives, including these:

- *1966.* The U.S. Congress passed the National Highway Safety Act, which established the U.S. Department of Transportation (DOT), a cabinet-level department. It provided matching grants to states for emergency medical services and forced them to develop effective EMS systems or risk losing federal highway construction funds. In 1969 the Emergency Medical Technician–Ambulance program was made public. The first EMT-I curriculum followed later.

- *1971.* The White House gave nearly $9 million to EMS model demonstration projects.

- *1972.* The Department of Health, Education, and Welfare funded a $16 million five-state initiative for the development of regional EMS systems. The next year, the Robert Wood Johnson Foundation provided approximately $15 million in grants for establishing regional EMS projects and communication systems.

Then, in 1973 the U.S. Congress passed the Emergency Medical Services Systems Act, which provided additional funding for a series of projects related to the delivery of trauma care. As a result, the development of regional EMS systems continued from 1974 through 1981. A total of $300 million was allocated to study the feasibility of EMS planning, operations, expansion, and research.

In order to be eligible for this funding, an EMS system had to include the following 15 components: manpower, training, communications, transportation, emergency facilities, critical-care units, public safety agencies, consumer participation, access to care, patient transfer, standardized record keeping, public information and education, system review and evaluation, disaster management plans, and mutual aid. Unfortunately, the designers of this legislation omitted two major components: system financing and **medical direction**. The Emergency Medical Services Systems Act was amended in 1976 and again in 1979, and a total of $215 million was appropriated over a seven-year period toward the establishment of regional EMS systems.

In 1981, the passage of the Consolidated Omnibus Budget Reconciliation Act (COBRA) essentially wiped out federal funding for EMS. The small amount of funding that remained was placed into state preventive-health and health-services block grants. The National Highway Traffic Safety Administration (NHTSA) attempted to sustain the efforts of the Department of Health and Human Services, but with its other EMS responsibilities and no additional funding, the momentum for continued development was lost.

In 1988, the Statewide EMS Technical Assessment Program was established by the NHTSA. It defines elements necessary to all EMS systems. Briefly, they are:

- *Regulation and policy.* Each state must have laws, regulations, policies, and procedures that govern its EMS system. It also is required to provide leadership to local jurisdictions.

Content Review

1973 EMSS ACT: 15 COMPONENTS OF EMS SYSTEMS
- Manpower
- Training
- Communications
- Transportation
- Emergency facilities
- Critical care units
- Public safety agencies
- Consumer participation
- Access to care
- Patient transfer
- Standardized record keeping
- Public information and education
- System review and evaluation
- Disaster management plans
- Mutual aid

medical direction medical policies, procedures, and practices that are available to providers either on-line or off-line.

Content Review

1988 NHTSA: "10 SYSTEM ELEMENTS"
- Regulation and policy
- Resources management
- Human resources and training
- Transportation
- Facilities
- Communications
- Trauma systems
- Public information and education
- Medical direction
- Evaluation

- *Resources management.* Each state must have central control of EMS resources so all patients have equal access to acceptable emergency care.
- *Human resources and training.* A standardized EMS curriculum should be taught by qualified instructors, and all personnel who transport patients in the prehospital setting should be adequately trained.
- *Transportation.* Patients must be safely and reliably transported by ground or air ambulance.
- *Facilities.* Every seriously ill or injured patient must be delivered in a timely manner to an appropriate medical facility.
- *Communications.* A system for public access to the EMS system must be in place. Communication among dispatchers, the ambulance crew, and hospital personnel must also be possible.
- *Trauma systems.* Each state should develop a system of specialized care for trauma patients, including one or more trauma centers and rehabilitation programs. It also must develop systems for assigning and transporting patients to those facilities.
- *Public information and education.* EMS personnel should participate in programs designed to educate the public. The programs are to focus on the prevention of injuries and how to properly access the EMS system.
- *Medical direction.* Each EMS system must have a physician as its medical director. This physician delegates medical practice to non-physician caregivers and oversees all aspects of patient care.
- *Evaluation.* Each state must have a quality improvement system in place for continuing evaluation and upgrading of its EMS system.

Many EMS providers today fail to realize that each component of the EMS system has gone through many stages of development. Nevertheless, in this technologically advanced country, there are still startling regional differences in the quality of prehospital care.

TODAY'S EMS SYSTEMS

Though EMS systems across the country and the world vary, certain elements are essential to ensure the best possible patient care.

LOCAL AND STATE-LEVEL AGENCIES

At the municipal and regional levels, an administrative agency manages the local EMS system's resources, developing operational protocols, and establishing standards and guidelines. The agency's planning board should include emergency physicians, the emergency nurse association, the firefighter association, state and local police, and "consumers." It develops a budget and selects a qualified administrative staff. The agency designates who may function within the system and develops policies consistent with existing state requirements and creates a quality assurance or quality improvement program.

State EMS agencies are typically responsible for allocating funds to local systems, sponsoring legislation concerning the prehospital practice of medicine, licensing, and certification, enforcing state EMS regulations, and appointing regional advisory councils.

In essence, EMS is made up of a series of systems within a system. The integration of these systems and the cooperation of all participants help to result in the best quality of emergency care.

MEDICAL DIRECTION

An EMS system must retain a **medical director**—a physician who is legally responsible for all clinical and patient-care aspects of the system. Prehospital medical care provided by non-physicians is considered an extension of the medical director's license; that is, prehospital care providers are the medical director's designated agents, regardless of who their employers may be.

All prehospital care providers are the medical director's designated agents, regardless of who their employer may be.

medical director a physician who is legally responsible for all of the clinical and patient-care aspects of an EMS system. Also referred to as *medical direction.*

The medical director's role in an EMS system is to:

- Educate and train personnel
- Participate in personnel and equipment selection
- Develop clinical protocols in cooperation with expert EMS personnel
- Participate in quality improvement and problem resolution
- Provide direct input into patient care
- Interface between the EMS system and other health-care agencies
- Advocate within the medical community
- Serve as the "medical conscience" of the EMS system, including advocating for quality patient care

In addition to the responsibilities listed above, the medical director is the ultimate authority for all on-line (direct) and off-line (indirect) medical direction.

On-Line Medical Direction

On-line medical direction occurs when a qualified physician gives direct orders to a prehospital care provider by either radio or telephone (Figure 1-2). Medical direction may be delegated to a mobile intensive care nurse (MICN), a physician assistant (PA), or an EMT-I. In all circumstances, ultimate on-line responsibility remains with the medical director.

On-line medical direction offers several benefits to the patient, including immediate medical consultation and use of telemetry to provide instant diagnostic information to the medical director. In most systems, on-line consultations can be recorded for review and quality improvement.

At the emergency scene, the provider with the most knowledge and experience in the delivery of prehospital emergency care should be in charge. When a non-affiliated physician, or **intervener physician,** is on scene and on-line medical direction does not exist, the EMT-I should relinquish responsibility to the physician. However, the intervener physician must first identify himself, demonstrate a willingness to accept responsibility, and document the intervention as required by the local EMS system. If his treatment differs from established protocol, the intervener physician must accompany the patient in the ambulance to the hospital. If an intervener physician is on scene and on-line medical direction does exist, the on-line physician is ultimately responsible. In case of a disagreement, the EMT-I must take orders from the on-line physician.

Off-Line Medical Direction

Off-line medical direction refers to medical policies, procedures, and practices that a system physician has set up in advance of a call. It includes "prospective medical direction," such as guidelines on the selection of personnel and supplies, training and education, and protocol development. It also includes "retrospective medical direction," such as auditing, peer review, and other quality assurance processes.

Protocols are the policies and procedures of an EMS system. They provide a standardized approach to common patient problems, a consistent level of medical care, and a standard for accountability. Based on such protocols, the on-line physician can assist prehospital personnel in interpreting the patient's complaint, understanding assessment findings, and providing the appropriate treatment. Protocols are designed around the four "Ts" of emergency care:

- *Triage*—guidelines that address patient flow through an EMS system, including how system resources are allocated to meet the needs of patients
- *Treatment*—guidelines that identify procedures to be performed upon direct order from medical direction and procedures that are pre-authorized protocols called **standing orders**
- *Transport*—guidelines that address the mode of travel (air vs. ground) based on the nature of the patient's injury or illness, his condition, the level of care required, and estimated transport time

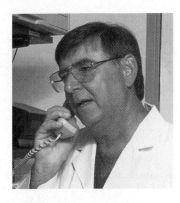

FIGURE 1-2 The medical director can provide on-line guidance to EMS personnel in the field.

on-line medical direction occurs when a qualified physician gives direct orders to a prehospital care provider by either radio or telephone.

intervener physician a licensed physician, professionally unrelated to patients on scene, who attempts to assist EMS providers with patient care.

Content Review

FOUR "Ts" OF EMERGENCY CARE
- Triage
- Treatment
- Transport
- Transfer

off-line medical direction refers to medical policies, procedures, and practices that medical direction has set up in advance of a call.

protocols the policies and procedures for all components of an EMS system.

standing orders preauthorized treatment procedures; a type of treatment protocol.

- *Transfer*—guidelines that address receiving facilities to ensure that the patient is admitted to the one most appropriate for definitive care

Protocols also are established for special circumstances, such as Do Not Resuscitate (DNR) orders, patients who refuse treatment, sexual abuse, abuse of children or elderly people, termination of CPR, and intervener physicians. Although protocols standardize field procedures, they should allow the EMT-I the flexibility to improvise and adapt to special circumstances.

PUBLIC INFORMATION AND EDUCATION

The public is an essential, yet often overlooked, component of an EMS system. EMS should have a plan to educate the public on recognizing an emergency, accessing the system, and initiating basic life support procedures.

Recognizing an emergency can save lives. For example, the American Heart Association (AHA) estimates that over 300,000 cardiac arrests per year occur before the patient reaches the hospital. Such arrests are called "sudden death" because most happen within two hours of the onset of cardiac symptoms. Many patients delay calling for help when symptoms occur. If the patient and bystanders are taught to recognize the emergency and call for help in time, many cases of sudden death could be prevented.

The second aspect of public education is system access. Citizens must know how to activate EMS in an emergency to avoid life-threatening delays. Whether access is by way of 9-1-1 or a local seven-digit phone number, the number should be well publicized, and citizens should be taught how to give the necessary information to the emergency medical dispatcher.

Finally, after recognizing an emergency and activating EMS, citizens must know how to provide basic life support assistance, such as CPR and bleeding control after major trauma. Abundant research indicates that a relationship exists between EMS response times and mortality (death) rates of patients. Communities have proven that when many citizens are trained in basic life support—and there is a rapid advanced life support (ALS) response—a larger number of patients can be successfully resuscitated.

Future public involvement may include bystander defibrillation. With the development of automated external defibrillator (AED) technology, it may soon be possible to place affordable, portable AEDs in the homes of cardiac patients as well as in all public places.

COMMUNICATIONS

The communications network is the heart of a regional EMS system. A communications plan should include:

- *Citizen access*. A well-publicized universal number, such as 9-1-1, provides direct citizen access to emergency services. Multiple community numbers add life-threatening minutes to emergency response times. Enhanced 9-1-1, or E-9-1-1, gives automatic locations of the caller, instant routing of the call to the appropriate emergency service (fire, police, or EMS), and instant callback capability.

- *Single control center* (Figure 1-3). One control center that can communicate with and direct all emergency vehicles within a large geographical area is best. Ideally, all public service agencies should be dispatched from the same communications center.

- *Operational communications capabilities*. With these, EMS dispatch can manage all aspects of system response and assess the system's readiness for the next response. Emergency units can communicate with each other and with other agencies during mutual aid and disaster operations. Hospitals also can communicate with other hospitals in the region to assess specialty capabilities.

- *Medical communications capabilities*. EMS providers can communicate with the receiving facility and, in many areas, transmit ECG telemetry signals to the on-line physician. Hospitals also can communicate with each other to facilitate patient transfer.

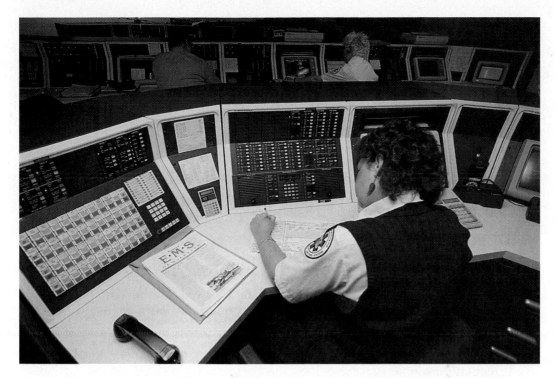

FIGURE 1-3 The ideal communications center can communicate with and control the movement of all emergency units within an EMS system.

- *Communications hardware.* Radios, consoles, pagers, cell phone transmission towers, repeaters, telephone landlines, and other telecommunications equipment are required.
- *Communications software.* This includes radio frequencies and, in many systems, satellite and high-tech computer programs that track ambulances. Procedures, policies consistent with FCC standards and local protocols, and back-up communications plans for disaster operations are essential.

EMERGENCY MEDICAL DISPATCHER (EMD)

The **emergency medical dispatcher** (EMD) is crucial to the operation of EMS. EMDs not only send ambulances to the scene, but also make sure that system resources are in constant readiness to respond. EMDs must be both medically and technically trained. The course should be standardized and include certification by a government agency.

EMS DISPATCH

Emergency medical dispatching is the nerve center of an EMS system. It should be under the full control of the medical director and the EMS agency. In general, EMS system status management relies on projected call volumes and locations to make strategic placement of ambulances and crews. This method helps to reduce response times. Another management method, "priority dispatching," was first used by the Salt Lake City Fire Department. Using a set of medically approved protocols, EMDs are trained to medically interrogate a distressed caller, prioritize symptoms, select an appropriate response, and give life-saving pre-arrival instructions.

In 1974, the Phoenix Fire Department introduced a pre-arrival instruction program developed by medically trained dispatchers. In that program, callers initiate life-saving first aid with the dispatcher's help while they wait for emergency units to arrive on scene. In 1985, the Seattle EMS system initiated a successful program of instructing callers in CPR. Pre-arrival instruction may result in increased liability, but the liability risk of not providing it may far outweigh the risk of providing it.

emergency medical dispatcher (EMD) EMS person medically and technically trained to assign emergency medical resources to a medical emergency.

An effective EMS dispatching system places the first responding units on scene within 4 minutes of onset of the emergency. The American Heart Association (AHA) reports that brain resuscitation will not be successful unless proper BLS intervention (CPR) occurs within 4 minutes. Studies also suggest that defibrillation within 8 minutes can reverse sudden-death mortality. So, the goal of emergency response is: BLS care in less than 4 minutes and ALS care in less than 8 minutes after the event. High-performance systems meet this standard more than 90% of the time.

EMS EDUCATION AND CERTIFICATION

EMS education includes both initial and continuing programs. *Initial education* programs are the original training courses for prehospital providers. *Continuing education* programs include refresher courses for recertification and periodic in-service training.

Initial Education

An EMT-I's initial education is completion of a course that follows the most recent *EMT-Intermediate: National Standard Curriculum* published by the U.S. DOT, which establishes the minimum content and sets a nationwide standard for EMT-I programs. The National Standard Curriculum is divided into three specific learning domains:

- *Cognitive,* which consists of facts, or information knowledge
- *Affective,* which requires students to assign emotions, values, and attitudes to that information
- *Psychomotor,* which consists of hands-on skills students learn while in laboratory and clinical settings

Once initial education is completed, the EMT-I will become either certified or licensed, depending on the state. **Certification** is the process by which an agency or association grants recognition to an individual who has met its qualifications. Many states certify EMTs.

Licensure is a process of occupational regulation. Through licensure, a governmental agency (usually a state agency) grants permission to engage in a given trade or profession to an applicant who has attained the degree of competency required to ensure the public's protection. Some states choose to license EMTs instead of certifying them. (Note that there is an unfounded general belief that a licensed professional has greater status than one who is certified or registered. However, a certification granted by a state, conferring a right to engage in a trade or profession, is in fact a license.)

Registration is accomplished by entering your name and essential information within a particular record. An EMT is registered so that the state can verify the provider's initial certification and monitor recertification. Almost every state has an EMS office that tracks the registration of emergency care providers. Although some states track only ALS providers, others maintain registers on the certifications of all provider levels.

Reciprocity is the process by which an agency grants automatic certification or licensure to an individual who has comparable certification or licensure from another agency. For example, some states grant reciprocity to EMTs who are certified in another state.

Certification Levels

In 1983, because of variations in state and regional EMS terminology, there were as many as 30 levels of prehospital care providers. Since then, the National Registry of EMTs has recognized—and the DOT has developed curricula for—four different levels of providers. They are:

- *First Responder.* Usually the first EMS-trained provider to arrive on scene, the First Responder's role is to stabilize the patient until more advanced EMS personnel arrive. He is trained to perform a general patient assessment and to provide emergency care such as bleeding control, spinal stabilization, and CPR. He also may assist in emergency childbirth. In some areas, he is trained in the administration of oxygen and in the use of an automated external defibrillator (AED).

---

certification the process by which an agency or association grants recognition to an individual who has met its qualifications.

licensure the process by which a governmental agency grants permission to engage in a given occupation to an applicant who has attained the degree of competency required to ensure the public's protection.

registration the process of entering your name and essential information within a particular record. In EMS this is done in order for the state to verify the provider's initial certification and to monitor recertification.

reciprocity the process by which an agency grants automatic certification or licensure to an individual who has comparable certification or licensure from another agency.

Content Review

EMS CERTIFICATION LEVELS

- First Responder
- EMT-Basic
- EMT-Intermediate
- EMT-Paramedic

- *Emergency Medical Technician-Basic (EMT-B).* This EMS provider is trained to do all that a First Responder can do, plus perform complex immobilization procedures, restrain patients, and drive and staff ambulances. The EMT-B also may assist in the administration of certain medications and, in some areas, perform endotracheal intubation.
- *Emergency Medical Technician-Intermediate (EMT-I).* The EMT-I should possess all EMT-B skills and be competent in advanced airway management, intravenous fluid therapy, and certain other advanced skills. In some states, the EMT-I may be trained as a cardiac technician and authorized to administer additional medications.
- *Emergency Medical Technician-Paramedic (EMT-P).* As the most advanced EMS provider, the paramedic is trained in all EMT-I skills, plus advanced patient assessment, trauma management, pharmacology, cardiology, and other medical skills. He should successfully complete advanced cardiac life support (ACLS) and pediatric advanced life support (PALS) courses offered by the AHA. Basic trauma life support (BTLS) or prehospital trauma life support (PHTLS) course completion is also desirable.

In addition to gaining knowledge and skills, the EMT-I should have or acquire the high regard for human dignity and passion for excellence expected of all **health-care professionals.**

health-care professionals properly trained and licensed or certified providers of health care.

profession refers to the existence of a specialized body of knowledge or skills.

professionalism refers to the conduct or qualities that characterize a practitioner in a particular field or occupation.

National Registry of EMTs

The National Registry of Emergency Medical Technicians (NREMT) prepares and administers standardized tests for the First Responder, EMT-B, EMT-I, and EMT-P. It establishes the qualifications for registration and serves as a major tool for reciprocity by providing a process for EMTs to become certified when moving from one state to another. The National Registry also develops and evaluates EMT training programs. Currently, the majority of states use National Registry examinations. Several states instead offer locally developed examinations.

Professional Organizations

Belonging to a professional organization is a good way to keep informed and share ideas. National EMS organizations include:

- National Association of Emergency Medical Technicians (NAEMT)
- National Association of Search and Rescue (NASAR)
- National Association of State EMS Directors (NASEMSD)
- National Association of EMS Physicians (NAEMSP)
- National Flight Paramedics Association (NFPA)
- National Council of State EMS Training Coordinators (NCSEMSTC)

These are just some examples of organizations through which EMS providers can enrich themselves and pursue their particular interests. Such organizations assist in the development of educational programs, operational policies and procedures, and the implementation of EMS.

Professional Journals

The following is just a partial list of the many journals that are available to keep the EMT-I aware of the latest changes in this ever-changing industry as well as offer an opportunity for EMS professionals to write and publish articles:

- *Annals of Emergency Medicine*
- *Emergency Medical Services*
- *Journal of Emergency Medical Services*
- *Journal of Emergency Medicine*
- *Journal of Pediatric Emergency Medicine*

- *Journal of Trauma*
- *Prehospital Emergency Care*

PATIENT TRANSPORTATION

Patients who are transported under the direction of an EMS system should be taken to the nearest appropriate medical facility whenever possible. Medical direction should designate that facility, based on the needs of the patient and the availability of services. In some cases, the patient's need for special services (such as care for burns) means designating a facility that is not nearby. At other times, the closest facility will be designated for stabilization of the patient while transfer is arranged. The ultimate authority for this decision remains with on-line medical direction.

Patients may be transported by ground or air. Today, trauma care systems use law enforcement, municipal, hospital-based, private, and military helicopter transport services to transfer patients. Fixed-wing aircraft also are used when patients must be transported long distances, usually more than 200 miles.

All transport vehicles must be licensed and meet local and state EMS requirements. In 1983, the American College of Surgeons Committee on Trauma recommended a standard set of equipment to be carried by providers of BLS services. In 1988, the American College of Emergency Physicians (ACEP) recommended a list of ALS supplies and equipment. These recommendations serve as guidelines for all prehospital EMS systems. Regional standardization of equipment and supplies is most effective in facilitating inter-agency efforts during disaster operations.

In 1974, in response to a request from the DOT, the General Services Administration developed the "KKK-A-1822 Federal Specifications for Ambulances." This was the first attempt at standardizing ambulance design. The act defined the following basic types of ambulances:

- *Type I.* A conventional cab and chassis on which a module ambulance body is mounted, with no passageway between driver and patient compartments.
- *Type II.* A standard van, body, and cab form an integral unit. Most have a raised roof.
- *Type III.* A specialty van with forward cab, integral body, and a passageway from driver's compartment to patient's compartment.

Only these certified ambulances may display the registered "Star of Life" symbol as defined by the NHTSA. The word "ambulance" should appear in mirror image on the front so that other drivers can identify the ambulance in their rear-view mirrors.

In 1980, the revision "KKK-A-1822A" aimed at improving ambulance electrical systems by designing a low-amp lighting system to replace antiquated light bars and beacons. In 1985, another revision "KKK-A-1822B" specified changes based on National Institute for Occupational Safety and Health (NIOSH) standards. These include reduced internal siren noise, high engine temperatures, and exhaust emissions; safer cot-retention systems; wider axles; hand-held spotlights; battery conditioners for longer life; and venting systems for oxygen compartments. The KKK-A-1822 specifications continue to be updated periodically as technology and standards change.

All ambulances purchased with federal funds must comply with these criteria. However, some states have adopted their own stricter criteria.

RECEIVING FACILITIES

Not all hospitals are equal in emergency and support service capabilities. So, how do you get the right patient to the right facility in an appropriate amount of time? EMS systems categorize hospitals according to their ability to receive and treat emergency patients. EMS coordinators use these categories to quickly identify the most appropriate facility for definitive treatment or life-saving stabilization. Regionalizing available services also helps give all patients reasonable access to the appropriate facility. Burn, trauma, pediatric, psychiatric, perinatal, cardiac, spinal, and poison centers are examples of specialty service facilities that offer high-level care for specific groups of patients in a wide region. Large EMS systems should designate a resource hospital that will coordinate specialty resources and ensure appropriate patient distribution.

To select the appropriate receiving facility for your patient, it is important to know which facilities in your area offer the following services:

- Fully staffed and equipped emergency department
- Trauma care capabilities
- Operating suites available 24 hours a day, 7 days a week
- Critical care units, such as post-anesthesia recovery rooms and surgical intensive care units
- Cardiac facilities with on-staff cardiologists
- Neurology department that provides a "stroke team"
- Acute hemodialysis capability
- Pediatric capabilities, including pediatric and neonatal intensive care units
- Obstetric capabilities, including facilities for high-risk delivery
- Radiological specialty capabilities, such as computerized tomography (CT) and magnetic resonance imaging (MRI)
- Burn specialization for infants, children, and adults
- Acute spinal-cord and head-injury management capability
- Rehabilitation staff and facilities
- Clinical laboratory services
- Toxicology, including hazardous materials (hazmat) decontamination facilities
- Hyperbaric oxygen therapy capability
- Microvascular surgical capabilities for replants
- Psychiatric facilities

Receiving facilities are categorized by the level of care they can provide. For example, the American College of Surgeons categorizes trauma centers by levels:

- *Level I*—provides the highest level of trauma care
- *Level II*—may not have specialty pediatrics or a neurosurgeon on site
- *Level III*—generally does not have immediate surgical facilities available

A fourth designation may be given to specialty referral centers, which offer unique services. They include burn, pediatric, psychiatric, perinatal, cardiac, spinal, and poison centers.

Ideally, all receiving facilities should have the following capabilities: an emergency department with an emergency physician on duty at all times, surgical facilities, a lab and blood bank, x-ray capabilities available around the clock, and critical and intensive care units. They should have a documented commitment to participate in the EMS system, a willingness to receive all emergency patients in transport regardless of their ability to pay, and medical audit procedures to ensure quality care and medical accountability. Finally, receiving facilities should exhibit a desire to participate in multiple-casualty preparedness plans.

MUTUAL AID AND MASS-CASUALTY PREPARATION

Since the resources of any one EMS system can be overwhelmed, a mutual-aid agreement ensures that help is available when needed. Such agreements may be among neighboring departments, municipalities, systems, or states. Cooperation must transcend geographical, political, and historical boundaries.

Each EMS system should have a disaster plan for catastrophes that can overwhelm available resources. There should be a coordinated central management agency, integration of all EMS system components, and a flexible communications system. Frequent drills should test the plan's effectiveness and practicality.

Each EMS system should have a disaster plan that is practiced frequently.

Legal Notes

Since the attacks on the United States on September 11, 2001, disaster response and EMS have taken on significantly more and different responsibilities. All EMS personnel must be prepared for disasters, regardless of the cause. Biological and chemical agents pose significant risks to EMS personnel. Preparation and education is the key to survival in the event they are encountered.

Excellence is the only acceptable quality of an EMS system.

Content Review

GUIDELINES FOR QUALITY IMPROVEMENT
- Leadership
- Information and analysis
- Strategic quality planning
- Human resources development and management
- EMS process management
- EMS system results
- Satisfaction of patients and other stakeholders

quality assurance (QA) a program designed to maintain continuous monitoring and measurement of the quality of clinical care delivered to patients.

continuous quality improvement (CQI) an evaluation program that emphasizes service and uses customer satisfaction as the ultimate indicator of system performance.

rules of evidence guidelines for permitting a new medication, process, or procedure to be used in EMS.

QUALITY ASSURANCE AND IMPROVEMENT

The only acceptable quality of an EMS system is excellence. In 1997, the NHTSA released a manual called *A Leadership Guide to Quality Improvement for Emergency Medical Services Systems.* Its guidelines are based on the following components:

- Leadership
- Information and analysis
- Strategic quality planning
- Human resources development and management
- EMS process management
- EMS system results
- Satisfaction of patients and other stakeholders

A **quality assurance (QA)** program monitors and measures the quality of clinical care delivered to patients through evaluation of objective data such as response times, adherence to protocols, patient survival, and other key indicators. QA programs document the effectiveness of the care provided. They also help to identify problems and selected areas that need improvement. A common complaint about QA programs is that they tend to identify only the problems and therefore focus only on punitive corrective action. Thus, prehospital personnel often view QA programs negatively.

As a result, many EMS systems have taken QA a step further with a **continuous quality improvement (CQI)** program. A CQI program emphasizes customer satisfaction and includes evaluations of such aspects as billing and maintenance. In contrast to QA programs, CQI focuses on recognizing, rewarding, and reinforcing good performance. The dynamic process of CQI includes six basic steps: researching and identifying systemwide problems; elaborating on the probable causes; listing possible solutions; outlining a plan of corrective action; providing the resources and support needed to ensure the plan's success; and reevaluating results continuously.

In general, EMS quality can be divided into two categories: "take-it-for-granted" quality and service quality.

"Take-It-for-Granted" Quality

People must be able to "take it for granted" that EMS will respond quickly to a 9-1-1 call and act at the highest level of professionalism, providing care that is safe, appropriate, and the best that is available.

When considering a new medication, process, or procedure, we must follow set rules before permitting its use in EMS. These rules, often called **rules of evidence,** were developed by Joseph P. Ornato, M.D., Ph.D. They include the following guidelines:

- *There must be a theoretical basis for the change.* That is, the change must make sense based on relevant medical science.
- *There must be ample research.* Any device or medication for patient care must be justified by adequate scientific human research.
- *It must be clinically important.* The device, medication, or procedure must make a significant clinical difference to the patient. For example, a defibrillator may mean the difference between living and dying for some patients, whereas color-coordinated stretcher linen has little clinical significance.
- *It must be practical, affordable, and teachable.* Some medical devices remain too expensive and too impractical for use in routine prehospital emergency care.

Another way to accomplish "take-it-for-granted" quality improvement is through the ongoing education of personnel. An EMT-I can improve his or her skills by reading, taking classes, soliciting feedback on clinical performance from receiving hospitals, and following up on patients. **Peer review**—the process of EMS personnel reviewing each other's patient reports, emergency care, and interactions with patients and families—is another way for an EMT-I to improve knowledge and skills.

Ethics are the standards that govern the conduct of a group or profession. Prehospital providers at all levels have an ethical responsibility to their patients and to the public. The public expects excellence from the EMS system, and we should accept no less than excellence from ourselves.

Service Quality

In the business world, service quality is called "customer satisfaction." This is the kind of quality that individual customers get excited about, feel good about, and tell stories about. These are the little extras that exceed a customer's expectations and elicit thank-you letters. Prime examples of customer satisfaction include patient statements such as: "You fed my cat before we left." "You remembered my name and introduced me to the nurse." "You held my hand." "You seemed like a friend when I needed one."

Customer satisfaction can be created or destroyed with a simple word or deed. A significant part of the way we communicate with one another is through body language and tone of voice. An EMT-I who genuinely cares about the patient communicates it in many subtle ways. From the patient's perspective this is much more important than IVs, backboards, and ECGs.

RESEARCH

The future enhancement of EMS is strongly dependent on the availability of quality research. The current trend of introducing "new and improved" ideas or new "high tech" equipment to existing procedures must be evaluated scientifically. Unfortunately, many EMS protocols and procedures in use today have evolved without clinical evidence of usefulness, safety, or benefit to the patient. One area that will rely heavily on research is funding. As managed care increases its influence, EMS systems will be forced to validate their effectiveness. Restrictions on reimbursement will determine the quality of EMS research. Outcome studies will also be required to justify funding and ensure the future of EMS.

Future EMS research must address the following issues: Which prehospital interventions actually reduce morbidity and mortality? Are the benefits of certain field procedures worth the potential risks? What is the cost-benefit ratio of sophisticated prehospital equipment and procedures? Is field stabilization possible, or should the patient be transported immediately in every case?

The EMT-I can play a valuable role in data collection, evaluation, and interpretation of research. The components of a research project include the following:

- Identify a problem, explain the reason for the proposed study, and state the hypothesis or a precise question.
- Identify the body of published knowledge on the subject.
- Select the best design for the study, clearly outline all logistics, examine all patient-consent issues, and get them approved through the appropriate investigational review process.
- Begin the study and collect raw data.
- Analyze and correlate your data in a statistical application.
- Assess and evaluate the results against the original hypothesis or question.
- Write a concise, comprehensive description of the study for publication in a medical journal.

Current EMS practice must be justified by hard clinical data derived from an objective, valid program of ongoing research. EMS providers at all levels share the responsibility for identifying research opportunities, conducting peer-review programs, and publishing the

peer review an evaluation of the quality of emergency care administered by an individual, which is conducted by that individual's peers (others of equal rank). Also, an evaluation of articles submitted for publication.

Customer satisfaction can be created or destroyed with a simple word or deed.

The future enhancement of EMS is strongly dependent on the availability of quality research.

Patho Pearls

For many years EMS has been based on anecdotes and unproven theories. Today, EMS personnel must base their practice on sound scientific evidence. Because of this, all EMTs must fundamentally understand EMS research.

results of their projects. As leaders in the prehospital care environment, EMT-Is should set an example in the development of and participation in research projects.

Evidence-Based Medicine

A movement has been building in the field of medicine. It is called *evidence-based medicine (EBM)*. This movement has been widely embraced by those in emergency medicine, so it is only logical that its principles are applied to EMS. Evidence-based medicine is the conscientious, explicit, and judicious use of the current best evidence in making decisions about the care of individual patients. It requires combining clinical expertise with the best available clinical evidence from systematic research.

To practice effective evidence-based medicine, EMS personnel must first be proficient in prehospital care and exercise sound clinical judgment. These traits can only be developed following a comprehensive initial education program and clinical experience and practice. To move to the next level, EMS personnel must be familiar with the current and past research pertinent to prehospital care—and be able to integrate that knowledge into the care of individual patients. Furthermore, EMS personnel must know how to read and interpret the scientific literature and determine whether information is sound.

A good EMT-I can become excellent by using both clinical expertise and the best available external evidence. External clinical evidence can invalidate previously accepted treatments and procedures and replace them with new ones that are more powerful, more effective, and much safer. In today's medical setting, neither clinical expertise nor external evidence alone is enough. There must always be a balance between the two.

Over the last decade or so, various EMS practices and procedures have been studied. Some treatments, such as the use of pneumatic antishock garments (PASG), did not stand up to the test. Other treatments, such as early defibrillation, were found to have a significant impact on survival. By using the best research data available, EMS was able to abandon a practice (PASG) that helped few, if any patients. It also was able to embrace a practice (early defibrillation) that has saved countless lives through diverse programs such as bystander defibrillation. Practicing evidence-based medicine ensures that we are providing our patients the best possible care at the lowest possible price.

SYSTEM FINANCING

At present in the United States, there is a wide variety of EMS system designs. EMS can be hospital-based, fire- or police-department based, a municipal service, a private commercial business, a volunteer service, or some combination. Major differences exist in methods of EMS system finance, too. They range from fully tax-subsidized municipal systems to all-volunteer squads supported solely by contributions.

EMS funding can come from many sources. The most common is fee-for-service revenue, which may be generated from Medicare, Medicaid, private insurance companies, specialty service contracts, or private paying patients. Most of these sources of revenue are referred to as "third-party payers," because payment comes from someone other than the patient. To date, almost all third-party payers require the patient to be transported or the EMS service will not be compensated for a response. Reimbursement may also be based on the level of care the patient receives during transport.

Because of the high costs of health care and complex billing and reimbursement systems, the "Public Utility Model" and the "Failsafe Franchise" are becoming increasingly popular. In these systems, a municipality establishes the design and standards for the contract bid, then periodically—usually every three or four years—holds a wholesale competition open to the market. The provider firm that wins the contract must manage services properly and efficiently throughout the contract term or face severe penalties, usually in the form of fines. The use of models such as these shifts the financial burden of operating an EMS system from the local community to the service franchise.

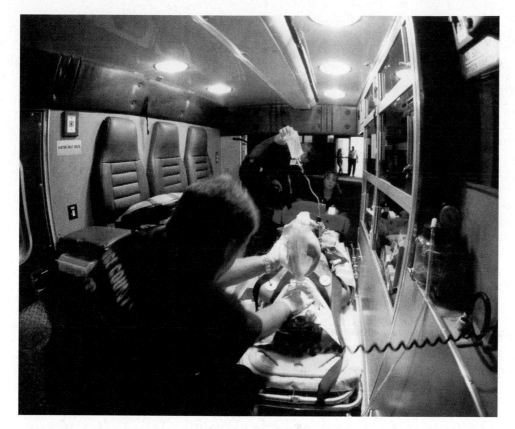

FIGURE 1-4 An EMT-I maintains a professional attitude while making medical and ethical decisions about severely injured and critically ill patients.

Part 3: Roles and Responsibilities of the EMT-Intermediate

The roles and responsibilities of the EMT-I are dramatically different than they were 10 years ago. Today, EMT-I emergency care is an enormous responsibility for which you must be mentally, physically, and emotionally prepared. You will be required to have a strong knowledge of **pathophysiology** and of the most current medical technology. You will have to be capable of maintaining a professional attitude while making medical and ethical decisions about severely injured and critically ill patients (Figure 1-4). You will be required to provide not only competent emergency care but also emotional support to your patients and their families.

pathophysiology the study of how disease affects normal body processes.

PRIMARY RESPONSIBILITIES

An EMT-I's responsibilities include emergency medical care for the patient and a variety of other responsibilities before, during, and after a call.

PREPARATION

Preparation includes making sure that inspection and routine maintenance have been completed on your emergency vehicle and on all equipment. It means restocking medications and IV solutions and checking their expiration dates. In addition, you must be very familiar with:

- All local EMS protocols, policies, and procedures
- Communications system hardware (radios) and software (frequency utilization and communication protocols)

> **Content Review**
>
> ### PRIMARY RESPONSIBILITIES
> - Preparation
> - Response
> - Scene size-up
> - Patient assessment
> - Patient management
> - Disposition and transfer
> - Documentation
> - Clean-up, maintenance, and review

- Local geography, including populations and alternative routes during rush hours
- Support agencies, including services available from neighboring EMS systems and the methods by which efforts and resources are coordinated

RESPONSE

During an emergency response, remember that personal safety is your number-one priority. If your ambulance crashes en route to an incident because of speeding or running red traffic lights, you will be of no benefit to the patient. Always follow basic safety precautions en route to an incident. Wear a seatbelt, obey posted speed limits, and monitor the road for potential hazards.

You must also get to the scene in a timely manner. Make certain you know the correct location of the incident and, en route, request any additional personnel or services that you think may be needed. Do not wait to ask for assistance until you get to a chaotic scene. Learn to anticipate potential high-risk situations based on dispatch information and experience. For example, if any of the following is reported to be on scene, you may need to call for assistance:

- Multiple patients
- Motor-vehicle collisions
- Hazardous materials
- Rescue situations
- Violent individuals (patients or bystanders)
- Reported use of a weapon
- Knowledge of previous violence

PATIENT ASSESSMENT AND MANAGEMENT

Your primary responsibilities as an EMT-I involve scene size-up and the assessment and management of the patient (Figure 1-5). These topics will be discussed fully in subsequent chapters. Keep in mind that your primary concern is the safety of yourself, your crew, the patient, and bystanders.

APPROPRIATE DISPOSITION

As noted earlier, the mode of transport and the selection of receiving facility are critical decisions to be made for your patient. For example, you might opt for ground or air transport. You might choose the nearest medical facility or a facility with special treatment capabilities such as burn care or hyperbaric oxygen therapy.

Most patients request transportation to the nearest medical facility. However, patients enrolled in managed-care programs, such as health maintenance organizations (HMOs) or designated provider groups, may request transport to a facility approved by their group, which may be a facility other than the nearest hospital. Other patients may ask you to transport them to a facility outside of your run area. Even though the requested facility may be appropriate for the patient, an equally appropriate hospital may be closer. Remember, you are responsible for patient care and, therefore, also ultimately responsible for selecting the transport destination. When in doubt, contact on-line medical direction for advice and support.

In some areas, EMT-Is provide **primary care.** They have well-defined protocols that allow them to treat patients at the scene and transfer them to facilities other than a hospital. Consider this example: a child has a simple 2-inch laceration on his arm. Instead of transporting the patient to a hospital—thereby using resources that are not needed for this patient and incurring a costly emergency department fee for the family—the EMT-I contacts medical direction and requests permission to transport the child to a local outpatient center.

Another type of disposition is "treat and release" in which EMT-Is assess the patient and provide emergency care. If they determine there is no need for further medical attention, they contact medical direction and request orders not to transport. In some systems, EMT-Is may then contact a specialized dispatch center where an office appointment is made with a local physician.

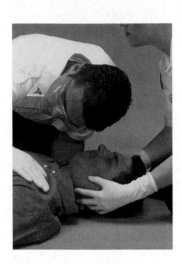

FIGURE 1-5 An EMT-I's responsibilities include personal safety, as well as assessment and management of the patient.

primary care basic health care provided at the patient's first contact with the health-care system.

Although disposition systems such as these are not widely accepted, the increasing numbers of people in managed-care programs (which generally attempt to achieve optimum care while controlling costs) may change that. Innovative programs such as these are setting standards for the future of EMS.

PATIENT TRANSFER

The managed-care environment has caused many people—both laypeople and health-care providers—to occasionally question whether certain actions that are intended to reduce the cost of medical care are actually in the patient's best interest. For example, to avoid the cost of duplicating equipment and services in a number of facilities that serve the same geographical area, managed-care systems have encouraged facilities to specialize and, often, to transfer patients to a facility that can provide the specific care needed.

Occasionally, there may be a question as to whether the approved transfer of a patient from one facility to another for cost reasons is in the patient's best interest. When you are assigned to transport a patient, you share responsibility—with the receiving and accepting physician—for the treatment and care of the patient. When you are in doubt about the patient's stability for the duration of transport, or about the capabilities of the receiving facility, contact medical direction.

Before removing the patient from a hospital, request a verbal report from the primary-care provider (usually a registered nurse or a physician). Also request a copy of essential parts of the patient's chart, including a summary of the patient's past and present medical history. However, if the results of diagnostic tests taken at the facility are not ready when you are prepared to leave, do not delay patient transport. The data can be sent by fax, E-mailed, or telephoned to the receiving facility.

Your first priority during transport is the patient. While en route, contact the receiving facility and provide them with an estimated time of arrival (ETA) and an update on the patient's condition. Upon arrival at your destination, seek out the contact person (usually a registered nurse or physician). Provide that person with an updated patient report, including any treatment or changes in status while en route. All documents provided by the sending facility should be turned over to the receiving care provider along with a copy of your run report. If required by your service, obtain appropriate billing/insurance information at this time.

DOCUMENTATION

Maintaining a complete and accurate written patient care report is essential to the flow of patient information, to research efforts, and to the quality improvement of your EMS system. Documentation will be discussed in detail in Chapter 11.

RETURNING TO SERVICE

Once you have completed patient care, turned the patient over to the hospital staff, and completed all documentation, immediately prepare to return to service (Figure 1-6). Clean and decontaminate the unit, properly discard disposable materials, restock supplies, and replace and stow away equipment. If necessary, refuel the unit on the way back to your station or post. Review the call with crew members, including any problems that may have occurred. Such a dialogue can lead to solutions that enhance the delivery of quality patient care. Finally, the EMT-I team leader should check crew members for signs of stress and assist anyone who needs help.

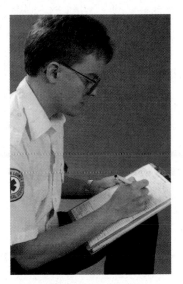

FIGURE 1-6 An EMT-I's responsibilities do not end with delivering the patient to the emergency department. Documentation, among other tasks, is as important as the call itself.

ADDITIONAL RESPONSIBILITIES

The role of the EMT-I involves duties in addition to those associated with emergency response. Those duties may include training civilians in CPR, EMS demonstrations and seminars, teaching first-aid classes, organizing prevention programs, and engaging in professional development activities. All involve taking an active role in promoting positive health practices in your community.

COMMUNITY INVOLVEMENT

Prehospital providers should take the lead in helping the public learn how to recognize an emergency, how to provide basic life support (BLS), and how to properly access the EMS system. A successful effort can save lives. Providing educational programs can also encourage positive health practices in the community, such as the AHA's "prudent heart living" campaign. EMS injury prevention projects, such as seat-belt awareness and the proper use of child safety seats, are essential to the reduction of long-term disability and accidental death.

In order to decide what injury prevention projects need to be developed in a community, EMS systems often conduct illness and injury risk surveys. For example, an EMS service reviews run reports for a 6-month period and finds they responded to 10 vehicle collisions at railroad crossings. A public safety campaign directed at the safe crossing of railroad tracks may be appropriate. Once an EMS service has identified a problem and target audience, they should seek community agencies, including the local political structure, in order to assist in the development, promotion, and delivery of the campaign.

Community involvement enhances the visibility of EMS, promotes a positive image, and puts forth EMS personnel as positive role models. It also creates opportunities to improve the integration of EMS with other public agencies through cooperative programs.

COST CONTAINMENT

Promoting wellness and preventing illness and injury will be important components of EMS in the future. Some systems have already begun to direct resources toward such programs, which decrease the need for emergency services. The theory is to reduce the cost of the services provided to the community by decreasing the burden on the system.

One strategy is to establish protocols that specify the mode of transportation for nonemergency patients. Some systems already operate vans rather than ambulances to transport such patients to and from nursing facilities or from their residences to a doctor's office. Though an additional expense to the system, this service reduces emergency equipment costs and the demand for emergency personnel. The result is a decrease in the overall operating expense, which results in an increase in revenue.

Another strategy used in many areas of the country is having EMS and hospitals team up to provide an alternative to the emergency department. They transport patients to freestanding outpatient centers or clinics, which ultimately reduces the cost of care to the patient and the system. The development of such alliances will undoubtedly continue. However, caution should be taken to ensure that the patient always receives the appropriate emergency care based on need, not cost.

CITIZEN INVOLVEMENT IN EMS

Citizen involvement in EMS helps to give "insiders" an outside, objective view of quality improvement and problem resolution. Whenever possible, members of the community should be used in the development, evaluation, and regulation of the EMS system. When considering the addition of a new service or the enhancement of an existing one, community members should help to establish what is needed. After all, they are your "customers," and their needs are your priority.

PROFESSIONALISM

profession refers to the existence of a specialized body of knowledge or skills.

professionalism refers to the conduct or qualities that characterize a practitioner in a particular field or occupation.

An EMT-I is a member of the health-care profession. The word **profession** refers to a specialized body of knowledge or skills. Generally self-regulating, a profession will have recognized standards, including requirements for initial and ongoing education. When you have satisfied the initial education requirements as an EMT-I, you may then be either certified or licensed. The EMS profession has regulations that ensure that members maintain standards. For the EMT-I, these regulations come in the form of periodic recertification with a specified amount of continuing education time.

The term **professionalism** refers to the conduct or qualities that characterize a practitioner in a particular field. Health-care professionals promote quality patient care and pride in their profession, setting and striving for the highest standards, and earning the respect of team members and the public. Attaining professionalism requires an understanding of what distinguishes the professional from the non-professional.

PROFESSIONAL ATTITUDES

A commitment to excellence is a daily activity. While on duty, health-care professionals place their patients first; non-professionals place their egos first. True professionals establish excellence as their goal and never allow themselves to become complacent about their performance. They practice their skills to the point of mastery and then keep practicing them to stay sharp and improve. They also take refresher courses seriously, because they know they have forgotten a lot and because they are eager for new information. Non-professionals believe their skills will never fade.

Professionals set high standards for themselves, their crew, their agency, and their system. Non-professionals aim for the minimum standard and can be counted on to take the path of least resistance. Professionals critically review their performance, always seeking ways to improve. Non-professionals look to protect themselves, hide their inadequacies, and place blame on others. Professionals check out all equipment before the emergency response. Non-professionals hope that everything will work, supplies will be in place, batteries will be charged, and oxygen levels will be adequate.

An EMT-I is responsible for acting in a professional manner both on and off duty. Remember, the community you serve will judge other EMS providers, the service you work for, and the EMS profession as a whole by your actions.

Professionalism is an attitude, not a matter of pay. It cannot be bought, rented, or faked. Although it is a young industry, EMS has achieved recognition as a bona fide allied health profession. Gaining professional stature is the result of many hard-working, caring individuals who refused to compromise their standards. Always strive to maintain that level of performance and commitment.

PROFESSIONAL ATTRIBUTES

Leadership

Leadership is an important but often forgotten aspect of EMT-I training. EMT-Is are important members of the advanced prehospital team (Figure 1-7). So, you must develop a leadership style that suits your personality and gets the job done. Although there are many successful styles of leadership, certain characteristics are common to all great leaders. They include:

- Self-confidence
- Established credibility
- Inner strength
- Ability to remain in control
- Ability to communicate

Content Review

PROFESSIONAL ATTRIBUTES
- Leadership
- Integrity
- Empathy
- Self-motivation
- Professional appearance and hygiene
- Self-confidence
- Communication skills
- Time-management skills
- Diplomacy in teamwork
- Respect
- Patient advocacy
- Careful delivery of service

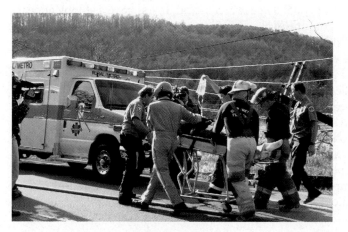

FIGURE 1-7 As a leader in EMS, you must interact with patients, bystanders, and other rescue personnel in a professional manner.

- Willingness to make a decision
- Willingness to accept responsibility for the consequences of the team's actions

The successful team leader knows the members of the crew, including each one's capabilities and limitations. Ask crew members to do something beyond their capabilities and they will question your ability to lead, not their ability to perform.

Integrity

The patient and other members of the health-care team assume that you, as an EMT-I, have integrity. The single most important behavior that you will be judged by is honesty. Your work will often put you in the patient's home or in charge of the patient's wallet and other personal possessions, such as jewelry and items left in a vehicle. You must be trustworthy. The easiest way to lose respect is to be dishonest. Additionally, in acting as an agent of the medical director, you are entrusted with carefully following protocols, providing the best possible care, and accurately documenting it.

Empathy

One of the most important components to successful interaction with a patient and family is empathy. To have empathy is to identify with and understand the circumstances, feelings, and motives of others. As a professional, you will often have to place your own feelings aside to deal with others, even when you are having a bad day. EMT-Is who act in a professional manner can show empathy by:

- Being supportive and reassuring
- Demonstrating an understanding of the patient's feelings and the feelings of the family
- Demonstrating respect for others
- Having a calm, compassionate, and helpful demeanor

Self-Motivation

You will often work without direct supervision, so it is up to you to be able to motivate yourself and establish a positive work ethic. Examples of a positive work ethic are:

- Completing assigned duties without being asked or told to do so
- Completing all duties and assignments without the need for direct supervision
- Correctly completing all paperwork in a timely manner
- Demonstrating a commitment to continuous quality improvement
- Accepting constructive feedback in a positive manner
- Taking advantage of learning opportunities

Appearance and Personal Hygiene

From the moment you arrive at the scene of an emergency, you are judged by the way you present yourself. Good appearance and personal hygiene are critical. If you have a sloppy appearance, your patient may suspect that your medical care will be sloppy, too. Slang, foul, abusive, or off-color language is not acceptable and will alienate you from your patients. Your appearance, as well as your behavior, are vital to establishing credibility and inspiring confidence.

Always wear a clean, pressed uniform. Multiple pagers and holsters with tape hanging from them, or rubber gloves pulled through a belt loop, simply do not give you a professional appearance. Also, avoid wearing an abundance of patches and pins on your uniform. Remember, it is the care you provide, not the patches and pins you wear, that will impress the patient. Keep hair off your collar. If facial hair is allowed, keep it neat and trimmed. A light-colored tee shirt may be worn under your uniform shirt, which should be buttoned up, with only the top collar button open. Jewelry, other than a wedding ring, a watch, or small plain earrings for a female, is unprofessional. Long fingernails that have the potential to puncture protective gloves also should be avoided.

Self-Confidence

The patient and family will not trust you if they sense you do not trust yourself. A lack of self-confidence shows and is the basis of many lawsuits. The easiest way to gain self-confidence is to accurately assess your strengths and limitations, then seek every opportunity to improve any weaknesses. Also, keep in mind that self-confidence does not equal cockiness. When a self-confident EMT-I is presented with a complex situation, he or she will ask for assistance.

Communication

Communication is a skill often underestimated in EMS services. Providing emergency care in the prehospital environment requires constant communication with the patient, family, and bystanders, as well as with other EMS providers and rescuers from other public agencies. Communication skills are discussed in detail in later chapters.

Time Management

The experienced EMT-I who plans ahead, prioritizes tasks, and organizes them to make maximum use of time will generally be more effective in the field. An EMT-I with good time-management skills is punctual for shifts and meetings and completes tasks such as paperwork and maintenance duties on or ahead of schedule.

Some simple time-management techniques that you can use are making lists, prioritizing tasks, arriving at meetings or appointments early, and keeping a personal calendar. By implementing just one or two of these techniques, you may find your schedule to be more manageable and less stressful.

Teamwork and Diplomacy

The EMT-I is a leader. Leadership implies the ability to work with other people—to foster teamwork. Teamwork requires diplomacy, or tact and skill in dealing with people, even when you are under siege from the patient or family. Diplomacy requires the EMT-I to place the interests of the patient or team ahead of his own interests. It means listening to others, respecting their opinions, and being open-minded and flexible when it comes to change. A strong leader of any team realizes that he will be successful only if he has the support of all team members. A confident leader will:

- Place the success of the team ahead of personal self-interest
- Never undermine the role or opinion of another team member
- Provide support for members of the team, both on and off duty
- Remain open to suggestions from team members and be willing to change for the benefit of the patient
- Openly communicate with everyone
- Above all, respect the patient, other health-care providers, and the community you serve

Respect

To respect others is to show and feel deferential regard, consideration, and appreciation for them. An EMT-I respects all patients, and provides the best possible care to each and every one of them, no matter what their race, religion, sex, age, or economic condition. Showing that you care for a patient's or family member's feelings, being polite, and avoiding the use of demeaning or derogatory language toward even the most difficult patients are simple ways to demonstrate respect.

Patient Advocacy

An EMT-I is an advocate for patients, defending them, protecting them, and acting in their best interests. Except when your safety is threatened, you should always place the needs of your patient above your own.

Careful Delivery of Services

Professionalism requires the EMT-I to deliver the highest quality of patient care with very close attention to detail. Examples of behaviors that demonstrate a careful delivery of service include:

- Mastering and refreshing skills
- Performing complete equipment checks
- Careful and safe ambulance operations
- Following policies, procedures, and protocols

CONTINUING EDUCATION AND PROFESSIONAL DEVELOPMENT

Only through continuing education and recertification can the public be assured that quality patient care is being delivered consistently. So after you are certified and/or licensed, you have an important responsibility to continue your personal and professional development. Remember, everyone is subject to the decay of knowledge and skills over time. So, use this as a rule of thumb: As the volume of calls decreases, training should correspondingly increase.

Refresher requirements and courses vary from state to state, but the goals are the same—to review previously learned materials and to receive new information. Since EMS is a relatively young industry, new technology and data emerge rapidly. Make a conscious effort to keep up. A variety of journals, seminars, computer news groups, and learning experiences are available to help. So are professional EMS organizations at the local, state, and national levels. Additionally, by participating in activities designed to address work-related issues—such as case reviews and other quality improvement activities, mentoring programs, research projects, multiple-casualty incident drills, in-hospital rotations, equipment in-services, refresher courses, and self-study exercises—you can expect substantial career growth.

Part 4: Well-Being of the EMT-Intermediate

> *Well-being is a fundamental aspect of top-notch performance.*
>
>

Well-being, or wellness, is a fundamental aspect of top-notch performance in EMS. It includes your physical well-being as well as your mental and emotional well-being. Part 4 discusses the many elements of well-being. If you learn now and enhance your knowledge later, you stand a good chance of enjoying a long and rewarding career of helping others—all because you helped yourself.

BASIC PHYSICAL FITNESS

The benefits of achieving acceptable physical fitness are well known. They include a decreased resting heart rate and blood pressure, increased oxygen-carrying capacity, increased muscle mass and metabolism, and increased resistance to illness and injury. Quality of life is enhanced as is self-image. Other benefits are improved mental outlook, reduced anxiety levels, and enhanced ability to maintain sound motor skills throughout life.

CORE ELEMENTS

Core elements of physical fitness are cardiovascular endurance (aerobic capacity), muscular strength, and flexibility. Like a three-legged stool, if any one of the three is deficient, the whole becomes unstable. Each is equally important.

Be careful about plunging into a well-intended effort to get in shape. For example, before starting an exercise or stretching regimen, it can be helpful to measure your current state of fitness. There are various methods of assessing the three core elements of fitness. Many EMS agencies have access to facilities with precise assessment methods and trained personnel. Take advantage of any available to you.

Content Review

BASICS OF PHYSICAL FITNESS
- Cardiovascular endurance
- Strength and flexibility
- Nutrition and weight control
- Disease prevention
- Freedom from harmful habits and addictions
- Back safety

Table 1-1   FINDING YOUR TARGET HEART RATE

1. Measure your resting heart rate. (You will use this total later).
2. Subtract your age from 220. This total is your estimated maximum heart rate.
3. Subtract your resting heart rate from your maximum heart rate, and multiply that figure by 0.7.
4. Add the figure you just calculated to your resting heart rate.

EXAMPLE: In a 44-year-old woman whose resting heart rate is 52, maximum heart rate would be 176 (220 − 44). Maximum heart rate minus resting heart rate is 124 (176 − 52). Multiply 124 by 0.7 for a value of 86.8. Resting heart rate plus the calculated figure is 138.8 (52 + 86.8). Rounded up, this person's target heart rate is 140 beats per minute.

Muscular strength is achieved with regular exercise that may be isometric or isotonic. *Isometric exercise* is active exercise performed against stable resistance, where muscles are exercised in a motionless manner. *Isotonic exercise* is active exercise during which muscles are worked through their range of motion. Weight lifting is an obvious way to achieve muscular strength, and it is excellent all-around training for the body. Rotate between training the muscles of your upper body and shoulders, chest and back, and lower body. Do abdominal exercises daily. Take time to get in-depth information about the best approach from a trainer or other knowledgeable person.

Cardiovascular endurance results from exercising at least three days a week vigorously enough to raise your pulse to its target heart rate (Table 1-1). There is no need to become a marathon runner to gain aerobic capacity. Try a brisk walk, or ride a stationary bike while watching TV. Make it a daily habit. Even modest exercise helps. Walking briskly from the outer reaches of the employee parking lot, using stairs whenever possible, and playing actively with your children all count toward physical fitness.

Flexibility seems to be the forgotten element of fitness. Without an adequate range of motion, your joints and muscles cannot be used efficiently or safely. A body builder with tight hamstrings may be as much at risk for back injury as anyone else. To achieve (or regain) flexibility, stretch the main muscle groups regularly. Try to stretch daily. Never bounce when stretching; this causes micro-tears in muscle and connective tissues. Hold a stretch for at least 60 seconds. A side benefit of good flexibility is prevention or reduction of back pain. Stretching is an excellent TV-time activity. If you are interested, consider studying yoga.

NUTRITION

Good nutrition is fundamental to your well-being because food is your fuel. In addition to eating balanced meals, you must also eat in moderation, limit fat consumption, and exercise. One key to eating well is to learn the major food groups and eat a variety of foods from them daily:

- *Grains/breads*. 6 to 11 servings per day, for complex carbohydrates, B vitamins, and fiber
- *Vegetables*. 3 to 5 servings per day, for fiber, iron, vitamins A and C, and folate
- *Fruits*. 2 to 4 servings per day, for vitamins A and C, potassium, and fiber
- *Dairy products*. 2 to 3 servings per day, for calcium, protein, and vitamins A and D
- *Meat/fish*. 2 to 3 servings per day, for protein, zinc, iron, and B vitamins

Avoid or minimize intake of fat, salt, sugar, cholesterol, and caffeine. For example, you can avoid a dose of fat by eating lean instead of marbled meat. An apple is far more nutritious than a slice of apple pie. In general, aim for a diet that is approximately 40% carbohydrates, 40% protein, and 20% fat. Food portions also have a significant impact on body weight. Even a well-planned, healthy diet can result in weight gain if the portions are too large. Note that snacking is a weight-gain trap. Plan to eat low-calorie snacks and to buy them before you get hungry. Food labels (Figure 1-8) contain abundant information about nutritional content.

Content Review

MAJOR FOOD GROUPS
- Grains/breads
- Vegetables
- Fruits
- Dairy products
- Meat/fish

Nutrition Facts

Serving Size 8 fl oz (240 mL)
Servings Per Container 8

Amount Per Serving

Calories 110   Calories from Fat 0

% Daily Value*

Total Fat 0g	0%
Sodium 0mg	0%
Potassium 450mg	13%
Total Carbohydrate 26g	9%
Sugars 22g	
Protein 2g	

Vitamin C 120% • Calcium 2%
Thiamin 10% • Niacin 4%
Vitamin B6 6% • Folate 15%

Not a significant source of saturated fat, cholesterol, dietary fiber, vitamin A and iron.

* Percent Daily Values are based on a 2,000 calorie diet.

FIGURE 1-8   Example of a standardized food label.

Learn to read them. Standardization of food labels has reduced much of the confusion. Be sure to check the serving size to avoid misinterpreting the food's overall nutritional value.

Eating on the run, as EMS providers must often do, can be less detrimental if you plan ahead and carry a small cooler filled with whole-grain sandwiches, cut vegetables, fruit, and other wholesome foods. If you must, stop at a local market instead of the fast-food place next door. Buy fresh fruit, yogurt, and sensible deli selections. They are more nutritious and much cheaper than fast-food options. Monitor your fluid intake. Your body needs plenty of fluids to flush food through your system and eliminate toxins. Fill a "go-cup" with fresh ice water when you stop by the emergency department instead of spending your money on soft drinks.

PREVENTING CANCER AND CARDIOVASCULAR DISEASE

Exercising and eating well can help you prevent both cancer and cardiovascular disease. Although for the typically youthful EMS provider, the likelihood of being hit by either of these diseases may seem remote, but it happens. You can do a lot to prevent it. Minimizing stress through healthy stress management practices, for example, can work wonders. Be sure to assess yourself and your family history.

Exercise improves cardiovascular endurance, helps lower blood pressure, and tips the balance of your body composition favorably—all good measures against cardiovascular disease. Know your cholesterol and triglyceride levels and keep them in check. For women who are menopausal, be informed about the risks and benefits of using hormone replacement therapy (particularly estrogen).

Diet can also do much to minimize the chances of getting certain cancers. Foods such as broccoli and high-fiber foods can help reduce the incidence of cancer; others, such as charcoal-cooked foods, can increase it. The connection between sun exposure and skin cancer is also well known. So take the precaution of using sunblocks and wear sunglasses and a hat when you can. In addition, watch out for the warning signs of cancer, such as blood in the stools (even in young people, especially men), a changing mole, unexplained weight loss, unexplained chronic fatigue, and lumps.

Be sure to include appropriate periodic risk-assessment screening and self-examination habits in your personal well-being program. That includes tests such as mammograms and prostate exams as you get older.

HABITS AND ADDICTIONS

Many people who work high-stress jobs overuse and abuse substances such as caffeine and nicotine. These bad habits are rampant in EMS. Each can contribute to long-term diseases such as cancer and cardiovascular disease. Choose a healthier life and avoid overindulging in these and other harmful substances such as alcohol. For example, smoking cessation programs are usually easily accessed locally or on the internet. Whatever it takes, the message is clear: get free of addictions, particularly those that threaten your well-being. Substance abuse programs, nicotine patches, and twelve-step groups all exist to help you help yourself. The first step has to be yours.

BACK SAFETY

EMS is a physically demanding endeavor. Of the movements needed (scrambling down embankments, climbing ladders or trees, squeezing into narrow spaces, and so on), none will be more frequent than lifting and carrying equipment and patients. To avoid back injury, you must keep your back fit for the work you do. You also must use proper lifting techniques each time you pick up a load, whether the load is heavy or light.

Back fitness begins with conditioning the muscles that support the spinal column. These are the "guy wires" that stabilize the spine, much the way cables help keep telephone poles upright. Note that the muscles of the abdomen are also crucial to overall spinal-column strength and safe lifting. Never perform old-fashioned sit-ups. They can seriously strain your lumbar spine. Instead, use abdominal crunches, which target only the stomach muscles. Consult an exercise coach or trainer for specifics.

Correct posture will minimize the risk of back injury (Figure 1-9). Good nutrition helps maintain healthy connective tissue and intervertebral discs. Excess weight contributes to

Pay particular attention to keeping your back fit for the work you do. Always use the proper techniques for lifting and moving patients and equipment.

Legal Notes

Back injuries represent one of the greatest risks to EMS providers and account for a significant monetary expenditure in worker compensation claims. Programs that will help minimize such injuries should be an ongoing aspect of any EMS system.

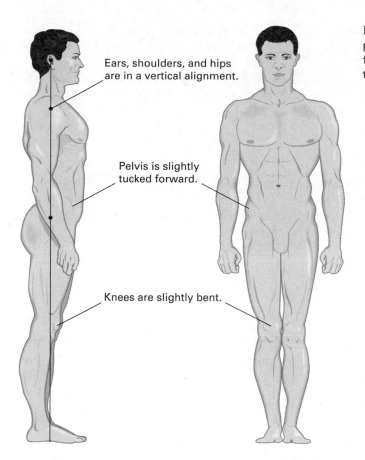

Ears, shoulders, and hips are in a vertical alignment.

Pelvis is slightly tucked forward.

Knees are slightly bent.

FIGURE 1-9A Correct standing posture. Note the straight line from the ear to the hip down to the arch of the foot.

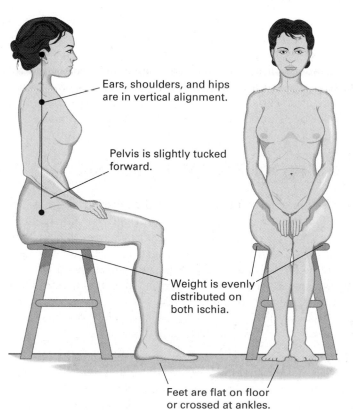

Ears, shoulders, and hips are in vertical alignment.

Pelvis is slightly tucked forward.

Weight is evenly distributed on both ischia.

Feet are flat on floor or crossed at ankles.

FIGURE 1-9B Correct sitting posture. Note the straight line from the ear through the shoulder and hip and from knee to the arch of the foot.

disc deterioration. So does smoking. Thus, proper weight management and smoking cessation are relevant to back health. Finally, adequate rest gives the spine non–weight-bearing time to nourish discs and repair itself.

Proper lifting techniques should ideally be taught by and practiced with a trainer who understands the variety of challenges faced by EMS providers. Important principles of lifting are as follows:

- Move a load only if you can safely handle it.
- Ask for help when you need it—for any reason.
- Position the load as close to your body and center of gravity as possible.
- Keep your palms up whenever possible.
- Do not hurry. Take the time you need to establish good footing and balance. Keep a wide base of support with one foot ahead of the other.
- Bend your knees, lower your buttocks, and keep your chin up. If your knees are bad, do not bend them more than 90 degrees.
- "Lock in" the spine with a slight extension curve and tighten the abdominal muscles to support spinal positioning.
- Always avoid twisting and turning.
- Let the large leg muscles do the work of lifting, not your back.
- Exhale during the lift. Do not hold your breath.
- Given a choice, push. Do not pull.
- Look where you are walking or crawling. Take only short steps if you are walking. Move forward rather than backward whenever possible.
- When rescuers are working together as a team to lift a load, only one person should be in charge of verbal commands.

Heed your own body's signals. You are stronger some days than others. Know when you are physically depleted due to exhaustion, lack of food, or minor illness. Use volunteers wisely, and be sure to ask if their backs are strong enough for the job.

Never reach for an item, or attempt to lift it, and twist at the same time. Most back injuries occur because of the cumulative effect of such low-level everyday stresses. Everything you do on behalf of back safety adds up to choices that can mean the difference between a long and rewarding career in EMS, or one shortened by an injury. Be careful!

PERSONAL PROTECTION FROM DISEASE

In recent years the emphasis on infection control has focused on the most devastating diseases, such as HIV/AIDS, hepatitis B and C, and tuberculosis—and rightly so. Fortunately, there is a lot you can do to minimize your risk of infection. A good first step is to develop a habit of doing the things promoted in this chapter. Eating well, getting adequate rest, and managing stress are among the building blocks of a good defense against infection. In addition, it is a good idea to periodically assess your risk for infection, such as noticing when you feel run down or when your hands are dangerously chapped.

INFECTIOUS DISEASES

infectious disease any disease caused by the growth of pathogenic microorganisms, which may be spread from person to person.

pathogens microorganisms capable of producing disease, such as bacteria and viruses.

Infectious diseases are caused by **pathogens** such as bacteria and viruses, which may be spread from person to person. For example, infection by way of *bloodborne pathogens* can occur when the blood of an infected person comes in contact with another person's broken skin (cuts, sores, chapped hands) or by way of parenteral contact (stick by a needle or other sharp object). Infection by *airborne pathogens* can occur when an infected person sneezes or coughs, causing body fluids in the form of tiny droplets to be inhaled or to come in contact with the mucous membranes of another person's eyes, nose, or mouth.

Table 1-2 COMMON INFECTIOUS DISEASES

Disease	Mode of Transmission	Incubation Period
Acquired immune deficiency syndrome (AIDS)	AIDS- or HIV-infected blood via intravenous drug use, semen and vaginal fluids, blood transfusions, or (rarely) needle sticks. Mothers also may pass HIV to their unborn children.	Several months or years
Hepatitis B, C	Blood, stool, or other body fluids, or contaminated objects.	Weeks or months
Tuberculosis	Respiratory secretions, airborne or on contaminated objects.	2 to 6 weeks
Meningitis, bacterial	Oral and nasal secretions.	2 to 10 days
Pneumonia, bacterial and viral	Oral and nasal droplets and secretions.	Several days
Influenza	Airborne droplets, or direct contact with body fluids.	1 to 3 days
Staphylococcal skin infections	Contact with open wounds or sores or contaminated objects.	Several days
Chicken pox (varicella)	Airborne droplets, or contact with open sores.	11 to 21 days
German measles (rubella)	Airborne droplets. Mothers may pass it to unborn children.	10 to 12 days
Whooping cough (pertussis)	Respiratory secretions or airborne droplets.	6 to 20 days

HIV/AIDS, hepatitis B and C, and tuberculosis are diseases of great concern because they are life threatening. However, one may be exposed to many different infectious diseases. See Table 1-2 for some common ones, their modes of transmission, and **incubation periods.**

Even when someone is carrying pathogens for disease, signs of an illness may not be apparent. For this reason, *you must consider the blood and body fluids of every patient you treat as infectious.* Safeguards against infection are mandatory for all medical personnel. They involve a strict form of infection control called body substance isolation (BSI).

INFECTION-CONTROL PRACTICES

Body Substance Isolation (BSI)

Body substance isolation (BSI) is a strategy that is based on the assumption that all blood and body fluids are infectious. It dictates that all EMS personnel take BSI precautions with every patient. To achieve this, appropriate **personal protective equipment (PPE)** should be available in every emergency vehicle. The minimum recommended PPE includes the following:

- *Protective gloves.* Wear disposable protective gloves before initiating any emergency care. When an emergency involves more than one patient, change gloves between patients. When gloves have been contaminated, remove and dispose of them properly as soon as possible (Figure 1-10).

- *Masks and protective eyewear.* These should be worn together whenever blood spatter is likely to occur, such as with arterial bleeding, childbirth, endotracheal intubation and other invasive procedures, oral suctioning, and clean-up of equipment that requires heavy scrubbing or brushing. Both you and your patient should wear masks whenever the potential for airborne transmission of disease exists.

- *HEPA and N-95 respirators.* Due to the resurgence of tuberculosis (TB), you must protect yourself from infection through the use of a high-efficiency particulate air (HEPA) respirator or an N-95 respirator. Wear one whenever

incubation period the time between contact with a disease organism and the appearance of the first symptoms.

body substance isolation (BSI) a strict form of infection control that is based on the assumption that all blood and body fluids are infectious.

personal protective equipment (PPE) equipment used by EMS personnel to protect against injury and the spread of infectious disease.

Assume all blood and body fluids are infectious, and take the proper BSI precautions whenever you treat a patient.

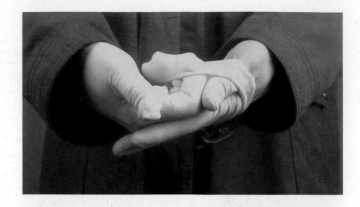

FIGURE 1-10A To remove gloves, first hook the gloved fingers of one hand under the cuff of the other glove. Then pull that glove off without letting your gloved fingers come in contact with the skin.

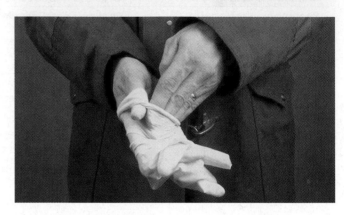

FIGURE 1-10B Then slide the fingers of the ungloved hand under the remaining glove's cuff. Push that glove off, being careful not to touch the glove's exterior with your bare hand.

you care for a patient with confirmed or suspected TB, especially during procedures that involve the airway, such as the administration of nebulized medications, endotracheal intubation, or suctioning.

- *Gowns.* Disposable gowns protect your clothing from splashes. If large splashes of blood are expected, such as with childbirth, wear an impervious gown.
- *Resuscitation equipment.* Use disposable resuscitation equipment as your primary means of artificial ventilation in emergency care.

Handwashing is perhaps the most important infection-control practice.

These garments and equipment will also assist you in achieving, to the extent possible, the universal precautions recommended by the Centers for Disease Control. Infectious diseases are minimized through the use of appropriate work practices and equipment especially engineered to minimize risk. For example, use disposable invasive equipment once, and then dispose of it properly. Launder reusable clothing with infection control in mind.

Probably the most important infection-control practice is handwashing as soon as possible after every patient contact and decontamination procedure. First, remove any rings or jewelry from your hands and arms. Then lather your hands vigorously front and back for at least 15 seconds up to 2 or 3 inches above the wrist. Lather and rub between your fingers and in the creases and cracks of your knuckles. Scrub under and around the fingernails with a brush. Rinse well under running water, holding your hands downward so that the water drains off your fingertips. Finally, dry your hands on a clean towel. Plain soap works perfectly well for handwashing. When soap is not available, use an anti-microbial handwashing solution or an alcohol-based foam or towelette.

Content Review

HANDWASHING

1. Lather with soap and water.
2. Scrub for at least 15 seconds.
3. Rinse under running water.
4. Dry on a clean towel.

Vaccinations and Screening Tests

Immunizations against many illnesses are available. Get them. Even "nuisance" illnesses can be avoided if you get vaccinated. Immunizations are available for rubella (German measles), measles, mumps, chicken pox, and other childhood diseases, as well as for tetanus/diphtheria, polio, influenza, hepatitis B, and Lyme disease. Some, such as tetanus, may require booster shots periodically, so monitor your personal medical history well. Also arrange for routine tuberculosis (TB) screenings.

Be sure to get all appropriate vaccinations, boosters, and screenings on a regular basis.

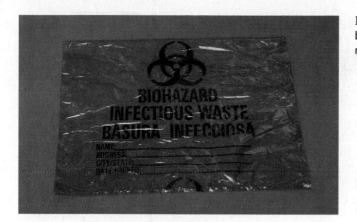

FIGURE 1-11 Dispose of biohazardous wastes in a properly marked bag.

Decontamination of Equipment

Any personal protective equipment (PPE) designed for a single use should be properly disposed of after use. The same is true of medical devices designed for a single use. Such materials should be discarded in a red bag marked with a biohazard seal (Figure 1-11). Needles and other sharp objects should be discarded in properly labeled, puncture-proof containers. Containers should be disposed of according to local guidelines.

Non-disposable equipment that has been contaminated must be cleaned, disinfected, or sterilized:

- **Cleaning** refers to washing an object with soap and water. After caring for a patient, wash your work areas down with approved soaps. Throw away single-use cleaning supplies in a proper biohazard container.

- **Disinfecting** includes cleaning with a disinfecting agent, which should kill many microorganisms on the surface of an object. Disinfect equipment that had direct contact with the intact skin of a patient, such as backboards and splints. Use a commercial disinfectant or bleach diluted in water (one part bleach to 100 parts water, or follow local guidelines).

- **Sterilizing** is the use of a chemical or a physical method such as pressurized steam to kill all microorganisms on an object. Items that were inserted into the patient's body (a laryngoscope blade, for example) should be sterilized by heat, steam, or radiation. There are also EPA-approved solutions for sterilization.

If your equipment needs more extensive cleaning, bag it and remove it to an area designated for this purpose. Disposable work gloves worn during cleaning and decontamination should be properly discarded. If your clothing has become contaminated, bag the items and wash them in accordance with local guidelines. After removing contaminated clothing, take a shower before dressing again.

Post-Exposure Procedures

By definition, an **exposure** is any occurrence of blood or body fluids coming in contact with non-intact skin, the eyes or other mucous membranes, or parenteral contact (needle stick). In most areas, an EMS provider who has had an exposure should (Figure 1-12):

- Immediately wash the affected area with soap and water.
- Get a medical evaluation.
- Take the proper immunization boosters.
- Notify the agency's infection-control liaison.
- Document the circumstances surrounding the exposure, including the actions taken to reduce chances of infection.

In general, the EMS provider should cooperate with the incident investigation and comply with all required reporting responsibilities and time frames.

cleaning washing an object with cleaners such as soap and water.

disinfecting cleaning with an agent that can kill some microorganisms on the surface of an object.

sterilizing use of a chemical or physical method such as pressurized steam to kill all microorganisms on an object.

exposure any occurrence of blood or body fluids coming in contact with non-intact skin, mucous membranes, or parenteral contact (needle stick).

Follow your EMS system guidelines on all management and documentation of any exposure to a patient's blood or body fluids.

INFECTIOUS DISEASE EXPOSURE PROCEDURE

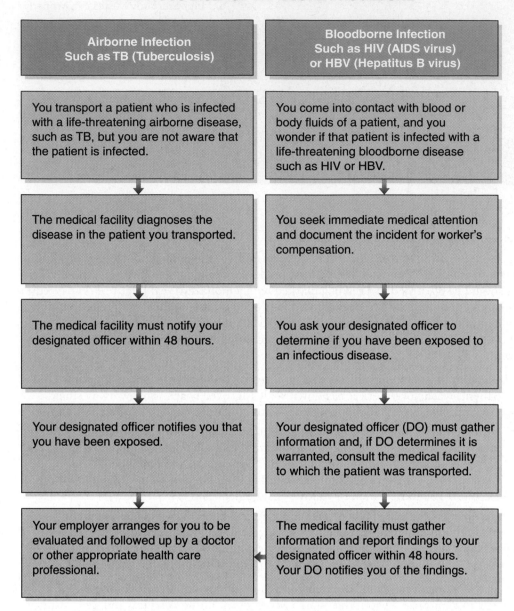

Airborne Infection Such as TB (Tuberculosis)	Bloodborne Infection Such as HIV (AIDS virus) or HBV (Hepatitus B virus)
You transport a patient who is infected with a life-threatening airborne disease, such as TB, but you are not aware that the patient is infected.	You come into contact with blood or body fluids of a patient, and you wonder if that patient is infected with a life-threatening bloodborne disease such as HIV or HBV.
The medical facility diagnoses the disease in the patient you transported.	You seek immediate medical attention and document the incident for worker's compensation.
The medical facility must notify your designated officer within 48 hours.	You ask your designated officer to determine if you have been exposed to an infectious disease.
Your designated officer notifies you that you have been exposed.	Your designated officer (DO) must gather information and, if DO determines it is warranted, consult the medical facility to which the patient was transported.
Your employer arranges for you to be evaluated and followed up by a doctor or other appropriate health care professional.	The medical facility must gather information and report findings to your designated officer within 48 hours. Your DO notifies you of the findings.

FIGURE 1-12 A federal regulation called the Ryan White Comprehensive AIDS Resources Emergency (CARE) Act outlines procedures to follow after an occupational exposure to HIV, hepatitis B, diphtheria, meningitis, plague, hemorrhagic fever, rabies, or tuberculosis.

DEATH AND DYING

As an EMT-I, you will encounter death much more frequently than other people do. Often you will see it as it happens. This can lead to a sense of cumulative overload, which you will need to recognize and deal with in a healthy manner.

LOSS, GRIEF, AND MOURNING

A long-standing taboo against discussing death and dying changed when pioneer Elisabeth Kübler-Ross braved the backlash to meet with terminally ill hospital patients to discuss their feelings about death and dying. Before then, it was assumed dying people did not want to talk about the experience. What Kübler-Ross learned is that there are five predictable stages of loss:

Content Review

STAGES OF LOSS
- Denial
- Anger
- Bargaining
- Depression
- Acceptance

- *Denial, or "not me."* This is the inability or refusal to believe the reality of the event. It is a defense mechanism, during which the patient puts off dealing with the inevitable end of life.

- *Anger, or "why me?"* The patient's anger is really frustration related to his inability to control the situation. That anger could focus on anyone or anything.

- *Bargaining, or "okay, but first let me . . ."* In the patient's mind, he tries to make a deal to "buy additional time" to put off or change the expected outcome.

- *Depression, or "okay, but I haven't . . ."* The patient is sad and despairing, often mourning things not accomplished and dreams that will not come true. The patient withdraws or retreats into a private world, unwilling to communicate with others.

- *Acceptance, or "okay, I'm not afraid."* The patient may come to realize his fate and achieve a reasonable level of comfort with the anticipated outcome. At this stage, the family may need more support than the patient.

A person experiencing any significant loss usually works through these stages, given enough time. Although there is a tendency to progress from one stage to the next in order, both dying patients and their loved ones experience the stages in their own unique ways. They may jump around among the stages, they may go back and forth, or they may never finish them. It is important for you to remain flexible in your expectations, so you can decide how best to help, if asked.

Given enough time, a person experiencing death or dying usually works through the five stages of loss.

Because EMT-Is encounter death and dying often, there is a mistaken belief that they handle it better. However, EMT-Is are human, too. Let yourself deal with death and dying when it occurs. Do not shirk the support of friends and family. Do not try to "tough it out." Use every opportunity to process a specific incident in a healthy, appropriate manner and grieve losses that have an impact on you.

Grief is a feeling. Mourning is a process. A grieving person feels mostly sadness or distress. A person in mourning is immersed in the process of displaying and ultimately dissipating the feelings of grief. The sense of loss is predictably most intense immediately after the news is received. Although numerous models for the mourning process exist, a good rule of thumb is that after the loss of a close friend or relative, a period of one year of mourning is normal.

Upon initially hearing the news of a death, a person experiences a "paralyzing, totally incapacitating surge of grief that is exactly comparable to the incapacitating pain of an acute eye or testicle blow in that the whole world shrinks down to that acute pain." Typically, the feeling lasts for 5 to 15 minutes. When you deliver the news of a death, remember that a survivor cannot function during this grief spike. After delivering the news, wait until it is past and the survivor is ready and able to receive information and make decisions.

A period of intense feelings that continues for around 4 to 6 weeks follows the grief spike. Feelings may include loss, anger, resentment, sadness, and even guilt, depending on the relationship and the circumstances surrounding the death. Gradually, the intensity and immediacy of the loss fades into a phase dominated by a sense of loneliness, which lasts about 6 months. Finally, a period of recovery ensues. The survivor begins to view the loss more objectively and rediscovers an interest in living. Key to the process of mourning is the passage of significant dates and anniversaries, such as birthdays, holidays, and the monthly (then annual) date when the loss occurred.

How different people cope with difficult moments, such as death, varies. If you are dealing with a child, understand that children's perceptions are different from an adult's. (See Table 1-3 for a summary.) This is true of all the special populations you will encounter, such as the elderly and people with mental disabilities. The elderly, for example, may be particularly concerned about the effects of the loss on other family members, about further loss of their own independence, and about the costs of a funeral and burial. There is a wide variety of responses to death among different peoples and cultures as well. Be flexible, and be ready for anything.

WHAT TO SAY

As Do Not Resuscitate orders and other out-of-hospital death situations increase, EMS personnel are more often placed in the position of telling people that someone has died. It

Table 1-3	NEEDS AND EXPECTATIONS OF CHILDREN REGARDING DEATH	
Age Range	Characteristics	Suggestions
Newborn to age 3	Senses that something has happened in family, and notices that there is much activity in the household. Realizes that people are crying and sad. Watch for irritability and changes in eating, sleeping, or other behavioral patterns.	Be sensitive to the child's needs. Try to maintain consistency in routines. Maintain consistency with significant people in child's life.
Ages 3 to 6	Believes death is a temporary state, and may ask continually when the person will return. Believes in magical thinking, and may feel responsible for the death or it is punishment for own behavior. May be fearful of catching the same illness and die, or may believe that everyone else he loves will die also. Watch for changes in behavior patterns with friends and at school, difficulty sleeping, and changes in eating habits.	Emphasize that the child was not responsible for the death. Reinforce that when people are sad, they cry, and that crying is normal and natural. Encourage the child to talk about and/or draw pictures of his feelings, or to cry.
Ages 6 to 9	May prefer to hide or disguise feelings to avoid looking babyish. Is afraid significant others will die. Seeks out detailed explanations for death, and differences between fatal illness and "just being sick." Has an understanding that death is real, but may believe that those who die are too slow, weak, or stupid. Fantasizes in an effort to make everything the way it was. Denial is most helpful coping skill.	Talk about the normal feelings of anger, sadness, and guilt. Share your own feelings about death. Do not be afraid to cry in front of the child. This and other expressions of loss help to give the child permission to express his feelings.
Ages 9 to 12	Begins to understand the irreversibility of death. May seek details and specifics of the situation, and may need repeated, explicit explanations. Hard-won sense of independence becomes fragile, and may show concern about the practical matters of his lifestyle. May try to act "adult," but then regress to earlier stage of emotional response. When threatened, expresses anger toward the ill/deceased, himself or other survivors.	Set aside time to talk about feelings. Encourage sharing of memories to facilitate grief response.
Ages 12 to 18	Demanding developmental processes are an awkward fit with need to take on different family roles. Retreats to safety of childhood. Feels pressure to act as an adult, while still coping with skills of a child. Suppresses feelings in order to "fit in," leaving teen isolated and vulnerable.	Encourage talking, but respect need for privacy. See if a trusted, reliable friend or adult can provide appropriate support. Locate support group for teens.

would be nice to have a script for those difficult moments, but the reality is that you have to assess the scene and the people in each situation to determine the safest and most compassionate way to deliver the sad news.

In terms of safety, you never know how people will respond, even if you know them. Most people accept the news quietly. However, some allow their grief to flood out of them in very physical ways, such as throwing things, kicking walls, or screaming and running in circles. Before speaking, consciously position yourself between them and the door or other escape route. Remember, initially the grief spike has its grip on the survivors. There is little you can do but give them a safe, private place to get through it. Also, for safety, do not deliver the news to a large group. Ask the primary people (no more than four or five) to step aside with you to a private place. Let them tell the others in their own way.

Find out who is who among the survivors. Do not make assumptions. Then address the closest survivor, preferably in a way that shows compassion. That is, avoid standing above the survivor. Instead, sit or squat so that your eyes are at the same level. If the survivor is alone, call for a friend, neighbor, clergy member, or relative. Wait to tell the survivor the news until that person has arrived.

Introduce yourself by name and function ("My name is Kate. I'm an EMT-Intermediate with West End Ambulance.) A careful choice of words is helpful. Although it may seem blunt, use the words "dead" and "died," rather than euphemisms which may be misinterpreted or misunderstood. Use gentle eye contact and, if appropriate, the power of touching an arm or holding a hand. Basic elements of your message should include:

- The loved one has died.

- There is nothing more anyone could have done.

- Your EMS service is available to assist the survivors if needed. (Sometimes, medical emergencies occur in survivors in the wake of such stressful news.)

- Information about local procedures for out-of-hospital death, such as the inspection of the scene by the medical examiner or coroner, and so on.

Do not include statements about God's will or relief from pain or any subjective assumption. You do not know the people well enough to know the details about their relationship or their religious preferences.

WHEN IT IS SOMEONE YOU KNOW

Many EMT-Is are called to serve in small communities, where calls often involve people they know. Elements of this are both rewarding and heart-wrenching. People may be greatly relieved to see a familiar, trusted face among the EMS team. There also is a lot of support for EMS in small communities, because the EMT-I is there to help others during their most fearful moments. However, being involved when the life of someone you know is threatened or lost can have a powerful impact on your own emotions. If it is too much, you must find a way to manage the stress. Oftentimes, you must grieve as well. Your well-being demands it.

STRESS AND STRESS MANAGEMENT

WHAT IS STRESS?

Many aspects of EMS are stressful. Stress, according to researcher Hans Selye, is "the nonspecific response of the body to any demand." The word **stress** also refers to a hardship or strain, or a physical or emotional response to a stimulus. A person's reactions to stress are individual. They are affected by previous exposure to the stressor, perception of the event, general life experience, and personal coping skills.

A stimulus that causes stress is known as a *stressor*. Stress is usually understood to generate a negative affect, or *distress*, in an individual. There is also "good" stress, which is called *eustress* (for example, seeing a lost loved one for the first time in years). However, even eustress generates physiological and psychological signs and symptoms.

Adapting to stress is a dynamic, evolving process. As a person adapts, he or she develops:

- *Defensive strategies*. Although sometimes helpful for the short term, these strategies deny and distort the reality of a stressful situation.

- *Coping*. This is an active process during which a person confronts the stressful situation and changes or adjusts as necessary. Coping may not serve as the best strategy for the long term.

- *Problem-solving skills*. These skills are regarded as the healthiest approach to everyday concerns. Reflected in the ability to analyze a problem and recognize multiple options and potential solutions, mastery generally comes only as a result of extensive experience with similar situations.

stress a hardship or strain; a physical or emotional response to a stimulus.

EMS has abundant stressors, which provide ample opportunities for the development of problem-solving skills. There are administrative stressors, such as waiting for calls, shift work, loud pagers, and inadequate pay. There are scene-related stressors, such as violent and abusive people, flying debris, vomit, loud noises, and chaos. There are emotional and physical stressors, such as fear, demanding bystanders, abusive patients, frustration, exhaustion, hunger or thirst, and lifting heavy objects.

Environmental stress may be in the form of siren noise, inclement weather, confined work spaces, and the frequent urgency of rapid scene responses and life-or-death decisions. In addition, the often difficult world of EMS can strain an EMT-I's family relationships and possibly lead to conflicts with supervisors and co-workers. Add this to the common personality traits of EMT-Is, which include a strong need to be liked and often unrealistically high self-expectations, and the combination can lead to disturbing feelings of guilt or anxiety. All these stressors take a toll on the EMT-I.

Your job in managing stress is to learn these things:

To manage stress, identify your own personal stressors, the amount of stress you can take before it becomes a problem, and what specific stress-management techniques work for you.

- *Your personal stressors.* Each person has an individual list. What is stressful to you may be enjoyable to someone else. What was stressful to you last year may be replaced by new stressors this year.

- *Amount of stress you can take before it becomes a problem.* Stress occurs in a tornado-like continuum. It starts with a few breezes, but it can increase in force until it is whirling out of control. Stopping the "storm" early is key to your well-being. You need to know which stress responses are early indicators for you, so you can deal with them at that point.

- *Stress management strategies that work for you.* Again, this is totally individual. Those who seek personal well-being must become well-versed about personally appropriate options.

If a person piles on stressor after stressor without regard for the consequences, the results are likely to be bad. Stress-related disease is avoidable if you make a habit of doing what is necessary to preserve your personal well-being.

There are three phases of a stress response: alarm, resistance, and exhaustion. At the end comes a period of rest and recovery.

Content Review

PHASES OF A STRESS RESPONSE
- Alarm
- Resistance
- Exhaustion

- *Stage I: Alarm.* The alarm phase is the "fight-or-flight" phenomenon. It occurs when the body physically and rapidly prepares to defend itself against a perceived threat. The pituitary gland begins by releasing adrenocorticotropic (stress) hormones. Hormones continue to flood the body via the autonomic nervous system, coordinated by the hypothalamus. Epinephrine and norepinephrine from the adrenal glands increase heart rate and blood pressure, dilate pupils, increase blood sugar and slow digestion, and relax the bronchial tree. This reaction ends when the event is recognized as not dangerous.

- *Stage II: Resistance.* This stage starts when the individual begins to cope with the stress. Over time, an individual may become desensitized or adapted to stressors. Physiological parameters, such as pulse and blood pressure, may return to normal.

- *Stage III: Exhaustion.* Prolonged exposure to the same stressors leads to exhaustion of an individual's ability to resist and adapt. Resistance to all stressors declines. Susceptibility to physical and psychological ailments increase. A period of rest and recovery is necessary for a healthy outcome.

It would be great if we could manage each stressor to the point of recovery before the next one hits, but that is not how it works. Typically, people are still dealing with one stress (or the same ongoing one, such as the chronic stress of shift work) when additional stressors pile on, resulting in cumulative stress. If stress accumulates without intervention, the consequences can be serious.

Shift Work

There will always be shift work in EMS. Because EMS is a 24-hour, 7-days-a-week endeavor, someone has to be functional at all times. This is inherently stressful because of disruptions in the biorhythms of the body, known as circadian rhythms, and sleep deprivation.

Circadian rhythms are biological cycles that occur approximately every 24 hours. These include hormonal and body temperature fluctuations, appetite and sleepiness cycles, and other bodily processes. When life patterns disrupt the circadian rhythms, biological effects can be stressful. For example, sleep deprivation is common among people who work at night. The inherent dangers to EMT-Is are clear. If you have to sleep in the daytime, here are some tips to minimize the stress:

- Sleep in a cool, dark place that mimics the nighttime environment.
- Stick to sleeping at your **anchor time** (times you can rest without interruption), even on days off. Do not try to revert to a daytime lifestyle on days off. For example, if you work 9 P.M. to 5 A.M. and your anchor time is 8 A.M. to noon, then go to bed early on days off and on workdays sleep from 8 A.M. to 3 P.M.
- Unwind appropriately after a shift in order to rest well. Do not eat a heavy meal or exercise right before bedtime.
- Post a "day sleeper" sign on your front door, turn off the phone's ringer, and lower the volume of the answering machine.

circadian rhythms physiological phenomena that occur at approximately 24-hour intervals.

anchor time set of hours when night-shift worker can reliably expect to rest without interruption.

Signs of Stress

A variety of factors can trigger a stress response. They include the loss of something valuable, injury or the threat of injury, poor health or nutrition, general frustration, and ineffective coping mechanisms. Remember, each individual is susceptible to different stressors and therefore has a different constellation of signs and symptoms.

These signs and symptoms (Table 1-4) are a blessing in a way, because they are the body's way of warning that corrective stress management is needed. The warnings typically are mild at first, but left uncorrected they will build in intensity until you are forced to rest. If it means having a heart attack or collapsing, that is what the body will do. So, pay attention. If you catch a warning sign of excessive stress early and manage it, there is no need to reach the extreme end-point commonly referred to as **burnout**.

burnout occurs when coping mechanisms no longer buffer stressors, which can compromise personal health and well-being.

Common Techniques for Managing Stress

There are two main groups of defense mechanisms and techniques for managing stress: beneficial and detrimental. Detrimental techniques may provide a temporary sense of relief, but they will not cure the problem. They only make things worse. They include substance abuse (alcohol, nicotine, illegal and prescription drugs), overeating or other compulsive behaviors, chronic complaining, freezing out or cutting off others and the support they could give you, avoidance behaviors, and dishonesty about your actual state of well-being ("I'm just fine!"). It is far better for you to spend your energy on beneficial techniques that serve to dissipate the accumulation of stress and promote actual recovery.

In situations where your stress response threatens your ability to handle the moment, you can:

- *Use controlled breathing.* Focus attention on your breathing. Take in a deep breath through your nose. Then exhale forcefully but steadily through your mouth so that you can hear the air rush out. Press all the air out of your lungs with your abdomen. Do this two or more times until you feel steadier. This technique helps to reduce your adrenaline levels and slows your heart rate so you can do your job appropriately.
- *Reframe.* Mentally reframe interfering thoughts such as "I can't do this" or "I'm scared." Be sure to deal with the thoughts later, or they will continue to interfere with the performance of your duties.

Table 1-4 WARNING SIGNS OF EXCESSIVE STRESS

Physical	Cognitive
Nausea/vomiting	Confusion
Upset stomach	Lowered attention span
Tremors (lips, hands)	Calculation difficulties
Feeling uncoordinated	Memory problems
Diaphoresis (profuse sweating), flushed skin	Poor concentration
	Difficulty making decisions
Chills	Disruption in logical thinking
Diarrhea	Disorientation, decreased level of awareness
Aching muscles and joints	Seeing an event over and over
Sleep disturbances	Distressing dreams
Fatigue	Blaming someone
Dry mouth	
Shakes	
Headache	
Vision problems	
Difficult, rapid breathing	
Chest tightness or pain, heart palpitations, cardiac rhythm disturbances	

Emotional	Behavioral
Anticipatory anxiety	Change in activity
Denial	Hyperactivity, hypoactivity
Fearfulness	Withdrawal
Panic	Suspiciousness
Survivor guilt	Change in communications
Uncertainty of feelings	Change in interactions with others
Depression	Change in eating habits
Grief	Increased or decreased food intake
Hopelessness	Increased smoking
Feeling overwhelmed	Increased alcohol intake
Feeling lost	Increased intake of other drugs
Feeling abandoned	Being overly vigilant to environment
Feeling worried	Excessive humor
Wishing to hide	Excessive silence
Wishing to die	Unusual behavior
Anger	Crying spells
Feeling numb	
Identifying with victim	

- *Attend to the medical needs of the patient.* Even if you know the people involved, do not let those relationships interfere with your responsibilities as an EMS provider. Later, when it is appropriate to do so, address your stress about the call.

For long-term well-being, one of the best stress management techniques is to take care of yourself—physically, emotionally, and mentally. Remember that regular exercise does not have to be extreme. Do something that you enjoy and find relaxing. At stressful times, pay especially close attention to your diet. If you smoke, make it a goal to quit.

Create a non-EMS circle of friends and renew old friendships or activities. Take a vacation or a few days off. Say "no!" to the next offer of an overtime shift. Listen to music, meditate, and learn positive thinking. Try the soothing techniques of guided imagery and progressive relaxation. Some EMT-Is have even quit EMS for a while. In general, you can make many choices. The key principle is to generate positive options for yourself and keep choosing them until you have recovered.

For long-term well-being, the best stress-management technique is to take care of yourself; that is, eat properly, exercise regularly, and take time off!

SPECIFIC EMS STRESSES

There are three types of clearly defined EMS stress:

- *Daily stress*. Most EMS stress is unrelated to critical incidents and disasters. Instead, it is related to such things as pay, working conditions, dealing with the public, administrative matters, and other hassles of day-to-day living. To help deal with daily stress, all emergency personnel should develop personal stress management strategies, such as a personal support system made up of co-workers, family, clergy, and others.

- *Small incidents*. Incidents involving only one or two patients, including those with injuries or deaths of emergency workers, are best handled by competent mental health personnel in an individual or small group setting. Mental health professionals should be familiar with EMS and be ready to respond when needed. They should then continue to screen affected emergency workers for signs and symptoms of abnormal response to stress and, if detected, refer them accordingly to other competent mental health professionals who use accepted techniques in treatment.

- *Large incidents and disasters*. Most EMS personnel will never encounter a disaster situation. However, all must be ready in case such a catastrophe occurs. The stress of large-scale disasters can be mitigated by a well-coordinated and organized response. Use of the Incident Command System (ICS) in large incidents and disasters serves to appropriately direct responding personnel. It also provides for rotating personnel through rehabilitation and surveillance stations. Those who are showing signs of stress or fatigue are removed from duty, at least temporarily. Here, too, there is a role for competent mental health professionals, who should be readily available to provide psychological first aid.

MENTAL HEALTH SERVICES

Mental health professionals can provide the information and education needed for rescuers to understand trauma, what to expect, and where to get help if needed. In addition, competent mental-health personnel should be available at all major incidents to provide "psychological first aid" to rescuers and victims. Psychological first aid includes:

- Listening
- Conveying compassion
- Assessing needs
- Ensuring that basic physical needs are met
- Not forcing personnel to talk
- Providing or mobilizing family or significant others
- Encouraging, but not forcing, social support
- Protecting rescuers and victims from additional harm

Psychological first aid is not a treatment or packaged proprietary intervention technique. It is an attempt to provide practical palliative care and contact while respecting the wishes of those who may not be ready to deal with the possible onslaught of emotional responses in the early days following an incident. It entails providing comfort, information, and meeting people's immediate practical and emotional needs.

DISASTER MENTAL HEALTH SERVICES

The emotional well-being of both rescuers and victims is an important concern in any multiple-casualty incident. In the past, Critical Incident Stress Management (CISM) was recommended for use in emergency services. However, recent evidence has clearly shown that CISM and Critical Incident Stress Debriefing (CISD), do not appear to mitigate the effects of traumatic stress and, in fact, may interfere with the normal grieving and healing process and should not be used.

However, there remains an important role for competent mental health professionals in any multiple-casualty incident. Mental health personnel should be available on scene to provide psychological first aid to all those affected by an incident—including EMS personnel. At the same time, they can survey rescuers and victims for the development of abnormal stress-related symptoms. In addition, mental health professionals should be available within two months following a critical incident to screen and assist anyone who may be developing stress-related symptoms. Persons so affected may be referred for additional counseling or mental health care.

GENERAL SAFETY CONSIDERATIONS

The topic of scene safety is vast and requires career-long attention. Considering the many problems that can occur, it is impressive how few injuries there are. Your risks include violent people, environmental hazards, structural collapse, motor vehicles, and infectious disease. Many of these hazards can be minimized with protective equipment, such as helmets, body armor, reflective tape for night visibility, footwear with ankle support, and BSI precautions against infectious disease. Whatever protective equipment you have should be used.

INTERPERSONAL RELATIONS

Safety issues that arise in out-of-hospital care often stem from poor interpersonal relations. EMT-Is are public ambassadors of health care. Interpersonal safety begins with effective communication. If you can build a rapport with the strangers you have been sent to serve, you will gain their trust. Suspicious, angry, upset people are far more likely to be defensive and inflict harm than those who see a reason to trust what you are doing.

Building rapport depends on the ability to put your personal prejudices aside. Everyone has prejudices. But as a representative of an institution far greater than yourself, you must never allow them to interfere with appropriate patient and bystander management. In fact, go beyond curbing prejudice, and challenge yourself to treat every person you meet with dignity and respect.

You can begin by taking time to pay attention to the rich array of cultural diversity and learning to see those differences as valuable and positive. In particular, learn about the different cultural backgrounds of people in your area and how to work with them effectively. For example, although you may like a lot of eye contact, understand that it is regarded as more polite in several cultures to avoid eye contact. Therefore, someone showing you esteem might avoid eye contact with you. This is not wrong. It is just different. Listen well to the stories of other people and see what you can learn. When a person can accept differences easily, it becomes easier to work toward win–win situations on the streets.

ROADWAY SAFETY

Roadways are unsafe places. There are good books, classes, and mentors to help you become aware of the various roadway hazards. Learn the principles of:

- Safely following an emergency escort vehicle
- Intersection management, when traffic is moving in several directions
- Noting hazardous conditions, such as spilled hazardous materials (gasoline, industrial chemicals, and so on), downed power lines, and proximity to moving traffic; also noting adverse environmental conditions

Treat every person you meet with dignity and respect, no matter what their race, sex, age, religion, economic background, or present condition.

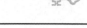

One of the greatest hazards in EMS is the motor vehicle. Be sure to obey roadway laws and follow all driving safety guidelines.

- Evaluating the safest parking place when arriving at a roadway incident
- Safely approaching a vehicle in which someone is slumped over the wheel
- Patient compartment safety—in particular, bracing yourself against sudden deceleration or swerving to avoid roadway hazards; and making a habit of hanging on consistently, especially when changing positions
- Safely using emergency lights and siren

An ambulance escort can create additional hazards. Inexperienced ambulance operators often follow the escort vehicle too closely and are unable to stop when the escort does. Inexperienced operators also may assume that other drivers know the ambulance is following an escort. In fact, other drivers do not know and often pull out in front of the ambulance just after the escort vehicle passes.

Multiple-vehicle responses can be just as dangerous, especially when responding vehicles travel in the same direction close together. When two vehicles approach the same intersection at the same time, they may not only fail to yield to each other, but also other drivers may yield for the first vehicle only, not the second one. Extreme caution must be taken when approaching intersections.

Certain equipment is intended to promote your safety on roadways. For example, to be visible to oncoming drivers, who may have dirty, smeared, pitted windshields and may not be sober, wear reflective tape and orange or lime-green safety vests. In fact, you also may be issued other protective gear, especially if you are in the fire service. Using respiratory protection, gloves, boots, turnout coat and pants (or coveralls), and other specialty safety equipment is the mark of an aware, professional EMT-I. Ask non-medical personnel to set out flares or cones, if needed. Leave some emergency lights flashing, although be careful not to blind oncoming drivers.

To park safely at a roadway incident, make it a habit to scan each individual setting. Notice curves, hilltops, volume, and the speed of surrounding traffic. Ideally, park in the front of a crash site on the same side of the street. This facilitates access to the patient compartment and equipment, and it protects you from traffic coming from behind. However, when responding to an incident such as "person slumped behind wheel," maintain the defensive advantage by staying behind the vehicle, and use spotlights to "blind" the person until you know there are no hostile intentions. Walk to the vehicle with cautious alertness until you are sure it is not a trap.

The use of seatbelts in the front of an ambulance should be an obvious habit, both for safety and for role modeling. Less obvious is the use of safety restraints in the patient compartment. An improper assumption is that the EMT-I is too busy attending the patient and passengers to wear a seatbelt. However, buckling into a seatbelt for a safer ride is, in fact, possible during much or most of ambulance transport times. Death and major disability is common when someone is in the patient compartment during a crash. For your well-being, wear a seatbelt whenever possible, even "in back."

Because ambulances represent help and hope, it is doubly tragic when an EMT-I crew is involved in a motor-vehicle crash caused by the misuse of lights and siren. Lights and siren are tools, not toys. They are the EMT-I's means for gaining quick access to people in dire need. Those who misuse the mandate to operate them chip away at the public's trust in EMS. Whether using lights and siren or not, in most states, the EMT-I has a legal responsibility to drive with "due regard for the safety of all others." As a professional, you are obligated to study and use safe driving practices at all times.

Part 5: Illness and Injury Prevention

How often do EMS crews respond to incidents that could easily have been prevented? How often have you thought to yourself "I wish there was something I could have done" in the wake of senseless circumstances surrounding an accidental injury or illness? But what if EMS personnel asked questions before an incident occurred? How many injuries could be prevented? How many lives could be saved? Part 5 focuses on these questions and discusses illness and injury prevention as an EMT-I's crucial duty and responsibility.

EPIDEMIOLOGY

Injury is one of our nation's most important health problems.

Injuries result from interaction with potential hazards in the environment, which means they may be predictable and preventable.

epidemiology the study of factors that influence the frequency, distribution, and causes of injury, disease, and other health-related events in a population.

years of productive life age at death subtracted from 65.

injury intentional or unintentional damage to a person resulting from exposure to mechanical or any other form of energy or from absence of essentials such as heat or oxygen.

injury risk a situation that puts people in danger of injury.

injury-surveillance program ongoing systematic collection, analysis, and interpretation of injury data important to public health practice.

teachable moment the time shortly after an injury when patients and observers may be more receptive to teaching about how similar injuries may be prevented in the future.

primary prevention keeping an injury or illness from ever occurring.

secondary prevention medical care after an injury or illness that helps to prevent further problems from occurring.

tertiary prevention rehabilitation activities after an injury or illness.

Injury is one of our nation's most important health problems. Consider the following facts offered by the U.S. Department of Transportation:

- Injury surpassed stroke as the third leading cause of death in the United States, and it is the leading cause of death in people ages one to forty-four.
- Injuries that are unintentional result in nearly 70,000 deaths and millions of nonfatal injuries each year. The leading causes of death from unintentional injuries are motor-vehicle collisions, fires, burns, falls, drownings, and poisonings.
- The estimated lifetime cost of injuries will exceed $114 billion.
- For every one death caused by injury, there are an estimated 19 hospitalizations and 254 emergency department visits.

Though many people believe that injuries "just happen," evidence shows that injuries result from interaction with potential hazards in the environment. Thus, it has been suggested that "MVAs" (motor-vehicle accidents) should be called "MVCs" (motor-vehicle collisions), since driving while intoxicated or at 80 mph and crashing is no accident. In other words, many injuries may be predictable and preventable. The study of the factors that influence the frequency, distribution, and causes of injury, disease, and other health-related events in a population is called **epidemiology.**

Concepts related to epidemiology that you should know include **years of productive life,** a calculation made by subtracting the age at death from 65. (For example, in a liability suit concerning the death of a 45-year-old person, a jury might assess damages based on the deceased's loss of 20 years as a wage-earner.) Another concept is **injury,** which refers to the intentional or unintentional damage to a person resulting from acute exposure to thermal, mechanical, electrical, or chemical energy or from the absence of such essentials as heat and oxygen. An accident is an unintentional injury, but an injury that is purposefully inflicted either on oneself (e.g., suicide) or on another person (e.g., homicide) is an intentional injury. Intentional injuries make up about a third of all injury deaths. Other categories of intentional injury include rape, assault, and domestic, elder, and child abuse.

Other concepts related to epidemiology include **injury risk,** which is a real or potentially hazardous situation that puts people in danger of sustaining injury. As medical professionals, EMS providers should assess every scene and situation for injury risk and maintain statistics as part of an **injury-surveillance program,** or the ongoing systematic collection, analysis, and interpretation of injury data essential to the planning, implementation, and evaluation of public health practice.

An injury-surveillance program must also include a component for the timely dissemination of data to those who need to know. The final link in the injury-surveillance chain is the application of these data to prevention and control. **Teachable moments** occur shortly after an injury when the patient and observers remain acutely aware of what has happened and may be more receptive to teaching about how similar injury or illness could be prevented in the future.

By becoming involved in injury prevention, EMS providers can focus on **primary prevention** or keeping an injury from ever occurring. Medical care and rehabilitation activities that help to prevent further problems from occurring are referred to, respectively, as **secondary prevention** and **tertiary prevention.**

PREVENTION WITHIN EMS

Even armed with the best equipment and technology, EMS providers cannot save every life. However, by working as partners in public health and safety, members of the EMS community can go beyond their normal daily routine and work with the public to prevent avoidable illness and injury.

EMS providers are widely distributed in the population, often reflecting the composition of their communities. They are often considered to be champions of the health-care consumer and are welcome in schools and other community institutions. Medical personnel are high-profile role models and, as such, can have a significant impact on the reduction of injury rates. In rural areas, EMS providers are sometimes the most medically educated individuals, often looked upon for advice and direction. Essentially, the more than 600,000 EMS providers in the United States comprise a great arsenal in the war to prevent injury and disease.

Organizational Commitment

EMS organizational commitment is vital to the development of prevention activities in the following areas:

- *Protection of EMS providers.* The leadership of EMS agencies must assure that policies are in place to promote response, scene, and transport safety. The appropriate personal protective equipment (PPE) should be issued to protect against exposure to bloodborne and airborne pathogens as well as environmental hazards. An overall commitment to safety and wellness should be emphasized and supported.
- *Education of EMS providers.* A "buy-in" from employees at every level is key to the success of any prevention program. EMS managers have the responsibility of instructing employees in the fundamentals of primary prevention. Public and private sector specialty groups may be called upon for specific training (Figure 1-13). EMS providers should also have the skills and training necessary to defend against violent patients or other hostile attackers. Classes in on-scene survival techniques should be commonplace in every EMS agency.
- *Data collection.* Monitoring and maintaining records of patient illnesses and injuries is essential in determining trends and in developing and measuring the success of prevention programs. Each agency should contribute data to local, regional, state, and national systems that track such information.

Content Review

Organizational Commitment

- Protect EMS providers
- Provide initial and continuing education
- Collect and distribute illness and injury data
- Empower EMS personnel

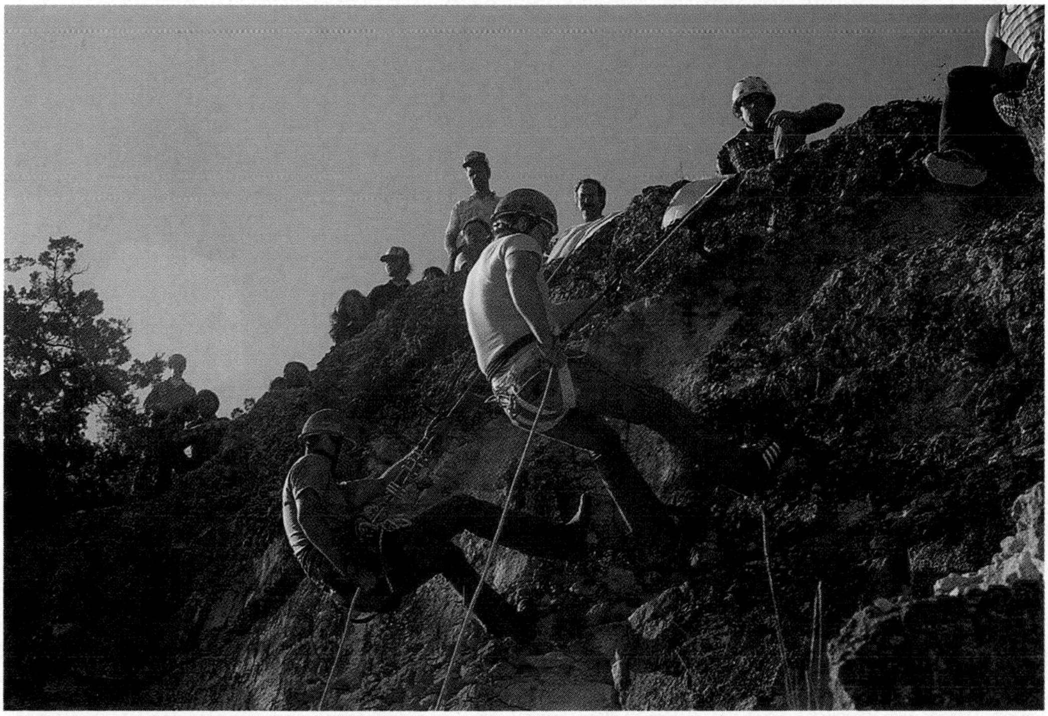

Figure 1-13 Training in specialized safety procedures should be available to you.

- *Financial support.* An agency's internal budget should reflect support for prevention strategies as a priority. If necessary, support must be sought from outside the organization. Large corporations are often willing to donate funds in exchange for stand-by coverage at an event or company function. State highway safety offices can offer funding for traffic-related projects, such as those involving child safety seats, seat belts, and drunk driving. Advertising agencies may contribute billboards for safety messages and public service announcements. Partnerships with local hospitals can result in advertising safety messages in newsletters and flyers. Community groups such as Mothers against Drunk Driving (MADD) and junior auxiliaries also are great resources for initiating community and school programs.

- *Empowerment of EMS providers.* Frontline personnel are the ultimate factor in achieving success in a prevention program. Managers should identify, encourage, and foster, and reward employee interest, support, and involvement. In addition, managers should rotate assignment to prevention programs and provide salary for off-duty injury prevention activities.

EMS PROVIDER COMMITMENT

Illness and injury prevention should begin at home and be carried over into the workplace. The priority for EMS providers is to protect themselves from harm. Employers have an obligation to provide a safe environment. Written guidelines and policies should promote wellness and safety among employees, emphasizing the following areas:

- Body substance isolation (BSI) precautions
- Physical fitness
- Stress management
- Seeking professional care and counseling
- Driving safely

SCENE SAFETY

Safety is always your first priority. Once your unit is dispatched to a call, evaluate the dispatch information before arrival. Focus your attention on response and equipment needed. Upon arrival, park the unit in the safest and most convenient place to load the patient as well as to leave the scene. Consider traffic, road conditions, and all other possible hazards. Directing traffic is primarily the responsibility of local law enforcement agencies. The safest method for traffic control at serious vehicle collisions is to stop all traffic and reroute it to different roads. This is for the safety of patients, bystanders, and rescue personnel.

Note that if you are called to an area with potential health hazards, such as an industrial park or a chemical plant or an area with high crime rates, approach the scene with caution. Be sure to protect yourself appropriately. If you do not have adequate protection or are not specifically trained to control specific hazards, never enter a hazardous scene. Call in specialized teams, such as a hazardous materials crew, if necessary. Law enforcement agencies should be contacted for any violent, potentially violent, or dangerous scene, including those involving domestic abuse or other crimes.

If the scene is safe to enter, be sure to wear reflective clothing to provide added protection on the scene. With BSI precautions in place, approach patients with your safety in mind. Determine the mechanisms of injury (forces that caused injury) or the nature of illness. Treat the patient according to protocol.

After patient care is addressed and a transport decision is made, make sure your unit is secure before departure. Have your partner check the outside of the unit to make certain that all doors are secured. The patient should be secured on an ambulance stretcher with at least three straps and shoulder straps if available. If a family member is allowed to accompany the patient, that person should be placed in the passenger seat in the front compartment with vehicle restraints in place.

Safety is always your first priority.

PREVENTION IN THE COMMUNITY

As a component of health care, EMS has a responsibility to not only prevent injury and illness among EMS workers, but also to promote prevention among the members of the public.

AREAS OF NEED

Infants and Children

Each year, nearly 290,000 infants are born weighing less than 5.5 pounds (2,500 grams), often as a result of inadequate prenatal care. Low birth weight is a key indicator of poor health at the time of birth. Babies born too small or too soon are far more likely to die in the first year of life. Annually, more than 4,000 die of low birth weight and prematurity. Among those who survive, an estimated 2% to 5% have a disability, and one quarter of the smallest survivors (born weighing less than 1,500 grams) have serious disabilities such as mental retardation, cerebral palsy, seizure disorders, or blindness.

One of every three deaths among children in the United States results from an injury. The number of injuries, of course, far exceeds the number of deaths. The most common causes of fatal injuries in children include motor-vehicle collisions, pedestrian or bicycle injuries, burns, falls, and firearms. Injuries generally can be classified into intentional events (such as shootings and assaults), unintentional events (such as motor-vehicle collisions), and alleged unintentional events (such as suspicious injury patterns that suggest possible abuse).

In motor-vehicle collisions, young children are easily thrown on impact. Because a young child's head is large in proportion to the body, an unrestrained child tends to fly head first into the windshield or out of the car when a collision occurs. The back seat is the best seat for children twelve years old or younger. In this location, the properly restrained child is least likely to sustain injuries in a crash. Car safety seats and seat belts can prevent most severe injuries to passengers of all ages if they are used correctly. Air bags are designed to save people's lives when used with seat belts, and they can protect drivers and passengers who are correctly buckled.

Infants and toddlers are commonly injured by cars backing up in driveways or parking lots. Children between the ages of five and nine who are struck by cars typically dart out in traffic. Children riding bicycles can be injured when they collide with cars or other fixed objects or when they are thrown from the bicycle. The most serious bicycle-related injuries are head injuries, which can cause death or permanent brain damage.

Falls are the most frequent cause of injury to children younger than six years old. About 200 children die from falls each year. Fire and burn injuries occur in the highest numbers in the very young. Most are caused by scalding from a hot liquid such as when children grab pot handles and spill the contents.

In this modern age of media and the internet, children and young adults are bombarded with an incredible amount of information and are often faced with some of the same stressors as adults. Sometimes those stressors become overwhelming. One of the most troubling recent trends is the number of violent acts among young people, occurring in the form of self-destructive behavior, gang violence, and assaults. In addition, firearm injury to children is becoming more common as a result of the accessibility of handguns. Injuries and deaths occur when children and adolescents take guns to school. The number of firearm deaths has doubled since 1953. About 15% of all firearm-related deaths are unintentional, often resulting from improper handling and lack of safety mechanisms.

Geriatric Patients

Falls account for the largest number of preventable injuries for persons more than 75 years of age. As a result of slower reflexes, failing eyesight and hearing, and arthritis, the elderly are at increased risk of injury from falls. Falls frequently result in fractures since the bones become weaker and more brittle with age.

The aging process also places the elderly at a greater risk for serious head injury as well as other injuries. Although many geriatric patients are completely coherent, many others have some degree of dementia. Alzheimer's disease is merely one of the mental conditions

EMS has a responsibility to prevent injury and illness not only among EMS personnel but also among members of the public.

Content Review

AREAS IN NEED OF PREVENTION ACTIVITIES

- Low birth weight
- Unrestrained children in cars
- Bicycle-related injuries
- Household fire and burn injuries
- Unintentional firearm-related deaths
- Alcohol-related motor-vehicle collisions
- Fall injuries in the elderly
- Workplace injuries
- Sports and recreation injuries
- Misuse or mishandling of medications
- Early discharge of patients

Cultural Considerations

Studies have shown that the incidence of EMS calls is higher in areas where there is poverty and many elderly. EMS personnel must recognize that this will be a significant part of the job.

that can affect the elderly. The associated confusion can contribute to dangerous behaviors such as wandering away from home or into a roadway.

Motor-Vehicle Collisions

As noted earlier, EMS and law enforcement have long referred to vehicular collisions as motor-vehicle accidents (MVAs). However, the term motor-vehicle collision (MVC) more accurately reflects the fact that no collision is an accident, something caused the crash to occur. Such crashes are responsible for more than half of all deaths from unintentional injuries. Alcohol use is a factor in about half of all motor-vehicle fatalities.

Work and Recreation Hazards

In the workplace, back injuries account for 22% of all disabling injuries. Injuries to the eyes, hands, and fingers are responsible for another 22%. Even the quietest office setting can be hazardous. Never underestimate the potential dangers in an area that appears to be safe. Copy machines, electrical cords, faulty wiring, and shoddy building construction can be hazardous.

Sports injuries are commonly seen in persons of all ages due to the increased popularity and participation in outdoor recreational activities. Football, soccer, baseball, as well as running, hiking, and biking are among popular sports that can result in fractures, dislocations, sprains, and strains.

Medications

When an illness or injury occurs and treatment is sought, medications are often part of the treatment regimen. These medications are occasionally taken improperly (too much or not enough), or they are taken by others, sometimes causing serious medical problems. Medications of any kind should be taken only by those for whom they are prescribed. They should be stored according to label directions. They should also be continued until the prescription is completed. Following the physician's, the pharmacist's, and the label directions is imperative.

Early Discharge

Managed-care organizations such as HMOs and insurance companies often mandate shorter hospital stays and early discharges from the hospital, urgent care centers, and other outpatient facilities. Such policies often result in more patients who are at home sooner with illnesses that are less completely treated. These patients may call 9-1-1 for supportive care and intervention.

IMPLEMENTATION OF PREVENTION STRATEGIES

The following is a list of prevention strategies that you should be able to implement:

- *Preserve the safety of the response team.* Always remember that your first priority is your safety and the safety of your fellow crew members. The next priorities are the patient and, finally, bystanders. Do what you can and what is within your training to maintain a safe and secure working area. Do not hesitate to contact back-up units and law enforcement personnel if necessary.

- *Recognize scene hazards.* Size up the scene for potential risks or dangers before entering. Be aware of your surroundings. Is there anyone or anything that could cause harm to you, your crew, or the patient? Does the mechanism that injured the patient still pose a threat to the rescuers? Are there any hazardous materials in the area? Has any crime been committed? Are there structural risks? Are there temperature extremes for which you are unprepared? Call for the appropriate assistance.

- *Document findings.* Document your patient-care findings at the end of every call. Note that EMS patient forms often can be designed to include specific data on injury prevention in order to benefit researchers and implement future prevention programs. Such a form should include space to describe scene conditions at the time of EMS arrival, the mechanism of injury, and any risks

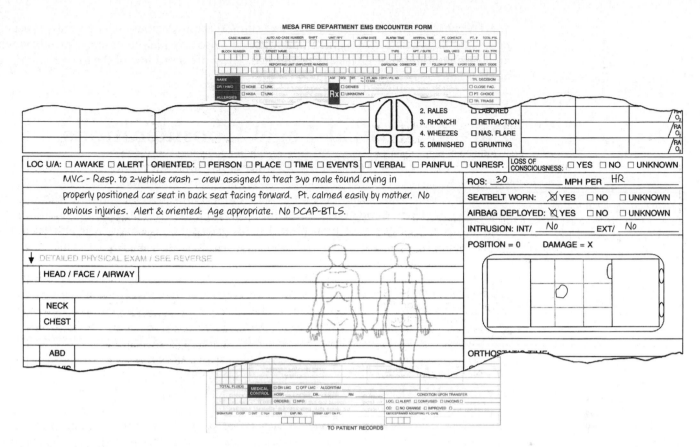

FIGURE 1-14 Documentation of primary and secondary injury prevention data.

that were overcome. If protective devices were used (or not used) during the emergency, these should be documented, too. (See Figure 1-14 for an example.)

- *Engage in on-scene education.* Take advantage of a teachable moment to decrease future emergency responses. Remain objective, non-judgmental, and non-threatening. Inform your listeners of how they can prevent the recurrence of a similar emergency and, if needed, instruct them on the use of protective devices.

- *Know your community resources.* Determine what your patient's needs are and how you may assist him. Your patient may require a referral to an outside agency such as a prenatal clinic, a social service organization that offers food, shelter, clothing, mental health resources or counseling, or other services. Your system may also allow for referral or transportation to a clinic, urgent care, or alternative form of health care. Be aware of the presence of both licensed and unlicensed day-care centers in your area. Encourage parents to provide pre-existing consent for treatment and transport in case of illness or injury at a day care facility. Follow local protocol to report suspected abuse situations. Consider developing a social service resource guide for your organization to provide solutions and ideas for these and other situations.

- *Conduct a community needs assessment.* Conducting a needs assessment will assist in identifying community priorities. Consider the following:

  - Childhood and influenza immunizations
  - Prenatal and well-baby clinics
  - Elder-care clinics
  - Defensive driving classes
  - Workplace safety courses
  - Health clinics (co-sponsored by local hospitals or health-care organizations)
  - Prevention information on your agency's website

The population served and its ethnic, cultural, and religious makeup may affect the needs and approaches that are most appropriate. Also consider community members who are learning disabled or physically challenged. These are just a few of the ideas that may be appropriate for your organization.

Part 6: Medical–Legal Considerations in Prehospital Care

Your best protection from liability is to perform systematic assessments, provide appropriate medical care, and maintain accurate and complete documentation.

To practice competent prehospital care today, EMT-Is must become familiar with the legal issues they are likely to encounter in the field. As an EMT-I, you must be prepared to make the best medical and the most appropriate legal decisions. Part 6 addresses general legal principals in addition to specific laws and legal concepts that affect the EMT-I's daily practice.

Note that since laws vary from state to state, and protocols can vary from county to county, the information contained here cannot be used as a substitute for competent legal advice. Just like the practice of medicine, the practice of law involves some art, some science, and is always heavily dependent on the unique facts present in each situation. If you are faced with a specific legal question, you must rely on the advice of your attorney.

LEGAL DUTIES AND ETHICAL RESPONSIBILITIES

liability legal responsibility.

As an EMT-I, you have specific legal duties. Failure to perform your job appropriately can result in civil or criminal liability. Your best protection from **liability** (legal responsibility) is to perform a systematic patient assessment, provide the appropriate medical care, and maintain accurate and complete documentation of all incidents.

An EMT-I also is responsible for meeting ethical standards. Ethical standards are not laws. They are principles that identify desirable conduct by members of a particular group. Your ethical responsibilities include:

- Promptly respond to the needs of every patient.
- Treat all patients and their families with courtesy and respect.
- Maintain mastery of your skills and medical knowledge.
- Participate in continuing education and refresher training.
- Critically review your performance and seek improvement.
- Report honestly and with respect for patient confidentiality.
- Work cooperatively and with respect for other emergency professionals.

In addition you will encounter moral issues. Morality concerns right and wrong as governed by individual conscience. Always strive to meet the highest legal, ethical, and moral standards when providing patient care.

THE LEGAL SYSTEM

Sources of Law

In the United States, there are four primary sources of law: constitutional law, common law, legislative (or statutory) law, and administrative (or regulatory) law.

constitutional law law based on the U.S. Constitution.

Constitutional law is based on the Constitution of the United States, which sets forth our basic governmental structures and protects people against governmental abuse. For example, the Fourth Amendment protects people from unreasonable searches and seizures.

common law law derived from society's acceptance of customs and norms over time. Also called *case law* or *judge-made law*.

Common law, also referred to as "case" or "judge-made" law, originated with the English legal system and is derived from society's acceptance of customs and norms over time. Common law changes and grows over the years. As a part of common law, precedents set by the courts are generally followed by other courts.

Legislative law (or statutory law) does not come from court decisions. It is created by law-making or legislative bodies. Statutes are enacted at the federal, state, and local levels by the legislative branches of government. Examples of legislative bodies include the U.S. Congress, state assemblies, city councils, and district boards. Legislative law takes precedence over common-law decisions.

Administrative law (or regulatory law) is enacted by an administrative or governmental agency at either the federal or state level. Administrative agencies, such as the Occupational Safety and Health Administration (OSHA), will take a statute enacted by a legislative body and will produce rules and regulations necessary to implement it. The agency is given the authority to make regulations based on that statute, enforce rules, regulations, and statutes under its authority, and hold administrative hearings to carry out penalties for any violations of its rules.

legislative law law created by law-making bodies such as Congress and state assemblies. Also called *statutory law*.

administrative law law that is enacted by governmental agencies at either the federal or state level. Also called *regulatory law*.

Categories of Law

The United States has two general categories of law: civil law and criminal law. **Criminal law** deals with crime and punishment. It is an area of law in which the federal, state, or local government will prosecute an individual on behalf of society for violating laws meant to protect society. Homicide, rape, and burglary are examples of criminal wrongs. Violations of criminal laws are punished by imprisonment, a fine, or combination of the two.

Civil law deals with noncriminal issues, such as personal injury, contract disputes, and matrimonial issues. In civil litigation, which involves conflicts between two or more parties, the plaintiff (person initiating the litigation) will seek to recover damages from the defendant (person against whom the complaint is made). **Tort law,** which is a branch of civil law, deals with civil wrongs committed by one individual against another (rather than against society). Tort law claims include negligence, medical malpractice, assault, battery, and slander.

Note that the United States has a federal court system and a state court system. The federal court system was created by the U.S. Constitution. Generally, only cases that involve a question of federal law or cases in which the parties are citizens of different states will be heard in a federal court. The state court system is the location for most of the cases in which an EMT-I may become involved. In trial courts, a judge or jury determines the outcome of individual cases. Appellate courts hear appeals of decisions by trial courts or other appeals courts. The decisions of appellate courts may set precedents for later cases.

criminal law division of the legal system that deals with wrongs committed against society or its members.

civil law division of the legal system that deals with noncriminal issues and conflicts between two or more parties.

tort law branch of civil law that deals with civil wrongs committed by one individual against another.

ANATOMY OF A CIVIL LAWSUIT

If you have ever been served with legal papers, you know that being sued or even being called to testify at a trial can be very unsettling. A basic understanding of the legal system can help. The following is a brief description of the components of a civil lawsuit:

- *Incident.* For example, a person is driving on a road and fails to see a stop sign. When he passes through the intersection, he hits another car and that driver sustains several injuries.

- *Investigation.* The injured driver's attorney makes a preliminary inquiry into the facts and circumstances surrounding the incident to determine if the case has merit.

- *Filing of the complaint.* The injured driver (now called the "plaintiff") commences the lawsuit by filing a complaint with the court. The complaint contains information such as the names of the parties, the legal basis for the claim, and the damages sought by the plaintiff. A copy of the complaint is served on the defendant.

- *Answering the complaint.* The defendant's attorney then prepares an answer, which addresses each allegation made in the complaint. The answer is then filed with the court, and a copy is given to the plaintiff's attorney.

- *Discovery.* Before any lawsuit appears in front of a judge or jury, both parties to an action participate in pre-trial discovery. This is the stage of the lawsuit

Content Review

COMPONENTS OF A CIVIL LAWSUIT
- Incident
- Investigation
- Filing of complaint
- Answering complaint
- Discovery
- Trial
- Decision
- Appeal
- Settlement

when all relevant information about the incident is shared so that parties can prepare trial strategies. Discovery may include:

- *Examination before trial,* which is also called a "deposition," allows a witness to answer questions under oath with a court stenographer present.

- *Interrogatory,* used by either side, is a set of written questions that requires written responses.

- *Requests for document production* entitles each side to request relevant documents, including the patient care report, records of the receiving hospital, any subsequent medical records, police records, and other records necessary to help prove or defend the lawsuit.

- *Trial.* A trial will be commenced at the lowest level of court in the state. In many states, they are called "superior" courts. At the trial, each side will be given the opportunity to present all relevant evidence and testimony from witnesses.

- *Decision.* After deliberations, the judge or jury determines the guilt or liability of the defendant and then decides the amount of damages to award the plaintiff.

- *Appeal.* After the jury's decision is entered by the court, either party may be entitled to an appeal. Generally, grounds for an appeal are limited to errors of law made by the court. Appeals will not be heard at the lower-level court, but by the higher-level appellate court.

- *Settlement.* This can occur at any stage of the lawsuit. Generally, the defendant will offer the plaintiff an amount of money that is less than the amount for which he is being sued. The plaintiff may then agree to accept the reduced amount on the condition, for example, that he will no longer pursue the case.

LAWS AFFECTING EMS AND THE EMT-INTERMEDIATE

Most of the laws that affect EMS and EMT-Is are state laws. Although these laws vary from state to state, they share common principles.

Scope of Practice

The range of duties and skills EMT-Is are allowed and expected to perform is called the **scope of practice.** Usually, the scope of practice is set by state law or regulation and by local medical direction. Often, a state will have a general "medical practice act" that governs the practice of medicine and all health-care professionals. These acts prescribe how and to what extent a physician may delegate authority to an EMT-I. As you learned earlier in this chapter, EMT-Is may function only under the direct supervision of a licensed physician through a delegation of authority. Generally, EMT-Is should follow orders given by on-line and off-line medical direction. However, you should not blindly follow orders that you know are medically inappropriate.

Circumstances in which an order from medical direction may be legitimately refused include: when you are ordered to provide a treatment that is beyond the scope of your training and inconsistent with established protocols or procedures, and when you are ordered to administer a treatment that you reasonably believe would be harmful to the patient. For example, imagine that an EMT-I is en route to the hospital with a 220-pound (100 kg) patient who is having 15 multi-focal premature ventricular contractions (PVCs) per minute. The treatment protocol for such a condition is to administer 1.0 to 1.5 mg/kg of lidocaine, or 100 to 150 mg to a 200-pound patient. The on-line physician orders the EMT-I to administer 1 gram (1,000 mg) of lidocaine. The EMT-I knows this amount of medication would seriously harm the patient. What should he do? He should first raise the concern with the physician. If the physician still insists, the EMT-I should refuse to follow the order and document the incident thoroughly on the patient care report.

In addition, every EMS system should have a policy in place to guide EMT-Is in dealing with intervener physicians (on-scene licensed physicians who are professionally unrelated to the patient and who are attempting to assist with patient care). Generally, such a policy requires that certain conditions be met before the EMT-I should allow the intervener physi-

scope of practice range of duties and skills EMT-Is are allowed and expected to perform.

You may function as an EMT-I only under the direct supervision of a licensed physician through a delegation of authority.

cian to assume control of patient care. That is, the physician must be properly identified to the EMT-I, licensed to practice medicine in the state, willing to accept the responsibility of continuing medical care until the patient reaches the hospital, and willing to document the intervention as required by the local EMS system.

Licensure and Certification

Other laws that directly affect the EMT-I's ability to practice relate to certification and licensure requirements. Certification refers to the recognition granted to an individual who has met predetermined qualifications to participate in a certain activity. It is usually given by a certifying agency (not necessarily a government agency) or professional association. For example, after completing an approved EMT-I program in the state of New York, a student who passes an approved written and practical examination will become a certified New York State EMT-I.

Licensure is a process used to regulate occupations. Generally, a governmental agency, such as a state medical board, grants permission to an individual who meets established qualifications to engage in a particular profession or occupation. Certification or licensure, or perhaps both, may be required by your state or local authorities for you to practice as an EMT-I.

Most states have laws that govern EMT-I practice and set forth the requirements for certification, licensure, recertification, and relicensure. It is your responsibility to understand fully the EMS laws and regulations in your state.

Motor-Vehicle Laws

As with other EMS-related laws, motor-vehicle laws vary from state to state. Generally, special motor-vehicle laws govern the operation of emergency vehicles and the equipment they carry. These laws apply to areas such as vehicle maintenance and use of the siren and emergency lights. It is important that you become familiar with the laws of your state. Keep up to date with local regulations, too.

Mandatory Reporting Requirements

Each state enacts different laws designed to protect the public. For example, most states have laws that require a health-care worker to report to local authorities any suspected spousal abuse, child abuse and neglect, or abuse of the elderly. In many states, violent crimes, such as sexual assault, gunshot wounds, and stab wounds must be reported to law enforcement. Emergencies that threaten public health, such as animal bites and communicable diseases, also must be reported to the proper authorities. The content of such reports and to whom they must be made is set by law, regulation, or policy. Become familiar with the circumstances under which you are required to make a report. If you fail to make a required report, you may be criminally and civilly liable for your inaction.

Legal Protection for the EMT-Intermediate

In addition to the laws that protect patients, legislative bodies have enacted laws to protect EMT-Is. For example, some jurisdictions have enacted laws that criminally punish a person who commits assault or battery against an EMT-I while he is providing medical care. Others have laws prohibiting the obstruction of EMT-I activity.

Immunity, or exemption from legal liability, is another form of protection. Governmental immunity is a judicial doctrine that prohibits a person from bringing a lawsuit against a government without its consent. However, most states today have waived their immunity rights, and courts are becoming increasingly likely to strike down the ones that still exist. This type of liability protection, even if allowed under law, generally serves to protect only the government agency, not the individual EMT-I. Therefore, you should not rely on governmental immunity to protect you from claims of negligence.

Virtually every state has **Good Samaritan laws,** which provide immunity to people who assist at the scene of a medical emergency. Though these laws vary from state to state, generally, they protect a person from liability if that person acts in good faith, is not negligent (most states will cover acts of simple negligence but not ones of gross negligence), acts within his scope of practice, and does not accept payment for services. The Good Samaritan laws of many states have been expanded to protect both paid and volunteer prehospital personnel.

Content Review

COMMONLY MANDATED REPORTS

- Spouse abuse
- Child abuse and neglect
- Elder abuse
- Sexual assault
- Gunshot and stab wounds
- Animal bites
- Communicable diseases

immunity exemption from legal liability.

Good Samaritan laws laws that provide immunity to certain people who assist at the scene of a medical emergency.

Legal Notes

Good Samaritan laws vary from state to state. Some provide protection for paid EMS personnel, while others exclude paid personnel. Learn the Good Samaritan laws in effect in the area where you work.

As an EMT-I, you should also become familiar with local laws and regulations governing the use of physical restraints for dangerous or violent patients. There also may be regulations governing entry into restricted areas such as military installations, nuclear power plants, and sites with hazardous materials. Since the laws affecting EMT-I practice vary from state to state, your agency should obtain the advice of an attorney in order to minimize potential exposure to liability.

Other laws are designed to protect the EMT-I in the event of exposure to bloodborne or airborne pathogens. For example, the Ryan White Comprehensive AIDS Resources Emergency Act (Ryan White CARE Act) requires hospitals and EMS agencies to create a notification system to provide information and assist the EMT-I when an exposure occurs. This law allows the EMT-I who has been exposed to certain diseases to have access to medical records in order to determine if the patient has tested positive for, or is exhibiting signs and symptoms of, an infectious disease. The Ryan White CARE Act is a federal law, but many states have enacted similar or even more comprehensive laws to protect EMT-Is who may have been exposed to infectious diseases. It is important for each agency to appoint an infection control officer and for this individual to implement protocols and an appropriate infection control plan.

LEGAL ACCOUNTABILITY OF THE EMT-INTERMEDIATE

As an EMT-I, you are required to provide a level of care to your patients that is consistent with your education and training and equal to that of any other competent EMT-I with equivalent training. You also are expected to perform your duties in a reasonable and prudent manner, as any other EMT-I would do in a similar situation. Any deviation from this standard might open you to allegations of negligence and liability for any resulting damages.

NEGLIGENCE AND MEDICAL LIABILITY

negligence deviation from accepted standards of care recognized by law for the protection of others against the unreasonable risk of harm.

Negligence is defined as a deviation from accepted standards of care recognized by law for the protection of others against the unreasonable risk of harm. It can result in legal accountability and liability. In the health-care professions, negligence is synonymous with malpractice.

Components of a Negligence Claim

In a negligence claim against an EMT-I, the plaintiff must establish and prove four particular elements in order to prevail: a duty to act, a breach of that duty, actual damages to the patient or other individual, and proximate cause (causation of damages).

duty to act a formal contractual or informal legal obligation to provide care.

First, the plaintiff must establish that the EMT-I had a **duty to act.** That is, he must prove that the EMT-I had a formal contractual or informal legal obligation to provide care. Note that the act of voluntarily assuming care of a patient may imply that there was a duty to act, which creates a continuing duty to act. For example, in some states if an off-duty EMT-I witnesses a person choking, he may be under no legal duty to act. However, if that EMT-I initiates care, then he has a duty to continue care. The rationale behind this rule is if bystanders see that a victim is being helped, they may walk away. If the EMT-I rendering assistance walks away after initiating treatment, but not completing it, the patient may actually be left in a worse condition than if the EMT-I never tried to help.

Duties that are expected of the EMT-I include:

- Duty to respond to the scene and render care to ill or injured patients
- Duty to obey federal, state, and local laws and regulations
- Duty to operate the emergency vehicle reasonably and prudently
- Duty to provide care and transportation to the expected standard of care
- Duty to provide care and transportation consistent with the EMT-I's scope of practice and local medical protocols
- Duty to continue care and transportation through to appropriate conclusions

Content Review

ELEMENTS OF NEGLIGENCE

- Duty to act
- Breach of that duty
- Actual damages
- Proximate cause

Second, the plaintiff must prove there was a **breach of duty** by the EMT-I. An EMT-I always must exercise the degree of care, skill, and judgment that would be expected under like circumstances by a similarly trained, reasonable EMT-I in the same community. The **standard of care** specific to the EMT-I's practice is generally established by court testimony and referenced to published codes, standards, criteria, and guidelines applicable to the situation. A breach of duty may occur by malfeasance, misfeasance, or nonfeasance:

- *Malfeasance,* or the performance of a wrongful or unlawful act by the EMT-I. For example an EMT-I commits malfeasance if he assaults a patient.

- *Misfeasance,* or the performance of a legal act in a manner that is harmful or injurious. For example, an EMT-I commits misfeasance when he inadvertently intubates a patient's esophagus, fails to confirm tube placement, and leaves the tube in place.

- *Nonfeasance,* or the failure to perform a required act or duty. For example, it would be an act of nonfeasance to fail to fully immobilize a collision patient who is complaining of neck and back pain.

In some cases, negligence may be so obvious that it does not require extensive proof. Unlike criminal cases, which require proof "beyond a reasonable doubt," civil cases require only a proof of guilt by a "preponderance of evidence." In most cases, the burden of proving negligence rests on the plaintiff. As a result, when it is difficult to do so, a plaintiff may sometimes invoke the doctrine of *res ipsa loquitur,* which is Latin for "the thing speaks for itself."

To support a claim of *res ipsa loquitur,* the complainant must prove that the damages would not have occurred in the absence of somebody's negligence, the instruments causing the damages were under the defendant's control at all times, and the patient did nothing to contribute to his own injury. After the doctrine of *res ipsa loquitur* is invoked in court, the burden of proof shifts from the plaintiff to the defendant.

For example, a classic situation in which *res ipsa loquitur* might be used occurs when a patient has an appendectomy and wakes to find that a surgical instrument has been left inside his abdomen. To prove negligence in this case, the plaintiff's attorney would show that the damage would not have occurred without the physician's negligence, that the surgical instrument was under the physician's control at all relevant times, and that the patient did not contribute to the injury. Many cases in which *res ipsa loquitur* would be successful are settled out of court.

Another situation in which little proof is required occurs when the EMT-I violates a statute and injury to a plaintiff results. Some laws state that if a statute is violated and an injury resulted, a person will be guilty of *negligence per se,* or automatic negligence. For example, if an EMT-I, who is driving in non-emergency mode, fails to stop at a red light and hits a pedestrian, the EMT-I's negligence is obvious. He violated vehicle and traffic statutes that prohibit a vehicle from running a red light, and he is therefore guilty of *negligence per se.*

After a duty to act and a breach of that duty have been proven, **actual damages** is the third required element of proof in a negligence claim. That is, the plaintiff must prove that he was actually harmed in a way that can be compensated by the award of damages. This is an essential component. A lawsuit cannot be won if the EMT-I's action caused no ill effects. The plaintiff must prove that he suffered compensable physical, psychological, or financial damage such as medical expenses, lost wages, lost future earnings, conscious pain and suffering, or wrongful death.

In addition, the plaintiff may seek punitive (punishing) damages. These are awarded only when a defendant commits an act of gross negligence or willful and wanton misconduct. An act of ordinary negligence, such as accidentally allowing an IV to infiltrate, will not support an award of punitive damages. If punitive damages are awarded to the plaintiff, most insurance policies will not cover them. Therefore, the EMT-I may become personally liable for any punitive damages awarded to the plaintiff.

Finally, to prove negligence, the plaintiff must show that the EMT-I's action or inaction was the **proximate cause** of the damages; that is, the action or inaction of the EMT-I immediately caused or worsened the damage suffered by the plaintiff. For example, a cardiac

breach of duty an action or inaction that violates the standard of care expected from an EMT-I.

standard of care the degree of care, skill, and judgment that would be expected under like or similar circumstances by a similarly trained, reasonable EMT-I in the same community.

Always exercise the care, skill, and judgment expected under like circumstances by a similarly trained, reasonable EMT-I in the same community.

actual damages refers to compensable physical, psychological, or financial harm.

proximate cause action or inaction of the EMT-I that immediately caused or worsened the damage suffered by the patient.

patient who breaks his arm during an ambulance collision while en route to the hospital will likely be able to prove that his injuries resulted from the incident; that is, the collision was the proximate cause of his injuries. However, a patient with a sprained wrist who happens to suffer a stroke while in the ambulance would have difficulty proving the ambulance ride was the proximate cause of the stroke.

Proximate cause may also be thought of in terms of "foreseeability." To show the existence of proximate cause, the plaintiff needs to prove that the damage to the patient was reasonably foreseeable by the EMT-I. This is usually established by expert testimony. For example, imagine that an EMT-I negligently crashes into a telephone pole with the ambulance. As a result, two people are injured—the patient who was in the back of the ambulance and, two blocks away, a baby who was dropped by his mother when the loud crash startled her. It should be easy for the patient to prove proximate cause, because it was reasonably foreseeable that an ambulance crash could hurt passengers. However, if the woman who dropped her baby sued the EMT-I, she probably would not be able to establish proximate cause. Although the crash was the reason her baby was injured, it was not a foreseeable injury resulting from the ambulance crash.

Defenses to Charges of Negligence

If you are accused of negligence as an EMT-I, you may be able to avoid liability if you can establish a defense to the plaintiff's claim. The following is a list of potential defenses to negligence:

- *Good Samaritan laws.* If the EMT-I can establish that his actions were protected by a Good Samaritan law, liability may be avoided. Note that such laws generally do not protect providers from acts of gross negligence, reckless disregard, or willful or wanton conduct, and they do not prohibit the filing of lawsuits.

- *Governmental immunity.* These laws do not offer much protection for the individual EMT-I accused of negligence. Though governmental immunity laws vary from state to state, the current legal trend is toward limiting this type of protection.

- *Statute of limitations.* This is a law that sets the maximum time period during which certain actions can be brought in court. After the time limit is reached, no legal action can be brought regardless of whether or not a negligent act occurred. Statutes of limitations vary from state to state, so carefully review the laws in your state. Note that they may vary for different negligent acts and for cases involving children.

- *Contributory or comparative negligence.* Some state laws will reduce or eliminate a plaintiff's award of damages if the plaintiff is found to have caused or worsened his own injury. For example, imagine that a patient involved in a car crash complained of neck pain but refused to let the EMT-I properly immobilize his spine. The EMT-I explained the risks of refusing treatment, but the patient signed a "release-from-liability" form anyway. Later, the patient learns that he has permanent spinal-cord damage and sues the EMT-I for negligence. Many courts will find that the EMT-I was not negligent because, by refusing necessary treatment, the patient contributed to the exacerbation of his own injury.

To protect yourself against claims of negligence, you should receive appropriate education, training, and continuing education; receive appropriate medical direction, both on-line and off-line; always prepare accurate, thorough documentation; have a professional attitude and demeanor at all times; always act in good faith; and use your own common sense. In addition, it is essential for all EMT-Is to be covered by liability insurance. Although many employers and agencies carry coverage, it is a good idea to obtain your own because your agency's coverage may be inadequate.

SPECIAL LIABILITY CONCERNS

Medical Direction

If an EMT-I makes a mistake in the field and is sued by the injured patient, it is possible that the patient will also sue the EMT-I's medical director and the on-line physician. The on-line physician may be liable to a patient for giving the EMT-I medically incorrect orders or advice, for the refusal to authorize the administration of a medically necessary medication, or for directing an ambulance to take a patient to an inappropriate medical facility.

An EMT-I's medical director may be liable to the patient for the negligent supervision of the EMT-I. In order for the patient to be successful in this type of claim, he would have to prove that the physician breached a duty to supervise the EMT-I and that breach was the proximate cause of the patient's injuries. Examples include: the medical director's failure to establish medication protocols or standing orders consistent with the current standards of medical practice for the EMT-I to use in the field; the medical director observed and then failed to correct an EMT-I's poor intubation technique; or the medical director received complaints of inappropriate care by an EMT-I and then failed to effectively investigate and resolve the problem.

Borrowed Servant Doctrine

As an EMT-I, you may find yourself in the position of supervising other emergency care providers, such as EMT-Bs or EMT-Is. When doing so, it will be your responsibility to make sure they perform their duties in a professional and medically appropriate manner. Depending on the degree of supervision and the amount of control you have, you may be liable for any negligent act they commit. This is called the "borrowed servant" doctrine. For it to apply, the EMT-I accused of negligence must have taken the employees of another employer under his control and exercised supervisory powers over them.

Civil Rights

In addition to suing you for negligence, a patient may be able to sue you under certain circumstances for violating his civil rights if you fail to render care for a discriminatory reason. As an EMT-I, you may not withhold medical care for reasons such as race, creed, color, gender, national origin, or in some cases, ability to pay. Also, all patients should be provided with appropriate care regardless of their status, condition, or disease (including AIDS/HIV, tuberculosis, and other communicable diseases).

Off-Duty EMT-Intermediates

Liability also may arise in a situation in which an off-duty EMT-I renders assistance at the scene of an illness or injury. Generally, any person who provides basic emergency first aid to another person would be protected from liability under a Good Samaritan law. However, when the off-duty EMT-I provides advanced life support, a problem may arise. In most states, EMT-Is cannot practice advanced skills unless they are practicing within an EMS system. To perform EMT-I skills and procedures that require delegation from a physician while off-duty may constitute the crime of practicing medicine without a license. Learn the law in your jurisdiction.

EMT-INTERMEDIATE AND PATIENT RELATIONSHIPS

The relationship you establish with your patient is a very important one. Not only must you provide the best medical care, you also have legal and ethical duties to protect the patient's privacy and treat him with honesty, respect, and compassion.

CONFIDENTIALITY

All records related to the emergency care rendered to a patient must be kept strictly confidential. Keeping patient **confidentiality** means that any medical or personal information

confidentiality the principle of law that prohibits the release of medical or other personal information about a patient without the patient's consent.

about a patient—including medical history, assessment findings, and treatment—will not be released to a third party without the express permission of the patient or legal guardian. However, there are specific circumstances under which a patient's confidential information may be released:

- *Patient consents to the release of his records.* A patient may request a copy of his medical records for any reason. If the patient is a child, consent for release of medical records must be obtained from the child's parent or other legal guardian. The request should be accepted only if it is in writing, specifically authorizes the agency to release the records, and contains the patient's signature (or other authorized signature). If the request so directs, it is permissible to forward the records to the patient's physician, insurance company, attorney, or any other party the patient specifies. Be sure your agency retains a copy of the consent document.

- *Other medical care providers have a need to know.* For example, it is not a breach of patient confidentiality to discuss the patient's condition with on-line medical direction or to give a patient report to an emergency department nurse upon arrival at the hospital. This is permitted because it allows medical care appropriate for the patient to be continued. It is not acceptable, however, to discuss confidential patient information with medical providers who have no responsibility for the patient's care.

- *EMS is required by law to release a patient's medical records.* Records may be requested by a court order that is signed by a judge, or they may be requested by subpoena (a command to appear at a certain time and place to give testimony). When an agency receives a court order or subpoena, it is good practice to consult with an attorney to make sure the order is valid and for assistance with compliance. Failure to comply with a court order or subpoena may result in severe penalties.

- *There are third-party billing requirements.* For EMS agencies that bill patients for services, it is generally necessary to release certain confidential information to receive reimbursement from private insurance companies, Medicaid, or Medicare. If possible, the agency should obtain patient authorization for this purpose.

The law provides penalties for the breach of confidentiality. The improper release of information may result in a lawsuit against the EMT-I for defamation (libel or slander), breach of confidentiality, or invasion of privacy. If found guilty, the EMT-I may be responsible for paying money damages to the patient.

Health Insurance Portability and Accountability Act (HIPAA)

The Health Insurance Portability and Accountability Act of 1996 (HIPAA) changed the methods EMS providers use to file for insurance and Medicare payments. It also adds important new layers of privacy protection for EMS patients. The privacy protections provide, among other things, that all EMS employees be trained in HIPAA compliance. Furthermore, EMS providers must develop administrative, electronic, and physical barriers to unauthorized disclosure of patients' protected health information. Disclosures of information—except for purposes of treatment, obtaining payment for services, health care operations, and disclosures mandated or permitted by law—must be preauthorized in writing. HIPAA requires providers to post notices in prominent places advising patients of their privacy rights and provides both civil and serious criminal penalties for violations of privacy.

Patients are given the right to inspect and copy their health records, restrict use and disclosure of their individually identifiable health information, amend their health records, require a provider to communicate with them confidentially, and account for disclosures of their protected health information except for treatment, payment, health care operations, and legally required reporting purposes. The requirements of HIPAA are detailed and every EMS provider must become familiar with them.

Legal Notes

HIPAA significantly enhances the confidentiality of medical records and mandates that EMS personnel be educated as to the requirements of the law.

Legal Notes

HIPAA also provides methods to assure that EMS personnel who have been exposed to a communicable disease are notified in a timely fashion.

DEFAMATION

Defamation occurs when a person makes an intentional false communication that injures another person's reputation or good name. A patient may sue an EMT-I for defamation if the EMT-I communicates an untrue statement about a patient's character or reputation without legal privilege or consent. Defamation can occur in written form or through verbal statements.

Libel is the act of injuring a person's character, name, or reputation by false statements made in writing or through the mass media with malicious intent or reckless disregard for the falsity of those statements. Allegations of libel can be avoided by completing an accurate, professional, and confidential patient care report. Do not use slang and value-loaded words or phrases in your report (for example, do not refer to a patient as "stupid" or use any derogatory race-based terms). Since many states consider the patient care report part of the public record, never write anything on it that could be considered libelous.

Slander is the act of injuring a person's character, name, or reputation by false or malicious statements spoken with malicious intent or reckless disregard for the falsity of those statements. An allegation of slander can be avoided by limiting oral reporting of a patient's condition to appropriate personnel only. Note that many EMS systems record ambulance-hospital radio transmissions, and scanners, which give the public access to EMS transmissions, are common in the United States. Therefore, information transmitted over the radio should be limited to essential matters of patient care. In most cases, the patient's name and insurance status should not be transmitted over the radio.

defamation an intentional false communication that injures another person's reputation or good name.

libel the act of injuring a person's character, name, or reputation by false statements made in writing or through the mass media with malicious intent or reckless disregard for the falsity of those statements.

slander the act of injuring a person's character, name, or reputation by false or malicious statements spoken with malicious intent or reckless disregard for the falsity of those statements.

INVASION OF PRIVACY

An EMT-I may be accused of invasion of privacy for the release of confidential information, without legal justification, regarding a patient's private life, which might reasonably expose the patient to ridicule, notoriety, or embarrassment. That includes, for example, the release of information regarding HIV status or other sensitive medical information. The fact that released information is true is not a defense to an action for invasion of privacy.

CONSENT

By law, you must get a patient's consent before you can provide medical care or transport. **Consent** is the granting of permission to treat. More accurately, it is the granting of permission to touch. It is based on the concept that every adult human being of sound mind has the right to determine what should be done with his own body. Touching a patient without appropriate consent may subject you to charges of assault and battery.

A patient must be **competent** in order to give or withhold consent. A competent adult is one who is lucid and able to make an informed decision about medical care. He understands your questions and recommendations, and he understands the implications of his decisions made about medical care. Although there is no absolute test for determining competency, keep the following factors in mind when making a determination: the patient's mental status, the patient's ability to respond to questions, statements regarding the patient's competency from family or friends, evidence of impairment from drugs or alcohol, or indications of shock.

consent the patient's granting of permission for treatment.

> *By law, you must get a patient's consent before you provide medical care or transportation.*
>

competent able to make an informed decision about medical care.

Informed Consent

Conscious, competent patients have the right to decide what medical care to accept. However, for consent to be legally valid, it must be **informed consent,** or consent given based on full disclosure of information. That is, a patient must understand the nature, risks, and benefits of any procedures to be performed. So, before providing medical care, you must explain the following to the patient in a manner he can understand:

- Nature of the illness or injury
- Nature of the recommended treatments
- Risks, dangers, and benefits of those treatments

informed consent consent for treatment that is given based on full disclosure of information.

- Alternative treatment possibilities, if any, and the related risks, dangers, and benefits of accepting each one
- Dangers of refusing treatment, including transport

Informed consent must be obtained from every competent adult before treatment may be initiated. Conscious, competent patients may revoke consent at any time during care and transport. In most states, a patient must be eighteen years of age or older in order to give or withhold consent. Generally, a child's parent or legal guardian must give informed consent before treatment of the child can begin.

Expressed, Implied, and Involuntary Consent

Three more types of consent are expressed, implied, and involuntary. **Expressed consent** is the most common. It occurs when a person directly grants permission to treat—verbally, non-verbally, or in writing. Often, the act of a patient requesting an ambulance is considered an expression of a desire to be treated. However, just because the patient consents to a ride to the hospital does not mean he has consented to all types of treatment (such as the initiation of an IV and/or the administration of medications). You must obtain consent for each treatment you plan to provide. Consent from the patient does not always need to be granted verbally. It may be expressed by allowing care to be rendered.

Unconscious patients cannot grant consent. When treating them or any patient who requires emergency intervention but is mentally, physically, or emotionally unable to grant consent, treatment depends on **implied consent** (sometimes called "emergency doctrine"). That is, it is assumed that the patient would want life-saving treatment if he were able to give informed consent. Implied consent is effective only until the patient no longer requires emergency care or until the patient regains competence.

Occasionally, a court will order patients to undergo treatment, even though they may not want it. This is called **involuntary consent.** It is most commonly encountered with patients who must be held for mental-health evaluation or as directed by law enforcement personnel who have the patient under arrest. It also is used on occasion to force patients to undergo treatment for a disease that threatens the community at large (tuberculosis, for example). Law-enforcement personnel often will accompany patients who are undergoing court-ordered treatment.

Consent issues also can arise when an EMT-I is called by law-enforcement officials to treat a sick or injured prisoner or arrestee. The officers may tell you that they have the legal authority to give consent to treatment for the patient simply because the patient is in police custody. However, a competent adult in police custody does not necessarily lose the right to make medical decisions for himself. In fact, many prisoners have successfully sued health-care providers for rendering treatment without consent. Generally, forced treatment is limited to emergency treatment necessary to save life or limb or treatment ordered by the court. Be sure that you are familiar with your local protocols and laws on this issue.

Special Consent Situations

In the case of a **minor** (depending on state law, this is usually a person under the age of 18), consent should be obtained from a parent, legal guardian, or court-appointed custodian. The same is true of a mentally incompetent adult. If a responsible person cannot be located, and if the child or mentally incompetent adult is suffering from an apparent life-threatening injury or illness, treatment may be rendered under the doctrine of implied consent.

Generally, an **emancipated minor** is considered an adult. This is a person under 18 years of age who is married, pregnant, a parent, a member of the armed forces, or financially independent and living away from home. As an adult, an emancipated minor may legally give informed consent. Anyone else under the age of 18 may not grant informed consent.

Withdrawal of Consent

A competent adult may withdraw consent for any treatment at any time. However, refusal must be informed. That is, the patient must understand the risks of not continuing treat-

expressed consent verbal, nonverbal, or written communication by a patient that he wishes to receive medical care.

implied consent consent for treatment that is presumed for a patient who is mentally, physically, or emotionally unable to grant consent. Also called *emergency doctrine.*

involuntary consent consent to treatment granted by the authority of a court order.

minor depending on state law, this is usually a person under the age of 18.

emancipated minor a person under 18 years of age who is married, pregnant, a parent, a member of the armed forces, or financially independent and living away from home.

REFUSAL OF TREATMENT AND TRANSPORTATION

I, THE UNDERSIGNED HAVE BEEN ADVISED THAT MEDICAL ASSISTANCE ON MY BEHALF IS NECESSARY AND THAT REFUSAL OF SAID ASSISTANCE AND TRANSPORTATION MAY RESULT IN DEATH, OR IMPERIL MY HEALTH. NEVERTHELESS, I REFUSE TO ACCEPT TREATMENT OR TRANSPORT AND ASSUME ALL RISKS AND CONSEQUENCES OF MY DECISION AND RELEASE GOLD CROSS AMBULANCE COMPANY AND ITS EMPLOYEES FROM ANY LIABILITY ARISING FROM MY REFUSAL.

____
SIGNATURE OF PATIENT

____
WITNESSED BY

____
DATE SIGNED

FIGURE 1-15 Example of a release-from-liability form.

ment or transport to the hospital in terms he can fully understand. A common example of a patient withdrawing consent occurs after a hypoglycemic patient regains full consciousness with the administration of dextrose. The patient should be encouraged—but may not be forced—to go to the emergency department. If he is competent, the patient may refuse transport. In such cases, advanced life support measures, such as IV fluids, which were initiated when the patient was unconscious, should be discontinued. The patient also should complete a release-from-liability form (Figure 1-15).

Sometimes patients choose to accept one recommended treatment, but refuse others. For example, a patient involved in a motor-vehicle crash may refuse to be fully immobilized but ask to be transported to the hospital. It is very important for you to do everything in your power to be sure he understands why spinal precautions are necessary and what may happen if they are not taken. If a competent adult continues to refuse care, be sure to thoroughly document his reason for refusal and your attempts to convince him to change his mind. Have the patient and a witness sign a release-from-liability form.

Refusal of Service

Not every EMS run results in the transportation of a patient to a hospital. Emergency care should always be offered to a patient, no matter how minor the injury or illness may be. However, often, the patient will refuse. If this occurs, you must:

- Be sure that the patient is legally permitted to refuse care; that is, the patient must be a competent adult.
- Make multiple and sincere attempts to convince the patient to accept care.
- Enlist the help of others, such as the patient's family or friends, to convince the patient to accept care.
- Make certain that the patient is fully informed about the implications of his decision and the potential risks of refusing care.
- Consult with on-line medical direction.
- Have the patient and a disinterested witness, such as a police officer, sign a release-from-liability form.
- Advise the patient that he may call you again for help if necessary.
- Attempt to get the patient's family or friends to stay with the patient.
- Document the entire situation thoroughly and accurately on your patient care report.

Remember, the refusal of care must be informed. That is, the patient must be told of and understand all possible risks of refusal. Decisions not to transport should involve medical

Refusal of care by a patient must be informed and properly documented.

Cultural Considerations

Religious and cultural beliefs impact a patient's health-care decisions. Some patients, such as Christian Scientists, prefer to use prayer instead of traditional health care and may refuse treatment on religious grounds. Likewise, Jehovah's Witnesses believe that blood transfusions are prohibited by biblical teachings.

direction. It is a good idea to put the patient directly on the phone with the on-line physician. If all efforts fail, be sure to thoroughly document the reasons for refusal and your efforts to change the patient's mind. If an on-line physician was involved, it is a good idea to obtain his signature on your patient care report.

Problem Patients

As an EMT-I, you will occasionally encounter a "problem patient," one who is violent, a victim of a drug overdose, an intoxicated adult or minor, or an ill or injured minor with no adult available to provide consent for medical treatment. Such a patient can present you with a medical–legal dilemma. For example, consider the patient who has allegedly taken an overdose of medication. Concerned family members may panic and activate the EMS system. However, upon your arrival at the scene, you find the patient alert, oriented, denying that he has taken any medication, and refusing to give consent for treatment or transport.

In a case such as this, attempt to develop trust and some rapport with the patient. If he continues to refuse, and remains alert and oriented, a refusal form should be completed and witnessed by a police officer. If the patient will not sign the form, have a police officer or family member sign it, indicating that the patient verbally refused care. If, however, the situation becomes dangerous, or you have reason to suspect the patient has tried to injure himself, police officers or family members should consider legal measures to force the patient to receive treatment.

The intoxicated person who refuses treatment and transport also poses a problem for the EMT-I. Every effort should be made to encourage the patient to accept care and transport to the hospital. If the patient refuses, explain to him in a calm and detailed manner the implications of refusal. However, if you determine that the patient cannot understand the nature of his illness or the consequences of his refusal, then he may not refuse treatment because he is not competent to do so. Involve law enforcement at this point. If the patient is competent to make such a decision, then have him sign a refusal form. Your conversation with the patient and his refusal should be witnessed by an impartial third party such as a police officer.

Regardless of the type of problem patient, always document the encounter in detail. Your records should include a description of the patient, the results of any physical examination (or reasons for the lack of one), important statements made by the patient and other persons at the scene, and the names and addresses of any witnesses. If you are going to include an important statement from the patient or witnesses in your patient care report, put the exact statement in quotation marks.

Ideally, a police officer should respond to the scene of all problem patients and should either sign the patient care report as a witness or, if the EMT-I's safety is at risk, accompany the patient and EMT-I to the emergency department.

LEGAL COMPLICATIONS RELATED TO CONSENT

There are many legal complications related to consent to treatment. If the EMT-I does not obtain the proper consent to treat or fails to continue appropriate treatment, he may be liable for damages based on a tort cause of action, such as abandonment, assault, battery, or false imprisonment.

Abandonment

Abandonment is the termination of the EMT-I-patient relationship without providing for the appropriate continuation of care while it is still needed and desired by the patient. You cannot initiate patient care and then discontinue it without sufficient reason. You cannot turn the care of a patient over to personnel who have less training than you without creating potential liability for an abandonment action. For example, an EMT-I who has initiated advanced life support should not turn the patient over to an EMT-Basic or a First Responder for transport.

Abandonment can occur at any point during patient contact, including in the field or in the hospital emergency department. Physically leaving a patient unattended, even for a short time, may also be grounds for a charge of abandonment. If, for example, you leave a patient at a hospital without properly turning over his care to a physician or nurse, you may be liable for abandonment. It is always a good idea to have the nurse or physician to whom you have passed responsibility for patient care sign your patient care report.

Assault and Battery

Failure to obtain appropriate consent before treatment could leave the EMT-I open to allegations of assault and battery. **Assault** is defined as unlawfully placing a person in apprehension of immediate bodily harm without his consent. For example, your patient states that he is scared of needles and refuses to let you start an IV. If you then show him an IV catheter and bring it toward his arm as if to start an IV, you may be liable for assault.

Battery is the unlawful touching of another individual without his consent. It would be battery to actually start an IV on a patient who does not consent to such treatment. An EMT-I can be sued for assault and battery in both criminal and civil contexts.

False Imprisonment

False imprisonment may be charged by a patient who is transported without consent or who is restrained without proper justification or authority. It is defined as intentional and unjustifiable detention of a person without his consent or other legal authority, and may result in civil or criminal liability. Like assault and battery, a charge of false imprisonment can be avoided by obtaining appropriate consent.

This is a particular problem with psychiatric patients. In most cases, you can avoid allegations of false imprisonment by having a law enforcement officer apprehend the patient and accompany you to the hospital. If no officer is available, you should attempt to consult with medical direction and carefully judge the risks of false imprisonment against the benefits of detaining and treating the patient. You should determine whether medical treatment is immediately necessary and whether the patient poses a threat to himself or to the public when you are making your decision to treat or transport.

Reasonable Force

If it is safe to do so, you may use a reasonable amount of force to control an unruly or violent patient. The definition of **reasonable force** depends on the amount of force necessary to ensure that the patient does not cause injury to himself, you, or others. Excessive force can result in liability for the EMT-I. Force used as punishment will be considered assault and battery for which the patient may be able to recover damages and the EMT-I may face criminal charges. When you believe it is necessary to use force, involve law enforcement if possible.

The use of restraints may be indicated for a combative patient. Restraints must conform to your local protocols. Restraining devices typically used by EMS providers include straps, jackets, and restraining blankets. In this circumstance, an EMS team's goal is to use the least amount of force necessary to safely control the patient while causing him the least amount of discomfort. If the use of restraints is indicated, involve law enforcement officials.

PATIENT TRANSPORTATION

The transportation of patients to a health-care facility is an integral part of the patient-care continuum. During transportation to a health-care facility, be sure to maintain the same level of care as was initiated at the scene. This means that if you, as an EMT-I, initiate advanced emergency care procedures, you must either ride with the patient to the hospital or ensure that another EMT-I will accompany the patient. If you fail to do so, and the patient is harmed as a result, you may be liable for abandonment.

One of the greatest areas of potential liability for EMT-Is is emergency vehicle operations. It is essential that you become familiar with your state and local laws. The laws that provide exceptions from driving rules and regulations may allow you, for example, to drive at a rate of speed in excess of a posted speed limit; but if you are negligent at any time during the operation of your vehicle, you will not be protected from liability.

Another issue that will arise is patient choice of destination. If you work in a small area with only one hospital, you are not likely to encounter difficulties. However, many EMT-Is work in areas that have many hospitals and medical centers to choose from. Over the past

assault an act that unlawfully places a person in apprehension of immediate bodily harm without his consent.

battery the unlawful touching of another individual without his consent.

false imprisonment international and unjustifiable detention of a person without his consent or other legal authority.

reasonable force the minimal amount of force necessary to ensure that an unruly or violent person does not cause injury to himself or others.

Legal Notes

Patient restraint has become a particularly thorny legal issue for EMS personnel. Because physical restraint has been associated with significant problems, all EMS systems must have detailed protocols and standing orders that deal with it specifically.

Be sure to maintain the proper level of care during transport of a patient to a health-care facility.

few years, increasing numbers of lawsuits involving facility selection have been brought by patients. Some have sued EMT-Is themselves, claiming negligence based on the failure to transport to the nearest or most appropriate hospital.

An additional issue you may need to address involves the patient's insurance company protocols. In some situations, it may be appropriate to respect a patient's choice of facility based on his insurance company's facility-choice protocols. Local restrictions by insurance companies and health-care maintenance organizations may determine under what conditions and to what facilities patient transport may be authorized and paid for. Although most areas are not yet being confronted with restrictions on service provision, it may be only a matter of time. However, never put patient care in jeopardy by transporting to a less appropriate facility because of insurance concerns.

In general, facility selection should be based on patient request, patient need, and facility capability. Local written protocols, the EMT-I, on-line medical direction, and the patient should all play a role in facility selection. The patient's preference, however, should be honored unless the situation or the patient's condition dictates otherwise.

RESUSCITATION ISSUES

Advances in medical technology have saved and prolonged thousands of lives. However, in some instances, the use of sophisticated medical technology may only prolong pain, suffering, and death. When a person is seriously injured or gravely ill, family members must make difficult decisions regarding the medical care to be provided, including the use or withdrawal of life-support systems.

Generally, you are under obligation to begin resuscitative efforts when summoned to the scene of a patient who is unresponsive, pulseless, and apneic (not breathing). There are times, however, when you will determine that resuscitation is not indicated. This occurs with patients who have a valid Do Not Resuscitate (DNR) order, with patients who are obviously dead (decapitated, for example), with patients with obvious tissue decomposition or extreme dependent lividity (gravitational pooling of blood in dependent areas of the body), or with a patient who is at a scene that is too hazardous to enter.

Always follow your state laws, local protocols, and medical direction. The role of medical direction should be clearly delineated and included in your agency's protocols. If you are authorized to determine that resuscitative efforts are not indicated, be sure to thoroughly document your decision and the criteria upon which it was based.

ADVANCE DIRECTIVES

To improve communication between patients, their family members, and physicians regarding such matters, the federal government enacted the Patient Self-Determination Act of 1990. This act requires hospitals and physicians to provide patients and their families with sufficient information to make informed decisions about medical treatment and the use of life-support measures, including CPR, artificial ventilation, nutrition, hydration, and blood transfusions.

Patients and their families are therefore more likely than ever to have prepared a written statement of the patient's own preference for future medical care, or an **advance directive.** An advance directive is a document created to ensure that certain treatment choices are honored when a patient is unconscious or otherwise unable to express his choice of treatments. They come in a variety of forms. The most common encountered in the field are living wills, durable powers of attorney for health care, and Do Not Resuscitate (DNR) orders.

The types of advance directives recognized in each state are governed by state law and local protocols. Medical direction must establish and implement policies for dealing with advance directives in the field. Those policies should clearly define the obligations of an EMT-I who is caring for a patient with an advance directive. They should also provide for reasonable measures of comfort to the patient and emotional support to the patient's family and loved ones. Some states do not allow EMT-Is to honor living wills in the field, but do allow them to honor valid Do Not Resuscitate (DNR) orders. Be sure you are familiar with your state law and local policies.

Content Review

ADVANCE DIRECTIVES
- Living wills
- Durable powers of attorney for health care
- DNR orders
- Organ donor cards

advance directive a document created to ensure that certain treatment choices are honored when a patient is unconscious or otherwise unable to express his choice of treatment.

Living Will

A **living will** is a legal document that allows a person to specify the kinds of medical treatment he wishes to receive should the need arise. For example, many states allow patients to include in living wills their wishes concerning dying in a hospital or at home, receiving CPR, and donation of their organs and other body parts. In addition, patients with prolonged illnesses sometimes invoke the right to choose a person who may make health-care decisions for them in the event that their mental functions become impaired. They might formalize this decision by way of a special notation in a living will. (They may also do this through execution of a document called a "Durable Power of Attorney for Health Care" or "Health Care Proxy.") Living wills, once signed and witnessed, are effective until they are revoked by the patient.

Be sure you know your local protocols concerning living wills. If any question arises on scene, contact medical direction for instructions.

Do Not Resuscitate (DNR) Orders

A **Do Not Resuscitate (DNR) order** is a common type of advance directive. Usually signed by the patient and his physician, the DNR order is a legal document that indicates to medical personnel which, if any, life-sustaining measures should be taken when the patient's heart and respiratory functions have ceased. DNR orders generally direct EMS personnel to withhold CPR in the event of a cardiac arrest. When you honor a DNR order, do not simply pack up your equipment and leave the scene. You still may have the patient's family and loved ones to attend to. Provide emotional support as appropriate.

DNR orders pose a particular problem in the field. EMT-Is are often called to nursing homes or residences where they find a patient in cardiac arrest and in need of resuscitation. As a rule, you are legally obligated to attempt resuscitation. If a physician has written a specific order to avoid it, the EMT-Is should not have been summoned. Even so, people tend to panic and will call for help. Valid DNR orders should be honored as your protocols allow. Note, however, that if there is any doubt as to the patient's wishes, resuscitation should be initiated.

Occasionally, you may be requested to treat a patient as a "slow code" or "chemical code only." This is not legally permitted. Cardiac resuscitation is an all-or-nothing proposition. Treating a cardiac arrest with only medications would mean abandoning airway management and defibrillation. To do so, even at the request of the family, amounts to negligence and must be avoided.

Potential Organ Donation

Over the past few years, advances in medicines have led to an increased number of organ transplants. As organs and tissues are in very high demand and short supply, many EMS systems are now becoming a vital link in the organ procurement and transplant process. Some have developed protocols that specifically address organ viability after a patient's death. These include providing circulatory support through IV fluids and CPR and ventilatory support via endotracheal tube. Whether or not your EMS has protocols in place for potential organ donation, it is important for you to consult with on-line medical direction when you have identified a patient as a potential donor.

DEATH IN THE FIELD

Whether you arrive at the scene of a patient who has died before your arrival or you make an authorized decision to terminate resuscitative efforts, a death in the field must be appropriately dealt with and thoroughly documented. Follow state and local protocols and contact medical direction for guidance.

Legal Notes

Some states require that relatives of a recently deceased person be asked about the possibility of organ donation. Become familiar with the laws in your state.

CRIME AND ACCIDENT SCENES

You may be called to treat a patient at a crime scene. You must not sacrifice patient care to preserve evidence or to become involved in detective work. You can best assist investigating officers by properly treating the patient and by doing your best to avoid destroying any potential evidence. As an EMT-I, your responsibilities at a crime scene include the following:

- If you believe a crime may have been committed on scene, immediately contact law enforcement if they are not already involved.
- Protect yourself and the safety of other EMS personnel. This should always be your primary consideration. You will not be held liable for failing to act if a scene is not safe to enter.
- Once a crime scene has been deemed safe, initiate patient contact and medical care.
- Do not move or touch anything at a crime scene unless it is necessary to do so for patient care. Observe and document the original placement of any items moved by your crew. If the patient's clothing has holes made by a gunshot or a stabbing, leave them intact if possible. If the patient has an obvious mortal wound, such as decapitation, try not to touch the body at all. Do your best to protect any potential evidence.
- If you need to remove items from the scene, such as an impaled weapon or bottle of medication, be sure to document your actions and notify investigating officers.

Treat the scene of an accident in the same way. Ensure your own safety and the safety of your crew and treat your patients as medically indicated.

DOCUMENTATION

The treatment of your patient does not end until you have properly documented the entire incident. A complete patient care report is your best protection in a malpractice action. In fact, a well-written report may actually discourage a plaintiff from filing a malpractice case in the first place. In general, a plaintiff's attorney will request copies of all medical records, including the EMT-I's report, before filing a lawsuit. If the EMT-I's report is sloppy, incomplete, or otherwise not well written, this may encourage the plaintiff to sue.

A well-documented patient care report has the following characteristics:

- *It is completed promptly after patient contact.* It should be made in the course of business, not long after the event. Any delay could cause you to forget important observations or treatments. If possible, a copy of the completed report should be left with the emergency department staff before you leave the hospital. This copy will become part of the patient's permanent medical records. Note: never delay patient care to attend to a patient care report.
- *It is thorough.* The main purpose is not simply to record patient data, it also is meant to support the diagnosis and treatment that you provided to the patient. All actions, procedures, and administered medications should be documented. Remember: "If you didn't write it down, you didn't do it."
- *It is objective.* Avoid the use of emotional and value-loaded words. They are irrelevant and also may be the cause of a libel suit.
- *It is accurate.* Be precise, avoiding abbreviations and jargon that are not commonly understood. Try to limit your report to information that you have personally seen or heard. If you document something that you do not have personal knowledge of, indicate the source of your information. Document your observations, not your assumptions, and do not draw a medical conclusion that you are not competent to make. For example, you cannot conclusively diagnose a patient as having pneumonia. You can, however, report your suspicion of pneumonia and document consistent findings.

- *It maintains patient confidentiality.* Follow your agency's policies regarding the release of patient information. Whenever possible, patient consent should be obtained before release of information.

Intentional alteration of a medical record amounts to an admission of guilt by the EMT-I. If a patient care report is found to be incomplete or inaccurate, a written amendment should be attached with the date and time the amendment was written, not the date of the original report. Send a copy of the addendum to the receiving hospital to become a part of the patient's medical records. Medical records need to be maintained for a period prescribed by state law. Become familiar with the record retention requirements in your state.

It is in your best interest to learn and follow all state laws and local protocols related to your practice as an EMT-I. Also be sure to receive good training and keep current by pursuing continuing education, reading industry journals, and obtaining recertification or relicensure as required by state law. Always act in good faith and use your common sense. High-quality patient care and high-quality documentation are always your best protection from liability.

Part 7: Ethics in Advanced Prehospital Care

When asked what the most difficult part of the job is, most EMT-Is do not say "ethics." Nonetheless, a significant percentage of advanced life support calls do pose possible ethical conflicts, such as calls involving choice of hospital destination, a patient refusing emergency care, or advance directives. So, whether or not you are consciously thinking about ethics, you are almost certain to be called upon to decide what is the ethical thing to do from time to time in the course of your work.

OVERVIEW OF ETHICS

Ethics and morals are closely related concepts. Morals are generally considered to be social, religious, or personal standards of right and wrong. **Ethics** more often refers to the rules or standards that govern the conduct of members of a particular group or profession. Both ethics and morals address a question Socrates asked: "How should one live?"

ethics the rules or standards that govern the conduct of members of a particular group or profession.

RELATIONSHIP OF ETHICS TO LAW AND RELIGION

Ethics and the law have a great deal in common, but they are distinct. In general, laws have a much narrower focus. Laws frequently describe what is wrong in the eyes of society. Ethics goes beyond what is wrong and examines what is right, or good. As a result, the law frequently has little or nothing to say about ethical problems. In fact, laws themselves can be unethical (such as the laws that once perpetuated racial segregation). Even though ethics and the law are different, ethical discussions can sometimes benefit from techniques developed in the law. In particular, the law emphasizes impartiality, consistency, and methods to identify and balance conflicting interests.

Just as ethics differs from the law, it also differs from religion. In a pluralistic society such as ours, ethics must be understood by and apply to people who hold a broad range of religious beliefs or no religious beliefs at all. Thus ethics cannot derive from a single religion. It is true, however, that religion can enhance and enrich one's ethical principles and values.

MAKING ETHICAL DECISIONS

There are many approaches to determining how a medical professional should behave. One approach is to say that each person must decide how to behave and whatever decision that person makes is okay. This is known as *ethical relativism*. However, people typically do not find ethical relativism satisfactory. For example, no reasonable person would say that it was acceptable for the Nazis to behave as they did. A similar approach is to say, "Just do what is right." This sounds fine, but different people have different beliefs about what is "right." Even the Golden Rule—"Do unto others as you would have them do unto you"—is not a sufficient guideline. What happens when the care provider's desires and values differ from the patient's? It becomes clear that reason and logic must be used and emotion must be excluded as much as possible from the decision-making process.

> *Reason must be used and emotion must be excluded as much as possible from the decision-making process.*
>

CODES OF ETHICS

Over the years, a number of organizations have drafted codes of ethics for the members of their organizations. The American Medical Association has a code of ethics for physicians. The American College of Emergency Physicians has a code of ethics specifically for emergency physicians. The American Nurses Association and Emergency Nurses Association both have codes for practitioners in their fields. In 1948, the World Medical Association adopted the "Oath of Geneva." The National Association of EMTs adopted a code of ethics for EMTs in 1978.

Most codes of ethics address broad humanitarian concerns and professional etiquette. Few provide solid guidance on the kind of ethical problems commonly faced by practitioners. For example, an EMT-I is expected to work in an uncontrolled environment that is sometimes dangerous. A person who is unwilling to enter a scene until every risk has been totally eliminated is not acting in accordance with the expectations of the profession. Conversely, an EMT-I is expected to refrain from entering a hazardous area until the risks have been made manageable. Common sense should help in resolving conflicts such as these.

THE FUNDAMENTAL QUESTIONS

The single most important question an EMT-I has to answer when faced with an ethical challenge is "What is in the patient's best interest?" Usually the answer is obvious, but not always. For example, what is in the best interest of a terminally ill patient who goes into cardiac arrest—to resuscitate, or not to start resuscitation in order to prevent further suffering?

An EMT-I must be very cautious in accepting a family's description of what a patient desires. The family is often under a great deal of stress when the EMT-I encounters them. The EMT-I must also realize that the family may not agree with the patient's desires. They may be led to substitute their own desires for the patient's.

> *The single most important question an EMT-I has to answer when faced with an ethical challenge is, "What is in the patient's best interest?"*
>

Under ideal circumstances, a written statement describing the patient's desires will be available. In many states, such a statement (which meets other specified state and local requirements) is required by law before an EMT-I may elect not to start resuscitation efforts. In less extreme circumstances, the patient may state verbally what he wishes you to do and not do. It may sometimes be difficult for an EMT-I to agree or to comply with a patient's wishes, but as long as the patient is competent and the desires are consistent with good practice, the EMT-I is obligated to respect the patient's wishes.

FUNDAMENTAL PRINCIPLES

A common approach to resolving problems in **bioethics** today is to employ four fundamental principles or values. These principles are beneficence, nonmaleficence, autonomy, and justice:

- **Beneficence** is related to a more familiar term, *benevolence*. Both come from Latin and concern doing good. However, benevolence means the desire to do good (usually the main reason people become EMT-Is), whereas *beneficence* means actually doing good (the EMT-I's obligation to the patient).

- **Nonmaleficence** means not doing harm. (*Maleficence* means doing harm, the opposite of *beneficence*.) Few medical interventions are without risk of harm. Under the principle of nonmaleficence, however, the EMT-I is obligated to minimize that risk as much as possible. This includes, for example, making the scene safe and protecting the patient from impaired or unqualified health-care providers. The Latin phrase, *primum non nocere,* which means "first, do no harm," sums up nonmaleficence very well.

- **Autonomy** refers to a competent adult patient's right to determine what happens to his own body, including treatment for medical illnesses and injuries. Under ordinary conditions, a patient must give consent before the EMT-I can begin treatment. There are, of course, exceptions to this (see the discussion of consent in this chapter), but the implication is that the EMT-I must be truthful in describing to the patient his condition and the risks and benefits of treatment. It also implies respect for the patient's privacy.

- **Justice** refers to the EMT-I's obligation to treat all patients fairly, without regard to sex, race, ability to pay, or cultural background, among other conditions.

RESOLVING ETHICAL CONFLICTS

The EMT-I needs to have a system for resolving ethical conflicts. One such method of resolving ethical issues is illustrated in the following scenario:

You represent your service at the regional EMS coordinating agency. The head nurse for the emergency department (ED) of a large hospital mentions how recent cutbacks in support staff have led to difficulty retrieving patients' medical records in a timely manner. This has led to a number of difficulties in treating patients. As a result, the ED was considering asking incoming ambulances to give patients' names and dates of birth on the radio. This would give the ED staff additional time to search for the patient's medical records.

You consider the issue's ethical aspects. First, you identify the problem: Is it justifiable to breach patient confidentiality in order to expedite the retrieval of medical records? Second, you list the possible actions that might be taken in this situation: provide all patients' names and dates of birth on the radio; continue, as now, to identify patients only by age and sex; or provide selected patients' names and dates of birth on the radio.

To reason out an ethical problem, first state the action in a universal form. Then list the implications or consequences of the action. Finally, compare them to relevant values, as follows:

1. *State the action in a universal form.* Describe what should be done, who should do it, and under what conditions. For example, EMS (who) will

bioethics ethics as applied to the human body.

beneficence the principle of doing good for the patient.

nonmaleficence the obligation not to harm the patient.

autonomy a competent adult patient's right to determine what happens to his own body.

First, do no harm.

justice the obligation to treat all patients fairly.

Content Review

SOLVING AN ETHICAL PROBLEM

1. State the action in a universal form.
2. List the implications or consequences of the action.
3. Compare them to relevant values.

volunteer names and dates of birth for all patients (what) on the radio (condition).

2. *List the implications, or consequences, of the action.* Positive consequences: The ED will be able to get records sooner for patients who have records at that hospital. There will be no change for most patients because hospital records are often irrelevant to emergency care. The ED admitting staff may be able to admit patients more quickly. Negative consequences: Patients' names and dates of birth will be broadcast to thousands of people listening with scanners. Long term, people with scanners will learn more about patients who go to the hospital via EMS. Because private information may be broadcast, patients may become reluctant to call EMS. Conceivably, there may be more burglaries at homes of patients who use EMS.

3. *Compare the consequences to relevant values.* A list of values that pertain to this case might include beneficence, nonmaleficence, autonomy, and confidentiality. That is, if EMS provided names and dates of birth for all patients on the radio, what would be the benefit to the patient (beneficence)? A few patients might be cared for sooner because their records arrived sooner. Most patients will see no benefit because they have no records at that hospital or time is not a significant issue (such as for a laceration that requires sutures). Autonomy suffers under this arrangement because the patient is not given the opportunity to consent (or decline). The patient's name and date of birth go out over the air without his permission. And, in this case, nonmaleficence and confidentiality are intertwined. There is potential for harm to the patient and to future patients who lose faith in the EMS system's ability to maintain privacy.

Since the possible consequences of providing all patients' names and dates of birth on the radio are not compatible with the values we consider important and relevant, you must go back and test another action using this same method.

What about the second option—simply to continue the current policy of identifying all patients over the radio only by age and sex? The consequences might be that people listening to scanners can learn about patients EMS is transporting but not their identities, and a few patients may get delayed care because their records do not arrive quickly enough. A comparison with relevant values reveals that patient confidentiality and patient confidence in EMS are unchanged, but the patients who might benefit from earlier arrival of their records may be suffering.

What about the third option—to provide names and dates of birth of selected patients, such as severely injured patients whose treatment must not be delayed? A comparison with relevant values shows that there is potential benefit for selected patients, a breach of confidentiality for those patients, but no breach of confidentiality for any other patients. So, the scenario may conclude as follows:

The third option sounds closer to being acceptable, but you wonder if there is a way to further limit loss of confidentiality. You suggest revising the rule to read, "EMS broadcasts the names and dates of birth of selected patients who (1) *meet predetermined criteria* (2) *when there is no other private means of communication available.*" This strictly limits the loss of confidentiality to patients who may benefit from it and encourages both EMS and the ED to find other less public means of identifying patients. For example, having someone at the scene telephone the ED to relay the patient's name and date of birth privately.

The method described above is useful when you come upon a new ethical problem and time is not an issue. In situations where time is limited, an abbreviated method can sometimes be used. First, ask yourself whether the current problem is similar to other problems for which you have already formulated a rule. If the answer is yes, follow that rule. If the answer is no, analyze the potential action against three tests suggested by Iserson: the impartiality test, the universalizability test, and the interpersonal justifiability test:

Content Review

QUICK WAYS TO TEST ETHICS
- Impartiality test
- Universalizability test
- Interpersonal justifiability test

- *Impartiality test*—asks whether you would be willing to undergo this procedure or action if you were in the patient's place. This is really a version of the Golden Rule (Do unto others as you would have them do unto you), which helps to reduce the possibility of bias.
- *Universalizability test*—asks whether you would want this action performed in all relevantly similar circumstances, which helps the EMT-I to avoid shortsightedness.
- *Interpersonal justifiability test*—asks whether you can defend or justify your actions to others. It helps to ensure that an action is appropriate by asking the EMT-I to consider whether other people would think the action reasonable.

When there is little time to consider a new ethical problem, these three questions can help an EMT-I navigate murky waters, allowing him to find an acceptable solution in a short time.

ETHICAL ISSUES IN CONTEMPORARY EMT-INTERMEDIATE PRACTICE

The preceding discussion described principles and methods for dealing with ethical issues. The following discussion is meant to help you apply those principles to several commonly encountered situations as well as some less common situations you may face.

ETHICS AND RESUSCITATION
Consider the following scenario:

You are leaving the emergency department in your ambulance when a woman jumps out of a window of the hospital and lands on the road in front of you. Your partner stops the vehicle, and you grab your kit. As you reach the patient, a breathless aide runs out the door and says, "Don't do anything! She's got a DNR order!" How does this affect the care you administer? Your instincts say, treat her now and let the hospital sort things out later if she survives.

In this case, your instincts are probably steering you in the right direction for a number of reasons. First, state law requires that you see the order and verify its legitimacy in some manner. In this case, the order is not available for you to see so you are under no legal obligation to withhold care.

Second, if the patient is alive (as she appears to be), even a valid DNR order would not prevent you from assessing the patient and administering basic care, including comfort care.

Third, the principle of nonmaleficence says do no harm. Refraining from helping her might cause irreversible harm, perhaps death. The principle of beneficence also urges you to help the patient. The potential conflict arises when you consider autonomy. The competent patient of legal age has a right to determine what happens to her body, but you are unable to verify her wishes regarding resuscitation.

The conclusion of the scenario is as follows:

You and your partner go ahead and assess the patient. She responds to verbal stimuli by moaning, her airway is open, ventilations are adequate, and she has several lacerations and apparent fractures. Since you are literally in front of the hospital, you limit your interventions to quick immobilization on a spine board with bleeding control and oxygen by mask. You rapidly move her to the ED and turn her over to the team there.

Later you discover that she had originally been admitted for evaluation of new-onset seizures. When the doctors told her she might have a brain tumor, she signed a DNR form. Fortunately, no tumor was found and her prognosis is actually quite good. The trauma team finds no life-threatening injuries from her fall and expects her to be able to begin psychiatric treatment before she leaves the hospital. This additional information makes you very glad you decided to go ahead with treatment.

More states are passing laws or regulations allowing prehospital personnel to withhold certain treatment when the patient has a DNR order. A valid order consists of a written statement describing interventions a particular patient does not wish to have that is recognized by the authorities of that state.

EMT-Is spend a great deal of time and energy learning how to assess and treat patients with life-threatening problems. It becomes difficult, then, for an EMT-I to watch someone die without doing something to try to stop it. You must nonetheless respect the patient's wishes when a competent patient has clearly communicated what he really wants. DNR orders make this easier because they typically must be signed or approved by a physician, increasing the likelihood that the decision was thoroughly thought through.

When there is no such order, however, it becomes more difficult for the EMT-I to determine what the patient's wishes truly are. Family members may be able to describe the patient's desires, but they can have conflicts of interest that make their statements less credible. For example, the patient may have accepted his impending death before his family has. They may want you to attempt resuscitation when that was clearly against the patient's expressed wishes. A less common situation is one in which the patient wishes all resuscitation efforts, but the family does not because they do not wish to prolong their own suffering or they have other less noble motivations.

In cases such as this, the general principle for EMT-Is to follow is, "When in doubt, resuscitate." This usually satisfies the principles of beneficence and nonmaleficence, admittedly perhaps at the expense of autonomy, but one of the biggest advantages to this approach is that, unlike the alternative, it is not irreversible. If you refrain from attempting resuscitation, it is certain that the patient will die. If you attempt resuscitation, there is no guarantee the patient will survive, but the patient can be removed from life-sustaining equipment later if that is deemed appropriate. Another advantage is that there will be more time later to sort out competing interests.

What about not attempting resuscitation when the situation appears to be futile? This option may appear attractive at first glance. After a little investigation, though, the issue becomes much more complex. How would a reasonable person or society define "futile"? Except at the extreme ends of the spectrum, there is no consensus on what constitutes a futile attempt at resuscitation. In addition, there is the issue of who would actually make the decision that a resuscitation attempt is futile in a particular case. Is it the experienced EMT-I who has seen very few lives saved under similar circumstances or the new EMT-I who is still excited about the prospect of saving lives every day? How can it be fair to have such wide disparities in such an important decision? Clearly, the concept of futility does not provide a useful guide for whether or not to attempt resuscitation.

Another related topic is what to do when an advance directive is presented to you after you have begun resuscitation. Once you have verified the validity of the order and the identity of the patient, you are obligated ethically (and perhaps legally, depending on your state) to cease resuscitation efforts. This can be a very difficult situation for you emotionally, but you have an obligation to respect the patient's autonomy and to stop doing something to him that he did not want. Follow your local protocols regarding procedures for cessation of resuscitation efforts.

ETHICS AND CONFIDENTIALITY

Consider this scenario:

You are called at one o'clock in the morning to a local hotel for a man reported to be unresponsive (but breathing) at the front desk. When you arrive, one of the guests at the hotel meets you and tells you he found the clerk slumped over in his chair, apparently unconscious, with what smelled like alcohol on his breath.

You approach the patient. His skin appears normal, and he is moving air well. He does not respond when you call him by the name on his name plate, Howard.

A general principle for EMT-Is to follow is, "When in doubt, resuscitate."

He has a strong, regular radial pulse that is within normal limits. You do not smell anything except for a faint minty odor. When you shake his shoulder and call his name again, he opens his eyes, looks around, and asks, "Who are you?"

You explain to Howard that you were called by a concerned guest who could not wake him up. Howard says he is fine now and does not want to go to a hospital. He is alert and oriented to person, place, and time. He denies any complaints, takes no medications, and has no past medical history. His vital signs are within normal limits. He denies any alcohol intake or use of any other drugs. The physical exam is unremarkable.

By your protocols and standard operating procedures, you have no reason to attempt to force the patient to go to a hospital. You complete the appropriate documentation for a refusal of transport and are leaving the lobby when the guest who called 9-1-1 stops you. "Aren't you going to take him to the hospital?" he asks. No, you reply, he does not want to go. "But what if there's a fire in the hotel and he's passed out and unable to help guests evacuate?"

This makes you stop and think, and you begin to weigh the rights of the hotel guests against the rights of your patient.

Your obligation to the patient is to maintain as confidential the information you obtained as a result of your participation in this medical situation. If you reported his condition to hotel management, what would you report? You have found no objective evidence that he is under the influence of alcohol or drugs. Depending on the state you are in, you may actually have a legal obligation to maintain confidentiality under circumstances such as these. On the other hand, what if there is an emergency in which the desk clerk's assistance is needed and he is unable to provide it? That is a conceivable but unlikely possibility. There is no clear and present danger that would require you to report.

There are a number of reasons to respect confidentiality in general. In an emergency, a patient assumes that he can be honest with these strangers who have come to help him because they will protect his privacy. If that trust was violated without sufficient cause, patients might very well be embarrassed or humiliated. This would undermine the public's trust in EMS. If word got around that private information was being made public, patients might not be forthcoming in giving their medical histories, potentially leading to disastrous consequences. For example, a man who had recently taken sildenafil (Viagra) for erectile dysfunction might deny taking it before you give him nitroglycerin. That drug interaction is potentially serious, possibly even fatal.

Nonetheless, there are times when it is appropriate and necessary to breach confidentiality. Every state has laws requiring the reporting of certain health facts such as births, deaths, particular infectious diseases, child neglect and abuse, and elder neglect and abuse. These last requirements have the most applicability to EMS. They are considered justifiable reasons to breach confidentiality because, in the eyes of society, the benefit to someone who is defenseless (protection from harm and perhaps even death) and to the public (a safer environment for children and the elderly) outweighs the right to privacy of a particular person. A valid court order is also considered a reasonable justification for breaching confidentiality. So is a clear threat by a patient to a specific person, as well as informing other health-care professionals who will care for the patient.

Clearly, patient confidentiality is an important principle, but not an inviolable one. When determining whether it is appropriate to breach confidentiality, take into account the probability of harm, the magnitude of the expected harm, and alternative methods of avoiding harm that do not require encroaching on confidentiality.

In the scenario above, factors do not justify breaching confidentiality. The person who called 9-1-1 for emergency assistance, however, is under no such obligation. The scenario comes to an end as follows:

You inform the hotel guest that you are unable to discuss the case with anyone because of confidentiality. However, you point out, the guest is not under the same obligation. He replies, "OK, you may not be able to do anything about it, but I'm calling the manager!"

ETHICS AND CONSENT

Consider this scenario:

> Bob, a 58-year-old male, has been having crushing substernal pain radiating to his left arm for several hours. He also is pale, sweaty, and nauseated. He denies shortness of breath. His condition remains unchanged after you give him oxygen and nitroglycerin. When you ask Bob which hospital he wants to go to, he tells you, "I'm not going to any hospital." Surprised, you find it difficult to understand why someone in this much pain would not want to go to a hospital. You try to enlist the help of relatives over the telephone (Bob lives alone), but they are unable to persuade the patient. He has no regular physician, so that option is not available to you. Finally, you decide to try on-line medical direction. While you are waiting for the physician to come to the phone, you wonder: If the patient continues to refuse, can you force him to go? How can you act in the best interest of a patient who refuses to accept what you feel certain is best for him?

A competent patient of legal age has the fundamental right to decide what health care he will receive and will not receive. This is at the core of patient autonomy. To exercise this right, a patient must have the information necessary to make an informed decision, the mental faculties to weigh the risks and benefits of various treatment options, and the freedom from restraints that might hamper his ability to exercise his options (such as threats).

It is sometimes appropriate to use the doctrine of implied consent to force the patient to go to the hospital. For the EMT-I to use this approach, the patient must be unable to give consent. Typically, the doctrine is invoked when the patient is unable to communicate, but it also can be employed when the patient is incapacitated because of drugs, illness, or injury. In this scenario, however, the patient shows no signs of being incapacitated. He is alert and oriented, making judgments and answering questions in a manner completely compatible with competence. The fact that the patient refuses something you recommend does not, in itself, indicate that he is incompetent.

Before you leave the patient, you must not only do the things you need to do to protect yourself legally, but you must also assure yourself that the patient truly understands the issues at hand and is able to make an informed decision. As difficult as it may be for you, if the patient is able to do these things, you may have to accept the patient's desires and leave him.

ETHICS AND ALLOCATION OF RESOURCES

EMT-Is do not usually think of themselves as guardians of finite resources, but occasionally they are. The most obvious example of this is when more patients are present than the EMT-I is able to manage, such as in a multiple-casualty incident. While learning how to provide emergency medical care for multiple patients at the same scene, you might ask: What are the ethics of triage?

There are several possible approaches to consider in parceling out scarce resources. Patients could all receive the same amount of attention and resources (true parity). They could receive resources based on need. Or they could receive what someone has determined they've earned.

The civilian method of triage, where the most seriously injured patients receive the most care, is based on need. This is intended to produce the most good for the most people. However, other methods of triage are in use. Military triage, for example, has traditionally concentrated on helping the least seriously injured because this approach produces the greatest number of soldiers who can return to duty. When the President or Vice President visits a town or city, there is typically an ambulance dedicated for the dignitary's use if needed. The ambulance is not to be used for anyone else. Because these officials are so important and because so many others need them, the typical order of care is changed.

A controversy exists in emergency medicine as to whether or not celebrities should be treated ahead of others. The argument for doing so typically emphasizes the disorder brought to the ED by the presence of a celebrity and the need to get the person out of the ED as quickly as possible to restore normal operation. The argument against takes the position that giving preferential treatment to a celebrity is an affront to justice and fairness.

All of these methods have their proponents for different situations. The key to resolving the issue of allocation of scarce resources is to examine the competing theories in light of the circumstances at hand.

ETHICS AND OBLIGATION TO PROVIDE CARE

Those who provide emergency care have a special obligation to help all those in need. Many other health-care professionals are free to pick and choose their patients, accepting only those who have health insurance or who can themselves pay for the services delivered by the health-care professional. This is not the case in emergency medicine. EMT-Is, like other emergency professionals, are obligated to provide medical care for those in need without regard to ability to pay. They also have an ethical obligation to prevent and report instances of patient "dumping," where those without insurance are transferred against their will to public or charity hospitals.

A particular issue arises regarding the patient who is a member of a managed care organization such as a health maintenance organization (HMO). The HMO may insist that the patient be treated at a particular facility with which it has a contract. This must not be allowed to interfere with the patient's emergency care. The EMT-I, like every other member of the EMS system, has an obligation to act in the patient's best interest, even when that goes against the HMO's economic interests.

Another situation is offering assistance when off duty. Although some states require EMTs, among others, to stop and render help when they come upon someone in need of emergency care, there is still a strong ethical obligation to do so. This does not extend to situations where the EMT-I would put himself in danger (such as, getting into a car teetering on the edge of a cliff), if assisting would interfere with important duties owed to others (such as leaving young children unattended in a car), or when someone else is already providing assistance. In return, society offers limited liability in the form of Good Samaritan statutes in every state in the United States.

ETHICS AND TEACHING

When patients call for EMS, they generally expect to receive care from qualified, credentialed individuals. EMS systems with students working in them should make sure students are clearly identified by the uniform they wear. The EMT-I acting as preceptor should also, when appropriate, inform patients of the presence of a student and request the patient's consent before the student performs a procedure. This sounds more cumbersome than it actually is. Patients who are unable to consent obviously do not fall into this category. Implied consent is invoked in this case. Patients who are able to consent are frequently very understanding of the student's need for experience. As long as the preceptor stresses that he is overseeing the student, the vast majority of patients usually consent.

Another issue related to students is how many attempts they should be allowed in order to perform procedures such as intravenous placement and endotracheal intubation before the preceptor steps in. Factors to consider include the student's skill level, the anticipated difficulty of the procedure, and the relative importance of the procedure. It is important to have a limit, at least initially, for the number of times a student will be allowed to attempt a procedure. Such a number will need to be decided by each system in consultation with the medical director.

ETHICS AND PROFESSIONAL RELATIONS

As a health-care professional, the EMT-I answers to the patient. As a physician extender, the EMT-I answers to a physician medical director. As an employee (or volunteer), the EMT-I answers to the EMS system. These competing interests can sometimes make life difficult. Each can lead to ethical challenges.

In general, there are three potential sources of conflict between EMT-Is and physicians. One possibility is a case in which a physician orders something the EMT-I believes is contraindicated. For example, suppose a physician ordered an EMT-I to transport a critical blunt-trauma patient without attempting any intravenous access, either at the scene or en route during the anticipated 45-minute transport. This order would run counter to standard medical practice.

Legal Notes

The EMT-I functions under the auspices of the EMS medical director as detailed in system protocols and standing orders. Providing ALS skills and interventions outside of your EMS system can lead to possible legal problems and litigation.

A different situation arises when the physician orders something the EMT-I believes is medically acceptable but not in the patient's best interests. For example, imagine you are transporting a patient with stable vital signs who is complaining of abdominal pain. In accordance with your protocols, you and your partner have each tried twice to start an IV line without success. The patient's veins are some of the worst you have ever seen, and you have no expectation that you will be successful on further attempts. The patient experienced considerable pain with each attempt and is now crying, asking you not to try any more. The physician, however, insists you continue attempts to gain access.

A third potential source of conflict is the situation in which the physician orders something the EMT-I believes is medically acceptable but morally wrong. For example, you are ordered to stop CPR on a young male found in cardiac arrest after blunt trauma. His initial rhythm of asystole has remained unchanged, and you know it is almost always associated with death. Nonetheless, although there is a very slim chance of recovery for the patient if you continue your resuscitation efforts, you would not be able to live with yourself if you did not at least try.

In each of the three cases, it is certainly appropriate for the EMT-I to start by confirming the order and asking the physician to repeat it. If the order is confirmed, the EMT-I would be prudent to ask the physician for an explanation, given the controversial nature of the orders. The next steps will depend on the physician's explanation, the patient's condition, the need for the intervention in the judgment of the EMT-I, the feasibility of performing the intervention (like gaining IV access), and the amount of time available to discuss the issue.

Ultimately, the EMT-I must determine for himself how the patient's interests are best served. This typically does not lead to conflict, but on occasion the EMT-I may run into situations like the ones described above. In these cases, the EMT-I must consider the competing interests of beneficence, nonmaleficence, autonomy, and justice; the roles of the physician and the EMT-I; the relative confidence (or lack thereof) the EMT-I has in his own medical and ethical judgment; how far the EMT-I is willing to go as an advocate for his patient; and the degree of risk acceptable to the EMT-I in contravening physician orders.

It is important for the EMT-I to understand that no matter what decision he makes, he will have to defend it. The explanation that he was just following the doctor's orders (or, conversely, just doing what he felt was right) will not be sufficient in and of itself. An EMT-I is expected to be more than a robot. He is expected to simultaneously be a physician extender, working under a physician's license, and a clinician with the ability and independence to recognize and question inappropriate orders. The EMT-I should also understand that he is not expected to act immorally. On the other hand, if the individual's morals are significantly out of step with the expectations of the profession, he needs to reconsider his profession.

Disagreements with physician orders happen rarely. Usually they are the result of poor communication (such as, saying one thing while meaning another or static interfering with the radio transmission) or lack of sufficient information. Conflicts with physicians that reach the level in the examples above are fortunately rare. When they happen, the EMT-I must be willing to be an advocate for the patient and act in the patient's best interests.

ETHICS AND RESEARCH

EMS research is only in its infancy, but it will clearly become more important and more common as the field establishes the foundation necessary to introduce, modify, and justify field interventions. As this occurs, EMT-Is will become instrumental in implementing research protocols and gathering data. It is essential that an EMT-I participating in a research project understand the importance of gaining expressed patient consent or following federal, state, and local regulations regarding implied consent.

The goal of patient care is to improve the patient's condition. The goal of research, on the other hand, is to help future generations. The two goals are not the same, so patients must be protected from untoward outcomes as much as possible.

One very important way of protecting the patient is by gaining the patient's expressed consent. There are several difficulties with this. One is the concern that a patient experiencing an emergency may not be able to truly consent because of the emotional pressures he is feeling. This pressure may occur in spite of the EMT-I's best efforts to explain matters calmly and impartially.

Another concern is with the patient who is unable to consent. An excellent example of this occurs in cardiac-arrest research. By the very nature of the problem being studied, the investigators will be unable to gather consent from the patient. In this case, the federal government has strict rules, for example, about community notification before the study begins and gaining consent from the patient or an appropriate family member as soon as possible after a patient is entered into the study. An EMT-I participating in such a study needs to be familiar with these rules and their implications.

Although many interventions have been tested and found to be life saving, there are unfortunately documented instances of patients denied treatment for life-threatening conditions in the name of research in the United States (e.g., the Tuskegee syphilis research project in which treatment for the disease was withheld). The EMT-I has an obligation to prevent such things from happening in EMS research.

SUMMARY

This is an exciting time for EMS and prehospital medicine. The EMT-I of the twenty-first century is a true health-care professional who can provide a significant impact on health care.

EMS has evolved over many years. Today, a comprehensive EMS system provides a continuum of care from First Responder to hospital and rehabilitative staff, from the mechanic who maintains the ambulance fleet to the emergency physician. It is a total team effort. The EMT-I is the leader of the prehospital emergency medical team. You must undertake the responsibility of preparing yourself to do the job and of continually updating your knowledge and skills. The best EMT-Is are those who make a commitment to excellence.

As an EMT-I, you must attend first to your own well-being in order to maintain the health and fitness to help others and to be a positive role model. Additionally, each member of EMS shares the responsibility of promoting wellness and preventing illness and injury among co-workers and in the community.

As an EMT-I, you also have the responsibility to know and follow the laws related to your profession and to behave ethically by acquiring a foundation in ethical values and having a system for making ethical decisions.

The best EMT-Is are those who make a commitment to excellence.

ON THE WEB

For additional practice and review, go to the companion website at www.prenhall.com/bledsoe and click on *Intermediate Emergency Care: Principles & Practice*.

CHAPTER 2

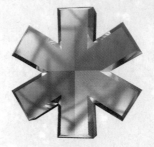

Overview of Human Systems

Objectives

Part 1: The Cell and the Cellular Environment (begins on page 83)

After reading Part 1 of this chapter, you should be able to:

1. Define the following terms: anabolism, anatomy, catabolism, homeostasis, metabolism, pathophysiology, physiology (p. 87).
2. Name the levels of organization of the body from simplest to most complex and explain each. (pp. 83–100)
3. Describe the general characteristics of each of the four major categories of tissues. (pp. 85–86)
4. Define each of the cellular transport mechanisms and give an example of the role of each in the body: diffusion, osmosis, facilitated diffusion, and active transport. (pp. 94–96)

5. Describe the water compartments and name the fluid in each. (pp. 89–91)
6. Explain how water moves between compartments. (pp. 94–96)
7. Explain the regulation of the intake and output of water. (pp. 91–94)
8. Describe the three buffer systems in body fluids. (pp. 97–100)
9. Explain the renal mechanisms for pH regulation of extracellular fluid. (pp. 97–100)
10. Describe the effects of acidosis and alkalosis. (pp. 97–100)

Part 2: Body Systems (begins on page 100)

After reading Part 2 of this chapter, you should be able to:

1. Identify the anatomical terms for the parts of the body, for the anatomical planes, and for describing location of body parts with respect to one another. (pp. 102, 115, 126, 133, 134, 139, 151, 164)

2. Review the body cavities and the major organs within each, including the abdomen and its underlying organs. (pp. 213–216)
3. Name the three major layers of the skin. (pp. 100–102)

Continued

4. Describe how glucose is converted to energy during cellular respiration. (pp. 180–181)
5. Describe the functions of the skeleton and explain how bones and joints are classified. (pp. 113–128)
6. List the three types of muscles and describe the structure and function of each. (pp. 130–134)
7. Describe the anatomy and physiology of the nervous system, including the meninges and cerebrospinal fluid. (pp. 136–137, 155–174)
8. Describe the structures of neurons, types of nerves, and the roles of polarization, depolarization, and repolarization in nerve impulse transmission. (pp. 155–174)
9. State the functions of hormones, including the hormones of the pancreas, and discuss the regulator processes of hormonal secretion. (pp. 174–183)
10. State the functions of epinephrine and norepinephrine and explain their relationship to the sympathetic division of the autonomic nervous system. (pp. 166–171)
11. Describe the characteristics and composition of blood, as well as the function of the red and white blood cells and platelets. (pp. 103–112)
12. State the importance of blood clotting. (pp. 110–113)
13. Describe the anatomy and physiology of the cardiovascular system, including the pericardium, the valves, and the major vessels and chambers. (pp. 183–200)
14. Describe coronary circulation, the cardiac cycle, and the parts of the cardiac conduction pathway. (pp. 186–192)
15. Explain how the nervous system regulates heart rate and the force of contractions. (pp. 188–192)

16. Explain the relationship among stroke volume, heart rate, and cardiac output. (pp. 195–199)
17. Describe the structure of arteries and veins and relate their structure to function. (pp. 193–195)
18. Describe the structure of capillaries and explain the exchange processes that take place there. (pp. 193–195)
19. Describe the pathway and purpose of pulmonary circulation. (pp. 199–200)
20. Describe the pathway and purpose of systemic circulation. (pp. 199–200)
21. Explain the factors that maintain and regulate blood pressure. (pp. 195–199)
22. Describe the functions of the lymphatic system. (p. 195)
23. Describe the immune response. (pp. 106–110)
24. Describe the anatomy and physiology of the respiratory system, including the nervous and chemical mechanisms that regulate it. (pp. 200–213)
25. Describe normal inhalation and exhalation. (pp. 206–208)
26. Differentiate between ventilation and respiration. (pp. 206–208)
27. Explain the diffusion of gases across the alveolar-capillary junction and how oxygen and carbon dioxide are transported in the blood. (pp. 209–211)
28. Describe the functions of the digestive system and name its major divisions. (pp. 216–218)
29. Explain why the respiratory system has an effect on pH and describe respiratory compensating mechanisms. (p. 211)

Case Study

Medic-1 is an Advanced Life Support (ALS) unit that serves a suburban community. Today, it is staffed by EMT-Intermediates Terry Martinez and Mark Westbrook. In addition, EMT-Intermediate (EMT-I) student Steve Matthews is riding as a part of his field internship. They have just backed into the station with three sacks of groceries when a frantic teen runs up to them. He says that his neighbor is having some sort of problem and wants them to come and take a look.

The crew gets back into the unit and drives the short distance to the scene. Upon arrival, they find a 34-year-old female seated in a porch swing in moderate distress. She is anxious and slightly confused. Between breaths, she complains of a tightness in her chest and difficulty swallowing. She denies any significant event that might have led to her symptoms. Her medical history is unremarkable as is her family history.

On physical exam, the EMT-Is find her to be cold, pale, and diaphoretic. Her voice is hoarse, and she is having obvious difficulty breathing. Her pulse is rapid and weak. They continue their assessment. Her airway is patent. Breath sounds are present but diminished at the bases. Scattered wheezes are heard throughout both lung fields. The peripheral pulses are weak, but equal. In addition, they note a characteristic "wheal and flare" rash, consistent with hives, on her chest and abdomen.

Based upon their assessment, the EMT-Is feel the patient's signs and symptoms are consistent with an anaphylactic reaction. As they begin treatment, Mark explains to Steve the underlying pathophysiology. "The patient's mental status change is most likely due to inadequate ventilation," he says. Mark also explains that, in many instances, an obvious cause for an anaphylactic reaction cannot be identified. Mark quickly describes how the body reacts to a foreign substance with an exaggerated immune response. The presence of the offending substance causes specialized cells to release histamine and other potent substances. These in turn cause the signs and symptoms seen. For example, histamine causes constriction of the bronchioles, resulting in wheezing and decreased air movement. It also causes the capillaries to become "leaky," causing the wheal and flare rash of urticaria (hives).

Based upon an understanding of the pathophysiological processes involved in the current emergency, the EMT-Is begin a treatment plan. First, they move the patient to the stretcher and begin assisting ventilations with a bag-valve-mask unit and 100% oxygen. An IV of normal saline is quickly placed in the patient's left forearm. The patient's blood pressure is 80/60, her pulse rate is 120 beats per minute, and her respiratory rate is 44 breaths per minute. Furthermore, her mental status is deteriorating.

Because of the rapid progression of the anaphylactic reaction, the EMT-Is administer 0.5 mg of epinephrine 1:10,000 intravenously per standing orders. They follow this with a 250 ml bolus of normal saline. Epinephrine reverses many of the adverse effects of histamine. The fluid bolus helps replace intravascular fluid lost to third spaces. Later, the patient receives 50 mg of diphenhydramine (Benadryl) intravenously. This is a potent antihistamine and serves to blunt the adverse effects of histamine and other substances released in the course of the anaphylactic reaction.

Upon arrival at the hospital, the patient is much improved. Her mental status is improved, and the hives have disappeared. She remains tachycardic from both the anaphylactic reaction and the epinephrine administered by the EMT-Is. While in the emergency department, she redevelops some wheezing as the effects of the epinephrine wear off. The emergency physician orders the administration of 0.5 mg of albuterol (Ventolin) in 2.5 mL of normal saline via a small volume nebulizer. The patient's wheezes disappear following the treatment. Because of the severe nature of the reaction, she is admitted to the emergency department's Clinical Decision Unit for 23 hours. She ultimately does well and goes home the next day with a prescription for an antihistamine and a steroid dose pack.

INTRODUCTION

An understanding of basic human anatomy and physiology is fundamental to EMT-Intermediate practice. Part 1 of this chapter presents an overview of organization of human body systems, including:

- The cell
- Tissues
- Organs, organ systems, and the organism
- System integration
- Fluids and electrolytes
- Acid-base balance

Part 2 describes the major body systems:

- Integumentary system
- Blood
- Musculoskeletal system
- Head, face, and neck
- Spine and thorax
- Nervous system
- Endocrine system
- Cardiovascular system
- Respiratory system
- Abdomen
- Digestive system and spleen
- Urinary system
- Reproductive system

Part 1: The Cell and the Cellular Environment

THE NORMAL CELL

The fundamental unit of the human body is the **cell** (Figure 2-1). It contains all necessary components to turn essential nutrients into energy, remove waste products, reproduce, and carry on other essential life functions.

cell the basic structural unit of all plants and animals. A membrane enclosing a thick fluid and a nucleus. Cells are specialized to carry out all of the body's basic functions.

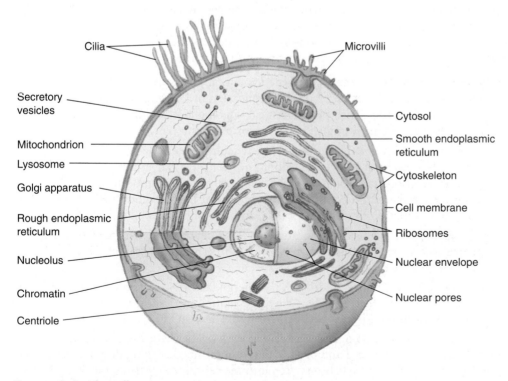

FIGURE 2-1 The cell.

The two kingdoms of cells are *prokaryotes* and *eukaryotes*. Prokaryotes are the cells of lower plants and animals such as blue-green algae and bacteria. Their structure is very simple, with an indistinct nucleus that is not encased in a membrane, and containing no other internal structures. Eukaryotes are the cells of higher plants and animals such as most algae, fungi, protozoa—and humans. Eukaryotes are, of course, more complex than prokaryotes. The cell structure discussed on the following pages relates to the eukaryotes.

CELL STRUCTURE

A cell is similar to a small, self-sustaining city. Within the cell, specialized structures perform specific functions. In a normal cell, all the structures and functions work together to maintain a normal, balanced environment. Each cell has three main elements: the cell membrane, the cytoplasm, and the organelles.

The Cell Membrane

The **cell membrane** (sometimes called the *plasma membrane*) is the outer covering that encircles and protects the cell.

The membrane is selectively permeable, or **semipermeable,** which means that it allows certain substances to pass from one side to another but does not allow others to pass. Vital functions of the cell membrane, made possible by its selective permeability, include electrolyte and fluid balance and the transfer of enzymes, hormones, and nutrients into and out of the cell. These functions will be discussed in greater detail later.

Without the cell membrane, the interior contents of a cell would become exposed to the extracellular environment and quickly die. That is why the bacterial cellular membrane is the site targeted by many antibiotic drugs—because destroying the cell membrane kills the cell.

Cytoplasm

Cytoplasm is the thick, viscous fluid that fills and gives shape to the cell, also called *protoplasm*. The clear liquid portion of the cytoplasm is called *cytosol*. Substances dissolved in the cytosol are mainly electrolytes, proteins, glucose (sugar), and lipids (fatty substances). Structures of various sizes and functions are dispersed throughout the cytosol.

Organelles

Structures that perform specific functions within the cell are called *organelles*. Six of the most important organelles are the nucleus, the endoplasmic reticulum, the Golgi apparatus, mitochondria, lysosomes, and peroxisomes. A brief discussion of a few of their functions provides an idea of the complex activity that takes place within a cell:

- *Nucleus.* The **nucleus** contains the genetic material, deoxyribonucleic acid (DNA), and the enzymes necessary for replication of DNA. DNA determines our inherited traits and also plays a critical ongoing role within our bodies. DNA must be constantly copied and transferred to the cells.

- *Endoplasmic reticulum.* The endoplasmic reticulum is a network of small channels that has both rough and smooth portions. Rough endoplasmic reticulum functions in the synthesis (building) of proteins. Smooth endoplasmic reticulum functions in the synthesis of lipids, some of which are used in the formation of cell membranes, and carbohydrates.

- *Golgi apparatus.* The Golgi apparatus is located near the nucleus of most cells. It performs a variety of functions including synthesis and packaging of secretions such as mucus and enzymes.

- *Mitochondria.* The mitochondria are the energy factories, sometimes called the "powerhouses," of the cells. They convert essential nutrients into energy sources, often in the form of **adenosine triphosphate (ATP).**

- *Lysosomes.* Lysosomes contain digestive enzymes. Their functions include protection against disease and production of nutrients, breaking down bacteria and organic debris that has been taken into the cells and releasing usable substances such as sugars and amino acids.

Content Review

MAIN ELEMENTS
OF THE CELL
- Cell membrane
- Cytoplasm
- Organelles

cell membrane the outer covering of a cell. Also called *plasma membrane.*

semipermeable able to allow some, but not all, substances to pass through. Cell membranes are semipermeable.

nucleus the organelle within a cell that contains the DNA, or genetic material; in the cells of higher organisms, the nucleus is surrounded by a membrane.

adenosine triphosphate (ATP) a high-energy compound present in all cells, especially muscle cells; when split by enzyme action, it yields energy. Energy is stored in ATP.

- *Peroxisomes.* Peroxisomes are similar to lysosomes. Especially abundant in the liver, they absorb and neutralize toxins such as alcohol.

A wide variety of other structures and functions exist within the cell. Within the nucleus, for example, there are one or more smaller organelles called *nucleoli* (plural of nucleolus). Another component of the nucleus is chromatin (tangles of chromosome filaments containing DNA). Additional organelles exist in the cytoplasm (cytosol) outside the nucleus, including the cytoskeleton (a structure of protein filaments that supports the internal structure of the cell), ribosomes (granular structures that manufacture proteins—some float free, others attach to the surface of the endoplasmic reticulum, which creates the "rough" endoplasmic reticulum), vesicles (which play a role in transferring and storing secretions from the rough endoplasmic reticulum and Golgi complex), and centrioles (which play a role in cell division). On the surface of some cells are microvilli (folds on the cell surface), and, on some cells, whiplike cilia and flagella (which move fluids across cell surfaces and move cells through the surrounding extracellular fluid).

CELL FUNCTION

All the cells of the human body have the same general structure and contain the same genetic material but, through a process called *differentiation,* or maturation, cells become specialized. Eventually, cells perform specific functions that are different from the functions performed by other cells.

There are seven major functions of cells:

- *Movement* is performed by muscle cells. Skeletal muscles move arms and legs. The smooth muscle around blood vessels causes them to dilate or constrict as necessary. Other smooth muscle moves food and wastes through the digestive tract. Cardiac muscle causes the chambers of the heart to contract. (See Muscle Tissue in the next section.)

- *Conductivity* is the function of nerve cells that creates and transmits an electrical impulse in response to a stimulus.

- *Metabolic absorption* is a function of cells of the intestines and kidneys, which take in nutrients that pass through the body.

- *Secretion* is performed by glands that produce substances such as hormones, mucus, sweat, and saliva.

- *Excretion* is a function all cells perform as they break down nutrients and expel wastes.

- *Respiration* is the function by which cells take in oxygen, which is used to transform nutrients into energy.

- *Reproduction* is the process by which cells enlarge, divide, and reproduce themselves, replacing dead cells and enabling new tissue growth and healing of wounds. Some cells, such as nerve cells, cannot reproduce; for instance, a severed spinal cord cannot repair itself.

TISSUES

Tissue refers to a group of cells that perform a similar function. The following are the four basic types of tissue:

- **Epithelial tissue** lines internal and external body surfaces and protects the body. In addition, certain types of epithelial tissue perform specialized functions such as secretion, absorption, diffusion, and filtration. Examples of epithelial tissue are skin, mucous membranes, and the lining of the intestinal tract.

- **Muscle tissue** has the capability of contraction when stimulated. There are three types of muscle tissue (see Figure 2-42 in the Musculoskeletal System section later in this chapter).
  - *Cardiac* muscle is tissue that is found only within the heart. It has the unique capability of spontaneous contraction without external stimulation.

Patho Pearls

Most medications used in emergency care act at the cellular level.

tissue a group of cells that perform a similar function.

epithelial tissue the protective tissue that lines internal and external body tissues. Examples: skin, mucous membranes, the lining of the intestinal tract.

muscle tissue tissue that is capable of contraction when stimulated. There are three types of muscle tissue: *cardiac* (myocardium, or heart muscle), *smooth* (within intestines, surrounding blood vessels), and *skeletal,* or *striated* (allows skeletal movement). Skeletal muscle is mostly under voluntary or conscious control; smooth muscle is under involuntary or unconscious control; cardiac muscle is capable of spontaneous or self-excited contraction.

connective tissue the most abundant body tissue; it provides support, connection, and insulation. Examples: bone, cartilage, fat, blood.

nerve tissue tissue that transmits electrical impulses throughout the body.

organ a group of tissues functioning together. Examples: heart, liver, brain, ovary, eye.

organ system a group of organs that work together. Examples: the cardiovascular system, formed of the heart, blood vessels, and blood; the gastrointestinal system, comprising the mouth, salivary glands, esophagus, stomach, intestines, liver, pancreas, gallbladder, rectum, and anus.

Content Review

ORGAN SYSTEMS

- Cardiovascular
- Respiratory
- Gastrointestinal
- Genitourinary
- Reproductive
- Nervous
- Endocrine
- Lymphatic
- Muscular
- Skeletal

– *Smooth* muscle is the muscle found within the intestines and encircling blood vessels. Smooth muscle is generally under the control of the involuntary, or autonomic, component of the nervous system.
– *Skeletal* muscle is the most abundant muscle type. It allows movement and is mostly under voluntary control.

- **Connective tissue** is the most abundant tissue in the body. It provides support, connection, and insulation. Examples of connective tissue include bones, cartilage, and fat. Blood is also sometimes classified as connective tissue.

- **Nerve tissue** is tissue specialized to transmit electrical impulses throughout the body. Examples of nerve tissue include the brain, spinal cord, and peripheral nerves.

ORGANS, ORGAN SYSTEMS, AND THE ORGANISM

A group of tissues functioning together is an **organ.** For example, the pancreas consists of epithelial tissue, connective tissue, and nervous tissue. Together, these tissues perform the essential functions of the pancreas. These functions include production of certain digestive enzymes and regulation of glucose metabolism.

A group of organs that work together is referred to as an **organ system.** The following are important organ systems:

- *Cardiovascular system.* The cardiovascular system consists of the heart, blood vessels, and blood. It transports nutrients and other essential elements to all parts of the body.

- *Respiratory system.* The respiratory system consists of the lungs and associated structures. It provides oxygen to the body, while removing carbon dioxide and other waste products.

- *Gastrointestinal system.* The gastrointestinal system consists of the mouth, salivary glands, esophagus, stomach, intestines, liver, pancreas, gallbladder, rectum, and anus. It takes in complex nutrients and breaks them down into a form that can be readily used by the body. It also aids in the elimination of excess wastes.

- *Genitourinary system.* The genitourinary system consists of the kidneys, ureters, bladder, and urethra. It is important in the elimination of various waste products. It also plays a major role in the regulation of water, electrolytes, blood pressure, and other essential body functions.

- *Reproductive system.* The reproductive system provides for reproduction of the organism. In the female, it consists of the ovaries, fallopian tubes, uterus, and vagina. In the male, it consists of the testes, prostate, seminal vesicles, vas deferens, and penis.

- *Nervous system.* The nervous system consists of the brain, spinal cord, and all of the peripheral nerves. It controls virtually all bodily functions and is the seat of intellect, awareness, and personality.

- *Endocrine system.* The endocrine system is a control system closely associated with the nervous system. It consists of the pituitary gland, pineal gland, pancreas, testes (male), ovaries (female), adrenal glands, thyroid gland, and parathyroid glands. There is evidence that other organs—such as the heart, kidney, and intestines—have endocrine functions. As noted earlier, the endocrine system exerts its effects through the release of chemical messengers called *hormones.*

- *Lymphatic system.* The lymphatic system is often considered a part of the cardiovascular system. It consists of the spleen, lymph nodes, lymphatic channels, thoracic duct, and the lymph fluid itself. It is important in fighting disease, in filtration, and in removing waste products of cellular metabolism.

- *Muscular system.* The muscular system is responsible for movement, posture, and heat production. It consists, primarily, of the skeletal muscles.

- *Skeletal system.* The skeletal system consists of the bones, cartilage, and associated connective tissue. It provides for support, protection, and movement. The bone marrow is the site for production of various blood cells, including the red blood cells and certain types of white blood cells.

The sum of all cells, tissues, organs, and organ systems is the **organism**. The failure of any component, from the cellular level to the organ-system level, can result in the development of a serious medical emergency.

SYSTEM INTEGRATION

The human body is not just a static structure of bones and cavities and tubes. It is a dynamic organization in which cells, tissues, organs, and organ systems perform functions essential to the preservation of the organism. **Homeostasis** is the term for the body's natural tendency to keep the internal environment and metabolism steady and normal. At the cellular level, the body will strive to maintain a very constant environment, because cells do not tolerate extreme environmental fluctuations.

A significant amount of energy is needed to maintain the order that is evident in the **anatomy** (structure) and **physiology** (function) of the organism. Potential energy is stored in the biochemical bonds of cells and tissues in plants and animals, and the kinetic energy necessary to maintain homeostasis is obtained by the breaking of those bonds. Food provides energy substrates such as sugar, fats, and proteins which, when broken down, produce the energy for the maintenance of homeostasis. **Metabolism** is the term used to refer to the building up (**anabolism**) and breaking down (**catabolism**) of biochemical substances to produce energy.

The body's cells interact and intercommunicate, similar to a multi-cellular "social" organism. Communication among the cells consists of electrochemical messages. When something interferes with the normal sending or receiving of these messages, a disease process can begin or advance.

Many intercellular messages are conveyed by substances secreted by various body glands. Endocrine glands, sometimes called *ductless glands* (including the pituitary, thyroid, parathyroid, adrenal glands, the Islets of Langerhans in the pancreas, the testes, and the ovaries), secrete hormones directly into the circulatory system, where they travel to the target organ or tissue. Exocrine glands secrete substances such as sweat, saliva, mucus, and digestive enzymes onto the epithelial surfaces of the body (the skin or linings of body cavities and organs) via ducts.

Several types of signaling take place among cells. Endocrine signaling (via hormones distributed throughout the body) is one mode of intercellular communication. Paracrine signaling (non-endocrine, non-hormonal) involves secretion of chemical mediators by certain cells that act only on nearby cells. In autocrine signaling, cells secrete substances that may act upon themselves. In synaptic signaling, cells secrete specialized chemicals called neurotransmitters, such as norepinephrine, acetylcholine, serotonin, and dopamine, which transmit signals across synapses, the junctions between neurons.

These chemical signals—in the form of hormones and neurotransmitters—are received by various kinds of receptors. Receptors can be nerve endings, sensory organs, or proteins that interact with and then respond to the chemical signals and other stimuli. Many of the medications administered by EMT-Is act upon these receptors. Chemoreceptors respond to chemical stimuli. Chemoreceptors within the brain respond to increasing levels of CO_2 in the cerebrospinal fluid, stimulating respiratory centers in the brainstem to increase the rate and depth of respirations. Baroreceptors respond to pressure changes. Baroreceptors in the arch of the aorta and in the carotid sinuses along the carotid artery sense changes in blood pressure, which then cause the cardiac centers in the medulla to alter the heart rate. Alpha and beta adrenergic receptors on the surfaces of cells in the bronchi, heart, and blood vessels respond to neurotransmitters and medications, resulting in a variety of cardiovascular and respiratory responses.

As the above examples demonstrate, when normal intercellular communication is interrupted and normal metabolism is disturbed, the body will respond in various ways to compensate and attempt to restore the normal metabolism, i.e., homeostasis.

organism the sum of all the cells, tissues, organs, and organ systems of a living being. Examples: the human organism, a bacterial organism.

The failure of any component of an organism—from the cellular level to the organ system level—can result in a serious medical emergency.

homeostasis the natural tendency of the body to maintain a steady and normal internal environment.

anatomy the structure of an organism; body structure.

physiology the functions of an organism; the physical and chemical processes of a living thing.

pathophysiology the study of how disease affects normal body processes.

metabolism the total changes that take place during physiological processes.

anabolism the constructive phase of metabolism in which cells convert non-living substances into living cytoplasm.

catabolism the destructive phase of metabolism in which cells break down complex substances into simpler substances with release of energy.

When something interferes with the electrochemical messages cells send to each other, a disease process can begin or advance.

neurotransmitter a substance that is released from the axon terminal of a presynaptic neuron upon excitation and that travels across the synaptic cleft to either excite or inhibit the target cell. Examples include acetylcholine, norepinephrine, and dopamine.

When normal metabolism is disturbed, the body attempts to restore normal metabolism, i.e., homeostasis.

Content Review

EFFECTS OF DISEASE

- Local (at the site of the illness or injury)
- Systemic (throughout the body)

negative feedback loop body mechanisms that work to reverse or compensate for, a pathophysiological process, (or to reverse any physiological process, whether pathological or nonpathological).

Each organ system plays a role in maintaining homeostasis. An example is the body's response to the accumulation of cellular carbon dioxide that occurs during exercise. The respiratory system immediately attempts to return the internal environment to its normal state by increasing the respiratory rate and depth to eliminate excess carbon dioxide—which is why runners pant.

The organization of the human body is very complex, with constant interactions occurring within and among the systems to maintain homeostasis. When disease interrupts these interactions, it can cause both local effects (at the specific site of the illness or injury) and systemic effects (throughout the body). When this happens, body cells and systems will respond to restore normal conditions.

To understand how human systems interact, physiologists sometimes view them from an engineering perspective. Various body systems respond to inputs, or stressors, that may be sensed by other systems. The system receiving the input responds in some fashion, creating an output. The portion of the system creating the output, be it a cell or an organ, is known as the *effector*. For example, consider a large laceration to an extremity with severe blood loss. The drop in blood pressure resulting from the blood loss is sensed by the baroreceptors, which in turn cause messages to be sent from the cardiac center in the medulla to the heart, resulting in an increase in the rate and strength of contractions in an attempt to restore normal blood pressure. By definition, the input would be the drop in pressure sensed by the baroreceptors; the effector would be the heart, which increased its rate in response to signals from the medulla; and the output would be the resultant increase in blood pressure.

This kind of feedback is essential for maintaining stability within a system and homeostasis for the organism. When the output of a system corrects the situation that created the input, it is said to loop, or feedback on the input, and a **negative feedback loop** exists—"negative" because the feedback negates the input caused by the original stressor. To elaborate on the example of the baroreceptors, the output or increase in blood pressure resulting from the increased heart rate feeds back on, or cancels out, the original input (low blood pressure), and the heart (effector) no longer has to maintain an elevated rate. This particular feedback loop is known as the baroreceptor reflex mechanism.

Unfortunately, the grim reality of this model is that blood loss often overwhelms the heart's ability to respond with an increased rate. At that point, the system has lost the ability to compensate, and, as an EMT-I, you must intervene by administering fluids and taking other necessary therapeutic measures. When the outputs of effector organs are ineffective in correcting the input condition, decompensation is said to have occurred.

Patho Pearls

Almost since the inception of advanced prehospital care, aggressive fluid resuscitation has always been a major component of trauma treatment. However, several recent studies have questioned the role of aggressive fluid resuscitation. Research has shown that fewer than 10% of trauma patients (blunt and penetrating) present with hypotension. Many of these are hypotensive for reasons other than blood loss (i.e., pneumothorax, gastric distension).

It has been demonstrated that the body has natural compensatory mechanisms that are activated when the blood pressure falls to between 70 and 85 torr. Even at this lowered blood pressure, cerebral and renal perfusion is maintained. Elevation of the blood pressure to pre-injury levels, through aggressive fluid resuscitation and PASG, can result in progressive re-bleeding at the injury site. In addition, as blood is lost, it is replaced with crystalloid solutions that do not contain any hemoglobin or clotting factors. Thus, over time, with aggressive fluid resuscitation, the blood becomes more dilute and its capacities to transport oxygen and initiate clotting are diminished.

Many trauma experts are now calling for trauma patients to be maintained in a region of "permissive hypotension," where fluids are judiciously given to maintain the systolic blood pressure between 70 and 85 torr. Like many issues in EMS, practices should only change when there is overwhelming scientific data. Soon, however, "permissive hypotension" may be the standard of care for trauma patients.

In the case of decompensation, the feedback system does not or cannot restore homeostasis. The opposite problem can also occur when the feedback system goes too far and overcompensates for the original problem. To prevent this, it is important for the body to have some way to stop the output and to restore the heart rate to normal, because the inability to control the pulse rate would cause instability in the cardiovascular system and danger to the organism. In fact, the body does have numerous means of controlling or halting output.

Biological systems generally employ negative feedback loops to maintain stability. Positive feedback systems do exist in human physiology. (Positive feedback enhances, rather than negates, the effects of input.) An example would be some short-lived positive feedback loops involved in follicular (egg) development in females. However, these loops work in conjunction with negative feedback loops to maintain stability.

Feedback activity must be orchestrated and synchronized to maintain homeostasis. Two systems work together to maintain homeostasis and to integrate the responses of different systems: the nervous system and the endocrine system. They are functionally and anatomically coupled to allow for this integration. For example, the pituitary gland of the endocrine system is joined with the hypothalamus of the nervous system by a stalklike structure called the *infundibulum*. This allows for rapid communication between these two body control systems.

There are important temporal differences in the responses of these two systems. Nervous system response is generally rapid in onset but short-lived. An example is the baroreceptor reflex mechanism, mentioned earlier, which is primarily mediated by the nervous system. Conversely, endocrine responses generally take longer—that is, they have a slower onset of action but a longer duration. For example, the pituitary gland secretes antidiuretic hormone (ADH) in response to low blood pressure. ADH acts on the renal (kidney) tubules, causing water to be reabsorbed into the blood instead of being eliminated from the body. This causes an increase in intravascular fluid volume that compensates for the decrease in intravascular volume caused by the blood loss. All these responses are stimulated by pathological alterations or events.

THE CELLULAR ENVIRONMENT: FLUIDS AND ELECTROLYTES

Many pathological conditions, both medical and traumatic, adversely affect the fluid and electrolyte balance of the body. Certain disease processes, such as diabetic ketoacidosis and heat emergencies, are associated with certain electrolyte abnormalities. Severe derangements in fluid and electrolyte status can result in death. For this reason, as an EMT-I, you need to have a good understanding of the fluids and electrolytes present in the human body.

Some fluid and electrolyte derangements can result in death.

WATER

Water is the most abundant substance in the human body. In fact, water accounts for approximately 60% of the total body weight (the average for all ages). The total amount of water in the body at any given time is referred to as the **total body water (TBW).** In an adult weighing 70 kilograms (154 pounds), the amount of total body water would be approximately 42 liters (11 gallons) (Figure 2-2).

Water is distributed into various compartments of the body (Table 2-1). These compartments are separated by cell membranes. The largest compartment is the intracellular compartment. This compartment contains the **intracellular fluid (ICF),** which is all of the fluid found inside body cells. Approximately 75% of all body water is found within this compartment. The extracellular compartment contains the remaining 25% of all body water. It contains the extracellular fluid (ECF), all of the fluid found outside the body cells.

There are two divisions within the extracellular compartment. The first contains the **intravascular fluid**—the fluid found outside of cells and within the circulatory system. It is essentially the same as the blood plasma. The remaining compartment contains the **interstitial fluid**—all the fluid found outside of the cell membranes, yet not within the

total body water (TBW) total amount of water in the body at a given time.

intracellular fluid (ICF) the fluid inside the body cells.

intravascular fluid the fluid within the circulatory system; blood plasma.

interstitial fluid the fluid in body tissues that is outside the cells and outside the vascular system.

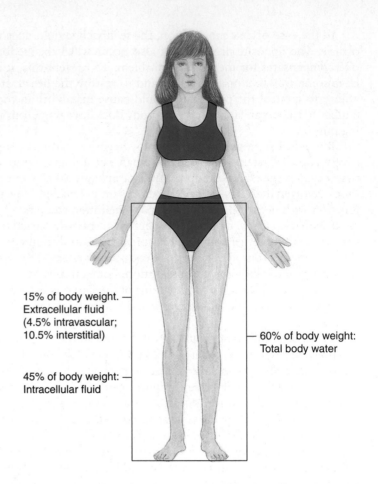

FIGURE 2-2 Percentage of body weight due to water as distributed into various fluid compartments.

15% of body weight. Extracellular fluid (4.5% intravascular; 10.5% interstitial)

45% of body weight: Intracellular fluid

60% of body weight: Total body water

Table 2-1	BODY FLUID COMPARTMENTS	
Compartment	Percentage of Total Body Water	Volume in 70 kg Adult
Intracellular fluid	75.0%	31.50 L
Extracellular fluid	25.0%	10.50 L
Interstitial fluid	17.5%	7.35 L
Intravascular fluid	7.5%	3.15 L

circulatory system. For example, minute amounts of fluid are found in the synovial fluid that lubricates the joints, the aqueous humor of the eye, secretions including saliva, gastric juices, bile, and so on.

Total body water (TBW) and its distribution vary with age and physiological condition. At birth, an infant's TBW is about 75% to 80% of its body weight, compared with the 65% TBW of the average adult. Infants have a higher TBW for two reasons. First, infants have less fat than adults. (Fat does not absorb water, so the less fat in the body, the more water.) Second, water is essential for the high rates of metabolism that are necessary to promote growth in the infant. The TBW slowly decreases to approximately 70% to 75% by age one. Diarrhea is especially worrisome in the infant, because it can mean the loss of a significant percentage of TBW. In addition, body systems that compensate for fluid loss are still immature, so that infants can rapidly become dangerously dehydrated and subject to electrolyte imbalances. By late childhood the TBW decreases to 65% to 70%.

By early adulthood, the TBW of males and females begins to differ. In adult males, TBW constitutes approximately 65% to 70% of the body weight, while in adult females the average TBW is 60% to 65%. The gender difference is the result of hormonal differences that result in the male's greater muscle mass and the female's greater percentage of body fat.

As the human body ages, the loss of muscle mass, increased percentage of fat, and the body's decreasing ability to regulate fluid levels lowers the TBW to around 45% to 55%. Due to a decreasing ability to regulate electrolytes and fluid levels, the elderly, like the very young, are at high risk for dehydration and disorders related to electrolyte imbalances.

Hydration

Water is the universal **solvent.** That is, most substances dissolve in water. When they do, various chemical changes take place. For this reason, the water content of the body is crucial to virtually all of the body's biochemical processes. Normally, the total volume of water in the body, as well as the distribution of fluid in the three body compartments, remains relatively constant. This occurs despite wide fluctuations in the amount of water that enters and is excreted from the body on a daily basis. The water coming into the body is referred to as *intake*. The water excreted from the body is referred to as *output*. To maintain relative homeostasis, the intake must equal the output, as shown below.

Intake

digestive system:	
liquids	1,000 mL
food (solids)	1,200 mL
metabolic sources:	300 mL
TOTAL:	2,500 mL

Output

lungs (water vapor):	400 mL
kidneys (urine):	1,500 mL
skin (perspiration):	400 mL
intestines (feces):	200 mL
TOTAL:	2,500 mL

Several mechanisms work to maintain a relative balance between input and output. For example, as explained earlier, when the fluid volume drops, the pituitary gland secretes antidiuretic hormone (ADH), which causes the kidney tubules to reabsorb more water into the blood and to excrete less urine. This process helps to restore the fluid volume to normal values.

Thirst also regulates fluid intake. The sensation of thirst normally occurs when body fluids decrease, stimulating the person to take in more fluids orally. Conversely, when too many fluids enter the body, the kidneys are activated and more urine is excreted, thus eliminating excess fluid. The body also maintains fluid balance by shifting water from one body space to another.

Dehydration The term **dehydration** refers to an abnormal decrease in the total body water, which can result from several factors:

- *Gastrointestinal losses* result from prolonged vomiting, diarrhea, or malabsorption disorders.
- *Increased insensible loss* is loss of water through normal mechanisms that is difficult to detect or measure (e.g., perspiration, water vapor from the lungs, saliva). These can be increased in fever states, during hyperventilation, or with high environmental temperatures.
- *Increased sweating* (also called perspiration or diaphoresis) can result in significant fluid loss. This can occur with many medical conditions or high environmental temperatures.
- *Internal losses* (commonly called "third space" losses) are losses of fluid into various body fluid compartments. In this situation, fluid is typically lost from the intravascular compartment into the interstitial compartment, effectively taking it out of the circulating volume. This can occur with peritonitis, pancreatitis, or bowel obstruction. It can also occur in poor nutritional states where not enough protein is present in the vascular system to retain water.
- *Plasma losses* occur from burns, surgical drains and fistulas, and open wounds.

solvent a substance that dissolves other substances, forming a solution.

Water is the universal solvent. Water is crucial to virtually all of the body's biochemical processes.

dehydration excessive loss of body fluid.

Patho Pearls

As a rule in the prehospital setting, any fluids administered to a patient should be isotonic crystalloids because an EMT does not know the patient's underlying fluid and electrolyte status.

Dehydration rarely involves only the loss of water. More commonly, electrolytes are also lost. At the hospital, fluid replacement will be based on both fluid and electrolyte deficits, once the patient's electrolyte abnormalities are determined through laboratory testing.

Clinically, the dehydrated patient will exhibit dry mucous membranes and poor skin **turgor.** Often the patient has excessive thirst. As it becomes more severe, dehydration will be accompanied by an increased pulse rate, decreased blood pressure, and orthostatic hypotension (increased pulse and decreased blood pressure on rising from a supine position). In infants, the anterior fontanelle may be sunken and the diaper may be dry or reveal the presence of highly concentrated (dark yellow, strong-smelling) urine. The absence of tears in a crying infant, a capillary refill time greater than two seconds, dry mucosa, and a decrease in urinary output are signs that indicate severe dehydration. The treatment for dehydration is replacement of fluid.

Overhydration Overhydration can occur as well. The major sign of overhydration is edema. Patients with heart disease may manifest overhydration much earlier than patients without heart disease. In severe cases of overhydration, overt heart failure may be present. Treatment is directed at removing the excessive fluid.

ELECTROLYTES

HOW TO READ CHEMICAL NOTATION

To describe chemical substances and reactions, scientists use chemical notation, a kind of "shorthand." Every chemical element has a one- or two-letter abbreviation. Just four elements—hydrogen, oxygen, carbon, and nitrogen—comprise over 99% of the body's atoms. These are called the major elements. Nine trace elements account for the remaining less than 1%.

Major Element	Symbol	Percent	Trace Element	Symbol
Hydrogen	H	62.0%	Calcium	Ca
Oxygen	O	26.0%	Chlorine	Cl
Carbon	C	10.0%	Iodine	I
Nitrogen	N	1.5%	Iron	Fe
			Magnesium	Mg
			Phosphorus	Ph
			Potassium	K
			Sodium	Na
			Sulfur	S

An atom is the smallest particle of an element. A molecule is a combination of atoms. The notation for a molecule combines the notations of the included elements. A subscript number after an element indicates the number of atoms of that element. If there is just one atom, there is no number. For example:

NaCl (Sodium chloride, or table salt. A sodium chloride molecule has 1 sodium atom and 1 chlorine atom.)

H_2O (Water. A water molecule has 2 hydrogen atoms and 1 oxygen atom.)

H_2CO_3 (Carbonic acid. A carbonic acid molecule has 2 hydrogen, 1 carbon, and 3 oxygen atoms.)

Ions

Each atom is made up of even smaller particles: electrons (which have a negative electrical charge), protons (which have a positive electrical charge), and neutrons (which are

(continued)

Dehydration usually involves loss of both water and electrolytes.
⟜⊸

turgor normal tension in a cell; the resistance of the skin to deformation. (In a normally hydrated person, the skin, when pinched, will quickly return to its normal formation. In a dehydrated person, the return to normal formation will be slower.)

overhydration the presence or retention of an abnormally high amount of fluid.

uncharged). Protons and neutrons are in the inner core, or nucleus, of the atom whereas electrons occupy outer orbits around the nucleus. Sometimes an atom of an element can lose one or more of its outer electrons or can capture one or more extra electrons from another element.

An ion is an atom that has lost one or more negatively charged electrons and now has a positive charge, or an atom that has gained one or more electrons and now has a negative charge. A superscript plus ($^+$) indicates a positively charged cation. A superscript minus ($^-$) indicates a negatively charged anion. For example:

Na$^+$ (A sodium ion has lost an electron and has a positive charge.)

Ca^{++} (A calcium ion has lost two electrons and has a double positive charge.)

Cl$^-$ (A chloride ion has gained an electron and has a negative charge.)

Electrolytes are substances that form ions when they break down, or dissociate, in water. Remember that the body and its blood are mostly water. The ions formed by dissociation of electrolytes in the body's fluids are a major factor in body metabolism.

Chemical Reactions

Notations for chemical reactions use a plus sign ($+$) to indicate substances that are combined and an arrow ($\rightarrow$) to show the direction of the reaction. The reactants are usually on the left, the product of the reaction on the right.

$$2H + O \rightarrow H_2O$$
(2 hydrogen atoms + 1 oxygen atom $\rightarrow$ 1 water molecule)

In some circumstances, a reaction may be reversible. That is, separate elements may synthesize (combine), or the synthesized substance may dissociate (break down) into separate components. A two-directional arrow ($\leftrightarrow$) shows that a reaction is reversible and can be read in either direction.

$$CO_2 + H_2O \leftrightarrow H_2CO_3$$
(carbon dioxide + water $\rightarrow$ carbonic acid)

or

(carbonic acid $\rightarrow$ water + carbon dioxide).

Notice that no atoms are gained or lost in a chemical reaction. In the example above, the two oxygen atoms in CO_2 and the single oxygen atom in H_2O combine to equal the three oxygen atoms in H_2CO_3. The hydrogen and carbon atoms are also equal on both sides of the reaction.

Up and down arrows ($\uparrow \downarrow$) are used to indicate an increase or decrease in the substance that follows the arrows. For example:

$$\uparrow H^+$$
(an increase in hydrogen ions)

$$\downarrow CO_2$$
(a decrease in carbon dioxide)

electrolyte a substance that, in water, separates into electrically charged particles.

dissociate separate; break down. For example, sodium bicarbonate, when placed in water, dissociates into a sodium cation and a bicarbonate anion.

ion a charged particle; an atom or group of atoms whose electrical charge has changed from neutral to positive or negative by losing or gaining one or more electrons. (In an atom's normal, non-ionized state, its positively charged protons and negatively charged electrons balance each other so that the atom's charge is neutral.)

cation an ion with a positive charge—so called because it will be attracted to a cathode, or negative pole.

anion an ion with a negative charge—so called because it will be attracted to an anode, or positive pole.

The various chemical substances present throughout the body can be classified either as electrolytes or non-electrolytes. **Electrolytes** are substances that **dissociate** into electrically charged particles when placed into water. The charged particles are referred to as **ions**. Ions with a positive charge are called **cations,** whereas ions with a negative charge are called **anions.**

An example of this would be the dissociation of the drug sodium bicarbonate when placed into water. Sodium bicarbonate is a neutral salt. When placed into water, it dissociates into two charged particles, as shown below.

$$NaHCO_3 \rightarrow Na^+ + HCO_3^-$$
sodium bicarbonate $\rightarrow$ sodium cation + bicarbonate anion
neutral salt $\rightarrow$ cation + anion

Sodium bicarbonate is an example of an electrolyte that is taken into the body as a medication. However, there are many naturally occurring electrolytes present in the body. The most frequently occurring cations include:

- *Sodium* (Na^+). Sodium is the most prevalent cation in the extracellular fluid. It plays a major role in regulating the distribution of water because water is attracted to and moves with sodium. In fact, it is often said that "water follows sodium." Sodium is also important in the transmission of nervous impulses. An abnormal increase in the relative amount of sodium in the body is called *hypernatremia*, whereas an abnormal decrease is referred to as *hyponatremia*.

- *Potassium* (K^+). Potassium is the most prevalent cation in the intracellular fluid. It is also important in the transmission of electrical impulses. An abnormally high potassium level is called *hyperkalemia*, whereas an abnormally low potassium level is referred to as *hypokalemia*.

- *Calcium* (Ca^{++}). Calcium has many physiological functions. It plays a major role in muscle contraction as well as nervous impulse transmission. An abnormally increased calcium level is called *hypercalcemia*, whereas an abnormally decreased calcium level is called *hypocalcemia*.

- *Magnesium* (Mg^{++}). Magnesium is necessary for several biochemical processes that occur in the body and is closely associated with phosphate in many processes. An abnormally increased magnesium level is called *hypermagnesemia*; an abnormally decreased magnesium level is called *hypomagnesemia*.

The most frequently occurring anions include:

- *Chloride* (Cl^-). Chloride is an important anion. Its negative charge balances the positive charge associated with the cations. It also plays a major role in fluid balance and renal function. Chloride has a close association with sodium.

- *Bicarbonate* (HCO_3^-). Bicarbonate is the principle **buffer** of the body. This means that it neutralizes the highly acidic hydrogen ion (H^+) and other organic acids. (Buffering will be discussed in more detail later in this chapter.)

- *Phosphate* (HPO_4^-). Phosphate is important in body energy stores. It is closely associated with magnesium in renal function. It also acts as a buffer, primarily in the intracellular space, in much the same manner as bicarbonate.

Many other compounds carry negative charges. Among these are some of the proteins, certain organic acids, and other compounds. Electrolytes are usually measured in milliequivalents per liter (mEq/L).

Non-electrolytes are molecules that do not dissociate into electrically charged particles. These include glucose, urea, proteins, and similar substances.

OSMOSIS AND DIFFUSION

As discussed earlier, the various fluid compartments are separated by cell membranes. These membranes are semipermeable, allowing the passage of certain materials while restricting the passage of others. Compounds with small molecules, such as water (H_2O), pass readily through the membrane; larger compounds, such as proteins, are restricted. This selective movement of fluids results from the presence of pores (openings) in the membrane. Electrolytes do not pass as readily as water through the membrane. This is due not so much to their size as to their electrical charge.

When solutions on opposite sides of a semipermeable membrane are equal in concentration, the relationship is said to be **isotonic**. When the concentration of a given solute (dissolved substance) is greater on one side of the membrane than on the other, it is said to be **hypertonic**. When the concentration is less on one side of the cell membrane, as compared with the other, it is referred to as **hypotonic**. This difference in concentration is known as the **osmotic gradient**.

buffer a substance that tends to preserve or restore a normal acid-base balance by increasing or decreasing the concentration of hydrogen ions.

isotonic equal in concentration of solute molecules; solutions may be isotonic to each other.

hypertonic having a greater concentration of solute molecules; one solution may be hypertonic to another.

hypotonic having a lesser concentration of solute molecules; one solution may be hypotonic to another.

osmotic gradient the difference in concentration between solutions on opposite sides of a semipermeable membrane.

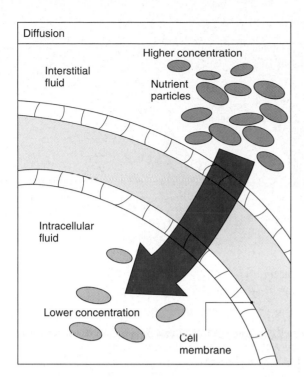

Diffusion

Interstitial fluid

Higher concentration

Nutrient particles

Intracellular fluid

Lower concentration

Cell membrane

FIGURE 2-3 Diffusion is the movement of a substance from an area of greater concentration to an area of lesser concentration.

The natural tendency of the body is to keep the balance of electrolytes and water equal on both sides of the cell membrane. This is an example of homeostasis. If one side of a cell membrane has an increased quantity of a given electrolyte (is hypertonic), there will be a shift of the electrolyte from that side and a shift of water from the other side to restore balance in concentration—the balanced state.

The tendency of molecules to move from an area of higher concentration to an area of lower concentration is referred to as **diffusion** and does not require energy (Figure 2-3). The diffusion of a solute (usually an electrolyte) across a cell membrane from the area of higher concentration to the area of lower concentration continues until the natural balance is again attained. This movement from an area of higher concentration to an area of lower concentration is termed a movement *with the osmotic gradient*.

Water also moves across the cell membrane so as to dilute the area of increased electrolyte concentration. The movement of water is more rapid than the movement of electrolytes. This form of diffusion (the passage of any solvent, usually water, through a membrane) is referred to as **osmosis** (Figure 2-4). It occurs in the direction opposite to the direction of solute movement. For example, if a semipermeable membrane separates solutions of water and sodium, and if the concentration of sodium is two times higher on one side of the membrane than on the other, then two things occur. Sodium diffuses from the area of higher concentration (the hypertonic side) to the area of lesser concentration (the hypotonic side). Concurrently, water diffuses in the opposite direction. That is, water leaves the hypotonic side and diffuses across the membrane to the hypertonic side. These actions continue until the concentration of water and sodium on both sides has equalized.

In addition to diffusion, two other mechanisms—active transport and facilitated diffusion—can transport substances across cell membranes. **Active transport** is the movement of a substance across the cell membrane *against the osmotic gradient* (that is, toward the side that already has more of the substance).

For example, the body requires cells of the myocardium to be negatively charged on the inside of the cells compared with the outside. However sodium, with its positive charge, tends to diffuse passively into the cell. This would destroy the negative charge inside the cell. In order to maintain the desired negative charge, sodium ions are actively pumped out of the cell, while potassium ions are pumped into the cell, by a mechanism known as the sodium-potassium pump. (Sodium and potassium ions are both positive, but more sodium ions are pumped out of the cell than potassium ions are pumped in, creating the desired negative charge inside the cell.)

diffusion the movement of molecules through a membrane from an area of greater concentration to an area of lesser concentration.

osmosis the passage of a solvent such as water through a membrane.

active transport movement of a substance through a cell membrane against the osmotic gradient; that is, from an area of lesser concentration to an area of greater concentration, opposite to the normal direction of diffusion.

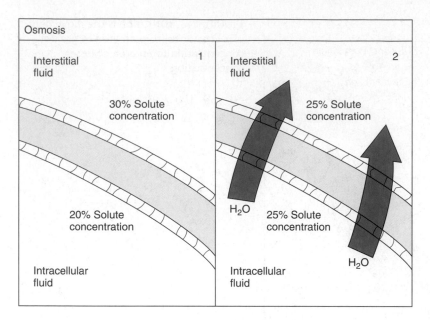

FIGURE 2-4 Osmosis is the movement of water from an area of higher WATER concentration to an area of lesser WATER concentration. Because water is a solvent, it moves from an area of lower SOLUTE concentration to an area of higher SOLUTE concentration.

Active transport is faster than diffusion, but it requires the expenditure of energy, which diffusion does not. Proteins are moved across the cell membrane in a similar fashion.

Certain molecules can move across the cell membrane by another process known as **facilitated diffusion.** Glucose is an example of such a molecule. Facilitated diffusion requires the assistance of "helper proteins," parts of a membrane transport system, on the surface of the cell membrane. These proteins, once activated, bind to the glucose molecule. Following binding, the protein changes its configuration and transports the glucose molecule to the inside of the cell, where it is released. Depending on the substance being transported, facilitated diffusion may or may not require energy.

Water Movement between Intracellular and Extracellular Compartments

The mechanisms by which water and solutes move across cell membranes, as described above, ensure that the **osmolality** of body water, both within and outside the cells, is normally in equilibrium. (The term *osmolality* refers to the concentration of solute per kilogram of water; a related term, **osmolarity**, refers to the concentration of solute per liter of water. The terms are often used interchangeably.) Sodium, the most abundant ion in the extracellular fluid, is responsible for the osmotic balance of the extracellular space. Potassium plays the same role in the intracellular space.

Generally, the osmolality of intracellular fluid does not change very rapidly. However, when there is a change in the osmolality of extracellular fluid, water will move from the intracellular to the extracellular compartment, or vice versa, until osmotic equilibrium is regained.

Water Movement between Intravascular and Interstitial Compartments

Within the extracellular compartment, movement of water between the plasma in the intravascular space and the interstitial space is primarily a function of forces at play in the capillary beds.

In general, the movement of water and solutes across a cell membrane is governed by **osmotic pressure.** Osmotic pressure is the pressure exerted by the concentration of solutes on one side of a semipermeable membrane, such as a cell membrane or the thin wall of a capillary. Osmotic pressure can be thought of as a "pull" rather than a "push," because a hypertonic concentration of solutes tends to pull water from the other side of the membrane.

facilitated diffusion diffusion of a substance such as glucose through a cell membrane that requires the assistance of a "helper," or carrier protein.

osmolality the concentration of solute per kilogram of water.

osmolarity the concentration of solute per liter of water (often used synonymously with *osmolality*).

osmotic pressure the pressure exerted by the concentration of solutes on one side of a membrane that, if hypertonic, tends to "pull" water (cause osmosis) from the other side of the membrane.

Generally, this is a two-way street as solutes move out of a space while water moves into the space to balance the concentration of solutes on both sides of the membrane. However, a somewhat different osmotic mechanism operates between the plasma inside a capillary and the interstitial space outside the capillary. Blood plasma generates **oncotic force,** which is sometimes called *colloid osmotic pressure.* Plasma proteins are colloids, large particles that do not readily move across the capillary membrane. They tend to remain within the capillary. At the same time, very little water is in the interstitial space. The small amount of water that does get into the interstitial space is usually taken up by the lymph system. Therefore, since little water is outside the capillary, and because plasma proteins do not readily move outside the capillary, the forces governing movement of water between the capillary and the interstitial space are almost all on one side, governed by the plasma on the inside of the capillary.

Another force inside the capillaries is **hydrostatic pressure,** which is the blood pressure, or force against the vessel walls, created by contractions of the heart. Hydrostatic pressure does tend to force some water out of the plasma and across the capillary wall into the interstitial space, a process that is called **filtration.** Hydrostatic pressure (a force that favors filtration, pushing water out of the capillary) and oncotic force (a force opposing filtration, pulling water into the capillary) together are responsible for **net filtration,** which is described in Starling's hypothesis:

Net filtration = (Forces favoring filtration) − (Forces opposing filtration)

Net filtration in a capillary is normally zero. It works this way: As plasma enters the capillary at the arterial end, hydrostatic pressure forces water to cross the capillary membrane into the interstitial space. This loss of water increases the relative concentration of plasma proteins. By the time the plasma reaches the venous end of the capillary, the oncotic force exerted by the increased concentration of plasma proteins is great enough to pull the water from the interstitial space back into the capillary. The outcome is that water is retained in the intravascular space and does not remain in the interstitial space.

ACID-BASE BALANCE

Acid-base balance is a dynamic relationship that reflects the relative concentration of hydrogen ions (H$^+$) in the body. Hydrogen ions are acidic and the concentration of these within the body must be maintained within fairly strict limits. Any deviation in the hydrogen ion concentration adversely affects all of the biochemical events that occur in the body. The hydrogen ion concentration is dynamic, changing from second to second.

THE pH SCALE

The total number of hydrogen ions present in the body at any given time is very high. Because of this, the **pH** system of measurement is used. The pH scale is inversely related to hydrogen ion concentration. That is, the greater the hydrogen ion concentration, the lower the pH. The lower the hydrogen ion concentration, the higher the pH.

The pH scale is logarithmic, each number representing a value ten times that of its neighboring number, so that pH 6 represents a hydrogen ion concentration 10 times as great as that represented by pH 7. The following formula represents pH:

$$pH = \log \frac{1}{[H^+]}$$

The pH scale ranges from 1 to 14. A pH of 1 means that only hydrogen ions are present. A pH of 14 means that virtually no hydrogen ions are present. The pH of water is 7.0, which is a neutral pH. The pH of the body is normally 7.35 to 7.45 (Table 2-2).

Because hydrogen ions are acidic, a pH below 7.35 is referred to as **acidosis.** A substance that produces negatively charged ions that can neutralize the positively charged hydrogen ions (or other acids) is called an *alkali* or base. An excess of alkaline (base) substances or a deficit of acids produces a pH above 7.45, which is referred to as **alkalosis.** In humans, a variation of only 0.4 of a pH unit in either direction from normal (6.9 or 7.8) can be fatal.

oncotic force a form of osmotic pressure exerted by the large protein particles, or colloids, present in blood plasma. In the capillaries, the plasma colloids tend to pull water from the interstitial space across the capillary membrane into the capillary. Oncotic force is also called *colloid osmotic pressure.*

hydrostatic pressure blood pressure or force against vessel walls created by the heart beat. Hydrostatic pressure tends to force water out of the capillaries into the interstitial space.

filtration movement of water out of the plasma across the capillary membrane into the interstitial space.

net filtration the total loss of water from blood plasma across the capillary membrane into the interstitial space. Normally, hydrostatic pressure forcing water out of the capillary is balanced by oncotic force pulling water into the capillary for a net filtration of zero.

pH abbreviation for *potential of hydrogen.* A measure of relative acidity or alkalinity. Since the pH scale is inverse to the concentration of acidic hydrogen ions, the lower the pH the greater the acidity and the higher the pH the greater the alkalinity. A normal pH range is 7.35 to 7.45.

acidosis a high concentration of hydrogen ions; a pH below 7.35.

alkalosis a low concentration of hydrogen ions; a pH above 7.45.

Table 2-2 THE pH SCALE AND HYDROGEN ION CONCENTRATIONS

pH		Example	H^+ Concentration*	
Acidic	0	Hydrochloric acid	10^{-0}	(1.0)
	1	Stomach secretions	10^{-1}	(0.1)
	2	Lemon juice	10^{-2}	(0.01)
	3	Cola drinks	10^{-3}	(0.001)
	4	White wine	10^{-4}	(0.0001)
	5	Tomato juice	10^{-5}	(0.00001)
	6	Coffee, urine, saliva	10^{-6}	(0.000001)
Neutral	7	Distilled water	10^{-7}	(0.0000001)
Basic	8	Blood, semen	10^{-8}	(0.00000001)
	9	Bile	10^{-9}	(0.000000001)
	10	Bleach	10^{-10}	(0.0000000001)
	11	Milk of magnesia	10^{-11}	(0.00000000001)
	12	Ammonia water	10^{-12}	(0.000000000001)
	13	Drain opener	10^{-13}	(0.0000000000001)
	14	Lye	10^{-14}	(0.00000000000001)

*Hydrogen ion concentrations are expressed in moles per liter, a quantity based on molecular weight.

Content Review

THREE MECHANISMS OF HYDROGEN ION REMOVAL
- Bicarbonate buffer system
- Respiration
- Kidney function

BODILY REGULATION OF ACID-BASE BALANCE

The body is constantly producing hydrogen ions (acids) through metabolism and other biochemical processes. To maintain the acid-base balance, these hydrogen ions must be constantly eliminated from the body. There are three major mechanisms to remove hydrogen ions from the body. The fastest mechanism is often referred to as the *buffer system* or the bicarbonate buffer system.

The two components of the bicarbonate buffer system are bicarbonate ion (HCO_3^-) and carbonic acid (H_2CO_3). These two compounds are in equilibrium with hydrogen ion (H^+), as follows: In some circumstances hydrogen ion combines with bicarbonate ion to produce carbonic acid. In other circumstances, carbonic acid dissociates into bicarbonate ion and hydrogen ion:

$$H^+ + HCO_3^- \leftrightarrow H_2CO_3$$

hydrogen ion + bicarbonate ion ↔ carbonic acid

In a healthy individual, for every molecule of carbonic acid, there are 20 molecules of bicarbonate ion. Any change in this 20:1 ratio is immediately corrected without significant change in the total body pH. This occurs in the following manner: An increase in hydrogen ion (acidosis) is corrected as the excess hydrogen ions combine with bicarbonate ions to form carbonic acid. (Thus an increase in hydrogen ion leads to an increase in carbonic acid—driving the equation above to the right.) Conversely, when there is a deficit in hydrogen ions (alkalosis), carbonic acid will dissociate into bicarbonate ion and hydrogen ion. (Thus a decrease in hydrogen ion leads to a decrease in carbonic acid—driving the equation above to the left.) (Figure 2-5)

Increased Acid:
$$\uparrow H^+ + HCO_3^- \rightarrow \uparrow H_2CO_3$$
Decreased Acid:
$$\downarrow H^+ + HCO_3^- \rightarrow \downarrow H_2CO_3$$

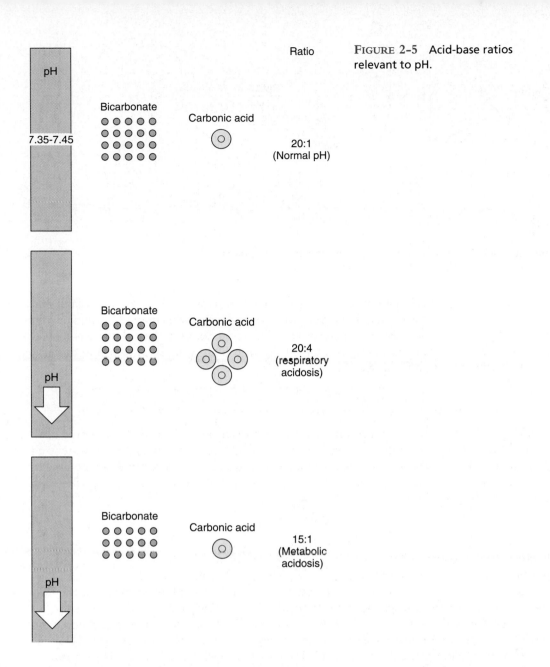

Ratio

FIGURE 2-5 Acid-base ratios relevant to pH.

pH

7.35-7.45

Bicarbonate

Carbonic acid

20:1
(Normal pH)

pH

Bicarbonate

Carbonic acid

20:4
(respiratory acidosis)

pH

Bicarbonate

Carbonic acid

15:1
(Metabolic acidosis)

Carbonic acid is a weak acid that is better tolerated by the body than pure hydrogen ion. However, the body carries this reaction further. Any increase in carbonic acid must also be eliminated.

The elimination of excess carbonic acid takes place as follows: Carbonic acid is unstable and eventually dissociates into carbon dioxide and water. This normally slow process is speeded by the blood's erythrocytes, which contain an enzyme called *carbonic anhydrase*. Carbonic anhydrase causes carbonic acid to be converted to carbon dioxide and water very rapidly—so rapidly that carbonic acid exists for only a fraction of a second before it is converted into carbon dioxide and water. Most buffering of acid in the body occurs in the erythrocytes.

The enzyme also works in a reverse fashion, which allows carbon dioxide and water to be quickly converted into carbonic acid. The reaction proceeds in accordance with LeChetalier's Principle. Given an excess of carbon dioxide on the right-hand side of the equilibrium, a stress is placed on it such that it must shift to the left, which is sometimes referred to as a mass action effect. The net effect of this is the generation of more hydrogen ion and

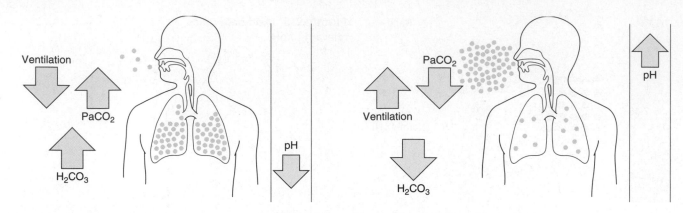

FIGURE 2-6 The respiratory component of acid-base balance.

acidosis. The clinical application of this is that when a patient is said to hypoventilate, that is, retain CO_2, then the accumulation (stress) of increased CO_2 forces the equilibrium to shift to the left, causing what is known as respiratory acidosis. So, with the aid of carbonic anhydrase, an equilibrium eventually is attained between hydrogen ion and carbon dioxide. The following equation illustrates this relationship.

$$H^+ + HCO_3^- \leftrightarrow H_2CO_3 \leftrightarrow H_2O + CO_2$$

hydrogen ion + bicarbonate ion $\leftrightarrow$ carbonic acid $\leftrightarrow$ water + carbon dioxide

Thus an increase in hydrogen ion (acid) would result in an increase in carbonic acid. With the aid of carbonic anhydrase, carbonic acid would quickly dissociate into water and carbon dioxide. Conversely (since the reaction can move in either direction), an increase in CO_2 causes an increase in hydrogen ion concentration and a decrease in pH (increase in acidity), as shown below.

$$\uparrow H^+ \leftrightarrow \uparrow CO_2$$

In conjunction with the bicarbonate buffer system described above, the body regulates acid-base balance by two other mechanisms, respiration and kidney function. Increased respirations cause increased elimination of CO_2, which results in a decrease in hydrogen ions and an increase in pH. Conversely, decreased respirations cause CO_2 to be retained. This causes an increase in hydrogen ions and a decrease in pH (Figure 2-6).

The kidneys also can regulate the pH by altering the concentration of bicarbonate ion (HCO_3^-) in the blood. Increased elimination of HCO_3^- results in a lowered pH. (There is less bicarbonate ion to combine with and eliminate hydrogen ion.) Conversely retention of HCO_3^- causes an increase in pH. (There is more bicarbonate ion to combine with and eliminate hydrogen ion.) In addition, the kidneys affect the acid-base balance by removing or retaining various chemicals. Normally, the kidneys remove larger metabolic acids, excreting them in the urine, resulting in an increase in pH.

Part 2: Body Systems

INTEGUMENTARY SYSTEM

Content Review

LAYERS OF THE SKIN
- Epidermis
- Dermis
- Subcutaneous tissue

The protective envelope we call the skin is a complex structure. Understanding how it is put together and how it functions will help you appreciate the importance of injuries to it and the value of their proper care.

THE SKIN

The epidermis, dermis, and subcutaneous tissue layers comprise what is commonly known as the skin (Figure 2-7). Each of these layers performs functions essential to helping the body maintain homeostasis and each plays an important role in the wound repair process.

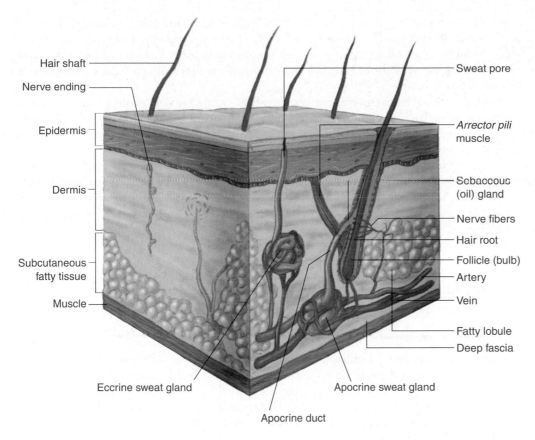

Labels on figure:
Hair shaft
Nerve ending
Epidermis
Dermis
Subcutaneous fatty tissue
Muscle
Eccrine sweat gland
Apocrine duct
Sweat pore
Arrector pili muscle
Sebaceous (oil) gland
Nerve fibers
Hair root
Follicle (bulb)
Artery
Vein
Fatty lobule
Deep fascia
Apocrine sweat gland

FIGURE 2-7 Layers and major structures of the skin.

Epidermis

The outermost skin layer is the **epidermis.** It is generated by a layer of cells just above the dermis (stratum germinativum). These cells divide rapidly, generating a movement of cells upward toward the epidermal surface. As the epidermis contains no vasculature, the further these cells are pushed away from the dermis, the less circulation they receive, and they eventually die. As they die, they flatten and interlock, providing a firm and secure barrier around the body (stratum corneum). The outermost cells are eventually abraded or washed away and then replaced, allowing the epidermis to maintain its thickness. It normally takes 2 weeks for a cell to move from the dermal border to the surface of the epidermis and another 2 to 4 weeks until it is abraded away. This outward movement of cells helps the body resist invasion by bacteria.

A waxy substance called **sebum** lubricates the surface of the epidermis. This lubrication acts much like oil on leather. It keeps the outer layers of the skin flexible, strong, and resistant to penetration by water. The epidermis is also responsible for the pigmentation that protects the skin from the harmful effects of ultraviolet radiation. The thickness of the epidermis varies greatly, depending on the amount of abrasion and pressure it receives. On the soles of the feet, it is very thick and strong, while over the eye it is microscopic in thickness and very delicate.

Dermis

Directly beneath the epidermis is the **dermis,** a connective tissue that helps contain the body and supports the functions of the epidermis. The upper layer of the dermis is the papillary layer, consisting of loose connective tissue, capillaries, and nerves supplying the epidermis. The reticular layer is the deeper dermis made up of strong connective tissue that integrates the dermis firmly with the subcutaneous layer below. This tissue also holds the skin firmly around the body and permits the stretching and flexibility necessary for articulation.

epidermis outermost layer of the skin composed of dead or dying cells.

sebum fatty secretion of the sebaceous gland that helps keep the skin pliable and waterproof.

dermis true skin, it is the layer of tissue producing the epidermis and housing the structures, blood vessels, and nerves normally associated with the skin. Also called the *corium.*

Patho Pearls

Goosebumps, also called gooseflesh, are a part of the body's response to cold and result from contraction of the *arrector pili* muscles in the skin.

The dermis contains blood vessels, nerve endings, glands, and other structures. It is here that **sebaceous glands** produce sebum and secrete it directly onto the surface of the skin or into hair follicles. **Sudoriferous glands** secrete sweat to help move heat out of and away from the body through evaporation. Hair follicles produce hair that helps to reduce surface abrasion and conserve heat.

The two types of sweat glands are *eccrine glands* and *apocrine glands*. Eccrine glands, also known as merocrine glands, open onto the skin surface and help control body temperature through water excretion. They are widely distributed but are most heavily concentrated in the axilla and genital areas. Apocrine glands are found exclusively in the armpits and genital region, and they open into hair follicles. These glands respond to emotional stress. During adolescence, the apocrine glands enlarge and actively increase the axillary sweating that causes adult body odor. Also during this period, the sebaceous glands increase their activity, giving the skin an oily appearance. This predisposes the teenager to acne problems.

As a person ages, sebaceous and sweat gland activity decreases. As a result, the skin becomes drier and produces less perspiration. The epidermis thins and flattens, and the dermis loses some of its vascularity. The skin wrinkles as it loses turgor. In warmer climates, the skin can become thickened, yellowed, and furrowed and take on a weather-beaten appearance. Elderly people develop a variety of spots on the thin skin of the backs of their hands and forearms. Whitish, depigmented marks are known as pseudoscars. Purple spots (purpura) caused by minor capillary bleeding may appear and fade after a few weeks.

In the dermis are several resident body cells responsible for initiating the attack on invading organisms, foreign materials, and damaged cells, and for beginning the repair of damaged tissue. The macrophages and lymphocytes (types of white blood cells) begin the inflammation response by killing invading bodies and triggering a call for other, similar cells. Mast cells control the microcirculation to tissues and respond to the initial invasion, increasing capillary flow and permeability. Fibroblasts lay down and repair protein strands to strengthen the wound site and begin restoring the skin's integrity.

Subcutaneous Tissue

Subcutaneous tissue is the body layer beneath the dermis. It is rich in fatty or adipose tissue, which helps it absorb the forces of trauma, protecting the tissues and vital organs beneath. Because of its fatty content, heat moves outward through the subcutaneous tissue three times more slowly than through muscles or other layers of the skin; hence it is of great value in conserving body temperature. The body directs blood below the subcutaneous tissue to conserve heat and above it through the dermis when it is necessary to radiate heat.

THE HAIR

Hair is a tactile sensory organ that also has a role in sexual stimulation and attraction. It covers the entire body except the palms, soles, and parts of the sex organs. Hair develops from the base of the hair follicle, where it is nourished by the papilla, a vast capillary network. An involuntary arrector pili muscle fiber attaches to the base of the hair shaft. When these arrectores pilorum contract, the hair stands erect and goose bumps appear on the skin.

The two types of hair are *vellus* and *terminal*. Vellus hair is short, fine, and lacking pigment (similar to "peach fuzz"). Terminal hair is coarser, thicker, and pigmented. It appears on the eyebrows and scalp, in the armpits and groin of both sexes, and on the faces and bodies of males.

With aging the hair turns gray from a decrease in pigmentation and its growth declines. A transition from terminal to vellus hair on the scalp causes baldness in both men and women. The opposite occurs in the nares and ears of men, where terminal hair replaces vellus hair. Both genders generally experience a decrease in body hair as they age. Loss of the lateral third of the eyebrow is also normal in the elderly.

THE NAILS

Nails are found at the most **distal** ends of fingers and toes and are primarily for protection. Nails are strong yet flexible and provide a sharp edge for scratching, scraping, and clawing. They are made up of the nail plate, the nail bed, the **proximal** nail fold, and the nail root

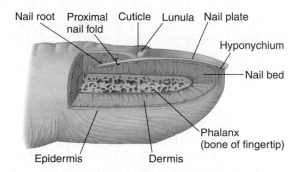

Nail root Proximal Cuticle Lunula Nail plate
        nail fold

Hyponychium

Nail bed

Phalanx
(bone of fingertip)

Epidermis Dermis

FIGURE 2-8 The nail.

(Figure 2-8). The angle between the proximal nail fold and the nail plate should be less than 180 degrees. Fingernails grow approximately 0.1 mm daily, slightly faster in the summertime. The nail plate lies on a highly vascular nail bed that gives the nail a pink appearance. Nail edges should be smooth and rounded. The nail plates should be smooth, flat, or slightly curved and should feel hard and uniformly thick. As a person ages, nail growth diminishes because of decreased peripheral circulation. The nails, especially the toenails, become hard, thick, brittle, and yellowish.

BLOOD

The **hematopoietic system** consists of blood (both cells and plasma), bone marrow, the liver, the spleen, and the kidneys. The cellular components of blood are formed by the differentiation of a **pluripotent stem cell** in a process termed **hematopoiesis.** In the fetus, hematopoiesis occurs first outside of the bone marrow (*extramedullary hematopoiesis*) in the liver, spleen, lymph nodes, and thymus. By the fourth month, the developing bone marrow begins to produce blood cells (*intramedullary hematopoiesis*). After birth, the bone marrow is the primary site of blood cell production and extramedullary hematopoiesis greatly diminishes, occurring mostly in the liver and spleen. By adulthood, hematopoiesis occurs exclusively in the bone marrow unless a pathological state exists.

In hematopoiesis, the stem cell reproduces to maintain a constant population of cells. Some stem cells then further differentiate into myeloid multipotent stem cells that, in turn, differentiate into unipotent progenitors. These unipotent progenitors ultimately mature into *basophils, eosinophils, neutrophils, monocytes* (types of white blood cells), *erythrocytes* (red blood cells), and *thrombocytes* (platelets.) Pluripotent stem cells may also differentiate into common lymphoid stem cells that ultimately mature into *lymphocytes* (another type of white cell). The kidney, and to a lesser extent the liver, produce **erythropoietin,** the hormone responsible for red blood cell production. The liver also removes toxins from the blood and produces many of the clotting factors and proteins in plasma. The spleen, an important part of the immune system, has cells that scavenge abnormal blood cells and bacteria.

Blood volume normally remains relatively constant at about 6% of total body weight. With an average of 80 to 85 mL of blood per kilogram of body weight, a person who weighs 75 kilograms has approximately 6 liters of blood. The body can easily handle up to about one-half liter of lost blood or fluid. An example is routine blood donations where healthy donors tolerate the blood loss without complication.

The major determinants of the blood volume are red cell mass and plasma volume. Red blood cells remain confined to the intravascular compartment. If their destruction remains constant, then only changes in the rate of production can alter the size of the circulating red cell mass. The plasma volume on the other hand can rapidly change due to fluid shifts between the intravascular and extravascular space. These fluid shifts help to preserve circulating blood volume in the event of acute hemorrhage. Other compensatory mechanisms include vasoconstriction, tachycardia, and increased cardiac contractility to maintain adequate tissue perfusion until significant losses overwhelm these measures. When these compensatory measures fail, the patient enters decompensated shock. Fortunately, a young, healthy individual can compensate for loss of as much as 25% to 30% of blood volume.

Content Review

HEMATOPOIETIC SYSTEM COMPONENTS
- Bone marrow
- Liver
- Spleen
- Kidneys
- Blood

hematopoietic system body system having to do with the production and development of blood cells, consisting of the bone marrow, liver, spleen, kidneys, and the blood itself.

pluripotent stem cell a cell from which the various types of blood cells can form.

hematopoiesis the process through which pluripotent stem cells differentiate into various types of blood cells.

erythropoietin the hormone responsible for red blood cell production.

Content Review

COMPONENTS OF BLOOD

- Plasma
- Formed elements
  - Red blood cells
  - White blood cells
  - Platelets

plasma thick, pale yellow fluid that makes up the liquid part of the blood.

COMPONENTS OF BLOOD

Blood consists of liquid, or plasma, and of formed elements—red blood cells, white blood cells, and platelets.

Plasma

Plasma is a thick, pale yellow fluid that is 90% to 92% water and 6% to 7% proteins. Fats, carbohydrates, electrolytes, gases, and certain chemical messengers comprise the remaining 2% to 3%. Plasma transports the cellular components of blood and dissolved nutrients throughout the body and, at the same time, transports waste products from cellular metabolism to the liver, kidneys, and lungs, where they can be removed from the body.

Most plasma components can move back and forth across the capillary membranes to the interstitial fluid. However, plasma proteins, such as albumin, are large molecules and have great difficulty diffusing across the membranes. This is fortunate, since they remain in the plasma to help retain water in the capillaries. As noted earlier, this is known as *oncotic force,* or *colloid osmotic pressure.* Plasma proteins perform many other functions, including clotting of blood, dismantling of clots, buffering of the blood's acid-base balance, transporting hormones and regulating their effects, and providing a source of energy.

Electrolytes are also found in the plasma. (As noted earlier, these are chemical substances that dissociate into charged particles in water.) They are essential for nerve conduction, muscle contraction, and water balance. They can easily diffuse across capillary membranes based on their concentration gradients. Carbohydrates in plasma are generally in the form of glucose, the primary energy source for all body tissues. Glucose is especially important to brain cells as they cannot obtain energy from fat metabolism. (Glucose cannot diffuse across most cell membranes without assistance from the hormone insulin.) Plasma also performs a role in gas transport. In addition to being carried by red blood cells, carbon dioxide and oxygen are dissolved and transported in plasma.

Red blood cells

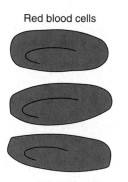

FIGURE 2-9   Red blood cells.

Red Blood Cells

The primary function of blood is to transport oxygen from the lungs to the tissues. At rest, the body consumes about 4 mL of oxygen per kilogram of body weight every minute. Because it stores little oxygen, the body would quickly succumb to anoxia without the continued transport provided by the blood.

The red blood cell (RBC), or **erythrocyte,** is a biconcave disc that does not have a nucleus when mature (Figure 2-9). It contains **hemoglobin** molecules that transport oxygen. Hemoglobin comprises four subunits of *globin,* each bonded to a *heme* (iron containing) molecule. Each globin subunit can bind with one oxygen molecule; thus, each complete hemoglobin molecule can carry up to four oxygen molecules. When all four subunits are carrying an oxygen molecule, the hemoglobin is 100% saturated. When fully saturated, each gram of hemoglobin can transport 1.34 mL of oxygen.

erythrocyte red blood cell.

hemoglobin oxygen-bearing molecule in the red blood cells. It is made up of iron-rich red pigment called *heme* and a protein called *globin.*

pO_2 partial pressure of oxygen (*partial pressure* is the pressure exerted by a given component of a gas containing several components).

pCO_2 partial pressure of carbon dioxide.

Oxygen Transport   The effectiveness of oxygen transport depends on many factors. Red blood cell mass (the number of red blood cells present) is obviously a factor in oxygen transport. The greater the number of red blood cells, the greater the potential oxygen carrying capacity. The percentage of oxygen bound to hemoglobin increases as the **pO_2** increases. This is illustrated in the oxygen-hemoglobin dissociation curve (Figure 2-10). Normal pO_2 is approximately 95 mmHg. Based on this, the oxygen-hemoglobin dissociation curve indicates that normal oxygen saturation is about 97%. Hemoglobin's affinity for oxygen is also a factor in oxygen transport. Several factors affect oxygen affinity, including pH, **pCO_2,** concentration of 2,3-DPG, and temperature.

The lower the pH (that is, the more acidic the blood), the more readily hemoglobin releases oxygen. This shifts the oxygen-hemoglobin dissociation curve to the right. In contrast, alkalosis makes hemoglobin bind to oxygen more tightly. This shifts the oxygen-hemoglobin dissociation curve to the left (Figure 2-11). The pCO_2 is directly related to the pH. Thus, in the lungs, as pCO_2 decreases with diffusion of CO_2 into the alveoli, the quantity of oxygen that binds with the hemoglobin increases. The opposite effect occurs when the blood reaches

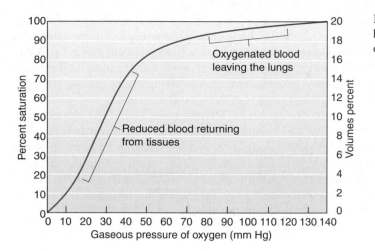

FIGURE 2-10 The oxygen-hemoglobin dissociation curve.

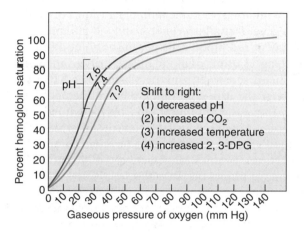

FIGURE 2-11 Effects of pH, increased carbon dioxide, temperature, and 2,3-DPG on the oxygen-hemoglobin dissociation curve.

Shift to right:
(1) decreased pH
(2) increased CO_2
(3) increased temperature
(4) increased 2, 3-DPG

the tissues. There, waste CO_2 from the tissues diffuses into the blood, causing the hemoglobin to give up more oxygen to the tissues. This is called the **Bohr effect.**

Except for hemoglobin, the most abundant chemical in red blood cells is **2,3-diphosphoglycerate (2,3-DPG).** During prolonged periods of hypoxia, the level of 2,3-DPG increases. This shifts the oxygen-hemoglobin dissociation curve to the right and can increase the pCO_2 in the plasma as much as 10% more than it otherwise would have been. However, the increased 2,3-DPG makes it more difficult for oxygen to combine with hemoglobin in the lungs. This effect casts doubt on whether 2,3-DPG's effect in hypoxia is as beneficial as was once thought.

An elevation in the body temperature causes a shift to the right of the oxygen-hemoglobin dissociation curve and a decrease in hemoglobin's affinity for blood. Conversely, a fall in body temperature causes hemoglobin to bind oxygen more tightly. During periods of hyperthermia and pyrexia (fever), hemoglobin's decreased affinity for oxygen enhances oxygenation of the peripheral tissues and end organs.

Exercise has several effects on oxygen affinity. First, exercise causes the production and release of carbon dioxide and other acids, especially from the large muscles. It also increases body temperature. Thus, both a decrease in pH and an increase in body temperature causes hemoglobin to release oxygen more readily. This serves to enhance peripheral tissue oxygenation during strenuous exercise and work.

Importantly, other substances can compete with oxygen for hemoglobin's binding sites. The greater a substance's affinity for the binding sites, the more readily the substance binds with hemoglobin. The classic example is carbon monoxide (CO). Carbon monoxide has 210–250 times oxygen's affinity for hemoglobin and competes for the same binding sites. In carbon monoxide poisoning, when CO binds to one of the hemoglobin molecule's four binding sites, the hemoglobin molecule is altered so that the remaining three oxygen molecules are held more tightly. This inhibits oxygen release in the peripheral tissues, contributing to hypoxia, acidosis, and eventually shock.

Bohr effect phenomenon in which a decrease in pCO_2/acidity causes an increase in the quantity of oxygen that binds with the hemoglobin; conversely, an increase in pCO_2/acidity causes the hemoglobin to give up a greater quantity of oxygen.

2,3-diphosphoglycerate (2,3-DPG) chemical in the red blood cells that affects hemoglobin's affinity for oxygen.

erythropoiesis the process of producing red blood cells.

hemolysis destruction of red blood cells.

sequestration the trapping of red blood cells by an organ such as the spleen.

hematocrit the packed cell volume of red blood cells per unit of blood.

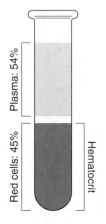

FIGURE 2-12 Hematocrit, including plasma.

Content Review

WHITE BLOOD CELLS
—BLASTS
- Myeloblasts
- Monoblasts
- Lymphoblasts

leukocyte white blood cell.

chemotaxis the movement of white blood cells in response to chemical signals.

phagocytosis process in which white blood cells engulf and destroy an invader.

Red Blood Cell Production Red blood cell production is termed **erythropoiesis.** Erythropoietin, a hormone produced primarily by the kidney, stimulates the bone marrow's production of erythrocytes. Erythropoietin is secreted when the renal cells sense hypoxia. This in turn stimulates the bone marrow to increase RBC production, resulting in increased red cell mass. Although a relatively slow process, this effectively increases the oxygen carrying capacity of blood, thereby increasing oxygen delivery to the tissues.

The red blood cell lives approximately 120 days. Hemorrhage, **hemolysis** (destruction of the RBC), or **sequestration** of the RBCs by the liver or spleen may significantly reduce its life span. Hemorrhage may occur outside the body or be hidden within a body cavity such as the peritoneum, retroperitoneum, or GI tract. Hemolysis may occur within the circulatory system in sickle cell disease and in rare autoimmune anemias. The spleen and liver contain specialized scavenger cells called *macrophages* (a type of white blood cell) that can remove damaged or abnormal red blood cells from the circulation.

Laboratory Evaluation of Red Blood Cells and Hemoglobin Red blood cells (RBC) are quantified or measured and reported in two ways, RBC count and hematocrit. The RBC count is the total number of RBCs reported in millions per cubic millimeter (mm^3) of blood. Normal values vary with age and sex but in general run between 4.2 and 6.0 million/mm^3.

The **hematocrit** is the packed cell volume of red blood cells per unit of blood (Figure 2-12). This measurement is obtained by placing a sample of blood in a centrifuge and spinning it at high speed so that the cellular elements separate from the plasma. The RBCs are the heaviest blood component since they carry the iron-containing pigment hemoglobin. They are forced to the bottom of the tube. Above the red blood cells are the white blood cells. On the top of the specimen is the plasma, which consists primarily of water. The RBCs' column height is divided by the blood's total column height (cellular component plus plasma) and reported as a percentage. Normal values range between 40% and 52%, with females generally running a few percentage points below males.

Another way to determine the status of red blood cells is to measure the concentration of hemoglobin present. This is typically expressed as the number of grams of hemoglobin present per deciliter of whole blood. The hemoglobin concentration decreases in two ways. First, when the number of red blood cells present is below normal, the hemoglobin is also below normal. In some cases, the red blood cell volume can be normal, but the amount of hemoglobin present may be decreased. In emergency medicine, it is commonplace to measure the hemoglobin in addition to the hematocrit (H&H). Both values indicate red blood cell volume and capability. The normal hemoglobin in a man is 12.0 to 15.0 g/dL; for a woman, it is 10.5 to 14.0 g/dL.

White Blood Cells

White blood cells (WBCs), called **leukocytes** or white corpuscles, circulate through the bloodstream and tissues, providing protection from foreign invasion. They are extremely mobile, traveling through the blood stream to wherever they are needed in order to fight infection.

A large population of leukocytes does not move freely within the blood stream but instead is attached to the blood vessels' walls. These *marginated* leukocytes may quickly return to the circulating pool in response to stress, corticosteroids, seizures, epinephrine, and exercise. This process is called *demargination*. Marginated leukocytes that attach more firmly to the vascular lining through *adhesion* may then leave the blood vessels by *diapedesis*. This enables the leukocytes to squeeze between the cells lining the blood vessels and to follow chemical signals (**chemotaxis**) to the infection site. There, they may engulf and destroy an invader by **phagocytosis** (Figure 2-13). Others stimulate either chemical or immune responses to fight infection.

Healthy people have from 5,000 to 9,000 white blood cells per microliter of blood. An infection can increase that number to more than 16,000. Such an increase is a classical sign of bacterial infection. White blood cells originate in the bone marrow from undifferentiated

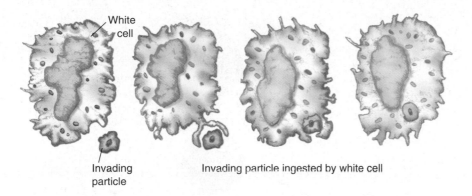

White cell

Invading particle

Invading particle ingested by white cell

FIGURE 2-13   White blood cells engulfing and destroying an invader in the process called *phagocytosis.*

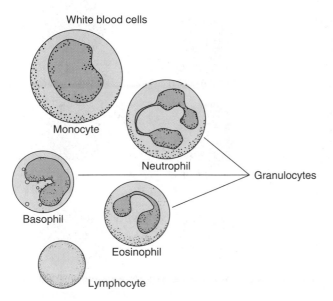

White blood cells

Monocyte

Neutrophil

Granulocytes

Basophil

Eosinophil

Lymphocyte

FIGURE 2-14   Types of white blood cells.

leukopoiesis the process through which stem cells differentiate into the white blood cells' immature forms.

stem cells. Through a process termed **leukopoiesis,** these stem cells respond to specific growth factors that allow them to differentiate into three main blasts (immature forms): myeloblasts, monoblasts, and lymphoblasts.

WBCs are categorized as *granulocytes, monocytes,* or *lymphocytes* (Figure 2-14).

Granulocytes   Granulocytic WBCs, so named for the granules they contain, form from stem cells that differentiate in the bone marrow in response to hormonal stimulation. These cells mature through several stages from myeloblast to promyelocyte, myelocyte, metamyelocyte, band form, and mature form (Figure 2-15). Their mature forms are classified by the type of stain they absorb: *basophils* absorb basic stains and have blue granules; *eosinophils* absorb acidic stains and contain red granules; *neutrophils* absorb neither acidic nor basic stains well and contain pale blue and pink granules.

Basophils are granulocytes that primarily function in allergic reactions. Within their granules they store all of the histamine in the circulating blood. In response to an allergic stimulus, the cells degranulate, releasing histamines that cause vasodilation, bronchoconstriction, rhinorrhea, increased vascular permeability, and increased neutrophil and eosinophil chemotaxis. Basophils also contain heparin, which breaks down blood clots.

Eosinophils are highly specialized members of the granulocytic series. They can inactivate the chemical mediators of acute allergic reactions, thereby modulating the anaphylactic

Content Review

WHITE BLOOD CELL CATEGORIES
• Granulocytes
• Monocytes
• Lymphocytes

Content Review

GRANULOCYTE CLASSIFICATIONS
• Basophils
• Eosinophils
• Neutrophils

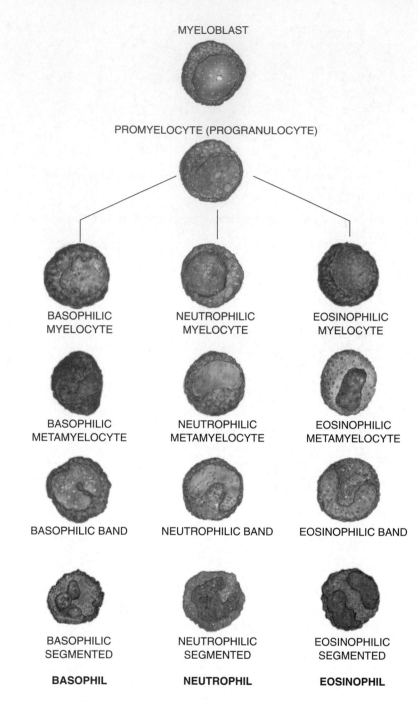

MYELOBLAST

PROMYELOCYTE (PROGRANULOCYTE)

| BASOPHILIC MYELOCYTE | NEUTROPHILIC MYELOCYTE | EOSINOPHILIC MYELOCYTE |

| BASOPHILIC METAMYELOCYTE | NEUTROPHILIC METAMYELOCYTE | EOSINOPHILIC METAMYELOCYTE |

| BASOPHILIC BAND | NEUTROPHILIC BAND | EOSINOPHILIC BAND |

| BASOPHILIC SEGMENTED | NEUTROPHILIC SEGMENTED | EOSINOPHILIC SEGMENTED |

BASOPHIL   **NEUTROPHIL**   **EOSINOPHIL**

FIGURE 2-15 Granulocyte maturation.

major basic protein (MBP) a larvacidal peptide.

neutropenia a low neutrophil count.

response. They also contain **major basic protein (MBP),** which they release in conjunction with an antibody response shown to fight parasitic infections.

Neutrophils primary function is to fight infection. They leave the blood stream by diapedesis and engulf and kill microorganisms that have invaded the body. Once they have phagocytized the microorganism, primary and secondary granules within the neutrophil fuse with the phagosome, and the organism is killed and digested. In severe infections the total neutrophil count may rise rapidly, with immature (band) forms apparent on the peripheral blood smear under microscopic examination. If the neutrophil count is low (**neutropenia**), the body cannot mount an appropriate response to infection, and the infection may overwhelm the body's defenses and kill the individual. Neutropenia may result from primary bone marrow disorders that decrease production, from overwhelming infection, viral syndrome, autoimmune disease, or drugs, and from nutritional deficiencies.

Monocytes   Monocytes are unique in that after their initial phase of maturation they are released into the circulation and can remain there as circulating monocytes or migrate to distant sites to further mature into free or fixed tissue macrophages. Macrophages, the "garbage collectors" of the immune system, engulf both foreign invaders and dead neutrophils. They also can attack tumor cells and participate in tissue repair. Monocytes and macrophages also secrete growth factors to stimulate production of granulocytes and red blood cells. Some macrophages are fixed within tissues, residing in the liver, spleen, lungs, and lymphatic system. These cells are part of the reticuloendothelial system. They remove foreign matter, cellular debris, and proteins from the blood. After engulfing foreign proteins or infectious agents, these fixed macrophages of the reticuloendothelial system can stimulate lymphocyte production in an immune response against these agents.

Lymphocytes   Lymphocytes are the primary cells involved in the body's immune response. They are located throughout the body in the circulating blood as well as in other tissues such as lymph nodes, circulating in lymph fluid, bone marrow, spleen, liver, lungs, intestine, and skin. Lymphocytes are characteristically small, round, white blood cells containing no granules on staining. However similar they may appear, these cells are highly specialized. They contain surface receptor sites specific to a single antigen (foreign protein) and stand ready to initiate the immune response to rid the body of that particular substance or infectious agent.

Immunity   The two basic subpopulations of lymphocytes are T cells and B cells. T cells mature in the thymus gland, located in the mediastinum, and then migrate throughout the body. They are responsible for developing cell-mediated immunity, also called *cellular immunity*. Once an antigen activates them, they generate other cells called *effector cells* that are responsible for delayed-type hypersensitivity reactions, tumor suppression, graft rejection (organ transplant rejections), and defense against intracellular organisms. B cells produce antibodies to combat infection, which is termed *humoral immunity*. They originate in the bone marrow and then migrate to peripheral lymphatic tissues. There they can be exposed to antigens from invading organisms and respond by producing the specific antibodies necessary to defend against them. Some of these B cells' lines are maintained and give the body a "memory" of the previous infection. When the body is subsequently exposed to the same antigen or infection, it generates a rapid response to quickly overwhelm the infection.

Autoimmune Disease   Autoimmune disease occurs when the body makes antibodies against its own tissues. These antibodies may be limited to specific organs, such as the thyroid, as occurs in *Hashimoto's thyroiditis*. Or, they may involve virtually every tissue type as in the antinuclear antibodies of *systemic lupus erythematosis (SLE)* that attack the body's cell nuclei. Several anemias result from autoimmunity. Mechanisms for the development of autoimmune disease include genetic factors and viral infections.

autoimmune disease condition in which the body makes antibodies against its own tissues.

Alterations in Immune Response   Several factors can alter the body's immune response. For example, patients who receive an organ transplant must take drugs that inhibit cellular immunity and prevent graft rejection. If they do not, the T cells will recognize the new organ as "not self" and begin the process of attacking it. This is called *rejection*. Unfortunately, organ recipient immunosuppressed patients are at risk for infections from many different organisms including bacteria, viruses, fungi, and protozoa. Human immunodeficiency virus (HIV) effectively destroys cell-mediated immunity by selectively attacking and ultimately killing T cells. This also leaves the patient at risk for opportunistic infections against which the body cannot defend itself, ultimately killing him. Patients who have cancer are often immunocompromised by the disease itself or by chemotherapy agents that also attack the bone marrow. These agents decrease leukocyte production to extremely low levels, leaving the body defenseless against infection. As an EMT-I, you must protect your immunosuppressed patients from undue exposure to infection by good hand-washing technique, correct IV technique, and proper wound care. If you have an infection, you must take precautions not to transmit it to your patients. If the infection is highly contagious, as in influenza or chicken pox, you may have to work in a non–patient-care setting.

Inflammatory Process   The **inflammatory process** is a nonspecific defense mechanism that wards off damage from microorganisms or trauma. It attempts to localize the damage

inflammatory process a non-specific defense mechanism that wards off damage from microorganisms or trauma.

thrombocyte blood platelet.

hemostasis the combined
mechanisms that work to
prevent or control blood loss.

while destroying the source, at the same time facilitating repair of the tissues. Causes of the inflammatory process may be an infectious agent, trauma, chemical, or immunologic. After local tissue injury occurs, the damaged tissues release chemical messengers that attract white blood cells (chemotaxis), increase capillary permeability, and cause vasodilation. If bacteria are present, responding neutrophils or macrophages phagocytize them and tissue repair begins. The greater capillary permeability and vasodilation allows increased blood flow to the area and enables fluid to leak out of the capillaries. The process of local inflammation results in redness, warmth, swelling, and usually pain. The pain serves as a reminder against overuse, allowing time for rest and repair. Systemic inflammation is an inflammatory reaction, often in response to a bacterial infection. Fever is a common symptom and likely occurs in response to chemical mediators that macrophages release in response to the infectious agent. These chemical mediators act on the brain and lead to stimulation of the sympathetic nervous system, which causes vasoconstriction, heat conservation, and fever. The macrophages also release factors that stimulate the release of leukocytes from the bone marrow, leading to an elevated white blood cell count.

Platelets

Platelets, or **thrombocytes,** are small fragments of large cells called *megakaryocytes.* Like the other blood cells described so far, megakaryocytes come from an undifferentiated stem cell in the bone marrow. The hormone *thrombopoietin* stimulates these stem cells to differentiate through several stages into megakaryocytes, which then mature and break up into platelets, small fragments without nuclei. The normal number of platelets ranges from 150,000 to 450,000 per microliter of blood. As they function to form a plug at an initial bleeding site and also secrete factors important in clot formation, too few platelets, a condition called *thrombocytopenia,* can lead to bleeding problems and blood loss. Too many platelets, *thrombocytosis,* may cause abnormal clotting, plugs in vessels, and emboli that may travel to the extremities, heart, lungs, or brain. Platelets survive from seven to ten days and are removed from circulation by the spleen.

Platelets are activated when they contact injured tissue. This contact stimulates an enzyme within the platelet, causing the surface to become "sticky," which in turn leads the platelets to aggregate and form a plug. Platelets also adhere to the damaged tissue to keep the plug in place. As the platelets aggregate, they release chemical messengers that also activate the blood clotting system.

HEMOSTASIS

Hemostasis—from *hemo* (blood) and *stasis* (standing still)—is the term used to describe the combined three mechanisms that work to prevent or control blood loss. These mechanisms include:

- Vascular spasms
- Platelet plugs
- Stable fibrin blood clots (coagulation)

When a blood vessel tears, the smooth muscle fibers (*tunica media*) in the vessel walls contract. This causes vasoconstriction and reduces the size of the tear. Less blood flows through the constricted area, effectively limiting blood loss, and the smaller tear makes it easier for a platelet plug to develop and stop blood loss. At any tear in a blood vessel, platelets aggregate and adhere to collagen, a connective tissue that supports the blood vessels. This forms a platelet plug, which acts much like bubble gum stuck into a hole. The plug is unstable, however, and would permit the vessel to bleed again if not for the formation of a stable fibrin clot. This process, blood coagulation, is initiated in part by the platelet plug (Figure 2-16).

Because of the smoothness of the *tunica intima,* the blood vessels' innermost lining, blood normally flows through the vessels without frictional damage to cells or platelets. Damage to cells or to the vessel lining, however, starts the coagulation cascade. This cascade, or sequence of events, can be activated either by damage to vessels (extrinsic pathway) or by trauma to blood from turbulence (intrinsic pathway). Either results in the cascade's progres-

Broken Blood Vessel Wall

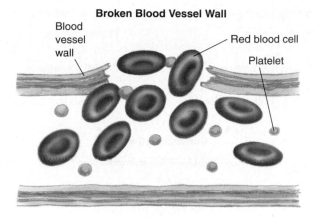

Blood vessel wall

Red blood cell

Platelet

FIGURE 2-16 Clot formation.

Clot Formation

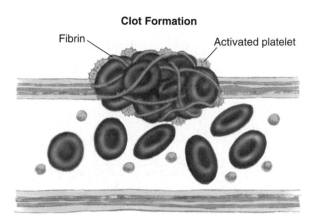

Fibrin

Activated platelet

sion to a clot. Most clotting proteins are produced in the liver and circulate in an inactive state. The best known of these are *prothrombin* and *fibrinogen*. The damaged cells send out a chemical message that activates a specific clotting factor. This activates each protein in turn, until a stable fibrin clot forms. To completely stop the bleeding, the coagulation cascade relies on the platelet plug and the clotting factors to interact. Once the bleeding stops, the inflammatory and healing processes can begin. The coagulation cascade can be summarized thus (Figure 2-17):

1. *Intrinsic pathway.* Platelets release substances that lead to the formation of prothrombin activator

    or

    Extrinsic pathway. Tissue damage causes platelet aggregation and the formation of prothrombin activator.

2. *Common pathway.* The prothrombin activator, in the presence of calcium, converts prothrombin to thrombin.

3. *Thrombin.* In the presence of calcium, thrombin converts fibrinogen to stable fibrin, which then traps blood cells and more platelets to form a clot.

The development of a clot does not end the coagulation cascade. What the body can do it usually can undo, given sufficient time. Once a fibrin clot is formed, it releases a chemical called *plasminogen*. Plasminogen is converted to *plasmin* and is then capable of dismantling, or lysing, a clot through the process of **fibrinolysis**. A clot's dismantling generally takes from hours to days. By that time, scarring has begun.

Thrombosis (clot formation), when it occurs in coronary arteries or cerebral vasculature, may lead to heart attack and stroke. To stimulate or speed fibrinolysis and thus breakdown

fibrinolysis the process through which plasmin dismantles a blood clot.

thrombosis clot formation, which is extremely dangerous when it occurs in coronary arteries or cerebral vasculature.

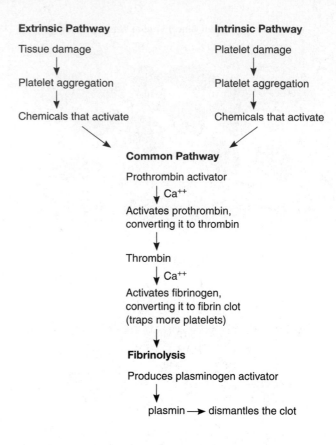

FIGURE 2-17 The coagulation cascade.

Extrinsic Pathway

Tissue damage

↓

Platelet aggregation

↓

Chemicals that activate

Intrinsic Pathway

Platelet damage

↓

Platelet aggregation

↓

Chemicals that activate

Common Pathway

Prothrombin activator

↓ Ca^{++}

Activates prothrombin, converting it to thrombin

↓

Thrombin

↓ Ca^{++}

Activates fibrinogen, converting it to fibrin clot (traps more platelets)

↓

Fibrinolysis

Produces plasminogen activator

↓

plasmin → dismantles the clot

clots, medical researchers have developed several thrombolytic agents. These agents may help reestablish blood flow to these vital organs, limiting or preventing tissue death, and thus helping to prevent the patient's disability or death. Thrombolytics are effective only against blockages whose components include a fibrin clot.

Patients who lack certain clotting factors can have bleeding disorders that may complicate their assessment and treatment. Other patients take medications that decrease the effectiveness of platelets or the coagulation cascade. Recall that an enzyme on a platelet membrane makes the membrane sticky. Certain medications such as aspirin, dipyridamole (Persantine), and ticlopidine (Ticlid) irreversibly alter the enzyme, thus decreasing the platelets' ability to aggregate and initiate the coagulation cascade. Other medications such as heparin and warfarin (Coumadin) cause changes within the clotting cascade that prevent clot formation. Heparin, in conjunction with antithrombin III (a naturally occurring thrombin inactivator), rapidly inactivates thrombin, which then prevents formation of the fibrin clot. Warfarin (Coumadin) blocks vitamin K activity necessary to generate the activated forms of clotting factors II, VII, IX, and X, effectively interrupting the clotting cascade.

Vitamin K (AquaMEPHYTON) enhances clotting. Certain byproducts of tobacco smoking (especially in females on birth control pills) also enhance clotting. Relative or complete immobility, trauma, polycythemia (high red blood cell count), and cancer may also lead to increased clotting as blood becomes relatively stagnant. This allows platelet activation to begin, which leads to clotting. To counteract the effects of decreased activity, many patients take aspirin or other antiplatelet inhibitors and wear compressive stockings to facilitate venous drainage from the lower extremities.

MUSCULOSKELETAL SYSTEM

The musculoskeletal system is a complex arrangement of levers and fulcrums, powered by biochemical motors, that provides motion and support for the body. It consists of two distinct subsystems, the skeleton and the muscles. The skeleton is the human body's superstructure, whereas the muscles supply the power of motion to this superstructure, the

Patho Pearls

Vitamin K is an antidote for toxicity due to the anticoagulant warfarin (Coumadin).

Patho Pearls

Medications and fluids can be administered by placing a needle into the medullary canal of selected bones (proximal tibia, sternum). This procedure, called *intraosseous therapy*, should be reserved for cases where other routes of venous access prove unavailable.

organs, and the other body components. These subsystems also produce body heat, store essential salts and energy sources, and create the majority of blood cells for transporting oxygen and combating disease.

The musculoskeletal system is covered by the skin and subcutaneous tissue. These elements protect the skeleton and muscles, as well as other body systems, from trauma, fluid loss, infection, and fluctuations in body temperature. The skin also provides some cushioning for the skeletal components, as on the soles of the feet during walking.

SKELETAL TISSUE AND STRUCTURE

As the body's living framework, the skeleton has a structure and design that permits it to perform a variety of functions and to repair itself as needed within limits. The skeleton is a complex, living system of cells, salt deposits, protein fibers, and other specialized elements. Besides giving the body its structural form, the skeleton serves four other important purposes:

- It protects the vital organs.
- It allows for efficient movement despite the forces of gravity.
- It stores many salts and other materials needed for metabolism.
- It produces the red blood cells used to transport oxygen.

Although the skeleton is not often thought of as alive, it is exactly that. Its cells live within a matrix of protein fibers and salt deposits. These living cells constantly change the structure and dynamics of the human frame. In fact, 20% of the total bone mass (salts, protein fiber, and bone cells) is replaced each year by the remodeling process.

Bone Structure

The structure of a typical bone consists of numerous aligned cylinders of bone. Minute blood vessels travel lengthwise along the bone through small tubes, called **haversian canals.** These blood vessels are surrounded by layers of salts deposited in collagen fibers. Bone cells called **osteocytes** are trapped within the matrix and maintain the collagen and the calcium, phosphate, carbonate, and other salt crystals. Other bone cells, osteoblasts and osteoclasts, deposit or dissolve these salt deposits as necessary. **Osteoblasts** lay down new bone in areas of stress during growth and during the bone repair cycle. **Osteoclasts** dissolve bone structures that are not carrying the pressures of articulation and support or when the body requires more salts for electrolyte balance. These three types of bone cells maintain a dynamic and efficient structure for supporting and moving the body.

A continuous blood supply brings oxygen and nutrients to the bones and removes carbon dioxide and waste products from them. The blood vessels enter and exit the bone shaft through **perforating canals** and distribute blood to both the bone tissue and the structures located within the medullary canal of the shaft and bone ends. As with any other body tissue, bone tissue becomes ischemic and will eventually die if the blood supply is reduced or cut off. The bone does not show evidence of such degeneration for quite some time, and certainly not during prehospital emergency care. However, the long-term effects of **devascularization** may be devastating.

The long bones, such as those of the forearm (humerus) and thigh (femur), best demonstrate the organization of bone tissue into structural body elements (Figure 2-18). The major areas and tissues of the long bones include the diaphysis, the epiphysis, the metaphysis, the medullary canal, the periosteum, and the articular cartilage.

Diaphysis   The **diaphysis** is the central portion or shaft of the long bone. It consists of a very dense and relatively thin layer of compact bone. Because of its tubular structure, the diaphysis efficiently supports weight yet is relatively light. Although the design of the bone shaft enables it to carry weight well, lateral forces may cause the shaft to break rather easily.

Epiphysis   Toward the ends of the long bone, its structure changes. The bone's diameter increases dramatically, and the underlying thin, hard, compact bone of the shaft changes to a network of skeletal fibers and strands. This network, called the **epiphysis,** spreads the stresses and pressures of weight bearing over a larger surface. The tissue of the epiphysis in

Some 20% of the total bone mass is replaced each year by the remodeling process.

haversian canals small perforations of the long bones through which the blood vessels and nerves travel into the bone itself.

osteocytes bone forming cell found in the bone matrix that helps maintain the bone.

osteoblasts cells that help in the creation of new bone during growth and bone repair.

osteoclasts bone cells that absorb and remove excess bone.

perforating canals structures through which blood vessels enter and exit the bone shaft.

devascularization loss of blood vessels from a body part.

diaphysis hollow shaft found in long bones.

epiphysis end of a long bone, including the epiphyseal, or growth plate and supporting structures underlying the joint.

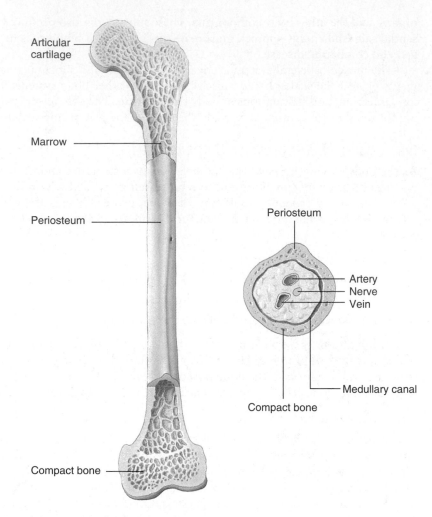

FIGURE 2-18 The internal anatomy of a long bone.

cancellous having a latticework structure, as in the spongy tissue of a bone.

articular surface surface of a bone that moves against another bone.

metaphysis growth zone of a bone, active during the development stages of youth. It is located between the epiphysis and the diaphysis.

epiphyseal plate area of the metaphysis where cartilage is generated during bone growth in childhood. Also called *growth plate.*

medullary canal cavity within a bone that contains the marrow.

yellow bone marrow tissue that stores fat in semi-liquid form within the internal cavities of a bone.

red bone marrow tissue within the internal cavity of a bone responsible for manufacture of erythrocytes and other blood cells.

periosteum the tough exterior covering of a bone.

cross-section resembles a rigid bony sponge and is called spongy or **cancellous** bone. Covering this network of fibers is a very thin layer of compact bone supporting the surface that meets and moves against another bone, the **articular surface.**

Metaphysis   The **metaphysis** is an intermediate region between the epiphysis and diaphysis. It is where the diaphysis's hollow tube of compact bone makes the transition to the bone-fiber honeycomb of the epiphysis's cancellous bone. In this region is the **epiphyseal plate,** also called the *growth plate.* During childhood, cartilage is generated here and the plate widens. Osteoblasts from the end of the diaphysis deposit salts within the cartilage's collagen matrix to create new bone tissue. This results in the lengthening of the infant's and then the child's bone. During the growth period, the epiphyseal plate is also weaker than the rest of the bone and associated joints and is thus a frequent site of fractures in pediatric patients.

Medullary Canal   The chamber formed within the hollow diaphysis and the cancellous bone of the epiphysis is called the **medullary canal.** The central medullary canal is filled with **yellow bone marrow** that stores fat in a semi-liquid form. The fat is a readily available energy source the body can use quickly and easily. **Red bone marrow** fills the cancellous bone chambers of the larger long bones, the pelvis, and the sternum. It is responsible for the manufacture of erythrocytes and other blood cells.

Periosteum   A tough fibrous membrane called the **periosteum** covers the exterior of the diaphysis. With extensive vasculature and innervation, it transmits sensations of pain when the bone fractures and then initiates the bone repair cycle. Blood vessels and nerves penetrate both the periosteum and compact bone by traveling through the small perforating canals. Tendons intermingle with the collagen fibers of the periosteum and with the collagen fibers of the bony matrix to form strong attachments.

Cartilage   A layer of connective tissue called **cartilage** is a continuous collagen extension of the underlying bone and covers a portion of the epiphyseal surface. It is a smooth, strong, and flexible material that functions as the actual surface of articulation between bones. Cartilage is very slippery and somewhat compressible. It permits relatively friction-free joint movement and absorbs some of the shock associated with activity, such as walking.

Classification of Bones   Bones are classified according to their general shape. Those previously described are considered long bones and include the humerus, radius, ulna, tibia, fibula, metacarpals (hand), metatarsals (foot), and phalanges (fingers and toes). The bones of the wrists and ankles, the carpals and tarsals, are short bones. The bones of the cranium, sternum, ribs, shoulder, and pelvis are classified as flat. Irregularly shaped bones include the bones of the vertebral column and the facial bones. Another special type of bone is the **sesamoid bone,** a bone that grows within tendinous tissue; one example is the kneecap, or patella.

Joint Structure

Bones move at, and are held together by, a relatively sophisticated structure called a **joint**.

Types of Joints   There are three basic types of joints, which are classified by the amount of movement they permit. **Synarthroses** are immovable joints, such as the sutures of the skull or the juncture between jaw and the teeth (which is called a *gomphosis*). **Amphiarthroses** are joints that allow some very limited movement. Examples include the joints between the vertebrae and between the sacrum and the ilium of the pelvis. **Diarthroses,** or **synovial joints,** permit relatively free movement. Such joints include the elbow, knee, shoulder, and hip.

Diarthroses are divided into three categories of joints based on the movements they allow (Figure 2-19). These include:

- *Monaxial joints*
  - Hinge joints permit bending in a single plane. Examples include the knees, elbows, and fingers.
  - Pivot joints are characterized by the articulation between the atlas (the first cervical vertebrae) and the axis of the spine. They allow the head to rotate through a wide range of motion.
- *Biaxial joints*
  - Condyloid, or gliding, joints provide movement in two directions. They are located at the joints of carpal bones in the wrist and between the clavicle and sternum.
  - Ellipsoidal joints provide a sliding motion in two planes, as between the wrist and the metacarpals.
  - Saddle joints allow for movement in two planes at right angles to each other. Examples are the joints at the bases of the thumbs.
- *Triaxial joints*. Ball-and-socket joints permit full motion in a cone of about 180 degrees and allow a limb to rotate. Examples include the hip and shoulder.

These joints permit various types of motion. **Flexion/extension** is the bending motion that reduces/increases the angle between articulating elements. **Adduction/abduction** is the movement of a body part toward/away from the **midline. Rotation** refers to a turning along the axis of a bone or joint. **Circumduction** refers to movement through an arc of a circle.

Ligaments   **Ligaments** are bands of connective tissue that hold bones together at joints. They stretch and permit motion at the joint while holding the bone ends firmly in position. The ends of the ligaments attach to the joint ends of each of the associated bones. Ligaments surround the articular region and cross it at many oblique angles. This arrangement ensures that the joint is held together firmly but flexibly enough to permit movement through a designed range of motion.

cartilage connective tissue providing the articular surfaces of the skeletal system.

sesamoid bone bone that forms in a tendon.

Bones are classified by shape.

joint area where adjacent bones articulate.

synarthroses joints that do not permit movement

amphiarthroses joints that permit a limited amount of independent motion.

diarthroses synovial joints.

synovial joint joint that permits the greatest degree of independent motion.

flexion bending motion that reduces the angle between articulating elements.

extension bending motion that increases the angle between articulating elements.

adduction movement of a body part toward the midline.

abduction movement of a body part away from midline.

midline an imaginary line drawn vertically through the middle of the body, dividing it into right and left.

rotation a turning along the axis of a bone or joint.

circumduction movement at a synovial joint where the distal end of a bone describes a circle but the shaft does not rotate; movement through an arc of a circle.

ligaments connective tissue that connects bone to bone and holds joints together.

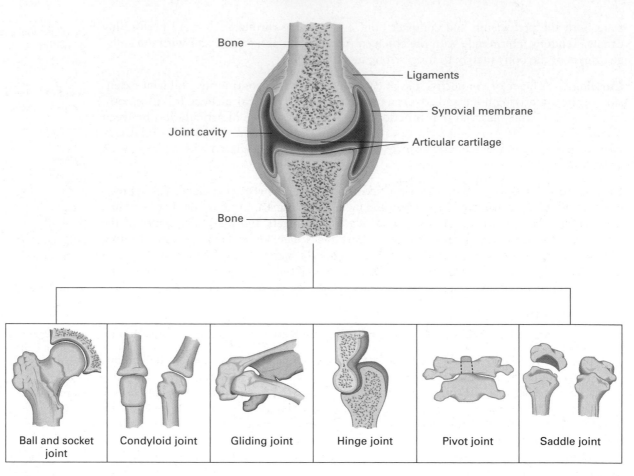

FIGURE 2-19 Types of joints.

Content Review

TYPES OF JOINTS

- Synarthroses—immovable
- Amphiarthroses—very limited movement
- Diarthroses (synovial joints)—relatively free movement:
  - Monaxial
  - Biaxial
  - Triaxial

---

joint capsule the ligaments surrounding a joint; *synovial capsule.*

---

synovial fluid substance that lubricates synovial joints.

---

bursae sacs containing synovial fluid, which cushions adjacent structures; singular *bursa.*

---

axial skeleton bones of the head, thorax, and spine.

Joint Capsule   The ligaments surrounding a joint form what is known as the **joint capsule** or *synovial capsule* (Figure 2-20). This chamber holds a small amount of fluid to lubricate the articular surfaces. This oily, viscous substance, known as **synovial fluid,** assists joint motion by reducing friction. Its lubrication reduces friction to about one fifth that of two pieces of ice sliding together. Small sacs filled with synovial fluid, known as **bursae,** are also located between tendons and ligaments or cartilage in the elbows, knees, and other joints to reduce friction and absorb shock. Synovial fluid flows into and out of the articular cartilage as the joint undergoes pressure and movement. The cartilage acts like a sponge, pushing out fluid as it is compressed and drawing in fluid when it is relaxed. This movement of synovial fluid circulates oxygen, nutrients, and waste products to and from the joint cartilage.

SKELETAL ORGANIZATION

The human skeleton is made up of approximately 206 bones (Figure 2-21). These bones form two major divisions, the axial and the appendicular skeletons.

The **axial skeleton** consists of the bones of the head, thorax, and spine. These bones form the axis of the body, protect the elements of the central nervous system, and make up the thoracic cage, which is the dynamic housing for respiration. The components of the axial skeleton will be discussed under the headings, "Head, Face, and Neck" and "Spine and Thorax."

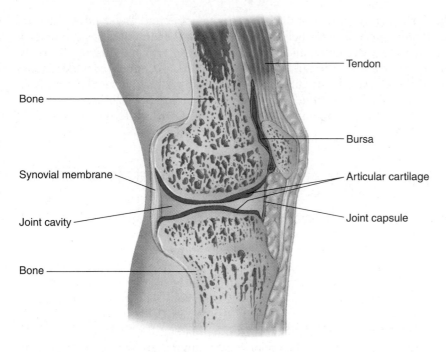

Bone

Synovial membrane

Joint cavity

Bone

Tendon

Bursa

Articular cartilage

Joint capsule

FIGURE 2-20 Structure of a joint.

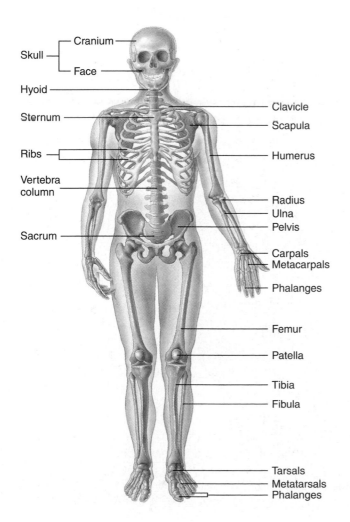

Skull
— Cranium
— Face

Hyoid

Sternum

Ribs

Vertebra column

Sacrum

Clavicle

Scapula

Humerus

Radius
Ulna
Pelvis

Carpals
Metacarpals

Phalanges

Femur

Patella

Tibia

Fibula

Tarsals
Metatarsals
Phalanges

FIGURE 2-21 The human skeleton.

The **appendicular skeleton** consists of the bones of the upper and lower extremities, including both the shoulder girdle and the pelvis, and excepting the sacrum. These bones provide the structure for the extremities and permit the major articulations of the body. Extremity long bones are similar in design and structure. Both upper and lower extremities are affixed to the axial skeleton and articulate with joints supported by several bones. Each of these extremities has a single long bone proximally and paired bones distally. The terminal member, the hand or foot, is made up of numerous bones with differing purposes, yet parallel designs.

Extremities

The extremities are the arms and legs, including the wrists and hands, elbows, shoulders, ankles and feet, knees, hips, and pelvis.

Wrists and Hands   The radius and ulna articulate with the carpal bones at the wrist, or radiocarpal joint (Figure 2-22). The carpals articulate with the metacarpals. The metacarpals articulate with the proximal phalanges at the metacarpophalangeal (MCP) joint. The proximal phalanges articulate with the middle phalanges at the proximal interphalangeal (PIP) joint. The middle phalanges articulate with the distal phalanges at the distal interphalangeal (DIP) joint. Movement at the wrist includes flexion, extension, radial deviation, and ulnar deviation. Movement at the MCP, PIP, and DIP joints includes flexion and extension. The MCP joints also allow abduction (spreading the fingers out) and adduction (bringing them back together). The major flexor muscles are the flexor carpi radialis and flexor carpi ulnaris (Figure 2-23). The major extensor muscles are the extensor carpi radialis longus, extensor carpi radialis brevis, and extensor carpi ulnaris.

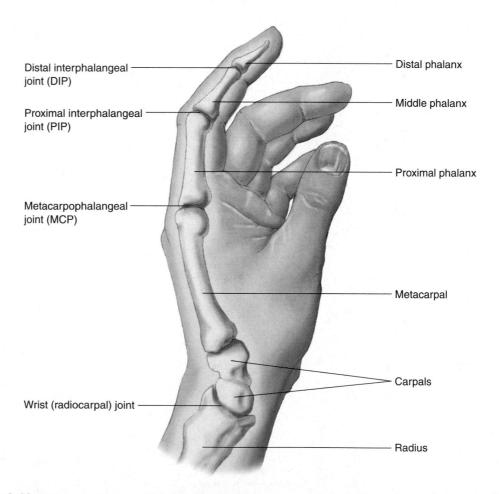

FIGURE 2-22   Bones and joints of the hand and wrist.

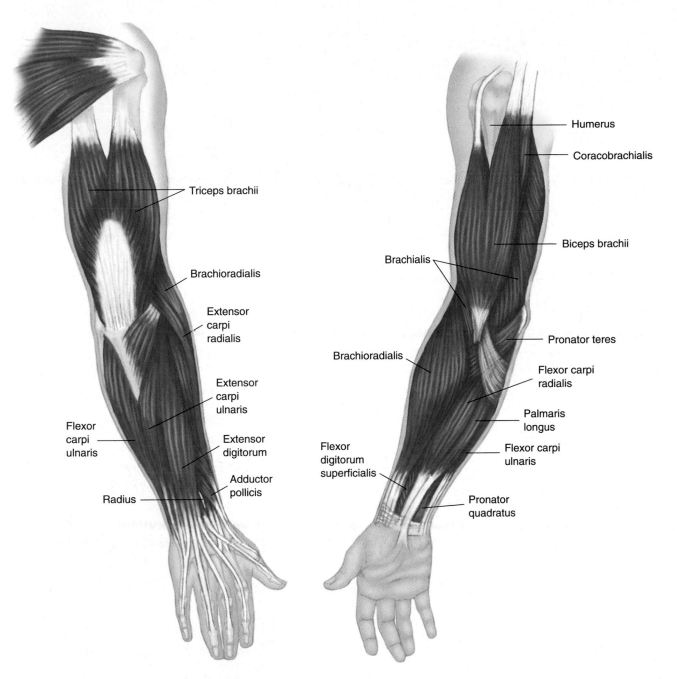

FIGURE 2-23 Muscles of the arm.

Elbows The lateral and medial epicondyles (large rounded edges) of the distal humerus, the olecranon process of the proximal ulna, and the proximal radius comprise the elbow joint (Figure 2-24). Between the olecranon process and skin lies a bursa. The ulnar nerve (funny bone) extends through the groove between the olecranon process and the medial epicondyle. The elbow is a hinge joint, allowing flexion and extension. The major flexor muscles are the biceps (Figure 2-25). The major extensor muscles are the triceps (Figure 2-26). Just below the elbow, the relationship of the radius and ulna to the pronator and supinator muscles allows the forearm to supinate (turn palm up) and pronate (turn palm down) (Figure 2-27).

Shoulders The shoulder girdle consists of articulations between the clavicle and the scapula and between the scapula and the head of the humerus (Figure 2-28). The sternoclavicular joint, which joins the clavicle and the manubrium, is the only bony link

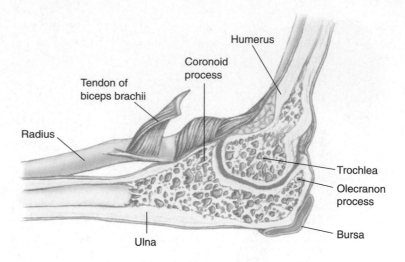

FIGURE 2-24 The elbow.

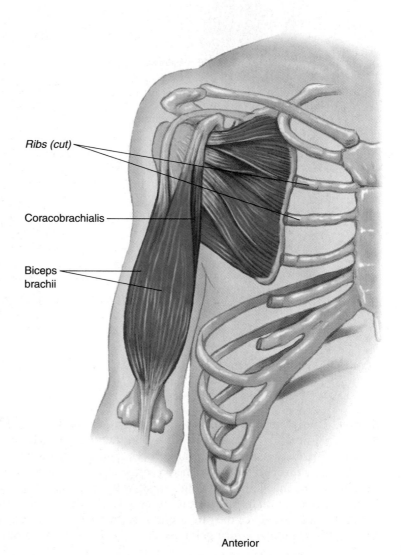

Anterior

FIGURE 2-25 Elbow flexors.

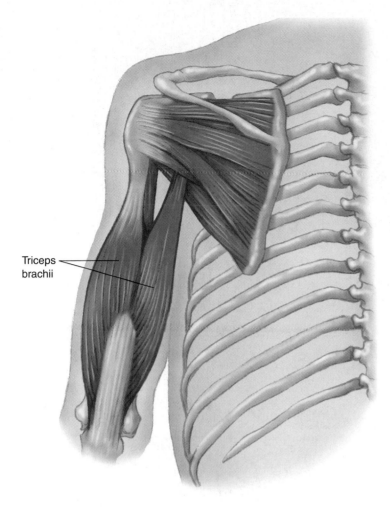

Triceps
brachii

Posterior

FIGURE 2-26 Elbow extensors.

between the upper extremity and the axial skeleton. Movement at this joint is largely passive and occurs as a result of active movements of the scapula. The distal clavicle articulates with the acromion, or acromion process, of the scapula at the acromioclavicular (AC) joint. The clavicle acts as a strut, keeping the upper limb away from the thorax and permitting a greater range of motion. The AC joint also helps provide stability to the upper limb, reducing the need for muscle energy to keep the shoulder in its proper alignment.

The glenohumeral joint is a ball-and-socket joint that allows flexion, extension, internal and external rotation, abduction, and adduction. It has the greatest range of motion of any joint in the body and as a result is the most frequent site for dislocation. The head of the humerus (ball) fits into the glenoid cavity (socket) of the scapula. The proximal humerus has two rounded protrusions called the greater and lesser *tubercles*. The biceps tendon runs through the bicipital groove between the greater and lesser tubercles and is easily palpable on the lateral surface of the shoulder. The glenohumeral joint is encapsulated and reinforced by the tendons and four muscles that make up the rotator cuff and by the large deltoid muscle (Figures 2-29 and 2-30). The muscles of the rotator cuff include the supraspinatus, the infraspinatus, the teres minor, and the subscapularis muscles.

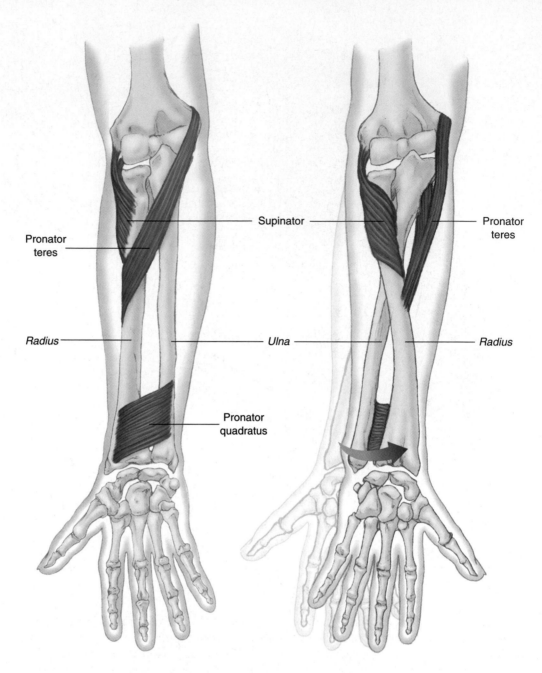

Pronator teres

Supinator

Pronator teres

Radius

Ulna

Radius

Pronator quadratus

FIGURE 2-27 Pronator-supinator muscles.

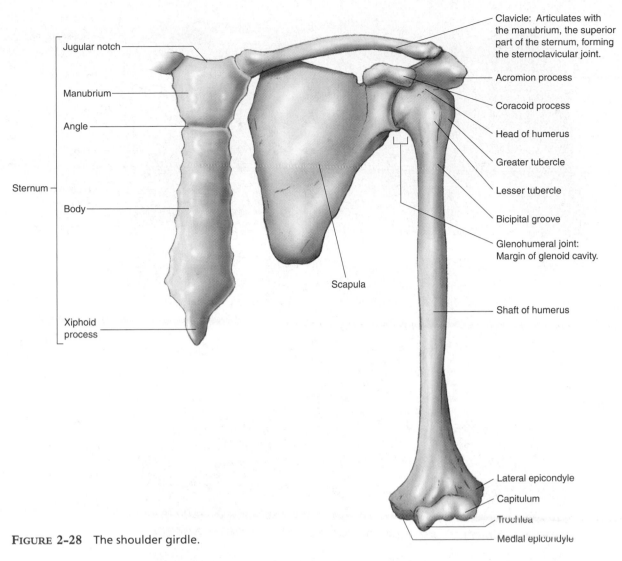

Jugular notch

Manubrium

Angle

Sternum

Body

Xiphoid
process

Scapula

Clavicle: Articulates with
the manubrium, the superior
part of the sternum, forming
the sternoclavicular joint.

Acromion process

Coracoid process

Head of humerus

Greater tubercle

Lesser tubercle

Bicipital groove

Glenohumeral joint:
Margin of glenoid cavity.

Shaft of humerus

Lateral epicondyle

Capitulum

Trochlea

Medial epicondyle

FIGURE 2-28 The shoulder girdle.

FIGURE 2-29 Shoulder girdle
ligaments.

Coracoacromial ligament

Acromioclavicular ligament

Acromion

Subacromial bursa

Tendon of
infraspinatus muscle

Glenohumeral ligaments

Glenoid fossa

Glenoid labrum

Articular capsule

Teres minor muscle

Clavicle

Coracoclavicular
ligament

Coracoid process

Subcoracoid bursa

Coracohumeral
ligament (cut)

Tendon of *biceps
brachii muscle*

Subscapular bursa

Subscapularis muscle

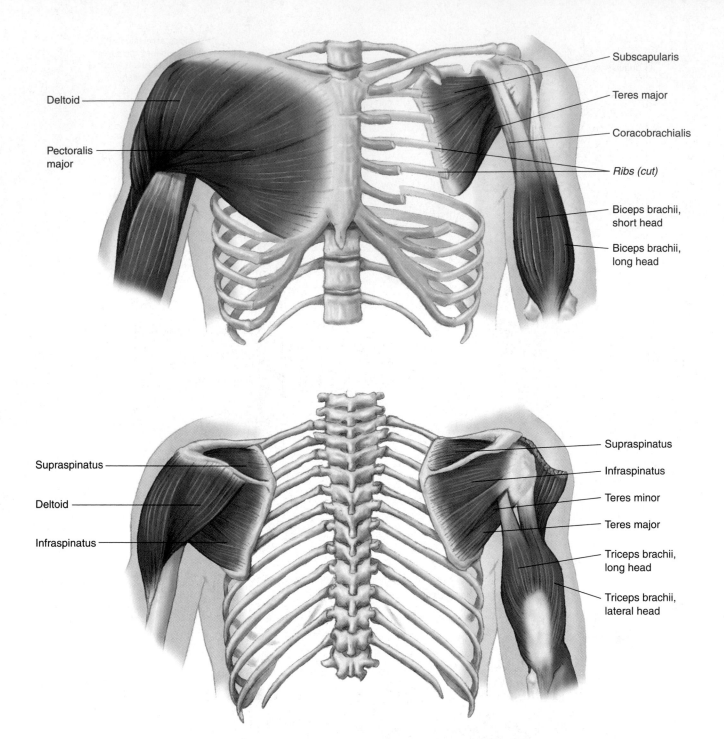

Deltoid

Pectoralis
major

Subscapularis

Teres major

Coracobrachialis

Ribs (cut)

Biceps brachii,
short head

Biceps brachii,
long head

Supraspinatus

Deltoid

Infraspinatus

Supraspinatus

Infraspinatus

Teres minor

Teres major

Triceps brachii,
long head

Triceps brachii,
lateral head

FIGURE 2–30 Shoulder muscles.

Ankles and Feet The foot comprises seven tarsal bones, five metatarsal bones, and fourteen phalanges (Figure 2-31). The talus, the calcaneus (heel), and the other tarsals articulate in a system of joints that allows inversion (lifting the inside of the foot) and eversion (lifting the outside of the foot). The most distal tarsals articulate with the metatarsals, which articulate with the proximal phalanges at the metatarsophalangeal joints.

   At the ankle joint, the distal tibia (medial malleolus) and the distal fibula (lateral malleolus) articulate with the talus (Figure 2-32). Ligaments stretching from each malleolus to the foot itself hold the ankle joint together. The strong Achilles tendon, which inserts on the calcaneus (heel), also helps maintain the ankle's integrity. Movement in the ankle is limited to dorsiflexion (raising the foot) and plantar flexion (lowering the foot). The major dorsiflexor

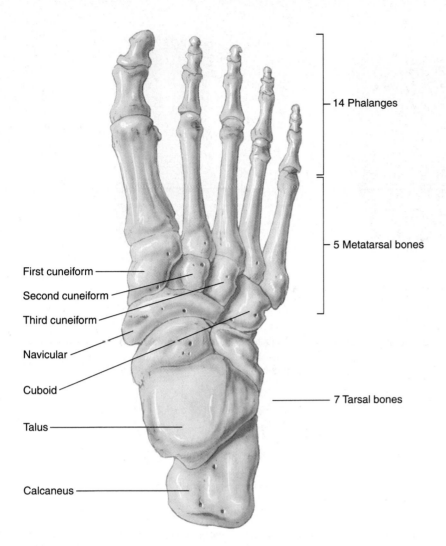

14 Phalanges

5 Metatarsal bones

First cuneiform

Second cuneiform

Third cuneiform

Navicular

Cuboid

7 Tarsal bones

Talus

Calcaneus

FIGURE 2-31 Bones of the foot.

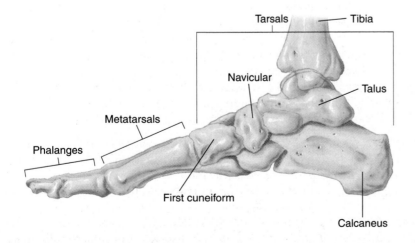

Tarsals   Tibia

Navicular

Talus

Metatarsals

Phalanges

First cuneiform

Calcaneus

FIGURE 2-32 The foot and ankle.

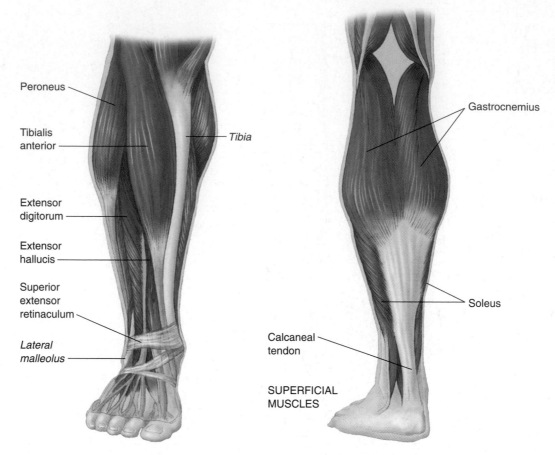

Peroneus

Tibialis anterior

Extensor digitorum

Extensor hallucis

Superior extensor retinaculum

Lateral malleolus

Tibia

Gastrocnemius

Soleus

Calcaneal tendon

SUPERFICIAL MUSCLES

FIGURE 2-33   The dorsiflexors.

FIGURE 2-34   The plantar flexors.

muscle is the tibialis anterior (Figure 2-33). The major plantar flexor is the gastrocnemius (calf muscle) (Figure 2-34).

Knees   The knee joint involves the distal femur, the proximal tibia, and the patella (Figure 2-35). The distal femur and the proximal tibia meet at this joint and are cushioned by the lateral meniscus and the medial meniscus, which form a cartilaginous surface for pain-free movement. The joint capsule contains synovial fluid. Several ligaments surround the knee joint and help maintain its integrity. The **medial** and **lateral** collateral ligaments provide side-to-side stability and are easily palpable. The **anterior** and **posterior** cruciate ligaments, which give the knee front-to-back stability, lie deep within the joint capsule and are not palpable.

The knee is a modified hinge joint, allowing flexion and extension, with some rotation during flexion. The major flexors are a group of three muscles (biceps femoris, semimembranosus, and semitendinosus) known as the hamstrings (Figure 2-36). The major extensors are a group of four muscles (vastus lateralis, vastus intermedius, vastus medialis, and rectus femoris) known as the quadriceps (Figure 2-37). The femur can rotate on the tibia slightly. The patella lies deep in the middle of the quadriceps tendon, which inserts on the tibial tuberosity below the knee. Concave areas at each side of the patella and below it contain synovial fluid.

Hips and Pelvis   The hip is the juncture of the lower extremities with the pelvis. The pelvis is a strong skeletal structure consisting of two symmetrical structures called the *inominates*. The sacrum of the spine is posterior to and joined to the inominates. Each inominate is constructed from one large flat bone, the ilium, the two irregular bones, the ischium and the pubis, all fused together.

The hip joint involves the head of the proximal femur (ball) and the acetabulum (socket) of the ischium (Figure 2-38). Although the hip is a ball-and-socket joint like the shoulder, the two are very different. Although the shoulder has a wide range of motion, the hip joint

medial toward the midline or center of the body.

lateral toward the left or right of the midline.

anterior toward the front of the body. *Opposite of* posterior.

posterior toward the back. *Opposite of* anterior.

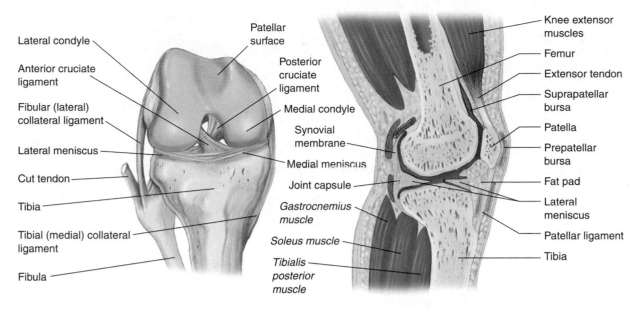

Lateral condyle

Anterior cruciate ligament

Fibular (lateral) collateral ligament

Lateral meniscus

Cut tendon

Tibia

Tibial (medial) collateral ligament

Fibula

Patellar surface

Posterior cruciate ligament

Medial condyle

Synovial membrane

Medial meniscus

Joint capsule

Gastrocnemius muscle

Soleus muscle

Tibialis posterior muscle

Knee extensor muscles

Femur

Extensor tendon

Suprapatellar bursa

Patella

Prepatellar bursa

Fat pad

Lateral meniscus

Patellar ligament

Tibia

FIGURE 2-35 The knee.

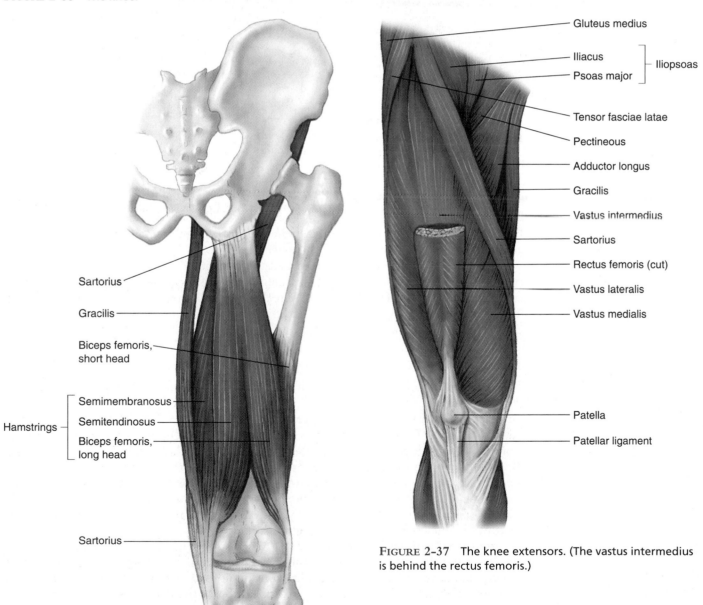

Sartorius

Gracilis

Biceps femoris, short head

Hamstrings

Semimembranosus

Semitendinosus

Biceps femoris, long head

Sartorius

FIGURE 2-36 The knee flexors.

Gluteus medius

Iliacus

Psoas major

] Iliopsoas

Tensor fasciae latae

Pectineous

Adductor longus

Gracilis

Vastus intermedius

Sartorius

Rectus femoris (cut)

Vastus lateralis

Vastus medialis

Patella

Patellar ligament

FIGURE 2-37 The knee extensors. (The vastus intermedius is behind the rectus femoris.)

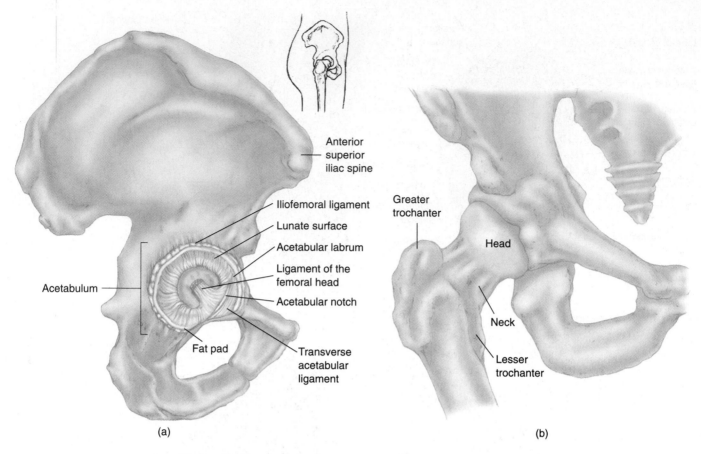

Anterior superior iliac spine

Iliofemoral ligament

Lunate surface

Acetabular labrum

Ligament of the femoral head

Acetabular notch

Acetabulum

Fat pad

Transverse acetabular ligament

Greater trochanter

Head

Neck

Lesser trochanter

(a)

(b)

FIGURE 2-38   The hip joint.

is restricted by many large ligaments, a bony ridge in the pelvis, and capsular fibers. Hip flexion, the most important movement, occurs via the iliopsoas muscle group (Figure 2-39). Other movements, though much more limited in range than the shoulder, include extension, abduction, adduction, and internal and external rotation.

A number of muscle groups control these movements. One of these is the gluteus, a series of adductor muscles and lateral rotators (Figure 2-40). Three bursa in the hip play an important role in pain-free movement. The iliopectineal bursa sits just anterior to the hip joint. The trochanteric bursa lies just to the side and behind the greater trochanter. The ischiogluteal bursa resides under the ischial tuberosity.

BONE AGING

> *Bones of the young child remain flexible and do not reach maximum strength until maturation, which is usually completed by 18 to 20 years of age.*

The bones, like all other body tissues, evolve during fetal development and after birth. Bone initially forms in the embryo as loose cartilaginous tissue. Before birth, the skeletal structure is predominantly cartilage, with very little ossified bone evident. This is one reason that infants are highly flexible yet unable to support themselves. Ossified bone begins to appear along the long bone shafts and then extends to the epiphyseal plates. It also develops within the epiphyses and grows outward to form the articular surfaces. Over time, the bone formation becomes complete to the epiphyseal plate, and the epiphysis is fully formed. The epiphyseal plate continues to generate cartilage, with the shaft and epiphyses growing from it. As the young adult reaches full height and the end of skeletal growth, the epiphyseal plates narrow, become bony, and cease to produce cartilage.

Associated with bone development and aging is the transition from flexible, cartilaginous bone to firm, strong, and fully ossified bone. Bones of the young child remain flexible and do not reach maximum strength until early adulthood. Although each bone matures at a different time, almost all maturation is complete by 18 to 20 years of age.

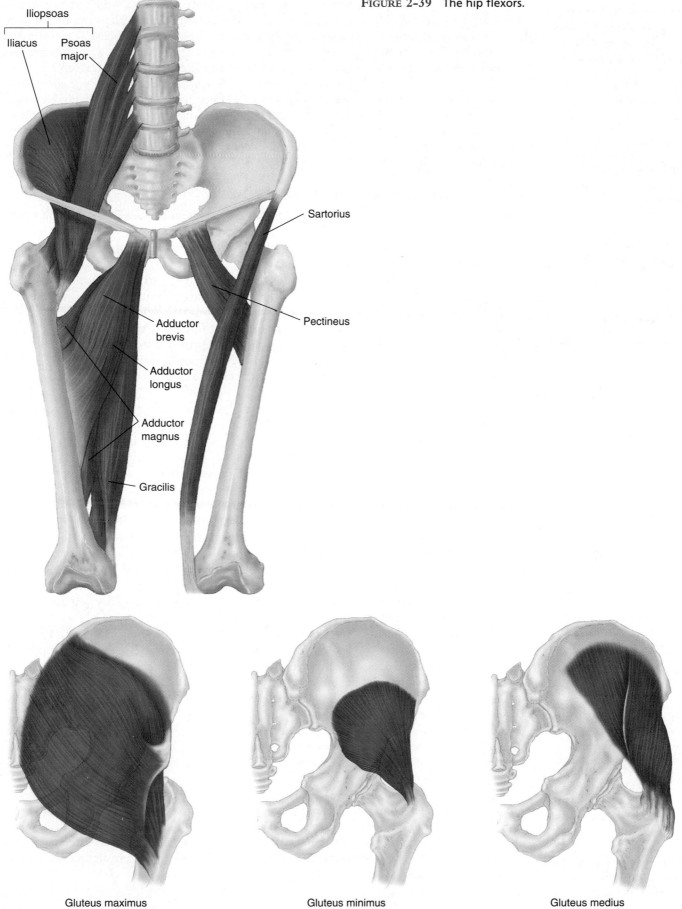

FIGURE 2-39   The hip flexors.

Iliopsoas

Iliacus

Psoas major

Sartorius

Pectineus

Adductor brevis

Adductor longus

Adductor magnus

Gracilis

Gluteus maximus

Gluteus minimus

Gluteus medius

FIGURE 2-40   The gluteus muscles.

Patho Pearls

Osteoporosis is common in post-menopausal women and a common contributing factor to fractures.

Content Review

TYPES OF MUSCLE
- Cardiac muscle
- Smooth muscle
- Skeletal muscle

---

fasciculus small bundle of muscle fibers.

---

origin attachment of a muscle to a bone that does not move (or experiences the least movement) when the muscle contracts.

---

insertion attachment of a muscle to a bone that moves when the muscle contracts.

---

opposition pairing of muscles that permits extension and flexion of limbs.

Around the age of 40 the body begins to lose its ability to maintain the bone structure. It is unable to rebuild the collagen matrix and the deposition of salt crystals is reduced from what it was in earlier years. The effects of these changes appear very slowly. They include a very gradual diminution of bone strength, an increase in bone brittleness, a progressive loss of body height, and some curvature of the spine. The incidence of bone fractures also increases, especially at the high stress points of the lumbar spine and the femur's surgical neck.

Age-related changes in the skeletal system also affect other body systems. For example, the cartilage of the costal-condral joints and the costal bones (the ribs) becomes less flexible, which leads to shallower, more energy-consuming respirations. Also, the intravertebral disks lose water content and become less flexible, more prone to herniation, and narrower, thus shortening the trunk.

MUSCULAR TISSUE AND STRUCTURE

More than 600 muscle groups make up the muscular system (Figure 2-41). As you might expect, a large number of EMS calls involve injuries to this extensive system. Injuries to it may result from excessive forces indirectly expressed to the muscles and their attachments or from direct trauma, either blunt or penetrating.

There are three types of muscle tissue within the body—cardiac, smooth, and skeletal (Figure 2-42). Of these, the most specialized is the cardiac muscle comprising the myocardium. It contracts rhythmically on its own (automaticity), emitting an electrical impulse in the process (excitability), and passing that impulse along to the other cells of the myocardium (conductivity). In this way, the heart provides its lifelong rhythmic contraction and pumping. Cardiac muscle can also be classified according to its structure, which combines characteristics of both skeletal and smooth muscle and is thus called *smooth-striated*.

The second muscle type is smooth, or involuntary, muscle, which is not under conscious control but functions at the direction of the autonomic nervous system. These muscles are found in the arterial and venous blood vessels, the bronchioles, the bowel, and many other organs. Smooth muscle contracts to reduce (or relaxes to expand) the lumen (diameter) of the vasculature, airways, or digestive tract. Smooth muscles have the ability to contract over a wide lateral distance, enabling them to accommodate great changes in length, such as those that occur during filling and evacuation of the bladder and contraction and dilation of the arterioles.

The final type of muscle tissue is skeletal (also called *striated* or voluntary). A person has conscious control over these muscles, which are associated with the mobility of the extremities and the body in general. Skeletal muscles are also controlled by the nerves of the somatic nervous system. The skeletal muscles are the largest component of the muscular system, comprising between 40% and 50% of the body's total weight. They are the type of muscle most commonly traumatized.

Skeletal muscles lie directly beneath a protective layer of skin and subcutaneous fat. Because of their hunger for oxygen during activity, they have a more than ample supply of blood vessels. Individual muscle cells layer together to form a muscle fiber, many fibers layer together to form a muscle **fasciculus**, and fasciculi layer together to form a muscle body, such as the triceps. A muscle body has a strength of about 50 pounds of lift per square inch of cross-sectional area.

Skeletal muscles attach to the bones at a minimum of two locations. These attachment points are called the **origin** and the **insertion**, depending upon how the bones move with contraction. The point of attachment that remains stationary as the muscle contracts is the origin. The attachment to the moving bone is the insertion.

Muscles usually pair, one on each side of a joint. This configuration is essential because muscles can actively contract, not lengthen. One muscle moves the extremity in one direction by contraction, while the opposing (and relaxed) muscle stretches. The opposing muscle can then in turn contract, stretching the first muscle and moving the extremity in the opposite direction. This arrangement, called **opposition**, permits the straightening (extension) and then bending (flexion) of the limbs.

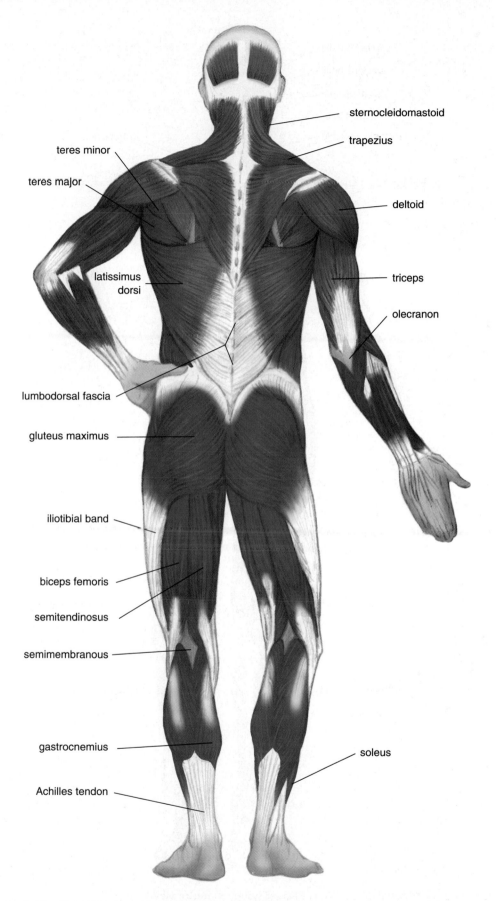

sternocleidomastoid

trapezius

teres minor

teres major

deltoid

latissimus dorsi

triceps

olecranon

lumbodorsal fascia

gluteus maximus

iliotibial band

biceps femoris

semitendinosus

semimembranous

gastrocnemius

soleus

Achilles tendon

FIGURE 2-41   The muscular system (posterior view).

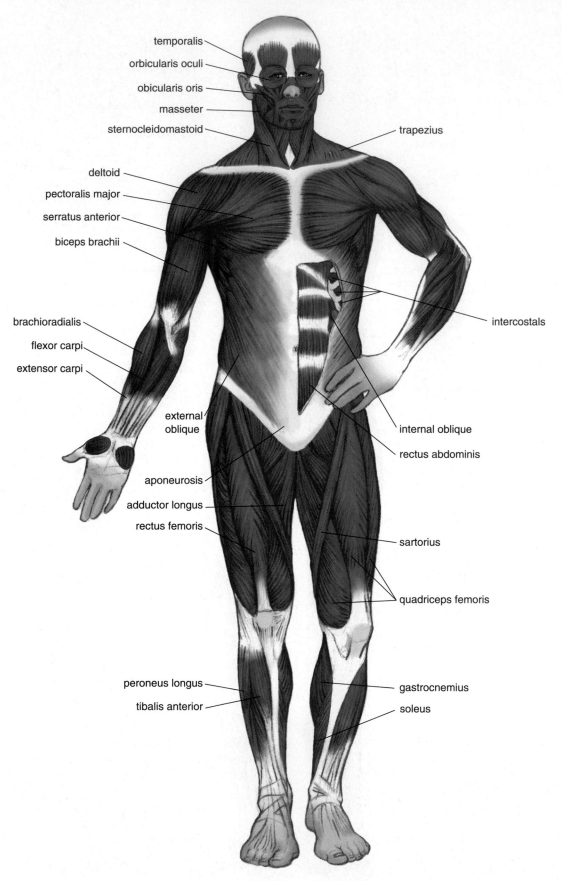

temporalis
orbicularis oculi
obicularis oris
masseter
sternocleidomastoid
trapezius
deltoid
pectoralis major
serratus anterior
biceps brachii
intercostals
brachioradialis
flexor carpi
extensor carpi
external oblique
internal oblique
rectus abdominis
aponeurosis
adductor longus
rectus femoris
sartorius
quadriceps femoris
peroneus longus
tibalis anterior
gastrocnemius
soleus

FIGURE 2-41 (CONTINUED) The muscular system (anterior view).

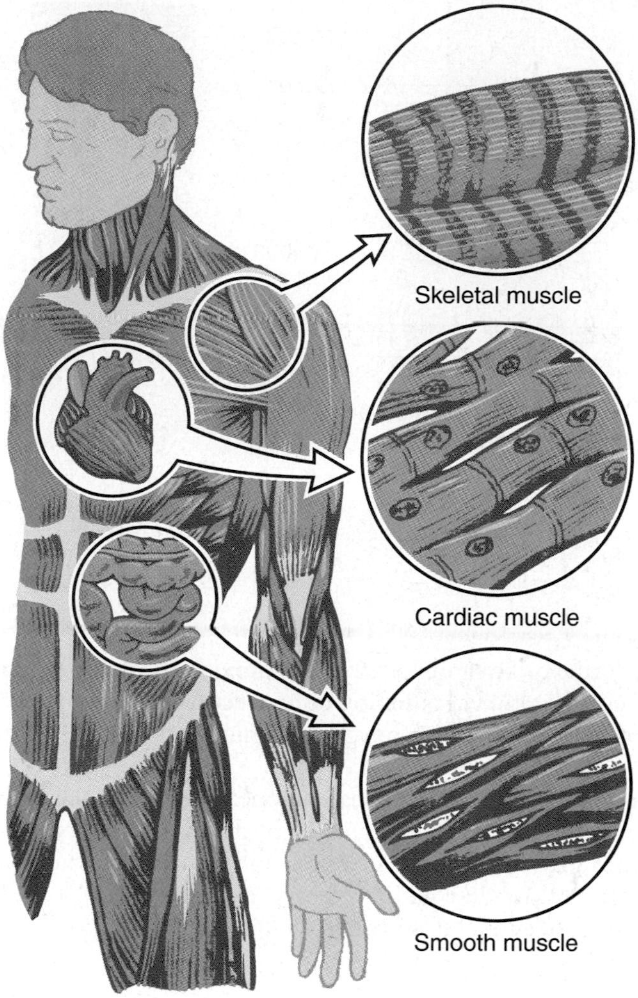

FIGURE 2-42 Three types of muscle.

Skeletal muscle

Cardiac muscle

Smooth muscle

With several muscles attached to a joint with different origins and insertions, the body enjoys a wide variety of motions. In the shoulder, for example, the humerus can travel through several types and ranges of motion. These include moving the extremity away from the body (*abduction*) and toward the body (*adduction*), turning the humerus (*rotation*) through about 60 degrees, and circling the entire extremity (*circumduction*) through a 180-degree arc.

Tendons are specialized bands of connective tissue that accomplish the attachment of muscle to bone at the insertion and, in some cases, at the origin (Figure 2-43). These very fibrous ribbons, actually parts of the muscles, are extremely strong and do not stretch. They are so strong that in some instances they will break an area of bone loose rather than tear. The Achilles tendon demonstrates the strength of this particular tissue. It can be felt as the band posterior to the malleoli of the ankle. This tendon is the muscle-controlled cord that allows a person to lift the entire body weight when standing on the toes.

The forearm demonstrates the sophistication of the muscle-tendon relationship. As the muscles controlling finger flexion contract, you can feel them tensing in the **dorsal** forearm. You can also visualize and palpate tendon movement in the distal forearm and wrist as the fingers flex and extend. It is easy to appreciate the damage a deep transverse laceration can cause to the underlying connective tissues and their control of distal skeletal structures. Tendons are often classified by the action they perform when the muscle associated with them contracts—for example, flexor or extensor, abductor or adductor, etc.

The muscle tissue is responsible not only for the body's movement but also for the production of heat energy. A chemical reaction between oxygen and simple sugars produces the energy of motion. Heat, water, and carbon dioxide are by-products of this reaction. More than half the energy created by muscle motion is heat that helps maintain body temperature.

dorsal toward the back or spine. *Opposite of* ventral.

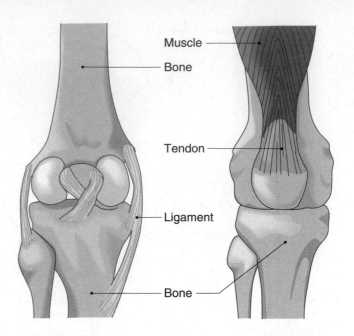

FIGURE 2-43 How muscle attaches to bone.

Muscle
Bone
Tendon
Ligament
Bone

The body then excretes water in the urine or sweat, expels carbon dioxide through respiration, and dissipates excess heat through the skin via radiation or convection. The body must constantly meet the requirements of muscle tissues for oxygen and nutrients and eliminate the waste products of those tissues, including heat.

Muscles are found in a condition of slight contraction called **tone.** Even while the body is at rest, the central nervous system sends some limited impulses to the muscle fibers causing a few to contract. These impulses give the muscles firmness and ensure that they are ready to contract when the need arises. Muscle tone may be very significant in a well-conditioned athlete or absent (flaccid muscle tone) in someone with peripheral motor nerve disruption.

tone state of slight contraction of muscles that gives them firmness and keeps them ready to contract.

HEAD, FACE, AND NECK

THE HEAD

The head is made up of three structures that cover the brain: the scalp, the cranium, and the meninges. Each of these structures provides essential protection from the environment and from trauma.

THE SCALP

The scalp is a strong and flexible mass of skin, fascia (bands of connective tissue), and muscular tissue that is able to withstand and absorb tremendous kinetic energy. The scalp is also extremely vascular in order to help maintain the brain at the body's core temperature. Scalp hair further insulates the brain from environmental temperatures and, to a lesser degree, from trauma.

The scalp is only loosely attached to the skull and is made up of the overlying skin and a number of thin layers of muscle and connective tissue underneath. Directly beneath the skin and covering the most **superior** surface of the head is a fibrous connective tissue sheet called the **galea aponeurotica.** Connected anteriorly to it and covering the forehead is a flat sheet of muscle, the frontal muscle. Connected posteriorly and covering the posterior skull surface is the occipitalis muscle. Laterally, the auricularis muscles cover the areas above the ears and between the lateral brow ridge and the occiput. A layer of loose connective tissue beneath these muscles and the galea and just above the periosteum is called the *areolar tissue.* It contains emissary veins that permit venous blood to flow from the dural sinuses into the venous vessels of the scalp. These emissary veins also exist in the upper reaches of the nasal cavity. These veins become potential routes for infection in scalp wounds or nasal in-

superior above; higher than; toward the head. *Opposite of inferior.*

galea aponeurotica connective tissue sheet covering the superior aspect of the cranium.

juries. A helpful way to remember the layers of skin protecting the scalp is the mnemonic SCALP: S—skin, C—connective tissue, A—aponeurotica, L—layer of subaponeurotica (areolar) tissue, P—the periosteum of the skull (the pericranium).

CRANIUM

The bony structure supporting the head and face is the skull. It can be subdivided into two components, the facial bones that form the skeletal base for the face and the vault for the brain, called the **cranium** (Figure 2-44). The cranium actually consists of several bones fused together at pseudo-joints called **sutures**. These bony plates are constructed of two narrow layers of hard compact bone, separated by a layer of cancellous bone. The plates form a strong, light, rigid, and spherical container for the brain. The cranium is, therefore, quite effective in protecting its contents from the direct effects of trauma. This vault, however, provides very little space for internal swelling or hemorrhage. Any expanding lesion within the cranium results in an increase in **intracranial pressure (ICP)**. This reduces cerebral perfusion and can severely damage the delicate brain tissue.

The cranial bones form regions that are helpful in describing the cerebral structures beneath. The anterior or frontal bone begins at the brow ridge and covers the upper and anterior surface of the brain. The parietal bones, one on either side, begin just behind the lateral brow ridge and form the skull above the external portions (pinnae) of the ears. The occipital bone forms the posterior and inferior aspect of the cranium, extending to and forming the foramen magnum. The temporal bones form the lateral cranial surfaces anterior to the ears. The ethmoid and sphenoid bones, which are very irregular in shape, form the portion of the cranium concealed and protected by the facial bones.

cranium vault-like portion of the skull encasing the brain.

sutures pseudo-joints that join the various bones of the skull to form the cranium.

intracranial pressure (ICP) pressure exerted on the brain by the blood and cerebrospinal fluid.

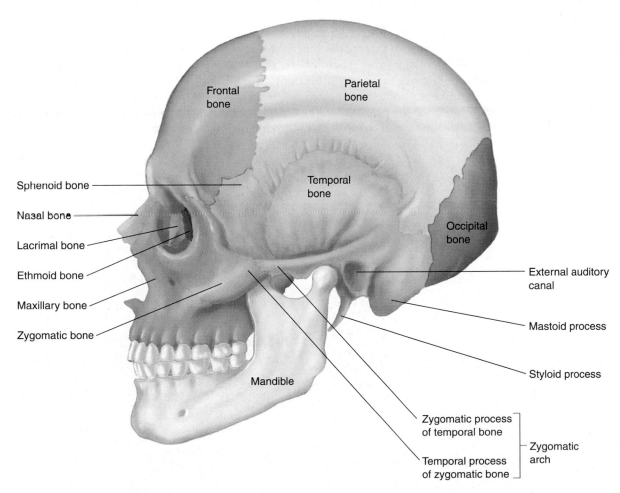

FIGURE 2-44 Bones of the human skull.

The base of the skull consists of portions of the occipital, temporal, sphenoid, and ethmoid bones. This area is important in cases of trauma because the openings, or foramina, for blood vessels, the spinal cord, the auditory canal, and the cranial nerves pass through it. These openings weaken the area, leaving it prone to fracture with serious trauma.

Other anatomical points of interest within the cranium are the cribriform plate and the foramen magnum. The cribriform plate is an irregular portion of the ethmoid bone and a portion of the base of the cranium. It and the remainder of the base of the cranium have rough surfaces against which the brain may abrade, lacerate, or contuse during severe deceleration. The foramen magnum is the largest opening in the skull. It is located at the base of the skull where it meets the spinal column and is where the spinal cord exits the cranium.

The Meninges

meninges three membranes that surround and protect the brain and spinal cord. They are the dura mater, pia mater, and arachnoid membrane.

dura mater tough layer of the meninges firmly attached to the interior of the skull and interior of the spinal column.

pia mater inner and most delicate layer of the meninges. It covers the convolutions of the brain and spinal cord.

arachnoid membrane middle layer of the meninges.

The final protective mechanisms for the brain and the spinal cord are the **meninges** (Figure 2-45). They are a group of three tissues between the cranium and the brain and the spinal column and cord. The outermost layer is the **dura mater** (tough mother), a tough connective tissue that provides protection for the central nervous system. The dura mater is actually two layers. The outer layer is the cranium's inner periosteum. The dural layer is made up of tough, continuous connective tissue that extends into the cranial cavity where it forms partial structural divisions (the falx cerebri and the tentorium cerebelli). Above the dura mater lie some of the larger arteries that provide blood flow to the surface of the brain. Between the dural layers lie the dural sinuses, major venous drains for the brain.

The meningeal layer closest to the brain and spinal cord is the **pia mater** (tender mother). It is a delicate tissue, covering all the convolutions of the brain and cord. Although more delicate when compared with the dura mater, the pia mater is still more substantial than brain and spinal cord tissue. The pia mater is a highly vascular tissue with large vessels that supply the superficial areas of the brain.

Separating the two layers of mater is a stratum of connective tissue called the **arachnoid membrane.** It covers the inner dura mater and suspends the brain in the cranial cavity with collagen and elastin fibers. The arachnoid membrane gets its name from its weblike appearance (arachnoid, meaning "spiderlike"). Beneath the arachnoid membrane is the subarachnoid space, which is filled with cerebrospinal fluid. This region provides cushioning for the brain when the head is subjected to strong forces of acceleration or deceleration.

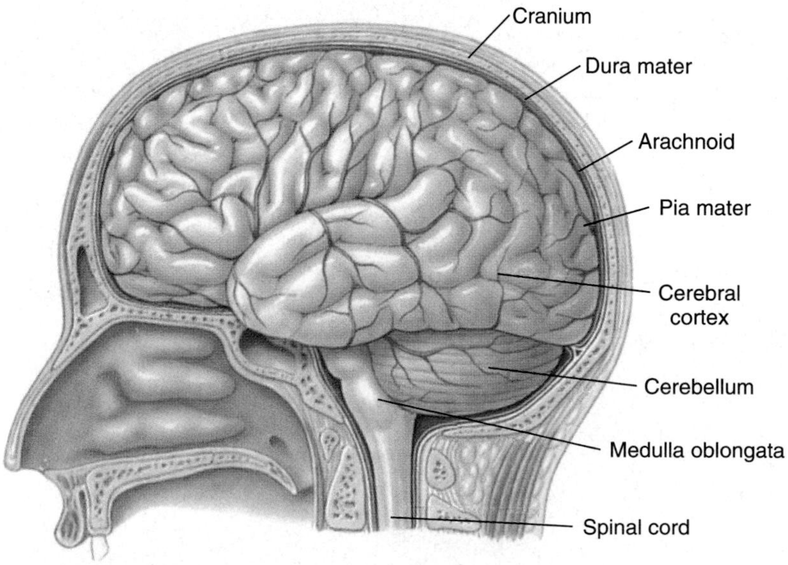

FIGURE 2-45 The meninges and skull.

Cerebrospinal Fluid

Cerebrospinal fluid is a clear, colorless solution of water, proteins, and salts surrounding the central nervous system that absorbs the shock of minor acceleration and deceleration. The brain constantly generates cerebrospinal fluid in the largest two of four spaces (or ventricles) within the substance of the brain. The fluid circulates through the ventricles, then through the subarachnoid space, where it is returned to the venous circulation through the dural sinuses. The cerebrospinal fluid provides buoyancy for the brain and actually floats it in a near-weightless environment within the cranial cavity. This fluid also is a medium through which nutrients and waste products such as oxygen, proteins, salts, and carbon dioxide are diffused into and out of the brain tissue.

The Brain

The brain occupies about 80% of the interior of the cranium. It is made up of three major structures essential to human function—the cerebrum, cerebellum, and the brainstem.

The **cerebrum** is the largest element of the nervous system and occupies most of the cranial cavity. It consists of an exterior cortex of gray matter (cell bodies) and is the highest functional portion of the brain. The central portion of the cerebrum is predominantly white matter, mostly communication pathways (axons). The cerebrum is the center of conscious thought, personality, speech, motor control, and of visual, auditory, and tactile (touch) perception. The cerebrum is regionalized into lobes roughly lying beneath the bones of the cranium (and given the same names). The frontal region is anterior and determines personality. The parietal region, which is superior and posterior, directs motor and sensory activities as well as memory and emotions. The occipital region, which is posterior and inferior, is responsible for sight. Laterally, the temporal regions are the centers for long-term memory, hearing, speech, taste, and smell.

A structure called the *falx cerebri* divides the cerebrum into right and left hemispheres. A dural partition, the falx cerebri, extends into the cranial cavity from the interior and superior surface of the cranium (Figure 2-46). Corresponding to the falx cerebri is a fissure in the cerebrum called the *central sulcus*. This fissure physically splits the cerebrum into the left and right hemispheres, each of which controls (for the most part) the activities of the opposite side of the body. The crossing of nerve impulses from one side to the other takes place just below the medulla oblongata. The tentorium cerebelli is a similar fibrous sheet within the occipital region, running at right angles to the falx cerebri. It separates the cerebrum from the cerebellum. The brainstem perforates the tentorium through an opening called the *tentorium incisura*.

The oculomotor nerve (CN-III), which controls pupil size, travels along the tentorium. It is likely to be compressed as intracranial pressure rises or the brain is displaced due to edema, a growing mass, or hemorrhage. This compression causes pupillary disturbances that manifest most commonly on the same side as the problem. If the pressure is great enough, it may affect both sides and both pupils may dilate and fix.

The left cerebral hemisphere is identified as the dominant hemisphere in most of the population, with the exception of a few left-handed individuals. It is responsible for mathematical computations (occipital region) and writing (parietal region) and is the center for language interpretation (occipital region) and speech (frontal region). The right, nondominant cerebral hemisphere processes nonverbal imagery (occipital region).

The **cerebellum** is located directly under the tentorium. It lies posterior and inferior to the cerebrum. The cerebellum "fine tunes" motor control and allows the body to move smoothly from one position to another. Additionally, it is responsible for balance and maintenance of muscle tone.

The **brainstem** is an important central processing center and the communication junction among the cerebrum, spinal cord, cranial nerves, and cerebellum. It includes the midbrain, the pons, and the medulla oblongata. The **midbrain** makes up the upper portion of the brainstem and consists of the hypothalamus, thalamus, and associated structures. The **hypothalamus** controls much of endocrine function, the vomiting reflex, hunger, thirst, kidney function, body

The crossing of nerve impulses from one side of the body to the other takes place just below the medulla oblongata.

cerebrospinal fluid fluid surrounding and bathing the brain and spinal cord (the elements of the central nervous system).

cerebrum largest part of the brain. It consists of two hemispheres separated by a deep longitudinal fissure. It is the seat of consciousness and the center of the higher mental functions such as memory, learning, reasoning, judgment, intelligence, and emotions.

cerebellum portion of the brain located dorsally to the pons and medulla oblongata. It plays an important role in the fine control of voluntary muscular movements.

brainstem the part of the brain connecting the cerebral hemispheres with the spinal cord. It is composed of the medulla oblongata, the pons, and the midbrain.

midbrain portion of the brain connecting the pons and cerebellum with the cerebral hemispheres.

hypothalamus portion of the brain important for controlling certain metabolic activities, including the regulation of body temperature.

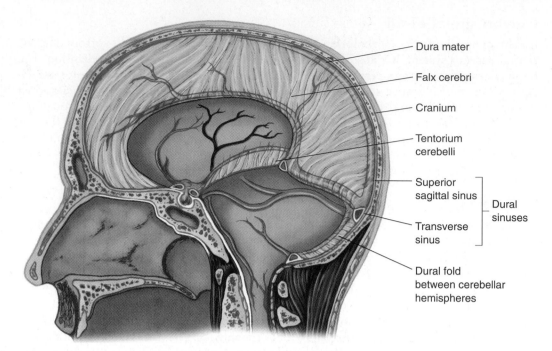

Dura mater

Falx cerebri

Cranium

Tentorium cerebelli

Superior sagittal sinus ⎤
⎥ Dural
⎥ sinuses
Transverse sinus ⎦

Dural fold between cerebellar hemispheres

FIGURE 2-46 The partitions extending into the skull, the falx cerebri, and tentorium cerebellum.

thalamus switching station between the pons and the cerebrum in the brain.

reticular activating system (RAS) a series of nervous tissues keeping the human system in a state of consciousness.

pons process of tissue responsible for the communication interchange among the cerebellum, the cerebrum, midbrain, and the spinal cord.

medulla oblongata lower portion of the brainstem containing the respiratory, cardiac, and vasomotor centers

Though the brain accounts for only 2% of the body's total weight, it consumes about 20% of the body's oxygen.

Patho Pearls

Rupture of a blood vessel at the base of the brain usually results in a subarachnoid hemorrhage as the blood remains below the level of the arachnoid membrane.

temperature, and emotions. The **thalamus** is the switching center between the pons and the cerebrum and is a critical element in the **reticular activating system (RAS)**, the system that establishes consciousness. This region also provides the major tracts, or pathways, for the optic and olfactory nerves.

The **pons** acts as the communication interchange among the various components of the central nervous system—the cerebellum, the cerebrum, midbrain, and the spinal cord. It is a bulb-shaped structure directly above the medulla oblongata and appears to be responsible for the sleep component of the reticular activating system.

The last nervous system structure still within the cranial vault is the **medulla oblongata.** It is recognizable as a bulge in the very top of the spinal cord. The medulla contains three important centers—the respiratory center, the cardiac center, and the vasomotor center. The cardiac center regulates the rate and strength of cardiac contractions. The vasomotor center controls the distribution of blood and maintains blood pressure. The respiratory center controls respiratory depth, rate, and rhythm.

In order to maintain its advanced functioning, the brain has a high metabolic rate. Though the brain accounts for only 2% of the body's total weight, it receives about 15% of the cardiac output and consumes about 20% of the body's oxygen. It requires this circulation whether it is at rest or engaged in active thought. Further, this blood supply must be constant because the brain has no stored energy sources. It needs constant supplies of glucose, thiamine (to help metabolize glucose), and oxygen and relies almost solely on aerobic metabolism. If the blood supply stops, unconsciousness follows within 10 seconds, and brain death will ensue within 4 to 6 minutes.

Central Nervous System Circulation

Four major arterial vessels provide blood flow to the brain. The first two are the internal carotid arteries. These vessels divide from the common carotid at the carotid sinus and then enter the cranium through its base. The two posterior vessels, the vertebral arteries, ascend along and through the vertebral column. They then enter the base of the skull, where they join and form a singular basilar artery.

The internal carotid and basilar arteries interconnect through the circle of Willis in the base of the brain. This structure is an arterial circle that ensures good circulation to the brain, even if one of the large feeder vessels is obstructed. Various arteries branch out from the circle of Willis and supply the substance of the brain itself.

Venous drainage occurs initially through bridging veins that drain the surface of the cerebrum. They "bridge" with the dural sinuses (large, thin-walled veins). These ultimately drain into the internal jugular veins and then into the superior vena cava.

Blood–Brain Barrier

The capillaries of the brain are special in that their walls are thicker and not as permeable as those found elsewhere in the body. They do not permit the interstitial flow of proteins and other materials as freely as do other body capillaries. This ensures that many substances found in the circulatory system, such as some hormones, do not affect the central nervous system cells. Lymphatic circulation is also lacking in the brain and is replaced by the cerebrospinal fluid flow system. This results in a very special and protected environment for central nervous system cells. If frank blood seeps into the central nervous system tissue, it acts as an irritant, initiating an inflammatory response, resulting in edema.

Cerebral Perfusion Pressure

Cerebral perfusion is exceptionally critical and depends on many factors. Primarily, the pressure within the cranium (intracranial pressure or ICP) resists blood flow and good perfusion to the central nervous system tissue. Usually the pressure is less than 10 mmHg and does not significantly impede blood flow as long as the mean arterial blood pressure (MAP is the diastolic blood pressure plus one third the pulse pressure) is at least 50 mmHg. The pressure moving blood through the cranium is the **cerebral perfusion pressure (CPP)**. This is calculated as the mean arterial pressure (MAP) minus the intracranial pressure (ICP). Changes in ICP are met with compensatory changes in blood pressure to ensure adequate cerebral perfusion pressure (CPP) and cerebral blood flow. This compensating reflex is called **autoregulation.**

Since the cranium is a fixed vault for the structures of the brain, its volume and the pressure within are shared by the occupants. Any expanding mass (tumor), hemorrhage, or edema within the cranium will displace some other occupant such as the cerebrospinal fluid or blood, since they are the only readily movable media. This displacement maintains the intracranial pressure (ICP) very effectively, up to a point. When the volumes of cerebrospinal fluid and venous blood are reduced to their limits, however, the ICP begins to rise. Autoregulation then raises the blood pressure to ensure there is enough differential (CPP) to provide good cerebral perfusion. However, this increase in blood pressure causes the ICP to rise still higher and cerebral blood perfusion to diminish even more. As this cycle of increasing ICP and increasing blood pressure continues, brain injury and death are close at hand.

Cranial Nerves

The cranial nerves are nerve roots originating within the cranium and along the brainstem. They comprise 12 distinct pathways that account for some of the more important senses, innervate the facial area, and control significant body functions.

Ascending Reticular Activating System

The ascending reticular activating system is a tract of neurons within the upper brainstem, the pons, and the midbrain that is responsible for the sleep-wake cycle. It is a complex control system that monitors the amount of stimulation the body receives and regulates important bodily functions such as respiration, heart rate, and peripheral vascular resistance. Injury to the midbrain may result in unconsciousness or coma, whereas injury to the pons may result in a protracted waking state.

THE FACE

Facial bones make up the anterior and **inferior** structures of the head and include the zygoma, maxilla, mandible, and nasal bones (Figure 2-47). The **zygoma** is the prominent bone of the cheek. It protects the eyes and the muscles controlling eye and jaw movement. The **maxilla** comprises the upper jaw, supports the nasal bone, and provides the lower border of the orbit. The nasal bone is the attachment for the nasal cartilage as it forms the shape of the nose. The last of the facial bones is the **mandible,** or jawbone. It resembles two horizontal "L's," which join anteriorly and hinge underneath the posterior zygomatic arch.

cerebral perfusion pressure (CPP) the pressure moving blood through the brain.

autoregulation process that controls blood flow to the brain tissue by causing alterations in the blood pressure.

$$CPP = MAP - ICP$$

inferior beneath; lower; toward the feet. *Opposite of superior.*

zygoma the cheekbone.

maxilla bone of the upper jaw.

mandible the jawbone.

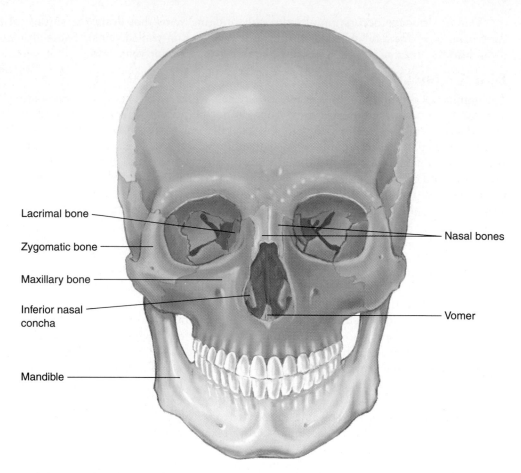

Lacrimal bone

Zygomatic bone

Maxillary bone

Inferior nasal
concha

Mandible

Nasal bones

Vomer

FIGURE 2-47 The facial bones.

Besides forming the beginning of the airway and the alimentary canal, the facial bones form supporting and protective structures for several sense organs, including the tongue (taste), eye (sight), and olfactory nerve (smell).

The facial region, like most other areas of the body, is covered with skin that serves to protect the tissue underneath from trauma and against adverse environmental effects. In the facial region, the skin is very flexible and relatively thin. It also has a very good vascular supply and hemorrhages freely when injured. Beneath the skin is a minimal layer of subcutaneous tissue and, beneath that, are the many small muscles that control facial expression and the movements of the mouth, eyes, and eyelids.

Circulation for the facial area is provided by the external carotid artery as it branches into the facial, temporal, and maxillary arteries. The facial artery crosses the mandible, then travels up and along the nasal bone. The maxillary artery runs under the mandible and zygoma, then provides circulation to the cheek area. The temporal artery runs anterior to the ear just posterior to the zygoma. Each major artery has an associated vein paralleling its path.

The most important cranial nerves traversing this area are the trigeminal (CN-V) and the facial (CN-VII). The trigeminal nerve provides sensation for the face and some motor control over eye movement. It also enables the chewing process. The facial nerve provides motor control to the facial muscles and contributes to the sensation of taste.

The nasal cavity is formed by the juncture of the ethmoid, nasal, and maxillary bones. It is a channel running posteriorly with a bony septum dividing it into left and right chambers and plates protruding medially from the lateral sides. These plates, called *turbinates,* form support for the vascular mucous membranes that serve to warm, humidify, and collect particulate matter from the incoming air. The lower border of the nasal cavity is formed by the bony hard palate and then, posteriorly, by the more flexible cartilaginous soft palate. The soft palate moves upward to close off the opening of the posterior nasal cavity during swallowing. The nasal bone lies anterior and inferior to the eyes and provides a base for the nasal cartilage. The nasal cartilage defines the shape of the nose and divides the nostrils and their openings, which are called the **nares.**

The oral cavity is formed by the concave shape of the maxillary bone, the palate, and the upper teeth meeting the mandible and the lower teeth. The floor of the chamber consists of musculature and connective tissue that span the mandible and support the tongue. The tongue is a large muscle that occupies much of the oral cavity, provides the taste sensation, and moves food between the teeth during chewing (mastication) and propels the chewed food posteriorly, then inferiorly during swallowing. The tongue connects with the hyoid bone, a free floating U-shaped bone located inferiorly and posteriorly to the mandible. The mandible articulates with the temporal bone at the temporomandibular joint, under the posterior zygoma, and is moved by the masseter muscles. The lip muscles (obicularis oris) are responsible for sealing the mouth during chewing and swallowing.

Special structures are found in and around the oral cavity. Salivary glands provide saliva, the first of the digestive juices. These glands are located just anterior and inferior to the ear, under the tongue, and just inside the inferior mandible. Specialized lymphoid nodules, the tonsils, are located in the posterior wall of the pharynx.

Prominent cranial nerves serving the oral area include the hypoglossal, the glossopharyngeal, the trigeminal, and the facial nerves. The hypoglossal nerve (CN-XII) directs swallowing and tongue movement. The glossopharyngeal nerve (CN-IX) controls saliva production and taste. The trigeminal nerve (CN-V) carries sensations from the facial region and assists in chewing control. The facial nerve (CN-VII) controls the muscles of facial expression and taste.

Posterior and inferior to the oral cavity is a collection of soft tissue called the *pharynx*. The process of swallowing begins in the pharynx once the bolus of food has been propelled back and down by the tongue. The epiglottis moves downward while the larynx moves up, sealing the lower airway opening. The food or liquid moves into the esophagus where a peristaltic wave begins its trip to the stomach. This area is of great importance because it maintains the critical segregation of materials between the digestive tract and the airway.

Sinuses are hollow spaces within the bones of the cranium and face that lighten the head, protect the eyes and nasal cavity, and help produce the resonant tones of the voice. They also strengthen this region against the forces of trauma.

The Ear

The outer, visible portion of the ear is termed the **pinna.** It is composed of cartilage and has a poor blood supply. It connects to the external auditory canal, which leads to the eardrum. The external auditory canal contains glands that secrete wax (cerumen) for protection. The ear's important structures are interior and exceptionally well protected from nearly all trauma (Figure 2-48). Only trauma involving great pressure differentials (e.g., blast and diving injuries) or basilar skull fractures are likely to damage this area.

The ear provides the body with two very useful functions, hearing and positional sense. The middle and inner ear contain the structures needed for hearing. Hearing occurs when sound waves cause the tympanic membrane (eardrum) to vibrate. The eardrum transmits the vibrations through three very small bones (the ossicles) to the cochlea, the organ of hearing. These vibrations stimulate the auditory nerve, which in turn transmits the signal to the brain.

The **semicircular canals** are responsible for sensing position and motion. They are three hollow, fluid-filled rings set at different angles. When the head moves, fluid in these rings shifts. Small cells with hairlike projections sense the motion and signal the brain to help maintain balance. This positional sense is present even when the eyes are closed. If injury or illness disturbs this area, it transmits excess signals to the brain. Patients then experience a continuous moving sensation known as vertigo.

The Eye

The eyes provide much of the input we use to interact with our environment. Although they are placed prominently on the face, the eyes are well protected from trauma by a series of facial bones. The frontal bones project above the globe of the eye, while the nasal bones and cartilage protect medially. The bone of the cheek, or zygoma, completes the physical protection both laterally and inferiorly. These bones collectively form the eye socket or **orbit.** The soft tissue of the eyelid and the eyelashes give additional protection to the critical ocular surface.

---

nares the openings of the nostrils.

pinna outer, visible portion of the ear.

semicircular canals the three rings of the inner ear. They sense the motion of the head and provide positional sense for the body.

orbit the eye socket.

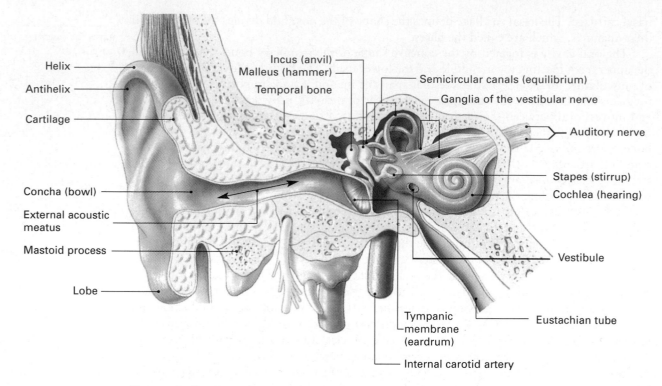

Helix
Antihelix
Cartilage

Concha (bowl)
External acoustic meatus
Mastoid process
Lobe

Incus (anvil)
Malleus (hammer)
Temporal bone

Semicircular canals (equilibrium)
Ganglia of the vestibular nerve
Auditory nerve

Stapes (stirrup)
Cochlea (hearing)

Vestibule

Tympanic membrane (eardrum)
Internal carotid artery

Eustachian tube

FIGURE 2-48 The anatomy of the ear.

vitreous humor clear watery fluid filling the posterior chamber of the eye. It is responsible for giving the eye its spherical shape.

retina light- and color-sensing tissue lining the posterior chamber of the eye.

aqueous humor clear fluid filling the anterior chamber of the eye.

iris pigmented portion of the eye. It is the muscular area that constricts or dilates to change the size of the pupil.

pupil dark opening in the center of the iris through which light enters the eye.

sclera the white portion of the eye.

cornea thin, delicate layer covering the pupil and the iris.

conjunctiva mucous membrane that lines the eyelids.

lacrimal fluid liquid that lubricates the eye.

The eye is a spherical globe, filled with liquid (Figure 2-49). Its major compartment (the posterior chamber) contains a crystal-clear gelatinous fluid called **vitreous humor.** Lining the posterior of the compartment is a light- and color-sensing tissue known as the **retina.** Images focused on the retina are transmitted to the brain via the optic nerve. The lens separates the posterior and anterior chambers. The lens is responsible for focusing light and images on the retina by the action of small muscles that change its thickness. A fluid called **aqueous humor,** which is similar to vitreous humor, fills the anterior chamber. The anterior chamber also contains the **iris,** the muscular and colored portion of the eye that regulates the amount of light reaching the retina. Light enters the eye through the dark opening in the center of the iris called the **pupil.**

By examining the eye, you can easily identify several of its components such as the colored iris and the central black pupil. Bordering the iris is the **sclera,** the white and vascular area that forms the remaining, underlying surface of the exposed eye. The **cornea,** a very thin, clear, and delicate layer, covers both the pupil and iris. Continuous with the cornea and extending out to the eyelid's interior surface is the **conjunctiva,** another delicate, smooth layer that slides over itself and the cornea when the eye closes or blinks.

The eye is bathed in **lacrimal fluid,** which is produced by almond-shaped lacrimal glands located along the brow ridge just lateral and superior to the eyeball. Lacrimal fluid flows through lacrimal ducts and then over the cornea. Because the cornea does not have blood vessels, the fluid provides crucial lubrication, oxygen, and nutrients. If injury or some other mechanism—for example, a contact lens left in an unconscious patient's eye—prevents this fluid from reaching the cornea, the surface of the eye may be damaged. The lacrimal fluid is drained from the eye into the lacrimal sac, located along the medial orbit, and empties then into the nose.

The last major functional elements of the eye are the muscles that move them and their controlling cranial nerves. These small muscles are attached to the eyeball in the region of the conjunctival fold and are hidden within the eye socket and under the zygomatic arch. The oculomotor (CN-III), trochlear (CN-IV), and abducens (CN-VI) nerves control these muscles, which in turn control the eye's motion. The oculomotor nerve controls pupil dilation, conjugate movement (movement of the eyes together), and most of the eye's normal

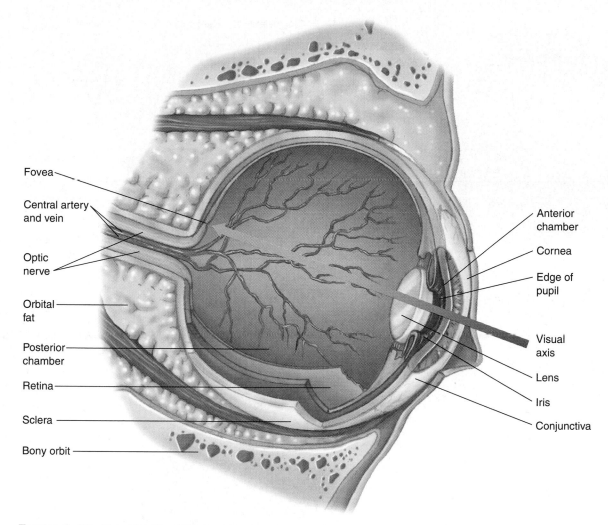

Fovea

Central artery and vein

Optic nerve

Orbital fat

Posterior chamber

Retina

Sclera

Bony orbit

Anterior chamber

Cornea

Edge of pupil

Visual axis

Lens

Iris

Conjunctiva

FIGURE 2-49   The anatomy of the eye.

range of motion. The trochlear nerve moves the eye downward and inward. The abducens nerve is responsible for eye abduction (outward gaze).

The Mouth

The lips mark the entrance to the mouth and play a role in the articulation of speech. The mouth houses the tongue, the gums (gingiva), and the teeth (Figure 2-50). The roof of the mouth is formed by the hard palate and the soft palate. The uvula is the peninsular extension of the soft palate that hangs in the back of the mouth. The oral cavity, lined with buccal (cheek/mouth) mucosa, is rich in mucous membranes. The parotid glands, just in front of the ears, and the submandibular glands, just beneath the mandible, secrete digestive enzymes and saliva into the oral cavity (Figure 2-51). The sublingual glands secrete enzymes just beneath the tongue. You can easily palpate these glands under the chin.

The tongue, a large, mobile muscle covered by mucous membranes, has many functions. It helps in chewing by keeping food on the teeth, and it assists in swallowing by moving the food into the oropharynx. It also contains the taste buds and is essential in forming words when we speak.

A highly vascular mucosa lines the gingiva, giving it a pink color. The teeth are anchored in bony sockets; only their white enamel-covered crowns are visible. An adult normally has 32 permanent teeth, including incisors, canines, premolars, and molars. The pharynx consists of three distinct areas: the nasopharynx (behind the nasal cavity), the oropharynx (back of the throat), and the laryngopharynx (just above the epiglottis). At the back of the throat on either side, the tonsils help separate the oropharynx (food processing) from the nasopharynx (air passage).

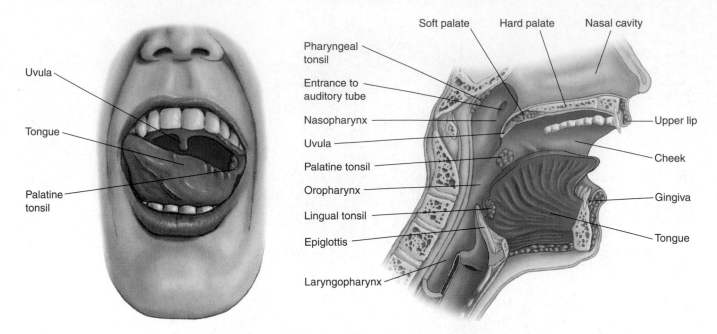

FIGURE 2-50 The mouth.

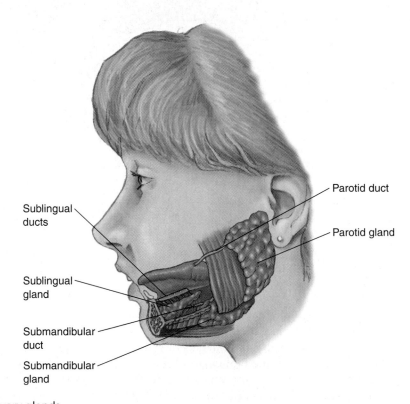

FIGURE 2-51 The salivary glands.

THE NECK

The neck (Figure 2-52) is the region that links the head to the rest of the body. Traveling through this anatomical area are blood for the facial region and brain, air for respiration, food for digestion, and neural communications to sense the body and its environment and to control both the voluntary and involuntary muscles and glands of the body. The neck also contains some of the important muscles used to provide head and shoulder movement as well as the thyroid and parathyroid glands of the endocrine system.

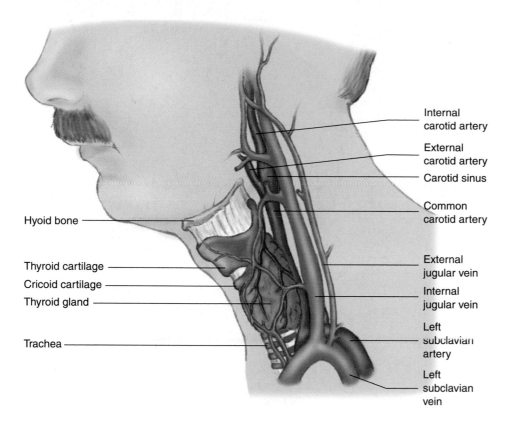

Hyoid bone

Thyroid cartilage

Cricoid cartilage

Thyroid gland

Trachea

Internal carotid artery

External carotid artery

Carotid sinus

Common carotid artery

External jugular vein

Internal jugular vein

Left subclavian artery

Left subclavian vein

FIGURE 2-52 The neck.

Vasculature of the Neck

The major blood vessels traversing the neck are the carotid arteries and the jugular veins. The carotid arteries arise from the brachiocephalic artery on the right and the aorta on the left. They travel upward and medially along the trachea and split into internal and external carotid arteries at about the level of the larynx's upper border. At this split are the carotid bodies and carotid sinuses, which are responsible for monitoring carbon dioxide and oxygen levels in the blood and the blood pressure, respectively. The jugular veins are paired on each side of the neck. The internal jugular vein runs in a sheath with the carotid artery and vagus nerve, whereas the external jugular vein runs superficially just lateral to the trachea. The jugular veins join the brachiocephalic veins just beneath the clavicles.

Airway Structures

The airway structures of the neck begin with the larynx. It is a prominent hollow cylindrical column made up of the thyroid and cricoid cartilages, atop the trachea. The thyroid opening is covered during swallowing by a cartilaginous and soft tissue flap, the epiglottis. The vocal cords, two folds of connective tissue sitting atop the opening of the larynx, further protect the airway. These cords vibrate with air passage and form sounds; they may also close in spasm to prevent foreign bodies from entering the lower airway. The cricoid cartilage is a circular ring between the thyroid cartilage and the trachea. The trachea is a series of C-shaped cartilages that maintain the tracheal opening. The posterior trachea shares a common border with the anterior surface of the esophagus. The trachea extends inferiorly to just below the sternum, where it bifurcates into the left and right mainstem bronchi at the carina.

Other Structures of the Neck

The cervical portion of the spinal column traverses the neck and provides the skeletal support for both the head and neck. It is also an attachment point for the ligaments that hold the column together and give it its strength and for the tendons that support and move the head and shoulders.

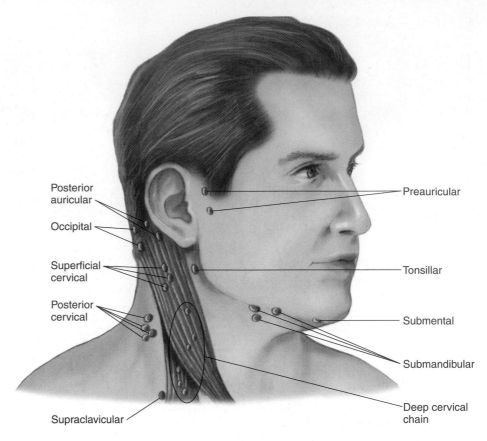

Posterior auricular

Occipital

Superficial cervical

Posterior cervical

Supraclavicular

Preauricular

Tonsillar

Submental

Submandibular

Deep cervical chain

FIGURE 2-53 The lymph nodes of the head and neck.

The cervical spine also contains the spinal cord. The spinal cord is the critical conduit for nervous signals between the brain and the body, and injury to it can be serious, even life threatening. From the spinal cord and between each vertebral junction, the peripheral nerve roots branch out. These structures direct signals to and receive signals from the limbs, internal organs, and sensory structures of the body. (The anatomy of the cervical spine is addressed in detail later in this chapter.)

Other structures within the neck include the esophagus, cranial nerves, thoracic duct, thyroid and parathyroid glands, and brachial plexus. The esophagus is a smooth muscle tube located behind the trachea that carries food and liquid to the stomach. Its anterior border is continuous with the posterior border of the trachea. Some cranial nerves, including the glossopharyngeal (CN-IX) and the vagus (CN-X), traverse the neck. The vagus nerve is essential for many parasympathetic activities including speech, swallowing, and cardiac, respiratory, and visceral function. The glossopharyngeal nerve innervates the carotid bodies and carotid sinuses, monitoring blood oxygen levels and blood pressure.

The **lymphatic system** helps drain fluid from the head and face and assists in fighting infection. A long chain of lymph nodes runs along the side of the neck, behind the ears, and under the chin (Figure 2-53). They are palpable when congested with infectious products. (The lymphatic system is discussed further in the Cardiovascular System section, later in this chapter.) The right and left thoracic ducts deliver lymph to the venous system at the juncture of the jugular and subclavian veins.

The thyroid gland sits over the trachea just below the cricoid cartilage and controls the rate of cellular metabolism as well as the systemic levels of calcium. The brachial plexus is a network of nerves in the lower neck and shoulder responsible for lower arm and hand function. Lastly, numerous muscles (including the sternocleidomastoid, platysma, and upper trapezius), fascia, and soft tissues are found in the neck.

lymphatic system a network of valveless vessels that drains fluid, called *lymph,* from the body tissues. Lymph nodes help filter impurities en route to the subclavian vein and thence to the heart.

SPINE AND THORAX

THE SPINE

The spine consists of a supporting skeletal structure, the vertebral column, and a central nervous system pathway, the spinal cord. These are important functional elements both for body posture and movement and for communication among the body's many systems. The vertebral column provides skeletal support for and permits movement of the head, assists in maintaining the shape of the thoracic cage, supports the upper body, and forms the posterior aspect of the pelvis. The spinal cord, contained and protected within the vertebral column, is the main communication conduit of the central nervous system. It is responsible for transmitting messages from the brain to the body organs and tissues and from the sensory nerves in the organs, skin, and other tissues back to the brain.

THE VERTEBRAL COLUMN

The vertebral column is a hollow skeletal tube made up of 33 irregular bones, called **vertebrae.** This column attaches to the head, to the bones of the rib cage, and to the pelvis. It provides the central skeletal support structure and a major portion of the axial skeleton. At the same time, the vertebrae provide a protective container for the spinal cord. Several components with differing functions may make up the structure of each individual vertebra.

vertebrae the 33 bones making up the vertebral column; singular *vertebra.*

The major weight-bearing component of a vertebra is the **vertebral body.** It is a cylinder of skeletal tissue made up of cancellous bone surrounded by a layer of hard, compact bone. It lies anterior to the other components of the vertebra.

vertebral body short column of bone that forms the weight-bearing portion of a vertebra.

The size of the vertebral body varies with its location along the spinal column (Figure 2-54). The first two cervical vertebrae (C-1 and C-2) do not have vertebral bodies because of their specialized functions. Below C-1 and C-2, the size of the vertebral bodies increases progressively moving down the spine because the vertebral column is supporting an increasing portion of the upper body's weight. The lumbar spine has the strongest and largest vertebral bodies due to the weight they bear. Because of the fused nature of the sacrum and coccyx, these regions have no discernable bodies.

A component of the vertebra posterior to the vertebral body is the **spinal canal,** which is the opening, or foramen, that accommodates the spinal cord. This opening is formed by small fused bony structures that are joined together to create a ring. The lateral structures of the ring are called **pedicles.** The two posterior structures are called **laminae.** The inferior surface of the pedicle contains a notch, called the *intervertebral foramen.* This notch permits the exit of a peripheral nerve root and spinal vein and the entrance of a spinal artery on each side of the spinal canal and at each vertebral junction.

spinal canal opening in the vertebrae that accommodates the spinal cord.

pedicles thick, bony struts that connect the vertebral bodies with the spinous and transverse processes and help make up the opening for the spinal canal.

A bony outgrowth called the **transverse process** is located at the juncture of the pedicle and lamina on each side of a vertebra. There is also a bony outgrowth where the laminae join, which is called the **spinous process.** The spinous process is the posteriorly and inferiorly oriented bony protrusion that you can feel along the spine.

laminae posterior bones of a vertebra that help make up the foramen, or opening, of the spinal canal.

The spinous and transverse processes are points of attachment for ligaments and tendons. Ligaments hold the vertebrae firmly together and in place while they permit limited motion. The tendons attach muscles to the vertebral column and permit these muscles to move the spine, other bones, and the body. This attachment of muscles and capsule of ligaments protects and strengthens the vertebral column against the forces of trauma.

transverse process bony outgrowth of the vertebral pedicle that serves as a site for muscle attachment and articulation with the ribs.

Between the vertebral bodies are cartilaginous **intervertebral disks.** These disks are formed of a strong yet somewhat flexible outer cover called the *annulus fibrosus* and a soft and gelatinous inner region called the *nucleus pulposus.* The intervertebral disks accommodate some motion of the adjacent vertebrae, limit bone wear, and absorb shock along the length of the spinal column. The intervertebral disks make up about 25% of the total length of the spinal column, and their degeneration accounts for much of the height loss associated with advancing age.

spinous process prominence at the posterior part of a vertebra.

The elements of the spinal column also have numerous articular surfaces. These surfaces are found on the vertebral bodies, the pedicles, and on the transverse and spinous processes. The articular surfaces enable the spinal column to move around the spinal cord without compressing it, permit articulation with the skull and ribs, and make possible the formation of the rigid, immobile joint of the pelvis.

intervertebral disk cartilaginous pad between vertebrae that serves as a shock absorber.

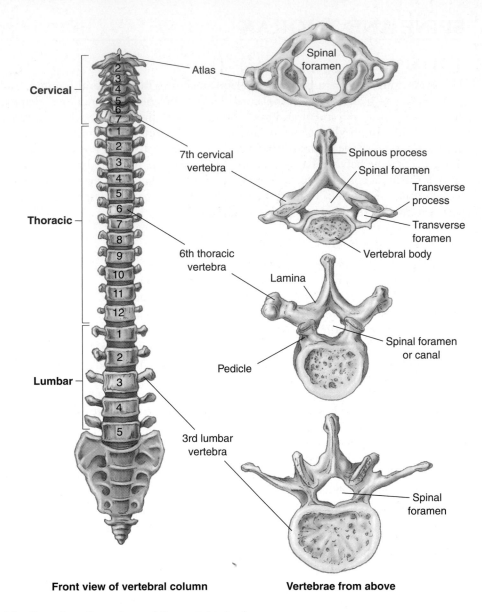

Cervical
1
2
3
4
5
6
7

Thoracic
1
2
3
4
5
6
7
8
9
10
11
12

Lumbar
1
2
3
4
5

Atlas — Spinal foramen

7th cervical vertebra

Spinous process
Spinal foramen
Transverse process
Transverse foramen
Vertebral body

6th thoracic vertebra

Lamina

Spinal foramen or canal

Pedicle

3rd lumbar vertebra

Spinal foramen

Front view of vertebral column   **Vertebrae from above**

FIGURE 2-54   Changing dimensions of the vertebral column.

The vertebral bodies are held firmly together by strong ligaments to ensure that the spinal foramen safely accommodates the spinal cord and that the body has a reasonable range of motion. The anterior longitudinal ligament extends along the anterior surfaces of the vertebral bodies. It provides the major stability of the spinal column and resists hyperextension. The posterior longitudinal ligament travels along the posterior surfaces of the vertebral bodies, within the spinal canal. This ligament helps to prevent hyperflexion; when it is disrupted, the result is, frequently, a spinal cord injury. Other ligaments encapsulate the spinous processes (interspinous ligaments) and the transverse processes. These ligaments strengthen and stabilize the column against excessive lateral bending, rotation, and flexion.

Divisions of the Vertebral Column

The vertebral column is divided into five regions: the cervical, the thoracic, the lumbar, the sacral, and the coccygeal (Figure 2-55). Each region is unique in its design and function and has a curve that reverses the curve of the spinal section(s) adjacent to it. The individual vertebrae of the column are identified by the first letter of their region and numbered from superior to inferior. For example, the most inferior of the seven cervical vertebrae is identified as C-7.

Content Review

DIVISIONS OF THE VERTEBRAL COLUMN
- Cervical spine
- Thoracic spine
- Lumbar spine
- Sacral spine
- Coccygeal spine

Cervical

I
II
III
IV
V
VI
VII

Cervical

I
II
III
IV
V
VI
VII
VIII
IX
X
XI
XII

Thoracic

Thoracic

Lumbar

I
II
III
IV
V

Lumbar

Sacral

Sacral

Coccygeal

Cervical Spine   The cervical spine consists of seven cervical vertebrae located between the base of the skull and the shoulders. The cervical spine is the sole skeletal support for the head, which weighs about 16 to 22 pounds.

The first two cervical vertebrae have a unique relationship with the head and each other that permits rotation to left and right and nodding of the head. The first cervical vertebra, C-1, is called the *atlas* (after the Greek god who held up the world) and supports the head. It is securely affixed to the occiput and permits nodding but does not accommodate any twisting or turning motion. It and the next vertebra, C-2, differ from most vertebrae in not having discernable vertebral bodies. Vertebra C-2, called the *axis*, has a small bony tooth, called the *odontoid process* or *dens*, that projects upward. This projection provides a pivotal point around which the atlas and head can rotate from side to side.

The remaining cervical vertebrae permit some rotation as well as flexion, extension, and lateral bending. The range of motion provided by the cervical spine is greater than allowed by any other portion of the spinal column. Yet, the portion of the spinal cord traveling through the cervical vertebrae is most critical to life functions. The last cervical vertebra

The range of motion provided by the cervical spine is the greatest allowed by any region, yet the cord in this region is critical to life functions.

(C-7) is quite noticeable as its spinous process is pronounced and can be felt as the first bony prominence along the spine and just above the shoulders.

Thoracic Spine The thoracic spine consists of 12 thoracic vertebrae. The first rib articulates individually with the first thoracic vertebra at two locations, with the transverse process and with the vertebral body. The next nine ribs articulate with the transverse process and the superior portion of the vertebral body as well as with the inferior portion of the vertebral body that is adjacent (superior) to it. This system of fixation limits rib movement and increases the strength and rigidity of the thoracic spine. The last two ribs articulate only with the vertebral bodies, which permits greater movement and flexibility.

Because the thoracic spine supports more of the human body than the cervical spine, the thoracic vertebral bodies are larger and stronger. The spinous and transverse processes are also larger and more prominent because they are associated with the musculature holding the upper body erect and with the movement of the thoracic cage during respiration.

Lumbar Spine The five bones of the lumbar spine each carry the weight of the head, neck, and thorax above them. They also bear the forces of bending and lifting above the pelvis. The vertebral bodies are largest in this region of the spinal column, and the intervertebral disks are also the thickest and bear the greatest stress. The lumbar pedicles and lamina are also thick, whereas the transverse and spinous processes are shorter and stouter than those in the thoracic spine. The spinal foramen is largest in the lumbar region.

Sacral Spine The sacral spine consists of five sacral vertebrae that fuse into the posterior plate of the pelvis. This plate, in conjunction with the two innominate bones of the pelvis, protects the urinary and reproductive organs and attaches the pelvis and lower extremities to the axial skeleton. The articulation with the pelvis occurs at the sacroiliac joint on the lateral surface of the sacrum. This joint is very strong and permits no movement. The upper body balances on the sacrum.

Coccygeal Spine The coccygeal spine is made up of three to five fused vertebrae that represent the residual elements of a tail. They comprise the short skeletal end of the vertebral column.

Curvature of the Spine The vertebral column curves through each region of the spine. The cervical and lumbar regions of the spine demonstrate concave curves, and the thoracic and sacral regions represent convex curves. These curves strengthen the spine and permit a greater range of supported motion.

The Spinal Meninges

The spinal meninges are similar to those covering and protecting the structures within the cranium. They consist of the dura mater, the arachnoid, and the pia mater. The meninges cover the entire spinal cord and the peripheral nerve roots as they leave the spinal column. However, the spinal meninges are not as strongly secured to the spinal column as the meninges are to the cranium. The dura mater is firmly attached to the base of the skull and to a collagen fiber called the *coccygeal ligament* at the top of the sacrum. These attachments and the dura mater's attachments associated with each pair of peripheral nerve roots help position the cord centrally within the spinal canal yet permit the column to move around the cord (Figure 2-56).

As it does in the brain, cerebrospinal fluid bathes the spinal cord by filling the subarachnoid space. The fluid provides a medium for the exchange of nutrients and waste products and absorbs the shocks of sudden movements. Cerebrospinal fluid is produced in the ventricles of the brain and then circulates through the ventricles and through the arachnoid space of the spinal meninges. The fluid is absorbed by specialized cells (the arachnoid villi) in the lower portion of the lumbar meninges, a region called the *spinal cistern*.

The distance between the spinal cord and the interior of the vertebral foramen varies in the different spinal regions. The region with the closest tolerance between the cord and the interior surfaces of the spinal foramen is the thoracic spine, where movement of the spinal column is most limited. Although this region is injured only infrequently, just a slight displacement into the vertebral foramen is likely to cause spinal cord injury. The greatest spacing between the cord and the interior of the vertebral column is found in upper lumbar and upper cervical (C-1 and C-2) regions.

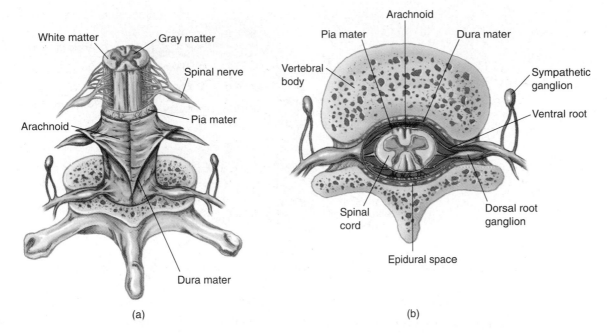

FIGURE 2-56 Structural protection of the spinal cord.

Injuries to the mid- or lower lumbar regions do not endanger the spinal cord because the cord ends at the L-1 level in mature adults. Injury to the lumbar spine can, however, damage the peripheral nerve roots there. The vertebral foramen below L-1 is filled with cerebrospinal fluid and is where the fluid may be most safely removed for diagnostic testing (spinal tap).

THE THORAX

The thoracic cage is the chamber that moves air in and out and where oxygen and carbon dioxide are exchanged to support the body's metabolism. It consists of the thoracic skeleton, diaphragm, and associated musculature. It is also the location of the heart, major blood vessels, and other important structures essential for body function. It contains the trachea, bronchi, and lungs, and the mediastinum. Finally, the dynamics of the chest, respiration, are controlled by a series of centers in the brain and blood vessels.

Thoracic Skeleton

The thoracic skeleton is defined by 12 pairs of C-shaped ribs, which articulate posteriorly with the thoracic spine and then extend in an anterior and inferior direction (Figure 2-57). The upper seven pairs join the sternum at their cartilaginous endpoints. The eighth through tenth ribs have cartilage at their distal anterior ends that join the cartilage of the seventh rib at the inferior margin of the sternum. The eleventh and twelfth ribs are often termed the floating ribs and have no anterior attachment.

The sternum completes the anterior bony structure of the thorax and is made up of three sections: the manubrium, the body of the sternum, and the xiphoid process. The manubrium is the superior portion of the sternum and is the medial endpoint of the clavicle and first rib. The sternal angle (also known as the angle of Louis) is the junction of the manubrium and the body of the sternum and is palpable through the skin as an elevation or prominence. This structure has clinical significance as it is the site of attachment of the second rib and quickly allows the EMT-I to identify the second intercostal space. This location is important because it is where to perform a needle decompression of the chest in the event of a tension pneumothorax. The xiphoid process is the most inferior portion of the sternum and meets the body at the junction of the costal cartilages of the lower ribs.

The thorax is divided by imaginary vertical lines used to describe positions lateral to the sternum. These lines include the **midclavicular line,** the anterior axillary line, the **midaxillary line,** and the posterior axillary line. When combined with a rib level, these lines

midclavicular line an imaginary line from the center of either clavicle down the anterior thorax.

midaxillary line an imaginary line from the middle of the armpit to the ankle; divides the body into anterior and posterior planes.

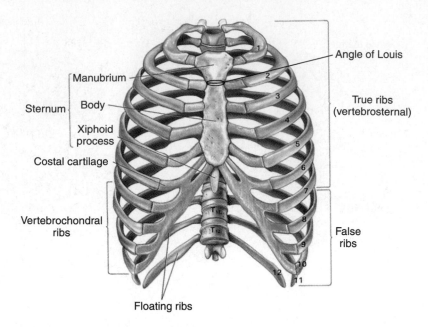

Manubrium

Sternum — Body

Xiphoid
process

Costal cartilage

Vertebrochondral
ribs

Floating ribs

Angle of Louis

True ribs
(vertebrosternal)

False
ribs

FIGURE 2-57   Skeletal components of the thorax.

serve as good landmarks for describing wounds, locating underlying structures, and for identifying locations to perform procedures. The space just inferior to each rib is called an *intercostal space* and is given the number of the rib above it. For example, the anterior axillary line extends from the anterior margin of the axilla (armpit) inferiorly along the thoracic wall. Its intersection with the fifth intercostal space is generally used in the emergency department to place a thoracostomy tube in patients with pneumothorax or hemothorax. It is not frequently used for prehospital needle decompression because this site is often obscured by the patient's arms or by immobilization devices and blankets.

The thoracic inlet is the superior opening in the thorax. It is narrow in comparison to the thoracic outlet, and is defined by the curvature of the first rib, with its posterior attachment at the first thoracic vertebra and ending anteriorly, at the manubrium. The thoracic outlet is formed posteriorly by the twelfth vertebra, laterally by the curvature of the twelfth rib, and extends anteriorly and superiorly along the costal margin to the **xiphisternal joint.**

The Diaphragm

The diaphragm is a muscular, dome-like structure that separates the abdominal cavity from the thoracic cavity. It is affixed to the lower border of the rib cage, while its central and superior margin may extend to the level of the fourth intercostal space anteriorly and the sixth intercostal space posteriorly during maximal expiration. This superior positioning may allow penetrating wounds of the lower half of the thorax to penetrate the diaphragm and enter the abdominal cavity. The aorta, esophagus, and inferior vena cava exit the thoracic cavity through separate openings in this structure. The diaphragm is a major muscle of respiration, contracting to displace the floor of the thoracic cavity downward during inspiration and relaxing and moving upward with expiration.

Associated Musculature

The chest wall musculature along with the shoulder musculature, clavicles, scapula, and humerus provide additional protection to the vital structures within the upper thorax (Figure 2-58). The clavicles articulate laterally with the acromion process of the scapula. The scapula covers the posterior and lateral aspects of the first six ribs and articulates with the humerus to complete the shoulder girdle.

Chest wall muscles between the ribs, called the *intercostal muscles,* along with the diaphragm and the sternocleidomastoid muscles are the major muscles of respiration. The sternocleidomastoid muscles raise the upper rib and sternum and, with the sternum, the anterior attachments of the next nine ribs. The intercostal muscles contract to further elevate

xiphisternal joint union between xiphoid process and body of the sternum.

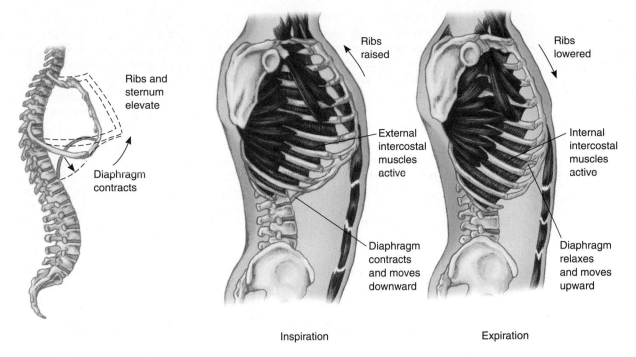

Ribs and
sternum
elevate

Diaphragm
contracts

Ribs
raised

External
intercostal
muscles
active

Diaphragm
contracts
and moves
downward

Ribs
lowered

Internal
intercostal
muscles
active

Diaphragm
relaxes
and moves
upward

Inspiration

Expiration

FIGURE 2-58   The diaphragm and muscles of the chest change its volume to effect respirations.

the ribs and increase the anterior-posterior dimension of the thorax. Simultaneously, the diaphragm, which forms the floor of the thorax, contracts and flattens to further increase the volume of the thoracic cavity. As the thoracic volume increases, the pressure within it becomes less than atmospheric. Air rushes in through the tracheobronchial tree and into the alveoli to equalize this pressure gradient, filling the lungs.

As the musculature relaxes, the diaphragm again intrudes upward into the thoracic cavity, the ribs and sternum move inferiorly, and the ribs move closer together in an inferior and posterior direction. This decreases the thoracic volume and increases the intrathoracic pressure. When the pressure within the thorax exceeds that of the surrounding atmosphere, air rushes out. Therefore exhalation in the resting state is largely a passive activity aided by the elastic recoil of the lungs. Gravity helps facilitate this action with downward displacement of the ribs in either the upright or supine position. This changing of volume to move air in and out is called the *bellows effect*.

The changing volume and pressure within the thoracic cage also assist with the pumping of blood to and venous return from the systemic circulation. The decreased intrathoracic pressure of inspiration helps move venous blood toward the thorax and heart, whereas the increased pressure of expiration helps move arterial blood away from the heart and thorax. The changing intrathoracic pressure affects the blood pressure and pulse strength. Normally, the systolic blood pressure and pulse strength fall during inspiration and rise during expiration.

The diaphragm is the primary muscle of respiration. The intercostal muscles are recruited to increase the depth of respiration. As the rate, depth, and work of respiration increase due to exercise or stress from trauma or infection, more accessory muscles of ventilation are recruited. These include the sternocleidomastoid and scalene muscles of the neck for inspiration and the anterior abdominal muscles to aid in forceful exhalation. The rhomboid muscles lift, abduct, and rotate the scapulae to help lift the upper chest with inspiration. The cough reflex, important to keeping the airways clear and alveoli expanded, depends on the addition of the latissimus dorsi muscles located along the posterior and lateral thoracic wall and the erector spinae muscles along the spine to allow for forceful contraction of the thorax.

Trachea, Bronchi, and Lungs

Contained within the thoracic cavity are the tracheobronchial tree and the lungs. The trachea is the hollow and cartilage-supported respiratory pathway through which air moves in

Normal inspiration is an active process, whereas normal expiration is a passive process.

pulmonary hilum central
medial region of the lung
where the bronchi and
pulmonary vasculature enter
the lung.

*The layers of the pleura
and the small volume of
fluid between them cause
the lungs to move with the
thoracic cage.*

and out of the thorax and lungs. It enters through the thoracic inlet and divides into the right and left mainstem bronchi at the carina, located in the upper central thorax. The right and left mainstem bronchi extend for about 3 centimeters and enter their respective lungs at the **pulmonary hilum.** The pulmonary hilum is also where the pulmonary arteries enter and the pulmonary veins exit the lungs and is the sole point of fixation of the lung in the thoracic cage. The bronchi then further divide into bronchioles, which ultimately terminate in the alveoli. The lungs contain millions of these tiny grape-shaped alveoli, which are the basic unit of structure and function in the lungs.

Each lung occupies one side of the thoracic cavity and is divided into lobes. The right lung has three lobes, the upper, middle and lower. The left lung has two lobes, the upper and lower. The left upper lobe contains the cardiac notch against which the heart rests. The lower section of the left upper lobe (the lingula), projects around the lateral border of the heart and corresponds to the middle lobe of the right lung.

The lungs are covered by the visceral pleura, a smooth membrane that lines the exterior of the lungs. It folds over on itself at the pulmonary hilum and then lines the inside of the thoracic cavity, becoming the parietal pleura. This dual layer forms a potential space called the *pleural space*. It contains a small amount of serous (pleural) fluid for lubrication and permits the lungs to expand and contract easily. This dual layer also creates the seal that causes the lungs to expand and contract with the changing volume of the thoracic cavity.

The trachea, bronchi, and lungs are discussed further in the Respiratory System section later in this chapter.

Mediastinum and Heart

The mediastinum (Figure 2-59) is the central space within the thoracic cavity bounded laterally by the lungs, inferiorly by the diaphragm, and superiorly by the thoracic outlet. The heart is located within and fills most of the mediastinum. (The heart is discussed in detail in the Cardiovascular System section, later in this chapter.) Through the mediastinum, the great vessels (see the next section) traverse to and from the heart, and the trachea and esoph-

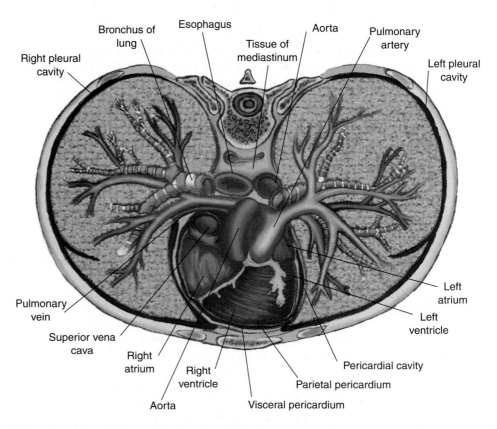

FIGURE 2-59 Structures of the mediastinum and thorax.

agus enter the thorax. The esophagus then courses anterior to the aorta before exiting through the diaphragm at the thoracic outlet (esophageal hiatus or foramen).

The vagus nerve, which provides parasympathetic innervation of thoracic and abdominal viscera, enters the thorax bilaterally through the thoracic inlet and traverses the mediastinum giving branches to the larynx, esophagus, trachea, bronchi, and heart. The vagus nerve then exits the thorax through the esophageal opening in the diaphragm to innervate the abdominal viscera. The phrenic nerve (originating from the third, fourth, and fifth cervical nerve roots) also enters the thorax through the thoracic inlet and traverses the thorax to innervate the diaphragm.

The thoracic duct (part of the lymphatic system) also traverses the thorax from the thoracic outlet where it enters through the aortic opening in the diaphragm. It typically crosses the midline from the right side of the aorta in the posterior mediastinum at the level of the fifth thoracic vertebra and then ascends above the level of the left clavicle before arching back downward to empty into the left internal jugular vein. The thoracic duct carries most of the body's lymphatic drainage (all but the right side of the head, neck, thorax, and right upper extremity).

Great Vessels

The **great vessels** are those large arteries and veins that enter and leave the heart and are found in the mediastinum. They are the aorta, the superior and inferior vena cava, the pulmonary arteries, and the pulmonary veins. Injury to these large vascular structures can lead to significant blood loss and death if the condition is not quickly recognized and repaired. The aorta, which is fixed at three positions within the thorax, is not only susceptible to penetrating injury, but also to blunt injury by rapid deceleration or shear forces. It is fixed at the annulus where it attaches to the heart, at the **ligamentum arteriosum** near the bifurcation of the pulmonary artery, and at the aortic hiatus where it passes through the diaphragm and enters the abdomen.

Other major vessels that branch from the great vessels in the upper thorax include the subclavian arteries and veins, the common carotid arteries, and the innominate artery (which is the first large branch off the aortic arch dividing into the right common carotid and right subclavian). The internal mammary vessels are inferior branches of the subclavians running along the anterior surface of the pleura, posterior to the costochondral (rib-cartilage) junction. They are often harvested for coronary artery bypass grafts. The intercostal arteries are branches of the thoracic aorta (except for the first two, which arise from branches of the subclavian) that run along the lower margins of the ribs along with the intercostal nerves. Finally, the bronchial arteries (one right and two left) are usually branches of the thoracic aorta that nourish the non-respiratory tissues of the lung.

Esophagus

The esophagus enters the thorax through the thoracic inlet with and just posterior to the trachea. It continues the length of the mediastinum and exits through the esophageal hiatus of the diaphragm. It is a muscular tube that is contiguous with the posterior wall of the trachea and conducts food and drink from the oral pharynx to the stomach. It moves food and liquid toward the stomach through a rhythmic muscular contraction called *peristalsis*. During vomiting, peristalsis reverses and propels the emesis up the esophagus.

NERVOUS SYSTEM

The nervous system is the body's principal control system. This network of cells, tissues, and organs regulates nearly all bodily functions via electrical impulses transmitted through nerves, all of which are highly susceptible to hypoxia (oxygen deficiency). The endocrine system is closely related to the nervous system. It exerts bodily control via hormones. You will learn more about this system later in this chapter. A third system, the circulatory system, assists in regulatory functions by distributing hormones and other chemical messengers.

The nervous system consists of two main divisions—the **central nervous system** and the **peripheral nervous system**. The central nervous system consists of the brain and the spinal cord. The peripheral nervous system is somewhat more complex. As you look at

great vessels the large arteries and veins located in the mediastinum that enter and exit the heart; the aorta, superior and inferior vena cava, pulmonary arteries, and pulmonary veins.

ligamentum arteriosum cord-like remnant of a fetal vessel connecting the pulmonary artery to the aorta at the aortic isthmus.

The nervous system is the body's principal control system.

central nervous system the brain and the spinal cord.

peripheral nervous system part of the nervous system that extends throughout the body and is composed of the cranial nerves arising from the brain and the peripheral nerves arising from the spinal cord. Its subdivisions are the somatic and the autonomic nervous systems.

FIGURE 2-60 Overview of the
nervous system.

FIGURE 2-60 Overview of the nervous system.

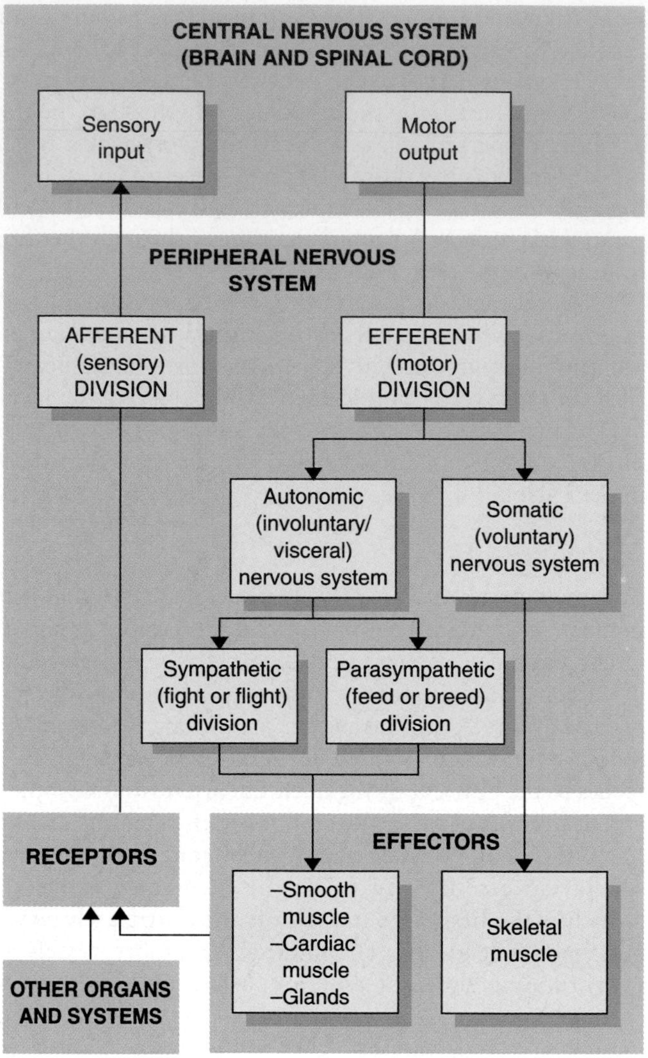

somatic nervous system part
of the nervous system
controlling voluntary bodily
functions.

autonomic nervous system
part of the nervous system
controlling involuntary bodily
functions. It is divided into the
sympathetic and the
parasympathetic systems.

sympathetic nervous system
division of the autonomic
nervous system that prepares
the body for stressful
situations. Mediated by the
neurotransmitters epinephrine
and norepinephrine, its
actions include increased heart
rate and dilation of the
bronchioles and pupils.

**parasympathetic nervous
system** division of the
autonomic nervous system
that is responsible for
controlling vegetative
functions. Mediated by the
neurotransmitter
acetylcholine, its actions
include decreased heart rate
and constriction of the
bronchioles and pupils.

neuron nerve cell; the
fundamental component of the
nervous system.

Figure 2-60, note that the peripheral nervous system is divided into two major subdivisions—the **somatic nervous system,** which governs voluntary functions (those we control consciously), and the **autonomic nervous system,** which has two subdivisions—the **sympathetic nervous system** and the **parasympathetic nervous system.** These two subdivisions of the autonomic nervous system work together to carry out involuntary physiological processes such as regulation of blood pressure, heart rate, and digestion.

You will learn more about these divisions of the nervous system as you continue through the next pages. As you read, it will be helpful if you think of the nervous system as a "living computer." The central nervous system is the central processing unit and the various divisions of the peripheral nervous system carry on the input and output processes.

FUNDAMENTAL UNIT: THE NEURON

The fundamental unit of the nervous system is the nerve cell, or **neuron.** The neuron includes the *cell body* (soma), containing the nucleus; the *dendrites,* which transmit electrical impulses to the cell body; and the *axons,* which transmit electrical impulses away from the cell body (Figure 2-61).

The transmission of impulses in the nervous system resembles the conduction of electrical impulses through the heart. In its resting state, the neuron is positively charged on the outside and negatively charged on the inside. When electrically stimulated, sodium rapidly surges into the cell and potassium rapidly leaves it so that there is no longer a difference in electrical charge between the inside and the outside. This "depolarization," or loss of the charge difference, is subsequently transmitted down the neuron at an extremely high rate of speed.

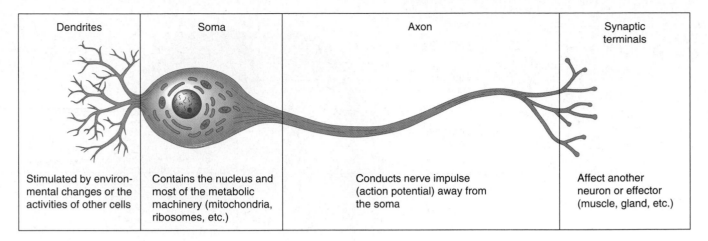

FIGURE 2-61 Anatomy of a neuron.

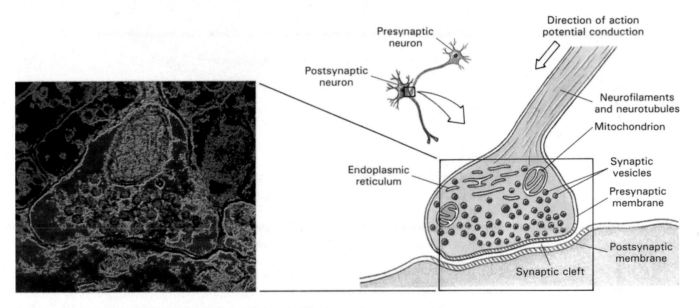

FIGURE 2-62 The synapse: (a) electron micrograph, (b) schematic.

The neuron joins with other neurons at junctions called *synapses* (Figure 2-62). The neurons never come into direct contact with each other at these synapses. Instead, upon reaching the synapse, the axon causes the release of a chemical *neurotransmitter*. This neurotransmitter, either acetylcholine or norepinephrine, then crosses the gap between the axon of the depolarized neuron and the dendrite of the adjacent neuron. The neurotransmitter stimulates the post-synaptic membrane of the connecting nerve. Acetylcholine is the neurotransmitter of the parasympathetic and voluntary (somatic) nervous systems. Norepinephrine is found in the synaptic terminals of sympathetic nerves. (See the later description of the divisions of the peripheral nervous system.)

CENTRAL NERVOUS SYSTEM

Knowledge of the anatomy and physiology of the central nervous system—the brain and the spinal cord—is essential to understanding and treating nervous system emergencies. Note that the basic structures of the central nervous system and some of the related terminology were presented earlier in the chapter under the headings "Head, Face, and Neck" and "Spine and Thorax."

Content Review

CENTRAL NERVOUS SYSTEM
- Brain
- Spinal cord

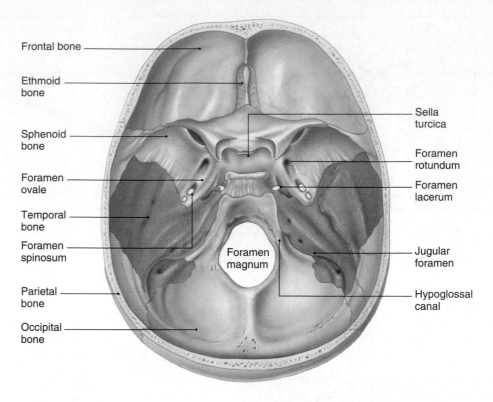

Frontal bone

Ethmoid bone

Sphenoid bone

Foramen ovale

Temporal bone

Foramen spinosum

Parietal bone

Occipital bone

Sella turcica

Foramen rotundum

Foramen lacerum

Foramen magnum

Jugular foramen

Hypoglossal canal

FIGURE 2-63 The bones of the skull.

Protective Structures

Most of the central nervous system is protected by bony structures. The brain lies within the cranial vault, protected by the skull. Covered by the scalp, the cranium consists of the bones of the head, excluding the facial bones. Bones composing the cranium include two single bones—the frontal and occipital bones—and a series of paired bones—the parietals, temporals, sphenoids, and ethmoids (Figure 2-63; also review Figure 2-44).

The spinal cord is housed inside and is protected by the spinal canal formed by the vertebrae of the spinal column. (Review Figure 2-54.)

Protective membranes called the *meninges* cover the entire central nervous system. Three layers of meninges pad, or cushion, the brain and spinal cord (Figure 2-64). The durable, outermost layer is referred to as the *dura mater.* The middle layer is a web-like structure known as the *arachnoid membrane.* The innermost layer, directly overlying the central nervous system, is called the *pia mater.* The space between the pia mater and the arachnoid membrane is referred to as the subarachnoid space, and the space between the dura mater and the arachnoid membrane is called the *subdural space.* The space outside the dura mater is called the *epidural space.* Both the brain and the spinal cord are bathed in *cerebrospinal fluid,* a watery, clear fluid that acts as a cushion to protect these organs from physical impact.

The Brain

The brain is the largest part of the central nervous system. The following information provides a general profile of the brain's anatomy and physiology.

Divisions of the Brain   Filling the cranial vault, the brain is divided into six major parts: the cerebrum, the diencephalon (which includes the thalamus and hypothalamus), the mesencephalon (midbrain), the pons, the medulla oblongata, and the cerebellum (Figure 2-65).

The cerebrum and diencephalon constitute the *forebrain:*

- *Cerebrum.* The cerebrum is in the anterior and middle area of the cranium. Containing two hemispheres, it is joined by a structure called the *corpus callosum.* The cerebrum governs all sensory and motor actions. It is the seat of

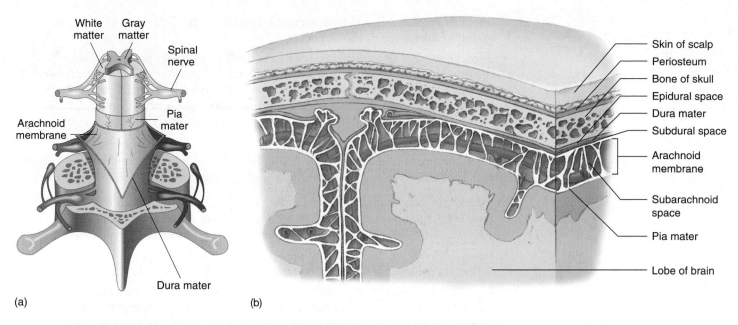

FIGURE 2-64 The meninges: (a) posterior view of the spinal cord showing the meningeal layers; (b) the meninges of the brain.

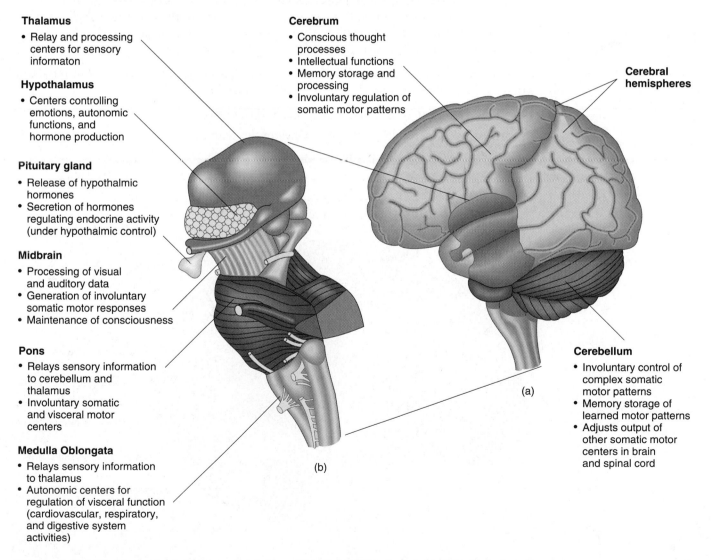

Thalamus
- Relay and processing centers for sensory informaton

Hypothalamus
- Centers controlling emotions, autonomic functions, and hormone production

Pituitary gland
- Release of hypothalmic hormones
- Secretion of hormones regulating endocrine activity (under hypothalmic control)

Midbrain
- Processing of visual and auditory data
- Generation of involuntary somatic motor responses
- Maintenance of consciousness

Pons
- Relays sensory information to cerebellum and thalamus
- Involuntary somatic and visceral motor centers

Medulla Oblongata
- Relays sensory information to thalamus
- Autonomic centers for regulation of visceral function (cardiovascular, respiratory, and digestive system activities)

Cerebrum
- Conscious thought processes
- Intellectual functions
- Memory storage and processing
- Involuntary regulation of somatic motor patterns

Cerebral hemispheres

Cerebellum
- Involuntary control of complex somatic motor patterns
- Memory storage of learned motor patterns
- Adjusts output of other somatic motor centers in brain and spinal cord

FIGURE 2-65 The human brain: (a) superficial view of the brain; (b) components of the brainstem.

intelligence, learning, analysis, memory, and language. The *cerebral cortex* is the outermost layer of the cerebrum.

- *Diencephalon.* Covered by the cerebrum, the diencephalon is sometimes called the *interbrain.* Inside it are the *thalamus, hypothalamus* (which is connected to the pituitary gland), and the *limbic system.* This area is responsible for many involuntary actions such as temperature regulation, sleep, water balance, stress response, and emotions. It plays a major role in regulating the autonomic nervous system.

The mesencephalon (midbrain), pons, and the medulla oblongata collectively form the brainstem. The brainstem and the cerebellum together constitute the *hindbrain:*

- *Mesencephalon,* or midbrain. The mesencephalon, located between the diencephalon and the pons, is responsible for certain aspects of motor coordination. The mesencephalon is the major region controlling eye movement.

- *Pons.* Between the midbrain and the medulla oblongata, the pons contains connections between the brain and the spinal cord.

- *Medulla oblongata.* The medulla oblongata is located between the pons and the spinal cord. It marks the division between the spinal cord and the brain. Major centers for controlling respiration, cardiac activity, and vasomotor activity are located here.

- *Cerebellum.* The cerebellum is located in the posterior fossa of the cranial cavity. It consists of two hemispheres closely related to the brainstem and higher centers. The cerebellum coordinates fine motor movement, posture, equilibrium, and muscle tone.

Patho Pearls

Aphasia, or the inability to speak, is more common in strokes that affect the left side of the brain, where major portions of the speech center are located.

Areas of Specialization   Several areas of specialization are recognized within the brain and have clinical application (Figure 2-66). These include:

- *Speech.* Located in the temporal lobe of the cerebrum.
- *Vision.* Located in the occipital cortex of the cerebrum.
- *Personality.* Located in the frontal lobes of the cerebrum.

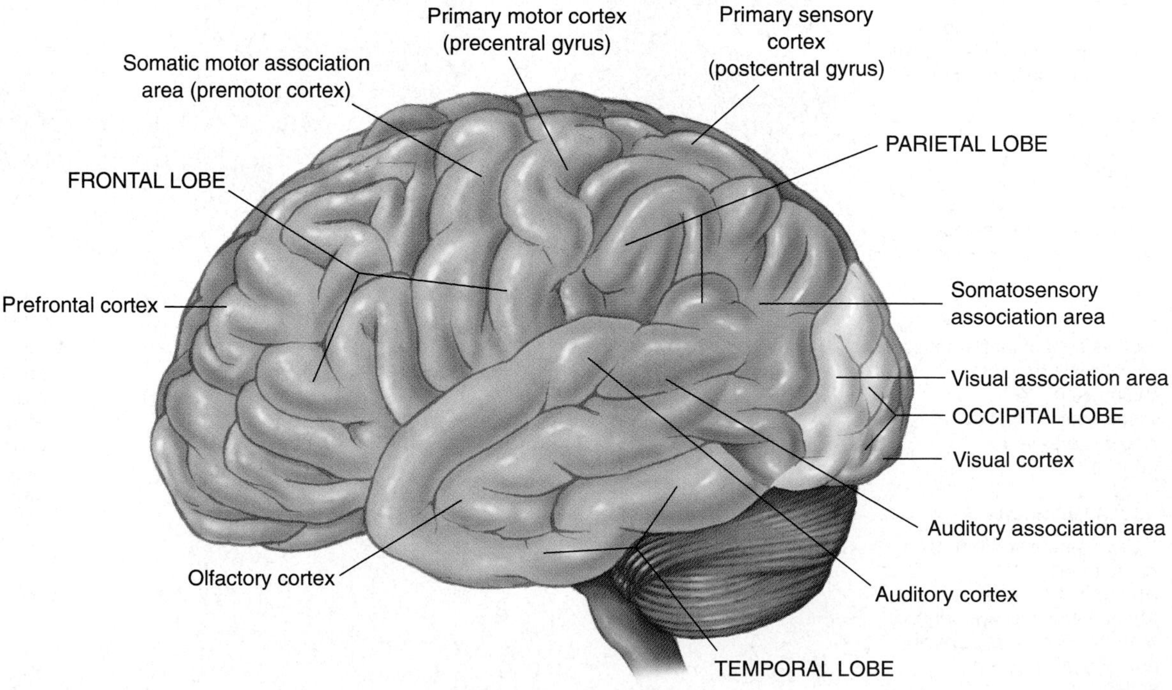

FIGURE 2-66   External anatomy of the brain.

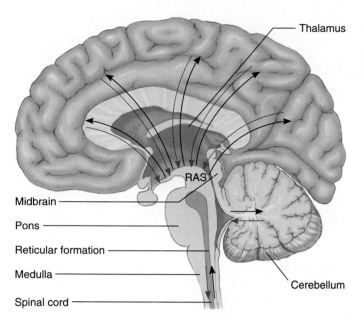

FIGURE 2-67 The reticular activating system (RAS), which sends and receives messages from various parts of the brain.

- *Balance and coordination.* Located in the cerebellum.
- *Sensory.* Located in the parietal lobes of the cerebrum.
- *Motor.* Located in the frontal lobes of the cerebrum.
- *Reticular activating system.* The reticular activating system (RAS) operates in the lateral portion of the medulla, pons, and especially the midbrain. The RAS sends impulses to and receives impulses from the cerebral cortex. It is a diffuse system of interlacing nerve cells responsible for maintaining consciousness and the ability to respond to stimuli (Figure 2-67).

Vascular Supply   The brain receives about 20% of the body's total blood flow per minute. Blood flow to the brain is provided by two systems. The *carotid system* is anterior, and the *vertebrobasilar system* is posterior. Both join at the *Circle of Willis* before entering the structures of the brain (Figure 2-68). The system is designed so that interruption of any part will not cause significant loss of blood flow to the tissues. Venous drainage of the brain is through the venous sinuses and the internal jugular veins.

Besides blood flow, cerebrospinal fluid bathes the brain and spinal cord. Several chambers within the brain, called *ventricles,* contain most of the intracranial volume of this fluid.

The Spinal Cord

The **spinal cord** is the central nervous system pathway responsible for transmitting sensory input from the body to the brain and for conducting motor impulses from the brain to the body muscles and organs. Through this pathway, the brain monitors and controls most body functions. Additionally, the spinal cord acts as a reflex center, intercepting sensory signals and initiating short-circuited (reflex) signaling to muscle bodies as needed. If this pathway is compromised, control of the body below the injury is lost.

In the fetus, the cord fills the entire length of the vertebral column. However, the growth of cord does not keep pace with the growth of the vertebral column. This discrepancy means that, as a person grows, the peripheral nerve roots are pulled into the spinal foramen. The sheath of the dura below L-2 is thus filled with numerous strands of peripheral nerves. The resulting structure resembles the tail of a horse and is called the *cauda equina* (Latin for horse's tail). In the adult, the spinal cord extends from the base of the brain (the medulla oblongata) to approximately the L-1 or L-2 level.

Like all central nervous system tissue, the spinal cord constantly needs oxygenated blood. This blood is supplied through paired spinal arteries that branch off the vertebral, cervical, thoracic, and lumbar arteries. These spinal arteries travel through intervertebral foramina, then split into anterior and posterior arteries. On the surface of the spinal cord

spinal cord central nervous system pathway responsible for transmitting sensory input from the body to the brain and for conducting motor impulses from the brain to the body muscles and organs.

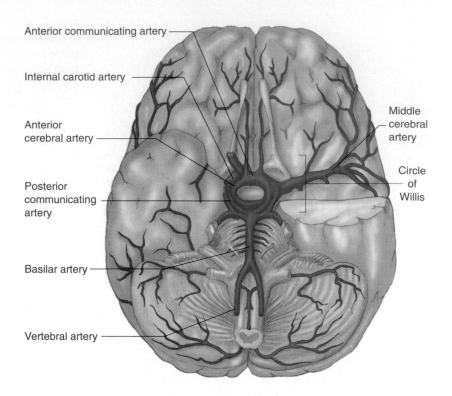

Anterior communicating artery

Internal carotid artery

Anterior cerebral artery

Posterior communicating artery

Basilar artery

Vertebral artery

Middle cerebral artery

Circle of Willis

FIGURE 2-68 An interior view of the brain showing the Circle of Willis, which is formed by the anterior and posterior communicating arteries.

anterior medial fissure deep crease along the ventral surface of the spinal cord that divides the cord into right and left halves.

posterior medial sulcus shallow longitudinal groove along the dorsal surface of the spinal cord.

gray matter areas in the central nervous system dominated by nerve cell bodies; the central portion of the spinal cord.

white matter material that surrounds gray matter in the spinal cord; made up largely of axons.

ascending tracts bundles of axons along the spinal cord that transmit signals from the body to the brain.

descending tracts bundles of axons along the spinal cord that transmit signals from the brain to the body.

there are numerous interconnections (anastomoses) between the arteries to provide a better chance for adequate circulation in case of vascular blockage or injury.

Anatomically, the spinal cord is a long cylinder divided into left and right halves by the **anterior medial fissure** and by the **posterior medial sulcus.** In cross section, the central part of the cord has a butterfly or H shape and appears gray in color. This **gray matter** is made up largely of neural cell bodies and plays an important role in the reflex system.

The remaining areas, or **white matter,** then form three bundles or columns of myelinated (covered with a protein sheath) nerve fibers on each side of the cord around the gray matter: the anterior white column, the lateral white column, and the posterior white column. This white matter is composed of nerve cell pathways, called *axons.* It contains bundles of axons that transmit signals upward to the brain in what are called **ascending tracts** and bundles that transmit signals downward to the body in what are called **descending tracts.** These tracts are paired, one ascending and one descending on each side, and injury may affect either or both.

A thorough discussion of organization and functions of the ascending and descending spinal tracts is beyond the scope of this textbook. However, knowing the functions of some motor and sensory pathways can aid you in recognizing spinal cord injury.

The important ascending (sensory) tracts or fasciculi include the fasciculus gracilis, fasciculus cutaneous, and the spinothalamic tracts. The fasciculus gracilis and fasciculus cutaneous carry sensory impulses of light touch, vibration, and positional sense from the skin, muscles, tendons, and joints to the brain. They are located on the posterior portion of the cord (posterior columns). Their injury causes disruption on the ipsilateral (same side) of the body because the left to right switching occurs at the medulla. The spinothalamic tracts include both lateral and anterior tracts. The anterior pathway conducts pain and temperature, whereas the lateral pathway conducts touch and pressure sensation. These pathways cross as they enter the cord, hence injury results in contralateral (opposite side) deficits.

The important descending (motor) spinal nerve tract is the corticospinal tract. It is responsible for voluntary and fine muscle movement on the ispilateral side of the body. This

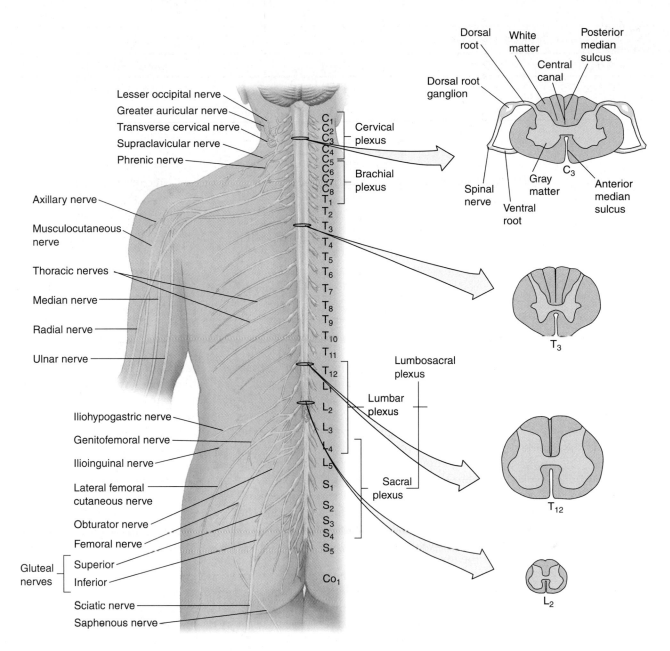

FIGURE 2-69 The spinal cord and spinal nerves.

pathway lies on the posterior and lateral portions of the cord. Two other descending tracts are the reticulospinal and rubrospinal tracts. The reticulospinal tract consists of three sub-tracts, one lateral, one medial, and one anterior. It is thought to be involved with sweating and the muscular activity associated with posturing. The rubrospinal tracts are lateral pathways that affect and control fine motor function of the hands and feet. Injury affects the ipsilateral side of the body with both of these pathways.

Spinal Nerves

Spinal nerves are the peripheral nerve roots that branch in pairs from the spinal cord (Figure 2-69). They travel through the intervertebral foramina and have both sensory and motor components. They provide the largest part of the innervation of the skin, muscles, and internal organs.

There are 31 pairs of spinal nerve roots. The first pair exits the spinal column between the skull and the first cervical vertebra. Each of the next seven pairs exits just below one of the cervical vertebrae and is identified as C-2 through C-8. (Although there are only seven

spinal nerves 31 pairs of nerves that originate along the spinal cord from anterior and posterior nerve roots.

Table 2-3   SPINAL NERVE PLEXUSES

Plexus	Origin	Nerve	Control	Result of Injury
Cervical	C-1 to C-5	Phrenic	Diaphragm	Respiratory paralysis
Brachial	C-5 to C-8, T-1	Axillary	Deltoid/skin of shoulder	Deltoid muscle paralysis
		Radial	Triceps/forearm	Wristdrop
		Median	Flexor muscles, forearm, arm	Decreased usage
		Musculocutaneous	Flexor muscles of arm	Decreased usage
		Ulnar	Wrist/hand	Claw hand; inability to spread fingers
Lumbar	T-12 to L-4	Femoral	Lower abdomen, gluteus, thighs	Inability to extend leg, flex hip
		Obturator	Abductor muscles Medial thigh	Decreased usage
Sacral	L-4 to 5-3	Sciatic	Lower extremity	Decreased usage

cervical vertebrae, there are eight cervical spinal nerves.) There are twelve pairs of thoracic nerves, five lumbar, five sacral, and one coccygeal. Each of these pairs originates just below the vertebra with whose name it is identified. Each spinal nerve pair has two dorsal and two **ventral** roots. The ventral roots carry motor impulses from the cord to the body, and the dorsal roots carry sensory impulses from the body to the cord. (C-1 and Co [coccygeal]-1 do not have dorsal [sensory] roots.)

ventral toward the front or toward the anterior part of the body. *Opposite of* dorsal.

The nerve roots often converge in a cluster of nerves called a *plexus* (Table 2-3). A plexus (or braiding) permits peripheral nerve roots to rejoin and function as a group. The cervical plexus, made up of the first five cervical nerve roots, innervates the neck and produces the phrenic nerve. The phrenic nerve (consisting of peripheral nerve roots C-3 through C-5) is responsible for diaphragm control. The brachial plexus joins the nerves controlling the upper extremity (C-5 through T-1). The lumbar and sacral plexuses control the innervation of the lower extremity.

dermatome topographical region of the body surface innervated by one nerve root.

The sensory components of the spinal nerves innervate specific and discrete areas of the body surface. These areas are called **dermatomes** and are distributed from the occiput of the head to the heel of the foot and buttocks (Figure 2-70). Key locations to recognize for assessment include the collar region (C-3), the little finger (C-7), the nipple line (T-4), the umbilicus (T-10), and the small toe (S-1).

myotome muscle and tissue of the body innervated by a spinal nerve root.

The motor components of the spinal nerve roots also innervate discrete tissues and muscles of the body in regions called **myotomes.** However, as the body grows and matures, some muscles merge and their control is not as specific as it is with the dermatomes. Key myotomes for neurological evaluation include arm extension (C-5), elbow extension (C-7), small finger abduction (T-1), knee extension (L-3), and ankle flexion (S-1). Evaluation of areas controlled by both dermatomes and myotomes can help you identify the spinal cord region associated with an injury.

The spinal cord also performs some primary processing functions, speeding body responses and helping the brain maintain balance and muscle tone. These responses, called *reflexes,* occur as special neurons in the cord, called *interneurons,* intercept sensory signals (Figure 2-71). For example, if you touch a hot stove, the severe pain sends an intense signal to the brain. This strong signal simultaneously triggers an interneuron in the spinal cord to direct a signal to the flexor muscles telling them to contract. The limb withdraws without waiting for the signal sent to the brain to reach it, be processed, and trigger a command to be sent back to the limb. The speed of this reflex action reduces the seriousness of injury. Other reflexes help stabilize the body if it stands in one position for a length of time. As the stretch receptors report the body is moving, the interneurons signal muscles to counteract

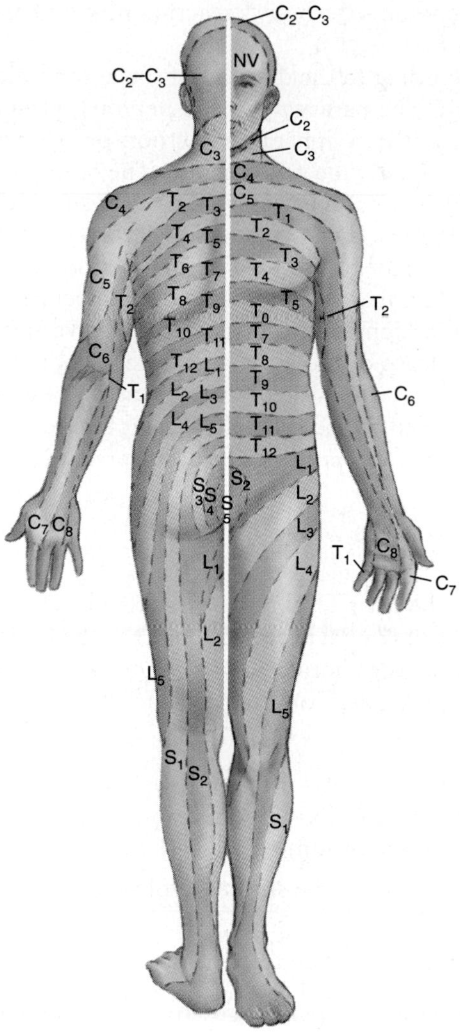

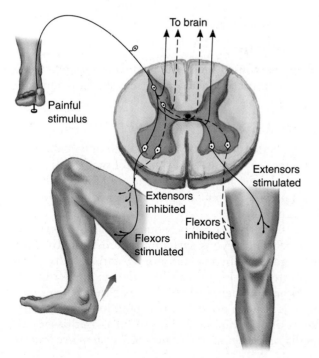

FIGURE 2-70 The dermatomes. Each dermatome corresponds to a spinal nerve.

C₂–C₃
C₂–C₃
NV
C₂
C₃
C₃
C₄
C₅
C₄ T₂ T₃ T₁
T₄ T₅ T₂
C₅ T₆ T₇ T₃
T₂ T₈ T₉ T₄
C₆ T₁₀ T₁₁ T₅ T₂
T₁ T₁₂ L₁ T₀
L₂ L₃ T₇ C₆
L₄ L₅ T₈
S₂ T₉
S₃ S₄ S₅ T₁₀
L₁ T₁₁
L₂ T₁₂
L₃ L₁
L₁ L₂
L₄ L₃
T₁ C₈
C₇ C₈ C₇
L₄
L₂
L₅
L₅
S₁ S₂
S₁

FIGURE 2-71 The reflex response.

To brain

Painful
stimulus

Extensors
stimulated

Extensors
inhibited

Flexors
inhibited

Flexors
stimulated

165

the movement to help maintain position. This again reduces the body's reaction time and allows the body to stand or maintain a steady position.

The spinal nerves can be further subdivided according to the division of the autonomic nervous system they serve and to their spinal origin. The parasympathetic nervous system controls rest and regenerative functions and consists of the peripheral nerve roots branching from the sacral region and the cranial nerves (predominantly the vagus nerve). The parasympathetic nervous system's major tasks are to slow the heart and increase digestive system activity; the system also plays a role in sexual stimulation. The sympathetic nervous system adjusts the body's metabolic rate to waking activity, provides "fight-or-flight" functions, and branches from nerves originating in the thoracic and lumbar regions. This system decreases organ and digestive activity through vasoconstriction, constricts the venous blood vessels, and affects the body's metabolic rate through the release of the adrenal hormones norepinephrine and epinephrine. In shock, the sympathetic nervous system causes systemic vasoconstriction to reduce the venous blood volume and increase peripheral vascular resistance. It also increases the heart rate to increase cardiac output in response to dropping preload and blood pressure.

PERIPHERAL NERVOUS SYSTEM

Consisting of the cranial and the peripheral nerves, the peripheral nervous system has both voluntary and involuntary components. The 12 pairs of **cranial nerves** originate in the brain and supply nervous control to the head, neck, and certain thoracic and abdominal organs (Figure 2-72). The peripheral nerves, as described previously, originate in the spinal cord and supply nervous control to the periphery.

The four categories of peripheral nerves are:

- *Somatic sensory.* These afferent nerves transmit sensations involved in touch, pressure, pain, temperature, and position (proprioception).
- *Somatic motor.* These efferent fibers carry impulses to the skeletal (voluntary) muscles.
- *Visceral (autonomic) sensory.* These afferent tracts transmit sensations from the visceral organs. Sensations such as a full bladder or the need to defecate are mediated by visceral sensory fibers.
- *Visceral (autonomic) motor.* These efferent fibers exit the central nervous system and branch to supply nerves to the involuntary cardiac muscle and smooth muscle of the viscera (organs) and to the glands.

Somatic (Voluntary) Nervous System

The voluntary component of the peripheral nervous system, often called the *somatic nervous system,* is responsible for the conscious control of movement, primarily controlling the skeletal muscles.

Autonomic (Involuntary) Nervous System

The involuntary component of the peripheral nervous system, commonly called the *autonomic nervous system,* is responsible for the unconscious control of many body functions, including those governed by the smooth muscle, cardiac muscle, and the glands. The two functional divisions of the autonomic nervous system are the sympathetic nervous system and the parasympathetic nervous system.

The autonomic nervous system arises from the central nervous system. The nerves of the autonomic nervous system exit the central nervous system and subsequently enter specialized structures called **autonomic ganglia.** In the autonomic ganglia, the nerve fibers from the central nervous system interact with nerve fibers that extend from the ganglia to the various target organs. Autonomic nerve fibers that exit the central nervous system and terminate in the autonomic ganglia are called **pre-ganglionic nerves.** Autonomic nerve fibers that exit the ganglia and terminate in the various target tissues are called **post-ganglionic nerves.** The ganglia of the sympathetic nervous system are located

---

cranial nerves 12 pairs of nerves that extend from the lower surface of the brain.

Content Review

PERIPHERAL NERVOUS SYSTEM
- Voluntary (somatic)
- Involuntary (autonomic)
  - Sympathetic
  - Parasympathetic

autonomic ganglia groups of autonomic nerve cells located outside the central nervous system.

pre-ganglionic nerves nerve fibers that extend from the central nervous system to the autonomic ganglia.

post-ganglionic nerves nerve fibers that extend from the autonomic ganglia to the target tissues.

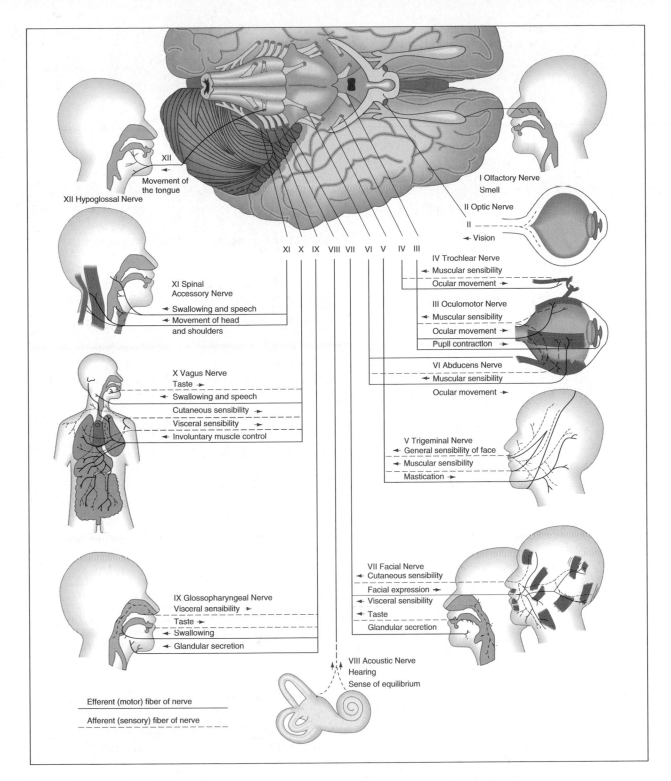

XII Hypoglossal Nerve
XII
Movement of the tongue

I Olfactory Nerve
Smell

II Optic Nerve
II
Vision

XI Spinal Accessory Nerve
Swallowing and speech
Movement of head and shoulders

IV Trochlear Nerve
Muscular sensibility
Ocular movement

III Oculomotor Nerve
Muscular sensibility
Ocular movement
Pupil contraction

X Vagus Nerve
Taste
Swallowing and speech
Cutaneous sensibility
Visceral sensibility
Involuntary muscle control

VI Abducens Nerve
Muscular sensibility
Ocular movement

V Trigeminal Nerve
General sensibility of face
Muscular sensibility
Mastication

VII Facial Nerve
Cutaneous sensibility
Facial expression
Visceral sensibility
Taste
Glandular secretion

IX Glossopharyngeal Nerve
Visceral sensibility
Taste
Swallowing
Glandular secretion

VIII Acoustic Nerve
Hearing
Sense of equilibrium

Efferent (motor) fiber of nerve
Afferent (sensory) fiber of nerve

XI X IX VIII VII VI V IV III

FIGURE 2-72   The cranial nerves.

close to the spinal cord. The ganglia of the parasympathetic nervous system are located close to the target organs (Figure 2-73).

The sympathetic and parasympathetic systems are antagonistic. In their normal state, they exist in balance with each other. During stress, the sympathetic system dominates. During rest, the parasympathetic system dominates.

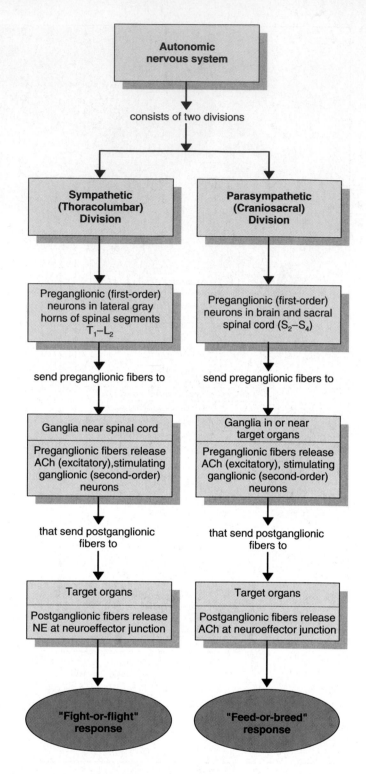

FIGURE 2-73 Components of the autonomic nervous system.

Sympathetic Nervous System   The sympathetic nervous system, often referred to as the "fight-or-flight" system, prepares the body for stressful situations. It is located near the thoracic and lumbar part of the spinal cord.

Pre-ganglionic nerves leave the spinal cord through the spinal nerves and end in the sympathetic ganglia. The two types of sympathetic ganglia are sympathetic chain ganglia and collateral ganglia (Figure 2-74). In addition, special pre-ganglionic sympathetic nerve fibers innervate the adrenal medulla. Post-ganglionic nerves that exit the sympathetic chain gan-

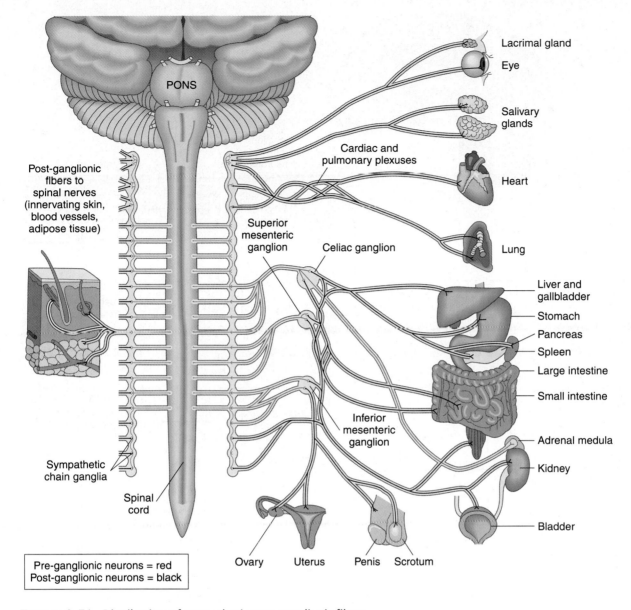

PONS

Lacrimal gland

Eye

Salivary glands

Cardiac and pulmonary plexuses

Heart

Post-ganglionic fibers to spinal nerves (innervating skin, blood vessels, adipose tissue)

Superior mesenteric ganglion

Celiac ganglion

Lung

Liver and gallbladder

Stomach

Pancreas

Spleen

Large intestine

Small intestine

Inferior mesenteric ganglion

Adrenal medula

Kidney

Sympathetic chain ganglia

Spinal cord

Ovary   Uterus   Penis   Scrotum

Bladder

Pre-ganglionic neurons = red
Post-ganglionic neurons = black

FIGURE 2-74 Distribution of sympathetic post-ganglionic fibers.

glia extend to several peripheral target tissues of the sympathetic nervous system. When stimulated, these fibers have several effects. They include:

- Stimulation of secretion by sweat glands
- Constriction of blood vessels in the skin
- Increase in blood flow to skeletal muscles
- Increase in the heart rate and force of cardiac contractions
- Bronchodilation
- Stimulation of energy production

The collateral ganglia are located in the abdominal cavity. Nerves leaving the collateral ganglia innervate many of the organs of the abdomen. Stimulation of these fibers causes several conditions. They include:

- Reduction of blood flow to abdominal organs
- Decreased digestive activity

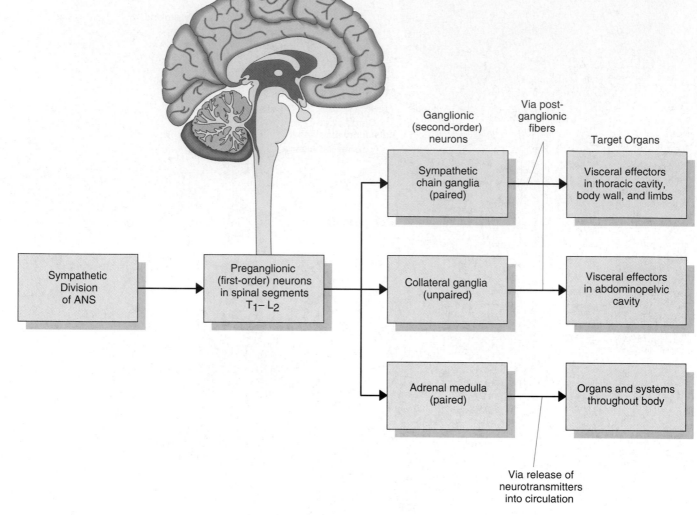

FIGURE 2-75 Organization of the sympathetic division of the autonomic nervous system.

- Relaxation of smooth muscle in the wall of the urinary bladder
- Release of glucose stores from the liver

Sympathetic nervous system stimulation also results in direct stimulation of the adrenal medulla, the inner portion of the adrenal gland (Figure 2-75). The adrenal medulla in turn releases the hormones norepinephrine (noradrenalin) and epinephrine (adrenalin) into the circulatory system. Approximately 80% of the hormones released by the adrenal medulla are epinephrine. Norepinephrine constitutes the remaining 20%. Once released, these hormones are carried throughout the body where they cause their intended effects by acting on hormone receptors. The release of norepinephrine and epinephrine by the adrenal medulla stimulates tissues that are not innervated by sympathetic nerves. In addition, it prolongs the effects of direct sympathetic stimulation. All of these effects serve to prepare the body to deal with stressful and potentially dangerous situations.

Sympathetic stimulation ultimately results in the release of the hormone norepinephrine from post-ganglionic, presynaptic nerves. The norepinephrine subsequently crosses the synaptic cleft and interacts with adrenergic receptors on the postsynaptic nerves. Shortly thereafter, the norepinephrine is either taken up by the presynaptic neuron for reuse or broken down by enzymes present within the synapse (Figure 2-76). Sympathetic stimulation also results in the release of the hormones epinephrine and norepinephrine from the adrenal medulla. In addition, both epinephrine and norepinephrine interact with specialized adrenergic receptors on the membranes of the target organs. These receptors are located

Content Review

TYPES OF SYMPATHETIC RECEPTORS

- Adrenergic
  - Alpha$_1$(α_1)
  - Alpha$_2$ (α_2)
  - Beta$_1$(β_1)
  - Beta$_2$(β_2)
- Dopaminergic

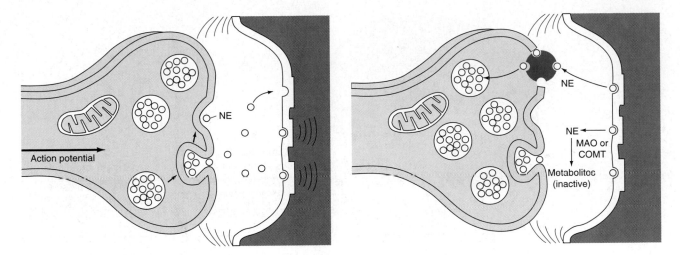

FIGURE 2-76 Physiology of an adrenergic synapse. Norepinephrine is released from the presynaptic nerve and stimulates receptors on the postsynaptic nerve. Subsequently, the norepinephrine is either taken up by the presynaptic nerve or deactivated by enzymes in the synapse.

throughout the body. Once stimulated by the appropriate hormone, they cause a response in the organ or organs they control.

The two known types of sympathetic receptors are the *adrenergic receptors* and the *dopaminergic receptors*. The adrenergic receptors are generally divided into four types. These four receptors are designated alpha$_1$ (α_1), alpha$_2$ (α_2), beta$_1$ (β_1), and beta$_2$ (β_2). The α_1 receptors cause peripheral vasoconstriction, mild bronchoconstriction, and stimulation of metabolism. The α_2 receptors are found on the presynaptic surfaces of sympathetic neuroeffector junctions. Stimulation of α_2 receptors is inhibitory. These receptors serve to prevent over-release of norepinephrine in the synapse. When the level of norepinephrine in the synapse gets high enough, the α_2 receptors are stimulated and norepinephrine release is inhibited. Stimulation of β_1 receptors causes increases in heart rate, cardiac contractile force, and cardiac automaticity and conduction. Stimulation of β_2 receptors causes vasodilation and bronchodilation. Dopaminergic receptors, although not fully understood, evidently cause dilation of the renal, coronary, and cerebral arteries.

Parasympathetic Nervous System   The parasympathetic nervous system, sometimes called the "feed-or-breed" system, is responsible for controlling vegetative functions, such as normal heart rate and blood pressure.

The parasympathetic nervous system arises from the brain stem and the sacral segments of the spinal cord. The pre-ganglionic neurons of the parasympathetic nervous system are typically much longer than those of the sympathetic nervous system, because the ganglia are located close to the target tissues. Parasympathetic nerve fibers that leave the brain stem travel within four of the cranial nerves including the oculomotor nerve (III), the facial nerve (VII), the glosso-pharyngeal nerve (IX), and the vagus nerve (X). These fibers synapse in the parasympathetic ganglia with short post-ganglionic fibers that then continue to their target tissues. Postsynaptic fibers innervate much of the body, including the intrinsic eye muscles, the salivary glands, the heart, the lungs, and most of the organs of the abdominal cavity. The sacral segment of the parasympathetic nervous system forms distinct pelvic nerves that innervate ganglia in the kidneys, bladder, sex organs, and the terminal portions of the large intestine (Figure 2-77). Stimulation of the parasympathetic nervous system results in the following conditions:

- Pupillary constriction
- Secretion by digestive glands
- Reduction in heart rate and cardiac contractile force
- Bronchoconstriction
- Increased smooth muscle activity along the digestive tract

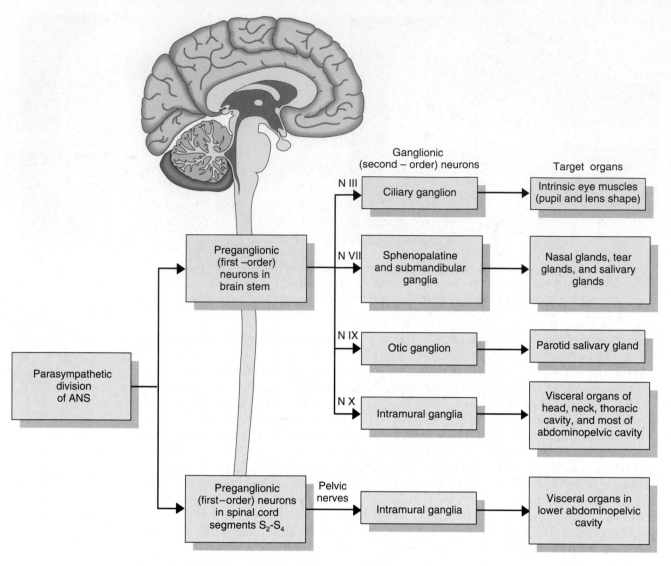

FIGURE 2-77 Organization of the parasympathetic division of the autonomic nervous system.

These and other functions facilitate the processing of food, energy absorption, relaxation, and reproduction (Figure 2-78).

All pre-ganglionic and post-ganglionic parasympathetic nerve fibers use acetylcholine as a neurotransmitter. Acetylcholine, when released by presynaptic neurons, crosses the synaptic cleft and activates receptors on the postsynaptic neurons or on the neuroeffector junction. Acetylcholine is also the neurotransmitter for the somatic nervous system and is present in the neuromuscular junction. Acetylcholine is very short-lived. Within a fraction of a second after its release, it is deactivated by another chemical called *acetylcholinesterase.* Acetic acid and choline, which are produced when acetylcholine is deactivated, are taken back up by the presynaptic neuron (Figure 2-79).

The parasympathetic system has two main types of ACh receptors, nicotinic and muscarinic. Knowing these receptors' locations and functions will greatly simplify learning the functions of drugs in this class. Nicotinic$_N$ (neuron) receptors are found in all autonomic ganglia, where acetylcholine serves as the presynaptic neurotransmitter of both the parasympathetic and sympathetic nervous systems. Nicotinic$_M$ (muscle) receptors are found at the neuromuscular junction and initiate muscular contraction as part of the somatic nervous system. Muscarinic receptors are found in many organs throughout the body and are

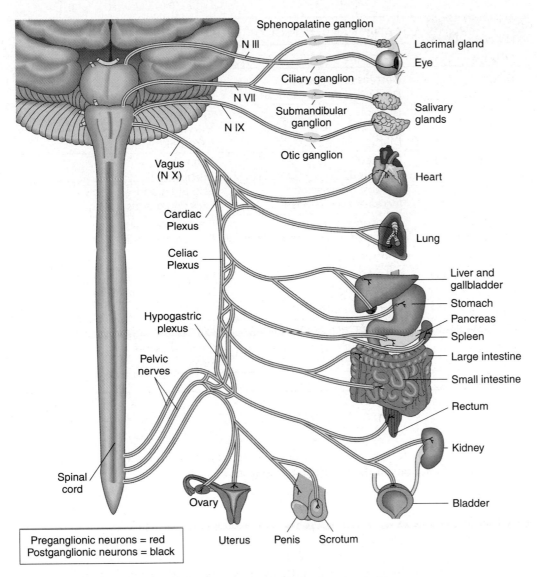

Preganglionic neurons = red
Postganglionic neurons = black

FIGURE 2–78   Distribution of the parasympathetic post-ganglionic fibers.

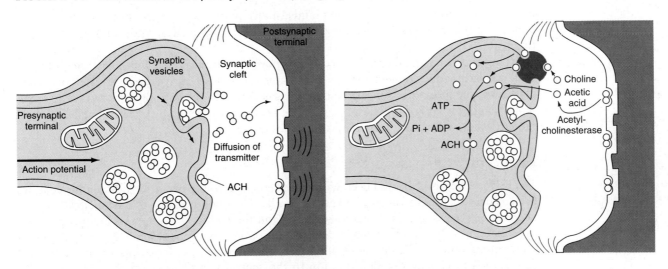

FIGURE 2–79   Physiology of a cholinergic synapse. Acetylcholine is released from the presynaptic nerve and stimulates receptors on the postsynaptic nerve. Subsequently, acetylcholinesterase breaks down the acetylcholine and the presynaptic nerve fiber takes up the products.

Table 2-4	LOCATION AND EFFECT OF MUSCARINIC RECEPTORS	
Organ	**Functions**	**Location**
Heart	Decreased heart rate	Sinoatrial node
	Decreased conduction rate	Atrioventricular node
Arterioles	Dilation	Coronary
	Dilation	Skin and mucosa
	Dilation	Cerebral
GI Tract	Relaxed	Sphincters
	Increased	Motility
	Increased salivation	Salivary glands
	Increased secretion	Exocrine glands
Lungs	Bronchoconstriction	Bronchiole smooth muscle
	Increased mucous production	Bronchial glands
Gallbladder	Contraction	
Urinary bladder	Relaxation	Urinary sphincter
	Contraction	Detrusor muscle
Liver	Glycogen synthesis	
Lacrimal glands	Secretion (increased tearing)	Eye
Eye	Contraction for near vision	Ciliary muscle
	Constriction	Pupil
Penis	Erection	

primarily responsible for promoting the parasympathetic response. Table 2-4 summarizes the locations and actions of the muscarinic receptors.

ENDOCRINE SYSTEM

There are eight major glands in the endocrine system: the hypothalamus, pituitary gland, thyroid gland, parathyroid glands, thymus, pancreas, adrenal glands, and gonads. The pineal gland is also an endocrine gland, but much of its function remains unclear. In addition to the endocrine glands, many body tissues have been found to have endocrine function. These include the kidneys, heart, placenta, and parts of the digestive tract.

The endocrine glands are located throughout the body (Figure 2-80). Although Figure 2-80 shows an adult, remember that the thymus is primarily active during childhood, when it plays a role in maturation of the immune system. By adulthood, the thymus is so small that it is not visualized on chest X-rays. The hormones secreted by endocrine glands, their target tissues, and their effects are listed in Table 2-5.

HYPOTHALAMUS

The hypothalamus is located deep within the cerebrum of the brain. Hypothalamic cells act both as nerve cells, or neurons, and as gland cells. The hypothalamus is the junction, or connection, between the central nervous system and the endocrine system. As neurons, many hypothalamic cells receive messages from the autonomic nervous system—peripheral nerves that, among other functions, detect internal conditions such as blood pressure or blood glucose level and convey that information to the central nervous system through nerve impulses. Some hypothalamic cells respond by producing nerve impulses that travel to cells in the posterior pituitary gland. Other hypothalamic cells respond as gland cells by producing and releasing hormones into the stalk of tissue that connects the hypothalamus and the anterior pituitary gland.

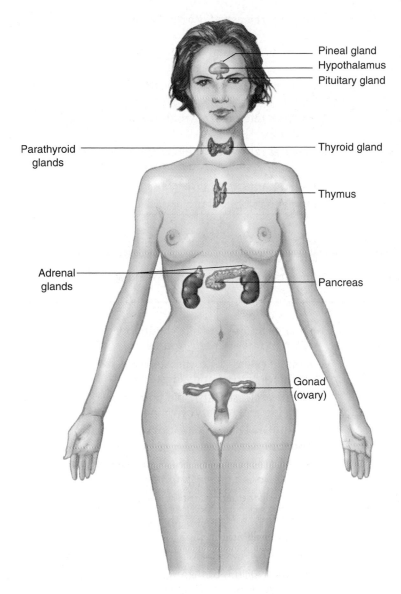

Pineal gland
Hypothalamus
Pituitary gland

Parathyroid glands

Thyroid gland

Thymus

Adrenal glands

Pancreas

Gonad (ovary)

FIGURE 2-80 The major glands of the endocrine system.

In response to impulses from the autonomic nervous system, the hypothalamus—and other organs of the endocrine system—can release the hormones that promote homeostasis:

- Growth hormone releasing hormone (GHRH)
- Growth hormone inhibiting hormone (GHIH)
- Corticotropin releasing hormone (CRH)
- Thyrotropin releasing hormone (TRH)
- Gonadotropin releasing hormone (GnRH)
- Prolactin releasing hormone (PRH)
- Prolactin inhibiting hormone (PIH)

Table 2-5 — ENDOCRINE SYSTEM: GLANDS, HORMONES, TARGET TISSUES, HORMONE EFFECTS

Gland and Major Hormone(s)	Target Tissues	Major Hormone Effect(s)
Hypothalamus		
Growth hormone releasing hormone (GHRH)	Anterior pituitary	Stimulates release of growth hormone
Growth hormone inhibiting hormone (GHIH) (or somatostatin)	Anterior pituitary	Suppresses release of growth hormone
Corticotropin releasing hormone (CRH)	Anterior pituitary	Stimulates release of adrenocorticotropin
Thyrotropin releasing hormone (TRH)	Anterior pituitary	Stimulates release of thyroid-stimulating hormone
Gonadotropin releasing hormone (GnRH)	Anterior pituitary	Stimulates release of luteinizing hormone and follicle-stimulating hormone
Prolactin releasing hormone (PRH)	Anterior pituitary	Stimulates release of prolactin
Prolactin inhibiting hormone (PIH)	Anterior pituitary	Suppresses release of prolactin
Posterior pituitary gland		
Antidiuretic hormone (ADH)	Kidneys	Stimulates increased reabsorption of water into blood volume
Oxytocin	Uterus and breasts of females, kidneys	Stimulates uterine contractions and milk release
Anterior pituitary gland		
Growth hormone (GH)	All cells, especially growing cells	Stimulates body growth in childhood; causes switch to fats as energy source
Adrenocorticotropic hormone (ACTH)	Adrenal cortexes	Stimulates release of corticosteroidal hormones cortisol and aldosterone
Thyroid-stimulating hormone (TSH)	Thyroid	Stimulates release of thyroid hormones thyroxine and triiodothyronine
Follicle-stimulating hormone (FSH)	Ovaries or testes	FSH stimulates development of sex cells (ovum or sperm)
Luteinizing hormone (LH)	Ovaries or testes	LH stimulates release of hormones (estrogen, progesterone or testosterone)
Prolactin (PRL)	Mammary glands	Stimulates production and release of milk
Thyroid gland		
Thyroxine, T4	All cells	Stimulates cell metabolism
Trilodothyronine, T3	All cells	Stimulates cell metabolism
Calcitonin	All cells	Stimulates calcium uptake by bones, decreasing blood calcium level
Parathyroid glands		
Parathyroid hormone (PTH)	Bone, intestine, kidneys	Stimulates calcium release from bone, calcium uptake from GI tract, calcium reabsorption in kidney, all increasing blood calcium level
Thymus		
Thymosin	White blood cells; primarily T lymphocytes	Stimulates reproduction and functional development of T lymphocytes

As indicated in Table 2-5, most hypothalamic hormones, including thyrotropin releasing hormone (TRH) and growth hormone releasing hormone (GHRH), stimulate secretion of pituitary hormones that rouse yet another endocrine gland or body tissue to increased activity. For example, in response to TRH the anterior pituitary releases thyroid stimulating hormone, and thyroid stimulating hormone then acts upon the thyroid gland to increase thyroid activity.

Gland and Major Hormone(s)	Target Tissues	Major Hormone Effect(s)
Pancreas		
Glucagon	All cells, particularly in liver, muscle, and fat	Stimulates hepatic glycogenolysis and gluconeogenesis, increasing blood glucose level
Insulin	All cells, particularly in liver, muscle, and fat	Stimulates cellular uptake of glucose, increased rate of synthesis of glycogen, proteins, and fats, decreasing blood glucose level
Somatostatin	Alpha and beta cells in the pancreas	Suppresses secretion of glucagon and insulin within islets of Langerhans
Adrenal medulla		
Epinephrine (or adrenaline)	Muscle, liver, cardiovascular system	Stimulates features of "fight-or-flight" response to stress
Norepinephrine	Muscle, liver, cardiovascular system	Stimulates vasoconstriction
Adrenal cortex		
Glucocorticoids		
Cortisol	Most cells, particularly white blood cells (cells responsible for inflammatory and immune responses)	Stimulates glucagon-like effects, acts as anti-inflammatory and immunosuppressive agent
Mineralocorticoids		
Aldosterone	Kidneys, blood	Contributes to salt and fluid balance by stimulating kidneys to increase potassium excretion and decrease sodium excretion, increasing blood volume
Androgenic hormones		
Estrogen	Most cells	See effects under Ovaries and Testes
Progesterone	Uterus	
Testosterone	Most cells	
Ovaries		
Estrogen	Most cells, particularly those of female reproductive tract	Stimulates development of secondary sexual characteristics, plays role in maturation of egg before ovulation
Progesterone	Uterus	Stimulates uterine changes necessary for successful pregnancy
Testes		
Testosterone	Most cells, particularly those of male reproductive tract	Stimulates development of secondary sexual characteristics, plays role in development of sperm cells
Pineal gland		
Melatonin	Exact action unknown	Releases melatonin in response to light, may help determine daily, lunar, and reproductive cycles, may affect mood

The pair of hypothalamic hormones—growth hormone releasing hormone (GHRH) and growth hormone inhibitory hormone (GHIH)—demonstrate a major trait of endocrine function: many hormonal activities are driven not by one hormone, but rather by two hormones with opposing effects. GHRH stimulates secretion of growth hormone, and GHIH suppresses secretion of growth hormone. The actual amount of growth hormone secreted by the anterior pituitary depends on the net amount of stimulation (Figure 2-81).

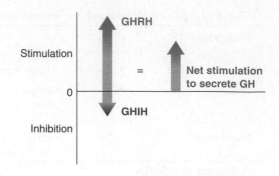

FIGURE 2-81 Regulation by hormone pairs. The net level of stimulation created by the opposing actions of growth hormone releasing hormone (GHRH) and growth-hormone inhibitory hormone (GHIH) determines the amount of growth hormone (GH) secreted by the anterior pituitary.

PITUITARY GLAND

The pituitary gland is only about the size of a pea. It is divided into posterior and anterior pituitary lobes. These tissues have different embryonic origins and different functional relationships with the hypothalamus. The *posterior pituitary gland* responds to nerve impulses from the hypothalamus, whereas the *anterior pituitary gland* responds to hypothalamic hormones that travel down the stalk that connects the anterior pituitary and hypothalamus. As you look at the target tissues of the anterior pituitary in Table 2-5, you will understand why physiologists once thought of the pituitary gland as the "master gland." Its hormones have a direct impact on endocrine glands throughout the body. The term is not used much anymore, because the dependence of the pituitary on the hypothalamus has been made clear.

As noted above, the pituitary gland has two lobes, the posterior and the anterior.

Posterior Pituitary

The posterior pituitary produces two hormones:

- *Antidiuretic hormone (ADH)*—causes retention of body water
- *Oxytocin*—causes uterine contraction and lactation

ADH, also known as vasopressin, causes the kidneys to increase water reabsorption. This retention of water, or antidiuretic effect, results in increased circulating blood volume and decreased urine volume. Increased secretion of ADH is part of the homeostatic mechanism that can counteract losses of blood volume up to about 25%. Clinically, you will see increased ADH secretion in early shock states associated with dehydration or hemorrhage. Note that the opposite effect, decreased secretion of ADH, occurs after ingestion of alcohol and when there is a significant rise in circulating blood volume.

Although it is unlikely that a disorder in ADH secretion will present as a medical emergency, you should understand such endocrine dysfunction when patients discuss their medical histories. *Diabetes insipidus,* a disorder marked by large volumes of urine, is caused by inadequate ADH secretion relative to blood volume. The resultant reduction of blood volume, or diuretic effect, appears as excessive urine production. In a 24-hour period, the kidneys normally produce 1 to 1.5 liters of urine. In diabetes insipidus, it is not uncommon for urine output to increase to almost 20 liters per day. You can remember the characteristic urine presentation of diabetes insipidus by remembering that dilute urine has an insipid, or neutral, odor (and taste).

Oxytocin, the natural form of the drug Pitocin, stimulates uterine contraction and lactation in women who have just delivered a baby. Oxytocin actually causes the "letdown" of milk by stimulating contractile cells within the mammary glands. An infant suckling at the breast stimulates receptors in the nipples that causes the release of oxytocin from the posterior pituitary. This, in turn, causes discharge of milk so that the infant can feed. Following delivery, it is recommended that the infant be placed on the breast to suckle, thus stimulating the release of oxytocin. In addition to stimulating milk letdown, the oxytocin stimulates uterine contraction, which can help minimize postpartum bleeding.

In both sexes, oxytocin has a mild antidiuretic effect, which is similar to that of ADH due to their chemical similarity. The relationship between oxytocin and ADH has direct application to emergency medicine. Women in preterm labor are often given an IV fluid bolus in an attempt to suppress uterine contractions without the use of drugs. This works in the following way: the administration of IV fluid bolus causes an increase in circulating blood volume, which is detected by autonomic nerves in the kidneys. An impulse is sent through the hypothalamus to the posterior pituitary, where it causes decreased secretion of ADH. This inhibition of ADH secretion in turn triggers decreased secretion of oxytocin, which contributes to the observed increase in urine production and, one hopes, the goal of suppression of preterm labor.

Anterior Pituitary

Because almost all of the anterior pituitary hormones regulate other endocrine glands, disorders directly involving the anterior pituitary are rarely a factor in endocrine emergencies. Table 2-5 lists the six hormones secreted by the anterior pituitary, as well as target tissues and hormone effects. As you can see, five of the six hormones regulate the activity of target glands, whereas the sixth affects almost all cells:

Five anterior pituitary hormones affect target glands:

- *Adrenocorticotropic hormone (ACTH)*—targets the adrenal cortexes
- *Thyroid-stimulating hormone (TSH)*—targets the thyroid
- *Follicle-stimulating hormone (FSH)*—targets the gonads, or sex organs
- *Luteinizing hormone (LH)*—also targets the gonads
- *Prolactin (PRL)*—targets the mammary glands of women

The sixth anterior pituitary hormone has a broader effect.

- *Growth hormone (GH)*—targets almost all body cells

GH has its most significant effects in children because it is the primary stimulant of skeletal growth. In adults, GH has several physiological effects, but the most significant is metabolic. GH causes adipose cells to release their stored fats into the blood and causes body cells to switch from glucose to fats as the primary energy source. The net effect is that the body uses up fat stores and conserves its sugar stores.

THYROID GLAND

The two lobes of the thyroid gland are located in the neck anterior to and just below the cartilage of the larynx, with one lobe on either side of the midline. The two lobes are connected by a small isthmus, or band of tissue, that crosses the trachea at the level of the cricoid cartilage. The thyroid produces three hormones:

- *Thyroxine (T4)*—stimulates cell metabolism
- *Triiodothyronine (T3)*—stimulates cell metabolism
- *Calcitonin*—lowers blood calcium levels

The thyroid is composed of tiny hollow sacs called *follicles*, which are filled with a thick fluid called *colloid*. The hormones thyroxine (T4) and triiodothyronine (T3) are produced within the colloid. When stimulated by the pituitary hormone TSH or by environmental conditions such as cold, the thyroid gland releases these hormones to increase the general rate of cell metabolism.

The thyroid gland also contains perifollicular cells called *C cells*, which produce a different hormone, calcitonin. Calcitonin lowers blood calcium levels by increasing uptake of calcium by bones and inhibiting breakdown of bone tissue. Parathyroid hormone has the opposite, or antagonistic, effect on the blood calcium level, which is covered in the following discussion of the parathyroid glands.

Disorders of excessive or deficient production of thyroid hormones T4 and T3 are called *hyperthyroidism* and *hypothyroidism*, respectively.

PARATHYROID GLANDS

Each parathyroid gland is to very small, with a maximum diameter of 5 mm and weight of only 35 to 40 mg. Normally, four parathyroid glands are located on the posterior lateral surfaces of the thyroid, one pair above the other. Sometimes more than four parathyroid glands are present, but only rarely are there fewer. The parathyroid glands secrete:

- *Parathyroid hormone (PTH)*—increases blood calcium levels

PTH increases blood calcium levels through actions on three different target tissues. In bone, the primary target, PTH causes release of calcium into the blood. In the intestines, PTH converts vitamin D into its active form, causing increased absorption of calcium. In the kidneys, PTH causes increased reabsorption of calcium. PTH is the antagonist of calcitonin, and the balance of PTH and calcitonin determines the level of blood calcium. The parathyroid glands rarely cause clinical problems. However, they can be accidentally damaged or removed during surgery or they may be damaged if the thyroid gland is irradiated. In either case, the loss of parathyroid function may result in hypocalcemia, low blood calcium levels.

THYMUS GLAND

The thymus is in the mediastinum just behind the sternum. It is fairly large in children but shrinks into a small remnant of fat and fibrous tissue in adults. Although the thymus is usually considered a lymphatic organ on the basis of its anatomy, its most important function is as an endocrine gland. During childhood, it secretes:

- *Thymosin*—promotes maturation of T lymphocytes

Thymosin is critical to maturation of T lymphocytes, the cells responsible for cell-mediated immunity. The T of T lymphocyte stands for thymus.

PANCREAS

The pancreas, located in the upper retroperitoneum behind the stomach and between the duodenum and spleen, is composed of both endocrine and exocrine tissues. The exocrine tissues, known as acini, secrete digestive enzymes essential to digestion of fats and proteins into a duct that empties into the small intestine.

The microscopic clusters of endocrine tissue found within the pancreas are known as *islets of Langerhans*. Although there are one to two million islets interspersed throughout the pancreas, they comprise only about 2% of its total mass. The three most important types of endocrine cells in the islets of Langerhans are termed alpha (α), beta (β), and delta (δ) (Figure 2-82). Each type produces and secretes a different hormone. In addition, the islets contain a much smaller number of cells called *polypeptide cells*. These cells produce pancreatic polypeptide (PP), the function of which is still unclear.

The alpha and beta cells produce two hormones essential for homeostasis of blood glucose:

- *Glucagon*—increases blood glucose
- *Insulin*—decreases blood glucose

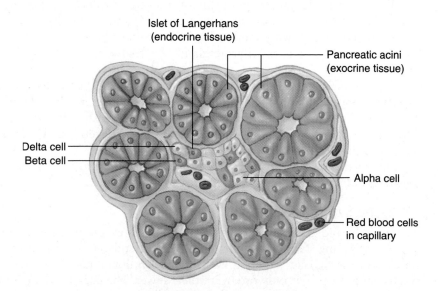

FIGURE 2-82 The internal anatomy of the pancreas.

Approximately 25% of islet tissue is made up of alpha cells. Alpha cells produce the hormone glucagon. When blood glucose level falls, alpha cells increase secretion of glucagon. Glucagon stimulates breakdown of glycogen, the complex carbohydrate that is the storage form of glucose, into individual glucose molecules that are released into the blood. This process, called **glycogenolysis,** takes place in more than one tissue, but activity in the liver is by far the most important in raising blood glucose level.

The liver is the largest and heaviest of the internal organs and so it has many cells that can contain glycogen. In addition, liver cells have the greatest capacity to store glycogen—liver cells can store 5% to 8% of their weight as glycogen. Compare this with the capacity of skeletal muscle (1% to 3%), another important storage tissue in the body. In addition to stimulating glycogenolysis, the hormone glucagon also stimulates liver breakdown of body proteins and fats with subsequent chemical conversion to glucose. This second process, which produces glucose from non-sugar sources, is called **gluconeogenesis.** Both processes contribute to homeostasis by raising the blood glucose level.

Beta cells make up about 60% of islet tissue, and they produce the hormone insulin. Insulin is the antagonist of glucagon: Insulin lowers the blood glucose level by increasing the uptake of glucose by body cells. In addition, insulin promotes energy storage in the body by increasing the synthesis of glycogen, protein, and fat. Because the liver removes circulating insulin within 10 to 15 minutes from time of secretion, it must be secreted constantly to sustain an appropriate balance of glucagon and insulin—a balance that results in a steady supply of glucose for immediate use as an energy source and for appropriate energy storage. Loss of functional beta cells leads to increased blood glucose levels as seen in diabetes.

Delta cells, which comprise about 10% of islet tissue, produce *somatostatin*. This hormone acts within islets to inhibit secretion of glucagon and insulin. Somatostatin also retards nutrient absorption from the intestines, although its mechanisms of action in the gut are poorly understood. As you look at Table 2-5, note that somatostatin is the same substance as growth-hormone inhibiting hormone (GHIH).

glycogenolysis the breakdown of glycogen to glucose, primarily by liver cells.

gluconeogenesis conversion of protein and fat to form glucose.

ADRENAL GLANDS

The paired adrenal glands are located on the superior surface of the kidneys. Each gland has two distinct anatomical divisions with different functions. The inner portion of the adrenal gland is called the *adrenal medulla,* and its cells behave both as nerve cells and as gland cells. The adrenal medulla is intimately related to the sympathetic component of the autonomic nervous system. When sympathetic nerves carry an impulse into the adrenal medulla, its cells respond by secreting the catecholamine hormones *epinephrine* (or adrenalin) and *norepinephrine* into the bloodstream. The outer portion of the adrenal gland is called the *adrenal cortex,* and it consists of endocrine tissue. The adrenal cortex secretes three classes of steroidal hormones that differ only slightly in chemical structure but have very distinct effects in the body:

- *Glucocorticoids,* of which cortisol is by far the most important, account for 95% of adrenocortical hormone production. Similar to glucagon, they increase the blood glucose level by promoting gluconeogenesis and decreasing glucose utilization as an energy source. If you recall that cortisone is a commonly used medical glucocorticoid, you will realize that this class of hormones also inhibits inflammatory reactions and immune-system responses, as well as potentiates the effects of catecholamines. The anterior pituitary hormone that promotes release, ACTH, is secreted in response to stress, trauma, or serious infection.

- *Mineralocorticoids,* of which aldosterone is the most important, contribute to salt and fluid balance in the body by regulating sodium and potassium excretion through the kidneys.

- *Androgenic hormones* have the same effects as those secreted by gonads, and they will be covered in that discussion.

You may see disorders related to deficient or excessive secretion of adrenal hormones present as medical emergencies.

GONADS

Some differences in the gonads are obvious: ovaries produce eggs, whereas testes produce sperm cells. However, the gonads of both sexes share one vital function: they are the endocrine glands chiefly responsible for the sexual maturation of puberty and any subsequent reproduction.

OVARIES

The ovaries, or female gonads, are paired organs about the size of an almond and are located in the pelvis on either side of the uterus. Under the regulation of the anterior pituitary hormones FSH and LH, the ovaries produce:

- *Estrogen*
- *Progesterone*

The hormone *estrogen* promotes the development and maintenance of secondary female sexual characteristics. Estrogen also plays a role in the egg development that precedes ovulation during each menstrual cycle. *Progesterone* is familiarly known as the "hormone of pregnancy" because it is necessary for implantation of the fertilized egg and maintenance of the uterine lining throughout pregnancy. Estrogen also serves to protect the female against heart disease. When estrogen levels fall at menopause, the female's risk of developing heart disease quickly increases to the level of the male's. In addition, the ovaries produce small amounts of *testosterone,* which influences some body changes associated with puberty.

TESTES

The male gonads, or testes, are located outside of the abdominal cavity in the scrotum. Under the regulation of the anterior pituitary hormones FSH and LH, the testes produce:

- *Testosterone*

The hormone testosterone promotes the development and maintenance of secondary male sexual characteristics and plays a role in development of sperm.

PINEAL GLAND

The pineal gland is located in the roof of the thalamus in the brain. Its function has remained somewhat elusive. However, it has been shown that the pineal gland releases the hormone melatonin in response to changes in light. For example, melatonin production is lowest during daylight hours and highest in the dark of the night. Because of this, the pineal is felt to help determine day-length and lunar cycles and plays a role in controlling the reproductive "biological clock." Melatonin may affect a person's mood. The pineal gland has been implicated in seasonal affective disorder (SAD), which is characterized by severe depression during the winter months. Further research will help clarify the role of melatonin.

OTHER ORGANS WITH ENDOCRINE ACTIVITY

We have discussed the principal glands of the endocrine system. Many tissues not considered part of the endocrine system have important endocrine functions. Organs in other systems secrete hormones directly into the blood. The placenta can be considered an endocrine gland because of its secretion of *human chorionic gonadotropin (hCG)* throughout gestation. It is the early secretion of hCG that is detected by at-home pregnancy tests. In the digestive tract, gastric and intestinal mucosa produce the hormones *gastrin* and *secretin,* both of which regulate digestive function.

Additionally, hormone-producing cells are located in the atrial walls of the heart. *Atrial natriuretic hormone (ANH)* is secreted by certain atrial cells in response to increased stretching of the atrial walls due to abnormally high blood volume or blood pressure. The hormone ANH is an antagonist to ADH and inhibits secretion of aldosterone, thus contributing to a homeostatic reduction in blood volume by increasing urine production.

The kidneys also have some endocrine function. Certain kidney cells will react to a decrease in blood volume or blood pressure by releasing the enzyme *renin.* Renin acts on angiotensinogen, converting it to angiotensin I. In the lungs, angiotensin I is converted to angiotensin II by angiotensin-converting enzyme (ACE). Angiotensin II stimulates the adrenal production of aldosterone, which causes water retention by the kidneys. This leads to increased blood volume and blood pressure. In addition to renin, the kidneys secrete the hormone erythropoietin that stimulates the production of red blood cells by the bone marrow.

CARDIOVASCULAR SYSTEM

Two major components of the cardiovascular system are the heart and the peripheral blood vessels.

ANATOMY OF THE HEART

The heart is a muscular organ, approximately the size of a closed fist. It is in the center of the chest in the mediastinum, anterior to the spine and posterior to the sternum (Figure 2-83). Approximately two-thirds of the heart's mass is to the left of the midline, with the remainder to the right. The bottom of the heart, or apex, is just above the diaphragm, left of the midline. The top of the heart, or base, lies at approximately the level of the second rib. The great vessels connect to the heart through the base.

TISSUE LAYERS

The heart consists of three tissue layers: endocardium, myocardium, and pericardium (Figure 2-84). The *endocardium* is the innermost layer. It lines the heart's chambers and is bathed in blood. The *myocardium* is the thick middle layer of the heart. Its cells are unique in that they physically resemble skeletal muscle but have electrical properties similar to smooth muscle. These cells also contain specialized structures that help to rapidly conduct electrical impulses from one muscle cell to another, enabling the heart to contract.

The *pericardium* is a protective sac surrounding the heart. It consists of two layers, visceral and parietal. The visceral pericardium, also called the *epicardium,* is the inner layer, in contact with the heart muscle itself. The parietal pericardium is the outer, fibrous layer. In the pericardial cavity, between these two layers, is about 25 mL of pericardial fluid, a

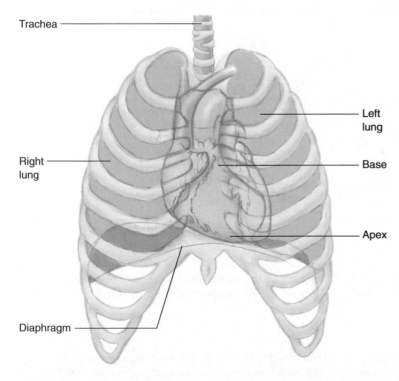

Trachea

Left lung

Right lung

Base

Apex

Diaphragm

FIGURE 2-83 Location of the heart within the chest.

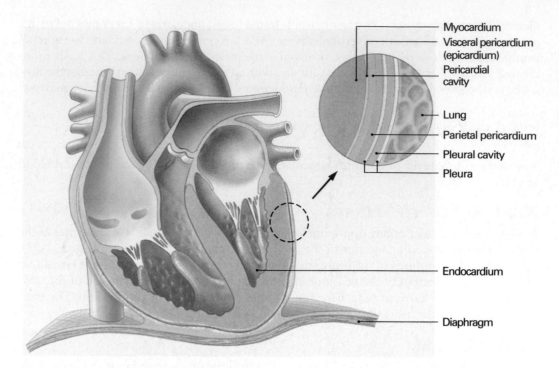

Myocardium
Visceral pericardium (epicardium)
Pericardial cavity
Lung
Parietal pericardium
Pleural cavity
Pleura

Endocardium

Diaphragm

FIGURE 2–84   Layers of the heart.

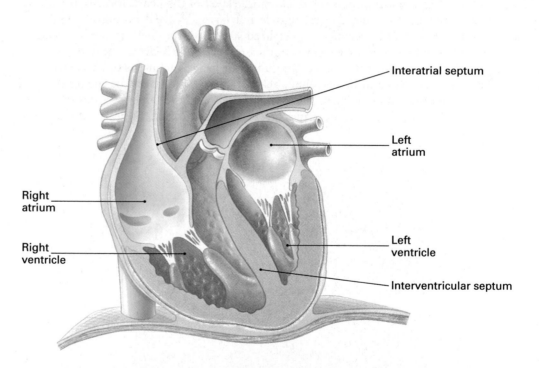

Interatrial septum

Left atrium

Right atrium

Left ventricle

Right ventricle

Interventricular septum

FIGURE 2–85   The chambers of the heart.

straw-colored lubricant that reduces friction as the heart beats and changes position. Certain disease processes and injuries can increase the amount of fluid in this sac, compressing the heart and decreasing cardiac output.

Chambers

The heart contains four chambers (Figure 2-85). The *atria,* the two superior chambers, receive incoming blood. The *ventricles,* the two larger, inferior chambers, pump blood out of the heart. The right and left atria are separated by the *interatrial septum.* The ventricles are

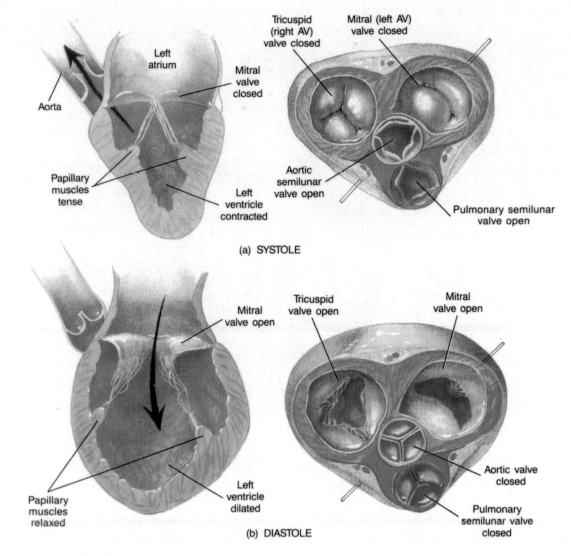

Labels in figure:
- Aorta
- Left atrium
- Tricuspid (right AV) valve closed
- Mitral (left AV) valve closed
- Mitral valve closed
- Papillary muscles tense
- Left ventricle contracted
- Aortic semilunar valve open
- Pulmonary semilunar valve open

(a) SYSTOLE

- Mitral valve open
- Tricuspid valve open
- Mitral valve open
- Papillary muscles relaxed
- Left ventricle dilated
- Aortic valve closed
- Pulmonary semilunar valve closed

(b) DIASTOLE

FIGURE 2–86   The valves of the heart.

separated by the *interventricular septum*. Both septa contain fibrous connective tissue as well as contractile muscle. The walls of the atria are much thinner than those of the ventricles and do not contribute significantly to the heart's pumping action.

Valves

The heart contains two pairs of valves, the *atrioventricular valves* and the *semilunar valves,* made of endocardial and connective tissue (Figure 2-86). The atrioventricular valves control blood flow between the atria and the ventricles. The right atrioventricular valve is called the *tricuspid valve* because it has three leaflets, or cusps. The left atrioventricular valve, called the *mitral valve,* has two leaflets. These valves are connected to specialized papillary muscles in the ventricles. When relaxed, these papillary muscles open the valves and allow blood flow between the two chambers. Specialized fibers called *chordae tendoneae* connect the valves' leaflets to the papillary muscles. They prevent the valves from prolapsing into the atria and allowing backflow during ventricular contraction.

The semilunar valves regulate blood flow between the ventricles and the arteries into which they empty. The left semilunar valve, or aortic valve, connects the left ventricle to the aorta. The right semilunar valve, or pulmonic valve, connects the right ventricle to the pulmonary artery. These valves permit one-way movement of blood and prevent backflow.

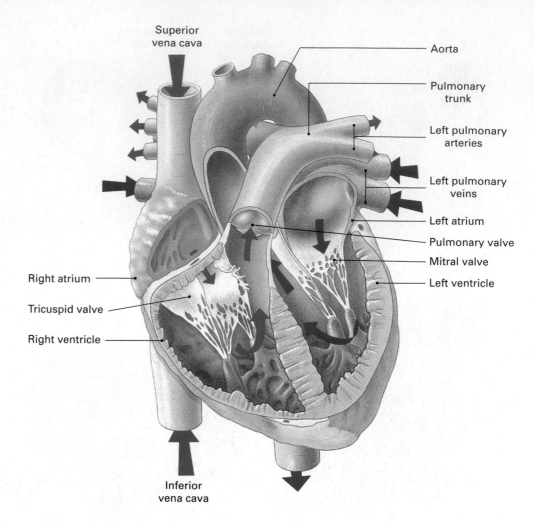

Superior
vena cava

Aorta

Pulmonary
trunk

Left pulmonary
arteries

Left pulmonary
veins

Left atrium

Pulmonary valve

Mitral valve

Left ventricle

Right atrium

Tricuspid valve

Right ventricle

Inferior
vena cava

FIGURE 2-87   Blood flow through the heart.

Blood Flow

The right atrium receives deoxygenated blood from the body via the superior and inferior venae cavae (Figure 2-87). The *superior vena cava* receives deoxygenated blood from the head and upper extremities, the *inferior vena cava* from the areas below the heart. The right atrium pumps this blood through the tricuspid valve and into the right ventricle. The right ventricle then pumps the deoxygenated blood through the pulmonic valve to the *pulmonary artery* and on to the lungs. (The pulmonary artery is the only artery in the body that carries deoxygenated blood.)

After the blood circulates through the lungs and becomes oxygenated, it returns to the left atrium via the *pulmonary veins.* (The pulmonary veins are the only veins in the body that carry oxygenated blood.) The left atrium sends this oxygenated blood through the mitral valve and into the left ventricle. Finally the left ventricle pumps the blood through the aortic valve to the aorta, which feeds the oxygenated blood to the rest of the body. Intracardiac pressures are higher on the left than on the right because the lungs offer less resistance to blood flow than the systemic circulation. Thus, the left myocardium is thicker than the right.

The major vessels of the body all branch off of the aorta, which has three main parts. The *ascending aorta* comes directly from the heart. The *thoracic aorta* curves inferiorly and goes through the chest (or thorax). The *abdominal aorta* goes through the diaphragm and enters the abdomen.

Coronary Circulation

Although the endocardium is bathed in blood, the heart does not receive its nutrients from the blood within its chambers but from the coronary arteries (Figure 2-88). The coronary

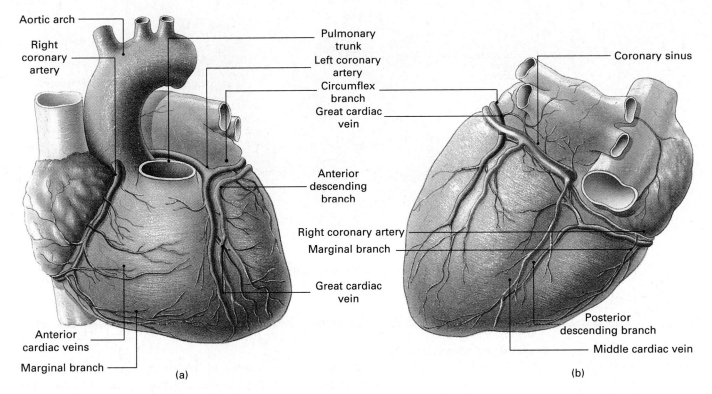

FIGURE 2-88 The coronary circulation: (a) anterior; (b) posterior.

arteries originate in the aorta, just above the leaflets of the aortic valve. The main coronary arteries lie on the surface of the heart, and small penetrating arterioles supply the myocardial muscle. The left coronary artery supplies the left ventricle, the interventricular septum, part of the right ventricle, and the heart's conduction system. Its two major branches are the *anterior descending artery* and the *circumflex artery.*

The *right coronary artery* supplies a portion of the right atrium and right ventricle and part of the conduction system. Its two major branches are the *posterior descending artery* and the *marginal artery.* (Although the blood supply to most people's hearts follows this pattern, anatomical variants do exist.) The coronary vessels receive blood during diastole, when the heart relaxes, because the aortic valve leaflets cover the coronary artery openings (ostia) during systole, when the heart contracts.

Blood drains from the left coronary system via the *anterior great cardiac vein* and the lateral marginal veins. These empty into the *coronary sinus.* The right coronary artery empties directly into the right atrium via smaller cardiac veins.

Many **anastomoses** (communications between two or more vessels) among the various branches of the coronary arteries allow collateral circulation. Collateral circulation is a protective mechanism that provides an alternative path for blood flow in case of a blockage somewhere in the system. This is analogous to a river's developing small tributaries to reach a larger body of water.

CARDIAC PHYSIOLOGY

The Cardiac Cycle

Although the heart's right and left sides perform different functions, they act as a unit. The right and left atria contract at the same time, filling both ventricles to their maximum capacities. Both ventricles then contract at the same time, ejecting blood into the pulmonary and systemic circulations. The pressure of the contraction closes the tricuspid and mitral valves and opens the aortic and pulmonic valves at the same time.

The **cardiac cycle** is the sequence of events that occurs between the end of one heart contraction and the end of the next. To evaluate heart sounds and read electrocardiographs, you must thoroughly understand the pumping action of the cardiac cycle (Figure 2-89). **Diastole,**

> **Patho Pearls**
>
> The coronary arteries are perfused during diastole.

anastomosis communication between two or more vessels.

cardiac cycle the period of time from the end of one cardiac contraction to the end of the next.

diastole the period of time when the myocardium is relaxed and cardiac filling and coronary perfusion occur.

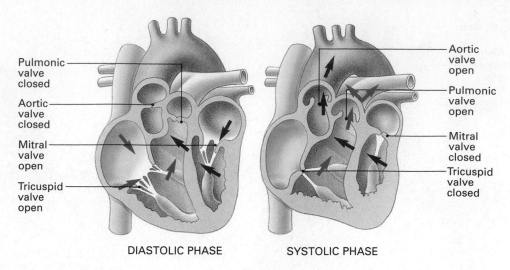

Pulmonic valve closed

Aortic valve closed

Mitral valve open

Tricuspid valve open

Aortic valve open

Pulmonic valve open

Mitral valve closed

Tricuspid valve closed

DIASTOLIC PHASE   SYSTOLIC PHASE

FIGURE 2–89   Relation of blood flow to cardiac contractions.

systole the period of the cardiac cycle when the myocardium is contracting.

the first phase of the cardiac cycle, is the relaxation phase. This is when ventricular filling begins. Blood enters the ventricles through the mitral and tricuspid valves. The pulmonic and aortic valves are closed.

During the second phase, **systole,** the heart contracts. The atria contract first, to finish emptying their blood into the ventricles. Atrial systole is relatively quick and occurs just before ventricular contraction; in healthy hearts, this atrial "kick" boosts cardiac output. The pressure in the ventricles now increases until it exceeds the pressure in the aorta and pulmonary artery. At this point blood flows out of the ventricles through the pulmonic and aortic valves and into the arteries. The pressure also closes the mitral and tricuspid valves and, if working properly, prevents backflow of blood into the atria. When pressures in the artery exceed the pressures in the ventricles, the valves close and diastole begins again.

Nervous Control of the Heart

The sympathetic and parasympathetic components of the autonomic nervous system work in direct opposition to one another to regulate the heart. In the heart's normal state the two systems balance. In stressful situations, however, the sympathetic system becomes dominant. During sleep the parasympathetic system dominates. The sympathetic nervous system innervates the heart through the *cardiac plexus,* a network of nerves at the base of the heart (Figure 2-90).

The sympathetic nerves arise from the thoracic and lumbar regions of the spinal cord, then leave the spinal cord and form the sympathetic chain, which runs along the spinal column. The cardiac plexus arises in turn from ganglia in the sympathetic chain and innervates both the atria and ventricles. The chemical neurotransmitter for the sympathetic nervous system, and thus for the cardiac plexus, is norepinephrine. Its release increases heart rate and cardiac contractile force, primarily through its actions on beta receptors.

As noted earlier, the sympathetic nervous system has two principal types of receptors, alpha and beta. Alpha receptors are located in the peripheral blood vessels and are responsible for vasoconstriction. Beta$_1$ receptors, primarily located in the heart, increase the heart rate and contractility. Beta$_2$ receptors, principally located in the lungs and peripheral blood vessels, cause bronchodilation and peripheral vasodilation. Medications specific to these various receptors cause different physiological effects. For instance, beta blockers slow the heart rate and lower blood pressure by blocking the beta1 receptors, whose job is to increase heart rate and contractility.

Parasympathetic control of the heart occurs through the vagus nerve (the tenth cranial nerve). The vagus nerve descends from the brain to innervate the heart and other organs. Vagal nerve fibers primarily innervate the atria, although some innervate the upper ventricles. The neurotransmitter for the parasympathetic nervous system, and thus the vagus nerve, is acetylcholine. Its release slows the heart rate and slows atrioventricular conduc-

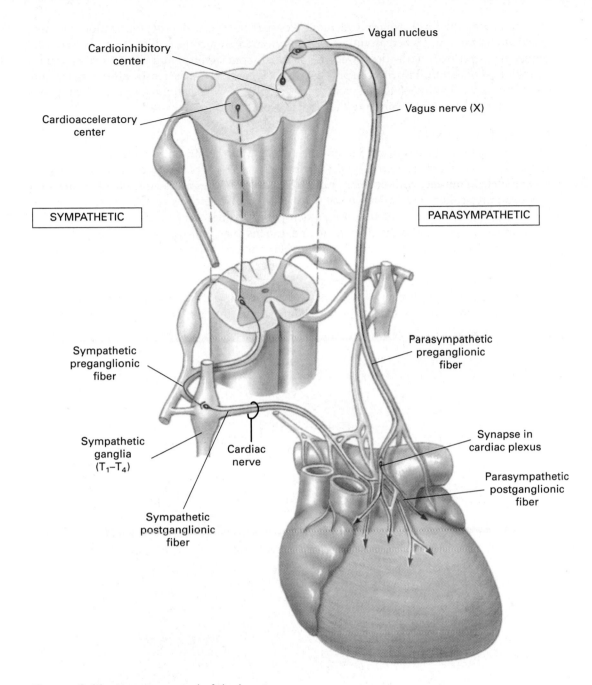

FIGURE 2-90 Nervous control of the heart.

tion. Several maneuvers can stimulate the vagus nerve, including Valsalva maneuver (forced expiration against a closed glottis, which can occur when lifting heavy objects), pressure on the carotid sinus (carotid sinus massage), and distention of the urinary bladder.

The terms *chronotropy, inotropy,* and *dromotropy* describe autonomic control of the heart. **Chronotropy** refers to heart rate. A positive chronotropic agent increases the heart rate. Conversely, a negative chronotropic agent decreases the heart rate. **Inotropy** refers to the strength of a cardiac muscular contraction. A positive inotropic agent strengthens the cardiac contraction, whereas a negative inotropic agent weakens it. **Dromotropy** refers to the rate of nervous impulse conduction. A positive dromotropic agent speeds impulse conduction, and a negative dromotropic agent slows conduction.

Role of Electrolytes   Cardiac function, both electrical and mechanical, depends heavily on electrolyte balances. Electrolytes that affect cardiac function include sodium (Na^+), calcium (Ca^{++}), potassium (K^+), chloride (Cl^-), and magnesium (Mg^{++}). Sodium plays a major role

chronotropy pertaining to heart rate.

inotropy pertaining to cardiac contractile force.

dromotropy pertaining to the speed of impulse transmission.

in depolarizing the myocardium. Calcium takes part in myocardial depolarization and myocardial contraction. Hypercalcemia can result in increased contractility, whereas hypocalcemia is associated with decreased myocardial contractility and increased electrical irritability. Potassium influences repolarization. Hyperkalemia decreases automaticity and conduction, whereas hypokalemia increases irritability. New research is also investigating the roles of magnesium and chloride in the cardiac cycle.

Electrophysiology

The heart has three types of cardiac muscle: atrial, ventricular, and specialized excitatory and conductive fibers. The atrial and ventricular muscle fibers contract in much the same way as skeletal muscle, with one major difference. Within the cardiac muscle fibers are special structures called **intercalated discs** (Figure 2-91). These discs connect cardiac muscle fibers and conduct electrical impulses quickly—400 times faster than the standard cell membrane—from one muscle fiber to the next. This speed allows cardiac muscle cells to function physiologically as a unit. That is, when one cell becomes excited, the action potential spreads rapidly across the entire group of cells, resulting in a coordinated contraction. This functional unit is a **syncytium**.

The heart has two syncytia—the *atrial syncytium* and the *ventricular syncytium*. The atrial syncytium contracts from superior to inferior, so that the atria express blood to the

intercalated discs specialized bands of tissue inserted between myocardial cells that increase the rate in which the action potential is spread from cell to cell.

syncytium group of cardiac muscle cells that physiologically function as a unit.

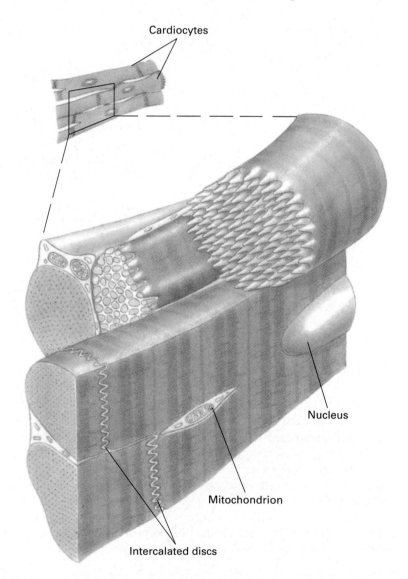

Cardiocytes

Nucleus

Mitochondrion

Intercalated discs

FIGURE 2-91   Microscopic appearance of cardiac muscle. The intercalated discs speed transmission of the electrical potential quickly from one cell to the next.

ventricles. The ventricular syncytium, on the other hand, contracts from inferior to superior, expelling blood from the ventricles into the aorta and pulmonary arteries. The syncytia are separated from one another by the fibrous structure that supports the valves and physically separates the atria from the ventricles. The only way an impulse can be conducted from the atria to the ventricles is through the *atrioventricular (AV) bundle.* Cardiac muscle functions according to an all-or-none principle. That is, if a single muscle fiber becomes *depolarized,* the action potential will spread through the whole syncytium. Stimulating a single atrial fiber will thus completely depolarize the atria, and stimulating a single ventricular fiber will completely depolarize the ventricles.

Cardiac Depolarization

Understanding **cardiac depolarization** is essential to interpreting electrocardiograms (ECGs). Normally, an ionic difference exists on the two sides of a cell membrane. The cell's sodium-potassium pump expels sodium (Na^+) from the cell. This leaves more negatively charged anions inside the cell than positively charged cations. Thus, the inside of the cell is more negatively charged than the outside. This difference, called the **resting potential,** can be measured experimentally by placing one probe inside the cell and another outside the cell and determining the difference in millivolts. The resting potential in a myocardial cell is approximately 290 mV (Figure 2-92).

When the myocardial cell is stimulated, the membrane surrounding the cell changes instantaneously to allow sodium ions to rush into the cell, bringing with them their positive charge. This charge is so strong that it gives the inside of the cell a positive charge approximately 120 mV greater than the outside. This influx of sodium and change of membrane

cardiac depolarization a reversal of charges at a cell membrane so that the inside of the cell becomes positive in relation to the outside; the opposite of the cell's resting state in which the inside of the cell is negative in relation to the outside.

resting potential the normal electrical state of cardiac cells.

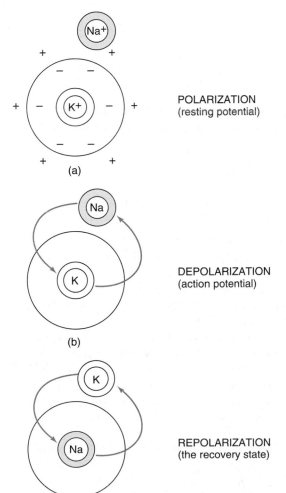

FIGURE 2-92 Schematic of ion shifts during depolarization and repolarization.

POLARIZATION
(resting potential)

(a)

DEPOLARIZATION
(action potential)

(b)

REPOLARIZATION
(the recovery state)

(c)

action potential the stimulation of myocardial cells, as evidenced by a change in the membrane electrical charge, that subsequently spreads across the myocardium.

repolarization return of a cell to its pre-excitation resting state.

polarity is the **action potential.** After the influx of sodium, a slower influx of calcium ions (Ca^{++}) through the calcium channels increases the positive charge inside the cell. Once depolarization occurs in a muscle fiber, it is transmitted throughout the entire syncytium, via the intercalated discs, until the entire muscle mass is depolarized. Contraction of the muscle follows depolarization.

The cell membrane remains permeable to sodium for only a fraction of a second. Thereafter, sodium influx stops and potassium escapes from inside the cell. This returns the charge inside the cell to normal (negative). In addition, sodium is actively pumped outside the cell, allowing the cell to **repolarize** and return to its normal resting state.

Cardiac Conductive System

The cardiac conductive system stimulates the ventricles to depolarize in the proper direction. As mentioned earlier, the atria contract from superior to inferior, the ventricles from inferior to superior. If the depolarization impulse originated in the atria and spread passively to the ventricles, then the ventricles would depolarize from superior to inferior and would be ineffective. The cardiac conduction system, therefore, must initiate an impulse, spread it through the atria, transmit it quickly to the apex of the heart, and thence stimulate the ventricles to depolarize from inferior to superior. To do this, the conduction system relies on specialized conductive fibers comprising muscle cells that transmit the depolarization potential through the heart much faster than can regular myocardial cells.

To accomplish their task, the cells of the cardiac conductive system have the important properties of excitability, conductivity, automaticity, and contractility:

excitability ability of the cells to respond to an electrical stimulus.

- **Excitability.** The cells can respond to an electrical stimulus, like all other myocardial cells.

conductivity ability of the cells to propagate the electrical impulse from one cell to another.

- **Conductivity.** The cells can propagate the electrical impulse from one cell to another.

automaticity pacemaker cells' capability of self-depolarization.

- **Automaticity.** The individual cells of the conductive system can depolarize without any impulse from an outside source. This property is also called *self-excitation.* Generally, the cell in the cardiac conductive system with the fastest rate of discharge, or automaticity, becomes the heart's pacemaker. As a rule, the highest cell in the conductive system has the fastest rate of automaticity. Normally, this cell is in the sinoatrial (SA) node, high in the right atrium; however, if one pacemaker cell fails to discharge and depolarize, then the cell with the next fastest rate becomes the pacemaker.

contractility ability of muscle cells to contract, or shorten.

- **Contractility.** Since the cells of the cardiac conductive system are specialized cardiac muscle cells, they retain the ability to contract.

Internodal atrial pathways connect the SA node to the AV node (Figure 2-93). These internodal pathways conduct the depolarization impulse to the atrial muscle mass and through the atria to the AV junction. The AV junction (the "gatekeeper") slows the impulse and allows the ventricles time to fill. Then, the impulse passes through the AV junction into the AV node and on to the AV fibers, which conduct the impulse from the atria to the ventricles. In the ventricles the AV fibers form the bundle of His.

The bundle of His subsequently divides into the right and left bundle branches. The right bundle branch delivers the impulse to the apex of the right ventricle. From there the Purkinje system spreads it across the myocardium. The left bundle branch divides into anterior and posterior fascicles that also ultimately terminate in the Purkinje system. At the same time that the impulse is transmitted to the right ventricle, the Purkinje system spreads it across the mass of the myocardium. Repolarization predominantly occurs in the opposite direction.

Each component of the conductive system has its own intrinsic rate of self-excitation:

SA node = 60 to 100 beats per minute

AV node = 40 to 60 beats per minute

Purkinje system = 15 to 40 beats per minute

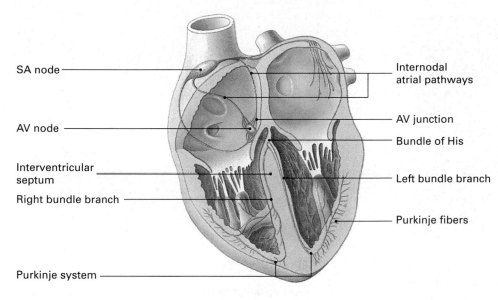

SA node

Internodal atrial pathways

AV node

AV junction

Bundle of His

Interventricular septum

Right bundle branch

Left bundle branch

Purkinje fibers

Purkinje system

FIGURE 2-93 The cardiac conductive system.

ANATOMY OF THE PERIPHERAL CIRCULATION

The peripheral circulation (Figure 2-94) transports oxygenated blood from the heart to the tissues and subsequently transports deoxygenated blood back to the heart. Oxygenated blood leaves the heart via the arterial system, while deoxygenated blood returns via the venous system. (As noted earlier, the exceptions to this rule are the pulmonary artery and the pulmonary veins.)

A capillary wall consists of a single layer of cells. The walls of arteries and veins, however, comprise several layers (Figure 2-95). The arteries' and veins' innermost lining, the *tunica intima,* is a single cell layer thick. The middle layer, the *tunica media,* consists of elastic fibers and muscle. It gives blood vessels their strength and recoil, which results from the difference in pressure inside and outside the vessel. The tunica media is much thicker in arteries than in veins. The outermost lining is the *tunica adventitia,* a fibrous tissue covering. It gives the vessel strength to withstand the pressures generated by the heart's contractions. The cavity inside a vessel is the *lumen.*

The vessels' diameters vary significantly and are directly related to the amount of blood they can transport. The larger the diameter, the greater the blood flow. In fact, according to **Poiseuille's law** the blood flow through a vessel is directly proportional to the fourth power of the vessel's radius. For example, a vessel with a relative radius of 1 would transport 1 mL per minute of blood at a pressure difference of 100 mmHg. If the vessel's radius were increased to 4, keeping the pressure difference constant, the flow would increase to 256 mL (4^4) per minute.

Poiseuille's law a law of physiology stating that blood flow through a vessel is directly proportional to the radius of the vessel to the fourth power.

Arterial System

The arterial system, which carries oxygenated blood from the heart, functions under high pressure. The larger arterial vessels are the arteries. The arteries branch into smaller structures called *arterioles,* which control blood flow to various organs by their degree of resistance. The arterioles continue to divide until they become capillaries, which are the connection points between the arterial and venous systems. The vascular system and the tissues are able to exchange gases, fluids, and nutrients through the very thin capillary walls.

Venous System

The venous system transports blood from the peripheral tissues back to the heart. It functions under low pressure with the aid of surrounding muscles and one-way valves within the veins. Blood enters the venous system through the capillaries, which drain into the venules. The venules, in turn, drain into the veins, the veins into the venae cavae, and the venae cavae into the atria.

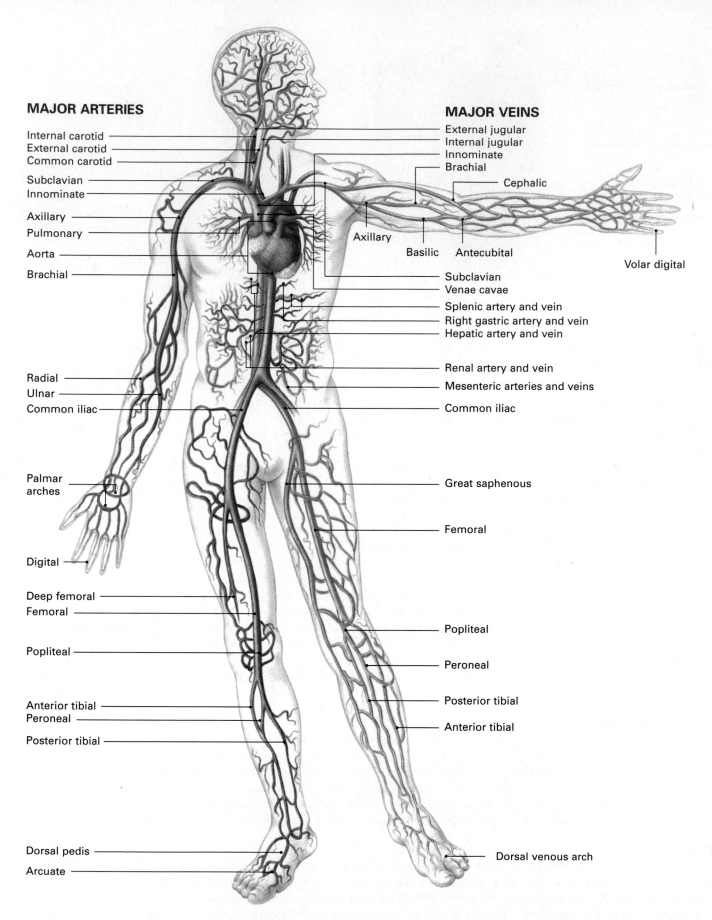

MAJOR ARTERIES

Internal carotid
External carotid
Common carotid

Subclavian
Innominate

Axillary
Pulmonary

Aorta

Brachial

Radial
Ulnar
Common iliac

Palmar
arches

Digital

Deep femoral
Femoral

Popliteal

Anterior tibial
Peroneal

Posterior tibial

Dorsal pedis
Arcuate

MAJOR VEINS

External jugular
Internal jugular
Innominate
Brachial

Cephalic

Axillary

Basilic   Antecubital

Volar digital

Subclavian
Venae cavae
Splenic artery and vein
Right gastric artery and vein
Hepatic artery and vein

Renal artery and vein
Mesenteric arteries and veins

Common iliac

Great saphenous

Femoral

Popliteal

Peroneal

Posterior tibial

Anterior tibial

Dorsal venous arch

FIGURE 2-94 The circulatory system.

194

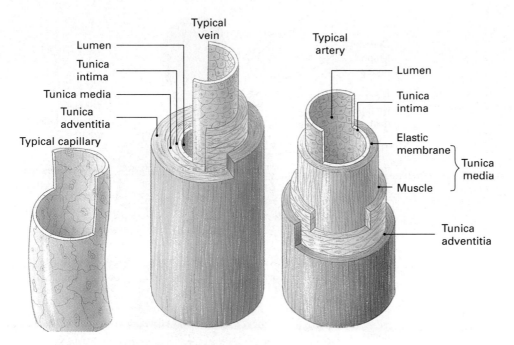

FIGURE 2-95   The layers of the peripheral arteries.

Lymphatic System

The lymphatic system is a network of valveless vessels that drains fluid, called *lymph,* from the body tissues and delivers it to the subclavian vein (Figure 2-96). Lymph nodes in the neck, the axilla, and the groin help filter impurities en route to the heart. The lymph system plays an important role in the body's immune system. It also plays an important role in our circulatory system.

When arterial blood flows into a capillary bed, hydrostatic pressure pushes fluid across the capillary membrane into the tissues. As the blood flows through the capillary bed, this pressure diminishes. Plasma proteins in the capillaries create an oncotic pressure gradient that draws fluid back into the blood stream. On the venous side of the capillary bed, the oncotic pressure drawing fluid in is greater than the hydrostatic pressure pushing fluid out. The net effect is that fluid returns to the capillary for its return to the heart. In a perfect system, whatever fluid enters the tissues at one end of the capillary bed should return to the circulation at the other end. In reality, some fluid usually remains in the tissues. The lymph system acts as an auxiliary drainage system, collecting the remaining fluid from the tissues and returning it to the heart.

PHYSIOLOGY OF PERFUSION

As discussed earlier, all body cells require a constant supply of oxygen and other essential nutrients, whereas waste products, such as carbon dioxide, must be constantly removed. It is the circulatory system, in conjunction with the respiratory and gastrointestinal systems, that provides the body's cells with these essential nutrients and removal of wastes. This is accomplished by the passage of blood through the capillaries, the small vessels that interface with body cells, whereas oxygen and carbon dioxide, nutrients and wastes, are exchanged by movement across the capillary walls and cell membranes. This constant and necessary passage of blood through the body's tissues is called **perfusion.** Inadequate perfusion of body tissues is **hypoperfusion,** which is commonly called *shock.*

Components of the Circulatory System

Perfusion depends on a functioning and intact circulatory system. The three components of the circulatory system are the pump (heart), fluid (blood), and container (blood vessels). A derangement in any one of these can adversely affect perfusion (Figure 2-97).

perfusion the supplying of oxygen and nutrients to the body tissues as a result of the constant passage of blood through the capillaries.

hypoperfusion inadequate perfusion of the body tissues, resulting in an inadequate supply of oxygen and nutrients to the body tissues. Also called *shock.*

All body cells require a constant supply of oxygen and other nutrients.

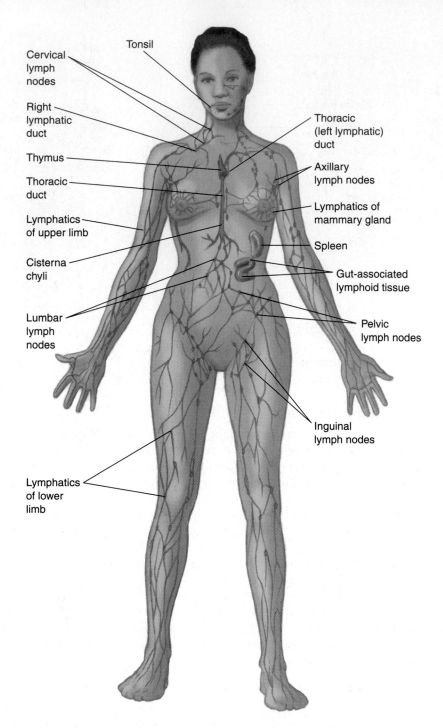

FIGURE 2-96 The lymphatic system.

Labels on figure:
- Tonsil
- Cervical lymph nodes
- Right lymphatic duct
- Thymus
- Thoracic duct
- Lymphatics of upper limb
- Cisterna chyli
- Lumbar lymph nodes
- Lymphatics of lower limb
- Thoracic (left lymphatic) duct
- Axillary lymph nodes
- Lymphatics of mammary gland
- Spleen
- Gut-associated lymphoid tissue
- Pelvic lymph nodes
- Inguinal lymph nodes

ejection fraction ratio of blood pumped from the ventricle to the amount remaining at the end of diastole.

stroke volume the amount of blood ejected by the heart in one cardiac contraction.

Content Review

FACTORS AFFECTING STROKE VOLUME
- Preload
- Cardiac contractility
- Afterload

The Pump The heart is the pump of the cardiovascular system. It receives blood from the venous system, pumps it to the lungs for oxygenation, and then pumps it to the peripheral tissues. The normal ventricle ejects about two-thirds of the blood it contains at the end of diastole. This ratio is the **ejection fraction.** The amount of blood ejected by the heart in one contraction is referred to as the **stroke volume.** Each time the ventricle pumps blood into the aorta, it generates a pressure wave along the major arteries, which we feel as a pulse. Stroke volume varies between 60 and 100 mL, with the average being 70 mL. The three factors affecting stroke volume are preload, cardiac contractile force, and afterload.

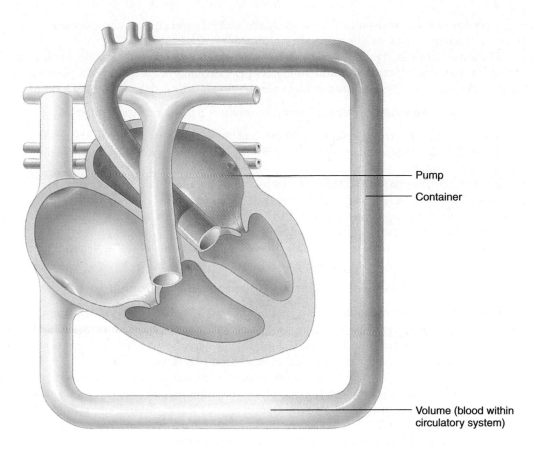

Pump

Container

Volume (blood within circulatory system)

FIGURE 2-97   Components of the circulatory system.

Preload is the amount of blood delivered to the heart during diastole (when the heart fills with blood between contractions). Preload depends on venous return. The venous system is a capacitance, or storage system. That is, it can be contracted or expanded, to some extent, as needed to meet the physiological demands of the body. When additional oxygenated blood is required, the venous capacitance is reduced, thus increasing the amount of blood delivered to the heart. The greater the preload, the greater the stroke volume.

Preload also affects **cardiac contractile force.** The greater the volume of preload, the more the ventricles are stretched. The greater the stretch, up to a certain limit, the greater will be the subsequent cardiac contraction. This phenomenon, known as **Starling's law of the heart,** can be illustrated through the example of a rubber band. The more the rubber band is stretched, the greater will be its velocity when released. Myocardial muscle, however, has its limits. If stretched too far, it will not contract properly and will weaken. Think of blowing up a tire. The tension in the walls increases as you put more air in the tire. If you were to put too much air in the tire, the tire would break or bulge from the side. If either of these happened, the tension in the wall would decrease, and if you filled the tire again it would not perform as well as before.

In addition, cardiac contractile force is affected by the circulating hormones called *catecholamines* (epinephrine and norepinephrine) controlled by the sympathetic nervous system. Catecholamines enhance cardiac contractile force by action on the beta-adrenergic receptors on the surface of the cells.

Finally, stroke volume is affected by afterload. **Afterload** is the resistance against which the ventricle must contract. This resistance must be overcome before ventricular contraction can result in ejection of blood. Afterload is determined by the degree of peripheral vascular resistance, which depends on the amount of vasoconstriction present. (The arterial system can be expanded and contracted to meet the metabolic demands of the body.) An increase

preload the pressure within the ventricles at the end of diastole, commonly called the *end-diastolic volume.*

cardiac contractile force force of the strength of a contraction of the heart.

Starling's law of the heart law of physiology stating that the more the myocardium is stretched, up to a certain limit, the more forceful is the subsequent contraction.

afterload the resistance against which the heart must pump.

in peripheral vascular resistance decreases stroke volume, and conversely, a decrease in peripheral vascular resistance allows stroke volume to increase.

The amount of blood pumped by the heart in one minute is referred to as the **cardiac output.** It is a function of stroke volume (milliliters per beat) and heart rate (beats per minute). Cardiac output is usually expressed in liters per minute. It can be defined by this equation:

$$\text{stroke volume (mL/b)} \times \text{heart rate (bpm)} = 5 \text{ cardiac output (mL/min)}$$

Since the average stroke volume is 70 mL and the normal heart rate is about 70 beats per minute, the average cardiac output is 4,900 mL per minute (rounded to 5,000 mL/min or 5 liters per minute).

The foregoing equation illustrates the factors that can affect cardiac output. An increase in stroke volume or an increase in heart rate can increase cardiac output. Conversely, a decrease in stroke volume (in turn governed by preload, contractile force, and afterload) or a decrease in heart rate can decrease cardiac output.

Blood pressure, the tension exerted by blood against the arterial walls, depends on both cardiac output and peripheral vascular resistance.

$$\text{blood pressure} = \text{cardiac output} \times \text{peripheral vascular resistance}$$

Peripheral vascular resistance is the pressure against which the heart must pump. Since the circulatory system is a closed system, increasing either cardiac output or peripheral vascular resistance increases blood pressure. Likewise, a decrease in cardiac output or a decrease in peripheral vascular resistance decreases blood pressure.

The body does its best to keep the blood pressure relatively constant by employing compensatory mechanisms and negative feedback loops to regulate the elements of the above formula. As noted earlier, baroreceptors in the carotid sinuses and in the arch of the aorta closely monitor blood pressure. If blood pressure increases, the baroreceptors send signals to the brain that cause the blood pressure to return to its normal values. This is accomplished by decreasing the heart rate, decreasing the preload, or decreasing peripheral vascular resistance.

The baroreceptors are also stimulated if the blood pressure falls. The heart rate is increased, as is the strength of the cardiac contractions. There is also arteriolar constriction, venous constriction (which results in decreased container size), and overall increased peripheral vascular resistance. Also, the adrenal medulla (the inner portion of the adrenal gland) is stimulated. This results in the secretion of epinephrine and norepinephrine, which further enhance the response.

The Fluid Blood is the fluid of the cardiovascular system. It is a viscous fluid; that is, it is thicker and more adhesive than water. As a result, blood flows more slowly than water. Blood, which consists of the plasma and the formed elements (red cells, white cells, and platelets), transports oxygen, carbon dioxide, nutrients, hormones, metabolic waste products, and heat.

An adequate amount of blood is required for perfusion. Since the cardiovascular system (the heart and blood vessels) is a closed system, the volume of blood present must be adequate to fill the container, as described below.

The Container Blood vessels (arteries, arterioles, capillaries, venules, and veins) serve as the container of the cardiovascular system. The blood vessels can be thought of as a continuous, closed, and pressurized pipeline by which blood moves throughout the body. Although the heart functions as the pump of the circulatory system, the blood vessels—under the control of the autonomic nervous system—can regulate blood flow to different areas of the body by adjusting their size as well as by selectively rerouting blood through the microcirculation.

Although the arteries and veins, like the heart, are subject to direct stimulation from sympathetic portions of the autonomic nervous system, the microcirculation (comprised of the small vessels: the arterioles, capillaries, and venules) is primarily responsive to local tissue needs. The capability of some vessels in the capillary network to adjust their diameter permits the microcirculation to selectively supply undernourished tissue, while temporarily bypassing tissues with no immediate need. Capillaries have a sphincter at the origin of the capillary (between arteriole and capillary), called the *pre-capillary sphincter,* and another at the end of the capillary (between capillary and venule), called the *post-capillary sphincter.* The pre-capillary sphincter responds to local tissue conditions, such as acidosis and hy-

cardiac output the amount of blood pumped by the heart in one minute.

blood pressure the tension exerted by blood against the arterial walls.

peripheral vascular resistance the resistance of the vessels to the flow of blood: increased when the vessels constrict, decreased when the vessels relax.

poxia, and opens as more arterial blood is needed. The post-capillary sphincter opens when blood is to be emptied into the venous system.

Blood flow through the vessels is regulated by two factors, peripheral vascular resistance and pressure within the system. Peripheral vascular resistance, as noted earlier, is the resistance to blood flow. Vessels with larger inside diameters offer less resistance, whereas vessels with smaller inside diameters offer greater resistance. Peripheral vascular resistance is governed by three factors—the length of the vessel, the diameter of the vessel, and blood viscosity.

There is very little resistance to blood flow through the aorta and arteries, but a significant change in peripheral resistance occurs at the arterioles and precapillary sphincters. This is because the inside diameter of the arteriole is much smaller, as compared with that of the aorta and arteries. Additionally, the arteriole has the ability to make a pronounced change in its diameter, as much as fivefold. It tends to do this in response to local tissue needs and autonomic nervous signals.

Contraction of the venous side of the vascular system results in decreased capacitance and increased cardiac preload. The arterial system, on the other hand, provides systemic vascular resistance. An increase in arterial tone increases resistance, which increases blood pressure.

Oxygen Transport

Oxygen is brought into the body via the respiratory system. During inspiration, approximately 500 to 800 mL of atmospheric air is taken in through the upper and lower airways, coming to rest in the alveoli of the lungs.

Surrounding the alveoli are capillaries that are perfused by the pulmonary circulation. The blood that comes into the pulmonary capillaries is oxygen-depleted blood that was returned from the body to the right atrium of the heart, then pumped by the right ventricle of the heart into the pulmonary arteries and thence into the pulmonary capillaries.

The air in the alveoli contains a concentration of about 13.6% oxygen. This is less than the 21% concentration of oxygen in atmospheric air because of various factors, including the fact that some air always remains in the alveoli from earlier respirations and oxygen is constantly being absorbed from this air. Nevertheless, alveolar air is far richer in oxygen than blood that enters the pulmonary capillaries.

Another way of stating this is that the *partial pressure of oxygen* present in air in the alveoli of the lungs is greater than the partial pressure of oxygen in the blood within the pulmonary circulation. (In a mix of gases, the portion of the total pressure exerted by each component of the mix is known as the partial pressure of that component.) For this reason, oxygen from the alveoli diffuses across the alveolar-capillary membrane and into the bloodstream—from the area of greater partial pressure to the area of lower partial pressure.

The red blood cells pick up this oxygen while passing through the pulmonary capillary bed. Oxygen binds to the hemoglobin molecule of the red blood cells, which serve as the primary carriers of oxygen within the bloodstream. Normally, between 95% and 100% of the hemoglobin is saturated with oxygen. The oxygen-enriched blood then circulates back to the heart through the venous side of the pulmonary circulation. Passing through the left atrium and into the left ventricle, the oxygen-enriched blood is pumped throughout the body via the systemic circulation.

Upon reaching capillaries throughout the body, the oxygen-rich blood interfaces with the tissues. The tissues contain cells that are oxygen-deficient as a result of normal metabolic activity. Since the partial pressure of oxygen is greater in the bloodstream than in the cells, oxygen will diffuse from the red blood cells across the capillary wall-cell membrane barrier, into the cells and tissues.

Overall, the movement and utilization of oxygen in the body depends on the following conditions:

- Adequate concentration of inspired oxygen
- Appropriate movement of oxygen across the alveolar/capillary membrane into the arterial bloodstream
- Adequate number of red blood cells to carry the oxygen

The precapillary sphincter responds to local tissue demands such as acidosis and hypoxia.

Content Review
MAJOR FUNCTIONS OF PERFUSION
- Oxygen transport
- Waste removal

Content Review
FICK PRINCIPLE
The movement and utilization of oxygen by the body is dependent upon:
- Adequate concentration of inspired oxygen
- Appropriate movement of oxygen across the alveolar/capillary membrane into the arterial bloodstream
- Adequate number of red blood cells to carry the oxygen
- Proper tissue perfusion
- Efficient off-loading of oxygen at the tissue level

- Proper tissue perfusion
- Efficient off-loading of oxygen at the tissue level

The dependence on this set of conditions for oxygen movement and utilization is known as the Fick Principle.

Waste Removal

The waste products of cellular metabolism are expelled from the cells and carried away by the blood. Carbon dioxide leaves the bloodstream during the oxygen-carbon dioxide exchange, which occurs through the alveolar/capillary membranes. Carbon dioxide is ultimately eliminated by exhalation from the lungs. Some cellular waste products are expelled into the interstitial fluid and picked up by the lymphatic system. These ultimately flow through the lymph channels into the thoracic duct. The thoracic duct empties the waste products into the venous side of the circulatory system. Other wastes are cleansed from the blood by the kidneys and excreted as urine. Finally, some cellular waste products are emptied into the gastrointestinal system and expelled in the feces.

There is some local control of both tissue perfusion and waste removal. When the amounts of metabolic waste products (such as lactic acid) increase, the tissues subsequently become acidotic. This local acidosis causes nearby precapillary sphincters to relax, thus opening the capillaries and increasing perfusion of the affected tissues. This provides increased capacity for waste elimination and response to local metabolic demands.

RESPIRATORY SYSTEM

The respiratory system provides a passage for oxygen, a gas necessary for energy production, to enter the body and for carbon dioxide, a waste product of the body's metabolism, to exit. This gas exchange, called **respiration,** requires a patent, open airway as well as adequate respiratory function. Many pathological processes can inhibit respiration. To understand the interventions that you will use to maintain adequate airway and ventilatory function, you must thoroughly understand the anatomy of the upper and lower airway.

UPPER AIRWAY ANATOMY

The upper airway extends from the mouth and nose to the larynx (Figure 2-98). It includes the nasal cavity, oral cavity, and pharynx. The larynx joins the upper and lower airways.

Content Review

UPPER AIRWAY COMPONENTS
- Nasal cavity
- Oral cavity
- Pharynx

nasal septum cartilage that separates the right and left nasal cavities.

sinus air cavity that conducts fluids from the eustachian tubes and tear ducts to and from the nasopharynx.

Nasal Cavity

The nasal cavity is the most superior part of the airway. The maxillary, frontal, nasal, ethmoid, and sphenoid bones comprise the lateral and superior walls of the nasal cavity. The hard palate forms the floor of the nasal cavity. The cartilaginous and highly vascular **nasal septum** separates the right and left nasal cavities.

Several different structures connect with the nasal cavity. These include the **sinuses,** the eustachian tubes, and the nasolacrimal ducts. The sinuses are air-filled cavities that are lined with a mucous membrane. There are four pairs of sinuses—the ethmoid sinuses, the frontal sinuses, the maxillary sinuses, and the sphenoid sinuses. The sinuses, named for the bone where they are contained, help reduce the overall weight of the head and are thought to assist in heating, purifying, and moistening the inhaled air. The sinuses help trap bacteria entering the nasal cavity. Because of this, they can become infected. Fractures of the upper sinuses (sphenoids) can occasionally cause cerebrospinal fluid (CSF) to leak from the cranial cavity into the nasal cavity. Clinically this presents with clear fluid draining from the nose (rhinorrhea) and can provide a direct route for the transmission of pathogens to the brain and associated structures.

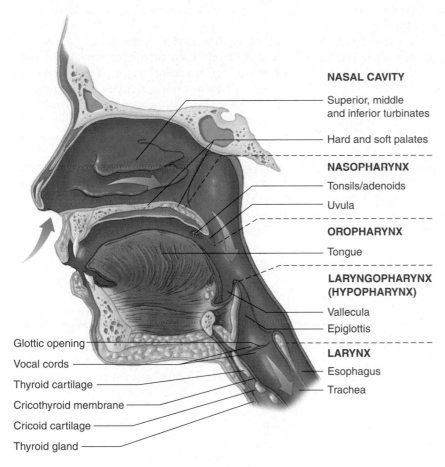

NASAL CAVITY

Superior, middle and inferior turbinates

Hard and soft palates

NASOPHARYNX

Tonsils/adenoids

Uvula

OROPHARYNX

Tongue

LARYNGOPHARYNX (HYPOPHARYNX)

Vallecula

Epiglottis

LARYNX

Esophagus

Trachea

Glottic opening

Vocal cords

Thyroid cartilage

Cricothyroid membrane

Cricoid cartilage

Thyroid gland

FIGURE 2-98 Anatomy of the upper airway.

The **eustachian tubes,** or auditory tubes, connect the ear with the nasal cavity and allow for equalization of pressure on each side of the tympanic membrane. Swallowing can assist in equalizing this pressure. The **nasolacrimal ducts** drain tears and debris the eyes into the nasal cavity. This can cause the nose to run when someone cries.

Air enters the nasal cavity through the external **nares** (nostrils). Nasal hairs just inside the external nares initially filter the incoming air. The air then proceeds into the nasal cavity, where it strikes three bony projections, the superior, middle, and inferior turbinates, or conchae. These shelflike structures, which are parallel to the nasal floor, serve as conduits into the sinuses, increase the surface area of the nasal cavity, and cause turbulent airflow. This turbulence helps to filter the air by depositing airborne particles on the **mucous membrane** lining the nasal cavity. Hairlike fibers called *cilia* propel those trapped particles to the back of the pharynx, where they are swallowed.

Because the mucous membrane is covered with **mucus** and has a rich blood supply, it also immediately warms and humidifies the air entering the nose. By the time the air reaches the lower airway, it is at body temperature (37°C), 100% humidified, and virtually free of airborne particles. Air proceeds from the nasal cavity through internal nares into the nasopharynx. The tissue of the nasal cavity is extremely delicate and vascular. Therefore, it is susceptible to trauma.

Oral Cavity

The cheeks, the hard and soft palates, and the tongue form the mouth, or oral cavity. The lips that surround the mouth's opening are fleshy folds of skin. Behind the lips lie the gums and teeth, normally numbering 32 in the adult. Significant force is required to avulse (dislodge) or fracture the teeth. Broken or dislodged teeth can potentially obstruct the airway.

eustachian tube a tube that connects the ear with the nasal cavity.

nasolacrimal duct narrow tube that carries into the nasal cavity the tears and debris that have drained from the eye.

nare nostril.

mucous membranes tissues lining body cavities that handle air transport; usually contain cells that secrete mucus.

mucus slippery secretion that lubricates and protects airway surfaces.

The hard palate anteriorly and the soft palate posteriorly form the top of the oral cavity and separate it from the nasal cavity.

The tongue, a large muscle on the bottom of the oral cavity, is the most common airway obstruction. It attaches to the mandible and the hyoid bone through a series of muscles and ligaments. The U-shaped hyoid bone is located just beneath the chin. The hyoid bone is unique. It is the only bone in the axial skeleton that does not articulate with any other bone. Instead, it is suspended by ligaments from the styloid process of the temporal bone and serves to anchor the tongue and larynx, as well as to support the trachea.

Pharynx

The **pharynx** is a muscular tube that extends vertically from the back of the soft palate to the superior aspect of the esophagus. It allows the air to flow into and out of the respiratory tract and food and liquids to pass into the digestive system. It contains several openings, including the internal nares, the mouth, the larynx, and the esophagus.

The pharynx is divided into three regions: the nasopharynx, the oropharynx, and the laryngopharynx (hypopharynx). The nasopharynx is the uppermost region, extending from the back of the nasal opening to the plane of the soft palate. The oropharynx extends from the plane of the soft palate to the hyoid bone. The adenoids, lymphatic tissue in the mouth and nose, filter bacteria. Either hypertrophy or swelling of the adenoids from infection may make them large enough to obscure your view. The laryngopharynx extends posteriorly from the hyoid bone to the esophagus and anteriorly to the larynx. The laryngopharynx is especially important in airway management.

Because the mouth and pharynx serve dual purposes for respiration and digestion, a number of mechanisms help prevent accidental blockage. To prevent foreign material from entering the trachea and lungs, sensitive nerves activate the body's cough and swallowing mechanisms as well as the **gag reflex.**

Located anteriorly in the hypopharynx is the epiglottis, a leaf-shaped cartilage that prevents food from entering the respiratory tract during swallowing. Just anterior and superior to the epiglottis is the **vallecula,** a fold formed by the base of the tongue and the epiglottis. It is an important landmark for **endotracheal intubation.** A series of ligaments and muscles connect the epiglottis to the hyoid bone and mandible. Immediately behind the hypopharynx are the fourth and fifth cervical vertebral bodies.

Larynx

The **larynx** is the complex structure that joins the pharynx with the trachea (Figure 2-99). Lying midline in the neck, it is attached to and lies just inferior to the hyoid bone and anterior to the esophagus. It consists of the thyroid and cricoid cartilage (both considered tracheal cartilage), glottic opening, vocal cords, arytenoid cartilage, pyriform fossae, and cricothyroid membrane.

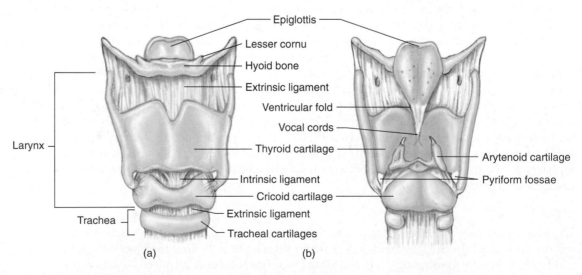

FIGURE 2-99 Internal anatomy of the upper airway.

The main laryngeal cartilage is the shield-shaped thyroid cartilage. Larger in males than in females, the thyroid cartilage forms the anterior prominence called the *Adam's apple*. The arytenoid cartilage, which forms a pyramid-shaped attachment for the vocal cords posteriorly, is an important landmark for endotracheal intubation. Posteriorly, smooth muscle closes a gap in the thyroid cartilage. Directly behind the Adam's apple, the thyroid cartilage houses the glottic opening, the narrowest part of the adult trachea, which is bordered by the vocal cords. The patency of the glottic opening, or **glottis**, depends heavily on muscle tone. On either side of the glottic opening are the pyriform fossae, recesses that form the lateral borders of the larynx. The thyrohyoid membrane attaches the upper end of the thyroid cartilage to the hyoid bone.

Within the laryngeal cavity lie the true vocal cords, white bands of cartilage that regulate the passage of air through the larynx and produce voice by contraction of the laryngeal muscles. The vocal cords can also close together to prevent foreign bodies from entering the airway. The passage of an endotracheal tube between the vocal cords interferes not only with the creation of sound, but also with the protective function of coughing.

Beneath the thyroid cartilage is the cricoid cartilage, which forms the inferior border of the larynx. Often it is considered the first tracheal ring. Unlike the thyroid and other tracheal cartilages, whose posterior surfaces are open and not fused, the cricoid cartilage forms a complete ring. The esophagus lies behind the cricoid cartilage, so pressure applied in a posterior direction to the anterior cricoid cartilage occludes the esophagus (**Sellick's maneuver**), thus inhibiting vomiting and subsequent **aspiration** during airway management. In children, the cricoid cartilage is the narrowest part of the laryngeal airway. The fibrous **cricothyroid membrane** connects the inferior border of the thyroid cartilage with the superior aspect of the cricoid cartilage. It is the site for surgical airway techniques.

A mucous membrane lines most of the larynx. Rich with nerve endings from the vagus nerve, it is so sensitive that any irritation sparks a cough, or forceful exhalation of a large volume of air. First, air is drawn into the respiratory passageways. Next, the glottic opening shuts tightly, trapping the air within the lungs. Then the abdominal and thoracic muscles contract, pushing against the diaphragm and increasing intrathoracic pressure. The vocal cords suddenly open, and a burst of air forces foreign particles out of the lungs. The laryngeal mucous membrane is so sensitive that its stimulation by a laryngoscope or endotracheal tube can cause bradycardia (slow pulse rate), hypotension (low blood pressure), and decreased respiratory rate.

Other structures proximate to the larynx are the thyroid gland, carotid arteries, and jugular veins. The thyroid gland is a "bow-tie" shaped endocrine gland located in the neck. It is highly vascular and lies inferior to the cricoid cartilage. It contains two lobes, one on each side of the trachea. These lobes are joined in the middle by the isthmus that extends across the trachea. The carotid arteries run closely along the trachea. Several branches of the carotid arteries cross the trachea. Likewise, the jugular veins lie very close to the trachea. Several branches of the jugular veins, such as the superior thyroid vein, cross the trachea.

LOWER AIRWAY ANATOMY

The lower airway extends from below the larynx to the alveoli (Figure 2-100). This is where the respiratory exchange of oxygen and carbon dioxide occurs. Helpful landmarks are the fourth cervical vertebra at the posterior superior border, and the xiphoid process anterior inferiorly, though the posterior lung extends beyond this inferiorly.

Trachea

As air enters the lower airway from the upper airway, it first enters and then passes through the **trachea.** The trachea is a 10–12 centimeter-long tube that connects the larynx to the two mainstem bronchi. It contains cartilaginous, C-shaped, open rings that form a frame to keep it open. The trachea is lined with respiratory epithelium containing cilia and mucus-producing cells. The mucus traps particles that the upper airway did not filter. The cilia then move the trapped particulate matter up into the mouth where it is swallowed or expelled.

glottis lip-like opening between the vocal cords.

Sellick's maneuver pressure applied in a posterior direction to the anterior cricoid cartilage that occludes the esophagus.

aspiration inhaling foreign material, such as vomitus, into the lungs.

cricothyroid membrane membrane between the cricoid and thyroid cartilages of the larynx.

Content Review

LOWER AIRWAY COMPONENTS

- Trachea
- Bronchi
- Alveoli
- Lung parenchyma
- Pleura

trachea a 10–12 cm-long tube-shaped structure that connects the larynx to the mainstem bronchi.

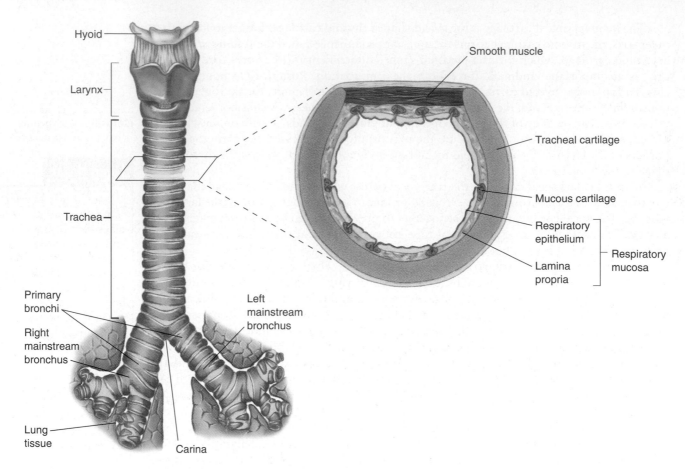

FIGURE 2-100 Anatomy of the lower airway.

The Bronchi

At the carina, the trachea divides, or bifurcates, into the right and left mainstem **bronchi.** The right mainstem bronchus is almost straight, whereas the left mainstem bronchus angles more acutely to the left. Because of this, the right mainstem is often the site of aspirated foreign bodies. In addition, when an endotracheal tube is inserted too far, it tends to enter the right mainstem bronchus, thus ventilating only the right lung. Mainstem bronchi enter the lung tissue at the hilum, and then divide into the secondary and tertiary bronchi. The secondary and tertiary bronchi ultimately branch into the bronchioles, or small airways.

The bronchioles are encircled with smooth muscle that contains beta$_2$ adrenergic receptors. When stimulated, these beta$_2$ receptors relax the bronchial smooth muscle, thus increasing the airway's diameter. This bronchodilation can increase the amount of air transported through the bronchiole. Conversely, parasympathetic receptors, when stimulated, cause the bronchial smooth muscles to contract, thus reducing the diameter of the bronchiole. This bronchoconstriction can inhibit the movement of air through the bronchiole.

After approximately 22 divisions, the bronchioles turn into the respiratory bronchioles. These structures contain only muscular connective tissue and have a limited capacity for gas exchange. The respiratory bronchioles terminate at the alveoli.

Patho Pearls

Invariably, when inserted too far, an endotracheal tube enters the right mainstem bronchus.

The Alveoli

The respiratory bronchioles divide into the alveolar ducts, which terminate in balloon-like clusters of **alveoli** called *alveolar sacs* (Figure 2-101). The alveoli contain an alveolar membrane that is only one or two cell layers thick. Because of this, the alveoli comprise the key functional unit of the respiratory system. Most oxygen and carbon dioxide gas exchanges take place here, although limited gas exchange may occur in the alveolar ducts and respiratory bronchioles. The alveoli become thinner as they expand. This facilitates diffusion of oxygen and carbon dioxide.

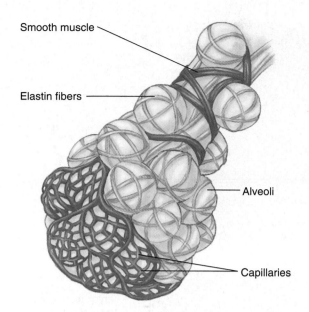

FIGURE 2-101   Anatomy of the alveoli.

Smooth muscle

Elastin fibers

Alveoli

Capillaries

The alveoli's surface area is massive, totaling more than 40 square meters—enough to cover half of a tennis court. These hollow structures resist collapse largely because of the presence of surfactant, a chemical that decreases their surface tension and makes it easier for them to expand. Alveolar collapse (**atelectasis**) can occur if surfactant is insufficient or if the alveoli are not inflated. No gas exchange takes place in atelectatic alveoli.

atelectasis alveolar collapse.

The Lung Parenchyma

The alveoli are the terminal end of the respiratory tree and the functional units of the lungs. As such, they are the core of the lung **parenchyma**. The lung parenchyma is arranged in two pulmonary lobules that form the anatomic division of the lungs. These lobules are further organized into lobes. The right lung has three lobes, the upper lobe, the middle lobe, and the lower lobe. The left lung, which shares thoracic space with the heart, has only two lobes, the upper lobe and the lower lobe.

parenchyma principle or essential parts of an organ.

The Pleura

Membranous connective tissue called **pleura** covers the lungs. The pleura consists of two layers, visceral and parietal. The visceral pleura envelopes the lungs and does not contain nerve fibers. In contrast, the parietal pleura lines the thoracic cavity and does contain nerve fibers. The potential space between these two layers, called the *pleural space,* usually holds a small amount of fluid that reduces friction between the pleural layers during respiration. Occasionally, the pleura can become inflamed, causing significant pain with respiration. This condition, called *pleurisy,* is a common cause of chest pain, particularly in cigarette smokers.

pleura membranous connective tissue covering the lungs.

THE PEDIATRIC AIRWAY

The pediatric airway is fundamentally the same as an adult's, but you will need to know the differences in relative size and position of some components. The airway is smaller in all aspects, particularly the diameters of the openings and passageways.

In the pharynx, the jaw is smaller and the tongue relatively larger, resulting in greater potential airway encroachment (Figure 2-102). The epiglottis is much floppier and rounder ("omega" shaped). The dental (alveolar) ridge and teeth are softer and more fragile than an adult's and potentially more subject to damage from airway maneuvers.

The larynx lies more superior and anterior in children and is funnel-shaped because the cricoid cartilage is undeveloped. Before the age of ten, the cricoid cartilage is the narrowest part of the airway. Most significantly, even a small foreign body or a limited degree of swelling in the pediatric airway can be life threatening. Because of this, young children tend to suffer more problems related to the trachea than do older children. A

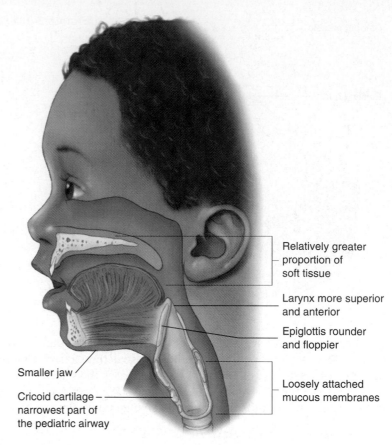

Relatively greater
proportion of
soft tissue

Larynx more superior
and anterior

Epiglottis rounder
and floppier

Loosely attached
mucous membranes

Smaller jaw

Cricoid cartilage –
narrowest part of
the pediatric airway

FIGURE 2-102   Anatomy of the pediatric airway.

common example is croup (laryngotracheobronchitis), a viral infection that causes the soft tissues below the glottis to swell. This can reduce the diameter of the airway, potentially causing serious problems.

The ribs and the cartilage of the pediatric thoracic cage are softer and more pliable. This lack of rigidity lessens the ability of the thoracic wall and accessory muscles to assist lung expansion during inspiration. As a result, infants and children tend to rely more on their diaphragms for breathing. Always pay close attention to these differences when treating pediatric patients, especially those with respiratory complaints.

PHYSIOLOGY OF THE RESPIRATORY SYSTEM

Just as successful airway management requires a firm understanding of airway anatomy, a good outcome for these patients requires a working knowledge of the mechanics of oxygenation and ventilation. Your knowledge of normal respiratory physiology will lay the groundwork for your comprehension of important **pathophysiology** and will help you to determine which actions will ensure optimal patient care.

pathophysiology the study of how disease affects normal body processes.

Respiration and Ventilation

Respiration is the exchange of gases between a living organism and its environment. Pulmonary, or external, respiration occurs in the lungs when the respiratory gases are exchanged between the alveoli and the red blood cells in the pulmonary capillaries through the capillary membranes (Figure 2-103). In addition, cellular, or internal, respiration occurs in the peripheral capillaries. It is the exchange of the respiratory gases between the red blood cells and the various body tissues. Cellular respiration in the peripheral tissue produces carbon dioxide (CO_2). The blood picks up this waste product in the capillaries and transports it as bicarbonate ions through the venous system to the lungs. Although respiration describes the process of gas exchange in the lungs and peripheral tissues, **ventilation** is the mechanical process that moves air into and out of the lungs. Ventilation is necessary for respiration to occur.

ventilation the mechanical process that moves air into and out of the lungs.

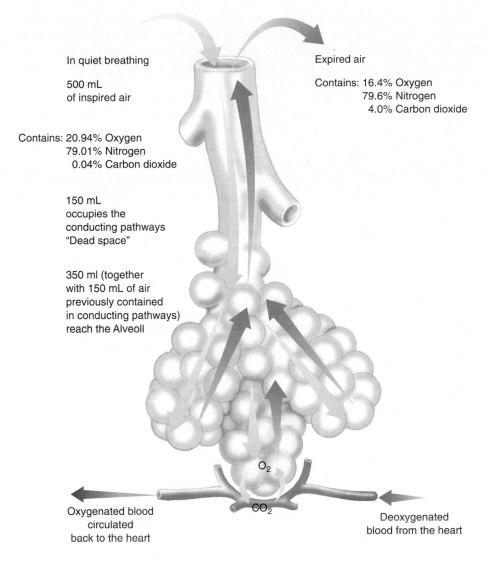

In quiet breathing

500 mL
of inspired air

Contains: 20.94% Oxygen
79.01% Nitrogen
0.04% Carbon dioxide

150 mL
occupies the
conducting pathways
"Dead space"

350 ml (together
with 150 mL of air
previously contained
in conducting pathways)
reach the Alveoll

Expired air

Contains: 16.4% Oxygen
79.6% Nitrogen
4.0% Carbon dioxide

O_2

CO_2

Oxygenated blood
circulated
back to the heart

Deoxygenated
blood from the heart

FIGURE 2-103   Diffusion of gases across an alveolar membrane.

Respiratory Cycle   Nothing within the lung parenchyma makes it contract or expand. Pulmonary ventilation, therefore, depends on changes in pressure within the thoracic cavity. These changes occur in a respiratory cycle involving coordinated interaction among the respiratory system, the central nervous system, and the musculoskeletal system.

The thoracic cavity is a closed space, opening to the external environment only through the trachea. The diaphragm separates the thoracic cavity from the abdomen. When the diaphragm contracts, it draws downward, away from the thoracic cavity, thus enlarging it. Likewise, when the muscles between the ribs, or intercostal muscles, contract, they draw the ribcage upward and outward, away from the thoracic cavity, further increasing its volume.

The respiratory cycle begins when the lungs have achieved a normal expiration and the pressure inside the thoracic cavity equals the atmospheric pressure. At this point, respiratory centers in the brain communicate with the diaphragm by way of the phrenic nerve, signaling it to contract and thus initiate the respiratory cycle. As the size of the thorax increases in relation to the volume of air it holds, pressure within the thorax decreases, becoming lower than atmospheric pressure. This negative intrathoracic pressure invites air into the thorax through the airway. Because the visceral and parietal pleura remain in contact with each other under normal circumstances, the highly elastic lungs immediately assume the thoracic cavity's internal contour. These combined factors move air into the lungs (inspiration). At the same time, the alveoli inflate with the lungs. They become thinner as they expand, allowing oxygen and carbon dioxide to diffuse across their membranes.

When the pressure in the thoracic cavity again reaches that of the atmosphere, the alveoli are maximally inflated. Pulmonary expansion stimulates microscopic stretch receptors in the bronchi and bronchioles. These receptors signal the respiratory center by way of the vagus nerve to inhibit inspiration, and the air influx stops. This process is primarily protective, as it prevents overinflation of the lungs.

At the end of inspiration, the respiratory muscles now relax, thus decreasing the size of the chest cavity, and in turn increasing the intrathoracic pressure. The naturally elastic lungs recoil, forcing air out through the airway (expiration) until intrathoracic and atmospheric pressure are equal once again. Normal expiration is a passive process, whereas inspiration is an active process, using energy. In respiratory inadequacy, when this process fails to provide satisfactory gas exchange, the patient may use accessory respiratory muscles such as the strap muscles of his neck and his abdominal muscles to augment his efforts to expand the thoracic cavity.

Pulmonary Circulation Respiration also requires an intact circulatory system. In fact, during each cardiac cycle, the heart pumps as much blood to the lungs as it pumps to the peripheral tissues. In the capillaries, these cells take oxygen from red blood cells coming from the arterial system and give up carbon dioxide to blood returning to the venous system. The venous system carries this deoxygenated blood to the right side of the heart, and the right ventricle pumps it into the pulmonary artery (Figure 2-104).

The pulmonary artery immediately branches into the right and the left pulmonary arteries, each supplying its respective lung. In turn, both branches quickly fan into smaller arteries that end in the pulmonary capillaries. These capillaries are spread over the surfaces of the alveoli, where the red blood cells exchange carbon dioxide for oxygen. The pulmonary capillaries recombine into larger veins, eventually terminating in the pulmonary vein. The pulmonary vein empties the oxygenated blood into the left atrium of the heart. Finally, the heart transports the oxygenated blood through the left ventricle and into the systemic arterial system via the aorta and its tributaries.

The lungs themselves receive little of their blood supply from the pulmonary arteries or veins. Instead, bronchial arteries that branch from the aorta supply most of their blood. Bronchial veins return this blood from the lungs to the superior vena cava.

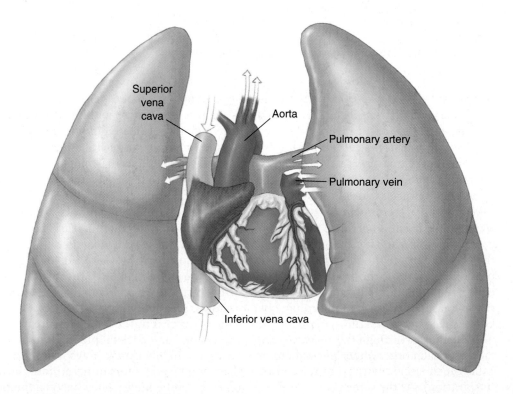

FIGURE 2-104 Pulmonary circulation.

Table 2-6 PARTIAL PRESSURES AND CONCENTRATIONS OF GASES

Gas	Partial Pressure Atmospheric (torr)	Partial Pressure Alveolar (torr)	Concentration Atmospheric	Concentration Alveolar
Nitrogen	597.0	569.0	78.62%	74.9%
Oxygen	159.0	104.0	20.84%	13.7%
Carbon dioxide	0.3	40.0	0.04%	5.2%
Water	3.7	47.0	0.50%	6.2%
TOTAL	760.0	760.0	100.00%	100.0%

Measuring Oxygen and Carbon Dioxide Levels

You can determine the amount of oxygen and carbon dioxide in the blood by measuring their partial pressures. **Partial pressure** is the pressure exerted by each component of a gas mixture. In other words, the partial pressure of a gas is its percentage of the mixture's total pressure. The partial pressure of oxygen at normal atmospheric pressure, for example, is the percentage of oxygen in atmospheric air (21%) multiplied by the atmospheric pressure at sea level (760 torr, or 14.7 pounds per square inch):

$$0.21 \times 760 \text{ torr} = 159.6 \text{ torr}$$

(Note that torr and mmHg are the same measures of pressure.) Earth's atmosphere consists of four major respiratory gases: nitrogen (N_2), oxygen (O_2), carbon dioxide (CO_2), and water vapor (H_2O). Although nitrogen is metabolically inert, it is needed to inflate gas-filled body cavities such as the chest. Table 2-6 lists these four respiratory gases' partial pressures and concentrations in the environment and in the alveoli.

Since alveolar partial pressure and arterial partial pressure are essentially the same in the normal lung, normal arterial partial pressures for oxygen and carbon dioxide may be expressed:

$$\text{Oxygen (PaO}_2) = 100 \text{ torr (average} = 80 - 100)$$

$$\text{Carbon dioxide (PaCO}_2) = 40 \text{ torr (average} = 35 - 45)$$

Alveolar partial pressures are abbreviated **PA** (PAO_2 and $PACO_2$) while arterial partial pressures are abbreviated **Pa** (PaO_2 and $PaCO_2$). Because these values are usually the same, however, they typically appear as the shortened notations PO_2 and PCO_2.

Diffusion   **Diffusion** is the movement of a gas from an area of higher concentration to an area of lower concentration, attempting to reach equilibrium. Diffusion transfers gases between the lungs and the blood and between the blood and the peripheral tissues. The rate of diffusion of a gas across the pulmonary membranes depends on the gas's solubility in water. For example, carbon dioxide is 21 times more soluble in water than oxygen and readily crosses the pulmonary capillary membranes. In the peripheral tissues, the gradient (direction of diffusion) for CO_2 is from the tissue, where its concentration is high, to the capillary blood, where its concentration is low.

In the lungs, oxygen dissolves in water at the alveolar membrane and leaves the area of higher concentration, the alveoli, and enters the area of lower concentration, the venous blood in the pulmonary capillaries. Concurrently, carbon dioxide leaves the area of higher concentration, the arterial blood, and enters the area of lower concentration, the alveoli. The blood returns from the pulmonary vein to the heart and then moves into the systemic circulation.

Oxygen Concentration in the Blood   Oxygen diffuses into the blood plasma, where most of it combines with hemoglobin and is measured as oxygen saturation (SpO_2). The remainder is dissolved in the blood and is measured as the PaO_2. Hemoglobin approaches 100% saturation when the PaO_2 of dissolved oxygen reaches 90–100 torr. Each gram of

partial pressure the pressure exerted by each component of a gas mixture.

PA alveolar partial pressure.

Pa arterial partial pressure.

diffusion movement of a gas from an area of higher concentration to an area of lower concentration.

saturated hemoglobin carries 1.34 milliliters of oxygen. Oxygen saturation is the ratio of the blood's actual oxygen content to its total oxygen-carrying capacity:

$$\text{Oxygen saturation} = O_2 \text{ content}/O_2 \text{ capacity} \times 100(\%)$$

The hemoglobin molecule carries the vast majority of oxygen in the blood (approximately 97%). Very little oxygen dissolves in the plasma. Since partial pressure measurements detect only the amount of oxygen dissolved in the plasma and do not always reflect the total oxygen saturation, they can be misleading. For example, a patient who has suffered carbon monoxide poisoning cannot transport enough oxygen to the peripheral tissues since carbon monoxide displaces oxygen from the hemoglobin molecule. But an arterial blood gas sample might reveal a normal or high PaO_2. This would indicate that adequate oxygen was reaching the blood. In fact, however, an inadequate amount of hemoglobin would be available to transport the oxygen to the peripheral tissues, thus resulting in peripheral hypoxia.

Several factors can affect oxygen concentrations in the blood:

- *Decreased hemoglobin concentration* (anemia, hemorrhage)
- *Inadequate alveolar ventilation* due to low inspired-oxygen concentration, respiratory muscle paralysis, and pulmonary conditions such as emphysema, asthma, or pneumothorax
- *Decreased diffusion across the pulmonary membrane* when diffusion distance increases or the pulmonary membrane changes; for example, when fluid enters the space between the alveolar membrane and the pulmonary capillary membrane, as in pneumonia, chronic obstructive pulmonary disease (COPD), or pulmonary edema (swelling).
- *Ventilation/perfusion mismatch* occurs when a portion of the alveoli collapses, as in atelectasis. Blood travels past these collapsed alveoli without oxygenation (shunting), without carbon dioxide, and without oxygen uptake. This can result from **hypoventilation,** which can occur secondary to pain or inability to inspire (traumatic asphyxia). When the lung collapses, as in **pneumothorax, hemothorax,** or a combination of the two, less surface area is available for gas exchange. Alternatively, a ventilation/perfusion mismatch can occur when blood is prevented from reaching the alveolar capillary membranes but alveolar ventilation remains adequate. This occurs when a blood clot travels to or is formed in the pulmonary arterial system, a condition known as pulmonary thromboembolism.

You can correct oxygen derangements by increasing ventilation, administering supplemental oxygen, using intermittent positive pressure ventilation (IPPV), or administering drugs to correct underlying problems such as pulmonary edema, asthma, or **pulmonary embolism.** The emergency being treated determines the desired fractional concentration of oxygen (**FiO₂**) to be delivered. It is crucial to remember not to withhold oxygen from any patient whose clinical condition indicates its need.

Carbon Dioxide Concentration in the Blood The blood transports carbon dioxide mainly in the form of bicarbonate ion (HCO_3^-). It carries approximately 70% as bicarbonate and approximately 20% combined with hemoglobin. Less than 7% is dissolved in the plasma. Several factors influence carbon dioxide's concentration in the blood, including increased CO_2 production and/or decreased CO_2 elimination:

- *Hyperventilation lowers CO_2 levels* and can be the result of an increased respiratory rate or deeper respiration, both of which increase the minute volume. (Minute volume is discussed more completely later.)
- *Increased CO_2 production* can be caused by:
  - Fever
  - Muscle exertion
  - Shivering
  - Metabolic processes resulting in the formation of metabolic acids

hypoventilation reduction in breathing rate and depth.

pneumothorax accumulation of air or gas in the pleural cavity.

hemothorax accumulation in the pleural cavity of blood or fluid containing blood.

pulmonary embolism blood clot that travels to the pulmonary circulation and hinders oxygenation of the blood.

FiO₂ concentration of oxygen in inspired air.

- *Decreased CO_2 elimination* (increased CO_2 levels in the blood) resulting from decreased alveolar ventilation is commonly caused by hypoventilation due to:
  - Respiratory depression by drugs
  - Airway obstruction
  - Impairment of the respiratory muscles
  - Obstructive diseases such as asthma and emphysema

Increased CO_2 levels (**hypercarbia**) are usually treated by increasing the rate and/or volume of ventilation and by correcting the underlying cause.

Regulation of Respiration

Respiratory Rate   The number of times a person breathes in one minute, the **respiratory rate,** is unique in that both voluntary and involuntary nervous system mechanisms control it. We do not ordinarily need to make a conscious effort to breathe; our brains automatically regulate this function. However, we can voluntarily override our involuntary respirations until physical and chemical mechanisms signal the nervous system's respiratory centers to provide involuntarily impulses and correct any breathing irregularities.

Nervous Impulses from the Respiratory Center   The main respiratory center lies in the medulla oblongata in the brainstem. Various neurons within the medulla initiate impulses that result in respiration. A rise in the frequency of these impulses increases the respiratory rate. Conversely, a decrease in their frequency decreases the respiratory rate. The medulla is connected to the respiratory muscles primarily via the vagus nerve. This is an involuntary pathway. If the medulla fails to initiate respiration, an additional control center in the pons, called the *apneustic center,* assumes respiratory control to ensure the continuation of respirations. A third center, the *pneumotaxic center,* also in the pons, controls expiration.

Stretch Receptors   During inspiration, the lungs become distended, activating stretch receptors. As the degree of stretch increases, these receptors fire more frequently. The impulses they send to the brainstem inhibit the medullary cells, decreasing the inspiratory stimulus. Thus, the respiratory muscles relax, allowing the elastic lungs to recoil and expel air from the body. As the stretch decreases, the stretch receptors stop firing. This process, called the *Hering-Breuer reflex,* prevents overexpansion of the lungs.

Chemoreceptors   Other involuntary respiration controls include central chemical receptors in the medulla and peripheral chemoreceptors in the carotid bodies and in the arch of the aorta. These chemoreceptors are stimulated by decreased PaO_2, increased $PaCO_2$, and decreased pH. (The pH scale expresses the degree of acidity or alkalinity. A lower pH indicates greater acidity; a higher pH indicates greater alkalinity. The general principles of pathophysiology chapter discusses pH in greater detail.) Cerebrospinal fluid (CSF) pH is the primary control of respiratory center stimulation. The CSF pH responds very quickly to changes in arterial PCO_2. Any increase in PCO_2 decreases CSF pH, which in turn stimulates the central chemoreceptors to increase respiration. Conversely, low $PaCO_2$ levels raise CSF pH, in turn decreasing chemoreceptor stimulation and slowing respiratory activity. Because $PaCO_2$ is inversely related to CSF pH, $PaCO_2$ is seen as the normal neuroregulatory control of respirations. Additionally, any increase in the arterial $PaCO_2$ stimulates the peripheral chemoreceptors to signal the brainstem to increase respiration, thus speeding CO_2 elimination from the body.

Hypoxic Drive   The body also constantly monitors the PaO_2 and the pH. In fact, **hypoxemia** (decreased partial pressure of oxygen in the blood) is a profound stimulus of respiration in a normal individual. People with chronic respiratory disease such as emphysema and chronic bronchitis tend to retain CO_2 and, therefore, have a chronically elevated $PaCO_2$. Chemoreceptors in the periphery eventually become accustomed to this chronic condition, and the central nervous system stops using $PaCO_2$ to regulate respiration. This activates a default mechanism called **hypoxic drive,** which increases respiratory stimulation when PaO_2 falls and inhibits respiratory stimulation when PaO_2 climbs. High-volume oxygen administration to people with this condition can cause respiratory arrest. Because high-flow oxygen can quickly double or even triple the PaO_2, peripheral chemoreceptors stop stimulating the respiratory centers, causing **apnea.** (Although this is a potential threat, it is never appropriate to withhold oxygen from a patient for whom oxygen therapy is indicated; if the respiratory effort becomes inadequate, ventilatory assistance will be necessary.)

Measures of Respiratory Function

The respiratory rate is the number of respiratory cycles per minute, normally 12 to 20 breaths per minute in adults, 18 to 24 in children, and 40 to 60 in infants. Several factors affect respiratory rate:

- Fever—increases rate
- Emotion—increases rate
- Pain—increases rate
- Hypoxia (inadequate tissue oxygenation)—increases rate
- Acidosis—increases rate
- Stimulant drugs—increase rate
- Depressant drugs—decrease rate
- Sleep—decreases rate

EMT-Is must fully understand ventilatory mechanics and capacities for the average adult's respiratory system. This knowledge enables you to adapt your mechanical ventilation techniques to your patient's size, lung compliance, need for hyperventilation, or other individual requirements. It is especially crucial in situations that call for advanced mechanical ventilator skills. Respiratory capacities and measurements with which you must be familiar include:

total lung capacity (TLC) maximum lung capacity.

tidal volume (V_T) average volume of gas inhaled or exhaled in one respiratory cycle.

minute volume (V_{min}) amount of gas inhaled and exhaled in one minute.

- **Total Lung Capacity (TLC).** This is the maximum lung capacity—the total amount of air contained in the lung at the end of maximal inspiration. In the average adult male, this volume is approximately 6 liters.

- **Tidal Volume (V_T).** The tidal volume is the average volume of gas inhaled or exhaled in one respiratory cycle. In the adult male this is approximately 500 mL (5 to 7 mL/kg).

- *Dead Space Volume (V_D).* The dead space volume is the amount of gas in the tidal volume that remains in air passageways unavailable for gas exchange. It is approximately 150 ml in the adult male. Anatomical dead space includes the trachea and bronchi. Obstructions or diseases such as chronic obstructive pulmonary disease or atelectasis can cause physiologic dead space.

- *Alveolar Volume (V_A).* The alveolar volume is the amount of gas in the tidal volume that reaches the alveoli for gas exchange. It is the difference between tidal volume and dead-space volume (approximately 350 ml in the adult male):

$$V_A = V_T - V_D$$

- **Minute Volume (V_{min}).** The minute volume is the amount of gas moved in and out of the respiratory tract in one minute:

$$V_{min} = V_T \times \text{respiratory rate}$$

- *Alveolar Minute Volume ($V_{A\text{-}min}$).* The alveolar minute volume is the amount of gas that reaches the alveoli for gas exchange in one minute:

$$V_{A\text{-}min} = (V_T - V_D) \times \text{respiratory rate}$$

or

$$V_{A\text{-}min} = V_A \times \text{respiratory rate}$$

- *Inspiratory Reserve Volume (IRV).* The inspiratory reserve volume is the amount of air that can be maximally inhaled after a normal inspiration.

- *Expiratory Reserve Volume (ERV).* The expiratory reserve volume is the amount of air that can be maximally exhaled after a normal expiration.

- *Residual Volume (RV)*. The residual volume is the amount of air remaining in the lungs at the end of maximal expiration.
- *Functional Residual Capacity (FRC)*. The functional residual capacity is the volume of gas that remains in the lungs at the end of normal expiration:

$$FRC = ERV + RV$$

- *Forced Expiratory Volume (FEV)*. The forced expiratory volume is the amount of air that can be maximally expired after maximum inspiration.

THE ABDOMEN

The abdominal cavity is bound by the diaphragm, superiorly; the pelvis, inferiorly; the vertebral column, the posterior and inferior ribs, and the back muscles (psoas and paraspinal muscles), posteriorly; the muscles of the flank, laterally; and the abdominal muscles, anteriorly (Figure 2-105). The cavity is divided into three spaces: the **peritoneal space** (containing those organs or portions of organs covered by the abdominal (peritoneal) lining); the **retroperitoneal space** (containing those organs posterior to the peritoneal lining); and the **pelvic space** (containing the organs within the pelvis). Anatomical landmarks of this area include the centrally located umbilicus (the navel), the xiphoid process (tip of the sternum) at the upper and central abdominal border, the bony ridges of the pelvis (the iliac crests) inferiorly and laterally, and the pubic prominence inferiorly.

The abdomen is divided into four subregions by imaginary vertical and horizontal lines intersecting at the umbilicus (naval) and forming the right and left upper and lower quadrants. The right upper quadrant contains the gallbladder, right kidney, most of the liver, some small bowel, a portion of the ascending and transverse colon, and a small portion of the pancreas. The left upper quadrant contains the stomach, spleen, left kidney, most of the pancreas, and a portion of the liver, small bowel, and transverse and descending colon. The right lower quadrant contains the appendix, and portions of the urinary bladder, small bowel, ascending colon, rectum, and female genitalia. The left lower quadrant contains the sigmoid colon and portions of the urinary bladder, small bowel, descending colon, rectum, and female genitalia.

peritoneal space division of the abdominal cavity containing those organs or portions of organs covered by the peritoneum.

retroperitoneal space division of the abdominal cavity containing those organs posterior to the peritoneal lining.

pelvic space division of the abdominal cavity containing those organs located within the pelvis.

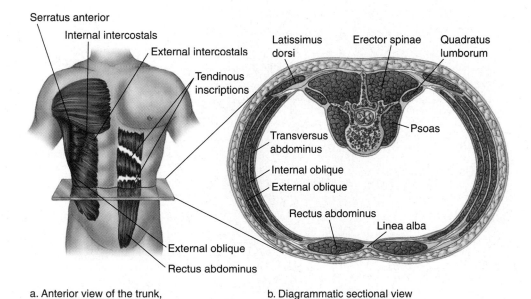

a. Anterior view of the trunk, showing superficial and deep members of the oblique and rectus groups.

b. Diagrammatic sectional view through the abdominal region.

FIGURE 2-105 Muscles protecting the organs of the abdominal cavity.

The major structures within the abdomen include the digestive tract, the accessory organs of digestion, the spleen, the structures and organs of the urinary system, and the female reproductive organs. (The male reproductive organs, or genitalia, are considered to be part of the urinary system. The female reproductive organs are separate from the urinary system, and include the reproductive organs within the abdomen as well as the external genitalia.)

ABDOMINAL VASCULATURE

The abdominal contents are supplied with blood via the abdominal aorta, which travels along and to the left of the spinal column. It sends forth many branches to discrete organs and the bowel (Figure 2-106). The abdominal aorta bifurcates at the upper sacral level into two large iliac arteries. These eventually become the femoral arteries as they traverse and then exit the pelvis. The attachment of these arteries to the pelvic structure is quite firm and may result in their tearing if the pelvis is fractured and displaced. The inferior vena cava is located along the spinal column and collects venous blood from the lower extremities and the abdomen, relatively parallel to the arterial system, returning it to the heart. The abdomen also houses a special circulatory system, the portal system. This venous subsystem collects venous blood and the fluid and nutrients absorbed by the bowel and transports them to the liver. The liver detoxifies the fluid, stores excess nutrients, adds nutrients when they are deficient, and then sends

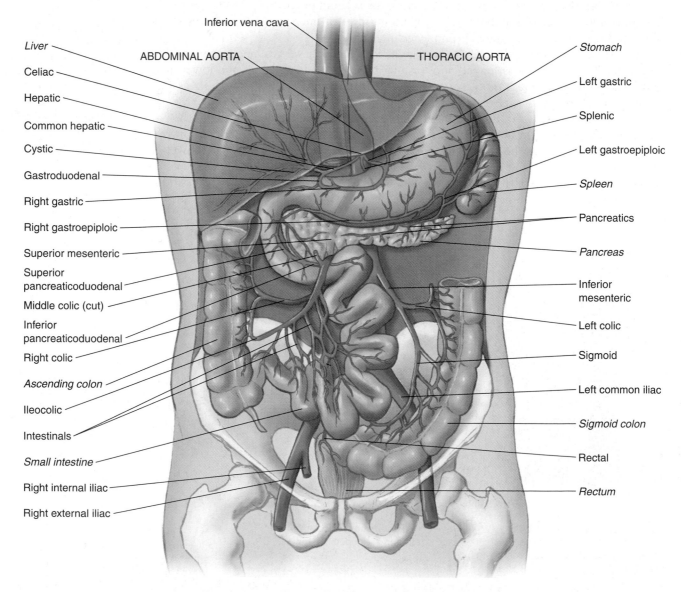

FIGURE 2-106 The abdominal arteries.

the blood/nutrient/fluid mixture into the inferior vena cava, just below the heart. There it mixes with venous blood and is circulated through the heart and then the rest of the body.

THE PERITONEUM

Many of the abdominal organs are covered by a serous membrane called the **peritoneum** (Figure 2-107). This tissue resembles the pleura of the lungs and functions in a similar manner. The parietal peritoneum covers the most of the interior surface of the anterior and lateral abdominal cavity, whereas the visceral peritoneum covers the individual organs. A small amount of fluid is found between the peritoneal layers and permits free movement of the bowel during digestion.

The digestive tract is restrained and prevented from tangling by a structure called the **mesentery.** The mesentery is a double fold of peritoneum containing blood vessels, lymphatic vessels, nerves, and fatty tissue. It suspends the bowel from the posterior abdominal wall. An additional fold of mesentery, called the *omentum,* also covers, insulates, and protects the anterior surface of the abdomen. The thickness of the omentum varies with the size and percentage of body fat of the patient. It may be several inches thick in the obese patient or very narrow in the thin and muscular patient.

Most of the abdominal structures are covered by peritoneum, with the exception of the kidneys, duodenum, pancreas, urinary bladder, the posterior portions of the ascending and descending colon, and the rectum. Most of the major vascular structures within the abdomen are also retroperitoneal. An organ's relation to the peritoneum becomes important in trauma because irritation of the peritoneum (peritonitis) presents with more apparent signs and symptoms than does hemorrhage or the release of other fluids into the retroperitoneal space.

The abdominal cavity is a dynamic place. The diaphragm moves up and down, displacing the abdominal contents with each breath. With deep expiration, the central portion of the diaphragm moves as far upward as the fourth intercostal space, anteriorly (the nipple line), and the seventh intercostal space (the inferior tips of the scapulae), posteriorly. (The edge of the diaphragm attaches to the border of the rib cage.) During forced and maximal expiration, the diaphragm moves as much as 3 inches (9 cm) inferiorly. This movement displaces the abdominal contents up and down with each breath.

peritoneum fine fibrous tissue surrounding the interior of most of the abdominal cavity and covering most of the small bowel and some of the abdominal organs.

mesentery double fold of peritoneum that supports the major portion of the small bowel, suspending it from the posterior abdominal wall.

Patho Pearls

In the prehospital setting, it is not necessary to accurately determine the exact cause of a patient's abdominal pain. You need to know only that the pain exists and the most likely cause.

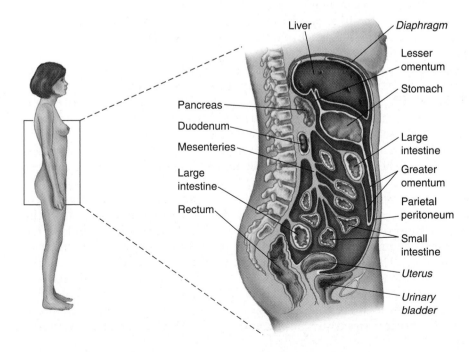

FIGURE 2-107 Reflections of the peritoneum.

Additionally, the volume of substance within the hollow organs varies—an empty (10 mL) versus a distended (500 mL) bladder or a full (1.5 liter) versus an empty stomach. The digestive tract is also suspended from the back of the abdominal cavity and is permitted some movement as it digests food. This dynamic movement becomes an important consideration when anticipating abdominal injury due to blunt or penetrating trauma.

DIGESTIVE SYSTEM

The digestive system includes the digestive tract and the accessory organs of digestion (Figure 2-108). The digestive tract (also called the *alimentary canal*) is the muscular tube that physically and chemically breaks down and absorbs the fluids and nutrients from the food consumed. The accessory organs of digestion include the liver, gallbladder, and pancreas. These organs prepare and store digestive enzymes and perform other important body functions.

DIGESTIVE TRACT

digestive tract internal passageway that begins at the mouth and ends at the anus; also called the *alimentary canal.*

The **digestive tract** is a thin, 25-foot-long hollow muscular tube responsible for churning the material to be digested, for excreting digestive juices to be mixed with it, and for absorbing nutrients and then water. Abdominal components of the digestive tract consist of the stomach, the small bowel (duodenum, jejunum, and ileum), the large bowel (or colon), the rectum, and the anus. These structures fill the anterior and lateral aspects of the abdominal cavity, except for the area occupied by the liver.

The esophagus enters the abdomen through the hiatus of the diaphragm (just posterior to the xiphoid process) and then deposits its contents into the stomach. The stomach is a J-shaped muscular container that mixes the ingested material with hydrochloric acid and enzymes (both produced in the gastric wall) into a thick fluid called **chyme.** The acid released by the stomach increases the gastric acidity (pH) to between 1.5 and 2.0. This is a very acidic fluid that would damage the stomach and the initial lining of the small bowel if not for the continuous production of a protective mucus. The stomach is highly variable in size, depending on the amount of material it contains. It can distend to hold as much as 1.5 liters of food after a large meal.

chyme semifluid mixture of ingested food and digestive secretions found in the stomach and small intestine.

Chyme is released in small boluses into the first component of the small bowel, the duodenum. The duodenum is approximately 1 foot in length and is where the digesting material is mixed with bile from the liver (stored in the gallbladder) and pancreatic digestive juices. These agents raise the pH of the chyme (returning it towards neutral) and help release the nutrients it contains.

peristalsis wave-like muscular motion of the esophagus and bowel that moves food through the digestive system.

The digesting food is propelled along the small and large bowel by waves of contraction called **peristalsis.** The muscles of the digestive tract constrict the bowel's lumen behind a mass of food, then progressively constrict the lumen in the direction of desired movement. The resulting rhythmic constriction moves the digesting material through the tract. As chyme enters the next two segments of the small bowel (the jejunum and the ileum), the mixing decreases and the nutrients, released by the physical and chemical digestion processes, are absorbed, directed to the liver for detoxification, and then released into the circulatory system.

As the food continues through the digestive tract, it arrives at the large bowel. Here masses of bacteria assist in releasing vitamins and fluid from the digesting food while the large bowel absorbs most of the remaining fluid content. The water serves to hydrate the body while the digestive juices are re-absorbed and reprocessed to rejoin the digestive process upstream again. The large bowel ascends superiorly along the right side of the abdomen (ascending colon), traverses the abdomen just below the liver and stomach (transverse colon), then descends along the left lateral abdomen (descending colon). It aligns with the rectum through the S-shaped sigmoid colon where the end waste products of the digestive process (feces) await excretion (defecation) through the terminal valve, the anus.

The Digestive System

ORGANS OF THE DIGESTIVE SYSTEM

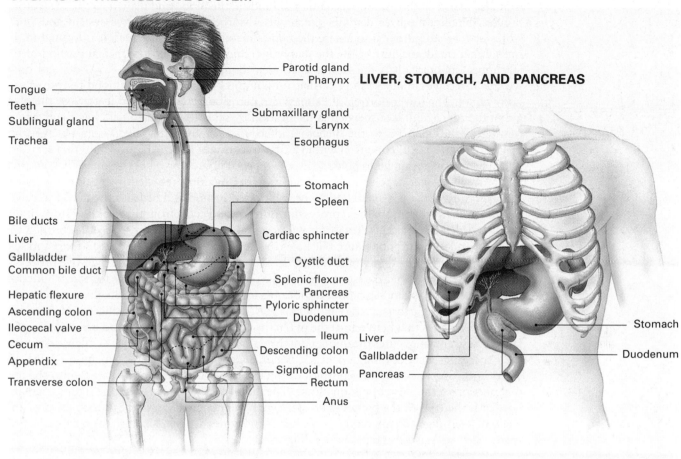

Parotid gland
Pharynx

Tongue
Teeth
Sublingual gland
Trachea

Submaxillary gland
Larynx
Esophagus

Stomach
Spleen

Bile ducts
Liver
Gallbladder
Common bile duct

Cardiac sphincter

Cystic duct
Splenic flexure

Hepatic flexure
Ascending colon
Ileocecal valve
Cecum
Appendix
Transverse colon

Pancreas
Pyloric sphincter
Duodenum
Ileum
Descending colon
Sigmoid colon
Rectum
Anus

LIVER, STOMACH, AND PANCREAS

Liver
Gallbladder
Pancreas

Stomach
Duodenum

LARGE INTESTINE

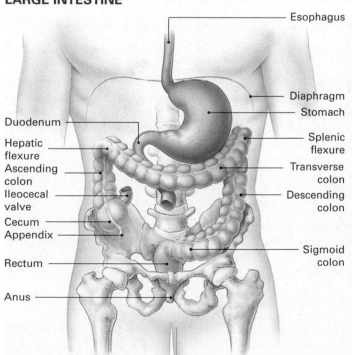

Esophagus

Duodenum

Hepatic flexure
Ascending colon
Ileocecal valve
Cecum
Appendix

Rectum

Anus

Diaphragm
Stomach

Splenic flexure

Transverse colon

Descending colon

Sigmoid colon

SMALL INTESTINE

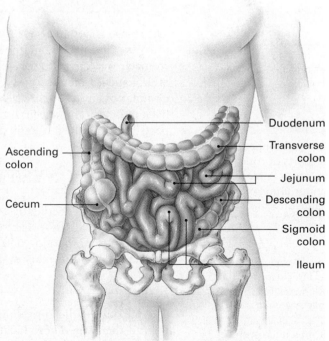

Ascending colon

Cecum

Duodenum

Transverse colon

Jejunum

Descending colon

Sigmoid colon

Ileum

FIGURE 2-108   The digestive tract and accessory organs.

ACCESSORY ORGANS OF DIGESTION

The liver is a vascular structure responsible for detoxifying the blood, removing damaged or aged erythrocytes, and storing glycogen and other important agents for body metabolism. The liver also assists in the osmotic regulation of fluids in the blood and plays a role in the clotting process. Finally, the liver detoxifies materials absorbed by the digestive system and either stores or releases nutrients to assure the body's metabolic needs are met. It is located in the right upper quadrant, just below the diaphragm and extends into the medial portion of the left upper quadrant. It is the largest abdominal organ, accounting for 2.5% of total body weight. It receives about 25% of cardiac output and holds the greatest blood reserve of any body organ. The lower portion of its mass can occasionally be palpated just below the margin of the rib cage. It is suspended in its location by several ligaments including the ligamentum teres, and connects to the omentum inferiorly. The liver is a solid organ but is rather delicate in nature. It is contained within a fibrous capsule (visceral peritoneum) that serves to retard hemorrhage and helps hold the liver together if injured by blunt trauma. When injured, the liver will regenerate to some degree but will not function as efficiently as before the injury.

The gallbladder is a small hollow organ located behind and beneath the liver. It receives bile (a waste product from the reprocessing of red blood cells) from the liver and stores it until it is needed during digestion of fatty foods. It then constricts and sends bile through the bile duct and into the duodenum. Bile helps the body by emulsifying (breaking apart and suspending) ingested fats that would otherwise remain as clumps during the digestive process.

The other accessory digestive organ is the pancreas. It is responsible for the production of glucagon and insulin, hormones responsible for the regulation of blood glucose levels and the transport of glucose across cell membranes. The pancreas also produces very powerful digestive enzymes that help return the pH of the chyme toward normal and break down proteins. These enzymes enter the duodenum through the common bile duct. Similar to the liver, the pancreas is a solid, though delicate, organ, encapsulated in a serous membrane. It is located in the medial and lower portion of the left upper quadrant and extends into the medial portion of the right upper quadrant. The duodenum wraps around the right pancreatic border. If the cells of the pancreas are damaged, the pancreatic enzymes become active and begin to "self-digest" pancreatic tissue. If these enzymes are released into the retroperitoneal space, they will also damage surrounding tissue.

THE SPLEEN

flanks the part of the back below the ribs and above the hip bones.

The spleen is not an accessory organ of digestion but rather a part of the immune system. It is a very vascular organ about the size of the palm of the hand and is located behind the stomach and lateral to the kidney in the left upper quadrant. The spleen performs some immunological functions and also stores a large volume of blood. It is the most fragile abdominal organ, though well protected in its location by the rib cage, spine, and **flank** and back muscles. The spleen, however, can be injured during blunt trauma, especially with impacts affecting the left flank and, when injured, it bleeds heavily.

Patho Pearls

During prolonged transports of critical patients, it is important to monitor urine output and document your findings.

URINARY SYSTEM

The urinary system contains four major structures, the kidneys, ureters, urinary bladder, and urethra (Figure 2-109). First the discussion will include the structures and functions of the urinary system, focusing on the kidneys. Then the text will cover the additional structures of the male genitourinary system.

kidney an organ that produces urine and performs other functions related to the urinary system.

KIDNEYS

The left kidney lies in the upper abdomen behind the spleen, and the right kidney lies behind the liver. These locations correspond to the left and right areas of the small of the back, or the flanks. A healthy **kidney** in a young adult is about the size of a fist and contains about one million **nephrons,** the microscopic structures that produce urine.

nephron a microscopic structure within the kidney that produces urine.

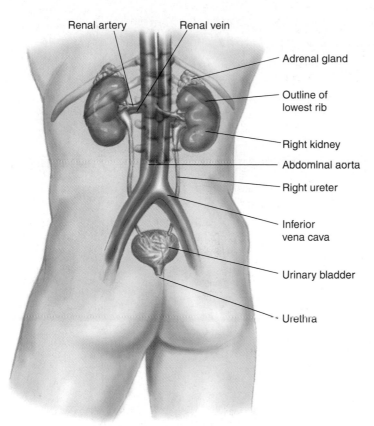

FIGURE 2-109 Anatomy of the urinary system, posterior view.

Renal artery

Renal vein

Adrenal gland

Outline of lowest rib

Right kidney

Abdominal aorta

Right ureter

Inferior vena cava

Urinary bladder

Urethra

With aging comes a normal loss of nephrons—10% per decade of life after age 40—so you should always be alert to the possibility of compromised kidney function in elderly patients.

Gross and Microscopic Anatomy of the Kidney

The renal artery and vein, as well as nerves, lymphatic vessels, and the ureter, pass into the kidney through the notched region called the **hilum.** The tissue of the kidney itself is visibly divided into an outer region, the **cortex,** and an inner region, the **medulla.** Medullary tissue is divided into fan-shaped regions, or **pyramids.** Each pyramid ends in a portion of tissue called the **papilla,** which projects into the hollow space of the **renal pelvis** (Figure 2-110). The spaces of the pelvis come together at the origin of the ureter. Urine forms in the cortical and medullary tissue of the kidney and leaves the kidney through the renal pelvis and ureter.

The functional unit of the kidney, the nephron, forms urine (Figure 2-111). Each nephron consists of a tubule divided into structurally different portions and capillaries that form a complex net of vessels covering the surface of the tubule. Blood that has entered the kidney through the renal artery flows through successively smaller vessels until it reaches a **glomerulus,** a cluster of capillaries surrounded by **Bowman's capsule,** the cup-shaped, hollow structure that is the first part of the nephron. Water and chemical substances enter the tubule through Bowman's capsule. After passage through successive parts of the tubule—the **proximal tubule, descending loop of Henle, ascending loop of Henle,** and **distal tubule**—urine drips into the **collecting duct** before entering the renal pelvis and ureter.

Kidney Physiology

The physiology of the kidneys is one of the most complex topics in human physiology. Its explanation often requires several book chapters. The following is a brief overview.

hilum the notched part of the kidney where the ureter and other structures join kidney tissue.

cortex the outer tissue of an organ such as the kidney.

medulla the inner tissue of an organ such as the kidney.

pyramids the visible tissue structures within the medulla of the kidney.

papilla the tip of a pyramid; it juts into the hollow space of the kidney.

renal pelvis the hollow space of the kidney that junctions with a ureter.

glomerulus a tuft of capillaries from which blood is filtered into a nephron.

Bowman's capsule the hollow, cup-shaped first part of the nephron tubule.

proximal tubule the part of the tubule beyond Bowman's capsule.

descending loop of Henle the part of the tubule beyond the proximal tubule.

ascending loop of Henle the part of the tubule beyond the descending loop of Henle.

distal tubule the part of the tubule beyond the ascending loop of Henle.

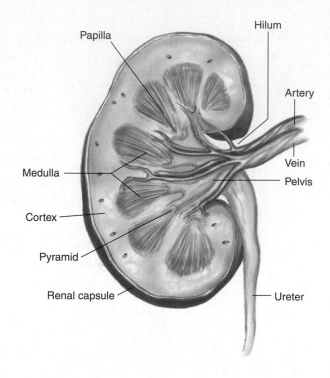

FIGURE 2-110 Cross section of the kidney.

Papilla

Hilum

Artery

Vein

Pelvis

Medulla

Cortex

Pyramid

Renal capsule

Ureter

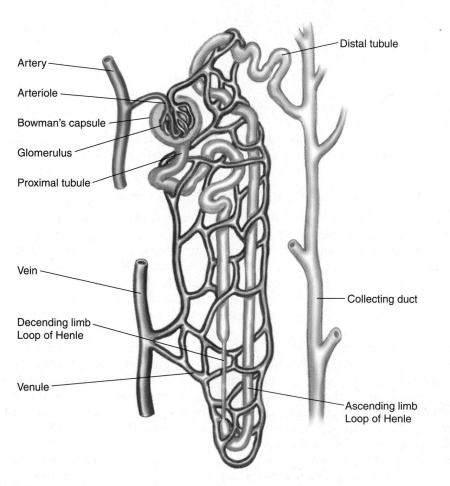

Artery

Arteriole

Bowman's capsule

Glomerulus

Proximal tubule

Vein

Decending limb
Loop of Henle

Venule

Distal tubule

Collecting duct

Ascending limb
Loop of Henle

FIGURE 2-111 Anatomy of the nephron.

Overview of Nephron Physiology   Forming and eliminating urine are the basis for two of the kidneys' major functions: (1) maintaining blood volume with proper balance of water, electrolytes, and pH and (2) retaining key compounds such as glucose while excreting wastes such as urea. A third function, controlling arterial blood pressure, relies both on urine formation and on a second mechanism that does not involve urine production. Last, kidney cells regulate erythrocyte development, but this process does not involve urine formation in any way.

Urine is produced through the interactions among capillary blood flowing over the nephron tubule, the fluid flowing inside the tubule, and the capillary and tubular cells themselves. Three general processes are involved in formation of urine: **glomerular filtration, reabsorption** of substances from the renal tubule into blood, and **secretion** of substances from blood into the renal tubule.

The first step in urine formation is filtration of blood. As blood flows through the capillaries of the glomerulus, water and numerous chemical materials are filtered out of the blood and into Bowman's capsule. Normally, the only blood elements that are not freely filtered into the capsule are blood cells and the plasma proteins, all of which are too large to pass through the pores formed by cell junctions in the capillary walls. Consequently, the fluid formed in the capsule—the **filtrate**—roughly resembles blood plasma except for the absence of proteins.

The rate at which blood is filtered, the **glomerular filtration rate (GFR)**, averages 180 liters/day, the equivalent of 60 complete passages of blood plasma through the glomerular filters. This remarkable efficiency underlies the kidneys' ability to excrete toxic or foreign substances such as urea or drug metabolites so quickly that the substances do not accumulate in the blood.

Filtration is a nonselective process based primarily on molecular size (electrical charge is a secondary factor), and it is essential to urine formation. In contrast, reabsorption of substances into the blood and secretion of substances into the renal tubule are highly selective processes. Almost all elements of filtrate are handled independently of the other elements. The processes of reabsorption and secretion are essential to forming urine with the correct composition and volume to compensate for current body conditions, that is, to maintain homeostasis.

Reabsorption and secretion involve intercellular transport, the movement of a molecule across a cell membrane to either enter or exit a cell. Similar to other intercellular transport processes, they occur in one of three ways: **simple diffusion,** facilitated diffusion, or active transport. Both simple and facilitated diffusion are passive processes in that neither requires the cell to spend energy. In simple diffusion, molecules small enough to pass through a cell membrane randomly move into and out of the cell. Because net movement is always from the region of higher concentration to that of lower concentration, simple diffusion leads toward equalization of molecular concentration on both sides of the membrane. Water molecules always move by simple diffusion. **Osmosis** is the process in which water molecules move so that the concentrations of particles dissolved in water (or **osmolarity**) approach equivalence on both sides of a membrane. A solution with a higher concentration than another solution is **hyperosmolar** to the other; a solution with a lower, more dilute concentration is **hypo-osmolar** to the other.

In **facilitated diffusion,** molecules still move from the region of higher concentration to that of lower concentration. However, a molecule-specific carrier in the membrane acts as a tunnel and speeds the movement of molecules through the membrane. The body cells' normal handling of glucose is an example of this process. When insulin binds to a glucose-specific carrier in the cell membrane, glucose can pass into the cell ten times faster than when insulin is not bound to the carrier.

Active transport is the only process that can produce a net movement of molecules from a region of lower concentration to one of higher concentration. This uphill movement against the concentration gradient is possible because energy is spent to drive the action of the molecule-specific carrier in the membrane. Active transport processes are vital to renal tubular physiology because they allow for the precise balance of reabsorption and secretion that results in independent, homeostatic handling of electrolytes and other substances such as glucose.

glomerular filtration the removal from blood of water and other elements, which enter the nephron tubule.

reabsorption the movement of a substance from a nephron tubule back into the blood.

secretion the movement of a substance from the blood into a nephron tubule.

filtrate the fluid produced in Bowman's capsule by filtration of blood.

glomerular filtration rate (GFR) the volume per day at which blood is filtered through capillaries of the glomerulus.

simple diffusion the random motion of molecules from an area of high concentration to an area of lower concentration.

osmosis the diffusion pattern of water in which molecules move to equalize concentrations on both sides of a membrane.

osmolarity the measure of a substance's concentration in water.

hyperosmolar a solution that has a concentration of the substance greater than that of a second solution.

hypo-osmolar a solution that has a concentration of the substance lower than that of a second solution.

facilitated diffusion a form of molecular diffusion in which a molecule-specific carrier in a cell membrane speeds the molecule's movement from a region of higher concentration to one of lower concentration.

active transport movement of a molecule through a cell membrane from a region of lower concentration to one of higher concentration; movement requires energy consumption within the cell.

Tubular Handling of Water and Electrolytes Tubular handling of water and electrolytes including sodium (Na^+), potassium (K^+), hydrogen (H^+), and chloride (Cl^-) is the basis for control of blood volume and maintenance of electrolyte balance, including pH. As you recall, Na^+ is the dominant cation in the body's extracellular fluids, including blood, whereas K^+ is the dominant cation in intracellular fluid. Appropriate retention of Na^+ in the body, along with osmotic retention of water, is key to maintaining blood volume. Selective retention of K^+ and H^+, along with anions such as Cl^-, maintains the balance of blood electrolytes and blood pH.

Filtrate formed in Bowman's capsule enters the proximal tubule (review Figure 2-111). The cells of the proximal tubule have an extensive brush border that maximizes contact between cell membrane and filtrate. They also have high concentrations of molecule-specific carriers in their membranes and maintain a high level of metabolic activity, producing energy that can support active transport. Under normal conditions, about 65% of filtered Na^+ and Cl^- is reabsorbed in the proximal tubule, along with osmotic reabsorption of about the same percentage of filtered water. Reabsorption takes place by both passive and active transport processes. Much of the active Na^+ reabsorption is coupled with secretion of H^+ into the tubule; H^+ secretion raises the pH of the arterial-derived blood flowing in capillaries surrounding the tubule. Further handling of H^+ as the filtrate moves through the tubule determines the pH both of the venous blood leaving the kidneys and of the urine excreted from the body.

As filtrate moves through the next part of the nephron, the loop of Henle, its volume and composition change further. Simple diffusion is the dominant process in the first part of the loop. By the time filtrate has moved through the descending limb of the loop, roughly another 20% of the filtrate's original water load has been reabsorbed. The cells of the second, ascending limb of the loop of Henle are normally virtually impermeable to water; however, passive and active reabsorption of significant amounts of electrolytes occurs in the same part of the tubule. This reabsorption of electrolytes without reabsorption of water produces a relatively dilute fluid that may exit the collecting duct as dilute urine. Healthy kidneys can produce urine with an osmolarity as low as one-sixth the osmolar concentration of blood plasma, an action termed **diuresis**. A number of hormones alter tubular handling of water and electrolytes (Table 2-7). Some increase the permeability of the distal tubule, collecting duct, or both, so that far more water is reabsorbed. **Antidiuresis,** the result of this hormonal activity, can form a very concentrated urine with an osmolarity as high as four times that of plasma.

The ability of healthy kidneys to handle significant swings in water and electrolyte intake is remarkably large. Studies have shown that an individual can increase his sodium intake to ten times the average amount or decrease it to roughly one-tenth the average, and the kidneys will still compensate properly. Blood volume and sodium content change only modestly from their baseline, normal levels.

diuresis formation and passage of a dilute urine, decreasing blood volume.

antidiuresis formation and passage of a concentrated urine, preserving blood volume.

Table 2-7	HORMONES THAT AFFECT TUBULAR HANDLING OF WATER AND KEY ELECTROLYTES	
Hormone	**Target Tissue**	**Effect(s)**
Aldosterone	Distal tubule, collecting duct	Increase in reabsorption of Na^+, Cl^-, and water
		Increase in secretion of K^+
Angiotensin II	Proximal tubule	Increase in reabsorption of Na^+, Cl^-, and water
		Increase in secretion of H^+
Antidiuretic hormone (ADH)	Distal tubule, collecting duct	Increase in reabsorption of water
Atrial natriuretic hormone (ANH)	Distal tubule, collecting duct	Decrease in reabsorption of Na^+ and Cl^-

Source: From Arthur C. Guyton and John E. Hall, *Textbook of Medical Physiology,* 9th ed. Philadelphia: W.B. Saunders, 1996.

Tubular Handling of Glucose and Urea   Glucose and urea represent substances that the kidneys handle in opposite fashion. Critical substances such as glucose are retained in the body, and wastes such as urea are excreted.

Glucose is freely filtered into Bowman's capsule as an element of filtrate. Normally, glucose is completely reabsorbed through an active transport process by the time filtrate leaves the proximal tubule. The body's absolute retention of glucose is usually maintained until the blood glucose level reaches about 180 mg/dL; above that level, glucose begins to be lost in urine. This pattern, in which glucose is completely reabsorbed until a ceiling, or threshold level of blood glucose is reached, is due to saturation of the active-transport process responsible for reabsorption of glucose. At excessively high blood glucose levels, so much glucose enters the filtrate that the proximal tubule's transport capacity to reabsorb it is insufficient. When this occurs, as in uncontrolled diabetes mellitus type I, the body loses not only glucose but also large amounts of water through **osmotic diuresis.**

Urea, a waste product, is also freely filtered into Bowman's capsule. However, tubular handling of this small molecule is very different from that of glucose. Urea is passively reabsorbed throughout most of the tubule, and about half of the filtered load will remain in urine. Thus, the kidneys' ability to excrete urea efficiently depends on the glomerular filtration rate, or GFR. If blood passes through the glomerular capillaries at an adequate rate, the net result of filtration and passive reabsorption keeps the blood level from rising toward a toxic level. The blood urea nitrogen (BUN) test directly measures blood concentration of urea and is an indirect indicator of GFR. **Creatinine,** another waste product of metabolism, has larger molecules than urea and is not reabsorbed. Because all of the filtered creatinine will be eliminated in urine, the blood concentration of creatinine is a direct indicator of GFR.

Control of Arterial Blood Pressure   The kidneys regulate systemic arterial blood pressure in several ways. Over the long term, they control the body's balance of water and electrolytes, thus maintaining blood volume at a healthy level. In addition, juxtaglomerular cells, specialized cells adjacent to glomerular capillary cells, respond to low blood pressure by releasing an enzyme called **renin.** Within seconds of its release renin produces significant amounts of the active hormone angiotensin I. As angiotensin I flows through the lungs, angiotensin converting enzyme (ACE) produces angiotensin II, the powerful vasoconstrictor that immediately raises arterial blood pressure. Angiotensin II acts both on kidney tubular cells (Table 2-7) and on adrenal cells, causing the latter to secrete aldosterone. The renin-angiotensin system has an important role in maintenance of blood pressure, as noted earlier.

Control of Erythrocyte Development   The kidneys produce 90% of the body's **erythropoietin,** a hormone that regulates the rate at which erythrocytes mature in bone marrow. The exact mechanism that produces erythropoietin is unclear. The impact of renal tissue death, however, is clear and profound; the nonkidney sources of erythropoietin can produce only about one-third to one-half the red cell mass (measured as hematocrit) needed by the body.

THE URETERS

Urine drains from the renal pelvis into the **ureter,** the long duct that runs from the kidney to the urinary bladder (review Figure 2-109). Each ureter is about 25 cm long, and like the kidney, is located in the retroperitoneum of the abdomen. A thin muscular layer in the walls of the ureters limit their ability to distend in response to internal pressure. The ureters' nerves derive from renal, gonadal, or hypogastric nerve trunks. The microscopic structure of the ureters and the nature of their nerve supply are important in understanding the symptoms caused by kidney stones lodged in a ureter.

THE URINARY BLADDER

The **urinary bladder,** the anteriormost organ in the pelvis of both men and women, stores urine. The muscular bladder usually contains at least a small amount of urine, which produces its roughly spherical shape. The bladder neck, through which urine passes during urination, is held in place by ligaments. In women, connective tissue loosely attaches the bladder's posterior wall to the anterior vaginal wall. In men, the wall of the bladder is structurally continuous with the prostate gland.

osmotic diuresis greatly increased urination and dehydration that results when high levels of glucose cannot be reabsorbed into the blood from the kidney tubules and the osmotic pressure of the glucose in the tubules also prevents water reabsorption.

creatinine a waste product caused by metabolism within muscle cells.

FUN and creatinine are both important indications of renal function.

renin an enzyme produced by kidney cells that plays a key role in controlling arterial blood pressure.

erythropoietin a hormone produced by kidney cells that stimulates maturation of red blood cells.

ureter a duct that carries urine from kidney to urinary bladder.

urinary bladder the muscular organ that stores urine before its elimination from the body.

THE URETHRA

The **urethra** is the duct that carries urine from the bladder to the exterior of the body. In women, the urethra is only about 3- to 4-cm long and opens to the external environment via a small orifice just anterior to that of the vagina. In men, the urethra is about 20-cm long and ends at the tip of the penis. The shorter ureter in the female is probably one reason the female urinary system is more vulnerable to bacterial infection from environmental (largely skin) sources. Because the male urethra carries both urine and male reproductive fluid, it can be an entryway for sexually transmitted diseases.

REPRODUCTIVE SYSTEM

It is important to have an understanding of both the female and the male reproductive systems.

FEMALE REPRODUCTIVE SYSTEM

The most important female reproductive organs are internal and are located within the pelvic cavity. These include the ovaries, fallopian tubes, uterus, and vagina, which are essential to reproduction. The external genitalia have accessory functions, in that they protect body openings and play an important role in sexual functioning.

External Genitalia

The female external genitalia are known collectively as the vulva, or pudendum (Figure 2-112). These external genitalia consist of highly-vascular tissues that protect the entrance to the birth canal. They include the perineum, mons pubis, labia, and clitoris.

The external genital organs begin to mature and take adult proportions during adolescence. Puberty also marks the appearance of breast buds, pubic hair, and the first period (menarche). The age in which sexual development occurs varies among individuals. As women

FIGURE 2–112   The vulva.

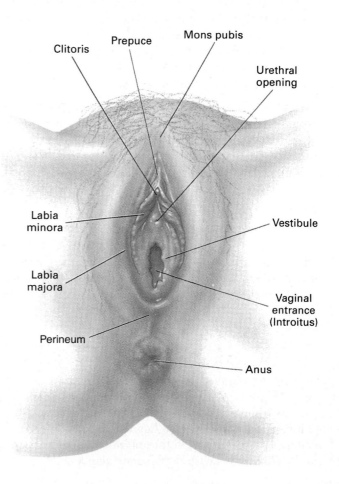

grow older, ovarian function diminishes, menstrual periods cease, and pubic hair becomes gray and sparse. The labia and clitoris become smaller; the vagina narrows and shortens and its lining (the mucosa) becomes thin, pale, and dry. The ovaries and uterus decrease in size.

Perineum   The **perineum** is a roughly diamond-shaped, skin-covered muscular tissue that separates the vagina and the anus. These tissues form a sling-like structure supporting the internal pelvic organs and are able to stretch during childbirth. This area is sometimes torn as a result of sexual assault or during childbirth. An *episiotomy,* or incision of the perineum, may be done to facilitate delivery of the baby and to prevent spontaneous tearing, which may cause significant injury to the perineum and adjacent structures. Sometimes the term perineum is used to include the entire vulvar area.

perineum muscular tissue that separates the vagina and the anus.

Mons Pubis   The **mons pubis** is a fatty layer of tissue over the pubic symphysis, the junction of pubic bones. During puberty, the hormone estrogen causes fat to be deposited under the skin, giving it a moundlike shape. This serves as a cushion that protects the pubic symphysis during intercourse. Also during puberty, the mons becomes covered with pubic hair and its sebaceous and sweat glands become more active.

mons pubis fatty layer of tissue over the pubic symphysis.

Labia   The **labia** are the structures that protect the vagina and the urethra. There are two distinct sets of labia. The labia majora are located laterally, whereas the labia minora are more medial. Both sets of labia are subject to injury during trauma to the vulvar area, such as occurs with sexual assault.

labia structures that protect the vagina and urethra, including the labia majora and the labia minora.

The *labia majora* are two folds of fatty tissue that arise from the mons pubis and extend to the perineum, forming a cleft. During puberty, pubic hair grows on the lateral surface, and sebaceous glands on the hairless medial surface begin to secrete lubricants. The labia majora serve to protect the inner structures of the vulva. The *labia minora,* lying medially within the labia majora, are two smaller, thinner folds of highly vascular tissue, well supplied with nerves and sebaceous glands, which secrete lubricating fluid. During sexual arousal the labia minora become engorged with blood.

The area protected by the labia minora is called the *vestibule.* The vestibule contains the urethral opening and the external opening of the vagina called the *vaginal orifice,* or *introitus.* The secretions of two pairs of glands (Skene and Bartholin) lubricate these structures during sexual stimulation. Located within the vestibule is the *hymen.* It is a thin fold of mucous membrane that forms the external border of the vagina, partly closing it.

Clitoris   The **clitoris** is highly innervated and richly vascular erectile tissue that lies anterior to the labia minora. This cylindrical structure is a major site of sexual stimulation and orgasm in women. The prepuce is a fold of the labia minora that covers the clitoris.

clitoris highly innervated and vascular erectile tissue anterior to the labia minora.

Internal Genitalia

The internal female reproductive organs are the vagina, the uterus, the fallopian tubes, and the ovaries (Figures 2-113 and 2-114).

Vagina   The **vagina** is an elastic canal made up primarily of smooth muscle, 9 to 10 cm in length, that connects the external genitalia to the uterus. It lies between the urethra/bladder and the anus/rectum. Lined with mucous membrane, the vagina extends up and back from the vaginal orifice to the lower end of the uterus (cervix). The vaginal walls are crisscrossed with ridges that allow them to stretch during childbirth, allowing passage of the fetus. The vagina's primary blood supply is the vaginal artery. The pudendal nerve innervates the lower third of the vagina and the external genitalia. The vagina has three functions:

vagina canal that connects the external female genitalia to the uterus.

- It is the female organ of copulation and receives the penis during sexual intercourse.
- Often called the *birth canal,* it forms the final passageway for the infant during childbirth.
- It provides an outlet for menstrual blood and tissue to leave the body.

Uterus   The **uterus** is a hollow, thick-walled, muscular, inverted–pear-shaped organ that connects with the vagina. It lies in the center of the pelvis and is flexed forward between the bladder and rectum above the vagina. Approximately 7.5 cm (3 inches) long and 5 cm (2 inches)

uterus hollow organ in the center of the abdomen that provides the site for fetal development.

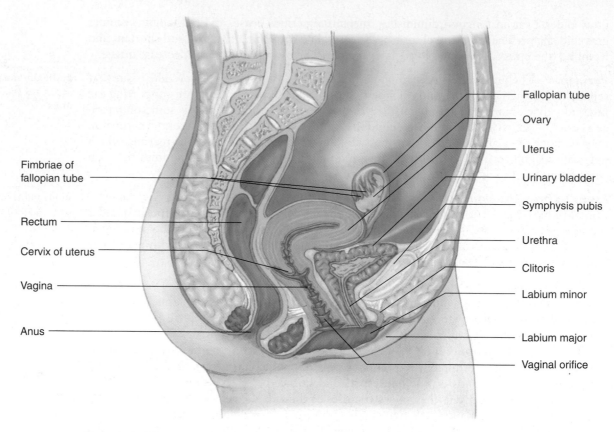

Fallopian tube
Ovary
Uterus
Urinary bladder
Symphysis pubis
Urethra
Clitoris
Labium minor
Labium major
Vaginal orifice

Fimbriae of
fallopian tube
Rectum
Cervix of uterus
Vagina
Anus

FIGURE 2-113 Cross-sectional anatomy of the female reproductive system.

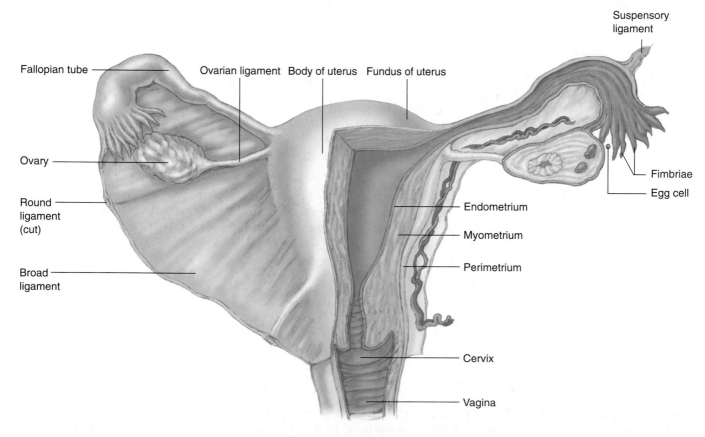

Fallopian tube
Ovarian ligament   Body of uterus   Fundus of uterus
Suspensory ligament
Ovary
Round ligament (cut)
Broad ligament
Fimbriae
Egg cell
Endometrium
Myometrium
Perimetrium
Cervix
Vagina

FIGURE 2-114 The uterus, fallopian tubes, and ovaries.

wide, the uterus is held loosely in position by ligaments, peritoneal folds, and the pressure of adjacent abdominal structures. The primary function of the uterus is to provide a site for fetal development. During pregnancy, the uterus stretches to a size capable of containing the fetus, placenta, and the associated membranes and amniotic fluid. At term, the gravid uterus measures approximately 40 cm (16 inches) in length. The uterus has an extensive blood supply, primarily from the uterine arteries, which are branches of the internal iliac artery. The autonomic nervous system innervates the uterus. In a non-pregnant state, the uterine cavity is flat and triangular.

The uterus has two major parts: the *body* (or corpus) and the *cervix*, or neck. The upper two-thirds of the uterus forms the body and is comprised of smooth muscle layers. The lower third is the cervix.

The rounded uppermost portion of the body of the uterus is the fundus, which lies above the point where the fallopian tubes attach. Measurement of fundal height (distance from the symphysis pubis to the fundus) may be used to estimate gestational age during pregnancy. The fundal height measured in centimeters is generally comparable to the weeks of gestation. For instance, if the fundal height is 30 cm, the gestational age is about 30 weeks. This method of assessing uterine size is most accurate from 22 to 34 weeks.

The body of the uterus has three layers of tissue that make up the uterine wall. The innermost layer or lining is called the **endometrium.** Each month, stimulated by estrogen and progesterone, the endometrium builds up in preparation for the implantation of a fertilized ovum. If fertilization does not occur, the lining degenerates and sloughs off. This sloughing of the uterine lining is referred to as the menses, or menstrual period.

endometrium the inner layer of the uterine wall where the fertilized egg implants.

The thick middle layer of the uterine wall, called the **myometrium,** is made up of three distinct layers of smooth muscle fibers. In the outer layer, primarily over the fundus, the fibers run longitudinally, which allows expulsion of the fetus following cervical dilation. The middle (and thicker) layer is made up of figure-eight patterns of interlaced muscle fibers which surround large blood vessels. The contraction of these fibers helps control post-delivery bleeding. The myometrial fibers also contract during menstruation to maximize the sloughing of the endometrium. It has been suggested that menstrual cramps are due to fatigue of the myometrial fibers. The innermost layer of the myometrium is composed of circular smooth muscle fibers that form sphincters at the point of fallopian tube attachment and at the internal opening of the cervix.

myometrium the thick middle layer of the uterine wall made up of smooth muscle fibers.

The outermost layer of the uterine wall is a serous membrane called the **perimetrium,** which partially covers the corpus of the uterus. The perimetrium, which is a layer of the visceral peritoneum that lines the abdominal cavity and abdominal organs, does not extend to the cervix. The most significant aspect of this partial coverage is that it allows surgical access to the uterus without the risk of infection that is associated with peritoneal incisions.

perimetrium the serosal peritoneal membrane which forms the outermost layer of the uterine wall.

The cervix, or neck of the uterus, extends from the narrowest portion of the uterus to connect with the vagina. That distance forms the cervical canal and is only approximately 2.5 cm (1 inch) in length. Elasticity characterizes the cervix. During labor, it dilates to a diameter of approximately 10 cm to allow delivery of the fetus.

Fallopian Tubes The two **fallopian tubes,** also called *uterine tubes,* are thin flexible tubes that extend laterally from the uterus and curve up and over each ovary on either side. Each tube is approximately 10 cm (4 inches) in length and about 1 cm in diameter (about the size of a pencil lead), except at its ovarian end which is trumpet shaped. Each fallopian tube has two openings, a fimbriated (fringed) end that opens into the abdominal cavity in the area adjacent to the ovaries and a minute opening into the uterus. The function of the tubes is to conduct the egg from the space around the ovaries into the uterine cavity via peristalsis (wavelike muscular contractions). Fertilization usually occurs in the distal third of the fallopian tube.

fallopian tubes thin tubes that extend laterally from the uterus and conduct eggs from the ovaries into the uterine cavity.

Ovaries The **ovaries** are the primary female gonads, or sex glands. The almond-shaped ovaries are situated laterally on either side of the uterus in the upper portion of the pelvic cavity. They have two functions: one function is the secretion of the hormones estrogen and progesterone in response to stimulation from follicle stimulating hormone (FSH) and luteinizing hormone (LH) secreted from the anterior pituitary gland. The second function of the ovaries is the development and release of eggs (ova) for reproduction.

ovaries the primary female sex glands that secrete estrogen and progesterone and produce eggs for reproduction.

The Menstrual Cycle

The female undergoes a monthly hormonal cycle, generally every 28 days, that prepares the uterus to receive a fertilized egg. The onset of the menstrual cycle, that is, the onset of ovulation at puberty, establishes female sexual maturity. This onset, known as **menarche**, usually begins between the ages of 10 and 14. At first, the periods are irregular. Later they become more regular and predictable. The length of the menstrual cycle may vary from 21 to 32 days. A "normal" menstrual cycle is what is normal for the woman in question. Because of this, it is important to inquire as to the normal length of the patient's menstrual cycle. Regardless of the length of the menstrual cycle, the period of time from ovulation to menstruation is always 14 days. Any variance in cycle length occurs during the preovulatory phase.

From puberty to menopause, the female sex hormones (estrogen and progesterone) control the ovarian-menstrual cycle, pregnancy, and lactation. These hormones are not produced at a constant rate, but rather their production surges and diminishes in a cyclical fashion. The secretion of estrogen and progesterone by the ovaries is controlled by the secretion of FSH and LH.

Proliferative Phase   The first two weeks of the menstrual cycle, known as the proliferative phase, are dominated by estrogen, which causes the uterine lining (endometrium) to thicken and to become engorged with blood. In response to a surge of LH at approximately day 14, **ovulation** (release of an egg) takes place.

At birth, each female's ovary contains some 200,000 ova within immature ovarian follicles known as graafian follicles. This is the female's lifetime supply of ova, which are gradually depleted through ovulation during her lifetime.

In response to FSH and increased estrogen levels, once during every menstrual cycle, a follicle reaches maturation and ruptures, discharging its egg through the ovary's outer covering into the abdominal cavity. The ruptured follicle, under the influence of LH, develops the corpus luteum, a small yellowish body of cells, which produces progesterone during the second half of the menstrual cycle. If the egg is not fertilized, the corpus luteum will atrophy about 3 days before the onset of the menstrual phase. If the egg is fertilized, the corpus luteum will produce progesterone until the placenta takes over that function.

The cilia (fine, hairlike structures) on the fimbriated ends of the fallopian tubes draw the egg into the tube and sweep it toward the uterus. If the woman has had sexual intercourse within approximately 24 hours of ovulation, fertilization may take place. If the egg is fertilized, it normally implants in the thickened lining of the uterus, where the fetus subsequently develops. If it is not fertilized, it passes into the uterine cavity and is expelled.

Secretory Phase   The stage of the menstrual cycle immediately surrounding ovulation is referred to as the secretory phase. If the egg is not fertilized, the woman's estrogen level drops sharply while the progesterone level dominates. Uterine vascularity increases during this phase in anticipation of implantation of a fertilized egg.

Ischemic Phase   If fertilization doesn't occur, estrogen and progesterone levels fall. Vascular changes cause the endometrium to become pale and small blood vessels to rupture.

Menstrual Phase   During the menstrual phase, the ischemic endometrium is shed, along with a discharge of blood, mucus, and cellular debris. This is known as **menstruation**. A "normal" menstrual cycle depends upon the regular pattern in the individual woman. The first day of the menstrual cycle is the day on which bleeding begins and the menstrual flow usually lasts from 3 to 5 days, although this varies from woman to woman. An average blood loss of about 50 mL is common. The absence of a menstrual period in any woman in the childbearing years (generally ages 12 to 55) who is sexually active and whose periods are usually regular should raise the suspicion of pregnancy.

Some women regularly experience marked physical signs and symptoms immediately before the onset of their menstrual period. These are collectively known as **premenstrual syndrome (PMS)**. Although you may hear crude jokes made about PMS, there is no denying the reality of the physical changes that accompany the changing hormonal levels. It is not uncommon for women to report breast tenderness or engorgement, transient weight

menarche the onset of menses, usually occurring between ages 10 and 14.

ovulation the release of an egg from the ovary.

menstruation sloughing of the uterine lining (endometrium) if a fertilized egg is not implanted. It is controlled by the cyclical release of hormones. Menstruation is also referred to as a *period.*

premenstrual syndrome (PMS) a variety of signs and symptoms, such as weight gain, irritability, or specific food cravings associated with the changing hormonal levels that precede menstruation.

gain or bloating as a result of fluid retention, excessive fatigue, and/or cravings for specific foods. Women who are prone to migraine headaches may see them increase during the premenstrual period. Other women may have only minimal physical symptoms, but are more affected by emotional responses such as irritability, anxiety, or depression. The severity of PMS varies with each individual and may require treatment focused on relief of symptoms.

Menopause, the cessation of menses, marks the cessation of ovarian function and the cessation of estrogen secretion. Menstrual periods generally continue to occur until a woman is 45 to 55, at which time they begin to decline in frequency and length until they ultimately stop. The end of reproductive life is also known as the climacteric, which is derived from Greek meaning "critical time of life." Occasionally, physicians use the term surgical menopause, which means that a woman's periods have stopped because of surgical removal of her uterus, ovaries, or both. The decrease in estrogen levels causes many women to experience hot flashes, night sweats, and mood swings during menopause. It is not uncommon for hormone replacement therapy (oral estrogen, or estrogen and progesterone) to be prescribed to help relieve these complaints and to provide other health benefits associated with continuing adequate levels of these hormones.

menopause the cessation of menses and ovarian function resulting from decreased secretion of estrogen.

The Pregnant Uterus

The dynamics of pregnancy greatly affect the anatomy of the female abdominal cavity (Figure 2-115). The uterus and its contents grow rapidly from the time of conception until delivery and are well protected during the first trimester (3 months) of pregnancy. During the second trimester (12 to 24 weeks), the progressive enlargement of the uterus displaces most of the abdominal contents upward as the growing uterus rises out of the pelvis and its upper border extends above the umbilicus. By 32 weeks and until the end of the pregnancy, the uterus fills the abdominal cavity to the level of the lower rib margin. This enlarging mass in the abdomen also increases the intra-abdominal pressure and displaces the diaphragm upward. This displacement reduces lung capacity at the same time that the physiologic changes of pregnancy increase the tidal volume.

Pregnancy also affects the maternal physiology by raising the circulatory volume by about 45% and, by the third trimester, raising the cardiac rate by about 15 beats per minute and the cardiac output by up to 40%. The increase in the vascular volume is accompanied by a less significant increase in the number of erythrocytes. The result is a relative anemia

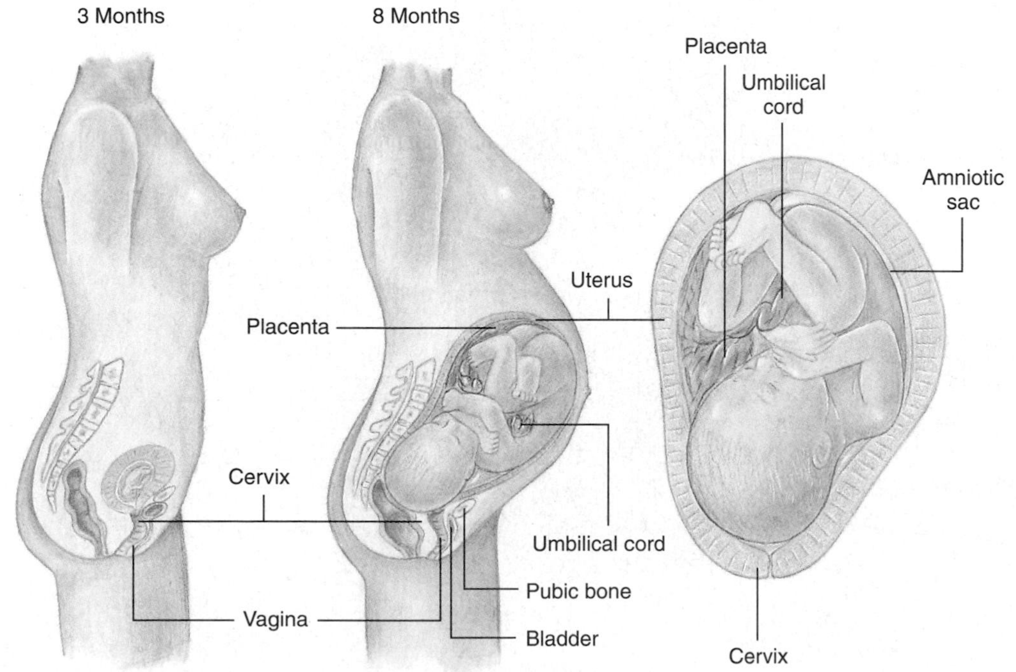

FIGURE 2-115 The pregnant uterus.

that becomes an important consideration with aggressive fluid resuscitation for the mother in shock. In the last trimester of pregnancy, the uterus is significant in both size and weight and may compress the vena cava, reducing venous return to the heart and inducing a temporary hypotension in the supine patient (supine hypotensive syndrome). Finally, the developing fetus means there are now two lives to protect when the mother suffers any trauma, especially involving the abdomen.

MALE REPRODUCTIVE SYSTEM

As noted earlier, the male reproductive organs are considered to be part of the urinary system (Figure 2-116). Like the female reproductive system, the male reproductive system includes both external and internal genitalia.

Testes

The **testes** are the primary male reproductive organs. They produce both the hormones responsible for sexual maturation and sperm cells, male sex cells. The testes lie outside of the abdomen in a muscular sac called the *scrotum*. Normal scrotal temperature is about 2°C to 3°C lower than abdominal temperature, which is critical for development of sperm.

Epididymis and Vas Deferens

Sperm cells pass from the testis into the **epididymis,** a small sac where they are stored. Each testis with its paired epididymis is palpable inside the scrotum. Sperm are channeled from the epididymis into the **vas deferens,** a muscular duct that carries them into the pelvis and through the substance of the prostate gland to its opening into the urethra. Sperm cells mix with special fluid before passing into the urethra for ejaculation, elimination from the body.

The vas deferens passes through an opening in the inguinal ligament known as the inguinal canal. The testicular blood supply also runs through this opening, an anatomical weak point that is the site of male hernias.

testes primary male reproductive organs that produce hormones responsible for sexual maturation and sperm; singular *testis.*

epididymis small sac in which sperm cells are stored.

vas deferens duct that carries sperm cells to the urethra for ejaculation.

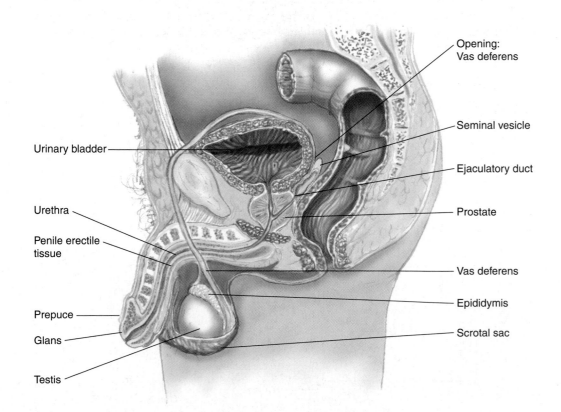

FIGURE 2-116 Anatomy of the male genitourinary system.

Prostate Gland

The **prostate gland** surrounds the male urinary bladder neck, and the first part of the urethra runs through its tissue. The prostate gland is a major source of the fluid that combines with sperm to form semen, the ejaculated male reproductive fluid. In emergency care, the prostate is probably most important in its role as part of the urinary system. Because the first part of the urethra passes through the prostate, enlargement of the prostate can narrow or obstruct the urethra and block urine flow.

prostate gland gland that surrounds the male urinary bladder neck and is a major source of the fluid that combines with sperm to form semen.

The Penis

The **penis** is the male organ of copulation. Its spongy internal tissues fill with blood to produce penile erection. The skin covering the end of the penis, the *foreskin,* is often surgically removed in infancy through circumcision; the difference in appearance is noticeable.

The male genital organs begin to mature and take adult proportions during adolescence. Puberty also marks a noticeable increase in the size of the testes. As in the female, the actual age in which sexual development occurs will vary widely. As men grow older, the penis decreases in size and the testes hang lower in the scrotum. The pubic hair becomes gray and sparse.

penis male organ of copulation.

SUMMARY

An understanding of human anatomy and physiology is basic to EMT-I practice. It starts with an understanding of the basic organization of the human body, beginning with the cell and moving on to more complex structures: the tissues, organs, organ systems, and system integration within the organism itself.

Also critical is an understanding of the important body systems including the integumentary system; blood; the musculoskeletal system; the head, face, and neck; the spine and thorax; the nervous, endocrine, cardiovascular, and respiratory systems; the abdomen, digestive system, and spleen; and the urinary and reproductive systems.

ON THE WEB

For additional practice and review, go to the companion website at www.prenhall.com/bledsoe and click on *Intermediate Emergency Care: Principles & Practice.*

Chapter 3

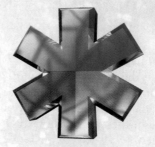

Emergency Pharmacology

Objectives

Part 1: Basic Pharmacology (begins on page 234)

After reading Part 1 of this chapter, you should be able to:

1. List the four main sources of drug products. (p. 235)
2. Discuss the standardization of drugs and how they are classified. (p. 238)
3. List the components of a drug profile. (p. 236)
4. Differentiate among the chemical, generic (nonproprietary), and trade (proprietary) names of a drug. (pp. 234–235)
5. Discuss the EMT-Intermediate's responsibilities and scope of management pertinent to the administration of medications, including special considerations for pregnant, pediatric, and geriatric patients. (pp. 238–241)
6. List and describe the general properties of drugs. (pp. 247–249)
7. List and describe liquid, solid, and gas drug forms. (pp. 246–247)
8. Differentiate between enteral and parenteral routes of drug administration. (pp. 245–246)
9. Describe mechanisms of drug action. (pp. 247–249)
10. List and differentiate the phases of drug activity, including the pharmaceutical, pharmacokinetic, and pharmacodynamic phases. (pp. 241–252)
11. Describe the processes called pharmacokinetics and pharmacodynamics, including theories of drug action, drug-response relationship, factors altering drug responses, predictable drug responses, iatrogenic drug responses, and unpredictable adverse drug responses. (pp. 241–252)
12. Discuss considerations for storing and securing drugs. (p. 247)

Part 2: Nervous System Components (begins on page 252)

After reading Part 2 of this chapter, you should be able to:

1. Review the specific anatomy and physiology pertinent to pharmacology. (pp. 252–258)

Part 3: EMT-Intermediate Medications (begins on page 259)

After reading Part 3 of this chapter, you should be able to:

1. List and describe the drugs that an EMT-Intermediate may administer in a pharmaco-logical management plan according to local protocol. (pp. 259–269)

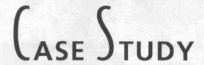

CASE STUDY

A police officer pulls a 27-year-old female driver off to the side of the road at the intersection of Quincy Place and Route 122. Because of the dangerous driving he witnessed and the driver's erratic behavior, unsteady gait, and slurred speech, the officer suspects that the driver is intoxicated. To be safe, the officer requests immediate EMS backup.

EMS 117 EMT-Intermediates (EMT-Is) arrive on scene in 2 minutes. They find a young woman arguing with the police officer. As they assess scene safety, they see the patient turn and lunge at the officer. The officer subdues the patient, who thrashes around briefly before losing consciousness.

At the officer's signal, the EMT-Is go in to do their jobs. They perform an initial assessment, quickly determining that the patient's airway is clear, and breathing and circulation are adequate. They do not detect any immediate life threats, and they begin to review possible causes of the altered mental status. To rule out hypoglycemia, they perform a rapid glucose determination using a glucometer. Then, while one EMT-I conducts a physical exam of the patient, the other notes that her blood sugar is 22 mg/dL. Per approved standing orders, an IV is established and 50 mL of 50% dextrose is administered. The patient quickly responds, becomes fully oriented, and thanks them for their help. She then mentions that she has been ill for a few days and has not been eating well.

The EMT-Is urge the patient to go to the hospital for additional evaluation. She declines, stating that she has recently scheduled a physician's appointment and that she is late for a meeting. They advise the patient of the risks of refusing care. Nevertheless, she continues to refuse assistance. The EMT-Is assure themselves that the patient is fully conscious, oriented, and capable of refusing consent. They instruct the patient to go immediately to the mini-mart across the street to get something to eat, and she agrees. They then aseptically discontinue the IV and have the patient sign a release-from-liability form, which is witnessed by the police officer. They return their equipment to the ambulance and notify the dispatcher that they are back in service.

INTRODUCTION

The use of herbs and minerals to treat the sick and injured has been documented as long ago as 2,000 B.C.E. Ancient Egyptians, Arabs, and Greeks probably passed formulations down through generations by word of mouth for centuries until they were finally recorded in pharmacopeias. By the end of the Renaissance, pharmacology was a distinct and growing discipline, separate from medicine. During the seventeenth and eighteenth centuries, tinctures of opium, coca, and digitalis were available. The related concept of vaccination with biological extracts began in 1796 with Edward Jenner's smallpox inoculations. By the nineteenth century, atropine, chloroform, codeine, ether, and morphine were in use. The discoveries of animal insulin and penicillin in the early twentieth century dramatically changed the treatment of endocrine/metabolic and infectious diseases. Now, at the beginning of the twenty-first century, recombinant DNA technology has produced human insulin and tissue plasminogen activator (tPA). These drugs have markedly changed the treatment of diabetes and cardiovascular disease.

Presently in the United States, the Food and Drug Administration (FDA) is allowing many previously prescription-only drugs to become available over the counter. This is due in part to a growing consumer awareness in health care and also in part to consumer marketing by the pharmaceutical industry. The industry is actively seeking drugs that appeal widely to the consumer for treatments and cures. Pharmaceutical research to limit aging or increase life span is growing rapidly. The federal government also offers incentives to pharmaceutical companies to research drugs for rare diseases. These so-called "orphan drugs" are often expensive to investigate and have a limited sales potential, making them less profitable to develop and manufacture than others.

General principles of pharmacology are presented in this chapter, which is divided into three parts:

> Part 1: Basic Pharmacology
>
> Part 2: Nervous System Components
>
> Part 3: EMT-Intermediate Medications

Part 1: Basic Pharmacology

Part 1 concerns the basics of pharmacology. Drug names (including chemical, generic, official, and brand names) will be explained. The sources of drugs, reference materials for drugs, components of a drug profile, and legal considerations will be described. A major focus of Part 1 will be the safe and effective administration of medications, including the "six rights" (right medication, dose, time, route, patient, and documentation) as well as special considerations in medication administration for pregnant, pediatric, and geriatric patients. Finally, basic concepts of pharmacology, specifically pharmacokinetics and pharmacodynamics, will be examined.

NAMES

drug chemical used to diagnose, treat, or prevent disease.

pharmacology the study of drugs and their interactions with the body.

Drugs are chemicals used to diagnose, treat, or prevent disease. **Pharmacology** is the study of drugs and their actions on the body. To study and converse about pharmacology, health care professionals must have a systematic method for naming drugs. The most detailed name for any drug is its chemical description, which states its chemical composition and molecular structure. Ethyl-1-methyl-4-phenylisonipecotate hydrochloride, for example, is a chemical name. A generic name is usually suggested by the manufacturer and confirmed by the United States Adopted Name Council. It becomes the FDA's official name when listed in the *United States Pharmacopeia (USP),* the official standard for information about pharmaceuticals in the United States. In the case of ethyl-1-methyl-4-phenylisonipecotate hydrochloride, the generic name is meperidine hydrochloride, USP. To foster brand loyalty among its customers, the manufacturer gives the drug a brand name (sometimes called a trade name or proprietary name)—in our example, Demerol. The brand name is a proper name and should be capitalized. Most manufacturers also register the name as a trademark, so the stylized ® or ™ may follow the name, as in Demerol®. Another example is the widely prescribed sedative Valium:

- *Chemical name:* 7-chloro-1, 3-dihydro-1-methyl-5-phenyl-2H-1, 4-benzodiazepin-2-one
- *Generic name:* diazepam
- *Official name:* diazepam, USP
- *Brand name:* Valium®

Content Review

DRUG NAMES
- Chemical name
- Generic name
- Official name
- Brand name

SOURCES

The four main sources of drugs are plants, animals, minerals, and the laboratory (synthetic). Plants may be the oldest source of medications; primitive people probably used them directly as herbal medicines. Indirectly, plant extracts such as gums and oils have long been a source of medications. Examples include the purple foxglove, a source of digitalis (a glycoside), and deadly nightshade, a source of atropine (an alkaloid). Animal extracts are another important source of drugs. For many years the primary sources of insulin for treating diabetes mellitus were the extracts of bovine (cow) and porcine (pig) pancreas. Minerals are inorganic sources of drugs such as calcium chloride and magnesium sulfate. Synthetic drugs are created in the laboratory. They may provide alternative sources of medications for those found in nature, or they may be entirely new medications not found in nature.

Cultural Considerations

Many cultures place great trust in the use of herbal and folk remedies. Some have proven beneficial by modern research. It is important to ask about them when you obtain your patient's history. Some folk medications can contain potentially toxic compounds such as lead or arsenic.

REFERENCE MATERIALS

Obtaining information on drugs can be difficult. Using multiple sources of information about drugs is usually a good idea. Every book about drugs, including this one, has a disclaimer regarding doses and current uses, referring the reader to local medical direction for the final word. Using multiple sources and comparing the authors' statements about a drug may lead you to the best available information. EMS providers generally like small, short guides that they can carry in a shirt pocket. These usually include important details about drugs that out-of-hospital providers administer along with a long list of commonly prescribed drugs and their classes. These EMS guides are useful if you clearly understand the drugs used in your system and have a working knowledge of commonly prescribed drug classes.

Drug inserts, the printed fact sheets that drug manufacturers supply with most medications, contain information prescribed by the U.S. FDA. The *Physician's Desk Reference*, a compilation of these drug inserts, also includes three indices and a section containing photographs of drugs. It is among the most popular references, but it contains only factual information and must be interpreted by informed readers. The American Hospital Formulary Service annually publishes *Drug Information* as a service to the American Society of Health System Pharmacists. It contains an authoritative listing of monographs on virtually every drug used in the United States. A less bulky reference to keep in an ambulance might be one of the many drug guides for nurses. They contain information on hundreds of drugs in a format similar to the EMS drug guides, but they also offer information on commonly prescribed drugs rather than only on emergency drugs. Also popular is the *Monthly Prescribing Reference*. Designed to assist physicians in prescribing medications, it can also help them determine which medications are available for treating specific diseases. The information it contains about new medications is especially useful. Most hospitals also maintain a listing of drugs, or formulary, that profiles the particular drugs they have available. The American Medical Association also publishes a useful reference, the *AMA Drug Evaluation*. The Internet provides an enormous amount of information, but you must be especially cautious when using it as a source, because it allows anyone with a computer to be a publisher, with no requirement for accuracy.

Content Review

SOURCES OF DRUG INFORMATION
- *United States Pharmacopeia (USP)*
- *Physician's Desk Reference*
- *Drug Information*
- *Monthly Prescribing Reference*
- *AMA Drug Evaluation*

It is helpful to carry a pharmaceutical reference in EMT-I response vehicles.

COMPONENTS OF A DRUG PROFILE

A drug's profile describes its various properties. As an EMT-I student, you will become familiar with drug profiles as you study specific medications. A typical drug profile contains the following information:

- *Names.* These most frequently include the generic and trade names, although the occasional reference includes chemical names.
- *Classification.* This is the broad group to which the drug belongs. Knowing classifications is essential to understanding the properties of drugs.
- *Mechanism of action.* The way in which a drug causes its effects; its pharmacodynamics.
- *Indications.* Conditions that make administration of the drug appropriate (as approved by the FDA).
- *Pharmacokinetics.* How the drug is absorbed, distributed, and eliminated; typically includes onset and duration of action.
- *Side effects/adverse reactions.* The drug's untoward or undesired effects.
- *Routes of administration.* How the drug is given.
- *Contraindications.* Conditions that make it inappropriate to give the drug. Unlike when the drug is simply not indicated, a contraindication means that a predictable harmful event occurs if the drug is given in this situation.
- *Dosage.* The amount of the drug that should be given.
- *How supplied.* This typically includes the common concentrations of the available preparations; many drugs come in different concentrations.
- *Special considerations.* How the drug may affect pediatric, geriatric, or pregnant patients.

Drug profiles may also include other components, such as its interactions with other drugs or with foods, when appropriate.

Know and obey the laws and regulations governing medications and their administration.

Content Review

DRUG LAWS AND REGULATIONS
- Federal law
- State laws and regulations
- Individual agency regulations

LEGAL

Knowing and obeying the laws and regulations governing medications and their administration will be an important part of your career. These laws and regulations come from three distinct authorities: federal law, state laws and regulations, and individual agency regulations.

FEDERAL LAW

Drug legislation in the United States has been aimed primarily at protecting the public from adulterated or mislabeled drugs. The *Pure Food and Drug Act of 1906,* enacted to improve the quality and labeling of drugs, named the *United States Pharmacopeia* as this country's official source for drug information. The *Harrison Narcotic Act of 1914* limited the indiscriminate use of addicting drugs by regulating the importation, manufacture, sale, and use of opium, cocaine, and their compounds or derivatives. The *Federal Food, Drug and Cosmetic Act of 1938* empowered the FDA to enforce and set premarket safety standards for drugs. In 1951, the *Durham-Humphrey Amendments* to the 1938 act (also known as the prescription drug amendments) required pharmacists to have either a written or verbal prescription from a physician to dispense certain drugs. It also created the category of over-the-counter (OTC) medications. The *Comprehensive Drug Abuse Prevention and Control Act* (also known as the Controlled Substances Act) of 1970 is the most recent major federal legislation affecting drug sales and use. It repealed and replaced the Harrison Narcotic Act.

The federal government strictly regulates controlled substances because of their high potential for abuse. Since not all drugs cause the same level of physical or psychological dependence, they do not all need to be regulated in the same way. To accommodate their

Table 3-1	SCHEDULES OF DRUGS ACCORDING TO THE CONTROLLED SUBSTANCES ACT OF 1970	

Schedule	Description	Examples
Schedule I	High abuse potential; may lead to severe dependence; no accepted medical indications; used for research, analysis, or instruction only	Heroin, LSD, mescaline
Schedule II	High abuse potential; may lead to severe dependence; accepted medical indications	Opium, cocaine, morphine, codeine, oxycodone, methadone, secobarbital
Schedule III	Less abuse potential than Schedule I and II; may lead to moderate or low physical dependence or high psychological dependence; accepted medical indications	Limited opioid amounts or combined with noncontrolled substances: Vicodin, Tylenol with codeine
Schedule IV	Low abuse potential compared to Schedule III; limited psychological and/or physical dependence; accepted medical indications	Diazepam, lorazepam, phenobarbital
Schedule V	Lower abuse potential compared to Schedule IV; may lead to limited physical or psychological dependence; accepted medical indications	Limited amounts of opioids; often for cough or diarrhea

differences, the Controlled Substance Act of 1970 created five schedules of controlled substances, each with its own level of control and record keeping requirements (Table 3-1). Most emergency medical services administer only a few controlled substances, usually a narcotic analgesic such as morphine sulfate and a benzodiazepine anticonvulsant such as diazepam.

The majority of the remaining drugs provided by an EMS are prescription drugs—those whose use the FDA has designated sufficiently dangerous to require the supervision of a health care practitioner (physician, dentist, and in some states, nurse practitioner or certified physician's assistant). For emergency medical services this means the physician medical director is in effect prescribing the drugs in advance, based on the assessments and judgments of EMS providers in the field.

Over-the-counter (OTC) medications are generally available in small doses and, when taken as recommended, present a low risk to patients. Of the few OTC drugs that EMS providers administer, acetaminophen and aspirin are probably the most common. Although laws vary from state to state, they still require most EMS providers to obtain a physician's order (either written, verbal, or standing) to administer OTC drugs.

Federal drug laws require that certain substances be appropriately secured, distributed, and accounted for. Because of the complexity of this issue and the large variability of drugs used in EMS systems across the country, specific answers to these concerns are not practical here. Consult your local protocols, laws, and most importantly, medical director for guidance in this area.

STATE LAW

State laws vary widely. Some states have legislated which medications are appropriate for an EMT-I to give, while others have left those decisions to local control. Local control varies as well. In some areas, regional EMS authorities set the local standards; in others the individual medical directors and department directors do. In all cases, however, the physician medical director can delegate to an EMT-I the authority to administer medications, either by written, verbal, or standing order. You must know the laws of the state where you practice.

LOCAL LAW

In each community, local leaders are responsible for ensuring public safety. Local EMS agencies have the responsibility to create local policies and procedures to ensure the public well being. An excellent example of a local procedure protecting the patient (and thereby the

Consult local protocols, laws, and, medical direction for guidance in securing and distributing controlled substances.

individual EMS provider and agency) would be a requirement to use a pulse oximeter whenever a patient is sedated or paralyzed. Although this requirement would not have the force of law, it would locally help to ensure that local EMS providers do not overlook hypoxia in these patients.

STANDARDS

Because some generic drugs affect patients differently than their brand name counterparts, standardization of drugs is a necessity. Despite FDA standards, drugs sold or distributed by various manufacturers may have biological or therapeutic differences. An **assay** determines the amount and purity of a given chemical in a preparation in the laboratory (in vitro). Although two generically equivalent preparations may contain the same amount of a given chemical (drug), they may have different therapeutic effects. This relative therapeutic effectiveness of chemically equivalent drugs is their **bioequivalence.** Bioequivalence is determined by a **bioassay,** which attempts to ascertain the drug's availability in a biological model (in vivo). Again, the *United States Pharmacopeia (USP)* is the official standard for the United States.

PATIENT CARE: SAFE AND EFFECTIVE ADMINISTRATION OF MEDICATIONS

An EMT-I is responsible for the standard of care for patients in his charge. He is, therefore, personally responsible—legally, morally, and ethically—for the safe and effective administration of medications. The following guidelines will help you to meet that responsibility:

- Know the precautions and contraindications for all medications you administer.
- Practice proper technique.
- Know how to observe and document drug effects.
- Maintain a current knowledge in pharmacology.
- Establish and maintain professional relationships with other health care providers.
- Understand the pharmacokinetics and pharmacodynamics.
- Have current medication references available.
- Take careful drug histories from patients including:
  - Name, strength, and daily dose of prescribed drugs
  - Over-the-counter drugs
  - Vitamins
  - Herbal medications
  - Folk-medicine or folk-remedies
  - Allergies
- Evaluate the compliance, dosage, and adverse reactions.
- Consult with medical direction when appropriate.

SIX RIGHTS OF MEDICATION ADMINISTRATION

No pharmacology chapter would be complete without discussing the six rights of medication administration. They include the right medication, the right dose, the right time, the right route, the right patient, and the right documentation.

Right Medication

When following a physician's verbal medication order, repeat the order back to him to confirm that you both intend the same thing for the patient. Inspect the label on the drug at least three times before giving the medication to the patient: first, as you remove the medication from the drug box or cabinet; second, as you draw the medication into the syringe or dole the tablet into a cup; and third, immediately before you administer the medication.

---

assay test that determines the amount and purity of a given chemical in a preparation in the laboratory.

bioequivalence relative therapeutic effectiveness of chemically equivalent drugs.

bioassay test to ascertain a drug's availability in a biological model.

Content Review

SIX RIGHTS OF MEDICATION ADMINISTRATION
- Right medication
- Right dose
- Right time
- Right route
- Right patient
- Right documentation

Failure to confirm the medication name is one of the most common medication administration errors. If you have any question about a drug, do not administer it without confirmation. Showing the medication container to your partner and asking for confirmation is an easy way to further ensure that you are giving the right drug.

Right Dose

To reduce medication errors, many drugs come in unit **dose packaging.** That is, the package contains a single dose for a single patient. Dosages of many emergency drugs, however, are based on patient weight, so a prefilled syringe may not contain the exact amount a patient needs. You will have to calculate the correct dose. One good practice for identifying potential medication errors is to consider the number of unit dose packages needed for a single dose. If your calculations tell you to open ten vials for one dose of medication, prudence requires you to check the calculation and dose carefully. The package may contain a unit dose of the wrong medication, or you may have miscalculated.

dose packaging medication packages that contain a single dose for a single patient.

Right Time

Although the EMT-I usually gives medications in urgent and emergent situations rather than on a schedule, timing can still be very important. Giving nitroglycerin tablets too soon may precipitate hypotension; if epinephrine is not repeated on time during cardiac arrest it may not help to lower the threshold for defibrillation. Take care to give medications punctually and to document their administration promptly.

Right Route

You often will have to choose from among several treatments for a particular problem. In these cases, knowing the principles of pharmacokinetics can help greatly in giving your patient the medication via the right route. For example, knowing that you should administer epinephrine intravenously rather than subcutaneously to the patient in anaphylactic shock because blood is being shunted away from the skin will guide you to the proper administration route.

Right Patient

As the EMT-I's role in health care expands, you will find yourself caring for more people than just "the patient in the back of the truck." You will deal with multiple patients, and the potential for giving medication to the wrong patient will be real. You will have to identify patients by name before administering medications.

Right Documentation

The drugs you administer in the field do not stop affecting your patients when they enter the hospital. As a result, you must completely document all of your care, especially any drugs you have administered, so that long after you have gone on to your next call, other providers will know what drugs your patient has had.

SPECIAL CONSIDERATIONS

Pregnant Patients

Any time you administer drugs to a woman of childbearing years, you must consider the possibility that she is pregnant. Treating pregnant patients clearly means treating two patients. Although emphasis appropriately seems to center on the mother during care, you must understand that many drugs that affect the mother also affect the fetus. A drug's possible benefits to the mother must clearly outweigh its potential risks to the fetus. For example, some situations such as cardiac arrest justify giving the mother medications that may harm the fetus because the drug's possible harm to the fetus is clearly outweighed by the fetus's certain death if the mother dies.

Pregnancy presents two particular pharmacological problems: changes in the mother's anatomy and physiology, and the potential for drugs to harm the fetus. Because the mother is supporting the fetus entirely, her heart rate, cardiac output, and blood volume will increase. This altered maternal physiology can affect the onset and duration of action of many medications. During the first trimester of pregnancy the ingestion of some drugs (**teratogenic drugs**) may potentially deform, injure, or kill the fetus. During the last trimester, drugs administered

Content Review

SPECIAL CONSIDERATIONS
- Pregnant patients
- Pediatric patients
- Geriatric patients

Patho Pearls

Some medications cross the placenta and affect the fetus. Because of this, it is prudent to ask whether a female patient might be pregnant before administering a medication.

teratogenic drug medication that may deform or kill the fetus.

Table 3-2	FDA PREGNANCY CATEGORIES
Category	Description
A	Adequate studies in pregnant women have not demonstrated a risk to the fetus in the first trimester or later trimesters.
B	Animal studies have not demonstrated a risk to the fetus, *but* there are no adequate studies in pregnant women. OR Adequate studies in pregnant women have not demonstrated a risk to the fetus in the first trimester and there is no risk in the last trimester, *but* animal studies have demonstrated adverse effects.
C	Animal studies have demonstrated adverse effects, *but* there are no adequate studies in pregnant women; however, benefits may be acceptable despite the potential risks. OR No adequate animal studies or adequate studies of pregnant women have been done.
D	Fetal risk has been demonstrated. In certain circumstances, benefits could outweigh the risks.
X	Fetal risk has been demonstrated. This risk outweighs any possible benefit to the mother. Avoid using in pregnant or potentially pregnant patients.

to the mother may pass through the placenta to the fetus. Some of these drugs will have unwanted effects on the fetus. Others may not be metabolized and/or excreted, possibly resulting in toxic accumulations. Additionally, a breast-feeding mother's milk may pass some drugs to her infant.

Under some conditions, of course, the health and safety of mother and fetus demand the use of drugs during the pregnancy. Examples include pregnancy-induced diabetes, hypertension, and seizure disorders. To help health care providers determine when drugs are needed during pregnancy, the FDA has developed the classification system shown in Table 3-2. Always consult medical direction for any questions about drug safety in pregnancy.

Pediatric Patients

Several physiological factors affect pharmacokinetics in newborns and young children. These patients' absorption of oral medications is less than an adult's due to various differences in gastric pH, gastric emptying time, and low enzyme levels. A newborn's skin is thinner than an older patient's and is therefore more permeable to topically administered drugs. This can result in unexpected toxicity. Older children still have less gastric acid than do adults, but their gastric emptying times reach an adult's around the sixth to eighth month of life. Because children up to a year old have diminished plasma protein concentrations, drugs that bind to proteins have higher **free drug availability**. That is, a greater proportion of the drug will be available in the body to cause either desired or undesired effects. Water distribution is different in the neonate as well. Neonates have a much higher proportion of extracellular fluid (nearly 80%) than adults (50% to 55%). This higher amount of water means a greater volume and, with less than expected protein binding, may require higher drug doses. The premature infant is especially susceptible to drugs penetrating the *blood-brain barrier* because immature connective tissues form a weaker obstacle.

The newborn's metabolic rates may be much lower than an adult's, but they rise rapidly and by a few years of age may triple an adult's. These metabolic rates then decline steadily until early adolescence, when they reach adult levels. A newborn's low metabolic rate and incompletely developed hepatic system result in a higher risk for toxic interactions. Neonates' metabolic pathways also are different from an adult's, meaning that some drugs will not have the expected effect or may have other unexpected effects. Finally, the imma-

free drug availability proportion of a drug available in the body to cause either desired or undesired effects.

Children are not small adults. Drug dosages must consider the various physiological differences.

Legal Notes

The dosing of medications for pediatric patients is based on their size and age. Thus, the dosage ranges vary significantly. It is difficult to memorize pediatric doses and best to carry a reference containing the various common ones.

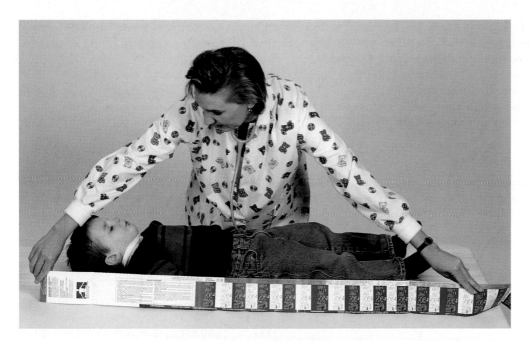

FIGURE 3-1   A Broselow tape is useful for calculating drug dosages for pediatric patients.

ture neonatal renal and hepatic system delays elimination of many drugs and their metabolites. Dosing schedules may have to be adjusted to accommodate longer half-lives until these systems mature at about six months to one year of age.

With all of these factors, a pediatric patient's drug function can differ radically from an adult's. Pediatric drug dosages must be individualized to minimize the risks of toxicity. Body surface area and weight are the two most common factors in calculating dosages. The Broselow tape gives a good approximation for children of average height/weight ratio. It bases its calculations on the child's height (length), and assumes the child's weight is at the fiftieth percentile for his height (Figure 3-1). The Broselow tape primarily addresses drugs administered in the critical care setting.

Geriatric Patients

Significant changes in pharmacokinetics may also occur in patients older than about 60 years. They may absorb oral medications slower due to decreased gastrointestinal motility. Decreased plasma protein concentration may alter distribution of drugs in their systems, leaving drugs free that would otherwise have been protein bound. Body fat increases and muscle mass decreases with age; therefore, lipid soluble drugs may have greater deposition, thereby lowering the amount of available drug. Absorption and distribution of intramuscular injections may alter if volumes are inappropriate for the remaining muscle mass. Because the liver primarily handles biotransformation, depressed liver function in an aging patient may delay or prolong drug action. The aging process may also slow elimination by the renal system.

Older patients are also more likely to be on multiple medications or to have multiple underlying disease processes. Various medication interactions can have a severe impact on patients. For example, sildenafil (Viagra) and nitroglycerin given together may cause severe hypotension. Underlying diseases may affect therapeutics in unexpected ways. Congestive heart failure, for instance, may cause congestion of the vasculature in the gastrointestinal (GI) tract, delaying the absorption of oral medications. The congestive heart failure patient may also have compromised renal function, delaying his elimination of drugs.

PHARMACOLOGY

Pharmacology is the study of drugs and their interactions with the body. Drugs do not confer any new properties on cells or tissues; they only modify or exploit existing functions.

Patho Pearls

The chance of a medication interaction increases significantly the greater the number of medications the patient is taking. Thus, proceed with caution when administering an emergency medication to a patient who routinely takes more than two.

Use caution when administering medications to older patients because they are likely to be on multiple medications.

They may be given for their local action (in which case systemic absorption of the drug is discouraged) or for systemic action. Although generally given for a specific effect, drugs tend to have multiple actions at multiple sites, so they must be thought of in terms of their systemic effects rather than in terms of an isolated single effect. Pharmacology's two major divisions are pharmacokinetics and pharmacodynamics. You have already learned that **pharmacokinetics** addresses how drugs are transported into and out of the body. **Pharmacodynamics** deals with their effects once they reach the target tissues.

PHARMACOKINETICS

Strictly defined, pharmacokinetics is the study of the basic processes that determine the duration and intensity of a drug's effect. These four processes are absorption, distribution, biotransformation, and elimination.

Review of Physiology of Transport

Pharmacokinetics depends on the body's various physiological mechanisms that move substances across the body's compartments. These mechanisms can be broken down into two broad categories based on their energy requirements and then further classified. A mechanism is referred to as **active transport** if it requires the use of energy to move a substance. This energy is achieved by the breakdown of high-energy chemical bonds found in chemicals such as adenosine triphosphate (ATP). ATP is broken down into adenosine diphosphate (ADP) liberating a considerable amount of biochemical energy. A common example of an active transport mechanism is the sodium-potassium (Na^+-K^+) pump. This is a protein pump that actively moves potassium ions into the cell and sodium ions out of the cell. Because this movement goes *against* the ions' concentration gradients, it must use energy.

Large molecules, such as glucose and most of the amino acids, do not readily pass through the cell membrane because of their size. These molecules are moved across the cell membrane with the help of special "carrier" proteins found on the surface of the target cells. These large molecules are "carried" across the cell membrane in a special transport process called **carrier-mediated diffusion** or **facilitated diffusion**. Once the molecule to be transported binds with the carrier protein, the configuration of the cell membrane changes, allowing the large molecule to enter the target cell. Insulin, an important hormone secreted by the endocrine pancreas, can increase the rate of carrier-mediated glucose transport from ten- to twenty-fold. This is the principle mechanism by which insulin controls glucose use in the body.

Most drugs travel through the body by means of **passive transport,** the movement of a substance without the use of energy. This requires the presence of concentration gradients in a solution. Diffusion and osmosis are forms of passive transport. **Diffusion** involves the movement of solute in the solution, whereas **osmosis** involves the movement of the solvent (usually water). In diffusion, the solute's molecules or ions move *down* their concentration gradients from an area of higher concentration to an area of lower concentration. Conversely, in osmosis the solvent's molecules move *up* the concentration gradient from an area of low solute concentration to an area of higher solute concentration. Another way of looking at this is to think of osmosis as simply the diffusion of solvent from an area of high solvent concentration to an area of low *solvent* concentration. A final type of passive transport is **filtration.** This is simply the movement of molecules across a membrane down a *pressure* gradient, from an area of high pressure to an area of lower pressure. This pressure typically results from the hydrostatic force of blood pressure.

Absorption

When a drug is administered to a patient it must find its way to the site of action. If a drug is given orally or injected into any place except the blood stream, its absorption into the blood stream is the first step in this process. (Since drugs given intravenously or intra-arterially enter directly into the blood stream no absorption needs to occur.) Several factors affect a drug's absorption. The body absorbs most drugs faster when they are given intramuscularly than when they are given subcutaneously. This is because muscles are more vascular than subcutaneous tissue. Of course, anything that slows blood flow delays absorption. Shock and hypothermia are just two examples. Conversely, processes such as fever and hyperthermia increase peripheral blood flow and speed absorption.

Drugs given orally (enterally) must first survive the digestive processes before being absorbed across the mucosa of the gastrointestinal system. If a drug is not soluble in water it will have difficulty being absorbed. Time-released medications take advantage of this with an enteric coating that slowly releases the medication. Some drugs have an enteric coating that will not dissolve in the more acidic environment of the stomach, but will dissolve in the alkaline environment of the duodenum. This allows a drug that would irritate the stomach or be destroyed by stomach acid to be passed through the stomach into the duodenum and absorbed there. Besides being able to survive stomach acid, a drug must also be somewhat lipid (fat) soluble in order to cross the cells' lipid two-layered (bilayered) membranes. Many drugs **ionize,** or become electrically charged or polar following administration. Generally speaking, ionized drugs do not absorb across the membranes of cells (lipid bilayers), but fortunately, most drugs do not fully ionize. Instead they reach an equilibrium between their ionized and non-ionized forms, and the non-ionized form can be absorbed. A drug's pH also affects the extent to which it ionizes. A drug that is a weak acid ionizes much more substantially in an alkaline environment than in an acidic environment; conversely, an alkaline drug ionizes more readily in an acidic environment than in an alkaline environment. For example, aspirin (an acidic drug) does not dissociate well in the stomach (an acidic environment) and is therefore readily absorbed there.

The nature of the absorbing surface and the blood flow to the administration site also affect drug absorption. The rate of absorption is directly related to the amount of surface area available for absorption. The greater the area, the faster the absorption. Much of the gastrointestinal system has multiple invaginations, or folds, that increase its surface area. Also, the greater the blood flow is to an area, the faster will be the rate of absorption. Again, the GI tract has a rich vascular system with many capillaries that perfuse its absorbing surfaces, allowing nutrients (and drugs) to diffuse into the blood stream.

Finally, the drug's concentration affects its absorption. Because drugs diffuse in the body, the higher their concentration, the more rapidly the body absorbs them. This principle is frequently used when giving a "loading dose" of a drug and following it with a "maintenance infusion." The loading dose is typically a larger dose of the same concentration of the drug. On occasion, a more concentrated solution of the drug is used as the loading dose. Regardless, the desired effect is to rapidly raise the amount of the drug in the system to a therapeutic level. This is typically followed by a continuous infusion of the drug at a lower concentration, or slower administration rate, to keep it at the therapeutic level.

Bioavailability is the measure of the amount of a drug that is still active after it reaches its target tissue. This is the bottom line as far as absorption is concerned. The goal of administering a drug is to ensure sufficient bioavailability of the drug at the target tissue in order to produce the desired effect, after considering all of the absorption factors.

Distribution

Once a drug has entered the blood stream, it must be distributed throughout the body. Most drugs pass easily from the blood stream, through the interstitial spaces, into the target cells. Some drugs, however, bind to proteins found in the blood, most commonly albumin, and remain in the body for a prolonged time. They thus have a sustained release from the blood stream and a prolonged period of action. The therapeutic effects of a drug are primarily due to the unbound portion of the drug in the blood. A drug that is bound to plasma proteins cannot cross membranes and reach the target cells. Thus, only the unbound drug is in equilibrium with the target cells and can cross the cell membranes.

Changing the blood stream's pH can affect the protein-binding action of a drug. Tricyclic antidepressants (TCAs), for instance, are strongly bound to plasma proteins. Making the blood more alkaline increases protein binding of the TCA molecules. Therefore, in addition to supportive therapy, serious overdoses of TCAs are treated by administering sodium bicarbonate. Sodium bicarbonate makes the blood more alkaline (raises the pH), causing increased binding of the TCA to serum proteins. Cumulatively, this decreases the amount of free drug in the blood, thus decreasing the adverse effects. Sodium bicarbonate administration also facilitates elimination of the drug through the urine.

ionize to become electrically charged or polar.

bioavailability amount of a drug that is still active after it reaches its target tissue.

The presence of other serum protein-binding drugs can also affect drug-protein binding. For example, the drug warfarin (Coumadin) is highly protein bound (99%). Its therapeutic effects are due to the one percent of the drug that is unbound and circulating in the blood stream. Aspirin molecules bind to the same binding site on the serum proteins as do warfarin molecules. Thus, when aspirin is administered to a patient on warfarin, it displaces some of the protein-bound warfarin, increasing the amount of free (unbound) warfarin in the blood. Even if it displaces only 1% of the total warfarin, it effectively doubles the available warfarin. This can lead to unwanted side-effects such as hemorrhage.

Albumin is one of the chief proteins in the blood that is available for binding with drugs. When albumin levels are low (hypoalbuminemia), as occurs in malnutrition, drugs that are normally protein bound rise to much greater blood levels than anticipated. For example, consider a patient who has been taking warfarin without difficulty. If he develops hypoalbuminemia, his normal dose of warfarin will result in much more of the drug being available in the body, possibly leading to dangerous bleeding.

Certain organs exclude some drugs from distribution. For example, the tight junctions of the capillary endothelial cells in the central nervous system (CNS) vasculature form a **blood-brain barrier.** These cells are packed together so tightly that only non-protein-bound, highly lipid-soluble drugs can cross into the CNS. The so-called **placental barrier** can likewise prevent drugs from reaching a fetus, although it is not the solid barrier that its name implies. The fetus is exposed to almost every drug that the mother takes. But because any drug must traverse the maternal blood supply and cross the capillary membranes into the placenta (fetal) circulation, delivering drugs to a fetus requires them to be lipid soluble, non-ionized, and non-protein bound. This may slow some drugs or reduce their placental transfer to benign levels.

Other drugs are deposited in specific tissues. For example, fatty tissue can serve as a drug depot, or reservoir. Because blood flow is lower in fatty areas than in muscular areas, fatty tissue is a relatively stable depot; it can neither absorb nor release a large amount of drug in a short time. Similarly, bones and teeth can accumulate high amounts of drugs that bind to calcium, especially tetracycline antibiotics.

Biotransformation

Like other chemicals that enter the body, drugs are metabolized, or broken down, into different chemicals (metabolites). The special name given to the **metabolism** of drugs is **biotransformation.** Biotransformation has one of two effects on most drugs: (1) it can transform the drug into a more or less active metabolite, or (2) it can make the drug more water soluble (or less lipid soluble) to facilitate elimination. Some drugs, such as lidocaine, are totally metabolized before elimination, others only partially, and still others not at all. The body transforms some molecules of most drugs and eliminate others without transformation. Protein-bound drugs are not available for biotransformation. Some so-called **prodrugs** (or parent drugs) are not active when administered, but biotransformation converts them into active metabolites.

Many biotransformation processes occur in the liver. The endoplasmic reticula of hepatocytes (liver cells) contain microsomal enzymes that perform much of the metabolizing. (Smaller quantities of these enzymes are also found in the kidney, lung, and GI tract.) Because the blood supply from the GI tract passes through the liver via the portal vein, all drugs absorbed in the GI tract pass through the liver before moving on through the systemic circulation. The first pass through the liver may partially or completely inactivate many drugs. This **first-pass effect** is why some drugs cannot be given orally but instead must be given intravenously to bypass the GI tract and prevent first-pass hepatic metabolism. It also is why drugs that can be given either orally or intravenously may require a much higher oral dose than IV dose. Because we can observe the extent of first-pass metabolism, we can predict how much to increase a dose of an oral medication to deliver an effective amount of the drug into the general circulation.

The liver's microsomal enzymes react with drugs in two ways: phase-I, or nonsynthetic reactions; and phase-II, or synthetic reactions. *Phase-I reactions* most often **oxidize** the par-

blood-brain barrier tight junctions of the capillary endothelial cells in the central nervous system vasculature through which only non–protein-bound, highly lipid-soluble drugs can pass.

placental barrier biochemical barrier at the maternal/fetal interface that restricts certain molecules.

metabolism the body's breaking down chemicals into different chemicals.

biotransformation special name given to the metabolism of drugs.

prodrug (parent drug) medication that is not active when administered, but whose biotransformation converts it into active metabolites.

first-pass effect the liver's partial or complete inactivation of a drug before it reaches the systemic circulation.

oxidation the loss of hydrogen atoms or the acceptance of an oxygen atom. This increases the positive charge (or lessens the negative charge) on the molecule.

ent drug, although they may reduce it or **hydrolyze** it. These nonsynthetic reactions make the drug more water soluble to ease excretion. A number of drugs and chemicals increase the activity of, or induce, the microsomal enzyme that causes phase-I reactions. This means that more enzyme is produced and drugs are metabolized more rapidly. Because the microsomal enzymes are nonspecific, they can be induced by one drug or chemical and then biotransform other drugs or chemicals. *Phase-II reactions,* which are also called conjugation reactions, combine the prodrug or its metabolites with an endogenous (naturally occurring) chemical, usually making the drug more polar and easier to excrete.

hydrolysis the breakage of a chemical bond by adding water, or by incorporating a hydroxyl (OH⁻) group into one fragment and a hydrogen ion (H⁺) into the other.

Elimination

Whether they are unchanged or metabolized before elimination, most drugs (toxins and metabolites) are excreted in the urine. Some are excreted in the feces or in expired air.

Renal excretion occurs through two major processes: glomerular filtration and tubular secretion. Glomerular filtration is a function of glomerular filtration pressure, which in turn results from blood pressure and blood flow through the kidneys. Conditions that affect blood pressure and blood flow can affect renal elimination. Specialized transport systems in the walls of the proximal kidney tubules secrete drugs into the urine. These "pumps" are active transport systems and require energy in the form of adenosine triphosphate (ATP) to function. Some are specialized and transport only specific chemicals, whereas others can transport a range of similar chemicals. When drugs compete for the same pump, toxicity or other unwanted effects can result; however, combinations of some drugs can take advantage of this specialization to prolong their circulation. For example, probenecid blocks renal tubular pumps and competes for them with many antibiotics, among them penicillin, ampicillin, and oxacillin. Probenecid thus is sometimes given with those antibiotics to increase and prolong their blood levels.

The same factors that affect absorption at any other site also affect reabsorption in the renal tubules. Of particular concern is the urine pH. Lipid soluble and non-ionized molecules are readily reabsorbed. Changing the urine pH (usually by administering sodium bicarbonate to make it more alkaline) can affect the reabsorption in the renal tubules. For example, if a drug becomes ionized in a more alkaline environment, then making the urine more alkaline interferes with reabsorption and causes more of the drug to be excreted. Some drugs and their metabolites can be eliminated in the expired air. This is the basis of the breath test that police use to determine a driver's blood alcohol level. Ethanol is released in the expired air in proportion to its concentration in the blood stream. Although the liver degrades most ingested ethanol, exhalation releases a measurable quantity. Drugs also can be excreted in the feces. In enterohepatic circulation, if a drug (or its metabolites) is excreted into the intestines from bile, the body may reabsorb the drug and experience a sustained effect. Additionally, drugs may be excreted through sweat, saliva, and breast milk. Excretion through sweat glands is rarely a significant mechanism for elimination. Excretion through mammary glands becomes a concern when nursing mothers take medications.

Drug Routes

The route of a drug's administration clearly has an impact on the drug's absorption and distribution. The route's impact on biotransformation and elimination may not be so clear. The blood stream more quickly absorbs and distributes water-soluble drugs if given in more vascular compartments than if given in less vascular compartments. Oral or nasogastric administration of alkaline drugs may allow the gastric acids to neutralize the drug and prevent its absorption. The liver's first-pass effect may biotransform some orally administered drugs and degrade them almost immediately.

enteral route delivery of a medication through the gastrointestinal tract.

Enteral Routes The **enteral routes** deliver medications by absorption through the GI tract, which goes from the mouth to the stomach and on through the intestines to the rectum. They may be oral, orogastric/nasogastric, sublingual, buccal, or rectal.

- *Oral (PO).* The oral route is good for self-administered drugs. Most home medications are administered by this route. The drug must be able to tolerate the acidic gastric environment and be absorbed. Few emergency drugs are administered through this route.

Content Review

DRUG ROUTES
- Enteral
- Parenteral

- *Orogastric/nasogastric tube (OG/NG).* This route is generally used for oral medications when the patient already has the tube in place for other reasons.
- *Sublingual (SL).* This is a good route for self-administration and excellent absorption from the sublingual capillary bed without the problems of gastric acidity or absorption.
- *Buccal.* Absorption through this route between the cheek and gum is similar to sublingual absorption.
- *Rectal (PR).* This route is usually reserved for unconscious or vomiting patients or patients who cannot cooperate with oral or IV administration (small children).

Parenteral Routes Broadly defined, **parenteral route** denotes any area outside of the GI tract; however, additional, specific criteria applies to parenteral drug administration. Parenteral routes typically use needles to inject medications into the circulatory system or tissues. Consequently, some forms of parenteral drug delivery afford the most rapid drug delivery and absorption:

- *Intravenous (IV).* With its rapid onset, this is the preferred route in most emergencies.
- *Endotracheal (ET).* This is an alternative route for selected medications in an emergency.
- *Intraosseous (IO).* The intraosseous route delivers drugs to the medullary space of bones. Most often used as an alternative to IV administration in pediatric emergencies, it also sees limited use in adults.
- *Umbilical.* Both the umbilical vein and umbilical artery can provide an alternative to IV administration in newborns.
- *Intramuscular (IM).* The intramuscular route allows a slower absorption than IV administration, as the drug passes into the capillaries.
- *Subcutaneous (SC, SQ, SubQ).* This route is slower than the IM route, because the subcutaneous tissue is less vascular than the muscular tissue.
- *Inhalation/nebulized.* This route, which offers very rapid absorption, is especially useful for delivering drugs whose target tissues are in the lungs.
- *Topical.* Topical administration delivers drugs directly to the skin.
- *Transdermal.* For drugs that can be absorbed through the skin, the transdermal route allows slow, continuous release.
- *Nasal.* Useful for delivering drugs directly to the nasal mucosa, the nasal route has an expanding role in delivering systemically acting drugs.
- *Instillation.* Instillation is similar to topical administration, but places the drug directly into a wound or an eye.
- *Intradermal.* For allergy testing, intradermal administration delivers a drug or biologic agent between the dermal layers.

Drug Forms

Drugs come in many forms. Solid forms, generally given orally, include:

- *Pills.* Drugs shaped spherically are easy to swallow.
- *Powders.* Although they are not as popular as they once were, some powdered drugs are still in use.
- *Tablets.* Powders that are compressed into a disklike form.
- *Suppositories.* Drugs mixed with a waxlike base that melts at body temperature, allowing absorption by rectal or vaginal tissue.
- *Capsules.* Gelatin containers filled with powders or tiny pills; the gelatin dissolves, releasing the drug into the GI tract.

parenteral route delivery of a medication outside of the gastrointestinal tract, typically using needles to inject medications into the circulatory system or tissues.

Most emergency medications are given intravenously to avoid drug degradation in the liver.

Liquid drugs are usually solutions of a solid drug dissolved in a solvent. Some can be given parenterally. Others must be given enterally.

- *Solutions*. The most common liquid preparations. Generally water based, some may be oil based.
- *Tinctures*. Prepared using an alcohol extraction process; some alcohol usually remains in the final drug preparation.
- *Suspensions*. Preparations in which the solid does not dissolve in the solvent; if left alone, the solid portion will precipitate out.
- *Emulsions*. Suspensions with an oily substance in the solvent, even when well mixed globules of oil separate out of the solution.
- *Spirits*. Solution of a volatile drug in alcohol.
- *Elixirs*. Alcohol and water solvent, often with flavorings added to improve the taste.
- *Syrups*. Sugar, water, and drug solutions.

Some drugs come in a gaseous form. The most common drug supplied this way is oxygen. EMT-Is may also find nitrous oxide (N_2O) used as an inhaled analgesic in ambulances and emergency departments.

Drug Storage

Certain guidelines should dictate the manner in which drugs are stored; their properties may be altered by the environment in which they are stored. Although some EMS units are parked in heated stations, others are kept outdoors and exposed to the elements. EMS systems must consider the storage requirements of all drugs and diluents when deciding operational issues such as vehicle design and posting policies (as occurs in system status management). This rapidly becomes a clinical issue because the actual potency of most medications is altered if they are not stored in proper conditions. Examples of variables to consider when determining the proper method of drug storage include temperature, light, moisture, and shelf-life.

PHARMACODYNAMICS

When we consider a drug's pharmacodynamics, or effects on the body, we are specifically interested in its mechanisms of action and the relationship between its concentration and its effect.

Actions of Drugs

Drugs can act in four different ways. They may bind to a receptor site, change the physical properties of cells, chemically combine with other chemicals, or alter a normal metabolic pathway. Each of these actions involves a physiochemical interaction between the drug and a functionally important molecule in the body.

Drugs that Act by Binding to a Receptor Site   Most drugs operate by binding to a **receptor**. Almost all drug receptors are protein molecules on the surfaces of cells. They are part of the body's normal regulatory stimulation/inhibition function and can be stimulated or inhibited by chemicals. Each different receptor's name generally corresponds to the drug that stimulates it. For example, if an opiate stimulates the receptor, then the receptor is an opioid receptor. When multiple drugs stimulate the same receptor, standard practice is to use the generic name.

The force of attraction between a drug and a receptor is their **affinity**. The greater the affinity, the stronger the bond. Different drugs may bind to the same type of receptor site, but the strength of their bond may vary. The binding site's shape determines its receptivity to other chemicals, whether they are drugs or endogenous substances. These binding sites are relatively specific—a nonopiate drug generally does not affect an opiate binding site, although occasionally a drug with a similar receptor binding site unexpectedly cross reacts. Receptors can also have subtypes. At least five subtypes of adrenergic receptors, for example, are important to EMT-I practice.

Content Review

TYPES OF DRUG ACTIONS
- Binding to a receptor site
- Changing the physical properties of cells
- Chemically combining with other chemicals
- Altering a normal metabolic pathway

receptor specialized protein that combines with a drug resulting in a biochemical effect.

affinity force of attraction between a drug and a receptor.

efficacy a drug's ability to cause the expected response.

second messenger chemical that participates in complex cascading reactions that eventually cause a drug's desired effect.

down-regulation binding of a drug or hormone to a target cell receptor that causes the number of receptors to decrease.

up-regulation a drug causes the formation of more receptors than normal.

agonist drug that binds to a receptor and causes it to initiate the expected response.

antagonist drug that binds to a receptor but does not cause it to initiate the expected response.

agonist-antagonist (partial agonist) drug that binds to a receptor and stimulates some of its effects but blocks others.

competitive antagonism one drug binds to a receptor and causes the expected effect while also blocking another drug from triggering the same receptor.

noncompetitive antagonism the binding of an antagonist causes a deformity of the binding site that prevents an agonist from fitting and binding.

irreversible antagonism a competitive antagonist permanently binds with a receptor site.

A drug's pharmacodynamics also involve its ability to cause the expected response, or **efficacy.** Just as different drugs may have different affinities for a site, they may also have different efficacies; that is, drug A may cause a stronger response than drug B. Affinity and efficacy are not directly related. Drug A may cause a stronger response than drug B, even though drug B binds to the receptor site more strongly than drug A.

When a drug binds with its specific type of receptor, a chemical change occurs that ultimately leads to the drug's effect. In most cases, drugs either stimulate or inhibit the cell's normal biochemical actions. In fact, a drug cannot impart a new function to a cell. Some drugs may interact with a receptor and directly result in the desired effect. Other drugs, however, may interact with a receptor and cause the release or production of a second compound. This secondary compound, or **second messenger,** includes such compounds as calcium or cyclic adenosine monophosphate (cAMP). The cAMP is the most common second messenger. It has a multitude of effects inside the cell. These secondary messengers are particularly important in the endocrine system, as they principally occur in endocrine glands. Once cAMP is formed inside the cell, it activates still other enzymes, usually in a cascading action. That is, the first enzyme activates another enzyme, which activates a third enzyme, and so forth. This is important in that it amplifies the action so that even a small amount of a drug (or hormone) acting on the cell surface can initiate a powerful, cascading, activating force for the entire cell.

The number of receptors on a target cell usually does not remain constant on a daily basis or even from minute to minute. This is because the receptor proteins are often destroyed during the course of their function. At other times, they are either reactivated or remanufactured by the protein-manufacturing mechanism of the cell. Binding of a drug (or hormone) to a target cell receptor causes the number of receptors to decrease. This process is **down-regulation** of the receptors. It results in a decreased responsiveness of the target cell to the drug or hormone as the number of available active receptors decreases. In other cases, but less commonly, a drug (or hormone) can cause the formation of more receptors than normal. This process, **up-regulation,** increases the target tissue's sensitivity to the particular drug or hormone.

Chemicals that stimulate a receptor site generally fall into two broad categories, agonists and antagonists. **Agonists** bind to the receptor and cause it to initiate the expected response. **Antagonists** bind to a site but do not cause the receptor to initiate the expected response. Some drugs, **agonist-antagonists** (also called **partial agonists**), may do both. Nalbuphine (Nubain), for instance, stimulates some of the opioid agonists' analgesic properties but partially blocks others such as respiratory depression.

Receptor-mediated drug actions work like a lock (the receptor) and key (the agonist). If you put the key in the lock and turn it, the lock will open. An antagonist is like a key that fits into the lock but will not turn and cannot open the lock. Target tissues generally have many receptors, so to take the analogy another step, imagine that to get maximum effect a single key (agonist) must move around and open many doors (trigger many biochemical responses). An agonist-antagonist would be a key that unlocks and opens a door but gets stuck in the lock. That is, the drug causes the expected effect, but that drug also blocks another drug from triggering the same receptor. This **competitive antagonism** is considered surmountable because a sufficiently large dose of the agonist can overcome the antagonism.

Noncompetitive antagonism can also occur. Continuing the lock, key, and door analogy, imagine the door is barred. This antagonism would be insurmountable; no amount of agonist could overcome it. Noncompetitive antagonism occurs because the binding of the antagonist at a different site causes a deformity of the binding site that actually prevents the agonist from fitting and binding. **Irreversible antagonism** may also occur when a competitive antagonist permanently binds with a receptor site. When this occurs, no amount of agonist stimulates the receptor. For the effects of such an antagonist to wear off, the body must create new receptors.

Two drugs may appear to be antagonists while actually acting independently. This physiologic antagonism can occur when one drug's effects counteract another's. Although neither agent chemically affects the other, their net effect is antagonistic. An example of a receptor, agonist, antagonist, and agonist-antagonist can be described using an opiate receptor. These receptors occur naturally in the brain and respond to natural endorphins. Morphine sulfate acts as an agonist. It binds to the opiate receptor and causes the expected response of pain relief. Naloxone (Narcan) acts as an antagonist. It binds to the opiate receptor, but does not initiate the pain relief. It prevents morphine sulfate from binding to the site and thus effectively blocks the morphine and its response. If the patient is given nalbuphine (Nubain), an agonist-antagonist, it binds to the opiate receptor and relieves pain, but it is less efficacious than morphine. The nalbuphine blocks morphine from the receptor like an antagonist, but stimulates the receptor on its own like an agonist, although to a lesser extent.

Drugs that Act by Changing Physical Properties   Some drugs change the physical properties of a part of the body. Drugs that change the osmotic balance across membranes are good examples of this type of drug action. The osmotic diuretic mannitol (Osmotrol), for instance, increases urine output by increasing the blood's osmolarity, or osmotic "pull." This increased osmolarity triggers the normal regulatory systems to decrease water reabsorption in the renal tubules, thereby reducing the total amount of water in the body.

Drugs that Act by Chemically Combining with Other Substances   Drugs that participate in chemical reactions that change the chemical nature of their substrates (the chemical or substance on which a drug acts) play a large role in EMT-I practice. For example, isopropyl alcohol, which is often used to disinfect skin before percutaneous needle insertion for phlebotomy or IV cannulation, denatures the proteins on the surface of bacterial cells. This ruptures the cells, destroying the bacteria. The antacids are another example. They act by chemically neutralizing the hydrochloric acid in the stomach. Sodium bicarbonate given intravenously chemically neutralizes some of the acids in the blood stream, effectively making the blood more alkalotic.

Drugs that Act by Altering a Normal Metabolic Pathway   Some anticancer and antiviral drugs are chemical analogs of normal metabolic substrates. In a process that has been dubbed a counterfeit incorporation mechanism, these drugs can be incorporated into the products of metabolism of cancer cells. Since these drugs are not really the expected substrate, the anticipated product either will not form or, if formed, will be substantially or completely inactive.

Responses to Drug Administration

When a drug is administered, a response is obviously anticipated. The actual response may be the one desired, or it may be an unintended **side effect**. Most, if not all, drugs have at least some minor side effects. Because our knowledge of pharmacology and physiology has not yet arrived at the point where we can engineer the perfect drug, we must weigh the need for the desired response against the dangers of side effects. In essence, every time we give a medication, we must carefully weigh the risks against the benefits. Although undesirable, side effects are predictable. Iatrogenic responses, on the other hand, are not predicted. In general, the term *iatrogenic* refers to a disease or response induced by the actions of a care provider. Derived from the Greek *iatros* (physician) and *gennan* (to produce), it literally means *physician produced*. Negligence is not the only cause of iatrogenic responses. Some common unintended adverse responses to drugs include:

- *Allergic reaction.* Also known as hypersensitivity; this effect occurs as the drug is antigenic and activates the immune system, causing effects that are normally more profound than seen in the general population.
- *Idiosyncrasy.* A drug effect that is unique to the individual; different than seen or expected in the population in general.
- *Tolerance.* Decreased response to the same amount of drug after repeated administrations.
- *Cross tolerance.* Tolerance for a drug that develops after administration of a different drug. Morphine and other opioid agents are common examples. Tolerance for one agent implies tolerance for others as well.
- *Tachyphylaxis.* Rapidly occurring tolerance to a drug. May occur after a single dose. This typically occurs with sympathetic agonists, specifically decongestant and bronchodilation agents.

side effect unintended response to a drug.

Always weigh the need for a drug's desired response against the dangers of its side effects.

Legal Notes

The use of medications is one area where an EMT-I or Paramedic differs from the EMT-Basic. Most EMT-Basic skills, if performed improperly or incorrectly, have the potential to harm the patient. However, many EMT-I and Paramedic skills, if performed improperly or incorrectly, can potentially kill the patient. The administration of emergency medications in the prehospital setting has saved countless lives. However, there have been instances where patients have received the wrong medication or an incorrect dose of the correct medication resulting in patient harm. Because of this, EMT-Is must be extremely vigilant in regard to medication administration. Be certain to always confirm orders and write them down. Follow the six "rights" of medication administration. Double check your drugs, the doses, the expiration dates, and the intended route of administration. Following administration, constantly monitor your patient for the desired effects of the medication as well as any possible side effects. Accurately document your findings, including any untoward effects. It is essential that you make prehospital medication administration as safe as possible for all involved—you and the patient.

- *Cumulative effect.* Increased effectiveness when a drug is given in several doses.
- *Drug dependence.* The patient becomes accustomed to the drug's presence in his body and will suffer from withdrawal symptoms upon its absence. The dependence may be physical or psychological.
- *Drug interaction.* The effects of one drug alter the response to another drug.
- *Drug antagonism.* The effects of one drug block the response to another drug.
- *Summation.* Also known as an additive effect. Two drugs that both have the same effect are given together, analogous to $1 + 1 = 2$.
- *Synergism.* Two drugs that both have the same effect are given together and produce a response greater than the sum of their individual responses, analogous to $1 + 1 = 3$.
- *Potentiation.* One drug enhances the effect of another. A common example is promethazine (Phenergan) enhancing the effects of morphine.
- *Interference.* The direct biochemical interaction between two drugs; one drug affects the pharmacology of another drug.

Drug-Response Relationship

To have its optimum desired or therapeutic effects, a drug must reach appropriate concentrations at its site of action. The magnitude of the response therefore depends on the dosage and the drug's course through the body over time. Factors that can affect the drug's concentration may be pharmaceutical (the dosage form's disintegration and the drug's dissolution), pharmacokinetic (the drug's absorption, distribution, metabolism, and excretion), or pharmacodynamic (drug-receptor interaction). To predict how the drug will affect different people, a **drug-response relationship** thus correlates different amounts of drug to the resultant clinical response.

Most of the information needed to describe drug-response relationships comes from **plasma-level profiles,** which describe the lengths of onset, duration, and termination of action, as well as the drug's minimum effective concentration and toxic levels. The **onset of action** is the time from administration until a medication reaches its **minimum effective concentration** (the minimum level of drug necessary to cause a given effect). The length of time the amount of drug remains above this level is its **duration of action. Termination of action** is measured from when the drug's level drops below the minimum effective concentration until it is eliminated from the body.

The ratio of a drug's lethal dose for 50% of the population (LD_{50}) to its effective dose for 50% of the population (ED_{50}) is its **therapeutic index** (TI) or LD_{50}/ED_{50}. The therapeutic index represents the drug's margin of safety. As the range between effective dose and lethal dose decreases, the value of TI decreases; that is, it becomes closer to one. TI values

---

drug-response relationship correlation of different amounts of a drug to clinical response.

plasma-level profile describes the lengths of onset, duration, and termination of action, as well as the drug's minimum effective concentration and toxic levels.

onset of action the time from administration until a medication reaches its minimum effective concentration.

minimum effective concentration minimum level of drug needed to cause a given effect.

duration of action length of time the amount of drug remains above its minimum effective concentration.

termination of action time from when the drug's level drops below its minimum effective concentration until it is eliminated from the body.

therapeutic index ratio of a drug's lethal dose for 50% of the population to its effective dose for 50% of the population.

of close to one indicate a very small margin of safety. In other words, the effective dose and lethal dose of a drug whose TI value is close to one are nearly the same. This drug would be very difficult to effectively dose without causing toxicity.

The last component of the drug-response relationship, the **biologic half-life,** is the time the body takes to clear one half of the drug. Although the rates of metabolism and excretion both affect it, a drug's half-life ($t_{1/2}$) is independent of its concentration. For example, if the concentration of a drug were 500 µg/dL after administration and 250 µg/dL in 10 minutes, then its half-life would be 10 minutes. After another 10 minutes, 125 µg/dL would remain.

Factors Altering Drug Response

Different individuals may have different responses to the same drug given. Factors that alter the standard drug-response relationship include the following:

- *Age.* The liver and kidney functions of infants are not yet fully developed, so the response to drugs may be altered. Likewise, as a person ages, the functions of these organs begins to deteriorate. As a result, infants and the elderly are most susceptible to having an altered response to a drug.

- *Body mass.* The more body mass a person has, the more fluid is potentially available to dilute a drug. A given amount of drug causes a higher concentration in a person with little body mass than in a much larger person. Thus, most drug dosages are stated in terms of body mass. For example, the standard dose of lidocaine for a patient in cardiac arrest is 1.5 mg/kg. A 100 kg patient will receive 150 mg of lidocaine, whereas a 50 kg patient will receive only 75 mg.

- *Sex.* Most differences in drug response due to sex result from the relative body masses of men and women. The different distribution and amounts of body fat also affect the amounts of drug available at any given time.

- *Environmental milieu.* Various stimuli in a patient's environment affect his response to a given drug. This is most clearly seen with drugs affecting mood or behavior. The same dose of an antianxiety medication such as diazepam (Valium) has different effects, depending on the patient's mood or surroundings. For example, if the patient were afraid of heights, his usual dose of diazepam would not be likely to help him remain calm while rappelling from the top of a tall building. Surrounding conditions may also affect the distribution or elimination of a drug. Heat, for example, causes vasodilation and increases perspiration, both of which may alter the rate at which the body distributes and eliminates a drug.

- *Time of administration.* If a patient takes a drug immediately after eating, its absorption is different than if he took the same drug before breakfast in the morning. Some drugs may cause nausea if taken on an empty stomach and must therefore be taken only after eating.

- *Pathologic state.* Several disease states alter the drug-response relationship. Most notable are renal and hepatic dysfunctions, both of which may lead to excess accumulation of a drug in the body. Renal failure is likely to decrease elimination of drugs. Hepatic failure may decrease or inhibit their metabolism, prolonging their duration of action. Acid-base disturbances may alter a drug's solubility or the extent to which it ionizes, thus changing its absorption rate.

- *Genetic factors.* Genetic traits such as the lack of specific enzymes or lowered basal metabolic rate alter drug absorption or biotransformation and thus modify the patient's response.

- *Psychological factors.* A patient's mental state can also affect his response to a drug. The best known example of this is the placebo effect. Essentially, if a patient believes that a drug has a given effect, then he is much more likely to perceive that the effect has occurred.

biologic half-life time the body takes to clear one half of a drug.

Content Review

FACTORS AFFECTING DRUG-RESPONSE RELATIONSHIP

- Age
- Body mass
- Sex
- Environment
- Time of administration
- Pathology
- Genetics
- Psychology

Drug Interactions

Drug interactions occur whenever two or more drugs are available in the same patient. The interaction can increase, decrease, or have no effect on their combined actions. Any number of variables may cause these drug-drug interactions, including:

- One drug could alter the rate of intestinal absorption.
- Two drugs could compete for plasma protein binding, resulting in one's accumulation at the other's expense.
- One drug could alter the other's metabolism, thus increasing or decreasing either's bioavailability.
- One drug's action at a receptor site may be antagonistic or synergistic to another's.
- One drug could alter the other's rate of excretion through the kidneys.
- One drug could alter the balance of electrolytes necessary for the other drug's expected result.

In addition to drug-drug interactions, other types of interactions are possible. They include a drug's effects on the rate of absorption of food and nutrients, alteration of enzymes, and food-initiated alteration of drug excretion. Alcohol consumption and smoking may also cause interactions with drugs. Finally, some drugs are incompatible with each other. As an example, catecholamines such as epinephrine precipitate in an alkaline solution such as sodium bicarbonate.

Part 2: Nervous System Components

Part 2 begins with a discussion of nervous system function with emphasis on the autonomic nervous system. Many of the medications used in emergency care act on the autonomic nervous system. Because of this, EMT-Is must understand its structure and function.

AUTONOMIC NERVOUS SYSTEM

Many medications used in prehospital care directly affect the autonomic nervous system. It is essential that you have a good understanding of this system and the ways in which emergency medications affect it. As you may recall from Chapter 2, the nervous system can be divided into the *central nervous system* (brain and spinal cord) and the *peripheral nervous system* (all the other nervous system structures). The peripheral nervous system has two components: the *somatic nervous system,* which controls voluntary functions, and the *autonomic (involuntary) nervous system,* which controls all involuntary functions. The autonomic nervous system also has two components: the *sympathetic nervous system* and the *parasympathetic nervous system.*

The sympathetic nervous system tends to increase autonomic functions, whereas the parasympathetic nervous system tends to slow them down. The sympathetic nervous system allows the body to function under stress and is often referred to as the "fight-or-flight" aspect of the system. In contrast, the parasympathetic nervous system—or the "rest-and-repose" or "feed-and-breed" aspect of the system—primarily controls vegetative functions such as digestion of food.

The parasympathetic and sympathetic nervous systems work in constant opposition to control organ responses. For example, the sympathetic nervous system stimulates specific receptors in the heart that increase the heart rate. At the same time, the parasympathetic nervous system stimulates receptors that decrease the heart rate. The net result is the resting heart rate. When the body's physiologic needs dictate an increased heart rate, sympathetic stimuli dominate parasympathetic effects. Conversely, when the body needs to rest (with a decreased heart rate), parasympathetic stimuli predominate.

BASIC ANATOMY AND PHYSIOLOGY

The autonomic nervous system arises from the central nervous system. The nerves of the autonomic nervous system exit the central nervous system and subsequently enter specialized structures called **autonomic ganglia.** In the autonomic ganglia, the nerve fibers from the central nervous system interact with nerve fibers that extend from the ganglia to the various target organs. Autonomic nerve fibers that exit the central nervous system and terminate in the autonomic ganglia are called **pre-ganglionic nerves.** Autonomic nerve fibers that exit the ganglia and terminate in the various target tissues are called **post-ganglionic nerves.** The ganglia of the sympathetic nervous system are located close to the spinal cord, whereas the ganglia of the parasympathetic nervous system are located close to the target organs (Figure 2-73, page 168).

No actual physical connection exists between two nerve cells or between a nerve cell and the organ it innervates. Instead, there is a space, or synapse, between nerve cells. The space between a nerve cell and the target organ is a **neuroeffector junction.** Specialized chemicals called **neurotransmitters** conduct the nervous impulse between nerve cells or between a nerve cell and its target organ.

Neurotransmitters are released from presynaptic neurons and subsequently act on postsynaptic neurons or on the designated target organ. When released by the nerve ending, the neurotransmitter travels across the synapse and activates membrane receptors on the adjoining nerve or target tissue. The neurotransmitter is then either deactivated or taken back up into the presynaptic neuron.

The two neurotransmitters of the autonomic nervous system are acetylcholine and norepinephrine. Acetylcholine is utilized in the pre-ganglionic nerves of the sympathetic nervous system and in both the pre-ganglionic and post-ganglionic nerves of the parasympathetic nervous system. Norepinephrine is the post-ganglionic neurotransmitter of the sympathetic nervous system. Synapses that use acetylcholine as the neurotransmitter are **cholinergic** synapses. Synapses that use norepinephrine as the neurotransmitter are **adrenergic** synapses.

DRUGS USED TO AFFECT THE PARASYMPATHETIC NERVOUS SYSTEM

The parasympathetic system uses acetylcholine (ACh) as a neurotransmitter. Acetylcholine released by presynaptic neurons activates receptors on the postsynaptic neurons or on the neuroeffector junction. Receptors that are specialized for acetylcholine are termed cholinergic receptors. Medications that stimulate them are known as cholinergics (**parasympathomimetics**), and those that block them are known as anticholinergics or cholinergic blockers (**parasympatholytics**).

Cholinergics

Cholinergic drugs act either directly or indirectly. Direct-acting cholinergics (also called cholinergic esters) simulate the affects of acetylcholine by directly binding with the cholinergic receptors. Drugs in this class generally produce the same effects as cholinergic stimulation, mostly focused on the muscarinic receptors. Their adverse effects are related primarily to decreased heart rate, decreased peripheral vascular resistance resulting in hypotension and excessive salivation, urination, defecation, and sweating. Vomiting and abdominal cramps may also occur. The acronym SLUDGE (*s*alivation, *l*acrimation, *u*rination, *d*efecation, *g*astric motility, *e*mesis) is helpful for remembering these effects.

The prototype direct-acting cholinergic is bethanechol (Urecholine). Its pharmacokinetics make it a good clinical substitute for acetylcholine. It is not broken down by cholinesterase, the enzyme responsible for destroying acetylcholine, and therefore it has a longer duration of action. Most of its effects are on muscarinic receptors in the urinary bladder and GI tract. It may be given orally or subcutaneously. Thus, it is used primarily to increase micturition (urination) and peristalsis. Adverse effects are rare but related to its parasympathomimetic effects. Another direct-acting cholinergic medication, pilocarpine, is used as a topical treatment for glaucoma.

Indirect-acting cholinergic drugs affect acetylcholinesterase. By inhibiting its actions in degrading acetylcholine, they prolong the cholinergic response. These drugs affect both

---

autonomic ganglia groups of autonomic nerve cells located outside the central nervous system.

pre-ganglionic nerves nerve fibers that extend from the central nervous system to the autonomic ganglia.

post-ganglionic nerves nerve fibers that extend from the autonomic ganglia to the target tissues.

neuroeffector junction specialized synapse between a nerve cell and the organ or tissue it innervates.

neurotransmitter chemical messenger that conducts a nervous impulse across a synapse.

cholinergic pertaining to the neurotransmitter acetylcholine.

adrenergic pertaining to the neurotransmitter norepinephrine.

parasympathomimetic drug or other substance that causes effects like those of the parasympathetic nervous system. Also called *cholinergic*.

parasympatholytic drug or other substance that blocks or inhibits the actions of the parasympathetic nervous system. Also called *anticholinergic*.

Content Review

SLUDGE EFFECTS OF CHOLINERGIC MEDICATIONS
- Salivation
- Lacrimation
- Urination
- Defecation
- Gastric motility
- Emesis

muscarinic and nicotinic receptors and therefore have little specificity. Their uses are limited primarily to treating myasthenia gravis, some types of poisoning, and glaucoma as well as for reversing nondepolarizing neuromuscular blockade.

The two basic types of indirect-acting cholinergic drugs are reversible inhibitors and irreversible inhibitors. Both types bind with cholinesterase (ChE), acting as a substitute for acetylcholine. In doing so, they prevent cholinesterase from destroying acetylcholine. The difference between the reversible and irreversible inhibitors is how long they remain bound with cholinesterase. The reversible inhibitors remain bound with cholinesterase much longer than acetylcholine but eventually release it. The irreversible inhibitors, too, will eventually release cholinesterase, but they remain bound for so long that, from a practical standpoint, they can be considered irreversible.

Neostigmine (Prostigmin) is the prototype reversible cholinesterase inhibitor. It is used to treat myasthenia gravis, an illness characterized by muscle weakness and progressive fatigue. This illness is an autoimmune disease that destroys the nicotinic$_M$ receptors at the neuromuscular junction. With fewer of these receptors, muscles cannot be stimulated as well and weakness occurs. Neostigmine treats the symptoms of myasthenia gravis by blocking the degradation of acetylcholine, thereby prolonging its effects and increasing motor strength. Its primary side effects are due to the stimulation of muscarinic receptors and include the SLUDGE responses. Fortunately, these responses may be treated effectively with a cholinergic blocker. Neostigmine can also reverse a nondepolarizing neuromuscular blockade. This use is fairly uncommon, however, because such blockades typically are administered only intentionally as part of anesthesia or before intubation.

Physostigmine (Antilirium) is another reversible cholinesterase inhibitor. Its mechanism is similar to that of neostigmine, with their primary difference being in their pharmacokinetics. Although neostigmine is poorly absorbed across the cell membrane, physostigmine crosses rapidly and therefore has a shorter onset and may be given in lower doses. Physostigmine's chief use is for reversing overdoses of atropine, an anticholinergic drug that blocks muscarinic receptors.

Irreversible cholinesterase inhibitors have only one clinical function, the treatment of glaucoma, and only one drug, echothiophate (Phospholine Iodide), has been approved for that purpose. Cholinesterase inhibitors, however, are very useful as insecticides (organophosphates), and unfortunately, their mechanism of action is also very attractive for makers of chemical weapons. They are the chief component in nerve gases such as VX and sarin. They cause extensive stimulation of cholinergic receptors, ultimately resulting in the SLUDGE response. Toxic levels may also affect nicotinic$_M$ receptors, leading to paralysis. Treatment for such toxic exposures involves drugs such as high doses of atropine or pralidoxime (Protopam, 2-PAM) to block the effects of the accumulating acetylcholine. Pralidoxime can encourage irreversible cholinesterase inhibitors to release cholinesterase.

Anticholinergics

Anticholinergic agents oppose the parasympathetic (cholinergic) nervous system. Just as there are multiple types of cholinergic receptors, there are multiple classes of cholinergic receptor antagonists. We will discuss agents that selectively block muscarinic and nicotinic receptors as well as nonselective blockers (ganglionic blockers). A special subclass of nicotinic receptors is neuromuscular blocking drugs.

Muscarinic Cholinergic Antagonists   Cholinergic antagonists block the effects of acetylcholine almost exclusively at the muscarinic receptors. They are often called anticholinergics or parasympatholytics. They work by competitively binding with muscarinic receptors without stimulating them. As a result, these receptors cannot bind with acetylcholine.

The prototype anticholinergic drug is atropine, which is widely used to block muscarinic receptors and is commonly administered in the field. Found in the plant *Atropa belladonna,* atropine is one of several drugs classified as belladonna alkaloids (scopolamine is also in this classification). Readily absorbed through both enteral and parenteral routes, it has therapeutic effects at dose-dependent levels at most sites with muscarinic receptors. At low doses, atropine decreases secretion from salivary and bronchial glands as well as from the sympathetically innervated sweat glands. At moderate doses, it increases heart rate and causes mydriasis (dilated pupils) and blurry vision. At higher doses, it decreases gastric motility and stomach acid secretion. Atropine is also useful in reversing overdoses of muscarinic agonists (cholinergics or cholinesterase inhibitors). Its side effects, which are predictable, include dry mouth, blurred vision and photophobia, urinary retention, increased intraocular pressure, tachycardia, constipation, and anhidrosis (decreased sweating), which may cause hyperthermia. A helpful mnemonic for remembering the effects of atropine overdose is "hot as hell, blind as a bat, dry as a bone, red as a beet, mad as a hatter."

Scopolamine is another belladonna anticholinergic. Its actions are similar to atropine, but unlike atropine, scopolamine causes sedation and antiemesis. Thus, its primary purpose is to prevent motion sickness. It is available as a transdermal patch.

Several synthetic medications mimic the effects of the belladonna alkaloids while minimizing their side effects. Ipratropium bromide (Atrovent), an inhaled anticholinergic, is effective in treating asthma because it relaxes the bronchial smooth muscle and causes bronchodilation. It is frequently administered along with an inhaled beta-adrenergic agonist. Because it is inhaled and has little systemic effect, ipratropium bromide avoids many of atropine's side effects.

Other anticholinergic drugs include dicyclomine (Bentyl) and benztropine (Cogentin).

Nicotinic Cholinergic Antagonists Nicotinic cholinergic antagonists block acetylcholine only at nicotinic sites. They include ganglionic blocking agents that block the nicotinic$_N$ receptors in the autonomic ganglia and neuromuscular blocking agents that block nicotinic$_M$ receptors at the neuromuscular junction.

Ganglionic Blocking Agents

Ganglionic blockade is produced by competitive antagonism with acetylcholine at the nicotinic$_N$ receptors in the autonomic ganglia. This can, in effect, turn off the entire autonomic nervous system. The two drugs in this class are trimethaphan (Arfonad) and mecamylamine (Inversine). Both are used to treat hypertension. The adverse effects of ganglionic blockade include signs associated with antimuscarinic drugs such as atropine—dry mouth, blurred vision, urinary retention, and tachycardia. Other adverse effects arising from the vasodilation and decreased preload caused by sympathetic blockage include profound hypotension, with orthostatic hypotension even more evident. Trimethaphan is administered primarily for hypertensive crisis when other treatments are ineffective. These agents are almost never used anymore because they are not selective and many superior agents are available.

Neuromuscular Blocking Agents

Neuromuscular blockade produces a state of paralysis without affecting consciousness. Imagine how terrifying it would be to be fully conscious and aware but completely paralyzed, unable to move or breathe. Neuromuscular blockade is caused by competitive antagonism of nicotinic$_M$ receptors at the neuromuscular junction. This is useful during surgery as part of anesthesia and during electroconvulsive therapy for depression. These agents are most often used in the field to facilitate intubation.

Neuromuscular blocking agents are either depolarizing or nondepolarizing, depending on their mechanism of action. Most are nondepolarizing; only one depolarizing drug, succinylcholine (Anectine), is commonly used in the clinical setting. Tubocurarine, although not frequently used clinically, is the oldest neuromuscular blocker and the prototype nondepolarizing agent. It produces neuromuscular blockade by binding with the nicotinic$_M$ receptor sites without causing muscle depolarization. Succinylcholine acts in the same manner, but like acetylcholine, it does cause muscle depolarization when it binds with the nicotinic$_M$ receptor. It is useful as a neuromuscular blocker because, in contrast to acetylcholine, which rapidly separates from the receptor, it remains bound, preventing the muscle's repolarization. Several nondepolarizing agents are available; the specific agent chosen depends on its rate of onset and duration of action. Succinylcholine has the shortest onset and duration of action because it has a naturally occurring enzyme, pseudocholinesterase, which degrades it.

Ganglionic Stimulating Agents

Nicotinic$_N$ receptors reside at the ganglia of both the parasympathetic and sympathetic nervous systems. The alkaloid nicotine stimulates these receptors. Nicotine is found in tobacco and, although it has no therapeutic uses, is of interest for two reasons. Historically,

Content Review

EFFECTS OF ATROPINE OVERDOSE
- Hot as hell
- Blind as a bat
- Dry as a bone
- Red as a beet
- Mad as a hatter

Neuromuscular blockers affect nicotinic$_M$ receptors.

nicotine, along with muscarine, led to a much better understanding of the specific receptors in the autonomic nervous system. Also it is one of the most abused drugs in the world.

Nicotine may cause a variety of responses, most of which are dose related. At low doses, like those from smoking, nicotine causes excitation at the autonomic ganglia. This affects both the parasympathetic and sympathetic nervous systems. The parasympathetic response causes increased salivation, peristalsis, and secretion of gastric acid. The sympathetic response causes the release of norepinephrine and epinephrine. These lead to increases in heart rate, myocardial contractility, vasoconstriction, and blood pressure, all of which increase the heart's workload. Sympathetic stimulation also increases awareness and suppresses fatigue and appetite.

DRUGS USED TO AFFECT THE SYMPATHETIC NERVOUS SYSTEM

sympathomimetic drug or other substance that causes effects like those of the sympathetic nervous system. Also called *adrenergic.*

sympatholytic drug or other substance that blocks the actions of the sympathetic nervous system. Also call *antiadrenergic.*

Medications that stimulate the sympathetic nervous system are **sympathomimetics.** Medications that inhibit the sympathetic nervous system are called **sympatholytics.** Some medications are pure alpha agonists; others are pure alpha antagonists. Some medications are pure beta agonists; others are pure beta antagonists. Medications such as epinephrine stimulate both alpha and beta receptors. Other medications, such as the bronchodilators, are termed beta selective, since they act more on beta$_2$ receptors than on beta$_1$ receptors.

The sympathetic nervous system releases norepinephrine from post-ganglionic end terminals and epinephrine from the adrenal medulla. These neurotransmitters bind with adrenergic receptors. (Epinephrine is also called adrenalin because of its release from the adrenal medulla; hence the term *adren*-ergic). There are two main types of adrenergic receptors, each with two subtypes. These receptors' effects depend primarily on their locations. Table 3-3 describes the chief locations and primary actions of each receptor.

The primary clinical purpose for medications that stimulate alpha$_1$ receptors is peripheral vasoconstriction. Constriction of the arterioles increases afterload, whereas constriction of venules increases preload (decreasing venous capacitance or "pooling"). Both of these effects increase systolic and diastolic blood pressure and represent the chief therapeutic indication for alpha$_1$ agonists. Stimulation of alpha$_1$ receptors locally may be useful in combination with local anesthetics. The main reason to add the alpha$_1$ agonist in this context is to cause local vasoconstriction so that the systemic absorption of the anesthetic decreases, and its duration increases. Alpha$_1$ agonists are also useful topically to decrease nasal congestion caused by dilation and engorgement of nasal blood vessels. The primary adverse

Table 3-3 LOCATION OF ADRENERGIC RECEPTORS AND EFFECTS OF STIMULATION

Receptor	Response to Stimulation	Location
Alpha 1 (α_1)	Constriction	Arterioles
	Constriction	Veins
	Mydriasis	Eye
	Ejaculation	Penis
Alpha 2 (α_2)	Presynaptic terminals inhibition*	
Beta 1 (β_1)	Increased heart rate	Heart
	Increased conductivity	
	Increased automaticity	
	Increased contractility	
	Renin release	Kidney
Beta 2 (β_2)	Bronchodilation	Lungs
	Dilation	Arterioles
	Inhibition of contractions	Uterus
	Tremors	Skeletal muscle
Dopaminergic	Vasodilation (increased blood flow)	Kidney

*Stimulation of α_2 adrenergic receptors inhibits the continued release of norepinephrine from the presynaptic terminal. It is a feedback mechanism that limits the adrenergic response at that synapse. These receptors have no other identified peripheral effects.

responses to alpha$_1$ agonist agents are hypertension and local tissue necrosis. If a medication with significant alpha$_1$ properties infiltrates the surrounding tissue or distal body parts such as fingers, toes, earlobes or nose, inadequate local blood flow due to profound vasoconstriction will likely kill the tissue. Also, alpha$_1$ stimulation may cause reflex bradycardia due to the feedback mechanism that regulates blood pressure. As baroreceptors detect a rise in blood pressure, heart rate decreases to compensate.

Alpha$_1$ antagonism is indicated almost exclusively for controlling hypertension. By preventing the peripheral vasoconstriction of alpha$_1$ stimulation, these agents decrease blood pressure. They are also useful in treating local tissue necrosis caused by infiltration of alpha$_1$ agonists. Injecting alpha$_1$ antagonists into the area surrounding the infiltration prevents tissue death from excessive vasoconstriction. The effects of pheochromocytoma, a tumor of the adrenal medulla that causes the release of large amounts of catecholamine, may be treated with an alpha$_1$ blocker. The most common adverse effects of alpha$_1$ antagonism are orthostatic hypotension and reflex tachycardia. Just as alpha$_1$ stimulation may increase blood pressure and cause a baroreceptor-mediated bradycardia, the hypotension from alpha$_1$ blockage may lead to reflex tachycardia from the same mechanism. Other side effects include nasal congestion and inhibition of ejaculation. These agents may also increase blood volume. This is ironic, since their primary indication is hypertension. As another feedback mechanism detects hypotension, the kidneys begin to reabsorb sodium and water to increase blood volume. This is typically addressed by use of a diuretic concomitant with the alpha$_1$ antagonist.

Beta$_1$ stimulation increases heart rate, contractility, and conduction. Its primary indications are cardiac arrest and hypotension resulting from inadequate pumping. During cardiac arrest, beta$_1$ activation may stimulate contractions or increase the force of any existing contractions. Even if the heart is only fibrillating, these agents may increase the effectiveness of electrical defibrillation. In cardiogenic shock, when the heart is not pumping with enough force to overcome the afterload created by peripheral vascular resistance, beta$_1$ agonists can adequately increase the contractions' force. The chief adverse effects of beta$_1$ agonists include tachycardia, dysrhythmias, and chest pain from increasing work load.

Beta$_1$ antagonists are among the most frequently prescribed medications in the United States. Their most common use is to control blood pressure. By blocking the effects of beta$_1$ stimulation, they decrease heart rate (chronotropy) and contractility (inotropy). These agents are also effective in treating supraventricular tachycardias because they decrease the rate of impulse generation at the SA node (negative chronotropic effects) while also slowing conductivity through the AV node (negative dromotropic effects). Blocking beta$_1$ stimulation also helps treat angina pectoris and reduces the recurrence of myocardial infarction. Its main adverse effects are symptomatic bradycardia, hypotension, and AV block.

Beta$_2$ agonists are used to treat asthma and other conditions with excessive narrowing of the bronchioles. By stimulating beta$_2$ receptors in the lungs, these agents relax the bronchial smooth muscle and cause bronchodilation. Beta$_2$ agonists can also cause uterine smooth muscle relaxation, which may help to suppress preterm labor. Their primary adverse effects are muscle tremors and "bleed over" effects on unintended beta$_1$ stimulation such as tachycardias.

Although beta$_2$ blockade serves no clinically useful purpose, nonselective beta blockers have side effects of beta$_2$ blockade. Chief among these is bronchoconstriction and inhibition of glycogenolysis, the release of stored glycogen by the liver and skeletal muscles. Beta$_2$ stimulation causes glycogenesis. Antagonizing the beta$_2$ receptors can inhibit this release. This is not typically a problem for most people, but it can be very problematic for diabetics. It not only makes hypoglycemia more likely but also masks one of its common early warning signs, tachycardia.

Adrenergic Agonists

Drugs that stimulate the effects of adrenergic receptors work either directly, indirectly, or through a combination of the two. The direct-acting agents bind with the receptor and cause the same response as the normal neurotransmitter. In fact, most of the drugs in this category either are synthetically produced versions of the naturally occurring neurotransmitter or are

Phentolamine (Regitine), an alpha antagonist, can be used to help minimize tissue necrosis following extravasation of an alpha$_1$ agonist such as dopamine or norepinephrine.

Content Review

COMMON CATECHOLAMINES

- Natural
  - Epinephrine
  - Norepinephrine
  - Dopamine
- Synthetic
  - Isoproterenol
  - Dobutamine

Patho Pearls

Many of the adrenergic agonists, particularly the decongestants and respiratory drugs, can result in tachyphylaxis. That is, repeated doses of the same drug have decreased effects. In these cases, it may be prudent to change to a similar drug in the same family. The effects of a different drug can often be significantly better.

derivatives of those synthetically produced versions. The indirect-acting agents stimulate the release of epinephrine from the adrenal medulla and of norepinephrine from the presynaptic terminals. In turn, the epinephrine and norepinephrine stimulate the adrenergic receptors. The mixed actions of direct–indirect acting medications combine these mechanisms.

The most frequently used adrenergic agents are chemically and functionally similar to the endogenous neurotransmitters. These drugs, which are called catecholamines, include norepinephrine, epinephrine, and dopamine. Synthetic catecholamines are also available. They include dobutamine and isoproterenol. Noncatecholamine adrenergic agents, including ephedrine, phenylephrine, and terbutaline, also affect the adrenergic receptors and have useful clinical applications.

Almost all of the drugs in this section act on more than one type of receptor. Their specificity varies and is important in determining their uses. Table 3-4 lists their actions on various receptors.

Adrenergic Antagonists

Unlike most adrenergic agonists, the majority of available adrenergic antagonists are remarkably selective in which receptor they affect. This selectivity, however, occurs only at therapeutic doses. At higher doses, most agents lose their selectivity and begin affecting other receptors as well.

The two basic subcategories of alpha-adrenergic antagonists are "noncompetitive, long-acting" and "competitive, short-acting." They differ chiefly in the stability of their bond with the receptor. The prototype noncompetitive, long-acting alpha antagonist is phenoxybenzamine (Dibenzyline). The prototype competitive, short-acting antagonist is prazosin (Minipress). Prazosin also is the prototype for all alpha-adrenergic antagonists. Phentolamine (Regitine) is an important nonselective alpha antagonist because of its effects in reversing tissue necrosis caused by catecholamine infiltration.

Beta-adrenergic antagonists are more commonly referred to as beta blockers. Propranolol (Inderal) is the prototype beta blocker. It is a nonselective antagonist, which means that it blocks both $beta_1$ and $beta_2$ receptors. It is used to treat tachycardia, hypertension, and angina, all results of $beta_1$ blockade. Because it is nonselective, it also has the side effects of $beta_2$ blockade—bronchoconstriction and inhibited glycogenolysis. Propranolol was the first clinically employed beta blocker, but its use has declined since the development of more selective $beta_1$ antagonists. The prototype of these cardioselective beta blockers is metoprolol (Lopressor). At normal doses, metoprolol is selective for only $beta_1$ receptors; therefore, it does not cause propranolol's problematic side effects for asthmatics and diabetics. Atenolol (Tenormin) is another commonly used cardioselective beta blocker.

Table 3-4 ADRENERGIC RECEPTOR SPECIFICITY

Medication	Receptor				
	Alpha$_1$	Alpha$_2$	Beta$_1$	Beta$_2$	Dopaminergic
Phenylephrine	✔				
Norepinephrine	✔	✔	✔		
Ephedrine	✔	✔	✔	✔	
Epinephrine	✔	✔	✔	✔	
Dobutamine			✔		
Dopamine*			✔		✔
Isoproterenol			✔	✔	
Terbutaline				✔	

*Receptor specificity is dose-dependent. The higher the dose, the less dopaminergic effects are seen.

Part 3: EMT-Intermediate Medications

ACETYLSALICYLIC ACID (ASA)—ASPIRIN

Class: Analgesic. Inhibitor of platelet function. Anti-inflammatory.

Actions: Blocks platelet aggregation.

Indications: Chest pain suggestive of myocardial ischemia. Signs and symptoms suggestive of recent ischemic stroke.

Contraindications: Patients with a known hypersensitivity to the drug.

Precautions: GI bleeding and upset stomach.

Side Effects: Heartburn; nausea and vomiting.

Dosage: 160 mg or 325 mg by mouth (chewed).

Onset: 5 to 30 minutes

Peak Effects: 15 minutes to 2 hours

Route: Oral

Pediatric Dosage: Not recommended

ADENOSINE (ADENOCARD)

Class: Antidysrhythmic

Actions: Slows atrioventricular conduction.
   Can interrupt reentrant pathways through the atrioventricular node.
   Slows sinoatrial node rate.

Indications: Symptomatic paroxysmal supraventricular tachycardia (including those caused by Wolff-Parkinson-White syndrome).

Contraindications: Second- or third-degree heart block.
   Sick sinus syndrome.
   Known hypersensitivity to the drug.

Precautions: Arrhythmias, including blocks, are common at the time of cardioversion.
   Hypotension.
   Use with caution in asthmatic patients.
   Side effects are usually short-lived and better tolerated by the patient if they are informed of possible side effects prior to administration of the drug.

Side Effects: Facial flushing, headache, chest pain, shortness of breath, dizziness, nausea. Asystolic period following administration.

Dosage: 6 mg given as a rapid IV bolus over a 1- to 2-second period; if, after 1 to 2 minutes, cardioversion does not occur, administer a 12 mg dose over 1 to 2 seconds. If unsuccessful, a third dose of 12 mg can be administered 1 to 2 minutes later.

Onset: Within 20 to 30 seconds

Peak Effects: Within 20 to 30 seconds

Route: IV; should be administered directly into a vein or into the medication administration port closest to the patient and followed by flushing of the line with IV fluid.

Pediatric Dosage: 0.1 mg/kg rapid IV push followed by saline flush.
   May double (0.2 mg/kg), if second dose needed.
   Maximum first dose: 6 mg
   Maximum second dose: 12 mg
   Maximum single dose: 12 mg

AMIODARONE (CORDARONE)

Class: Antidysrhythmic

Actions: Prolongs the duration of the action potential and refractory period.
   Acts on all cardiac tissues.
   Blocks sympathetic stimulation.

Indications: Life-threatening ventricular and supraventricular dysrhythmias such as ventricular fibrillation (VF) and ventricular tachycardia (VT).

Contraindications: Severe sinoatrial (SA) node dysfunction.
   Second- and third-degree AV block.
   Hemodynamically significant bradycardia.

Precautions: Heart failure.

Side Effects: Nausea, hypotension, anorexia, malaise, fatigue, tremors, pulmonary toxicity, ventricular ectopic beats.

Dosage: Cardiac arrest from VF and VT: 300 mg.
   Recurrent VF or VT: 150 mg.
   Maximum Dose: 2.2 grams over 24 hours.

Onset: Immediate

Peak Effects: 30 to 45 minutes

Route: IV

Pediatric Dosage: 5 mg/kg IV (maximum dose: 15 mg/kg)

ATROPINE SULFATE

Class: Parasympatholytic (anticholinergic)

Actions: Blocks acetylcholine receptors. Increases heart rate. Decreases gastric secretions.

Indications: To increase heart rate and cardiac output in symptomatic bradycardia.
   Bradyasystolic cardiac arrest.
   Antidote for organophosphate poisoning.

Contraindications: None in the emergency setting.

Precautions: Use with caution in patients with signs of myocardial ischemia.

Side Effects: Palpitations, tachycardia, headache, dizziness, anxiety, dry mouth, pupillary dilation, blurred vision, urinary retention (especially in older men).

Dosage: Symptomatic bradycardia: 0.5 to 1.0 mg IVP (may repeat in 3 to 5 minutes to a maximum of 0.04 mg/kg).
   Bradyasystolic arrest: 1.0 mg IVP (may repeat every 3 to 5 minutes to maximum of 0.04 mg/kg).
   Organophosphate poisoning: 2 to 5 mg IV or IM every 10 to 15 minutes.

Onset: 30 to 90 seconds

Peak Effects: 20 to 60 minutes

Route: IV

Pediatric Dosage: 0.02 mg/kg IV (Minimum dose is 0.1 mg.)

BRONCHODILATORS

BETA AGONISTS

Beta agonists are the mainstay of acute therapy for asthma, emphysema, chronic bronchitis, and other forms of obstructive respiratory disease. The beta agonists are all chemically related to epinephrine. Thus, they act on adrenergic receptors. The drugs used in respiratory care are selective for $beta_2$ adrenergic receptors found primarily in pulmonary tissues. This serves to decrease the side effects such as palpitations and tremulousness. The respiratory beta agonists primarily differ in their onset of action, duration of effect, and tendency to cause side effects.

ALBUTEROL (VENTOLIN, PROVENTIL)

Class: Sympathomimetic bronchodilator

Actions: Selective $beta_2$ adrenergic agonist that causes relaxation of bronchial smooth muscle, thus decreasing airway resistance and increasing vital capacity.

Indications: Bronchospasm associated with reversible obstructive airway disease (asthma, chronic bronchitis, emphysema).

Contraindications: Patients with known hypersensitivity to drug.

Precautions: Use with caution in patients with cardiac ischemia.
Try to measure peak flow before and after treatment.

Side Effects: Tremors, anxiety, dizziness, headache, insomnia, nausea, palpitations, tachycardia, hypertension.

Dosage: Metered-dose inhaler: 90 mcg (two sprays).
Nebulizer: 2.5 mg in 2.5 to 3.0 mL normal saline. Repeat as needed.

Onset: 5 to 15 minutes

Peak Effects: 1 to 1.5 hours

Route: Inhalation

Pediatric Dosage: 0.15 mg/kg in 2.5 to 3.0 mL normal saline via nebulizer. Repeat as needed.

LEVALBUTEROL (XOPENEX)

Class: Sympathomimetic bronchodilator

Actions: Selective $beta_2$ adrenergic agonist that causes relaxation of bronchial smooth muscle thus decreasing airway resistance and increasing vital capacity. Levalbuterol is a chemical variant of albuterol with greater affinity for the $beta_2$ adrenergic receptors.

Indications: Bronchospasm associated with reversible obstructive airway disease (asthma, chronic bronchitis, emphysema).

Contraindications: Patients with known hypersensitivity to the drug.

Precautions: Use with caution in patients with cardiac ischemia.
Try to measure peak flow before and after treatment.

Side Effects: Tremors, anxiety, dizziness, headache, insomnia, nausea, palpitations, tachycardia, hypertension.

Dosage: Nebulizer: 0.63 mg in 3.0 mL normal saline every 6 to 8 hours.

Onset: 5 to 15 minutes

Peak Effects: 1 to 1.5 hours

Route: Inhalation

Pediatric Dosage: <12 years: 0.31 mg in 3.0 mL normal saline three times a day.

ISOETHARINE (BRONKOSOL)

Class: Sympathomimetic bronchodilator

Actions: Selective beta$_2$ adrenergic agonist that causes relaxation of bronchial smooth muscle, thus decreasing airway resistance and increasing vital capacity.

Indications: Bronchospasm associated with reversible obstructive airway disease (asthma, chronic bronchitis, emphysema).

Contraindications: Patients with known hypersensitivity to the drug.

Precautions: Use with caution in patients with cardiac ischemia. Try to measure peak flow before and after treatment.

Side Effects: Tremors, anxiety, dizziness, headache, insomnia, nausea, palpitations, tachycardia, hypertension.

Dosage: Metered-dose inhaler: 1 to 2 inhalations.
Nebulizer: 0.5 mL in 2 to 3 mL normal saline. Repeat as needed.

Onset: Immediate

Peak Effects: 5 to 15 minutes

Route: Inhalation

Pediatric Dosage: 0.01 mL/kg of 1% solution (maximum 0.5 mL) diluted in 2 to 3 mL normal saline.

METAPROTERENOL (ALUPENT)

Class: Sympathomimetic bronchodilator

Actions: Selective beta$_2$ adrenergic agonist that causes relaxation of bronchial smooth muscle thus decreasing airway resistance and increasing vital capacity.

Indications: Bronchospasm associated with reversible obstructive airway disease (asthma, chronic bronchitis, emphysema).

Contraindications: Patients with known hypersensitivity to the drug.

Precautions: Use with caution in patients with cardiac ischemia. Try to measure peak flow before and after treatment.

Side Effects: Tremors, anxiety, dizziness, headache, insomnia, nausea, palpitations, tachycardia, hypertension.

Dosage: Metered-dose inhaler: 0.65 mg (2 sprays).
   Nebulizer: 0.2 to 0.3 mL in 2.5 to 3.0 mL normal saline.

Onset: 1 minute

Peak Effects: 1 hour

Route: Inhalation

Pediatric Dosage: 0.1 to 0.2 mL/kg of 5% solution in 2.5 to 3.0 mL normal saline.

TERBUTALINE

Class: Sympathomimetic bronchodilator

Actions: Selective beta$_2$ adrenergic agonist that causes relaxation of bronchial smooth muscle, thus decreasing airway resistance and increasing vital capacity.

Indications: Bronchospasm associated with reversible obstructive airway disease (asthma, chronic bronchitis, emphysema). To suppress preterm labor.

Contraindications: Patients with known hypersensitivity to the drug.

Precautions: Use with caution in patients with cardiac ischemia. Try to measure peak flow before and after treatment.

Side Effects: Tremors, anxiety, dizziness, headache, insomnia, nausea, palpitations, tachycardia, hypertension.

Dosage: Subcutaneous: 0.25 mg every 15 to 30 minutes up to 0.5 mg in 4 hours.
   Metered-dose inhaler: 2 sprays 60 seconds apart

Onset: <15 minutes

Peak Effects: 30 to 60 minutes

Route: Subcutaneous Inhalation

Pediatric Dosage: Subcutaneous: 0.005 to 0.01 mg/kg (max 0.4 mg) every 15 to 20 minutes up to 2 doses.

PARASYMPATHOLYTICS

Parasympatholytic agents inhibit actions of the parasympathetic nervous system. When stimulated, the parasympathetic nervous system causes bronchoconstriction and an increase in bronchial and airway secretions. Parasympatholytic agents block these effects and cause bronchodilation and drying of airway secretions through a mechanism different than those of the beta agonists.

IPRATROPIUM (ATROVENT)

Class: Parasympatholytic bronchodilator

Actions: Anticholinergic agent, chemically related to atropine, which acts directly on bronchial smooth muscle causing bronchodilation. It also dries airway secretions.

Indications: Bronchospasm associated with reversible obstructive airway disease (asthma, chronic bronchitis, emphysema) and acute attacks of bronchospasm.

Contraindications: Persons with known hypersensitivity to the drug or atropine.

Precautions: Should not be used as primary treatment of bronchospasm. It should be used in conjunction with beta agonists or similar bronchodilators.

Side Effects: Blurred vision, bitter taste, dry mouth, nausea, constipation, hoarseness, urinary retention.

Dosage: Metered-dose inhaler: 2 sprays.
    Nebulizer: 0.5 mg in 2.5 to 3.0 mL normal saline.

Onset: 5 to 15 minutes

Peak Effects: 1.5 to 2.0 hours

Route: Inhalation

Pediatric Dosage: 0.125 to 0.250 mg in 2.5 to 3.0 mL of normal saline, or 1 to 2 inhalations from metered-dose inhaler.

DEXTROSE—50% (D50W)

Class: Carbohydrate

Actions: Dextrose (*d-glucose*) is the principal form of sugar used by the body to create energy.

Indications: To increased blood sugar levels in documented hypoglycemia.

Contraindications: None in a patient with documented hypoglycemia.

Precautions: Can cause tissue damage and necrosis at injection site. Can cause severe neurological symptoms (Wernicke's encephalopathy, Korsakoff's psychosis) in patients who are thiamine deficient.

Side Effects: Warmth or pain at injection site.

Dosage: 25 grams IV push

Onset: <1 minute

Peak Effects: Variable

Route: IV

Pediatric Dosage: 2 mL/kg of 25% solution (D25W)

DIAZEPAM (VALIUM)

Class: Sedative-hypnotic, anticonvulsant, anti-anxiety (benzodiazepine)

Actions: Exact sedative mechanism unknown.
    Suppresses spread of seizure activity across the motor cortex.

Indications: Status epilepticus.
    Acute anxiety.
    Premedication for painful procedures.

Contraindications: Patients with hypersensitivity to the drug. Shock. Coma.

Precautions: Use IV diazepam with extreme caution in the elderly, the very ill, and patients with COPD.

Side Effects: Drowsiness, fatigue, confusion, dizziness, hypotension, tachycardia, blurred vision, nausea, respiratory depression.

Dosage: Seizures: 5 to 10 mg IV/IM
    Anxiety: 2 to 5 mg IM
    Premedication: 5 to 15 mg IV

Onset: 1 to 5 minutes (IV)

Peak Effects: 15 minutes (IM)

Route: IV, IM

Pediatric Dosage: Seizures: 0.5 to 2.0 mg IV/IM
  Anxiety: 0.5 to 2.0 mg IM
  Premedication: 0.2 to 0.5 mg/kg IV

DIPHENHYDRAMINE (BENADRYL)

Class: Antihistamine (H_1 receptor antagonist)

Actions: Blocks H_1 histamine receptors with significant anticholinergic activities.

Indications: Allergic conditions.
  Anaphylaxis (after epinephrine).
  Extrapyramidal reactions.

Contraindications: Hypersensitivity to the drug or similar drugs.
  Pregnancy.

Precautions: Use with caution in asthma, seizure disorders, hypertension, and in older adults and young children.

Side Effects: Drowsiness, dizziness, disturbed coordination, palpitations, tachycardia, dry mouth, urinary retention, wheezing.

Dosage: 25 to 50 mg IM/IV

Onset: 15 to 30 minutes

Peak Effects: 1 to 4 hours

Route: IV/IM

Pediatric Dosage: 2 to 6 years: 6.25 mg IV/IM
  6 to 12 years: 12.5 to 25 mg IV/IM

EPINEPHRINE 1:1,000

Class: Sympathomimetic

Actions: Acts on both alpha and beta adrenergic receptors and imitates the actions of the sympathetic nervous system. Epinephrine 1:1,000 contains 1 milligram of epinephrine in 1 mL of solvent.

Indications: Allergic reactions.
  Reversible bronchospasm associated with asthma, chronic bronchitis, and emphysema.

Contraindications: Patients with hypersensitivity to the drug.

Precautions: Avoid accidental IV injection.
  Repeated injections can cause tissue necrosis.

Side Effects: Nervousness, restlessness, anxiety, tremors, palpitations, hypertension, MI, dysrhythmias, nausea, vomiting.

Dosage: 0.3 to 0.5 mg SQ

Onset: 3 to 10 minutes

Peak Effects: 20 minutes

Route: Subcutaneous

Pediatric Dosage: 0.01 mg/kg SQ

EPINEPHRINE 1:10,000

Class: Sympathomimetic

Actions: Acts on both alpha- and beta-adrenergic receptors and imitates the actions of sympathetic nervous system. Epinephrine 1:10,000 contains 1 mg of epinephrine in 10 mL of solvent.

Indications: Cardiac arrest.
Severe anaphylaxis.

Contraindications: Patients with hypersensitivity to the drug.

Precautions: Repeated injections can cause tissue necrosis.
Monitor vital signs and ECG.

Side Effects: Nervousness, restlessness, anxiety, tremors, palpitations, hypertension, MI, dysrhythmias, nausea, vomiting.

Dosage: Cardiac arrest: 1 mg IV every 3 to 5 minutes. 2 to 2.5 mg of epinephrine 1:1,000 diluted in 10 mL normal saline via ET tube.

Onset: < 2 minutes

Peak Effects: < 5 minutes

Route: IV, ET, IO

Pediatric Dosage: Cardiac arrest: 0.01 mg/kg epinephrine 1:10,000 IV/IO for initial dose. For subsequent doses: 0.1 mg/kg epinephrine 1:1,000 IV/IO.

FUROSEMIDE (LASIX)

Class: Loop diuretic

Actions: Inhibits reabsorption of sodium and chloride in the Loop of Henle.
Venodilator thus decreasing cardiac preload.

Indications: Acute pulmonary edema.
Congestive heart failure.

Contraindications: Patients with known hypersensitivity to the drug or to the sulfonamides.

Precautions: Use with caution in infants, elderly patients, and cardiogenic shock associated with MI.

Side Effects: Postural hypotension, dizziness, fluid and electrolyte imbalances, nausea, pruritis.

Dosage: 40 to 120 mg IV

Onset: Vasodilation: 5 to 10 minutes
Diuresis: 5 to 30 minutes

Peak Effects: Vasodilation: 30 minutes
Diuresis: 20 to 60 minutes

Route: IV, IM

Pediatric Dosage: 1 mg/kg slow IV

GLUCAGON

Class: Hormone

Actions: Increases blood glucose level by causing breakdown and release of stored glycogen and inhibiting the conversion of glucose to glycogen.

Increases heart rate, AV conduction, and myocardial contractility in a manner similar to catecholamines, but through a different mechanism.

Indications: Hypoglycemia. Beta blocker overdose.

Contraindications: Patients with known hypersensitivity to the drug.

Precautions: May be ineffective in patients with inadequate liver glycogen stores (i.e., alcoholism, malnutrition).

Side Effects: Dizziness, hypotension, nausea and vomiting.

Dosage: Hypoglycemia: 1.0 mg IM/SQ, may repeat every 15 to 20 minutes.

Beta blocker overdose: 50 to 150 mcg/kg IV over 1 minute.

Onset: 5 to 20 minutes

Peak Effects: 30 minutes

Route: IV, IM, SQ

Pediatric Dosage: Hypoglycemia: Neonates/infants: 0.025–0.3 mg/kg IM/IV/SC (max. dose 1 mg). Children: 0.03–0.1 mg/kg IM/IV/SC (max. dose 1 mg).

Beta blocker overdose: 50 to 150 mcg/kg IV over 1 minute.

LIDOCAINE (XYLOCAINE)

Class: Antidysrhythmic

Actions: Suppresses automaticity in the His/Purkinje system.
Elevates threshold for ventricular dysrhythmias.
Lowers threshold for defibrillation and cardioversion.

Indications: To convert ventricular fibrillation and ventricular tachycardia in cardiac arrest to a sinus rhythm.

To convert ventricular tachycardia with pulse to a sinus rhythm.

Contraindications: Patients with a history of hypersensitivity to the drug. Supraventricular dysrhythmias. High-grade heart blocks. Sinus bradycardia.

Precautions: Use with caution in patients with renal or liver disease, CHF, marked hypoxia, respiratory depression, and shock.

Side Effects: Drowsiness, dizziness, restlessness, confusion, bradycardia, conduction disorders, blurred vision, nausea, vomiting.

Dosage: VF/VT cardiac arrest: 1.0 to 1.5 mg/kg IV. Repeat every 3 to 5 minutes as needed up to 3 mg/kg. Following conversion, begin infusion at 2 to 4 mg/minute.

VT with pulse: 1.0 to 1.5 mg/kg slow IV. May repeat at one-half dose every 5 to 10 minutes until conversion (up to 3 mg/kg). Following conversion, begin infusion at 2 to 4 mg/minute.

Onset: < 3 minutes

Peak Effects: 5 to 7 minutes

Route: IV (bolus and infusion)

Pediatric Dosage: VF/VT cardiac arrest: 1 mg/kg IV. Repeat every 3 to 5 minutes as needed up to 3 mg/kg. Following cardioversion, begin infusion at 20 to 50 mcg/kg/minute. VT with pulse: 1.0 mg/kg IV followed by infusion at 20 to 50 mcg/kg/minute.

MORPHINE SULFATE

Class: Narcotic analgesic

Actions: Acts on opiate receptors in the brain that cause analgesia and sedation.

Indications: Moderate to severe pain.
To reduce preload in acute MI and pulmonary edema.

Contraindications: Known hypersensitivity to opiates.
Undiagnosed head injury.

Precautions: Do not administer to patients who are hypotensive or volume depleted.
Do not use in asthma, COPD, or severe respiratory failure.

Side Effects: Sedation, rash, respiratory depression, dysphoria, bradycardia, syncope, constipation, dry mouth.

Dosage: Pain: 2.5 to 15 mg IV; 5 to 20 mg IM/SQ.
To decrease preload: 1 to 2 mg IV every 5 to 6 minutes as needed.

Onset: IV (immediate)
IM (15 to 30 minutes)

Peak Effects: IV (20 minutes)
IM (30 to 60 minutes)

Route: IV, IM, SQ

Pediatric Dosage: 0.1 to 0.2 mg/kg IM/SC

NALOXONE (NARCAN)

Class: Narcotic antagonist

Actions: Blocks opiate receptors thus negating effects of opiates.

Indications: Narcotic overdose.

Contraindications: Patient hypersensitivity to the drug.
Do not use in non–opiate-induced respiratory depression.

Precautions: Titrate the dose to increase respirations.
Giving a large dose will induce an acute narcotic withdrawal syndrome.

Side Effects: Primarily due to narcotic withdrawal (tremors, agitation, runny nose, diarrhea).

Dosage: 0.4 to 2.0 mg IV/IM (2.0 to 2.5 times dose for ET). May be repeated every 2 to 3 minutes up to 10 mg.

Onset: IV: <2 minutes
IM/ET: 2 to 10 minutes

Peak Effects: IV: <2 minutes
IM/ET: 2 to 10 minutes

Route: IV, IM/ET

Pediatric Dosage: 0.01 mg/kg IV/IM (2.0 to 2.5 times dose ET). May be repeated every 2 to 3 minutes up to 10 mg.

NITROGLYCERIN (NITROSTAT)

Class: Nitrate

Actions: Potent vasodilator with anti-anginal, anti-ischemic, and antihypertensive effects.

Indications: To increase coronary perfusion and decrease chest pain in angina and MI. To reduce preload in acute pulmonary edema.

Contraindications: Patients with hypersensitivity to the drug.

Precautions: Use with caution in patients with head injuries, increased intracranial pressure, shock, and patients taking sildenafil (Viagra).

Side Effects: Headache, dizziness, postural hypotension, tachycardia, nausea, vomiting.

Dosage: 0.4 mg SL. May repeat every 3 to 5 minutes up to 3 tablets.
$\frac{1}{2}$ to 1 inch of ointment applied to chest wall.
0.4 mg (1 spray). May repeat every 3 to 5 minutes up to 3 sprays.

Onset: SL: 1 to 3 minutes
Topical: 20 to 30 minutes

Peak Effects: SL: 5 to 10 minutes
Topical: 1 to 4 hours

Route: SL, topical, sublingual spray

Pediatric Dosage: Not indicated

VASOPRESSIN (PITRESSIN)

Class: Hormone

Actions: Inhibits water secretion in the kidney.
Potent vasoconstrictor in higher doses (non-adrenergic).

Indications: To increase peripheral vascular resistance in CPR (as an alternative to epinephrine or after epinephrine has been used).

Contraindications: None in the emergency setting.

Precautions: Few in the emergency setting.

Side Effects: Infrequent with low dose.

Dosage: Cardiac arrest: 40 IU IV (single-dose only)

Onset: 5 minutes

Peak Effects: 10 to 20 minutes

Route: IV

Pediatric Dosage: Not indicated

Pharmacology is a cornerstone of prehospital practice. As an EMT-I, you must have a solid understanding of its foundations (legal issues, terminology, drug forms, and routes), pharmacokinetics, and pharmacodynamics if you are to practice your profession safely. Additionally, as an EMT-I, you must understand not only the medications you personally administer, but also the medications that your patients are taking on an ongoing basis. Although you are not likely to remember everything in this chapter after only one reading—with diligent study and practice—you can master this information.

This chapter has barely broken the surface of pharmacology. To continue your education, you should take the time to understand the mechanisms and interactions of the medications your patients are taking. If you do not already know them (you will not in the majority of cases as you begin your career), look them up. Many very useful drug references are available today. Most are small and can be easily carried with you on your unit or in your station.

Finally, pharmacology is a dynamic field with new discoveries being made every day. If you take your responsibilities as an EMT-I seriously and remain current on the latest changes in this field, you can be sure that you can give your patients the care they deserve. Please refer to the *Drug Guide for Paramedics* that is available from Brady.

ON THE WEB

For additional practice and review, go to the companion website at www.prenhall.com/bledsoe and click on *Intermediate Emergency Care: Principles & Practice*.

CHAPTER 4

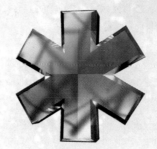

Venous Access and Medication Administration

Objectives

Part 1: Principles and Routes of Medication Administration (begins on page 274)

After reading Part 1 of this chapter, you should be able to:

1. Review the specific anatomy and physiology pertinent to medication administration. (pp. 274–303)
2. Discuss the legal aspects of medication administration, including the "six rights" of drug administration. (pp. 274–276)
3. Discuss medical asepsis, the differences between clean and sterile techniques, the use of antiseptics and disinfectants. (pp. 275–276)
4. Describe how body substance isolation (BSI) precautions relate to medication administration. (p. 275)
5. Describe the indications, equipment, techniques, precautions, and general principles of administering medications by the inhalation route. (pp. 280–283).
6. Differentiate among the different dosage forms of oral medications, and describe the

equipment and general principles of their administration. (pp. 284–288)
7. Describe the indications, equipment, techniques, precautions, and general principles of rectal medication administration. (pp. 288–298)
8. Describe the equipment, techniques, complications, and general principles for the preparation and administration of parenteral medications. (pp. 289–303)
9. Describe proper disposal of contaminated items and sharps. (p. 276)
10. Synthesize a pharmacological management plan including medication administration. (pp. 273–275)
11. Integrate pathophysiological principles of medication administration with patient management. (pp. 273–275)

Continued

Part 2: Intravenous Access, Blood Sampling, and Intraosseous Infusion (begins on page 303)

After reading Part 2 of this chapter, you should be able to:

1. Describe the indications, equipment, techniques, precautions, and general principles of peripheral venous cannulation. (pp. 303–330)
2. Describe the indications, equipment, techniques, precautions, and general principles of

intraosseous needle placement and infusion. (pp. 333–339)

3. Describe the purpose, equipment, techniques, complications, and general principles for obtaining a blood sample. (pp. 330–333)

Part 3: Medical Mathematics (begins on page 339)

After reading Part 3 of this chapter, you should be able to:

1. Review mathematical principles, equivalents, and conversions (pp. 339–342)
2. Calculate oral and parenteral drug dosages for all emergency medications administered

to adults, infants, and children. (pp. 343–345)

3. Calculate intravenous infusion rates for adults, infants, and children. (pp. 345–346)

CASE STUDY

It is early February, and clouds heavy with snow loom not far in the distance. EMT-I Susan Adams watches the sky and hopes that her shift will end before the storm hits. Suddenly the tones drop, alerting her and her partner, EMT-I Todd Michaels, to a 28-year-old female patient with shortness of breath. After acknowledging the call and confirming the location in the map book, Susan and Todd get under way. In preparation, Susan dons gloves and eye protection. Additionally, she reviews the likely causes of shortness of breath in a 28-year-old patient.

As Susan and Todd pull up to the residence, they observe a well-kept house. A woman frantically waves them inside, shouting that her daughter cannot breathe. Quickly, they grab the airway kit, cardiac monitor, and drug bag and then cautiously enter the residence.

Once inside, Susan and Todd begin to size up the scene. Immediately to their left, they find the female patient seated on a chair in a tripod position. Quick observation reveals her to be in considerable respiratory distress and exhibiting cyanosis around the lips and in the extremities. Even without a stethoscope, Susan detects expiratory wheezing.

Susan promptly introduces herself and Todd to the patient and asks what is wrong. The patient can barely talk, and Susan cannot obtain a specific chief complaint. Recognizing a life-threatening situation, she gains consent for treatment and turns her attention to the initial assessment.

The patient is responsive but exhibits lethargy and fatigue from hypoxia and the increased work of breathing. Inspection of the oral cavity reveals no foreign bodies or other obstructions. Susan deems the patient able to maintain her airway and foregoes a nasopharyngeal airway adjunct.

The patient presents tachypneic at 36 breaths per minute. Tidal and minute volume are shallow. Todd obtains a pulse oximetry reading of 86% on room air. A quick two-point auscultation reveals expiratory wheezing in the upper lobes of both the right and left lungs. The patient will not tolerate the assistance of ventilations with a bag-valve mask, so Susan applies a nonrebreathing face mask with 15 liters per minute of supplemental oxygen.

Without missing a beat, Susan proceeds to evaluate the circulatory system. The patient's radial pulse is weak and rapid, with accompanying cool, diaphoretic skin. Again Susan notes cyanosis.

Realizing the situation is critical, Susan turns to the patient's mother as Todd applies the cardiac monitor and obtains vital signs. When Susan asks about a history of asthma, the mother confirms it and adds that this partic-

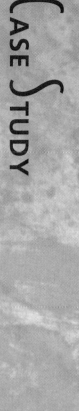
ular episode has been occurring over the past day and a half. Her daughter's metered dose inhaler of Alupent has not provided relief as it has in the past. Aside from the Alupent and asthma, the patient has no other medical history. She has no allergies and has not eaten or drunk anything today.

Confident that she is dealing with an asthmatic patient, Susan performs the detailed physical exam. She notes bilateral distention of the jugular veins and retractions at the suprasternal notch and intercostal spaces, along with nasal flaring and pursed lips. Quickly she auscultates breath sounds from the posterior thorax in a six-point pattern. She observes bilateral expiratory wheezing in the apices of the lungs, with no net air movement in the bases.

Todd informs Susan of the patient's vital signs: pulse, 116 beats per minute; respirations, 56 per minute; and blood pressure, 152/94 mmHg. With the initial assessment and SAMPLE history obtained, Susan begins emergency interventions. The cardiac monitor displays sinus tachycardia with no ectopy.

As Todd obtains a venous blood sample and establishes an IV line, Susan assembles a nebulizer to administer 2.5 mg of Albuterol. She gives the nebulizer complete with medication to the patient for self-administration. Following standing orders, Susan draws 0.5 mg of epinephrine 1:1,000 from a glass ampule with a syringe and hypodermic needle. Then she cleanses the site and delivers the subcutaneous injection into the tissue on the back of the patient's left arm. Todd prepares the cot and loads the patient for transport.

En route to the hospital, Susan performs the ongoing assessment by evaluating the components of the initial assessment and the effects of all interventions. The patient now is more alert and breathing easier. Her pulse oximetry reads 92%, and her expiratory wheezing has subsided significantly. Susan notes air movement in the bases of the lungs. Additionally, the cyanosis and diaphoresis have almost subsided, and vital signs have returned to normal limits. Because the pulse oximeter reading is still low and some residual wheezing persists, Susan gives another nebulized treatment of 2.5 mg of Albuterol. She alerts the receiving hospital by cellular telephone.

Once at the hospital, Susan and Todd turn over care to the emergency department staff. Later, they find out that the woman was admitted for overnight observation with the diagnosis of acute exacerbation of asthma. She is doing fine and is expected to be released in the morning.

INTRODUCTION

Medications, or **drugs,** are foreign substances placed into the human body. They serve a variety of purposes, including controlling specific diseases such as hypertension and helping the body cure diseases such as cancer and infection.

Medication administration will be an important part of the medical care you provide as an EMT-Intermediate (EMT-I). You may have to use medications to correct or prevent many life-threatening situations. You may also use them to stabilize or comfort a patient in distress. In addition to your knowledge of particular medications and their properties from the previous chapter on pharmacology, you must also be thoroughly skilled in drug administration. Specific drugs require specific routes and administration techniques. Their effectiveness depends directly upon their correct route of delivery. Incorrect or sloppy drug administration can have tremendous legal implications for the EMT-I. More importantly, it equates to poor care that can harm or even kill the patient.

This chapter discusses the routes and techniques you will use to correctly deliver your patient's medications. It is divided into three parts:

Part 1: Principles and Routes of Medication Administration

Part 2: Intravenous Access, Blood Sampling, and Intraosseous Infusion

Part 3: Medical Mathematics

medications/drugs foreign substances placed into the human body.

Part 1: Principles and Routes of Medication Administration

As an EMT-I, you are responsible for ensuring that all emergency drugs are in place and ready for immediate use. Therefore you must know your local drug distribution system. You will have to know where to obtain and replace each drug as it expires or is used, because another patient may require it at any time. You also will have to thoroughly document the administration and restocking of narcotics, because many local, state, and federal agencies mandate such record keeping. Always be certain that you correctly give all drugs in the right dose. Medication errors may prove disastrous in terms of patient care and legal responsibility. Your knowledge of drug indications, contraindications, side effects, dosages, and routes of administration is crucial to effective patient care.

You can attain effective pharmacologic therapy and eliminate medication errors by following the six rights of drug administration:

- Right person
- Right drug
- Right dose
- Right time
- Right route
- Right documentation

Your knowledge of drug indications, dosages, and routes of administration is of paramount importance.

If you ever doubt the use or dosage of a medication, contact medical direction immediately.

In the field, you will be responsible for the safe and appropriate delivery of medications. If you ever doubt the use or dosage of a medication, contact medical direction immediately. You must repeat back, or echo, all drug orders issued by direct medical command. For example, if medical direction ordered you to administer 25 grams of 50% dextrose, you would echo, "Medic 101 copies the medication order for 25 grams of 50% dextrose to be administered slow IV push." By echoing, you confirm your reception and understanding of the order. If medical direction has issued an inappropriate medication or dosage, echoing may bring it to light and elicit an immediate correction. If you still find the order questionable after echoing, diplomatically request clarification or ask about the intent.

Pharmacological therapy permits you to function as an extension of the physician. No room exists for medication errors, as once a drug is given it is difficult if not impossible to retrieve. In addition, withholding a needed medication can have catastrophic consequences. Concentration and knowledge are the keys to this component of advanced prehospital care.

MEDICAL DIRECTION

An EMT-I does not practice autonomously. You will operate under the license of a medical director who is responsible for all of your actions. This responsibility extends to the administration of medications.

The medical director determines which medications you will use and the routes by which you will deliver them. Some states have a "state drug list" whereby the medications a service carries are dictated by law or a legislative or regulatory agency. Some EMS services may offer two levels of advanced life support, that provided by the EMT-I and that provided by a paramedic. In these cases, there may be two separate medication lists for each level of provider. It is your responsibility to be familiar with medications approved for use by EMT-Is. Although some medications can be administered via off-line medical direction (written standing orders), you will need specific authorization for others after consulting on-line or direct medical direction. You must strictly abide by all of your medical director's guidelines.

Knowing all drug administration protocols is essential, especially which drugs to administer under standing orders and which to deliver only after getting authorization from medical direction. You can ill afford to waste valuable time looking up procedures and directives for the critical patient who requires immediate drug therapy. Furthermore, because inappropriate drug delivery can have serious consequences, you may face severe legal ramifications, even if your patient suffers no harm.

BODY SUBSTANCE ISOLATION

Establishing routes for drug delivery presents the constant potential for exposure to blood and other body fluids. Always take appropriate **body substance isolation (BSI) precautions** to decrease your risk of exposure. The type of BSI you use will vary according to the delivery route and your patient's condition. At a minimum, you should wear gloves. Optimally, you will also wear goggles and a mask. Remarkably, the simplest form of BSI is often the most neglected: handwashing. Washing your hands before and after patient contact is one of the most effective ways to decrease your exposure to infectious material. Chapter 1 includes a thorough discussion of BSI precautions.

body substance isolation (BSI) precautions a strict form of infection control that is based on the assumption that all blood and body fluids are infectious.

MEDICAL ASEPSIS

Medical **asepsis** (*a-*, without; *sepsis,* infection) describes a medical environment free of pathogens. Many prehospital procedures, especially those related to drug administration, place the patient at increased risk for infection. The external environment is full of microorganisms, many of them pathogenic. Techniques such as intravenous access or endotracheal intubation can allow pathogens to enter the patient's body, where they may cause **local** or **systemic** complications.

asepsis a condition free of pathogens.

local limited to one area of the body.

systemic throughout the body.

STERILIZATION

The most aseptic environment is a sterile one. A **sterile** environment is free of all forms of life. Generally, environments are sterilized with extensive heat or chemicals. A sterile environment is difficult to attain in the prehospital setting. Consequently, you must practice medically clean techniques to minimize your patient's risk of infection. **Medically clean** techniques involve the careful handling of sterile equipment to prevent contamination. For example, much of the equipment used for drug administration is packaged sterilely. Once you open the package, you must use a medically clean technique to keep the equipment clean and uncontaminated until you use it. If you drop a piece of equipment on a dirty surface, you should discard it and obtain a new piece. Other medically clean techniques, including handwashing, glove changing, and discarding equipment in opened packages, help prevent equipment and patient contamination. Remember, too, that many patients have lowered immunity levels or carry infectious diseases. Thus, keeping the ambulance and equipment clean is another essential medically clean procedure.

sterile free of all forms of life.

medically clean careful handling to prevent contamination.

DISINFECTANTS AND ANTISEPTICS

When administering medications, you must use disinfectants and antiseptics to ensure local cleanliness. Do not confuse disinfectants and antiseptics; the distinction is important. **Disinfectants** are toxic to living tissue. You will therefore use them only on nonliving surfaces or objects such as the inside of an ambulance or laryngoscope blades after use. Never use disinfectants on living tissue. **Antiseptics** are not toxic to living tissue. They destroy or inhibit pathogenic microorganisms already on living surfaces and are generally used to cleanse the local area before needle puncture. Common antiseptics include alcohol and iodine preparations used either alone or together. Frequently, antiseptics are diluted disinfectants.

disinfectant cleansing agent that is toxic to living tissue.

antiseptic cleansing agent that is not toxic to living tissue.

DISPOSAL OF CONTAMINATED EQUIPMENT AND SHARPS

Blood and body fluid can harbor infectious material that endangers the health-care provider, family, bystanders, or the patient himself. Many times, the patient is infected with pathogenic organisms long before signs and symptoms appear. Therefore, you must treat all blood and body fluids as potentially infectious.

Drug administration commonly involves needles in direct contact with the patient's blood and body fluid. Once used, a needle presents a significant risk. Inadvertent needle sticks, the most common accident in health care as a whole, can transmit diseases between the patient and the EMT-I. Properly handling needles and other sharps before and after patient use can prevent many of these accidental needle sticks. To minimize or eliminate the risk of an accidental needle stick, take these precautions:

- *Minimize the tasks you perform in a moving ambulance.* Use needles as sparingly as possible in the back of a moving ambulance. When appropriate, perform all interventions involving needles on scene. If en route, it may be occasionally necessary to have the driver pull the ambulance to the side of the road and stop briefly. Most EMT-Is become quite proficient at completing these procedures in a moving ambulance.

- *Immediately dispose of used sharps in a sharps container.* A **sharps container** is a rigid, puncture-resistant container clearly marked as biohazardous. You can deposit whole needles and prefilled syringes in it, thus eliminating the need for bending or cutting. Some sharps containers have adapters that permit the easy removal of needles from blood-draw equipment and syringes. You should also dispose of items such as used ampules in the sharps container. Avoid dropping sharps onto the floor for later disposal. In the heat of the moment, you may forget the sharp or mentally misplace it.

- *Recap needles only as a last resort.* If you absolutely must recap a needle, never use two hands to do so. Place the sharp on a stationary surface, and replace the cap with one hand. Although the one-hand method is still hazardous, it at least reduces the chance for an accidental needle stick.

By law, every medical organization must have a biological hazard exposure plan. Be familiar with yours. If you are exposed to blood or other body substances, follow the plan and immediately notify the appropriate resources. Remember that prevention is the best medicine.

MEDICATION ADMINISTRATION AND DOCUMENTATION

When administering medications, proper and thorough documentation is extremely important. You must record all information concerning the patient and the medication, including:

- Indication for drug administration
- Dosage and route delivered
- Patient response to the medication—both positive and negative

You must also document the patient's condition and vital signs before medication administration, as well as after. In addition to communicating all information to those to whom you transfer care, you must record it on a copy of the patient care report.

In emergent and nonemergent situations alike, you will administer a variety of medications through a variety of delivery routes. The routes of drug administration fall into four basic categories: percutaneous, pulmonary, enteral, and parenteral. Technically, drug deliveries through the rectum and pulmonary system are **topical** applications; however, accepted practice classifies these routes separately. Which route you use will depend on the drug you are administering and your patient's status.

PERCUTANEOUS DRUG ADMINISTRATION

Content Review

PERCUTANEOUS ROUTES
- Transdermal
- Mucous membrane

Percutaneous medications are applied to and absorbed through the skin or mucous membranes. They are easy to administer and bypass the digestive tract, making their absorption more predictable.

TRANSDERMAL ADMINISTRATION

Medications given by the **transdermal** (*trans-*, across; *dermal*, skin) route promote slow, steady absorption. Nitroglycerin, hormones, and analgesics are commonly administered transdermally. Transdermal delivery can also produce localized effects, as with anti-inflammatories and other bacteriostatic and softening agents. Applying medication locally avoids passing larger quantities of the medication through the entire body, where it is not needed. Transdermal medications include lotions, ointments, creams, foams, wet dressings, adhesive backed applications, and suppositories.

transdermal absorbed through the skin.

To administer a transdermal medication, use the following technique:

1. Take BSI precautions. Gloves avoid contaminating the medication and inadvertently getting it on your skin.
2. Clean and dry your patient's skin at the administration site.
3. Apply medication to the site as specified by the manufacturer. Avoid overdosing or underdosing when using lotion, ointment, cream, or foam.
4. Leave the medication in place for the required time. Monitor the patient for desirable or adverse effects.

You may need to place a dressing over the medication to protect the site and quantity of drug. Carefully follow all recommendations. Administration may vary subtly, depending on the form of medication and the specific manufacturer's instructions.

Several factors can affect how quickly the skin absorbs transdermal medications. Thin skin, overdose, or penetrating solvents can increase the absorption rate. Conversely, thick skin, scar tissue, or peripheral vascular disease can decrease the rate. If these factors are present, consider alternative sites or dosage adjustments.

MUCOUS MEMBRANES

Content Review

MUCOUS MEMBRANE MEDICATION SITES
- Tongue
- Cheek
- Eye
- Nose
- Ear

The mucous membranes absorb medications at a moderate to rapid rate. Similar to transdermal administration, drug delivery through the mucous membranes avoids the digestive tract and complications associated with that route. You can deliver drugs through the mucous membranes at several sites. However, specific drugs are made for specific sites and generally are not interchangeable.

Sublingual

Sublingual drugs are absorbed through the mucous membranes beneath the tongue (*sub-*, below; *lingual*, tongue). The sublingual region is extremely vascular and permits rapid absorption with systemic delivery. These medications are generally dissolvable tablets or sprays. One commonly administered sublingual medication is nitroglycerin.

sublingual beneath the tongue.

To administer a medication via the sublingual route, follow these steps:

1. Take appropriate BSI precautions.
2. Confirm the indication, medication, dose, sublingual route, and expiration date.
3. Have your patient lift his tongue toward the top and back of his oral cavity.
4. Place the pill or direct spray between the underside of the tongue and the floor of the oral cavity. Have your patient relax his tongue and mouth. If administering a pill, instruct the patient to let the pill dissolve and not to swallow.
5. Monitor the patient for desirable or adverse effects.

Buccal

buccal between the cheek and gums.

The **buccal** region lies in the oral cavity between the cheek and gums. Buccal medications are generally tablets. Hormonal and enzyme preparations are typically given buccally.

To administer a medication buccally, follow these steps:

1. Take appropriate BSI precautions.
2. Confirm the indication, medication, dose, buccal route, and expiration date.
3. Place the medication between the patient's cheek and gum. Instruct the patient to allow the pill or other preparation to dissolve. Ensure that the patient does not swallow the medication.
4. Monitor the patient for desirable or adverse effects.

Ocular

ocular medication drug administered through the mucous membranes of the eye.

Ocular medications are topical medications that are administered through the mucous membranes of the eye. These are typically local medications for alleviating eye pain, treating infection, decreasing intraocular pressure, or lubricating the eyelid. Medications delivered by way of the eye are labeled for ophthalmic use and packaged as drops or ointments.

If medication is to be administered only to one eye, be sure to medicate the correct eye. The following abbreviations designate right, left, or both eyes:

o.d.	right eye (*oculus dexter*)
o.s.	left eye (*oculus sinister*)
o.u.	both right and left eyes (*oculus uterque*)

To administer a medication via eye drops, use the following technique (Figure 4-1):

1. Use gloves and other appropriate BSI precautions.
2. Have your patient lie supine or lay his head back and look toward the ceiling.
3. Pull the lower eyelid downward to expose the conjunctival sac. Never touch the eye.
4. Use a medicine dropper to place the prescribed dosage on the conjunctival sac. Never administer medications directly on the eye unless specifically instructed.
5. Instruct the patient to hold his eye(s) shut for one to two minutes.

Legal Notes

Eye drops are for single patient use. Once administered, the container must be properly disposed of. Never re-use ophthalmic medications.

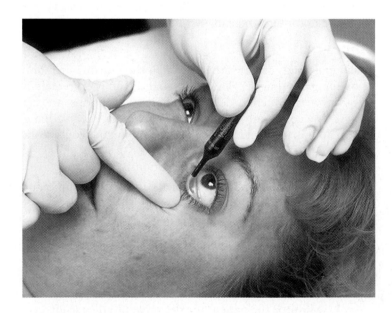

FIGURE 4-1 Eye drop administration. Use a medicine dropper to place the prescribed dosage on the conjunctival sac.

Ocular medications may also be packaged as ointments. To apply an ointment, follow the same procedure as above, but carefully squeeze the ointment onto the conjunctival sac. If you administer too much medication, carefully blot away the excess drops or ointment with sterile gauze. The ointment will melt as it warms to body temperature and will spread smoothly across the surface of the eye.

Nasal

The mucous membranes of the nose are another port for topical medication delivery. Given through the nares (nostrils), these **nasal medications** are usually drops or sprays intended for local effect. They commonly treat nasal congestion, hemorrhage, and infection.

nasal medication drug administered through the mucous membranes of the nose.

To administer a medication via the nose, use the following technique (Figure 4-2):

1. Use gloves and other appropriate BSI precautions.
2. Have the patient blow his nose and tilt his head backward.
3. Use a medicine dropper or squeezable nebulizer to administer the medication into the appropriate nare(s) according to the manufacturer's instructions.
4. Hold the nare(s) shut and/or tilt the head forward to distribute the medication.
5. Monitor the patient for desirable and undesirable effects.

Aural

Some medications are delivered to the mucous membranes of the ear and ear canal through drops or medicated gauze. These drugs primarily treat local infections and ear pain. Use the following technique to administer medicated drops (Figure 4-3):

1. Use gloves and other appropriate BSI precautions.
2. Confirm the indication, medication, dose, and expiration date.
3. Determine the correct ear for administration.
4. Have the patient lie in the lateral recumbent position with the affected ear upward.
5. Manually open the ear canal: for adult patients, pull the ear up and back; for pediatric patients, pull it down and back.
6. Administer the appropriate dose of medication with a medicine dropper.
7. Have the patient continue to lie with his ear up for ten minutes.
8. Monitor the patient for desirable and undesirable effects.

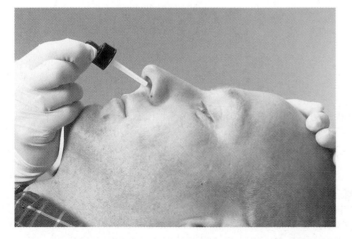

FIGURE 4-2 Nasal medication administration.

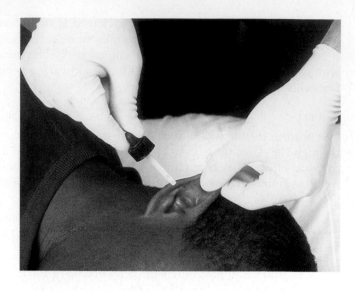

FIGURE 4-3 Aural medication administration. Manually open the ear canal and administer the appropriate dose.

Using medicated gauze or cotton is generally reserved for the hospital setting. If your local protocols permit you to administer these medications, follow the procedure outlined above, gently inserting the gauze into the ear instead of instilling medicated drops. Avoid tightly packing the ear canal.

PULMONARY DRUG ADMINISTRATION

inhalation drawing of medication into the lungs along with air during breathing.

injection placement of medication in or under the skin with a needle and syringe.

nebulizer inhalation aid that disperses liquid into aerosol spray or mist.

Special medications can be administered into the pulmonary system via **inhalation** or **injection.** Generally gases, fine mists, or liquids, these drugs include those that promote bronchodilation for respiratory emergencies. Other inhaled drugs are mucolytics, antibiotics, and topical steroids. Inhalation can also be used for humidification and pulmonary decongestion.

NEBULIZER

Typically, drugs administered by inhalation are delivered with the aid of a small volume **nebulizer.** A nebulizer uses pressurized oxygen to disperse a liquid into a fine aerosol spray or mist. Inhalation carries the aerosol into the lungs. Figure 4-4 illustrates a typical nebulizer. The specific design depends upon the manufacturer, but they all work on the same principle and typically have the same parts, as follows:

- Mouthpiece
- Medication reservoir
- Oxygen port
- Relief valve
- Oxygen tubing
- Oxygen source

To administer a drug with a nebulizer, follow these steps:

1. Put the medication in the medication reservoir. If the medication is not diluted, combine it with 3 to 5 cc sterile saline solution. This will allow adequate aerosolization. Screw the reservoir in place.
2. Assemble the nebulizer.
3. Attach oxygen tubing to the oxygen port and oxygen source.
4. Set the oxygen source regulator for 5 to 8 liters per minute.
   Note: Never set the oxygen pressure outside of this range. Less than 5 liters per minute will not create enough pressure to aerosolize the medication.

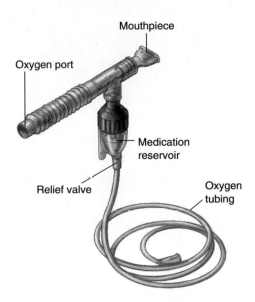

FIGURE 4-4 Small volume nebulizer.

Mouthpiece

Oxygen port

Medication reservoir

Relief valve

Oxygen tubing

More than 8 liters per minute will create too much pressure and destroy the oxygen tubing or nebulizer at its weakest point. Furthermore, because of pressure restrictions, do not attach the nebulizer to an oxygen humidifier.

5. Place the nebulizer in the patient's mouth. Instruct him to exhale and then seal his lips around the mouthpiece. Now have him hold the nebulizer and slowly inhale as deeply as possible. Upon maximum inhalation, instruct the patient to hold in the medication for one to two seconds before exhaling. This permits maximum deposition and absorption. Continue this process until the medication is completely gone. Typically, this takes three to five minutes.

Nebulizers also come preattached to an oxygen face mask in both pediatric and adult sizes (Figure 4-5). Use nebulization facemasks for pediatric or adult patients who cannot hold the nebulizer. Nebulizers for those who require long-term therapy may be powered by a battery or other energy source.

For a nebulizer to be effective, the patient must have an adequate tidal volume and respiratory rate. If the tidal volume is shallow or respiratory rate low, the medication will not move from the nebulizer into the lungs. For patients with a poor tidal and/or respiratory rate who cannot pull the medication into their lungs, you can connect nebulizers to a bag-valve mask and/or endotracheal tube.

METERED DOSE INHALER

Inhaled medications are also delivered through **metered dose inhalers (MDI)**. These small, handheld devices produce a medicated spray for inhalation. Patients with conditions such as asthma or chronic obstructive pulmonary disease (COPD) use MDIs to deliver a specific, or metered, dose of medication. An MDI consists of two parts: a medication canister and a plastic shell and mouthpiece (Figure 4-6). Some MDIs are equipped with a spacer. The spacer is a cylindrical canister between the inhaler and the mouthpiece. Prior to self-administration, the patient will depress the inhaler, sending a measured dose of drug into the spacer. The patient will then breathe in and out of the spacer through the mouthpiece, thus inhaling the drug into the lungs. This system is particularly useful for patients who have a hard time operating and inhaling the MDI. This is common in the elderly and in young children. The spacer, when used in conjunction with an MDI, is very effective.

Metered dose inhalers are usually self-administered. However, if your patient is incapacitated, you may have to physically assist with the administration or educate the patient or his caregivers in its use. To assist a patient in the use of an MDI, follow this technique:

1. Insert the medication canister into the plastic shell.
2. Remove the cap from the mouthpiece.

metered dose inhaler handheld device that produces a medicated spray for inhalation.

Legal Notes

Metered dose inhalers (MDIs) are for single patient use. Once administered, the container must be properly disposed of. Never re-use MDIs. Because of the cost, most EMS services use small-volume nebulizers instead of MDIs.

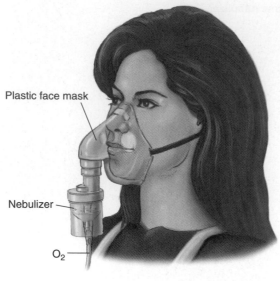

Plastic face mask

Nebulizer

O₂

(a) Nebulizer with attached face mask

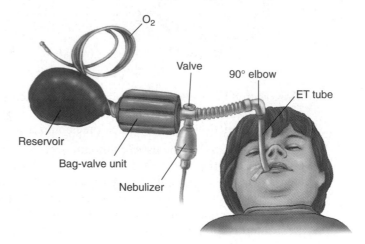

O₂

Valve

90° elbow

ET tube

Reservoir

Bag-valve unit

Nebulizer

(c) Nebulizer with bag-valve unit

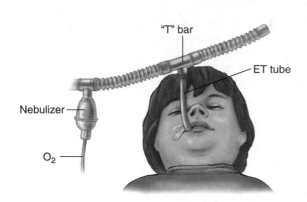

"T" bar

ET tube

Nebulizer

O₂

(b) Nebulizer with endotracheal tube

FIGURE 4–5   Nebulizer with attached face mask, bag-valve mask, and endotracheal tube.

3. Gently shake the MDI for 2–5 seconds.

4. Instruct the patient to maximally exhale.

5. Place the mouthpiece in the patient's mouth and have him form a seal with his lips.

6. As the patient inhales, press the canister's top downward to release the medication.

7. Have the patient hold his breath for several seconds.

8. Remove the inhaler from the patient's mouth and instruct him to breathe slowly.

9. If a second dose is necessary, wait according to the manufacturer's instructions. Then repeat.

10. In an acute respiratory emergency involving a patient with an MDI, always use a nebulizer instead of the MDI. Whereas the MDI delivers a small amount of medication, the nebulizer delivers larger quantities of medication mixed with water and oxygen.

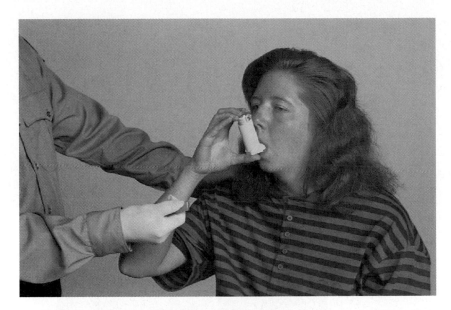

FIGURE 4-6 Metered dose inhaler.

Nebulizers and MDIs offer several advantages. In respiratory emergencies, less medication is needed because it reaches its exact site of action. The lower dosage is less likely to promote side effects, and if the patient has an adverse reaction, implementing or discontinuing drug delivery is easy. Furthermore, because the patient can hold the nebulizer, he will benefit from feeling more in control of his overall therapy. Most importantly, if your patient is hypoxic you can administer inhaled medications with supplemental oxygen.

The nebulizer and MDI also have disadvantages. Moving the aerosolized medication into the lungs depends on adequate ventilation. For the patient with a poor tidal and minute volume, nebulized medications are ineffective, as the drug cannot reach its site of action. In these cases, you should use the nebulizer in conjunction with a bag-valve mask and/or endotracheal tube. Additionally, the patient must exhibit an adequate level of consciousness and manual dexterity to hold the nebulizer and follow instructions correctly.

ENDOTRACHEAL TUBE

When you have not yet established an IV you can administer certain medications such as lidocaine (Xylocaine), epinephrine, atropine, and naloxone (Narcan) through an endotracheal tube. Delivering liquid medications into the lungs permits rapid absorption through the pulmonary capillaries. In fact, some authorities believe pulmonary absorption is as fast as intravenous absorption.

When using an endotracheal tube, you must increase conventional IV dosages from two to two and one-half times. You also should dilute the medication in normal saline to create 10 ml of solution and then quickly inject it down the endotracheal tube. Several ventilations must follow to aerosolize the medication and enhance its absorption. Ideally, you can pass a commercially manufactured catheter through the endotracheal tube and inject the medication through it. If CPR is underway, stop compressions while you administer the medication and ventilate for aerosolization.

ENTERAL DRUG ADMINISTRATION

Enteral drug administration is the delivery of any medication that is absorbed through the gastrointestinal (GI) tract. The GI tract, or alimentary canal, travels from the mouth to the stomach and on through the intestines to the rectum (Figure 4-7). You can administer enteral medications orally, through a gastric tube, or rectally.

Several advantages make the GI tract the most common route for medication delivery. Aside from sheer convenience, it is the least expensive route, and its use requires little

Content Review

ENDOTRACHEAL MEDICATIONS
- Lidocaine
- Epinephrine
- Atropine
- Naloxone

enteral drug administration the delivery of any medication that is absorbed through the gastrointestinal tract.

Content Review

ENTERAL ROUTES
- Oral
- Gastric tube
- Rectal

Legal Notes

Many types of tubes and access devices are used in modern health care. Never assume that a tube exiting the abdomen is a gastric tube. Only use tubes that are clearly marked as gastric tubes. If you are uncertain, withhold medication or fluid administration.

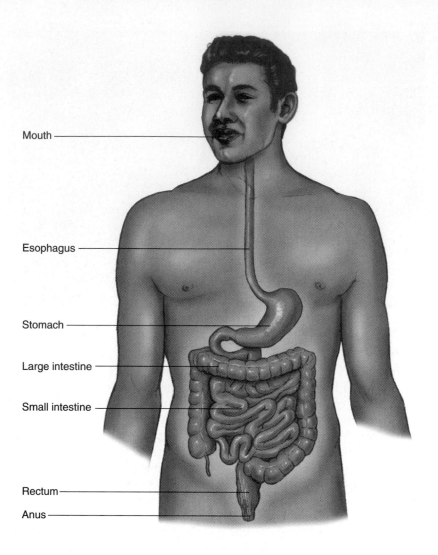

Mouth

Esophagus

Stomach

Large intestine

Small intestine

Rectum

Anus

FIGURE 4-7 Gastrointestinal tract.

equipment and minimal training. In some instances, after you have delivered a drug, you may be able to retrieve it by inducing vomiting, by removing it from the rectum, or simply by having the patient spit it out.

Conversely, enteral drug administration poses several disadvantages. Physical activity, emotions, or food can significantly alter the GI tract's chemical and physical environment, making absorption unreliable. In addition, as all blood from the stomach and small intestine must pass through the hepatic circulatory system (portal circulation), the liver's condition can reduce the medication's effectiveness. A dysfunctional liver can significantly alter drug distribution and, in extreme cases, metabolize therapeutic medications into inert or harmful substances. Furthermore, a patient resistant to or *noncompliant* in taking medications makes administration via the enteral route very difficult.

ORAL ADMINISTRATION

oral drug administration the delivery of any medication that is taken by mouth and swallowed into the lower GI tract.

Oral drug administration denotes any medication taken by mouth (oral) and swallowed into the GI tract. From the GI tract, the medication is absorbed and distributed throughout the body. When administering a medication by the oral route, you must be sure that the patient has an adequate level of consciousness to support his airway. Administering an oral medication to a patient who cannot support his airway may result in an airway occlusion or aspiration into the lungs. If aspiration into the lungs occurs, aspiration pneumonia and its deadly consequences may occur.

Medications for oral delivery come in a variety of forms, either solid or liquid, as follows:

- *Capsules*. Capsules contain liquid, dry, or beaded medication in a soluble casing. For maximum effectiveness, the patient must swallow them whole.
- *Tablets*. Tablets comprise medicated powder compressed into a small, solid disk. Typically, tablets may be scored to permit breaking in half or quarters when lesser dosages are required.
- *Pills*. Pills, comprised of medicated powder compressed into a small disk, are the same as tablets. In the past, the term pill was used to denote a solid medication taken by mouth. Over time, *tablet* has become the accepted term.
- *Enteric-coated/time-release capsules and tablets*. These forms of medication release the drug gradually as layers of the capsule or tablet slowly erode. Time-release capsules or tablets must be swallowed whole.
- *Elixirs*. Elixirs are liquid medications combined with alcohol or placed in a sweetened fluid.
- *Emulsions*. Emulsions are medications combined with a fat or oil emulsifier.
- *Lozenges*. Lozenges are solid forms of medication that slowly dissolve in the mouth, thus permitting gradual swallowing.
- *Suspensions*. A suspension is a liquid that contains small particles of solid medication.
- *Syrups*. A syrup is a concentrated solution of sugar in water or another liquid to which a medication is added.

Equipment for Oral Administration

Administering oral medications is simple and easy. The basic equipment that you may need depends on the medication and the patient's status:

- *Soufflé cup*. A soufflé cup is a paper or plastic cup. Placing a solid medication in a soufflé cup makes it easy to see and minimizes contact with the provider's hands.
- *Medicine cup*. A medicine cup is a plastic or glass cup with volumetric measurements on the side. It facilitates giving specific amounts of liquid medication. When you pour medication into the cup, the liquid does not form a flat surface but clings to the sides at a higher level, forming a *meniscus*. To compensate for the meniscus, measure the medication toward the center, at its lowest level.
- *Medicine dropper*. A medicine dropper has markings for measuring liquid volumes. You will use it for special medications and to administer medications to children or patients who cannot tolerate other forms of oral medication.
- *Teaspoon*. You will use these accurately sized measuring spoons to administer liquid medications. A teaspoon normally holds 5 mL of fluid; however, the volume of household teaspoons varies significantly. To ensure accurate medication administration, use a measured teaspoon or syringe.
- *Oral syringe*. Oral syringes are calibrated plastic syringes without a hypodermic needle. They are considered the most accurate oral means of administering liquid-based medications. When administering a medication with the oral syringe, place the end of the syringe in the patient's mouth and deliver only as much medication as the patient can safely swallow. Several administrations may be necessary to deliver a complete dose.
- *Nipple*. For the neonate or infant, liquid medication can be delivered with a plastic nipple.

Patho Pearls

Most people assume that a teaspoon holds 5 mL of liquid. However, most kitchen teaspoons vary in the quantity they hold and thus should not be used for medication administration.

General Principles of Oral Administration

To administer medications orally, use the following technique:

1. Take appropriate BSI precautions.
2. Note whether to administer the medication with food or on an empty stomach.
3. Gather any necessary equipment such as a soufflé cup or teaspoon. Mix liquids or suspensions or otherwise prepare medications as needed.
4. Have your patient sit upright (when not contraindicated).
5. Place the medication into your patient's mouth. Allow self-administration when possible; assist when needed.
6. Follow administration with 4–8 ounces of water or other liquid. Swallowing a liquid pushes the medication into the stomach.
7. Ensure that the patient has swallowed the medication and it is not hidden in his mouth. For some pediatric and psychiatric patients, you may have to visually confirm that the patient has swallowed the medication by inspecting the oral cavity.

GASTRIC TUBE ADMINISTRATION

For patients who have difficulty swallowing or whose nutritional status is poor, you may place a *gastric tube* to support or completely supplement nutritional requirements. Gastric tubes are also used in instances of drug overdose, trauma, and upper GI bleeding. They may be surgically inserted directly into the stomach through the abdomen or indirectly through the nose (nasogastric tube) or mouth (orogastric tube). Placing a gastric tube through the abdominal wall is reserved for the hospital setting. In some EMS systems, EMT-Is insert orogastric or nasogastric tubes in the field for emergencies. A properly placed gastric tube allows enteral medication delivery. Activated charcoal for toxic ingestion is commonly administered through a nasogastric or orogastric tube. Other medications, many used in the nonacute setting, also are administered via the gastric tube. With modification, most oral medications can be administered this way. However, you should avoid administering time-release capsules and enteric-coated tablets through a gastric tube, because crushing them for delivery destroys their slow-release mechanism. Also, ensure that the medication has been sufficiently crushed so not to become trapped and occlude the gastric tube.

To administer a medication via a gastric tube, use the following technique (Procedure 4-1):

1. Confirm proper tube placement. Disconnect the tube from the drainage or suction unit or clamping device. Clamp the tube from the drainage or suction unit to avoid gastric contents spilling from either device. Attach a cone-tipped syringe to the proximal end of the gastric tube. Gently inject air while auscultating over the stomach. Following this, withdraw the plunger while observing for the presence of gastric fluid or contents, which indicates appropriate placement. Leave the tube disconnected from the drainage or suction unit.

2. Irrigate the gastric tube. To irrigate the gastric tube, draw up 50 to 100 mL of normal saline into a cone-tipped syringe. Insert the syringe into the open end of the gastric tube. With the syringe tip pointed at the floor, gently inject the saline into the tube. If the saline encounters resistance, look for problems such as tube kinking. Also, have the patient lie on his left side and reattempt injection. If the saline still meets resistance, reattach the tube to the drainage or suction unit and contact medical direction for further directives.

3. Prepare the medication(s) for delivery. Crush tablets or empty capsules into 30 cc of warm water. Ensure that all particles are small so that they will not occlude the tube. You may administer liquid medications without further preparation.

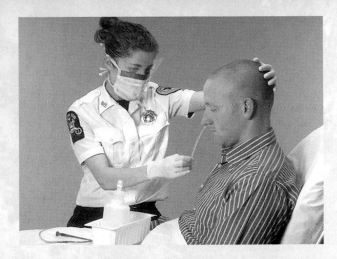

4-1a Confirm proper tube placement.

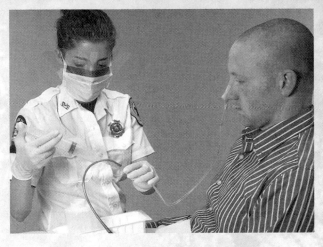

4-1b Withdraw the plunger while observing for the presence of gastric fluid or contents.

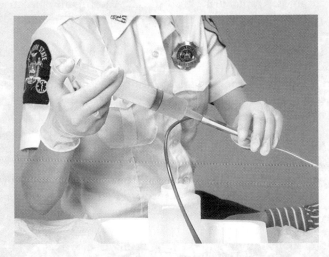

4-1c Instill medication into the gastric tube.

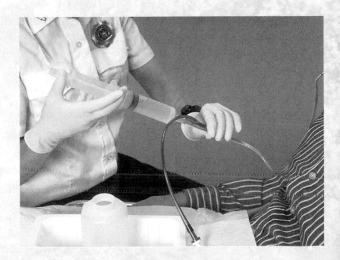

4-1d Gently inject the saline.

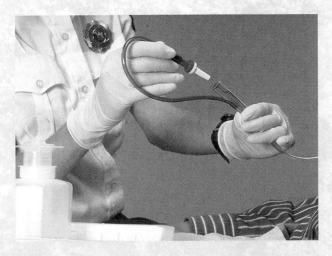

4-1e Clamp off the distal tube.

4. Draw the medication into a 30 to 50 mL cone-tipped syringe and place the tip into open gastric tube. Gently administer the medication into the gastric tube. Forceful application may create considerable distention and patient discomfort.

5. Draw 50 to 100 mL of warm normal saline into a cone-tipped syringe and attach it to the open end of the gastric tube. Gently inject the saline. This facilitates the medication's passage into the stomach and rinses the tube, ensuring that the patient receives the entire dose. Repeated administrations may be necessary.

6. Clamp the distal tube. Use a commercially manufactured device or hemostat to clamp shut the distal portion of the gastric tube for approximately 30 minutes after you administer the medication. Do not reattach to the drainage or suction unit. This will prevent the medication's inadvertent removal from the stomach.

If you must refill the syringe in order to administer the full dosage of medication, do not allow it to empty completely before you detach it from the gastric tube. This prevents drawing air into the syringe and then introducing it into the stomach, which causes discomfort.

RECTAL ADMINISTRATION

hepatic alteration change in a medication's chemical composition that occurs in the liver.

The rectum's extreme vascularity promotes rapid drug absorption. Additionally, because medications given rectally do not pass through the liver, they are not subject to **hepatic alteration;** thus their absorption is more predictable.

In the emergency setting, you may give certain drugs rectally if you cannot establish an IV line or use the oral route. These include diazepam (Valium) for protracted seizures or aspirin for cardiac or neurologic emergencies. In the nonacute setting, you may administer sedatives, antiemetics, or other specially prepared medications rectally.

Rectal administration may prove advantageous with the unconscious or pediatric patient, or when administering drugs with an objectionable taste or odor. Unfortunately, drug absorption may be erratic if gross fecal matter exists. In addition, some drugs may cause considerable anal or rectal irritation.

Rectal medications come in a variety of forms. In the emergency setting, they are typically liquid, thus permitting easy administration and rapid absorption. To administer a rectal medication in the emergent setting follow this technique:

1. Confirm the indication for administration and dose, and draw the correct quantity of medication into a syringe.

2. Place the hub of a 14-gauge Teflon catheter (removed from the angiocatheter) on the end of a needleless syringe (Figure 4-8).

3. Insert the Teflon catheter into the patient's rectum and inject the medication. Try to keep the medication in the lower part of the rectum. Administration higher in the rectum may result in the medication's being absorbed by veins that deliver the drug to the portal circulation.

4. Withdraw the catheter and hold the patient's buttocks together, permitting retention and absorption.

An alternative technique requires a small endotracheal tube instead of the Teflon angiocatheter. Remove the 15/22-mm BVM adapter and connect a syringe to the proximal end of the tube (Figure 4-9). Lubricate the tube and insert it into the rectum. Inject the medication, remove the tube, and hold the buttocks together.

In the nonemergent setting, suppositories or enemas are common methods for rectal administration. Because your responsibilities as an EMT-I may include nonemergent clinical settings, you should master these techniques. Additionally, the rectal route may prove beneficial for a pediatric patient who resists oral administration or for whom IV access proves impractical.

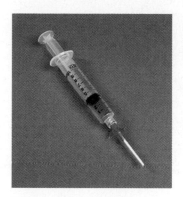

FIGURE 4-8 Catheter placement on needleless syringe.

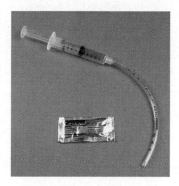

FIGURE 4-9 Syringe attached to endotracheal tube.

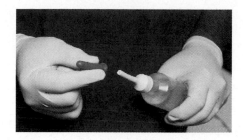

FIGURE 4-10 Prepackaged enema container.

Suppositories are medications packaged in a soft, pliable form. Generally refrigerated until they are used, they begin to melt at body temperature in the rectum. Some are lubricated to ease insertion. Suppositories can be lubricated by running a small amount of lukewarm tap water over the suppository before insertion. To administer a suppository, manually insert it into the rectum. Hold the buttocks shut for 5 to 10 minutes to allow for retention and absorption.

An **enema** is typically a liquid **bolus** of medication that is injected into the rectum. Medications given via this route are typically referred to as small volume enemas. They are typically prepackaged in a squeezable container with a rectal tip (Figure 4-10).

To administer a medicated small volume enema, use the following technique:

1. Take BSI precautions, and confirm the need for administration via a small-volume enema.
2. Place the patient on his left side. Flex his right leg to expose the anus.
3. Insert the prelubricated rectal tip into the anus and advance 3 to 4 inches.
4. Gently squeeze the medicated solution of the bottle into the rectum and colon.
5. Hold the buttocks together to enhance absorption into the rectal and intestinal tissue.

Only those medications with specific guidelines for rectal administration should be delivered by this route. Do not administer rectal medications in the presence of diarrhea, rectal bleeding, hemorrhoids, or any other situation involving severe anal irritation.

PARENTERAL DRUG ADMINISTRATION

Parenteral denotes any drug administration outside of the GI tract. Broadly, this encompasses pulmonary and some topical forms of medication delivery; however, additional, specific criteria apply to parenteral administration. Typically, the parenteral route involves the use of needles as medications are injected into the circulatory system or tissues. Consequently, some forms of parenteral drug delivery afford the most rapid drug delivery and absorption.

SYRINGES AND NEEDLES

Frequently, giving medications via the parenteral route requires a syringe and hypodermic needle.

Syringe

A **syringe** is a plastic tube with which liquid medications can be drawn up, stored, and injected. Syringes range in size from 1 cc to 100 cc and greater. Remember that medication

suppository medication packaged in a soft, pliable form, for insertion into the rectum.

enema a liquid bolus of medication that is injected into the rectum.

bolus concentrated mass of medication.

Do not administer rectal medications in the presence of diarrhea, rectal bleeding, hemorrhoids, or any other situation involving severe anal irritation.

parenteral drug administration outside of the GI tract.

syringe plastic tube with which liquid medications can be drawn up, stored, and injected.

FIGURE 4-11 Syringe.

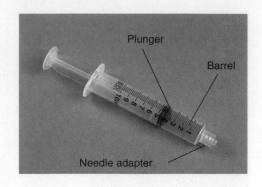

dosages are generally given by weight (g/mg/μg), syringes represent volume. Therefore you must be prepared to mathematically convert these measurements.

Two major components of a syringe are a barrel and a plunger (Figure 4-11). The tube-like barrel, or body, functions as a reservoir for medication. Markings on its side calibrate its overall volume. Smaller syringes are calibrated in 0.10-mL intervals, larger syringes in 1.0-mL intervals.

The plunger is a device that fits into the barrel. At one end it has a handle for pulling or pushing. At the opposite end, a rubber stopper fits snugly into the barrel. Pulling on the plunger draws material into the barrel; pushing on it expels material from the barrel. The rubber end forms a tight seal from which the fluid medication cannot escape. The junction of the fluid and rubber stopper measures the total volume of liquid in the syringe. The barrel's maximum volume should correspond closely to the volume of medication needed. For example, to administer 2 mL of medication, a 3-mL syringe would prove most appropriate.

An adapter at the syringe's distal end is compatible with the hub of an IV catheter or, as many cases will require, a hypodermic needle.

Hypodermic Needle

hypodermic needle hollow metal tube used with the syringe to administer medications.

The **hypodermic needle** is a hollow metal tube used with the syringe to administer medications. It is sharp enough to easily puncture tissues, blood vessels, or IV medication ports.

The hypodermic needle's primary components include a hilt and shaft. The hilt is a threaded plastic tube that screws securely onto the syringe's distal adapter. The shaft is a thin metal tube through which medications can flow from the syringe into the delivery site. A bevel at the shaft's distal end accounts for its sharpness (Figure 4-12).

gauge the diameter of a needle.

Hypodermic needles come in a variety of gauges and lengths. A needle's **gauge** describes its diameter. Generally, hypodermic needle gauges range from 18 to 27. The gauge and actual diameter are inversely related: the higher the gauge, the smaller the diameter. Thus a 25-gauge needle's diameter is smaller than that of an 18-gauge needle. Conversely, a 20-gauge needle's diameter is larger than that of a 22-gauge needle. Hypodermic needle lengths generally range from 3/8 to 1 1/2 inches. The package label lists the size of the syringe and the gauge and length of the hypodermic needle.

Because syringes and hypodermic needles frequently involve invasive procedures, they are packaged sterile. Never use a syringe or a hypodermic needle from a package that has been opened or tampered with. Used hypodermic needles are sharp and present a biohazard. Dispose of them immediately after you complete any task involving their use.

MEDICATION PACKAGING

All medications delivered by the parenteral route are liquids. They are packaged in a variety of containers with which you must be familiar, because obtaining medication from each type requires a different procedure. The kinds of parenteral drug containers include:

- Glass ampules
- Single and multidose vials
- Nonconstituted drug vials
- Prefilled syringes
- Intravenous medication fluids

FIGURE 4-12 Hypodermic needle.

You also must be thoroughly familiar with the information included on the labels of all medication containers:

- *Name of medication.* The label lists both the generic and trade name of the medication. Always ensure that you have selected the right medication.

- *Expiration date.* All medications have an expiration date after which they cannot be used. Never use an expired medication.

- *Total dose and concentration.* The total dose of drug is the total weight (g/mg/μg) of medication in the container. The concentration represents the weight of the drug per volume of fluid. For example, if 10 mg of a drug were packaged in 10 mL of fluid, the total dose would be 10 mg, and the concentration would be 10 mg/10 mL or 1 mg/mL. Beware! Identical drugs can be packaged in different dosages and concentrations.

These labels are printed directly on the vial, ampule, prefilled syringe, or IV medication bag. Always use them to confirm the correct medication.

Glass Ampules

An **ampule,** or amp, is a breakable glass vessel containing liquid medication. It has a cone-shaped top, thin neck, and circular tubular base for storing the medication (Figure 4-13). The thin neck is a vulnerable point where you intentionally break the ampule to retrieve its contents. Ampules usually range in volume from 1 to 5 mL. The least expensive form of drug packaging, they contain single doses of medication.

To obtain medication from a glass ampule, you will need a syringe and needle. Use the following technique (Procedure 4-2):

1. Confirm medication indications and patient allergies.
2. Confirm the ampule label (medication name, dose, and expiration).
3. Hold the ampule upright and tap its top to dislodge any trapped solution.
4. Place gauze around the thin neck and snap it off with your thumb.
5. Place the tip of the hypodermic needle inside the ampule and withdraw the medication into the syringe.
6. Reconfirm the indication, drug, dose, and route of administration.
7. Administer the medication appropriately via the indicated route.
8. Properly dispose of the needle, syringe, and broken glass ampule.

Always use the label printed directly on the container to confirm the correct medication.

ampule breakable glass vessel containing liquid medication.

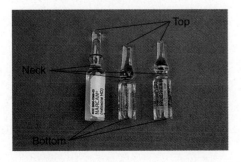

FIGURE 4-13 Ampules.

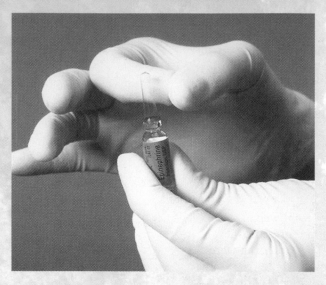

4-2a Hold the ampule upright and tap its top to dislodge any trapped solution.

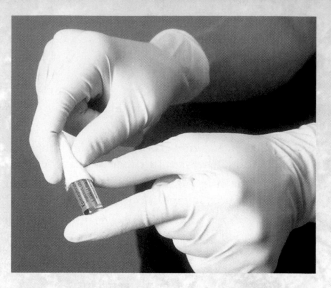

4-2b Place gauze around the thin neck.

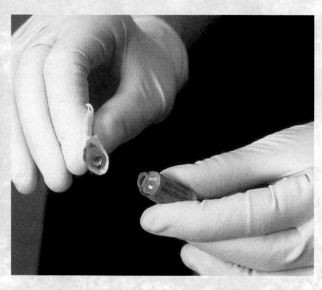

4-2c Snap it off with your thumb.

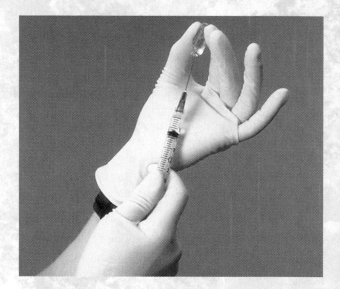

4-2d Draw up the medication.

Single and Multidose Vials

Vials are plastic or glass containers with a self-sealing rubber top (Figure 4-14). Vials may contain single or multiple doses of medication; the self-sealing rubber top prevents leakage from punctures and permits multiple access with a syringe and hypodermic needle. The medication inside the vial is packaged in a vacuum.

To obtain medication from a vial, follow these steps (Procedure 4-3):

1. Confirm medication indications and patient allergies.
2. Confirm the vial label (name, dose, and expiration).
3. Determine the volume of medication to be administered.
4. Prepare the syringe and hypodermic needle. Because the vial is vacuum packed, you will have to replace the volume of medication removed with air in order to maintain equilibrium in the vial. Withdraw the plunger to draw a volume of air into the syringe equal to the volume of medication to be administered. This technique permits easy medication retrieval from the vial.
5. Cleanse the vial's rubber top with an antiseptic alcohol preparation.
6. Insert the hypodermic needle into the rubber top and inject the air from the syringe into the vial. Then withdraw the appropriate volume of medication.
7. Reconfirm the indication, drug, dose, and route of administration.
8. Administer appropriately via the indicated route.
9. Properly dispose of the needle, syringe, and vial.

vial plastic or glass container with a self-healing rubber top.

Self-sealing rubber top

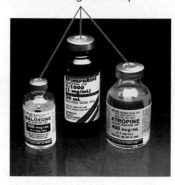

FIGURE 4-14 Vials.

Nonconstituted Drug Vial

The **nonconstituted drug vial** extends the viability and storage time of drugs that have a short shelf life or are unstable in liquid form. The nonconstituted drug vial actually consists of two vials, one containing a powdered medication and one containing a liquid mixing solution (Figure 4-15). To prepare the drug you must mix it, or reconstitute it, by withdrawing the liquid solution from its vial and placing it in the powdered medication's vial. In a **Mix-o-Vial** system, the two vials are joined and you must squeeze them together to break the seal and mix.

To prepare a medication from a nonconstituted drug vial, use the following technique (Procedure 4-4):

1. Confirm medication indications and patient allergies.
2. Confirm the vial's label (name, dose, expiration date).
3. Remove all solution from the vial containing the mixing solution, using the same procedure as you would to withdraw medication from a single or multidose vial.
4. With an alcohol preparation, cleanse the top of the vial containing the powdered drug and inject the mixing solution.
5. Gently agitate or shake the vial to ensure complete mixture.
6. Determine the volume of newly constituted medication to be administered.
7. Prepare the syringe and hypodermic needle. Because the vial is vacuum packed, you will have to replace the volume of medication removed with air to retain equilibrium in the vial. By withdrawing the plunger, place into the syringe a volume of air equal to the volume of medication that will be removed. This technique permits easy medication retrieval from the vial.
8. Cleanse the medication vial's rubber top with an antiseptic alcohol preparation.
9. Insert the hypodermic needle into the rubber top and withdraw the appropriate volume of medication.
10. Reconfirm the indication, drug, dose, and route of administration.

nonconstituted drug vial/ Mix-o-Vial vial with two containers, one holding a powdered medication and the other holding a liquid mixing solution.

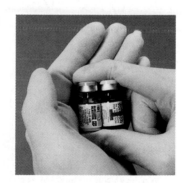

FIGURE 4-15 The nonconstituted drug vial actually consists of two vials, one containing a powdered medication and one containing a liquid mixing solution.

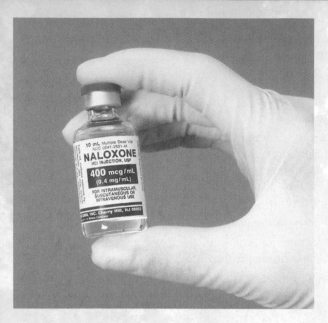

4-3a Confirm the vial label.

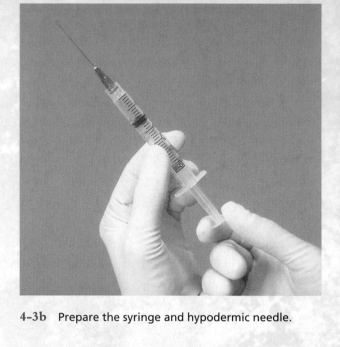

4-3b Prepare the syringe and hypodermic needle.

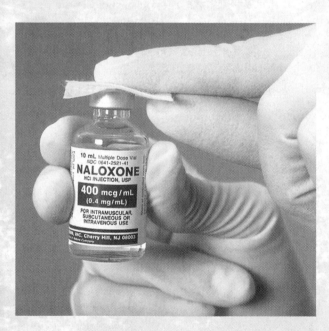

4-3c Cleanse the vial's rubber top.

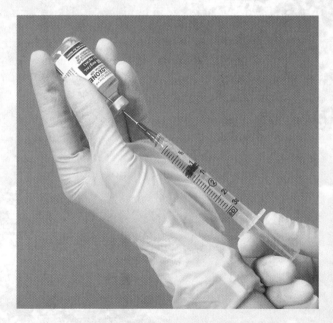

4-3d Insert the hypodermic needle into the rubber top and inject the air from the syringe into the vial.

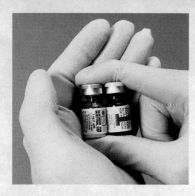

4-4a Nonconstituted drugs come in separate vials. Confirm the labels.

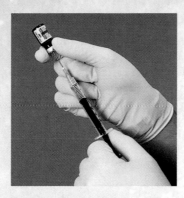

4-4b Remove all solution from the vial containing the mixing solution.

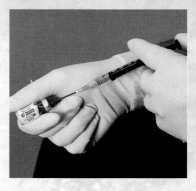

4-4c Cleanse the top of the vial containing the powdered drug and inject the solution.

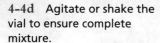

4-4d Agitate or shake the vial to ensure complete mixture.

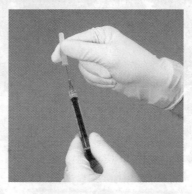

4-4e Prepare new syringe and hypodermic needle.

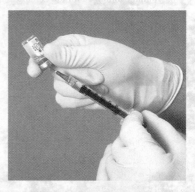

4-4f Withdraw the appropriate volume of medication.

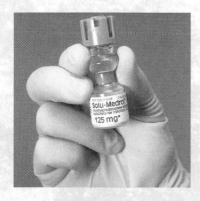

4-4g In the Mix-o-Vial system, the vials are joined at the neck. Confirm the labels.

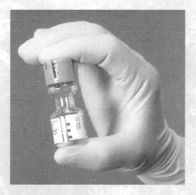

4-4h Squeeze the vials together to break the seal. Agitate or shake to mix completely.

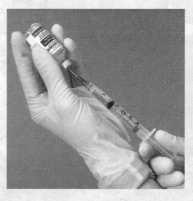

4-4i Withdraw the appropriate volume of medication.

11. Administer appropriately via the indicated route.
12. Monitor the patient for the desired effects.
13. Properly dispose of the needle and syringe.

In some instances you may have to place multiple medications into one syringe for a single delivery. For example, meperidine (Demerol) and promethazine (Phenergan) may be delivered in this manner. Meperidine, an analgesic, can cause nausea and vomiting when administered. To decrease the incidence of nausea and vomiting, you can simultaneously administer promethazine, an antiemetic. To perform this task, draw all medications in the appropriate order according to the procedures discussed. Always anticipate total volume and select an appropriate syringe size. To avoid complications, you must always be aware of drug incompatibilities.

Prefilled or Preloaded Syringes

Prefilled or **preloaded syringes** are packaged in tamper-proof containers with the medication already in the syringe. Because the syringe is prefilled, you do not need to draw the medication from another source. Generally, prefilled syringes contain standard dosages, thus decreasing the chance of dosage error.

The prefilled syringe consists of two parts: a syringe and a glass tube prefilled with liquid medication. The plastic syringe is similar to those described earlier; however, it does not have a plunger. Rather, you screw the prefilled glass tube into the syringe barrel and secure it (Figure 4-16). Pushing the glass container into the syringe barrel expels the medication through the attached hypodermic needle.

Follow these steps to administer a medication from a prefilled syringe:

1. Confirm medication indications and patient allergies.
2. Confirm the prefilled syringe label (name, dose, and expiration date).
3. Assemble the prefilled syringe. Remove the pop-off caps and screw together.
4. Reconfirm the indication, drug, dose, and route of administration.
5. Administer appropriately via the indicated route.
6. Properly dispose of the needle and syringe.

Intravenous Medication Solutions

Medicated solutions are another form of parenteral medication. They are packaged in an IV bag and administered as an intravenous (IV) **infusion**. IV medication solutions may be premixed or you may have to mix them. The section on IV drug infusions later in this chapter discusses their actual preparation and administration.

PARENTERAL ROUTES

Parenterally administered drugs can be absorbed locally or systemically. Additionally, depending on the route of administration, their absorption rate may be slow, sustained, or rapid. Parenteral delivery bypasses the digestive tract, thus making the drug's absorption, action, and onset more predictable. Because parenteral routes use hypodermic needles that contact body fluids, the risk of disease transmission is ever present.

FIGURE 4-16   Prefilled syringes.

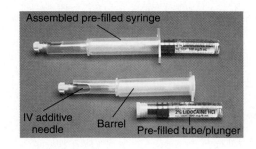

Parenteral drug delivery employs the following routes:

- Intradermal injection
- Subcutaneous injection
- Intramuscular injection
- Intravenous access
- Intraosseous infusion

Specific medications require specific routes of parenteral delivery; therefore you must be competent with every route. In this section we will discuss the specialized equipment, medications, and routes for intradermal, subcutaneous, and intramuscular injections. Because of their complexity, we will discuss intravenous access and intraosseous infusions separately in the following sections.

Whether you are administering a parenteral injection or an IV bolus or infusion, you should explain the entire procedure to the patient to help alleviate his anxiety. Finally, remember that hypoperfusion (hypovolemia or peripheral vascular disease, for instance), may significantly reduce parenteral absorption.

Intradermal Injection

Using a syringe and hypodermic needle, **intradermal** injections deposit medication into the dermal layer of the skin (*intra-*, within; *derma,* skin). The amount of medication placed in the dermal layer is quite small, typically less than 1 mL (Figure 4-17).

Capillaries in the dermis afford a very slow rate of absorption, with little or no systemic distribution. Rather, the bulk of medication remains localized in the area of administration. Intradermal delivery proves useful for allergy testing and tuberculin skin testing and for administering local anesthetics during suturing, wound debridement, and IV establishment.

The forearm and upper back are preferred sites for intradermal injections. These areas have little hair and are highly visible. Additionally, you should look for sites free of superficial blood vessels, which increase the chance for systemic absorption.

To administer an intradermal injection, you will need the following equipment:

- BSI protection
- Alcohol or betadine antiseptic preparations
- Packaged medication
- Tuberculin syringe (1 cc)
- 25–27 gauge needle, 3/8 to 1 inch long
- Sterile gauze and adhesive bandage

To administer an intradermal injection, follow these steps:

1. Assemble and prepare the needed equipment.
2. Take BSI precautions, and confirm the drug, indication, dosage, and need for intradermal injection.

intradermal within the dermal layer of the skin.

Capillaries in the dermis afford a very slow rate of absorption, with little or no systemic distribution.

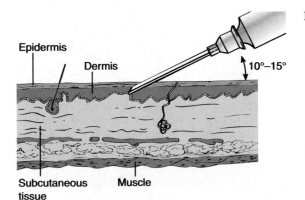

FIGURE 4-17 **Intradermal injection.**

3. Draw up medication as appropriate.

4. Prepare the site with alcohol or betadine. The intended site must be cleansed of pathogens, therein decreasing the likelihood of infection. Generally, you will use alcohol or betadine antiseptics. To appropriately cleanse the site, start at the site itself and work outward with an expanding circular motion. This motion will push pathogens away from the intended site of puncture.

5. Pull the patient's skin taut with your nondominant hand.

6. Insert the needle, bevel up, just under the skin, at a 10- to 15-degree angle.

7. Slowly inject the medication, look for a small bump or wheal to form as medication is deposited and collects in the intradermal tissue.

8. Remove the needle and dispose of it in the sharps container.

9. Place the adhesive bandage over the site; use the gauze for hemorrhage control if needed.

Do not rub or massage the injection site. This promotes systemic absorption and nullifies the advantage of localized effect.

Subcutaneous Injection

subcutaneous the layer of loose connective tissue between the skin and muscle.

The subcutaneous tissue has few blood vessels and thus promotes slow, sustained absorption, which prolongs a drug's effect on the body.

Subcutaneous injections place medication into the subcutaneous tissue (*sub-*, below; *cutaneous,* skin). The subcutaneous layer consists of loose connective tissue between the skin and muscle (Figure 4-18). The subcutaneous tissue has few blood vessels and thus promotes slow, sustained absorption, which prolongs a drug's effect on the body. Like intradermal injections, no more than 1.0 mL of medication is administered subcutaneously. Administering more than 1.0 mL of medication can cause irritation and, possibly, an abscess.

Administer subcutaneous injections where you can easily pinch the skin on the upper arms, thighs, or occasionally, the abdomen (Figure 4-19). Easily pinched skin contains more subcutaneous tissue and readily separates from the muscle. All sites should be free of superficial blood vessels, nerves, and tendons. Additionally, avoid areas with tattoos or bruising.

To perform a subcutaneous injection, you will need the following equipment:

- BSI protection
- Alcohol or betadine antiseptic preparations
- Packaged medication
- Syringe (1 to 3 cc)
- 24 to 26-gauge hypodermic needle, 3/8 to 1 inch long
- Sterile gauze and adhesive bandage

FIGURE 4-18 **Subcutaneous injection.**

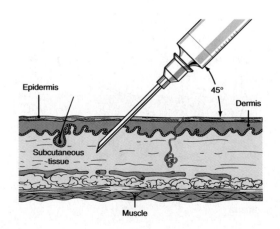

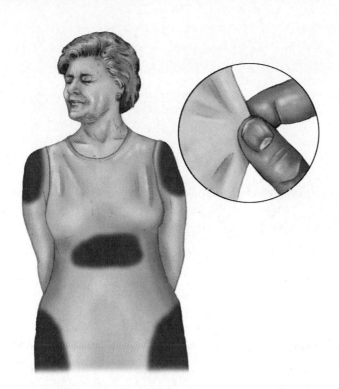

FIGURE 4-19 Subcutaneous injection sites (shown in red).

To administer a subcutaneous injection, use the following technique (Procedure 4-5):

1. Assemble and prepare equipment.
2. Take BSI precautions, and confirm the drug, indication, dosage, and need for subcutaneous injection.
3. Draw up the medication as appropriate.
4. Prepare the site with alcohol or betadine as described for an intradermal injection.
5. Gently pinch a 1-inch fold of skin.
6. Insert the needle just into skin at a 45-degree angle with the bevel up.
7. Pull the plunger back to aspirate tissue fluid.
8. If blood appears, the hypodermic needle is in a blood vessel, and absorption will be too rapid. Start the procedure over with a new syringe.
9. If no blood appears, proceed with step 10.
10. Slowly inject the medication.
11. Remove the needle and dispose of it in a sharps container.
12. Place an adhesive bandage over the site; use the gauze for hemorrhage control if needed.
13. Monitor the patient.

After you give the injection, gently rubbing or massaging the site will help initiate systemic absorption.

Some authorities recommend using an air plug in the syringe. This is approximately 0.1 mL of air that follows the injection and pushes the medication further into the subcutaneous tissue, thus preventing leakage or medication loss. To place an air plug in the syringe, aspirate approximately 0.1 mL of air into the barrel after you have drawn up the medication. Pointing the needle downward and perpendicular to the ground, tap the syringe with your finger to dislodge the air pocket. It will float to the top of the plunger, and from there it will follow the medication into the subcutaneous tissue.

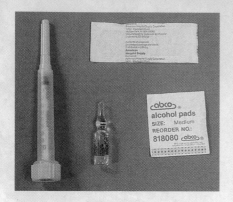

4-5a Prepare the equipment.

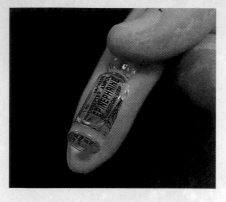

4-5b Check the medication.

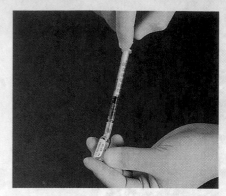

4-5c Draw up the medication.

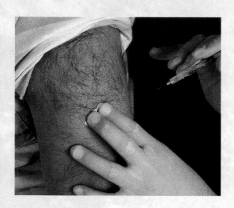

4-5d Prep the site.

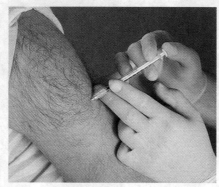

4-5e Insert the needle at a 45-degree angle.

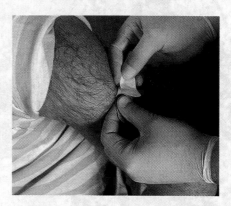

4-5f Remove the needle and cover the puncture site.

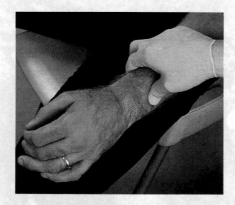

4-5g Monitor the patient.

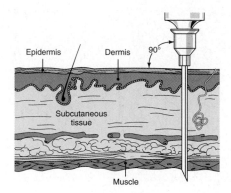

FIGURE 4-20   Intramuscular injection.

Epidermis   Dermis   90°

Subcutaneous tissue

Muscle

You can also deliver a subcutaneous injection into the sublingual region, or fleshy tissue below the tongue. To administer a subcutaneous injection, place the hypodermic needle of a small, medication-filled syringe into the sublingual tissue and then inject the medication as appropriate. Epinephrine in severe cases of asthma or anaphylaxis can be administered in this manner.

Intramuscular Injection

Intramuscular injections deposit medication into muscle (*intra-*, within; *muscular,* muscle). Muscle is extremely vascular and permits systemic delivery at a moderate absorption rate. Drug absorption through muscle is also relatively predictable. To reach the muscle, a needle must penetrate the dermal and subcutaneous tissue (Figure 4-20).

Several sites are used for intramuscular injections (Figure 4-21). Depending on the site, varying quantities of medication can be delivered. These sites and their correlating volumes of medication include:

- *Deltoid.* The deltoid muscle is 3 to 4 fingerbreadths below the acromial process (the bony bump on the shoulder). It is highly vascular and permits easy access. You can deliver up to 2.0 mL into this muscle.

- *Dorsal gluteal.* The dorsal gluteal muscle, or buttock, is a common administration point for intramuscular injections. Injections at this site can deliver 5.0 mL of medication or more. They cause little discomfort, but avoid the large sciatic nerve, which is the leg's major motor nerve. Damage to the sciatic nerve can decrease mobility or totally paralyze the leg. To help prevent neurological complication, envision an imaginary quadrant over the buttock; administer all injections in the upper and outer quadrant.

- *Vastus lateralis.* The vastus lateralis muscle of the thigh is another common site for intramuscular injection, especially for pediatric patients. As at the dorsal gluteal muscle, injections here can deliver 5 mL of medication or more. To deliver medication at this site, imagine a grid of nine boxes. Administer injections in the middle, outer box, or anterolateral part of the muscle.

- *Rectus femoris.* The rectus femoris lies over the femur and is closely associated with the vastus lateralis muscle. For intramuscular injection in the rectus femoris, place the medication into the center of the muscle at approximately mid-shaft of the femur. Up to 5 mL of drug volume can be administered into the rectus femoris.

When choosing a site, avoid bruised or scarred areas. Areas free of superficial blood vessels are most desirable.

To perform an intramuscular injection, you will need the following equipment:

- BSI protection
- Alcohol or betadine antiseptic preparation
- Packaged medication
- Syringe (1 to 5 mL, depending on dosage)

intramuscular within the muscle.

Muscle is extremely vascular and permits systemic delivery at a moderate absorption rate.

Content Review

INTRAMUSCULAR INJECTION SITES
- Deltoid
- Dorsal gluteal
- Vastus lateralis
- Rectus femoris

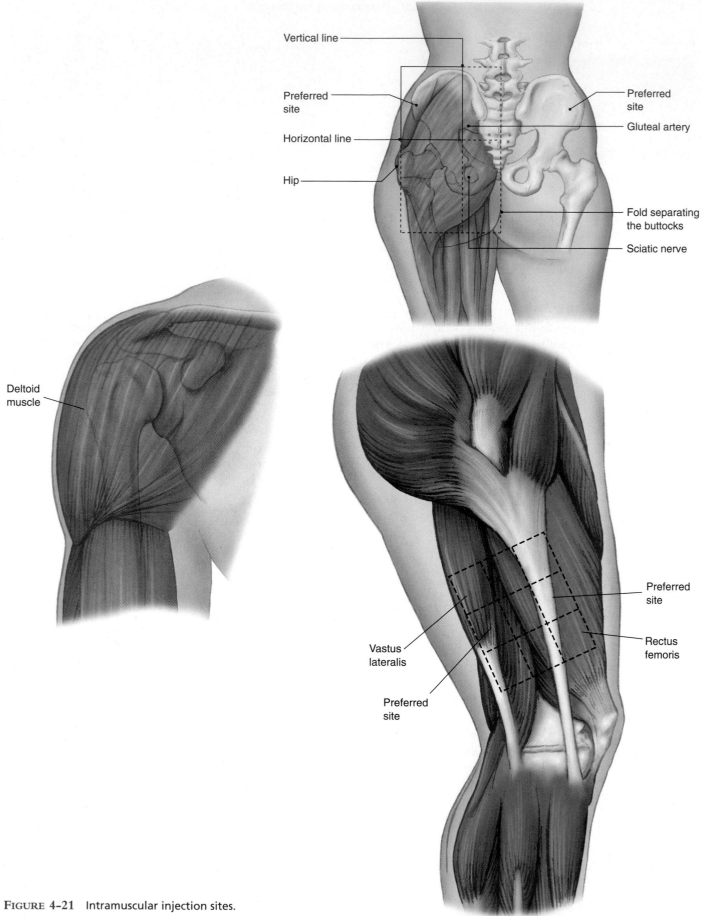

Vertical line

Preferred site

Horizontal line

Hip

Preferred site

Gluteal artery

Fold separating the buttocks

Sciatic nerve

Deltoid muscle

Preferred site

Rectus femoris

Vastus lateralis

Preferred site

FIGURE 4-21   Intramuscular injection sites.

- 21 to 23-gauge hypodermic needle, 3/8 to 1 inches long
- Sterile gauze and adhesive bandage

Follow these steps to administer an intramuscular injection (Procedure 4-6):

1. Assemble and prepare the needed equipment.
2. Take BSI precautions, and confirm the drug, indication, dosage, and need for intramuscular injection.
3. Draw up medication as appropriate.
4. Prepare the site with alcohol or betadine as described for an intradermal injection.
5. Stretch the skin taut over the injection site with your nondominant hand.
6. Insert the needle just into skin at a 90-degree angle with the bevel up.
7. Pull back the plunger to aspirate tissue fluid.
   - If blood appears, the hypodermic needle is in a blood vessel, and absorption of the medication will be too rapid. Start the procedure over with a new syringe.
   - If no blood appears proceed with step 8.
8. Slowly inject the medication.
9. Remove the needle and dispose of it in the sharps container.
10. Place an adhesive bandage over site; use gauze for hemorrhage control if needed.
11. Monitor the patient.

After administration, gently rubbing or massaging the site helps initiate systemic absorption. Do not massage the site, however, if you have administered heparin or another anticoagulant. Again, some authorities recommend a 0.1 mL air plug as described under subcutaneous injection.

Intravenous and Intraosseous Routes

Two important parenteral drug administration routes—intravenous access and intraosseous infusion—are discussed in detail in Part 2.

Part 2: Intravenous Access, Blood Sampling, and Intraosseous Infusion

This part of the chapter includes a discussion of IV access, including types of venous access and the variety of equipment required, where and how to establish access, flow rates, and possible complications. We will also detail intravenous administration of medications (bolus and infusion). Venous blood sampling techniques will also be covered.

Additionally, you will find information on intraosseous medication administration, including techniques, possible complications, and contraindications. Intraosseous administration is a route most often used in pediatric patients under five years of age.

INTRAVENOUS ACCESS

Intravenous (IV) access (*intra-*, within; *venous,* vein) or **cannulation,** is a routine EMT-I procedure. Circulating blood transports chemicals, proteins, and fluids throughout the body. Venous circulation can likewise deliver medications and fluids into the body and provides an invaluable tool for treating the sick and injured.

intravenous access
(**cannulation**) surgical puncture of a vein to deliver medication or withdraw blood.

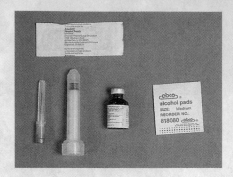

4-6a   Prepare the equipment.

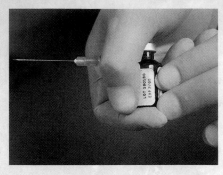

4-6b   Check the medication.

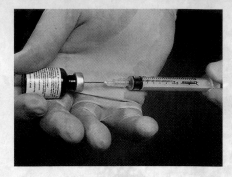

4-6c   Draw up the medication.

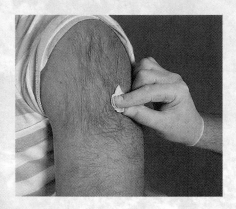

4-6d   Prepare the site.

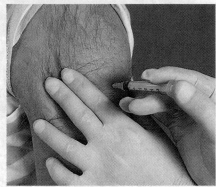

4-6e   Insert the needle at a 90-degree angle.

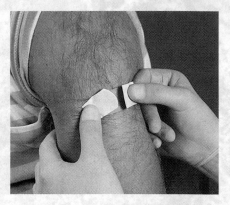

4-6f   Remove the needle and cover the puncture site.

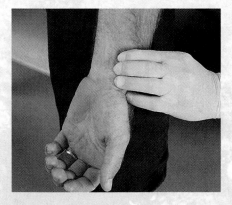

4-6g   Monitor the patient.

The following situations indicate intravenous access:

- Fluid and blood replacement
- Drug administration
- Obtaining venous blood specimens for laboratory analysis

Because veins are easier to locate and penetrate, venous access is preferable to arterial access. Additionally, venous circulation pressure is lower than arterial and presents fewer hemorrhage control complications.

TYPES OF INTRAVENOUS ACCESS

Medical care providers use two types of intravenous access, peripheral and central. As an EMT-I, you will most often perform peripheral IV access. Central venous access is rarely, if ever, performed in the prehospital setting.

Peripheral Venous Access

Although challenging, **peripheral venous access** is relatively easy to master. As the name implies, it uses peripheral veins. Common sites include the arms and legs and, when necessary, the neck. Figure 4-22 illustrates the specific veins commonly accessed on the hand, forearm, and leg.

peripheral venous access surgical puncture of a vein in the arm, leg, or neck.

Because some patients' veins may not be readily visible, you must know venous topography. In these cases, you will have to locate veins based on anatomical layout and palpation. Exhaust all possibilities on the arms before trying to locate the veins of the legs. Leg veins are more difficult to access and present complications more frequently. For neonates and infants, you may access veins in the scalp. Chapter 31, "Pediatric Emergencies," explains that technique.

When establishing a peripheral IV, start at the distal end of the extremity and work proximally. Once you have attempted cannulation, the disruption in blood flow hinders using veins distal to that site. However, the purpose of access also determines site selection. For example, rapid fluid administration requires larger veins, such as the antecubital fossa, as opposed to the smaller veins of the hand. The external jugular vein is considered a peripheral vein and can be accessed when other peripheral sites are not available.

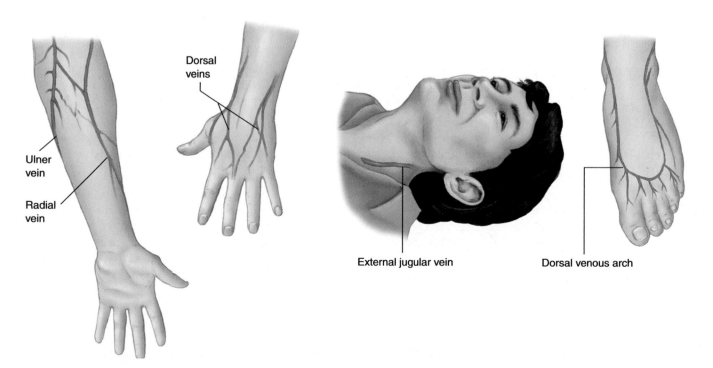

Dorsal veins

Ulner vein

Radial vein

External jugular vein

Dorsal venous arch

FIGURE 4-22   Peripheral IV access sites: veins of the arm, hand, neck, and foot.

central venous access surgical puncture of the internal jugular, subclavian, or femoral vein.

intravenous fluid chemically prepared solution tailored to the body's specific needs.

colloid intravenous solutions containing large proteins that cannot pass through capillary membranes.

crystalloid intravenous solutions that contain electrolytes but lack the larger proteins associated with colloids.

isotonic state in which solutions on opposite sides of a semi-permeable membrane are in equal concentration.

The major advantage of peripheral venous access is that it is relatively simple to perform because visualizing and accessing the veins is usually easy. Additionally, you can access peripheral veins while simultaneously doing other life-sustaining procedures such as CPR or endotracheal intubation. Conversely, peripheral veins collapse in hypovolemia or circulatory failure, thus becoming difficult to locate and access. Furthermore, the peripheral veins of geriatric patients, pediatric patients, or those with peripheral vascular disease may be fragile and difficult to cannulate. Finally, peripheral veins may roll and elude IV placement.

Central Venous Access

Central venous access is not within the scope of EMT-I practice. However, you may encounter patients who have indwelling central venous catheters in place. Protocols in some EMS systems allow EMT-Is to access existing central lines during emergency care. Always follow local protocols regarding central line access. For more information about central venous access, consult a text on advanced venipuncture techniques.

EQUIPMENT AND SUPPLIES FOR VENOUS ACCESS

Intravenous Fluids

Intravenous fluids are chemically prepared solutions tailored to the body's specific needs. They replace the body's lost fluids and/or aid the delivery of IV medications. They also can keep a vein patent when no fluid or drug therapy is required.

Intravenous fluids come in four different forms: colloids, crystalloids, blood, and oxygen-carrying fluids.

Colloids   Colloidal solutions contain large proteins that cannot pass through the capillary membrane. Consequently, they remain in the circulatory system for a long time. In addition, **colloids** have osmotic properties that attract water into the circulatory system. A small quantity of colloid can significantly increase intravascular volume (volume of blood and fluid contained within the blood vessels). Common colloids include:

- *Plasma protein fraction (plasmanate).* Plasmanate is a protein-containing colloid. Its principle protein, albumin, is suspended with other proteins in a saline solvent.
- *Salt-poor albumin.* Salt-poor albumin contains only human albumin. Each gram of albumin retains approximately 18 mL of water in the blood stream.
- *Dextran.* Dextran is not a protein but a large sugar molecule with osmotic properties similar to albumin. It comes in two molecular weights: 40,000 and 70,000 daltons. Dextran 40 has from two to two and one-half times the colloidal osmotic pressure of albumin. Anaphylactic reaction is a possible side effect.
- *Hetastarch (Hespan).* As with Dextran, hetastarch is a sugar molecule with osmotic properties similar to protein. Hetastarch does not appear to share the side effects of Dextran.

Although colloids help maintain vascular volume, using them in the field is not practical. Their high cost, short shelf life, and specific storage requirements suit them better to the hospital setting. However, the EMT-I who works in an emergency department, aeromedical service, or at a multiple-casualty incident may have to administer colloidal solutions.

Crystalloids   **Crystalloids** are the primary out-of-hospital IV solution. Crystalloids contain electrolytes and water but lack colloids' larger proteins and larger molecules. The many preparations of crystalloid solutions are classified by their tonicity (number of particles per unit volume) relative to that of body plasma:

- *Isotonic solutions.* **Isotonic** solutions have a tonicity equal to blood plasma. In a normally hydrated patient, they will not cause a significant fluid or electrolyte shift.

- *Hypertonic solutions.* **Hypertonic** solutions have a higher solute concentration than do the cells. When administered to the normally hydrated patient, they cause fluid to shift out of the intracellular compartment and into the extracellular compartment. Later, solute diffuses in the opposite direction.

- *Hypotonic solutions.* **Hypotonic** solutions have a lower solute concentration than do the cells. When administered to a normally hydrated patient, they cause fluid to move from the extracellular compartment and into the intracellular compartment. Later, the solutes move in the opposite direction.

The particular type of IV solution you select depends on your patient's needs. The three most commonly used IV fluids in prehospital care are the following:

- *Lactated Ringer's.* Lactated Ringer's solution is an isotonic electrolyte solution. It contains sodium chloride, potassium chloride, calcium chloride, and sodium lactate in water.

- *Normal saline solution.* Normal saline is an isotonic electrolyte solution containing 0.90% sodium chloride in water.

- *5% dextrose in water (D_5W).* D_5W is a hypotonic glucose solution used to keep a vein patent and to supply calories needed for cellular metabolism. Although D_5W initially increases circulatory volume, glucose molecules rapidly diffuse across the vascular membrane and increase the free water.

Both lactated Ringer's and normal saline solutions are used for fluid replacement because of their immediate ability to expand the circulating volume. However, due to the movement of electrolytes and water, two-thirds of either solution will be lost to the extravascular space within one hour. Crystalloids such as normal saline mixed with D_5W or half-strength normal saline (0.45%) are combinations or modifications of the above solutions.

Occasionally, you will have to warm or cool the IV fluid. A hypothermic patient may benefit from having a crystalloid warmed before and during fluid administration. Warm fluids assist in elevating the patient's core temperature. Conversely, cool fluids may benefit the patient with an increased core temperature. You can cool or warm fluids by storing them in a special temperature-controlled compartment or by using the heater or air conditioner in the ambulance, helicopter, or mobile intensive care unit. Commercial fluid heaters are available. Their use is detailed later in this chapter. Some fluids, such as blood and some colloids, require constant storage in a cool environment.

Blood The most desirable fluid for replacement is whole blood. Unlike colloids and crystalloids, the hemoglobin in blood carries oxygen. Blood, however, is a precious commodity and must be conserved so that it can be of benefit to the most people. Its use in the field is generally limited to aeromedical services or mass casualty incidents. The universal compatibility of O-negative blood makes it ideal for administration in the field.

Oxygen-Carrying Solutions In development are fluids that can carry oxygen and offload it for cellular use. These fluids, which remain experimental at present, show promise for treating hypovolemia in the field.

Packaging of Intravenous Fluids Most IV fluids and blood are packaged in soft plastic or vinyl bags of various sizes (50, 100, 250, 500, 1,000, 2,000, and 3,000 mL) (Figure 4-23). Some contain medication that is incompatible with plastic or vinyl and must be packaged in glass bottles.

The IV-fluid container provides the following important information:

- *Label.* A label on every IV bottle or bag lists the fluid type and expiration date. As with any other medication, IV solutions have a shelf life; do not use them after their expiration date. Discard any fluid that appears cloudy, discolored, or laced with particulate. Additionally, avoid using any fluid whose sealed packaging has been opened or tampered with.

- *Medication administration port.* A medication port on IV-solution bags or bottles permits you to inject medication into the fluid for infusion.

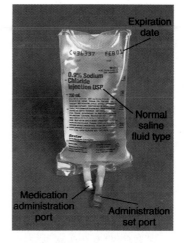

FIGURE 4-23 IV solution containers.

- *Administration set port.* The administration set port is where you place the spike from the IV administration tubing.

Administration Tubing

administration tubing flexible, clear plastic tubing that connects the solution bag to the IV cannula.

cannula hollow needle used to puncture a vein.

microdrip tubing administration tubing that delivers a relatively small amount of fluid.

macrodrip tubing administration tubing that delivers a relatively large amount of fluid.

IV **administration tubing** connects the solution bag to the IV **cannula** that is inserted into the patient's vein. Administration tubing is made of very flexible clear plastic. You must select from several types of administration tubing according to the patient's need. All tubing is packaged in a sterile container. If the container is opened or appears damaged, select another administration set. Any pathogens on the tubing will enter the patient, possibly causing long-term complications.

Microdrip and Macrodrip Tubing   **Microdrip** administration tubing delivers relatively small amounts of fluid to the patient. It is more appropriate when you need to restrict the overall fluid volume a patient will receive. **Macrodrip** administration tubing delivers relatively large amounts of fluid. It is more appropriate when volume replacement is necessary, as in shock, fluid replacement, or hypotension.

To effectively deliver IV fluids, you must be thoroughly familiar with the microdrip and macrodrip administration sets, their components, and their subtle differences (Figure 4-24):

FIGURE 4-24 **Macrodrip and microdrip administration sets.**

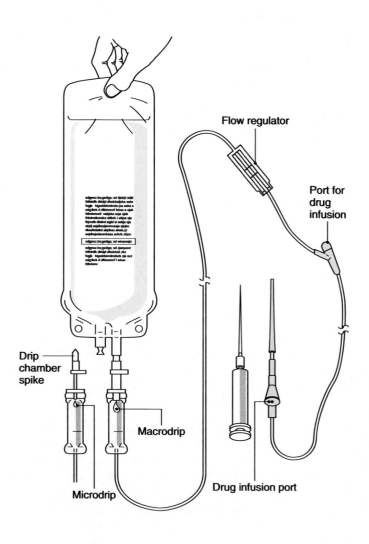

- *Spike.* The **spike** is a sharp-pointed plastic device that you insert into the administration set port on the IV-solution bag. A plastic sheath covering the spike keeps it sterile. When the sheath is removed, you must use a medically clean technique to avoid contaminating the spike. If the spike becomes contaminated, discard the administration set and start over with new tubing.

- *Drip chamber.* The **drip chamber** is a clear plastic chamber that allows you to view the **drip rate.** The drip chamber is squeezable; when compressed, it collects fluid from the IV-solution bag and acts as a reservoir for administration. For optimal fluid delivery, the drip chamber should be about one-third full; a line on the chamber marks the correct fluid level.

- *Drop former.* Inside the drip chamber is a **drop former.** In microdrip administration tubing, the drop former is a hollow metal stylet. In macrodrip tubing, it is a large circular opening at the top of the drip chamber. The drop former regulates each drop's size. The narrow metal stylet in the microdrip tubing creates smaller drops; the wider opening in the macrodrip tubing creates larger drops. In either case, the drop former's precise calibration allows you to calculate fluid volumes by counting drops, or **gtts:**
  - Microdrip 60 gtts = 1 mL
  - Macrodrip 10 gtts = 1 mL

  Depending on the manufacturer, macrodrip sets may equate 15 or 20 gtts to 1 mL. You must know drops per milliliter to calculate flow rates or medicated infusion dosages.

- *Tubing.* IV administration tubing is clear and very flexible. Thus, you can watch the solution flow through the administration set, and you can manipulate the tubing in tight situations. Some medications, such as IV nitroglycerin, are chemically incompatible with regular tubing and require special tubing.

- *Clamp.* IV administration tubing has a simple plastic clamp. When slid over the tubing, the clamp completely stops the flow of solution from the IV bag to the patient. It prevents both the entrainment of air into the tubing when changing IV bags and the backflow of medication when administering medications. You can also use it to stop infusion without disturbing the flow-regulator setting.

- *Flow regulator.* The flow regulator is a dial enclosed in a triangular plastic casing. It allows infinite control of flow rates ranging from a continuous stream to completely stopped. Rolling the dial towards the IV solution bag increases the drip frequency; rolling the dial towards the patient decreases the drip frequency.

- *Medication injection ports.* The **medication injection ports** have a self-sealing membrane into which you can insert a hypodermic needle for drug administration. Their design varies, depending on the manufacturer. When possible, use the medication port nearest the patient.

- *Needle adapter.* The **needle adapter** is a rigid plastic device at the administration tubing's distal end. It is specifically constructed to fit into the hub of an IV cannula. Similar to the spike, the needle adapter is sterile and covered by a protective cap. If it becomes contaminated at any time, start over with a new administration set.

IV Extension Tubing **Extension tubing** is IV tubing used to extend the original macrodrip or microdrip setup. Its packaging clearly marks it as such. Like administration sets, extension tubing is sterile and must be handled accordingly.

Extension tubing also permits the EMT-I to change the original administration tubing or the IV solution bag with little difficulty. For example, if you have to switch from a macrodrip set to a microdrip set, you can close the clamp on the extension and detach the primary tubing. Once you have flushed the new tubing with fluid, place the needle adapter into the

spike sharp-pointed device inserted into the IV solution bag's administration set port.

drip chamber clear plastic chamber that allows visualization of the drip rate.

drip rate pace at which the fluid moves from the bag into the patient.

drop former device that regulates the size of drops.

gtts drops (Latin *guttae*, drops [*gutta*, drop]).

medication injection port self-healing membrane into which a hypodermic needle is inserted for drug administration.

needle adapter rigid plastic device specifically constructed to fit into the hub of an intravenous cannula.

extension tubing IV tubing used to extend a macrodrip or microdrip setup.

receiving port on the extension tubing and release the clamp. You can now resume fluid therapy without risking complications or having to painfully reinitiate a second IV line.

Electromechanical Pump Tubing   Mechanical infusion devices may require specially manufactured pump tubing. Typically, pump tubing has special components that attach directly to the pump. Additionally, bladders and relief points permit you to void possible air bubbles. Many specific models of electromechanical infusion pumps require specific pump tubing. When using a mechanical infusion pump, be sure to have the appropriate tubing on hand.

Measured Volume Administration Set   The **measured volume administration set** can deliver specific volumes of fluid with or without medication. It is especially advantageous for pediatric patients, patients with renal failure, or other patients who cannot tolerate fluid overload.

The measured volume administration set consists of either microdrip or macrodrip tubing, with the addition of a large **burette chamber** marked in 1.0 mL increments. The burette chamber holds between 120 and 150 mL of fluid. Its components include:

- Flanged spike
- Clamp
- Airway handle
- Medication injection port
- Burette chamber
- Float valve
- Drip chamber
- Flow regulator
- Medication injection port
- Needle adapter

When opened, the airway handle on top of the burette chamber permits air to be displaced or replaced as fluid enters or exits the chamber. If a medication must be mixed in a specific amount of IV solution, you can add it through the medication administration port after correctly filling the chamber.

Blood Tubing   Administering whole blood or blood components requires **blood tubing,** which contains a filter that prevents clots and other debris from entering the patient. Without exception, all blood must be filtered. Blood that is stored or delivered over an extended period is prone to form fibrin clots or to accumulate other debris. If these clots or debris enter the circulatory system, they can travel in the form of an embolus.

Some aeromedical and facility-based EMT-Is administer blood, primarily during transport, and must be familiar with blood tubing. Although most ambulances do not carry blood, EMT-Is may initiate normal saline with blood tubing in anticipation that whole blood or blood products will be required immediately in the emergency department. Blood tubing comes in two configurations, straight and Y. Y tubing has two administration ports, one for blood and one for IV normal saline solution. Typically, blood is administered with normal saline. Fluids similar to lactated Ringer's increase the potential for blood coagulation. The two-port design permits immediate access to normal saline if the blood supply is exhausted or must be shut down, as for a transfusion reaction. When you use Y blood tubing, establish a traditional IV by connecting a bag of normal saline to the tubing. Attach the blood to the second port when needed, while maintaining strict medical asepsis. Using the flow regulator, discontinue the normal saline while opening the clamp regulating the flow of blood. Straight blood tubing has only one reservoir. Therefore, only blood is attached to the tubing. A medication administration port close to the needle adapter allows you to piggyback a secondary line of normal saline into the tubing.

Miscellaneous Administration Sets   Some tubing now has a manual dial that can set drops per minute or specific flow rates. Some manufacturers have created a single drip chamber that can create either microdrips or macrodrips.

---

measured volume administration set IV setup that delivers specific volumes of fluid.

burette chamber calibrated chamber of berutrol IV administration tubing that enables precise measurement and delivery of fluids and medicated solutions.

blood tubing administration tubing that contains a filter to prevent clots or other debris from entering the patient.

Intravenous Cannulas

The IV cannula permits actual puncture and access into a patient's vein. The distal portion of the administration tubing connects to the IV cannula. The three basic types of IV cannulas are:

- Over-the-needle catheter
- Hollow-needle catheter
- Plastic catheter inserted through a hollow needle

Over-the-Needle Catheter Often called an **angiocatheter,** the semi-flexible **over-the-needle catheter** encloses a sharp metal stylet (needle) (Figure 4-25).

- *Metal stylet (needle).* The metal stylet punctures the skin and blood vessel. Blood flows through the hollow stylet to the flashback chamber.
- *Flashback chamber.* Blood in the clear plastic flashback chamber confirms placement of the stylet in the vein.
- *Teflon catheter.* The Teflon catheter slides over the metal stylet into a successfully punctured vein.
- *Hub.* Located on the back of the Teflon catheter, the hub receives the needle adapter of the administration tubing once removed from the metal stylet.

For peripheral venous access, the over-the-needle catheter is preferred since it is easy to place and anchor and permits freer movement of the patient.

Hollow-Needle Catheter For pediatrics or other patients with tiny, delicate veins, use **hollow-needle catheters** (Figure 4-26). These catheters do not have a Teflon tube; rather, the metal stylet itself is inserted into the vein and secured there. Because the sharp metal stylet can easily damage the vein, you must insert it very carefully. Some hollow-needle catheters have wings for guidance and securing into a vein. These hollow-needle catheters are referred to as winged catheters or butterfly catheters.

Catheter Inserted Through the Needle The **catheter inserted through the needle** is also called an **intracatheter.** It consists of a Teflon catheter inserted through a large metal stylet

over-the-needle catheter/angiocatheter semi-flexible catheter enclosing a sharp metal stylet.

hollow-needle catheter stylet that does not have a Teflon tube but is itself inserted into the vein and secured there.

catheter inserted through the needle (intracatheter) Teflon catheter inserted through a large metal stylet.

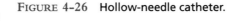

FIGURE 4-25 Over-the-needle catheter.

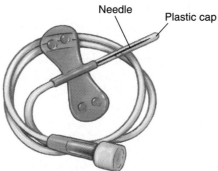

FIGURE 4-26 Hollow-needle catheter.

FIGURE 4-27 Catheter inserted through the needle.

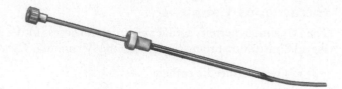

(Figure 4-27). Used in the hospital setting to implement central lines, its proper placement requires great skill, as discussed previously.

The size of an IV cannula is expressed as its gauge. The *larger* the gauge, the *smaller* the diameter of the stylet and catheter. For example, a 22-gauge cannula is smaller than a 14-gauge cannula. The larger diameter, 14-gauge catheter allows greater flow rates than the smaller diameter 22-gauge cannula. When establishing venous access, choose the cannula size most appropriate for the patient condition. Typical uses for the various sizes of cannulas are:

- *22-gauge.* Small gauges are used for fragile veins such as those of the elderly or children.
- *20-gauge.* Moderate gauges are used for the average adult who does not need fluid replacement.
- *18-gauge, 16-gauge, or 14-gauge.* Larger gauge cannulas are used to increase volume or to administer viscous medications such as dextrose. Blood can be administered only through a cannula that is 16-gauge or larger.

The largest gauge cannula that will fit into a vein is not always appropriate. A cardiac patient with large veins should not receive a 14-gauge cannula for medication administration, just as a multi-systems trauma patient with good veins should not receive a 22-gauge cannula for fluid administration. Remember that IV access is painful and causes discomfort not only to those receiving it but also to family members watching a loved one in distress.

Miscellaneous Equipment

The **venous constricting band** is a flat rubber band applied proximal to the intended puncture site. It impedes venous return, thereby engorging veins and making them easier to see. This helps you to select the best site and makes venipuncture easier. Never restrict arterial blood flow with the constricting band, and never leave it in place longer than two minutes.

IV access is an invasive procedure; therefore you must use medically clean techniques, including antiseptic preparations, to prevent infection. Applying alcohol and betadine before and after venipuncture decreases the chance of infection.

Once you have established an IV, you must secure it. Medical tape and an adhesive bandage are inexpensive and easy to apply. You can also apply clear membranes over the site. Commercial devices manufactured specifically for this task are also available. Have gauze on hand for hemorrhage control if IV cannulation is unsuccessful or if blood leaks from around the site.

Obtaining a venous blood specimen at the time of venipuncture saves the patient from being stuck with a needle again later. This chapter's section on venous blood sampling discusses this technique in detail.

INTRAVENOUS ACCESS IN THE HAND, ARM, AND LEG

As an EMT-I, you will most often establish peripheral IVs in the hand, arm, or leg. The veins in these places are relatively easy to locate and accessing them causes the patient less pain. In addition, the likelihood of complications is less with these veins than with the external jugular vein (discussed later) or central IV initiation. Therefore, the veins of the hand, arm, and leg are the primary sites for IV initiation.

To establish a peripheral IV in the hand, arm, or leg, use the following technique (Procedure 4-7):

1. Confirm indication and type of IV setup needed. Gather and arrange all supplies and equipment beforehand to make the process easy and accessible.

IV access is painful and causes discomfort not only to those receiving it but also to family members watching a loved one in distress.

venous constricting band flat rubber band used to impede venous return and make veins easier to see.

Never leave the constricting band in place more than 2 minutes.

Legal Notes

In order to minimize the chances of a catheter sheer reaching the patient's central circulation, always leave the venous constricting band in place until you have completely removed the needle from the catheter.

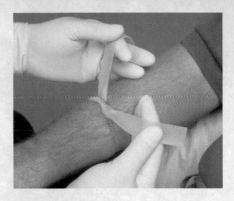

4-7a   Place the constricting band.

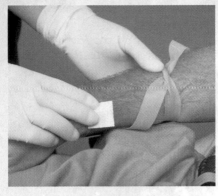

4-7b   Cleanse the venipuncture site.

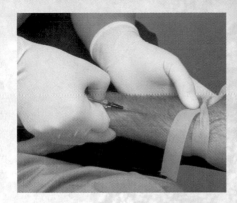

4-7c   Insert the IV cannula into the vein.

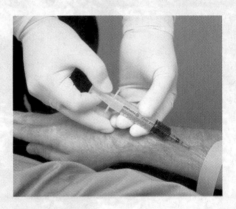

4-7d   Withdraw any blood samples.

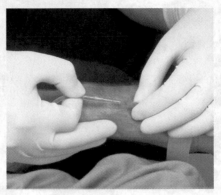

4-7e   Connect the IV tubing.

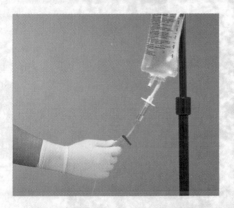

4-7f   Turn on the IV and check the flow.

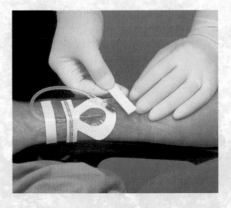

4-7g   Secure the site.

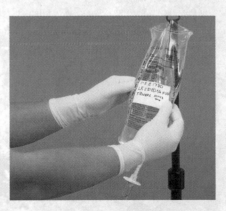

4-7h   Label the IV solution bag.

- IV fluid
- Administration set
- Intravenous cannula
- Tape or commercial securing device
- Venous blood drawing equipment
- Venous constricting band
- Antiseptic swab (betadine/alcohol)

When appropriate, explain the entire process to the patient. Take the proper BSI precautions, including gloves and goggles, because IV access is invasive and presents the potential for blood exposure.

2. Prepare all needed equipment. Examine the IV fluid for clarity and expiration date. Insert the administration tubing spike in the IV solution bag's administration set port. Squeeze fluid from the IV fluid container into the drip chamber until it reaches the fill line. Open the clamp and/or flow regulator to flush the solution through the administration tubing and expel trapped air bubbles. Shut down the flow regulator and replace the cap over the needle adapter. Remember that the IV administration set is sterile; if any contamination occurs you must replace the set with a new one.

3. Select the venipuncture site. Acceptable sites have clearly visible veins and are free of bruising or scarring. Straight veins are easier to cannulate than crooked ones.

4. Place the constricting band proximal to the intended site of puncture. Tighten it enough to impede venous blood flow without restricting arterial blood passage. Never leave the constricting band in place more than two minutes, because intrinsic changes will occur in the slowed venous blood.

5. Cleanse the venipuncture site. You must cleanse the intended site of pathogens to decrease the likelihood of infection. Alcohol and betadine are the most commonly used antiseptics. Start at the site itself and work outward in an expanding circle. This pushes pathogens away from the puncture site.

6. Insert the IV cannula into the vein. With your nondominant hand, pull all local skin taut to stabilize the vein and prevent it from rolling. With the distal bevel of the metal stylet up, insert the cannula into the vein at a 10- to 30-degree angle. Continue until you feel the cannula "pop" into the vein or see blood in the flashback chamber. The metal stylet is now in the vein; however, the Teflon catheter is not. To place the catheter into the vein, carefully advance the cannula approximately 0.5 cm further. (If you are using a butterfly cannula, it has no Teflon catheter, and you must carefully advance the needle itself.)

7. Holding the metal stylet stationary, slide the Teflon catheter over the needle into the vein. Place a finger over the vein at the catheter tip and tamponade (press gently downward to occlude the vein), thus preventing blood from flowing from the catheter and/or air from entraining into the circulatory system. Carefully remove the metal stylet and promptly dispose of it in the sharps container. Remove the venous constricting band.

8. Obtain venous blood samples as discussed in the section on venous blood sampling.

9. Attach the administration tubing to the cannula. Remove the protective cap from the needle adapter and tightly secure the needle adapter into the cannula hub. Open the flow regulator and allow the fluid to run freely for several seconds. Adjust the flow rate. Do not let go of the cannula and administration tubing until you have secured them as explained in step 10.

10. Apply antibiotic ointment to the site and cover it with an adhesive bandage or other commercial device. Loop the distal tubing and secure with tape.

This makes the medication administration port more accessible and attaches the device to the patient more securely. Continue by taping the administration tubing to the patient, proximal to the venipuncture site.

11. Label the IV solution bag with the following information:
    - Date and time initiated
    - Person initiating the IV access

12. Continually monitor the patient and flow rate.

Intravenous Access in the External Jugular Vein

The external jugular vein is a large peripheral blood vessel in the neck, between the angle of the jaw and the middle third of the clavicle. It connects into the central circulation's subclavian vein. Because it lies so close to the central circulation, cannulation here offers many of the same benefits afforded by central venous access. Fluids and medications rapidly reach the core of the body from this site.

Consider accessing the external jugular only after you have exhausted other means of peripheral access or when a patient requires immediate fluid administration. This is an extremely painful site to access, so you typically will reserve its use for patients with a decreased or total loss of consciousness.

Cannulating the external jugular vein requires essentially the same equipment as other forms of peripheral IV access, plus a 10-mL syringe. You will not need a constricting band. To access the external jugular, use the following technique (Procedure 4-8):

1. Prepare all equipment as for peripheral IV access in an arm, hand, or leg. In addition, fill the 10-mL syringe with 3 to 5 mL of sterile saline. Attach the distal part of the syringe to the flashback chamber of a large bore, over-the-needle catheter. Take the proper BSI precautions.

2. Place the patient supine and/or in the Trendelenburg position. This position increases blood flow to the chest and neck, thus distending the vein and making it easier to see. In addition, the supine-Trendelenburg position decreases the chance of air entering the circulatory system during cannulation.

3. Turn the patient's head to the side opposite of access. This maneuver makes the site easier to see and reach; do not perform it if the patient has traumatic head and/or neck injuries.

4. Cleanse the site with antiseptics. Start at the site of intended puncture and work outward 1 to 2 inches in ever increasing circles.

5. Occlude venous return by placing a finger on the external jugular just above the clavicle. This should distend the vein, again allowing greater visualization and ease of puncture. Never apply a venous constricting band around the patient's neck.

6. Position the IV cannula parallel with the vein, midway between the angle of the jaw and clavicle. Point the catheter at the medial third of the clavicle and insert it, bevel up, at a 10- to 30-degree angle.

7. Enter the external jugular while withdrawing on the plunger of the attached syringe. You will see blood in the syringe or feel a pop as the cannula enters the vein. Once inside the vein, advance the entire angiocatheter another 0.5 cm so the tip of the Teflon catheter lies within the lumen of the vein. Then slide the Teflon catheter into the vein and remove the metal stylet as previously described. Immediately dispose of the metal stylet.

8. Obtain venous blood samples as discussed in the section on venous blood sampling.

9. Attach the administration tubing to the IV catheter. Allow the IV solution to run freely for several seconds. Set the flow rate and secure as appropriate.

10. Monitor the patient for complications.

Consider accessing the external jugular only after you have exhausted other means of peripheral access or when a patient requires immediate fluid administration.

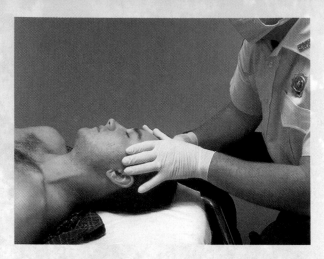

4-8a   Place the patient in a supine or Trendelenburg position.

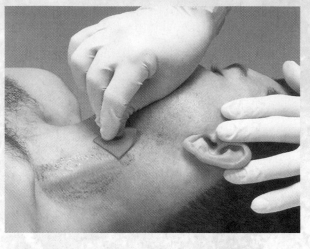

4-8b   Turn the patient's head to the side opposite of access and cleanse the site.

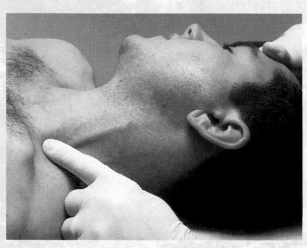

4-8c   Occlude venous return by placing a finger on the external jugular just above the clavicle.

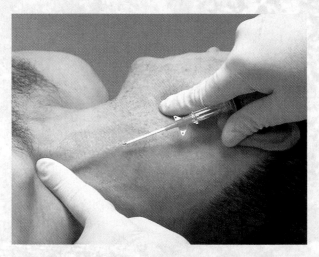

4-8d   Point the catheter at the medial third of the clavicle and insert it, bevel up, at a 10- to 30-degree angle.

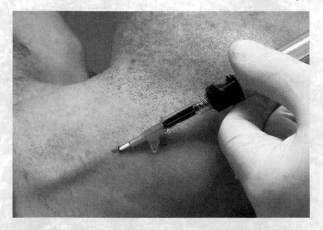

4-8e   Enter the external jugular while withdrawing on the plunger of the attached syringe.

Although using the external jugular vein has advantages, it also has distinct drawbacks. You may inadvertently puncture the airway or damage the nearby arterial vessels. Additionally, this is a painful entry site for the conscious patient. To minimize risks, perform the procedure very carefully.

INTRAVENOUS ACCESS WITH A MEASURED VOLUME ADMINISTRATION SET

When using a measured volume administration set, follow this procedure (Procedure 4-9):

1. Prepare the tubing by closing all clamps and insert the flanged spike into the IV solution bag's spike port.

2. Open the airway handle. Open the uppermost clamp and fill the burette chamber with approximately 20 mL of fluid. Squeeze the drip chamber until the fluid reaches the fill line. Open the bottom flow regulator to purge air through the tubing. When all air is purged, close the bottom flow regulator.

3. Continue to fill the burette chamber with the designated amount of solution.

4. Close the uppermost clamp and open the flow regulator until you reach the desired drip rate. Leave the airway handle open, so that air replaces the displaced fluid.

To refill the burette chamber, open the uppermost clamp until you have delivered the desired volume; then repeat step 4.

You can also use measured volume administration sets for continuous fluid administration. Fill the burette chamber with at least 30 mL of solution and close the airway handle. Leave the uppermost clamp open and adjust the rate with the lower flow regulator.

INTRAVENOUS ACCESS WITH BLOOD TUBING

To establish an IV with blood tubing, use the following procedure:

1. Prepare the tubing by closing all clamps and insert the flanged spike into the spike port of the blood and/or normal saline solution (Y-configured tubing).

2. Squeeze the drip chamber until it is one-third full and blood covers the filter. Repeat for the normal saline if you are using Y tubing.

3. If you are using straight tubing, piggyback a secondary line of normal saline into the blood tubing, unless you plan to piggyback the straight blood tubing into a large bore primary line.

4. Flush all tubing with normal saline and blood as appropriate.

5. Attach blood tubing to the intravenous cannula or into a previously established IV line.

6. Ensure patency by infusing a small amount of normal saline. Shut down when you have confirmed patency.

7. Open the clamp(s) and/or flow regulator(s) that allows blood to move from the bag to the patient. Adjust the flow rate accordingly.

8. When blood therapy is complete or must be discontinued, shut down the flow regulator from the blood supply and open the regulator(s) for the normal saline solution.

FACTORS AFFECTING INTRAVENOUS FLOW RATES

If an IV does not flow properly, check for the following problems and correct them as appropriate.

- *Constricting band.* Has the venous constricting band been removed? This is probably the most common mistake both in and out of the hospital. Additionally, ensure that the patient is not wearing restrictive clothing that interferes with venous blood flow.

> **Content Review**
>
> **IV TROUBLESHOOTING**
> - Constricting band still in place?
> - Edema at puncture site?
> - Cannula abutting vein wall or valve?
> - Administration set control valves closed?
> - IV bag too low?
> - Completely filled drip chamber?

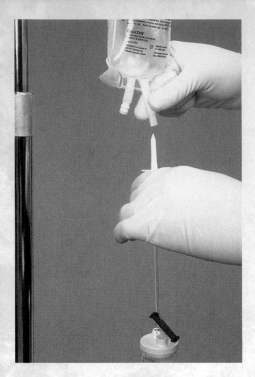

4-9a Spike the solution bag.

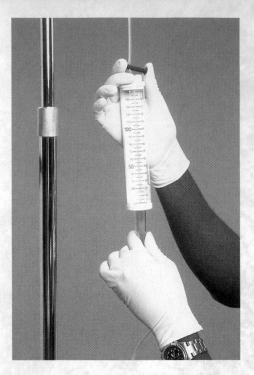

4-9b Open the uppermost clamp and fill the burette chamber with the desired volume of fluid.

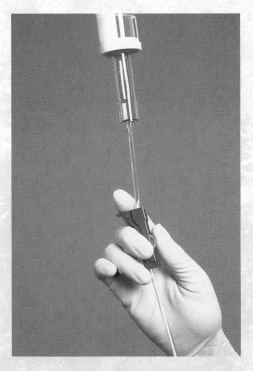

4-9c Close the uppermost clamp and open the flow regulator.

- *Edema at the puncture site.* Swelling at the IV site indicates fluid collection caused by infiltration. This **extravasation** occurs if you accidentally puncture the vein more than once, thus allowing IV solution and blood to escape from the second puncture and accumulate in the surrounding tissue. An infiltrated IV site is not usable.

- *Cannula abutting the vein wall or valve.* If the distal tip of the cannula butts against a wall or valve, carefully reposition it. You may have to untape and retape the cannula once you have achieved an adequate flow rate. Additionally, you may need to use an arm board to keep the patient's extremity straight, because flexion may kink the vein at the site and impede the solution's flow.

- *Administration set control valves.* Ensure that the flow regulator is open. Be sure to check the flow regulator and clamps of both the primary and any secondary or extension tubing.

- *IV bag height.* When you move the patient, you may raise the cannulation site above the IV solution bag. This interrupts the solution's gravitational flow from the bag into the patient.

- *Completely filled drip chamber.* Is the drip chamber completely filled? You can easily correct this by inverting the bag and squeezing the fluid from the drip chamber back into the bag.

- *Catheter patency.* A blood clot at the end of the Teflon catheter or needle may obstruct the flow of solution from the IV solution bag into the body. If the flow slows, increase the IV drip rate to keep the catheter or needle clear. If the flow stops completely, cleanse the medication administration port closest to the IV entry site with alcohol preparations and insert a syringe and hypodermic needle. Gently aspirate back on the syringe until the blood clot is pulled into the syringe. Never flush an IV that has stopped running because of a clot. Flushing forces the clot into the circulatory system and can cause occlusions in the heart or lungs.

If flow remains inadequate after you have eliminated all of these possible causes, lower the IV bag below the insertion site. If blood flows into the IV administration tubing, the site is patent and the problem lies elsewhere. If the problem persists, remove the IV and reestablish it on another extremity, using all new equipment. If you do not observe blood return, the site is inoperable.

COMPLICATIONS OF PERIPHERAL INTRAVENOUS ACCESS

Even though it is a routine procedure, IV access is not trouble free. It can cause a number of complications.

Pain

Pain at the puncture site occurs during needle penetration or with extravasation. To minimize pain, use a smaller gauge catheter or use a 1% lidocaine solution (without epinephrine) to anesthetize the overlying skin before insertion.

Local Infection

Local infection occurs if you do not properly cleanse the site and thus introduce pathogens through the puncture. This complication does not become apparent until after the IV has been established for several hours.

Pyrogenic Reaction

Pyrogens (foreign proteins capable of producing fever) in the administration tubing or IV solution can cause a pyrogenic reaction. The abrupt onset of fever (100°F to 106°F), chills, backache, headache, nausea, and vomiting characterize these reactions. Cardiovascular collapse may also result.

Typically, a pyrogenic reaction occurs within one-half to one hour after you initiate an IV. If you suspect a pyrogenic reaction, immediately terminate the IV and reestablish access in the opposite side with new equipment and fluid.

extravasation leakage of fluid or medication from the blood vessel that is commonly found with infiltration.

Content Review

IV ACCESS COMPLICATIONS

- Pain
- Local infection
- Pyrogenic reaction
- Catheter shear
- Inadvertent arterial puncture
- Circulatory overload
- Thrombophlebitis
- Thrombus formation
- Air embolism
- Necrosis
- Anticoagulants

pyrogen foreign protein capable of producing fever.

Typically, pyrogenic reactions occur secondary to the use of IV solutions that have been contaminated with a microorganism or other foreign matter. Pyrogenic reactions underscore the need to discard any fluid that is cloudy or any equipment that has been opened.

Allergic Reaction

A patient receiving IV therapy may develop an allergic reaction. Most often allergic reactions accompany the administration of blood or colloidal (protein-containing) solutions. In addition, some patients may react to the latex in some types of IV administration tubing.

The sudden onset of hives (urticaria), itching (pruritis), localized or systemic edema, or shortness of breath may signify an allergic reaction. If you suspect an allergic reaction, stop the IV infusion and remove the IV catheter. Treat the patient as discussed in Chapter 22 on allergies and anaphylaxis.

Catheter Shear

embolus foreign particle in the blood.

A catheter shear can occur if you pull the Teflon catheter through or over the needle after you have advanced it into the vein. The soft plastic catheter will easily snag on the metal stylet's sharp point and shear off, thus forming a plastic **embolus.** Therefore, never draw the Teflon catheter over the metal stylet after you have advanced it.

Inadvertent Arterial Puncture

Because arteries may lie close to veins, accidental arterial puncture may occur. Arterial blood is bright red and characteristically spurts with each contraction of the heart. When an arterial puncture occurs, immediately remove the catheter and apply direct pressure to the site for at least five minutes. Do not release the pressure until the hemorrhage has stopped.

Circulatory Overload

circulatory overload an excess in intravascular fluid volume.

Circulatory overload occurs if you administer too much fluid for the patient's condition. You must monitor flow rates carefully, especially for patients with medical conditions such as kidney failure or heart failure who are intolerant of excessive fluid. Continually examine the patient for signs of circulatory overload (rales, tachypnea, dyspnea, and jugular venous distention, as discussed in Chapter 7 on physical exam techniques). If you encounter circulatory overload, adjust the flow rate.

Thrombophlebitis

thrombophlebitis inflammation of the vein.

Thrombophlebitis, or inflammation of the vein, is particularly common in long-term IV therapy. Redness and edema at the puncture site are typical signs of thrombophlebitis. This complication may also present as pain along the course of the vein, sometimes accompanied by inflammation and tenderness. Typically, thrombophlebitis does not occur until several hours after IV initiation. When you suspect thrombophlebitis, terminate the IV and apply a warm compress to the site.

Thrombus Formation

thrombus blood clot.

A **thrombus,** or blood clot, can form if IV access injures the vessel wall. A thrombus may form around the catheter and occlude the movement of fluid between the IV and the blood vessel. If you suspect a thrombus, restart the IV using new equipment. Do not attempt to dislodge the clot with a fluid bolus, because this may create an embolus that causes neurological or pulmonary complications.

Air Embolism

air embolism air in the vein.

Air embolism occurs when air enters the vein. Air embolus is most likely to occur during central venous access or when administration tubing has not been properly flushed. Failure to tamponade larger veins during cannulation may allow air into the vein.

Necrosis

necrosis the sloughing off of dead tissue.

Necrosis, or the sloughing off of dead tissue, occurs later in IV therapy as medication has extravasated into the interstitial space.

Anticoagulants

Anticoagulant drugs such as aspirin, Coumadin, or heparin increase the chance of bleeding and impede hemorrhage control during IV establishment. They drastically increase the complications of hematoma or infiltration.

anticoagulant drug that inhibits blood clotting.

CHANGING AN IV BAG OR BOTTLE

You may sometimes have to change an IV bag or bottle. This generally occurs when only 50 ml of solution remain and you must continue therapy after those 50 ml are depleted. Changing the solution bag or bottle is a sterile process. If the equipment becomes contaminated you should dispose of it.

To change the IV solution bag or bottle, use the following technique:

1. Prepare the new IV solution bag or bottle by removing the protective cover from the IV tubing port.
2. Occlude the flow of solution from the depleted bag or bottle by moving the roller clamp on the IV administration tubing.
3. Remove the spike from the depleted IV bag or bottle. Be careful not to drop or contaminate the spike in any way.
4. Insert the spike into the new IV bag or bottle. Ensure that the drip chamber is filled appropriately.
5. Open the roller clamp to the appropriate flow rate.

If air becomes entrained within the administration tubing during this process, cleanse the medication administration port below the trapped air and insert a hypodermic needle and syringe. Pull the plunger back to aspirate the trapped air into the syringe. After you have removed the air, adjust the IV flow rate as needed.

INTRAVENOUS DRUG ADMINISTRATION

Medications can be delivered through an existing IV line. As the IV line is seated directly into a vein, the blood rapidly absorbs these medications and distributes them throughout the body. IV administration avoids many of the barriers to drug absorption in other routes. For example, drugs given via the GI tract face enzymes and other chemicals that may deactivate, exacerbate, or in some other way alter the medication being administered. Likewise, local tissues can absorb drugs administered via the subcutaneous or intramuscular routes, thus preventing the total dosage from reaching the blood stream for delivery. The two methods for administering drugs through an IV line are IV bolus and IV infusion.

Intravenous Bolus

An IV bolus involves injecting the circulatory system with a concentrated dose of drug through the medication administration port of an established IV. This procedure requires the following equipment:

- BSI protection
- Alcohol antiseptic preparation
- Packaged medication
- Syringe (size depends on the volume of drug you administer)
- 18- to 20-gauge hypodermic needle, 1 to 1 1/2 inches long
- Existing IV line with medication port

To administer an IV medication bolus, use the following technique (Procedure 4-10):

1. Ensure that the primary IV line is patent.
2. Confirm the drug, indication, dosage, and need for an IV bolus.
3. Draw up the medication or prepare a prefilled syringe as appropriate.

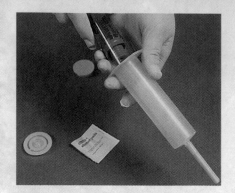

4-10a   Prepare the equipment.

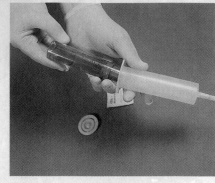

4-10b   Prepare the medication.

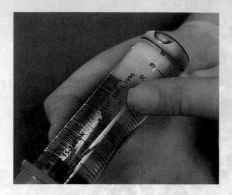

4-10c   Check the label.

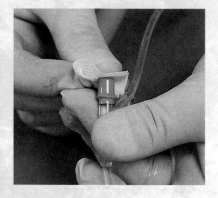

4-10d   Select and clean an administration port.

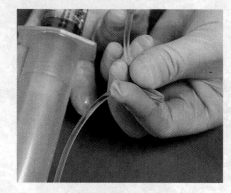

4-10e   Pinch the line.

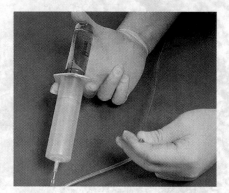

4-10f   Administer the medication.

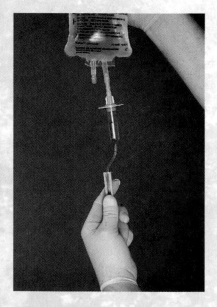

4-10g   Adjust the IV flow rate.

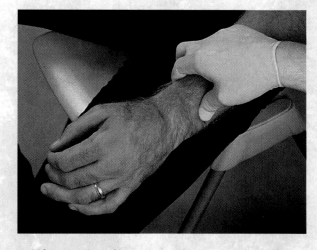

4-10h   Monitor the patient.

4. Cleanse the medication port nearest the IV site with an alcohol antiseptic preparation.

5. Insert a hypodermic needle through the port membrane.

6. Pinch the IV line above the medication port. This prevents the medication from traveling toward the fluids bag, forcing it instead toward the patient.

7. Inject the medication as appropriate.

8. Remove the hypodermic needle and syringe and release the tubing.

9. Open the flow regulator to allow a 20-cc fluid flush. The fluid will push the medication into the patient's circulatory system.

10. Dispose of the hypodermic needle and syringe as appropriate. Monitor the patient for desired or undesired effects.

Intravenous Drug Infusion

Many cardiac drugs and antibiotics are given as IV infusions (IV piggybacks). Intravenous drug infusions deliver a steady, continual dose of medication through an existing IV line. You may give them either as an initial dosage or to maintain drug levels after delivering an initial bolus.

Piggybacking IV infusions through an existing IV line gives you greater control over medication delivery and allows you easily to discontinue the infusion when therapy is complete or must be stopped. Never administer IV infusions as a primary IV line.

IV infusions are contained in bags or bottles of IV solution. If the IV infusion is premixed, read the label on the bag for the following information:

Never administer IV infusions as a primary IV line.

• Name of medication

• Total dosage in weight mixed in bag

• Concentration (weight per single cc)

• Expiration date

If the infusion is not premixed, make a label listing this information and attach it to the bag (Figure 4-28). Additionally, note the date and time you mixed the infusion, and initial it.

Use the following technique to administer a medication as an IV infusion (Procedure 4-11):

1. Establish a primary IV line and assure patency.

2. Confirm administration indications and patient allergies.

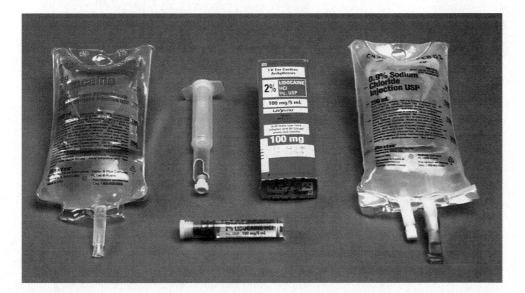

FIGURE 4–28   If an IV solution is not premixed, you will have to mix and label it yourself.

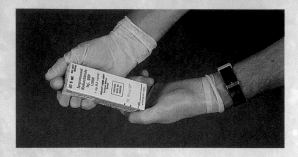

4-11a Select the drug.

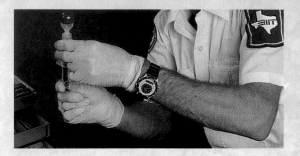

4-11b Draw up the drug.

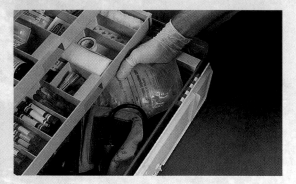

4-11c Select IV fluid for dilution.

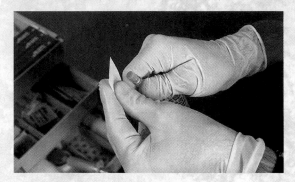

4-11d Clean the medication addition port.

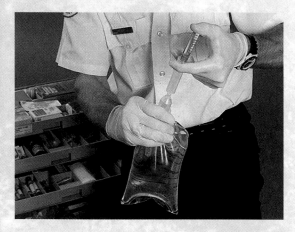

4-11e Inject the drug into the fluid.

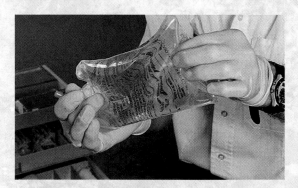

4-11f Mix the solution.

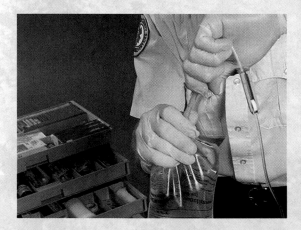

4-11g Insert an administration set and connect to main IV line with needle.

3. Prepare the infusion bag or bottle. (If the infusion is premixed, continue to step 4.)
   a. Draw up the appropriate quantity of medication from its source with a syringe.
   b. Cleanse the IV bag or bottle's medication port with an alcohol antiseptic wipe.
   c. Insert the hypodermic needle into the medication port and inject the medication.
   d. Gently agitate the bag or bottle to mix its contents.
   e. Label the bag or bottle.

4. Connect administration tubing to the medication bag or bottle and fill the drip chamber to fluid line. Most infusions require microdrip tubing. If you use a mechanical infusion pump, you may need to use special tubing.

5. Place the hypodermic needle on the administration tubing's needle adapter and flush the tubing with solution. (The needle adapter typically accepts a 20-gauge needle.)

6. Cleanse the medication administration port on the primary line with alcohol and insert the secondary line's hypodermic needle. Secure the hypodermic needle and the secondary administration line with tape or another securing device.

7. Reconfirm the indication, drug, dose, and route of administration.

8. Shut down the primary line so that no fluid flows from the primary solution bag.

9. Adjust the secondary line to the desired drip rate. If you are using a mechanical infusion pump set it accordingly.

10. Properly dispose of the needle and syringe.

When the infusion is complete, shut down the secondary line with the flow regulator or a clamp. Open the primary line and adjust it to the indicated drip rate. Remove the hypodermic needle from the medication administration port and properly dispose of all contents. If required by your local protocols, retain the medication bag to verify administration and for quality assurance.

You can also use measured volume administration tubing to administer medicated infusions. First, fill the burette chamber of a measured volume administration device with a specific volume of fluid. Then inject the drug through the medication injection site on top of the burette chamber. You must adjust the flow rate to deliver the precise amount of medication required. In addition, you can mix the medication within the IV bag or bottle as previously described and use the measured volume administration tubing solely for administering the infusion rather than for mixing it.

Heparin Lock and Saline Lock

When a patient requires occasional IV medication drips or boluses but does not need continuous fluid, heparin locks are used. A **heparin lock** is a peripheral IV port that does not use a bag of fluid. Like a typical IV start, it places an IV cannula into a peripheral vein; however, instead of IV administration tubing, it has attached short tubing with a clamp and a distal medication port (Figure 4-29). A heparin lock decreases the risk of accidental fluid overload and electrolyte derangement. You also may withdraw blood samples from the lock if it is in a suitable vein. For short-term use, saline locks may be used. Sterile saline is injected following the drug. Saline remains in the lock to keep it open. For long-term use, a heparin lock is preferred. Although it functions the same as a saline lock, a heparin lock is filled with a low concentration solution of heparin, which aids in keeping any blood that gets into the device from clotting. Typically, a drug is administered through the heparin lock. This is followed by a saline flush to ensure that no drug remains in the lock or hub. Then, the lock and hub are filled with a heparin solution. This aids in keeping the IV site open for a long period of time.

heparin lock peripheral IV port that does not use a bag of fluid.

FIGURE 4-29 Heparin lock.

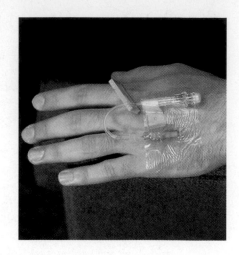

Initiating a heparin lock requires the following equipment:

- IV cannula
- Heparin lock
- Syringe with 3- to 5-cc sterile saline or commercial saline injection device
- Tape or commercial securing device
- Venous blood drawing equipment
- Venous constricting band
- Antiseptic swab (betadine/alcohol)

To place a heparin lock, follow these steps:

1. Select the venipuncture site.
2. Place the constricting band proximal to the puncture site.
3. Cleanse the venipuncture site with alcohol or betadine antiseptics.
4. Insert the IV cannula into the vein.
5. Slide the Teflon catheter into the vein.
6. Carefully remove the metal stylet and promptly dispose of it into the sharps container. Remove the venous constricting band.
7. Obtain venous blood samples, as explained under Venous Blood Sampling later in this chapter.
8. Attach the heparin lock tubing to the angiocatheter hub.
9. Cleanse the medication port and inject 3 to 5 mL of sterile saline into the lock. Easy flow of the saline without edema at the puncture site indicates patency. If you encounter resistance or if edema forms, restart the procedure with new equipment.
10. Apply antibiotic ointment to the site and cover with an adhesive bandage or other commercial device. Secure the tubing to the patient.

To administer an IV medication bolus through a heparin lock, assemble the following equipment and supplies:

- BSI protection
- Alcohol antiseptic preparation
- Packaged medication
- Syringe (the size depends on the volume being administered)
- 18- to 20-gauge hypodermic needle, 1 to 1 1/2 inches long

After you have gathered all equipment and supplies, use the following technique to administer an IV medication bolus with a heparin lock:

1. Confirm the drug, indication, dosage, and need for an IV bolus.
2. Draw up the medication or prepare a prefilled syringe as appropriate.
3. Cleanse the medication port nearest the IV site with alcohol antiseptic preparation.
4. Ensure that the plastic clamp is open.
5. Insert the hypodermic needle through the port membrane.
6. Inject the medication as appropriate.
7. Remove the hypodermic needle and dispose of it in the sharps container.
8. Follow the medication administration with a 10 to 20 mL saline flush from another syringe.
9. Properly dispose of the hypodermic needle and syringe. Monitor the patient for desired or undesired effects.

If fluid administration becomes necessary, you can unscrew the medication port and insert IV administration tubing. Periodically flush with sterile saline or heparin to prevent clot formation and occlusion at the Teflon catheter's distal end.

Venous Access Device

A **venous access device** is a surgically implanted port that permits repeated access to the central venous circulation. Implanted just under the skin, venous access devices are constructed of a plastic or stainless steel injection port and flexible catheter. The injection port, which lies just beneath the skin, contains a self-sealing septum that allows repeated penetration and access into the venous circulation. The self-sealing septum is connected to a flexible catheter that is placed within the lumen of a central vein, most often the superior vena cava.

Typically, patients with venous access devices have chronic illnesses that require repeated IV access for medication administration, long-term IV therapy, or blood sampling. Generally, venous access devices are placed on the anterior chest near the third or fourth rib lateral to the sternum. A venous access device is apparent as a raised circle just beneath the skin.

Use of an indwelling central venous access device requires special training. Delivering a medication through the venous access device requires a special needle specific for the venous access device in question. A common needle, the **Huber needle,** has an opening on the side of its shaft instead of at the tip. When placed into the injection port, this configuration allows easy administration of medication into the venous access device. Never access a venous access device unless you have the specific needle unique for the particular device. Always ask the patient, family, or nursing staff about the type of venous access device. Often, they have a supply of needles for the device.

To administer fluids, medication, or blood through a venous access device, you must first prepare the site using the following technique:

1. Take BSI precautions.
2. Fill a 10-mL syringe with approximately 7 mL of normal saline.
3. Place a 21- or 22-gauge Huber needle (or other specialized needle) on the end of the syringe.
4. Cleanse the skin over the injection port with povidone-iodine or alcohol preparations.
5. Stabilize the site with one hand while inserting the Huber needle at a 90-degree angle. Gently advance it until it meets resistance. This signals that the needle has contacted the floor of the injection port.

venous access device surgically implanted port that permits repeated access to central venous circulation.

Huber needle needle that has an opening on the side of the shaft instead of the tip.

6. Pull back on the plunger and observe for blood return. The presence of blood confirms placement.

7. Slowly inject the normal saline to ensure patency.

To administer the medication by intravenous bolus, use the following technique:

1. Prepare the medication, fluid, or blood for administration.

2. Attach a 21- or 22-gauge Huber needle (or other specialized needle) to the end of the syringe.

3. Cleanse the skin over the injection port with povidone-iodine or alcohol preparations.

4. Insert the needle into the injection port at a 90-degree angle until the needle cannot be further advanced. Pull back on the plunger of the syringe and observe for the return of blood. The presence of blood confirms proper placement.

5. Inject the medication as appropriate.

6. Remove and dispose of the syringe appropriately.

7. With another syringe and attached specialized needle, administer a bolus of heparinized saline to clear the catheter of any blood clots or other obstruction.

If the venous access device is not patent or access proves difficult, contact medical direction for further directives.

To administer IV fluids, use the following technique:

1. Prepare a primary IV line. Be sure to prime or flush the air from the administration tubing.

2. Attach a 21- or 22-gauge Huber needle (or other specialized needle) to the primary IV administration tubing. Insert a 10-mL syringe and hypodermic needle filled with 7 mL of normal saline solution into the tubing medication delivery port nearest the venous access device.

3. Cleanse the skin over the injection port with povidone-iodine or alcohol preparations.

4. Insert the needle into the injection port at a 90-degree angle until it encounters resistance.

5. Pinch the administration tubing above the medication administration port and pull back on the syringe plunger. Observe for the return of blood. The presence of blood confirms proper placement.

6. Gently inject the 7 mL of normal saline solution.

7. Set the primary line to the appropriate flow rate.

If administering a secondary medicated infusion, continue as follows:

1. Prepare a secondary line containing the fluid, blood, or medicated solution for infusion.

2. Attach a hypodermic needle to the needle adapter of the secondary line. Insert the secondary line into a medication administration port on the primary tubing.

3. Shut down the primary line and infuse the medicated solution as appropriate. Look for ease of administration as a sign of patency.

4. When infusion is complete, administer a bolus of heparinized saline to clear the catheter of any blood clots or other obstruction.

Using a venous access device is a very sterile procedure. You must take care to cleanse the site before delivering medications. Other complications of using a venous access device include infection, thrombus formation, and dislodgment of the catheter tip from the vein.

Electromechanical Infusion Devices

Electromechanical infusion devices permit the precise delivery of fluid and/or medications through electronic regulation. Anytime that IV infusion occurs, electromechanical infusion pumps provide optimal delivery. Infusion devices are classified as either infusion controllers or infusion pumps.

Infusion Controllers   **Infusion controllers** are gravity-flow devices that regulate the fluid's passage through the pump. Because infusion controllers do not use positive pressure, they will not force fluids into the **extravascular** space if you infiltrate the vein.

Infusion Pumps   **Infusion pumps** deliver fluids and medications under positive pressure (Figure 4-30). This pressure can cause complications such as hematoma or extravasation if you infiltrate the vein. Some infusion pumps contain a pressure monitor, which warns you if increased resistance is encountered with infiltration.

Syringe-type infusion pumps are gaining popularity for medical transport. Syringe pumps deliver their medications from a medical syringe without a hypodermic needle instead of from IV solution bags, fluids, or liquid medications (Figure 4-31). You place the syringe containing the medications in the pump, which uses computerized mechanics to gradually depress the plunger at the correct rate. These compact pumps prove advantageous during transport.

infusion controller gravity-flow device that regulates fluid's passage through an electromechanical pump.

extravascular outside the vein.

infusion pump device that delivers fluids and medications under positive pressure.

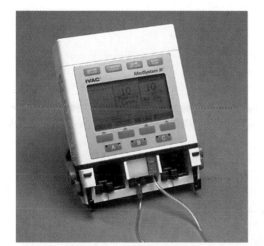

FIGURE 4-30   Infusion pump.

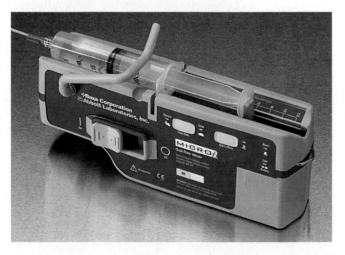

FIGURE 4-31   Syringe-type infusion pump.

Manufacturers make many different electromechanical infusion pumps. Depending on the maker, pump compatibility may require specialized administration tubing. With some computerized pumps, you can enter the basic information and then the pump will perform all medical calculations internally and automatically set the drip rate. Most infusion pumps contain internal monitoring devices that sound an alarm for problems such as infiltration, occlusion, or fluid source depletion. Electronic devices are prone to malfunction, so you must be prepared to perform all calculations and set the drip rate manually.

VENOUS BLOOD SAMPLING

The laboratory analysis of blood can provide valuable information about the sick and/or injured patient. The concentrations of electrolytes, gases, hormones, or other chemicals in blood can often shed light on the underlying causes of vague complaints such as dizziness or generalized weakness. Additionally, blood evaluation can confirm suspected conditions. For example, elevated cardiac enzymes in a patient's blood can confirm a suspected myocardial infarction.

In the field, you often will be the first to assess and treat an ill or injured patient. Many of your interventions can alter the blood's composition and erase important information. If you obtain venous blood samples before performing those interventions, they will enable the physician to evaluate the patient's original status.

Venous blood is commonly obtained via venipuncture. Thus, EMT-Is, who routinely initiate IV access, can simultaneously obtain blood samples. Doing so saves considerable hospital time and avoids multiple needle sticks.

You should obtain venous blood in the following situations:

- During peripheral access
- Before drug administration
- When drug administration may be needed

Never stop to draw blood if it will delay critical measures such as drug administration in cardiac arrest or transport in a multi-systems trauma.

Equipment for Drawing Blood

You will need the following equipment to obtain venous blood.

Blood Tubes **Blood tubes** are made of glass and have color-coded, self-sealing rubber tops. Blood tube sizes for adults generally range from 5 to 7 mL; for pediatric patients, from 2 to 3 mL (Figure 4-32). They are vacuum packed, and some contain a chemical anticoagulant. The different colored tops correspond to specific anticoagulants. A label on every blood tube identifies the type of additive and its expiration date. Do not use a blood tube after its expiration date, because both the anticoagulant and the vacuum lose their effectiveness.

Using blood tubes in their correct order is essential. If you do not follow the proper sequence, the various anticoagulants will cause cross contamination, skewing the results and

Never stop to draw blood if it will delay critical measures.

blood tube glass container with color-coded, self-sealing rubber top.

FIGURE 4-32 **Blood tubes.**

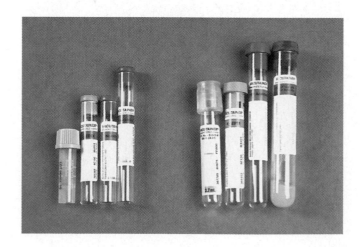

Table 4-1	BLOOD TUBE SEQUENCE	
	Anticoagulant	**Color of Top**
1.	None	Red
2.	Citrate	Blue
3.	Heparin	Green
4.	EDTA	Purple
5.	Fluoride	Gray

rendering the blood useless. Table 4-1 lists anticoagulants, the order in which you should use them, and the colors of their tops.

Miscellaneous Equipment   Depending on the technique used to obtain venous blood, you will also need syringes, hypodermic needles, and commercially manufactured plastic sleeves called vacutainers.

Obtaining Venous Blood

Obtaining venous blood is a simple process; however, if the blood is to remain useable, you must pay strict attention to detail. You can obtain blood either from an angiocath or directly from the vein. The technique you choose depends on the situation. In either case, venous blood samples are best obtained from sturdy veins such as the cephalic, basilic, or median. Smaller veins such as those on the back of the hand are more likely to collapse during retrieval, making the procedure difficult to complete.

Obtaining Venous Blood from an IV Angiocath   The most convenient way to obtain venous blood is through an angiocath at the time of peripheral vascular access. In addition to blood tubes, you will need a tube holder (Figure 4-33). The tube holder is commonly referred to as a **vacutainer**. A special adapter called a Leur lock fits into the tube holder. The **Leur lock** has a rubber-covered needle used to puncture the self-sealing top of the blood tube. The remaining portion of the Leur lock protrudes from the tube holder and fits snugly into the hub of the angiocath.

vacutainer device that holds blood tubes.

Leur lock adapter with a rubber-covered needle used to puncture a blood tube's self-sealing top.

To obtain blood directly from the angiocath, use the following procedure:

1. Assemble and prepare all equipment. Inspect the blood tubes for expiration or damage and insert the Leur lock into the vacutainer. *Note:* Never place blood tubes into the assembled vacutainer and Leur lock until you are ready to draw blood. This destroys the vacuum and renders the blood tube useless.
2. Establish IV access with the angiocatheter. Do not connect IV administration tubing.
3. Attach the end of the Leur adapter to the hub of the cannula.
4. In correct order, insert the blood tubes so that the rubber-covered needle punctures the self-sealing rubber top. Blood should be pulled into the blood tube.

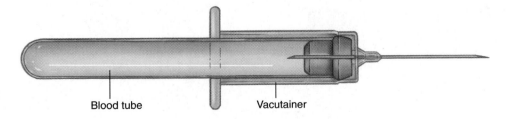

Blood tube   Vacutainer

FIGURE 4-33   Vacutainer with Leur-sampling needle.

5. Fill all blood tubes completely, because the amount of anticoagulant is proportional to the tube's volume. Gently agitate the tubes to mix the anticoagulant evenly with the blood.

6. Tamponade the vein and remove the vacutainer and Leur lock. Attach the IV and ensure patency.

7. Properly dispose of all sharps.

8. Label all blood tubes with the following information:
   - Patient's first and last name
   - Patient's age and gender
   - Date and time drawn
   - Name of the person drawing the blood

If commercial equipment is not available, use a 20-mL syringe (Figure 4-34). Attach the syringe's needle adapter to the angiocath hub and gently pull back the plunger. Blood will fill the syringe. When the syringe is full, remove it from the angiocath and place the IV line into the angiocath. Carefully attach a hypodermic needle to the syringe to puncture the tops of the blood tubes. In the appropriate order, place the collected blood into the blood tubes and gently agitate. When finished, properly dispose of all sharps and label the blood tubes.

Obtaining Blood Directly from a Vein   When IV access is difficult or unobtainable, you may draw blood directly from the vein with a hypodermic needle. This technique is useful for routine sampling that will not require further IV access. To draw blood directly from a vein, you will need the same equipment as for obtaining blood from an angiocath. Instead of a Leur lock, however, you will use a **Leur-sampling needle** (Figure 4-35). A Leur-sampling needle is similar to the Leur lock, but instead of an angiocath adapter it has a long, exposed needle. The Leur-sampling needle screws into the vacutainer, and you insert the exposed needle directly into the vein. You will also need a constricting band and antiseptic wipes.

To obtain blood directly from a vein, use the following procedure:

1. Assemble and prepare all equipment. Inspect the blood tubes for expiration or damage, and insert the Leur lock into the vacutainer.

Leur-sampling needle long, exposed needle that screws into the vacutainer and is inserted directly into the vein.

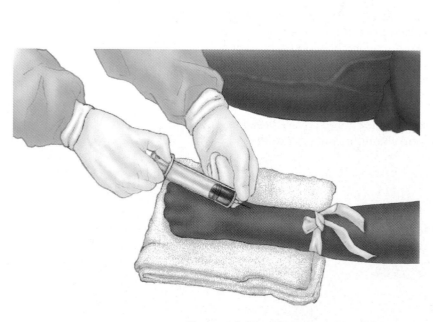 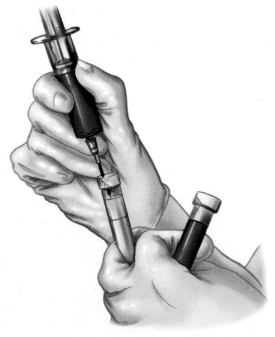

FIGURE 4-34   Obtaining a blood sample with a 20-mL syringe.

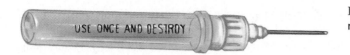

FIGURE 4-35   Leur-sampling
needle.

2. Apply the constricting band and select an appropriate puncture site.

3. Cleanse the site with alcohol or betadine.

4. Insert the end of the Leur-sampling needle into the vein and remove the constricting band.

5. In the correct order, insert each blood tube so that the rubber-covered needle punctures the self-sealing rubber top. Blood should be pulled into the tube.

6. Gently agitate the tube to evenly mix the anticoagulant with the blood. Completely fill all blood tubes, because the anticoagulant is proportional to the volume of the tube.

7. Place sterile gauze over the site and remove the sampling needle. Properly dispose of all sharps.

8. Cover the puncture site with gauze and tape or an adhesive bandage.

9. Label all blood tubes with the following information:
   - Patient's first and last name
   - Patient's age and gender
   - Date and time drawn
   - Person drawing the blood

Again, if commercial equipment is not available, you may use a 20-mL syringe. When using a syringe, attach an 18-gauge hypodermic needle to the end of the syringe and insert it into the vein. Gently pull back the plunger to fill the syringe with blood. When the syringe is full, remove the syringe and dress the puncture site. In the appropriate order, inject the collected blood into the blood tubes and gently agitate. When you have finished, properly dispose of all sharps and label the blood tubes.

Complications from drawing blood include damage to the vein wall, inadvertent removal of the IV angiocath, and hemoconcentration and hemolysis of the blood sample. **Hemoconcentration** occurs when the constricting band is left in place too long, elevating the numbers of red and white blood cells in the sample. **Hemolysis** is the destruction of red blood cells. When red blood cells are destroyed, they release hemoglobin and potassium, thus rendering the blood unusable. Causes of hemolysis include vigorously shaking the blood tubes after they are filled, using too small a needle for retrieval, or too forcefully aspirating blood into or out of a syringe.

hemoconcentration elevated numbers of red and white blood cells.

hemolysis the destruction of red blood cells.

REMOVING A PERIPHERAL IV

You should remove any IV that will not flow or has fulfilled its need. To do so, completely occlude the tubing with the flow regulator and/or clamp. Remove all tape or other securing devices from the tubing and patient. Place a sterile gauze pad over the puncture site. Apply pressure to the gauze with the fingers or thumb of your nondominant hand. With your dominant hand, grasp the cannula at its hub and swiftly remove it, pulling straight back. The site may bleed, so apply direct pressure with the gauze for five minutes. Immediately dispose of all materials in the appropriate biohazard container. Apply an adhesive bandage or tape clean gauze over the site to protect against infection.

Remove any IV that does not flow or has fulfilled its need.

INTRAOSSEOUS INFUSION

Intraosseous infusions involve inserting a rigid needle into the cavity of a long bone (*intra*, within; *os*, bone). The bone marrow contains a network of venous sinusoids that drain into the nutrient and emissary veins. These sinusoids accept fluids and drugs during intraosseous infusion and transport them to the venous system. Any solution or drug that can be administered by IV, either bolus or infusion, can be administered by the intraosseous route.

intraosseous within the bone.

Generally, you will use intraosseous infusions for the critical patient less than five years old when you cannot establish peripheral IV access. Less commonly, you may apply intraosseous infusions to adult patients. These patients have different access sites than pediatric patients, and rapid volume administration is not nearly as effective. Situations that might require an intraosseous route include shock, status epilepticus, trauma, and cardiac arrest, and critical pediatric patients where rapid IV access cannot be obtained. Initiate intraosseous lines only after 90 seconds or three unsuccessful attempts to establish peripheral IV access.

ACCESS SITE

The bone most commonly used for intraosseous access is the tibia. Pediatric access uses the proximal tibia. Adult and geriatric access uses the distal tibia. To properly locate appropriate sites and avoid complications, you must understand the anatomy and physiology of the tibia (Figure 4-36). The tibia is a long bone that transfers weight from the femur to the foot. In conjunction with the fibula, it permits walking. Its three main sections are the diaphysis,

FIGURE 4-36   Tibia.

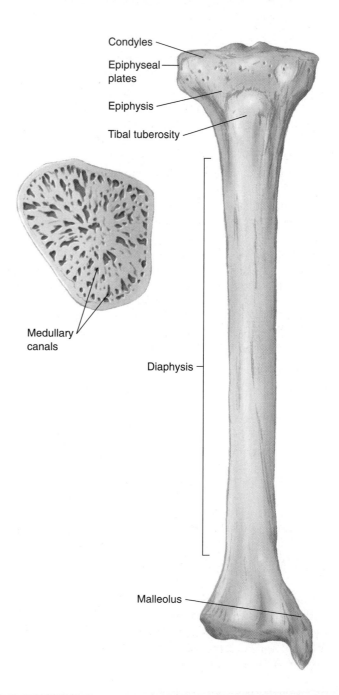

Condyles
Epiphyseal plates
Epiphysis
Tibal tuberosity
Medullary canals
Diaphysis
Malleolus

which is the middle, and the two epiphyses, one at either end. Epipheseal disks, or growth plates, between the diaphysis and the epiphyses, allow the tibia to grow and develop and are present in children. Damage to these disks during intraosseous access can cause long-term growth complications or abnormalities.

Within the diaphysis, the medullary canal holds the vascular bone marrow. When placed correctly, the distal part of the intraosseous needle is situated in the medullary canal. On either side of the proximal tibia are the medial and lateral condyles. You can identify the proximal epiphysis by palpating the condyles.

Between the condyles, on the top of the anterior tibial crest, is a palpable bump called the tibial tuberosity. The tibial tuberosity lies at the level of the epipheseal growth plate, for which it provides an excellent reference. Consequently, the tibial tuberosity is extremely important in locating the appropriate pediatric intraosseous access site.

At the distal end of the tibia lie the lateral malleolus and the medial malleolus. They mark the distal epipheseal portion of the tibia and are important landmarks for intraosseous placement in the adult or geriatric patient.

For the pediatric patient (under five years old), you will establish intraosseous access on the medial aspect of the proximal tibia (Figure 4-37a). This site is from two to three fingerbreadths below the tibial tuberosity. At this level, place the needle on the flat area medial to the anterior tibial crest. For adult or geriatric patients, place the needle at the distal part of the tibia, one to two fingerbreadths above the medial malleolus (Figure 4-37b).

EQUIPMENT FOR INTRAOSSEOUS ACCESS

Intraosseous placement requires a specially designed needle and a 10-mL syringe. Manufactured specifically for intraosseous access, an intraosseous needle is a 14- to 18-gauge hollow cannula with a sharp metal **trocar** inside (Figure 4-38). The trocar gives strength for puncture and prevents occlusion during insertion. Upon placement, the trocar is removed. The intraosseous needle has a plastic handle for insertion and an adjustable plastic disk to stabilize the needle once it is in place. You will attach a 10-mL syringe with 3 to 5 mL of sterile saline to the intraosseous needle. The syringe and saline are used similarly to IV access

trocar a sharp, pointed instrument.

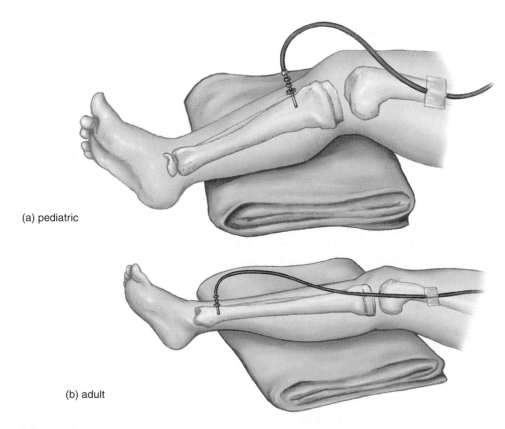

(a) pediatric

(b) adult

FIGURE 4-37 Pediatric and adult intraosseous needle placement sites.

FIGURE 4-38   Intraosseous needle.

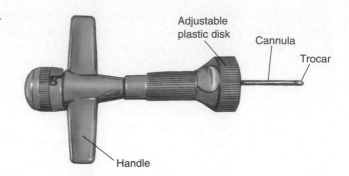

FIGURE 4-38   Intraosseous needle.

Adjustable plastic disk

Cannula

Trocar

Handle

of the external jugular vein. A large-bore spinal needle with a trocar in place is an acceptable substitute for an intraosseous needle.

Other equipment for intraosseous placement is similar to that for a peripheral IV access line (fluid, administration tubing, tape, antiseptics, and gauze). However, you will not use a constricting band or traditional cannula. Depending on the specific intraosseous needle, you may need an adapter to connect the administration tubing and the needle.

PLACING AN INTRAOSSEOUS INFUSION

To place an intraosseous line use the following technique (Procedure 4-12):

1. Determine the indication for intraosseous access.

2. Assemble and check all equipment.

3. Position the patient. Rotate the leg toward the outside to expose the medial, proximal aspect of the tibia.

4. Locate the access site. Palpate the tibia and use all landmarks.
    – *Pediatric.* Locate the tibial tuberosity. Move from one to two fingerbreadths below the tibial tuberosity and find the flat expanse medial to the anterior tibial crest.
    – *Adult or geriatric.* Find the medial malleolus. Move from one to two fingerbreadths below the medial malleolus and locate the flat expanse medial to the anterior tibial crest.

5. Cleanse the site with alcohol or betadine. Start at the puncture site and work outward in an expanding circular motion.

6. Perform the puncture. Holding the needle perpendicular to the puncture site, insert it with a twisting motion until you feel a decrease in resistance or a "pop." When this occurs, the needle is in the medullary canal. Do not advance it any further. Generally, you will need to insert the needle only 2 to 4 mm for entry.

7. Remove the trocar and attach the saline-filled syringe. Slowly pull back the plunger to attempt aspiration into the syringe. Easy aspiration of bone marrow and blood confirms correct medullary placement.

8. Once you have confirmed placement, rotate the plastic disk toward the skin to secure the needle.

9. Remove the syringe and attach the prepared administration tubing and solution. Set the appropriate flow rate.

10. Secure the needle as if securing an impaled object by surrounding it with bulky dressings and taping them securely in place. Commercial devices are available.

11. Periodically flush the needle to keep it patent.

Any solution or drug that can be administered by IV bolus or continuous infusion can also be delivered by the intraosseous route. Use the medicinal administration port on the

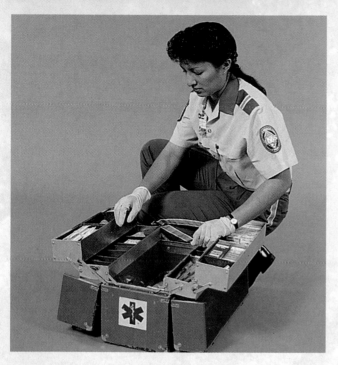

4-12a　Select the medication and prepare equipment.

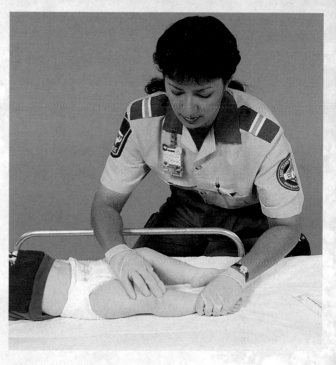

4-12b　Palpate the puncture site and prep with an antiseptic solution.

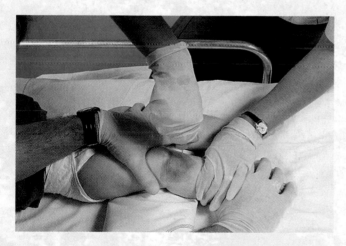

4-12c　Make the puncture.

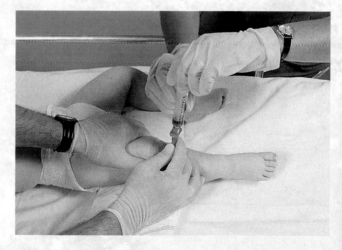

4-12d　Aspirate to confirm proper placement.

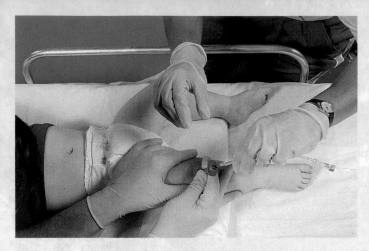

4-12e Connect the IV fluid tubing.

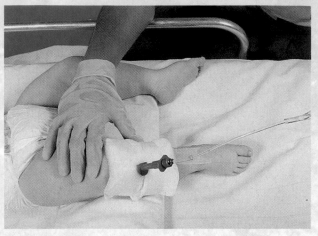

4-12f Secure the needle appropriately.

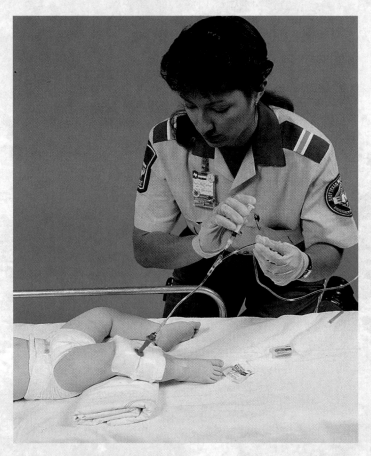

4-12g Administer the medication. Monitor the patient for effects.

primary administration tubing with the techniques described earlier under Intravenous Drug Administration.

When an intraosseous infusion is complete, shut down the secondary line with the flow regulator or a clamp. Open the primary line and adjust it to the indicated drip rate. Remove the hypodermic needle from the medication administration port and properly dispose of all contents if the infusion has been exhausted.

INTRAOSSEOUS ACCESS COMPLICATIONS AND PRECAUTIONS

Intraosseous access poses serious potential complications similar to those of peripheral access: local infection, thrombophlebitis, air embolism, circulatory overload, and allergic reactions, plus the following:

- *Fracture.* Too large a needle or too forceful an insertion can fracture the tibia, particularly in very young children.
- *Infiltration.* Infiltration occurs when IV solution collects in the local tissues instead of in the intramedullary canal. Infiltration may occur if you run fluids through an incorrectly placed needle or if a fracture has occurred. An infusion that does not run freely or the formation of an edema at the puncture site indicates infiltration. If infiltration occurs, immediately discontinue infusion and restart on the other leg.
- *Growth plate damage.* An improperly located puncture may damage the growth plate and result in long-term growth complications.
- *Complete insertion.* To avoid complete puncture (needle passing through both sides of the tibia), stop advancing the needle once you feel the pop. If complete puncture occurs, remove the needle with a reverse twisting motion and start again on the other leg. Apply direct pressure and a sterile dressing over the site(s) for at least five minutes.
- *Pulmonary embolism.* If bone, fat, or marrow particles enter the circulatory system, pulmonary embolism may result. Use proper technique and watch for signs associated with pulmonary embolism (sudden onset of chest pain or shortness of breath).

CONTRAINDICATIONS TO INTRAOSSEOUS PLACEMENT

Do not attempt intraosseous placement in the following situations:

- Fracture to the tibia or femur on the side of access
- Osteoporosis
- Establishment of a peripheral IV line

Part 3: Medical Mathematics

Proper drug administration requires basic mathematical proficiency. Because drug dosages are not always standardized, you may have to calculate amounts according to the patient's age, weight, or other medically related criteria. To properly prepare and administer medications, you must understand roman numerals and be proficient in multiplication, division, fractions, decimal fractions, proportions, and percentages. If you are deficient in one or more of these areas, refer to any text on basic and intermediate math.

METRIC SYSTEM

The metric system's three fundamental units are grams, meters, and liters. Prefixes denote values greater or less than the basic unit. Table 4-2 lists metric prefixes.

> **Content Review**
>
> ### INTRAOSSEOUS ACCESS COMPLICATIONS
> - Fracture
> - Infiltration
> - Growth plate damage
> - Complete insertion
> - Pulmonary embolism
> - Infection

> *You must continually refresh your intraosseous access skills so that you can perform this technique properly when needed.*
>
>

> **Content Review**
>
> ### FUNDAMENTAL METRIC UNITS
> - Grams—mass
> - Meters—distance
> - Liters—volume

Table 4-2	METRIC PREFIXES	
Prefix	**Multiplier**	**Abbreviation**
kilo-	1,000	(k)
hecto-	100	(h)
deka-	10	(D)
deci-	1/10 or 0.1	(d)
centi-	1/100 or 0.01	(c)
milli-	1/1,000 or 0.001	(m)
micro-	1/1,000,000 or 0.000001	(mcg or μg)

The most commonly used prefixes in pharmacology are *kilo-, centi-, milli-,* and *micro.* The prefix *milli- (m)* refers to 1/1,000. Thus, a milliliter equals 1/1,000 of a liter. Similarly, a milligram is 1/1,000 of a gram. The prefix *micro-* expresses 1/1,000,000. A microgram is 1/1,000,000 of a gram.

CONVERSION BETWEEN PREFIXES

If you know the prefixes and their numerical equivalents, you can easily convert measurements to smaller or larger units. To convert a measurement to a smaller unit, multiply the original measurement by the numerical equivalent of the smaller measurement's prefix.

Example 1: Convert 3 grams to milligrams.

Milligrams (1/1,000) are smaller than grams; therefore, multiply 3 by 1,000:

$$3 \text{ (grams)} \times 1,000 \text{ (milli)} = 3,000$$
$$3 \text{ grams} = 3,000 \text{ milligrams}$$

Example 2: Convert 2.67 liters to milliliters.

Milliliters (1/1,000) are smaller than a liter; therefore multiply 2.67 by 1,000:

$$2.67 \text{ liters} \times 1,000 \text{ (milli)} = 2,670$$
$$2.67 \text{ liters} = 2,670 \text{ milliliters}$$

To convert a measurement to a larger unit, divide the original measurement by the numerical equivalent of the smaller measurement's prefix.

Example 3: Convert 1,600 micrograms to grams.

A microgram is 1/1,000,000 the size of a gram; therefore, divide 1,600 by 1,000,000:

$$1,600/1,000,000 = 0.0016 \text{ grams}$$
$$1,600 \text{ micrograms} = 0.0016 \text{ grams}$$

When converting a measurement to or from a prefix that is not the fundamental unit, first convert the existing measurement to the fundamental measurement. Then convert the fundamental measurement to the desired unit.

Example 4: Convert 5.6 milligrams to micrograms.

First, convert the 5.6 milligrams to grams:

$$5.6 \text{ milligrams}/1,000 = 0.0056 \text{ grams (g)}$$
$$5.6 \text{ milligrams} = 0.0056 \text{ grams}$$

Now, convert 0.0056 grams to micrograms as previously described:

$$0.0056 \text{ (grams)} \times 1,000,000 = 5,600 \text{ micrograms}$$
$$5.6 \text{ milligrams} = 5,600 \text{ micrograms}$$

Table 4-3	METRIC EQUIVALENTS	
Household	**Apothecary**	**Metric**
1 gallon	4 quarts	3.785 liters
1 quart	1 quart	0.946 liters
16 ounces	approximately 1 pint	473 milliliters (mL)
1 cup	approximately ½ pint	approximately 250 mL
1 tablespoon		approximately 16 mL
1 teaspoon		approximately 4–5 mL

For the beginner, this technique avoids confusion. The more experienced provider will be able to make a direct conversion from milligrams to micrograms.

HOUSEHOLD AND APOTHECARY SYSTEMS OF MEASURE

In the past, pharmacology traditionally used the household and apothecary systems to measure drug dosages. Gradually, the metric system has replaced those systems, but you may occasionally encounter their remnants. Table 4-3 gives the metric equivalents of the household and apothecary units you will most likely encounter.

WEIGHT CONVERSION

Some medication dosages are calculated according to kilograms of body weight. To convert pounds to kilograms use the following formula:

$$\text{kilograms} = \text{pounds}/2.2$$

Example 5: How many kilograms does a 182-pound person weigh?

$$\text{kilograms} = 182 \text{ lbs}/2.2$$
$$\text{kilograms} = 82.7$$

TEMPERATURE

The international thermometric scale measures temperature in degrees Celsius. Although degrees Celsius is often cited interchangeably with degrees centigrade, the two scales are slightly different. For practical purposes, however, you can think of them both as dividing the interval between the freezing and boiling points of water into 100 equal parts, with 0°C being the freezing point and 100°C being the boiling point. The household measurement system, on the other hand, divides the interval between the freezing and boiling points of water into 180 equal parts, with 32°F being the freezing point and 212°F being the boiling point. When taking a body temperature, use the following formulas to convert between degrees Fahrenheit and degrees Celsius:

$$°F = 9/5°C + 32$$
$$°C = 5/9 \, (°F - 32)$$

Example 6: Convert 98.2°F to °C

$$°C = 5/9 \, (98.2 - 32)$$
$$°C = 5/9 \, (66.2)$$
$$°C = 36.8$$
$$98.2°F = 36.8°C$$

Example 7: Convert 28.4°C to °F

$$°F = 9/5 \, (28.4) + 32$$
$$°F = 51.12 + 32$$
$$°F = 83.1$$
$$28.4°C = 83.1°F$$

unit predetermined amount of medication or fluid.

Converting between the different prefixes and different systems of measurement is crucial in calculating drug dosages. You should continually practice all conversions, not only during your formal education, but also throughout your career in the emergency medical services.

UNITS

Some medications are measured in **units.** Penicillin, heparin, and insulin are administered in units. Units do not convert between the metric, household, and apothecary systems.

MEDICAL CALCULATIONS

stock solution standard concentration of routinely used medications.

Frequently you will have to apply basic mathematical principles to calculate specific quantities before administering medications and fluids. In prehospital care, the following forms of medications often require calculation:

- Oral medications
- Liquid parenteral medications
- IV fluid administration
- IV medication infusions

Most medications are provided in **stock solution.** Therefore you must calculate the exact amount of medication to remove from the stock for administration. To calculate basic drug dosage, you will need three facts:

- Desired dose
- Dosage on hand
- Volume on hand

desired dose specific quantity of medication needed.

concentration weight per volume.

dosage on hand the amount of drug available in a solution.

volume on hand the available amount of solution containing a medication.

The **desired dose** is the specific quantity of medication needed. Most dosages are expressed as a weight (grams, milligrams, or micrograms). Dosages may be standard or calculated according to body weight or age.

All liquid medications are packaged as concentrations. **Concentration** refers to weight per volume. A liquid medication's concentration is the drug's weight (grams, milligrams, or micrograms) per volume of liquid (mL) in which it is dissolved. For example, 50% dextrose (D_{50}) is packaged as a concentration of 25 grams (weight) dextrose in 50 mL (volume) of water. From the concentration, you can determine the **dosage on hand** (weight) and the **volume on hand.** For 50% dextrose, the dosage on hand is 25 grams and the volume on hand is 50 mL. Concentrations are identified on all drug packaging and labels.

Because you cannot see the desired dose dissolved in liquid, you must convert its weight to volume, a readily visible measurement, using the following formula:

$$\text{volume to be administered} = \frac{\text{volume on hand (desired dose)}}{\text{dosage on hand}}$$

Legal Notes

The administration of medications in an emergency setting increases the chances of accidental needle-stick injuries for all involved. It is paramount that EMT-Is anticipate potential dangers and avoid them. For example, the natural instinct of many people following pain (such as occurs with a medication injection) is to withdraw. This sudden movement can cause an accidental needle-stick injury. Likewise, the combative or agitated patient poses a significant risk for all. Always make sure that medication administration is safe. If it is not, defer administration until additional resources or personnel are available. Your safety and the safety of your partner come first.

To use this formula, you must express all weight and volume measurements with the same metric prefix. For example, if the desired dose is expressed in *milli*grams, the dosage on hand must also be expressed in *milli*grams, volume on hand in *milli*liters.

CALCULATING DOSAGES FOR ORAL MEDICATIONS

The following example illustrates how to calculate the volume of a specific drug dosage:

Example 1: A physician orders you to administer 90 mg of acetaminophen to a pediatric patient. The liquid acetaminophen is packaged as a concentration of 500 mg in 8 mL of solution. How much of the medication will you administer?

Because you cannot see the 90 mg of acetaminophen, you must convert this weight to a volume. To do so you need these facts:

$$\text{desired dose} = 90 \text{ mg}$$
$$\text{dosage on hand} = 500 \text{ mg}$$
$$\text{volume on hand} = 8 \text{ mL}$$

Use the formula to calculate the dosage's volume:

$$\text{volume to be administered} = \frac{\text{volume on hand (8 mL)} \times \text{desired dose (90 mg)}}{\text{dosage on hand (500 mg)}}$$

$$\text{volume to be administered} = (8 \times 90)/500$$
$$\text{volume to be administered} = 720/500$$
$$\text{volume to be administered} = 1.44$$

Administer 1.44 mL of solution to deliver 90 mg of acetaminophen.

Another way to calculate drug dosages is the ratio (fraction) and proportion method. A ratio (fraction) illustrates a relationship between two numbers. A proportion is the comparison of two numerically equivalent ratios. Using the variable x, the above problem can be stated:

$$8 \text{ mL}/500 \text{ mg} = x \text{ mL}/90 \text{ mg}$$

To solve the problem, cross multiply the numerals:

$$8/500 = x/90$$
$$720/500 = x$$
$$1.44 = x$$
$$x = 1.44 \text{ mL}$$

> **Math Summary 1**
>
> $$x \text{ mL} = \frac{8 \text{ mL} \times 90 \text{ mg}}{500 \text{ mg}}$$
>
> $$x \text{ mL} = \frac{720}{500}$$
>
> $$x \text{ mL} = 1.44$$

> **Math Summary 2**
>
> $$\frac{500 \text{ mg}}{8 \text{ mL}} = \frac{90 \text{ mg}}{x \text{ mL}}$$
>
> $$x \text{ mL} = \frac{720}{500}$$
>
> $$x \text{ mL} = 1.44 \text{ mL}$$

CONVERTING PREFIXES

The following example shows how to calculate the volume to be administered when the desired dose, the dosage on hand, and the volume on hand are not all expressed in metric units with the same prefix.

Example 2: A physician orders you to give 250 mg of a drug via IV bolus. The multidose vial contains 2 grams of the drug in 10 mL of solution. How much of the medication should you administer?

Because the desired dose is expressed as *milli*grams, the dosage on hand must be converted from grams to milligrams. In the metric system, 2 grams equal 2,000 milligrams. You now know:

$$\text{desired dose} = 250 \text{ mg}$$
$$\text{dosage on hand} = 2{,}000 \text{ mg}$$
$$\text{volume on hand} = 10 \text{ mL}$$

$$x \text{ mL} = \frac{10 \text{ mL} \times 250 \text{ mg}}{2{,}000 \text{ mg}}$$

$$x \text{ mL} = \frac{2{,}500}{2{,}000}$$

$$x \text{ mL} = 1.25$$

Now you can use the formula to calculate the volume to be administered:

$$\text{volume to be administered} = \frac{\text{volume on hand (10 mL)} \times \text{desired dose (250 mg)}}{\text{dosage on hand (2,000 mg)}}$$
$$\text{volume to be administered} = (10 \times 250)/2{,}000$$
$$\text{volume to be administered} = 2{,}500/2{,}000$$
$$\text{volume to be administered} = 1.25$$

Administer 1.25 mL of solution to deliver 250 mg medication.

You can also solve this problem using the ratio proportion as follows:

$$10 \text{ mL}/2{,}000 \text{ mg} = x \text{ mL}/250 \text{ mg}$$
$$2{,}500 = 2{,}000x$$
$$2{,}500/2{,}000 = x$$
$$1.25 = x$$
$$x = 1.25 \text{ mL}$$

Math Summary 4

$$\frac{2{,}000 \text{ mg}}{10 \text{ mL}} = \frac{25 \text{ mg}}{x \text{ mL}}$$

$$x \text{ mL} = \frac{250}{2{,}000}$$

$$x \text{ mL} = 1.25 \text{ mL}$$

Tablets also come in stock doses. If the dosage of one tablet or pill is more than needed, divide the tablet or pill to make the correct dose. Do not divide enteric or time-release capsules.

CALCULATING DOSAGES FOR PARENTERAL MEDICATIONS

You can use the same formula to calculate specific doses and volume for parenteral medication delivery.

> **Example 3:** A physician wants you to administer 5 mg of medication subcutaneously. The ampule contains 10 mg of the drug in 2 mL of solvent. How much medication should you use?

$$\text{desired dose} = 5 \text{ mg}$$
$$\text{dosage on hand} = 10 \text{ mg}$$
$$\text{volume on hand} = 2 \text{ mL}$$
$$\text{volume to be administered} = \frac{\text{volume on hand (2 mL)} \times \text{desired dose (5 mg)}}{\text{dosage on hand (10 mg)}}$$
$$\text{volume to be administered} = (2 \times 5)/10$$
$$\text{volume to be administered} = 10/10$$
$$\text{volume to be administered} = 1 \text{ mL}$$

Administer 1 mL of solution to deliver 5 mg of the medication.

Using the ratio and proportion method, the problem is solved as follows:

$$2 \text{ mL}/10 \text{ mg} = x \text{ mL}/5 \text{ mg}$$
$$10/10 = x$$
$$1 = x$$
$$x = 1.0 \text{ mL}$$

Math Summary 5

$$\frac{10 \text{ mg}}{2 \text{ mL}} = \frac{5 \text{ mg}}{x \text{ mL}}$$

$$x \text{ mL} = \frac{10}{10}$$

$$x \text{ mL} = 1.0 \text{ mL}$$

CALCULATING WEIGHT-DEPENDENT DOSAGES

Occasionally, you will have to calculate the desired dose according to the patient's weight.

> **Example 4:** You must administer 1.5 mg/kg of lidocaine via IV bolus to a patient in stable ventricular tachycardia. The concentration of lidocaine is 100 mg in a prefilled syringe containing 10 mL of solution. The patient weighs 158 lbs.

Start by converting the patient's weight to kilograms:

$$\text{kilograms} = \text{pounds}/2.2$$
$$\text{kilograms} = 158 \text{ lbs.}/2.2$$
$$\text{kilograms} = 71.82$$

The patient weighs approximately 72 kg.

Calculate the desired dose:

$$1.5 \text{ mg} \times 72 \text{ kg} = 108 \text{ mg}$$

You now know these three facts:

$$\text{desired dose} = 108 \text{ mg}$$
$$\text{dosage on hand} = 100 \text{ mg}$$
$$\text{volume on hand} = 10 \text{ mL}$$

Use the same formula as before to calculate the volume to be administered:

$$\text{volume to be administered} = \frac{\text{volume on hand } (10 \text{ mL}) \times \text{desired dose } (108 \text{ mg})}{\text{dosage on hand } (100 \text{ mg})}$$

$$\text{volume to be administered} = (10 \times 108)/100$$
$$\text{volume to be administered} = 1{,}080/100$$
$$\text{volume to be administered} = 10.8$$

Administer 10.8 mL of solution to deliver 108 mg of lidocaine.

After you have calculated the desired dose, you can solve this problem using the ratio and proportion method as previously illustrated.

Math Summary 6

$$x \text{ mL} = \frac{10 \text{ mL} \times 108 \text{ mg}}{100 \text{ mg}}$$

$$x \text{ mL} = \frac{1{,}080}{700}$$

$$x \text{ mL} = 10.8 \text{ mL}$$

CALCULATING INFUSION RATES

To deliver fluid or medication through an IV infusion, you must calculate the correct infusion rate in drops per minute. To do so you must know the administration tubing's drip factor, as well as the volume on hand, desired dose, and dosage on hand.

Medicated Infusions

To calculate the correct IV infusion rate, use the following formula:

$$\text{drops/minute} = \frac{\text{volume on hand} \times \text{drip factor} \times \text{desired dose}}{\text{dosage on hand}}$$

Example 5: A physician wants you to administer 2 mg per minute of lidocaine to a patient. To prepare the infusion, you mix 2 g of lidocaine in an IV bag containing 500 mL of 5% dextrose in water (D_5W). You will use a microdrip administration set (60 gtts/mL). Calculate the infusion rate.

$$\text{desired dose} = 2 \text{ mg}$$
$$\text{dosage on hand} = 2{,}000 \text{ mg } (2 \text{ grams})$$
$$\text{volume on hand} = 500 \text{ mL}$$
$$\text{drip factor} = 60 \text{ gtts/mL}$$

$$\text{drops/minute} = \frac{\text{volume on hand } (500 \text{ mL}) \times \text{drip factor } (60 \text{ gtts/mL}) \times \text{desired dose } (2 \text{ mg})}{\text{dosage on hand } (2{,}000 \text{ mg})}$$

$$\text{drops/minute} = (500 \times 60 \times 2)/2{,}000$$
$$\text{drops/minute} = 60{,}000/2{,}000$$
$$\text{drops/minute} = 30$$

Run the infusion at 30 drops/minute to infuse 2 mg lidocaine per minute.

Math Summary 7

$$\frac{100 \text{ mg}}{10 \text{ mL}} = \frac{108 \text{ mg}}{x \text{ mL}}$$

$$x \text{ mL} = \frac{1{,}080}{100}$$

$$x \text{ mL} = 10.8 \text{ mL}$$

Math Summary 8

$$x \text{ drops/min} = \frac{500 \text{ mL} \times 60 \text{ gtts/mL} \times 2 \text{ mg}}{500 \text{ mg}}$$

$$x \text{ drops/min} = \frac{60{,}000}{2{,}000}$$

$$x \text{ drops/min} = 30$$

Fluid Volume Over Time

Fluids with or without medications may require administration over a specific period of time. To deliver the fluid correctly you must calculate volume/time. This calculation, requires the following information:

- volume to be administered
- drip factor of the administration set (gtts/ml)
- total time of infusion (minutes)

infusion rate speed at which a medication is delivered intravenously.

To calculate the **infusion rate,** use this formula:

$$\text{drops/minute} = \frac{\text{volume to be administered (drip factor)}}{\text{time in minutes}}$$

Example 6: A physician tells you to administer 500 mL of normal saline solution to a patient over 1 hour (60 minutes). The administration tubing is a macrodrip set with a drip factor of 10 gtts/mL. At what drip rate would you run this infusion?

$$\text{volume to be administered} = 500 \text{ mL}$$
$$\text{administration set drip factor} = 10 \text{ gtts/mL}$$
$$\text{total time of infusion} = 60 \text{ minutes}$$

Calculate the infusion rate:

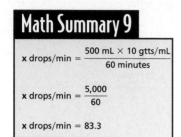

Math Summary 9

$$x \text{ drops/min} = \frac{500 \text{ mL} \times 10 \text{ gtts/mL}}{60 \text{ minutes}}$$

$$x \text{ drops/min} = \frac{5,000}{60}$$

$$x \text{ drops/min} = 83.3$$

$$\text{drops/minute} = \frac{(500 \text{ mL}) \ (10 \text{ gtts/mL})}{60 \text{ minutes}}$$
$$\text{drops/minute} = (500 \times 10)/60$$
$$\text{drops/minute} = 5,000/60$$
$$\text{drops/minute} = 83.3$$

Set the flow rate at approximately 83 drops per minute to infuse 500 mL of normal saline in almost exactly 60 minutes.

You can use the same formula to determine how long it will take to use all the fluid in a container.

Example 7: You are transporting a patient with an IV antibiotic. The infusion rate is 45 gtts/minute and the administration tubing is a microdrip set (60 gtts/mL). 150 mL remain in the 500 mL bag of D₅W. How long until the antibiotic will complete infusion?

Use the same formula as in Example 6; however, in this instance you will find time in minutes.

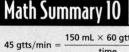

Math Summary 10

$$45 \text{ gtts/min} = \frac{150 \text{ mL} \times 60 \text{ gtts/mL}}{\text{time}}$$

$$45 = \frac{9,000}{x}$$

$$x = \frac{9,000}{45}$$

$$x = 200 \text{ minutes}$$

$$45 \text{ drops/minute} = \frac{(150 \text{ mL}) \ (60 \text{ gtts/mL})}{\text{time}}$$
$$45 = (150 \times 60)/\text{time}$$
$$45 = 9,000/\text{time}$$
$$\text{time} = 9,000/45$$
$$\text{time} = 200$$
$$45 \text{ drops/minute} = 200 \text{ minutes}$$

The antibiotic will complete infusion in 200 minutes, or 3 hours and 20 minutes.

Calculating Dosages and Infusion Rates for Infants and Children

Infants and children cannot tolerate underdoses or overdoses of medication and fluids. When you administer infusions to pediatric patients, you must calculate exact flow rates. Because infants and children differ drastically from adults in size and internal development, their dosages often depend on weight. Most weight-dependent dosages express the patient's weight in kilograms, so you must make the appropriate conversion from pounds as discussed earlier. Occasionally, you may encounter a medication that is based on body surface area (BSA). Chemotherapeutic agents for children are often based on BSA. Although you will not initiate such drugs, you may encounter them on critical care transports either by ground or air. Many aids for calculating pediatric drug doses and infusion rates are available, including charts, forms, and length-based resuscitation tapes. Even though these devices are helpful, you should not rely on them exclusively. They are no substitute for knowledge.

SUMMARY

Drug administration is a fundamental skill used in the treatment of the sick and injured. For medications to be effective, they must be safely delivered into the body by the appropriate route. Many different routes for drug delivery are available to the EMT-I; however, specific drugs require specific routes for administration.

It is your responsibility to be familiar with all routes of drug delivery and the techniques for establishing and using them. You will use some routes of medication administration infrequently, and they will quickly fade from memory. Nonetheless, someone's well-being may depend on your ability to use such a route in an emergency. Therefore, periodic review of all routes used in medication administration is highly recommended. In addition, you must accurately calculate many drug dosages. Dosage errors and inappropriate medication administration harm patient care and cast serious doubt on your ability.

ON THE WEB

For additional practice and review, go to the companion website at www.prenhall.com/bledsoe and click on *Intermediate Emergency Care: Principles & Practice.*

CHAPTER 5

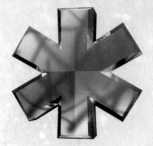

Airway Management and Ventilation

Objectives

After reading this chapter, you should be able to:

1. Review the anatomy and physiology of the respiratory system, specifically the upper and lower airways. (See Chapter 2)
2. Define the terms hypoxia (p. 354), hypoxemia (p. 352), pulsus paradoxus (p. 355), gag reflex (p. 370), and gastric distention. (p. 367)
3. Explain the primary objective of airway maintenance. (p. 350)
4. Identify commonly neglected prehospital skills related to airway. (pp. 358–360)
5. List factors that decrease oxygen concentrations in the blood and increase or decrease carbon dioxide production in the body. (p. 352)
6. Describe how to measure oxygen and carbon dioxide in the blood. (pp. 357–360)
7. List causes of upper airway obstruction and respiratory disease and describe the modified forms of respiration. (pp. 350–352, 354)
8. Identify types of oxygen cylinders and pressure regulators (including a high-pressure regulator and a therapy regulator) and explain safety considerations of oxygen storage and delivery. (p. 360)
9. Describe supplemental oxygen delivery devices, including their indications, contraindications, advantages, disadvantages, complica-

tions, liter flow range, and concentrations of delivered oxygen. (pp. 360–361)
10. Describe the use, advantages, and disadvantages of an oxygen humidifier. (p. 361)
11. Explain the risk of infection to EMS providers associated with ventilation. (pp. 366, 367, 368, 379, 396)
12. Describe the indications, contraindications, advantages, disadvantages, complications, and techniques for ventilating a patient: mouth-to-mouth; mouth-to-nose; mouth-to-mask; one, two, and three person bag-valve-mask; flow-restricted, oxygen-powered ventilation device; and automatic transport ventilator (ATV). (pp. 361–365)
13. Compare the ventilation techniques used for an adult patient to those used for pediatric patients. (pp. 363–364)
14. Define, identify, and describe a tracheostomy, a laryngectomy, a stoma, a tracheostomy tube, and how to ventilate and manage the airway of a patient with a stoma. (pp. 397–398)
15. Describe a complete airway obstruction and related maneuvers. (pp. 350–352)
16. Define and explain the implications of partial airway obstruction with good and poor air exchange. (pp. 350–351)

CASE STUDY

Ellis County Unit 947 is dispatched to a motor-vehicle collision on rural County Road 664, approximately 8 miles from town. This particular stretch of road is well known to EMS personnel because of a number of serious incidents over the last several months. The road contains numerous sharp curves and is under construction in several locations. Today, Unit 947 is staffed by EMT-Intermediates (EMT-Is) Crystal Jernigan and Charles Allen. In addition, EMT-I student Sharon Rodriquez is assigned to the unit for her field internship.

Upon arrival at the scene, they find one vehicle that has apparently run off the road and struck a telephone pole. Witnesses to the collision estimate the vehicle was traveling at approximately 45 miles per hour before striking the pole. The lone 24-year-old male occupant was ejected from the vehicle and lies face down in a ditch approximately 50 feet from the car. After ensuring scene safety and taking appropriate body substance isolation (BSI) precautions, Crystal assesses the patient. She finds him to be unresponsive. Charles and Sharon help her to log-roll the patient to a supine position with cervical-spine precautions applied. Sharon holds in-line cervical spine stabilization while Crystal opens the airway with the modified jaw-thrust technique.

The patient exhibits agonal respirations. In addition, gurgling noises are heard with each breath. After suctioning bloody secretions from his mouth, Crystal attempts to insert an oropharyngeal airway. However, the patient's teeth are tightly clenched and the airway will not allow the tube to pass. Crystal provides ventilatory support with a bag-valve-mask unit and 100% oxygen. The Glasgow Coma Score is 5. In anticipation of endotracheal intubation, the cardiac monitor and pulse oximeter are applied. An IV of normal saline is established. The equipment and supplies are readied. As they prepare for the procedure, Charles applies Sellick's maneuver while Sharon continues to hold cervical-spine stabilization. Crystal inserts the tube without difficulty. Proper placement is assured by seeing the tube pass through the vocal cords, the presence of condensation inside the tube, bilateral equal breath sounds, the absence of sounds over the epigastrium, and a positive change in the end-tidal CO_2 detector.

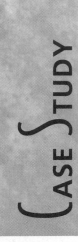

CASE STUDY

While Crystal secures the tube, the initial assessment is completed, and a rapid trauma exam is conducted. The patient is placed into a cervical collar and secured to a backboard while assessment and treatment continue. The patient has no obvious injuries. His blood pressure is 150/90, and his pulse rate is 64. Respirations are being assisted at a rate of 24 breaths per minute. With mechanical ventilation, pulse oximetry reveals an oxygen saturation reading of 98%. The finger-stick glucose test is 88 mg/dL. ALS unit 947 transports the patient to the emergency department without further incident.

Following the initial emergency department assessment, a nonenhanced computed tomography (CT) scan of the brain is obtained. The patient is found to have a large subdural hematoma that requires emergency surgical drainage. Following surgery, the patient regains consciousness. He spends 24 hours in the ICU and is then moved to a regular hospital room. The EMT-Is stop by the hospital and visit on their next duty shift. The patient has no recall of the crash whatsoever. The last thing he remembers is looking on the floor of the car for a CD that he dropped. One week after the crash, he is discharged with no neurological deficits.

Airway management and ventilation are the first and most critical steps in the initial assessment of every patient.

Your deliberate and precise use of simple, basic airway skills is the key to successful airway management and good patient outcome.

pneumothorax the presence of gas or air in the plural cavity.

Blockage of the airway is an immediate threat to the patient's life and a true emergency.

Content Review

CAUSES OF AIRWAY OBSTRUCTION
- Tongue
- Foreign bodies
- Trauma
- Laryngeal spasm and edema
- Aspiration

upper airway obstruction an interference with air movement through the upper airway.

INTRODUCTION

Airway management and ventilation are the first and most critical steps in the initial assessment of every patient you will encounter. You must immediately establish and maintain an open airway while providing adequate oxygen delivery and carbon dioxide elimination for all patients. Without adequate airway maintenance and ventilation, the patient will succumb to brain injury or even death in as little as 6 to 10 minutes. Early detection and intervention of airway and breathing problems, including bystander action, are vital to patient survival.

Your deliberate and precise use of simple, basic airway skills is the key to successful airway management and good patient outcome. Once you have applied the basic airway techniques to properly provide oxygenation and ventilation for your patient, you can use more sophisticated airway maneuvers and skills to further stabilize his airway. You must continually monitor and reassess the airway, being careful to watch for displacement of the endotracheal tube, mucous plugging, equipment failure, or the development of a **pneumothorax.**

This chapter provides the information and skills you will need to manage even the most difficult airway. It begins with an overview of respiratory problems and then explores the initial assessment and management of the airway and ventilation. (You may wish to review airway anatomy and physiology in Chapter 2 at this time.)

RESPIRATORY PROBLEMS

Respiratory emergencies can pose an immediate life threat to the patient. You must calmly and quickly assess the severity of his illness or injury while considering the potential causes of and treatment for his respiratory distress. Often, he will give you little help either because of anxiety or difficulty speaking. His respiratory difficulty may be due to airway obstruction, injury to upper or lower airway structures, inadequate ventilation caused by worsening of an underlying lung disease and fatigue, or central nervous system problems that threaten the airway or respiratory effort.

AIRWAY OBSTRUCTION

Blockage of the airway is an immediate threat to the patient's life and a true emergency. **Upper airway obstruction** may be defined as an interference with air movement through the upper airway. The tongue, foreign bodies, vomitus, blood, or teeth can all obstruct the upper airway.

Airway obstruction may be either partial or complete. Partial obstruction allows either adequate or poor air exchange. Patients with adequate air exchange can cough effectively; those with poor air exchange cannot. They often emit a high-pitched noise while inhaling

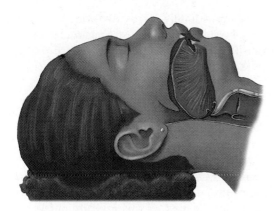

FIGURE 5-1 The tongue as an airway obstruction.

(stridor), and their skin may have a bluish appearance (cyanosis). They also may have increased breathing difficulty, which can manifest as choking, gagging, dyspnea, or dysphonia (difficulty speaking). When you cannot feel or hear airflow from the nose and mouth, or when the patient cannot speak (**aphonia**), breathe, or cough, his airway is completely obstructed. He will quickly become unconscious and die if you do not relieve the obstruction. In the absence of breathing, difficulty ventilating the patient indicates complete airway obstruction.

aphonia inability to produce speech sounds from larynx.

The Tongue

The tongue is the most common cause of airway obstruction (Figure 5-1). Normally, the submandibular muscles directly support the tongue and indirectly support the epiglottis. Without sufficient muscle tone, though, the relaxed tongue falls back against the posterior pharynx, thus occluding the airway. This may produce snoring respiratory noises. At the same time, the epiglottis also may block the airway at the larynx. This at least diminishes airflow into the respiratory system, and the patient's breathing efforts may inadvertently suck the base of his tongue into an obstructing position. The patient's tongue can block his airway whether he is lateral, supine, or prone; however, the blockage depends on the position of the patient's head and jaw, so simple airway maneuvers such as the jaw-thrust can usually open his airway.

The tongue is the most common airway obstruction.

Foreign Bodies

Large, poorly chewed pieces of food can obstruct the upper airway by becoming lodged in the hypopharynx. These cases often involve alcohol consumption and denture dislodgement. Because they frequently occur in restaurants and are mistaken for heart attacks, they are commonly called "café coronaries." The patient may clutch his neck between the thumb and fingers, a universal distress signal. Children, especially toddlers, often aspirate foreign objects, because they have the tendency to put objects into their mouths.

Trauma

In trauma, particularly when the patient is unresponsive, loose teeth, facial bone fractures, and avulsed or swollen tissue may obstruct the airway. Secretions such as blood, saliva, and vomitus may compromise the airway and risk aspiration. Additionally, penetrating or blunt trauma may obstruct the airway by fracturing or displacing the larynx, allowing the vocal cords to collapse into the tracheal lumen.

Laryngeal Spasm and Edema

Because the glottis is the narrowest part of an adult's airway, edema (swelling) or laryngospasm (spasmotic closure of the vocal cords) is potentially lethal. Even moderate edema can severely obstruct airflow and cause asphyxia (the inability to move air into and out of the respiratory system). Just beneath the mucous membrane that covers the vocal cords is a layer of loose tissue where blood or other fluids can accumulate, resulting in swelling (laryngeal edema) after an injury. This swelling will be slow to subside. Causes of laryngeal spasm and laryngeal edema include trauma, anaphylaxis, epiglottitis, and inhalation of superheated air, smoke, or toxic substances. The most common cause of laryngospasm is

Since the glottis is the narrowest part of an adult's airway, edema or spasm of the vocal cords is potentially lethal.

overly aggressive intubation. It often occurs, too, immediately on **extubation**, especially when the patient is semiconscious. Some authors suggest that laryngeal spasm can sometimes be partially overcome by strengthening ventilatory effort or forceful upward pull of the jaw, although the success of these maneuvers is quite variable.

Aspiration

Vomitus is the most commonly aspirated material. Patients most at risk for this are those with altered mental status who are so obtunded (drowsy) that they cannot adequately protect their airways. This can occur with hypoxia, central nervous system toxins, or brain injury, among other causes. In addition to obstructing the airway, aspiration's other effects also significantly increase patient mortality. Vomitus consists of food particles, protein-dissolving enzymes, hydrochloric acid, and gastrointestinal bacteria that have been regurgitated from the stomach into the hypopharynx and oropharynx. If this mixture enters the lungs, it can result in increased interstitial fluid and pulmonary edema. The consequent marked increase in alveolar/capillary distance seriously impairs gas exchange, thus causing **hypoxemia** and hypercarbia. Aspirated materials can also severely damage the delicate bronchiolar tissue and alveoli. Gastrointestinal bacteria can produce overwhelming infections. These complications occur in 50% to 80% of patients who aspirate foreign matter.

hypoxemia decreased partial pressure of oxygen in the blood.

INADEQUATE VENTILATION

Insufficient **minute volume** respirations can compromise adequate oxygen intake and carbon dioxide removal. Also, oxygenation may be insufficient when conditions increase metabolic oxygen demand or decrease available oxygen. A reduction of either the rate or the volume of inhalation leads to a reduction in minute volume. In some cases, the respiratory rate may be rapid but so shallow that little air exchange takes place.

minute volume amount of gas inhaled and exhaled in one minute.

Among the causes of such decreased ventilation are depressed respiratory function from impairment of respiratory muscles or nervous system, bronchospasm from intrinsic disease, fractured ribs, pneumothorax, **hemothorax**, drug overdose, renal failure, spinal or brainstem injury, or head injury. In some conditions, such as sepsis, the body's metabolic demand for oxygen can exceed the patient's ability to supply it. Additionally, the environment may contain a decreased amount of oxygen, as in high-altitude conditions or a house fire, which also produces toxic gases such as cyanide and carbon monoxide. These situations of inadequate ventilation can lead to hypercarbia and hypoxia.

hemothorax accumulation in the pleural cavity of blood or fluid containing blood.

RESPIRATORY SYSTEM ASSESSMENT

Vigilance is the key to airway management in every patient. The trauma patient whose airway and breathing initially looked fine on exam may become symptomatic with the pneumothorax that was not initially evident. The asthma patient who initially responded to nebulizer treatment may have a sudden bronchospasm and worsen acutely. Minute-by-minute reassessment of the adequacy of every patient's airway and breathing is essential. The changes may be subtle increases in respiratory rate, worsening or onset of irregularity, or increased difficulty speaking.

Vigilance is the key to airway management in every patient.

INITIAL ASSESSMENT

The purpose of the initial assessment is to identify any immediate threats to the patient's life, specifically airway, breathing, and circulation problems (**ABCs**). First, assess the airway to ensure that it is patent. Snoring or gurgling may indicate potential airway problems. Next determine the adequacy of breathing. If the patient is comfortable, with a normal respiratory rate, alert, and speaking without difficulty, you may generally assume that breathing is adequate.

ABCs airway, breathing, and circulation.

Patients with altered mental status warrant further evaluation. Feel for air movement with your hand or cheek. Look for the chest to rise and fall normally with each respiratory cycle. Listen for air movement and equal bilateral breath sounds. The absence of breath sounds on one side may indicate a pneumothorax or hemothorax in the trauma patient. In an adult patient, the respiratory rate generally ranges between 12 and 20 breaths per minute. Breathing should be spontaneous, effortless, and regular. Irregular breathing suggests a significant problem and usually requires ventilatory support. Observe the chest wall for any asymmetrical movement. This condition, known as **paradoxical breathing**, may suggest a **flail chest**. Patients who show increased respiratory effort, insisting on upright, sniffing, or semi-Fowler's positioning, or those refusing to lie supine, should be considered to be in significant respiratory distress.

If the patient is not breathing, or if you suspect airway problems, open the airway using the head-tilt/chin-lift or jaw-thrust maneuver, as described later in this chapter. If trauma is possible, use the jaw-thrust maneuver while stabilizing the cervical spine in a neutral position. Once the airway is open, reevaluate the breathing status. If breathing is adequate, provide supplemental oxygen and assess circulation. Consider the use of airway adjuncts, as discussed later. If breathing is inadequate or absent, begin artificial ventilation (Figure 5-2). When assisting a patient's breathing with a ventilatory device (bag-valve mask or mechanical ventilation device), or after placing an airway adjunct, (nasopharyngeal airway or oropharyngeal airway), or endotracheally intubating, monitor the chest's rise and fall to determine correct usage and placement. (These ventilatory devices and mechanical airways are discussed in detail later in this chapter.)

paradoxical breathing assymetrical chest wall movement that lessens respiratory efficiency.

flail chest defect in the chest wall that allows a segment to move freely, causing paradoxical chest wall motion.

FOCUSED HISTORY AND PHYSICAL EXAMINATION

After you complete the initial assessment and correct any immediate life threat, conduct a focused history and physical exam while continuously monitoring the patient's airway, breathing, and circulation.

Focused History

The time when the patient and his family noted the onset of symptoms is important information, as is whether the acute event occurred suddenly or gradually. Identifying possible triggers such as allergens or heat also can help the patient avoid them in the future. Additionally, the symptoms' course of development since onset will help direct diagnosis and treatment. Have they been progressively worsening, recurrent, or continuous? Associated symptoms further help to assess the cause of the patient's problem. Has he had fever or chills, productive cough, chest pain, nausea or vomiting, or diaphoresis? Does he think his voice sounds normal?

The patient's past medical history will put his present complaints into perspective and help identify the risk factors for a variety of likely diagnoses. Determine whether the present episode is similar to any past episodes of shortness of breath, what medical evaluations have been done, and what they have found. Has the patient ever been admitted to the hospital for his complaints? Has he ever been intubated?

The recent history leading to the onset of symptoms is also important. Did the patient run out of medication? Has he been noncompliant with (not taken) his medications? Did he drink too much fluid or alcohol? Did he have a seizure or vomit? Did he eat something that might induce an allergy? Did he receive any trauma? If an injury is involved, evaluate the

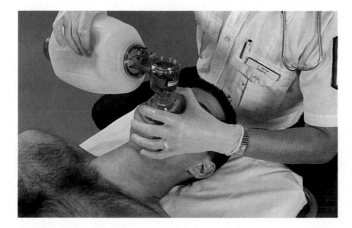

FIGURE 5-2 Bag-valve mask ventilation.

mechanism of injury. Keep in mind that blunt trauma to the neck may have injured the larynx. Anything that makes the patient's condition better (ameliorates) or worse (exacerbates, aggravates) is also significant.

Physical Examination

Your physical examination of a patient with respiratory problems should continue with the evaluation of his airway, breathing, and circulation begun during your initial assessment. Now you will use the physical examination techniques of inspection, auscultation, and palpation to evaluate his injury or illness in more detail and determine your plan of action.

Inspection   Begin the physical assessment by inspecting the patient. Evaluate the adequacy of his breathing. Note any obvious signs of trauma. Always remember to assess the skin color as an indicator of oxygenation status. Early in respiratory compromise, the sympathetic nervous system will be stimulated to help offset the lack of oxygen. When this happens, the skin will often appear pale and diaphoretic. **Cyanosis** (bluish discoloration) is another sign of respiratory distress. When oxygen binds with the hemoglobin, the blood appears bright red. Deoxygenated hemoglobin, on the other hand, is blue and gives the skin a bluish tint. This is not a reliable indicator, however, since severe tissue hypoxia is possible without cyanosis. In fact, cyanosis is considered a late sign of respiratory compromise. When it does appear, it usually affects the lips, fingernails, and skin. A red skin rash, especially if accompanied by hives, may indicate an allergic reaction. A cherry-red skin discoloration on rare occasions may be associated with carbon monoxide poisoning, as can bullae (large blisters).

Observe the patient's position. Tripod positioning (seated, leaning forward, with one arm forward to stabilize the body) may indicate chronic obstructive pulmonary disease (COPD) or asthma exacerbation; orthopnea (increased difficulty breathing while lying down) may indicate congestive heart failure or asthma.

Next, inspecting for **dyspnea**—an abnormality of breathing rate, pattern, or effort—is essential. Dyspnea may cause or be caused by **hypoxia**. Prolonged dyspnea without successful intervention can lead to **anoxia** (the absence or near-absence of oxygen), which without intervention is a premorbid (occurring just before death) event, as the brain can survive only 4 to 6 minutes in this state. Remember that all interventions are useless if you do not establish a patent airway.

Also observe for the following modified forms of respiration:

* *Coughing*—forceful exhalation of a large volume of air from the lungs. This performs a protective function in expelling foreign material from the lungs.
* *Sneezing*—sudden, forceful exhalation from the nose. It is usually caused by nasal irritation.
* *Hiccoughing* (hiccups)—sudden inspiration caused by spasmodic contraction of the diaphragm with spastic closure of the glottis. It serves no known physiological purpose. It has been associated occasionally with acute myocardial infarctions on the inferior (diaphragmatic) surface of the heart.
* *Sighing*—slow, deep, involuntary inspiration followed by a prolonged expiration. It hyperinflates the lungs and reexpands atelectatic alveoli. This normally occurs about once a minute.
* *Grunting*—a forceful expiration that occurs against a partially closed epiglottis. It is usually an indication of respiratory distress.

Note any decrease or increase in the respiratory rate, which is one of the earliest indicators of respiratory distress. Also, look for use of the accessory respiratory muscles—intercostal, suprasternal, supraclavicular, and subcostal retractions—and the abdominal muscles to assist breathing. This indicates increased respiratory effort secondary to respiratory distress. In infants and children, nasal flaring and grunting indicate respiratory distress. COPD patients having difficulty breathing will purse their lips during exhalation. Monitor

cyanosis bluish discoloration of the skin due to reduced hemoglobin in the blood.

dyspnea an abnormality of breathing rate, pattern, or effort.

hypoxia state in which insufficient oxygen is available to meet the oxygen requirements of the cells.

anoxia the absence or near-absence of oxygen.

the patient's blood pressure, including any differences noted during expiration versus inspiration. Patients with severe COPD may sustain a drop in blood pressure during inspiration. This drop is due to increased pressure within the thoracic cavity that impairs the ability of the ventricles to fill. Thus, decreased ventricular filling leads to decreased blood pressure. A drop in blood pressure of greater than 10 torr is termed **pulsus paradoxus** and may be indicative of severe obstructive lung disease.

pulsus paradoxus drop in blood pressure of greater than 10 torr during inspiration.

Determine if the pattern of respirations is abnormal—deep or shallow in combination with a fast or slow rate. Some common abnormal respiratory patterns include:

- *Kussmaul's respirations*—deep, slow or rapid, gasping breathing, commonly found in diabetic ketoacidosis
- *Cheyne-Stokes respirations*—progressively deeper, faster breathing alternating gradually with shallow, slower breathing, indicating brainstem injury
- *Biot's respirations*—irregular pattern of rate and depth with sudden, periodic episodes of apnea, indicating increased intracranial pressure
- *Central neurogenic hyperventilation*—deep, rapid respirations, indicating increased intracranial pressure
- *Agonal respirations*—shallow, slow, or infrequent breathing, indicating brain anoxia

Finally, observing altered mentation may be key in determining if breathing is adequate or if significant hypoxia may be present. If the patient's mental status is not normal, you must determine his usual baseline mental status before you can make this assessment.

Auscultation   Following inspection, listen at the mouth and nose for adequate air movement. Then listen to the chest with a stethoscope (auscultate) (Figure 5-3). In a prehospital setting, you should auscultate the right and left apex (just beneath the clavicle), the right and left base (eighth or ninth intercostal space, midclavicular line), and the right and left lower thoracic back or right and left midaxillary line (fourth or fifth intercostal space, on the lateral aspect of the chest). When the patient's condition permits, you can monitor six locations on the posterior chest, three right, and three left. The posterior surface is preferable because heart sounds do not interfere with auscultation at this location. However, because patients are usually supine during airway management, the anterior and lateral positions

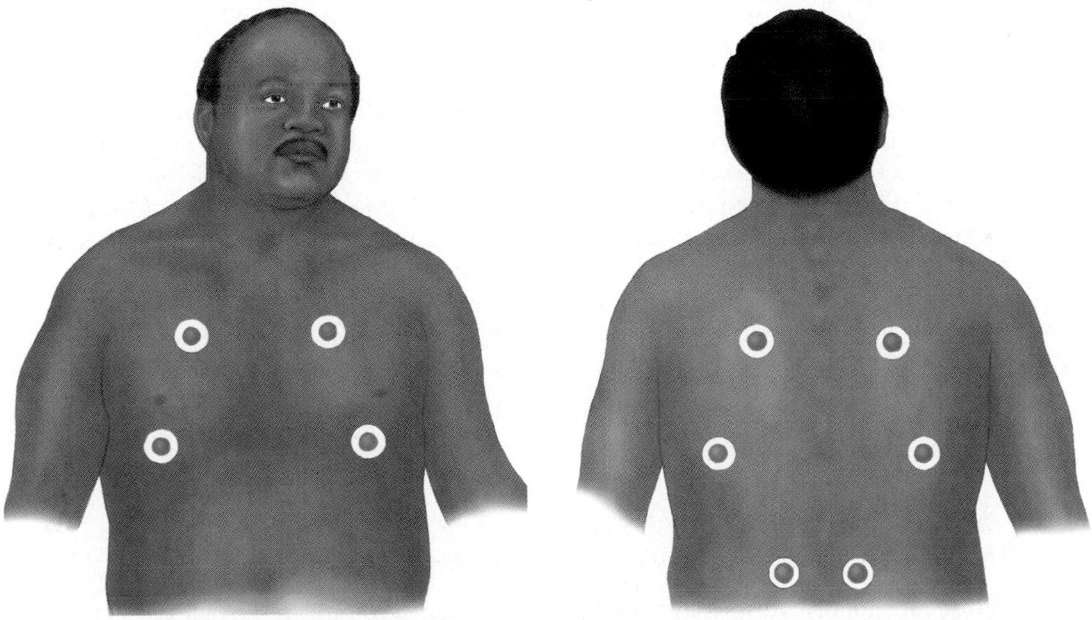

FIGURE 5-3   Positions for auscultating breath sounds.

usually prove more accessible. Breath sounds should be equal bilaterally. Sounds that point to airflow compromise include:

- *Snoring*—results from partial obstruction of the upper airway by the tongue
- *Gurgling*—results from the accumulation of blood, vomitus, or other secretions in the upper airway
- *Stridor*—a harsh, high-pitched sound heard on inhalation, associated with laryngeal edema or constriction
- *Wheezing*—a musical, squeaking, or whistling sound heard in inspiration and/or expiration, associated with bronchiolar constriction
- *Quiet*—diminished or absent breath sounds are an ominous finding and indicate a serious problem with the airway, breathing, or both

Beware of the quiet chest.

Sounds that may indicate compromise of gas exchange include:

- *Crackles* (rales)—a fine, bubbling sound heard on inspiration, associated with fluid in the smaller bronchioles
- *Rhonchi*—a coarse, rattling noise heard on inspiration, associated with inflammation, mucus, or fluid in the bronchioles

When you assess the effectiveness of ventilatory support or the correct placement of an airway adjunct, remember that air movement into the epigastrium may sometimes mimic breath sounds. Thus, listening to the chest should be only one of several means that you use to assess air movement. Another method of checking correct placement of an airway adjunct is to auscultate over the epigastrium; it should be silent during ventilation. When you provide ventilatory support, watch for signs of gastric distention. They suggest inadequate hyperextension of the neck, undue pressure generated by the ventilatory device, or improper placement of airway adjuncts.

Palpation   Finally, palpate the patient. First, using the back of your hand or your cheek, feel for air movement at the mouth and nose. (If an endotracheal tube is in place, you can check for air movement at the tube's adapter.) Next, palpate the chest for rise and fall. In addition, palpate the chest wall for tenderness, symmetry, abnormal motion, crepitus, and subcutaneous emphysema.

compliance the stiffness or flexibility of lung tissue.

When ventilating with a bag-valve device, gauge airflow into the lungs by noting compliance. **Compliance** refers to the stiffness or flexibility of the lung tissue, and it is indicated by how easily air flows into the lungs. When compliance is good, airflow meets minimal resistance. When compliance is poor, ventilation is harder to achieve. Compliance is often poor in diseased lungs and in patients suffering from chest wall injuries or tension pneumothorax. If a patient shows poor compliance during ventilatory support, look for potential causes. Upper airway obstructions, which cause difficulty with mechanical ventilation, can mimic poor compliance. If ventilating the patient is initially easy but then becomes progressively more difficult, repeat the initial assessment and look for the development of a new problem, possibly related to the mechanical airway maneuvers. The following questions will aid this assessment:

- Is the airway open?
- Is the head properly positioned in extension (nontrauma patients)?
- Is the patient developing tension pneumothorax?
- Is the endotracheal tube occluded (a mucous plug or aspirated material)?
- Has the endotracheal tube been inadvertently pushed into the right or left mainstem bronchus?
- Has the endotracheal tube been displaced into the esophagus?
- Is the mechanical ventilatory equipment functioning properly?

A fall in pulse rate in a patient with airway compromise is an ominous finding.

Pulse rate abnormalities may also suggest respiratory compromise. Tachycardia (an abnormally fast pulse) usually accompanies hypoxemia in an adult, whereas bradycardia (an abnormally slow pulse) hints at anoxia with imminent cardiac arrest.

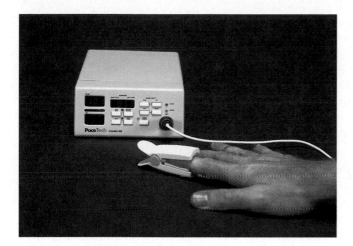

FIGURE 5-4 Pulse oximeter.

Noninvasive Respiratory Monitoring

Several available devices will help you measure the effectiveness of oxygenation and ventilation. Those measurements used most commonly in prehospital care are pulse oximetry, capnography, and esophageal detection devices. Peak expiratory flow testing can also be useful in the prehospital setting for some respiratory diseases.

Pulse Oximetry **Pulse oximetry** is widely used in prehospital emergency care. A pulse oximeter measures hemoglobin oxygen saturation in peripheral tissues (Figure 5-4). It is non-invasive (does not require entering the body), rapidly applied, and easy to operate. Pulse oximetry readings are accurate and continually reflect any changes in peripheral oxygen delivery. In fact, oximetry often detects problems with oxygenation faster than assessments of blood pressure, pulse, and respirations.

> **pulse oximetry** a measurement of hemoglobin oxygen saturation in the peripheral tissues.

To determine peripheral oxygen saturation, you place a sensor probe over a peripheral capillary bed such as a fingertip, toe, or earlobe. In infants, you can wrap the sensor around the heel and secure it with tape. The sensor contains two light-emitting diodes and two sensors. One diode emits near-red light, a wavelength specific for oxygenated hemoglobin; the other emits infrared light, a wavelength specific for deoxygenated hemoglobin. Each hemoglobin state absorbs a certain amount of the emitted light, preventing it from reaching the corresponding sensor. Less light reaching the sensor means more of its type of hemoglobin is in the blood. The oximeter then calculates the ratio of the near-red and infrared light it has received to determine the oxygen saturation percentage (SaO_2).

Pulse oximeters display the SaO_2 and the pulse rate as detected by the sensors. They show the SaO_2 either as a number or as a visual display that also shows the pulse's waveform. The relationship between SaO_2 and the partial pressure of oxygen in the blood (PaO_2) is very complex. However, the SaO_2 does correlate with the PaO_2. The greater the PaO_2, the greater will be the oxygen saturation. Since hemoglobin carries 98% of oxygen in the blood and plasma carries only 2%, pulse oximetry accurately analyzes peripheral oxygen delivery.

Pulse oximetry is often called the "fifth vital sign." When available, you should use it in virtually any situation to determine the patient's baseline value, to guide patient care, and to monitor the patient's responses to your interventions. As a guide, normal SaO_2 varies between 95% and 99%. Readings between 91% and 94% indicate mild hypoxia and warrant further evaluation and supplemental oxygen administration. Readings between 86% and 91% indicate moderate hypoxia. You should generally give these patients 100% supplemental oxygen, exercising caution in those with COPD. Readings of 85% or lower indicate severe hypoxia and warrant immediate intervention, including the administration of 100% oxygen, ventilatory assistance, or both. Your goal is to maintain the SaO_2 in the normal range (95% to 99%).

False readings with pulse oximetry are infrequent. When they do occur, the oximeter often generates an error signal or a blank screen. Causes of false readings include carbon monoxide poisoning, high-intensity lighting, and certain hemoglobin abnormalities. The absence of a pulse in an extremity also will cause a false reading. In hypovolemia and in severely anemic patients, the pulse oximetry reading may be misleading. Although the SaO_2 reading may be normal, the total amount of hemoglobin available to carry oxygen may be so markedly decreased that the patient remains hypoxic at the cellular level.

Pulse oximetry provides key information about the patient and is an important part of emergency care, including prehospital care. However, it is only one more assessment tool and does not replace other physical assessment or monitoring skills. Do not depend solely on pulse oximetry readings to guide care. Always consider and treat the whole patient.

Capnography Capnography is the measurement of exhaled carbon dioxide concentrations. The devices that make such measurements are called capnometers or end-tidal carbon dioxide ($ETCO_2$) detectors. Their use in prehospital care has increased significantly, most commonly to assess proper placement of an endotracheal tube. The absence of carbon dioxide from the exhaled air strongly indicates that the tube is in the esophagus; its presence indicates proper tracheal placement. Capnography can be used to ensure proper tube placement following insertion and to monitor tube placement during ventilation and CPR.

Capnometers are available either as disposable colorimetric devices or as electronic monitors (Figures 5-5 and 5-6). They are attached either in-line or alongside the endotracheal tube and the ventilation device. A color change in the colorimetric device or a light on the electronic monitor confirms proper tube placement. On the colorimetric device, the low CO_2 content of inspired air makes the device purple, whereas the higher CO_2 content of expired air makes it yellow. Some electronic devices now combine pulse oximetry, $ETCO_2$ detection, blood pressure, pulse rate, respiratory rate, and temperature monitors in one unit (Figure 5-7).

Although capnography is accurate, the $ETCO_2$ level falls precipitously during cardiac arrest. Therefore, these patients may not cause a color change on the $ETCO_2$ detector despite proper placement of the endotracheal tube.

Capnography is being used with increasing frequency to monitor non-intubated patients as well. It can provide important information in regard to patient condition, especially in cases of bronchospastic disease (asthma, COPD) where it can help determine early whether a patient's respiratory status is changing. Likewise, capnography can also monitor perfusion status and provide an early indication of impending shock. As with pulse oximetry, you should use a capnometer only with other methods of assessing endotracheal placement. It does not replace actually visualizing the endotracheal tube's passage through the vocal cords.

Esophageal Detector Device The esophageal detector device (EDD) is a simple and inexpensive tool to help determine whether an endotracheal tube is in the trachea or the esophagus. It uses the anatomical principle that the trachea is a rigid tube and will not collapse with negative pressure, whereas the esophagus is a collapsible tube that flattens with negative pressure and does not allow air to enter the syringe. The EDD may be either a rigid syringe or a bulb syringe (Figure 5-8). Once the patient is intubated, attach the EDD to the

capnography the measurement of exhaled carbon dioxide concentration.

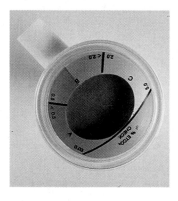

FIGURE 5-5 Colorimetric end-tidal CO_2 detector.

FIGURE 5-6 Electronic end-tidal CO_2 detector.

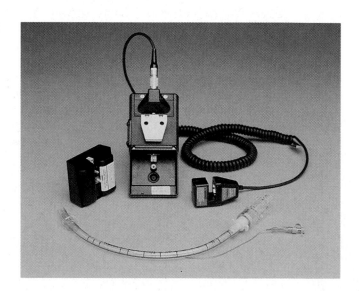

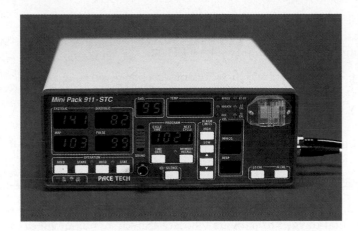

FIGURE 5-7 Combined devices check pulse oximetry, ETCO₂, blood pressure, pulse, respiratory rate, and temperature.

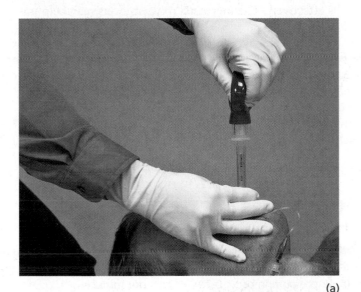

(a)

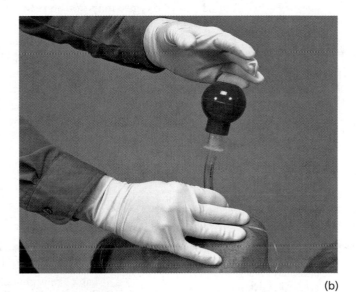

(b)

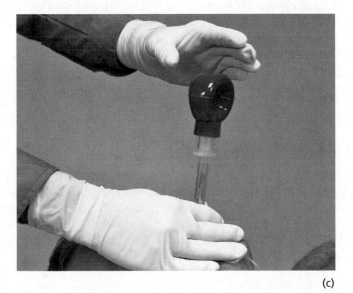

(c)

FIGURE 5-8 An esophageal intubation detector—bulb style. **a.** Squeeze the device and then attach it to the endotracheal tube. **b.** If the bulb refills easily upon release, it indicates correct placement. **c.** If the bulb does not refill, the tube is improperly placed.

proximal end of the endotracheal tube (ETT). Then you quickly pull back the syringe, aspirating air from the endotracheal tube. Air withdrawn easily confirms ETT placement in the trachea. If air is difficult or impossible to withdraw, the ETT is in the esophagus.

Peak Expiratory Flow Testing   Peak expiratory flow testing uses a disposable plastic chamber into which the patient exhales forcefully after maximal inhalation. It can be used as a crude measure of respiratory efficacy. Improving measurements can indicate good response to treatment.

OXYGENATION

Oxygen is an important drug, and you must thoroughly understand its indications and precautions. Administering supplemental oxygen to patients who are frankly hypoxic will diminish the hypoxia's secondary effects on organs such as the brain and the heart. Provide supplemental oxygen to patients who are in shock or at risk of shock, regardless of their oxygen saturation. Although the patient may be oxygenating his arterial blood well, the oxygen may not be reaching his cells effectively. The increased oxygen levels may help improve perfusion.

Never withhold oxygen from any patient for whom it is indicated. However, use caution with COPD patients. These patients lose the impulse to breathe at normal or supranormal oxygen levels. Their normal respiratory regulatory mechanism (elevated $PaCO_2$) has failed, and their impulse to breathe is triggered by a low PaO_2, or hypoxia. This is termed hypoxic drive. As a general approach, slowly increase these patients' oxygen until their breathing is less labored and they are more comfortable, though not necessarily back to their baseline. Watch your patient closely to be sure his decreased breathing effort does not signal impending respiratory failure. If this occurs, be ready to support the patient's ventilations, using basic maneuvers, adjuncts, and bag-valve mask (BVM).

OXYGEN SUPPLY AND REGULATORS

Oxygen is supplied either as a compressed gas or a liquid. Compressed gaseous oxygen is stored in an aluminum or steel tank in 400 liter (D), 660 liter (E), or 3,450 liter (M) volumes. To calculate how long the oxygen will last:

$$\text{tank life in minutes} = (\text{tank pressure in psi} \times 0.28) + \text{liters per minute}$$

Liquid oxygen is cooled to aqueous form and warmed back to its gaseous state for delivery. Although liquid oxygen requires less storage space than an equal amount of compressed oxygen, you must keep it upright and accommodate other special requirements for its storage and transfer.

Regulators for oxygen tanks are either **high-pressure regulators,** which are used to transfer oxygen at high pressures from tank to tank, or **therapy regulators,** which are used for delivering oxygen to patients. The default pressure for therapy regulators is 50 psi, which is controlled within the regulator to allow for adjustable low-flow oxygen delivery.

OXYGEN DELIVERY DEVICES

Oxygen delivery to patients is measured in liters of flow per minute (L/min). A number of delivery devices are available; the patient's condition dictates which method you use. You must continually reassess the patient who requires oxygen therapy to be certain that the method of delivery and flow rate are adequate. You should not use these devices for patients with poor respiratory effort, severe hypoxia, or apnea or for patients who exhibit mouth breathing.

Nasal Cannula

The **nasal cannula** is a catheter placed at the nares. It provides an optimal oxygen supplementation of up to 40% when set at 6 L/min flow. At flow rates above 6 L/min, the nasal mucous membranes become very dry and easily break down. Patients generally tolerate the

---

Never withhold oxygen from any patient for whom it is indicated.

high-pressure regulator regulator used to transfer oxygen at high pressures from tank to tank.

therapy regulator pressure regulator used for delivering oxygen to patients.

Continually reassess the patient who requires oxygen therapy to be certain that the method of delivery and flow rate are adequate.

Content Review

OXYGEN DELIVERY DEVICES
• Nasal cannula
• Venturi mask
• Simple face mask
• Partial rebreather mask
• Nonrebreather mask
• Small-volume nebulizer
• Oxygen humidifier

nasal cannula catheter placed at the nares.

nasal cannula well. It is indicated for low to moderate oxygen requirements and long-term oxygen therapy.

Venturi Mask

The **venturi mask** is a high-flow face mask that uses a venturi system to deliver relatively precise oxygen concentrations, regardless of the patient's rate and depth of breathing. As oxygen passes into the mask through a jet orifice in the base of the mask, it entrains room air. The device then delivers the resulting mixture to the patient. Some venturi masks have dial selectors to control the amount of ambient air taken in; others have interchangeable caps. Either type can deliver concentrations of 24%, 28%, 35%, or 40% oxygen. The liter flow depends on the oxygen concentration desired. The venturi mask is particularly useful for COPD patients, who benefit from careful control of inspired oxygen concentration.

venturi mask high-flow face mask that uses a venturi system to deliver relatively precise oxygen concentrations.

The venturi mask is particularly useful for COPD patients, who benefit from careful control of inspired oxygen concentrations.

Simple Face Mask

The simple face mask is indicated for patients requiring moderate to high oxygen concentrations. Side ports allow room air to enter the mask and dilute the oxygen concentration during inspiration. Flow rates generally range from about 6 to 10 L/min, providing 40% to 60% oxygen at the maximum rate, depending on the patient's respiratory rate and depth. Delivery of volumes beyond 10 L/min does not enhance oxygen concentration.

Partial Rebreather Mask

The partial rebreather mask is indicated for patients requiring moderate to high oxygen concentrations when satisfactory clinical results are not obtained with the simple face mask. One-way discs that cover the partial rebreather mask's side ports prevent the inspiration of room air. Minimal dilution occurs with inspiration of residual expired air along with the supplemental oxygen. Maximum flow rate is 10L/min.

Nonrebreather Mask

The nonrebreather mask has one-way side ports as well, but also has an attached reservoir bag to hold oxygen ready to inhale. It provides the highest oxygen concentration of all oxygen delivery devices available, 80% to 95% at 15 L/min. It is not indicated as continuing support for poor respiratory effort and severe hypoxia; however, you should place it initially to preoxygenate these patients while you prepare them for intubation, unless initial ventilatory support with BVM and 100% oxygen is indicated.

Small-Volume Nebulizer

Nebulizer chambers containing 3 to 5 cc of fluid are attached to a face mask that allows for delivery of medications in aerosol form (nebulization). Pressurized oxygen or air enters the chamber to create a mist, which the patient then inspires. Oxygen is the usual carrier, but in many COPD cases, supplemental oxygen by nasal cannula with nebulization using air is preferred.

Oxygen Humidifier

You can provide humidified oxygen to the patient by attaching a sterile water reservoir to the oxygen outlet. Humidified oxygen benefits patients with croup, epiglottitis, or bronchiolitis, as well as those patients receiving long-term oxygen therapy.

VENTILATION

Many of your cases in the field will call for ventilatory support. These situations range from apneic patients to less obvious instances when patients are experiencing depressed respiratory function. Remember that an unconscious patient's respiratory center may not function adequately. A significant decrease in the patient's rate or depth of breathing will lead to decreased respiratory minute volume, hypercarbia, hypoxia, and a lowered pH. If you do not

Content Review

VENTILATION METHODS
- Mouth-to-mouth/ mouth-to-nose
- Mouth-to-mask
- Bag-valve mask
- Flow-restricted, oxygen-powered ventilation device
- Automatic transport ventilator

tidal volume average volume of gas inhaled or exhaled in one respiratory cycle.

correct this, respiratory or cardiac arrest may occur. Effective ventilatory support requires a **tidal volume** of at least 800 mL of oxygen at 12 to 20 breaths per minute.

When providing ventilatory support, you must generate enough force to overcome the elastic resistance of the lungs and chest wall, as well as the frictional resistance in the respiratory passageways, without overinflating the lungs. This is similar to blowing up a balloon; you must overcome the balloon's resistance in order to inflate it. Keep in mind that air travels the path of least resistance. If you do not maintain a tight seal between the ventilation mask and your patient's face, air flows out of the gaps rather than through the respiratory passageways.

Effective artificial ventilation requires a patent airway, an effective seal between the mask and the patient's face, and delivery of adequate ventilatory volumes. Use care when you attempt to generate enough pressure to ventilate the lungs. Too much pressure may lead to gastric distention and regurgitation. Also, be certain that you allow the patient to exhale between delivered breaths.

MOUTH-TO-MOUTH/MOUTH-TO-NOSE VENTILATION

Mouth-to-mouth and mouth-to-nose ventilation are the most basic methods of rescue ventilation. Both are indicated in the presence of apnea when no other ventilation devices are available. They require no special equipment, yet both allow an adequate seal between the rescuer and the patient and can provide effective ventilatory support, with adequate tidal volumes and oxygenation; however, the capacity of the person delivering the ventilations limits both methods. Also, both methods provide only limited oxygen—the rescuer's expired air contains only 17% oxygen. The major drawback is its potential for exposing either the rescuer or the patient to communicable diseases through contact with blood and other body fluids. Take care not to hyperinflate the patient's lungs or to hyperventilate yourself.

MOUTH-TO-MASK VENTILATION

The pocket mask is a clear plastic device that is placed over an apneic patient's mouth and nose. It prevents direct contact between you and your patient's mouth, thus reducing the risk of contamination and subsequent infection. It may be easier to obtain a good seal on the patient's face using a mask. However, the mask is only useful if it is readily available. Do not use it in awake patients.

A variety of pocket masks are available. Some are reusable, others are disposable. Most are small and compact enough to fit in a pocket or purse, and you should always carry one. Because of the increasing risks of infectious diseases, you should use a disposable mask whenever you ventilate a patient. These devices usually have a one-way valve that prevents you from contacting the patient's expired air. The valve may also provide an inlet for supplemental oxygen; mouth-to-mask ventilation combined with an oxygen flow rate of 10 L/min can deliver an inspired oxygen concentration of approximately 50%. To apply the mouth-to-mask technique, position the head to open the airway by one of the previously discussed methods, position the mask to obtain a good seal, and provide adequate ventilatory volumes. As with mouth-to-mouth and mouth-to-nose methods, hyperinflation of the patient's lungs, gastric distention in the patient, and hyperventilation in the rescuer are potential complications.

BAG-VALVE DEVICES

bag-valve mask ventilation device consisting of a self-inflating bag with two one-way valves and a transparent plastic face mask.

For patients with apnea or an unsatisfactory respiratory effort, prehospital and emergency department personnel most commonly use the bag-valve device. When used correctly, the bag-valve device assists in ventilating patients by expanding the lungs and improving alveolar ventilation, thus preventing hypoxia. When using the bag-valve device with the mask, the EMT-I must still open the airway with either the jaw-thrust or head-tilt/chin-lift maneuver. Do not use the device in awake patients who cannot tolerate the procedure.

The **bag-valve mask** (BVM) consists of an oblong, self-inflating, silicone or rubber bag with two one-way valves (an air/oxygen-inlet valve and a patient valve) and a transparent plastic face mask, which is available in three sizes: neonatal, child, or adult. Some BVMs have a built-in colorimetric capnometer (Figure 5-9). With the increasing risks of transmitting infectious diseases, BVMs should be disposable. Do not reuse them.

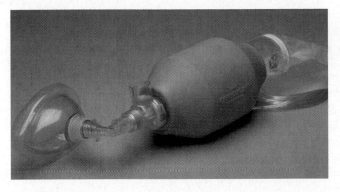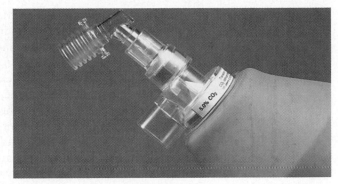

FIGURE 5-9   Bag-valve mask with a built-in colorimetric capnometer.

You can use BVMs with or without oxygen. Without oxygen they deliver only room air (21% oxygen) to the patient; with oxygen attached, the deliverable amount of oxygen increases from 60% to 70%. The bag-valve device also has an adjunct oxygen reservoir or corrugated tubing that can deliver 90% to 95% oxygen when coupled with an oxygen source. If possible, connect all patients who require a bag-valve device to an oxygen reservoir with oxygen at 15 L/min.

BVMs for pediatric cases may have a pop-off valve. BVMs for adults should not have pop-off valves, because patients with high airway resistance and poor lung compliance will activate the pop-off valve, thus preventing effective ventilation.

One, two, or three rescuers may perform BVM ventilation. One-person BVM ventilation is the most difficult method to master because obtaining and maintaining the mask seal can be challenging. You must not only keep the airway open with a jaw-thrust or chin-lift but also at the same time keep the mask sealed well and squeeze the BVM to deliver an adequate tidal volume. Two-person BVM ventilation is the most efficient method, providing superior mask seal and tidal volumes when applied correctly. It requires the availability of an adequate number of trained medical personnel. Three-person BVM ventilation also provides excellent mask seal and volume delivery, but it requires more personnel, and it crowds access to the patient's airway.

To perform the two-person BVM method, the first rescuer maintains the mask seal while the second squeezes the bag. With the three-person BVM method, the first rescuer applies manual airway maneuvers, the second maintains the mask seal, and the third squeezes the bag. Observe the patient for chest rise, development of gastric distention, and changes in compliance of the bag with ventilation. Complications of BVM ventilation include inadequate volume delivery if there is a poor mask seal or improper technique, barotrauma from overinflation of the lungs, and gastric distention.

Ventilation of Pediatric Patients

The differences in the pediatric patient's anatomy require some variation in ventilation technique. First, a child's relatively flat nasal bridge makes achieving mask seal more difficult. Pressing the mask against the child's face to improve the seal can obstruct his airway, which is more compressible than an adult's. You can best achieve the mask seal with the two-person BVM technique, using a jaw-thrust to maintain an open airway.

For BVM ventilation, the bag size depends on the child's age. Full-term neonates and infants require a pediatric BVM with a capacity of at least 450 mL. For children up to eight years of age, the pediatric BVM is preferred, though for patients in the upper age range you can use an adult BVM with a capacity of 1,500 mL if you do not maximally inflate it. Children older than eight years require an adult BVM to achieve adequate tidal volumes. Additionally, be certain that the mask fits properly, from the bridge of the nose to the cleft of the chin. If a length-based resuscitation tape (Broselow tape) is available, you can use it to help determine the proper size.

To achieve a proper mask seal, place the mask over the patient's mouth and nose; avoid compressing the eyes. Using one hand, place your thumb on the mask at the apex and your index finger on the mask at the chin (C-grip). Apply gentle pressure downward on the mask to establish an adequate seal. Maintain the airway by lifting the bony prominence of the chin with the remaining fingers forming an E under the jaw; avoid placing pressure on the soft area under the chin. You may use the one-rescuer technique, although the two-rescuer technique is more effective.

Ventilate according to current standards, obtaining chest rise with each breath. Begin the ventilation and say "squeeze," providing just enough volume to initiate chest rise—be very careful not to overinflate the child's lungs. Allow adequate time for exhalation, saying "release, release." Continue ventilations, saying "squeeze, release, release." To assess adequacy of ventilations, look for adequate chest rise, listen for lung sounds at the third intercostal space, midaxillary line, and assess for clinical improvement (skin color and heart rate).

FLOW-RESTRICTED, OXYGEN-POWERED VENTILATION DEVICES (DEMAND VALVES)

The **demand valve device,** also called the manually triggered, oxygen-powered ventilation device or flow-restricted, oxygen-powered ventilation device, will deliver 100% oxygen to a patient at its highest flow rates (40 L/min maximum). Flow is restricted to 30 cm H_2O or less to diminish gastric distention that can occur with its use. The device is rugged, compact, and easy to handle. It also includes an easy-to-locate manual control button. In addition, the entire device can be attached to a face mask or a mechanical airway (Figure 5-10).

The complete system consists of high-pressure tubing that connects to an oxygen supply, and a valve that is activated by a push button or lever. When the valve is opened, oxygen flows to the patient. Most of these units also contain an inspiratory release valve that makes them useful in treating spontaneously breathing patients who need high oxygen concentrations. The slight negative pressure created by inhalation opens the valve. The greater the inspiratory effort, the higher the flow. When inhalation ceases, so does oxygen flow. This helps decrease the likelihood of overinflation during ventilation of a patient with respiratory effort. The indications for use of oxygen-powered ventilation devices include the need for high-volume, high-oxygen-concentration delivery in awake, compliant patients. You may use it in unconscious patients, but be extremely cautious, because you cannot measure delivered volumes or feel lung compliance. The demand valve device is easy to use and provides high oxygen concentrations. However, the demand valve device has several drawbacks. During ventilation, it does not give the rescuer a sense of chest compliance; thus, you

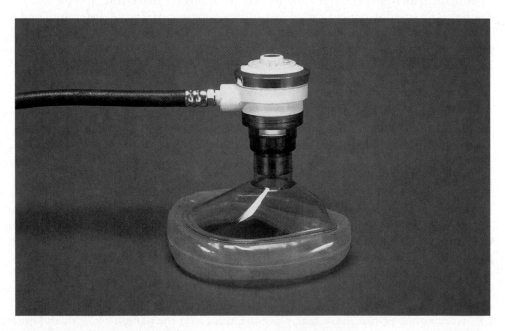

FIGURE 5-10 Demand valve and mask.

must take care not to overinflate the lungs. The high pressures that the device generates may injure the lungs, which can lead to pneumothorax and subcutaneous emphysema. Also, the demand valve resuscitator may open the esophagus, causing gastric distention in patients who have not been intubated. Finally, the high flow rate of the demand valve resuscitator will quickly drain a portable oxygen cylinder. You will have to use another means of ventilatory support if the cylinder requires changing during patient management.

The demand valve resuscitator is not recommended for use with patients under the age of 16. Because of the sudden high pressures that this device can produce, you should use it with extreme caution in intubated patients or those with chest trauma.

AUTOMATIC TRANSPORT VENTILATOR

Several compact mechanical ventilators are available for prehospital care. Designed for convenience and easy use during patient care and transport, these lightweight and durable portable devices offer a number of advantages. They maintain minute volume better than bag-valve devices, and they tolerate temperatures ranging from $-30°F$ to $125°F$ with great dependability. In cardiac arrest, the automatic ventilator allows you to interpose chest compressions between mechanical breaths. They are mechanically simple and adapt to a portable oxygen supply.

The compact ventilator typically comes with two or three controls: one for the ventilatory rate, the other for tidal volume (Figure 5-11). It also has a standard 15/22 mm adapter, so that you can attach it to a variety of airway devices. Some of these automatic units deliver controlled ventilation only. Others function as intermittent mandatory ventilators, reverting to controlled mechanical ventilation in patients who are not breathing. Tidal volume in most is adjustable, whereas the ventilatory rate may be either fixed or adjustable. The inspired oxygen concentration is usually fixed at 100%, but it may be adjustable.

Many of these ventilators have a pop-off valve that prevents pressure-related injury. When airway pressure exceeds a preset level (typically 60 cm H_2O), the valve opens, venting some of the tidal volume. This feature can hinder ventilating patients with cardiogenic pulmonary edema, adult respiratory distress syndrome (ARDS), pulmonary contusion, bronchospasm, or other disorders in which high airway pressures must be overcome. Consider using a bag-valve device if this problem occurs. Also, these devices generally have no alarms to warn of possible tube displacement or barotrauma.

As a rule, you should not use mechanical ventilators in children less than five years old, awake patients, or patients with obstructed airways or increased airway resistance, as described above. Otherwise, when indicated, the device can prove a valuable tool. In intubated patients, the mechanical ventilator allows you to perform other vital tasks. Its disadvantages are that it can be difficult to secure and proper functioning depends on oxygen tank pressure.

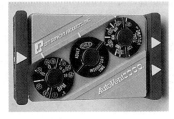

FIGURE 5-11 Portable mechanical ventilator.

SUCTIONING

Anticipating complications when managing the patient's airway is the key for successful outcomes. You must be prepared to **suction** all airways in order to remove blood or other secretions and for the patient who vomits. Suctioning equipment must be readily available for all patients, to prevent a simple vomiting episode from becoming a complicated aspiration episode that increases the patient's risk for greater morbidity or mortality.

SUCTIONING EQUIPMENT

Many different suctioning devices are available. They may be handheld, oxygen powered, battery operated, or mounted (nonportable). To suit the prehospital environment, your equipment should be lightweight, portable, durable, generate a vacuum level of at least 300 mmHg when the distal end is occluded, and allow a flow rate of at least 30 L/min when the tube is open. In addition to a portable device, the ambulance should have a mounted, vacuum-powered suction device that can generate stronger suction and can be a backup device in case of equipment failure. The most commonly used suction catheters are either

suction to remove with a vacuum-type device.

Table 5-1	TYPES OF SUCTIONING CATHETERS	
Hard/Rigid Catheter	**Soft Catheters**	
A large tube with multiple holes at the distal end	Long, flexible tube; smaller diameter than hard-tip catheters	
Suctions larger volumes of fluid rapidly	Cannot remove large volumes of fluid rapidly	
Standard size	Various sizes	
Used in oropharyngeal airway only	Can be placed in the oropharynx, nasopharynx, or down the endotracheal tube	
Removes larger particles	Suction tubing without catheter (facilitates suctioning of large debris)	

hard/rigid catheters ("Yankauer" or "tonsil tip") or soft catheters ("whistle tip"). Table 5-1 summarizes their differences.

Because suctioning reduces a patient's access to oxygen, limit each attempt to 15 seconds. If possible, hyperventilate the patient with 100% oxygen before and after each effort. Clear any fluids from the upper airway first, because assisted breathing may cause aspiration. Do not apply suction while inserting the catheter. Apply suction only as you withdraw the catheter after properly positioning it.

Complications of suctioning are related to hypoxia from prolonged suctioning attempts without proper ventilation. The decrease in myocardial oxygen supply can cause cardiac dysrhythmias. Suctioning can also stimulate the vagus nerve, causing bradycardia and hypotension, or the anxiety of being suctioned can cause hypertension and tachycardia. Stimulation of the cough reflex will cause a patient to cough, causing an increase in intracranial pressure and reducing cerebral blood flow.

SUCTIONING TECHNIQUES

You must have suction equipment beside any patient who has airway compromise and will need airway management. Do the following to suction a patient:

1. Wear protective eyewear, gloves, and face mask.
2. Preoxygenate the patient; this may require hyperventilating him.
3. Determine the depth of catheter insertion by measuring from the patient's earlobe to his lips.
4. With the suction turned off, insert the catheter into your patient's pharynx to the predetermined depth.
5. Turn on the suction unit and place your thumb over the suction control orifice; limit suction to 15 seconds.
6. Continue to suction while withdrawing the catheter. When using a whistle-tip catheter, rotate it between your fingertips.
7. Hyperventilate the patient with 100% oxygen.

In many cases you will suction extremely viscous, or thick, secretions, which can obstruct the flow of fluid through the tubing. To reduce this problem, suction water through the tubing between suctioning attempts. This dilutes the secretions and facilitates flow to the suction canister. Most suction units have small water canisters for this purpose.

Tracheobronchial Suctioning

You may have to suction some patients through an endotracheal tube or a tracheostomy tube to remove secretions or mucous plugs that can cause respiratory distress. Suctioning these patients risks hypoxia, so oxygenating them before and after the procedure is essential. If possible, use sterile technique to avoid contaminating the pulmonary system. Use only the soft-tip catheter to avoid damaging any structures and be certain to prelubricate it. Once you have preoxygenated the patient with 100% oxygen, lubricate the catheter tip with a water-soluble gel and gently insert it until you feel resistance. Then apply suction for only 10 to 15 seconds while extracting the catheter. Ventilation and oxygenation are mandatory immediately after each suctioning attempt. You may have to inject 3 to 5 mL of sterile water into the endotracheal tube to help loosen thick secretions.

GASTRIC DECOMPRESSION

A common problem with ventilating a nonintubated patient is **gastric distention,** which occurs when the procedure's high pressures trap air in the stomach. As the stomach expands with this trapped air, the risk of vomiting rises. The enlarged stomach also pushes against the diaphragm, inhibiting the lungs' expansion and increasing their resistance to ventilation. Once the patient has gastric distention, you should place a tube in his stomach for gastric decompression, using either the nasogastric or orogastric approach.

gastric distention inflation of the stomach.

Nasogastric tube placement is generally preferred in alert patients because it allows them to talk, whereas orogastric tube placement is recommended in patients with facial fractures to avoid placing the tube through a skull fracture into the brain. Indications for gastric tube placement include the need for decompression because of the risk of aspiration or difficulty ventilating. In addition, large-bore gastric tubes are occasionally placed for gastric lavage in hypothermia and some overdose emergencies. The possibility of esophageal bleeding dictates extreme caution in patients with esophageal disease or trauma. Avoid placing gastric tubes in the presence of an esophageal obstruction because of the increased risk of esophageal perforation. Both routes effectively accomplish gastric decompression; the orogastric route adds the advantage of allowing the use of a larger bore tube for lavage. Disadvantages of both routes include discomfort to patients and minor interference with orotracheal intubation. When no contraindication exists (such as facial fractures), nasogastric tube placement for gastric decompression is generally preferred. Both routes put the patient at risk for vomiting, misplacement into the trachea, or trauma and bleeding from poor technique.

Always wear protective eyewear, gloves, and face shield whenever you place a nasogastric or orogastric tube. Do the following to place a nasogastric or orogastric tube:

1. Place the patient's head in a neutral position while preoxygenating.
2. Determine the length of tube insertion by measuring from the epigastrium to the angle of jaw, then to the tip of the nares.
3. If the patient is awake, use a topical anesthetic to the nares or oropharynx. Suppress the gag reflex with a topical anesthetic applied into the posterior oropharynx or with IV lidocaine.
4. Lubricate the distal tip of the gastric tube and gently insert the tube into the nares and along the nasal floor or, alternately, into the oral cavity at midline. Advance the tube gently. If the patient is awake, encourage swallowing to facilitate the tube's passage.
5. Advance to the predetermined mark on the tube.
6. Confirm placement by injecting 30 to 50 mL of air while listening to the epigastric region for air sounds. If the patient develops an inability to speak after gastric tube placement, malposition of the tube through the vocal cords and into the trachea has occurred, so you must remove the tube.
7. Apply suction. Note gastric contents that pass through the tube.
8. Secure the tube in place.

BASIC AIRWAY MANAGEMENT

Deciding if a patient has a patent airway is the most important step in the initial assessment. Airway management is one of the few prehospital interventions known to improve patient survival rates. Once you have determined that intervention is needed, you must use simple manual airway maneuvers and equipment before proceeding with more advanced techniques such as endotracheal intubation, placement of the Esophageal Tracheal CombiTube (ETC), or laryngeal mask airway (LMA). Always provide supplemental oxygen to all patients for whom it is indicated; never withhold it even from the COPD patient. Be sure to always wear protective eyewear and gloves to avoid contact with the patient's body fluids. If you suspect cervical spine injury, perform modified airway techniques with appropriate cervical spine stabilization. Once you have secured the airway, frequently reassess for an adequate airway and ventilation.

MANUAL AIRWAY MANEUVERS

Manual maneuvers are the simplest airway management techniques and are highly effective but often neglected in prehospital care. The head-tilt/chin-lift and the jaw-thrust are safe and dependable maneuvers for relieving obstruction by the tongue. Perform one of these techniques on all unconscious patients but not on responsive patients. If you suspect cervical spine injury, perform the modified jaw-thrust with in-line stabilization of the cervical spine.

Head-Tilt/Chin-Lift

In the absence of cervical spine trauma, the head-tilt/chin-lift is the best technique for opening the airway in an unresponsive patient who is not protecting his own airway. The head-tilt is hazardous to patients with cervical spine injuries; do not use it for those patients. Do the following to perform the head-tilt/chin-lift:

1. Place the patient supine and position yourself at the side of the patient's head.
2. Place one hand on the patient's forehead and, using firm downward pressure with your palm, tilt the head back.
3. Put two fingers of the other hand under the bony part of the chin and lift the jaw anteriorly to open the airway.

Caution: Avoid compressing the soft tissues of the neck and chin.

Jaw-Thrust Maneuver

A jaw-thrust maneuver is also acceptable for an unresponsive patient without the risk of cervical spine injury who cannot protect his airway. Do the following to perform a jaw-thrust:

1. Place the patient supine and kneel behind his head.
2. Apply fingers on each side of the jaw at the mandibular angles.
3. Lift the jaw forward (anterior) with a gentle tilting of the patient's head to open the airway.

For trauma patients, maintain the cervical spine in neutral position and use either the jaw-thrust without head-tilt or the modified jaw-thrust. You can perform both of these maneuvers with a cervical collar in place:

1. *Jaw-thrust without head-tilt:* lift the jaw by grasping under the chin and behind the teeth, without tilting the head. Use extreme caution with this technique, as even unresponsive patients can clench their teeth shut; do not use this method if the patient's mouth resists opening.
2. *Modified jaw-thrust:* lift the jaw using fingers behind the mandibular angles; do not tilt the head. Use this method if the patient's mouth resists opening.

Although they are simple and effective, none of these manual airway maneuvers protects the airway from aspiration. Additionally, the jaw-thrust and modified jaw-thrust are

 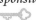

difficult to maintain for an extended time. The jaw-thrust is impossible to maintain if the patient becomes responsive or combative. Using them with a BVM is often difficult and typically requires a second rescuer. Finally, maintaining the jaw-thrust requires you to keep your thumb in the patient's mouth.

Sellick's Maneuver

To help prevent regurgitation and reduce gastric distention, Sellick's maneuver applies gentle pressure posteriorly on the anterior cricoid cartilage (Figures 5-12 and 5-13). Since the esophagus lies just behind the cricoid cartilage, this maneuver effectively closes the esophagus to pressures as high as 100 cm/H_2O. It also facilitates intubation by moving the larynx posterior, bringing it into view.

To locate the cricoid cartilage, palpate the thyroid cartilage (Adam's apple) and feel the depression just below it (cricothyroid membrane). The prominence just inferior to this depression is the ring of cricoid cartilage. Using the thumb and index finger of one hand, apply pressure to the anterior and lateral aspects of the cricoid cartilage just next to the midline. In infants, use one fingertip and apply gentle downward pressure, taking care to avoid excessive pressure.

When you use this technique during BVM ventilation and endotracheal intubation, a second rescuer is required, and you must remember that the patient will likely regurgitate when you release cricoid pressure. Ideally, therefore, once you have applied Sellick's maneuver, you must maintain it until endotracheal intubation is confirmed and personnel are

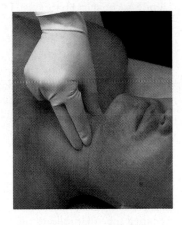

FIGURE 5-12 Sellick's maneuver (cricoid pressure).

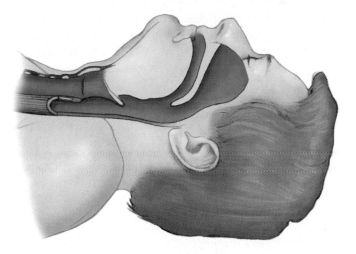

FIGURE 5-13a Airway before applying Sellick's maneuver.

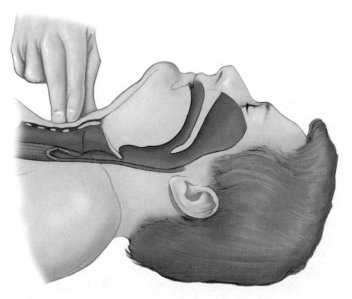

FIGURE 5-13b Airway with Sellick's maneuver applied. (Note compression of the esophagus.)

Always attempt any appropriate manual maneuver before placing a mechanical airway.

nasopharyngeal airway uncuffed tube that follows the natural curvature of the nasopharynx, passing through the nose and extending from the nostril to the posterior pharynx.

French unit of measurement approximately equal to one-third meter.

gag reflex mechanism that stimulates retching, or striving to vomit, when the soft palate is touched.

Never use a nasopharyngeal tube when you suspect a basilar skill fracture, because it can inadvertently pass into the cranial vault.

ready to suction the oropharynx or place a nasogastric tube to decompress the stomach. Additionally, use caution in any patient with a suspected cervical spine injury, because movement of the neck in these patients could cause further spinal cord injury. Complications of Sellick's maneuver include esophageal rupture from unrelieved gastric pressure and obstruction of the trachea or laryngeal trauma from excessive manual pressure.

BASIC MECHANICAL AIRWAYS

In the absence of trauma, secretions, foreign bodies, and edema, basic manual airway maneuvers should clear the tongue from the air passages. However, the tongue often falls back to block the airway again. Two available airway adjuncts—the nasopharyngeal airway and the oropharyngeal airway—correct this. These adjuncts cannot replace good head positioning, but they do help to lift the base of the tongue forward and away from the posterior oropharynx, establishing a patent airway. Always attempt any appropriate manual maneuvers before placing a mechanical airway.

Nasopharyngeal Airway

The **nasopharyngeal airway** is an uncuffed tube made of soft rubber or plastic. The nasopharyngeal airway follows the natural curvature of the nasopharynx, passing through the nose and extending from the nostril to the posterior pharynx just below the base of the tongue. It varies from 17- to 20-cm long, and its diameter ranges from 20 F to 36 F (**French**). A funnel-shaped projection at its proximal end helps prevent the tube from slipping inside a patient's nose and becoming lost or aspirated. The distal end is beveled to facilitate passage. You will use the nasopharyngeal airway to relieve soft tissue upper airway obstruction in cases where an oropharyngeal airway is not advised. Specific indications for the use of the nasopharyngeal airway include obtunded patients (with or without a suppressed **gag reflex**) and unconscious patients. If the patient does not tolerate the nasopharyngeal airway, you should remove it.

The nasopharyngeal airway's advantages are:

- It can be rapidly inserted and safely placed blindly.
- It bypasses the tongue, providing a patent airway.
- You may use it in the presence of a gag reflex.
- You may use it when the patient has suffered injury to his oral cavity (anything from trauma to the mandible to significant soft tissue damage to the tongue or pharynx).
- You may suction through it.
- You may use it when the patient's teeth are clenched.

Disadvantages of the nasopharyngeal airway are:

- It is smaller than the oropharyngeal airway.
- It does not isolate the trachea.
- It is difficult to suction through.
- It may cause severe nosebleeds if inserted too forcefully.
- It may cause pressure necrosis of the nasal mucosa.
- It may kink and clog, obstructing the airway.
- Inserting it is difficult if nasal damage (old or new) is present.
- You may not use it if the patient has or is suspected to have a basilar skull fracture.

Do not use the nasopharyngeal airway in patients who are predisposed to nosebleeds or who have a nasal obstruction. Also never use it when you suspect a basilar skull fracture, because the tube can inadvertently pass into the cranial vault.

The properly sized nasopharyngeal tube is slightly smaller in diameter than the patient's nostril, and in adults it is equal to or slightly longer than the distance from the patient's nose to his earlobe. Selecting the appropriate size is important. Too small a tube will not extend

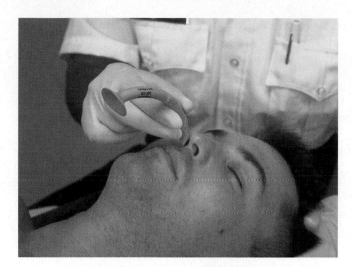

FIGURE 5-14 Nasopharyngeal airway.

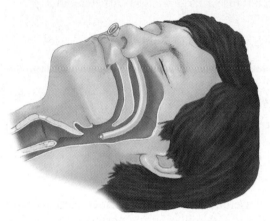

FIGURE 5-15 Nasopharyngeal airway, inserted.

past the tongue; too long a tube may pass into the esophagus and result in hypoventilation and gastric distention with artificial ventilation (Figures 5-14 and 5-15). Do the following to insert the nasopharyngeal airway:

1. If the patient has no history of trauma, hyperextend his head and neck.
2. Ensure or maintain effective ventilation. If indicated, hyperventilate the patient with 100% oxygen.
3. Lubricate the exterior of the tube with a water-soluble gel to prevent trauma during insertion. If possible, use a lidocaine gel in the alert or responsive patient; its anesthetic effect on the mucosa will make insertion more comfortable.
4. Push gently up on the tip of the nose and pass the tube into the right nostril. If the septum is deviated and you cannot easily insert the tube into the right nostril, use the left nostril. With the bevel oriented toward the septum, insert the tube gently along the nasal floor, parallel to the mouth. Avoid pushing against any resistance, because this may cause tissue trauma and airway kinking.
5. Verify appropriate position of the airway. Clear breath sounds and chest rise indicate correct placement. Also, feel at the airway's proximal end for airflow on expiration.
6. Hyperventilate the patient with 100% oxygen, if indicated.

Although semi-conscious patients tolerate a nasopharyngeal airway better than an oropharyngeal airway, it too may cause vomiting and laryngospasm. Insertion of the nasopharyngeal airway may injure the nasal mucosa, leading to bleeding, aspiration of clots, and the need for suctioning. Forceful insertion of the airway may lacerate the adenoids, causing considerable bleeding.

Oropharyngeal Airway

The **oropharyngeal airway** is a noninvasive semicircular plastic or rubber device designed to follow the palate's curvature. It holds the base of the tongue away from the posterior oropharynx, thus preventing it from obstructing the glottis. Its use is indicated in patients with no gag reflex.

When properly positioned, this device has several advantages:

- It is easy to place using proper technique.
- Air can pass around and through the device.
- It helps prevent obstruction by the teeth and lips.
- It helps manage unconscious patients who are breathing spontaneously or need mechanical ventilation.
- It makes suction of the pharynx easier, because a large suction catheter can pass on either side of the device.
- It serves as an effective bite block in case of seizures or to protect the endotracheal tube.

Disadvantages of the oropharyngeal airway are:

- It does not isolate the trachea or prevent aspiration.
- It cannot be inserted when the teeth are clenched. It may obstruct the airway if not inserted properly.
- It is easily dislodged.
- Return of the gag reflex may produce vomiting.

Never use an oropharyngeal airway in conscious or semi-conscious patients who have a gag reflex, since it may cause vomiting or laryngospasm.

Do not use an oropharyngeal airway in conscious or in semi-conscious patients who have a gag reflex, because it may cause vomiting (by stimulating the posterior tongue gag reflexes) or laryngospasm.

Oropharyngeal airways are available in sizes ranging from no. 0 (for neonates) to no. 6 (for large adults). Selecting the proper size is important. If the airway is too long, it can press the epiglottis against the entrance of the larynx, resulting in airway obstruction. If it is too small, it will not adequately hold the tongue forward. To measure for the appropriate oropharyngeal airway, place the flange beside the patient's cheek, parallel to the front of the teeth. A properly sized airway will extend from the patient's mouth to the angle of his jaw (Figure 5-16). Do the following to place the oropharyngeal airway:

1. If the patient has no history of trauma, hyperextend his head and neck. Open the mouth and remove any visible obstructions.
2. Ensure or maintain effective ventilation; if indicated, hyperventilate the patient with 100% oxygen.
3. Grasp the patient's jaw and lift anteriorly.
4. With your other hand, hold the airway device at its proximal end and insert it into the patient's mouth. Make sure the curve is reversed, with the tip pointing toward the roof of the mouth.
5. Once the tip reaches the level of the soft palate, gently rotate the airway 180 degrees until it comes to rest over the tongue.
6. Verify appropriate position of the airway. Clear breath sounds and chest rise indicate correct placement.
7. Hyperventilate the patient with 100% oxygen, if indicated.

Make sure the airway is correctly positioned. Improper placement can obstruct the airway by pushing the tongue back against the posterior oropharynx (Figure 5-17). The device's advancing out of the mouth during ventilatory efforts indicates improper placement.

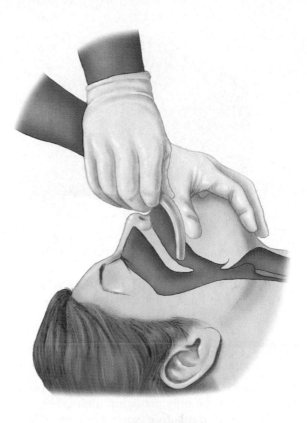

FIGURE 5-16a Insert the oropharyngeal airway with the top facing the palate.

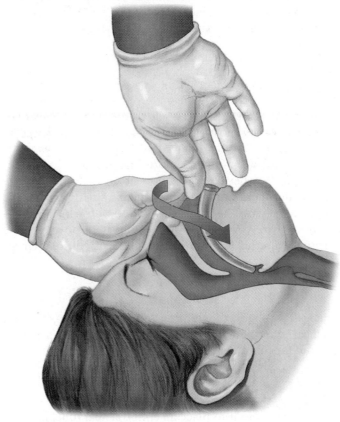

FIGURE 5-16b Rotate the airway 180-degrees into position.

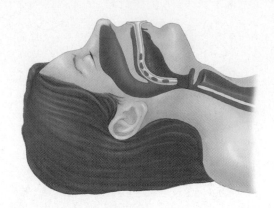

FIGURE 5-17 Improper placement of oropharyngeal airway.

Improper technique can also cause dental or pharyngeal trauma. An alternative insertion method useful in both pediatric and adult patients is to press the tongue upward and forward with a tongue blade. Then, the airway can be advanced until the flange is seated at the teeth. This is the preferred method of airway insertion in infants and children.

ADVANCED AIRWAY MANAGEMENT

Endotracheal intubation is clearly the preferred method of advanced airway management in prehospital emergency care, since it allows the greatest control of the airway.

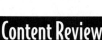

Inserting advanced mechanical airways requires special training. The preferred method of airway management is endotracheal intubation, as it is the only procedure that effectively isolates the trachea. In some EMS systems, endotracheal intubation is not available. These systems use other airway devices such as the Esophageal Tracheal CombiTube (ETC), pharyngeo-tracheal lumen (PtL) airway, or laryngeal mask airway (LMA).

ENDOTRACHEAL INTUBATION

Endotracheal intubation involves inserting an endotracheal tube into the trachea to provide the patient with a definitive, protected airway. It is clearly the preferred method of advanced airway management in prehospital emergency care, because it allows the greatest control of the airway with a BVM unit or ventilator. Under most circumstances, it requires direct visualization of the larynx with a laryngoscope, though alternative methods are available. Successfully accomplishing endotracheal intubation requires more training than other techniques, and you must maintain ongoing proficiency to ensure patient safety. To ensure the quality of your judgment and skill, you must continuously review field intubations and the criteria for performing them. You must also remember that, although endotracheal intubation affords the most effective airway control, you are bypassing important physiological functions of the upper airway—warming, filtering, and humidifying the air before it enters the lower airway.

EQUIPMENT

The equipment needed for endotracheal intubation includes a laryngoscope (handle and blade), an appropriate-size endotracheal tube, a 10-mL syringe, a stylet, a BVM, a suction device, a bite block, Magill forceps, and tape or a commercial tube-holding device.

Laryngoscope

laryngoscope instrument for lifting the tongue and epiglottis to see the vocal cords.

The **laryngoscope** is an instrument for lifting the tongue and epiglottis out of the way so that you can see the vocal cords. You will typically use it to place an endotracheal tube, but you may also use it with Magill forceps to retrieve a foreign body obstructing the upper airway.

A laryngoscope consists of a handle and a blade. The handle may be either reusable or disposable. It houses batteries that power a light in the blade's distal tip. This light illuminates the airway, making it easier to see upper airway structures. The point attaching the handle and the blade is called the fitting. It locks the blade in place and provides electrical contact between the batteries and the bulb (Figure 5-18).

Content Review

ENDOTRACHEAL INTUBATION EQUIPMENT
- Laryngoscope (handle and blade)
- Endotracheal tube
- 10-mL syringe
- Stylet
- Bag-valve mask
- Suction device
- Bite block
- Magill forceps
- Tape or tube-holding device

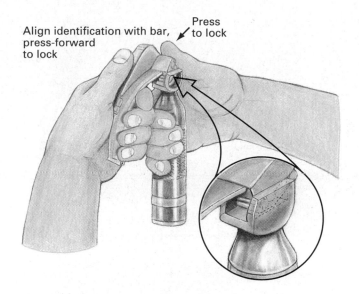

Align identification with bar, press-forward to lock

Press to lock

FIGURE 5-18 Engaging the laryngoscope blade and handle.

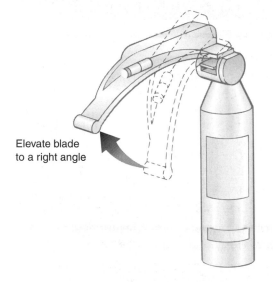

FIGURE 5-19 Activating the laryngoscope light source.

Elevate blade to a right angle

To prepare for intubation, attach the indentation on the proximal end of the laryngoscope's blade to the bar of the handle. It will click into place when properly seated. To determine if the laryngoscope is functional, raise the blade to a right angle with the handle until it clicks into place (Figure 5-19). The light should turn on and be bright and steady. A yellow, flickering light will not sufficiently illuminate the anatomical structures. If the light fails to go on, the problem may be either dead batteries or a loose bulb. Every airway kit should include spare parts. Infrequently, the contact points or the wire that runs through the blade to the bulb will fail.

Like the handle, the blade may be reusable or disposable. Two common types of blades are the curved blade (MacIntosh blade) and the straight blade (often referred to as the Miller, Miller-Abbott, Wisconsin, or Flagg blade). Laryngoscope blades range in size from 0 for infants to 4 for large adults (Figure 5-20).

The curved blade is designed to fit into the vallecula (Figure 5-21). When you lift its handle anteriorly, the blade elevates the tongue and, indirectly, the epiglottis, allowing you to see the glottic opening. Because the curved blade does not touch the larynx, it should not traumatize or stimulate the very sensitive gag receptors on the posterior surface of the epiglottis. The curved blade also permits more room for viewing and ETT insertion. The straight blade, on the other hand, is designed to fit under the epiglottis (Figure 5-22). When you lift its handle anteriorly, the blade directly lifts the epiglottis out of the way.

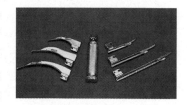

FIGURE 5-20 Laryngoscope blades.

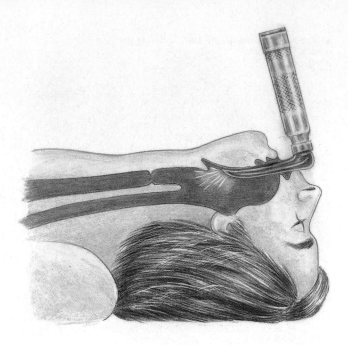

FIGURE 5-21 Placement of the MacIntosh blade into the vallecula.

FIGURE 5-22 Placement of the Miller blade under the epiglottis.

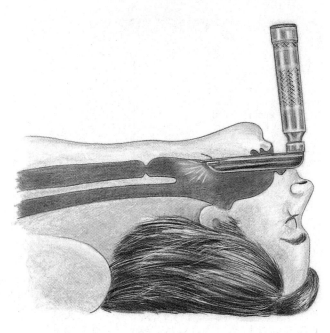

Which blade you use is largely a matter of individual preference, but you should be skilled with both in order to accommodate patients' anatomical differences. A straight blade is better for endotracheal intubation in infants, because it stabilizes their floppier epiglottises and provides greater displacement of their relatively larger tongues. It also is better for the occasional adult patient with a floppy epiglottis or large tongue.

Endotracheal Tubes

ETT endotracheal tube.

The endotracheal tube (**ETT**) is a flexible, translucent tube open at both ends and available in lengths ranging from 12 to 32 cm, with centimeter markings along its length (Figure 5-23). The proximal end has a standard 15 mm inside diameter/22 mm outside diameter connector that attaches to the ventilatory device, usually a BVM. The ETT is available with internal tube diameters ranging from 2.5 to 4.5 mm (uncuffed) and from 5.0 to 9.0 mm (cuffed). The distal end has a beveled tip to facilitate smooth movement through airway passages. When present, an inflatable 5- to 10-mL cuff at the distal end of ETT sizes from 5.0 to 9.0 mm provides a seal between the ETT and the trachea. A thin inflation tube runs the

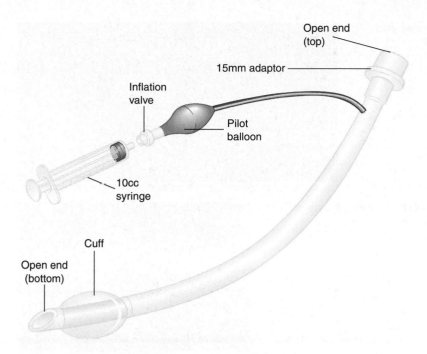

FIGURE 5-23 ETT and syringe.

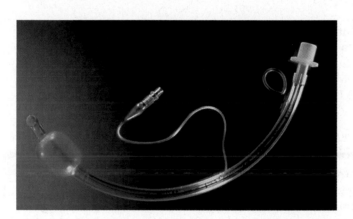

FIGURE 5-24 Endotrol ETT.

length of the main tube from the distal cuff to a syringe. A one-way valve at the proximal end of the inflation tube permits the syringe to push air into the distal cuff or pull it out, but prevents air from escaping the cuff when the syringe is removed. A pilot balloon at the inflation tube's proximal end indicates whether the distal cuff is properly inflated. The pilot balloon should be partially inflated but soft to avoid overinflating the distal cuff and inadvertently pressuring the tracheal mucosa. This could cause ischemia of the tracheal wall. Always check the distal cuff for leaks before insertion.

Suppliers typically prewrap an ETT in a curved shape. This is because the trachea lies anteriorly in the neck, and the tube must be directed upward to enter the glottic opening. On the Endotrol ETT, an O-shaped ring attaches to a plastic wire that runs the length of the tube and terminates distally (Figure 5-24). Pulling the ring bends the distal end of the tube upward and directs it into the glottic opening. This can facilitate placement of the tube without the need for a stylet.

Endotracheal tubes come in a variety of sizes. Markings on the tubes indicate their internal diameter in millimeters. The typical tube sizes for average-sized adult patients are 7.0 to 9.0 mm (females, 7.0 to 8.0 mm; males, 7.5 to 8.5 mm). A generally acceptable size for both male and female adults is 7.5 mm.

Stylet The malleable **stylet** is a plastic-covered metal wire used to direct the ETT anteriorly by bending its distal end into a J or hockey-stick shape (Figures 5-25 and 5-26). It is

stylet plastic-covered metal wire used to bend the ETT into a J or hockey-stick shape.

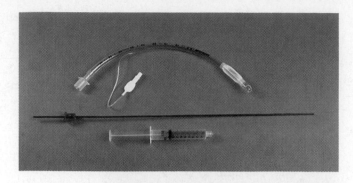

FIGURE 5-25 ETT, stylet, and syringe, unassembled.

FIGURE 5-26 ETT, stylet, and syringe, assembled for intubation.

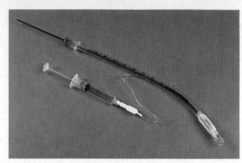

particularly useful in patients with extremely anterior laryngeal anatomy or those with short, fat necks for which head positioning can be difficult. Although using stylets is not mandatory, many EMT-Is prefer to use them in the prehospital setting because they afford greater control of the ETT. The wire stylet may damage tissues during intubation if it extends past the distal end of the ETT; therefore, you should keep it recessed at least 2 cm from the tip of the tube.

10-mL Syringe   The syringe allows you to inflate the distal cuff just enough to avoid air leaks around the ETT without causing tracheal ischemia.

Tube-Holding Devices   Tie-downs or tape secure the endotracheal tube once it is in the trachea. The reasons for securing the ETT are twofold. First, moving the patient about during resuscitation or transportation can easily dislodge the tube. Even if the ETT is not actually dislodged, its movement can still cause cardiovascular stimulation, an elevation in intracranial pressure, or injury to the tracheal mucosa. Second, the person providing ventilatory support may inadvertently push down on the ETT, forcing it into the right or left mainstem bronchus. Using tape requires extra care, because it can loosen when either the patient's face or the tube is moist. A number of commercial tube-holding devices are available.

Magill forceps scissor-style clamps with circular tips.

Magill Forceps   The **Magill forceps** are scissor-style clamps with circular tips. You will use them to remove foreign bodies or to redirect the endotracheal tube during intubation (Figure 5-27).

Lubricant   Water-soluble lubricants facilitate inserting the ETT. Do not use petroleum-based lubricants; they may damage the ETT and cause tracheal inflammation.

Suction Unit   A suction unit helps to remove secretions and foreign materials from the oropharynx during intubation attempts. It is a vital element that you must never forget.

Capnometer or Other Confirmation Device   These adjuncts to intubation are becoming the standard of care in most areas. You must be familiar with the devices, their role in intubation, and the requirements of your local protocols for their use.

Additional Airways   You should also have an oropharyngeal airway available during endotracheal intubation. You will occasionally use it as a block to prevent the patient from biting down on and collapsing the ETT.

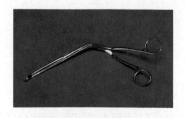

FIGURE 5-27 Magill forceps.

Protective Equipment Endotracheal intubation, like many airway procedures, carries the risk of exposure to body substances. Because of this, it is essential to take body substance isolation (BSI) precautions. These include, but are not limited to, gloves, mask, protective eyewear, and possibly a gown. Remember, personal safety comes first!

Endotracheal Intubation Indications

Monitoring success rates for particular skills is not hard with an appropriate quality assurance program. Evaluating your ability to judge which patients should be intubated is considerably more difficult. Often the patient's condition may warrant trying nebulizer treatments or supplemental oxygen before deciding to intubate. A patient's continued distress and failure to respond to treatment clearly indicate intubation. In conjunction with the medical director, you are responsible for continually improving your judgment regarding the use of advanced airway management techniques. This includes recognizing subtle indicators that the patient's condition is worsening, before the onset of respiratory arrest.

Endotracheal intubation provides a definitive, secure, open airway for patients who are experiencing, or are likely to experience, upper airway compromise. Some of the indications for endotracheal intubation in these patients include respiratory or cardiac arrest; unresponsiveness without a gag reflex; inability to protect the airway, resulting in an increased risk of aspiration; and obstruction due to foreign bodies, trauma, burns, or anaphylaxis. Endotracheal intubation also improves oxygenation and ventilation in patients with extreme lower airway difficulty. Some lower airway indications include severe respiratory distress due to diseases such as asthma, COPD, CHF, or pneumonia, as well as pneumothorax, hemothorax, or hemopneumothorax with respiratory difficulty. Clearly, then, endotracheal intubation may be indicated in breathing and apneic patients, though caution must be used in any patient with an intact gag reflex.

Do not attempt endotracheal intubation in the prehospital setting if epiglottitis is present, unless airway failure is imminent. Attempts to manipulate the airway in epiglottitis are very likely to result in vigorous laryngospasm. The most prudent management of epiglottitis is oxygenation of the patient without agitation. The preferred treatment for epiglottitis is rapid transport to the operating room for endotracheal intubation under more controlled conditions. This is carried out with the necessary equipment for emergency tracheostomy opened and ready for immediate use. Sometimes, these patients steadily worsen, and loss of their airway is imminent and inevitable. In this case, the benefits from endotracheal intubation outweigh the risks. Regardless, the most experienced member of the crew should perform the procedure. Also, it is important to remember that there may be significant laryngeal edema and it may be necessary to insert a smaller than normal endotracheal tube. This should be kept in mind before undertaking this procedure. Always follow local protocols and contact medical direction regarding endotracheal intubation in cases where epiglottitis is present or suspected.

Advantages of Endotracheal Intubation

Advantages of endotracheal intubation include the following:

- Isolates the trachea and permits complete control of the airway.
- Impedes gastric distention by channeling air directly into the trachea.
- Eliminates the need to maintain a mask seal.
- Offers a direct route for suctioning of the respiratory passages.
- Permits administration of the medications lidocaine, epinephrine, atropine, and naloxone via the endotracheal tube. (Use the mnemonic LEAN to remember these medications.)

Disadvantages of Endotracheal Intubation

Disadvantages of endotracheal intubation include the following:

- Requires considerable training and experience.
- Requires specialized equipment.

You are responsible for continually improving your judgment regarding airway management.

Content Review

ENDOTRACHEAL INTUBATION INDICATORS

- Respiratory or cardiac arrest
- Unconsciousness or obtusion without gag reflex
- Risk of aspiration
- Obstruction due to foreign bodies, trauma, burns, or anaphylaxis
- Respiratory extremis due to disease
- Pneumothorax, hemothorax, or hemopneumothorax with respiratory difficulty

Content Review

COMPLICATIONS OF ENDOTRACHEAL INTUBATION

- Equipment malfunction
- Teeth breakage and soft-tissue laceration
- Hypoxia
- Esophageal intubation
- Endobronchial intubation
- Tension pneumothorax

- Requires direct visualization of the vocal cords.
- Bypasses the upper airway's function of warming, filtering, and humidifying the inhaled air.

Complications of Endotracheal Intubation

Intubation presents a number of potential complications. Properly attending to detail and taking appropriate precautions will help you to avoid these problems.

Equipment Malfunctions Equipment malfunctions consume valuable time when you are establishing a definitive airway and effective oxygenation and ventilation. Having a pre-assembled airway kit that is checked regularly lessens the chances of this occurring. Ideally someone should check the airway kit daily to be sure that all needed supplies are present and that the bulb, batteries, and blade are in good working condition.

Teeth Breakage and Soft-Tissue Lacerations Endotracheal intubation can injure the lips and teeth, but you can eliminate this hazard by carefully using the laryngoscope as an instrument, not a tool. When inserting the blade into the mouth and pharynx, guide it gently into place, avoiding pressure on the teeth. When manipulating the jaw anteriorly, use gentle traction upward and toward the feet rather than rotating and flexing your wrist, which will make the laryngoscope function as a lever. All levers require a fulcrum—and the only fulcrums available in your patient's mouth is his upper incisors. A rotating/flexing action may thus break teeth. To avoid this hazard, lift the laryngoscope's handle (exposing the epiglottis) after you have applied the blade to the base of the tongue. After this, keep your wrist straight and do any lifting with your shoulder and arm.

If you use the laryngoscope too roughly, you can lacerate the patient's lips, tongue, or pharyngeal structures, producing profuse bleeding that is hard to control. This can also happen if you direct the tube away from midline into the pyriform sinuses or allow the stylet to protrude from the distal end of the ETT. In the larynx and lower airway, you might damage the vocal cords, cause laryngeal edema, or tear the trachea if you are not careful. A gentle technique and attention to detail are the keys to avoiding these complications.

Legal Note

Although negligence and malpractice lawsuits against EMS personnel are still relatively uncommon, many of those that do arise involve issues related to airway management. Improper airway management—such as failure to recognize a displaced endotracheal tube—can result in death or serious disability. Because of this, EMT-Is must take great care to make certain that airway management procedures are proper.

Always remain competent in endotracheal intubation. If you work in a system where there is limited opportunity for its use, then you should increase your in-service education and possibly arrange to spend some time in the hospital performing intubations.

Always make sure that all airway equipment is functioning properly. This includes checking ET tube cuffs, laryngoscope light bulbs, mechanical ventilation devices, and other adjuncts. These must be kept in a readily accessible location and checked on a regular basis.

After performing endotracheal intubation, it is essential to confirm and document proper tube placement by at least three methods. Esophageal detector devices are good, but end-tidal carbon dioxide detectors and capnometry are better. Following intubation, periodically and religiously check and confirm continued proper tube placement. These findings should be documented. If there is a doubt in regard to tube placement, the tube should be checked or removed and mechanical ventilation continued.

Remember, the greatest chances of tube displacement occur with patient movement. This is especially so when the stretcher with the patient is moved out of the ambulance. When a one-person stretcher is lowered to a level position, care must be taken to ensure that the ET tube has not been dislodged.

The skill of endotracheal intubation does not end after successful placement of the tube. Continuous and vigilant monitoring of tube placement should occur until the patient is turned over to the hospital staff.

Hypoxia   Delays in oxygenation, either from interruption of basic airway techniques and BVM ventilation with 100% oxygen or from prolonged intubation attempts, can produce profound, life-threatening hypoxia. Each patient's unique anatomy and unusual clinical situations can challenge even the most experienced EMT-I. One basic rule that helps avoid hypoxia during intubation is to limit each intubation attempt to no more than 30 seconds before reoxygenating the patient. To gauge this interval, some EMT-Is hold their breath from the time they stop ventilating the patient until they start again.

To avoid hypoxia during intubation, limit each intubation attempt to no more than 30 seconds before reoxygenating the patient.

If you cannot pass the tube through the vocal cords on the first attempt, at least identify your landmarks and note any unique or difficult features that you may need to address. For example, too much edema might indicate a smaller ETT. Or the patient's larynx might be more anterior than you realized from his external anatomy, and you will need to use a different blade or change the ETT angle. You can then pass the tube on a subsequent attempt, after hyperventilating the patient with basic airway techniques and 100% oxygen using a BVM device.

Esophageal Intubation   Misplacement of the ETT into the esophagus deprives the patient of oxygenation and ventilation. It is potentially lethal, resulting in severe hypoxia and brain death if you do not recognize it immediately. It also directs air into the stomach, encouraging regurgitation, which can lead to aspiration. Indicators of esophageal intubation include:

Esophageal intubation is lethal if you do not recognize it immediately.

- Absence of chest rise and absence of breath sounds with mechanical ventilation
- Gurgling sounds over the epigastrium with each breath delivered
- Distention of the abdomen
- Absence of breath condensation in the endotracheal tube
- Persistent air leak, despite inflation of the tube's distal cuff
- Cyanosis and progressive worsening of the patient's condition
- Phonation (noise made by the vocal cords)
- No color change with colorimetric ETCO$_2$ detector
- Falling pulse oximetry reading

If you have any suspicion that the tube is in the esophagus, remove it immediately. Hyperventilate the patient with 100% oxygen and attempt endotracheal intubation with another tube.

Endobronchial Intubation   If you pass the endotracheal tube successfully through the vocal cords and advance it too far, it likely will enter either the right or left mainstem bronchus. As discussed earlier, the ETT may be misplaced to either side, but it is more likely to pass into the right mainstem, which angles away from the trachea less acutely than does the left. In either case, the ETT ventilates only one lung and the result is hypoventilation and hypoxia from inadequate gas exchange. Also, when the bag-valve device **insufflates** enough air for two lungs into the smaller area of only one lung, it can create enough pressure to cause barotrauma such as a pneumothorax, worsening the patient's condition.

insufflate to blow into.

You can avoid inserting the ETT too far by following these guidelines:

1. Advance the distal cuff no more than 1 to 2 cm past the vocal cords.
2. Once the tube is positioned, hold it in place with one hand to prevent it from being pushed any farther.
3. Inflate the cuff and firmly secure the tube in place with tape or a commercial tube-holding device.
4. Note the number marking on the side of the ETT where it emerges from the patient's mouth at the teeth, gums, or lips. This will allow you to quickly recognize any changes in tube placement. Approximate ETT depth for the average adult is 21 cm at the teeth for women and 23 cm at the teeth for men, though this will vary.

Findings in endobronchial intubation include:

- Breath sounds present on one side of the chest but diminished or absent on the other
- Poor compliance (resistance to ventilations with the bag-valve device)
- Cyanosis, cardiac dysrhythmias, or other evidence of hypoxia

To resolve the problem, loosen or remove any securing devices and withdraw the ETT until breath sounds are present and equal bilaterally. Be certain to deflate the cuff when pulling back on the ETT.

Tension Pneumothorax   Any tear in the lung parenchyma can cause a pneumothorax. If this is allowed to progress untreated, a tension pneumothorax (an accumulation of air or gas in the pleural cavity) may develop. A tension pneumothorax is a large pneumothorax that affects other structures in the chest. An expanding tension pneumothorax will adversely affect the other lung, the heart, and the structures of the mediastinum. It eventually displaces these structures away from the side of the chest with the tension pneumothorax. In addition to mainstem bronchus intubation, tension pneumothorax can result if you use too much of the bag-valve device's volume on a small adult or child or use the full bag-valve device volume against diseased lungs with poor compliance. Tension pneumothorax is marked by progressively worsening compliance (more difficulty in ventilating), diminished unilateral breath sounds, hypoxia with hypotension, and distended neck veins. Often the trachea will deviate from the side of the chest with the pneumothorax. Also, the marked increase in intrathoracic pressure resulting from the tension pneumothorax can prevent the ventricles from adequately filling. This causes a decrease in cardiac output and worsens the patient's overall condition. If you suspect tension pneumothorax, needle decompression of the chest is indicated, as described in Chapter 17 on thoracic trauma.

Orotracheal Intubation

The most widely preferred and, therefore, the most commonly used path for endotracheal intubation is the orotracheal route. Many medical personnel favor this route because it involves direct visualization of the vocal cords and a clear view of the ETT's passage through them. It is thus the most accurate method of intubation and the least likely to induce trauma to the airway. To perform orotracheal intubation in the absence of suspected trauma (Procedure 5-1):

1. Place the patient in a supine position.
2. After using basic manual and adjunctive airway maneuvers to open the airway and ventilate, hyperventilate the patient with 100% oxygen.
3. While your partner ventilates the patient, prepare your intubation equipment, including suction, and be certain that all needed equipment is present and in good working order. Assemble and check the laryngoscope blade and handle to be certain you have a steady, bright light—then close the handle. Insert the stylet into the ETT, making sure to keep the distal end of the stylet at least 2 cm proximal to the distal tip of the ETT. You may choose to bend the distal end of the ETT into a hockey-stick shape just proximal to the distal cuff to help direct the ETT anteriorly. Apply water-soluble lubricant to the distal end of the ETT and reinsert. Leaving the ETT partially in its packaging until you are ready to insert it helps keep it as clean as possible. Fill the 10-mL syringe with 5 to 10 mL of air and attach it to the valve at the proximal end of the ETT, using a twisting motion to lock it in place. Check the cuff for air leaks.
4. Turn on the suction and attach an appropriate tip.
5. Position the patient's head and neck. Remove any dentures or partial dental plates. To visualize the larynx, you must align the three axes of the mouth, the pharynx, and the trachea. To do this, place the patient's head in a "sniffing position" by flexing the neck forward and the head backward. Inserting a

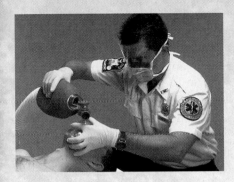

5-1a Hyperventilate the patient.

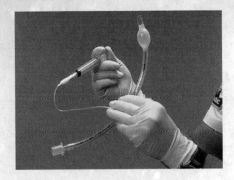

5-1b Prepare the equipment.

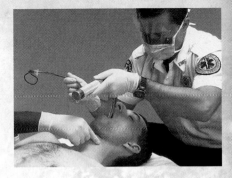

5-1c Apply Sellick's maneuver and insert laryngoscope.

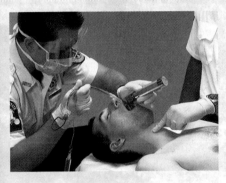

5-1d Visualize the larynx and insert the ETT.

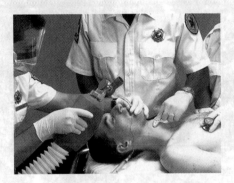

5-1e Inflate the cuff, ventilate, and auscultate.

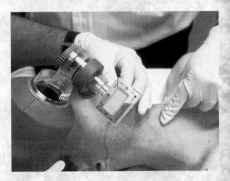

5-1f Confirm placement with an ETCO$_2$ detector.

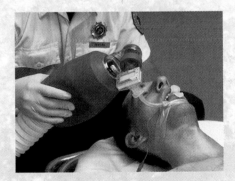

5-1g Secure the tube.

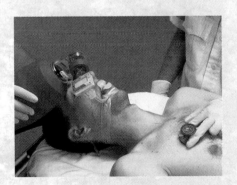

5-1h Reconfirm ETT placement.

rolled towel or sheet under the patient's shoulders or the back of the head may help. Establishing this position is extremely difficult in patients with short, fat necks or whose motion is limited by such conditions as arthritis.

6. Hold the laryngoscope in your left hand whether you are right or left handed. Most laryngoscopes are designed for right-handed people; that is, the right-handed person must hold the laryngoscope in his left hand in order to manipulate the endotracheal tube with his right.

7. If you have not already done so, have your partner apply Sellick's maneuver (cricoid pressure) and maintain it until you confirm ETT placement in the trachea.

8. Insert the laryngoscope blade gently into the right side of the patient's mouth. With a gentle sweeping action, displace the tongue to the left. This pushes the tongue out of your line of vision and allows more room to manipulate the endotracheal tube.

9. Move the blade slightly toward the midline. Advance the MacIntosh (curved) blade until the distal end is at the base of the tongue in the vallecula; advance the Miller (straight) blade until the distal end is under the epiglottis. As you advance the blade, move the patient's lower lip away from the blade using the index finger of your right hand.

10. Lift the laryngoscope handle slightly upward and toward the feet to displace the jaw. Be careful not to put pressure on the teeth. At this point, you can see any vomitus, blood, or secretions in the posterior pharynx. You likely will have to suction the airway clear. If the secretions are thick or copious, you may need to remove the suction tip and use the suction hose.

11. Upon lifting the jaw, determine if the laryngoscope blade is in proper position. You may need to adjust it before you can visualize the vocal cords. If you cannot see landmarks clearly, gently withdraw the blade, slowly and slightly. This may bring the vocal cords into view. If it does not, you might need to gently advance the blade farther into the hypopharynx.

12. Keeping your left wrist straight, use your left shoulder and arm to continue lifting the mandible and tongue to a 45-degree angle to the ground (up and toward the feet) until the glottis is exposed (Figure 5-28). Often you may not see the entire glottis, but you should see at least its posterior third or half. If the larynx lies anteriorly, a slight increase in your partner's pressure on the Sellick's maneuver should improve your view of the vocal cords. Occasionally, your partner will need to lessen the cricoid pressure slightly to allow you to visualize the vocal cords. Be ready to instruct him to apply more or less cricoid pressure.

13. Hold the ETT in your right hand with your fingertips as you would a dart or a pencil; this gives you control to gently maneuver the ETT. Advance the tube through the right corner of the patient's mouth, and direct it toward the midline.

14. Directly visualizing the vocal cords, pass the ETT gently through the glottic opening until its distal cuff disappears beyond the vocal cords; then advance it another 1 to 2 cm.

15. Hold the tube in place with your hand to prevent its displacement. Do not let go under any circumstance until it is taped or tied securely in place. Attach a bag-valve device to the 15/22 mm connector on the tube; have the capnometer attached to the bag-valve device as your local protocols require.

16. Inflate the distal cuff with 5 to 10 mL of air. To avoid tracheal trauma or ischemia from excessive cuff pressure, apply only enough pressure to prevent air leakage around the ETT during ventilation. Listen for any air leak and adjust the cuff's pressure as needed. When cuff pressure is correct, remove the syringe, using a twisting motion to prevent any air leak.

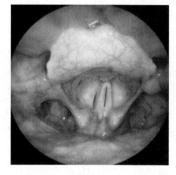

FIGURE 5-28 Glottis visualized through laryngoscopy.

17. Check for proper tube placement. While listening for equal bilateral breath sounds over the chest, watch to see that the chest rises and falls symmetrically. Listen over the epigastrium to be certain you hear no gastric sounds. Look for moisture condensation in the exhaled breath; it should appear in the ETT during each exhalation.

18. Hyperventilate the patient with 100% oxygen. Gently insert an oropharyngeal airway to serve as a bite block.

19. Secure the ETT with umbilical tape while maintaining ventilatory support. Loop the tape around the tube at the level of the patient's teeth, attaching it tightly to the tube without kinking or pinching it. Then wrap the tape around the patient's head and tie it at the side of his neck. Alternatively, use a commercial tube-holding device.

20. Repeat step 17 periodically to confirm proper ETT placement. Also repeat step 17 after any major patient movement or movement of his head or neck. (Neck manipulation can displace the tube up to 5 cm.) Continue to support the tube manually while maintaining ventilatory support.

Verification of Proper Endotracheal Tube Placement   Continuously checking and rechecking tube placement is an important responsibility during endotracheal intubation. The hypervigilance with which you must monitor the patient's clinical condition cannot be overemphasized. You can employ a number of methods in the field to confirm correct ETT placement. You should put them to maximum use, but do not become overly reliant on technology. The patient's clinical condition should be the deciding factor in your patient management decisions.

The most reliable method of confirming proper ETT placement is direct visualization of its passage through the vocal cords. This requires the proper use of a laryngoscope and continued visualization of the vocal cords throughout intubation. If you do this, you have little chance of inadvertently intubating the esophagus.

Following ETT placement, watch to be sure that the patient's chest rises with ventilations. If the ETT is misplaced in the esophagus, the chest will not rise. You also should auscultate for breath sounds. Their equal presence over both sides (apices and bases) of the chest and their absence over the epigastrium helps to confirm proper ETT placement. Conversely, their absence over the chest and their presence over the epigastrium indicate an esophageal intubation. Breath sounds present on one side but absent or diminished on the other indicate that the ETT may be advanced too deeply into one of the mainstem bronchi, that bronchial obstruction may be present, or that a pneumothorax is present. Absent breath sounds bilaterally may indicate esophageal intubation.

It is essential that endotracheal tube placement be verified by a secondary method. Capnometers and esophageal detector devices can be used for this. Adequate levels of exhaled carbon dioxide, as detected by a capnometer, confirm proper endotracheal tube placement. The ability to withdraw air readily from an esophageal detector device's syringe further confirms placement of the ETT in the trachea. Resistance to air withdrawal, or the creation of a vacuum, denotes esophageal intubation. Capnometers offer a distinct advantage over esophageal detector devices in that they can remain in place during ongoing patient care to monitor the status of the ETT during mechanical ventilation and during other procedures such as CPR.

Also observe the endotracheal tube's contents. Exhaled air approaches 100% humidity. Usually, the ambient relative humidity is less than 100%. Thus, condensation inside the ETT suggests its proper placement. Because the gastric sphincter relaxes in critically ill patients and the high pressures of a BVM create gastric distention, patients frequently vomit and aspirate during resuscitation. If you misplace the ETT into the esophagus, you may observe an efflux of gastric contents through the ETT, particularly with subsequent ventilation attempts. Because aspiration into the trachea also may have occurred, you might see vomitus in the ETT even with proper endotracheal intubation; nonetheless, this finding always should raise suspicion of esophageal intubation and prompt further investigation.

It is important to ensure proper endotracheal tube placement. Allegations of improperly placed endotracheal tubes are a major reason for EMT-I malpractice suits. Because of this, it

The hypervigilance with which you must monitor the patient's clinical condition cannot be overemphasized.

is important to verify and document proper endotracheal tube placement. In fact, it is ideal to verify and document at least three different indicators of proper placement. These may include:

- Visualization of the tube passing between the cords
- Presence of bilateral breath sounds
- Absence of breath sounds over the epigastrium
- Positive end-tidal CO_2 change on a capnometer
- Verification of endotracheal placement by an esophageal detector device
- Presence of condensation inside the endotracheal tube
- Absence of vomitus inside the endotracheal tube
- Absence of phonation, or vocal sounds, once the tube is placed

In addition, an increase in the oxygen saturation helps support proper placement of the endotracheal tube. Likewise, a rise and fall of the chest indicates endotracheal intubation. Worsening gastric distention may indicate possible esophageal placement. Any gastric distention should be investigated. Remember, though, it is not uncommon for gastric distention to develop prior to endotracheal intubation due to mechanical ventilation. Even in experienced hands, it is very difficult to avoid gastric distention with mechanical ventilation until an endotracheal tube is placed.

Appropriate treatment of a trauma patient's other injuries is meaningless if you do not ensure a patent airway and adequate oxygenation and ventilation.

Trauma Patient Intubation   Airway management and ventilatory support in the trauma patient are essential for a successful outcome. Appropriate treatment of all other injuries is meaningless if you do not ensure a patent airway and adequate oxygenation and ventilation.

The trauma patient presents a number of obstacles to effective airway management and ventilation. Some of them may be the need for extrication, blood in the oropharynx, distorted anatomy due to injury, and the need to protect the cervical spine. Getting an adequate seal on a mask is very difficult when the patient is being extricated or has significant facial trauma. You must keep the cervical spine in a neutral, in-line position throughout your management of all patients with known or suspected cervical spine trauma. Digital intubation, transillumination intubation, and nasotracheal intubation provide potential solutions for some patients when trauma complicates airway management, but visualizing the vocal cords is still preferable. You can do this effectively using direct laryngoscopy-assisted orotracheal intubation with manual in-line stabilization of the cervical spine (Procedure 5-2).

To perform orotracheal intubation with in-line stabilization:

1. After basic manual and adjunctive airway maneuvers, have your partner maintain in-line stabilization while kneeling at the patient's side, facing his head. This is done by placing both hands over the patient's ears with the little, ring, and middle fingers under the occiput, the index fingers anterior to the ears, and the thumbs on the face over the maxillary sinuses.

2. Apply slight pressure in a caudal direction (toward the feet) to support and immobilize the head.

3. Proceed gently with orotracheal intubation, remembering the need to minimize movement of the cervical spine.

Pediatric Intubation

Pediatric airway emergencies generally produce more anxiety than adult emergencies among both medical care providers and family. It is important to take appropriate steps to separate the parent from the pediatric patient with significant respiratory distress or apnea to effectively manage the airway. Although the indications, procedures, and precautions for airway management in children are fundamentally the same as in adults, you must take additional precautions and remember several significant differences. These concerns revolve around variances in anatomy, as discussed in Chapter 2. To review the anatomical features of the pediatric airway:

- Structures are proportionally smaller and more flexible than an adult's.
- Tongue is larger in relation to the oropharynx.

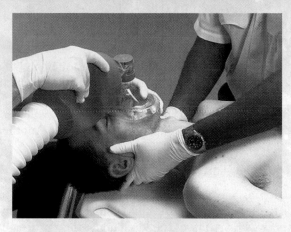

5-2a   Hyperventilate the patient and apply manual C-spine stabilization.

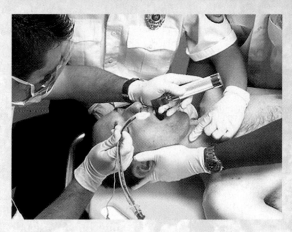

5-2b   Apply Sellick's maneuver and intubate.

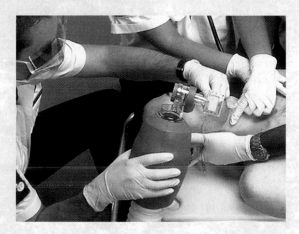

5-2c   Ventilate the patient and confirm placement.

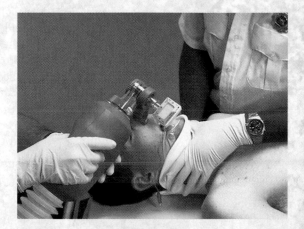

5-2d   Secure the ETT and place a cervical collar.

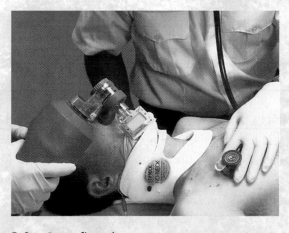

5-2e   Reconfirm placement.

- Epiglottis is floppy and round ("omega" shaped).
- Glottic opening is higher and more anterior in the neck.
- Vocal cords slant upward, toward the back of the head, and are closer to the base of the tongue.
- Narrowest part of the airway is the cricoid cartilage, not the glottic opening as in adults.

A straight laryngoscope blade is preferred for most pediatric patients, although straight or curved may be useful for adolescents. Also, selecting the appropriate tube diameter for children is critical. Too large a tube can cause tracheal edema and/or damage to the vocal cords, while too small a tube may not allow exchange of adequate ventilatory volumes. Table 5-2 lists general guidelines for selecting ETT size according to the child's age. Another guide for children's sizes is:

$$\text{ETT size (mm)} = (\text{Age in years} + 16) \div 4$$

Correct tube size for an eight-year-old, for instance, would be $(8 + 16) \div 4$, or 6 mm. You can also measure tube size by matching it to the diameter of the child's smallest finger. Usually you will use noncuffed endotracheal tubes with infants and children under the age of eight years, because the round narrowing of these patients' cricoid cartilage forms a suitable cuff.

The depth of insertion of the distal tip for pediatric endotracheal tubes should be 2 to 3 cm below the vocal cords, since deeper insertion may result in mainstem intubation or injury to the carina. The uncuffed ETT has a black glottic marker at its distal end that should be placed at the level of the vocal cords. The cuffed ETT should be placed so that the cuff is just below the vocal cords. For detailed guidelines regarding depth of insertion for different age groups, refer to Table 5-2. Alternately, you can use the formula $(3 \times \text{ETT inside diameter}) - 1$.

Also remember that infants and small children have greater vagal tone than adults. Therefore, laryngoscopy and passage of an endotracheal tube are more likely to precipitate a vagal response, dramatically slowing the child's heart rate and decreasing cardiac output and blood pressure.

The indications for endotracheal intubation in a pediatric patient are the same as those for adults:

- Ventilatory support with a BVM is inadequate.
- Cardiac or respiratory arrest.
- It is necessary to provide a route for drug administration (LEAN) or ready access to the airway for suctioning.
- Prolonged artificial ventilation is needed.

Additionally, if local protocols allow, you may use endotracheal intubation in a child with epiglottitis if his condition is rapidly deteriorating.

To perform endotracheal intubation on a pediatric patient (Procedure 5-3):

1. After initiating basic manual and adjunctive maneuvers, hyperventilate the patient with 100% oxygen, using the appropriately sized BVM.

Table 5-2 APPROXIMATE SIZE OF ETT FOR PEDIATRICS

Patient's Age	ETT Size	Type	Depth of ETT Insertion	Laryngoscope Blade Size
Premature infant	2.5–3.0	Uncuffed	8 cm	0 straight
Full-term infant	3.0–3.5	Uncuffed	8–9.5 cm	1 straight
Infant to one year	3.5–4.0	Uncuffed	9.5–11 cm	1 straight
Toddler	4.0–5.0	Uncuffed	11–12.5 cm	1–2 straight
Preschool	5.0–5.5	Uncuffed	12.5–14 cm	2 straight
School age	5.5–6.5	Uncuffed	14–20 cm	2 straight
Adolescent	7.0–8.0	Cuffed	20–23 cm	3 straight or curved

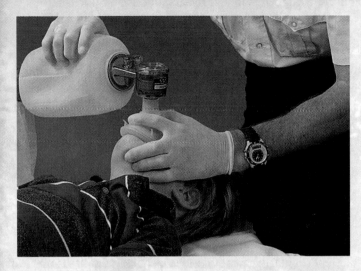

5-3a Hyperventilate the child.

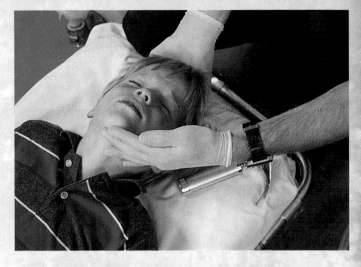

5-3b Position the head.

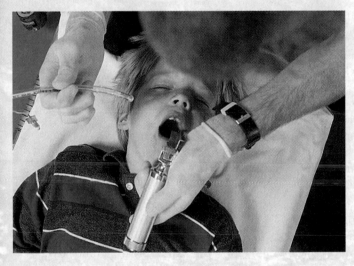

5-3c Insert the laryngoscope.

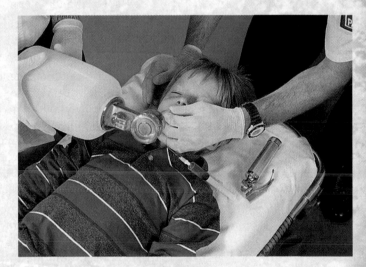

5-3d Insert the ETT and ventilate the child.

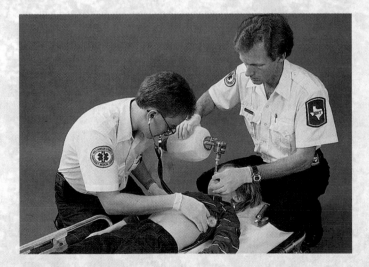

5-3e Confirm placement and secure the ETT.

2. Prepare and check your equipment. As stated earlier, a straight blade laryngoscope is usually preferred in infants and small children, since it provides greater displacement of the tongue and better visualization of the epiglottis. Also, with children younger than eight years old, use an uncuffed endotracheal tube. Because of the short distance between the mouth and the trachea, you rarely need a stylet to position the tube properly. Remember to lubricate the ETT with water-soluble gel.

3. Place the patient's head and neck in an appropriate position. You should maintain a pediatric patient's head in a sniffing position (perhaps by placing a towel under his head), unless you know of or suspect trauma. In case of trauma, proceed with manual in-line stabilization of the cervical spine.

4. Have your partner apply gentle cricoid pressure (Sellick's maneuver).

5. Hold the laryngoscope in your left hand and insert it gently into the right side of the patient's mouth. With a sweeping action, displace the tongue to the left.

6. Move the blade slightly toward the midline and then advance it until the distal end reaches the base of the tongue.

7. Look for the tip of the epiglottis, and position the laryngoscope properly. Keep in mind that a child—particularly an infant—has a shorter airway and a higher glottis than an adult. Because of this, you may see the cords much sooner than you expect.

8. If you cannot see the glottis, bring the blade gently and slowly out until the vocal cords fall into view. Lift the epiglottis gently with the tip of the laryngoscope. Be certain not to use the teeth or gums as a fulcrum.

9. Grasp the endotracheal tube in your right hand and, under direct visualization of the vocal cords, insert it through the right corner of the patient's mouth into the glottic opening. Pass it through until the distal 10 mm or distal cuff of the ETT disappears 2 to 3 cm beyond the vocal cords. In some cases, advancing an endotracheal tube is difficult at the level of the cricoid. Do not force the ETT through this region, because it may cause laryngeal edema and bleeding.

10. Hold the tube in place with your left hand and attach an infant- or child-sized bag-valve device to the 15/22 mm connector and deliver several breaths, checking for proper tube placement. Watch for the chest to rise and fall symmetrically with each ventilation. Auscultate for equal, bilateral breath sounds at the lateral chest wall, high in the axilla. Breath sounds over the epigastrium should be absent with ventilations. The patient should improve clinically, with pinker color and increased heart rate. Additionally, use the capnometer as previously discussed.

11. If the tube has a distal cuff, inflate it with just enough air to prevent any air leaks.

12. Secure the ETT with tape or a commercial device as with an adult patient, note placement of distance marker at teeth/gums, recheck for proper placement, and continue ventilatory support. Periodically reassess ETT placement, and watch the patient carefully for any clinical signs of difficulty. As with the adult patient, allow no more than 30 seconds to pass without ventilating your patient.

Field Extubation

Infrequently, an intubated patient will awaken and be intolerant of the ETT. If the patient is clearly able to maintain and protect his airway and accomplish adequate spontaneous respirations and is not under the influence of any sedating agents, and if reassessment indicates the problem that led to endotracheal intubation is resolved, extubation may be indicated. However, you must consider the high risk of laryngospasm, involuntary closure of the glottis, upon extubation, especially in the awake patient. Laryngospasm may prohibit successful reintubation attempts. Additionally, in repeat attempts at rapid sequence intubation the medications will produce variable responses and do not ensure relaxation of the laryngospasm. The need for field extubation is extremely rare.

To perform field extubation:

1. Continue blood and body fluid precautions. Ensure patient's oxygenation. A crude method for accomplishing this in the field is to be certain that the patient's mental status, skin color, and pulse oximetry are optimal on room air with the ETT in place.
2. Prepare intubation equipment and suction.
3. Confirm patient responsiveness.
4. Suction the patient's oropharynx.
5. Deflate the ETT cuff.
6. Remove the ETT upon cough or expiration.
7. Provide supplemental oxygen as indicated.
8. Reassess the adequacy of the patient's ventilation and oxygenation.

ESOPHAGEAL TRACHEAL COMBITUBE

The **Esophageal-Tracheal CombiTube** (ETC) is a dual-lumen airway with a ventilation port for each **lumen**. The longer, blue port is the distal port; the shorter, clear port is the proximal port, which terminates in the hypopharynx. The ETC has two inflatable cuffs—a 15 mL cuff just proximal to the distal port and a 100 mL cuff just distal to the proximal port.

It is inserted blindly through the mouth into the posterior oropharynx and then gently advanced. When inserted one port enters the trachea and the other enters the esophagus (Figures 5-29 and 5-30). To determine which port has entered the trachea and is to be ventilated, first ventilate the longer external port, since esophageal insertion is highly likely. Now auscultate the chest. If you hear breath sounds over the chest and none over the stomach, continue ventilating through the longer external port. If you hear ventilation sounds

Esophageal Tracheal CombiTube (ETC) dual-lumen airway with a ventilation port for each lumen.

lumen the tunnel through a tube.

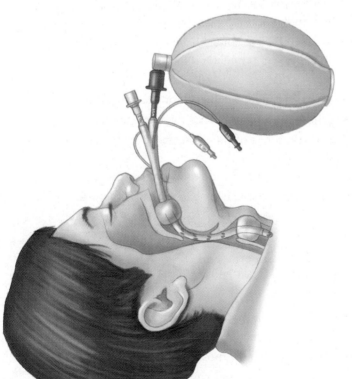

FIGURE 5-29 ETC airway—tracheal placement.

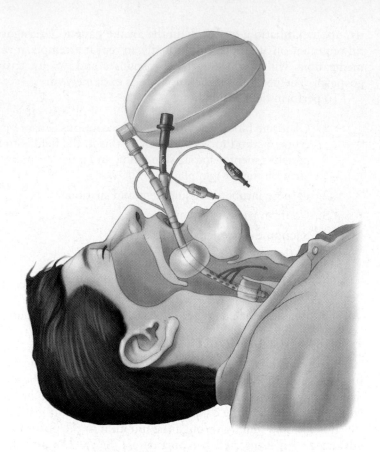

FIGURE 5-30 ETC airway—
esophageal placement.

over the stomach without breath sounds over the chest, stop ventilating through the longer port and attach the bag-valve device to the shorter port. The distal cuff isolates the distal port, and the larger proximal cuff isolates the proximal port, encouraging air that is insufflated into the hypopharynx to enter the trachea.

Advantages of the Esophageal Tracheal CombiTube

Advantages of the ETC include the following:

- It provides alternate airway control when conventional intubation techniques are unsuccessful or unavailable.
- Insertion is rapid and easy.
- Insertion does not require visualization of the larynx or special equipment.
- The pharyngeal balloon anchors the airway behind the hard palate.
- The patient may be ventilated regardless of tube placement (esophageal or tracheal).
- It significantly diminishes gastric distention and regurgitation.
- It can be used on trauma patients, since the neck can remain in neutral position during insertion and use.
- If the tube is placed in the esophagus, gastric contents can be suctioned for decompression through the distal port.

Disadvantages of the Esophageal Tracheal CombiTube

Disadvantages of the ETC include the following:

- Suctioning tracheal secretions is impossible when the airway is in the esophagus.
- Placing an endotracheal tube is very difficult with the ETC in place.
- It cannot be used in conscious patients or in those with a gag reflex.
- The cuffs can cause esophageal, tracheal, and hypopharyngeal ischemia.
- It does not isolate and completely protect the trachea.

- It cannot be used in patients with esophageal disease or caustic ingestions.
- It cannot be used with pediatric patients.
- Placement of the CombiTube is not foolproof—errors can be made if assessment skills are not adequate.

Inserting the Esophageal Tracheal CombiTube

Do the following to insert the ETC:

1. Complete basic manual and adjunctive maneuvers and provide supplemental oxygen and ventilatory support with a BVM and hyperventilation.
2. Place the patient supine and kneel at the top of his head.
3. Prepare and check the equipment.
4. Place the patient's head in neutral position. Stabilize the cervical spine if cervical injury is possible.
5. Insert the ETC gently at midline through the oropharynx, using a tongue-jaw-lift maneuver, and advance it past the hypopharynx to the depth indicated by the markings on the tube. The black rings on the tube should be between the patient's teeth.
6. Inflate the pharyngeal cuff with 100 mL of air and the distal cuff with 10 to 15 mL of air.
7. Ventilate through the longer blue proximal port with a bag-valve device connected to 100% oxygen, while auscultating over the chest and stomach. If you hear bilateral breath sounds over the chest and none over the stomach, secure the tube and continue ventilating.
8. If you hear gastric sounds over the chest instead of breath sounds, change ports and ventilate through the clear connector. Confirm breath sounds over the chest with no gastric sounds. Use multiple confirmation techniques as previously discussed (visualize, auscultate, use a capnometer, monitor clinical improvement).
9. Secure the tube and continue ventilating with 100% oxygen.
10. Frequently reassess the airway and adequacy of ventilation.

PHARYNGO-TRACHEAL LUMEN AIRWAY

The **pharyngo-tracheal lumen airway** (PtL) is a two-tube system (Figure 5-31). The first tube is short, with a large diameter; its proximal end is green. A large cuff encircles the tube's lower third. When inflated, the cuff seals the entire oropharynx. Air introduced at this tube's proximal end will enter the hypopharynx. The second tube is long, with a small diameter, and clear. It passes through and extends approximately 10 cm beyond the first tube. This second tube may be inserted blindly into either the trachea or the esophagus. A distal cuff, when inflated, seals off whichever anatomical structure the tube has entered. When the second tube enters the trachea, you will ventilate the patient through it.

Each of the PtL's tubes has a 15/22 mm connector at its proximal end, allowing the attachment of a standard ventilatory device. A semi-rigid plastic stylet in the clear plastic tube allows redirection of the oropharyngeal cuff while the other cuff remains inflated. An adjustable, cloth neck strap holds the tube in place. When the long, clear tube is in the esophagus, deflating the cuff in the oropharynx allows you to move the device to the left side of the patient's mouth. This may permit endotracheal intubation while continuing esophageal occlusion. However, placement of an endotracheal tube with a PtL already in place is difficult at best.

Advantages of the Pharyngo-Tracheal Lumen Airway

Advantages of the PtL airway include the following:

- Can function in either the tracheal or esophageal position.
- Has no face mask to seal.

pharyngo-tracheal lumen airway (PtL) a two-tube system.

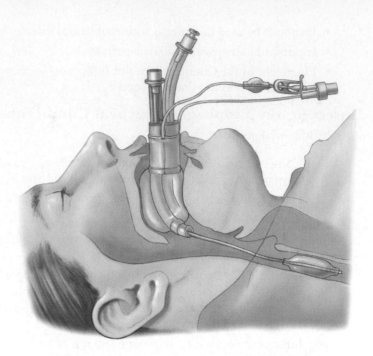

FIGURE 5-31 Pharyngo-tracheal lumen airway.

- Does not require direct visualization of the larynx and, thus, does not require the use of a laryngoscope or additional specialized equipment.
- Can be used in trauma patients, since the neck can remain in neutral position during insertion and use.
- Helps protect the trachea from upper airway bleeding and secretions.

Disadvantages of the Pharyngo-Tracheal Lumen Airway

Disadvantages of the PtL airway include the following:

- It does not isolate and completely protect the trachea from aspiration.
- The oropharyngeal balloon can migrate out of the mouth anteriorly, partially dislodging the airway.
- Intubation around the PtL is extremely difficult, even with the oropharyngeal balloon deflated.
- It cannot be used in conscious patients or those with a gag reflex.
- It cannot be used in pediatric patients.
- It can only be passed orally.

Inserting the Pharyngo-Tracheal Lumen Airway

Do the following to insert the PtL airway:

1. Complete basic manual and adjunctive maneuvers and provide supplemental oxygen and ventilatory support with a BVM and hyperventilation.
2. Place the patient supine and kneel at the top of his head.
3. Prepare and check the equipment.
4. Place the patient's head in the appropriate position. Hyperextend the neck if there is no risk of cervical spine injury. Maintain neutral position with stabilization of the cervical spine if cervical spine injury is possible.
5. Insert the PtL gently, using the tongue-jaw-lift maneuver.
6. Inflate the distal cuffs on both PtL tubes simultaneously with a sustained breath into the inflation valve.

7. Deliver a breath into the green oropharyngeal tube. If the patient's chest rises and you auscultate bilateral breath sounds, the long clear tube is in the esophagus. Inflate the pharyngeal balloon and continue ventilations via the green tube.

8. If the chest does not rise and you auscultate no breath sounds, the long clear tube is in the trachea. Remove the stylet from the clear tube and ventilate the patient through that tube.

9. Attach the bag-valve device to the 15-mm connector, secure the tube, and continue ventilatory support with 100% oxygen.

10. Multiple placement confirmation techniques are again essential, as are good assessment skills. Misidentification of placement has been reported. Frequently reassess the airway and adequacy of ventilation.

If the patient regains consciousness or if the protective airway reflexes return, remove the PtL. It is best to remove the PtL before endotracheal intubation.

Complications of PtL placement include:

- Pharyngeal or esophageal trauma from poor technique
- Unrecognized displacement of the long tube from the trachea into the esophagus
- Displacement of the pharyngeal balloon

LARYNGEAL MASK AIRWAY (LMA)

The laryngeal mask airway (LMA) may assist with ventilations in the unconscious patient without laryngeal reflexes when tracheal intubation is unsuccessful. First introduced in 1983 in the United Kingdom, it was approved for use in the United States in 1991. The LMA is an effective airway and a safe alternative to endotracheal intubation. It has an inflatable distal end (similar to a small face mask), which is placed in the hypopharynx and then inflated (Figure 5-32). The size of the distal end is large enough to prevent it from passing into the esophagus during insertion. A bag-valve device or mechanical ventilator at the proximal end assists respirations (similar to an endotracheal tube). The laryngeal

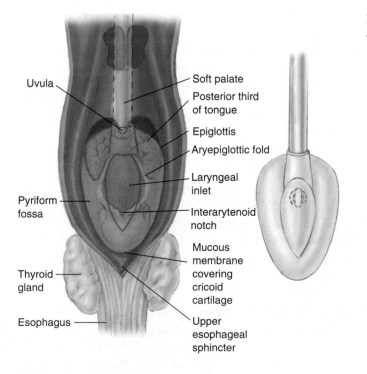

FIGURE 5-32 Laryngeal mask airway.

Uvula
Soft palate
Posterior third of tongue
Epiglottis
Aryepiglottic fold
Laryngeal inlet
Pyriform fossa
Interarytenoid notch
Mucous membrane covering cricoid cartilage
Thyroid gland
Esophagus
Upper esophageal sphincter

mask airway is supplied in five sizes. The LMA can be resterilized following the manufacturer's recommendations, but the number of times it can be resterilized is somewhat limited.

Advantages of the Laryngeal Mask Airway

The LMA can be rapidly placed without the need to visualize the airway. The incidence of coughing and sore throat is less than with endotracheal intubation. The LMA may actually be easier to use than a face mask for simple mechanical ventilation. As with endotracheal intubation, the LMA may cause minor changes in blood pressure and heart rate in the patient

Disadvantages of the Laryngeal Mask Airway

The LMA's disadvantage is that it does not isolate the trachea; therefore, it does not protect the airway from regurgitation and aspiration. Endotracheal intubation cannot be carried out with the LMA in place. Also, it cannot be used in a patient who has a gag reflex or is semiconscious. You must weigh these disadvantages against the benefits of establishing a patent airway.

Inserting the Laryngeal Mask Airway

Do the following to insert the laryngeal mask airway:

1. Take BSI precautions.
2. Complete basic manual and adjunctive maneuvers and provide supplemental oxygen and ventilatory support with a BVM and hyperventilation.
3. Place the patient in a supine position and kneel at the top of his head.
4. Prepare and check the equipment.
5. Place the patient's head in the sniffing position (unless there is possible spinal injury, whereupon you should stabilize the cervical spine).
6. Fully deflate the cuff.
7. Position the tube for insertion.
8. Lubricate the dorsal (posterior) surface of the cuff with a water-based lubricant.
9. Flatten the mask tip against the patient's hard palate before sliding it downward into position. The curved portion of the LMA points toward the patient and away from you.
10. Avoid accidental aspiration of lubricant by *not* placing lubricant on the ventral (anterior) surface of the cuff.
11. The LMA tube and cuff are advanced until the tip is in the esophagus. Use your index finger to push at the junction of the tube and the mask to advance the airway. Stop when resistance is encountered. Note that the black line is located on the posterior surface of the LMA to conform correct positioning of the tube. If this line is twisted to the anterior or either side, then the LMA is incorrectly positioned.
12. Avoid the epiglottis by pressing downward and backward against the posterior wall of the pharynx during insertion.
13. Verify position by direct visualization or with a laryngoscope.
14. Inflate the cuff with approximately 20 mL of air. The soft tissues over the larynx should rise. If there is substantial resistance to inflation, then the position of the LMA should be reassessed.
15. Attach the bag-valve unit and begin ventilation with 100% oxygen. Watch for rise and fall of the chest.
16. Secure the LMA tube in much the same way as you would an endotracheal tube. Consider continuous capnometry if available.
17. Frequently reassess the airway and adequacy of ventilation.

MANAGING PATIENTS WITH STOMA SITES

Often patients who have had a laryngectomy (removal of the larynx) or tracheostomy (surgical opening into the trachea) breathe through a **stoma,** an opening in the anterior neck that connects the trachea with the ambient air. These patients frequently have tracheostomy tubes, which consist of an inner and outer cannula, in place to keep the soft tissue stoma open (Figure 5-33).

A patient with a stoma often has problems with excessive secretions. A laryngectomy produces a less effective cough, making it more difficult to clear secretions. If these secretions organize, they form a mucous plug that can occlude the stoma and, thus, the airway. A stoma apparatus generally has a fixed outer portion and an inner cannula. The inner cannula can be easily removed and cleaned, then replaced. Timely replacement of the outer cannula is important if it must also be removed, because the stoma can constrict within just a few hours to prohibit its replacement without dilation.

As the external stoma site narrows, so can the inner tracheal diameter; either can produce potentially life-threatening stenosis (constricting or narrowing of the passage). Any acute inflammation that leads to soft tissue swelling can worsen this by further reducing the stoma and tracheal diameter. Further, this stenosis may make the cannula very difficult or impossible to replace. In this case, choose the largest diameter ETT that will pass through the stoma to maintain the airway before complete obstruction occurs. Lubricate the ETT, instruct the patient to exhale, and gently insert the ETT approximately 1 to 2 cm beyond the distal cuff. Inflate the cuff. Then confirm comfort, patency, and proper placement. Be

stoma opening in the anterior neck that connects the trachea with ambient air.

Timely replacement of a stoma device's outer cannula is important because the stoma can constrict within just a few hours to prohibit its replacement without dilation.

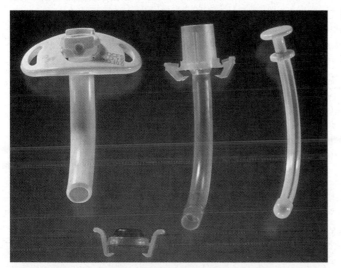

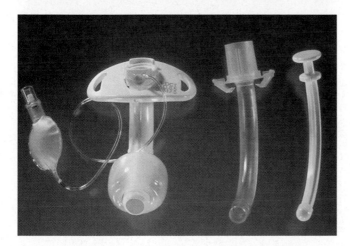

FIGURE 5-33 Tracheostomy cannulae.

certain to suspect and check for improper placement into the surrounding subcutaneous tissue, which will produce a false lumen. Subcutaneous emphysema as well as the lack of clinical improvement in the patient, indicates a false lumen.

You must use extreme caution with any suctioning, since this process can itself cause soft tissue swelling. Begin by preoxygenating the patient with 100% oxygen. Inject 3 mL sterile saline down the trachea through the stoma. Instruct the patient to exhale. Then gently insert the catheter until resistance is met. While the patient coughs or exhales, suction the airway during withdrawal of the catheter.

When the patient with a stoma requires ventilatory assistance, the bystander may use the mouth-to-stoma technique and rescue personnel will generally use a BVM device. If you use the mouth-to-stoma technique, it is preferable to use a pocket mask to cover the stoma for protection from communicable disease. For either technique, locate the stoma site and expose it. Obtain a tight seal around the stoma site and check for adequate ventilation. Be sure to seal the mouth and nose if you note air leaking from these sites.

Summary

Airway assessment and maintenance is the most critical step in managing any patient. If you do not promptly establish a definitive airway and provide proper ventilation, the patient's outcome will be poor. Frequently reassessing the airway is mandatory to ensure that the patient has not decompensated, requiring additional airway procedures. Successful management of all airways requires the EMT-I to follow the proper management sequence.

Basic airway and management skills can make the difference between a successful outcome and a poor patient prognosis. Once you have mastered these basic skills and made them a part of airway management in every patient, you should learn and utilize advanced skills such as intubation. You must maintain proficiency in all airway skills, especially the more advanced techniques, through ongoing continuing education, physician medical direction, and testing with each EMS service. If you cannot do this, it is in the patient's best interest to focus on less sophisticated airway skills. If you anticipate that every airway will be complicated, apply basic airway skills before using advanced procedures, perform frequent reassessments, and give the patient his best chance for meaningful survival.

On the Web

For additional practice and review, go to the companion website at www.prenhall.com/bledsoe and click on *Intermediate Emergency Care: Principles & Practice*.

CHAPTER 6

History Taking

Objectives

After reading this chapter, you should be able to:

1. Describe the factors that influence the EMT-Intermediate's ability to collect medical history. (pp. 401–405, 413–416)
2. Describe the structure, purpose, and techniques for obtaining a patient history. (pp. 401–416)
3. Discuss the importance of using open-ended and closed questions. (p. 403)
4. Describe the use of and differentiate between facilitation, reflection, clarification, empathetic responses, confrontation, and interpretation. (pp. 404–405)
5. List the components of a history of an adult patient. (p. 406)
6. List and describe the strategies to overcome situations that represent special challenges in obtaining a medical history. (pp. 413–416)

CASE STUDY

En route to a call, EMT-Intermediate (EMT-I) John Mason reviews the key elements of a medical interview in his head. This is his first shift with his paramedic partner, and he wants to make a good impression. He is told that he will assess all patients this morning. As they approach the scene, John quickly sizes it up. Nothing seems unusual. To the best of his knowledge, the scene is safe.

According to the dispatch information, John and his partner are responding to an elderly man with abdominal pain. Upon first meeting, John notices that his patient is in no real distress and appears stable. John does an initial assessment and then begins taking a patient history. He introduces himself and his partner and asks for his patient's name, which he will use throughout the interview.

John begins with a general question, "What seems to be the problem today, Mr. Saban?"

"My stomach hurts," Mr. Saban replies.

John begins exploring the history of the present illness with questions, including: "What were you doing when it started? Did it come on suddenly? Does anything make it worse or better? Can you describe how it feels? Can you point to the area that hurts? Does the pain travel anywhere else? How bad is it? On a scale of 1 to 10, with 10 being the worst pain you have ever felt, how would you rate this pain? When did it start? Is it constant or does it come and go? Are you nauseous and have you vomited? Have you experienced a change in your bowel habits? Do you have any difficulty breathing?"

It seems that Mr. Saban's pain came on suddenly after he ate that afternoon. He describes the pain as sharp in the upper right quadrant that radiates to the right shoulder area. As Mr. Saban answers John's questions, John leans forward, listening intently and often repeating Mr. Saban's words. John's partner watches and seems pleased.

As John continues, he begins forming a differential field diagnosis, which includes hepatitis, acute myocardial infarction, pneumonia, aneurysm, gallbladder disease, gastritis, pancreatitis, and peptic ulcer disease. John asks, "Mr. Saban, have you ever been treated for this problem in the past? Are you being treated for any other problems right now? Do you have diabetes, heart disease, breathing problems, kidney problems, or stomach problems? Have you been injured recently? Have you had any surgeries? Does this problem usually happen right after eating? Are you taking any medications for it right now? Are you allergic to any medications? Do you smoke? Do you drink? How often do you drink? Did you drink any alcohol today? Does this problem get worse when you drink? What did you eat today?"

John learns that Mr. Saban commonly has experienced pain after eating fatty foods. When John learns that his patient also drinks moderately every other day, he begins thinking about gallbladder disease. He decides to proceed to the review of body systems, beginning with the gastrointestinal (GI) system. He learns that Mr. Saban often has indigestion and protracted episodes of pain and that his stools are clay colored. He also has noticed a yellowish tint to his eyes and that he feels feverish. Mr. Saban denies vomiting blood or having blood in his stools. Hearing this, John suspects that his patient has an acute gallbladder problem. He conducts a focused physical exam and takes vital signs.

En route to St. Joseph's Hospital, John conducts a detailed physical exam while his partner observes. At the hospital John reports to the ED attending, Dr. Zehner, who agrees with his preliminary diagnosis of gallbladder disease. Following an assessment that includes laboratory testing and an ultrasound, Dr. Zehner calls for the surgical service. After the call, John's partner critiques him and reviews the key points of taking a patient history with him. He is extremely pleased with the orderly fashion in which John was able to obtain important information that allowed him to focus the physical exam and led to his correct field diagnosis. Having done well, John looks forward to his next opportunity to conduct a patient assessment.

INTRODUCTION

In the majority of medical cases, you will base your field diagnosis on the patient history. Clearly, how you conduct the patient interview and the questions you ask will determine how much relevant medical information your patient reveals. In medical cases, obtaining an adequate history of your patient's chief complaint, recent illnesses, and significant past medical history is as important as, if not more important than, the physical exam. The information you gather will direct the physical exam and reveal clues to your patient's problem. Although we present the history by itself in this chapter, you will most likely conduct it simultaneously with parts of the physical exam.

The ability to elicit a good history is the foundation for providing good care to patients you have never met before. To conduct a good interview you must gain your patient's trust in just a very short time. Then you must ask the right questions, listen intently to your patient's answers, and respond accordingly. In this chapter we will discuss both the verbal and nonverbal components of taking a comprehensive medical history.

We present the medical history in its entirety, as a well structured, yet flexible, tool having several component procedures that are conducted in order. In reality, your patient's answers will alter the sequence of your questioning, and some of the information in this chapter will not readily adapt itself to prehospital emergency medicine. As you gain clinical experience, you will learn which components of the history are appropriate to the particular situations you encounter. Whether your patient is critical or stable, the situation determines the length and completeness of the interview. For example, complicated medical cases require a close investigation of your patient's chief complaint and past medical history. Trauma cases, on the other hand, are generally sudden events not precipitated by medical conditions and require only a modified approach to history taking.

The interview is the focal point of your relationship with your patients. It establishes the bonding necessary for effective and efficient patient care. By asking a series of well-designed questions you begin to build a profile of your patients. You also should have a good understanding of their problems and a list of causes (**differential field diagnosis**) to explain their signs and symptoms. Often, learning about your patient's history, medications, and even their lifestyle will reveal clues to your final field diagnosis.

differential field diagnosis the list of possible causes for your patient's symptoms.

ESTABLISHING PATIENT RAPPORT

Your patients will form an opinion about you within the first few minutes, so you must establish a positive rapport quickly. This is not always easy. The situation, the patient, and the conditions will determine your ability to establish rapport. You can do several things, however, to facilitate this task. By asking them the right questions you will discover their chief complaint and their symptoms. By responding to them with empathy, you will win their trust and encourage them to discuss freely their problems with you. Their answers will also help you decide which areas require in-depth investigation and on which body systems to focus.

SETTING THE STAGE

Sometimes you will assess a patient from a long-term care facility. If your patient's chart is available, as in a nursing home or extended care facility, review it before conducting the interview. Quickly note his age, sex, race, marital status, address, and occupation. The insight into your patient's life experiences that you begin developing with this information may provide subtle clues to help steer your questioning. Determine any past medical problems or previous referrals for the same condition. Note any treatments rendered and their effects. On emergency scenes, review the first responder's run sheet. Look for the chief complaint, a brief history, including a current medication list, and vital signs. Be careful not to let your patient's chart, his past medical history, or someone else's first impression bias your possible field diagnoses. Always accept such information gratefully, but briefly reconfirm it with the patient and conduct your interview with an open mind.

If possible, conduct the interview in a quiet room, alone, with no distractions. Since you are asking your patient to divulge very intimate information, privacy encourages open communication. It should be a place where you and your patient can sit down and comfortably talk about his current problem and past experiences. Unfortunately, on emergency runs, you conduct the patient interview in a variety of settings beyond your control—from the kitchen floor to a busy street corner or a crowded bus. Often the back of your ambulance is where your patient will disclose important personal information to you. Some patients, however, will still be reluctant to reveal intimate information to a nonphysician in the emergency setting. EMT-Is are often surprised at the hospital when their patients tell a different story to the physician in the emergency department, but this is common. To maximize your chances of obtaining a good history, practice the following techniques for developing better patient rapport.

FIRST IMPRESSION

When you arrive on the scene, your patient, his family, and bystanders will form an impression of you. You have only a few precious minutes to make that impression a positive one. If you expect your patient to trust you with very private information, you must establish a positive, trusting rapport. Present yourself as a caring, compassionate, competent, and confident health-care professional. Because this first impression will be based largely on your appearance, your uniform and grooming will play an important role in the EMT-patient relationship. Your appearance should suggest neatness, cleanliness, pride, and professionalism. Your uniform should be clean and pressed, your shoes or boots polished, your hands and nails clean, and your hair well groomed.

Your voice, body language, gestures, and especially eye contact should communicate that you care about your patient's problems. Your questioning process should make the patient comfortable, confident in your care, and supportive of your control of the situation. Position yourself at his eye level and focus your attention on him. Give his requests and concerns high priority, even if they are not medically significant. For example, if your patient complains of being cold, cover him with a blanket. Beyond making him feel warmer, it may also increase his confidence in your desire and ability to help. If you cannot care for a complaint immediately, express your concern and reassure him you will either take care of it shortly or get him to a setting where it can be cared for.

A calm, reassuring voice and demeanor can put even the most apprehensive patient at ease. Remember that although his problems may not seem extraordinary to you, they may be extremely disturbing to him. You are accustomed to handling emergency situations; he is not. You are not horrified by a gory scene; he probably is. You deal with life-threatening emergencies everyday; he probably never does. Understanding these differences helps you to display an appropriate demeanor and begin your interview.

INTRODUCTIONS

Immediately make eye contact with your patient and maintain it as you conduct the interview. Eye contact is the most important form of nonverbal communication. It tells your patient, "I am sincerely interested in you and your problems." Always keeping in mind that your personal safety takes the highest priority in any emergency, quickly determine whether you should enter your patient's personal space (1½ to 4 feet). Then kneel, crouch, or sit beside him and address him from eye level or lower to reassure him that he still has some control. Avoid standing over him, which appears threatening or indifferent.

Wear an identification badge. Introduce yourself by name, title, and agency. For example, "Hi, my name is Jay. I'm an Emergency Medical Technician with Brewerton Ambulance. What's your name?" Use your patient's name frequently during the interview. Ask him what he wishes to be called—for instance, "Mr. MacCormack," "Nicholas," or "Nick"—and respect his wishes. Avoid using slang terms, such as honey, toots, dude, chief, pops, or babe, which your patient might construe as disrespectful and demeaning. Note that this short verbal exchange can reveal a wealth of information on your patient's respiratory status, level of consciousness, hearing, and speech abilities, and on any language barriers.

Be aware of other forms of nonverbal communication. Your job is to gain your patient's trust and cooperation in order to assess and care for him effectively. You do so by demonstrating sincerity through both verbal and nonverbal communication. Patients will detect inconsistencies in what you say and how you say it. Your tone of voice, facial expressions, and body language convey your true attitudes. Your actions must match your words. Touch is a powerful communication tool. Used properly, it conveys compassion, caring, and reassurance to an already apprehensive patient. Make contact by shaking hands or offering a comforting touch (Figure 6-1). This yields the additional benefit of enabling you to begin your assessment. For example, touching your patient's wrist allows you to make personal contact while quietly assessing his pulse and skin condition. Of course, you should try to get a sense of how your patient reacts to touch. It may make some patients feel threatened or uncomfortable. Avoid touching hostile, paranoid, or combative patients.

Unless your patient is in critical condition, work efficiently but do not rush. As you ask questions, you can delegate other personnel to conduct a focused physical exam, take vital signs, place oxygen, set up an IV, and get the stretcher. Your role as interviewer is to establish patient contact and learn the history.

Be aware of your patient's comfort. If the setting does not lend itself to personal questions, move your patient to a more suitable location. For example, teenage girls usually will not truthfully answer questions about pregnancy with their parents nearby. Other patients

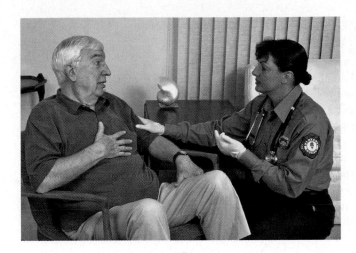

FIGURE 6-1 Use an appropriate compassionate touch to show your concern and support.

may not reveal relevant items about their medical history with bystanders listening. Sometimes moving your patient to the ambulance offers the needed privacy. If your patient is in obvious distress, try to alleviate his pain or discomfort while you interview him. For example, you may control minor bleeding and cover a wound that causes your patient distress. You might also immobilize a painful fracture site while you conduct the interview. Watch also for subtle signs of discomfort such as squirming, grimacing, and wincing.

ASKING QUESTIONS

Remembering everything your patient tells you is impossible. Taking notes is acceptable, and most patients will not mind you doing so. If your patient becomes concerned about the notes, simply explain why you are taking them and reassure him that your interactions are confidential. Make sure you maintain contact with your patient. Avoid focusing so closely on the clipboard questionnaire that you ignore your patient, with whom you are trying to establish a caring rapport. Jot down pieces of information crucial to your verbal and written reports such as a past history, medications, and vital signs.

Asking questions in a way that elicits accurate information from your patients is an art. To gather the patient history, you can use a combination of open-ended and closed questions. EMT-Is must understand these two very different types of questions. Open-ended questions allow your patient to explain how he feels in detail, in his words, instead of giving "yes" or "no" answers. His responses are usually more accurate and complete. "How would you describe the pain in your chest?" or "Where do you hurt?" are open-ended questions. They deal in generalizations, allowing your patient to respond freely and without limits. Some patients may wander off course when answering open-ended questions, and occasionally you will need to refocus the interview.

Closed questions elicit a short answer to a very direct question. They limit your patient's response to one or two words. They are appropriate when time or your patient's mental status or condition does not allow open-ended questions. For example, if your patient is gasping for breath while you are trying to determine the cause, phrase your questions for one-word answers or a nod or shake of the head: "Does your pain radiate to the shoulder?" or "Do you take diuretics?" Closed questions may be the most effective and efficient way to get your patients to describe their symptoms in exact terms. The disadvantages of such questions are that you may inadvertently lead your patient toward certain answers or elicit information that is too limited.

Some patients have difficulty describing their symptoms. In these cases, ask questions with multiple-choice options. For example, "Is your pain sharp, dull, burning, pressure-like, stabbing, or like something else?" Other patients may become confused, especially when more than one person is asking them questions. Avoid this by limiting the interview to one person, asking one question at a time, and allowing time for your patient to answer. Do not rush. You can become an efficient history taker by knowing which questions will elicit the most important information and by maintaining your patient's attention.

LANGUAGE AND COMMUNICATION

Use appropriate language during the interview. Nothing distances you from your patient more quickly than sophisticated medical terminology. "Have you ever had a heart attack?" is better than "Have you ever had an MI?" Effective communication means connecting with your patient. Most of your patients will not understand medical terms. Use an appropriate level of questions, but do not appear condescending. Other barriers to communication include cultural differences, language differences, deafness, speech impediments, and even blindness. When you encounter such obstacles, try to enlist someone who can communicate with your patient and act as an interpreter. An alternative is to adopt a conservative approach toward assessment, field diagnosis, and treatment.

Listening is an important part of the interview. The old saying, "Listen to your patient; he will tell you what is wrong," explains why it is crucial for a skilled clinician to be a good listener. Listen closely to what your patients tell you. Be careful not to develop tunnel vision from dispatch information. Begin your assessment without any preconceived notions about your patient's injury or illness. Also watch for subtle clues that your patient may not be telling the truth. For example, your patient tells you that his chest pain went away, but his facial expressions and body language suggest otherwise. Developing good communication skills takes time and practice.

Avoid working your way in strict order down any prearranged list of questions (such as those in this chapter). Use these lists as a guide only. Listen to your patients and watch for clues to important signs, symptoms, emotions, or other factors. Then modify your questions to follow those clues. The following practices promote **active listening**.

active listening the process of responding to your patient's statements with words or gestures that demonstrate your understanding.

Content Review

ACTIVE LISTENING SKILLS
- Facilitation
- Reflection
- Clarification

Facilitation

Maintain sincere eye contact, use concerned facial expressions, and lean forward while you listen. Cues such as "Mm-hmm," "Go on," or "I'm listening" all help your patient to open up. Sometimes strategic silence is also helpful.

Reflection

Repeat your patient's words. This encourages him to provide more details. Just make sure not to disturb his train of thought. For example:

Patient:	I can't breathe.
You:	You can't breathe?
Patient:	No, it feels like I can't take in a full breath because my chest hurts.
You:	Your chest hurts, too?
Patient:	Yes, it started this morning when I was working in the yard. I usually take a Nitro but I'm all out.

This simple reflection encouraged the patient to reveal facts about his history of heart disease. If you had merely investigated the chief complaint of dyspnea, discovering its true cause may have taken longer. Since the primary problem is not always the chief complaint, allowing your patient to take the lead is sometimes advantageous.

Clarification

In crisis, patients often cannot clearly describe what they feel. They will use vague, general words. Do not hesitate to ask for clarification. For example:

You:	Do you have any allergies?
Patient:	Yes, the last time I took penicillin I had a bad reaction.
You:	Can you describe the reaction?
Patient:	Well, I got itchy all over with a rash.
You:	Did you have any difficulty breathing or feel like you were choking?
Patient:	Oh, no, just the itching and rash.

By asking for clarification you distinguish between a simple allergic reaction and life-threatening anaphylaxis.

TAKING A HISTORY ON SENSITIVE TOPICS

EMT-I students normally have difficulty questioning their patients about embarrassing, sensitive, or very personal topics such as sexual activities, death and dying, drug and alcohol use, physical deformities, bodily functions, and domestic violence. Even though you may feel uneasy discussing these matters, you may learn important information about your patient's illness. To become more comfortable dealing with these subjects, watch experienced clinicians discuss them with their patients. Familiarize yourself with and practice some opening questions on sensitive topics that both put your patient at ease and encourage him to talk about it. If a particular area makes you most uncomfortable, attend a lecture or seminar and learn how professionals deal with this subject daily. Make the unfamiliar familiar and it will seem less imposing.

Look at two sensitive topics: physical violence and the sexual history. Your patient may not want to reveal a history of physical abuse. You should consider it when any of the following conditions are present:

- Injuries that are inconsistent with the story given
- Injuries that embarrass your patient
- Delay between the time of the injury and seeking help
- Past history of "accidents"
- Suspicious behavior of the supposed abuser

To earn your patient's trust, try to make him or her feel that the problem is not uncommon and that you understand the reasons. For example, you can ask your female patient, "Sometimes when husbands and wives argue a lot, it leads to physical fighting. I noticed you have some bruises. Can you tell me what happened? Did someone hit you?" With active listening techniques, such questioning will help establish a rapport that encourages open communication.

Taking a sexual history can be the most embarrassing and uncomfortable topic for an inexperienced health-care provider. The sexual history is normally taken later during the history but can be a part of the present illness or past history, depending on your patient's chief complaint. For example, if your patient complains of a genitourinary problem, a sexual history becomes important during questioning about the present illness. If your patient has a history of sexually transmitted disease, then a sexual history is relevant to the past history. Whenever you begin the sexual history, it is helpful to prepare your patient with introductory statements and questions such as, "Now I need to ask you some questions about your sexual health and activity. It may help me determine the cause of your problem and provide better care for you. This information will be strictly confidential. May I begin?" If your patient consents, proceed as follows: "Are you sexually active? Have you had sex with anyone in the last six months? Do you have more than one partner? Do you have sex with men, women, or both? Do you take precautions to avoid infection or unwanted pregnancy? Do you have any problems or concerns about your sexual function?" This may seem very uncomfortable for you but with time and clinical experience you will develop a sense of where and when these questions are appropriate. It is critical that you remain calm, objective, and nonjudgmental regardless of how your patient answers.

A COMPREHENSIVE PATIENT HISTORY

This section presents the components of a comprehensive patient history in a systematic order. In practice, you will ultimately select only those components that apply to your patient's situation and status. For example, if you help conduct preemployment physical exams for a corporation, you may use the entire form. On the other hand, if you respond to a gasping

Common sense and clinical experience will determine how much of the history to use.

Content Review

ELEMENTS OF THE PATIENT HISTORY

- Preliminary data
- Chief complaint
- Present illness/injury
- Past history
- Current health status
- Review of systems

patient in acute pulmonary edema, you will focus on the present illness. Common sense and clinical experience will determine how much of the following history to use.

PRELIMINARY DATA

For documentation, always record the date and time of the physical exam. Determine your patient's age, sex, race, birthplace, and occupation. This provides a starting point for the interview and establishes you as the interviewer. Who is the source of the information you receive about your patient? Is it the competent patient himself, his spouse, a friend, or a bystander? Are you receiving a report from a first responder, the police, or another healthcare worker? Do you have the medical record from a transferring facility? After you have gathered the information, you should establish its reliability, which will vary according to the source's knowledge, memory, trust, and motivation. Again, reconfirm the information with the patient, if possible. This is a judgment call based on your experience. For example, if the patient information you received from a particular first responder has been accurate in the past, you probably will trust it again. On the other hand, if the nurse at a physician's office has repeatedly provided you with erroneous information, you probably will doubt her accuracy.

CHIEF COMPLAINT

chief complaint the reason the ambulance was called in the patient's own words.

The history begins with an open-ended question about your patient's chief complaint. The **chief complaint** is the pain, discomfort, or dysfunction that caused your patient to request help. In a medical case, it may be a woman's call for help because she has chest pain. In a trauma case, it may be a bystander's call for assistance to a "man down" or a police officer's reporting an injury in an auto collision. Your patient may have called for more than one symptom. It is important to begin with a general question that allows your patient to respond freely. For example, "Why did you call us today?" or "What seems to be the problem?" Avoid the tunnel vision that often biases EMT-Is who focus on dispatch information that may or may not accurately describe the situation. As you interview and assess your patient, the chief complaint becomes more specific.

primary problem the underlying cause of the patient's symptoms.

The chief complaint differs from the **primary problem**. Although the chief complaint is a sign or symptom noticed by the patient or a bystander, the primary problem is the principal medical cause of the complaint. For example, your patient's chief complaint may be leg pain, but the primary problem is a tibia fracture. When possible, report and record the chief complaint in your patient's own words. For example, "I am having a hard time breathing" is better than "the patient has dyspnea." For the unconscious patient, the chief complaint becomes what someone else identifies or what you observe as the primary problem. In some trauma situations, for instance, the chief complaint might be the mechanism of injury such as "a gunshot wound to the chest," or "a fall from 25 feet."

PRESENT ILLNESS

Once you have determined the chief complaint, explore each of your patient's other complaints in greater detail. Be naturally inquisitive when exploring the events surrounding them. A practical template for exploring each one follows the mnemonic OPQRST—ASPN, an acronym for *Onset, Provocation, Quality, Region/Radiation, Severity, Time, Associated Symptoms,* and *Pertinent Negatives.* This line of questioning provides a full, clear, chronological account of your patient's symptoms.

Content Review

PRESENT ILLNESS: OPQRST-ASPN

- *O*nset of problem
- *P*rovocative/*P*alliative factors
- *Q*uality
- *R*egion/*R*adiation
- *S*everity
- *T*ime
- *A*ssociated *S*ymptoms
- *P*ertinent *N*egatives

Onset Did the problem develop suddenly or gradually? What was your patient doing when the symptoms started? In medical emergencies, investigate your patient's activities at the time of, or shortly before, the signs or symptoms developed. In some cases, especially trauma, you may have to gather information from a few weeks before the onset of symptoms. For example, the signs and symptoms of a subdural hematoma may not appear until weeks following an injury. Was the patient exercising or exerting himself, or at rest or sleeping? Was he eating or drinking? If so, what? In trauma cases, ensure that a medical problem did not cause the accident. For example, the sudden onset of an illness such as a seizure or syncope may have caused a fall.

Provocation/Palliation   What provokes the symptom (makes it worse)? Does anything palliate the symptom (make it better)? In many illnesses, certain factors such as motion, pressure, and jarring may increase or decrease pain, discomfort, or dysfunction. Does eating, movement, exertion, stress, or anything else provoke the current problem? Positioning also may be a factor. Your patient may wish to curl up and lie on his side to reduce abdominal pain. Congestive heart failure patients will sit bolt upright to ease respiration. They also may sleep with several pillows raising their upper body to relieve **paroxysmal nocturnal dyspnea** (PND), a sleep-disturbing breathing difficulty caused by fluid that accumulates in the lungs when they are supine. Ask your patient how breathing affects the discomfort. Deep breathing may increase the pain of a patient with an acute abdomen. A patient with pleuritic or rib-fracture pain will not breathe deeply, whereas breathing may not affect the pain of angina. Any patient with respiratory pain will breathe with shallower but more frequent breaths.

> **paroxysmal nocturnal dyspnea** sudden onset of shortness of breath at night.

   If your patient took a medication shortly before you arrived, its effect or lack of effect may help determine the problem. Drugs such as bronchodilators, hypoglycemic agents, antihypertensives, and anticonvulsants are commonly prescribed and taken at home. Investigate any medication used to relieve a problem and note its effectiveness. Ask about any activity, medication, or other circumstance that either alleviates or aggravates the chief complaint.

Quality   How does your patient perceive the pain or discomfort? Ask him to explain how the symptom feels and listen carefully to his answer. Does your patient call his pain crushing, tearing, oppressive, gnawing, crampy, sharp, dull, or otherwise? Quote his descriptors precisely in your report.

Region/Radiation   Where is the symptom? Does it move anywhere else? Identify the exact location and area of pain, discomfort, or dysfunction. Does your patient complain of pain "here," while holding a clenched fist over the sternum, or does he grasp the entire abdomen with both hands and moan? If your patient has not done so, ask him to point to the painful area. Identify the specific location or the boundary of the pain if it is regional.

   Determine if the pain is truly pain (occurring independently) or **tenderness** (pain on palpation). Also determine if the pain moves or radiates. Localized pain occurs in one specific area, whereas radiating pain travels away from the source, in one, many, or all directions. Evaluate moving pain's initial location and progression and any factors that affect its movement.

> **tenderness** pain that is elicited through palpation.

   Note any pain that may be referred from other parts of the body. **Referred pain** is felt in a part of the body away from the source of the disease or problem. The heart and diaphragm are two areas that most commonly produce referred pain. Cardiac problems such as myocardial infarction or anginal pain are usually referred to the left arm, with occasional referral to the neck, jaw, and back. Pain associated with irritation of the diaphragm (most commonly blood in the abdomen of the supine patient) generally is referred to the clavicular region.

> **referred pain** pain that is felt at a location away from its source.

Severity   How bad is the symptom? Severity is the intensity of pain or discomfort felt by your patient. Ask him how bad the pain feels, and then have him compare it to other painful problems he has experienced. Sometimes a patient can describe the severity of the pain on a scale from 1 to 10, with 10 being the worst pain he has ever felt. Also notice the amount of discomfort your patient's condition causes. How easy is it to distract your patient from his concern over the pain? Is your patient very still and resistive to your touch? Is he writhing about? The answers should give you a good idea of the intensity of your patient's pain.

Time   When did the symptoms begin? Is a symptom constant or intermittent? How long does it last? How long has this symptom affected your patient? For several days, hours, or just a few minutes or seconds? When did any previous episodes occur? How does this episode's length vary from earlier ones?

Associated Symptoms   What other symptoms commonly associated with the chief complaint in certain diseases can help rule in your field diagnosis? For example, if the chief complaint is chest pain, ask, "Are you short of breath? Are you nauseous? Have you vomited?

Are you dizzy or light-headed?" The presence of these symptoms would help support a field diagnosis of cardiac chest pain.

Pertinent Negatives Are any likely associated symptoms absent? Their absence is as important to the field diagnosis as their presence, because they help rule out a particular disease or injury. Note any element of the history or physical exam that does not support a suspected or possible field diagnosis. For example, it is significant if your patient who complains of chest pain denies shortness of breath, nausea, and lightheadedness.

PAST MEDICAL HISTORY

The past medical history may provide significant insights into your patient's chief complaint and your field diagnosis.

The past medical history may provide significant insights into your patient's chief complaint and your field diagnosis. Look in-depth at your patient's general state of health, childhood and adult diseases, psychiatric illnesses, accidents or injuries, surgeries, and hospitalizations. They may reveal general or specific clues that will help you to correctly assess his current problem. Your patient's condition, the situation, and time constraints determine how much information you can and should gather on the scene. For example, asking about childhood diseases may not be relevant for your acute cardiac or trauma patient.

General State of Health How does your patient perceive his general state of health?

Childhood Diseases What childhood diseases did your patient have? Did he have mumps, measles, rubella, whooping cough, chickenpox, rheumatic fever, scarlet fever, or polio? Again, this line of questioning's relevance depends on the patient and the situation.

Adult Diseases Is your patient a diabetic? Does he have a history of heart disease, breathing problems, high blood pressure, or similar conditions? A preexisting medical problem may contribute to your patient's current problem or influence his care during the next few hours. To discover significant preexisting medical problems, ask if your patient has recently seen a physician or been hospitalized. If so, for what conditions? If you discover a preexisting problem, investigate its effects on your patient. When did the problem last affect him? Is your patient on any special diets or prescribed medications or restricted in activity? Even with the trauma patient, do not forget that a medical problem may have led to an accident or may complicate the effects of trauma. Also, obtain the name of your patient's physician since it may be helpful to the emergency department staff.

Psychiatric Illnesses Does your patient have a history of mental illness? Has he ever been diagnosed with depression, mania, schizophrenia, or other problems? Is he being treated for a mental illness? If so, what medications is he taking? Has he ever had thoughts of suicide? Has he ever attempted suicide? Tailor these questions for patients you suspect of having a mental illness.

Accidents or Injuries Has your patient ever had a serious accident or injury requiring hospitalization? Has he had a previous injury that could be a factor in his current problem? For example, a seemingly minor head injury one week ago may present now as a subdural hematoma in your unconscious elderly patient. Keep this line of questioning to relevant information only. An old football injury or childhood laceration is probably not influencing your patient's chest pain and respiratory distress today. But his pneumonectomy (surgical removal of a lung) probably is the reason for the absence of lung sounds on his right side.

Surgeries or Hospitalizations Has your patient had any other hospitalizations or surgeries not already mentioned? Again, these may offer some insight into your suspected field diagnosis. For example, your patient is an 85-year-old man with a long history of congestive heart failure and no history of chronic lung disease. He suddenly presents with severe difficulty in breathing and audible wheezing. You should suspect the obvious—a cardiac problem. Do not look for the five-legged cat.

CURRENT HEALTH STATUS

The current health status assembles all the factors in your patient's present medical condition. Here, you try to gather information that completes the puzzle surrounding your patient's primary problem. Look for clues and correlations among the various sections of this part of the history. For example, your patient is a heavy smoker, has many allergies to inhaled particles, works in a coal mine, and frequently uses bronchodilating medications. He now complains of shortness of breath and expiratory wheezing. He is probably having an exacerbation of his chronic lung disease.

Current Medications Is your patient taking any medications? These include over-the-counter drugs, prescriptions, home remedies, vitamins, and minerals. If so, why? Your patient's explanation may not be medically accurate, but it may help to determine underlying conditions. For example, your 65-year-old patient tells you she takes a "water pill." You can safely assume she takes a diuretic and has a history of renal or cardiac problems. A medication not taken as prescribed may be responsible for the current medical problem—possibly caused by under- or over-medication. A recently prescribed medication may cause an allergic or untoward (severe and unexpected) reaction. It also may be expired and no longer effective. Even for trauma, emergency department personnel will need to know what medications your patient is taking. For example, if your patient takes warfarin, an anticoagulant, it would interfere with the normal clotting process and actually promote bleeding. If practical, bring your patient's medications to the hospital (Figure 6-2).

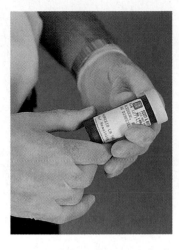

FIGURE 6-2 When practical, take your patient's medications with you to the hospital.

Allergies Does your patient have any known allergies, especially to penicillin, the "caine" family (local anesthetics), tetanus toxoid, or narcotics? These agents are occasionally given in emergency situations. What type of reaction did your patient have to the medication? For example, was it just a mild allergic reaction with a rash and itching or localized swelling or anaphylactic shock? Knowledge of your patient's allergies may prevent additional complications during the emergency department visit, especially if he becomes disoriented or unconscious during transport. If your patient is short of breath with wheezing, ask about environmental allergies. In cases of possible anaphylaxis, ask about allergies to drugs, to foods such as shellfish, nuts, and dairy products, and to insect bites and stings.

Tobacco Does your patient use tobacco? If so, what kind (cigarettes, cigars, pipe, smokeless, or other), how much, and for how long? To quantify his smoking history, multiply the number of packs smoked per day by the number of years he has smoked. The result is his pack/year history. For example, if your patient smoked two packs of cigarettes per day for 25 years, he is a 50 pack/year smoker. Anything over 30 packs/year is considered significant.

Alcohol, Drugs, and Related Substances Alcohol and drugs are often contributing factors in, if not the primary cause of, your patient's medical problems. Your job is not to pass judgment, but to gather data that will help direct your patient's medical treatment. Remaining nonjudgmental will aid you in your questioning. Start with a general question such as "How much alcohol do you drink?" If you suspect a drinking problem may be a factor, you can use the CAGE questionnaire (an alcoholism screening instrument) to determine the presence of alcoholism. Reserve this line of questioning for the chronic patient in a controlled setting. It would be inappropriate in a bar with an unruly, intoxicated patient.

Content Review

CAGE QUESTIONNAIRE
- **C**ut down
- **A**nnoyed
- **G**uilty
- **E**ye-opener

> The CAGE Questionnaire
>
> Have you ever felt the need to **C**ut down on your drinking?
>
> Have you ever felt **A**nnoyed by criticism of your drinking?
>
> Have you ever had **G**uilty feelings about drinking?
>
> Have you ever taken a drink first thing in the morning as an **E**ye-opener?
>
> Two or more "yes" answers suggest alcoholism and further lines of inquiry.

Ask about blackouts, accidents, or injuries that happened while drinking. Also ask about alcohol-related job losses, marital problems, and arrests while under the influence of alcohol. Similarly, ask about drug use. For example, "Do you use marijuana, cocaine, heroin, sleeping pills, or painkillers? How much do you take? How do these drugs make you feel? Have you had any bad reactions?" Because your patients realize you are not judging their substance abuse, they may feel more comfortable telling you about their patterns of use.

Diet Ask about your patient's normal daily intake of food and drink. Perhaps the 78-year-old retiree just moved to the Arizona desert and underestimated the increased fluid loss due to sweating. He does not realize he needs to increase his daily fluid intake, and now he is weak and dizzy from dehydration. Are there any dietary restrictions or supplements? Ask specifically about his use of foods with stimulating effects such as coffee, tea, cola drinks, and other beverages containing caffeine. For example, a 23-year-old patient with a rapid heart beat (200 beats per minute) drinks continuous cups of coffee each morning at her highly stressful job.

Screening Tests   Ask about certain screening tests that may have been done for your patient. Some examples include a purified protein derivative (PPD) test for suspected tuberculosis, Pap smears and mammograms for female problems, stool testing for occult blood, and cholesterol tests. Record the dates of the tests and their results.

Immunizations   Ask your patient about his immunizations for diseases such as tetanus, pertussis, diphtheria, polio, measles, rubella, mumps, influenza, hepatitis B, and pneumococcal vaccine. For example, ask the parent of a child suspected of epiglottitis if he had the hemophilus influenza B vaccine, which is a common cause for epiglottitis in children.

Sleep Patterns   Ask your patient what time he normally goes to bed and arises. Does he take daytime naps? Does he have problems falling asleep or staying asleep?

Exercise and Leisure Activities   Does your patient exercise regularly or lead a sedentary existence? Sometimes your patient's lifestyle will support your field diagnosis.

Environmental Hazards   Ask about possible hazards in the home, in school, and at the workplace. For example, your patient may live or work in an area with high levels of toxic substances. Many health problems can be traced to these environmental causes.

Use of Safety Measures   In an auto collision, was the patient using a seat restraint system? Were all passengers belted in? Did the air bag deploy? Such information aids you and the emergency department staff in determining the extent of damage caused by a particular mechanism of injury. For bicycle, in-line skate, and skateboard injuries, ask about the use of helmets and knee and elbow pads.

Since many disease processes are hereditary, it is important to learn the medical history of immediate family members.

Family History   Since many disease processes are hereditary, the medical history of immediate family members is important. In the nonemergency setting you may explore deep into the family tree and chart the medical history of grandparents, parents, aunts, and uncles. In the emergency setting, learning that your 45-year-old patient with chest pain had a father and brother who both died of heart attacks in their late forties is important information. Look for a family history of diabetes, heart disease, high cholesterol, high blood pressure, stroke, kidney disease, tuberculosis, cancer, arthritis, anemia, allergies, asthma, headaches, epilepsy, mental illness, alcoholism, drug addiction, and any symptoms similar to the patient's.

Home Situation and Significant Others   Who lives at home with your patient? Ask him about his home life—or lack of one. Ask about friends, family, support groups, loved ones. Find out if he has a support network and whom it includes. Who takes care of him when he needs help? Loneliness and isolation may complicate your patient's physical symptoms.

Daily Life   Ask your patient to describe his typical day. When does he get up? What does he do first? Then what? Such questions reveal a lot about your patient's state of mind and general wellness. Is he busy, active, and motivated to get up in the morning? Does he merely exist from the time he awakens and go through life with no purpose or direction? Is he under high levels of stress from morning to night in a job that requires him to take his problems home with him? Find out what kind of life your patient leads. It may reveal a lot about his illness.

Important Experiences   Ask about your patient's upbringing and home life growing up. How much schooling does he have? Was he in the military? What kinds of jobs has he held? What is his financial situation? Is he married, single, divorced, or widowed? What does he do for fun and relaxation? Is he retired or looking forward to retirement? Again, the answers give you a broader picture of your patient.

The renowned Canadian physician Sir William Osler once said, "Listen to the patient, and he will tell you what is wrong." This admonition is as true today as it was 100 years ago. A great deal of information can be determined from a skillful history taking. As you listen to a patient's medical history, try to understand the underlying pathophysiological processes that might cause the symptoms the patient describes. This will help you to fully comprehend the disease process or processes affecting the patient. For example, consider the following case.

Mrs. J. Franklin is a 72-year-old pensioner, twice widowed, who lives in an older section of town. She summons EMS with what initially seem like vague complaints. She reports to the dispatcher, when queried, that she is "just sick." You arrive and begin an assessment starting with a pertinent history. The patient reports that her symptoms began about two weeks ago after several family members came to her house with dinner, which included a baked ham. Since that time, she has developed some fatigue, progressive dyspnea, and occasional chest pain. She now reports that she often wakes up at 3:00 A.M. with breathing trouble that resolves when she walks around the room or sleeps with three pillows. She also cannot tie her shoes, and she missed church last Sunday for this very reason. Her medications have remained unchanged and include furosemide, nitroglycerin paste, digoxin, aspirin, and lisinopril.

Clearly, there are physiological cues in the patient's medical history. The symptoms began with a ham dinner. You learn that she kept the ham and has been eating it daily. The ham is salt cured. Thus, her sodium intake may have increased. Her medications have remained unchanged. Her symptoms seem to indicate worsening heart failure with episodes consistent with both left and right ventricular failure. Her nighttime dyspnea and orthopnea are consistent with left heart failure, whereas her inability to tie her shoes could be due to peripheral edema from right heart failure. The fatigue could be attributed to both. Thus, your physical examination should either support or contradict your history findings.

In fact, it was learned later that the patient's heart failure had always been somewhat tenuous and the sodium load she received from the ham was all that was necessary to cause congestive heart failure. She did well with two days of hospitalization, diuretic administration, and sodium restriction.

Dr. Osler was correct. The history is often the most important part of patient assessment.

Religious Beliefs   Some religions forbid certain treatments and have guidelines regarding the management of illness and injury. For example, some forbid whole blood transfusions. Knowing if your patient is guided by these beliefs can help you understand and care for him better. These questions require some expression of sensitivity, or it might be best to ask broadly if he has any limitations in medical care.

Patient's Outlook   Find out what your patient thinks and how he feels about the present and future.

REVIEW OF SYSTEMS

The **review of systems** is a series of questions designed to identify problems your patient has not already mentioned. It is a system-by-system list of questions that are more specific than those asked during the basic history. Again, the patient's chief complaint, condition, and clinical status determine how much, if any, of the review of systems you will use. For example, if your patient complains of chest pain, you may want to review the respiratory, cardiac, gastrointestinal, and hematological systems. If your patient complains of a headache, you may want to review the **HEENT** (head, eyes, ears, nose, and throat), neurological, peripheral vascular, and psychiatric systems. Let your patient lead you through the history. The following sampling includes a few of the many questions that you might ask.

review of systems a list of questions categorized by body system.

HEENT memory aid for head, eyes, ears, nose, and throat.

General   What is your patient's usual weight, and has the patient experienced any recent weight changes? Has he had weakness, fatigue, or fever?

Skin   Has your patient noticed any new rashes, lumps, sores, itching, dryness, color change, or changes in nails or hair? Could cosmetics or jewelry have caused these problems?

Head, Eyes, Ears, Nose, and Throat (HEENT)   Has your patient had headaches or recent head trauma? How is his vision? Does he wear glasses or contact lenses? When was his last eye exam? Has he experienced any of the following: pain, redness, excessive tearing, double vision, blurred vision, spots, specks, flashing lights? Has he ever had glaucoma or cataracts? How is his hearing? Does he use hearing aids? Has he ever experienced ringing in the ears (**tinnitus**), vertigo, earaches, infection, or discharge? Does he have frequent colds, nasal stuffiness, nasal discharge, hay fever, nose bleeds, sinus problems? Does he wear dentures? When was his last dental exam? Describe the condition of his teeth and gums. Do his gums bleed? Does he get a sore tongue, dry mouth, frequent sore throats, or hoarseness? Does he have lumps or swollen glands? Has he ever had a goiter, neck pain, difficulty swallowing, or stiffness?

Respiratory   Has your patient ever had wheezing, coughing up blood (**hemoptysis**), asthma, bronchitis, emphysema, pneumonia, tuberculosis, or pleurisy? When was his last chest X-ray? Is he coughing now? If so, can you describe the sputum?

Cardiac   Has your patient ever had heart trouble, high blood pressure, rheumatic fever, heart murmurs, chest pain or discomfort, palpitations, shortness of breath (**dyspnea**), shortness of breath while lying flat (**orthopnea**), or peripheral edema? Has he ever been awakened from sleep with shortness of breath (paroxysmal nocturnal dyspnea)? Has he ever had an electrocardiogram (ECG) or other heart tests?

Gastrointestinal   Has your patient ever had trouble swallowing, heartburn, loss of appetite, nausea/vomiting, regurgitation, vomiting blood (**hematemesis**), or indigestion? How often does he have a bowel movement? Describe the color and size of his stools. Have there been any changes in his bowel habits? Has he had rectal bleeding or black, tarry stools, hemorrhoids, constipation, or diarrhea? Has he had abdominal pain, food intolerance, or excessive belching or passing of gas? Has he had jaundice, liver or gallbladder problems, or hepatitis?

Urinary   How often does your patient urinate? Has he ever had excessive urination (**polyuria**), excessive urination at night (**nocturia**), burning or pain while urinating, blood in the urine (**hematuria**), urgency, reduced caliber or force of urine flow, hesitancy, dribbling, or incontinence? Has he ever had a urinary tract infection or stones?

Male Genital   Has your patient ever had a hernia, discharge from or sores on the penis, testicular pain, or masses? Has he ever had a sexually transmitted disease? If so, how was it treated?

Female Genital   At what age did your patient have her first menstrual period? Describe the regularity, frequency, duration, and amount of bleeding of her periods. When was her last menstrual period? Does she bleed between periods or after intercourse? Has she ever had difficulty with her period (**dysmenorrhea**) or premenstrual tension? At what age did she become menopausal? Were there symptoms or bleeding? Has she ever had any vaginal discharge, lumps, sores, or itching? Has she ever had a sexually transmitted disease? If so, how was it treated? How many times has she been pregnant? How many deliveries? Any abortions (spontaneous or induced)? Some health-care personnel use the G-P-A-L system to document a patient's history of pregnancy:

Gravida	How many times pregnant?
Para	How many viable births?
Abortions	How many abortions?
Living	How many living children?

Has she ever had complications of pregnancy? Does she use birth control? If so, what type? If postmenopausal, is she on hormone replacement therapy?

Peripheral Vascular   Has your patient ever had intermittent calf pain while walking (**intermittent claudication**), leg cramps, varicose veins, or blood clots?

Musculoskeletal   Has your patient ever experienced muscle or joint pain, stiffness, arthritis, gout, or backache? Describe the location or symptoms.

---

tinnitus the sensation of ringing in the ears.

hemoptysis coughing up blood.

dyspnea the sensation of having difficulty breathing.

orthopnea difficulty in breathing while lying in a supine position.

hematemesis vomiting blood.

polyuria excessive urination.

nocturia excessive urination at night.

hematuria blood in the urine.

dysmenorrhea menstrual difficulties.

intermittent claudication intermittent calf pain while walking that subsides with rest.

Neurologic Has your patient ever experienced any of the following: fainting, blackouts, seizures, speech difficulty, vertigo, weakness, paralysis, numbness or loss of sensation, tingling, "pins and needles," tremors, or other involuntary movements?

Hematologic Has your patient ever been anemic? Has he ever had a blood transfusion? If so did he have a reaction to it? Does he bruise or bleed easily?

Endocrine Has your patient ever had thyroid trouble? Did he ever experience heat or cold intolerance, or excessive sweating? Does he have diabetes? Has he ever had excessive thirst, hunger, or urge to urinate?

Psychiatric Is he nervous? Is he under much stress and tension? Has he ever been depressed? Has he ever thought of committing suicide?

SPECIAL CHALLENGES

No matter how long you practice as an EMT-I, some patients will present with special circumstances that challenge your skills. Your ability to deal with them will improve with time and practice.

SILENCE

Silence can become very uncomfortable if you are impatient. Why has your patient suddenly become silent? This question has no single answer. His silence can have many meanings and many uses. It may result from an organic brain condition that prevents him from forming thoughts. Or it may be due to dysarthria (difficulty in speaking due to muscular impairment). Maybe he is just collecting his thoughts or trying to remember details. Or maybe he is deciding whether he trusts you. He might be clinically depressed, or perhaps, he simply deals with situations by being quiet.

What do you do during the silence? Stay calm and observe your patient's nonverbal clues. Is he in pain? Is he scared? Is he on the verge of becoming hysterical or combative, or is he about to cry? You can encourage him to continue speaking by confronting him with your perceptions. For example, "I see you are obviously very upset about this. Do you want to talk about it?" If you sense your patient is not responsive to your questions, perform a brief orientation exam. Speak to him in a loud voice and call him by name. Shake him gently if he does not respond. If this does not elicit a response, assume a neurological problem and proceed accordingly.

Sometimes your behavior might have caused the silence. Are you asking too many questions too quickly? Have you offended your patient? Have you frightened him? Have you been insensitive? Have you failed to respond to your patient's needs? If your patient suddenly becomes silent, try to determine why, what is happening, and what you should do about it.

OVERLY TALKATIVE PATIENTS

The patient who rambles on can be just as frustrating to deal with as the one who will not talk at all. Why is your patient talking so fast and so much? Some patients react to stress this way. Maybe he has a lot to say. Maybe he needs someone to talk to; some lonely patients take any opportunity to communicate with another human being. What can you do in the emergency setting when time is scarce? This problem has no perfect solution. You can lower your goals and accept a less comprehensive history. You can briefly give your patient free rein. You can focus on the important areas and ask closed questions about them. You can interrupt him frequently and summarize what he says. Above all, try not to become impatient.

PATIENTS WITH MULTIPLE SYMPTOMS

Patients often present with multiple complaints. For example, your elderly patient may present you with a barrage of symptoms from an extensive medical history. Your challenge is to discover the chief complaint and why she called you today. If she complains of symptoms that suggest multiple disease states, the challenge is compounded. In these types of cases, you must sort through a multitude of information quickly and recognize patterns that lead you to a correct field diagnosis.

Some patients will answer "Yes" to every question you ask. They have every symptom you mention; although possible, this phenomenon is not probable. Your patient might simply misunderstand or be trying hard to cooperate. More than likely he has an emotional problem and requires a psychosocial assessment. Document your findings on your prehospital care report and request a psychological referral. Asking your patient what single complaint led him to call for help today often helps.

ANXIOUS PATIENTS

Anxiety is a natural reaction to stress. People who face serious illness or injury can be expected to exhibit some degree of anxiety. Sometimes this manifests itself as simple nervousness, tenseness, sweating, or trembling. Some patients will become silent, while others will ramble. Still others may exhibit anxiety attacks marked by a rapid heart rate, nausea and vomiting, chest pain, and shortness of breath. When you detect signs of anxiety, encourage your patient to speak freely about it. For example, you can say, "I see you are concerned about this. Do you want to talk about it?"

PATIENTS NEEDING REASSURANCE

Appropriate reassurance is a cornerstone of patient care. You must be careful, however, not to be overly reassuring or to prematurely reassure your anxious patient. It is natural to say, "Relax, everything is going to be all right. We are going to take care of you and get you to the hospital. Just relax and you will be all right." But your patient may have anxiety about something of which you are not aware. For instance, if your chest pain patient is anxious, you might naturally assume he is apprehensive about dying. In reality he may be anxious about something entirely different. He may be embarrassed about his anxieties, and instead of helping him deal with them, you have helped him cover them up. Now he may decide you are not interested in what is really bothering him and block further communication. Listen carefully to your patient before offering reassurance.

ANGER AND HOSTILITY

Often you will encounter angry patients or their families. They might be angry for many reasons. Your patient is sick, perhaps dying. The family is anticipating their future loss. Often they will lash out at the easiest target, which may be you. Sometimes you cannot do anything quickly enough or well enough for them. Understand that their anger is a natural part of the grieving process and they may be merely venting their frustration. Unfortunately you find yourself at the receiving end of their outbursts. Try to accept their feelings without getting defensive or angry in return.

INTOXICATION

Dealing with belligerent, intoxicated patients challenges even the most experienced EMT-I. These patients are irrational, they disrupt your control of the scene, and they rarely allow you to examine them. First and foremost, make sure your environment is safe. If your patient acts violently, call for the police before attempting any interaction. As you approach your patient, introduce yourself and offer a handshake. Avoid any challenging body language or remarks. Appear friendly and nonjudgmental, but always stay alert for a potential violent outburst. If your patient is shouting or cursing, do not try to get him to stop or to lower his voice. Listen to what he says, not how he says it, and try to understand his situation before making a clinical judgment. Sometimes a genuine offer of a place to sit helps calm an agitated, intoxicated person. Then you can begin your assessment.

CRYING

Sometimes your patients will cry. This can make any EMT-I uncomfortable. Crying is just another form of venting, an important clue to your patient's emotions. Accept it as a natural release and do not try to suppress it. Be patient, allow your patient to cry, and then offer a supportive remark. Quiet acceptance and supportive remarks will open the lines of communication once your patient composes himself.

DEPRESSION

Depression is a common problem and is also frequently misdiagnosed or ignored. It often presents with symptoms such as insomnia, fatigue, weight loss, or mysterious aches and pains. Depression is potentially lethal, so you must recognize the signs and evaluate the severity just as you would chest pain or shortness of breath. Ask your patient if he has ever thought about committing suicide, if he is currently thinking about suicide, if he has the means to commit suicide, and if he has ever attempted it. The more exact and precise his suicide plan, the more likely he is to carry it out.

depression a mood disorder characterized by hopelessness and malaise.

SEXUALLY ATTRACTIVE OR SEDUCTIVE PATIENTS

Occasionally you will encounter a patient who is attracted to you or to whom you are attracted. These feelings are natural. The key is not to allow these feelings to affect your behavior. Always keep your relationship professional. If necessary, clearly tell any patient who behaves seductively that you are there on a professional basis, not a personal one. Afterward, determine if how you dressed, what you did, or what you said helped your patient get the wrong impression about your relationship. Did you send the wrong signals? Whenever possible, always have a partner with you to avoid any accusations of improper behavior or touching.

CONFUSING BEHAVIORS OR HISTORIES

You may encounter a patient whose story you just cannot follow. No matter what you ask, the answers leave you confused and frustrated. You cannot seem to develop a clear picture about your patient's problems. In fact, his answers do not even seem to make any sense. For example, you ask, "When did your headache begin?" and he answers, "My head feels like a squirrel." In these cases, the problem is most likely psychotic (mental illness) or organic (**dementia** or **delirium**). Also consider head injury or other physiological conditions such as stroke.

dementia a deterioration of mental status that is usually associated with structural neurological disease.

Many psychotic patients live and function in their communities, with varying degrees of success. Some will provide an accurate past history; others will not. If your patient's behavior seems distant, aloof, inappropriate, or even bizarre, suspect a mental illness such as schizophrenia. It may be helpful to focus your assessment on this patient's mental status, with special emphasis on thought, perceptions, and mood.

delirium an acute alteration in mental functioning that is often reversible.

Delirium and dementia are disorders relating to cognitive function. Delirium is common in the acutely ill or intoxicated patient; dementia occurs more frequently in the elderly. These patients often cannot provide clear, accurate histories. Their descriptions of their symptoms and their accounts of how things happened are vague and inconsistent. They may appear inattentive to your questions and hesitant in their answers. They may even make up stories to fill in the gaps in their memories. In these cases, do not spend too much time trying to get a detailed history, because you will only become more frustrated. Focus on the mental status exam, with special emphasis on level of response, orientation, and memory.

LIMITED INTELLIGENCE

You can usually obtain an adequate history from a patient with limited intelligence. Do not assume that he will not be able to provide accurate information concerning his current or past medical status. Also, do not overlook obvious omissions because your patient appears to be giving you a good story. Try to evaluate your patient's education and mental abilities. If you suspect severe mental retardation, obtain the patient's history from family or friends. Above all, show a genuine interest in your patient and try to establish a positive relationship. Then, communication can still happen.

LANGUAGE BARRIERS

Few things are more frustrating than responding to an automobile collision with several patients who speak a language you do not understand. It is almost impossible to get an accurate history of the event. In these cases, try to locate an interpreter. Sometimes a family member speaks both languages and is willing to translate for you. Often, however, family

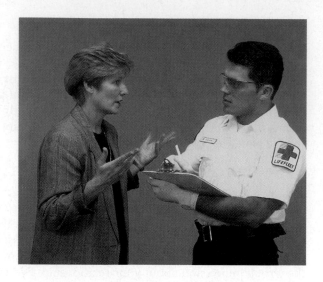

Figure 6-3 If the patient cannot provide useful information, gather it from family members or bystanders.

members cause more confusion by paraphrasing what the patient and you are saying. Instead of hearing your patient's exact words, you hear the translator's version, and the true meanings become vague. Do not waste time using your broken foreign language from high school, because you will invariably confuse everyone involved.

HEARING PROBLEMS

The challenge of communicating with a hearing-impaired person is much like that of overcoming a language barrier. Some options, however, afford a degree of flexibility. You can try handwritten questions, but they can be time consuming. Sign language is effective if the patient practices it and you find a proficient interpreter. If your patient reads lips, you must modify your communication techniques accordingly. Always face him directly in a well-lit setting, and speak slowly in a low-pitched voice. Avoid covering your mouth and trailing off the end of your sentences. If your patient has one good ear, use that to your advantage. If he wears a hearing aid, make sure it is working. If he has eyeglasses, make sure he wears them. Augment your speech with hand gestures and facial expressions.

BLINDNESS

Blind patients present special problems. They need you to identify yourself immediately, since they cannot see your uniform. Always announce yourself and explain who you are and why you are there. If possible, take your patient's hand to establish a personal contact and to show him where you are. Remember that nonverbal communications such as hand gestures, facial expressions, and body language are useless in these cases. Your voice is your only tool for effective communication.

TALKING WITH FAMILIES OR FRIENDS

You will often encounter patients who cannot give you any useful information. In these cases, find a third party who can augment the patient history and offer a useful adjunct to the patient's answers (Figure 6-3). The typical case is the postictal patient who cannot describe his seizure activity to you. Another example is learning from his friend that your patient's wife died in an automobile collision just three weeks ago. Now you better understand why your patient appears depressed and suicidal. Make sure that patient confidentiality is a priority when you accept personal information from a family member, friend, or bystander. Patient assessment is a comprehensive history and physical exam process.

SUMMARY

This chapter dealt with taking a good history. Although it presented the patient history in its entirety, common sense will determine which parts are appropriate for a given situation. Most of a prehospital care provider's work is patient contact. It is making a connection with people in crisis. Patients most often comment on the attitudes of their health-care providers. How well did they relate to them? Did they make them feel at ease? Did they care for them? Patients rarely comment on a caregiver's technical skills. Top-notch EMT-Is are technically skillful and treat all their patients with dignity and compassion. This begins with the history.

Good patient interaction can lead to good patient outcomes, improved patient satisfaction, and better adherence to treatment. As an EMT-I, you have the first opportunity to treat your patient when he enters the health-care environment. Let his first impression of the health-care industry be your caring, compassionate, professional demeanor. Conducting effective and efficient interviews and communicating with your patient are essential to good medical practice. Medical interviewing is a basic clinical skill that must be learned and practiced, much like airway management.

ON THE WEB

For additional practice and review, go to the companion website at www.prenhall.com/bledsoe and click on *Intermediate Emergency Care: Principles & Practice*.

Chapter 7

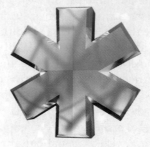

Techniques of Physical Examination

Objectives

After reading this chapter, you should be able to:

1. Define and describe the techniques of inspection, palpation, percussion, auscultation. (pp. 420–424)

2. Review the significance of and the procedures for taking vital signs. (pp. 424–427)

3. Describe the evaluation of mental status. (pp. 468–469)

4. Evaluate the importance of a general survey. (pp. 430–436)

5. Describe the examination of the following body regions, differentiate between normal and abnormal findings, and define the significance of abnormal findings:
   - skin, hair, and nails (pp. 436–437)
   - head, scalp, and skull (pp. 437–439)
   - eyes, ears, nose, mouth, and pharynx (pp. 439–443)
   - neck (pp. 443–445)
   - thorax (anterior and posterior) (pp. 445–450)
   - arterial pulse including rate, rhythm, and amplitude (pp. 449–450)
   - jugular venous pressure and pulsations (pp. 449–450)
   - heart (pp. 450–452)
   - abdomen (pp. 452–454)
   - male and female external genitalia (pp. 465–467)
   - peripheral vascular system (pp. 465–467)
   - extremities (pp. 454–462)
   - nervous system (pp. 467–472)

6. Describe the assessment of respiration and the characteristics of breath sounds. (pp. 424–426)

7. Describe percussion of the chest and differentiate among the percussion notes and their characteristics. (pp. 445–449)

8. Describe the general guidelines of recording examination information. (pp. 476–477)

9. Discuss the examination considerations for an infant or child. (pp. 472–476)

Case Study

The overnight crew at Station 51 tonight is EMT-Intermediate (EMT-I) Tony Morano and his EMT-Basic partner, Dan Lingwood. Early into their shift they are called to a "man-down" at Cirrincione's, a popular Italian restaurant featuring Sicilian cuisine. Also dispatched is a paramedic ambulance from a neighboring town. Upon arrival, Tony and his partner find Nick Scalisi, an agitated male in his early 70s who "just can't seem to stand up." Mr. Scalisi is alert and oriented. He complains of general weakness and of being unable to stand without wobbling or to walk a straight line.

Tony begins to elicit a history from Mr. Scalisi's wife. She claims he has been having these problems off and on for the past few days but that this is worse. Mr. Scalisi denies any chest pain, shortness of breath, dizziness, or nausea. His past history includes coronary artery disease, hypertension, and congestive heart failure. He takes nitroglycerin as needed, furosemide, aspirin, digoxin, captopril, and a potassium supplement. He and his wife have not yet eaten tonight. Tony tells his partner to get the stretcher and continues his assessment, which includes a focused physical exam and vital signs.

Because they have a 35-minute ride to McGivern General Hospital, Tony decides to perform a detailed physical exam en route. His patient appears to be an otherwise healthy 72-year-old man. He is well dressed and well groomed. His vital signs are blood pressure—150/86; heart rate—88, strong and regular; respirations—18; skin—warm, dry, and pink. Tony finds no evidence of head trauma. His patient's ears, nose, and throat are normal. He shows no facial drooping or slurred speech. His pupils are equal and reactive to light and accommodation. Extraocular muscles are intact. Tony notes nystagmus with his patient's left lateral gaze. His patient's trachea is midline, and his chest and abdomen appear normal. His distal extremities are warm and pink. His peripheral pulses are strong.

Tony decides to conduct a neurological examination. His patient's mental status is normal. He is alert and oriented to person, place, and time. His responses are appropriate and timely, and he does not drift off the topic or lose interest. His posture is somewhat slumped, and he has trouble maintaining his balance when standing. He also complains of difficulty buttoning his shirt. He has no tremors or fasciculations. His facial expressions are appropriate for the situation. His speech is inflected, clear and strong, fluent and articulate, and he can vary his volume. He expresses his thoughts clearly and speaks spontaneously with a clear and distinct voice. His present state of uncoordinated movement and imbalance agitates him, yet he organizes his thoughts and speaks logically and coherently.

Satisfied that Mr. Scalisi's mental status is normal, Tony continues with the motor function exam. Mr. Scalisi's general posture is slumped to the left. He has no tremors except at the very end of fine motor movements. His overall muscle bulk, tone, and strength appear normal.

Tony then asks his patient to perform a series of tests aimed at evaluating coordination. First, he asks him to tap the distal joint of his thumb with the tip of his index finger as rapidly as possible. Next, he asks him to place his hand palm-up on his thigh, quickly turn it over palm-down, and then repeat this movement as rapidly as possible for 15 seconds. Mr. Scalisi cannot perform these tests with his left hand. Nor can he perform point-to-point testing on his left side, and he has tremors at the far point. Finally, he cannot perform the heel-to-shin movement on his left side.

When the paramedic crew arrives, they are surprised at the completeness of the exam conducted by this crew. Concurring with Tony's field diagnosis of stroke, the paramedic contacts McGivern General Hospital and gives his report to Dr. Fullagar, a very impressed emergency physician. Computed tomography and magnetic resonance imaging results confirm a left cerebellar stroke.

INTRODUCTION

Patient assessment formally starts with the history, but the physical exam begins when you first set eyes on your patient.

Although assessment of a medical patient formally starts with the history, the physical examination actually begins when you first set eyes on your patient. Upon meeting him you immediately assess his general appearance, level of consciousness, breathing effort, and skin color. If you initially use touch as a reassuring gesture, you can also assess skin condition and peripheral pulses. Your physical assessment continues throughout the history as you ask questions and observe your patient's body language, facial expressions, and general demeanor. Thus, you cannot draw an exact dividing line between the history and the physical exam. In emergency street medicine, the two usually occur simultaneously.

This chapter presents more techniques of physical exam than you would ever use for a single patient. However, the purpose of the physical exam is to investigate areas that you suspect are involved in your patient's primary problem. On an emergency run, you limit the exam to only those aspects that you decide are appropriate. Practice and clinical experience will dictate your ability to apply the skills you learn in this section to real situations.

The purpose of the physical exam is to investigate areas that you suspect are involved in your patient's primary problem.

PHYSICAL EXAMINATION APPROACH AND OVERVIEW

EXAMINATION TECHNIQUES

Four techniques—inspection, palpation, auscultation, and percussion—are the foundation of the formal physical exam. Each can reveal information essential to a patient assessment.

Inspection

Content Review

PHYSICAL EXAM TECHNIQUES
- Inspection
- Palpation
- Percussion
- Auscultation

Inspection is the process of informed observation (Figure 7-1). A simple, noninvasive technique that clinicians often take for granted, it is also one of their most valuable tools in appraising patient condition. With a keen eye, you can evaluate your patient's condition in great detail.

Inspection begins when you first meet your patient and continues while you take his history. Often, this first impression forms the basis for your history because you will judge your patient's clinical status immediately. Notice how he presents himself. Is he conscious and alert or unconscious and flaccid? Is he lying on the floor, sitting upright, or limping badly

inspection process of informed observation.

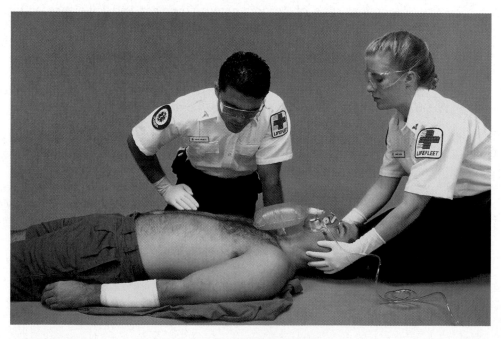

FIGURE 7-1 Inspect your patient's body for signs of injury or illness.

on one foot? Is he breathing normally or gasping for each breath? You can learn a great deal about your patient's neurological, musculoskeletal, and respiratory systems just by careful observation. Watch for changes in his emotional and mental status throughout the history and physical exam.

During the formal physical exam, consciously evaluate each body area, looking for discoloration, unusual motion, or deformity. Pay special attention to areas where you most expect to find signs and where the patient complains of symptoms. For example, if your patient struck his chest against a bent steering wheel, you would expect to see chest wall abnormalities. Remember that you may not notice the skin color changes that follow a significant contusion until after your patient arrives at the emergency department.

Effective inspection depends on good lighting, adequate time, and a curiosity for looking beyond the obvious. During your inspection, draw on your past clinical experiences to identify the signs of illness and injury. Knowing what you are looking for is essential. Do not hurry. Give yourself enough time to inspect and then to process what you see. Inspection is an ongoing process that should not end until you transfer your patient to emergency department staff. Finally, while respecting your patient's modesty and dignity, never allow clothing to obstruct your examination.

Palpation

Palpation is usually the next step in assessing your patient, although sometimes you will inspect and palpate your patient simultaneously. **Palpation** involves using your sense of touch to gather information. With your hands and fingers you can determine a structure's size, shape, and position. You also can evaluate its temperature, moisture, texture, and movement. You can check for growths, swelling, tenderness, spasms, rigidity, pain, and crepitus. When you become skilled at this procedure, you can detect a distended bladder, an enlarged liver, a laterally pulsating abdominal aorta, or the position of a fetus.

Certain parts of your hands and fingers are better than others for specific types of palpation. For example, the pads of your fingers are more sensitive than the tips for detecting position, size, consistency, masses, fluid, and crepitus; therefore, you would use them to palpate lymph nodes or rib fractures (Figure 7-2). The palm of your hand is better for sensing vibrations such as fremitus. Because its skin is thinner and more sensitive, the back of your hand or fingers is better for evaluating temperature.

palpation using your sense of touch to gather information.

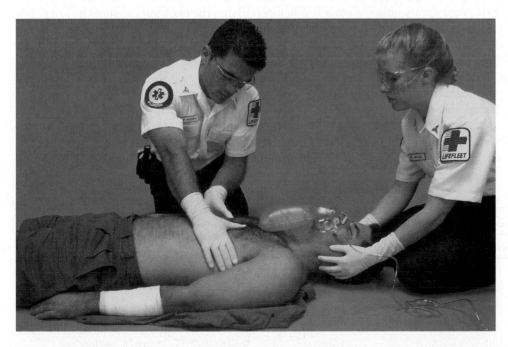

FIGURE 7-2 Palpate with the pads of your fingers to detect masses, fluids, and crepitus.

Palpation may be either deep or light. You control its depth by applying pressure with your hand and fingers. Since deep palpation may elicit tenderness or disrupt tissue or fluid, you should always perform light palpation first. Use light palpation to assess the skin and superficial structures. Press in approximately 1 centimeter. Apply the same gentle pressure you use to feel a pulse. Too much pressure dulls your sensitivity and can injure your patient.

To assess visceral organs such as those in the abdomen, use deep palpation. Apply pressure by placing the fingers of the opposite hand over the sensing fingers and gently pressing in about 4 centimeters. This will increase your sensitivity to any masses, guarding, or other abdominal pathology. Feel for areas of warmth that might reflect injury before significant edema or discoloration occur. Observe how your patient responds with facial expressions while you palpate tender areas. Even if he is unconscious, he may respond to pain with facial expressions or purposeful or purposeless motion.

Palpation begins your physical invasion of your patient. Three common sense tips will help make it therapeutic and respectful. Keep your hands warm, keep your fingernails short, and be gentle to avoid discomfort or injury to your patient.

To make palpation therapeutic and respectful, keep your hands warm, keep your fingernails short, and be gentle.

Percussion

percussion the production of sound waves by striking one object against another.

Percussion is the production of sound waves by striking one object against another. In this technique, you strike a knuckle on one hand with the tip of a finger on the opposite hand. The impact causes vibrations that produce sound waves from 4 to 6 centimeters deep in the underlying body tissue. We hear these sound waves as percussion tones. The density of the tissue through which the sound must travel determines the degree of percussion. The denser the medium, the quieter the tone. The tone's resonance or lack of resonance indicates whether the underlying region is filled with air, air under pressure, fluid, or normal tissue. Listen to each sound and evaluate its meaning (Table 7-1).

Move across the area that you are percussing and compare sounds with what you know to be normal there. For example, in the chest you expect to hear the resonant sound of a healthy lung filled with air and tissue. In a pneumothorax or emphysema, however, you may hear the hyperresonant sound of air trapped in the chest. In a hemothorax, you may hear the dull sound of blood in the same area.

Percussion is simple. Place one hand on the area of the body you wish to percuss. Use a finger of that hand (usually the middle finger) as the striking surface. Sharply tap the distal knuckle of that finger with the tip of your other middle finger (Figure 7-3). The tap should come from snapping the wrist, not the forearm or shoulder. Snap the finger back quickly to avoid dampening the sound. When percussing the chest, make sure the finger lies between the ribs and parallel to them. In this way you will percuss the tissue underneath the ribs, not the ribs themselves.

You must practice percussion on healthy people in order to recognize abnormalities in sick or injured patients.

A wall in your home is a good place to practice your percussion skills. As you percuss the air-filled area between wall studs, you will hear a hollow, resonant sound. Wall spaces filled with insulation will sound less resonant. When you percuss over a stud, you will notice a flatter, dull sound. You can apply this principle to the percussion of body cavities. Compare the sounds on the affected side with those on the unaffected side. The key is knowing what is normal, so above all you must practice percussion on healthy people in order to recognize abnormalities in sick or injured patients.

Table 7-1 PERCUSSION SOUNDS

Sound	Description	Intensity	Pitch	Duration	Location
Tympany	Drumlike	Loud	High	Medium	Stomach
Hyperresonance	Booming	Loud	Low	Long	Hyperinflated lung
Resonance	Hollow	Loud	Low	Long	Normal lung
Dull	Thud	Medium	Medium	Medium	Solid organs, liver
Flat	Extremely dull	Soft	High	Short	Muscle, atelectasis

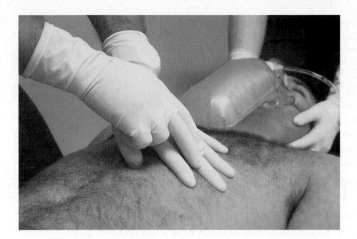

FIGURE 7-3 Percuss your patient to evaluate vibrations and sounds.

Unfortunately at most emergency scenes, especially those in the street, noise prevents percussing your patient effectively. Your clinical experience and common sense will tell you when to use this valuable assessment technique.

Auscultation

Auscultation involves listening for sounds produced by the body, primarily the lungs, the heart, the intestines, and major blood vessels. It is difficult to master. You may hear some sounds clearly, such as stridor, the high-pitched squeal of a partially obstructed upper airway. Most, however, require a stethoscope. You should perform auscultation in a quiet environment. Unfortunately, this is not always practical in emergency services. Hearing the low amplitude heart and lung sounds against on-scene noise or in-transit background noise may be especially difficult.

For your patient's comfort, warm the end piece of your stethoscope with your hands before auscultating. To auscultate, hold the end piece of your stethoscope between your second and third fingers and press the diaphragm firmly against your patient's skin (Figure 7-4). If you are using the bell side, place it evenly and lightly on the skin. Avoid touching the tubing with your hands or allowing it to rub any surfaces. Make sure the earpieces point anteriorly before you put them in your ears.

Listen for the presence of sound and its intensity, pitch, duration, and quality. When reporting and recording lung sounds, always note abnormal sounds (crackles, wheezes), their locations (bilateral, right lower lobe, bases), and their timing during the respiratory cycle (inspiratory, end-expiratory). Sometimes, closing your eyes helps you concentrate on the sounds by eliminating visual stimuli. Try to isolate and concentrate on one sound at a time. Generally, auscultate after you have used other assessment techniques. The only exception is the abdomen, which you should auscultate before palpation and percussion. An EMT-I should be proficient in auscultating blood pressure, lung sounds, and heart

auscultation listening with a stethoscope for sounds produced by the body.

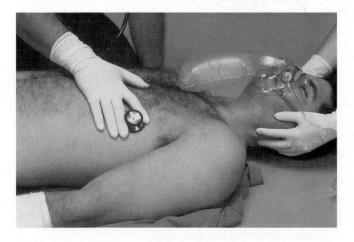

FIGURE 7-4 Auscultate body sounds with the stethoscope.

Measure vital signs early in the physical exam and, in emergency situations, repeat them often and look for trends.

Content Review

NORMAL ADULT VITAL SIGNS

- Pulse rate: 60–100
- Respiratory rate: 12–20
- Systolic BP ranges:
  –Male: 120–150
  –Female: 110–140 before menopause; 120–150 after menopause
- Body temperature: 98.6°F (37°C)

pulse rate number of pulses felt in 1 minute.

pulse rhythm pattern and equality of intervals between beats.

pulse quality strength, which can be weak, thready, strong, or bounding.

bradycardia pulse rate lower than 60.

tachycardia pulse rate higher than 100.

respiration exchange of oxygen and carbon dioxide in the lungs and at the cellular level.

respiratory rate number of times patient breathes in 1 minute.

tachypnea rapid breathing.

sounds. As with any other physical assessment tool, you cannot detect abnormalities unless you know what is normal. Take every opportunity to auscultate lung and heart sounds regularly.

Measurement of Vital Signs

The four basic vital signs in medicine are pulse, respiration, blood pressure, and body temperature. Although any complete physical examination should include all four, the first three are most important in prehospital care. They are the primary indicators of your patient's health. Measure them early in the physical examination and, in emergency situations, repeat them often and look for trends. For example, in a serious head injury, watch for your patient's systolic blood pressure to rise, his pulse pressure to widen, and his pulse rate to fall. These trends suggest an increase in intracranial pressure, a serious medical emergency. Conversely, a falling blood pressure with an increasing pulse rate may indicate shock. As an EMT-I, you should become an expert at taking vital signs on patients of every age.

Pulse   As the heart ejects blood through the arteries, a pulse wave results. Each pulse beat corresponds to a cardiac contraction and results from the ejected blood's impact on the arterial walls. The pulse is a valuable indicator of circulatory function. Your patient's pulse rate, rhythm, and quality indicate his hemodynamic (circulatory) status and the critical nature of his condition. **Pulse rate** refers to the number of pulsations felt in 1 minute. It can be slow (bradycardic), normal, or fast (tachycardic). **Pulse rhythm** refers to the pulse's pattern and the equality of intervals between beats. It can be regular, regularly irregular, or irregularly irregular. **Pulse quality** refers to the pulse's strength. Terms such as bounding or thready are used to describe the pulse's quality.

The normal pulse rate for an adult is 60 to 100 beats per minute. Rates below 60 are bradycardic; rates above 100 are tachycardic. **Bradycardia** may indicate an increase in parasympathetic nervous system stimulation. It might also be the result of a head injury, hypothermia, severe hypoxia, or drug overdose. Bradycardia is sometimes a normal finding in the well-conditioned athlete. Treat bradycardia only if it compromises your patient's cardiac output and general circulatory status. **Tachycardia** usually indicates an increase in sympathetic nervous system stimulation with which the body is compensating for another problem such as blood loss, fear, pain, fever, or hypoxia. It is an early indicator of shock and may indicate ventricular tachycardia, a life-threatening cardiac dysrhythmia.

The pulse's rhythm, when present, may be regular, regularly irregular, irregularly irregular, or grossly chaotic. Irregular pulse rates may be due to extra beats, skipped beats, or pacemaker problems and usually indicate a cardiac abnormality. The rhythm's effect on cardiac output determines if intervention is necessary.

The pulse's quality can be weak, strong, or bounding. Weak, thready pulses indicate a decreased circulatory status such as shock. Strong, bounding pulses may indicate high blood pressure, heat stroke, or increasing intracranial pressure. The pulse location may be another indicator of your patient's clinical status. The presence of a carotid pulse generally means that his systolic blood pressure is at least 60 mmHg. The presence of peripheral pulses indicates a higher blood pressure; their absence suggests circulatory collapse. Practice locating each of the pulse locations (Figure 7-5). As with other vital signs, take your patient's pulse frequently in the emergency setting and note any trends.

Respiration   Since oxygen and carbon dioxide exchange is essential to sustain life, **respiration** must occur continuously and must be effective. The lungs supply the arteries with oxygen and maintain the blood's pH by eliminating or retaining carbon dioxide. These two functions occur during respiration. Continuously observe your patient's respiratory rate, effort, and quality. Look for subtle signs of distress. Recognize when your patient requires rapid intervention such as aggressive airway management, positive pressure ventilation, and oxygenation. These interventions, some invasive, often make the difference between life and death.

Your patient's **respiratory rate** is the number of times he breathes in one minute. In general the normal respiratory rate for a healthy adult at rest is 12 to 20 breaths per minute. Rapid breathing (**tachypnea**) can be the result of hypoxia, shock, head injury, or anxiety.

Peripheral Pulse Sites

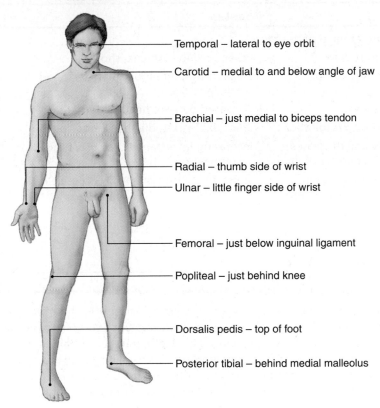

Temporal – lateral to eye orbit

Carotid – medial to and below angle of jaw

Brachial – just medial to biceps tendon

Radial – thumb side of wrist

Ulnar – little finger side of wrist

Femoral – just below inguinal ligament

Popliteal – just behind knee

Dorsalis pedis – top of foot

Posterior tibial – behind medial malleolus

FIGURE 7-5   Know each pulse location.

Slow breathing (**bradypnea**) can be caused by drug overdose, severe hypoxia, or central nervous system insult. Very rapid or very slow breathing rates require rapid intervention to ensure that the adequate exchange of gases continues.

Your patient's **respiratory effort** is how hard he works to breathe. Normal inhalation involves using the respiratory muscles (diaphragm and intercostals) to increase the chest's inner diameter. It is an active process that requires energy. The increasing space creates negative pressure, similar to a vacuum, that draws air into the lungs. Exhalation is the passive process of the respiratory muscles' elastic recoil. This normally effortless process can become difficult with some respiratory conditions. For example, an airway obstruction may compromise inhalation. The resultant increased breathing effort is evident in accessory muscle use, retractions, and possibly abnormal breath sounds.

Diseases such as asthma and emphysema, where the smaller airways collapse and trap air in the distal airways, may obstruct exhalation. Exhalation then becomes an active process that leads to respiratory distress and failure. Some injuries can decrease the respiratory effort. Rib fractures, for example, cause a decrease in chest wall expansion because it hurts to breathe. A pneumothorax decreases effective gas exchange because the air enters the pleural space instead of the alveoli. Children become tired and decrease their respiratory effort, making their condition even worse. Evaluating your patient's respiratory effort provides invaluable information about his respiratory status.

The **quality of respiration** refers to its depth and pattern. The depth, or **tidal volume**, of respiration is the amount of air your patient moves in and out of his lungs in one breath. The normal depth for a healthy adult at rest should be approximately 500 mL, just enough to cause the chest to rise. The tidal volume may increase during exercise or anxiety. It may decrease in the presence of a rib injury when every breath hurts.

Recognizing when your patient's respiration requires rapid intervention can make the difference between life and death.

bradypnea slow breathing.

respiratory effort how hard a patient works to breathe.

Very rapid or very slow breathing rates require rapid intervention to ensure that an adequate exchange of gases continues.

quality of respiration depth and pattern of breathing.

tidal volume amount of air one breath moves in and out of the lungs.

Table 7-2 BREATHING PATTERNS

	Condition	Description	Causes
∿∿∿∿	Eupnea	Normal breathing rate and pattern	
∿∿∿∿∿	Tachypnea	Increased respiratory rate	Fever, anxiety, exercise, shock
∼∼∼	Bradypnea	Decreased respiratory rate	Sleep, drugs, metabolic disorder, head injury, stroke
―――――	Apnea	Absence of breathing	Deceased patient, head injury, stroke
⋁⋀⋁⋀	Hyperpnea	Normal rate, but deep respirations	Emotional stress, diabetic ketoacidosis
⅏⎯⋀⋀⋀⎯⅏	Cheyne-Stokes	Gradual increases and decreases in respirations with periods of apnea	Increasing intracranial pressure, brain-stem injury
⋀⎯⋀⋀⎯⋀	Biot's	Rapid, deep respirations (gasps) with short pauses between sets	Spinal meningitis, many CNS causes, head injury
⋀⋀⋀⋀⋀⋀	Kussmaul's	Tachypnea and hyperpnea	Renal failure, metabolic acidosis, diabetic ketoacidosis
⌢⌢⌢⌢	Apneustic	Prolonged inspiratory phase with shortened expiratory phase	Lesion in brainstem

Assess your patient's respiratory depth by inspecting and palpating the chest wall for symmetrical chest expansion, by feeling and listening for air movement and noise from the nose and mouth, and by auscultating for lung sounds. The depth may be shallow, normal, or deep. Once again, you must know what is normal in order to recognize inadequate respiratory depth. The respiratory pattern should be regular. Variations in respiratory pattern can be associated with specific diseases (Table 7-2). Some irregular patterns such as Cheyne-Stokes may indicate serious brain or brain stem problems.

Blood Pressure   **Blood pressure** is the force of blood against the arteries' walls as the heart contracts and relaxes. It is equal to cardiac output times the systemic vascular resistance. Any alteration in the cardiac output or the vascular resistance will alter the blood pressure. An important indicator of your patient's condition, blood pressure is measured during both systole and diastole. **Systolic blood pressure** (the higher numerical value) measures the maximum force of blood against the arteries when the ventricles contract. **Diastolic blood pressure** (the lower numerical value) measures the pressure against the arteries when the ventricles relax and are filling with blood. The diastolic blood pressure is a measure of systemic vascular resistance and correlates well with changes in vessel size. The sounds of the blood hitting the arterial walls are called the **Korotkoff sounds.**

Many factors may influence your patient's blood pressure. Anxiety, for example, may cause it to rise. His position (sitting, lying, standing) also may affect the measurement. If your patient has recently been smoking, exercising, or eating, you must wait at least 5 to 10 minutes to allow his blood pressure to return to a resting level before you measure it. Because of these many intangibles, you should never use blood pressure as the single indicator of your patient's condition. Always correlate it with his other clinical signs of end-organ **perfusion** such as level of response, skin color, temperature, and condition, and peripheral pulses.

The average blood pressure in the healthy adult is 120/80. Females usually have a lower blood pressure until menopause. **Pulse pressure** is the difference between the systolic and diastolic pressures. For example, a blood pressure of 120/80 represents a pulse pressure of 40 mmHg. A normal pulse pressure is generally 30 to 40 mmHg. In certain conditions, such as pericardial tamponade or tension pneumothorax, the pulse pressure will narrow. In others, such as increasing intracranial pressure or fever, the pulse pressure will widen. Again, take your physiologically unstable patient's blood pressure as often as every 5 minutes to chart trends.

What is normal? This question has no easy answer. Generally, systolic blood pressure in adults ranges from 100 to 135 mmHg, diastolic from 60 to 80 mmHg. **Hypertension** in adults is defined as a pressure higher than 140/90. A blood pressure of 130/70, however,

blood pressure force of blood against artery walls as the heart contracts and relaxes.

systolic blood pressure force of blood against arteries when ventricles contract.

diastolic blood pressure force of blood against arteries when ventricles relax.

Korotkoff sounds sounds of blood hitting arterial walls.

perfusion passage of blood through an organ or tissue.

pulse pressure difference between systolic and diastolic pressures.

hypertension blood pressure higher than normal.

may represent hypertension if a patient's usual pressure is 90/60 or **hypotension** if his usual pressure is 170/90. The numbers are not as important as detecting trends and assessing end-organ perfusion. Do not define hypotension by numbers but by whether perfusion is adequate to sustain life.

Hypertension can result from cardiovascular disease, kidney disease, stroke, or head injury, where it is a classic sign of increasing intracranial pressure. It may be a predisposing factor to, and preexist in, stroke or cardiovascular disease. Did the hypertension occur before or after the condition? Hypotension usually indicates shock due to cardiac insufficiency (cardiogenic shock), low blood volume (hypovolemic shock), or massive vasodilation (vasogenic shock). Orthostatic hypotension is a decrease in your patient's blood pressure when he stands or sits up.

If you suspect shock due to blood or fluid volume loss and you do not suspect a spinal injury, perform a tilt test. Take your patient's pulse and blood pressure while he is supine. Then have him sit up and dangle his feet, then stand. In 30 to 60 seconds retake his vital signs. The healthy patient's vital signs should not change. The tilt test is positive either if his pulse rate increases 10 to 20 beats per minute or if his systolic blood pressure drops 10 to 20 mmHg. (Research has found that an increase in heart rate is a more sensitive indicator of hypovolemia than a decrease in systolic blood pressure.) This finding is common in patients suspected of hypovolemia.

Body Temperature   The body works hard to maintain a temperature of approximately 98.6°F (37°C). This temperature reflects the balance between heat production and heat loss through the skin and respiratory system. Even a slight variance can mean that significant events are happening within the body or on the body from environmental factors. Assess your patient's temperature to approximate his internal core temperature.

An increase in body temperature (**hyperthermia**) can result from environmental extremes, infections, drugs, or metabolic processes. Ordinarily the body's cooling mechanisms maintain a steady core temperature. In an extremely hot and humid environment or in cases such as heat stroke, the cooling mechanisms can fail and the core temperature can rise despite an internal thermostat that wants to maintain a normal temperature. Fever, on the other hand, results when the body tries to make its internal environment inhospitable to invading organisms. It often presents with a history of illness. The skin is somewhat dry until the fever breaks and the body's cooling mechanisms begin to take effect. As the body temperature rises, it begins to threaten body processes, specifically those of the brain. A temperature of up to 102°F (38°C) increases metabolism markedly. As body temperature rises above 103°F (39°C), the neurons of the brain may denature. At temperatures above 105°F (41°C), brain cells die and seizures may occur.

Extreme cold also affects body temperature. When peripheral vasoconstriction and shivering mechanisms can no longer balance heat production and loss, core temperature drops (**hypothermia**). At a body temperature of 93°F (34°C), normal body warming mechanisms begin to fail. As the core temperature drops below 90°F (31°C), shivering stops, heart sounds diminish and cardiac irritability increases. If the temperature drops much below 70°F (22°C), your patient will present with a deathlike appearance and, possibly, irreversible asystole (absence of heartbeat).

A variety of methods can provide accurate temperature readings. You can use glass thermometers to take oral, rectal, or axillary temperatures. A rectal thermometer is the preferred device for children younger than six years old and for patients with an altered level of consciousness. An axillary temperature reading is the least accurate of the three methods.

EQUIPMENT

To conduct a comprehensive physical examination, you will need a stethoscope, a sphygmomanometer, a penlight, tongue blades, and other equipment.

Stethoscope

The **stethoscope** is a basic tool used to auscultate most sounds (Figure 7-6). It transmits sound waves from the source through an end piece and along rubber tubes to the ear. One

---

hypotension blood pressure lower than normal.

Never use blood pressure as the single indicator of your patient's condition. Always correlate it with other clinical signs of end-organ perfusion.

Even a slight variance in body temperature can mean that significant events are happening within the body.

hyperthermia increase in body's core temperature.

hypothermia decrease in body's core temperature.

Content Review

PHYSICAL EXAM EQUIPMENT
- Stethoscope
- Sphygmomanometer
- Penlight
- Tongue blades
- Battery-operated thermometer

stethoscope tool used to auscultate most bodily sounds.

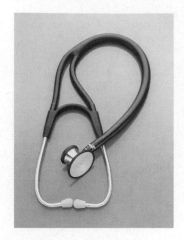

FIGURE 7-6 Use a stethoscope to auscultate most sounds.

side of the end piece is a rigid diaphragm that best transmits high-pitched sounds such as heart sounds and blood pressure sounds. The diaphragm also screens out low-pitched sounds such as lung sounds and bowel sounds. The other side of the end piece is a bell that uses the skin as a diaphragm. The sounds that the bell transmits vary with the amount of pressure exerted. For example, with light pressure the bell picks up low-pitched sounds; with firm pressure it acts like the diaphragm and transmits high-pitched sounds. Whether you use the bell or the diaphragm depends on which sounds you are auscultating. To hear blood pressure or heart sounds, for instance, use the diaphragm; to hear lung sounds, use the bell side.

Accurate auscultation depends in part on the quality of your instrument. Your stethoscope should have the following important characteristics:

- Rigid diaphragm cover
- Thick, heavy tubing that conducts sound better than thin, flexible tubing
- Short tubing (30 to 40 cm) to minimize distortion
- Earpieces that fit snugly—large enough to occlude the ear canal—and are angled toward the nose to project sound toward the eardrum
- Bell with a rubber-ring edge to ensure good contact with the skin

Sphygmomanometer

The circumstances and the patient care setting determine what type of equipment you use to measure blood pressure (Figure 7-7). Intensive care unit staff commonly use intra-arterial

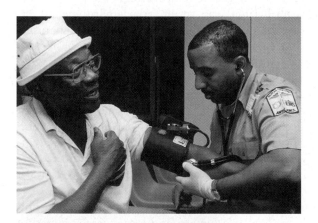
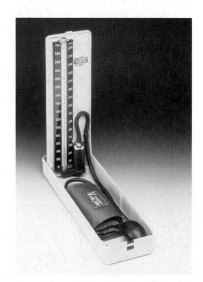
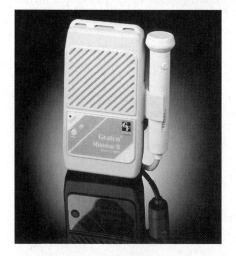
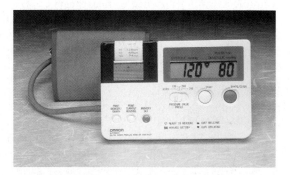

FIGURE 7-7 Use a blood pressure device suited to the circumstances. Clockwise from upper left: aneroid sphygmomanometer; mercury sphygmomanometer; digital electronic, and Doppler device.

pressure devices for critically ill patients who need continuous monitoring. When a noisy environment makes auscultation difficult or when the sounds are especially weak, a Doppler device that amplifies the sounds is useful. You will see these devices in the emergency department, newborn nursery, emergency vehicles, and labor and delivery suites. The most familiar blood-pressure measuring device is the aneroid **sphygmomanometer.** You will use it with your stethoscope to auscultate the sounds of the blood moving through an artery, usually the brachial artery. Because your patient's blood pressure is important in evaluating his condition, you must be able to measure it accurately.

A sphygmomanometer includes a bulb, a cuff, and a manometer. The cuff has an airtight, flat, rubber bladder enclosed within a fabric cover. Cuffs are available in various sizes and designs. Flexible tubing attaches the rubber bulb to the cuff. Squeezing the bulb pumps air into the cuff's bladder. A control valve allows you to inflate and deflate the cuff. To inflate the cuff, close the valve by turning it clockwise; to deflate the cuff, open the valve by turning it counterclockwise.

The **manometer** is a pressure gauge with a scale calibrated in millimeters of mercury (mmHg). Each line represents 2 mmHg. The heavy lines are 10 mmHg of mercury apart. The aneroid manometer displays the scale on a circular dial. As the pressure in the bladder changes, the needle moves and indicates the pressure reading at a given moment. When you use an aneroid sphygmomanometer, keep the dial in plain sight. The aneroid types lose their calibration, so you will need to calibrate them periodically against a mercury-type device.

The mercury sphygmomanometer displays the scale along a glass tube connected to a reservoir of mercury. As pressure in the cuff increases, the mercury in the tube rises. When using a mercury sphygmomanometer, keep the scale at eye level and vertical. Available as portable, wall-mounted, or floor units, mercury sphygmomanometers are more accurate than aneroid, but they are impractical for prehospital use.

Additional Equipment

Besides the above items, you will need sterile tongue blades to inspect inside the mouth and to initiate a gag reflex, a penlight to test your patient's pupillary responses, and a thermometer to measure body temperature. The danger of breakage limits the usefulness of a glass thermometer in the prehospital setting. In addition, a glass thermometer's inability to record temperatures below 96°F (36°C) prevents it from helping you evaluate the hypothermic patient. Available battery-operated devices measure temperature orally, rectally, and in the ear canal. If your service operates in areas of low environmental temperatures, equip your ambulance with a low-reading thermometer.

THE GENERAL APPROACH

How you approach your patient can set the stage for an efficient and effective patient assessment. Most patients are apprehensive about a physical examination. They feel exposed and vulnerable, and they fear painful procedures. This anxiety is multiplied in an emergency. You must recognize your patient's apprehension and take steps to alleviate it. Display confidence and skill while you complete your history and physical exam.

If you systematically assess your patient's complaints and efficiently perform your duties, he should feel safe. Then add the personal touches of active listening, a reassuring voice, and gestures that convey your sincere compassion and interest. Most patients will respond favorably. Let your patient know that you are not just checking off items on a diagnostic list; you are conducting a personal examination of his problems.

Proficiency will come only with clinical practice. In time, you will become adept at focusing the exam on your patient's chief complaint and present illness. In the emergency setting, no matter how nervous and apprehensive you may be, never let your patient see anything but a calm, professional, confident demeanor. This will help alleviate his anxiety about disclosing personal information to, and being examined by, a nonphysician. Try to remain objective, even when confronted by alarming or disgusting information. A bad bed sore, a perverted sexual story, or black tarry stools (melena) can test even the most experienced clinician's composure. Simply thinking about how embarrassed your patient must be may help you keep your composure.

sphygmomanometer blood pressure measuring device composed of a bulb, cuff, and manometer.

Because your patient's blood pressure is important in evaluating his condition, you must be able to measure it accurately.

manometer pressure gauge with a scale calibrated in millimeters of mercury (mmHg).

How you approach your patient, both in the emergency setting and elsewhere, can set the stage for an efficient and effective patient assessment.

OVERVIEW OF A COMPREHENSIVE EXAMINATION

The key to an effective, comprehensive exam is integrating each individual section into a unified patient assessment.

This section gives an overview of a physical exam. Later in the chapter each component will be described in detail. The key to an effective comprehensive exam is to integrate each individual section into a unified patient assessment. (Chapter 8 provides a template for conducting a problem-oriented patient assessment on both medical and trauma patients.)

As an EMT-I, you will determine which physical exam techniques to use. You will base your decision on your patient's presenting problem and clinical status. For example, if you are assessing a child just struck by an automobile and lying unconscious in the street, you will narrow your focus to the child's injuries. A physical examination should include a general survey and a detailed assessment of anatomical regions.

THE GENERAL SURVEY

A general survey is the first part of a physical examination. It begins with noting your patient's appearance and goes on to include vital signs and other assessments.

Appearance

A thorough evaluation of your patient's appearance can provide a great deal of valuable information about his health. Note his level of consciousness, posture, and any obvious signs of distress, such as sitting upright gasping for each breath or slumped to one side. Is his motor activity normal or does he have noticeable tremors or paralysis? Observe his general state of health, his dress, grooming, and personal hygiene. Obvious odors can also furnish significant information.

Level of Consciousness Is your patient awake? Is he alert? Does he speak to you in a normal voice? Are his eyes open and does he respond to you and others in the environment? If he is not apparently awake, speak to him in a loud voice. If he does not respond to your verbal cues, shake him gently. If he still does not respond, apply a painful stimulus such as pinching a tendon, rubbing his sternum, or rolling a pencil across a nail bed. Note his response.

Signs of Distress Is your patient in distress? For example, does he have a cardiac or respiratory problem, as evidenced by labored breathing, wheezing, or a cough? Is he in pain, as evidenced by wincing, sweating, or protecting the painful area? Is he anxious, as evidenced by his facial expression, cold moist palms, or nervous fidgeting?

Content Review

GENERAL SURVEY

- Appearance
- Vital signs
- Additional assessments:
  - Pulse oximetry
  - Cardiac monitoring
  - Blood glucose determination

Cultural Considerations

The physical examination process often includes viewing parts of the body generally shielded from the view of strangers. Because of this, some patients may be particularly sensitive about revealing various aspects of the body to a stranger—even an EMT.

The way in which you approach a patient for physical assessment must take into consideration the patient's cultural beliefs. In some cultures, especially certain Arab cultures, it is forbidden for a woman to reveal her face or body to a man who is not her husband. This constraint certainly makes a detailed physical exam difficult. Sometimes, in fact, an examination cannot be completed because of patient refusal. In some instances, an examination may only be allowed if the examiner is of the same gender as the patient. Likewise, seemingly innocent comments by rescuers—such as "You have a pretty face. Let me take a look at your head"—can be insulting or even offensive. It implies that flattery can convince them to consent to something that is not allowed by their culture, religion, or both.

If you work in an area where there is considerable cultural diversity, it is important to understand the cultural beliefs and practices of the groups you may encounter. More importantly, you must respect these cultural beliefs and, in turn, the patients will respect you.

Apparent State of Health   Is your patient healthy, robust, and vigorous? Or is he frail, ill-looking, or feeble? Does he have an obvious abnormality? Base your evaluation of his general state of health on your observations throughout the interview and physical examination.

Vital Statistics   Vital statistics, weight and height, are used widely in clinical medicine. Accurately measuring your patient's weight and height with a scale, however, is not a practical prehospital assessment procedure. You will occasionally estimate your patient's weight to administer medications of which the dose is weight dependent. You also may use a **Broselow tape** to measure your infant patient's length. The Broselow tape provides information concerning drug dosages, airway management adjuncts, and intravenous calculations based on your patient's height.

vital statistics height and weight.

Note your patient's general stature. Is he lanky and slender, short and stocky, muscular and symmetrical? Does he have any obvious deformities or disproportionate areas? Is he extremely thin or obese? If obese, is the fat evenly distributed or is it concentrated in his trunk? Has he gained or lost weight recently?

Broselow Tape a measuring tape for infants that provides important information about airway equipment and medication doses based on the patient's length.

Skin Color and Obvious Lesions   Is your patient's skin pale, suggesting decreased blood flow or anemia? Does he have central (lips, oral mucosa) or peripheral (nail beds, hands) cyanosis, the bluish color resulting from decreased oxygenation of the tissues? Does he have the yellow color of jaundice or high carotene levels? Note any rashes, bruises, scars, or discoloration.

Posture, Gait, and Motor Activity   Observe your patient's posture and presentation. Is he sitting straight up and forward, bracing his arms (tripodding)? This suggests a serious breathing problem such as acute pulmonary edema or airway obstruction. Does one side of his body droop and seem immobile, suggesting a stroke? Does he sit quietly or does he seem restless? Does he have tremors or other involuntary movements?

Dress, Grooming, and Personal Hygiene   Does your patient dress appropriately for the climate and situation? Are his clothes clean and properly fastened? Are they conventional for his age and social group? Abnormalities in dress might suggest the cold intolerance of hypothyroidism or the hiding of a skin rash or needle marks, or they might simply reflect personal preference. Look at his shoes. Are they clean? Do they have holes, slits, open laces, or other alterations to accommodate painful foot conditions such as gout, bunions, or edema? Does he wear a slipper, or slippers, instead of shoes? Is he wearing unusual jewelry such as a copper bracelet for arthritis or a medical information tag? Do his grooming and hygiene seem appropriate for his age, lifestyle, occupation, and social status? Does his lack of concern over appearance (overgrown nails and hair, for instance) suggest a long illness or depression?

Odors of Breath or Body   Does your patient have any unusual or striking body or breath odors? The acetone breath of a diabetic, the bitter-almond breath of a cyanide poisoning, the putrid smell of bacterial infection, or the obvious smell of alcohol may give important clues to the underlying problem. Avoid tunnel vision when you smell alcohol, which often masks other serious illnesses such as liver failure or injuries such as a subdural hematoma.

Facial Expression   Watch your patient's facial expressions throughout your interaction. His face should reflect his emotions during the interview and physical exam. The patient with hyperthyroidism may stare intently. The Parkinson's patient's face may appear immobile.

Vital Signs

Take a complete set of vital signs to include pulse, respiration, blood pressure, and temperature.

Pulse   To take the pulse of a conscious adult or large child, the most accessible and commonly used location is the radial artery. With the pads of your first two or three fingers, compress the radial artery onto the radius, just below the wrist on the thumb side (Procedure 7-1a). In the unconscious patient, begin by checking his carotid pulse. To locate the carotid pulse, palpate medial to and just below the angle of the jaw. Locate the thyroid cartilage

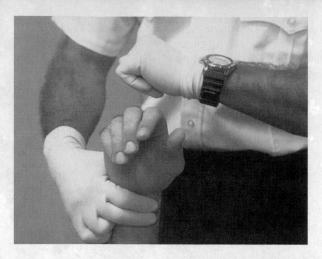

7-1a Assess the pulse as an indicator of circulatory function.

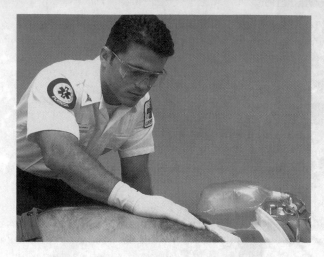

7-1b Count your patient's respirations.

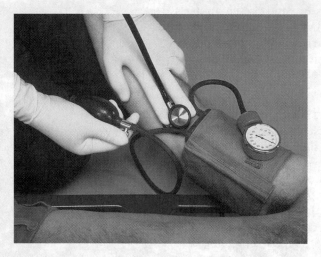

7-1c Assess blood pressure with a sphygmomanometer and stethoscope.

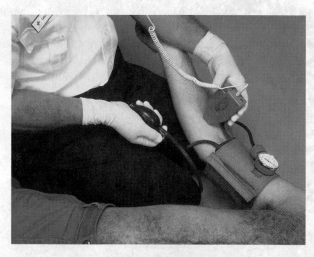

7-1d If you cannot hear blood pressure with a stethoscope, use an ultrasonic Doppler.

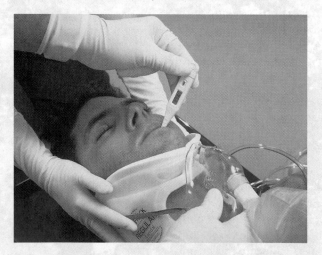

7-1e Use a battery-operated oral thermometer to take your patient's temperature.

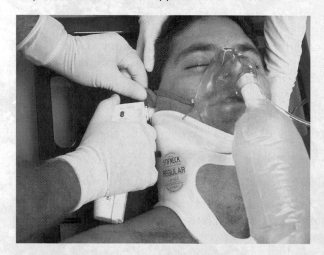

7-1f Use a specially designed, battery-operated thermometer to measure temperature inside the ear.

(Adam's apple) and slide your fingers laterally until they are between the thyroid cartilage and the large muscle in the neck (sternocleidomastoid). In infants and small children, use the brachial artery or auscultate for an apical pulse. Remember that auscultating an apical pulse does not provide information about your patient's hemodynamic status. To locate the brachial artery, feel just medial to the biceps tendon. Auscultate the apical pulse just below the left nipple. First, note your patient's pulse rate by counting the number of beats in 1 minute. If his pulse is regular, you can count the beats in 15 seconds and multiply that number by four. If his pulse is irregular, you must count it for a full minute to obtain an accurate total. Note also the pulse's rhythm and quality.

Respiration   To measure your patient's respiratory rate, place one hand on your patient's chest and count the breaths he takes in thirty seconds (Procedure 7-1b). Multiply that number by two. Because your patient may consciously or subconsciously control his breathing, try to evaluate it without his knowing. Also assess his respiratory effort and quality of respiration.

Blood Pressure   To measure your patient's blood pressure, first choose the arm you will use. Remove any clothing that covers the upper arm; do not take the blood pressure over clothing, if possible. Look for a dialysis shunt in patients with renal failure. Do not take a blood pressure in that arm. Place the arm in a slightly flexed position, palm up and fingers relaxed. Support the upper arm at the level of your patient's heart.

Use the correct size cuff to obtain an accurate measurement. Its width should be one-half to one-third the circumference of your patient's arm. For most adults, unless they are obese or extremely slim, the large size cuff (15-cm wide) will suffice. If your patient has an obese arm, use a larger cuff. If the larger cuff is still too small, use your patient's forearm and place your stethoscope over the radial artery. For all patients, use a cuff that covers approximately two thirds of his upper arm or thigh. Using a cuff that is too wide, too narrow, too long, or too short will result in an inaccurate measurement.

Turn the control valve counterclockwise to open it; squeeze all the air out of the bladder before applying the cuff. Locate the brachial artery by palpating on the medial side of the antecubital space until you feel a pulse. Place the lower edge of the cuff one inch above the antecubital space. Find the center of the bladder (usually marked on the cuff with an arrow) and place it directly over the artery. Fasten the cuff so it is smooth and fits tightly enough to obtain an accurate reading. If you have difficulty inserting a finger between the cuff and your patient's arm, it is snug enough. Also make sure the rubber tubing is clear of the cuff. Check the placement of the manometer so you can see it easily.

Now palpate the radial artery. With your other hand, turn the control valve completely clockwise and squeeze the bulb rapidly to inflate the cuff to approximately 30 mmHg over the point where the radial pulse disappears. Place your stethoscope directly over the brachial artery and hold it firmly in place without pressing on the artery (Procedure 7-1c). Turn the control valve counterclockwise slowly and steadily to deflate the cuff at a rate of 2 to 3 mmHg per heart beat. Deflating too slowly or too rapidly causes an inaccurate reading.

As you slowly deflate the cuff, watch the manometer and listen for the Korotkoff sounds. When you hear the first pulse beat, note the reading on the manometer dial or mercury column. This is the systolic pressure. Continue deflating the cuff until the pulsations diminish or become muffled. This is the diastolic pressure.

If you do not obtain a reading, wait 30 seconds to allow the blood pressure to normalize before inflating the cuff again. Sometimes you can palpate the artery during the deflation. The point at which you feel the pulse return marks the systolic reading. You cannot evaluate the diastolic pressure with the palpation method. To take your patient's blood pressure with a Doppler, follow the same procedure as for the palpation method, but instead of palpating for the return of the pulse, place the Doppler device over the palpated artery and listen for the "whooosh" of flowing blood indicating the systolic measurement (Procedure 7-1d). Record the blood pressure on your patient's chart. Include the systolic and diastolic pressures (for instance, 134/78), the arm used (right or left), and your patient's position (lying, sitting, or standing).

Temperature The type of glass thermometer you use determines how long you must leave it in place to get an accurate reading. To take your patient's temperature orally with a glass thermometer, place the thermometer under his tongue for at least 3 to 4 minutes. It may provide a false reading if your patient has swallowed liquid or smoked within 15 to 30 minutes. To use a rectal thermometer, lubricate it well and then insert it 1 1/2 inches into the rectum; leave it in place for at least 2 to 3 minutes. If you use an axillary thermometer, it must remain under your patient's armpit at least 10 minutes. If your service uses battery-operated devices, become familiar with them and follow the manufacturer's instructions for their use (Procedure 7-1e). For example, when using the tympanic membrane device, place the speculum into the ear canal, push the button and hold it for 2 to 3 seconds, then remove the device (Procedure 7-1f). The temperature is then displayed on a digital readout.

Additional Assessment Techniques

Additional assessment techniques include pulse oximetry, cardiac monitoring, and blood glucose determination.

Pulse Oximetry The **pulse oximeter** is a noninvasive device that measures the oxygen saturation of your patient's blood. It can reliably indicate your patient's cardiorespiratory status because it may tell you how well he is oxygenating the most peripheral vessels of his circulatory system. It also quantifies the effectiveness of your interventions such as oxygen therapy, medications, suctioning, and ventilatory assistance. For example, on room air, your patient's reading is 92%; after two minutes of high-flow, high-concentration oxygen therapy, it is 99%, showing a definite improvement.

The pulse oximeter has a probe-sensor and a monitoring unit with digital readouts. Attach the probe-sensor clip to your patient's finger, toe, or earlobe (Figure 7-8). The probe directs two lights (one red and one infrared) through a small area of tissue. The lights penetrate the tissue and are absorbed. Since saturated and desaturated hemoglobin absorb the lights differently, the sensors can determine their individual concentrations. The result is a measurement of your patient's oxygen saturation, or SaO_2.

Normal oxygen saturation at sea level should be between 96% and 100%. Generally, if the reading is below 95%, suspect shock, hypoxia, or respiratory compromise. Provide your patient with the appropriate airway management and supplemental oxygen and watch him carefully for further changes. Any reading below 90% requires aggressive airway management, positive pressure ventilation, or oxygen administration. The unresponsive patient may require invasive airway management and positive pressure ventilation.

Several factors affect the accuracy of a pulse oximetry reading. The sensors can accurately measure the oxygen saturation only if blood flow through the tissue is adequate. Most pulse oximeters display a digital readout of the pulse rate; others display a pulsation wave. In either case, if the display does not match your patient's actual pulse, the SaO_2 reading will be erratic. If your patient has decreased blood flow through the tissue, as in hypovolemia or hypothermia, you will obtain a false reading.

pulse oximeter noninvasive device that measures the oxygen saturation of blood.

FIGURE 7-8 Pulse oximetry allows you to determine quickly and accurately your patient's oxygenation status.

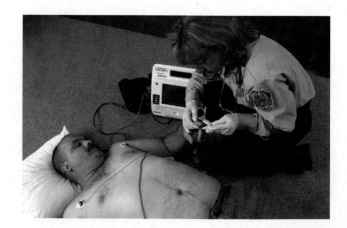

In cases of carbon monoxide (CO) poisoning, your saturation readings will be high while your patient's tissues are severely ischemic. This is because the CO molecule saturates the hemoglobin molecule 200 times more easily than does oxygen and the pulse oximetry probe cannot distinguish between hemoglobin that is bound to carbon monoxide and hemoglobin that is bound to oxygen. Your patient's hemoglobin is in fact saturated, but with carbon monoxide, not oxygen. Other than these limitations, the pulse oximeter, when teamed with other patient assessment techniques, can be a useful tool in the prehospital setting.

Cardiac Monitoring   The **cardiac monitor** is essential in assessing and managing the patient who requires advanced cardiac life support (ACLS) (Figure 7-9). The simplest prehospital machines monitor the electrical activity of the heart in three "leads" or positions. These "limb leads" adequately identify life-threatening cardiac rhythms. Also available for paramedic use are twelve-lead ECGs. They are essential in gathering data to confirm a myocardial infarction.

> **cardiac monitor** machine that displays and records the electrical activity of the heart.

Other features of cardiac monitors include pacing capabilities and the "quick-look" paddles and the "hands-off" defibrillation pads used in cardiac arrest. The paddles, which are placed on the patient's chest, allow you to check the cardiac rhythm and deliver a rapid electrical countershock. The hands-off defibrillation pads have two large electrodes that you attach to the chest wall. These replace the paddles and allow you to deliver a countershock without fear of injuring yourself.

All monitor-defibrillators can deliver a synchronized countershock in the presence of an unstable tachycardia. Most have a transcutaneous pacemaker that is placed externally on the chest and provides an electrical impulse to stimulate cardiac contraction in cases of bradycardia and heart blocks. This is a temporary measure until a permanent pacemaker can be implanted. Finally, some ECG machines have a "code summary" feature that prints out the electrical record of events and their times. This helps you document your patient's progress while in your care.

The cardiac monitor is a useful tool for measuring electrical activity, but it has one major disadvantage. It cannot tell you if the heart is pumping efficiently, effectively, or at all. The ECG reading does not necessarily correlate with the mechanical function of the heart. Electrical activity can exist with no mechanical contraction. Always assess your patient and compare what you see on the monitor with the rate and quality of the pulse.

> *Always compare what you see on a cardiac monitor with what you feel for a pulse.*
>
>

Blood Glucose Determination   In cases of altered mental status due to diabetic emergencies, seizures, and strokes, you will want to measure your patient's blood glucose level. The arrival of inexpensive, handheld **glucometers** makes this test easy to perform in the field. Most diabetic patients do it several times each day at home by themselves.

> **glucometer** tool used to measure blood glucose level.

To perform this procedure you will need a glucometer with test strips, a finger stick device with sterile lancets, alcohol wipe, and tissue or gauze pads. Simply place a drop of your patient's capillary blood from a finger stick onto a chemical reagent strip (Figure 7-10). Following the manufacturer's instructions, place the test strip in the glucometer and wait for the reading to appear. This procedure takes less than 1 minute to perform.

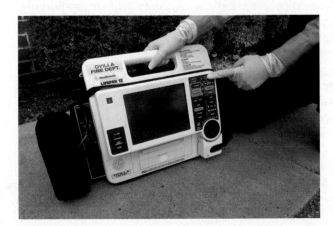

FIGURE 7-9   The cardiac monitor is essential to managing advanced cardiac life support.

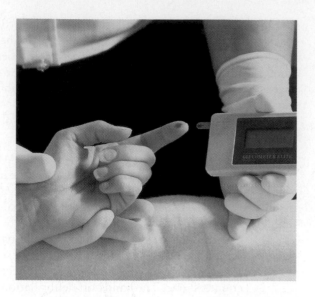

FIGURE 7-10 Use a glucometer to determine your patient's blood glucose.

Since all glucometers work differently, you must read the manufacturer's instructions carefully. The slightest mistake can alter the measurement's accuracy. For example, make sure the code numbers on the test strips match those on the digital reading. Also make sure you do not allow alcohol to contaminate the blood. Glucometers are moderately accurate when used properly and calibrated daily.

ANATOMICAL REGIONS

After you complete the general survey, you will examine the body regions and systems in more detail. Again, the specific situation and your experience and common sense will determine whether you conduct a thorough examination, as you would when performing physicals for an insurance company, or narrow the focus of your examination, as you might in an emergency setting.

SKIN

Although you will observe your patient's skin throughout your assessment, a comprehensive physical exam must also include a concentrated inspection of all areas of the skin. The skin provides data on a variety of systemic problems in addition to skin-related disorders. Examining the skin requires good light and a keen eye. The characteristics of normal skin vary with your patients' racial, ethnic, and familial backgrounds. Evaluate its color, moisture, temperature, texture, mobility and turgor, and any lesions. Always wear protective gloves if your patient has any areas of open skin, exudative lesions, or rashes.

Color Normal skin color in light-skinned people is pink, indicating adequate cardiorespiratory function and vascular integrity. This means that the capillaries in the skin are well oxygenated. The bright red oxyhemoglobin in the oxygen-rich blood circulating through the capillary beds gives the epidermis its pink appearance. A pale color suggests decreased blood flow through the skin. This is typical in hypothermia, hypovolemia, and compensatory shock, where blood flow through the distal capillary beds is severely diminished. It also is common in anemia, in which your patient's red blood cell count is low. As the hemoglobin loses its oxygen to the tissues, it changes to the darker, blue deoxyhemoglobin. Increased deoxyhemoglobin causes cyanosis, a bluish skin color. Cyanosis means that less oxygen is available at the tissue level.

Evaluate skin color where the epidermis is thinnest. This includes the fingernails and lips and the mucous membranes of the mouth and conjunctiva. In dark-skinned people, evaluate the sclera, conjunctiva, lips, nail beds, soles, and palms. Note any discoloration caused by vascular changes underneath the skin. *Petechiae* are small, round, flat, purplish spots caused by capillary bleeding from a variety of etiologies. *Ecchymosis* is a blue-black bruise resulting from trauma or bleeding disorders. Jaundice first appears in the sclera and then, in the late stages of liver disease, all over the skin. If only your patient's palms, soles, and face are yellow, he may have *carotanemia,* a harmless nutritional condition caused by eating a diet high in carrots and yellow vegetables or fruits.

Moisture Inspect and palpate the skin for dryness, increased sweating, and excessive oiliness. Dry skin, common during the cold winter months and in the elderly, may be the result of other conditions. Excessive oiliness, especially where the sebaceous glands are concentrated in the face, neck, back, chest, and buttocks, may suggest acne or hyperthyroidism. Increased sweating may indicate a sympathetic nervous system response to anxiety, fear, or exertion.

Temperature Use the backs of your fingers to feel the skin temperature in several different locations. Compare symmetrical body areas. Generalized warming or cooling suggests an environmental, infectious, or thyroid problem. Localized warmth may indicate bleeding or swelling.

Texture Feel your patient's skin. Is it rough or smooth? Are there large patches or small areas of scaling? Observe the skin's thickness. Thin and fragile skin is a sign of debilitating disease in the elderly. Thick skin often occurs with eczema and psoriasis. Inspect the palms and soles for calluses.

Mobility and Turgor Test the skin's **turgor** and elasticity by picking up a fold of skin over a bony prominence and then releasing it. Normal skin immediately returns to its original state. Poor turgor (tenting) results from dehydration. Test the skin's mobility by moving it over the bony prominence. Decreased mobility suggests edema or scleroderma, a progressive skin disease.

turgor normal tension in the skin.

Lesions A skin **lesion** is any disruption in normal tissue. Skin lesions can take any shape, color, or arrangement. Note their anatomical location and distribution. Are they generalized or localized? Do they involve exposed surfaces or areas that fold over? Do they relate to possible irritants such as wristbands, bracelets, or necklaces? Are they linear, clustered, circular, or dermatomal (following a sensory nerve pathway)? What type are they? Inspect and feel all skin lesions carefully.

lesion any disruption in normal tissue.

   When you detect a skin lesion, use anatomical landmarks to describe its exact location on the skin's surface. Describe its shape in terms such as oval, spherical, irregular, or tubular. Sometimes sketching an outline of the lesion is helpful. Record the size of the mass in centimeters, carefully measuring its length, width, and depth. Describe the consistency of the mass exactly as it feels to you (for instance, soft, firm, edematous, cystic, or nodular). Of particular concern is its mobility. If the mass is affixed to a specific structure, suspect a malignancy. Note any pain or tenderness surrounding the mass. Pulsation in the mass is another significant finding. For example, a mass that pulsates in all directions suggests an aneurysm.

NAILS

Inspect and palpate the fingernails and toenails. Observe the color beneath the transparent nail. Normally it is pink in light-skinned people and black or brown in dark-skinned people. Note if the nails appear blue-black or purple, brown, or yellow-gray. Look for lesions, ridging, grooves, depressions, and pitting. Depressions that appear in all nails are usually caused by a systemic disease. Gently squeeze the nail between your thumb and forefinger to test for adherence to the nail bed. A boggy nail suggests the clubbing seen in systemic cardiorespiratory diseases. The condition of the fingernails also can provide important insight into your patient's self-care and hygiene. Check the toenails for any deformity or injury such as being ingrown.

HEAD

You can also examine the skull when you inspect and palpate the scalp and hair. Look for any wounds or active bleeding. Observe the general size and contour of the skull. Palpate the cranium from front to back (Procedure 7-2a). It should be symmetrical and smooth.

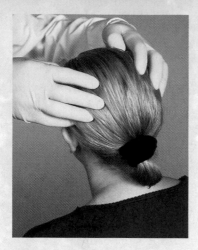

7-2a Palpate the cranium from front to back.

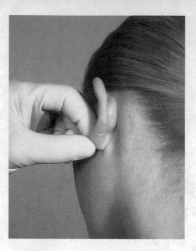

7-2b Inspect the mastoid process.

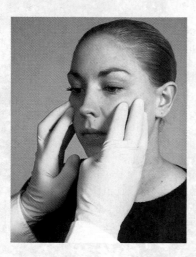

7-2c Palpate the facial bones.

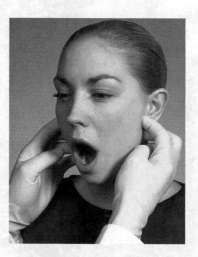

7-2d Palpate the temporo-mandibular joint.

Note any tenderness or deformities (depressions or protrusions). An indentation in the skull may suggest a depressed skull fracture. Note any areas of unusual warmth.

Inspect the face. Is it symmetrical? Are there any involuntary movements? Note any masses or edema. Observe the bony orbits of the eye for periorbital ecchymosis, a bluish discoloration also known as "raccoon eyes." Also check the mastoid process for discoloration (Procedure 7-2b). These are classic signs of a basilar skull fracture. They normally will not appear on the scene but will present hours after the injury occurs. Palpate the facial bones for stability and note any crepitus or loose fragments (Procedure 7-2c). Note whether your patient's facial expressions change appropriately with his mood.

Evaluate the temporomandibular joint (TMJ). Place the tip of your index finger into the depression in front of the tragus (the cartilaginous projection just in front of the ear's outer opening) and ask your patient to open his mouth (Procedure 7-2d). The tips of your fingers should drop into the joint space. Palpate the joint for tenderness, swelling, and range of motion. Sometimes, you may hear a clicking or snapping. This is neither unusual nor problematic unless it is accompanied by pain, swelling, and crepitus. Test for range of motion by asking your patient to open and close his mouth, jut and retract his jaw, and move it from side to side. Finally, assess the skin of the face for color, pigmentation, texture, thickness, hair distribution, and lesions.

EYES

First examine the external eyes. Place yourself directly in front of your patient. Inspect his eyes for symmetry in size, shape, and contour. Do they look alike? Do they protrude (proptosis)? Are they properly aligned? Note the eyelids' position relative to the eyeballs. They should cover the upper quarter of the iris. Are the eyes totally exposed or do the eyelids droop (ptosis)? Have your patient close his eyes. Do they close completely? Do you see any edema, inflammation, or mass? Note the eyelid's color. It should be pink, indicating good central oxygenation. If the lid is pale, your patient could be in shock or anemic. If cyanotic, he could have central hypoxemia. Are there any lesions?

Carefully observe the lids' shape and inspect their contours for any growths. If you see any drainage, note its color and consistency. Do the eyelashes turn inward to scrape against the eyeball or outward to prevent the complete closure of the eye? Are they clean and free from debris? Is there a stye (reddened swelling of the inner eyelid)? Quickly assess the regions of the lacrimal sacs and glands for swelling, excessive tearing, or dryness of the eyes.

Now ask your patient to look up while you pull down both lower eyelids to inspect the sclera and conjunctiva (Procedure 7-3a). Be careful not to put pressure on the eyeball. Ask your patient to look left and right, up and down. The conjunctiva should be clear and transparent, with no redness or cloudiness. Redness or a cobblestone appearance suggests an allergic or infectious conjunctivitis. Bright red blood in a sharply defined area surrounded by normal tissue, not extending into the iris, indicates a hemorrhage under the conjunctiva. Look for any nodules, swelling, or discharge. The normal sclera is white. A yellow sclera suggests the jaundice of liver disease.

Inspect the size, shape, and symmetry of the pupils. Are they unusually large (excessive dilation) or unusually small (excessive constriction)? Are they equal? Some patients (20%) have unequal pupils, a condition known as anisocoria; if the difference in the pupil's size is less than two millimeters and they react normally to light, anisocoria is benign. To test the pupils, first shine a light into one eye and observe that eye's reaction (Procedure 7-3b). This tests the eye's direct response. The pupil should constrict. Repeat this test for the other eye. Now shine a light into one eye and observe the other eye's reaction. This tests the eye's consensual response. Both eyes should react simultaneously to the light. Repeat this test for the other eye.

Normal pupils react to light equally and briskly. A sluggish pupil suggests increased intracranial pressure. Bilateral sluggishness may indicate global hypoxia to the brain tissue or an adverse drug reaction. Constricted pupils suggest an opiate overdose, whereas fixed and dilated pupils usually mean brain death.

Then, have your patient follow your finger as you move it in an H pattern in front of him (Procedure 7-3c). This tests the integrity of the extraocular muscles. Normal eye movements to follow your finger will be conjugate (together). Nystagmus is a fine jerking of the eyes; it may be normal if noted at the far extremes of the test.

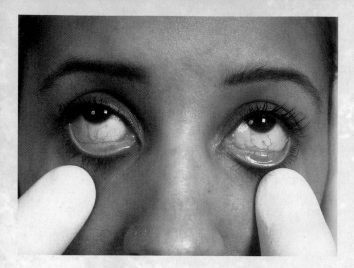

7-3a   Inspect the external eye.

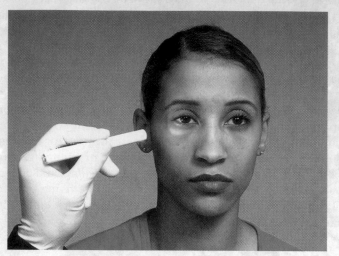

7-3b   Test each pupil's reaction to light.

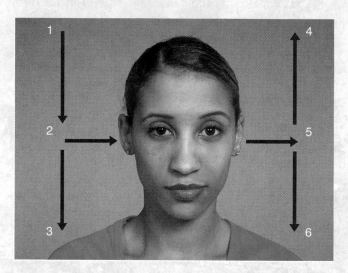

7-3c   Move your finger in an H pattern to test your patient's extraocular muscles.

EARS

Begin examining the external ears from in front of your patient. Are they symmetrical? Then examine each ear separately. Inspect the auricles for size, shape, symmetry, landmarks, color, and position on the head. Observe the surrounding area for deformities, lumps, skin lesions, tenderness, and erythema (redness). Pull the helix upward and outward and note any tenderness or discomfort (Procedure 7-4a). Press on the tragus and on the mastoid process (Procedure 7-4b). Pain or tenderness in any of these areas suggests infection such as otitis or mastoiditis. Discoloration in this area is known as Battle's sign, a common, but late, finding in a basilar skull fracture. An earache may arise from the ear itself or be referred from another place through adjoining and shared sensory nerve pathways. Sources of referred pain may include sinus problems, a bad tooth, **TMJ** pain, the common cold, a sore throat, and the cervical spine.

TMJ temporomandibular joint.

Inspect for discharge (otorrhea) from the ear canal (Procedure 7-4c). The discharge may contain mucus, pus, blood, or cerebrospinal fluid that may have leaked from the skull through a fracture in its base. Injuries to the ear itself can result from blunt trauma to the side of the head, causing temporary or permanent damage to the outer or middle ear. A ruptured eardrum can result from sticking a sharp object into the ear canal or from a pressure wave caused by an explosion.

NOSE

Check your patient's nose from the front and from the side and note any deviation in shape or color. Also note any nasal flaring, an indication of respiratory distress. Palpate the external nose for depressions, deformities, and tenderness (Procedure 7-5). With your penlight, examine the nasal mucosa for evidence of drainage and note the color, quantity, and consistency of the discharge. Rhinitis (a runny nose) may produce a watery, clear fluid, as seen in seasonal allergies. If the discharge appears thick and yellow, suspect an infection. Epistaxis (a nosebleed) may be caused by trauma or a septal defect.

MOUTH

Assess the mouth from anterior to posterior, starting with the lips. Note their condition and color. They should be pink, smooth, and symmetrical and devoid of lesions, swelling, lumps, cracks, or scaliness. Gently palpate the lips with the jaw closed and note any lesions, nodules, or fissures, especially at the corners (Procedure 7-6a). Observe the undersurfaces of the upper and lower lips (Procedure 7-6b). They should be wet and smooth. Look for any of the lip abnormalities in Table 7-3.

To examine the mouth you will need a bright light and a tongue blade. Holding the tongue blade like a chopstick will give you good downward leverage. Examine the oral mucosa for color, ulcers, white patches, and nodules. The oral mucosa should appear pinkish-red, smooth, and moist. Note the color of the gums and teeth. The gums should be pink with a clearly defined margin surrounding each tooth. Inspect the teeth for color, shape, and position. Are any missing or loose? Suspect periodontal disease if the gums are swollen, bleed easily, and are separated from the teeth by large crevices that trap food. Use a tongue blade to move the lateral lip to one side while you examine the buccal mucosa and parotid glands (Procedure 7-6c). Note the buccal mucosa's color and texture.

Table 7-3	LIP ABNORMALITIES
Lips	**Cause**
Dry, cracked	Dehydration, wind damage
Swelling/edema	Infection, allergic reaction, burns
Lesions	Infection, irritation, skin cancer
Pallor	Anemia, shock
Cyanosis	Respiratory or cardiac insufficiency

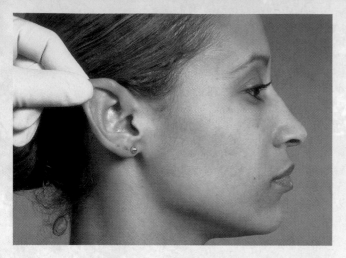

7-4a   Examine the external ear.

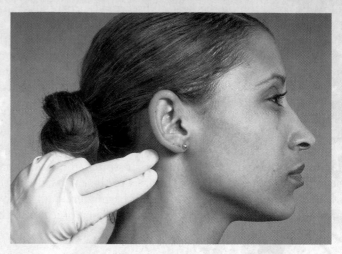

7-4b   Press on the mastoid process.

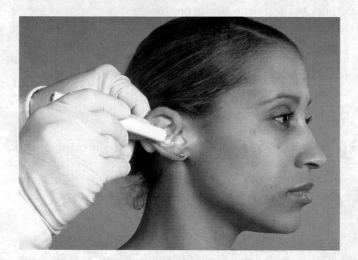

7-4c   Inspect the ear canal for drainage.

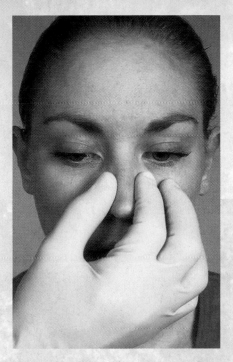

7-5   Palpate the external nose.

Ask your patient to stick his tongue straight out and then to move it from side to side. Coating of the tongue indicates dehydration. Note its color and normally velvety surface. Hold the tongue with a 2 inch × 2 inch gauze pad and a gloved hand to manipulate it for inspection (Procedure 7-6d). Make sure to inspect the sides and bottom of the tongue because malignancies are more likely to develop there, especially in patients over age 50 who smoke, chew tobacco, or drink alcohol (Procedure 7-6e). The undersurface should be smooth and pink; often you can see the bluish discoloration of dilated veins or the yellowish tint of early jaundice.

Note any odors from your patient's mouth. The smell of alcohol, feces (bowel obstruction), acetone (diabetic ketoacidosis), gastric contents, or the bitter-almond smell of cyanide poisoning may all provide important clues to your patient's problem. Also look for any fluids or unusual matter in your patient's mouth. For example, coffee-grounds-like material suggests bleeding in the upper GI area. Pink-tinged sputum indicates acute pulmonary edema, whereas green or yellow phlegm suggests a respiratory infection. Pay special attention to anything in your patient's mouth that can eventually obstruct his upper airway, including dentures or missing teeth.

Pay special attention to anything in your patient's mouth that could eventually obstruct the upper airway.

NECK

Briefly inspect your patient's neck for general symmetry and visible masses. Note any obvious deformity, deviation, tugging, masses, surgical scars, gland enlargement, or visible lymph nodes. Examine closely any penetrating injuries to the neck that may have damaged the trachea or major blood vessels; handle gently to avoid dislodging a clot that has halted bleeding. Immediately cover any open wounds with an occlusive dressing to prevent air

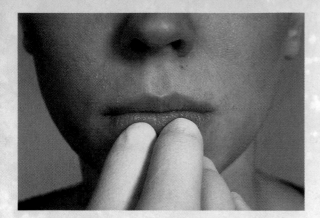

7-6a   Palpate the lips.

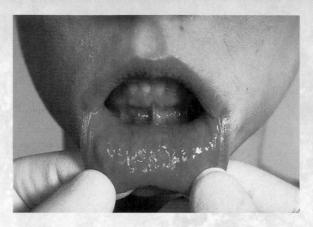

7-6b   Inspect the lips' undersurfaces.

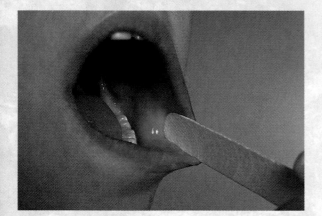

7-6c   Examine the buccal mucosa.

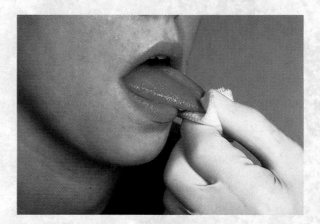

7-6d   Inspect the tongue using a gauze pad and gloved hand.

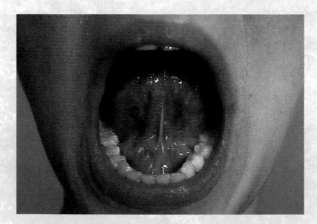

7-6e   Inspect under the tongue.

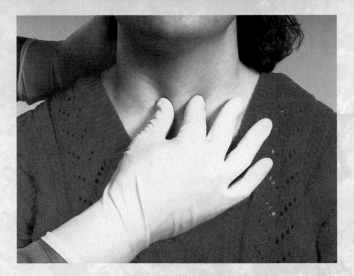

7-7a   Assess the trachea for midline position.

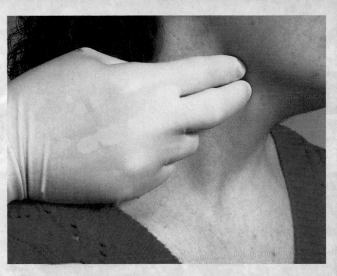

7-7b   Palpate the carotid pulse.

from entering a lacerated jugular vein during inspiration. Look for jugular vein distention while your patient is sitting upright and at a 45-degree incline. Palpate the trachea for midline position (Procedure 7-7a). Then gently palpate the carotid arteries and note their rate and quality of their pulses (Procedure 7-7b). Inspect and palpate for subcutaneous emphysema, the presence of air just below the skin. This generally suggests a tear in the tracheobronchial tree or a pneumothorax.

CHEST AND LUNGS

To assess the chest and thorax you will need a stethoscope with a bell and diaphragm. Have your patient sit upright, if possible, and expose his entire chest. At the same time, try to maintain your female patient's dignity when assessing her thorax and lungs by keeping her breasts covered. Perform your exam in the standard sequence—inspect, palpate, percuss, auscultate—and compare the findings from side to side. Always try to visualize the underlying lobes of the lungs during your exam.

Observe your patient's breathing. Look for signs of acute respiratory distress. Now count the respiratory rate and note his breathing pattern. Obviously prolonged inhalation or exhalation indicates difficulty moving air in or out of the lungs. Do you hear sounds of an upper airway obstruction (inspiratory stridor) or a lower airway obstruction (expiratory wheezing, rhonchi)? Any gross abnormalities in the respiratory rate or pattern require rapid emergency intervention.

Inspect the anterior chest wall and assess its symmetry. Funnel chest (pectus excavatum) is a condition in which the lower portion of the sternum is depressed (Figure 7-11). With a pigeon chest (pectus carinatum), the sternum curves outward. Do both sides of your patient's chest wall rise in unison? Note whether he is using neck muscles during inhalation or abdominal muscles during exhalation. If his skin retracts in the area above his clavicles (supraclavicular), at the notch above his sternum (suprasternal), and between his ribs (intercostal), suspect a ventilation problem. If multiple ribs are fractured, creating a "floating

Any gross abnormalities in the respiratory rate or pattern require rapid emergency intervention.

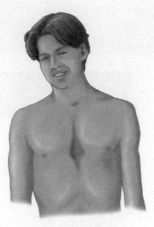
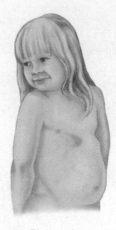
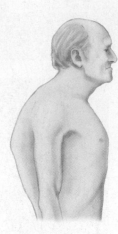

Funnel chest   Pigeon chest   Barrel chest

FIGURE 7-11   Chest wall abnormalities.

segment" or "traumatic flail chest," you may find paradoxical (opposite) movement of that part of the chest wall during breathing.

Now look at his chest from the side. Normally an adult's thorax is twice as wide as it is deep. That is, the transverse diameter of the chest wall is usually twice the antero-posterior diameter. In infants, the elderly, or patients with chronic pulmonary disease, however, the antero-posterior diameter is increased, giving them a barrel chest appearance.

Posterior Chest Examination

Next examine the posterior chest. Ask your patient to fold his arms across his chest and breathe normally during the exam. This moves his scapulae out of the way and allows more access to his posterior lung fields. Inspect his posterior chest for deformities and symmetrical movement as he breathes. Some patients may exhibit thoracic kyphoscoliosis, an abnormal spinal curvature that deforms the chest and makes your lung exam more challenging. Inspect the intercostal spaces for retractions or bulging; both are abnormal. Retractions may appear when airflow is impeded during inspiration. Bulging may appear when airflow is impeded during exhalation. Respiratory movement should be smooth and effortless. When it is not, suspect underlying respiratory disease or structural impairment.

Palpate the rib cage for rigidity. Feel for tenderness, deformities, depressions, loose segments, asymmetry, and crepitus. Then evaluate for equal expansion. First, locate the level of the posterior tenth rib. To do this, find the lowest rib and simply move up two more ribs. An alternate method for locating the posterior tenth rib is to palpate the spinous processes. Ask your patient to touch his chin to his chest. The most prominent spinous process is the seventh cervical vertebra. Locate it and count down to T-10 in the midline. Now place your hands parallel to the tenth rib on your patient's back with your fingers spread. Lightly grasp his lateral rib cage with your spread hands (Procedure 7-8a). Ask him to inhale deeply. Normally the distance between your thumbs will increase symmetrically by 3 to 5 centimeters during deep inspiration. If you detect decreased thoracic expansion or feel unilateral delay, suspect a disorder of the underlying lung, pleura, or diaphragm.

Percuss your patient's posterior chest to determine whether the underlying tissues are air filled, fluid filled, or solid. Also percuss to determine the position and boundaries of the diaphragm and underlying organs. Percuss both sides of the chest symmetrically from the apex to the base at 5-centimeter intervals, avoiding bony areas such as the scapulae (Procedure 7-8b). Percuss at least twice in each area and compare both sides of the thorax. Identify and note any area of abnormal percussion. For example, a hyperresonant sound in the right chest may indicate a pneumothorax, whereas a dull sound in the same area may indicate a hemothorax. Assess the percussion sounds according to their quality, intensity, pitch, and duration. Practice percussing the chest so that you become familiar with the normal resonance of the lungs and be able to identify abnormal sounds.

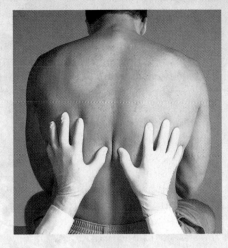

7-8a Palpate the posterior chest for excursion.

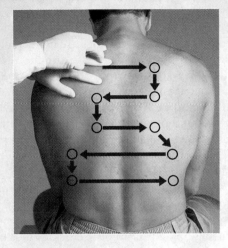

7-8b Percuss the posterior chest.

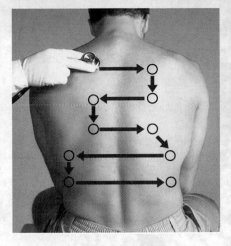

7-8c Auscultate the posterior chest.

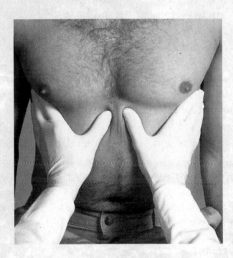

7-8d Palpate the anterior chest for excursion.

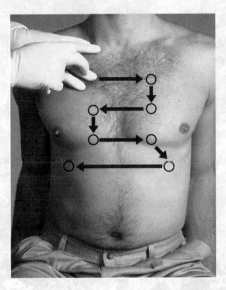

7-8e Percuss the anterior chest.

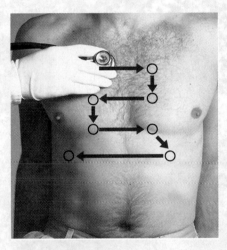

7-8f Auscultate the anterior chest.

crackles light crackling, popping, nonmusical sounds heard usually during inspiration.

wheezes continuous, high-pitched musical sounds similar to a whistle.

rhonchi continuous sounds with a lower pitch and a snoring quality.

stridor predominantly inspiratory wheeze associated with laryngeal obstruction.

pleural friction rub the squeaking or grating sound of the pleural linings rubbing together.

Auscultate your patient's chest for normal breath sounds, adventitious breath sounds, and voice sounds. Auscultate all lung fields and compare side-to-side. Evaluate the normal breath sounds produced by airflow through the upper and lower airways. These include tracheal, bronchial, bronchovesicular, and vesicular breath sounds (Table 7-4). Besides the normal breath sounds already mentioned, you also may hear adventitious sounds. These include crackles, wheezes, rhonchi, stridor, and pleural rubs.

Also known as "rales," **crackles** are light crackling, popping, nonmusical sounds heard usually during inspiration. They are produced by air passing through moisture in the broncho-alveolar system or from the abrupt opening of closed alveoli. Early inspiratory crackles, associated with chronic bronchitis and heart failure, begin shortly after inspiration starts, and they stop soon thereafter. These are coarse crackles—loud, low pitched, and long, similar to the sound of water boiling. They are often audible at the mouth.

Late inspiratory crackles, associated with congestive heart failure and interstitial lung diseases, begin in the first half of the inspiratory phase and continue into late inspiration. They are fine crackles—soft, high pitched, and very brief, similar to the sound of Rice Krispies crackling in milk. They commonly appear first at the base of the lungs and move upward as your patient's condition worsens. Usually, you can expect them to shift to dependent regions with changes in your patient's position. For example, if your heart failure patient is sitting up, expect to hear crackles first in the bases. If he is bedridden, expect to hear crackles first in the back.

Wheezes are continuous, high-pitched musical sounds similar to a whistle. They result when air moves through partially obstructed smaller airways. Their causes include asthma, bronchospasm, and foreign bodies. You may hear them without a stethoscope or by auscultating the chest during any or all phases of the respiratory cycle. They often originate in the small bronchioles and first appear at the end of exhalation. The closer to inspiration they appear, the worse your patient's condition.

Rhonchi are continuous sounds with a lower pitch and a snoring quality. They are caused by secretions in the larger airways, a common finding in bronchitis (diffuse) and pneumonia (localized). Rhonchi usually appear in early exhalation but may occur in early inspiration as well.

Stridor is a predominantly high-pitched inspiratory sound. It indicates a partial obstruction of the larynx or trachea.

Pleural friction rubs are the squeaking or grating sounds of the pleural linings rubbing together. They occur where the pleural layers are inflamed and have lost their lubrication. Pleural rubs are common in pneumonia and pleurisy (inflammation of the pleura). Because these sounds occur whenever your patient's chest wall moves, they appear during the entire respiratory cycle.

You may hear no breath sounds in some areas. This may result from effusion (fluid in the pleural space causing a decrease in functional lung tissue) or consolidation (infectious pus causing collapsed alveoli). In either case, note the area's size and intervene appropriately to ensure adequate ventilation and oxygenation of your patient.

Auscultate the posterior chest systematically. Have your patient fold his arms across his chest and breathe through his mouth more deeply and slowly than usual. Auscultate the same areas you percussed and compare the bilateral findings (Procedure 7-8c). Listen for at

Table 7-4 NORMAL BREATH SOUNDS

Sound	Description	Location	Duration
Tracheal	Very loud, harsh	Over the trachea	Nearly equal inspiratory and expiratory phases
Bronchial	Loud, high pitch, hollow	Over the manubrium	Prolonged expiratory phase
Bronchovesicular	Soft, breezy, lower pitch	Between the scapulae/ 2nd–3rd ICS lateral to the sternum	Approximately equal inspiratory and expiratory phases
Vesicular	Soft, swishy, lowest pitch	Lung periphery	Prolonged inspiratory phase

least one full breath at each location. Be alert for patient discomfort or hyperventilation. Note the pitch, intensity, and duration of each inspiratory and expiratory sound. If the sounds are decreased, suspect impaired airflow or poor sound transmission. If the sounds are absent, suspect no airflow. Note whether you hear sounds where you normally should. For example, when you auscultate over the peripheral lung fields, you should not hear tracheal, bronchial, or bronchovesicular breath sounds. Listen carefully and note what you hear, where you hear it, and when you hear it during the respiratory cycle. Also note whether the sounds change when your patient coughs or changes position.

Anterior Chest Examination

Your examination of the anterior chest will be similar to your examination of the posterior chest. Begin by having your patient lie supine with his arms relaxed but slightly abducted at his sides. Look for any gross deformities or asymmetrical movements. Does the chest wall rise symmetrically? Is there accessory muscle use? Look for abnormal retractions in the suprasternal, supraclavicular, and intercostal areas. Also check for calloused elbows from tripodding (leaning with elbows on a table or chair arms), and finger clubbing—both common signs of chronic lung disease. Is the trachea midline or deviated; does it tug during inhalation? In cases of tension pneumothorax the trachea will deviate away from the affected side. In cases of pulmonary fibrosis and atelectasis, it will tug toward the affected side during inhalation.

Palpate the anterior chest for deformities and areas of tenderness. Check for chest expansion by placing your thumbs along the costal margins on both sides and gently grasping the lateral rib cage (Procedure 7-8d). Ask your patient to inhale deeply. Normally your thumbs will separate symmetrically, and the distance between them will increase from 3 to 5 centimeters. If you detect decreased thoracic expansion or feel unilateral delay, suspect a disorder of the underlying lung, pleura, or diaphragm.

Percuss your patient's anterior chest to help determine whether the underlying tissues are air filled, fluid filled, or solid and to determine the position and boundaries of the diaphragm and underlying organs. Percuss each side of your patient's anterior chest from its apex to its base at 5-centimeter intervals at the mid-clavicular lines (Procedure 7-8e). Percuss at least twice in each area and compare both sides of the thorax. Identify and note any area of abnormal percussion. Remember that when percussing the right chest, you will hear dullness at the upper border of the liver. On the left side, you will hear the normal resonance of the lung change to tympany when you reach the stomach. You also will percuss an area of cardiac dullness from the third to the fifth intercostal spaces.

Finally, auscultate the anterior and lateral thorax systematically. Have your patient breathe through his mouth more deeply and slowly than usual. Auscultate the same areas you percussed and compare symmetrical areas (Procedure 7-8f). Listen for at least one full breath at each location. Be alert for patient discomfort or hyperventilation. As with posterior chest auscultation, note the pitch, intensity, and duration of each inspiratory and expiratory sound and whether you heard sounds where you should normally expect them. Listen for adventitious sounds.

CARDIOVASCULAR SYSTEM

To assess cardiac function, you must understand the cardiac cycle. During **diastole**, the heart's resting period, the ventricles relax. The pressure in the atria is greater than the pressure in the ventricles. This opens the tricuspid valve on the right side and the mitral valve on the left, allowing blood from the atria to fill the ventricles. During **systole** the ventricles contract and the tricuspid and mitral valves close, preventing backflow into the atria. The vibrations of these valves' closings generate the first heart sound—S_1, or the "lub." The increased pressure in the right ventricle opens the pulmonic semilunar valve, sending deoxygenated blood to the lungs. The increased pressure in the left ventricle opens the aortic semilunar valve, sending freshly oxygenated blood to the body. At the end of systole, as pressure in the ventricles falls, the pulmonic and aortic semilunar valves close tightly to prevent backflow. These vibrations generate the second heart sound—S_2, or the "dub." This cycle repeats approximately 60 to 100 times per minute in the healthy adult at rest. Extra sounds

diastole phase of cardiac cycle when ventricles relax.

systole phase of cardiac cycle when ventricles contract.

Content Review

HEART SOUNDS
- S_1—"lub"
- S_2—"dub"

known as heart murmurs result when valves do not fully open or close, causing turbulent flow that an experienced clinician can detect.

Begin your cardiovascular assessment by inspecting for signs of arterial insufficiency or occlusion in your patient's trunk and extremities. Look for skin pallor and other signs of decreased perfusion. Now assess the arterial pulses. Inspect the carotid arteries for visible pulsations just medial to the sternocleidomastoid muscles. Palpate the carotid arteries at the level of the cricoid cartilage to avoid pressing on the carotid sinus (Procedure 7-9a). Never palpate both carotid arteries simultaneously; doing so may decrease cerebral blood flow. Assess the carotid pulse for rate, rhythm, and quality. Does its quality vary? Do the variations correspond to respiration? For example, in pulsus paradoxus, the amplitude of the pulse diminishes with inspiration and increases with exhalation. Do you feel a vibration or humming (**thrills**) when you palpate the carotid artery? If so, auscultate the area with your stethoscope for **bruits**, the sounds of turbulent blood flow around a partial obstruction (Procedure 7-9b).

If you have not already taken your patient's blood pressure, do so now. Also check for jugular venous pressure, which approximates your patient's right atrial pressure. Position your patient supine, with his head elevated to about 30 degrees. Examine the external jugular veins for equality of distention. Abnormal bilateral distention indicates fluid-volume overload or that something such as congestive heart failure or cardiac tamponade is blocking venous return to the heart. Unilateral distention suggests a localized problem.

With your patient's head still raised to about 30 degrees, inspect and palpate the chest for the apical impulse (PMI) (Procedure 7-9c). When examining a woman with large breasts, gently displace the left breast upward and laterally, if needed, or ask her to do this for you. First, look for a pulsation at the cardiac apex, normally at the fifth intercostal space just medial to the mid-clavicular line. This pulsation represents the PMI. It helps you locate the left ventricle's apex.

If you cannot see the pulsation, ask your patient to exhale and stop breathing for a few seconds. Lateral displacement of the PMI indicates an enlarged right ventricle. The PMI may be displaced upward and to the left in pregnant women. If your patient is obese or has a very muscular chest wall or a barrel chest you may not detect the PMI. Percussion may help if you have difficulty palpating the PMI. Start lateral and work your way toward the midline (Procedure 7-9d). When you hear a change from resonance (lung) to dull (heart), you have located the PMI.

Using the diaphragm of your stethoscope, auscultate your patient's anterior chest for normal heart sounds and for abnormal or extra heart sounds (Procedure 7-9e). You may hear extra or abnormal heart sounds, depending on your patient's age and condition. Simply report what you hear to the emergency physician.

ABDOMEN

To examine the abdomen, you need good lighting, a relaxed patient, and exposure from above the xiphoid process to the symphysis pubis. Make sure your patient does not have a full bladder. Make him comfortable in the supine position with one pillow under the head and another under the knees. Have him place his hands at his sides. This helps relax his abdominal muscles, making the examination easier for you and more comfortable for him.

Ask your patient to point out any areas of pain or tenderness. Examine these areas last. Use warm hands and a warm stethoscope and keep your fingernails short. If your hands are cold, palpate your patient through his clothes until your hands warm up. Begin your exam slowly and avoid any quick, unexpected movements. Monitor your patient's facial expressions for pain and discomfort. During the exam, distract him with conversation or questions. Use inspection and palpation to perform the exam. When you examine the abdomen you will assess the gastrointestinal organs and other nearby organs and structures. Inspect the skin of the abdomen and flanks for scars, dilated veins, stretch marks, rashes, lesions, and pigmentation changes. Look for discoloration over the umbilicus (**Cullen's sign**) or over the flanks (**Grey-Turner's sign**); these are late signs suggesting intra-abdominal bleeding. Assess the size and shape of your patient's abdomen to determine whether it is scaphoid (concave), flat, round, or distended. Ask the patient if this is its usual size and shape. Note its symmetry. Check for bulges, hernias, or distended flanks. **Ascites** appear as bulges in the

---

thrill vibration or humming felt when palpating the pulse.

bruit sound of turbulent blood flow around a partial obstruction.

Cullen's sign discoloration around the umbilicus (occasionally the flanks) suggestive of intra-abdominal hemorrhage.

Grey-Turner's sign discoloration over the flanks suggesting intra-abdominal bleeding.

ascites bulges in the flanks and across the abdomen, indicating edema caused by congestive heart failure.

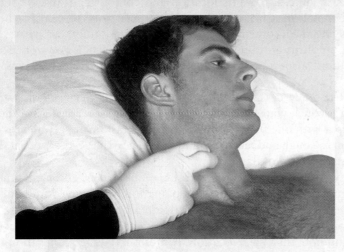

7-9a   Assess the carotid pulse.

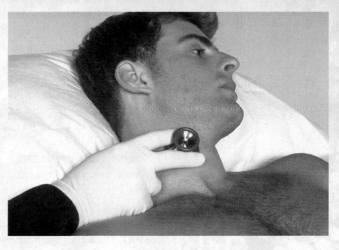

7-9b   Auscultate for bruits.

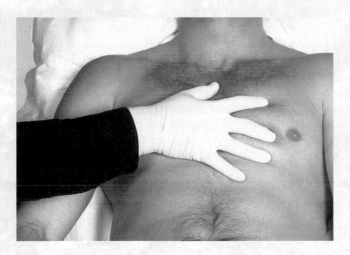

7-9c   Palpate for the apical impulse (PMI).

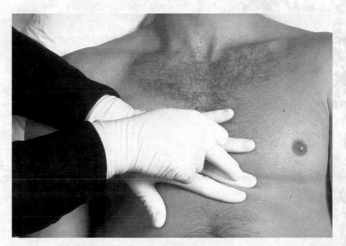

7-9d   Percuss for the PMI.

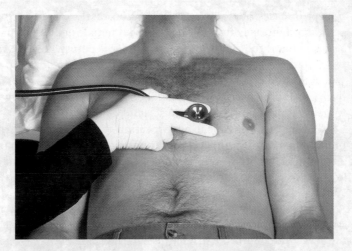

7-9e   Auscultate for heart sounds.

flanks and across the abdomen and indicates edema caused by congestive heart failure. A distended bladder or pregnant uterus can cause a suprapubic bulge. Bulges in the inguinal or femoral areas suggest a hernia.

Now look at your patient's umbilicus. Note its location and contour and observe for any signs of herniation or inflammation. Check for any visible pulsation, peristalsis (the wavelike motion of organs moving their contents through the digestive tract), or masses. You may see the normal pulsation of the aorta just lateral to the umbilicus. If you notice a bounding or exaggerated pulsation, suspect an aortic aneurysm. Visible peristalsis may indicate a bowel obstruction.

Palpate the abdomen to detect tenderness, muscular rigidity, and superficial organs and masses. Before you begin palpation, ask your patient if he has any pain or tenderness. If he does, ask him to point to the area with one finger. Palpate that area last, using gentle pressure with a single finger. Ask him to cough and tell you if and where he experiences any pain. If coughing causes pain, suspect peritoneal inflammation.

Now ask your patient to take slow, deep breaths with his mouth open, and have him flex his knees to relax his abdominal muscles. Perform light palpation by moving your hand slowly and just lifting it off the skin (Procedure 7-10a). Palpate all areas in the same sequence you used for auscultation and percussion. Watch your patient's face for signs of discomfort. Identify any masses and note their size, location, contour, tenderness, pulsations, and mobility. Abdominal pain on light palpation suggests peritoneal irritation or inflammation. If you feel rigidity or guarding while palpating, determine whether it is voluntary (patient anticipates the pain or is not relaxed) or involuntary (peritoneal inflammation).

Next, palpate the abdomen deeply to detect large masses or tenderness. Use one hand on top of another and push down slowly (Procedure 7-10b). Assess for rebound tenderness by pushing down slowly and then releasing your hand quickly off the tender area. If the peritoneum is inflamed, your patient will experience pain when you let go. Alternatively, hold your hand 1 centimeter above your patient's abdomen at rest. Then ask him to push his abdomen out to touch your hand. Limitation by pain suggests peritoneal irritation.

If you note a protruding abdomen with bulging flanks and dull percussion sounds in dependent areas, you might perform two tests for ascites. First assess for areas of tympany and dullness while your patient is supine. Then ask him to lie on one side. Percuss again, noting once more any areas of tympany and dullness. If your patient has ascites, the area of dullness will shift down to the dependent side and the area of tympany will shift up. To test for fluid wave, ask an assistant to press the edge of his hand firmly down the midline of your patient's abdomen (Procedure 7-10c). With your fingertips, tap one flank and feel for the impulse's transmission to the other flank through excess fluid. If you detect the impulse easily, suspect ascites.

FEMALE GENITALIA

Except in cases of trauma or abuse, you rarely would be expected to examine the female genitalia. Before examining the external female genitalia, make sure that the room is warm and quiet and that your patient's bladder is empty. Be sure to maintain privacy during this examination. To reduce any anxiety or embarrassment your patient may feel, explain what you are doing during the exam. Expose her body areas only as necessary, be sensitive to her feelings, and project a professional demeanor. Place a pillow under her head and shoulders to help relax her abdominal muscles.

Begin your assessment by inspecting your patient's external genitalia. Look at the mons pubis, labia, and perineum for abnormalities such as inflammation, swelling, or lesions. These abnormalities may signal a sebaceous cyst or a sexually transmitted disease such as syphilis or herpes simplex virus infection. Check the bases of the pubic hair for signs of lice such as excoriation, or small, itchy, red maculopapules.

Now retract the outer labia and inspect the inner labia and urethral meatus (opening). Assess for vaginal discharge. The normal discharge is clear or cloudy and has little or no odor. A white, curdlike discharge with no odor or a yeasty, sweet odor may suggest a fungal infection (candidiasis). A yellow, green, or gray discharge with a foul or fishy odor may suggest a bacterial infection (gonorrhea or *Gardnerella*). Examining the external female genitalia can be an embarrassing, uncomfortable experience, especially for male clinicians.

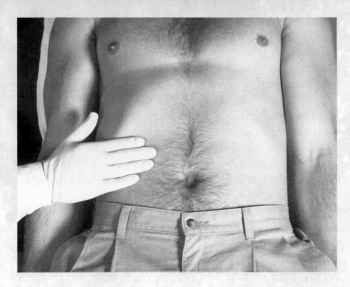

7-10a Light abdominal palpation.

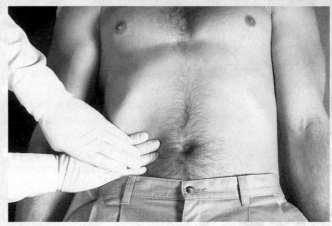

7-10b Deep abdominal palpation.

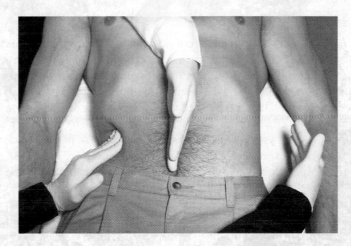

7-10c Test for ascites.

Remember it is probably twice as awkward for your patient. It is customary for male clinicians to have a female partner present during the examination.

MALE GENITALIA

Except for trauma, you rarely would be expected to inspect the male genitalia. Before examining the male genitalia make sure that the room is warm and quiet and that your patient's bladder is empty. Be sure to maintain privacy during this examination. To reduce any anxiety or embarrassment your patient may feel, explain what you are doing during the exam. Expose his body areas only as necessary, be sensitive to his feelings, and project a professional demeanor.

Begin your assessment by inspecting your patient's penis and scrotum. Note any inflammation and inspect the skin around the base of the penis for abnormalities such as lesions that may be caused by sexually transmitted diseases. Also check the bases of the pubic hair for signs of lice such as excoriation or small, itchy, red maculopapules. Next inspect the glans for signs of degeneration or other abnormalities. If the foreskin is present, ask your patient to retract it. Note any abnormalities and the location of the urethral meatus. Inspect the anterior surface of the scrotum and note its contour. Then lift the scrotum to inspect its posterior surface and note any swelling or lumps. Expect acute epididymitis or testicular torsion if your patient has scrotal swelling and lower abdominal pain. Testicular torsion requires immediate intervention.

Assess any discharge from the urethral meatus. Normally no discharge is present. A profuse, yellow discharge may be a sign of gonorrhea. A scant, clear or white discharge may suggest a nongonococcal urethritis. Examining the male genitalia can be an embarrassing, uncomfortable experience, especially for female clinicians. Remember it is probably twice as awkward for your patient. It is customary for female clinicians to have a male partner present during the examination.

EXTREMITIES

An examination of the extremities must include a detailed assessment of function and structure.

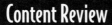

Content Review

STEPS IN EVALUATING JOINTS

1 Inspection
2 Palpation
3 Passive range of motion
4 Range of motion against gravity
5 Range of motion against resistance

An examination of the extremities must include a detailed assessment of function and structure. Inspect and palpate your patient's joints, their structure, their range of motion, and the surrounding tissues. Begin your assessment with a general observation of posture, build, and muscular development. Watch how your patient's body parts move and observe their resting positions. Begin the exam with your patient sitting to evaluate his head, neck, shoulders, and upper extremities. Then have him stand to assess his chest, back, and ilium; ask him to walk so that you can assess his gait. Finally, ask him to lie down to examine his hips, knees, ankles, and feet.

Inspect for swelling in or around joints, changes in the surrounding tissue, redness of the overlying skin, deformities, and symmetry of impairment. Swelling may be caused by trauma to the area or by excess synovial fluid in the joint space or tissues surrounding the joint. Tissue changes may include muscle atrophy, skin changes, and subcutaneous nodules resulting from rheumatoid arthritis or rheumatic fever. Skin redness may suggest inflammation or arthritis. Deformities may be produced by restricted range of motion, misalignment of the articulating bones, dislocation (complete separation of bone ends), or subluxation (partial dislocation). Symmetrical impairment is usually associated with a disorder such as rheumatoid arthritis.

Inspect and palpate each body part, then test its range of motion and muscle strength as explained in the Motor System section later in this chapter. Examine each joint and compare joints on opposite sides for equal size, shape, color, and strength. Swelling in a joint usually involves the synovial membrane or a bursa, which will feel spongy on deep palpation within the joint space. It also may involve the surrounding structures such as ligaments, cartilage, tendons, or the bones themselves. Redness of the overlying skin suggests a nontraumatic joint inflammation such as arthritis, gout, or rheumatic fever. Palpate for tenderness in and around the joint. Try to identify the specific structure that is tender, such as a ligament or tendon. Some common causes of a tender joint include arthritis, tendinitis, bursitis, or osteomyelitis. With the back of your hand, feel over the tender area for increased heat, which suggests arthritis.

After you have inspected and palpated each body part with your patient at rest, assess range of motion. Test each joint for passive range of motion, range of motion against gravity, and range of motion against resistance. First test the joint's passive range of motion by moving it in the directions that it normally allows. For example, test the elbow, a hinge joint, for flexion and extension. Note any resistance and whether the range of motion is within normal limits. Now test range of motion against gravity by asking your patient to perform the same movements by himself. Again, note the range of motion and any difficulties. Finally, test range of motion against resistance. Have your patient perform the same movements while you apply resistance.

Passive and active range should be equal. A discrepancy indicates either a muscle weakness or a joint problem. If your patient has difficulty with passive and active tests, suspect a joint problem. If he has difficulty only with active tests, suspect a weakened muscle or nerve disorder. A decreased range of motion could indicate arthritis or injury, whereas an increased range of motion suggests a loosening of the structures that support the joint.

Listen for **crepitation** (or **crepitus**), the crunching sounds of unlubricated parts rubbing against each other, while you manipulate the joint. Crepitus may indicate an inflamed joint or osteoarthritis. An obvious traumatic deformity could indicate a sprained ligament, a dislocation, or a bone fracture. In these cases, modify your manipulation and range of motion exam accordingly. Nontraumatic deformities are caused by arthritis or the misalignment of bones. Avoid manipulating a painful joint.

crepitation (or **crepitus**) crunching sounds of unlubricated parts in joints rubbing against each other.

Wrists and Hands

Begin by inspecting your patient's hands and wrists. Next palpate them by feeling the medial and lateral aspects of the **DIP joints** and then the **PIP joints** with your thumb and forefinger (Procedure 7-11a). Note any swelling, sponginess, bony enlargement, or tenderness. Then palpate the tops and bottoms of these joints in the same manner. Now ask your patient to flex his hand slightly so you can examine each MCP. Compress the **MCP joints** by squeezing the hand from side-to-side between your thumbs and fingers and note any swelling, tenderness, or sponginess (Procedure 7-11b). Finally, palpate each wrist joint with your thumbs and note any swelling, sponginess, or tenderness (Procedure 7-11c). If your patient has had swelling of both his wrists or finger joints for several weeks, suspect an inflammatory condition such as rheumatoid arthritis.

DIP joints distal interphalangeal joints.

PIP joints proximal interphalangeal joints.

MCP joints metacarpophalangeal joints.

To assess range of motion, ask your patient to make a fist with each hand and then open his fist and extend and spread his fingers. He should be able to make a tight fist and spread his fingers smoothly and easily. Next ask him to flex and then extend his wrist. Normal flexion is 90 degrees, extension 70 degrees (Procedure 7-11d). Check for radial and ulnar deviation by asking your patient to flex his wrist and move his hands medially and laterally. Normal radial movement is 20 degrees, ulnar movement 45 degrees (Procedure 7-11e).

If your patient complains of hand pain and numbness, especially at night, suspect carpal tunnel syndrome, the painful inflammation of the median nerve. To detect additional signs of this disorder, hold your patient's wrists in acute flexion for 60 seconds (Procedure 7-11f). In carpal tunnel syndrome, he will develop numbness or tingling in the areas innervated by the median nerve—the palmar surface of his thumb, index, and middle fingers, and part of his ring finger. Throughout these maneuvers watch for deformities, redness, swelling, nodules, or muscular atrophy.

Elbows

To examine the elbow, support your patient's forearm with your hand so that his elbow is flexed about 70 degrees (Procedure 7-12a). Inspect the elbow joint and note any deformities, swelling, or nodules. Palpate the joint structures for tenderness, swelling, or thickening. Press on the medial and lateral epicondyles (Procedure 7-12b). Inflammation of either the medial epicondyle (tennis elbow) or of the lateral epicondyle (golfer's elbow) suggests tendinitis at those muscle insertion sites. To assess range of motion, ask your patient to flex and extend his elbow (Procedure 7-12c). Normally he will flex his elbow up to 160 degrees and return it back to the neutral position. Then ask him to keep his elbows flexed and his arms at his sides. Now have him turn his palms up and then down. Normally both supination and pronation are 90 degrees (Procedure 7-12d).

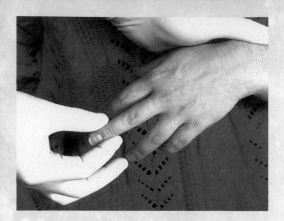

7-11a Palpate the DIP and PIP joints.

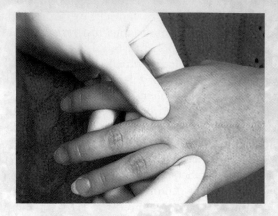

7-11b Palpate the MCP joint.

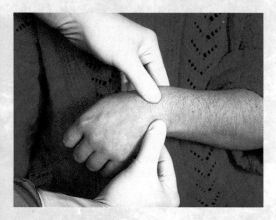

7-11c Palpate the wrist.

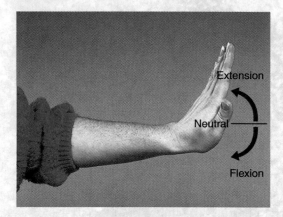

7-11d Assess wrist flexion and extension.

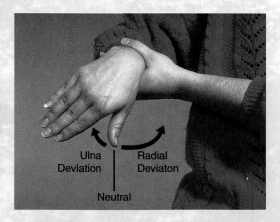

7-11e Assess radial and ulnar deviation.

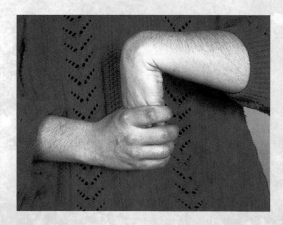

7-11f Test for carpal tunnel syndrome.

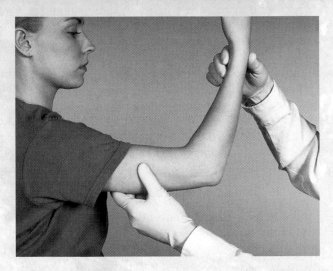

7-12a Inspect the elbow.

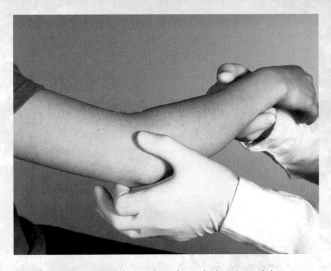

7-12b Palpate the lateral and medial epicondyles.

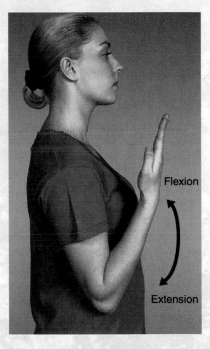

Flexion

Extension

7-12c Assess elbow flexion and extension.

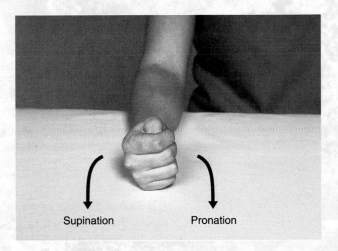

Supination

Pronation

7-12d Assess supination and pronation of the wrist.

Shoulders

To assess your patient's shoulders look at them from the front and then look at his scapulae from the back. Inspect the entire shoulder girdle for swelling, deformities, or muscular atrophy. Before you palpate, ask your patient if he has any pain in his shoulders. If so, have him point to it with one finger; palpate this area last. Palpate the shoulders with your fingertips, moving along the clavicles out toward the humerus (Procedure 7-13a). Palpate the sternoclavicular joint, acromioclavicular joint, subacromial region, and the bicipital groove for tenderness (biceps tendinitis) or swelling (bursitis). Now palpate over the greater tubercle of the humerus as you abduct the arm at the shoulder. Then palpate the scapulae.

To assess range of motion ask your patient to raise both arms forward and then straight overhead (flexion) (Procedure 7-13b). Expect to see forward flexion of 180 degrees. Next ask him to extend both arms behind his back (extension). Normal extension is 50 degrees. Now have him raise both arms overhead from the side (abduction) (Procedure 7-13c). Normal abduction is 180 degrees. Then ask him to lower his arms and swing them as far as he can across his body (adduction). Normal shoulder adduction is 75 degrees. Finally have him adduct his shoulders to 90 degrees, pronate, and flex his elbows 90 degrees to the front of his body. Now ask him to rotate his shoulders to the "goal post" position (external rotation) (Procedure 7-13d). Normal external rotation is 90 degrees. Finally, ask him to place both hands behind the small of his back (internal rotation). Normal internal rotation is 90 degrees. During these motions, cup your hands over your patient's shoulders and note any crepitus.

Ankles and Feet

Inspect the foot and ankle for obvious deformities, nodules, swelling, callouses, or corns. Palpate the anterior aspect of each ankle joint with your thumbs and note any sponginess, swelling, or tenderness (Procedure 7-14a). Feel along the Achilles tendon for tenderness or nodules. Exert pressure between your thumbs and fingers on each metatarsophalangeal joint (Procedure 7-14b). Acute inflammation of these joints suggests gout. Tenderness is an early sign of rheumatoid arthritis.

To test range of motion, ask your patient to bring his foot upward (dorsiflexion) (Procedure 7-14c). Normal dorsiflexion is 20 degrees. Then have him point it downward (plantar flexion). Normal plantar flexion is 45 degrees. Next, while stabilizing the ankle with one hand, grasp the heel with the other hand and invert the foot, then evert it (Procedure 7-14d). Normal inversion is 30 degrees; normal eversion 20 degrees. These four movements test the ankle joint's stability. A sprained ankle will cause your patient pain when the injured ligament is stretched or torn. Since the lateral ligaments are smaller and weaker than the medial ligaments, lateral sprains are more common, causing severe pain upon inversion and plantar flexion. In arthritis, pain and tenderness will accompany movement in any direction. Finally, flex and extend the toes (Procedure 7-14e). Expect a great range of motion in these joints, especially the big toes.

Knees

Inspect your patient's knees for alignment and deformities. Look for the concave areas that usually appear on each side of the patella and just above it. The absence of these concavities indicates swelling in the knee or the surrounding structures. If swelling is present, milk the medial aspect of the knee firmly upward two or three times to displace the fluid. Then press the knee just behind the lateral margin of the patella and watch for a return of fluid (a positive sign for effusion) (Procedure 7-15a). Feel for any thickening or swelling around the patella; these suggest synovial thickening or effusion. Compress the patella and move it against the femur (Procedure 7-15b). Note any pain or tenderness.

To test for range of motion, have your patient flex his knee to 90 degrees. Press your thumbs into the joint and palpate along the tibial margins from the patellar tendon laterally. Palpate along the course of each ligament and note any points of tenderness. If your patient has tenderness, expect damage to the meniscus or to lateral ligaments. If you feel irregular bony ridges, suspect osteoarthritis. Now test for stability of the medial and collateral ligaments by moving the knee joint from side to side with the knee flexed to 30 degrees

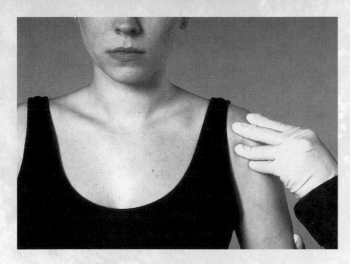

7-13a   Palpate the shoulder with your fingertips.

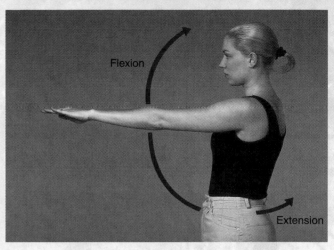

7-13b   Assess shoulder flexion and extension.

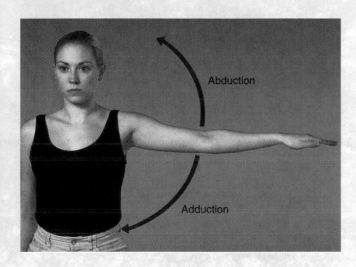

7-13c   Assess shoulder abduction and adduction.

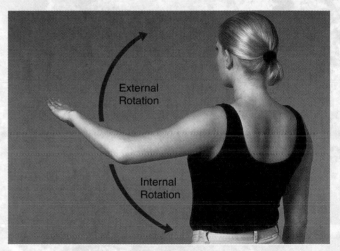

7-13d   Assess internal and external shoulder rotation.

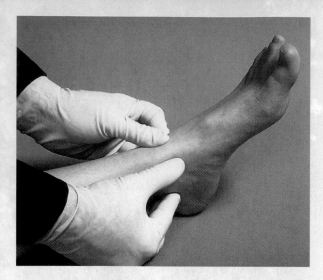

7-14a Palpate the ankle and foot.

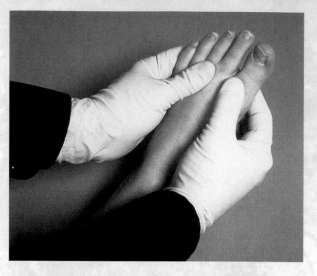

7-14b Palpate the metatarsal-phalangeal joints.

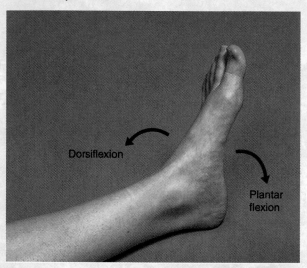

7-14c Assess dorsiflexion and plantar flexion.

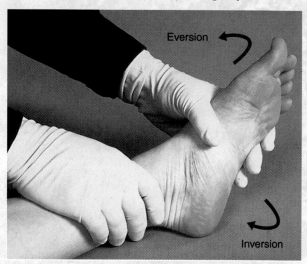

7-14d Assess inversion and eversion of the foot.

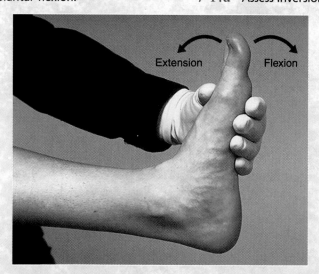

7-14e Test flexion and extension of the toes.

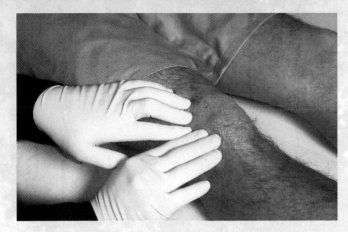

7-15a   Palpate the knee.

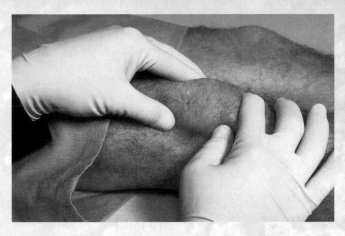

7-15b   Palpate the patella.

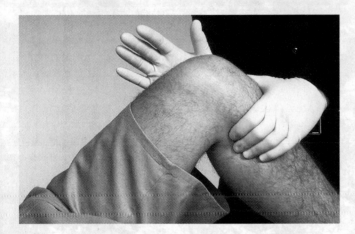

7-15c   Test the collateral ligaments of the knee.

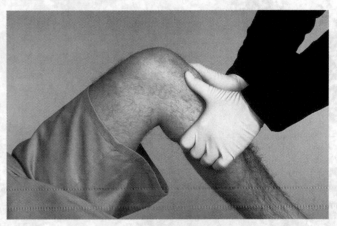

7-15d   Test the cruciate ligaments of the knee.

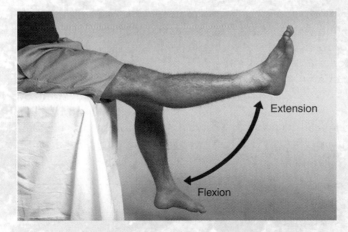

7-15e   Assess knee flexion and extension.

(Procedure 7-15c). There should be little movement if the joint is stable. Evaluate the anterior and posterior cruciate ligaments by using the "drawer" test. Try to move the knee joint anterior and posterior, similar to opening and closing a drawer (Procedure 7-15d). Again, if the ligaments are strong, there should be little movement.

Now have your patient sit at the edge of the exam table with his lower legs dangling. Ask him to extend his leg. Normal extension is 90 degrees (Procedure 7-15e). Ask him to roll over and try to touch his foot to his back. Normal flexion is 135 degrees. With your patient standing, inspect the posterior surface of his legs, especially the popliteal region behind his knees. Note any deformity or abnormalities such as bowlegs, knock-knee, or flexion contracture, the inability to fully extend the knee.

Hips

Inspect the hips for deformities, symmetry, and swelling. Palpate for tenderness all around the joint, including the three bursa and greater trochanter of the femur (Procedure 7-16a). Test the hip's range of motion with your patient supine. Ask him to raise his knee to his chest and pull it firmly against his abdomen. Observe the degree of flexion at the knee and hip (normally 120 degrees) (Procedure 7-16b). Now flex the hip at 90 degrees and stabilize the thigh with one hand while you grasp the ankle with the other. Swing the lower leg medially to evaluate external rotation and laterally to evaluate internal rotation (Procedure 7-16c). Normal external rotation is 40 degrees, normal internal rotation 45 degrees. Arthritis restricts internal rotation. To test for hip abduction, have your patient extend his legs. Then while you stabilize the anterior superior iliac spine with one hand, abduct the other leg until you feel the iliac spine move. This marks the degree of hip abduction, which is normally 90 degrees (Procedure 7-16d). If your patient complains of hip pain or if range of motion is limited, palpate the three bursa for swelling (bursitis) and tenderness.

SPINE

To assess your patient's spine, first inspect his head and neck for deformities, abnormal posture, and asymmetrical skin folds. The head should be erect and the spine straight. Ask your patient to bend forward slightly while you visually identify the spinous processes, the paravertebral muscles, the scapulae, the iliac crests, and the posterior iliac spines (usually marked by dimples). Draw imaginary horizontal lines across the shoulders and iliac crests. Now draw an imaginary vertical line from T1 to the space between the buttocks (gluteal cleft). Any deviations suggest a variety of pathologies.

Next, observe your patient from the side. Evaluate the curves of the cervical, thoracic, and lumbar spine and note any irregularities. Common abnormalities of the spine include lordosis, scoliosis, and kyphosis (Table 7-5). Using the pads of your fingers, palpate the spinous processes for tenderness (Procedure 7-17a). Feel the supporting structures for muscle tone, symmetry, size, and tenderness or spasms. If your patient exhibits tenderness of the spinous processes and paravertebral muscles, suspect a herniated intervertebral disk, most commonly found between L4 and S1.

Now test range of motion. First, test for flexion by asking your patient to touch his chin to his chest (Procedure 7-17b). Flexion is normally 45 degrees. Next, ask him to bend his head backward. This tests extension, which normally is up to 55 degrees. Now test for rotation by asking your patient to touch his chin to each shoulder (Procedure 7-17c).

Table 7-5	SPINAL CURVATURES
Condition	**Description**
Normal	Concave in cervical and lumbar regions, convex in thorax
Lordosis	Exaggerated lumbar concavity (swayback)
Kyphosis	Exaggerated thoracic concavity (hunchback)
Scoliosis	Lateral curvature

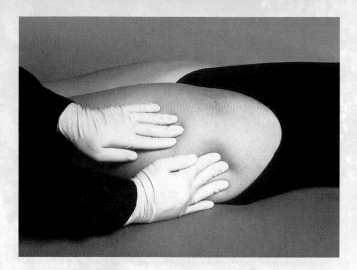

7-16a   Palpate the hip.

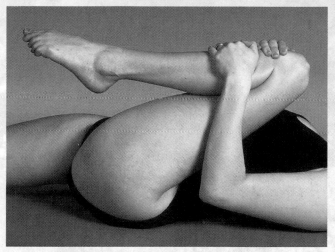

7-16b   Assess hip flexion with knee flexed.

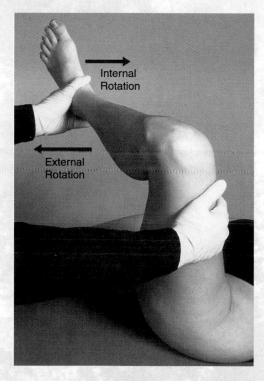

Internal
Rotation

External
Rotation

7-16c   Assess external and internal rotation
of the hip.

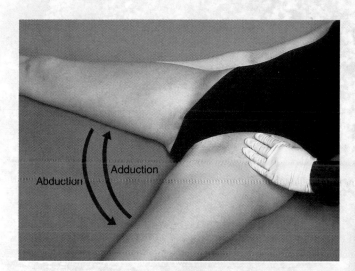

Adduction

Abduction

7-16d   Assess hip abduction and adduction.

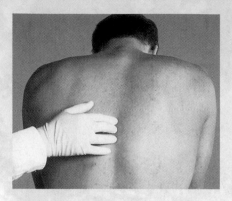

7-17a   Palpate the spine.

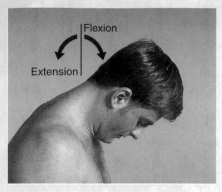

7-17b   Test flexion and extension of the head and neck.

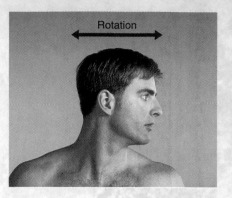

7-17c   Test rotation of the head and neck.

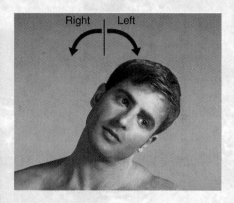

7-17d   Assess lateral bending of the head and neck.

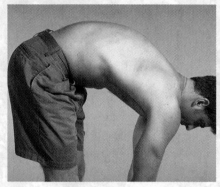

7-17e   Assess flexion of the lower spine.

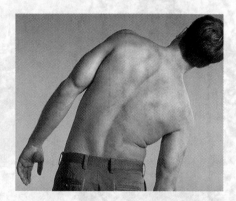

7-17f   Assess lateral bending of the lower spine.

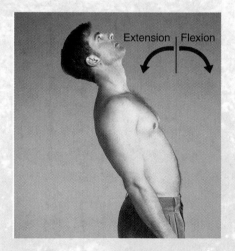

7-17g   Assess spinal extension.

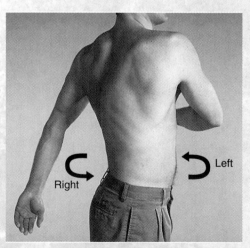

7-17h   Assess spinal rotation.

Normal rotation is 70 degrees on each side. Finally ask him to touch his ears to his shoulders without raising his shoulders. This assesses lateral bending, which normally is 40 degrees on each side (Procedure 7-17d). Now test for flexion of the lower spine with your patient standing. Ask him to bend and touch his toes (Procedure 7-17e). Note the smoothness and symmetry of movement, the range of motion, and the curves in the lumbar region. Normal flexion ranges from 75 degrees to 90 degrees. If the lumbar area remains concave or appears asymmetrical during this exam, your patient may have a muscle spasm. Next stabilize your patient's pelvis with your hands and have him bend sideways; normal lateral bending is 35 degrees on each side (Procedure 7-17f). To assess hyperextension, ask him to bend backward toward you; normal hyperextension is 30 degrees (Procedure 7-17g). Finally test spinal rotation by asking your patient to twist his shoulders one way, then the other. Normally they will rotate 30 degrees to each side (Procedure 7-17h).

If your patient complains of lower back pain radiating down the back of one leg, assess it by having him lie supine on the table. Ask him to raise his straightened leg until he feels pain. Note the angle of elevation at which the pain occurs, as well as the quality and distribution of the pain. Now dorsiflex your patient's foot. If this causes a sharp pain that radiates from your patient's back down his leg, suspect compression of the nerve roots of the lower lumbar region. Repeat this test with the other leg. Increased pain in the affected leg when the opposite leg is raised confirms the finding.

PERIPHERAL VASCULAR SYSTEM

To assess your patient's peripheral vascular system, inspect both arms from the fingertips to the shoulders. Note their size and symmetry. Observe swelling, venous congestion, the color of the skin and nail beds, and the skin texture. Yellow or brittle nails or poor color in the fingertips indicates chronic arterial insufficiency. Palpate the peripheral arteries to evaluate pulsation and capillary refill and to assess skin temperature (Procedure 7-18a and 7-18b). To palpate a peripheral pulse, lightly place your fingerpads over the artery's pulse point. Slowly increase the pressure until you feel a maximum pulsation. Note the rate, regularity, equality, and quality of the pulses. Count the number of beats in 1 minute. Then determine whether the pulse is regular, regularly irregular, or irregularly irregular. Finally, assess the quality of the pulse by noting its amplitude and contour; rate its quality from 0 to 3+ as shown in Table 7-6. Determine if it is absent, normal, weak, or bounding, and note any thrills (humming vibrations that feel similar to the throat of a purring cat). Thrills suggest a cardiac murmur or vascular narrowing. Expect the pulse of a normal adult to range between 60 and 100 beats per minute with a regular rhythm and normal amplitude.

Compare peripheral pulses bilaterally. If you detect a weak or absent pulse in one extremity, suspect an arterial occlusion proximal to the pulse point. Also compare distal and proximal pulses for equality. If you cannot palpate a distal artery, move proximally to another artery. For example, if you cannot palpate the radial artery, move to the brachial artery in the antecubital area.

Next, assess the feet and legs. Have your patient lie down and ask him to remove his socks. Inspect the legs from the feet to the groin. Note their size and symmetry. Evaluate the presence of swelling, venous congestion, the color of the skin and nail beds, and the skin texture. Note any venous enlargement. Evaluate scars, pigmentation, rashes, and ulcers. Palpate and compare the femoral pulses (Procedure 7-18c). Note the rate, regularity, equality, and quality of the pulses. Palpate the popliteal pulse behind the knee, the dorsalis pedis

Table 7-6	ASSESSING A PERIPHERAL PULSE
Score	Description
0	Absent pulse
1+	Weak or thready
2+	Normal
3+	Bounding

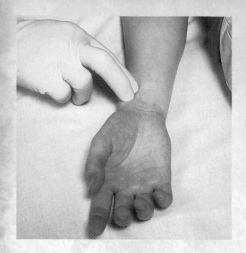

7-18a Palpate the radial artery.

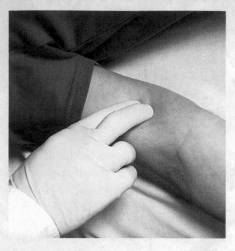

7-18b Palpate the brachial artery.

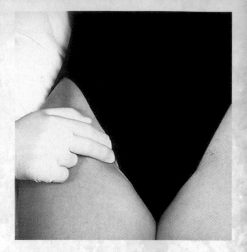

7-18c Palpate and compare the femoral arteries.

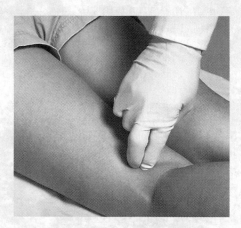

7-18d Palpate the popliteal pulse.

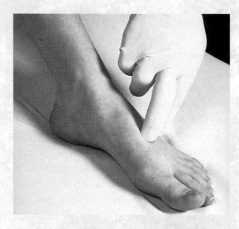

7-18e Palpate the dorsalis pedis pulse.

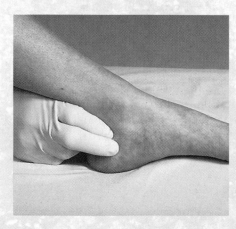

7-18f Palpate the posterior tibial pulse.

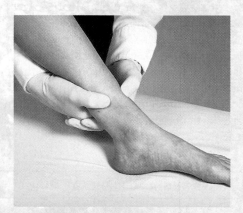

7-18g Palpate for edema.

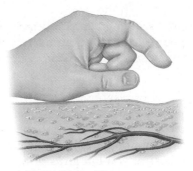
+1 Slight pitting edema

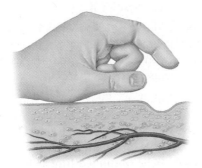
+4 Deep pitting edema

FIGURE 7-12   Assessing for edema.

pulse on top of the foot, and the posterior tibial pulse just behind the medial malleolus (Procedure 7-18d through 7-18f). Feel the temperature of the legs, feet, and toes with the back of your fingers and compare both sides. Unilateral coldness indicates an arterial occlusion. Bilateral coldness is due to an environmental problem, bilateral occlusion (saddle embolus) or to a general circulatory problem (shock).

Observe the legs for edema, the presence of an abnormal amount of fluid in the tissues. Compare one leg and foot with the other. Note their relative size and symmetry. Are veins, tendons, and bones easily visible under the skin? Edema will usually obscure these structures. Palpate for pitting edema by pressing firmly with your thumb for 5 seconds over the top of the foot, behind each medial ankle, and over the shins (Procedure 7-18g). **Pitting** is a depression left by the pressure of your thumb. Normally there should be no depression. If edema is present, evaluate the degree of pitting that can range from slight to marked (Figure 7-12). You can grade the depth of the pitting according to the appropriate scale in Table 7-7. Expect the pit to disappear within 10 seconds after you release the pressure. Bilateral edema suggests a central circulatory problem such as congestive heart failure or renal failure; unilateral edema suggests a lower extremity circulation abnormality such as deep vein thrombosis or venous occlusion. Note the extent of the edema. How far up the leg does it spread? The higher the edema, the more severe the problem.

pitting depression that results from pressure against skin when pitting edema is present.

NERVOUS SYSTEM

A comprehensive physical exam includes a thorough evaluation of your patient's mental status and thought processes. On the scene of an emergency, you would limit your mental exam to level of consciousness and basic orientation questions such as "What is your name?" "Where are you right now?" "What day is it today?" If you are conducting a full physical exam or evaluating someone with altered mentation, some or all of the following techniques will be useful.

When you conduct a neurological exam, you are attempting to answer two vital questions. First, are the findings symmetrical or unilateral? Second, if the signs are unilateral, is the site of origin in the central nervous system (brain and spinal cord) or in the peripheral nervous system (everything else).

A neurological exam attempts to answer two vital questions: are the findings symmetrical or unilateral, and if unilateral, where do they originate?

Content Review

AREAS OF NEUROLOGICAL EXAM
- Mental status and speech
- Motor system
- Sensory system

Table 7-7	PITTING EDEMA SCALE
Score	**Description**
1+	¼ inch or less
2+	¼ to ½ inch
3+	½ to 1 inch
4+	1 inch or more

Mental Status and Speech

Generally you will evaluate your patient's mental status and speech when you begin your interview. During this time you will assess his level of response, general appearance and behavior, and speech. If you detect abnormalities, continue your assessment with more specific questioning or testing as presented here.

Appearance and Behavior   First, assess your patient's level of response. Is he alert and awake? Does he understand your questions? Are his responses appropriate and timely, or does he drift off the topic easily or lose interest? If you detect an abnormality, continue with more specific questions. Is he lethargic (drowsy, but answers questions appropriately before falling asleep again)? Is he obtunded (opens his eyes and looks at you but gives slow, confused responses)? Sometimes you must arouse your patient repeatedly by gently shaking him or shouting his name. If he does not respond to your verbal cues, assess him with painful stimuli for coma or stupor. The stuporous patient is arousable for short periods but is not aware of his surroundings. The comatose patient is in a state of profound unconsciousness and is totally unarousable.

If your patient is awake and alert, observe his posture and motor behavior. Does he lie in bed or prefer to walk around? His posture should be erect and he should look at you. A slumped posture and a lack of facial expression may indicate depression. Excessive energetic movements or constantly watchful eyes suggest tension, anxiety, or a metabolic disorder. Watch the pace, range, and character of his movements. Are they voluntary? Are any parts immobile? Do posture and motor activity change with the environment? Some possible findings are listed in Table 7-8.

Observe your patient's grooming and personal hygiene. How is he dressed? Are his clothes clean, pressed, and properly fastened? Is his appearance appropriate for the season, climate, and occasion? A deterioration in grooming and personal hygiene in the previously well-groomed person may suggest an emotional problem, a psychiatric disorder, or an organic brain disease. Patients with obsessive-compulsive behavior may exhibit excessive attention to their appearance. Note your patient's hair, teeth, nails, skin, and beard. Are they well-groomed? Compare one side to another. One-sided neglect may suggest a brain lesion.

Also observe your patient's facial expressions. Are they appropriate? Do they vary when he talks with others and when the topic changes or is his face immobile throughout the interaction? Can he express happiness, sadness, anger, or depression? Patients with Parkinson's disease have facial immobility, with a mask-like appearance.

Speech and Language   Note your patient's speech pattern. Normally a person's speech is inflected, clear and strong, fluent and articulate, and varies in volume. It should express thoughts clearly. Is your patient excessively talkative or silent? Does he speak spontaneously or only when you ask him a direct question? Is his speech slow and quiet, as in depression? Is it fast and loud, as in a manic episode? Does he speak clearly and distinctly? Does he have dysarthria (defective speech caused by motor deficits), dysphonia (voice changes caused by vocal cord problems), or aphasia (defective language caused by neurologic damage to the brain)? With expressive aphasia his words will be garbled; with receptive aphasia, his words will be clear but unrelated to your questions. Your patient with aphasia may have such difficulty talking that you mistakenly suspect a psychotic disorder.

Mood   Observe your patient's verbal and nonverbal behavior for clues to his mood. Note any mood swings or behaviors that suggest anxiety or depression. Is he sad, elated, angry,

Table 7-8	POSTURE AND BEHAVIOR
Motor Activity	**Meaning**
Tense posture, restlessness, fidgeting	Anxiety
Crying, hand wringing, pacing	Agitated, depression
Hopeless, slumped posture, slowed movements	Depression
Singing, dancing, expansive movements	Manic

enraged, anxious, worried, detached, or indifferent? Assess the intensity of your patient's mood. How long has he been this way? Is his behavior normal for the circumstances? For example, anxiety is normal for someone having a heart attack; if your heart attack patient did not act frightened and concerned, that would be abnormal. If your patient is depressed, is he suicidal? If you suspect the possibility of suicide, ask him directly, "Have you ever thought of committing suicide? Are you currently thinking of committing suicide?"

Motor System

Inspect your patient's general body structure, muscle development, positioning, and coordination. What is his position at rest? Is he erect or does he slump to one side, suggesting unilateral paralysis or weakness? Note any obvious asymmetries, deformities, or involuntary movements. Are there tremors, tics, or fasciculations (twitches)? If so, note their location, rate, quality, rhythm, amplitude, and relation to your patient's posture, activity, fatigue, emotion, and other factors. For example, if your patient's hand begins to shake only when you ask him to perform a task with it such as writing his name or lifting a spoon, this suggests a postural tremor. Conversely, a tremor at rest that may disappear with voluntary movement suggests Parkinson's disease. To assess involuntary movement, observe your patient throughout the exam.

To determine your patient's muscle bulk, observe the size and contour of his muscles. Look for atrophy, a decrease in bulk and strength; hypertrophy, an increase in bulk and strength; or pseudohypertrophy, an increase in bulk and decrease in strength, as in muscular dystrophy. Flattened or concave contours, especially with fasciculations, may result from lower motor neuron disease. Some degree of muscle atrophy may be a normal part of the aging process or may result from the effects of diabetes on the peripheral nervous system. Look for signs of general muscle atrophy by checking for flattening of the thenar (thumb) muscle and for furrowing between the metacarpals. Unilateral muscle atrophy in the hands suggests median or ulnar nerve paralysis.

To assess muscle tone, feel the muscle's resistance to passive stretching in the extremities. Ask your patient to relax one of his arms. Then put the arm, wrists, and hands through a moderate range-of-motion exam (Procedure 7-19a). Repeat the exam in the lower extremities. If you detect decreased resistance, shake the hand loosely back and forth. It should move freely, but it should not be floppy (flaccid). Increased resistance may be caused by tension. Does the resistance persist throughout the motion (lead-pipe rigidity), or does it vary? If the resistance increases at the extreme limits of the movement, it is called spasticity. A ratchetlike jerkiness in the resistance is known as "cog-wheel rigidity," a common finding in a patient faking his symptoms or trying to resist your examination. Table 7-9 describes some common muscle tone findings.

Now focus on your patient's muscle strength. First, assess the strength of his grip. Test both grips simultaneously and compare them. Cross your middle finger over the top of your index finger to prevent your fingers from being hurt; then ask your patient to squeeze them as hard as possible (Procedure 7-19b). Normally you will have difficulty removing

Table 7-9	MUSCLE TONE
Finding	**Description**
Spasticity	Increased tone when passive movement applied, especially at the end of range. Common in stroke.
Rigidity	Increased rigidity throughout movement (lead-pipe). Common in Parkinson's disease and extrapyramidal reactions. Cog-wheel motion is a patient-applied resistance.
Flaccidity	Loss of muscle tone causing limb to be loose. Common in stroke, spinal cord lesion, and Guillain-Barré syndrome.
Paratonia	Sudden changes in tone with passive movement. Can be increased or decreased resistance. Common in dementia.

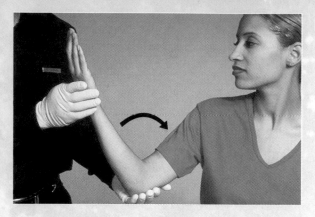

7-19a   Assess the elbow's range of motion.

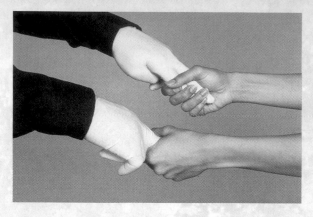

7-19b   Test your patient's grip.

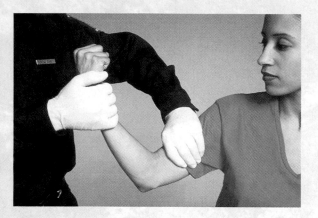

7-19c   Test arm strength.

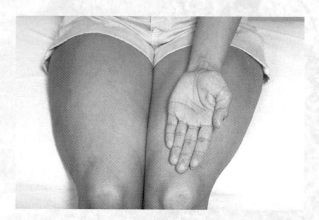

7-19d   Test for coordination with rapid alternating movements.

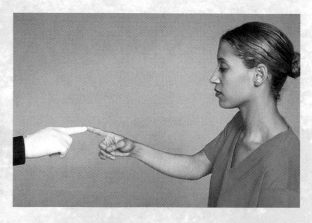

7-19e   Test coordination with point-to-point testing.

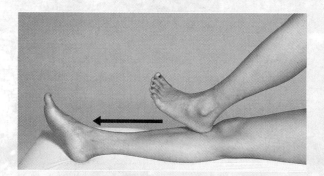

7-19f   Assess coordination with heel-to-shin testing.

Table 7-10 MUSCLE STRENGTH TESTS

Muscles	Nerves	Test
Biceps	C5, C6	Flexion of the elbow
Triceps	C6, C7, C8	Extension of the elbow
Wrist extensors	C6, C7, C8, radial nerve	Extension of the wrist
Fingers	C8, T1, ulnar nerve	Finger abduction
Thumb	C8, T1, median nerve	Thumb opposition
Iliopsoas	L2, L3, L4	Hip flexion
Hip extensor	S1	Hip extension
Hip abductors	L4, L5, S1	Hip abduction
Hip adductors	L2, L3, L4	Hip adduction
Quadriceps	L2, L3, L4	Knee extension
Hamstrings	L4, L5, S1, S2	Knee flexion
Feet	L4, L5	Dorsiflexion
Calf muscles	S1	Plantar flexion

Table 7-11 MUSCLE STRENGTH SCALE

Score	Description
5	Active movement against full resistance with no fatigue
4	Active movement against some resistance and gravity
3	Active movement against gravity
2	Active movement with gravity eliminated
1	Barely palpable muscle contraction with no movement
0	No visible or palpable muscle contraction

your fingers from your patient's grip. Continue testing all of the muscle groups listed in Table 7-10. While assessing muscle strength remember that each patient's age, gender, size, and muscular training will affect your exam results. When comparing sides, your patient's dominant side will be stronger. Test for muscle strength by having your patient move actively against your resistance (Procedure 7-19c). If the muscle is too weak to perform against resistance, have him try the movement against gravity or with gravity eliminated (you support the limb). Grade muscle strength on a scale from 1 to 5 (Table 7-11).

To assess your patient's coordination, test for rapid alternating movements. These maneuvers can be difficult to describe, so you should always demonstrate them to your patient. Ask him to repeat them as rapidly as possible while you observe for speed, rhythm, and smoothness. He should repeat all movements with both sides of the body. Keep in mind that his dominant hand usually will perform better than his nondominant hand. If his movements are slow, irregular and clumsy, suspect cerebellar or extrapyramidal tract disease or upper motor neuron weakness.

First, have your patient tap the distal joint of his thumb with the tip of his index finger as rapidly as possible. Then ask him to place his hand, palm up, on his thigh, quickly turn it over palm down, and return it palm up (Procedure 7-19d). Have him repeat this movement as quickly as possible for 15 seconds; evaluate both hands. Next have him perform point-to-point testing. Ask him to alternate touching your index finger and his nose several times while you observe for accuracy and smoothness (Procedure 7-19e). Note any tremors or difficulty performing this task, indicating cerebellar disease; evaluate both hands. Now assess for point-to-point testing in his legs. Ask him to touch his heel to the opposite knee, then run it down his shin to his big toe (Procedure 7-19f). Note the smoothness and accuracy of his actions. Repeat the test with the other leg. To test your patient's position sense, have him close his eyes and repeat this test for both legs. Abnormalities suggest cerebellar disease.

Sensory System

To assess the sensory system, test for pain, light touch, temperature, position, vibration, and discriminative sensations. Remember to compare distal areas to proximal areas, to compare symmetrical areas bilaterally, and to scatter the stimuli to assess most of the dermatomes. Ask your patient to close his eyes for each of these tests. To test for pain sensation, touch your patient's skin with a sharp object and ask him to tell you whether it is sharp or dull. Compare areas as you move along the different regions, intermittently substituting a dull object for the sharp one. To test for light touch, softly touch him with a fine piece of cotton. Ask him to tell you whenever he feels the cotton. An abnormality suggests a peripheral neuropathy. Test for temperature sensation by touching his skin with a vial filled with either hot or cold liquid.

PHYSICAL EXAMINATION OF INFANTS AND CHILDREN

Conducting a physical examination of a sick or injured child can challenge any clinician. Your success will depend on several factors. First, you must be familiar with the anatomical differences between children and adults. Second, you must understand the physical and psychological developmental stages of the different age groups. Most importantly, you must practice these skills daily.

BUILDING PATIENT AND FAMILY RAPPORT

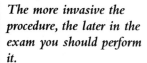

Children are not small adults, and you must not treat them as if they were.

Children are not small adults, and you must not treat them as if they were. Children are naturally apprehensive of strangers and new things. A sick or injured child is a frightened child. He fears pain, separation from his family, and unfamiliar surroundings. Dealing with these fears paves the way for a successful encounter with the child and his parents. You are a stranger. In uniform, you become even more ominous. Gaining your pediatric patient's trust becomes a vital part of your assessment. Unless he requires emergency critical care, take time to establish a rapport with him. This will help to ensure continuous cooperation.

The more invasive the procedure, the later in the exam you should perform it.

Although different age groups have specific fears and characteristics, the following general rules apply to pediatrics as a whole. Remain calm and confident. Be direct and honest about what you are doing, especially if you are performing a painful procedure. If possible, do not separate the child from his parents. Instead, elicit their help in obtaining the history and allow them to help hold the child while you conduct your exam. The more invasive the procedure, the later in the exam you should perform it—unless, of course, your patient is critically ill or injured. (Never delay important procedures or techniques on the critically ill or injured child.) Once your patient begins crying and resisting, the more difficult the rest of your exam will be, if not impossible. Finally, provide continuous reassurance and feedback to your patient and his family members. This helps reduce everyone's anxiety over what is wrong, what you are doing, and what comes next.

Position yourself at the child's eye level, use a soft voice, and smile a lot. Often a small toy, such as a teddy bear, can distract your patient while you examine him. If you are using diagnostic equipment, allow the child to handle it while you explain how it works. Make sure your movements are slow and deliberate, and explain everything you are doing.

ANATOMY AND THE PHYSICAL EXAM

To assess a child properly, you must understand his unique anatomy (Figure 7-13). The anatomical differences among age groups will alter your interpretation of physical findings. For example, since an infant's skin is thinner and contains less subcutaneous fat, you can expect environmental temperature extremes to affect him more severely.

This section deals with examining infants and children in the clinical situation. The pediatric chapter, Chapter 31, discusses a more detailed pediatric assessment.

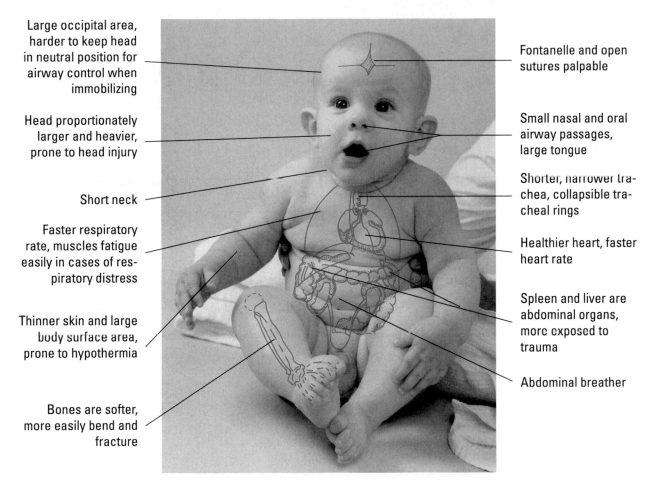

Large occipital area, harder to keep head in neutral position for airway control when immobilizing

Head proportionately larger and heavier, prone to head injury

Short neck

Faster respiratory rate, muscles fatigue easily in cases of respiratory distress

Thinner skin and large body surface area, prone to hypothermia

Bones are softer, more easily bend and fracture

Fontanelle and open sutures palpable

Small nasal and oral airway passages, large tongue

Shorter, narrower trachea, collapsible tracheal rings

Healthier heart, faster heart rate

Spleen and liver are abdominal organs, more exposed to trauma

Abdominal breather

FIGURE 7-13 Pediatric anatomy and physiology. You must understand a child's unique anatomy to assess him properly.

General Appearance

Especially in the emergency setting, note whether your patient looks toxic (sick). A toxic child appears not to recognize or respond to his parents. He may look tired and have a decreased respiratory effort and may have mottled skin or a generalized rash. He may be gray or cyanotic and look very sick, usually from some type of bacterial process. These children, who present with the signs and symptoms of respiratory failure or shock, usually require rapid transport while you provide aggressive resuscitation procedures (advanced airway management, oxygenation and ventilation, IV access, and rapid fluid administration).

Head and Neck

The bones of the skull are soft and the fontanelles ("soft spots," spaces between a child's cranial bones) stay opened until about 18 months (Figure 7-14). From this time until about age five, cartilage connects the sutures. This allows the skull to expand as the brain grows. Check the sutures for bulging (increased intracranial pressure) or sunkenness (dehydration). In infants, a soft bulging spot following a history of trauma suggests a head injury with increasing intracranial pressure. The same finding associated with a fever suggests meningitis.

Because a child's airways are so much smaller than an adult's, a minor obstruction can create an acute respiratory problem. Watch the child's face for signs of distress and increased respiratory effort, such as nasal flaring. Children in acute respiratory distress will appear anxious and not interested in their surroundings. Also watch for retractions and head bobbing. Listen for stridor, wheezing, and grunting as further signs of severe breathing problems. As the child speaks, listen for hoarseness (upper airway obstruction)

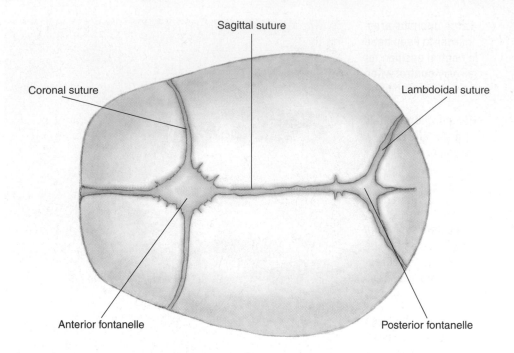

FIGURE 7-14   Fontanelle of the infant skull.

Hoarseness, suggesting an upper airway obstruction, or moaning, suggesting decreased consciousness, requires intervention and rapid transport.

or moaning (decreasing level of consciousness). These findings always require appropriate intervention and rapid transport. Remember, a crying or screaming child has a patent airway.

Observe the child's face for signs of pain and discomfort as you continue your examination. Inspect his eyes as you would an adult's. Assess the outer ear for position. The top of the ear should be on a horizontal line with the outer corner of the eye.

Inspect the child's mouth much the same as you would for the adult. A young child's mouth is small, but the tongue is relatively large, so examining his oral cavity will be a challenge. Examine the nose using a penlight. To examine the mucous membrane, tip the child's head back and use the penlight to inspect for color or swelling.

Evaluate the child's neck for stiffness, which—when associated with a fever—suggests meningitis.

Chest and Lungs

The rib cage in infants and small children is elastic and flexible. Because it is composed of more cartilage than bone at this age, rib fractures are rare. On the other hand, lung contusions are common, because the lung tissue is very fragile. Small children also have a mobile mediastinum with a greater tendency to develop a tension pneumothorax. The chest muscles are not well developed, so children are mostly diaphragm breathers until about age seven.

The chest muscles are considered accessory muscles in the young child; to evaluate his breathing, observe both the chest and abdomen for movement. A child in severe respiratory distress may exhibit a "see-saw" pattern in which his sternum and abdomen rise and fall in opposition to each other. Count the respiratory rate without touching your patient, if possible. Assess the rate, quality, and depth of his respirations. Normal respiratory rates vary with age, but generally they decrease as the child grows older. Table 7-12 gives normal vital signs for the various pediatric age groups. Auscultate for breath sounds with the bell of your stethoscope at the mid-axillary lines (Figure 7-15). Use this location to avoid hearing transmitted breath sounds from the opposite lung fields.

Cardiovascular

Unless the child has a congenital defect, his heart will be strong and healthy. His heart rate will vary with age, but generally it will decrease as he gets older. If the child is alert and uncooperative, measure his pulse rate by listening to the heart. Place your stethoscope between

Table 7-12	NORMAL PEDIATRIC VITAL SIGNS		
Age Group	Respiratory Rate	Heart Rate	Systolic Blood Pressure
Newborn	30–60	100–180	60–90
Infant	30–60	100–160	87–105
Toddler	24–40	80–110	95–105
Preschooler	22–34	70–110	95–110
School age	18–30	65–110	97–112
Adolescent	12–26	60–90	112–128

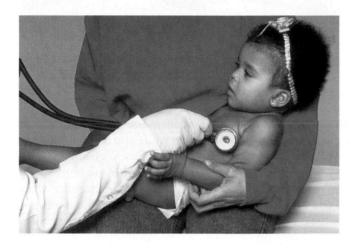

FIGURE 7-15 Place your stethoscope along your young patient's mid-axillary line.

the sternum and nipple on your patient's left side. Children have thin chest walls, so you will usually be able to observe the apical impulse of the heart. Remember that tachycardia or bradycardia can both be a response to hypoxia in infants and young children. Bradycardia is the initial response to this condition in the newborn; without aggressive intervention, cardiopulmonary arrest will soon follow. Blood pressure will vary in children, but generally it will rise as they grow older. Children respond to hypovolemia by increasing cardiac function.

Tachycardia or bradycardia both can be a response to hypoxia in infants and young children. Without aggressive intervention cardiopulmonary arrest will soon follow.

Abdomen

A child's liver and spleen are proportionally larger and more vascular than an adult's. Thus they extend beyond the rib cage and are more exposed. Likewise, the child's immature abdominal muscles provide less protection than an adult's. Inspect the abdomen first for movement. Normally only respiratory movements should be visible; peristalsis is not normally observable. Next, assess contour. The abdomen normally bulges by the end of inspiration. Note any asymmetry. Inspect the groin area for inguinal hernias, common in male children. Finally, look at the umbilicus for any hernias, common in children under three years.

Before you begin palpating the abdomen, make sure the child is comfortable. Bend his knees to relax the abdominal muscles and make palpation easier. Your hands should be warm. If the child is ticklish, cover his hands with yours as you palpate. Begin with light palpation and gradually increase the pressure (Figure 7-16). Palpate all four quadrants. Deep palpation is performed next. You are feeling for masses and tenderness. The child's facial expression is a better guide to pain than his words, since he may interpret your pressure as pain.

Musculoskeletal

Evaluate pulses, sensation, movement, and warmth in all four extremities. Check for capillary refill and feel for peripheral pulses (Figure 7-17). Evaluate the skin, which reveals important clues in children. Its color, turgor, moisture, and temperature are key indicators of his cardiovascular system's condition. Unlike the adult's, the child's capillary refill time

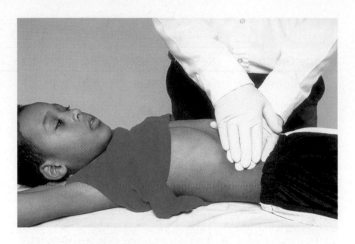

FIGURE 7-16 Gradually increase the pressure when palpating a young patient's abdomen.

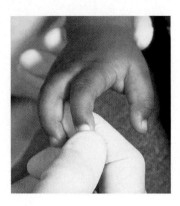

FIGURE 7-17 Pressing a child's fingernail is one of several ways to assess capillary refill. The child's capillary refill time is a good indicator of the child's peripheral perfusion status.

accurately reflects his peripheral perfusion status. When examining the musculoskeletal system, remember the growth and posture at different stages of the child's development. For example, a toddler walks with a broad base for support and is likely to appear bowlegged. A teenager with poor posture may suffer from a skeletal problem such as scoliosis.

Palpate the upper and lower extremities for swelling, tenderness, and contractions. Next have the child demonstrate the range of motion of his joints while you feel for smoothness of movement. Examine all joints. Check muscle strength in all muscle groups by asking the child to prevent you from moving a part of his body. A child's bones are more likely to break at the ends, where growth takes place. Until the child reaches adolescence, when these areas become as strong as the rest of the bone, injuries that occur near the joints are more likely to damage the bone than the ligaments or tendons. Assess the child's muscle coordination by having him stand and then hop on one foot. Repeat this for the other foot. Children usually enjoy this aspect of the physical examination. You can also have the child skip or jump.

Nervous System

The child's general behavior, level of consciousness, and orientation are signs of cerebral function. You have asked the parents to comment on their child's behavior during the history taking. You have observed the child's behavior throughout the examination and already have learned much about his cerebral function by interacting with him. Now test specific functions such as language and recall. You can test for cerebellar function with several games that children usually enjoy. First, as you move your finger, ask the child to touch his nose and then your finger. Consistent past-pointing should arouse your suspicion. An alternate test is to have the child pat his knees alternately with the palms and backs of his hands. Check for sensation over the child's face, trunk, arms, and leg. Check for hot and cold sensation by alternately touching the skin with warm and cold test tubes. Ask the child to close his eyes and tell you which he feels.

Remember, the most important characteristic of a physical assessment is thoroughness. Be systematic in your approach and, with practice, you will be able to do a complete and accurate physical assessment.

The most important characteristic of a physical assessment is thoroughness.

RECORDING EXAMINATION FINDINGS

The patient record is only as good as the accuracy, depth, and detail you provide.

After you perform the history and physical examination, it is time to record the findings on your patient's chart or permanent medical record. The information you enter enables you and other members of the health-care team to identify health problems, make a diagnosis, plan the appropriate care, and monitor your patient's response to treatment. The patient record is only as good as the accuracy, depth, and detail you provide.

All health-care clinicians follow a standard format when charting patient information. Using it and appropriate medical terminology will allow everyone to easily read and understand your assessment findings. Although your first attempts at writing a complete history and physical exam will be lengthy and possibly disorganized, clinical experience will eventually lead to a more efficient and organized record.

Your patient's chart is a legal document, and any information you enter may be used in court. Proper documentation is vital to your protection. Present the data legibly, accurately, and truthfully. The information should represent the findings of your history and physical examination—no more, no less. State your assessment, your analysis of the problem, and your management plan clearly and exactly. No question should ever arise about your assessment or care of your patient if you document it properly.

Be sure to include all data about your assessment. You cannot formulate an impression unless you have clearly spelled out the positive and negative details on which it was made. Remember that the absence of a sign or symptom (pertinent negative) may be just as important as its presence. Record everything in writing. If you do not document a neurological exam, you will never convince anyone that you performed it, especially not a plaintiff's lawyer or a jury. Be complete but avoid unnecessary words. For example, say "pale," not "pale in color." Also avoid lengthy repetitive phrases such as "patient states." Use accepted abbreviations and symbols whenever possible. Avoid using vague adjectives such as good, normal, and poor, because they are open to interpretation by other providers. Document what your patient tells you, not what you infer or interpret. Use direct quotes whenever possible.

The universally accepted organization for patient charts follows the subjective, objective, assessment, and plan (SOAP) format. Use this format when writing your patient's chart. Subjective information is what your patient tells you. It is composed of the chief complaint, the history of present illness, the past history, the current health status, and the review of systems. Objective information includes the data collected from the general survey, vital signs, head-to-toe anatomical exam, systems-oriented exam, and neurological exam, including the mental status. These are the data you gathered by inspection, palpation, percussion, auscultation, and other techniques of physical examination. Objective information also includes the results of any laboratory tests. The assessment summarizes the relevant data for each problem identified in the history and physical exam. The plan outlines your management strategy in three categories: diagnostic (how you will assess progress), therapeutic (any treatments), and educational (what you need to teach your patient). Chapter 11, "Documentation," deals with prehospital documentation in detail.

> *Record* everything *in writing.*

SUMMARY

This chapter has presented both a regional and a systems approach to physical examination. The setting, chief complaint, and clinical status of your patient will dictate how much of the physical exam you actually use. If you are at the scene of a critically ill or injured patient, you will assess only those areas relevant to the situation. If your patient presents with a minor, isolated musculoskeletal injury, you may focus your exam on that area and system. As you become more experienced, making these decisions will become easier.

ON THE WEB

For additional practice and review, go to the companion website at www.prenhall.com/bledsoe and click on *Intermediate Emergency Care: Principles & Practice.*

CHAPTER 8

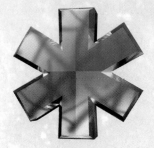

Patient Assessment in the Field

Objectives

After reading this chapter, you should be able to:

1. Recognize hazards/potential hazards associated with medical and trauma scenes. (pp. 481–488)
2. Identify unsafe scenes and describe methods for making them safe. (pp. 481–488)
3. Discuss common mechanisms of injury/nature of illness. (pp. 489–491)
4. Discuss the reason for identifying the total number of patients at the scene. (pp. 488–489)
5. Organize the management of a scene following size-up. (pp. 481–488)
6. Explain the reasons for identifying the need for additional help or assistance during the scene size-up. (pp. 481, 484–488)
7. Summarize the reasons for forming a general impression of the patient. (pp. 491–493)
8. Discuss methods of assessing mental status/levels of consciousness in the adult, infant, and child. (pp. 493–494)
9. Discuss methods of assessing and securing a patient's airway. (pp. 494–496)
10. State reasons for taking spinal precautions for the trauma patient. (pp. 492–493)
11. Describe methods for assessing respiration. (pp. 496–497)
12. Describe methods for assessing circulation, including assessing for external bleeding. (p. 497)
13. Describe normal and abnormal findings when assessing skin color, temperature, and condition. (p. 497)
14. Explain the reason and process for prioritizing a patient for care and transport. (pp. 500–501)
15. Describe orthostatic vital signs and evaluate their usefulness in assessing a patient in shock. (p. 516)
16. Describe the physical examination of a medical patient. (pp. 511–517)
17. Differentiate between an assessment for a patient who has an altered mental status and an assessment of other medical patients. (pp. 511–517)
18. Discuss the reasons for reconsidering the mechanism of injury. (pp. 503–505)
19. Explain why patients should receive a rapid trauma assessment and recite examples. (p. 503)
20. Describe the physical examination of a trauma patient. (pp. 503–510)

CASE STUDY

En route to the scene, EMT-Intermediates (EMT-Is) Chris Johnson and Nick Farina prepare for the worst. The initial report from bystanders at the scene says that a woman jumped from a fourth-floor balcony at the downtown shopping mall. She reportedly landed four stories below on the marble floor and lies bleeding with multiple injuries. If this is true, Chris thinks, she and Nick will likely find a significant mechanism of injury and serious injuries.

Upon arrival, Chris's worst fears come true. A woman in her 30s lies on the floor in a pool of blood with signs of obvious multiple trauma. Immediately, Chris directs Nick to stabilize the woman's head and neck and manually open her airway with a jaw-thrust. Nick, also a part-time respiratory therapist, is well suited for the job.

Chris begins the initial assessment by evaluating the patient's level of consciousness. She quickly notes that the patient is unresponsive to all stimuli. She then assesses the airway, which is noisy with gurgling blood. She immediately suctions the oropharynx and listens for air movement. The patient has shallow respirations at a rate of 38 per minute. Nick inserts an oropharyngeal airway and begins ventilation with a bag-valve mask (BVM) and supplemental oxygen at a rate of 12 per minute while Chris continues her assessment.

Because the patient exhibits signs of severe respiratory distress, Chris decides to assess her neck and chest before proceeding with the initial assessment. She quickly exposes the patient's chest and notices deformity to the right side with probable multiple rib fractures. She auscultates the chest and, noticing decreased breath sounds on the right side, suspects a pneumothorax or pulmonary contusion. Chris feels for radial and carotid pulses. She notes the absence of a radial pulse and the cool, pale look of the patient's skin. The carotid pulse is weak at a rate of approximately 130 beats per minute. Nick comments that the patient is in shock. Chris designates her as a priority 1, indicating rapid transport to the appropriate medical facility.

While Nick continues to maintain manual stabilization of the patient's neck, Chris begins a rapid trauma assessment. She starts at the head and quickly palpates a depressed skull fracture. Chris notes that her patient's trachea is midline and jugular veins are flat, temporarily ruling out a tension pneumothorax. She notices a rigid, distended abdomen and suspects intra-abdominal bleeding, which is most likely causing the profound shock. Next, Chris palpates the pelvis and notes an unstable pelvic ring, indicating

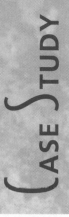
fracture. She also notes severe deformity and angulation to both femurs, suggesting bilateral fractures. As additional help from the fire department arrives, Chris instructs them to immobilize her patient with the pneumatic antishock garment while she prepares the back of the ambulance for transport.

During the four-minute ride to Memorial Hospital, Chris reassesses the patient's mental status and ABCs. She notes the following: heart rate, 130 and weak; blood pressure, 76/40; respirations, 38 and shallow. Chris decides to start two large-bore intravenous (IV) lines to begin fluid resuscitation. Nick performs the procedure and runs both lines wide-open. Chris contacts the hospital and gives a quick report to Dr. Prasad, the attending physician. Upon arrival, they transfer their patient to the emergency department staff and watch as an experienced team of trauma specialists prepares their patient for a quick ride to surgery.

INTRODUCTION

patient assessment problem-oriented evaluation of patient and establishment of priorities based on existing and potential threats to human life.

Patient assessment means conducting a problem-oriented evaluation of your patient and establishing priorities of care based on existing and potential threats to human life. In the previous two chapters you studied the techniques of performing a history and physical exam. As an EMT-I, you will certainly never perform all of the components of a history and physical exam in the acute setting. It is too time consuming and yields too much irrelevant information. Instead you will use your foundation of knowledge, skills, and tools to assess the acutely ill or injured patient. With time and clinical experience you will learn which components of the comprehensive exam apply to your particular patient.

Now you can use the pertinent components of the history and physical exam to perform patient assessments—problem-oriented assessments based on your patient's chief complaint. The basic components of patient assessment include the initial assessment; the focused history and physical exam, including vital signs; an ongoing assessment; and in some cases, a detailed physical exam.

Your patient's condition will determine which components you use and how you use them. For example, for trauma patients with a significant mechanism of injury, you will perform an initial assessment followed by a rapid trauma assessment (a head-to-toe exam aimed at traumatic signs and symptoms) and, if time allows, a detailed physical exam en route to the hospital. For patients with minor, isolated trauma, an initial assessment followed by a focused physical exam is warranted. For the responsive medical patient, you will conduct an initial assessment followed by a focused history and physical exam. Finally, for the unresponsive medical patient, you will perform an initial assessment followed by a rapid medical assessment (a head-to-toe exam aimed at medical signs and symptoms). In all cases, you will perform an ongoing assessment en route to the hospital to detect changes in patient condition.

The initial assessment's goal is to identify and correct immediately life-threatening conditions. These include airway compromise, inadequate ventilation, and major hemorrhage. During this rapid evaluation you use a variety of maneuvers and special equipment to manage any life threats as you find them. Immediately following the initial assessment you will establish the priorities of care. People such as the trauma patient with unstable vital signs and the unresponsive medical patient require a rapid head-to-toe exam and immediate transport to the hospital. Patients with minor, isolated trauma and most medical emergencies allow time to perform further assessments and provide care before transport.

Content Review

COMPONENTS OF PATIENT ASSESSMENT
- Initial assessment
- Focused history and physical exam
- Ongoing assessment
- Detailed physical exam

ALS advanced life support.

Your proficiency in performing a systematic patient assessment will determine your ability to deliver the highest quality of prehospital advanced life support (**ALS**) to sick and injured people. EMT-I patient assessment is a straightforward skill, similar to the assessment you might have performed as an EMT-Basic. It differs, however, in depth and in the kind of care you will provide as a result. Your assessment must be thorough, because many advanced life-support procedures are potentially dangerous. Safely and appropriately performing advanced procedures such as administration of drugs, defibrillation, synchronized cardioversion, or endotracheal intubation will depend on your assessment and correct field diagnosis. If your assessment does not reveal your patient's true problem, the consequences can be devastating.

As always, common sense dictates how you proceed in the field. When you assess the responsive medical patient, the history reveals the most important diagnostic information and takes priority over the physical exam. For the trauma patient and the unresponsive medical patient, the reverse is true. Yet trauma may cause a medical emergency, and conversely, a medical emergency may cause trauma. Only by performing a thorough patient assessment can you discover the true cause of your patient's problems. This chapter provides problem-oriented patient assessment templates based on the information and techniques presented in the previous two chapters. You will need to refer to those chapters for the details of taking a history and conducting a physical exam.

SCENE SIZE-UP

Scene size-up is the essential first step at any emergency. Before you enter a scene, take the necessary time to judge the situation. Fire officials drive just past a burning house so they can see three of its sides before they make strategic decisions. Follow their lead. Never rush into any situation; first stop and look around (Figure 8-1).

Upon arrival, determine whether the scene is safe. Does the situation require special body substance isolation (BSI) precautions? Is the mechanism of injury or the nature of illness obvious? Are there multiple patients? Do you need immediate additional resources? After an initial scene assessment, if necessary, report to your dispatcher what you have, what you need, and what you are doing. This way, you keep everyone informed and your dispatcher can send any necessary additional support.

Although size-up is your initial responsibility, remember that it is also an ongoing process. Emergency scenes are dynamic and can change suddenly. An injury to a child can erupt into a violent domestic dispute if one parent blames the other. A hazardous material

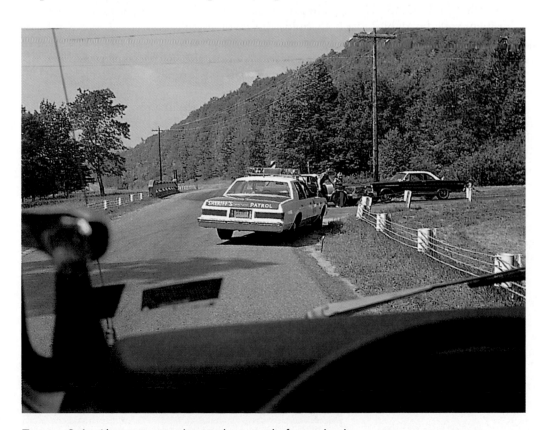

FIGURE 8-1 Always stop to size up the scene before going in.

If your assessment does not reveal your patient's true problem, the consequences can be devastating.

Only by performing a thorough patient assessment can you discover the true cause of your patient's problems.

Content Review

COMPONENTS OF SCENE SIZE-UP

• Body substance isolation
• Scene safety
• Location of all patients
• Mechanism of injury
• Nature of illness

Never rush into any situation; first stop and look around.

spill can ignite. An improperly stabilized car can shift. Always be alert for subtle signs of danger and avoid becoming a patient yourself.

Sizing up the scene gives you important information that will guide your actions. In trauma, a brief size-up of the accident scene reveals the mechanism of injury. From this, you can estimate the degree of energy transfer and possible seriousness of injuries. In a medical emergency, you can sometimes determine the nature of your patient's illness from clues at the scene. The smell of lower gastrointestinal (GI) bleeding, the sound of a hissing oxygen tank, or the sight of drug paraphernalia provides clues and an initial insight into your patient's situation. Learn to use all your senses when sizing up the scene.

The components of a scene size-up include:

- Body substance isolation (BSI) precautions
- Scene safety
- Location of all patients
- Mechanism of injury
- Nature of the illness

BODY SUBSTANCE ISOLATION

Body fluids frequently contain health-threatening pathogens. The best defense against bloodborne, body-fluidborne, and airborne agents is to take appropriate body substance isolation (BSI) precautions. Your goal is to prevent infectious disease from spreading to yourself or to others. Make sure that personal protective equipment such as gloves, masks, gowns, and eye protection is available on every emergency vehicle, and take the appropriate precautions on every emergency call (Figure 8-2). Your patient's clinical condition and the procedures you perform will determine the required precautions.

Most body isolation procedures are simply common sense. Wash your hands thoroughly before and after treating each patient whenever possible (Figure 8-3). This simple technique is the most effective method of preventing disease transmission between patients and their health-care workers. Wear latex or vinyl gloves anytime you expect to contact blood or other body fluids. This includes the mucous membranes, any areas with broken skin, or items soiled with blood or body fluids. Since you often cannot wash your hands before examining your patient, you should wear gloves also to avoid exposing your patient to your germs. If you are managing multiple patients, you should attempt to change gloves between patients in order to prevent cross-contamination. Discard all contaminated gloves in the appropriate biohazard bag (Figure 8-4).

Always use all the equipment recommended for a particular procedure or patient to maximize your protection against communicable diseases. If blood, vomit, or secretions might splash near your eyes, nose, or mouth, wear a face mask and protective eyewear. Such situations may include arterial bleeding, childbirth, invasive procedures such as endotracheal intubation, and oral suctioning, as well as during clean-up when heavy scrubbing is

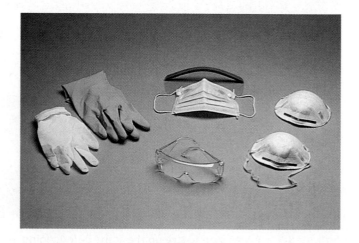

FIGURE 8-2 Always wear the appropriate personal protective equipment (PPE) to prevent exposure to contagious diseases.

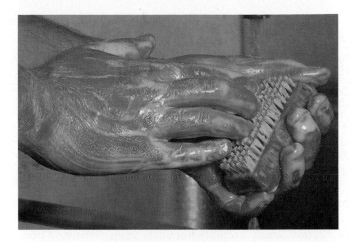

FIGURE 8-3 Careful, methodical handwashing helps reduce exposure to contagious disease.

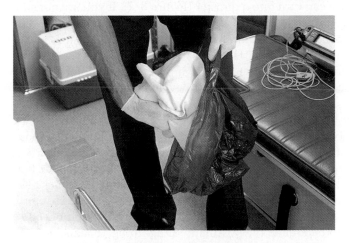

FIGURE 8-4 Place all contaminated items in the appropriate biohazard bag.

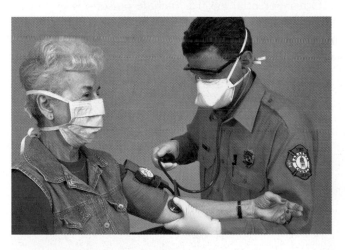

FIGURE 8-5 With a suspected tuberculosis patient, you may place a surgical-type mask on the patient while you wear a NIOSH-approved respirator. Monitor the patient's airway and breathing carefully.

necessary. If you expect large blood splashes, such as in emergency childbirth, wear a gown to protect your clothing.

Consider masking both yourself and your patient whenever the potential for airborne transmission of disease exists (Figure 8-5). The National Institute of Occupational Safety and Health has designed high-efficiency particulate air (HEPA) respirators to filter out the tuberculosis bacillus (TB). Always wear a properly fitted HEPA mask if you are managing a patient with suspected TB, especially when performing procedures such as endotracheal intubation, oral suctioning, and administering nebulized medications. These procedures present a high risk for the transmission of airborne particles.

SCENE SAFETY

scene safety doing everything possible to ensure a safe environment.

Scene safety simply means doing everything possible to ensure a safe environment for yourself, your crew, other responding personnel, your patient, and any bystanders—in that order. Your personal safety is the top priority at any emergency scene. Make sure you are not injured while providing care. If you become a patient yourself, you will do your own patient little good. You must determine that no hazards may endanger the lives of people on the scene. If your scene is unsafe, either make it safe or wait until someone else does (Figure 8-6).

Your personal safety is the top priority at any emergency scene.

As the first unit on the scene, you may overestimate your capability to manage a rescue situation. Do not attempt a hazardous rescue unless you are properly clothed, equipped, and trained. Individual acts of courage are sometimes necessary, but modern rescue operations emphasize safety first, not heroics. Foolish heroics often end in tragedy. If in doubt, it is better to err on the side of caution than to risk personal harm.

Content Review

ORDER OF PRIORITIES FOR SCENE SAFETY

1. You
2. Your crew
3. Other responding personnel
4. Your patient
5. Bystanders

Many factors can make an emergency scene unsafe. Through experience you will learn to identify them quickly. Do not become complacent. Sometimes even the most non-threatening, harmless-looking scene can turn into a disaster (Figure 8-7). If you are not sure the scene is safe, do not enter. As you approach a scene, immediately evaluate the surrounding area. Is it as your dispatcher's information has led you to expect, or does something just not look right? What do the bystanders' faces tell you? Are they angry, scared, or panicked? Be alert for situations that look or feel suspicious. If necessary, wait until law enforcement personnel secure the scene. Use all your senses to evaluate a scene and learn to trust your intuition. If your instincts tell you not to enter or to get out, follow them. They are the subconscious sum of your experiences. Listen to them; they are probably correct.

Listen to your instincts; they are probably correct.

Carefully look for and identify on-scene hazards before even attempting to reach your patient. To do otherwise places you, other rescuers, and your patient at risk. Remember that you may find such dangers at either medical or trauma scenes. Potential hazards include fire, structural collapse, traffic, unstable surfaces, and broken glass or jagged metal. Other risks involve hazardous materials—chemical spills, radiation, or gas leaks that might ignite or explode. A simple spark can set off a gas leak or oil spill. Electrical wires threaten both fire and electric shock. Look around to determine the possibility of lightning, avalanche, rock slides, cave-ins, or similar dangers. Other potential hazards include poisonous or caustic substances; biological agents; germ-infested materials; confined spaces such as vessels,

In every case, let common sense dictate scene management.

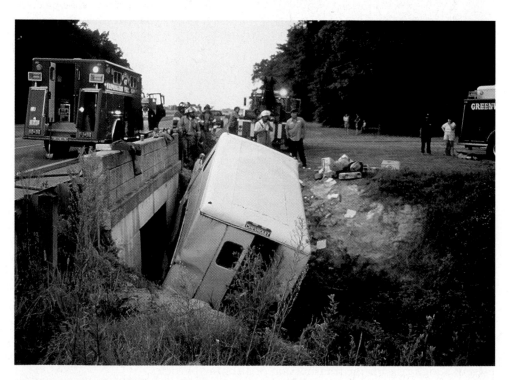

FIGURE 8-6 Look for potential hazards during scene size-up.

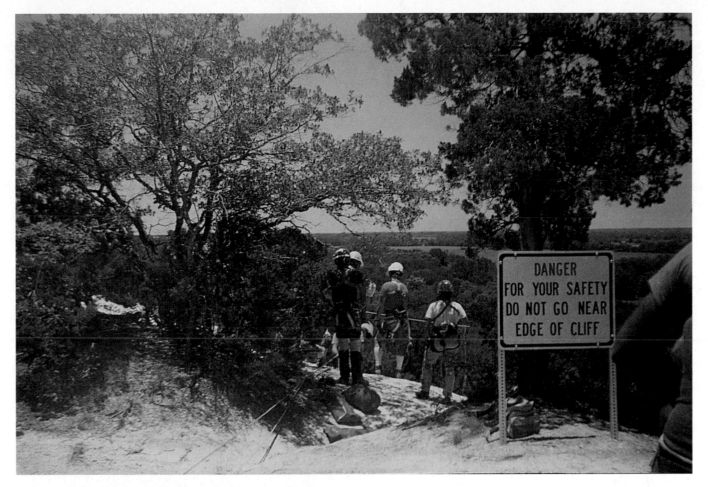

FIGURE 8-7 Even the most peaceful-looking scene can pose potential dangers.

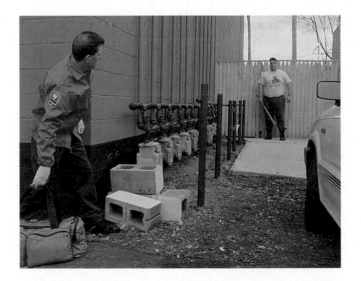

FIGURE 8-8 Wait for the police before entering a potentially hazardous scene.

trenches, mines, silos, or caves; and extreme heights. In every case, let common sense dictate scene management.

Crime scenes pose a special threat. When responding to a call in which the initial dispatch includes words such as shooting, stabbing, or domestic dispute, wait for law-enforcement personnel to secure the scene before entering (Figure 8-8). In fact, do not even enter the neighborhood, because sitting in your ambulance on the scene may undermine an already unstable environment. If possible, turn off your lights and siren and stage your vehicle a few blocks away, where it is not visible from the scene.

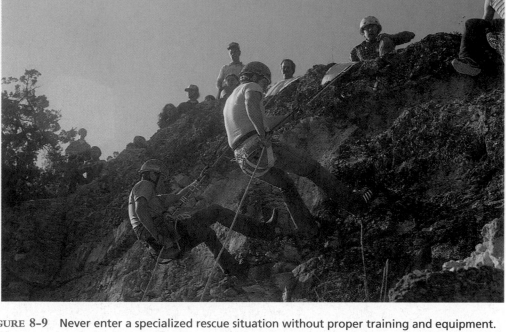

FIGURE 8-9 Never enter a specialized rescue situation without proper training and equipment.

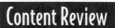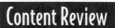
Content Review

MINIMUM RESCUE OPERATION EQUIPMENT

- Four-point suspension helmets
- Eye goggles and industrial safety glasses
- High-quality hearing protection
- Leather work gloves
- High-top, steel-toed boots
- Insulated coveralls
- Turnout gear

Content Review

MINIMUM PATIENT SAFETY EQUIPMENT

- Construction-type hard hats
- Eye goggles
- Hearing and respiratory protection
- Protective blankets
- Protective shielding

Safe, orderly, and controlled incident management is essential for everyone's safety.

Crash scenes requiring heavy-duty rescue procedures, scenes where toxic substances are present, crime scenes with a potential for violence, or scenes with unstable surfaces such as slippery slopes, ice, or rushing water all call for specialized crews, additional medical supplies, and sophisticated equipment (Figure 8-9). Do not even consider entering such situations unless you have the proper clothing, equipment, and training to work in them. Because getting backup requires extra time, this phase is critical. A prompt call to your dispatch center can save critical minutes in a life-threatening situation.

Without the appropriate protective gear, you will jeopardize your safety and your patient's. To participate in a rescue operation, you should have at least the following equipment immediately available: four-point suspension helmets; eye goggles or industrial safety glasses; high-quality hearing protection; leather work gloves; high-top, steel-toed boots; insulated coveralls; and turnout gear (Figure 8-10). Only personnel thoroughly trained in hazardous material (hazmat) suits or self-contained breathing apparatus (SCBA) should use them (Figure 8-11). These items are often supplied on specialty support vehicles such as hazmat response units and heavy-rescue trucks (Figure 8-12).

After you ensure that responding personnel have adequate safety equipment to manage the rescue scene, consider patient safety. Many considerations for rescuer safety also apply to patients. Additionally, patient safety equipment should at least include construction-type hard hats, eye goggles, hearing and respiratory protection, protective blankets, and protective shielding. You will need these to protect your patient during rescue operations (Figure 8-13). Patient safety also includes simple measures such as removing them from unstable environments such as temperature extremes, smoky rooms, or hostile crowds. For example, the simplest way to begin managing a patient suffering from hypothermia is to move him into a warm environment.

Safe, orderly, and controlled incident management is essential for everyone's safety. Call for specialty personnel to stabilize wreckage or turn off electrical power. Make sure someone routes traffic safely around a vehicle collision. Control bystanders and spot potential human hazards. Be certain that a hostile crowd or someone who assaulted your patient is not ready to attack you. Scenes involving toxic exposures, environmental hazards, and violent patients are especially worrisome. When possible, have law-enforcement personnel establish a tape line to cordon off the hazard zone to protect bystanders who do not realize the potential dangers of watching operations (Figure 8-14).

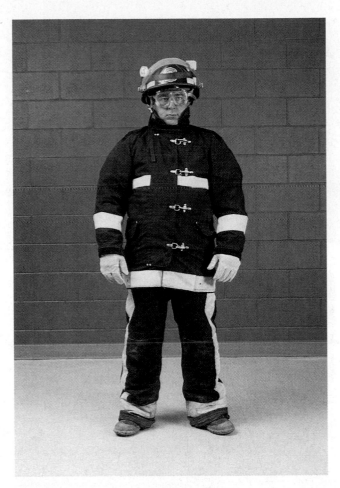

FIGURE 8–10   Full protective gear, including eye protection, helmet, turnout gear, and gloves.

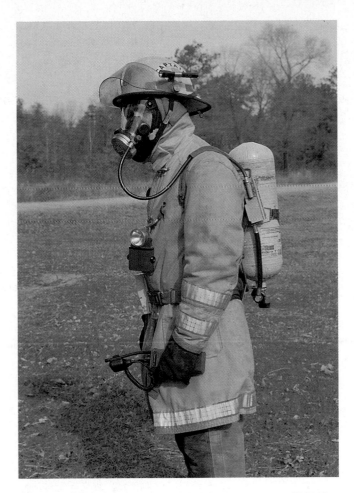

FIGURE 8–11   Self-contained breathing apparatus (SCBA).

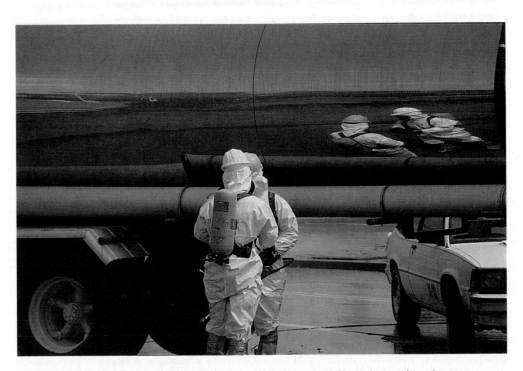

FIGURE 8–12   Hazardous materials responses require special training and equipment.

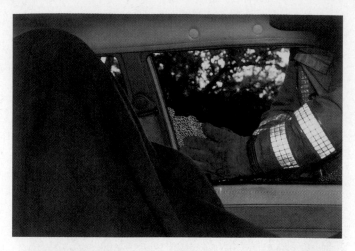

FIGURE 8-13 Protect the patient from hazards at the scene.

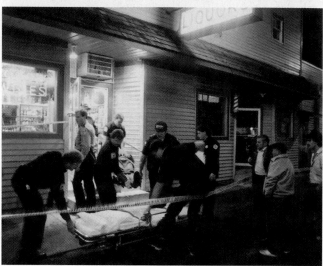

FIGURE 8-14 Tape lines help to keep bystanders out of hazardous scenes.

LOCATION OF ALL PATIENTS

Search the area to locate all patients.

Scene size-up also includes a search of the area to locate all of the patients. Ask yourself if other persons could be involved in the incident or affected by the medical problem. Determine where you are most likely to find the most seriously affected patients and how many patients will need transport. The mechanism of injury or the nature of the illness can help you determine the number of patients. For example, a two-car collision must include at least two drivers. Clues such as diaper bags, child auto seats, toys, coloring books, clothing, or twin spider-web impact marks in the windshield should lead you to search for more patients, especially children, than those who may be readily apparent. Some medical situations such as carbon monoxide poisoning can affect an entire household. A hazardous liquid spill in the chemistry lab can affect students and staff in an entire wing of a school.

Call for assistance early; it is wise to overestimate when asking for help.

If you find more patients than you can safely and effectively manage, call for assistance early. If possible, you should do this before you make contact with any patients, because you are less likely to call for help once you become involved with patient care. Often, as you proceed into a scene, more patients become apparent. It is wise to overestimate when asking for help at the scene.

Initiate the mass-casualty plan according to your local protocols (Figure 8-15). Again, try not to become involved in patient care, because two important functions must occur in the initial stages of any mass-casualty incident—command and triage. If you and your partner find yourselves in a situation that overwhelms your resources, one of you should establish command while the other begins triaging patients. The command person performs a scene size-up, determines the needs of the incident, makes a radio report requesting the necessary additional help, and directs on-coming crews to their duties (Figure 8-16). The triage

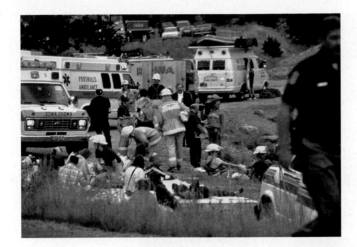

FIGURE 8-15 Follow local protocols when you respond to a mass-casualty incident.

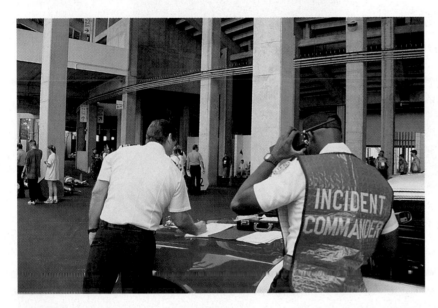

FIGURE 8-16 The incident commander directs the response and coordinates resources at a mass-casualty incident.

person performs a triage exam on all patients and prioritizes them for immediate or delayed transport (Figure 8-17). He may perform simple life-saving procedures such as opening the airway or controlling bleeding, but as a rule he should not stop to provide intensive care for any one patient.

MECHANISM OF INJURY

The **mechanism of injury** is the combined strength, direction, and nature of forces that injured your patient. It is usually apparent through careful evaluation of the trauma scene and can help you anticipate both the location and the seriousness of injuries. Identify the forces involved, the direction from which they came, and the bodily locations affected (Figure 8-18). For example, in a fall injury, how high was the patient, what did he land on, and what part of his body hit first? If your patient jumped from a height and landed on his feet, expect lower extremity, pelvic, and lumbar spine injuries.

In an automobile crash, the mechanism of injury is the process by which forces are exchanged between the automobile and what it struck, between your patient and the automobile's interior, and among the various tissues and organs as they collide with one another within the patient. Close inspection of the automobile and the forces, or various collisions, can lead to an **index of suspicion** (a prediction of injuries based on the mechanism of injury) for possible injuries. What does the car look like? If the windshield is cracked, expect head

mechanism of injury combined strength, direction, and nature of the forces that injured your patient.

index of suspicion your anticipation of possible injuries based on your analysis of the event.

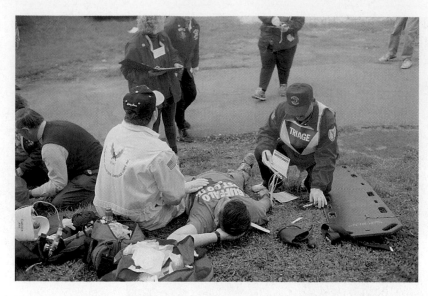

FIGURE 8-17   The triage person examines and prioritizes patients.

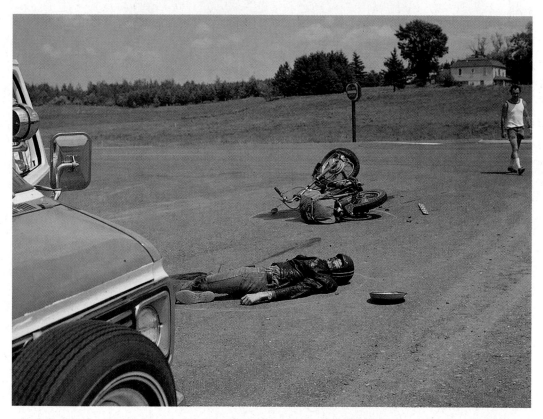

FIGURE 8-18   With trauma, try to determine the mechanism of injury during scene size-up.

and neck injuries. If the steering wheel is bent, expect chest and abdominal injuries. With a major intrusion into the passenger compartment, expect major trauma.

Expect a pedestrian struck by a car to have fractures of the lower extremities. If the auto was moving at 20 miles per hour, expect less severe fractures than if it were moving at 55 miles per hour. Also, internal injuries are less likely at lower speeds than at higher speeds. By evaluating the strength and nature of impact, you can anticipate which organs are injured and the degree of their damage.

For a gunshot patient, determine the type of gun used, the range of the shot, and if an exit wound exists. This information will enable you to estimate the damage along the bul-

Often the mechanism of injury is the only clue to the possibility of serious internal injury.

let's path and to formulate an index of suspicion for your patient's possible injuries. Expect the internal injuries from serious blunt trauma to be more extensive and severe than those you see externally. Often the mechanism of injury is the only clue to the possibility of serious internal injury.

NATURE OF THE ILLNESS

Determine the nature of the illness from bystanders, family members, or your patient himself. If he is alert and oriented, he is usually the best source of information about his problem. If he is unresponsive, disoriented, or otherwise unable to provide information, rely on family members, bystanders, or visual cues for this information.

The scene can give additional clues to your patient's condition. How is he positioned? Does he sit bolt upright gasping to breathe? Are pill bottles or drug paraphernalia nearby? Is medical-care equipment such as an oxygen tank, a nebulizer, or a glucometer in the room? For example, if you respond to a difficulty breathing call and your patient is using his nebulizer when you arrive, suspect a history of pulmonary disease such as asthma, emphysema, or chronic bronchitis. If your patient is an agitated 17-year-old with a rapid pulse and you notice crack cocaine ampules on the floor, suspect a substance abuse problem.

Sometimes the nature of the illness is not readily apparent. Your patient with severe breathing difficulty, for instance, may be suffering from respiratory disease, a cardiac problem, an allergic reaction, or a toxic exposure. Remember that the nature of your patient's illness may be very different from his chief complaint.

INITIAL ASSESSMENT

The **initial assessment** exemplifies the basis of all prehospital emergency medical care. Its goal is to identify and correct immediately life-threatening patient conditions of the <u>A</u>irway, <u>B</u>reathing, or <u>C</u>irculation (**ABCs**). If you find these conditions during this part of your assessment, treat them at once. For example, open a closed airway, provide ventilation, or control hemorrhage before moving on. Immediately following the initial assessment, decide priority regarding immediate transport or further on-scene assessment and care.

The initial assessment consists of the following steps:

- Forming a general impression
- Stabilizing the cervical spine as needed
- Assessing a baseline mental status
- Assessing the airway
- Assessing breathing
- Assessing circulation
- Determining priority

The initial assessment should take less than 1 minute, unless you have to intervene with life-saving measures. Perform the initial assessment as part of your ongoing assessment throughout the patient contact, especially after any major intervention or whenever your patient's condition changes.

FORMING A GENERAL IMPRESSION

The **general impression** is your initial, intuitive evaluation of your patient. It will help you determine his general clinical status (stable vs. unstable) and priority for immediate transport. Base your first impression on the information you gather from the environment, the mechanism of injury, the nature of the illness, the chief complaint, and your instincts.

Your patient's age, gender, and race often influence your index of suspicion. Very old and very young patients are more apt to have severe complications from injury or illness. For example, age is a factor in burn mortality, along with degree and body percentage. A 25-year-old patient with third degree burns over 50% of his body will have a 75% chance of mortality. A 45-year-old patient with the same burns will have a 95% chance of mortality.

Remember that the nature of your patient's illness may be very different from his chief complaint.

initial assessment prehospital process designed to identify and correct life-threatening airway, breathing, and circulation problems.

ABCs airway, breathing, and circulation.

Content Review

STEPS OF INITIAL ASSESSMENT

1. Form general impression
2. Stabilize cervical spine as needed
3. Assess mental status
4. Assess airway
5. Assess breathing
6. Assess circulation
7. Assign priority

The initial assessment should take less than one minute, unless you have to intervene with life-saving measures.

general impression your initial, intuitive evaluation of your patient.

Patient assessment actually starts as soon as you approach the scene. Clues about the patient's underlying pathophysiology might be evident from such things as positioning of the vehicle, downed power lines, or the appearance and actions of bystanders. However, your safety, and that of your fellow rescuers, is always paramount. Never approach a scene that appears unsafe. With time, you will develop a "sixth sense" about emergency scenes and bystanders.

As you begin the patient encounter, process all that you see into your patient assessment and care. For example, consider this scenario:

A car with two 16-year-old girls fails to negotiate a turn on a country road and overturns into a flowing creek adjacent to the road. Although the ambient temperature is in the 60s, you know that the temperature of the water in this area often is in the 40s. Thus, you should immediately suspect the possibility of hypothermia.

As the girls are removed from entrapment, no obvious injuries are noted. Vital signs are normal other than a slight tachycardia. However, peripheral pulses are weak and the skin is pale and cool. Is it shock? Is it hypothermia? Is it both? Your index of suspicion is high for both hypothermia and blunt force trauma. You follow local protocols in regard to immobilization, fluid therapy, and monitoring. Once in the ambulance and wrapped in a blanket, both girls start to show signs that blood flow to the skin is improving. By the time you reach the hospital, their skin has a normal color and their pulse rate is normal.

Following a comprehensive assessment in the emergency department, the girls are discharged to their parents with no apparent injuries. Thus, your instincts were right. The potential of shock was a greater risk to the girls than hypothermia, and you had to treat based on this risk. But, hypothermia turned out to be the principal problem. Integrating information from the scene size-up, patient history, and patient examination gave you a clear picture of the patient's underlying pathophysiological process.

Suspect a female of childbearing age with lower abdominal pain and vaginal bleeding to have a life-threatening gynecological emergency known as ruptured ectopic pregnancy. African-Americans have a higher incidence of hypertension and cardiovascular disease than do members of other racial groups.

Determine whether your patient's problem results from trauma or from a medical problem. Sometimes this will not be readily apparent. For example, did your patient slip and fall or get dizzy and fall? Note your patient's face and his posture and decide whether rapid intervention or a more deliberate approach is warranted. With experience you will be able to recognize even the subtlest clues of a patient in critical condition. Generally, the more serious the condition, the quieter your patient will be. Look at, listen to, and smell the environment. Gather as many clues as possible as you enter the scene.

Take the necessary body substance isolation (BSI) precautions with every patient. Then, if your patient is alert, identify yourself and begin to establish a rapport. For example, "Hello, I'm Darlene Button, an EMT-I with Brewerton Ambulance. I'm here to help you." This establishes your level of training, authority, and reason for being at your patient's side. It also allows your patient to refuse care. As discussed in Chapter 1 on medical/legal aspects of prehospital care, you cannot provide care without either implied or informed consent.

Reassure your patient. Listen to him and do not trivialize his complaints. Frequently we forget how significant an injury or illness, even a minor one, seems to a patient. With your experience, his problem may seem small, but for your patient it is a real concern. The ill or injured patient may worry about the long-term consequences for work, childcare, and finances. Understand these fears and support your patient psychologically as well as physiologically.

Listen to your patient and do not trivialize his complaints.

If the mechanism of injury is significant or if your patient is unresponsive, have your partner manually stabilize your patient's head and neck (Figure 8-19a). Do this before establishing his mental status and continue manual stabilization until you fully immobilize him to a long spine board. If your patient is awake, explain what you are doing and ask him not to move his neck. You do not want him to turn his head when you try to assess mental status. Ask your partner to maintain your patient's head in a neutral position as you begin your assessment. If your patient is a small child, place a small towel or pad beneath the shoulders to maintain proper alignment of the cervical spine (Figure 8-19b). This will com-

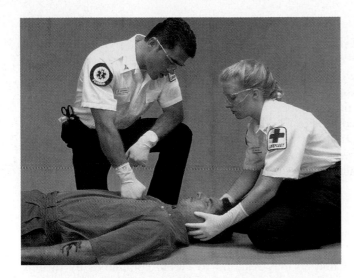

FIGURE 8-19A Manually stabilize the head and neck on first contact with the patient.

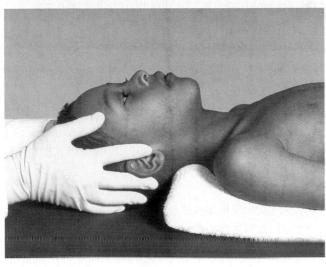

FIGURE 8-19B Place a folded towel under your young patient's shoulders to maintain proper alignment of the cervical spine.

pensate for the large occiput of the child's head, which normally would flex his neck when he was placed on a flat surface.

MENTAL STATUS

Your assessment of baseline mental status is crucial for all patients. For example, when you deliver your head injury patient to the emergency department, the neurosurgeon will want a chronological report of your patient's mental status from the time you arrived on the scene. This vital information helps the surgical team diagnose a deteriorating brain injury. If the patient was alert and oriented when you arrived, then became sleepy en route, and within 30 minutes was responsive only to deep pain stimuli, the suspicion for epidural hematoma is high. Rapid surgical intervention can save lives in most cases if the diagnosis is made quickly. Your baseline mental status documentation is critical to these patients' emergency care. Establishing a baseline mental status is also crucial in assessing the variety of medical situations that cause altered levels of response. Drug overdoses, poisonings, diabetic emergencies, sepsis, hypoxia, and hypovolemia are just a few of the many conditions that result in altered mentation. For the stroke patient, identifying the time of the symptom onset is critical for the emergency physician, who must consider administering clot-dissolving drugs within the 3-hour window of opportunity. This is possible only with your accurate assessment of the patient's change in mental status.

To record your patient's mental status, use the mnemonic AVPU: your patient is Alert, responds to Verbal stimuli, responds only to Painful stimuli, or is Unresponsive. Perform this exam by starting with verbal, and then moving to painful stimuli only if he fails to respond to your verbal cues.

Your assessment of baseline mental status is crucial for all patients with serious head trauma.

Content Review

AVPU

- **A**lert
- **V**erbal stimuli
- **P**ainful stimuli
- **U**nresponsive

Alert

An alert patient is awake, as evidenced by open eyes. He may be oriented to person (who he is), place (where he is), and time (day, month, and year) and give organized, coherent answers to your questions. He also may be disoriented and confused. For example, the patient with a suspected concussion will often be dazed and confused. The hypoxic or hypoglycemic patient may be combative. The shock patient may be restless and anxious. If his eyes are open and he appears awake, he is categorized as alert. Children's responses to your questions vary with their age-related physical and emotional development. Infants and young children are usually curious but cautious when a stranger approaches. Their level of response may not indicate the gravity of their condition. In fact, the quiet child is usually the seriously injured or ill child.

Verbal

If a patient appears to be sleeping but responds when you talk to him, he is responsive to verbal stimuli. He can respond by speaking, opening his eyes, moaning, or just moving. Note the level of his verbal response. Does he speak clearly, mumble inappropriate words, or make incomprehensible sounds? Children may respond to verbal commands by turning their heads or stopping activity. For infants you may have to shout to elicit a response.

Pain

If your child or adult patient does not respond to verbal stimuli, try to elicit a response with painful stimuli. Pinch his fingernails or rub your knuckles on his sternum and watch for a response. Again, he may respond by waking up, speaking, moaning, opening his eyes, or moving. Note the type of his motor response to the painful stimuli. Is his response purposeful or nonpurposeful? If he tries to move your hand away or to move himself away from the pain, it is purposeful. **Decorticate** (arms flexed, legs extended) or **decerebrate** (arms and legs extended) posturing is nonpurposeful and suggests a serious brain injury. For the infant, flick the soles of the feet and expect crying as the appropriate response.

Unresponsive

The unresponsive patient is comatose and fails to respond to any noxious stimulus. The AVPU scale describes your patient's general mental status. Avoid using terms such as semiconscious, lethargic, or stuporous since they are broadly interpreted and you have not had a chance to conduct a comprehensive neurological exam at this point. Your patient's response to stimulation will tell you a great deal about his condition. Any alteration or deterioration in mental status may indicate an emergent or already serious problem. A patient with an impaired mental status may have lost, or be in danger of losing, the ability to protect his airway. Take immediate steps to protect your patient's airway by proper positioning, use of airway adjuncts, or intubation, as appropriate. Provide oxygen to any patient with diminished mental status and seek out its cause.

AIRWAY ASSESSMENT

If your patient is responsive and can speak clearly, you can assume that his airway is patent. If your patient is unconscious, however, his airway may be obstructed. The supine unconscious patient's tongue often obstructs his upper airway. Because the mandible, tongue, and epiglottis are all connected, gravity allows these structures to block your patient's upper airway as his facial muscles relax.

You can open your patient's airway with one of two simple manual maneuvers, the jaw-thrust and the head-tilt/chin-lift. For the trauma patient with a suspected cervical spine injury, use the jaw-thrust to avoid movement of the cervical spine. Place your thumbs on your patient's cheeks and lift up on the angle of the jaw with your fingers. For all other patients, use the head-tilt/chin-lift. Place one hand on your patient's forehead and lift up under the chin with the fingers of your other hand. To open the airways of infants and young children, apply a gentle and conservative extension of the head and neck. These patients' upper airway structures are very flexible and are easily kinked when their necks are flexed or hyperextended. You must constantly readjust their airways to maximize patency.

To assess your patient's airway, look for chest rise while you listen and feel for air movement. If the airway is clear, you should hear quiet air flow and feel free air movement. A

---

decorticate arms flexed, legs extended.

---

decerebrate arms and legs extended.

Any alteration in mental status may indicate an emergent or already serious problem.

You must constantly adjust the airway of infants and young children in order to maximize patency.

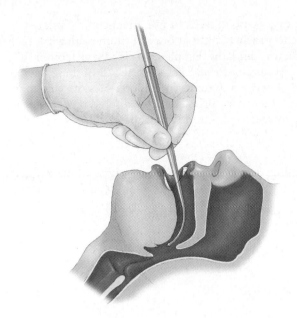

FIGURE 8-20 Suction fluids from your patient's airway.

noisy airway is a partially obstructed airway. Snoring occurs when the tongue partially blocks the upper airway. In this case, reposition the head and neck and reevaluate. Gurgling indicates that fluid, such as blood, secretions, or gastric contents, is blocking the upper airway. Gently open and examine the mouth for foreign bodies you can remove easily and quickly. Use aggressive suctioning to remove blood, vomitus, secretions, and other fluids (Figure 8-20).

The high-pitched inspiratory screech of stridor is caused by a life-threatening upper airway obstruction that may be due to a foreign body, severe swelling, allergic reaction, or infection. If you suspect a foreign body obstruction and your patient exhibits poor air movement, a weak cough, or a diminishing mental status, immediately deliver abdominal thrusts (Heimlich maneuver) to dislodge the object. If your patient is less than one year old, use back blows and chest thrusts instead of abdominal thrusts. If those maneuvers are ineffective, remove the object under direct laryngoscopy with Magill forceps.

Other causes of stridor require vastly differently approaches. Upper respiratory infections such as croup or epiglottitis require blow-by oxygen and a quiet ride to the hospital; respiratory burns demand rapid endotracheal intubation; and anaphylaxis necessitates vasoconstrictor medications. Since these vastly different management techniques are potentially life threatening when applied inappropriately, your correct field diagnosis is critical. If your patient presents with stridor, take time to evaluate the history and clinical signs and symptoms for foreign-body obstruction (sudden onset while eating), epiglottitis (fever, illness, drooling, inability to swallow), respiratory burns (history of facial burns, hoarseness), and anaphylaxis (hives, history of allergies).

The softer, expiratory whistle of wheezing is caused by constricted bronchioles, the smaller, lower airways. You will hear it in cases such as asthma, bronchitis, emphysema, or other causes of bronchospasm. Bronchiolitis, a lower respiratory infection, often causes these sounds in infants and young children. Wheezing patients require a bronchodilator medication to dilate the bronchioles and reduce airway resistance.

A patient who is not moving air is in respiratory arrest. Immediately provide ventilation with a BVM. Ventilate adult patients at a minimum of 12 breaths per minute and all children at a minimum of 20 breaths per minute. If you cannot ventilate the lungs, reposition the head and neck and try again. If there is still no air movement, assume a complete obstruction and begin measures to correct it.

Once you have cleared the airway, keeping it open may require constant attention. In these cases, insert a basic airway adjunct to help keep the tongue from blocking the upper airway. If your patient is unconscious and lacks a gag reflex, insert an oropharyngeal airway. If he has a gag reflex or significant orofacial trauma, insert a nasopharyngeal airway. Be cautious using a nasopharyngeal airway if you suspect a basilar skull fracture. If he has

Stridor signals a potentially life-threatening airway obstruction.

Once you have cleared the airway, keeping it open may require constant attention.

no gag reflex and cannot protect his airway, you will need to use advanced techniques to maintain airway patency. These include endotracheal intubation, multilumen airways such as the pharyngo-tracheal lumen (PtL) airway and the Esophageal Tracheal CombiTube (ETC). The multilumen airways are not appropriate for use in children. All of these devices for maintaining upper airway patency are described in detail in Chapter 5 on airway management and ventilation. If your patient has an airway problem or an altered mental status, administer high-flow, high-concentration oxygen by nonrebreather mask.

BREATHING ASSESSMENT

Assess your patient for adequate breathing. Immediately note any signs of inadequate breathing. These include:

- Altered mental status, confusion, apprehension, or agitation
- Shortness of breath while speaking
- Retractions (supraclavicular, suprasternal, intercostal)
- Asymmetrical chest wall movement
- Accessory muscle use (neck, abdominal)
- Cyanosis
- Audible sounds
- Abnormally rapid, slow, or shallow breathing
- Nasal flaring

Assess the respiratory rate and quality. Normal respiratory rates vary according to your patient's age. Abnormally fast or slow rates (Table 8-1) actually decrease the amount of air that reaches the alveoli for gas exchange. For patients with abnormally fast or slow respiratory rates and decreased tidal volumes, provide positive pressure ventilation with, for example, a BVM and supplemental oxygen, to ensure full lung expansion and maximum oxygenation. Note the respiratory pattern. Rapid (tachypneic), deep (hyperpneic) respirations are a compensatory mechanism and suggest the body is attempting to rid itself of excess acids. They may indicate a diabetic problem, severe acidosis, or head injury. They also may result from hyperventilation syndrome or from simple exertion. Kussmaul's respirations (deep, rapid breathing) accompanied by a fruity breath odor are a classic sign of a patient in a diabetic coma. In either case, always ensure an adequate inspiratory volume and administer high-flow, high-concentration oxygen. Cheyne-Stokes respirations, a series of increasing and decreasing breaths followed by a period of apnea, most likely result from a brainstem injury or increasing intracranial pressure. Biot's respirations, identified by short, gasping, irregular breaths, may signify severe brain injury. Again, ensure adequate inspiratory volume and provide ventilation with supplemental oxygen as needed.

If your trauma patient's breathing is inadequate, immediately conduct a rapid trauma assessment of the neck and chest before moving on to circulation. Identify and correct any

Content Review

SIGNS OF INADEQUATE BREATHING

- Altered mental status
- Shortness of breath
- Retractions
- Asymmetrical chest wall movement
- Accessory muscle use
- Cyanosis
- Audible sounds
- Abnormal rate or pattern
- Nasal flaring

If your patient's breathing is inadequate, immediately conduct a rapid trauma assessment of the neck and chest and provide positive pressure ventilation with supplemental oxygen.

Table 8-1	RESPIRATORY RATES	
Age	**Low Rate**	**High Rate**
Newborn	30	60
Infant (<1 year)	30	60
Toddler (1–2 years)	24	40
Preschooler (3–5 years)	22	34
School age (6–12 years)	18	30
Adolescent (13–18 years)	12	26
Adult (>18 years)	12	20

life-threatening conditions such as a sucking chest wound, a flail chest, or a tension pneumothorax. If your patient exhibits adequate breathing, move directly to circulation.

CIRCULATION ASSESSMENT

The **circulation assessment** consists of evaluating the pulse and skin and controlling hemorrhage. Go directly to the wrist and feel for a radial pulse (Procedure 8-1a). Its presence suggests a systolic blood pressure of at least 80 mmHg. If the radial pulse is absent, check for a carotid pulse (Procedure 8-1b). The carotid pulse's presence suggests a systolic blood pressure of at least 60 mmHg. In the infant, palpate the brachial pulse (Procedure 8-1c) or, if necessary, auscultate the apical pulse. If the pulse is absent in the adult patient, begin chest compressions immediately, evaluate the cardiac rhythm, and provide prompt defibrillation as needed. In the child, immediately begin cardiopulmonary resuscitation (CPR).

Assess your patient's pulse for rate and quality as detailed in Chapter 7. The normal heart rate varies with your patient's age (Table 8-2). Very fast rates (tachycardia) and very slow rates (bradycardia) may indicate a life-threatening cardiac dysrhythmia. Note the quality of the pulse. The normal pulse should be regular and strong. An irregular pulse may indicate a cardiac dysrhythmia requiring advanced cardiac life-support procedures. In head injury, heat stroke, or hypertension, you will often find a strong, bounding pulse. A weak, thready pulse usually indicates poor perfusion due to fluid loss, pump failure, or massive vasodilation.

Stop your patient's bleeding if you haven't already done so (Procedure 8-1d). Major bleeding usually originates with trauma, but it also can result from a medical emergency. For example, vaginal bleeding, rectal bleeding, and even a nosebleed associated with hypertension can result in life-threatening blood loss. For external bleeding, employ any appropriate measures for hemorrhage control, including direct pressure and elevation, pressure dressings, pressure points, and the last-resort tourniquet. Internal bleeding is not easily controlled in the prehospital setting and demands initiating transport as soon as possible.

Assess the skin for temperature, moisture, and color (Procedure 8-1e). Peripheral vasoconstriction decreases peripheral perfusion to the skin early in shock. The skin may appear mottled (blotchy), cyanotic (bluish), pale, or ashen. It may also feel cool and moist (clammy). This often indicates that warm, circulating blood has been shunted away from the skin to the core of the body to maintain perfusion of vital organs. If you find any of these signs, suspect conditions related to or caused by poor perfusion. In infants and young children capillary refill is a reliable indicator of circulatory function (Procedure 8-1f). In adults, smoking, medications, cold weather, or chronic conditions of the elderly may affect capillary refill, so you should always also consider the other indicators of circulatory function.

If your patient shows signs of circulatory compromise, consider elevating his legs to support venous return to the vital organs (Procedure 8-1g). Keep him warm, and on adult patients only, apply and inflate the pneumatic antishock garment as indicated by your local protocol (Procedure 8-1h). Chapter 15 on hemorrhage and shock explains this procedure fully. Consider starting large-bore IV lines en route to the hospital and infusing fluids to augment your patient's circulating blood volume (Procedure 8-1i).

circulation assessment
evaluating the pulse and skin and controlling hemorrhage.

Internal bleeding is not easily controlled in the prehospital setting and demands initiating transport as soon as possible.

Table 8-2 NORMAL PULSE RATE RANGES

Age	Low Rate	High Rate
Newborn	100	180
Infant (<1 year)	100	160
Toddler (1–2 years)	80	110
Preschooler (3–5 years)	70	110
School age (6–12 years)	65	110
Adolescent (13–18 years)	60	90
Adult (>18 years)	60	100

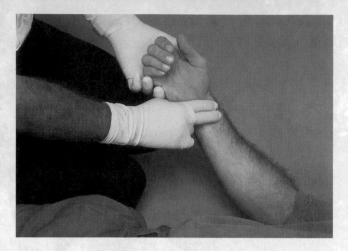

8-1a   To assess an adult's circulation, feel for a radial pulse.

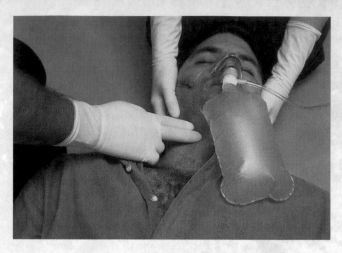

8-1b   If you cannot feel a radial pulse, palpate for a carotid pulse.

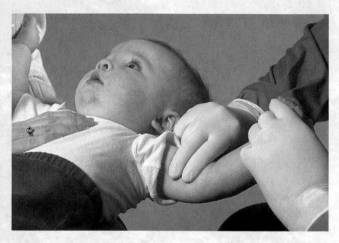

8-1c   To assess an infant's circulation, palpate the brachial pulse.

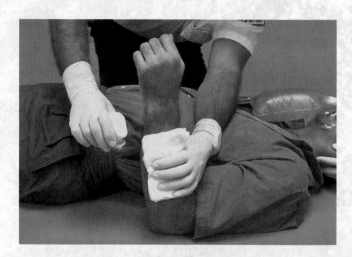

8-1d   Control major bleeding.

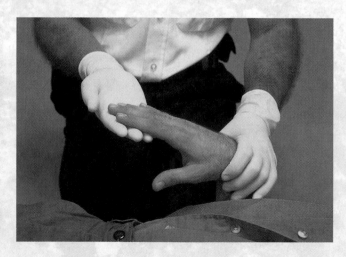

8-1e   Assess the skin.

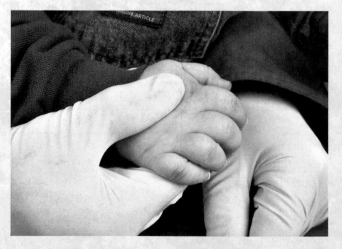

8-1f   Capillary refill time provides important information about the circulatory status of infants and young children.

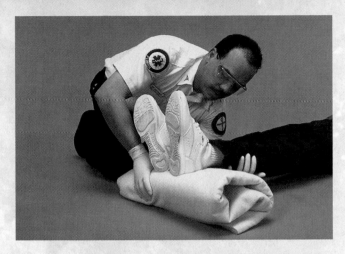

8-1g Elevate your patient's feet if you suspect circulation compromise.

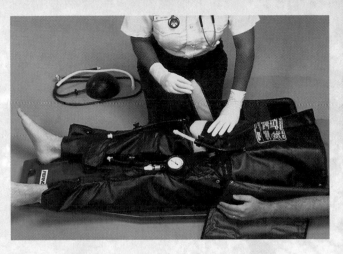

8-1h Apply a pneumatic antishock garment according to your local protocol.

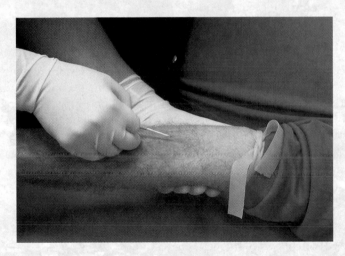

8-1i En route to the hospital, establish an IV.

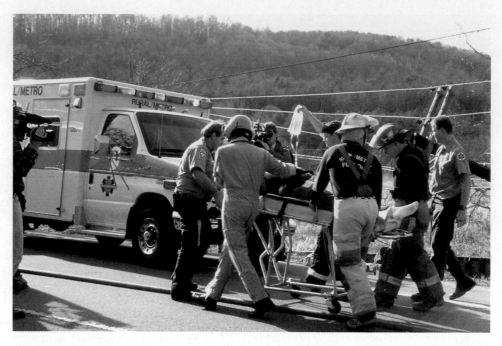

FIGURE 8-21 Expedite transport for a high-priority patient and continue assessment and care en route.

PRIORITY DETERMINATION

Do not delay transport for detailed assessments and procedures that you can provide en route to the hospital.

Once you have conducted an initial assessment, determine your patient's priority. If his initial assessment suggests a serious illness or injury, conduct a rapid head-to-toe assessment to identify other life threats and transport him immediately to the nearest appropriate facility that can deliver definitive care (Figure 8-21). Do not delay transport for detailed assessments and procedures that you can provide en route to the hospital.

Consider top priority and rapid transport for the following patients:

- Patients with a poor general impression
  - Apnea
  - Pulselessness
  - Obvious severe distress
- Patients with altered mental status
- Patients with airway compromise
  - Obstructive sounds such as gurgling, snoring, or stridor
  - Vomitus, secretions, blood, or foreign bodies obstructing the airway
  - Inability to protect the airway (absence of a gag reflex)
- Patients with abnormal breathing
  - Rates less or greater than normal for age
  - Absent or diminished air movement and breath sounds
  - Retractions
  - Accessory muscle use
- Patients with poor circulation
  - Weak or absent peripheral pulses
  - Pulse rates less or greater than normal for age
  - Irregular pulse
  - Pale, cool, diaphoretic skin
  - Uncontrolled bleeding
- Obvious serious or multiple injuries

In these cases, decide whether to stabilize your patient on the scene or expedite transport and initiate advanced life-support procedures en route. On the way to the hospital you

Content Review

TOP PRIORITY PATIENTS
- Poor general impression
- Unresponsive
- Responsive but cannot follow commands
- Difficult breathing
- Signs and symptoms of hypoperfusion
- Complicated childbirth
- Chest pain and blood pressure below 100 systolic
- Uncontrolled bleeding
- Severe pain
- Multiple injuries

can conduct a detailed history and physical exam and provide additional care as time allows. If your patient is stable, before transport you can conduct a focused history and physical exam—a problem-oriented patient assessment—followed by a detailed physical exam either at the scene or during transport as the situation requires, if time allows.

The initial assessment is the crucial first-step in providing life-saving measures to seriously ill or injured patients. It should take you less than 1 minute to perform, yet it will provide you with enough vital information to confirm your priority determination.

FOCUSED HISTORY AND PHYSICAL EXAM

The **focused history and physical exam** is the second stage of patient assessment. It is a problem-oriented process based on your initial assessment and your patient's chief complaint. How you conduct the focused history and physical exam will depend on which of four general categories your patient's initial presentation falls under:

- Trauma patient with a significant mechanism of injury or altered mental status
- Trauma patient with an isolated injury
- Responsive medical patient
- Unresponsive medical patient

Each type of patient requires a vastly different approach.

THE MAJOR TRAUMA PATIENT

The **major trauma patient** is one who has sustained a significant mechanism of injury or has an altered mental status from the incident. For serious trauma patients, you will conduct an initial assessment followed by a rapid trauma assessment, package your patient, provide rapid transport to the emergency department, and perform an ongoing assessment en route, in that order. If time allows, you can also perform a detailed assessment.

Mechanism of Injury

Begin the focused history and physical exam for major trauma patients by reconsidering the mechanism of injury (Figure 8-22). Although trauma poses a serious threat to life, its appearance often masks your patient's true condition. Extremity injuries, for example, are frequently obvious and grotesque, yet they rarely cause death. Conversely, life-threatening problems such as internal bleeding and rising intracranial pressure often occur with only

focused history and physical exam problem-oriented assessment process based on initial assessment and chief complaint.

major trauma patient person who has suffered significant mechanism of injury.

Content Review

MAJOR TRAUMA PATIENT
- Initial assessment
- Rapid trauma assessment
- Packaging
- Rapid transport and ongoing assessment

Your assessment of trauma patients must look beyond obvious injuries to the mechanism of injury.

Content Review

PREDICTORS OF SERIOUS INTERNAL INJURY
- Ejection from vehicle
- Death in same passenger compartment
- Fall from height greater than 20 feet
- Rollover of vehicle
- High-speed collision
- Vehicle-pedestrian collision
- Motorcycle crash
- Penetration of object into head, chest, or abdomen

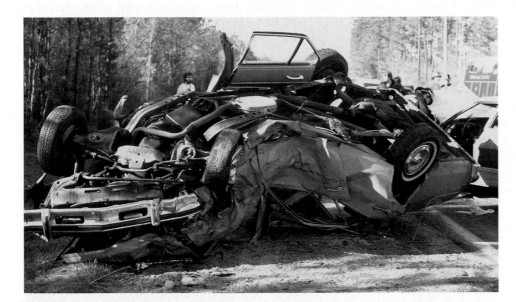

FIGURE 8-22 Evaluate the trauma scene to determine the mechanism of injury.

Content Review

ADDITIONAL PREDICTORS FOR INFANTS AND CHILDREN

- Fall from height greater than 10 feet
- Bicycle collision
- Medium-speed vehicle collision

subtle signs and symptoms. Your assessment of trauma patients must look beyond obvious injuries to the mechanism of injury for evidence that suggests life-threatening situations. Certain mechanisms predictably cause serious internal injury:

- Ejection from a vehicle
- Fall from height greater than 20 feet
- Rollover of vehicle
- High-speed vehicle collision with resulting severe vehicle deformity
- Vehicle-pedestrian collision
- Motorcycle crash
- Penetration of object into the head, chest, or abdomen

Additional considerations for infants and children include:

- Fall from height greater than 10 feet
- Bicycle collision
- Medium-speed vehicle collision with resulting severe vehicle deformity

The presence of these mechanisms suggests a high index of suspicion for serious injury. Quickly transport patients to a trauma center when either the mechanism of injury or your patient's clinical presentation indicates a likelihood of internal injury.

Other significant mechanisms of injury can result from seat belts, airbags, and child safety seats. Do not rule out serious injury just because your patient wore a seat belt. Seat belts can actually cause injuries, even when worn properly. Always ask your patient if he wore a seat belt and look for bruises across the chest or around the waist. If present, expect hidden internal injuries.

In general, airbags have been effective devices in preventing serious injury by protecting passengers from hitting the windshield, steering wheel, and dashboard. They deploy only when the front of the car hits another object. But they are not without complication. For example, they are designed to cushion the chests of large adults. If the passenger is a child or a short adult, the airbag will hit him in the face, causing injury. Also, airbags are designed to deflate automatically within seconds after inflation, which may allow passengers to be propelled into the steering wheel or dashboard. For this reason, they may not be effective without the seat belt. Always lift the deployed bag and inspect the steering wheel for deformity. If you discover a bent steering wheel, suspect serious internal injury (Figure 8-23).

A child safety seat, when used appropriately, also can save a life. But if the safety seat is not securely fastened to the car seat, it can come loose and be thrown when the collision occurs, causing severe head, neck, and body cavity trauma to its occupant. If the safety seat is used in the car's front seat, the child can suffer a serious injury when the airbag deploys.

Quickly transport patients with a high likelihood of internal injury to an appropriate medical facility.

Do not rule out serious injury just because your patient wore a seat belt.

Always lift a deployed airbag and inspect the steering wheel for deformity.

FIGURE 8-23 A bent steering wheel signals potentially serious injuries. *(Courtesy of Edward T. Dickinson, MD)*

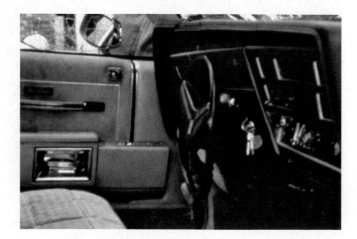

If your initial assessment rules out any immediate life-threatening condition, examine the suspected area of trauma. Physical signs of trauma such as abrasions or contusions confirm your index of suspicion. If you do not identify any physical evidence, reexamine the mechanism of injury and evaluate your patient's vital signs. You will miss many serious injuries if your index of suspicion is too low.

It is always best to err on the side of caution.

Usually, you will distinguish between those patients who need on-the-scene stabilization and those who need rapid transport after your initial assessment and rapid trauma assessment. Whether to transport your patient immediately or to attempt more extensive on-the-scene assessment and care is among your most difficult decisions, but the care you provide will be more effective if you decide quickly. As a rule, patients who experience the mechanisms of injury listed earlier or who display serious clinical findings should be transported quickly with IV access and other procedures attempted en route. Remember, you often arrive at the patient's side only minutes after the incident. He may not yet have lost enough blood internally to demonstrate signs of shock or progressive head injury. If in doubt, transport to an appropriate medical facility without delay. It is always best to err on the side of caution.

Rapid Trauma Assessment

After you finish your initial assessment, conduct a **rapid trauma assessment** to identify all other life-threatening conditions. Every trauma patient with a significant mechanism of injury, altered mental status, or multiple body-system trauma should receive a rapid trauma assessment. If your patient is responsive, ask him about symptoms as you proceed with your exam. Do not, however, focus totally on the areas your patient identifies as his chief problem. A patient with multiple injuries usually complains about his most painful injury. Sometimes, this may not be his most serious problem. Assess your patient systematically and avoid the tunnel vision invited by dispatch information, first responder reports, and your patient's chief complaint.

rapid trauma assessment quick check for signs of serious injury.

Assume that any trauma patient has a spinal injury if he has injuries above the shoulders, has a significant mechanism of injury, or complains of weakness, numbness, or spinal pain. Maintain spinal immobilization throughout your rapid trauma exam.

Avoid the tunnel vision invited by dispatch information, first responder reports, and your patient's chief complaint.

As you proceed through the exam and discover additional information about your patient, reconsider your decision to transport. Things can change unexpectedly, especially with children. For example, your child patient who appeared stable suddenly deteriorates, requiring you to expedite transport to the closest appropriate facility. The hallmark of an experienced EMT-I is the ability to improvise, adapt to new situations, and overcome obstacles that hinder good patient care.

The rapid trauma assessment is not a detailed physical exam but a fast, systematic assessment for other life-threatening injuries. Since you perform it before packaging your patient for transport, you must conduct it quickly. First, reassess your patient's mental status using the AVPU mnemonic and compare your findings with the baseline mental status from your initial assessment. Pay special attention to the head, neck, chest, abdomen, and pelvis. Injuries in these areas can occur with limited signs and symptoms, yet they may rapidly lead to patient deterioration and death. When inspecting an area for injury, keep in mind that the discoloration of contusions will develop over time and may not be apparent at first. Remember, your major concern may not be the injury you see but the internal injuries beneath the superficial wounds. Palpate to identify other signs such as tenderness, deformity, crepitation, symmetry, subcutaneous emphysema, or paradoxical movement. Compare muscle tone and tissue compliance from one side of the body or from one limb to another.

The mnemonic DCAP-BTLS may be helpful. The letters represent eight common signs of injury for which you are looking during most of this assessment: Deformities, Contusions, Abrasions, Penetrations, Burns, Tenderness, Lacerations, and Swelling.

Head Assess the head for DCAP-BTLS and crepitation (Procedure 8-2a). The scalp is extremely vascular and lacks the protective vasospasm mechanism that helps control bleeding. Thus even the most minor lacerations tend to bleed profusely. Inspect the scalp for lacerations that are hidden under hair matted with clotted blood. Look for blood flowing into the hair, and examine your gloved fingers periodically for blood or other body fluids (Procedure 8-2b).

Content Review

DCAP-BTLS

- **D**eformities
- **C**ontusions
- **A**brasions
- **P**enetrations
- **B**urns
- **T**enderness
- **L**acerations
- **S**welling

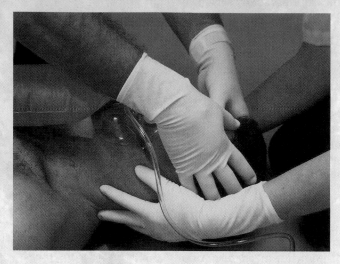

8-2a The first step in the rapid trauma assessment is to palpate the head.

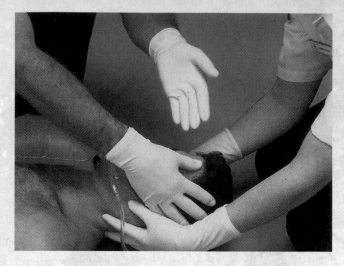

8-2b Periodically examine your gloves for blood.

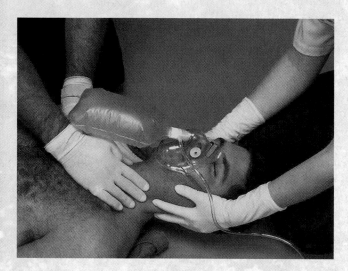

8-2c Inspect and palpate the entire neck. Pay particular attention to tracheal deviation and subcutaneous emphysema.

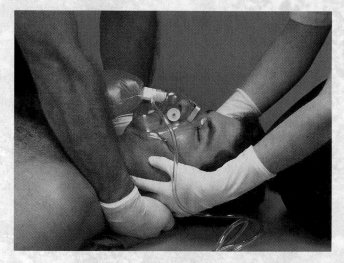

8-2d Inspect and palpate the posterior neck. Note any tenderness, irregularity, or edema.

If you detect uncontrolled bleeding from the scalp, apply a direct pressure dressing immediately. A simple scalp laceration can cause a life-threatening hemorrhage.

Palpate the skull for open wounds, depressions, protrusions, lack of symmetry, and any unusual warmth. Use cupped hands and do not probe with your fingers. If you feel a depression, stop palpating it, as this risks pushing a broken piece of bone into the brain. If you find an impaled object, stabilize it in place with bulky dressings. If your patient presents with an altered mental status and any abnormality in the structure of the skull, consider this a serious emergency and expedite transport while you continue your assessment and treatment.

Neck Inspect and palpate the neck for DCAP-BTLS and crepitation (Procedure 8-2c). Immediately cover any lacerations that may involve the major blood vessels such as the carotid arteries and jugular veins with an occlusive dressing. This is a high-pressure area and your patient can suffer significant blood loss quickly. Because inspiration generates negative pressures in the chest, the jugular veins may draw in air. This can result in a massive air embolus that prevents the heart from pumping blood.

Immediately cover any neck lacerations that may involve the major blood vessels.

Examine the jugular veins for abnormal distention. In a patient lying supine without circulatory compromise, these veins should distend slightly. If they do not, your patient may be hypovolemic. In the **semi-Fowler's position** (sitting up at a 45-degree angle), the veins should not distend. Distention beyond 45-degree angle is significant because something is inhibiting blood return to the chest. In the trauma patient, this may be the result of cardiac tamponade or tension pneumothorax.

semi-Fowler's position sitting up at a 45-degree angle.

Inspect and palpate the position of the trachea. It should lie midline and remain fixed during the breathing cycle. Tugging to one side during inspiration suggests a pneumothorax on that side. Displacement to one side may indicate a tension pneumothorax on the opposite side as the entire mediastinum is pushed away from the injury.

Finally, inspect and palpate the neck for **subcutaneous emphysema,** the crackling sensation caused by air just underneath the skin. This condition is the result of air leaking from the respiratory tree into the tissues of the neck. It strongly indicates a serious neck or chest injury.

subcutaneous emphysema crackling sensation caused by air just underneath the skin.

Now palpate the posterior neck for evidence of spinal trauma (Procedure 8-2d). Gently feel the spinous processes and note any deformities, swelling, and tenderness. If you feel a muscle spasm, consider it a reflex sign following injury somewhere along the spinal column. When a corroborating mechanism of injury is present, suspect a significant spinal injury requiring immobilization. At this point you can apply a cervical spinal immobilization collar (CSIC). Have someone maintain head and neck stabilization even after applying the collar until your patient is fully fastened to the long board.

Chest Look for signs of acute respiratory distress. If your patient has an upper airway obstruction, he may need to create tremendous negative pressures within his chest just to draw in air. To do so he will use accessory muscles in his neck and chest to help lift the chest wall. These negative pressures may cause suprasternal, supraclavicular, and intercostal retractions. A patient with a lower airway obstruction may have difficulty moving air out. To do so, he may use his abdominal muscles to force the diaphragm upward and inward. He also may purse his lips during exhalation in an attempt to maintain a back pressure to keep the airways open. Infants and small children grunt to maintain this back pressure. Accessory muscle use always indicates a patient in respiratory distress due to a difficulty in moving air. Assist these patients with positive pressure ventilation and supplemental oxygen as needed.

Quickly inspect and then palpate the chest. Begin palpating at the clavicles and work down and around the rib cage, checking for stability. Palpate the clavicles over their entire length, bilaterally (Procedure 8-3a). These bones, which fracture more frequently than any other bone in the human body, are located directly over the subclavian artery and vein and the superior-most aspect of the lung. Their fracture and displacement may lacerate the vessels or puncture lung tissue, leading to hemothorax, pneumothorax, hypovolemia, or all three.

Be especially careful when palpating the ribs. Beneath each rib lie an artery, a vein, and a nerve that overaggressive palpation can easily damage. Classical soft-tissue injury signs may not be present because the ecchymotic coloration of bruising likely will not have had time to develop. Look for erythema caused by impact to the ribs. The first three ribs are well supported by muscles, ligaments, and tendons. Because of the energy required to fracture

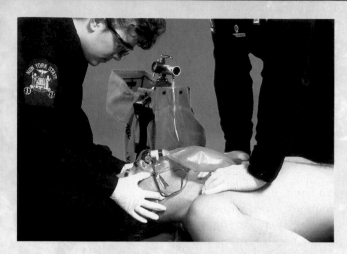

8-3a Palpate the clavicles.

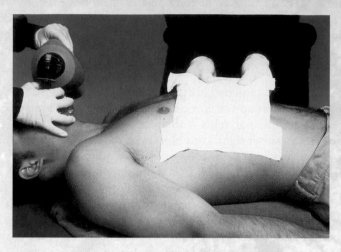

8-3b Stabilize flail chest.

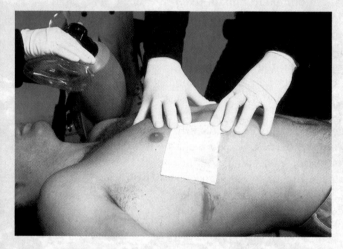

8-3c Seal any sucking chest wound with tape on three sides.

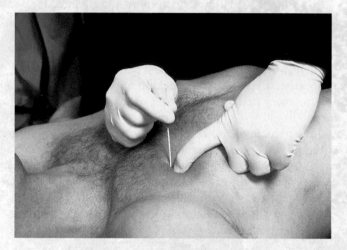

8-3d Perform needle decompression to relieve tension pneumothorax if authorized.

them, you should suspect major damage to the underlying organs, especially vascular structures, when they are broken.

If you notice the crackling of subcutaneous emphysema during chest palpation, suspect pneumothorax or a tracheo-bronchial tear. This condition results when air collects in the soft tissues. Subcutaneous air normally flows from the upper chest to the neck and head. In some cases, it drastically changes the patient's facial features before your eyes.

Observe for equal, symmetrical, effortless chest rise. The chest should rise with inhalation and fall with exhalation. An abnormality in the chest wall may inhibit this process. For example, a patient with a rib fracture hesitates to expand his chest because it hurts. The fracture of two or more adjacent ribs in two or more places causes an unstable flail (floating) segment, which may be evidenced by paradoxical chest wall movement. Paradoxical movement may not appear early in a flail segment because the muscles surrounding the fractured ribs may contract spasmodically, securing the ribs in place. As the muscles fatigue and relax, the flail segment becomes obvious in the paradoxical movement. A flail chest greatly reduces air movement. The underlying lung contusion and subsequent decreased tidal volume limit the air available for gas exchange. To ensure enough air movement for adequate gas exchange, assist ventilation with a BVM and supplemental oxygen. If the flail segment is loose, stabilize it to the chest wall with a large pad and tape (Procedure 8-3b).

Inspect your patient's chest front and back for open wounds. The lungs expand because they adhere to the inner chest wall. This adherence is made possible by the presence of two thin membranes, the visceral pleura, which covers the lungs, and the parietal pleura, which covers the inner chest wall. A film of liquid between these two layers creates a negative-pressure bond that forces the lungs to expand with the chest wall. Any opening in this system can disrupt adherence and cause the lung to collapse. Since air follows the path of least resistance, it may enter the chest cavity through the hole instead of through the respiratory tract. Thus, you should seal any open wounds with an occlusive dressing such as petroleum jelly gauze at the end of exhalation. Tape the dressing on three sides only to create a one-way valve effect, allowing air to escape but not be drawn in (Procedure 8-3c). Remember to check carefully under the armpits and back for knife and small-caliber gunshot wounds. You can easily miss these because the elastic skin closes quickly over the wound and limits external bleeding.

Auscultate both lungs quickly at each mid-axillary line for equal and adequate air movement. Unequal air movement may indicate the presence of a collapsed lung from a pneumothorax or hemothorax. Absent sounds on one side and diminished sounds on the other may suggest a life-threatening condition known as tension pneumothorax. This condition also presents with severe respiratory distress, accessory muscle use, retractions, tachycardia, hypotension, narrowing pulse pressure, and distended neck veins. Tracheal deviation may be a late sign of tension pneumothorax. If authorized, perform needle decompression immediately. Insert a large-bore IV catheter into the pleural space at the second intercostal space over the tip of the rib, midclavicular line, allowing the trapped air to escape and release the tension (Procedure 8-3d). Only through practice and repetition will you gain the confidence to recognize the difference between adequate and diminished lung sounds. Again, for patients with inadequate lung sounds, administer 100% oxygen and assist ventilation with a BVM as needed.

Abdomen   Inspect and palpate the abdomen for DCAP-BTLS and crepitation. Note any areas of bruising and guarding. Exaggerated abdominal-wall motion to assist respiration may result from spinal injury, airway obstruction, or respiratory muscle failure. Solid organs such as the kidneys, liver, and spleen can bleed enough blood into the abdominal cavity to cause profound shock.

Two characteristic areas for bruising are over the umbilicus (**Cullen's sign**) and over the flanks (**Grey-Turner's sign**). Both signs indicate intra-abdominal hemorrhage but usually will not occur until hours after the injury. Perform deep palpation over each quadrant and note any tenderness, rigidity, and guarding. Be careful, because deep palpation sometimes can aggravate the problem. Avoid spending time needlessly trying to make a specific diagnosis. You need only to recognize the possibility that an intra-abdominal hemorrhage exists and that your patient requires immediate transport to an appropriate medical facility for surgery.

Avoid spending time needlessly trying to make a specific diagnosis during rapid trauma assessment of the abdomen.

Cullen's sign bruising over the umbilicus.

Grey-Turner's sign bruising over the flanks.

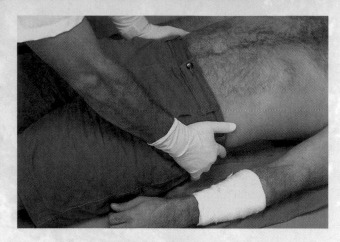

8-4a Assess the integrity of the pelvis by gently pressing medially on the pelvic ring.

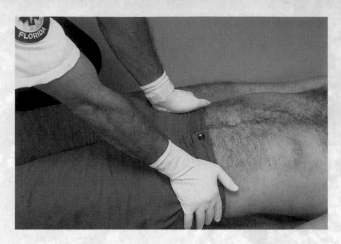

8-4b Compress pelvis posteriorly.

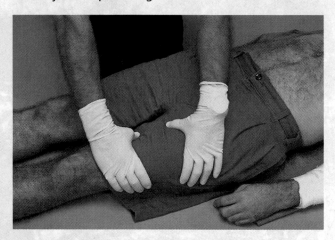

8-4c Palpate the legs.

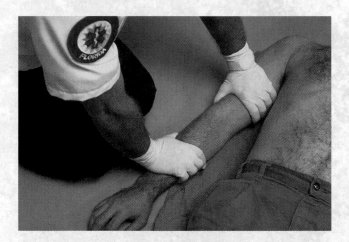

8-4d Palpate the arms.

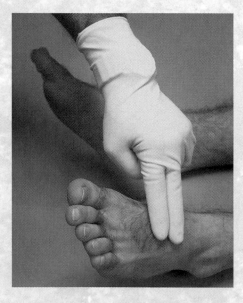

8-4e Palpate the dorsalis pedis pulse to evaluate distal circulation.

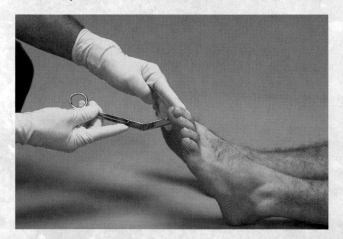

8-4f Assess distal sensation and motor function.

When injured, hollow organs such as the stomach and intestines spill their toxic contents into the abdomen, irritating the peritoneum, the inner-abdominal lining. Testing for rebound tenderness will help you determine if your patient's peritoneum is irritated. Gently palpate an area and let your hand up quickly. If your patient experiences pain with this release, it is likely due to peritoneal irritation. If you suspect intra-abdominal hemorrhage, provide oxygen and expedite transport. En route to the hospital, provide IV fluid resuscitation as needed.

Pelvis Examine the pelvis for DCAP-BTLS and crepitation. The importance of a stable pelvic ring cannot be overemphasized. A patient with a pelvic fracture or dislocation risks lacerating the iliac arteries and veins, major blood vessels running through that area. He can easily lose a significant amount of blood into the pelvic cavity.

Evaluate the pelvic ring at the iliac crests and symphysis pubis. With the palms of your hands, direct pressure medially and posteriorly (Procedure 8-4a and 8-4b). Then press posteriorly on the symphysis pubis, being careful not to entrap the penis or cause injury to the urinary bladder. Any pain, instability, or crepitus suggests a pelvic fracture. Always immobilize the pelvis before transport to prevent movement and a possible circulatory catastrophe. The pneumatic antishock garment may be used to immobilize an unstable pelvic fracture.

Examine the genital area for signs of incontinence, bleeding or priapism.

Extremities Inspect and palpate all four extremities for DCAP-BTLS and crepitation (Procedure 8-4c and 8-4d). Splint fractures en route to the hospital if your patient is unstable. Do not spend time splinting fractures on the scene.

Do not spend time splinting an unstable patient's fractures on the scene.

Before placing your patient on a backboard and immobilizing his spine, evaluate distal neurovascular function by checking for pulses, sensation, and the ability to move (Procedure 8-4e and 8-4f). If you cannot locate a pulse, determine the adequacy of perfusion by assessing the temperature, color, and condition of the skin of the extremity. Assume vascular compromise if pulse is absent, the extremity is cool, or the skin is ashen or cyanotic. The inability to feel and move both legs indicates complete spinal cord disruption. Diminished sensation or diminished motor ability may indicate a partial disruption. Weakness or disability on only one side of the body suggests brain injury due to a stroke or head injury. Evaluate these functions again after spinal immobilization to make certain they have not changed. Report and record all extremity function tests. Check for medical identification devices, which identify a medical condition that may complicate the injury (Figure 8-24).

Posterior Body If you suspect a spinal injury, carefully maintain manual stabilization of the head and spine as you log-roll the patient onto his side. Then inspect and palpate the posterior trunk for DCAP-BTLS and crepitation (Figure 8-25). Particularly note any tenderness in the spinal area. Palpate the buttocks to rule out hemorrhage, contusion, or other injury. Though predominantly soft tissue, this area is a large mass and can conceal considerable internal blood loss. Next, place the long spine board snugly against your patient's body and maintain alignment of the head and spine as you log-roll him into a supine position on the spine board. He is now ready to be secured to the spine board and transported.

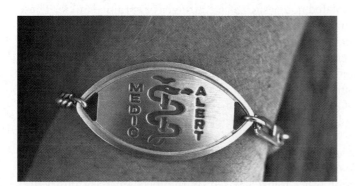
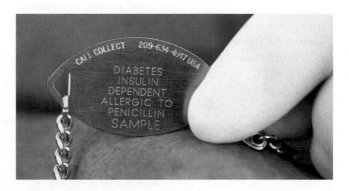

FIGURE 8-24 An example of a medical identification device, Medic Alert tags can give important information about the patient's condition and medical history.

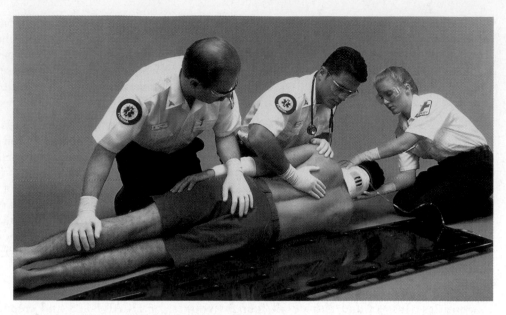

FIGURE 8-25 Inspect and palpate the posterior body.

Focus your minor-trauma assessment on the specific injury and conduct a DCAP-BTLS exam in that area.

Vital Signs

Take a baseline set of vital signs, either at the scene or during transport, as your patient's condition and circumstances allow. These vital signs include respiration rate and quality, pulse rate and quality, blood pressure, and skin temperature and condition. During your EMT-Basic training, you may have learned to include pupils as part of your vital sign check. Including a basic pupil response check (direct response to light) as part of your baseline and serial vital sign assessment is acceptable; however, during the detailed physical exam you may perform an expanded assessment of the pupils as outlined in Chapter 7.

History

The history consists of four elements: the chief complaint, the history of present illness, the medical history, and the current health status. (Refer to Chapter 6 for a detailed description of taking a history.) For major trauma cases when time is critical, use an abbreviated format that forms the acronym SAMPLE: **S**ymptoms, **A**llergies, **M**edications, **P**ast medical history, **L**ast oral intake, and **E**vents preceding the incident. This handy mnemonic is especially useful for eliciting a quick history from your trauma patient. If your patient cannot provide this information, elicit it from family, friends, and bystanders.

THE ISOLATED-INJURY TRAUMA PATIENT

Some trauma patients sustain an isolated injury such as a cut finger or sprained ankle. These patients have no significant mechanism of injury and show no signs of systemic involvement such as poor peripheral perfusion, altered mental status, tachycardia, or breathing problems. They do not require an extensive history or comprehensive physical exam. To treat the trauma patient with an isolated injury, first ensure his hemodynamic status via the initial assessment. Then conduct your focused history and physical exam on the specific isolated injury. Use the mnemonic DCAP-BTLS to evaluate the injured area and take a full set of vital signs. Then, if time allows, this is an excellent opportunity to use some of the advanced assessment techniques you learned in Chapter 7. After your exam of the isolated injury, take a SAMPLE history. Remember that some trauma patients may complain of an isolated problem but actually have more significant injuries. Avoid tunnel vision and develop a low threshold for suspecting other injuries based on the mechanism of injury and your patient's story.

1. Your patient is a young football player who twisted his knee and lies on the ground, complaining loudly of knee pain. After a quick initial assessment and DCAP-BTLS assessment, you conclude that your patient is in stable condition with no signs or symptoms of systemic involvement and good distal neurovascular function. Before splinting your patient's leg, you decide to elicit more information through a detailed exam of the knee. You inspect the normal concavities for evidence of excessive fluid in the joint by "milking" the knee joint on one side and looking for a fluid wave on the opposite side. Next you palpate the medial and lateral collateral ligaments for tenderness. Then, if doing so does not cause your patient undue pain, you examine the stability of the collateral ligaments with the "side-to-side" test and the cruciate ligaments with the "drawer test." Finally, you assess the knee's passive range of motion (flexion and extension) and note any limitations.

2. Your patient sustains a laceration to the palm of his hand from a bread knife. After you have controlled the bleeding and ensured no systemic involvement or major loss of blood, you decide to examine the hand further before bandaging it. You conduct a DCAP-BTLS exam and note that distal neurovascular function is intact. Knowing that the flexor tendons all run through the palm of the hand, you examine each tendon's function through a full range of motion exam. You ask your patient to make a fist, then open his hand and extend all of his fingers. You note any abnormalities, pain, or limitations in the range of motion.

3. Your patient is a teenager who was punched in the eye during a minor altercation with a classmate. After determining that he had no loss of consciousness and that he is alert and oriented with stable vital signs, equal and reactive pupils, and no signs or symptoms of serious head injury, you may conduct a more detailed exam of the injured eye. First you inspect the external structures for discoloration, deformity, or swelling and find all three. You palpate the orbit of the eye for tenderness and deformity. You look for evidence of hyphema (blood in the anterior chamber), indicating severe blunt trauma. With a penlight, you check for direct and consensual response to light. Finally, you assess the integrity of the extraocular muscles with the H test.

THE RESPONSIVE MEDICAL PATIENT

Assessing the responsive patient with a medical emergency is entirely different from assessing the trauma patient for two reasons. First, the history takes precedence over the physical exam. This is because, in the majority of cases, you will formulate your field diagnosis from your patient's story. The physical exam serves mostly to support your diagnostic impression. Second, your physical exam is aimed at identifying signs of medical complications such as inflammation, infection, and edema rather than signs of injury. The focused physical exam evaluates pertinent areas suggested by the history. Remember that you will begin treatment as you conduct your assessment. For example, while interviewing your patient who complains of chest pain, simultaneously take vital signs, administer oxygen, provide cardiac monitoring, and start an IV if appropriate (Figure 8-26). The following focused history and physical exam pertains to the responsive medical patient. For a more detailed description of the information and techniques outlined here, refer to Chapters 6 and 7.

History

Conscious, alert patients can usually tell you a great deal about their illness. Remember the old medical adage, "Listen to your patient; he will tell you what is wrong." Ask questions and then listen intently to your patient's answers. Since children may not be able to describe their illness and medical history clearly, look to their parents or guardians for this information. Elderly patients may pose several obstacles to the clear communication of medical

Listen to your patient; he will tell you what is wrong.

Content Review

HISTORY OF RESPONSIVE MEDICAL PATIENT
- Chief complaint
- History of present illness
- Past history
- Current health status

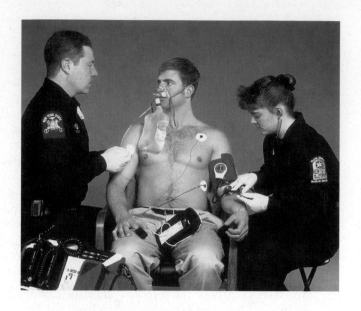

Figure 8-26 Begin treatment while you assess your responsive medical patient.

information. They are more likely to be confused, to have poor short-term and long-term memory, and to have hearing, speech, or sight difficulties. Obtaining an accurate history from such patients requires patience, empathy, and outstanding communication skills.

The history consists of four elements: the chief complaint, the history of the present illness, the past history, and the current health status.

Chief Complaint   The **chief complaint** is the pain, discomfort, or dysfunction that caused your patient to request help. Ask your patient, "What seems to be the problem?"

History of Present Illness   Discover the circumstances surrounding the chief complaint, following the mnemonic OPQRST—ASPN:

Onset	What was your patient doing when the problem/pain began? Did emotional or environmental factors contribute to the problem?
Provocation/Palliation	What makes the problem/pain worse or better?
Quality	Can your patient describe the problem/pain?
Region/Radiation	Where is the problem/pain and does it radiate anywhere?
Severity	How bad is the problem/pain? Can your patient rate it on a scale of 1 to 10?
Time	When did the problem/pain begin? How long does the pain last?
Associated Symptoms	Is your patient having any other problems?
Pertinent Negatives	Are any likely associated symptoms absent?

Past Medical History   The past medical history may provide significant insights into your patient's chief complaint and your field diagnosis. It includes your patient's general state of health, childhood and adult diseases, psychiatric illnesses, accidents and injuries, surgeries and hospitalizations. If your history taking reveals significant medical problems, investigate in more detail. Note when your patient first recognized the problem and how it affected him. How frequently did it happen and what medical care did he seek? Was the treatment effective or did the problem recur?

Current Health Status   The current health status assembles all of the factors regarding your patient's medical condition. It tries to gather information that completes the puzzle surrounding your patient's primary problem. The elements of the current health status include current medications, allergies, tobacco use, alcohol and substance abuse, diet, screening ex-

---

chief complaint the pain, discomfort, or dysfunction that caused your patient to request help.

Content Review

OPQRST-ASPN
- **O**nset
- **P**rovocation/Palliation
- **Q**uality
- **R**egion/Radiation
- **S**everity
- **T**ime
- **A**ssociated **S**ymptoms
- **P**ertinent **N**egatives

Content Review

PAST MEDICAL HISTORY
- General state of health
- Childhood and adult diseases
- Psychiatric illnesses
- Accidents and injuries
- Surgeries and hospitalizations

ams, immunizations, sleep patterns, exercise and leisure activities, environmental hazards, the use of safety measures, and any pertinent family or social history. Look for clues and correlations among the various sections of this part of the history. If your patient is critical and your time is limited, use the abbreviated SAMPLE format to elicit the history.

Focused Physical Exam

Once you have obtained the history, begin a focused physical exam based on the information you elicited from your patient. Let the diagnostic impression you formed during the history guide your examination. For example, if you suspect a myocardial infarction, examine areas pertinent to a patient having a heart attack—cardiac and respiratory systems, chest, neck, and peripheral perfusion. It would be pointless and impractical to test for nasal drainage, extraocular movements, or the elbow's range of motion. Use those exam techniques presented in Chapter 7 that pertain to your patient's special situation and clinical status.

Three common presentations among your responsive medical patients will be cardiac chest pain/respiratory distress, altered mental status, and acute abdomen. The following sections outline problem-oriented physical exams for those complaints. Note that for each of these cases, the focused physical exam is different. As you gain clinical experience you will be able to quickly assess your patient's pertinent areas according to your suspected field diagnosis. Likewise, clinical judgment and the seriousness of your patient's condition will determine which exam techniques you use on the scene and which you use en route to the hospital.

Chest Pain/Respiratory Distress   For a patient complaining of chest pain or respiratory distress, assess the following:

HEENT (Head, Eyes, Ears, Nose, and Throat)   Note the color of the lips. Lip cyanosis is an ominous sign of central circulatory hypoxia. For a patient complaining of chest pain or respiratory distress, assess the following: Examine the oral mucosa for pallor suggesting decreased circulation as in shock. Inspect any fluids in the mouth. Pink, frothy sputum (the result of plasma proteins' mixing with air and red blood cells in the alveoli) is a classic sign of acute pulmonary edema. Always keep the mouth clear of any fluids that may block the upper airway by aggressive suctioning. Note any swelling, redness, or hives, suggesting an allergic reaction.

Neck   Observe the neck for accessory muscle use and retractions, signs of acute respiratory distress. Retractions in the supraclavicular (above the clavicles) and suprasternal (above the sternum) notches indicate your patient is having difficulty inhaling. Palpate the carotid arteries for rate, quality, and equality; if you detect weak or unequal pulses, auscultate for bruits. Examine the jugular veins for abnormal distention. In a patient lying supine without circulatory compromise, these veins should distend slightly. This is normal. If the jugular veins do not distend in the supine position, your patient may be hypovolemic. In the semi-Fowler's position (sitting up at a 45-degree angle), the veins should disappear. Distention beyond 45 degrees is significant because something is inhibiting blood return to the chest. This may be the result of cardiac tamponade, tension pneumothorax, or right heart failure. Inspect and palpate the position of the trachea. It should lie midline and remain fixed during the breathing cycle. Tugging to one side during inspiration suggests a pneumothorax on that side. Displacement to one side may indicate a tension pneumothorax on the opposite side as the entire mediastinum is displaced.

Chest   Assess the respiratory rate and pattern again and administer oxygen or ventilation as needed. Note the length of the inspiratory and expiratory phases. A prolonged inspiratory phase suggests an upper airway obstruction. A prolonged expiratory phase suggests a lower airway obstruction such as in asthma and emphysema. Inspect and palpate the chest wall for symmetry of movement and intercostal retractions. A barrel chest suggests a history of emphysema. Look for the classic midline scar from open-heart surgery or the typical bulge of an implanted pacemaker or defibrillator.

Auscultate all lung fields (anterior to posterior, apices to bases) and compare side-to-side. Report and record the sounds you hear (crackles, wheezes), where you hear them (in the bases, apices, diffuse), and when they occur during the respiratory cycle (inspiratory, expiratory). For example, if your patient has bilateral inspiratory rales, you might suspect congestive heart failure or pulmonary edema. If he has diffuse expiratory wheezing, you might suspect the bronchospasm associated with asthma or chronic obstructive pulmonary disease. The presence of both would suggest acute pulmonary edema. A localized wheeze might indicate a pulmonary embolism, a foreign body aspiration, or an infection. Percuss the chest and back for hyperresonance (asthma, emphysema, pneumothorax) and dullness (pulmonary edema, pleural effusion, pneumonia).

Cardiovascular   Inspect for signs of arterial insufficiency or occlusion in your patient's trunk and extremities. Look for skin pallor and other signs of decreased perfusion. Inspect and palpate the chest for the point of maximum impulse (PMI). Assess central and peripheral pulses for equality, rate, regularity, and quality. Auscultate for heart sounds, identifying S_1, S_2, and any additional sounds.

Abdomen   Look for exaggerated abdominal muscle use during exhalation, a sign of lower airway obstruction as seen in asthma and emphysema. Inspect and palpate the abdomen for distention due to air or fluid. Ascites is an accumulation of fluid within the abdominal cavity caused by increased pressure in the systemic circulation as seen in patients with right heart failure. It is also common in patients with cirrhosis of the liver, where portal circulation (to and from the liver) is increased. Inspect and palpate the flanks and presacral area for edema in bed-ridden patients suspected of having congestive heart failure. Check for unusual pulsation of the descending aorta, just left of the umbilicus. Palpate for liver enlargement or upper quadrant tenderness suggesting ulcer disease, gallbladder disease, or pancreas problems, all of which can be confused as chest pain.

Extremities   Perform neurovascular checks on both hands and feet. These consist of checking for pulses, sensation, and the ability to move. Pay special attention to the equality of pulses in all extremities. Unequal pulses in the upper extremities suggest a thoracic aneurysm; unequal pulses in the lower extremities suggest an abdominal aneurysm. Assume vascular compromise if the pulse is absent, the limb is cool, or the skin is cyanotic or ashen. In cardiac and respiratory emergencies, evaluate the lower extremities for pitting edema. Depress the skin on the tibial plateau (Figure 8-27). If the depression remains after you remove your finger, pitting edema exists. This is a sign of chronic fluid retention as seen in heart and renal failure. Examine the fingernails for pitting. Check the wrists for medical identification devices such as Medic Alert tags.

Altered Mental Status   For a patient with an altered mental status, assess the following:

HEENT   Inspect and palpate the head to rule out any evidence of trauma. For example, the stroke patient may have suffered a skull fracture from falling on the floor. Palpate the fontanels of the infant for sunkenness (dehydration) and bulging (increasing intracranial pressure). Examine the face for symmetry. Unilateral facial drooping may indicate a stroke or inflammation of the facial nerve (Bell's palsy). Examine the pupils for direct and consensual response to light. One pupil getting larger or reacting more slowly to light could indicate a deteriorating brain pathology such as a stroke. A small portion of the population,

FIGURE 8-27   Check for peripheral edema.

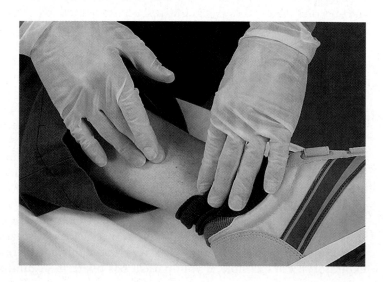

however, has unequal pupils, a benign condition known as anisocoria. Bilaterally sluggish pupils usually suggest decreased blood flow to the brain and hypoxia. Fixed and dilated pupils indicate severe brain anoxia. Your patient's pupils also may dilate from sympathomimetic or anticholinergic drug use. Pinpoint pupils suggest a narcotic drug overdose or pontine hemmorhage (bleeding within the pons). Test the integrity of the extraocular muscles with the H test. Normally your patient will move his eyes conjugately (together) to follow your finger. He may exhibit a nystagmus, a fine jerking of the eyes. At the far extremes of the test, nystagmus may be normal, but if you observe it during all extraocular movements it suggests pathology. Examine the conjunctiva for redness (irritation), pallor (hypoperfusion), or cyanosis (hypoxia). Inspect the sclera for jaundice.

Chest   Inspect, palpate, and auscultate the chest for any signs of cardiorespiratory involvement.

Abdomen   Look for evidence of trauma or internal bleeding.

Pelvis   Look for evidence of incontinence.

Extremities   Perform neurovascular checks on both hands and feet. These consist of checking for pulses, sensation, and the ability to move. Assume vascular compromise if the pulse is absent, the limb is cool, or the skin is cyanotic or ashen. Since the motor and sensory nerves run along different pathways in the spinal cord, you must check your patient's extremities both for mobility and for sensation of light touch and pain. As with trauma patients, the inability to feel and move both legs indicates complete spinal cord disruption. Diminished sensation or diminished motor ability indicates a partial disruption. Weakness or disability on only one side suggests brain dysfunction such as a stroke. Report and record all extremity function tests.

Posterior Body   Inspect the posterior body for deformities of the spine. Also check for evidence of incontinence. In the supine patient, inspect the flanks for presacral edema.

Neurological   Reassess your patient's level of consciousness and compare his response to your earlier findings. Note his speech pattern and any deficits in speech or language. Observe mood swings or behaviors that suggest anxiety or depression. Determine your patient's person, time, and place orientation. Does he know his name, the day of the week, and where he is? Inspect general body structure, muscle development, positioning, and coordination. Note any obvious asymmetries, deformities, or involuntary movements. Assess muscle tone by feeling the muscle's resistance to passive stretching in the extremities. Note the degree of resistance. Test for muscle strength by applying resistance during the range of motion evaluation. Assess for coordination and cerebellar function, using rapid alternating movements and point-to-point testing. Note seizure activity tremors.

Acute Abdomen   For a patient complaining of abdominal pain, assess the following:

HEENT   Notice any unusual odors coming from your patient's mouth. The smell of alcohol does not rule out a serious medical condition. The sweet smell of ketones suggests diabetes. A fecal odor may indicate a lower-bowel obstruction. The acidic smell of gastric contents means that your patient has vomited and may again. Inspect any fluids in the mouth. Coffee-ground emesis (vomiting) results from blood mixing with stomach acids and suggests upper GI bleeding. Fresh blood usually means recent hemorrhage from the upper GI tract.

Chest   Listen to breath sounds. Crackles may indicate pneumonia, a cause of upper abdomen pain.

Abdomen   Look for discoloration over the umbilicus (Cullen's sign) or over the flanks (Grey-Turner's sign) suggesting intra-abdominal bleeding. Check for any visible pulsation, peristalsis, or masses. If you notice a bounding or exaggerated pulsation, suspect an aortic aneurysm. Visible peristalsis may indicate a bowel obstruction. Palpate the abdomen to detect tenderness, muscular rigidity, and superficial organs and masses. The normal abdomen is soft and non-tender. Abdominal pain on light palpation suggests peritoneal irritation or inflammation. If you feel rigidity or guarding while palpating, determine whether it is voluntary (patient anticipates the pain or is not relaxed) or involuntary (peritoneal inflammation). Then palpate the abdomen deeply to detect large masses or tenderness. If the peritoneum is inflamed, your patient experiences pain when you let go.

Posterior Body   Inspect the posterior body for evidence of rectal bleeding.

Baseline Vital Signs

Prehospital medicine employs four basic vital signs: blood pressure, pulse, respiration, and temperature. As mentioned earlier, you may add a basic pupil assessment to this list. Your patient's vital signs are your windows to what is happening inside his body. They provide a unique, objective capsule assessment of his clinical status. Vital signs indicate severe illness and the urgency to intervene. Subtle alterations in these vital signs are often the only indication that your patient's condition is changing. They can warn you that your patient is deteriorating, or they can reassure you that he is responding to therapy.

Of the physical assessment techniques, taking accurate sets of vital signs reveals the most important information. As an EMT-I, you must assess these signs on every patient you evaluate. If your patient is with you for an extended time, measure and record his vital signs at intervals as his clinical condition dictates. Always reevaluate the vital signs after invasive procedures such as endotracheal intubation or fluid resuscitation and after any sudden change in your patient's condition. Accurate records of these numbers are invaluable when documenting your patient assessment.

If you suspect your patient of being hypovolemic, consider performing an orthostatic vital sign exam, commonly known as the tilt test. Take your patient's pulse and blood pressure while he is supine. Then have him sit up and dangle his feet. Finally, tell him to stand. Then in 30 to 60 seconds retake the vital signs. They should not change in the healthy patient. An increase in the pulse rate of 10 to 20 beats per minute or a drop in blood pressure of 10 to 20 mmHg, is a positive tilt test. This is a common finding in patients suspected of hypovolemia. Chapter 7 describes vital sign evaluation in detail.

Additional Assessment Techniques

Additional techniques include pulse oximetry, cardiac monitoring, and blood glucose determination. Refer to Chapter 7 for detailed descriptions of these techniques.

Pulse Oximetry   The pulse oximeter is a noninvasive device that measures the oxygen saturation of your patient's blood. It is usually a good indicator of cardiorespiratory status because it tells you how well your patient is oxygenating the most distal ends of his circulatory system. It also quantifies the effectiveness of your interventions such as oxygen therapy, medications, suctioning, and ventilatory assistance. Normal oxygen saturation at sea level should be between 96% and 100%. Generally, if the reading is below 95%, suspect shock, hypoxia, or respiratory compromise. Provide your patient with the appropriate airway management, supplemental oxygen, and watch him carefully for further changes. Any reading below 90% requires aggressive airway management, positive pressure ventilation, or oxygen administration.

Cardiac Monitoring   The cardiac monitor, which measures electrical activity, is essential in assessing and managing the patient who requires advanced cardiac life support (ACLS) measures. You should apply it to any patient you suspect of having a serious illness or injury. Its one major disadvantage, however, is that it cannot tell you if the heart is pumping efficiently, effectively, or at all. Always assess your patient and compare what you see on the monitor with what you feel for a pulse.

Blood Glucose Determination   In cases of altered mental status, such as diabetic emergencies, seizures, and strokes, measure your patient's blood sugar level. The arrival of inexpensive, hand-held glucometers makes this test simple and easy to perform in the field.

Emergency Medical Care

After conducting your physical exam, provide the necessary emergency medical care authorized by your medical director via standing orders. Then contact the on-line medical direction physician to request further orders. For example, you may administer 50% dextrose to an adult patient (25% dextrose to a pediatric patient) with documented hypoglycemia (Figure 8-28), intubate a patient in severe respiratory distress, or apply external cardiac pacing to a patient with third-degree heart block. Always base your emergency care on your patient's signs and symptoms as obtained with a thorough focused history and

---

Always reevaluate vital signs after invasive procedures and after any sudden change in your patient's condition.

Apply the cardiac monitor to any patient you suspect of having a serious illness or injury.

Always base care of responsive medical patients on signs and symptoms as obtained from a thorough focused history and physical exam.

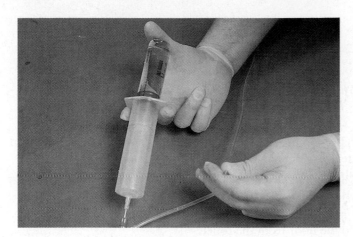

FIGURE 8-28 Administer 50% dextrose to a patient in insulin shock.

physical exam. Finally, en route to the hospital conduct an ongoing assessment as described later in this chapter.

Again, if time allows, in certain situations you may wish to selectively use some of the advanced assessments described in Chapter 7. For example, en route to the hospital you might conduct a more in-depth neurological exam for your patient who complains of strokelike symptoms. This encompasses a full mental status assessment including orientation, appearance and behavior, speech and language, mood; a motor system assessment including muscle bulk, tone, and strength; a sensory exam including sharp and dull identification, temperature discrimination. For your patient with upper respiratory distress and influenza symptoms you may decide to examine the posterior pharynx and tonsils for redness and exudates. For your patient suspected of having acute appendicitis, you may wish to use the psoas test. Ask your patient to bring his right knee to his chest, contracting the iliopsoas muscle group. This motion usually causes pain because the muscles rub against the inflamed appendix. Your clinical experience and judgment will guide these types of decisions. The scope of EMT-I practice is changing, not in procedures but in assessment capabilities. You will learn much more than your predecessors about anatomy and physiology, pathophysiology, and patient assessment. In time, you will learn which exam techniques yield the most relevant information and use them in your daily practice.

THE UNRESPONSIVE MEDICAL PATIENT

Since he cannot tell you what is wrong, the unresponsive medical patient requires an entirely different approach than the responsive patient. Assess the unresponsive medical patient much as you would a trauma patient. Begin with the initial assessment; then conduct a rapid head-to-toe exam known as the rapid medical assessment; and finally take a brief history from family or friends. This approach to the unresponsive medical patient also will help you to detect whether trauma may be involved.

After conducting the initial assessment, position your patient so that his airway is protected. If the cervical spine is not involved, place your patient in the recovery position, laterally recumbent. This will prevent secretions from obstructing his airway. Now begin the rapid medical assessment. The rapid medical assessment is similar to the rapid trauma assessment, except that you will look for signs of illness, not injury. Assess the head, neck, chest, abdomen, pelvis, extremities, and posterior aspect of the body. Perform the entire exam with the unresponsive patient. Then, assess baseline vital signs: pulse, blood pressure, respiration, and temperature. Finally, obtain a history from bystanders, family members, friends, or medical identification devices or services. If possible it should include the chief complaint, history of the present illness, past medical history, and current health status.

Evaluate your data and provide emergency medical care while performing additional tests such as cardiac monitoring, blood glucose determination, and pulse oximetry as needed. Consider your unresponsive patient unstable and expedite transport to the hospital, performing an ongoing assessment every 5 minutes en route.

Content Review

UNRESPONSIVE MEDICAL PATIENTS
- Initial assessment
- Rapid medical assessment
- Brief history

Expedite transfer of unresponsive medical patients to the hospital and perform an ongoing assessment every 5 minutes en route.

IN THE FIELD

The rapid assessment is not a comprehensive history and physical exam, but a practical, systematic assessment aimed at quickly identifying the cause of your patient's unresponsive condition. Your care for a patient with a coma of unknown origin, for example, might go something like this:

You are dispatched to an "unconscious person" in a residential area. Your patient is an elderly man who presents laterally recumbent on his bathroom floor. You conduct an initial assessment while your partner elicits information from the patient's wife:

General:	Your patient appears pale and diaphoretic, moaning unintelligibly. You find no apparent signs of trauma, and he appears to have slumped to the floor from the toilet.
Mental Status:	You establish your patient's mental status using the AVPU scale. He responds to your voice but cannot answer your questions.
Airway:	You open your patient's airway with a head-tilt/chin-lift maneuver and observe his breathing. His airway is clear. His breathing is rapid and shallow, but not labored. You ask another rescuer to administer positive pressure ventilation with supplemental oxygen while you continue with your assessment.
Circulation:	You palpate his radial pulse and note its absence. His carotid pulse is slow, irregular, and weak. His skin is pale, cool, and clammy, indicating poor peripheral perfusion.

You give this patient a high priority because of an altered mental status, rapid, shallow breathing, and poor peripheral perfusion. You suspect shock and begin a rapid medical assessment.

HEENT:	You note lip cyanosis, a sign of central hypoxia. You see no lip pursing, nasal flaring, or other signs of increased breathing effort such as retractions or accessory muscle use. You smell no unusual odors or fluids from the mouth. The face is symmetrical; the pupils are equal and round, but react to light sluggishly. The trachea is midline, there is no jugular vein distention.
Chest:	You note symmetrical chest wall movement and an equal and adequate rise and fall of the chest with each ventilation. You note some crackles in the lung bases. Your patient has no surgical scars.
ABD:	You see no ascites or abdominal distention, no rigidity or guarding, no rebound tenderness, no needle marks, no surgical scars or pulsating masses.
Pelvis:	You see no evidence of incontinence or of rectal bleeding.
Extremities:	No finger clubbing, no medical identification, no needle marks. Peripheral circulation is poor with no radial or pedal pulses. You note some pitting edema in lower extremities.
Posterior:	You note some edema in your patient's flanks.
Vital Signs:	Heart rate, 46 and regular; BP, 78/38; respirations, 36 and shallow.
Additional:	ECG monitor shows third-degree AV block; pulse oximetry, 92% on room air, 99% with oxygen; blood glucose, 110.

Your patient's wife reveals his long history of heart disease and a long list of cardiac medications. Your field diagnosis is cardiogenic shock due to the bradycardic rate of the third-degree block. While your partner initiates an IV, you set up for immediate external cardiac pacing.

DETAILED PHYSICAL EXAM

The **detailed physical exam** uses many components of the comprehensive evaluation presented in the previous two chapters. It is a careful, thorough process of eliciting the history and conducting a physical exam. The detailed physical exam is a luxury, designed for use en route to the hospital, if time allows, for patients with significant trauma or serious medical illnesses. Ironically, with critical patients you usually will not have time to perform this in-depth exam because you will be preoccupied with performing ongoing assessments and providing emergency care. So you will seldom, if ever, perform a complete exam in the field. In fact, physicians in the emergency department rarely perform a detailed exam on their critical patients. It is too comprehensive and time-consuming and yields little relevant information.

In the emergency setting, use a modified approach. You can individualize the exam to your patient's particular situation in many ways. For example, for the multi-trauma patient, perform a head-to-toe survey that is more detailed and slower than the rapid trauma assessment yet focuses on injury. For the 17-year-old football player who presents with shoulder pain, you may perform the entire portion of the shoulder exam. Palpating the abdomen and auscultating heart sounds would yield little useful information. For your stable patient who complains of abdominal pain, you may conduct an extensive history as detailed in Chapter 6, instead of the abbreviated SAMPLE history. Often you will elicit vital information from a seemingly obscure question during the review of systems. Again, clinical experience and your patient's condition will determine how you proceed with the detailed exam.

When you conduct the detailed exam you will use components of the history and physical exam presented in Chapters 6 and 7. Refer to those chapters for a complete description of the components outlined in this section. Interview your patient to ascertain the history, and then conduct a systematic head-to-toe physical exam. Place special emphasis on those areas suggested by your patient's chief complaint and present problem. Remember that the physical exam can be an anxiety-provoking experience for both the patient and the examiner. Using a professional, calm demeanor will minimize this anxiety.

DETAILED PHYSICAL EXAM FOR A MULTI-TRAUMA PATIENT

The following example illustrates how you might conduct a detailed physical exam for a multi-trauma patient en route to the hospital.

Head Palpate the cranium from front to back for symmetry and smoothness (Procedure 8-5a). Note any tenderness, deformities, and areas of unusual warmth. Inspect and palpate the facial bones for stability and note any crepitus or loose fragments (Procedure 8-5b). Any instability or asymmetry of the eye orbits, nasal bones, maxilla, or mandible suggests a facial bone fracture. In these cases, pay careful attention to the upper airway for obstruction from blood, bone chips, and teeth. Suction these patients aggressively to keep the upper airway clear.

When the base of the skull is fractured, blood and fluid from the brain can seep into the soft tissues around the eyes and ears and can drain from the ears or nose. Observe the bony orbits of the eye and the mastoid process behind the ears for discoloration. **Periorbital ecchymosis** (raccoon's eyes) is a black and blue discoloration surrounding the eye sockets. **Battle's sign** is a similar discoloration over the mastoid process just behind the ears (Procedure 8-5c). They are both late signs and usually are not visible on the scene unless a previous injury exists. Evaluate the temporomandibular joint for tenderness, swelling, and range of motion.

Eyes Examine the external structure of the eyes for symmetry in size, shape, and contour. Inspect the sclera and conjunctiva for discoloration, swelling, and exudate. Inspect the eyes for discoloration, foreign bodies, or blood in the anterior chamber (hyphema). Hyphema suggests that a tremendous blunt trauma to the anterior part of the eye has occurred. Check the pupils for equality in size and reaction to light (Procedure 8-5d). Bilaterally sluggish pupils usually suggest decreased cerebral perfusion and hypoxia. Fixed and dilated pupils indicate severe cerebral anoxia. Unequal pupils may indicate a variety of pathologies, including brain lesions, meningitis, drug poisoning, third-nerve paralysis, and increasing intracranial pressure.

detailed physical exam careful, thorough process of eliciting the patient's history and conducting a physical exam.

In the emergency setting, individualize the exam to your patient's particular situation.

Aggressively suction patients with facial fractures to keep the upper airway clear.

periorbital ecchymosis black and blue discoloration surrounding the eye sockets.

Battle's sign black and blue discoloration over the mastoid process.

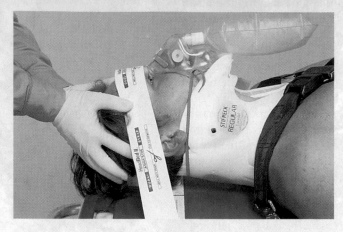

8-5a   Inspect and palpate the cranium from front to back.

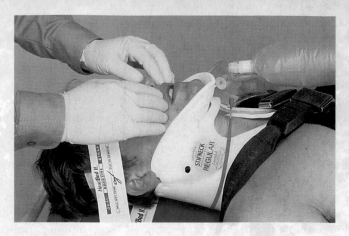

8-5b   Inspect and palpate the facial bones.

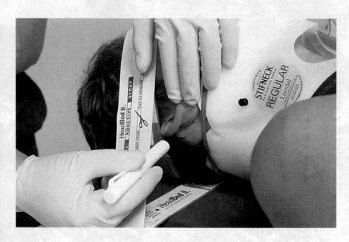

8-5c   Inspect the mastoid process for Battle's sign.

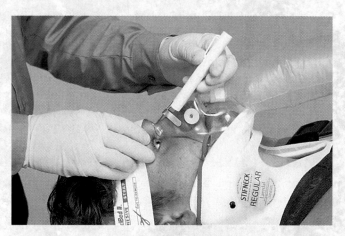

8-5d   Check the pupils for reaction to light.

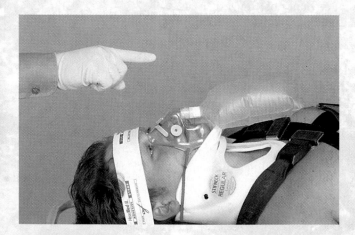

8-5e   Check for extraocular movement.

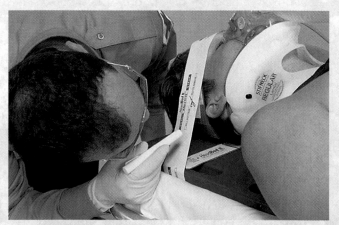

8-5f   Inspect the ear canal for drainage.

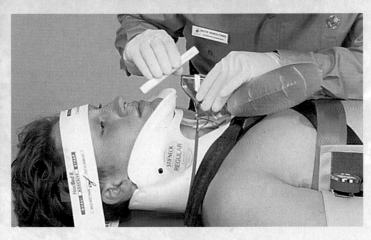

8-5g   Examine the nasal mucosa for drainage.

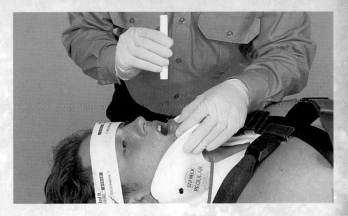

8-5h   Examine the oral mucosa for pallor.

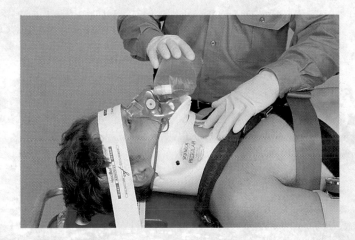

8-5i   Palpate the trachea for midline position.

Examine the eyes for conjugate movement, their ability to move together. Muscle or nerve damage to the eyes and certain drugs can cause dysconjugate gaze, in which the eyes seem to look in different directions. Check for extraocular movements. Note any inability of the eyes to follow your finger as you draw a large imaginary H in front of them; this indicates either nerve damage or an orbital fracture impinging on the extraocular muscles (Procedure 8-5e).

Ears   Examine the external ears and observe the surrounding area for deformities, lumps, skin lesions, tenderness, and erythema. Examine the ear canal for drainage (Procedure 8-5f). A basilar skull fracture can cause blood and clear cerebrospinal fluid to leak into the auditory canals and flow to the outside. Do not try to block this flow; just cover it with sterile gauze to prevent an easy route for infection.

Nose and Sinuses   Check your patient's nose from the front and from the side and note any deviation in shape or color. Palpate the external nose for depressions, deformities, and tenderness. Examine the nares for flaring, a sign of respiratory distress, especially in small children. Pay special attention to infants less than three months old. They are mainly nose breathers and need a clear, unobstructed nasal cavity for respiration. Examine the nasal mucosa for evidence of drainage and note the color, quantity, and consistency of the discharge (Procedure 8-5g). A clear, runny discharge may indicate leaking cerebral spinal fluid (CSF) from a basilar skull fracture.

The nasal cavity has a rich blood supply to warm the inspired air. Unfortunately, this can make bleeding in the nasal cavity severe and very difficult to control. If unconscious, these patients require aggressive suctioning. The patient who swallows this blood may complain later of nausea and vomiting.

Lip cyanosis is an ominous sign of central circulatory hypoxia.

Mouth and Pharynx   Note the condition and color of the lips. Lip cyanosis is an ominous sign of central circulatory hypoxia. Examine the oral mucosa for pallor suggesting poor perfusion as in shock (Procedure 8-5h). Ask your patient to extend his tongue straight out and have your patient say "aaaahhhh" while you examine the back of his throat. Note any odors or fluids coming from your patient's mouth; they can provide clues to infection, poisoning, and metabolic processes such as diabetic ketoacidosis.

Neck   Briefly inspect the neck for general symmetry. Note any obvious deformity, deviation, tugging, masses, surgical scars, gland enlargement, or visible lymph nodes. Examine any penetrating injuries to the neck closely for injury to the trachea or major blood vessels. Look for jugular vein distention while your patient is sitting up and at a 45-degree incline. Palpate the trachea for midline position (Procedure 8-5i). Then, palpate the carotid arteries and note their rate and quality.

Chest and Lungs   Observe your patient's breathing. Look for signs of acute respiratory distress. Count his respiratory rate and note his breathing pattern. Inspect the anterior and posterior chest walls for symmetrical movement. Note the use of neck muscles (sternocleidomastoids, scalene muscles) during inhalation or abdominal muscles during exhalation. Accessory muscle use suggests partial airway obstruction and difficulty moving air. Inspect the intercostal spaces for retractions or bulging.

Palpate the rib cage for rigidity (Procedure 8-6a). Feel for tenderness, deformities, depressions, loose segments, asymmetry, and crepitus. Evaluate for equal expansion. Percuss the chest symmetrically from the apices to the bases. Identify and note any area of abnormal percussion. Auscultate all lung fields and compare side-to-side (Procedure 8-6b).

Percussion can also provide evidence regarding chest pathology. If the region is hyperresonant, the thorax may contain air under pressure (tension pneumothorax). If the region is dull to percussion, it may be filled with blood (hemothorax) or other fluid (pleural effusion). Be sure to compare the sounds left-to-right and, during examination of the posterior body, front-to-back to confirm your evaluation.

Cardiovascular System   Look for skin pallor and other signs of decreased perfusion. Inspect and palpate the carotid arteries for rate, rhythm, and quality or amplitude. Inspect and palpate the chest for the PMI. Auscultate for normal, abnormal, and extra heart sounds.

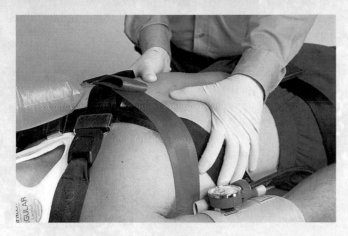

8-6a   Palpate the rib cage.

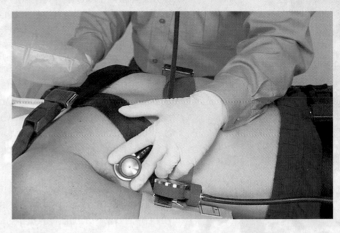

8-6b   Auscultate the lungs.

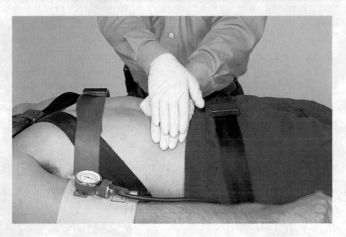

8-6c   Palpate the abdomen.

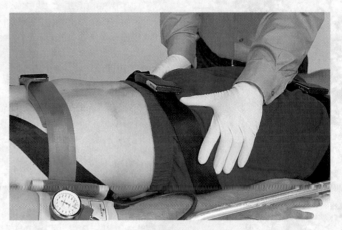

8-6d   Evaluate the pelvis.

Abdomen Inspect the skin of the abdomen and flanks for scars, dilated veins, stretch marks, rashes, lesions, and pigmentation changes. Look for Cullen's sign or Grey-Turner's sign suggesting intra-abdominal bleeding. Assess the size and shape of your patient's abdomen and note its symmetry. Palpate the abdomen to detect tenderness, muscular rigidity, and superficial organs and masses (Procedure 8-6c). Assess for rebound tenderness, a classic sign of peritoneal irritation, by pushing down slowly and then releasing your hand quickly off the tender area.

Pelvis Reevaluate the pelvic ring at the iliac crests and symphysis pubis (Procedure 8-6d). With the palms of your hands, direct pressure medially and posteriorly. Then press posteriorly on the symphysis pubis, being careful not to entrap the penis or cause injury to the urinary bladder. Any pain, instability, or crepitus suggests a pelvic fracture. Always immobilize the pelvis before transport to prevent movement and a possible circulatory catastrophe. If your patient presents in shock with an unstable pelvis, apply and inflate the pneumatic antishock garment.

Genitalia The external genitalia are extremely vascular and can bleed profusely when lacerated. Control hemorrhage in this area with direct pressure. Examine the male organ for priapism, a painful, prolonged erection usually caused by spinal cord injury or blood disturbances. Suspect a major spinal cord injury in any patient with a priapism. The female genitalia are somewhat well-protected from all but penetrating injury.

If you suspect your patient may have been raped or sexually abused, limit your assessment and management to only those techniques that are essential to patient stabilization. If possible, have a member of the same sex treat these patients. This may relieve any hostilities and anxiety that might be directed toward a caregiver of the opposite sex. Encourage the patient not to bathe. One of your most important tasks is to provide emotional support and reassurance.

Peripheral Vascular System Inspect all four extremities, noting their size and symmetry. Palpate the peripheral arteries for pulse rate and quality. Assess the skin for temperature, moisture, color, and capillary refill.

Musculoskeletal System Reinspect and palpate all four extremities. Inspect and palpate your patient's joints, their structure, their range of motion, and the surrounding tissues. Inspect for swelling in or around joints, changes in the surrounding tissue, redness of the overlying skin, deformities, and symmetry of impairment. Compare both sides for equal size, shape, color, and strength. Palpate for tenderness in and around the joint. Try to identify the specific structure that is tender, such as a ligament, or tendon.

Test for range of motion passively and against gravity and resistance. Difficulty during passive range of motion tests suggests a joint problem. Difficulty with gravity or against resistance suggests a muscular weakness or nerve problem. Listen for crepitation, the crunching sounds of unlubricated parts rubbing against each other, while you manipulate the joint. Perform distal neurovascular checks.

Nervous System A nervous system exam covers mental status and speech, the motor system, and the sensory system.

Mental Status and Speech First, assess your patient's level of consciousness and compare his response to your earlier findings. Observe his posture and motor behavior and his grooming and personal hygiene. Note his speech pattern and use of language. Observe your patient's mood from his verbal and nonverbal behavior. Assess his thoughts, perceptions, insight and judgment, memory, attention, and learning ability.

Motor System Inspect your patient's general body structure, muscle development, positioning, and coordination. Note any obvious asymmetries, deformities, or involuntary movements. Assess muscle tone by feeling the muscle's resistance to passive stretching in the extremities. Test for muscle strength by applying resistance during the range of motion evaluation. Assess for coordination and cerebellar function, using rapid alternating movements and point-to-point testing.

Sensory System Test for pain, light touch, and temperature. Compare distal areas to proximal areas, symmetrical areas bilaterally, and scatter the stimuli to assess most of the dermatomes. Assess your patient's ability to distinguish sharp from dull sensations.

One of your most important tasks for possible victims of rape or sexual abuse is to provide emotional support and reassurance.

Content Review

NERVOUS SYSTEM EXAM
- Mental status and speech
- Motor system
- Sensory system

VITAL SIGNS

Take another set of vital signs and compare them to earlier sets to detect any trends, patterns that indicate either an improvement or deterioration in your patient's condition. These trends include a rising or falling pulse rate and blood pressure; an increasing or decreasing respiratory rate and effort; changing skin temperature, color, and condition; and changing pupillary equality and response to light. Such trends may suggest specific pathologies, which you will learn in Chapters 12 to 18 on trauma emergencies and Chapters 19 to 28 on medical emergencies.

RECORDING EXAM FINDINGS

Record all exam findings on the appropriate run sheet or chart. Remain objective and nonjudgmental when recording the data. Chapter 11, "Documentation," gives detailed instructions on writing patient care reports.

ONGOING ASSESSMENT

En route to the hospital, conduct an ongoing series of assessments to detect trends, determine changes in your patient's condition, and assess the effectiveness of your interventions. Patient condition can change suddenly. You must steadfastly reassess mental status, airway patency, breathing adequacy, circulation, and any deterioration in areas already compromised (Procedure 8-7a). Conduct your ongoing assessment every 15 minutes for stable patients, every 5 minutes for unstable patients. Compare your findings to the baseline findings and note any trends.

MENTAL STATUS

Recheck your patient's mental status by performing the AVPU exam frequently during transport. Any deterioration in mental status is cause for great concern. The brain demands a constant supply of oxygen and glucose and a constant elimination of waste products. When it is deprived of either, even briefly, expect rapid mental status changes. A falling level of response indicates either direct or indirect brain pathology. For example, following a head injury, your patient who was alert and oriented at the scene gradually becomes sleepy and eventually unarousable. You should suspect a life-threatening increase in intracranial pressure (pressure inside the enclosed skull) and expedite transport to the appropriate medical facility. Or your patient with an intra-abdominal hemorrhage becomes increasingly less arousable due to the decreased oxygenated blood flow to the brain (indirect pathology). Or sometimes patients improve following your interventions. After you administer 50% dextrose to your hypoglycemic diabetic patient, for instance, he becomes alert and begins talking.

AIRWAY PATENCY

The patency of your patient's airway can change instantly. Bleeding, vomiting, and even secretions can suddenly obstruct the upper airway. Be prepared to suction your patient quickly. Respiratory burns and anaphylaxis can cause life-threatening swelling in a matter of minutes. Croup and epiglottitis also can quickly deteriorate into total upper airway occlusion.

Endotracheal intubation is the best way to secure the airway in patients with no gag reflex. But endotracheal tubes can become dislodged easily during transport. Recheck for tube placement frequently during transport and every time you move your patient onto a backboard, onto the stretcher, or onto the hospital gurney.

The price of proper airway management is eternal vigilance and a pessimistic outlook—anything that can go wrong will go wrong. Be prepared for the worst.

BREATHING RATE AND QUALITY

A change in respiratory rate or quality might indicate improvement or deterioration. A sudden increase in rate or respiratory effort suggests deterioration. For example, a patient has a serious problem if he suddenly gasps for air, has retractions, and uses his accessory neck muscles. Sometimes the signs are not so obvious. Subtle increases in respiratory rate can suggest

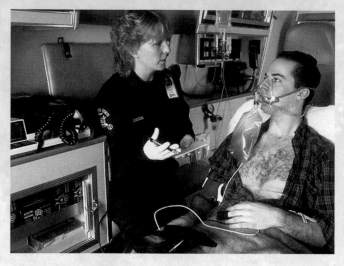

8-7a Reevaluate the ABCs.

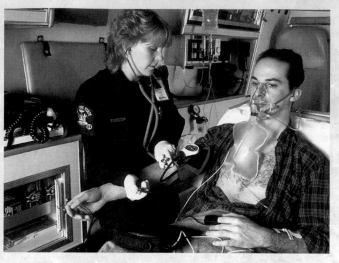

8-7b Take all vital signs again.

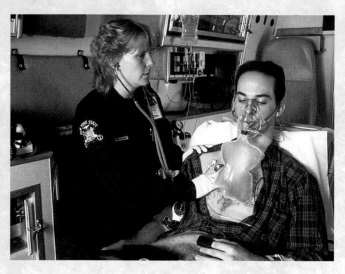

8-7c Perform your focused assessment again.

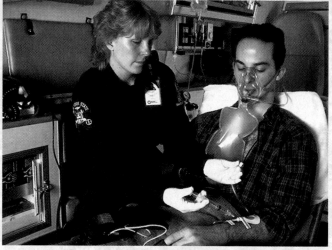

8-7d Evaluate the effects of your interventions.

a developing problem. A decrease in rate and effort could mean that your treatments are effective and your patient is improving. For example, after you administer an albuterol treatment, your patient breathes easier and his lung sounds improve. In infants and young children, however, a decrease in rate and effort may mean that your patient is exhausted and requires aggressive intervention. If, while assisting ventilation with a BVM, your partner suddenly complains that squeezing the bag is becoming more difficult, consider the possibility that a tension pneumothorax is developing or that bronchospasm or laryngospasm may be occurring. Airway and breathing management require constant reevaluation.

PULSE RATE AND QUALITY

Check central and peripheral pulses and compare the findings to earlier measurements. A rising pulse rate could indicate shock, hypoxia, or cardiac dysrhythmia. A falling rate could mean the terminal stage of shock or a rise in intracranial pressure. A sudden change in rate or regularity may suggest a cardiac dysrhythmia. The loss of peripheral pulses could mean decompensating shock.

SKIN CONDITION

Similar to mental status, the skin quickly reflects the body's hemodynamic status. Reevaluate your patient's skin color, temperature, and condition. Cyanosis suggests decreased oxygenation. Lip cyanosis indicates central hypoxia (overall oxygen status), whereas peripheral cyanosis indicates decreased oxygen to the tissues. Pallor and coolness suggest decreased circulation to the skin, as seen in shock. If your patient suddenly develops hives after you administer a medication, suspect an allergic reaction. A localized redness and warmth could indicate bleeding under the skin or vasodilation. Cyanosis and coolness in a lower extremity suggest a peripheral vascular problem such as an arterial occlusion. A deep vein thrombosis will result in redness, swelling, and warmth in the lower leg.

TRANSPORT PRIORITIES

Sometimes stable patients suddenly deteriorate en route to the hospital. For example, the formerly conscious and alert head-injury patient now responds only to pain. Or your stable cardiac patient suddenly develops a life-threatening dysrhythmia. Or your patient suddenly cannot breathe because his simple pneumothorax has developed into a tension pneumothorax. In these cases, while you provide life-saving treatments, change your transport decision to a higher priority. By the same token, if your unstable patient becomes stable, you may wish to downgrade your priority transport decision and decrease the danger and liability of driving with lights and siren on.

VITAL SIGNS

Reassessing vital signs reveals trends clearly (Procedure 8-7b). A rising pulse rate combined with a falling blood pressure indicates shock. A decreasing pulse rate combined with a rising blood pressure, associated with an irregular respiratory pattern, suggests a rise in intracranial pressure. Any change in heart rate could indicate a cardiac dysrhythmia. A narrowing pulse pressure with a weakening pulse indicates cardiac tamponade, a tension pneumothorax, or hypovolemic shock. Reevaluate your critical patient's vital signs every 5 minutes and look for changes.

Reevaluate your critical patient's vital signs every 5 minutes.

FOCUSED ASSESSMENT

Elicit your patient's chief complaint again to determine if the problem still exists or if other problems have arisen. Often following trauma your patient will develop more complaints en route to the hospital as the excitement of the incident begins to wear off. Patients often focus on their major injuries and might not even be aware of other problems. Repeat your focused assessment as your patient's chief complaint dictates (Procedure 8-7c).

EFFECTS OF INTERVENTIONS

Evaluate the effects of any interventions (Procedure 8-7d). Did the albuterol treatment help open the lower airways? Did the oxygen and nitroglycerin relieve the chest pain? What are the affects of the fluid challenge? Is the pneumatic antishock garment inhibiting your patient's breathing? Did your intervention help or harm your patient? Is he getting better or worse? Know the expected therapeutic benefits of your interventions, and then evaluate whether they worked. For example, you administer lidocaine to convert ventricular tachycardia. Following administration, observe your patient's electrocardiogram for changes while noting any harmful side effects such as nausea, vomiting, or seizures.

MANAGEMENT PLANS

Have the courage to admit your plan is not working and the flexibility to change it.

Evaluate whether your care is working. If it is not, consider another management plan. Develop the courage to admit your plan is not working and the flexibility to change your course of action. For example, your patient, an elderly man with a history of congestive heart failure (CHF) and chronic obstructive pulmonary disease (COPD), presents with severe difficulty breathing and audible wheezing. You suspect he is having an exacerbation of his COPD and administer two nebulizer treatments and begin transporting. En route, however, he is not improving, and now you also can hear crackles bilaterally. At this point, you suspect he is in CHF and change your management to administering nitroglycerin, furosemide, and morphine.

Your ability to reassess your patient, reevaluate your field diagnosis, and alter your management plan will optimize patient care.

Patients often present with multiple complaints, symptoms, and histories. Formulating a definitive diagnosis is difficult without the hospital's labs, X-rays, and other assessment tools. However, your ability to reassess your patient, reevaluate your field diagnosis, and alter your management plan will optimize patient care.

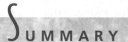
SUMMARY

Patient assessment is the key to providing effective prehospital emergency medical care. Its components include the initial assessment, the focused history and physical exam, vital signs, ongoing assessment, and the detailed physical exam. The initial assessment is designed to identify life-threatening airway, breathing, and circulation problems. The focused history and physical exam is designed to identify the signs and symptoms surrounding your patient's chief complaint. It is a problem-oriented approach that is easily modified to match your patient's clinical situation. The ongoing assessment is designed to reevaluate your patient for changes in status en route to the hospital. The detailed physical exam is a comprehensive head-to-toe evaluation designed to identify any conditions not already found. Although more suited to a clinical setting, it is intended to be done en route to the hospital if time allows.

The four general types of patients require distinctly different assessment approaches. The trauma patient with a significant mechanism of injury should receive an initial assessment, a rapid trauma assessment, and rapid transport. The patient with isolated, minor trauma, such as a cut finger or sprained ankle, should receive a physical exam focused on his particular problem or area. The responsive medical patient requires an initial assessment, a history and physical exam that focuses on his chief complaint, and vital signs. The unresponsive medical patient requires an initial assessment, followed by a rapid head-to-toe medical assessment and rapid transport. You will perform detailed history and physical exam techniques en route to the hospital if time and your patient's condition allow.

The assessment templates in this chapter are only guidelines. They do not dictate an exact procedure for assessing every patient. Instead, they provide general chronological guides to help you make critical transport and management decisions. As an EMT-I, you will be expected to use clinical judgment when deciding which assessment tools to use for your particular patient and situation. With time and experience, you will become adept at assessing real patients in crisis. The more effective and efficient you become with this process, the better your patient care will be.

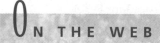
ON THE WEB

For additional practice and review, go to the companion website at www.prenhall.com/bledsoe and click on *Intermediate Emergency Care: Principles & Practice*

CHAPTER 9

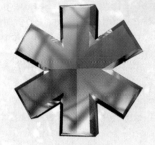

Clinical Decision Making

Objectives

After reading this chapter, you should be able to:

1. Compare the factors influencing medical care on scene to other medical settings. (pp. 531-532)
2. Differentiate among critical life-threatening, potentially life-threatening, and non–life-threatening patient presentations. (p. 532)
3. Evaluate the benefits and shortfalls of protocols, standing orders, and patient-care algorithms. (pp. 532–534)
4. Define the components, stages, and sequences of the critical thinking process for EMT-Intermediates and apply the fundamental elements. (pp. 534–540)

5. Describe the effects of the "fight-or-flight" response and its positive and negative effects on an EMT-Intermediate's decision making. (pp. 537–538)
6. Develop strategies for effective thinking under pressure. (pp. 537–538)
7. Summarize the "six Rs" of putting it all together: read the patient, read the scene, react, reevaluate, revise the management plan, review performance. (p. 540)

CASE STUDY

On a hot, muggy Friday evening the call comes in for a car vs. pedestrian. Reports from the scene are that a 14-year-old girl was struck by a car while in-line skating and lies in the street with blood coming from her mouth. The first emergency responder to arrive is Assistant Chief Tom Shoemaker who secures the scene, confirms the initial report, and calls for Air-One, the county helicopter. As the fire department rescue rolls out the door, the ambulance follows with EMT-I Sue McGivern and her sister Karen, an EMT-Basic.

   Upon arrival, Sue instructs Fred Jordan from rescue to stabilize the patient's head and neck while she begins an initial assessment. Her patient's name is Marcie. She is alert and oriented but does not remember what

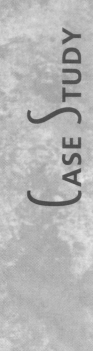
happened to her. She presents with obvious trauma to the mouth—all of her front teeth are missing or loose and she has minor bleeding. After the initial assessment and a rapid trauma assessment, Marcie appears hemodynamically stable. Sue decides to transport her by ground to a local community hospital. The rescue team immobilizes Marcie on a full backboard and quickly transports her.

En route to the hospital, Fred rides along to maintain verbal contact with Marcie and evaluate her mental status for changes. Sue begins her ongoing assessment and notes a declining mental status. Within minutes, Marcie becomes sleepy but is easily arousable by verbal stimuli. Sue decides to transport her to University Hospital, a level-one trauma center with a specialized pediatric emergency department. This is a longer transport, but Sue believes her patient may be developing increasing intracranial pressure.

Marcie begins complaining of wanting to vomit. Sue and Fred quickly log roll her onto her side, but her nausea subsides. In the ED, Marcie vomits the frank blood she swallowed from her dental trauma, and her level of consciousness deteriorates further. Within minutes she becomes responsive only to deep pain. The emergency physician, Dr. Olsson, asks Sue for a chronological report on Marcie's mental status. Sue reports that she was alert and oriented 30 minutes earlier and then became responsive only to verbal commands approximately 15 minutes ago. They quickly transfer Marcie for a computerized tomography (CT) scan, which reveals an epidural hematoma from lacerating the middle meningeal artery and some minor bleeding from the middle cerebral artery.

INTRODUCTION

As an EMT-I, you inevitably will face your moment of truth—a critical decision that can mean the difference between life and death.

As an EMT-I, you eventually may face your "moment of truth." You will confront a situation that requires you to make a critical decision. Often, you will have several options, but choosing the best one may mean the difference between life and death. And you may be all alone. You may be the highest trained provider on the scene and responsible for that decision. That you someday will have to make a decision on which your patient's life depends is a sobering thought.

In the 1970s, with rare exceptions, advanced prehospital providers made few critical decisions. They usually worked under rigidly written protocols developed by their medical director. Mostly, they were required to contact the medical direction physician who, after hearing their report, would diagnose the patient's problem and order treatment. They were no more than technicians who needed only good psychomotor skills to conduct patient assessments and follow orders. As prehospital care has evolved, EMT-Is now do much more than collect data for the physician to evaluate. You not only will have to gather information, but analyze it, form a field diagnosis, and devise a management plan. In some cases you will do these things before contacting your medical direction physician.

To fill the role of an EMT-I, you will need to develop your critical decision-making skills, which will help you to think rationally about what you are doing. Because patients seldom present with the classic textbook signs and symptoms, you will encounter situations that appear totally unfamiliar. These cases will call for you to use sound judgment in devising a management plan that meets your patient's needs. Making such decisions requires **clinical judgment,** using your knowledge and experience to make critical decisions regarding patient care. No one can teach you clinical judgment; you must develop it from experience. Unfortunately, experience often includes making bad decisions. We learn from our mistakes, if someone points them out and explains them to us. Your hospital and field preceptors will do this for you during this program.

In addition, your instructors also will place you in as many problem-solving situations as possible to begin developing your clinical judgment. The number and type of supervised patient contacts you make during this program will determine how much clinical judgment you develop as a student. The more types of cases you see during your clinical rotations, the more clinically competent you will be when you complete your education.

clinical judgment the use of knowledge and experience to diagnose patients and plan their treatment.

EMT-INTERMEDIATE PRACTICE

As an EMT-I, you must gather, evaluate, and synthesize much information in very little time. You will obtain this information using your senses (sight, smell, hearing, and touch) during the history and physical exam. Analyzing these data will involve the total of your education, training, and clinical experience. For example, as you enter a patient's home, the sound of his gasping for breath with audible wheezes startles you. Having heard wheezing before and having learned in class that it results from a variety of problems will help you to make what is called a differential diagnosis. The differential diagnosis is a preliminary list of possible causes for your patient's problem. For example, a differential diagnosis for diffuse wheezing might include asthma, emphysema, bronchitis, acute pulmonary edema, and anaphylaxis. Now you conduct a history and physical exam and arrive at a **field diagnosis,** or impression.

field diagnosis prehospital evaluation of the patient's condition and its causes.

Your next step will involve applying your clinical experience and exercising independent decision making as you develop and implement a management plan. For example, your gasping and wheezing patient is a young male who presents with a rapid onset of severe difficulty breathing. He has a history of asthma and allergies to nuts and you are not sure which problem caused this episode. You gather more information and learn that he did accidentally eat a piece of coffee cake that may have had a nut-based filling. You also notice hives forming quickly on his arms and face and that his voice is becoming more hoarse. Upon obtaining a blood pressure of 86/42, you make an initial field diagnosis of anaphylactic shock. You immediately administer oxygen. You then contact your medical direction physician who orders you to administer epinephrine subcutaneously to reduce the tissue swelling that threatens to close off his airway. You also prepare to support his breathing with a bag-valve mask (BVM) and endotracheal tube if necessary. Managing this critical patient requires you to think clearly and work effectively under pressure. Few prehospital situations create more pressure than a patient struggling to breathe.

The prehospital emergency medical setting is unlike any other medical care environment. EMT-Is carry out the same tasks as other clinicians. They assess patients, obtain vital signs, start IVs, manage airways, and perform other invasive procedures. The difference is that EMT-Is perform these procedures in various uncontrolled and unpredictable environments under circumstances that do not exist in other clinical settings and without information gathered from laboratory results and X-ray. For example, starting an IV line in a well-lit, quiet hospital room is not a major challenge. But starting one while balancing yourself in the back of a rapidly moving ambulance is. Often you will use your skills in seemingly unmanageable circumstances. The key is to block out the distractions and focus on the task.

Patho Pearls

In EMS education, emphasis is on when and where to apply an emergency intervention or administer a drug. With experience, you will learn that it is equally important to determine when not to apply an intervention or administer a drug. This is a trait that all skilled EMT-Intermediates must develop.

Above all, trauma is a surgical disease. Definitive care of the trauma patient often must occur in the operating room. Despite our best attempts and technology, certain trauma patients will only benefit from rapid transport to a trauma center followed by emergency surgery to correct the problem. Attempts at stabilization in the field often delay the patient from receiving what they actually need—rapid transport and surgical intervention.

It is easy to get caught up in the technology and care practices of modern EMS. However, it is important to realize that EMS, like many things in medicine, has its limitations. Sometimes, as the saying goes, discretion is the better part of valor. When faced with a critical trauma patient, the best care sometimes may simply be rapid immobilization and transport with any prehospital interventions provided en route. Making this decision will become easier with experience.

PATIENT ACUITY

Not everyone who calls 9-1-1 has a life-threatening emergency. Just the opposite is true. The vast majority of EMS patients are people who want transportation to the hospital for non–life-threatening problems. For others, the emergency department is their only health-care option, even for a sore throat. The spectrum of care in the prehospital setting includes three general classes of patient **acuity:** those with obvious critical life threats, those with potential life threats, and those with non–life-threatening presentations. Patients with obvious life-threatening conditions include major multi-system trauma; devastating single-system trauma; end-stage disease presentations such as liver or renal failure when the patient is in the last days of his terminal illness and is close to death; and acute presentations of chronic diseases such as asthma or emphysema. These patients present with serious airway, breathing, circulation, or neurological problems and often require aggressive resuscitation. Potential life-threatening conditions include serious multisystem trauma and multiple disease etiologies such as a diabetic with cardiac complications. Non–life-threatening presentations include isolated minor illnesses and injuries. You will be expected to manage cases in all three categories. In a typical 12-hour shift you may treat a patient in cardiac arrest; deliver a baby; control a lacerated, spurting artery; and transfer an elderly woman back to her nursing home. The wide range of patient types, degrees of severity, and complicating environmental factors makes out of hospital care a unique form of emergency medicine.

Arriving at a management plan for patients with minor medical and traumatic events requires little critical thinking or clinical judgment. For example, if your patient has a fractured tibia, you will splint the leg and transport him to the emergency department for X-rays and casting. You have no real life-saving decisions to make. On the opposite end of the acuity spectrum, patients with obvious life threats such as cardiac arrest and major trauma also require few critical decisions because caring for them is largely routine and standardized. For cardiac arrest, you perform CPR and work through the protocol associated with your patient's cardiac rhythm. For major trauma, you manage the ABCs while providing rapid transport to a trauma center.

Patients who fall between minor medical and life threatening on the acuity spectrum pose the greatest challenge to your critical thinking abilities. These patients might become unstable at any moment. For example, if your patient is an infant with signs of respiratory distress, you must recognize the signs of early respiratory failure and take precautionary measures to keep him from deteriorating to respiratory arrest. In these cases, you use your knowledge of pediatric respiratory assessment, your skills in airway and breathing management, and your clinical judgment to determine how and when to intervene. You will constantly reassess and revise your interventions as needed. One of the most important decisions you will make is whether to transport your patient immediately to the hospital, wait on the scene for a paramedic, or meet up with one en route. Your ability to evaluate factors such as patient condition, time to a paramedic vs. time to the hospital, weather conditions, terrain, etc. will determine the effectiveness of the decision you make. You must develop the ability to think quickly and clearly during times of great turmoil.

PROTOCOLS AND ALGORITHMS

EMT-Is function in EMS under the license of a medical director. Every state has enacted legislation allowing EMT-Is to practice medicine in the field and describing the scope of their practice. Within these laws, state and local EMS medical directors devise protocols that detail exactly what EMT-Is can do. **Protocols** are standards that include general and specific procedures for managing certain patient conditions. For example, every system will develop standards for managing asthma, congestive heart failure, and tension pneumothorax. Each will also develop protocols for special situations such as physician-on-scene, radio failure, and termination of resuscitation. **Standing orders** authorize you to perform certain procedures before contacting your medical direction physician. For example, you may administer oxygen, start an intravenous (IV) line, and administer aspirin and nitroglycerin to a patient with cardiac chest pain. For repeat nitro orders, you may have to consult the physician. Patient care **algorithms** are flow charts with arrows, lines, and boxes arranged

---

acuity the severity or acuteness of your patient's condition.

Patients who fall between minor medical and life-threatening on the acuity spectrum pose the greatest challenge to your critical thinking abilities.

protocol standard that includes general and specific principles for managing certain patient conditions.

standing orders treatments you can perform before contacting medical direction.

algorithm schematic flow chart that outlines appropriate care for specific signs and symptoms.

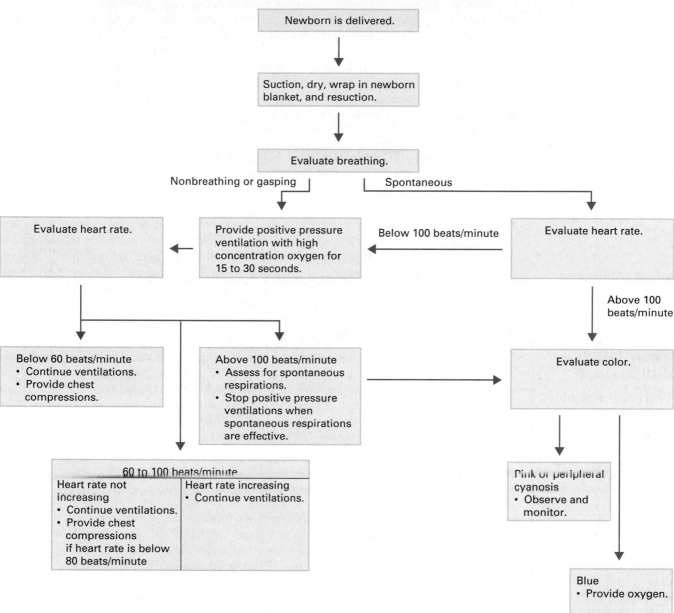

RESUSCITATION OF A NEWBORN

Newborn is delivered.

↓

Suction, dry, wrap in newborn blanket, and resuction.

↓

Evaluate breathing.

Nonbreathing or gasping | Spontaneous

Evaluate heart rate. ← Provide positive pressure ventilation with high concentration oxygen for 15 to 30 seconds. ← Below 100 beats/minute ← Evaluate heart rate.

Above 100 beats/minute ↓

Below 60 beats/minute
• Continue ventilations.
• Provide chest compressions.

Above 100 beats/minute
• Assess for spontaneous respirations.
• Stop positive pressure ventilations when spontaneous respirations are effective.

→ Evaluate color.

60 to 100 beats/minute

Heart rate not increasing	Heart rate increasing
• Continue ventilations. • Provide chest compressions if heart rate is below 80 beats/minute	• Continue ventilations.

Pink or peripheral cyanosis
• Observe and monitor.

Blue
• Provide oxygen.

FIGURE 9-1   To use a patient-care algorithm, follow the arrows to your patient's symptoms and provide care as indicated.

schematically (Figure 9-1). To use them, you simply start at the top and follow wherever your patient's signs and symptoms lead.

Protocols, standing orders, and patient-care algorithms provide a standardized approach to emergency patient care. However, they address only "classic" patients. Unfortunately, many patients present with atypical signs and symptoms, often requiring you to use clinical judgment and instinct to develop a management plan. Patients frequently present with nonspecific complaints that do not match any specific algorithm. Sometimes your patients just do not clearly describe what is bothering them. Another limitation of protocols is that they cannot adequately cover multiple disease etiologies such as the patient with chronic obstructive pulmonary disease and congestive heart failure. When your patient with

Do not allow the linear thinking, or "cookbook medicine" that protocols promote to restrain you from consulting with medical direction.

this multiple history presents with severe difficulty breathing, you must quickly identify the underlying condition that is causing the current problem and follow the appropriate protocol. Nor do protocols deal with managing more than one patient problem at a time in possible multiple treatment situations. For example, your stroke patient also presents with shock as well as bilateral wrist fractures and a fractured hip from the fall. Protocols are standards designed to promote consistent patient care in common situations. They are written also to allow you, in consultation with the medical direction physician, to use clinical judgment to provide optimum care in unusual situations. The linear thinking, or "cookbook medicine," that protocols promote should not restrict you from consulting with your medical direction physician in difficult or unusual cases.

CRITICAL THINKING SKILLS

The ability to think under pressure and make decisions cannot be taught; it must be developed. As an EMT-I, you may be a team leader on emergency scenes. In that role you must make sound, reasonable decisions regarding your patient's care. Several aspects of this program will help you to develop this essential skill. In the classroom you will work on case histories. In the labs you will practice patient scenarios on moulaged victims. In the hospital you will assess and help manage real patients in the emergency department and critical care units. In the field internship, you will assess and manage patients in the streets. In all of these settings you will begin developing clinical judgment.

FUNDAMENTAL KNOWLEDGE AND ABILITIES

First, you must have an excellent working knowledge of anatomy and physiology and of the pathophysiology of your patient's disease or injury. To assess and manage a patient who has difficulty breathing, for instance, you must know which organs and body systems are involved in breathing. You must understand the process of normal breathing and each body system's role in that effort. You must recall the factors that inhibit normal breathing and recognize the signs and symptoms of respiratory distress. For example, a patient might wheeze because of lower airway obstruction from secretions, bronchoconstriction, lung tissue edema, or any combination of these conditions. All reduce the inner diameter of the airways, restricting airflow and making moving air in and out of the lungs difficult. Managing this patient requires knowledge of the respiratory and cardiovascular causes of wheezing, because their treatments are vastly different. Respiratory causes for generalized wheezing include asthma and bronchitis, which you would manage with bronchodilators. Cardiac causes for wheezing include congestive heart failure, which you would manage with vasodilators and diuretics. Without a good working knowledge of these diseases, you might make a mistaken and potentially devastating field diagnosis.

You also must be able to focus on many specific data. When you conduct a patient assessment, you will evaluate all relevant information while focusing on specific important findings. You will be inundated with information requiring you to establish relationships and form conclusions. A patient who presents with difficulty breathing and wheezing would require an in-depth history and focused examination of his cardiac and respiratory systems. You also would assess other systems relative to his chief complaint (HEENT, musculoskeletal, neurological, and lymphatic), while remaining focused on the primary problem (cardiorespiratory). Although his chief complaint is difficulty breathing, his primary problem might be cardiac, muscular, infectious, allergic, or neurological.

You must be able to organize the information you obtain and form concepts from it. Initially you elicit your patient's chief complaint and begin to formulate a **differential field diagnosis.** As you conduct the history and a clearer picture of your patient's problem emerges, you narrow your differential field diagnosis to the most probable disease. For example, your patient has severe difficulty breathing and inspiratory stridor. Your differential field diagnosis might include foreign body obstruction, epiglottitis, respiratory burns, anaphylaxis, laryngeal trauma, and throat cancer. Then you learn that he is hoarse and febrile, has had a sore throat for two days, and in the past 6 hours has had increasing difficulty swal-

Content Review

DECISION-MAKING REQUIREMENTS

- Knowing anatomy, physiology, and pathophysiology
- Focusing on large amounts of data
- Organizing information
- Identifying and dealing with medical ambiguity
- Differentiating between relevant and irrelevant data
- Analyzing and comparing similar situations
- Explaining decisions and constructing logical arguments

differential field diagnosis the list of possible causes of your patient's symptoms.

lowing. You now suspect epiglottitis. This ability to formulate a working field diagnosis is essential for EMT-Is.

You must be able to identify and deal with medical ambiguity. Many patients present with vague signs and symptoms. It is not unusual for a patient to complain of "just not feeling right." He will provide you with an imprecise story and you will be unable to arrive at a specific field diagnosis. In these cases, your field diagnosis will have to be generalized as "abdominal pain" or "general illness." Often it will be almost impossible to definitively diagnose your patient without laboratory results, X-rays, and other tests.

You must be able to differentiate between relevant and irrelevant data. You will have to sift the important data from the many bits of information you receive during your patient assessment. A positive family history for sudden cardiac death is relevant for your patient with chest pain; for your patient with a fractured arm it is not. Pupil and extraocular movement exams are relevant for trauma and for patients with an altered mental status; for a patient with asthma or arthritis they are not. When you contact the medical direction physician, you will report critical information only. Likewise, in your written documentation you will record relevant information and omit the rest.

You must be able to analyze and compare similar and contrasting situations. What were the similarities among your last three anaphylactic shock patients? Did all three have hives, hoarse speech, severe difficulty breathing, and hypotension? Did they all have a history of allergies? Can you depend on any patterns of presentation for future calls such as this? Have some patient presentations been unusual? Have any patients presented with signs of anaphylaxis but had a different diagnosis? For example, your patient is a 45-year-old woman who presents with hives and severe itching. Your initial impression may be anaphylaxis, but further investigation reveals no other difficulty breathing or hypotension. You now change your impression to allergic reaction. You must be able to recall the factors that help rule in or rule out a particular disease or injury.

You must be able to explain your decisions and construct logical arguments. Often, the emergency physician will want to know what you were thinking when you made your field diagnosis. You must be able to express yourself rationally while you make your case. These are the times when you demonstrate your professionalism to other health-care providers. Observe the following conversation:

> *Physician:* Why did you think your patient just had an allergic reaction and not anaphylaxis? How can you rule out anaphylaxis in the field?
>
> *EMT-I:* Well, she generalized hives and itching after eating shellfish. But she had no difficulty breathing, her lungs were clear, her voice had no hoarseness, and her vital signs were normal.
>
> *Physician:* OK, I agree, good job!

Through interactions such as this, you establish credibility with the emergency physician. The next time you contact him regarding a patient, he is more apt to trust your assessment and judgment.

USEFUL THINKING STYLES

As an EMT-I, you will face confusing emergencies that would challenge even the most knowledgeable, analytical health-care provider. You must be able to stay calm and not panic. Your self-control in the face of extreme chaos will set the example for other team members to follow. Even when you are struggling to maintain your composure—especially then—never let others know. The key is focusing on the task and blocking out the distractions. Be like the duck—cool and calm on the water's surface, while paddling furiously underneath.

Assume and plan for the worst, and always err on the side of benefiting your patient. For example, if you are deliberating whether to immobilize your patient, initiate advanced life-support procedures, or administer oxygen, just do it! It is better to err by providing care than by withholding it. Be pessimistic! Anticipate all potential bad side effects of your treatments and have a "plan B" as an alternative. For example, as you deliver a bronchodilating drug to your severe asthmatic patient, anticipate that it will not work and mentally prepare

Content Review

FACILITATING BEHAVIORS
• Stay calm
• Plan for the worst
• Work systematically
• Remain adaptable

Be like the duck—cool and calm on the water's surface, while paddling furiously underneath.

Except for safety concerns, never allow anything to distract you from your most important job—assessing and caring for your patient.

to intubate him and perform positive pressure ventilation while you arrange for immediate transportation.

Establish and maintain a systematic assessment pattern. Practice your assessments until they become second nature, and you will avoid skipping and missing steps. Be disciplined and stay focused, especially when you are confronted with a complex emergency scene. For example, your patient lies moaning on the ground in a pool of blood. Bystanders are screaming at you to help him; others are trying to tell you what happened. The police are gathering the story and trying unsuccessfully to talk with your patient. You must gain control of this scene. You do so by focusing on your patient and performing a systematic assessment. Use common mnemonics (MS-ABC, OPQRST, SAMPLE) or make up your own to help you remember the key elements of your assessment. Except for safety concerns, never allow anything to distract you from your most important job—assessing and caring for your patient.

The different situations you encounter require a variety of management styles. Adapting your styles of situation analysis (reflective vs. impulsive), data processing (divergent vs. convergent), and decision making (anticipatory vs. reactive) to each situation will enable you to provide the best possible care in every case.

Reflective vs. Impulsive

reflective acting thoughtfully, deliberately, and analytically.

Some situations call for you to be **reflective,** to take your time, and to figure out what is wrong. You have a patient who complains of "not feeling well." She has a long history of cardiac, renal, respiratory, and diabetic problems. Since she is in no real distress and her vital signs are stable, you can take your time to determine her primary problem. Other situations call for immediate action. They require you to make an instinctive, **impulsive** decision and manage your patient's life-threatening condition. For example, if your patient presents apneic and pulseless, you will immediately begin CPR and prepare for defibrillation. If he presents with a spurting artery, you will at once take measures to control the hemorrhage. If he is choking and has a weak, ineffective cough, you will quickly perform the Heimlich maneuver. You have to think and act fast in these situations.

impulsive acting instinctively without stopping to think.

Divergent vs. Convergent

divergent taking into account all aspects of a complex situation.

To process the data you receive from your patient and the scene, you can use either a divergent or a convergent approach. The **divergent** approach considers all aspects of a situation before arriving at a solution. It is insightful and works well when you are confronted with complex scenarios. For example, your emotionally distraught, stable patient presents with multiple problems and a long, complicated medical history. You need to consider the physical, emotional, and psychological aspects of his condition before making a field diagnosis and management plan. Likewise, extricating a victim from a wooded scene requires you to weigh a variety of environmental and medical factors before selecting a mode of transport.

convergent focusing on only the most important aspect of a critical situation.

On the other hand, the **convergent** approach focuses narrowly on a situation's most significant aspects. This technically oriented approach relies heavily on step-by-step problem solving and is best suited for simple, uncomplicated situations that require little thought or reflection. For example, you have an unresponsive, apneic, pulseless patient who presents in ventricular fibrillation. Your immediate concern is simple and straightforward—you manage the ABCs and defibrillate him as quickly as possible. Experienced EMT-Is employ both approaches effectively in the appropriate situations.

Anticipatory vs. Reactive

Whenever possible, anticipate problems and act before they occur.

Your decision-making process can be either anticipatory or reactive. You either anticipate the possible ramifications of your actions in a proactive way or you react to events as you encounter them. For example, your patient presents with a severe laceration and severe blood loss. The bleeding is controlled. Now you can either anticipate his going into shock and begin measures before it happens, or you can wait until he shows signs of shock and then act. Unfortunately, by then it is often too late to do anything about it. Whenever possible, it is best to anticipate problems and act before they occur.

THINKING UNDER PRESSURE

When you must make a critical decision, physical influences may help or hinder your ability to think clearly. Your **autonomic nervous system,** which controls your involuntary actions, may respond by secreting "fight-or-flight" hormones. These hormones will enhance your vision and hearing and will improve your reflexes and muscle strength. However, they may also impair your ability to think critically and diminish your ability to assess and concentrate. In these instances you will revert to your most basic instincts. Many inexperienced EMT-Is have been mentally paralyzed by a complicated, critical call. With experience, you will learn to manage your nervousness and maintain a steadfast, controlled demeanor.

One way to enhance your ability to remain in control is to raise your technical skills to a **pseudo-instinctive** level. This means that you do not have to concentrate on them to perform them. For example, you do not think about tying your shoes, you just tie them. Such "muscle memory" is essential when performing emergency medical skills. When you set up for an albuterol nebulizer treatment, for instance, you automatically fit together the pieces of the device and administer the treatment without hesitation. This way you can concentrate on your patient's condition, controlling the scene, and managing the multitude of items that usually complicate any emergency call. Concentrating on more than one thing simultaneously is difficult, if not impossible.

MENTAL CHECKLIST

Thinking under pressure is not easy. Maintaining your composure, especially during a chaotic, complicated call is key to developing a management plan for the best patient outcome. Developing a routine mental checklist is a good way to stay focused and systematic. Pilots work through their preflight checklists routinely before ever turning over their engines. Medical clinicians develop acronyms and other mnemonics to remember critical elements during stressful incidents. For example, when conducting an initial assessment, use MS-ABC. Use OPQRST to elicit your patient's present history, or use SAMPLE when time is critical. You can adopt the following checklist any time you must make a critical decision:

- *Scan the situation.* Stand back and scan the situation. Sometimes you can miss subtle signs if you focus too narrowly on one aspect of your patient's problem. Look for environmental factors and other not-so-obvious clues. For example, your patient lies unconscious and cyanotic on the floor. You rule out any airway, breathing, or circulation problems. No medical history is available, and no medication bottles are present. When you detect a fruity odor on your patient's breath, you suspect diabetic coma.

- *Stop and think.* Do not do anything without stopping and weighing your actions. Consider all of your options before you act. Remember that for every action there is a reaction. Know what reactions to expect and anticipate their possible harmful effects. For example, after administering albuterol, monitor your patient closely for the expected benefits (ease of breathing) and early signs of toxicity (rapid pulse, tremors, nervousness).

- *Decide and act.* Once you have assessed the situation, make your decision and act confidently. Announce your management plan to your crew with a combination of authority, confidence, and respect. Convey the feeling that you know your actions are correct and will work. This confidence helps reassure your patient, his family, your crew, and other responders even in the most stressful situations.

- *Maintain control.* To maintain clear, efficient control of the scene and everyone involved, you must first control yourself. Many situations will challenge your inner strength and self-control. You will eventually be in charge of a scene where everyone seems out of control. These chaotic incidents can occur anywhere and anytime. Your job is to remain steadfast under fire.

autonomic nervous system part of the nervous system that controls involuntary actions.

pseudo-instinctive learned actions that are practiced until they can be done without thinking.

Maintaining your composure, especially during a chaotic, complicated call is key to developing a management plan for the best patient outcome.

Content Review

MENTAL CHECKLIST
- Scan the situation
- Stop and think
- Decide and act
- Maintain control
- Reevaluate

- *Reevaluate.* Regularly reevaluate your plan's effects and revise it accordingly. Never assume that your plan is working to perfection. Anticipate ways your patient might deteriorate and devise alternate plans. Conduct an ongoing assessment en route to the hospital and be prepared to revise your management plan. For example, if you notice increased lung congestion after administering fluids, stop the infusion.

THE CRITICAL DECISION PROCESS

Understanding the **critical thinking** process is essential for an EMT-I. Your ability to analyze data effectively and devise a practical management plan optimizes patient care. You can conduct the most comprehensive history and physical exam, but if you cannot analyze the data and devise the proper management plan, your efforts will be fruitless. The critical-thinking process has five steps: forming a concept, interpreting the data, applying the principles, evaluating the results, and reflecting on the incident. To explain the critical decision-making process, we will consider a 19-year-old female patient with a sudden onset of sharp pain to her lower right quadrant with some vaginal bleeding.

FORM A CONCEPT

The first step in critical decision making is to gather information and form a concept of your patient and the scene. You will get this information by assessing the general environment and the immediate surroundings. Note the mechanism of injury, if applicable. Then observe your patient's mental status, skin color, positioning, and note any deformities or asymmetry. In our sample case, your patient presents at home, sitting on a sofa. At first glance, she appears pale, diaphoretic, and anxious. Next you conduct an initial assessment, focusing on the MS-ABCs. Your initial goal is to identify and manage critical life threats. In this case, your general impression is of an alert and oriented but anxious young woman in moderate distress who presents with a clear airway; good air movement, as evidenced by her ability to converse in complete sentences; a strong, rapid, regular pulse; and cool, moist skin.

Now you ascertain your patient's chief complaint, history of present illness, past history, and current health status, while observing her affect (her general demeanor and attitude) and her degree of distress. You determine that her chief complaint is right lower quadrant pain that began suddenly 30 minutes ago. She also states she began bleeding at around the same time. She denies any nausea, vomiting, or diarrhea. You learn she has a past history of pelvic inflammatory disease and an active, unprotected sex life with multiple partners. Her last menstrual period was 6 weeks ago. She has had four pregnancies but no viable births. She appears in moderate distress.

Finally, you conduct a focused physical exam of the appropriate areas. This includes any diagnostic testing, such as an electrocardiogram, pulse oximetry, and blood glucose testing. You take a full set of vital signs, which can help you identify most life-threatening conditions. Remember that your patient's age, underlying physical and medical condition, and current medications can influence her vital signs. For example, the use of beta blockers could cause a general decrease in her pulse and blood pressure. Your patient has some deep palpation tenderness in the lower right quadrant but no rebound tenderness, and the rest of her abdomen is soft and nontender. She has minor bleeding at this time and has used only one sanitary pad since the bleeding began. Her vital signs are: pulse, 110 and regular; respirations, 20 and not labored; BP, 120/86.

INTERPRET THE DATA

After you assess the patient you will interpret all of your data in light of your knowledge and experience. In this case, your knowledge base includes female reproductive anatomy, the physiology of a normal pregnancy, and the pathophysiology of pregnancy complications along with their classic signs and symptoms. It also involves the anatomy, physiology, and pathophysiology of the cardiovascular system and the signs and symptoms of shock. Your experience base includes every patient you have assessed and managed with a similar presentation. Your attitude toward managing patients with these symptoms also becomes a factor, because your experience may prejudice you. Consider all of the data and determine the most common and statistically probable conditions that fit your patient's initial presentation. This is your differential field diagnosis. Then, consider the most serious condition that fits your patient's situation. In our example, a field diagnosis of a ruptured ectopic pregnancy is obvious. When a clear medical diagnosis is elusive, base your treatment on the presenting signs and symptoms.

APPLY THE PRINCIPLES

With your field diagnosis in mind, you devise a management plan that covers all contingencies. You will use written protocols, standing orders, and all the interventions at your disposal to manage your patient's particular problem. Sometimes patients present with atypical signs and symptoms. For example, a patient who presents with a sore throat and cough may actually be having a heart attack and congestive heart failure. Other times a protocol for your patient's problem simply may not exist. For example, your system may not have a protocol for facilitated intubation in head injuries. In these cases, consult with your medical direction physician for guidance in providing optimum care to your patient. The physician's emergency medical expertise and experience can be invaluable to you and your patient in unusual and difficult cases.

In our example, although your patient presents with relatively normal vital signs and is fully alert and oriented, you are very concerned. A basic principle of medicine is that all females of child-bearing age with lower abdominal pain are pregnant until proven otherwise. You initiate advanced life support precautions en route to the hospital, including high-flow, high-concentration oxygen and two large-bore IV lines. Her presentation leads you to expect the worst. If her fallopian tube ruptures and begins to hemorrhage, she will need rapid fluid resuscitation and general shock management. Your experience includes similar patients who suddenly suffered a life-threatening hemorrhage from a ruptured fallopian tube. Again, your attitude becomes a factor in that you will not allow her stable presentation to undermine your initial instinct—that she is potentially in serious trouble.

EVALUATE

During the ongoing assessment you reassess your patient's condition and the effects of your standing order/protocol interventions. In other words, you determine if your treatment is improving your patient's condition and status. For example, has the albuterol helped your patient's breathing? Did the nitro and oxygen relieve the chest pain? Is the hemorrhage under control? Reflect on your actions and either continue your original plan, discontinue treatment, or take a completely different approach. You may alter your initial impression if your patient's condition worsens or if you discover new information. If time and circumstances allow a detailed exam, you may discover less obvious problems.

In our sample case, your patient remains in potentially unstable condition. Your repeat assessment shows her vital signs are holding with the infusion of IV fluids. She is alert and not as anxious as before, and her skin is becoming warm and normal in color. You deliver her to the emergency department in stable, but guarded, condition.

REFLECT

After the call, discuss your field diagnosis and care with the emergency physician. Compare your field diagnosis with his diagnosis. Conduct a run critique with your crew and discuss ways to improve your assessment and management of this case and future cases. Add this data to your information and experience base for future calls. Make every patient contact a learning experience. In this case, the emergency physician confirms your field diagnosis with lab tests and an ultrasound.

Make every patient contact a learning experience.

Content Review

THE SIX Rs

- **R**ead the scene
- **R**ead the patient
- **R**eact
- **R**eevaluate
- **R**evise the management plan
- **R**eview your performance

A helpful mnemonic for the critical decision making process is the "six Rs":

1. *Read the scene.* Observe the general environmental conditions, the immediate surroundings, and any mechanism of injury.

2. *Read the patient.* Observe his level of consciousness, skin color, position, location, and any obvious deformity or asymmetry. Talk to him to determine the chief complaint and whether it is a new problem or a worsening of a preexisting condition. Touch him to evaluate skin temperature and condition, pulse rate and quality. Auscultate for problems with the upper and lower airways. Identify any life threats with the ABCs and take a full set of vital signs.

3. *React.* Address any life threats as found, determine the most common and serious existing conditions, and treat him accordingly.

4. *Reevaluate.* Conduct a focused and detailed physical assessment, note any response to your initial management interventions, and discover other less obvious problems.

5. *Revise the management plan.* Change or stop interventions that are not working or are causing your patient's condition to worsen, or try something new.

6. *Review your performance at run critique.* Be honest and critically evaluate your performance, always looking for better ways to manage a particular case presentation.

SUMMARY

Clinical decision making is an essential EMT-I skill that you will develop with time and experience. The prehospital environment is unlike any other medical care setting and you will have to make decisions in less than optimum and sometimes dangerous conditions. You may find yourself as the highest level of provider on the scene. Most times you will have the benefit of consulting with your medical direction physician in difficult and unusual situations; other times you may not. Your ability to gather information, analyze it, and make a critical decision may someday be the difference between your patient's life and death. This is inevitable. How well you prepare for that challenge will determine your ultimate success. The process begins in your EMT-I training program. You must develop a good working knowledge of anatomy, physiology, pathophysiology, and the principles of emergency medicine. In time, through repeated patient contacts, you will develop the clinical judgment needed to make effective patient care decisions.

The critical decision-making process involves a series of steps that experienced clinicians do almost unconsciously. First you gather information (history and physical exam) to form an initial impression and then interpret it against your knowledge and experience to develop a working field diagnosis. Next you apply the principles of emergency medicine to devise and implement a management plan and evaluate the effects of your treatments. Then you reevaluate and revise your plan as necessary. Finally you compare the findings with the emergency physician's diagnosis and discuss alternate ways to manage similar patients. With every patient contact, your experience grows and your clinical judgment improves. This is the essence of EMT-I practice.

ON THE WEB

For additional practice and review, go to the companion website at www.prenhall.com/bledsoe and click on *Intermediate Emergency Care: Principles & Practice.*

CHAPTER 10

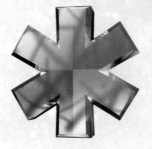

Communications

Objectives

After reading this chapter, you should be able to:

1. Identify the role and importance of verbal, written, and electronic communications in the provision of EMS. (pp. 543–549)
2. Describe the phases of communications necessary to complete a typical EMS response. (pp. 546–549)
3. Identify the importance of proper verbal communications and terminology during an EMS response. (pp. 543–544)
4. List factors that impede and enhance effective verbal and written communications. (pp. 543–546)
5. Explain the value of data collection during an EMS response. (p. 545)
6. Recognize the legal status of verbal, written, and electronic communications related to an EMS response. (pp. 554, 555, 557)
7. Identify current technology used to collect and exchange patient and/or scene information electronically. (pp. 549–553)
8. Identify the various components of the EMS communications system and describe their function and use. (pp. 543, 546–549)
9. Identify and differentiate among the following communications systems: simplex (p. 550); multiplex (p. 551); duplex (p. 551); trunked (p. 551); digital communications (p. 552); cellular telephone (p. 553); facsimile (pp. 552–553); computer (p. 553).
10. Describe the functions and responsibilities of the Federal Communications Commission. (p. 557)
11. Describe the role of emergency medical dispatch and the importance of prearrival instructions in a typical EMS response. (pp. 543, 547)
12. List appropriate caller information gathered by the emergency medical dispatcher. (p. 547)
13. Describe the structure and importance of the verbal communication of patient information to the hospital and medical direction. (pp. 554–556)
14. Diagram a basic communications system. (p. 544)
15. Organize a verbal radio report for electronic transmission to medical direction. (pp. 554–556)

CASE STUDY

On a warm, dry Sunday afternoon, a 31-year-old male loses control of his motorcycle and strikes a highway sign. Several people witness the incident. The first bystander to reach the patient rushes to his automobile to dial 9-1-1 on his cellular telephone. Emergency medical dispatcher Vern Holland takes the necessary information and dispatches a basic life support (BLS) engine company and an advanced life support (ALS) ambulance. As Holland dispatches the emergency units, his partner, dispatcher Fred Hughes, instructs the caller in basic emergency care. The units receive the call via a computer printout of essential information.

The responders quickly arrive at the scene and initiate the appropriate care. Because the patient has a severe head injury, the crew performs only a limited assessment and immediately initiates transport. As the ambulance departs, they relay the following to Dr. Jorol, the medical direction physician:

Ambulance:	Manlius Ambulance to Mercy Hospital.
Dr. Jorol:	Go ahead, Manlius.
Ambulance:	We are leaving the scene of a motorcycle crash on I-90. We have one patient, a male who is in his 30s, the rider of a motorcycle that went off the roadway and struck a sign. He responds to pain only, with obvious facial and chest trauma. There is a large laceration above the right eye with an exposed skull fracture. There is also blood draining from the right ear. Vital signs are: blood pressure 110/60, pulse 110 and regular, respirations 10 and labored. Pupils are dilated and minimally reactive, yet equal. Palpation of the cervical spine does not reveal any obvious deformity. There is no tracheal deviation. Breath sounds are symmetrical, yet diminished. There is subcutaneous emphysema on the right side of his chest and several palpable rib fractures. The abdomen is soft, and the pelvis appears stable. There may be some lower-extremity fractures. A rigid C-collar is in place and the spine has been stabilized. An endotracheal tube has been placed. Respirations are being assisted with a BVM using supplemental oxygen. We will attempt an IV en route. Our ETA is 20 minutes.
Dr. Jorol:	We copy, Manlius. Attempt an IV en route, but expedite transport and notify us of any further problems.
Ambulance:	We copy. Attempt an IV en route, and we will notify you with any changes.
Dr. Jorol:	The patient will be going into Trauma Room One. The trauma team will be in the ED awaiting your arrival.
Ambulance:	Copy that, Mercy. Manlius clear.

Upon arrival, the trauma team and a neurosurgeon meet the patient. Despite comprehensive care, the patient dies as a result of his head injury. However, at the family's request, the patient's organs are harvested. They are sent to cities more than 1,500 miles away and are used in two transplant operations.

INTRODUCTION

Knowledge of communications plays an important role in your EMT-Intermediate (EMT-I) training. All aspects of prehospital care require effective, efficient communications. During a routine transfer or a life-threatening emergency run, you will communicate with a wide variety of people. They will include:

- *Emergency medical dispatcher (EMD),* whose job it is to manage an entire system of EMS response and readiness, not just your call. You will transmit administrative information such as "responding," "arrived," "transporting," and "back-in-service." The EMD must know the location of all his resources to manage the system effectively. On a serious emergency call, the EMD can be your best ally by securing for you the resources you need to manage your incident.

- *Patient, his family, bystanders, and others,* who may at times not understand what you are doing and become obstructive. Quite often, people misconstrue your actions and words. You must try to keep them well informed.

- *Personnel from other responding agencies,* such as the police department, fire department, or mutual aid ambulances who may not share your priorities at the scene. You must communicate effectively with other responders to coordinate and implement your treatment plan. You will accomplish this face-to-face and via the radio. These communications require you to exhibit confidence and authority.

- *Other health-care professionals*—staff from physicians' offices, health-care facilities, and nursing homes—who usually do not understand the extent of your training or abilities. Often, uninformed staff will call you "ambulance drivers." In these cases, you must exhibit professionalism and a calm demeanor while you ask pertinent questions and discuss the case intelligently.

- *Medical direction physician,* who has extended his license to you in the field. The physician's expertise and advice can be a tremendous resource for you during the call. You will need to communicate patient information and scene assessment effectively to him. He can prepare for your arrival if you have communicated to him the needs of your patient. For example, you are transporting a patient with a serious head injury who exhibits a decreasing level of consciousness. By reporting this information, the emergency department (ED) can arrange for the trauma team, including a neurosurgeon, to meet you in the ED upon arrival. In such cases, good communication results in good patient care.

You must interact effectively with everyone involved in the call to coordinate a unified effort resulting in top-quality patient care. EMS is the ultimate team endeavor. Your performance as an EMT-I is just one component in a series of interactions that ensure continuous first-rate care. From the call taker to the rehabilitation specialist, all the players in this continuum are equally important—only their roles differ. Communication is not merely one aspect of an EMS response; it is the key link in the chain that results in the best possible patient outcome. Effective communication optimizes patient care during every phase of the EMS response.

> Communication is the key link in the chain that results in the best possible patient outcome.

VERBAL COMMUNICATION

Factors that can enhance or impede effective communication may be either **semantic** (the meaning of words) or technical (communications hardware). Communication requires a mutual language. For example, a city unit and a county unit that use different **10-code systems** will find it difficult to communicate effectively. A 10-10 may mean a working fire in one system and a cardiac emergency in another. Thus, many EMS systems have changed from using 10-codes to plain English.

semantic related to the meaning of words.

10-code system radio communications system using codes that begin with the word *ten.*

When reporting your patient's condition to the medical direction physician, you should use terminology that is widely accepted by both the medical and emergency services communities. Using a 10-code system with which the ED staff is unfamiliar would be inappropriate. Telling the medical direction physician that you have a victim of a 10-21-Golf (assault with a gun) may be meaningless. Conversely, if the medical direction physician asks you for your pregnant patient's EDC (due date) or her LMP (last menstrual period) and you do not know those acronyms, you have failed to communicate. The receiver must be able to decode the sender's message.

Your communication network must consist of reliable equipment designed to afford clear communication among all agencies within the system. This becomes a challenge in systems that cover large geographical areas or where terrain interferes with transmission and reception. If you want to communicate with a unit across the county but your radio is not powerful enough to transmit that far, communication will be difficult, if not impossible. A system that covers a large geographical expanse can place repeaters strategically throughout its service area. These devices receive transmissions from a low-powered source and rebroadcast them at a higher power (Figure 10-1).

Your regional EMS system may consist of many agencies that have conducted business for decades on different **radio bands** and **radio frequencies.** City units may transmit on **ultrahigh frequency** (UHF) radio waves because they penetrate concrete and steel well and are less susceptible to interference. County units may use a low-band frequency because those waves travel farther and better over varied terrain. In any event, communicating between agencies will be difficult unless all units share a common frequency. This is rarely the case. The spectrum of communications equipment currently ranges from antiquated radios to mobile data terminals mounted inside emergency vehicles. Geographically integrating communications networks would enable routine and reliable communication among EMS, fire, law enforcement, and other public safety agencies. This would in turn facilitate coordinated responses during both routine and large-scale operations. Developing the necessary hardware (equipment and network) and software (language) will be essential to improving emergency communications.

Your communication network must consist of reliable equipment designed to afford clear communication among all agencies within the system.

radio band a range of radio frequencies.

radio frequency the number of times per second a radio wave oscillates.

ultrahigh frequency radio frequency band from 300 to 3,000 megahertz.

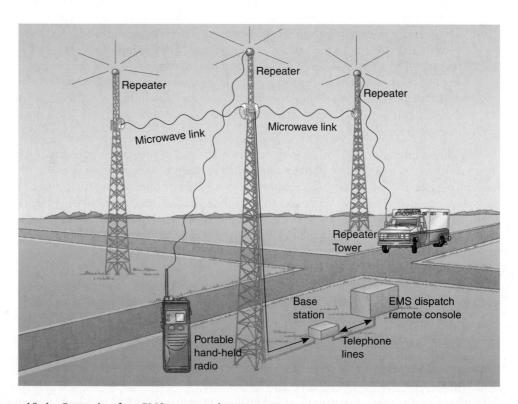

FIGURE 10-1   Example of an EMS system using repeaters.

WRITTEN COMMUNICATION

Written records are another important aspect of EMS communications. Your **prehospital care report (PCR)** is a written record of events that includes administrative information such as times, location, agency, and crew, as well as medical information. It will be used by hospital staff, agency administrators, system quality-assurance/improvement committees, insurance and billing departments, researchers, educators, and lawyers. The data collected from your PCR can help to monitor and improve patient care through medical audits, research, education, and system policy changes. Furthermore, your written documentation becomes a legal record of the incident and may become part of your patient's permanent medical record. All legal rules regarding confidentiality and disclosure pertain to your PCR.

The same factors that influence verbal communication also affect written communication. Be objective, write legibly, thoroughly document your patient's assessment and care, and use terminology that is widely accepted in the medical community (Figure 10-2). Finally, your PCR illustrates your professionalism. A sloppy, incomplete PCR suggests sloppy, inefficient care. The chapter on documentation deals with PCRs and other written communications in much greater detail.

TERMINOLOGY

Every industry develops its own terminology. Doing so makes communication within the industry clearer, more concise, and unambiguous. The airline industry, for example, uses the term *payload* to describe the total weight of everything (passengers, fuel, luggage, and other items) on an airplane. Musical composers and arrangers use words like *fortissimo, allegro,* and *a cappella* to describe a specific tempo or style.

The medical field also uses an extensive list of terms, acronyms, and abbreviations that allow quick, accurate communication of complex information. (The documentation chapter includes an extensive table of standard charting abbreviations.) An emergency physician may request a CBC (complete blood count), ABGs (arterial blood gases), or a CIP (cardiac injury profile)—common terms describing diagnostic tests run on acutely ill patients. The emergency services industry has further developed its own terms for radio communication (Table 10-1). These words or phrases shorten air time and transmit thoughts and ideas quickly. For

prehospital care report (PCR) the written record of an EMS response.

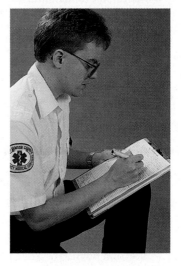

FIGURE 10-2 The prehospital care report is as important as the run itself. Complete it promptly, accurately, and legibly.

Table 10-1 COMMON RADIO TERMINOLOGY

Term	Meaning
Copy, 10-4, roger	I understand
Affirmative	Yes
Negative	No
Stand by	Please wait
Repeat	Please repeat what you said
Landline	Telephone communication
Rendezvous	Meet with
LZ	Landing zone (helicopter)
ETA	Estimated time of arrival
Over	I am finished with my transmission
Mobile status	On the air, driving around
Stage	Wait before entering a scene
Clear	End of transmission
Unfounded	We cannot find the incident/patient
Be advised	Listen carefully to this

Using industry terminology appropriately provides a common means of communicating with other emergency care professionals.

A brilliant assessment and management plan is futile if you cannot communicate it to others.

Content Review

EMS RESPONSE COMMUNICATIONS

- Detection and citizen access
- Call taking and emergency response
- Prearrival instructions
- Call coordination and incident recording
- Discussion with medical direction physician
- Transfer communications
- Back in service, ready for next call

PSAP public safety answering point.

example, *copy, 10-4,* and *roger* mean, "I heard you and I understand what you said." Using industry terminology appropriately is an important part of effective communication. It provides a common means of communicating with other emergency care professionals.

THE EMS RESPONSE

Your ability to communicate effectively during a stressful EMS response determines the success or failure of your efforts. A brilliant assessment and management plan is futile if you cannot communicate it to others. Dealing effectively with your patient and bystanders requires a variety of communication skills such as empathy, confidence, self-control, authority, and patience. Your clinical experience will suggest which skills to use in any particular situation. For example, you might use confidence and an authoritative posture when dealing with unruly bystanders. On the other hand, you would need to be gentle and empathetic with a child or an elderly grandmother. If you were in charge of an incident, you would have to communicate your authority within the structure of the emergency scene to providers from other responding agencies. Delegating tasks, listening to initial reports, and coordinating the scene require effective communication and interpersonal skills.

The sequence of an EMS response illustrates the importance of communications in prehospital care. A typical EMS response includes the following chain of events.

Detection and Citizen Access To begin the response to any emergency once it has occurred, someone must detect the problem and summon EMS (Figure 10-3). Any citizen with an urgent medical need should have a simple and reliable mechanism for accessing the EMS system. In the United States, most people access EMS by telephone; thus, a well-publicized universal telephone number such as 9-1-1 provides direct citizen access to the communications center. At enhanced 9-1-1 (E-9-1-1) communication centers, a computer displays the caller's telephone number and location. The centers also have instant call-back capabilities, should the caller hang up too soon. The 9-1-1 system has been available since the late 1960s. Most of the population in the United States has access to a 9-1-1 system. Highway call boxes, citizens band (CB) radio, and amateur radio all provide alternate means of accessing emergency help in some regions.

Calls to 9-1-1 usually connect the caller to a public safety answering point (**PSAP**), which then directs the caller to the appropriate agency for dispatch and response. In some

FIGURE 10–3 The response begins when someone detects an emergency and summons EMS support.

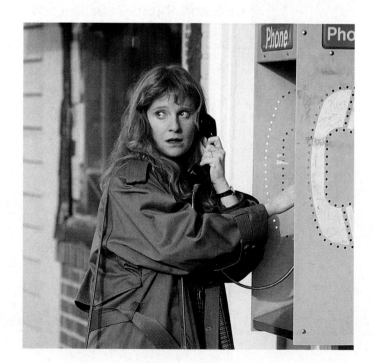

systems, the PSAP call taker will elicit the information and determine the nature of the response. In others, he will simply answer with the question, "Is this a police, fire, or medical emergency?" and transfer the caller to the appropriate dispatcher, who will then elicit the information. Many systems use computerized technology at the PSAP to connect the caller automatically with the appropriate agency. Some even provide language translation. Future global positioning systems will allow the dispatcher to pinpoint a cellular-phone caller's location. Additionally, automakers are installing communications computers in some automobiles. When involved in an accident, these "black boxes" automatically provide the dispatcher with the location, speed, type of collision, projected damage, and suspected severity of injury.

In some systems, all public safety agencies are located within the same facility. In others, they are connected electronically. No one way is best. If the public receives timely, appropriate responses to all emergency calls, the system is effective.

Call Taking and Emergency Response   The emergency medical dispatcher (**EMD**) is the public's first contact with the EMS system and plays a crucial role in every EMS response. The most important information the call taker must obtain is the address of the incident, the caller's name, the call-back number, and other pertinent factors. Ideally, he also will ascertain the nature of the emergency and other pertinent factors.

EMD emergency medical dispatcher.

In a coordinated system known as **priority dispatching**, medical dispatchers interrogate a distressed caller using a set of medically approved questions to elicit essential information about the chief complaint (Figure 10-4). Then, the dispatcher follows established guidelines to determine the appropriate level of response (Figure 10-5). These predetermined guidelines are based on criteria approved by the medical director. For example, an elderly man with a history of heart problems who is complaining of chest pain radiating to his left arm may indicate a priority-one response (life-threatening emergency, lights, and siren). In some systems, the appropriate response may include a fire department basic life support first responding unit, a paramedic engine company, and a transporting ambulance. Other systems may require a basic, intermediate-level, or paramedic ambulance. This form of call screening, when done appropriately, saves time and money because only the necessary resources are sent. It also limits the liability associated with lights and siren response to possible life-threatening incidents. Many private and public EMS systems throughout the United States use the priority dispatching system.

priority dispatching system using medically approved questions and predetermined guidelines to determine the appropriate level of response.

Prearrival Instructions   Many EMS systems provide **prearrival instructions**, a service that is considered the standard of care. Prearrival instructions complement the call screening process in a priority dispatch system. As the dispatcher sends the appropriate response, the caller remains on the line and receives prearrival instructions for suitable emergency measures such as cardiopulmonary resuscitation or hemorrhage control. During prearrivals, the

prearrival instructions dispatcher's instructions to caller for appropriate emergency measures.

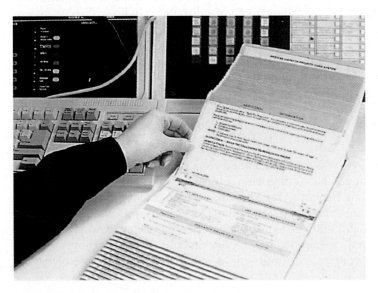

FIGURE 10-4   Priority dispatching and prearrival medical instruction have enhanced the efficiency of the EMS system.

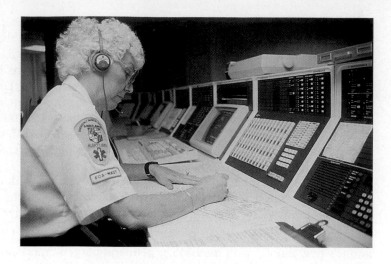

FIGURE 10-5 The dispatcher determines the appropriate level of response according to the established guidelines.

dispatcher also can obtain further information for the responding units. In the case of cardiac arrest, the dispatcher can relay information concerning the presence of a living will, a "Do Not Resuscitate" (DNR) form, or other advanced directives. In another case, a unit en route to a baby who had stopped breathing could reduce their response speed if they learned that the child had started breathing and was conscious. Prearrival instructions have saved many lives since 1974. They also are useful for comforting a distressed caller or providing emotional support to bystanders, family members, or the patient himself.

Call Coordination and Incident Recording   After sending the appropriate response and providing prearrival instructions, the emergency medical dispatcher's main duties are support and coordination. He will provide the responding units with any additional resources needed and record information about the call such as times, locations, and units involved. Your dispatcher can be your best friend. He can assign the resources you need to manage an incident—additional medical personnel to help with a cardiac arrest, for instance, or the fire department to provide specialized rescue. He also may facilitate communication with other agencies, hospitals, communication centers, and support services.

Discussion with Medical Direction Physician   After conducting your assessment and initiating care as outlined by your local protocols, you will contact the medical direction physician to discuss the case. Following consultation, he may give you further orders for interventions such as medications or other medical procedures. The many ways to conduct this communication include the radio, telephone, and cellular phone. Taping these communications for use later is advisable. For example, if a discrepancy arose as to your orders, you could always refer to the tape for evidence. At this point, you continue treatment and prepare your patient for transport. You will contact your dispatcher, who will record when you leave the scene and when you arrive at your destination.

Transmitting clear, concise, controlled reports will encourage your medical direction physicians to trust your assessments and on-scene treatment plans.

⚷

Your professional relationship with your medical direction physicians must be based on trust. Transmitting clear, concise, controlled reports will encourage your medical direction physicians to accept your assessments and on-scene treatment plans. Your ability to communicate effectively on the radio is an integral part of your professional reputation. The general radio procedures and standard format sections later in this chapter offer guidelines for communicating with your medical direction physician and transmitting patient information (Figure 10-6).

Transfer Communications   As you transfer care of your patient to the receiving facility staff, you must give the receiving nurse or physician a formal verbal briefing (Figure 10-7). This report should include your patient's vital information, chief complaint and history, physical exam findings, and any treatments rendered. Do not assume that the receiving nurse heard your radio report and knows of your patient. Some systems require the receiving nurse to sign the prehospital care report (PCR) to verify and document the transfer of care. In any case, don't leave your patient until you have completed some type of formal

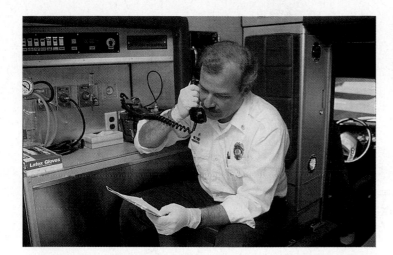

FIGURE 10-6 You will discuss each case with the medical direction physician and follow his instructions for patient care.

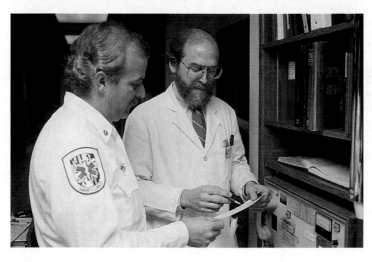

FIGURE 10-7 On arrival at the emergency department, you will give receiving personnel a formal, verbal briefing.

transfer of care, because you may be charged with abandonment. Many systems likewise require the medical direction physician to sign the PCR for any medications administered by EMT-Is, especially if they included controlled substances such as morphine or diazepam. In all cases, end your documentation with transfer of care information on your PCR.

> *Never leave your patient until you formally transfer responsibility for his care.*

COMMUNICATION TECHNOLOGY

EMS systems can use all of today's various communication technologies. These include the more traditional forms of radio communication as well as innovations in radio technology and other media.

RADIO COMMUNICATION

Many types of radio transmission are possible, with new technologies being developed every day. Usage may vary from system to system. This section discusses some of the more common technologies in use today.

Biotelemetry

Vital patient information, such as ECGs, can be transmitted over the radio by a process called **biotelemetry** (Figure 10-8). In the ambulance, ECG voltage is converted from an electrical impulse to audio tones by way of a modulator. The audio tones are then transmitted to the hospital over the radio. At the hospital, the transmission is converted to electrical impulses by a demodulator and displayed on an oscilloscope, on electrocardiogram (ECG) paper, or both. Telemetry is subject to interference by such things as muscle tremor, loose

biotelemetry the process of transmitting physiological data, such as an ECG, over distance, usually by radio.

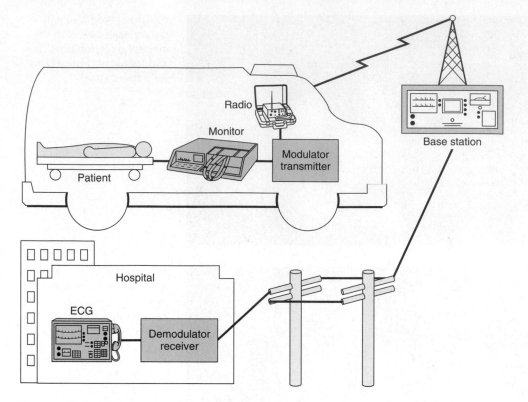

FIGURE 10-8 Biotelemetry allows the transmission of patient data, such as the ECG, from the scene to the hospital.

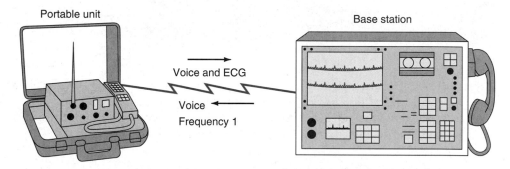

FIGURE 10-9 Simplex communications systems transmit and receive on the same frequency.

electrodes, 60-cycle interference (from other electrical sources), fluctuations in transmitter power, and by transmitting voice communications while telemetry is in progress.

Some systems use telemetry for every patient; others never use it. Use of telemetry alone, without field interpretation, is inappropriate. Always verify your interpretation with the medical direction physician, either over the radio or after arrival at the hospital. Check with your local system's protocols for the appropriate local use of biotelemetry.

Simplex

simplex communication system that transmits and receives on the same frequency.

The most basic communications systems use **simplex** transmissions. These systems transmit and receive on the same frequency and thus cannot do both simultaneously (Figure 10-9). After you transmit a message, you must release the transmit button and wait for a response. This slows communication because you have to wait for all traffic to stop before you can speak. It also makes the system more formal and prevents open discussion. Simplex communication systems are most effective on the scene, when the incident commander or EMS dispatcher must transmit orders or directions without interruption. Most dispatch systems and on-scene communications use simplex transmissions.

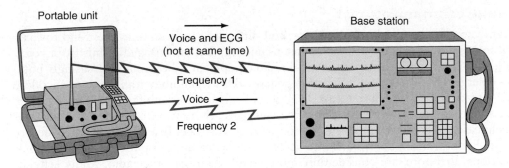

FIGURE 10-10   Duplex communications systems use two frequencies for each channel.

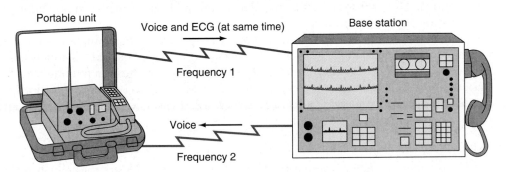

FIGURE 10-11   Multiplex systems can transmit voice and data at the same time.

Duplex

Duplex transmissions allow simultaneous two-way communications by using two frequencies for each channel (Figure 10-10). Each radio must be able to transmit and receive on each channel. For example, on channel one, a hospital base station might transmit on 468.000 megahertz (MHz) and receive on 478.000 MHz. Field radios would then transmit on 478.000 MHz and receive on 468.000 MHz—just the opposite. Either party could then transmit and receive on the same channel simultaneously.

Duplex systems work similar to telephone communications. Many areas use them for communications between the field provider and the medical direction physician. The major advantage of the duplex system is that one party does not have to wait to speak until the other party finishes his transmission. This allows a much freer discussion and consultation between physician and EMT-I. For example, the medical direction physician can interrupt your report with an important question or concern. On the other hand, this ability to interrupt can be a disadvantage when abused.

Duplex systems all allow you to transmit either voice messages or data such as ECG strips.

duplex communication system that allows simultaneous two-way communications by using two frequencies for each channel.

Multiplex

Multiplex systems are duplex systems with the additional capability of transmitting voice and data simultaneously (Figure 10-11). This enables you to carry on a conversation with the medical direction physician while you are transmitting an ECG strip. Speaking while you are transmitting the ECG strip, however, causes much interference on the ECG strip.

multiplex duplex system that can transmit voice and data simultaneously.

Trunking

Many communications systems operating in the 800 MHz range use **trunking** to hasten communications. Trunked systems pool all frequencies. When a radio transmission comes in, a computer routes it to the first available frequency. The computer routes the next transmission to the next available frequency, and so on. When a transmission terminates, that frequency becomes available and reenters the pool of unused frequencies. Trunking thus frees the dispatcher or field unit from having to search for an available frequency.

trunking communication system that pools all frequencies and routes transmissions to the next available frequency.

Digital Communications

digital communications data or sounds are translated into a digital code for transmission.

Voice transmission can be time-consuming and difficult to understand. The trend toward combining radio technology with computer technology has encouraged a shift from voice (analog) to **digital communications**. Digital radio equipment is becoming increasingly popular in emergency services communication systems. This technology translates, or encodes, sounds into digital code for broadcast. Digital transmission is much faster and much more accurate than analog transmission. Since the messages are transmitted in condensed form, they help ease the overcrowding of radio frequencies. Also, because you need a decoder to translate digital transmissions back into voice, scanners cannot monitor them. Your communications, therefore, are considerably more secure than over the radio. Many cellular phone companies now use digital transmissions. Future technology will link patient-monitoring devices to a small computer equipped with a radio for transmission.

mobile data terminal vehicle-mounted computer keyboard and display.

The **mobile data terminals** in many emergency vehicles are a basic form of digital communications. They are mounted in the vehicle cab and wired to the radio. When a data transmission such as the address of the incident comes in, the terminal displays the message on a screen or prints it in hard copy. Responders can reply by punching a button to send a message such as "en route," "arrived," or "transporting to the hospital." Though somewhat restrictive and primitive, these terminals have reduced on-air time to a minimum even in the busiest systems. It is important to remember, however, that voice communications will always have a place in emergency services. Crews will always need to speak to one another, to physicians and nurses, or to dispatchers.

ALTERNATIVE TECHNOLOGIES

Among the more common alternatives to radio communications are the cellular telephone, the facsimile machine, and the computer.

Cellular Telephone

cellular telephone system telephone system divided into regions, or cells, that are served by radio base stations.

Many EMS systems have found that **cellular telephones** are a cost-effective way to transmit essential patient information to the hospital (Figure 10-12). Cellular technology is available in even the most remote areas of the country. A cellular telephone service is divided into regions called cells. These cells are radio base stations, with which the mobile telephone communicates. When the transmission leaves one cell's range, another cell picks it up immediately, without interruption.

Like duplex radio transmissions, cellular phones make communication less formal, promote discussion, and reduce on-line times. They further allow the medical direction physician to speak directly with the patient and offer the further advantages of being widely available and highly reliable. Because the ECG signal is digitized, the hospital receives a better signal than if it were transmitted over radio waves. The telephones themselves are inexpensive, but cellular telephone systems charge a monthly fee for their use. Their major disadvantage is that each cell can handle only a limited number of calls. Geography can interfere with the signal of the cellular telephone, and in large metropolitan areas the cells often fill up and become unavailable, especially during peak hours. Other disadvantages are that anyone with a scanner can monitor conversations on analog cellular phones; cellular phones require an external antenna; and the cellular phone system will deny access to a cell if you do not know or forget the personal identification number (PIN). Despite their limitations, cellular telephones have become a popular medium for dispatching, on-scene, and medical direction communications.

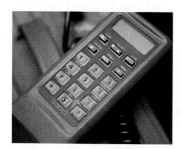

FIGURE 10-12 Cellular telephones have made it possible to transmit high-quality facsimiles, computer data, and 12-lead ECGs.

Facsimile

facsimile machine device for electronically transmitting and receiving printed information.

A **facsimile machine** (fax) provides a quick way to send printed information. This machine "reads" the printed information, digitizes it line-by-line, and transmits it to another machine, which then decodes it and prints a facsimile of the original. A fax machine enables health-care agencies to exchange medical information immediately. Future systems will allow EMS responders to access a patient's medical record from a general database; responders or data-base operators will be able to send the same information to the receiving facility. With some electronic run sheet systems, you will be able to transmit your patient information to the receiving hospital long before you arrive. This technology's one obvious limitation is that both the sending and the receiving agency must have access to a fax machine and a telephone line.

Computer

Computers have entered every aspect of our daily lives. In emergency services communications, they have revolutionized system management and incident data collection. Most dispatchers no longer enter data via pen and pencil, time-stamping machines, or typewriters. They can make a permanent record of any incident's events in real time. Computers also make research faster and easier. For example, if you wanted to determine which day of the week most cardiac calls happen, what time of day is busiest, or which area of a city needs more coverage, you could retrieve the pertinent data from your computerized records immediately. You can program your system to provide whatever type of data you want, in whatever format you desire. It also eliminates the need to enter retrospective data when conducting research. For example, the times, locations, and particulars of a call will be in the computer files for immediate retrieval during a research project. Limitations of a computer include its own power, speed, and capacity, as well as the operator's ability. Also, rigidly programmed machines that function only in certain restrictive ways can limit your flexibility.

NEW TECHNOLOGY

New technology is being developed every day. The National Aeronautics and Space Administration (NASA) has pioneered communications that allow television viewers to hear and see astronauts in space. Ground crews can monitor each astronaut's biological function and maintain a permanent record throughout the trip. And NASA has been doing this for decades.

In comparison with other industries, public safety communication systems are nearly archaic. Most EMS agencies still document patient assessment and care with hand-written run sheets, and some use radio equipment so old that replacement tubes are no longer available. But times are changing rapidly. Time constraints, storage space, and congested radio traffic necessitate developing new systems that will allow EMT-Is to transmit, receive, and store vital patient information quickly and reliably. Someday computer-based technology, digital satellite transmission, and electronic storage and retrieval of patient information will replace radio communications, written documentation, and file cabinets filled with EMS run sheets. These newer technologies are costly, but they do exist.

Current documentation systems already allow you to record all aspects of your EMS response electronically through use of a **touch pad**. With pen-based reporting systems you can record patient information on a handheld computer. These systems do away with written documentation and capture information in real time, eliminating the need to estimate times after the call. Some systems integrate diagnostic technology and enable you to transmit ECG and pulse oximetry readings to the hospital before arrival. Such advanced knowledge of diagnostic test results from the field may radically change a medical direction physician's decisions and reduce the time needed to make an in-hospital diagnosis and begin therapy. Some systems allow paramedics to transmit a 12-lead ECG, for example. This reduces the time before the paramedic in transit or receiving emergency department personnel can begin cardiac muscle-saving thrombolytic therapy for the patient with a suspected myocardial infarction. Other systems allow you to receive important medical information from your patient's permanent record while on the scene or in transit. For instance, at the home of a patient with an altered mental status and no family to relate his history, you might access his medical records and obtain his history via a computerized database. In this type of system, the transferring facility, the receiving hospital, and you can all access this information simultaneously.

A disadvantage of electronic recording systems is the absence of a "paper record" of the incident, should the information be accidentally erased or destroyed. The legal guidelines that apply to written and spoken communication also apply to electronic reporting. You must maintain patient confidentiality, you must be objective, and you must not **slander** or **libel** another person.

touch pad computer on which you enter data by touching areas of the display screen.

slander to orally defame another person.

libel to defame another person in writing.

protocol predetermined, written guidelines for patient care.

REPORTING PROCEDURES

As an EMT-I, you must effectively relay all relevant medical information to the receiving hospital staff. Initially, you might do this over the radio or by cellular telephone. Later, when you deliver your patient to the emergency department, you can give additional information in-person to the appropriate receiving hospital personnel.

One of your most important skills will be gathering essential patient information, organizing it, and relaying it to the medical direction physician. The medical direction physician will then issue appropriate orders for patient care. The amount and type of information you relay to the medical direction physician depends on the type of technology you use, your patient's priority, and your local communication **protocols**. For example, if communications in your region are not secured (private) you must limit the type of information you can communicate without breaching patient confidentiality. The acuteness of your patient's clinical status and the amount of local radio traffic also may determine the length of your report. For a critical patient you may give a brief report while you tend to your patient's medical needs. For a complicated medical emergency, you may wish to communicate a greater share of the results of your history and physical exam to the medical direction physician.

STANDARD FORMAT

Communicating patient information to the hospital or to the medical direction physician is a crucial function within the EMS system. Verbal communications, which may occur via radio or landline, give the hospital enough information on your patient's condition to prepare for his care. These communications also should initiate the medical orders you need to treat your patient in the field. A standard format for transmitting patient assessment information helps achieve those goals in several ways. First, it adds to the medical communications system's efficiency. Second, it helps the physician to assimilate information about the patient's condition quickly. Third, it ensures that medical information is complete. In general, your verbal reports to medical direction should include the following information:

- Identification of unit and provider
- Description of scene
- Patient's age, sex, and approximate weight (for drug orders)
- Patient's chief complaint and severity
- Brief, pertinent past history of the present illness or injury (OPQRST)
- Pertinent medical history, medications, and allergies (SAMPLE)
- Pertinent physical exam findings
- Treatment given so far/request for orders

Legal Notes

Many modern EMS communications systems use encryption or similar technologies to ensure privacy and security. However, certain EMS communications, including some cell phone communications, can be monitored by persons with scanners or similar devices, which are becoming as sophisticated as the radios themselves. Because of this, radios once thought secure, in fact, may not be. Furthermore, in many emergency departments, EMS radios are within earshot of patients, staff, and visitors. Thus, you should always assume that any EMS radio communication may be heard by someone other than the intended recipient. Because of this, you must carefully limit any information that might identify a particular patient. This includes such things as name, race, financial (insurance) status, and similar descriptors. Transmission of such information does not enhance patient care and may actually violate patient confidentiality laws including HIPAA and similar statutes. Always carefully plan your radio communications—especially when they deal with a particular patient.

- Estimated time of arrival at the hospital
- Other pertinent information

The formats and contents of reports for medical and trauma patients differ to include only the information relevant to either type of emergency. Reports for medical patients emphasize the history in the beginning of the report; reports for trauma patients emphasize the injuries and the physical exam.

After transmitting your report, you will await further questions and orders from the medical direction physician. Upon arrival, your spoken report will give essential patient information to the provider assuming care. It should include a brief history, pertinent physical findings, treatment, and responses to that treatment.

GENERAL RADIO PROCEDURES

Using the radio properly makes your communications skillful and efficient. All of your transmissions must be clear and crisp, with concise, professional content (Figure 10-13). Always follow these guidelines for effective radio use:

1. Listen to the channel before transmitting to ensure that it is not in use.
2. Press the transmit button for 1 second before speaking.
3. Speak at close range, approximately 2 to 3 inches, directly into, or across the face of, the microphone.
4. Speak slowly and clearly. Pronounce each word distinctly, avoiding words that are difficult to understand.
5. Speak in a normal pitch, keeping your voice free of emotion.
6. Be brief. Know what you are going to say before you press the transmit button.
7. Avoid codes unless they are part of your EMS system.
8. Do not waste air time with unnecessary information.
9. Protect your patient's privacy. When appropriate:
   - Use telephone rather than radio.
   - Turn off external speaker.
   - Do not use your patient's name; doing so violates Federal Communications Commission regulations.
10. Use proper unit or hospital numbers, and correct names or titles.
11. Do not use slang or profanity.
12. Use standard formats for transmission.
13. Be concise in order to hold the attention of the person receiving your radio report.
14. Use the **echo procedure** when receiving directions from the dispatcher or orders from the physician. Immediately repeating each statement confirms accurate reception and understanding.
15. Always write down addresses, important dispatch communications, and physician orders.
16. When completing a transmission, obtain confirmation that your message was received and understood.

Occasionally, communications equipment will not function properly. Even a weak battery can disrupt clear communication. If you are far from the base station, particularly if you have a portable radio, try to broadcast from higher terrain. Structures that contain steel and concrete can interfere with radio transmission. Simply moving outside the building or near a window may improve it. If that does not work, try using a telephone.

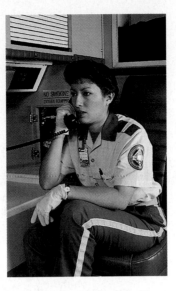

FIGURE 10-13 The professionalism of your communications reflects on the professionalism of your patient care.

echo procedure immediately repeating each transmission received during radio communications.

MODEL VERBAL REPORTS

The following examples demonstrate professional verbal reports for a medical patient and for a trauma patient. Neither report takes more than 45 seconds, and each gives the medical direction physician enough information to make an initial diagnosis and prepare for arrival. As you read them, consider how they follow the principles of effective communication discussed throughout this chapter, and note their differences in format and information.

Content Review

ELEMENTS OF MEDICAL PATIENT REPORT

- EMT-I identification
- Patient identification
- Subjective data
- Objective data
- Plan

Medical Patient

EMT-I Identification:	This is Brewerton ambulance, EMT-Intermediate Button.
Patient Identification:	We have a 63-year-old, 70-kg alert male, patient of Dr. Fullagar.
Subjective Data:	He complains of sudden onset of substernal chest pain radiating to the neck for the past half hour. He also complains of shortness of breath and nausea. He has a past history of cardiac problems and takes nitroglycerin, Isordil, and Procardia XL.
Objective Data:	He appears in moderate distress at this time, clutching his chest, but is able to speak in full sentences. Vitals are BP, 138/80; pulse, 88 and regular; respirations, 24 and slightly labored; skin warm and dry. He has clear lung sounds bilaterally, no JVD, peripheral edema or ascites. ECG shows sinus rhythm with an occasional unifocal PVC. Pulse oximetry is 92% on room air.
Plan:	We have him on oxygen at 15 liters per minute via nonrebreather mask, we have a saline lock in place, and have given him two baby aspirin. We are 5 minutes from our rendezvous point with Rural-Metro ambulance. Their paramedic will contact you for further orders.

Content Review

ELEMENTS OF TRAUMA PATIENT REPORT

- EMT-I identification
- Patient identification
- Mechanism of injury
- Injuries
- Plan

Trauma Patient

EMT-I Identification:	This is DeWitt Rescue 7, EMT-Intermediate Griffin.
Patient Identification:	We have a 23-year-old unresponsive female.
Mechanism of Injury:	She was the unbelted driver in a high-speed, head-on, one-car versus telephone pole collision with severe damage to the car and intrusion into the passenger compartment.
Injuries:	She has major head and chest trauma and shows signs of decompensated shock. Vitals are BP, 76 by palpation; pulse, 120 weak and regular, carotid only; respirations, 40 and shallow; skin cool, pale, and clammy. She has a depressed skull fracture in the left parietal region, and a right-sided flail chest. Her pupils are unequal and slow to react, no drainage from the ears or nose, no Battle's sign or raccoon's eyes. Trachea is midline, no JVD. She shows paradoxical chest wall movement and is cyanotic with diminished lung sounds on the right side. Pulse oximetry is 88% on room air.
Plan:	We have the patient fully immobilized, have stabilized the flail segment and are assisting ventilation with a bag-valve mask and supplemental oxygen. We have an IV of normal saline running wide open and are starting a second line. Our ETA is 20 minutes.

REGULATION

The **Federal Communications Commission** (FCC) controls and regulates all nongovernmental communications in the United States. This includes AM and FM radio, television, aircraft, marine, and mobile land frequency ranges. The FCC has designated frequencies within each radio band for special use. They include public safety frequencies in both the **very high frequency** band (VHF) and the ultrahigh frequency band (UHF). The primary functions of the FCC include:

- Licensing and allocating radio frequencies
- Establishing technical standards for radio equipment
- Licensing and regulating the technical personnel who repair and operate radio equipment
- Monitoring frequencies to ensure appropriate usage
- Spot-checking base stations and dispatch centers for appropriate licenses and records

The FCC requires all EMS communications systems to follow appropriate governmental regulations and laws. You must stay abreast of and obey any FCC regulations that apply to your communications.

Federal Communications Commission (FCC) agency that controls all nongovernmental communications in the United States.

very high frequency radio frequency band from 30 to 300 megahertz.

SUMMARY

As one of the fundamental aspects of prehospital care, accurate communications help ensure an EMS system's efficiency. Communications begin when the citizen accesses the EMS system and end when you complete your patient report. Your spoken messages must be understandable, and your written messages must be legible. All of your communications must be concise and complete and conform to national and local protocols. The more sophisticated and advanced your EMS system grows, the more sophisticated and advanced its communications—and, accordingly, your communications skills—must become.

ON THE WEB

For additional practice and review, go to the companion website at www.prenhall.com/bledsoe and click on *Intermediate Emergency Care: Principles & Practice*.

Chapter 11

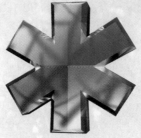

Documentation

Objectives

After reading this chapter, you should be able to:

1. Identify the general principles regarding the importance of EMS documentation and ways in which documents are used. (pp. 560–561)
2. Identify and properly use medical terminology, medical abbreviations, and acronyms. (pp. 563, 564–567)
3. Explain the role of documentation in agency reimbursement. (p. 560)
4. Identify and eliminate extraneous or nonprofessional information. (p. 571)
5. Describe the differences between subjective and objective elements of documentation. (pp. 571–573)
6. Evaluate a finished document for errors and omissions and proper use and spelling of abbreviations and acronyms. (pp. 568, 570)
7. Evaluate the confidential nature of an EMS report. (p. 580)

8. Describe the potential consequences of illegible, incomplete, or inaccurate documentation. (pp. 568, 570)
9. Describe the special documentation considerations concerning patient refusal of care and/or transport. (pp. 576–577)
10. Demonstrate how to properly record direct patient or bystander comments. (p. 568)
11. Describe the special considerations concerning mass casualty incident documentation. (p. 578)
12. Demonstrate proper document revision and correction. (pp. 570–571)
13. Apply the principles of documentation to computer charting, as access to this technology becomes available. (p. 580)
14. Assume responsibility for self-assessment of all documentation. (p. 580)

Case Study

Tom Brewster is nervous. He has never been to a deposition before, and though everyone has assured him that he is not the target of any legal action, he wonders what the lawyers want from him.

As he sits outside the conference room, he goes over the call in his head. It was about 2:30 in the morning. Eric Billings, his partner, and he had just finished cleaning up from a patient with gastrointestinal (GI) bleeding when they were dispatched to a single vehicle crash. The driver had gone off the eastbound side of the road, crossed a ditch, and smashed into a tree. The driver had been lucky. He was out of the car, standing on the shoulder of the road, and did not seem to have any serious injuries. He told Tom and Eric, "I think I'm fine. I just fell asleep and ran off the road." Still, they had performed an initial assessment followed by a rapid trauma assessment, immobilized the man, administered oxygen, and transported him to the emergency department. Tom rode in the back with the patient. On the way to the hospital he checked the patient's glucose level, started an intravenous (IV) as a precaution, and applied a cardiac monitor.

Everything was normal, Tom now thinks. "What did I miss?" He has reread his prehospital care report a hundred times. Though it has been 3 years, he now remembers almost every detail of the call. Until 2 weeks ago, he had almost completely forgotten about it. All too soon, the lawyers call Tom into the conference room, introduce themselves, and swear him to honesty. One of the lawyers begins, "Do you recall the crash that occurred on the evening in question?"

"Yes, I do," Tom replies. He recounts that upon their arrival at the scene, the driver was out of the vehicle. Tom states that they managed him like any other trauma patient and that he had no obvious injuries or indications of illness.

"Did the gentleman tell you he is diabetic?"

"No," Tom answers, "but we checked his blood sugar level, and it was normal."

"Did he tell you he has heart problems?"

"No," Tom says again, "but we did put him on the heart monitor, and his rhythm was normal."

"Did he tell you he ran off the road because he passed out?"

"No, he told me he fell asleep." Tom feels better. He has the answer to every question, and he has the prehospital care report (PCR) to back him up.

After a few more questions, the lawyers dismiss Tom and allow him to leave. He has no idea what they were getting at, but he knows that he answered every question honestly. He wonders if he would have had all the answers if the case had been from 6 or 8 years ago. He has really worked on his documentation in the last few years, and he knows he would have never remembered all those details without the help of his PCR.

Six weeks later Tom gets a letter from the lawyer thanking him for his testimony. It turns out the patient was suing his private doctor for not "recognizing his obvious diabetes and heart problems. He claimed these illnesses caused him to be involved in the motor-vehicle crash, and it resulted in serious injury." Tom's testimony—and his PCR—had been pivotal in getting the case dismissed.

INTRODUCTION

In this age of litigation, treating your patient and documenting his care are separate but equally important duties. Your written **prehospital care report (PCR)** is the only truly factual record of events. When written correctly it accurately describes your assessment and care throughout the emergency call. It documents exactly what you did, when you did it, and the effects of your interventions. It can be your best friend or your worst enemy in a court proceeding.

Your PCR is your sole permanent, complete written record of events during the ambulance call. The dispatch center may have a record of the call times and audio tapes of radio transmissions, and your patient will have his memory of the call. You and other responders also may have some recollections about the call. Your PCR, however, will always be considered the most comprehensive and reliable record of the event. In addition, it reflects your professionalism. A well-written, thorough PCR suggests a thorough, efficient assessment and quality care. A sloppy, incomplete PCR suggests sloppy, inefficient care.

prehospital care report (PCR) the written record of an EMS response.

Document exactly what you did, when you did it, and the effects of your interventions.

Your PCR reflects your professionalism.

USES FOR DOCUMENTATION

Your PCR is a valuable resource for a variety of people. They include medical professionals, EMS administrators, researchers, and occasionally, lawyers.

MEDICAL

Hospital staff (nurses and physicians) may need more information from you than they can get before you have to take another call. For example, they may want a chronological account of your patient's mental status from the time you arrived on the scene. Your PCR can tell the emergency department staff of your patient's condition before he arrived at the hospital. It serves as a baseline for comparing assessment findings and detecting trends that indicate improvement or deterioration. The surgical staff will want to know the mechanism of injury and other pertinent findings during your initial assessment of your patient and the scene.

Your PCR is an important document that helps ensure your patient's continuity of care.

If your patient is admitted to the hospital, the floor or intensive care unit staff may need more information about his original condition than he can remember. In addition, your PCR provides them with information from people at the scene to whom they might not have access—family, bystanders, first responders, or other witnesses. Knowing about the circumstances that led to the event or the mechanism of injury may also help rehabilitation specialists to provide better therapy. Your PCR becomes an important document that helps ensure your patient's continuous effective care (Figure 11-1).

ADMINISTRATIVE

response time time elapsed from when a unit is alerted until it arrives on scene.

EMS administrators must gather information for quality improvement and system management. Information regarding **response times,** call location, the use of lights and siren, and date and time is vital to evaluating your system's readiness to respond to life-threatening emergencies. It also is essential to providing information of community needs. The quality improvement or quality assurance committee use PCRs to identify problems with individual EMT-Is or with the EMS system. In some agencies, the billing department needs to determine which services are billable. Insurance carriers may need to know more about the illness or injury to process the claim. Some states use your PCR data to allocate funding for regional systems.

RESEARCH

Your PCR provides the basis for continuously improving patient care in your EMS system.

Your PCR may give researchers useful data about many aspects of the EMS call. For example, they may analyze your recorded data to determine the efficacy of certain medical devices or interventions such as drugs and invasive procedures. They also may use the data to cut costs, alter staffing, and shorten response times. Some systems use computerized or elec-

Prehospital Care Report

Agency Name	ARLINGTON RESCUE
Dispatch Information	CARDIAC
Call Location	124 CYPRUS ST 2nd FLOOR

MILEAGE	
END	2 4 4 9 6
BEGIN	2 4 4 7 6
TOTAL	0 0 0 2 0

CHECK ONE ☑ Residence ☐ Health Facility ☐ Farm ☐ Indus. Facility ☐ Other Work Loc. ☐ Roadway ☐ Recreational ☐ Other

LOCATION CODE 0 1 2 4

CALL TYPE AS REC'D
☑ Emergency
☐ Non-Emergency
☐ Stand-by

MECHANISM OF INJURY
☐ MVA (✓ seat belt used) N/A
☐ Fall of _____ feet
☐ Unarmed assault
☐ GSW
☐ Knife
☐ Machinery
☐ _____

USE MILITARY TIMES

CALL REC'D	0 7 0 5
ENROUTE	0 7 0 7
ARRIVED AT SCENE	0 7 1 9
FROM SCENE	0 7 3 8
AT DESTIN	0 7 5 4
IN SERVICE	0 8 1 0
IN QUARTERS	0 8 3 2

FIGURE 11-1 Run data in a prehospital care report is vital to your agency's efforts to improve patient care.

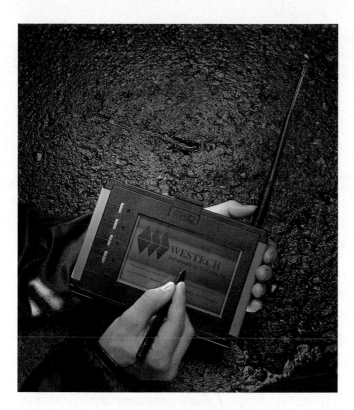

Figure 11-2 The hand-held electronic clipboard enables you to enter your prehospital care report directly into a computer.

tronic PCRs and a computerized database to analyze the data (Figure 11-2). Regardless of the method you use, your written documentation provides the basis for continuously improving patient care in your EMS system.

LEGAL

Your PCR becomes a permanent part of your patient's medical record. Lawyers may refer to it when preparing court actions, and in a legal proceeding it might be your sole source of information about the case. You may be called upon to testify in a case where your PCR becomes the central piece of evidence in your testimony. Or your PCR may serve as evidence in a criminal case and help determine whether the accused is innocent or guilty. Each state has its own laws regarding the length of time the hospital must keep its records.

Always write your PCR as if you knew you would have to refer to it someday in a court proceeding. Describe your patient's condition when you arrived and during your care, and note his status upon arrival at the hospital. Always document his condition before and after any interventions, and avoid writing any subjective opinions such as "the patient is intoxicated, obnoxious, and looks like a crack-addict." After your PCR is written, ask your partner to review it for completeness and accuracy. A complete, accurate, and objective account of the emergency call may be your best and only defense against a plaintiff's attorney who will try to find inconsistencies and ambiguities in your account.

GENERAL CONSIDERATIONS

Every EMS system has its own specific requirements for documentation. The type of call record used also varies from system to system. Some systems use reports with check boxes, some **bubble sheets,** which are computer scannable reports on which you record patient information by filling in boxes or "bubbles" (Figure 11-3). Still others may use computerized documentation. The particular type of operational data collected, such as time intervals, will also differ among systems. For example, proprietary EMS agencies may require more billing information than community-based volunteer agencies. The general characteristics of a well-written PCR, though, remain constant among all agencies and systems.

A complete, accurate, and objective account of the emergency call may be your best and only defense in court.

Content Review

CHARACTERISTICS OF A WELL-WRITTEN PCR
- Appropriate medical terminology
- Correct abbreviations and acronyms
- Accurate, consistent times
- Thoroughly documented communications
- Pertinent negatives
- Relevant oral statements of witnesses, bystanders, and patient
- Complete identification of all additional resources and personnel

bubble sheet scannable run sheet on which you fill in boxes or circles ("bubbles") to record assessment and care information.

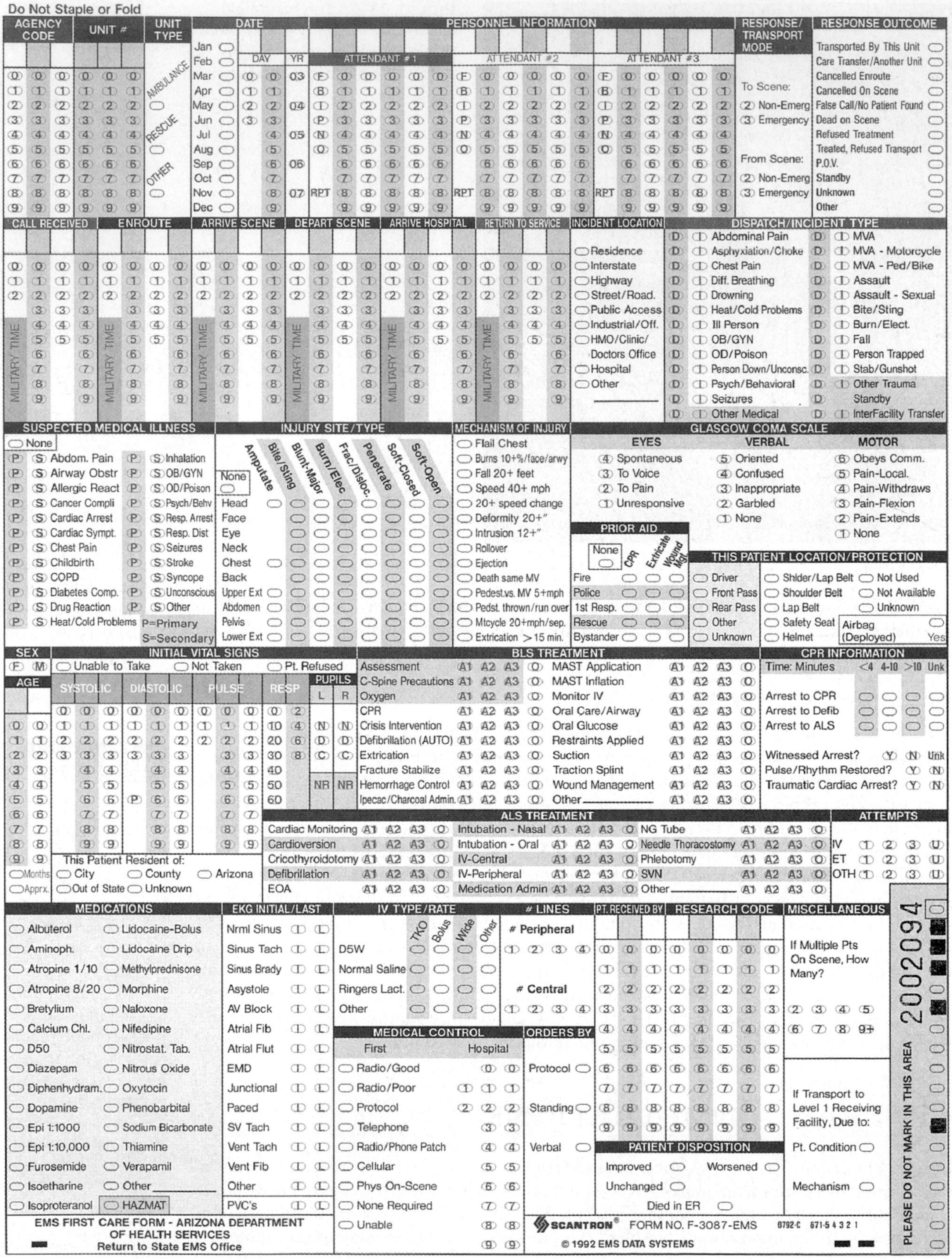

Do Not Staple or Fold

AGENCY CODE | UNIT # | UNIT TYPE: AMBULANCE, RESCUE, OTHER

DATE: Jan, Feb, Mar, Apr, May, Jun, Jul, Aug, Sep, Oct, Nov, Dec; DAY; YR 03, 04, 05, 06, 07

PERSONNEL INFORMATION: ATTENDANT #1, ATTENDANT #2, ATTENDANT #3 (F, B, I, P, N, O, RPT)

RESPONSE/TRANSPORT MODE: To Scene: (2) Non-Emerg, (3) Emergency; From Scene: (2) Non-Emerg, (3) Emergency

RESPONSE OUTCOME: Transported By This Unit; Care Transfer/Another Unit; Cancelled Enroute; Cancelled On Scene; False Call/No Patient Found; Dead on Scene; Refused Treatment; Treated, Refused Transport; P.O.V.; Standby; Unknown; Other

CALL RECEIVED | ENROUTE | ARRIVE SCENE | DEPART SCENE | ARRIVE HOSPITAL | RETURN TO SERVICE (MILITARY TIME)

INCIDENT LOCATION: Residence; Interstate; Highway; Street/Road.; Public Access; Industrial/Off.; HMO/Clinic/ Doctors Office; Hospital; Other

DISPATCH/INCIDENT TYPE: Abdominal Pain; Asphyxiation/Choke; Chest Pain; Diff. Breathing; Drowning; Heat/Cold Problems; Ill Person; OB/GYN; OD/Poison; Person Down/Unconsc.; Psych/Behavioral; Seizures; Other Medical; MVA; MVA - Motorcycle; MVA - Ped/Bike; Assault; Assault - Sexual; Bite/Sting; Burn/Elect.; Fall; Person Trapped; Stab/Gunshot; Other Trauma; Standby; InterFacility Transfer

SUSPECTED MEDICAL ILLNESS: None; Abdom. Pain; Airway Obstr; Allergic React; Cancer Compli; Cardiac Arrest; Cardiac Sympt.; Chest Pain; Childbirth; COPD; Diabetes Comp.; Drug Reaction; Heat/Cold Problems; Inhalation; OB/GYN; OD/Poison; Psych/Behv; Resp. Arrest; Resp. Dist; Seizures; Stroke; Syncope; Unconscious; Other; P=Primary S=Secondary

INJURY SITE/TYPE: Amputate; Bite/Sting; Blunt-Major; Burn/Elec; Frac/Disloc.; Penetrate; Soft-Closed; Soft-Open; None; Head; Face; Eye; Neck; Chest; Back; Upper Ext; Abdomen; Pelvis; Lower Ext

MECHANISM OF INJURY: Flail Chest; Burns 10+%/face/arwy; Fall 20+ feet; Speed 40+ mph; 20+ speed change; Deformity 20+"; Intrusion 12+"; Rollover; Ejection; Death same MV; Pedest.vs. MV 5+mph; Pedst. thrown/run over; Mtcycle 20+mph/sep.; Extrication >15 min.

GLASGOW COMA SCALE: EYES: (4) Spontaneous; (3) To Voice; (2) To Pain; (1) Unresponsive. VERBAL: (5) Oriented; (4) Confused; (3) Inappropriate; (2) Garbled; (1) None. MOTOR: (6) Obeys Comm.; (5) Pain-Local.; (4) Pain-Withdraws; (3) Pain-Flexion; (2) Pain-Extends; (1) None

PRIOR AID: None; CPR; Extricate; Wound Mgt.; Fire; Police; 1st Resp.; Rescue; Bystander

THIS PATIENT LOCATION/PROTECTION: Driver; Front Pass; Rear Pass; Other; Unknown; Shlder/Lap Belt; Shoulder Belt; Lap Belt; Safety Seat; Helmet; Not Used; Not Available; Unknown; Airbag (Deployed) Yes

SEX: F M | AGE: Months, Apprx.

INITIAL VITAL SIGNS: Unable to Take; Not Taken; Pt. Refused; SYSTOLIC; DIASTOLIC; PULSE; RESP; PUPILS L R (N, D, C, NR)

This Patient Resident of: City; County; Arizona; Out of State; Unknown

BLS TREATMENT: Assessment; C-Spine Precautions; Oxygen; CPR; Crisis Intervention; Defibrillation (AUTO); Extrication; Fracture Stabilize; Hemorrhage Control; Ipecac/Charcoal Admin.; MAST Application; MAST Inflation; Monitor IV; Oral Care/Airway; Oral Glucose; Restraints Applied; Suction; Traction Splint; Wound Management; Other (A1 A2 A3 O)

CPR INFORMATION: Time: Minutes <4 4-10 >10 Unk; Arrest to CPR; Arrest to Defib; Arrest to ALS; Witnessed Arrest? Y N Unk; Pulse/Rhythm Restored? Y N; Traumatic Cardiac Arrest? Y N

ALS TREATMENT: Cardiac Monitoring; Cardioversion; Cricothyroidotomy; Defibrillation; EOA; Intubation - Nasal; Intubation - Oral; IV-Central; IV-Peripheral; Medication Admin; NG Tube; Needle Thoracostomy; Phlebotomy; SVN; Other (A1 A2 A3 O)

ATTEMPTS: IV; ET; OTH (1 2 3 U)

MEDICATIONS: Albuterol; Aminoph.; Atropine 1/10; Atropine 8/20; Bretylium; Calcium Chl.; D50; Diazepam; Diphenhydram.; Dopamine; Epi 1:1000; Epi 1:10,000; Furosemide; Isoetharine; Isoproterenol; Lidocaine-Bolus; Lidocaine Drip; Methylprednisone; Morphine; Naloxone; Nifedipine; Nitrostat. Tab.; Nitrous Oxide; Oxytocin; Phenobarbital; Sodium Bicarbonate; Thiamine; Verapamil; Other; HAZMAT

EKG INITIAL/LAST: Nrml Sinus; Sinus Tach; Sinus Brady; Asystole; AV Block; Atrial Fib; Atrial Flut; EMD; Junctional; Paced; SV Tach; Vent Tach; Vent Fib; Other; PVC's

IV TYPE/RATE: TKO; Bolus; Wide; Other; D5W; Normal Saline; Ringers Lact.; Other

LINES: # Peripheral; # Central

MEDICAL CONTROL: First; Hospital; Radio/Good; Radio/Poor; Protocol; Telephone; Radio/Phone Patch; Cellular; Phys On-Scene; None Required; Unable

ORDERS BY: Protocol; Standing; Verbal

PT. RECEIVED BY | RESEARCH CODE

PATIENT DISPOSITION: Improved; Worsened; Unchanged; Died in ER

MISCELLANEOUS: If Multiple Pts On Scene, How Many? 2 3 4 5 6 7 8 9+; If Transport to Level 1 Receiving Facility, Due to: Pt. Condition; Mechanism

PLEASE DO NOT MARK IN THIS AREA 2002094

EMS FIRST CARE FORM - ARIZONA DEPARTMENT OF HEALTH SERVICES Return to State EMS Office

SCANTRON® FORM NO. F-3087-EMS 0792-C 671-5 4 3 2 1

© 1992 EMS DATA SYSTEMS

FIGURE 11-3 This prehospital care report's format allows a computer to scan its information.

MEDICAL TERMINOLOGY

An essential component of good documentation is the appropriate use of medical terminology. Medical terms, though sometimes difficult to spell, transform your report into a universally accepted medical document. Learning the meanings and correct spellings of the medical terms that you use in your PCRs is essential. Misused or misspelled words reflect poorly on your professionalism and may confuse the report's readers.

If you do not know how to spell a word, look it up or use another word. Many EMT-Is carry pocket-size medical dictionaries in their ambulances for this purpose. Using plain English is acceptable when you do not know the appropriate medical term or its correct spelling. "Chest" is just as accurate as "thorax" and better than "thoracks." "Belly" is not as professional as "abdomen," but it is still better than "abodemin."

If you do not know how to spell a word, look it up or use another word.

ABBREVIATIONS AND ACRONYMS

Medical abbreviations and acronyms allow you to increase the amount of information you can write quickly on your report (Table 11-1 on pages that follow). They also pose problems, however, because they can have multiple meanings. For instance, their meanings can vary in different areas of medicine. Is "CP" chest pain, cardiovascular perfusion, or cerebral palsy? Is "CO" cardiac output or carbon monoxide? Is "BLS" basic life support or burns, lacerations, and swelling? These are all common abbreviations with more than one accepted meaning. Furthermore, many abbreviations are specific to one community. You must be familiar with those used in your local EMS system.

You must be familiar with the acronyms and abbreviations of your local EMS system.

Abbreviations and acronyms can cause considerable confusion when someone unfamiliar with the call reads your report. Health-care professionals who are not familiar with local customs or with emergency medicine might not understand them. One way to clarify the meaning of a new abbreviation or acronym is to write it out the first time you use it, followed by the abbreviation or acronym in parenthesis. After that, you can use the abbreviation alone throughout the report. The following examples illustrate how abbreviations and acronyms can shorten your narratives. In standard English the report might be written:

> The patient is a 54-year-old conscious and alert male who complains of sudden onset of chest pain and shortness of breath, which started 20 minutes ago. He has taken 2 nitroglycerin with no relief. He denies any nausea, vomiting, or dizziness. He has a past history of coronary artery disease, a heart attack 3 years ago, and high blood pressure. He takes nitroglycerin as needed, Procardia XL, hydrochlorothiazide, and potassium. He has no known drug allergies.

Using abbreviations and acronyms, the same report might be written:

> Pt. is 54 y/o CAO male c/o sudden onset CP/SOB × 20 min. Pt took NTG × 2 s̄ relief. Ø n/v, dizziness. PH: CAD, AMI × 3y, HTN. Meds: NTG prn, Procardia XL, HCTZ and K⁺; NKDA.

TIMES

Incident times are another important but perilous part of the PCR. The times you record on your PCR are considered the official times of the incident. For medical and legal purposes, you must ensure their accuracy.

The PCR typically has spaces for the time the call was received, the dispatch time, the time of arrival at the scene, time of departure from the scene, time of arrival at the hospital, and time back in service. Other time intervals are important, as well. The time you and your crew arrived at the patient's side is often very different from the time the ambulance arrived at the scene—when your patient is on the fourth floor of a building without an elevator, for example, or in a field several hundred yards from the road. Whatever the reason, document in your report any significant discrepancies between your arrival at the scene and your arrival at the patient. The times of vital signs assessment, medication administration, certain medical procedures as local protocols require, and changes in patient condition are also important and require accurate documentation.

Table 11-1 STANDARD CHARTING ABBREVIATIONS

Patient Information/Categories

Asian	A	Medications	Med
Black	B	Newborn	NB
Chief complaint	CC	Occupational history	OH
Complains of	c/o	Past history	PH
Current health status	CHS	Patient	Pt
Date of birth	DOB	Physical exam	PE
Differential diagnosis	DD	Private medical doctor	PMD
Estimated date of confinement	EDC	Review of systems	ROS
Family history	FH	Signs and symptoms	S/S
Female	♀	Social history	SH
Hispanic	H	Visual acuity	VA
History	Hx	Vital signs	VS
History and physical	H&P	Weight	Wt
History of present illness	HPI	White	W
Impression	IMP	Year-old	y/o
Male	♂		

Body Systems

Abdomen	Abd	Gynecological	GYN
Cardiovascular	CV	Head, eyes, ears, nose, and throat	HEENT
Central nervous system	CNS	Musculoskeletal	M/S
Ear, nose, and throat	ENT	Obstetrical	OB
Gastrointestinal	GI	Peripheral nervous system	PNS
Genitourinary	GU	Respiratory	Resp

Common Complaints

Abdominal pain	abd pn	Lower back pain	LBP
Chest pain	CP	Nausea/vomiting	n/v
Dyspnea on exertion	DOE	No apparent distress	NAD
Fever of unknown origin	FUO	Pain	pn
Gunshot wound	GSW	Shortness of breath	SOB
Headache	H/A	Substernal chest pain	sscp

Diagnoses

Abdominal aortic aneurysm	AAA	Insulin-dependent diabetes mellitus	IDDM
Abortion	Ab	Intracranial pressure	ICP
Acute myocardial infarction	AMI	Mass casualty incident	MCI
Adult respiratory distress syndrome	ARDS	Mitral valve prolapse	MVP
Alcohol	ETOH	Motor vehicle crash	MVC
Atherosclerotic heart disease	ASHD	Multiple sclerosis	MS
Chronic obstructive pulmonary disease	COPD	Non–insulin-dependent diabetes mellitus	NIDDM
Chronic renal failure	CRF	Organic brain syndrome	OBS
Congestive heart failure	CHF	Otitis media	OM
Coronary artery bypass graft	CABG	Overdose	OD
Coronary artery disease	CAD	Paroxysmal nocturnal dyspnea	PND
Cystic fibrosis	CF	Pelvic inflammatory disease	PID
Dead on arrival	DOA	Peptic ulcer disease	PUD
Delirium tremens	DTs	Pregnancies/births (gravida/para)	G/P
Deep vein thrombosis	DVT	Pregnancy-induced hypertension	PIH
Diabetes mellitus	DM	Pulmonary embolism	PE
Dilation and Curettage	D&C	Rheumatic heart disease	RHD
Duodenal ulcer	DU	Sexually transmitted disease	STD
End-stage renal failure	ESRF	Transient ischemic attack	TIA
Epstein-Barr virus	EBV	Tuberculosis	TB
Foreign body obstruction	FBO	Upper respiratory infection	URI
Hepatitis B virus	HBV	Urinary tract infection	UTI
Hiatal hernia	HH	Venereal disease	VD
Hypertension	HTN	Wolff-Parkinson-White syndrome (disease)	WPW
Infectious disease	ID		
Inferior wall myocardial infarction	IWMI		

Table 11-1 **STANDARD CHARTING ABBREVIATIONS** (continued)

Medications

Angiotensin-converting enzyme	ACE	Lactated Ringer's, Ringer's Lactate	LR, RL
Aspirin	ASA	Magnesium sulfate	Mg^{++}
Bicarbonate	HCO_3^-	Morphine sulfate	MS
Birth control pills	BCP	Nitroglycerin	NTG
Calcium	Ca^{++}	Nonsteroidal antiflammatory agent	NSAID
Calcium channel blocker	CCB	Normal saline	NS
Calcium chloride	$CaCl_2$	Penicillin	PCN
Chloride	Cl^-	Phenobarbital	PB
Digoxin	Dig	Potassium	K^+
Dilantin (phenytoin sodium)	DPH	Sodium bicarbonate	$NaHCO_3$
Diphendydramine	DPHM	Sodium chloride	NaCl
Diphtheria-pertussis-tetanus	DPT	Tylenol	APAP
Hydrochlorothiazide	HCTZ		

Anatomy/Landmarks

Abdomen	Abd	Lymph node	LN
Antecubital	AC	Medial collateral ligament	MCL
Anterior axillary line	AAL	Metacarpalphalangeal (joint)	MCP
Anterior cruciate ligament	ACL	Metatarsalphalangeal (joint)	MTP
Anterior-posterior	A/P	Midaxillary line	MAL
Distal interphalangeal (joint)	DIP	Posterior axillary line	PAL
Dorsalis pedis (pulse)	DP	Posterior cruciate ligament	PCL
Gallbladder	GB	Proximal interphalangeal (joint)	PIP
Intercostal space	ICS	Right lower lobe	RLL
Lateral collateral ligament	LCL	Right lower quadrant	RLQ
Left lower lobe	LLL	Right middle lobe	RML
Left lower quadrant	LLQ	Right upper lobe	RUL
Left upper lobe	LUL	Right upper quadrant	RUQ
Left upper quadrant	LUQ	Temporomandibular joint	TMJ
Left ventricle	LV	Tympanic membrane	TM
Liver, spleen, and kidneys	LSK		

Physical Exam/Findings

Arterial blood gas	ABG	Hemoglobin	Hgb
Bilateral breath sounds	BBS	Inspiratory	Insp
Blood sugar	BS	Jugular venous distention	JVD
Breath sounds	BS	Laceration	lac
Cardiac injury profile	CIP	Level of consciousness	LOC
Central venous pressure	CVP	Moves all extremities (well)	MAEW
Cerebrospinal fluid	CSF	Nontender	NT
Chest X-ray	CXR	Normal range of motion	NROM
Complete blood count	CBC	Palpation	Palp
Computerized tomography	CT	Passive range of motion	PROM
Conscious, alert, and oriented	CAO	Point of maximal impulse	PMI
Costovertebral angle	CVA	Posterior tibial (pulse)	PT
Deep tendon reflexes	DTR	Pulse	P
Dorsalis pedis (pulse)	DP	Pupils equal and reactive to light	PEARL
Electrocardiogram	EKG, ECG	Pupils equal, round, reactive to light	
Electroencephalogram	EEG	and accomodation	PERRLA
Expiratory	Exp	Range of motion	ROM
Extraocular movements (intact)	EOMI	Respirations	R
Fetal heart tones	FHT	Tactile vocal fremitus	TVF
Full range of motion	FROM	Temperature	T
Full-term normal delivery	FTND	Unconscious	unc
Heart rate	HR	Urinary incontinence	UI
Heart sounds	HS		
Heel-to-shin (cerebellar test)	H→S		

(continued)

Table 11-1 | STANDARD CHARTING ABBREVIATIONS (continued)

Miscellaneous Descriptors

After (post-)	p̄	Not applicable	n/a
After eating	pc	Number	No or #
Alert and oriented	A/O	Occasional	occ
Anterior	ant.	Pack years	pk/yrs, p/y
Approximate	≈	Per	/
As needed	prn	Positive	+
Before (ante-)	ā	Posterior	post.
Before eating (*ante cibum,* before meal)	a.c.	Postoperative	PO
Body surface area (%)	BSA	Prior to arrival	PTA
Celsius	°C	Radiates to	→
Change	Δ	Right	Ⓡ
Decreased	↓	Rule out	R/O
Equal	=	Secondary to	2°
Fahrenheit	°F	Superior	sup.
Immediately	stat	Times (for 3 hours)	× (×3h)
Increased	↑	Unequal	≠
Inferior	inf.	Warm and dry	W/D
Left	Ⓛ	While awake	WA
Less than	<	With (*cum*)	c̄
Moderate	mod.	Without (*sine*)	s̄
More than	>	Zero	0
Negative	−		
No, not, none	∅		

Treatments/Dispositions

Advanced cardiac life support	ACLS	Nasogastric	NG
Advanced life support	ALS	Nasopharyngeal airway	NPA
Against medical advice	AMA	No transport—refusal	NTR
Automated external defibrillator	AED	Nonrebreather mask	NRM
Bag-valve mask	BVM	Nothing by mouth	NPO
Basic life support	BLS	Occupational therapy	OT
Cardiopulmonary resuscitation	CPR	Oropharyngeal airway	OPA
Carotid sinus massage	CSM	Oxygen	O₂
Continuous positive airway pressure	CPAP	Per square inch	psi
Do not resuscitate	DNR	Physical therapy	PT
Endotracheal tube	ETT	Positive end-expiratory pressure	PEEP
Estimated time of arrival	ETA	Short spine board	SSB
External cardiac pacing	ECP	Therapy	Rx
Intermittent positive-pressure ventilation	IPPV	Treatment	Tx
Long spine board	LSB	Turned over to	TOT
Nasal cannula	NC	Verbal order	VO

Medication Administration/Metrics

Centimeter	cm	Keep vein open	KVO
Cubic centimeter	cc	Kilogram	kg
Deciliter	dL	Liter	L
Drop(s)	gtt(s)	Liters per minute	LPM, L/min
Drops per minute	gtts/min	Microgram	mcg
Every	q	Milliequivalent	mEq
Grain	gr	Milligram	mg
Gram	g, gm	Milliliter	mL
Hour	h, hr, or °	Millimeter	mm
Hydrogen-ion concentration	pH	Millimeters of mercury	mmHg
Intracardiac	IC	Minute	min
Intramuscular	IM	Orally	po
Intraosseous	IO	Subcutaneous	SC, SQ
Intravenous	IV	Sublingual	SL
Intravenous push	IVP	To keep open	TKO
Joules	j		

Table 11-1 STANDARD CHARTING ABBREVIATIONS (continued)

Cardiology

Atrial fibrillation	AF	Paroxsysmal atrial tachycardia	PAT
Atrial tachycardia	AT	Paroxsysmal supraventricular tachycardia	PSVT
Atrioventricular	AV	Premature atrial contraction	PAC
Bundle branch block	BBB	Premature junctional contraction	PJC
Complete heart block	CHB	Premature ventricular contraction	PVC
Electromechanical dissociation	EMD	Pulseless electrical activity	PEA
Idioventricular rhythm	IVR	Supraventricular tachycardia	SVT
Junctional rhythm	JR	Ventricular fibrillation	VF
Modified chest lead	MCL	Ventricular tachycardia	VT
Normal sinus rhythm	NSR	Wandering atrial pacemaker	WAP

One common problem with documenting times is inconsistencies among the dispatch center clock, the ambulance clock, and your watch. Imagine a report that documents that the ambulance arrived on scene at 20:32 according to the dispatch time, that CPR was started at 20:29 according to your watch, and the first defibrillation was administered at 20:43 according to the defibrillator's internal clock. Although we may recognize this phenomenon and tend to discount the accuracy of the recorded times, they are nonetheless the official, legal times. So, whenever possible record all times from the same clock. When that is not possible, be sure that all the clocks and watches you use are synchronized. If they cannot be synchronized and the documented times seem to conflict with each other, explain this in your narrative. A simple statement such as, "All time intervals on the scene were documented using my watch, all other times are those reported by the dispatch center," will suffice.

Whenever possible, record all times from the same clock.

COMMUNICATIONS

Your communications with the hospital are another important item to document. Though your system may make voice recordings of those communications, the recordings are usually not kept indefinitely. Again, the PCR will likely be the only permanent record of your discussion with the medical direction physician. Specifically, you should document any medical advice or orders you receive and the results of implementing that advice and those orders. In some situations you might need to document what you reported to the physician and/or discussed with him, so the reader will be able to understand the decision-making process. Finally, always document the physician's name on your PCR and, if possible, have him sign it to verify your treatments.

Document any medical advice or orders you receive and the results of implementing that advice and those orders.

PERTINENT FINDINGS AND NEGATIVES

The patient assessment and medical interventions are the essence of the EMS event and become the core of your PCR. We will discuss specific approaches to documenting assessment and interventions later in this chapter, but some general rules apply regardless of the method.

Document all findings of your assessment, even those that are normal. Although the positive findings are usually of most interest, some negative findings—known as pertinent negatives—are also important. For example, if your respiratory distress patient does not have swollen ankles or crackles, that helps rule out a field diagnosis of congestive heart failure. If he does, that helps rule it in. If your patient with a broken leg cannot feel or move his foot, it suggests he may have a serious neurologic injury. If his has motor and sensory function, it suggests that he doesn't have a neurologic problem. You should include such information in your report.

Document all findings of your assessment, even those that are normal.

The pertinent findings and negatives vary for each chief complaint. In general, if a positive assessment finding for any given chief complaint would be important, a negative finding also is pertinent. Even though negative findings do not warrant medical care or intervention, your seeking them demonstrates the thoroughness of your examination and history of the event.

ORAL STATEMENTS

Also essential to every PCR, regardless of approach, are the statements of witnesses, bystanders, and your patient. They help document the mechanism of injury, your patient's behavior, the events leading up to the emergency, and any first aid or medical care others rendered before you arrived. They also may include information regarding the disposition of personal items such as wallets or purses. At crime scenes, document safety-related information such as weapons disposition. Your PCR may be the only written report of what happened to a murder weapon. Other details such as where you first saw a victim, what position he was in, and the time you arrived on the scene may be crucial evidence someday in a criminal proceeding.

Whenever possible, quote the patient—or other source of information—directly. Clearly identify the quotation with quotation marks, and identify its source. For example:

> Bystanders state the patient was "acting bizarre and threatening to jump in front of the next passing car."

ADDITIONAL RESOURCES

Document all of the resources involved in the event. If an air-medical service transported your patient, your documentation should include your assessment and all interventions up to the point when you transferred care. Identify the air-medical service and your patient's ultimate destination, if you know it. If other EMS, fire, rescue/extrication, or law enforcement agencies were involved in the call, document their roles. This can be particularly important in mutual aid calls, when many different agencies cooperate in your patient's care. Also include personnel from the coroner's or medical examiner's office for dead-on-arrival (DOA) scenes.

If a physician stops to help, identify him by name and document his qualifying credentials. If one of your medical direction physicians is on the scene and directs care, document his activities. Likewise document the names, credentials, and activities of any other medically qualified personnel present who offer to help. Your clinical experience and local protocols will determine how you integrate qualified health-care workers into your emergency scene. Document that integration carefully.

ELEMENTS OF GOOD DOCUMENTATION

A well-written PCR is accurate, legible, timely, unaltered, and professional. Each of these traits is essential.

COMPLETENESS AND ACCURACY

The accurate PCR should be precise but comprehensive. Include all of the relevant information that anyone might be expected to want later, and exclude superfluous information. For example, if your patient's foot was run over by a lawn mower, reporting that his great toe on that foot had been amputated six years ago would be important; documenting that he had his tonsils removed when he was three years old probably would not. That you applied direct pressure to the bleeding foot is pertinent; that the lawn mower was a John Deere model 6354 is not.

Many PCRs provide check boxes and a space for written narratives (Figure 11-4). You should complete both the narrative and check-box sections of every PCR. All check-box sections of a document must show that you attended to them, even if you did not use a given section on a call. The check boxes can help ensure that routine, common information is recorded for every call, but no PCR has a check box for every possible chief complaint, assessment finding, or intervention.

The narrative is the core of the documentation. Even if you document something in a check box, repeating that information in the narrative might be worthwhile. By doing so, you can expand on the yes-or-no limitations of the check box to explain the timing, the assessment findings, the circumstances, or the changes in patient condition associated with the indicated action.

Remember that proper spelling, approved abbreviations, and proper acronyms also affect your PCR's accuracy. Misspelled words lose their meaning, many abbreviations are not

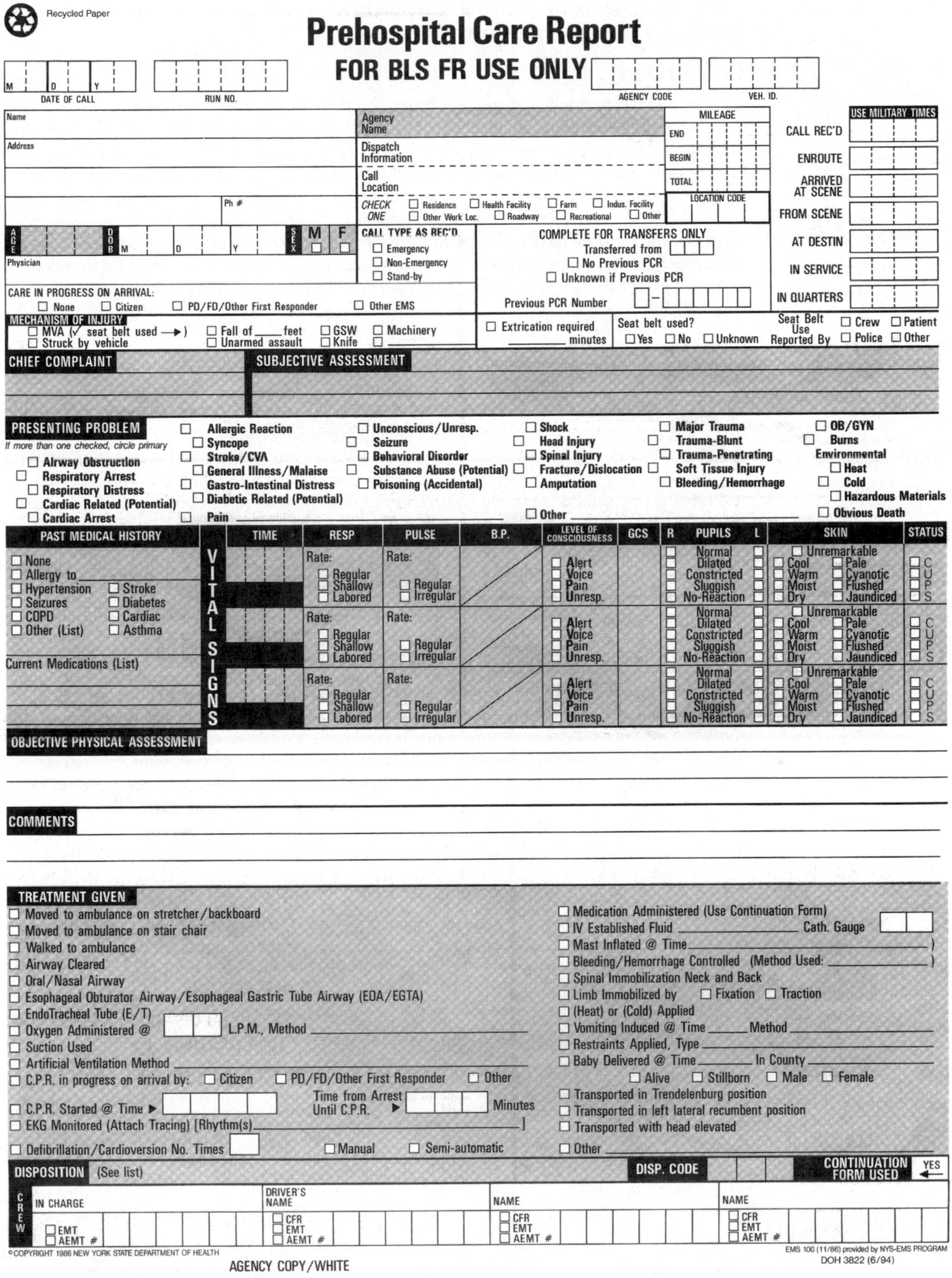

Recycled Paper

Prehospital Care Report

FOR BLS FR USE ONLY

M D Y DATE OF CALL | RUN NO. | AGENCY CODE | VEH. ID.

Name | Agency Name | MILEAGE: END / BEGIN / TOTAL | USE MILITARY TIMES: CALL REC'D / ENROUTE / ARRIVED AT SCENE / FROM SCENE / AT DESTIN / IN SERVICE / IN QUARTERS

Address | Dispatch Information

Call Location

Ph #

CHECK ONE ☐ Residence ☐ Health Facility ☐ Farm ☐ Indus. Facility ☐ Other Work Loc. ☐ Roadway ☐ Recreational ☐ Other | LOCATION CODE

AGE | DOB M D Y | SEX M ☐ F ☐

CALL TYPE AS REC'D ☐ Emergency ☐ Non-Emergency ☐ Stand-by

COMPLETE FOR TRANSFERS ONLY: Transferred from ☐ No Previous PCR ☐ Unknown if Previous PCR; Previous PCR Number

Physician

CARE IN PROGRESS ON ARRIVAL: ☐ None ☐ Citizen ☐ PD/FD/Other First Responder ☐ Other EMS

MECHANISM OF INJURY: ☐ MVA (✓ seat belt used →) ☐ Struck by vehicle ☐ Fall of ___ feet ☐ Unarmed assault ☐ GSW ☐ Knife ☐ Machinery ☐ ___

☐ Extrication required ___ minutes | Seat belt used? ☐ Yes ☐ No ☐ Unknown | Seat Belt Use Reported By ☐ Crew ☐ Patient ☐ Police ☐ Other

CHIEF COMPLAINT | SUBJECTIVE ASSESSMENT

PRESENTING PROBLEM (*If more than one checked, circle primary*): ☐ Airway Obstruction ☐ Respiratory Arrest ☐ Respiratory Distress ☐ Cardiac Related (Potential) ☐ Cardiac Arrest ☐ Allergic Reaction ☐ Syncope ☐ Stroke/CVA ☐ General Illness/Malaise ☐ Gastro-Intestinal Distress ☐ Diabetic Related (Potential) ☐ Pain ___ ☐ Unconscious/Unresp. ☐ Seizure ☐ Behavioral Disorder ☐ Substance Abuse (Potential) ☐ Poisoning (Accidental) ☐ Shock ☐ Head Injury ☐ Spinal Injury ☐ Fracture/Dislocation ☐ Amputation ☐ Other ___ ☐ Major Trauma ☐ Trauma-Blunt ☐ Trauma-Penetrating ☐ Soft Tissue Injury ☐ Bleeding/Hemorrhage ☐ OB/GYN ☐ Burns Environmental ☐ Heat ☐ Cold ☐ Hazardous Materials ☐ Obvious Death

PAST MEDICAL HISTORY: ☐ None ☐ Allergy to ___ ☐ Hypertension ☐ Seizures ☐ COPD ☐ Other (List) ☐ Stroke ☐ Diabetes ☐ Cardiac ☐ Asthma

Current Medications (List)

VITAL SIGNS	TIME	RESP	PULSE	B.P.	LEVEL OF CONSCIOUSNESS	GCS	R PUPILS L	SKIN	STATUS
		Rate: ☐ Regular ☐ Shallow ☐ Labored	Rate: ☐ Regular ☐ Irregular		☐ Alert ☐ Voice ☐ Pain ☐ Unresp.		☐ Normal ☐ Dilated ☐ Constricted ☐ Sluggish ☐ No-Reaction	☐ Unremarkable ☐ Cool ☐ Warm ☐ Moist ☐ Dry ☐ Pale ☐ Cyanotic ☐ Flushed ☐ Jaundiced	☐ C ☐ U ☐ P ☐ S
		Rate: ☐ Regular ☐ Shallow ☐ Labored	Rate: ☐ Regular ☐ Irregular		☐ Alert ☐ Voice ☐ Pain ☐ Unresp.		☐ Normal ☐ Dilated ☐ Constricted ☐ Sluggish ☐ No-Reaction	☐ Unremarkable ☐ Cool ☐ Warm ☐ Moist ☐ Dry ☐ Pale ☐ Cyanotic ☐ Flushed ☐ Jaundiced	☐ C ☐ U ☐ P ☐ S
		Rate: ☐ Regular ☐ Shallow ☐ Labored	Rate: ☐ Regular ☐ Irregular		☐ Alert ☐ Voice ☐ Pain ☐ Unresp.		☐ Normal ☐ Dilated ☐ Constricted ☐ Sluggish ☐ No-Reaction	☐ Unremarkable ☐ Cool ☐ Warm ☐ Moist ☐ Dry ☐ Pale ☐ Cyanotic ☐ Flushed ☐ Jaundiced	☐ C ☐ U ☐ P ☐ S

OBJECTIVE PHYSICAL ASSESSMENT

COMMENTS

TREATMENT GIVEN

☐ Moved to ambulance on stretcher/backboard
☐ Moved to ambulance on stair chair
☐ Walked to ambulance
☐ Airway Cleared
☐ Oral/Nasal Airway
☐ Esophageal Obturator Airway/Esophageal Gastric Tube Airway (EOA/EGTA)
☐ EndoTracheal Tube (E/T)
☐ Oxygen Administered @ ___ L.P.M., Method ___
☐ Suction Used
☐ Artificial Ventilation Method ___
☐ C.P.R. in progress on arrival by: ☐ Citizen ☐ PD/FD/Other First Responder ☐ Other
☐ C.P.R. Started @ Time ▶ ___ Time from Arrest Until C.P.R. ▶ ___ Minutes
☐ EKG Monitored (Attach Tracing) [Rhythm(s) ___]
☐ Defibrillation/Cardioversion No. Times ___ ☐ Manual ☐ Semi-automatic
☐ Medication Administered (Use Continuation Form)
☐ IV Established Fluid ___ Cath. Gauge
☐ Mast Inflated @ Time ___)
☐ Bleeding/Hemorrhage Controlled (Method Used: ___)
☐ Spinal Immobilization Neck and Back
☐ Limb Immobilized by ☐ Fixation ☐ Traction
☐ (Heat) or (Cold) Applied
☐ Vomiting Induced @ Time ___ Method ___
☐ Restraints Applied, Type ___
☐ Baby Delivered @ Time ___ In County ___ ☐ Alive ☐ Stillborn ☐ Male ☐ Female
☐ Transported in Trendelenburg position
☐ Transported in left lateral recumbent position
☐ Transported with head elevated
☐ Other ___

DISPOSITION (See list) | DISP. CODE | CONTINUATION FORM USED YES

CREW: IN CHARGE ☐ EMT ☐ AEMT # | DRIVER'S NAME ☐ CFR ☐ EMT ☐ AEMT # | NAME ☐ CFR ☐ EMT ☐ AEMT # | NAME ☐ CFR ☐ EMT ☐ AEMT #

©COPYRIGHT 1986 NEW YORK STATE DEPARTMENT OF HEALTH

EMS 100 (11/86) provided by NYS-EMS PROGRAM DOH 3822 (6/94)

AGENCY COPY/WHITE

FIGURE 11-4 Complete both the narrative and check-box sections of every PCR.

universally recognized, and several acronyms have more than one meaning. Make sure that the meaning of any abbreviation or acronym is clear.

LEGIBILITY

Your handwriting must be neat enough so that other people can read and understand the report.

Poor penmanship and illegible reports lead to poor documentation. Some EMS providers say, "I wrote it, and I can read it. That's all that matters." This is simply not true. The PCR does not exist solely for its author's reference. It is a permanent record that many different people use. Your handwriting must be neat enough that other people can read and understand the report, especially the narrative. It must also be neat enough that you can read and understand it yourself many years from now, long after the event has faded from your memory. Your writing must be heavy enough to transfer to any carbon copies. Using a ball-point pen whenever possible makes carbon copies more legible and makes it difficult for someone to tamper with the document. Clearly mark the check boxes to eliminate any doubt that a check mark is not just a meaningless scratch. Always remember that other members of the health-care team may use the report for medical information, research, or quality improvement.

TIMELINESS

Ideally, you should complete your report immediately after you complete the emergency call.

As a rule, you should avoid writing your report in the ambulance during transport of your patient for two reasons. First, the bumpy ride makes it difficult to write neatly. More importantly, your time is better spent communicating with your patient and conducting ongoing assessments. Most hospitals have an area where you can sit and complete your paperwork.

Ideally, you should complete your report immediately after you complete the emergency call, when the information is fresh in your mind and you can check with your partner or patient if you have any questions about the events. At times you may be too busy to complete the entire documentation immediately following a call. If so, make notes on scratch paper and write enough of the report that you will be able to finish it completely and accurately later. The sooner you finish it, the more details you are likely to recall and the better the report will be.

Never try to hide an error.

ABSENCE OF ALTERATIONS

Mistakes happen. During a busy shift or in the middle of the night you will check the wrong box, misspell a word, or omit important information. You will be thinking of one medication and write another's name on your report. If you make a mistake writing your report, simply cross through the error with one line and initial it (Figure 11-5). Some systems may expect you to date the correction, as well. Do not scribble over or blacken out any area of the call report. Never try to hide an error. Such foolish tactics only raise the reader's curiosity about what you wrote originally. After crossing out the error, continue with the correct information. If you find the error after you've already written several more sentences, submit an **addendum.**

addendum addition or supplement to the original report.

Whenever possible, have everyone involved in the call read or reread the PCR before you submit it. Make all corrections before you submit the report to the hospital or to the EMS administrative offices. Do not make changes on the original report after you have submitted it. If for any reason you need to make corrections after you have submitted the report, or some portion of it, place an addendum. Simply note on the original report, "See addendum," and attach the addendum to the original report. Write the addendum on a separate sheet of paper or on an official form if one exists. Likewise, if more information comes to your attention after you have submitted the report, write a supplemental narrative on a separate report form.

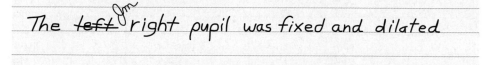

FIGURE 11-5 The proper way to correct a prehospital care report is to draw a single line through the error, write the correct information beside it, and initial the change.

Write any addendum to your report as soon as you realize that you made an error or that additional information is needed. Note the purpose of the revision and why the information did not appear on your original report. The addendum should document the date and time that it was written, the reason it was written, and the pertinent information. Only the original author of a report should attach an addendum, as it is part of the official call record. Agencies should have separate forms for other EMS personnel, supervisors, or citizens who, for some reason, want to contribute to the documentation.

PROFESSIONALISM

Write your report in a professional manner. Remember that someday it may be scrutinized by hospital staff, quality improvement committees, supervisors, lawyers, and the news media. Your patient's family may request, and is entitled to, a copy of your report from your agency. Write cautiously and avoid any remarks that might be construed as derogatory. **Jargon** can be confusing and does little to enhance your image. Do not describe a patient well known to EMS providers as a "frequent flyer." Never include slang, biased statements, or irrelevant opinions. Include only objective information. "The patient smelled of beer and had slurred speech and difficulty walking" are factual statements. "The patient was very drunk" is an inference; even if accurate, it is still just your opinion. **Libel** and **slander** are, respectively, writing or speaking false and malicious words intended to damage a person's character. Always write and speak carefully. A seemingly innocent phrase or comment can come back to haunt you.

> *Write cautiously and avoid any remarks that might be construed as derogatory.*

jargon language used by a particular group or profession.

libel writing false and malicious words intended to damage a person's character.

slander speaking false and malicious words intended to damage a person's character.

NARRATIVE WRITING

The narrative is the part of the written report in which you depict the call at length. Less structured than the check-box or fill-in sections of your report, the narrative allows you the freedom to describe your assessment findings in detail. When other people read your report, they usually will rely on your written narrative for the most relevant information. For example, as you transfer care to the emergency department nurse, she will usually scan your PCR for information concerning your patient's history, vital signs, and physical exam.

NARRATIVE SECTIONS

Any patient documentation includes three sections of importance—the subjective narrative, the objective narrative, and the assessment/management plan.

Subjective Narrative

The subjective part of your narrative typically contains any information that you elicit during your patient's history. This includes the chief complaint (CC), the history of present illness (HPI), the past history (PH), the current health status (CHS), and the review of systems (ROS). In trauma, this also includes the mechanism of injury, as told to you by your patient or bystanders. The following is a typical subjective narrative on a patient complaining of shortness of breath:

CC: The patient is a 74-year-old conscious black female who complains, "I can't catch my breath."

HPI: Gradual onset of severe shortness of breath for the past 3 hours; began while sitting in living room watching television; nothing provokes or relieves the dyspnea; her son states this is worse than usual for her. She has had a 3-day history of some vague chest discomfort. She denies any chest pressure, nausea, or dizziness.

PH: She has a 5-year history of heart problems and congestive heart failure; hospitalized for this problem 3 times in the past 5 years; no surgeries.

CHS: Meds: Isosorbide, nitroglycerin, furosemide, digoxin, potassium; No known drug allergies; 50 pack/year smoker; non-drinker; non-drug abuser.

ROS: Resp: Unproductive cough for 1 day; audible wheezing; no hx of COPD or asthma; last chest X-ray 1 year ago. Card: no palpitations, pressure, or pain; + orthopnea; + paroxysmal nocturnal dyspnea; + edema for past few days; past ECG 1 year ago. GU: No changes in urinary patterns. Per. Vasc: + pitting edema for few days; cold feet.

Objective Narrative

The objective part of your narrative usually includes your general impression and any data that you derive through inspection, palpation, auscultation, percussion, and diagnostic testing. This includes vital signs, physical exam, and tests such as cardiac monitoring, pulse oximetry, and blood glucose determination.

To document your physical exam you can use either of two approaches—head-to-toe or body systems. Although the medical community accepts both extensively, EMS more often uses the head-to-toe approach.

Head-to-Toe   The head-to-toe approach is well suited for any call when you perform an entire physical exam, because you document your findings in the same order that you conducted the exam—from head-to-toe. Remember that even though you may have conducted your pediatric assessment from toe-to-head, you should document it in head-to-toe order. This style encourages you to be systematic and thorough. It is appropriate for major trauma and serious medical emergencies, when you examine every body area and system. Include all circulatory and neurological findings within the body area you are documenting. For example, when recording findings in the extremities, include distal neurovascular function. When documenting the head, include the results of cranial nerve testing. The following illustrates the head-to-toe approach for a patient from an automobile collision:

General:	The patient presents in the front seat of the car, in moderate distress with bruises to his forehead and some facial lacerations. Pt. is alert and oriented to self, time, and place.
Vital signs:	Pulse—100 strong, regular radial; BP—110/88; Resp—24 non-labored; skin pale and cool.
HEENT:	Depression to right frontal bone, minor bleeding controlled prior to arrival; no drainage from ears, nose. No periorbital ecchymosis or Battle's sign; pupils equal and reactive to light; extraocular movements intact, cranial nerves II—XII intact.
Neck:	Trachea midline; no jugular vein distention; 1 cervical spine tenderness.
Chest:	Equal expansion; bruises across the chest wall; no deformities; equal bilateral breath sounds.
Abdomen:	Soft, non-tender.
Pelvis:	Unstable pelvic ring; pain upon palpation.
Extremities:	+ Circulation, sensory, and motor function in all four extremities; no deformities noted.
Posterior:	No injuries noted.
Labs:	Sinus tachycardia no ectopy, pulse oximetry 97% on supplemental oxygen.

Body Systems   The body systems approach focuses on body systems instead of body areas. It is best suited to screening and preadmission exams in which you conduct a comprehensive exam involving all body systems. Each body system has different key components that you should assess and document.

When you use the body systems approach in emergency medicine, you usually will focus only on the system, or systems, involved in the current illness or injury. For example, a patient having an asthma attack would require an in-depth evaluation of the respiratory system. Another patient with lower abdominal pain would need a close examination of the gastrointestinal system. Neither patient would require a full head-to-toe physical exam but, instead, intensive documentation of the affected body system or systems. The body systems approach can be one of the most comprehensive approaches to documentation.

The following illustrates a body systems approach for a patient with chest pain and shortness of breath:

General:	Patient is a healthy-looking female who presents sitting upright in her chair, able to speak in phrases only.
Vital Signs:	Pulse—90; BP—170/80; Resp—28 labored; skin—warm and diaphoretic
HEENT:	+ Lip cyanosis and pursing; some nasal flaring; pink, frothy sputum; jugular veins distended.
Respiratory:	Good respiratory effort; accessory neck muscle use; trachea midline; + intercostal, supraclavicular, suprasternal retractions; = chest expansion; diffuse crackles and wheezing in all lung fields, decreased breath sounds.
Per. Vasc.:	+ Ascites fluid wave; + 2 pitting edema in lower extremities; strong peripheral pulses.
Labs:	Sinus tachycardia with occasional unifocal premature ventricular contractions. Pulse oximetry—92% room air; 97% on supplemental oxygen.

Assessment/Management

In the assessment/management section, you document what you believe is your patient's problem. This is also known as your **field diagnosis,** or impression. For example, your field diagnosis for a patient with chest pain may be "possible angina or rule/out myocardial infarction." You do not have to make an exact diagnosis. When you are not sure, simply document what you suspect is the general problem. Sometimes, for instance, your field impression might be "rule out acute abdomen, or seizures." *Rule out* identifies possible diagnoses that you believe the emergency physician should evaluate.

field diagnosis what you believe is your patient's problem, based on your history and physical exam.

Record your complete management plan from start to finish. This includes how you packaged and moved your patient to the ambulance. Did you carry him on a stair-chair or on a backboard fully immobilized or did he walk? List any interventions you completed before contacting your medical control physician. For example, did you control bleeding with direct pressure? Did you start an IV? Then describe any orders from the medical control physician, and always include his name. Describe how you transported your patient and the effects of any interventions such as drug administration or other invasive procedures. Include the results of ongoing assessments and any changes in your patient's condition. Finally, describe your patient's condition when you transferred care to the emergency department staff. The following example is a management plan for a trauma patient with a pelvic fracture whose condition deteriorates en route to the hospital.

Record your complete management plan from start to finish.

On-Scene	
Extrication:	Rapid extrication from vehicle, placed supine on backboard
Airway:	Airway cleared with suctioning, nasopharyngeal airway inserted
Breathing:	Oxygen @ 15 liters/min via nonrebreather mask
Circulation:	Foot of stretcher raised 30°; bleeding from arm laceration controlled with dry sterile dressing and direct pressure; PASG applied; IV—16 ga., left antecubital area—normal saline run KVO per Dr. Johnson.

Transport

Transported by ground ambulance to University Hospital with full body immobilization supine on long spine board; ETA 10 minutes.

Ongoing: Patient becomes restless and anxious; VS: pulse—120 weak carotid only; BP—50 palpated; Resp—28; skin: cool, pale, clammy with some mottling; PASG inflated; initial IV run wide open; second IV 16 ga. right antecubital normal saline—run wide open.

Arrival

Patient transferred to ED staff restless; VS: pulse—120; BP—80 palpated; Resp—26; skin—mottled and cool.

GENERAL FORMATS

The mnemonics SOAP and CHART identify two common patterns for organizing a narrative report. These acronyms provide templates for most medical and trauma reports. They help you to arrange your history, physical exam, and management plan into a logical, readable structure. They are widely used because they group information in categories that differentiate between subjective and objective information. For example, someone wanting only to determine your patient's medications can find that list easily in either the SOAP or CHART format. Either pattern is acceptable and effective when used consistently.

SOAP

SOAP stands for *S*ubjective, *O*bjective, *A*ssessment, and *P*lan. The detailed SOAP format includes:

Subjective:
- Chief complaint
- History of present illness
- Past history
- Current health status
- Family history
- Psychosocial history
- Review of systems

Objective:
- Vital signs
- General impression
- Physical exam
- Diagnostic tests

Assessment:
- Field diagnosis

Plan:
- Standing orders
- Physician orders
- Effects of interventions
- Mode of transportation
- Ongoing assessment

Chart

CHART stands for *C*hief complaint, *H*istory, *A*ssessment, *R*x (treatment), and *T*ransport. The detailed CHART format includes:

Chief Complaint

History:
- History of present illness
- Past history
- Current health status
- Review of systems

Assessment:
- Vital signs
- General impression

Content Review

NARRATIVE FORMATS
- SOAP
- CHART
- Patient management
- Call incident

Content Review

SOAP
- *S*ubjective
- *O*bjective
- *A*ssessment
- *P*lan

Content Review

CHART
- *C*hief complaint
- *H*istory
- *A*ssessment
- *R*x (treatment)
- *T*ransport

- Physical exam
- Diagnostic tests
- Field diagnosis

Rx:
- Standing orders
- Physician orders

Transport:
- Effects of interventions
- Mode of transportation
- Ongoing assessment

Other Formats

Like patient assessment itself, documentation is not "one-size-fits-all." No one narrative format is ideal for all situations. Two additional formats—patient management and call incident—are appropriate in certain circumstances.

No single narrative format is ideal for all situations.

Patient Management   The patient management format is preferred for some critical patients, such as those in cardiac arrest, when you focus on immediately managing a variety of patient problems and not on conducting a thorough history and physical exam. This format is a chronological account from the time you arrived on the scene until you transferred care to someone else. It emphasizes your assessment and management of the conditions you found. Simply begin your chart with a description of the event and any other pertinent information and then document your management, starting with your airway, breathing, and circulation (ABCs) assessment. Record everything in real time and in absolute chronological order, and always include the results of your interventions. A patient management chart would look like this:

Use the patient management format for critical patients when you focus on immediately managing a variety of patient problems.

Patient is an 89-year-old Hispanic male who was found by his wife unconscious on the floor immediately after collapsing. He presents pulseless and apneic.

Time	Intervention
1320	Airway cleared with suctioning; quick look—ventricular fibrillation.
1321	Defibrillation @ 200, 300, 360 joules—no change.
1322	CPR begun; oropharyngeal airway inserted, ventilation with BVM @ 12/min with supplemental oxygen.
1324	IV 18-gauge left antecubital area—normal saline KVO; epinephrine 1:10,000 1 mg IVP.
1325	Defibrillation @ 360 joules—no change; lidocaine 100 mg IVP.
1327	Defibrillation @ 360 joules—patient converts to normal sinus rhythm rate of 72 with strong peripheral pulses; BP—110/76, no spontaneous respirations. ET tube inserted. + lung sounds bilaterally with BVM.
1328	Ventilation continued @ 12/min via BVM; lidocaine infusion 2 mg/min.
1332	Patient transferred to ambulance on stretcher—transported to University Hospital.
1335	Patient has spontaneous respirations @ 20/min, + bilateral breath sounds; becoming more awake; HR—72; BP—120/76.
1340	Arrived at UH—Patient is conscious, alert, and oriented with retrograde amnesia.

Call Incident   The call incident approach simply emphasizes the mechanism of injury, the surrounding circumstances, and how the incident occurred. Use this approach to begin documenting a trauma call with a significant mechanism of injury. It is most suitable when the events surrounding the call might be significant. It would be inappropriate for a man sitting in his living room with chest pain or for someone who simply cut his finger with a carving knife. You may use this style in both the subjective and objective sections of your PCR. The following example shows call incident documentation for a motor-vehicle crash:

Use the call incident approach to begin documenting a trauma call with a significant mechanism of injury.

Subjective: The patient is a 46-year-old conscious and alert white male who was an unrestrained driver in a low-speed, head-on, two-car motor-vehicle crash, moderate front-end damage, no passenger compartment intrusion, deformity to windshield, dashboard, and steering wheel. Patient states he "reached for cigarette on floor and when he looked up, there was another vehicle in front of him." He denies any loss of consciousness and can recall all details prior to and immediately following the crash. Patient complains of pain to the head, neck, chest, and hip from being thrown against the dashboard and windshield.

Objective: The patient presents in the front seat of the car, appears in moderate distress with bruises to his forehead, facial lacerations, and a deformed left leg. His left leg is pinned underneath the dashboard with his left foot hooked around the brake pedal. Upon arrival, fire department rescue personnel were holding manual stabilization of his head and neck and stabilizing the vehicle.

These are not the only systems of documentation. Indeed, you may use some combination of these systems or develop a unique format for your regional system. The important thing is for your documentation to be complete, accurate, and consistent. By using the same system to document every call, you will be less likely to accidentally overlook or omit something.

SPECIAL CONSIDERATIONS

Some circumstances create special problems for EMS documentation. Patient refusals, calls where transport is unnecessary, multiple patients, and mass casualties are among the more common examples. In these and other unusual circumstances, take extra care to document everything that happened during the call.

PATIENT REFUSALS

Patients retain the right to refuse treatment or transportation if they are competent to make that decision.

against medical advice (AMA) your patient refuses care even though you believe he needs it.

Two types of patients might refuse care. The first type is the person who is not seriously ill or injured and simply does not want to go to the hospital. For example, the belted driver of a minor automobile crash has an abrasion on his knee from striking the dashboard. He is alert and oriented, has no other injuries, and claims he will seek medical attention if it bothers him later. This type of patient usually signs your PCR in a special place marked "Refusal of Care," and you return to service.

The second type of patient is more worrisome. This patient refuses care even though you feel he needs it. This is known as **against medical advice (AMA).** Some legal experts regard AMA as your failure to convince your patient to accept necessary treatment and transport. Such patient refusals are particularly troublesome because they have the most potential to end badly. Still, patients retain the right to refuse treatment or transportation if they are competent to make that decision and are not actively suicidal. Although you cannot make a legal determination of competence (sometimes it takes a court decision), document that you believe your patient was competent to refuse care. Though specific laws vary from state to state, your patient will demonstrate competence by his understanding of the circumstances and the risks associated with refusing care and by accepting those risks and the responsibility for refusing care. Assess your patient as thoroughly as possible, with special emphasis on his mental status and behavior. Pay extra attention to any patient suspected of being under the influence of drugs or alcohol. Clearly document that your patient has an adequate mental status and understands your field diagnosis, alternative treatments, and the consequences of refusing care. Also record his reason for refusing care (Table 11-2).

Even after you document your patient's competence, most patient refusals require more thorough documentation than the typical EMS run because the opportunity for and consequences of abandonment charges are tremendous. Simply having your patient sign

Table 11-2	REFUSAL OF CARE DOCUMENTATION CHECKLIST

❏ Thorough patient assessment

❏ Competency of patient

❏ Your recommendation for care and transport

❏ Explanation to the patient about possible consequences of refusing care, including possibility of death, if appropriate

❏ Other suggestions for accessing care

❏ Willingness to return if patient changes mind

❏ Patient's understanding of statements and suggestions and apparent competence to refuse care based on that understanding

your PCR is not sufficient. Again, document that you described your patient's injuries to him and that he understood the risks of refusing treatment and transport. Inform him of potential complications from injuries that might not be obvious. Discuss those associated risks also and document this discussion. Also document any involvement of your patient's family or friends. Since ruling out serious injury is all but impossible in the field, you may need to make clear the possibility of your patient's dying. Although this might seem extreme, it plainly conveys that the risks are serious. A patient who was informed that he was at risk of dying, refused care, and subsequently had his leg amputated because of an infection would have a hard time convincing a jury that he did not think the risks were serious.

In many systems, you must contact the medical direction physician before allowing a patient to refuse transport. If you confer with a physician, document any information, advice, or orders that the physician gives you. If your patient speaks directly to the physician, document that as well. Once more, document that your patient understands the circumstances and the risks and still chooses to refuse transport. Note that you instructed him to call an ambulance or go to the emergency department if his condition worsens, or if he just changes his mind. You can ask a bystander or law enforcement officer to witness the patient refusal, although this is not always required.

Your documentation also should include a complete narrative with quotations and statements from others on the scene. For example, if your patient's wife and son plead with him to go to the hospital, include their comments in your report. If your system uses a specific form for patient refusals, complete that paperwork as well (Figure 11-6). The additional form, however, is not a substitute for a complete documentation of the circumstances.

SERVICES NOT NEEDED

Some systems allow you to determine that your patient does not need ambulance transport. Although such policies reduce ambulance utilization rates, the risks of denying transport are even greater than those of patient refusals. In these cases, the documentation must clearly demonstrate that transport was unnecessary. As with patient refusals, document any discussion you have with the emergency department physician and any advice you give to your patient.

Transportation may not be needed for other reasons, as well. Ambulances are often called to minor accidents where no injuries have occurred. When this happens, first responders such as the fire department rescue unit or a police agency might cancel the ambulance. If the ambulance is canceled en route, document the canceling authority and the time of notification. If you arrive on the scene and find no patients, document that. If, when you arrive, you are canceled by on-scene personnel, document that you made no patient contact and record the person and agency who canceled you. The difference is considerable between "no patients found" and "only minor injuries, patients refusing transport." Although they might refuse transport, evaluate people with even the most minor injuries. Consider them patients and document them accurately.

The risks of denying transport are even greater than those of patient refusals.

FIGURE 11-6   One example of a refusal-of-care form.

MASS CASUALTY INCIDENTS

Multiple patients, mass casualties, and disasters all present special documentation problems. The number of patients needing care and transport during such situations may overwhelm you. Often, more than one ambulance crew cares for the many patients. Some EMS personnel may fill only support roles and never actually provide patient care. Obtaining complete patient information might be impossible, and completing documentation for one patient before going on to care for others might be impractical.

In these situations, you must weigh your patients' needs against the demand for complete documentation. Document as much as possible—as quickly as possible—on your PCR. You can complete the documentation later as an addendum. If you cannot remember the particulars of a specific patient or transport, do not guess. Document only what you know to be factual and accurate. A simple note at the end of the documentation explaining the circumstances will account for any missing information.

Some EMS agencies use special forms for multiple patient events, and most provide a general incident report form or record that anyone connected with the call may complete. You should become familiar with local policies and procedures for documenting these situations. Many systems use **triage tags** to record vital information on each patient quickly. A triage tag has just enough room for your patient's vital information—name, major injuries, vital signs, treatment, and priority (urgent, non-urgent). You affix it to your patient, and it remains there throughout the event; you can transfer its information to your PCR later. Whatever your local policies, document as completely and accurately as possible without detracting from patient care.

Whatever your local policies regarding multiple patients and mass casualties, document as completely and accurately as possible without detracting from patient care.

triage tags tags containing vital information, affixed to your patient during a multi-patient incident.

CONSEQUENCES OF INAPPROPRIATE DOCUMENTATION

Inappropriate documentation can have both medical and legal consequences. The medical consequences of inadequate documentation are potentially the most serious. Health-care providers across several disciplines may refer to your PCR in planning their care for a patient. Do not guess about your patient's medical problems if you are not certain. An inaccurate or incomplete report can affect patient care for many hours, even days, after the ambulance call ends. Failing to document a medication allergy or documenting an incorrect medical history could have grave consequences. If no one can read your sloppy report, it is useless despite the importance of its information. Good documentation now enables good care later.

The potential legal consequences of inadequate documentation are enormous. If poor documentation results in inappropriate care, you may be held responsible. Or if the documentation does not make it clear that you informed a patient of the risks when he refused transport, you may be legally accountable for any harmful consequences. If the documentation does not explicitly say the patient in ventricular fibrillation was defibrillated immediately, you might be accused of providing inadequate care. Even though you did everything appropriately, poor, incomplete, or inaccurate documentation will encourage anyone who

Good documentation now enables good care later.

Poor, incomplete, or inaccurate documentation encourages frivolous lawsuits; good documentation discourages them.

is pursuing a frivolous lawsuit. Good documentation discourages such actions. Always remember that if it is not documented, you did not do it.

Inaccurate, incomplete, illegible documentation also reflects poorly on the EMS provider writing the report. Missing information, misspelled words, and poor penmanship give the impression of a sloppy, incompetent provider. Good documentation, on the other hand, enhances the EMS provider's professional stature.

ADDITIONAL RESPONSIBILITIES

As an EMT-I, you will assume responsibility for your documentation. Although documentation is often a begrudged task, it is one of the most important parts of an EMS call. Ensuring that your documentation is complete, accurate, legible, and appropriate is one of your professional responsibilities. As a professional, you should recognize this responsibility and set a positive example for others as you fulfill it.

Your report's confidentiality cannot be overemphasized. Confidentiality is your patient's legal right. Do not discuss your report with anyone not medically connected directly with the case. Generally, you are allowed to share patient information with another health-care provider who will continue care, with third-party billing companies, with the police if it is relevant to a criminal investigation, and with the court if it issues a subpoena. Your report also may be used for quality assurance or research. In these cases, block out the patient's name.

Computer charting will certainly become common in the future. Several systems now on the market allow you to enter data electronically, transmit that information to the receiving facility, and immediately receive a printed report. When you use such systems, remember that the principles of effective documentation still apply.

∫UMMARY

Regardless of the system you use for documentation, all EMS records should possess the same basic attributes. Appropriate terminology, proper spelling, accepted abbreviations and acronyms, and accurate times are essential. A description of the patient assessment and interventions, including pertinent negatives and communications with on-line physicians, is equally important. Finally, all of the personnel and resources involved in a call must be documented. The record must be accurate and precise, free of jargon, and neatly written. Corrections should be made properly, including the use of an addendum when appropriate.

Prehospital-care providers may use many systems of documentation, including the CHART and SOAP formats. Whatever system you use, it is best if you use the same one consistently. This results in more reliable, complete documentation and reduces the chances of omitting important information. Any of the existing documentation systems can incorporate a head-to-toe assessment of the patient. Special situations such as multiple patients and refusals of transportation require extra attention. They are often the most difficult calls to document, yet they are also the calls for which good documentation can be most valuable. A complete narrative—in addition to any check boxes or filled-in "bubbles"—is the best way to ensure that all the necessary information is documented.

Although EMS providers frequently dislike documentation, it is one of the most important parts of the EMS call. Ensuring that the documentation is complete, accurate, legible, and appropriate is one of an EMS provider's professional responsibilities. Your PCR is the only permanent record of the ambulance call and the only permanent reflection of your professionalism.

ON THE WEB

For additional practice and review, go to the companion website at www.prenhall.com/bledsoe and click on *Intermediate Emergency Care: Principles & Practice.*

CHAPTER 12

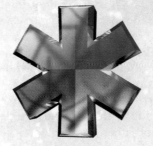

Trauma and Trauma Systems

Objectives

After reading this chapter, you should be able to:

1. Describe the prevalence and significance of trauma. (pp. 583–584)
2. List the components of a comprehensive trauma system. (pp. 584–586)
3. Identify the characteristics of and criteria for transport to community, area, and regional trauma centers. (pp. 584–586)
4. Identify the trauma triage criteria. (pp. 584–586)
5. Describe how trauma emergencies differ from medical emergencies in the scene size-up, patient assessment, prehospital emergency care, and transport. (pp. 586–589)
6. Explain the "Golden Hour" concept and describe how it applies to prehospital emergency care. (p. 588)
7. Explain the value and describe the criteria and procedure of air medical service in trauma patient care and transport. (p. 588)

CASE STUDY

On a warm, sunny midsummer day, the annunciator sounds and requests that the fly car with EMT-Intermediate (EMT-I) Earl Antak and the Hamilton Area Volunteer Ambulance respond to a bicycle/auto collision three miles south of Amble Corners. It is a 10-minute trip for Earl, and about the same for the volunteer ambulance. While the vehicles are en route, the dispatcher radios that the sheriff's department is on scene and that they have reported an unresponsive bicyclist.

Arriving at the location of the accident, Earl notes that members of the sheriff's department have secured the scene and are directing traffic. As he begins the scene size-up, he notices that several other cars are parked along the shoulder of the highway. Earl also sees a bicycle with a mangled front wheel resting against the open door of one of the cars. An officer from the sheriff's department is attending a young adult who is lying on the roadside about 45 feet in front of the car. As Earl studies the scene more closely, he observes that the car's open door has been bent forward and that glass from the car is strewn along the highway.

The officer tells Earl that the person he is attending is named John. He reports that John was unresponsive when the officer arrived, but is now responsive but somewhat confused. Earl's general impression is that the patient is a well-developed male in his early 20s. He is wearing a bicycle helmet, shorts, and a tee shirt. He has several abrasions to his right shoulder, arm, and forearm as well as to his right thigh. His helmet is badly scraped and deformed. Earl asks the officer to continue holding manual stabilization of the patient's head and neck while an EMT-I applies a cervical collar.

Earl's initial assessment reveals that John is responsive and oriented to person, but not to place or time. John reports that he was riding along at about 22 miles per hour when "this lady opened her door right in front of me." He flew through the window of that door and onto the pavement. He asks, "How's my bike?" His pulse rate is about 100 and his respirations are about 22 and full. Both lung fields are clear, and his skin is warm and very wet. Earl applies oxygen via nonrebreather mask at 15 liters per minute.

The rapid trauma assessment reveals a small deformity just medial to the right upper anterior shoulder and some crepitus and pain with any movement of the right shoulder. He has a large abrasion to the right thigh. The upper and lower extremities have reduced sensation to pain and touch, good pulses and temperature, bilaterally equal but limited strength, and no pain with motion, except in the right upper extremity (suspected clavicle fracture). There are no signs of soft-tissue injuries to the head, and John denies any pain other than to his right shoulder and thigh, a twinge in his neck, and a sensation of "pins and needles" in his extremities. When vital signs are taken, John's pulse is still 100, his respirations are still 22 and full, and his blood pressure is 132/84.

As the volunteer ambulance arrives, Earl uses his cell phone to contact medical direction for trauma center assignment. He is directed to Mt. Sinai Hospital, the closest Level 2 trauma center, and speaks to the trauma triage nurse. Earl tells the nurse that John meets the system's trauma triage criteria—unresponsiveness and a serious mechanism of injury—and relates his assessment findings and the patient's vital signs. Since the ground transport time is projected to be 35 minutes, he requests a helicopter intercept.

After about 8 minutes at the patient's side, Earl and the EMTs from the volunteer ambulance have applied a cervical collar, immobilized John onto a spine board, and loaded him into the ambulance. As transport begins, Earl establishes a 16-gauge intravenous (IV) access site, begins to administer normal saline at a to-keep-open rate, and continues to provide ongoing assessment. He notices that John can no longer remember what happened.

A few minutes later, the ambulance intercepts with a Central State Medivac helicopter at the predesignated landing zone, a parking lot at the county's community college. The flight paramedic greets Earl, takes his report, and quickly begins her assessment. She readies John for flight, and Earl helps load him into the helicopter. Within minutes of the ambulance's arrival, the helicopter takes off en route to the hospital.

Later that day, Earl gets a follow-up phone call from the flight paramedic, thanking him for providing good care for John and a good patient report. She says that John had a fracture of the right clavicle, an epidural bleed, which was managed by surgery, and a confirmed C2 and C3 fracture. Because of John's age and physical condition, he is expected to recover quickly.

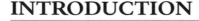

trauma a physical injury or wound caused by external force or violence.

Trauma is the leading killer of persons under age 44 in the United States.

INTRODUCTION

Trauma is a physical injury or wound caused by external force or violence. It is currently the number four killer of people in the United States behind cardiovascular disease, stroke, and cancer. It is, however, the leading cause of death of persons under age 44. As such, trauma steals the greatest number of productive years from its victims. It also may be the most expensive medical problem because of the productivity losses it causes in its victims and the high cost of initial care, rehabilitation, and often life-long maintenance of those victims.

Trauma accounts for about 150,000 deaths per year, with auto crashes responsible for about 44,000 and gunshot wounds another 38,000. Other deaths are attributed to falls, blasts, stabbings, crush injuries, and sports injuries. In addition to the great death toll from trauma, many more of its victims are injured and carry life-long physical reminders of their experiences with it.

Your role in trauma care, as a member of the Emergency Medical Services team, is to understand the structure and objectives of the trauma care system, to promote injury prevention, and to provide the seriously injured trauma patient with proper assessment, aggressive care, and rapid transport to the most appropriate facility. The remainder of this chapter will help you with these responsibilities as it further defines trauma, explains the components of trauma care systems, identifies the capabilities of different levels of trauma centers, and more fully defines your role as a care provider in the trauma system.

TRAUMA

The types of trauma can range from slight abrasions or scratches to the fatal, multiple-system injuries that might result from a high-speed automobile-versus-pedestrian collision. Trauma is broken down into two major categories, blunt and penetrating. **Penetrating trauma** occurs when an arrow, bullet, knife, or other object enters the body and exchanges energy with human tissue, thereby causing injury. **Blunt trauma** is injury that occurs as the energy and forces of collision with an object—not the object itself—enter the body and damage tissue. These two categories of trauma are discussed in greater detail in the next two chapters of this book.

penetrating trauma injury caused by an object breaking the skin and entering the body.

blunt trauma injury caused by the collision of an object and the body, into which the object does not enter.

Although trauma poses a serious threat to life, its presentation often masks the patient's true condition. Extremity injuries, for example, infrequently cause death. Yet they are often obvious and grotesque (Figure 12-1). On the other hand, life-threatening problems, such as internal bleeding and shock, may occur with only subtle signs and symptoms. When assessing a trauma patient, you must look beyond obvious injuries for evidence that suggests a life-threatening condition. When such a condition is found, you must ensure your patient has rapid access to the trauma system.

Life-threatening problems, such as internal bleeding and shock, can occur with only subtle signs and symptoms.

Serious and life-threatening injury occurs in fewer than 10% of trauma patients. In most patients with life-threatening injury, however, the injury is internal and is likely to involve the head or body cavity hemorrhage. Prehospital care can neither properly nor definitively stabilize these patients and their injuries in the field. The best care you can offer as an EMT-I is to secure the airway, ensure adequate respirations, control any significant external hemorrhage, and rapidly transport the patient to definitive trauma care. That care is only available at a specialized treatment facility with rapid access to surgery—a trauma center.

When assessing a trauma patient, look beyond obvious injuries for evidence that suggests a life-threatening condition.

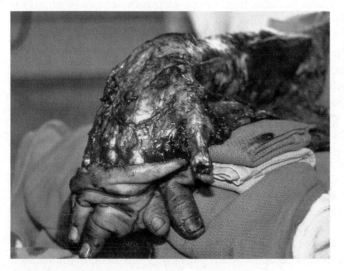

FIGURE 12-1 In prehospital care, it is essential that gruesome, non–life-threatening injuries do not distract you from more subtle, life-threatening problems. *(Courtesy of Edward T. Dickinson, MD)*

Some 90% of trauma patients do not have serious, life-threatening injuries. You can best care for these patients by providing thorough on-scene assessment and stabilization followed by conservative transport to the nearest general hospital or other appropriate health-care facility.

It is essential that you determine the difference between trauma patients with serious, life-threatening conditions and those less seriously injured patients during your assessment. You will be aided in making this determination by using guidelines known as trauma triage criteria. These criteria involve consideration of the mechanisms by which patients are injured and of the physical or clinical findings indicating internal injury. Using these criteria, which will be discussed in detail later in this chapter, will help you properly direct patients as they enter the trauma care system.

THE TRAUMA CARE SYSTEM

In the mid-to-late 1960s, several medically oriented groups investigated the death toll on U.S. highways. Their studies revealed that victims of vehicle crashes suffered not only from the injuries received in the crashes but also from the lack of an organized approach to bringing these victims into the health-care system. The studies also demonstrated that most hospitals were inadequately equipped and staffed to care for the victims of these crashes. These investigations led to passage of the Highway Safety Act of 1966 and to the development of today's EMS system.

More than two decades later, the American College of Surgeons, recognizing that the system of caring for severely injured trauma victims was still inadequate, successfully worked to achieve passage of the Trauma Care Systems Planning and Development Act of 1990. This act helped establish guidelines, funding, and state-level leadership and support for the development of trauma systems.

The trauma system is predicated on the principle that serious trauma is a surgical disease. This means that the proper care for serious internal trauma is often immediate surgical intervention to repair internal hemorrhage sites. Although patients with life-threatening injuries account for less than 10% of all trauma patients, immediate surgical care of these patients can drastically reduce trauma mortality and morbidity.

Care for seriously injured trauma patients is expensive and complicated. A well-designed EMS system will allocate limited resources in a way that provides the most efficient and effective care for these patients. Such a system utilizes hospitals with special resources and commitment to trauma patient care. These hospitals are designated as trauma centers.

TRAUMA CENTER DESIGNATION

The current model for a trauma system includes three levels of **trauma center**, with an increased ability and commitment to provide trauma care at each level (Table 12-1).

The Level I, or regional, trauma center is a hospital, usually a university teaching center, that is prepared and committed to handle all types of specialty trauma (Figure 12-2). These centers provide neurosurgery, microsurgery (limb reattachment), pediatric care, burn care, and care for multi-system trauma. They also provide leadership and resource support to other levels of the regional trauma system through system coordination and continuing medical and public education programs. When population density does not permit a commitment to the requirements of a Level I trauma center, a Level II trauma center may act as the regional trauma center.

The Level II, or area, trauma center, has an increased commitment to trauma care, but not as great as a Level I facility. It has surgical care capability available at all times for incoming trauma patients. Level II centers can handle all but the most seriously injured specialty and multi-system trauma patients. Staff at these facilities can stabilize those patients in preparation for transport to a Level I trauma center.

The Level III, or community, trauma center is a general hospital with a commitment to special staff training and resource allocation for trauma patients. These centers are located

Serious trauma is a surgical disease; its proper care is immediate surgical intervention to repair internal hemorrhage sites.

trauma center a hospital that has the capability of caring for acutely injured patients; trauma centers must meet strict criteria to use this designation.

The modern trauma system includes three levels of trauma center, each with an increased ability and commitment to providing trauma care.

Table 12-1	**CRITERIA FOR TRAUMA CENTER DESIGNATION**

Level I—Regional Trauma Center

Commits resources to address all types of specialty trauma 24 hours a day, 7 days a week.

Level II—Area Trauma Center

Commits the resources to address the most common trauma emergencies with surgical capability available 24 hours a day, 7 days a week; will stabilize and transport specialty cases to the regional trauma center.

Level III—Community Trauma Center

Commits to special emergency department training and has some surgical capability, but will usually stabilize and transfer seriously injured trauma patients to a higher level trauma center as needed.

Level IV—Trauma Facility

In remote areas, a small community hospital or medical care facility may be designated a trauma receiving facility, meaning that it will stabilize and prepare trauma patients with moderate to serious injuries for transport to a higher level facility.

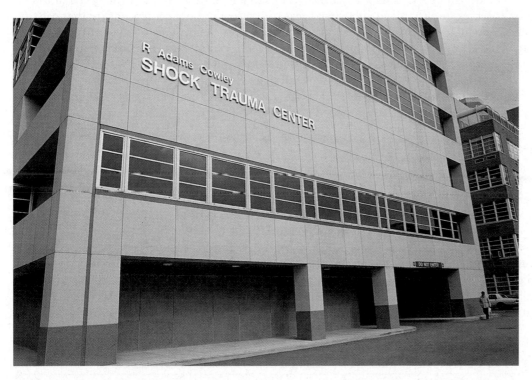

FIGURE 12-2   The R. Adams Cowley Shock Trauma Center in Baltimore, Maryland, is an example of a Level I trauma facility.

in smaller cities situated in generally rural areas. They are well prepared to care for most trauma victims and to stabilize and triage more seriously injured ones for transport to higher level trauma centers.

In some remote areas, there is provision for an additional level of trauma center. In these areas, seriously injured trauma patients may be taken to a Level IV trauma facility for stabilization and care before transport, often by helicopter, to a more distant, higher-level trauma center. In these areas, the incidence of trauma does not support the resource allocation necessary to meet the requirements of a trauma center; by default, some other type of health-care facility is identified as a trauma transport destination.

The design of a trauma system should be flexible in order to meet the needs of the region it serves. In urban and suburban areas, just a few trauma centers ensure that each receives adequate patient volume to maintain staff proficiency and to ensure that resources are being effectively used. In rural regions, a Level III center may act as the regional trauma center because the incidence of serious trauma does not support any greater commitment. In some areas, a Level IV facility may be all that is available and thus becomes the default destination for seriously injured trauma patients. Consult your Emergency Medical Services system plan to determine the intended patient flow patterns in your region.

SPECIALTY CENTERS

Beyond classification as trauma centers, certain medical facilities may be designated as specialty centers. Such facilities may include neurocenters, burn centers, pediatric trauma centers, and centers specializing in hand and limb reattachment by microsurgery. One other specialty service is hyperbaric oxygenation, which is important in the treatment of carbon monoxide poisoning and problems related to SCUBA diving.

Specialty centers have made a commitment of trained personnel, equipment, and other resources to provide services not usually available at a general or trauma hospital. These centers are also more likely to provide a higher level of intensive care and state-of-the-art injury management than that found in other facilities. Be aware of the specialty services available in your system as well as the protocols defining when patients should be directed to them.

YOUR ROLE AS AN EMT-INTERMEDIATE

As an EMT-I, your tasks in the trauma system are likely to include triage of trauma patients against standards established by your medical direction authority (trauma triage criteria) and ensurance of the rapid assessment, care, and transport of patients to the closest appropriate medical facility (Figure 12-3). For those patients that meet trauma triage criteria, the appropriate facility is the nearest trauma center.

trauma triage criteria
guidelines to aid prehospital personnel in determining which trauma patients require urgent transportation to a trauma center.

Trauma triage criteria are guidelines established to help you determine which patients require the services of a trauma center and which do not. The presence of certain mechanisms of injury and clinical findings has been proven, by research, to accurately reflect the potential for serious injury and the need for the intensive services available only at a trauma center. Compare your patient's mechanism of injury and any physical assessment findings to these pre-established criteria. These criteria are listed in detail later in this chapter. If your patient meets any of the criteria, rapid transport is required.

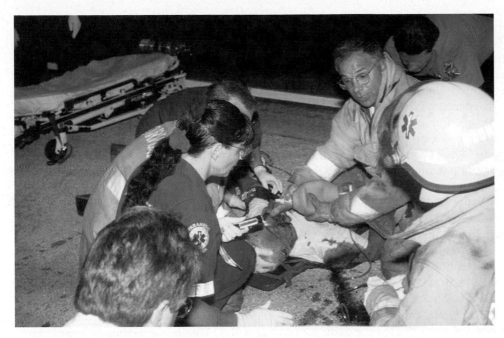

FIGURE 12-3 Your role as an EMT-Intermediate is to ensure the trauma patient's ABCs and prepare for rapid transport.

MECHANISM OF INJURY ANALYSIS

To help determine the **mechanism of injury,** mentally recreate the accident from evidence available at the scene. You should identify the forces involved in the incident, the direction from which they came, and the areas of the patient's body affected by these forces. In an automobile collision, for example, the mechanism of injury includes the energy exchange process between the auto and what it struck, between the patient and the auto's interior, and among the various tissues and organs as they collide, one with another, within the patient. Close inspection of the mangled auto reveals evidence about the collision and the forces at work in it. (See Chapter 13, "Blunt Trauma," and Chapter 14, "Penetrating Trauma.")

You will begin your consideration of the mechanism of injury during the scene size-up. Later, you should reconsider the mechanism of injury as the first step of the focused history and physical exam for the trauma patient.

INDEX OF SUSPICION

The information you gather during your consideration and reconsideration of the mechanism of injury suggests an **index of suspicion** for possible injuries. This index is an anticipation of possible injuries based on analysis of the event. For example, a pedestrian struck by a car can be expected to have lower extremity fractures. Further, if the auto were moving at 20 miles per hour, fracture severity would be less than if it were moving at 55 miles per hour. Also, the probability of internal injury at lower speeds is less than it would be at higher speeds. By evaluating the strength of the impact and its nature, you can anticipate the structures and organs damaged and the degree to which they have been damaged.

In addition to developing an index of suspicion for specific injuries, you will also examine the trauma patient for physical signs of injury, both during the initial assessment and during the rapid trauma assessment or the focused history and physical exam. The physical signs suggesting serious trauma include the signs and symptoms of shock and those of internal head injury. Since shock and head injury are the great killers in trauma, be watchful for the earliest evidence of their existence. Remember, the body compensates well for the internal loss of blood and hides serious signs of injury until late in the shock process. If you have any reason to suspect that a patient has sustained serious internal injury, move to enter that patient rapidly into the trauma system. Otherwise, provide frequent ongoing assessment to ensure that progressive signs of shock and internal head injury are discovered as early as possible.

mechanism of injury the processes and forces that cause trauma.

Consideration of the mechanism of injury begins during the scene size-up. The mechanism of injury should be reconsidered as the first step of the focused history and physical exam for trauma patients.

index of suspicion the anticipation of injury to a body region, organ, or structure based on analysis of the mechanism of injury.

If you have any reason to suspect that the patient has sustained serious internal injury, move to enter him or her rapidly into the trauma system.

THE GOLDEN HOUR

Golden Hour the 60-minute period after a severe injury; it is the maximum acceptable time between the injury and initiation of surgery for the seriously injured trauma patient.

Time is a very important consideration in the survival of seriously injured trauma patients. Research has demonstrated that patient survival rates increase dramatically as time from the trauma incident to the beginning of surgery decreases. The current goal for incident-to-surgery time is 1 hour, often referred to as the **Golden Hour.**

Factors such as the location of the incident and time needed to extricate a patient all consume a portion of the Golden Hour. Many of these factors are beyond your control; for that reason, it is vital to keep time spent on factors over which you do have control to the minimum. Ideally, you should provide the initial and rapid trauma assessments, emergency stabilization, patient packaging, and initiation of transport in less than 10 minutes. When distances or traffic conditions present prolonged ground transport times, reduce transport times by using an air medical service if possible.

Initial patient assessment, emergency stabilization, patient packaging, and initiation of transport should ideally take less than 10 minutes.

Air medical service, usually provided by helicopter, has added a weapon in the fight against time for the seriously injured trauma patient (Figure 12-4). The helicopter travels much faster than ground transport and in a straight line from the crash scene to the trauma center.

Be aware, however, that air medical transport is not appropriate in all cases. Trauma patients must be in relatively stable condition for it to be used. Additionally, the limited space within the aircraft and its associated engine noise make in-flight care difficult. Further, combative patients may endanger the safety of the flight crew and the aircraft. Adverse weather conditions can also limit the use of air medical transport. Finally, air medical transport services are very expensive and can be used most effectively only as part of a comprehensive EMS trauma system. Follow local protocols about when and how to request air medical transport.

DECISION TO TRANSPORT

The decision either to transport a patient immediately or to attempt more extensive on-scene care is among the most difficult you must make. The trauma triage criteria are designed to help you with this decision. As a rule, transport patients who experience certain mechanisms of injury or display key clinical findings quickly, with IV access and other time-consuming procedures attempted en route. Indicators for immediate transport are given in Table 12-2.

In applying trauma triage criteria, it is best to err on the side of caution.

In applying trauma triage criteria, it is best to err on the side of caution. If a patient does not fit the stated criteria, be suspicious. Remember, you often arrive at the patient's side only minutes after the accident. The patient may not yet have lost enough blood internally to exhibit signs of shock or progressive head injury. If in doubt, transport to a trauma center without delay.

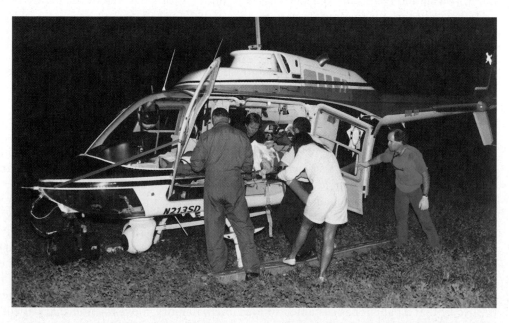

FIGURE 12-4 An air medical services helicopter can significantly reduce transport time from the scene to the trauma center.

Table 12-2	TRAUMA TRIAGE CRITERIA INDICATING NEED FOR IMMEDIATE TRANSPORT

Mechanism of Injury

- Falls from a height greater than 20 feet (3 times the victim's height)
- Pedestrian/bicyclist versus auto collisions
  —Struck by a vehicle traveling over 5 mph
  —Thrown or run over by vehicle
- Motorcycle impact at greater than 20 mph
- Ejection from a vehicle
- Severe vehicle impact
  —Speed at impact greater than 40 mph
  —Intrusion of more than 12 inches into occupant compartment
  —Vehicle deformity greater than 20 inches
- Rollover with signs of serious impact
- Death of another occupant in the vehicle
- Extrication time greater than 20 minutes

Significant mechanism of injury considerations with infants and children include the following:

- Fall from a height greater than 10 feet (3 times the victim's height)
- Bicycle/vehicle collision
- Vehicle collision at medium speed
- Vehicle collision where the infant or child was unrestrained

Physical Findings

- Revised Trauma Score less than 11
- Glasgow Coma Scale less than 14
- Systolic blood pressure less than 90
- Respiratory rate less than 10 or greater than 29
- Pulse less than 50 or greater than 120
- Penetrating trauma (except distal extremities)
- Two or more proximal long-bone fractures
- Flail chest
- Pelvic fractures
- Limb paralysis
- Burns to more than 15 percent of body surface area
- Burns to face or airway

These criteria are designed for the "over-triage" of trauma patients. They ensure that patients with very subtle signs and symptoms, yet with significant and serious injuries, are not missed during assessment. Use of these criteria means that you will transport some patients to trauma centers unnecessarily. However, transporting a patient who may not need the resources of a trauma center is far better than not transporting a patient who truly needs the care available only there.

INJURY PREVENTION

One of the best, most cost-effective ways of reducing mortality and morbidity is to prevent trauma in the first place. Several injury prevention programs have been very effective. Programs promoting seat belt use and awareness of the dangers of drinking and driving have encouraged teenagers and adults to drive more safely and responsibly. Other programs, such

One of the best and most cost-effective ways of reducing mortality and morbidity is to prevent trauma from happening in the first place.

as "let's not meet by accident," increase society's awareness of trauma systems as well as an appreciation for safety-oriented behaviors. Safety programs for users of boats and firearms also raise safety awareness and assist in injury prevention. The EMS system has a responsibility to support such programs and to promote their development where they do not exist. As an EMS provider, you should participate and encourage your peers to participate.

Technical developments such as better highway design, airbag restraint systems, and vehicles constructed to absorb the energy of crashes have also played major parts in greatly reducing the yearly highway death toll. EMT-Is have a responsibility to support the development and use of these new designs and technologies as a way of further reducing trauma deaths and injuries.

DATA AND THE TRAUMA REGISTRY

trauma registry a data retrieval system for trauma patient information, used to evaluate and improve the trauma system.

As with all EMS, research is the only way to recognize those trauma care practices and procedures that benefit patients and those that do not. In the trauma system, the **trauma registry** is a uniform and standard set of data collected by regional trauma centers. The data is analyzed to determine how well the system is performing and to identify factors that may contribute to or lessen chances of patient survival.

It is important that you do all that you can to support this research effort by ensuring that your prehospital care reports accurately and completely describe the findings of your assessments, the care you provide to patients, the results of ongoing assessments, and the times associated with calls. You should also consider taking part in and supporting prehospital research projects if the opportunity presents itself.

QUALITY IMPROVEMENT

Trauma system Quality Improvement (QI), or Quality Management (QM) is another way of examining system performance with the aim of providing better patient care. In the QI process, committees look at selected care modalities (called indicators) to determine if designated standards of care are being met. For trauma system QI, the committees would study the application of trauma triage criteria, performance of field skills, and amounts of time spent in various aspects of response, care, and transport of patients. QI committees may also look at select calls to determine if their documentation accurately reflects the results of assessment and the care given. If the system standards are not being met, the committees may suggest such steps as continuing education programs or modification of protocols. As a member of the trauma system, you should become actively involved in such programs and encourage the participation of your peers.

SUMMARY

Trauma remains one of the greatest tragedies of our modern society. It accounts for large numbers of deaths and disabling injuries and often affects individuals who are in their most productive years of life. A well-designed and well-implemented trauma system offers a way of lessening the impact of these traumas.

As an EMT-I, you are a part of the trauma system. You are charged with evaluating trauma patients by comparing their mechanisms of injury and the physical signs of their injuries with pre-established trauma triage criteria to determine which patients should enter the trauma system and which could be best cared for at a general hospital. In the presence of severe, life-threatening trauma, you must ensure rapid assessment, on-scene care, and appropriate transport to provide your patients with the best chances for survival.

ON THE WEB

For additional practice and review, go to the companion website at www.prenhall.com/bledsoe and click on *Intermediate Emergency Care: Principles & Practice.*

Chapter 13

Blunt Trauma

Objectives

After reading this chapter, you should be able to:

1. Identify and explain by example the laws of inertia and conservation of energy. (p. 594)

2. Define kinetic energy and force as they relate to trauma. (pp. 594–595)

3. Describe the organ collisions that occur with blunt trauma in vehicle crashes. (pp. 597–598)

4. Describe the effects of restraint systems—including seat belts, airbags, and child safety seats—on injury patterns in vehicle crashes. (pp. 598–601)

5. Compare and contrast the types of vehicle impacts and their expected injuries. (pp. 601–613)

6. Discuss the benefits of auto restraints and motorcycle helmet use. (pp. 601–605, 610–612)

7. Describe the mechanisms of injury associated with falls, crush injuries, and sports injuries. (pp. 619–622)

8. Identify common blast injuries and any special considerations regarding their assessment and proper care. (pp. 613–619)

9. Identify and explain any special assessment and care considerations for patients with blunt trauma. (pp. 598–622)

10. Given several preprogrammed and moulaged blunt trauma patients, provide the appropriate scene size-up, initial assessment, rapid trauma or focused physical exam and history, detailed exam, and ongoing assessment and provide appropriate patient care and transportation. (pp. 593–622)

Case Study

A call comes in to City Ambulance Unit 2 staffed by EMT-I Kris and BLS provider Bob. The dispatcher reports multiple injuries in a two-car collision at the freeway interchange. Because of backed-up traffic, the dispatcher tells the unit to use the exit ramp.

Police arrive at the scene and provide Unit 2 with an update while it is en route. A green auto traveling at freeway speed has plowed into a red car stalled at the interchange. The wreck involves three injured parties, one in the red car and two in the green.

When Unit 2 arrives on scene, the police have secured it and are directing traffic around the vehicles involved. Kris and Bob approach the vehicles and begin the scene size-up, noting that about 100 yards now separate the two vehicles. The green car has severe front-end damage. Two "spider-web" cracks appear across the windshield, the steering column is deformed, and the older car has no airbags. The police officer in charge reports that both people in the car had failed to wear seatbelts. The red car has severe rear-end damage, but the windshield is intact. The driver in this vehicle wore a seatbelt, and the headrest is in the up position. Before acting, Kris calls for another unit to back Unit 2. Kris and Bob now proceed to the green car, where they expect to find the worst injuries.

Kris and Bob perform initial assessments on the two occupants of that vehicle. The driver has suffered chest trauma caused by impact with the steering wheel. Although she is experiencing difficult and painful breathing, her airway is clear. She is oriented to time and place and denies any period of unconsciousness. Her pulses are strong, regular, and at a moderate rate. The physical exam reveals a forehead contusion, a reddened anterior chest with crepitus, and clear breath sounds bilaterally.

The passenger is unresponsive and cannot be aroused. She has shallow, rapid breaths and a rapid, barely palpable pulse. Her forehead is badly contused with moderate bleeding. Her thighs appear noticeably shortened. The rapid trauma assessment reveals instability of the pelvis and both femurs.

A police officer who has been trained as a First Responder indicates that the driver of the red car is conscious and alert. Although "shaken up," he has a blood pressure of 126/84 and a pulse of 86. He is breathing normally at a rate of 20. As the EMT-I in charge, Kris asks the officer to stay with the driver until the second ambulance arrives.

Meanwhile, Bob has told the driver of the green car not to move. He stabilizes the passenger's head manually while Kris applies oxygen and a cervical collar. Next, Kris prepares a long spine board with straps and a pneumatic anti-shock garment (PASG). They place the passenger on the board, strap her securely, and affix her head with a cervical immobilization device. Then they load her into the ambulance.

When the second ambulance arrives, Kris briefs the members of that crew and assigns the remaining patients, the two drivers. Kris and Bob then rush the passenger, who is the most critical victim, to a nearby trauma center. En route, vital signs are taken quickly and reveal a blood pressure of 82 by palpation and a weak radial pulse of 130. The legs look ashen, feel cool to the touch, and show no palpable pulses. Capillary refill time is 3 seconds in the upper extremities and longer in the lower ones. The pulse oximeter reading is 92%.

Kris gives a brief report to medical direction and receives orders in response. Bob inflates the PASG. Kris starts two large-bore IVs and runs fluids using pressure infusers. Kris readies intubation equipment and hyperventilates the patient using the bag-valve mask. The ambulance stops briefly while Kris attempts orotracheal intubation, with the patient's head held fixed in the neutral position. When the effort proves unsuccessful, Kris withdraws the tube, hyperventilates the patient again, and tries digital intubation. The technique works. Lung sounds are clear, chest excursion improves, and oximetry readings begin to rise.

The patient arrives at the trauma center with just under 1,500 mL of fluid infused and the PASG fully inflated. The operating room has been prepared for her. Doctors clear the C-spine by X-ray, repair vascular injuries associated with the pelvic fracture, and infuse six units of typed and cross-matched whole blood. The patient recovers after a few weeks of hospitalization and will walk again with only slight reminders of the injuries and care she received.

Based on the speed of impact and the vehicle damage, the second ambulance crew decides to transport the other two patients to the trauma center. The driver of the green car has two fractured ribs, a C-spine cleared by x-ray and CT scan, and no neurologic deficit. She stays overnight for observation and is released the next afternoon with some medication for rib fracture pain. The other driver has a clear C-spine and returns home shortly after the emergency department evaluation.

INTRODUCTION

Blunt trauma is the most common cause of trauma death and disability. It results from an energy exchange between an object and the human body, without intrusion of the object through the skin (Figure 13-1). The energy exchange causes a chain reaction among various body tissues that crushes and stretches their structures, resulting in injury beneath the surface. Blunt trauma is especially confounding because the true nature of the injury is often hidden, and evidence of the serious injury is very subtle or even absent.

To properly care for victims of blunt trauma, you should understand the injury process and its results. This study, called kinetics of trauma, gives insight into the events that produce injury, known as the mechanism of injury. This insight then helps you develop an index of suspicion, an anticipation of the nature and severity of likely injuries. Armed with an index of suspicion, you then better focus your trauma patient assessment, triage, and care because you know what happened and the injuries the event is likely to have produced.

This chapter looks at the kinetics of blunt trauma, vehicular collisions, blast injuries, and other types of blunt trauma to help you better understand the prevalent mechanisms of injury and their physiological results.

Blunt trauma is the most common cause of trauma death and disability.

Blunt trauma can be deceptive because the true nature of the injury is often hidden and evidence of its seriousness is very subtle or even absent.

KINETICS OF BLUNT TRAUMA

Kinetics is a branch of physics dealing with forces affecting objects in motion and the energy exchanges that occur as objects collide. These collisions, or impacts, are the events that induce injury in patients. An understanding of kinetics helps you appreciate and anticipate

kinetics the branch of physics that deals with motion, taking into consideration mass and force.

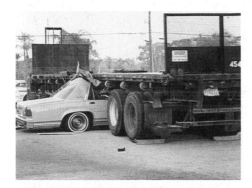

FIGURE 13–1 Blunt trauma is the most common cause of injury and trauma-related death. It is a physical exchange of energy from an object or surface transmitted through the skin into the body's interior.

Patho Pearls

The principles of physics play a significant role in the pathophysiology of both blunt and penetrating injuries. In blunt trauma, the energy tends to be more widely distributed than with penetrating injuries. Also, as discussed in this chapter, solid organs are at greater risk of injury following blunt trauma than hollow organs, because they tend to absorb more of the energy of impact.

Any patient who has sustained a blunt-force injury to the abdomen should increase your index of suspicion of solid organ injury. Injuries to the liver, spleen, pancreas, or even the kidneys can result in massive blood loss. Once at the trauma center, surgeons may elect to manage some blunt-force injuries conservatively, whereas others will require immediate surgical repair. However, it is important to remember that some hollow organs will begin to react in a way similar to solid organs when they are full or distended. For example, the urinary bladder may be full at the time of injury. Blunt-force trauma may result in its rupture with subsequent spillage of urine into the abdomen. Likewise, immediately after a meal, the stomach may be full and rupture or tear, spilling its contents into the abdomen.

Thus, questions about recent meals, alcohol and fluid intake, and similar factors must be taken into consideration when caring for a victim of blunt trauma.

the results of auto and other impacts. The two basic principles of kinetics are the law of inertia and the law of energy conservation. Further, the kinetic energy and force formulas quantify the energy exchange process between the moving object and the human body. These laws and formulas best describe what happens during impact and help in our understanding of blunt trauma.

INERTIA

The law of **inertia,** as described by Sir Isaac Newton and also known as Newton's first law, helps explain what happens during blunt trauma. The first part of his first law states: "A body in **motion** will remain in motion unless acted upon by an outside force." As an example, think of identical autos moving at 55 miles per hour. One car brakes for a red light; the other rams into a bridge abutment. An "outside force" stops the motion of both vehicles, but with very different results. In the first case, the car's brakes absorb the energy of motion. In the second, the front bumper and grill, the frame, and eventually the occupants of the car absorb the energy as the car stops.

The second part of the law states: "A body at rest will remain at rest unless acted upon by an outside force." Examples of this include an auto accelerating from a stop sign or a stopped vehicle propelled forward by a rear-end collision. In the first case, the auto engine provides the force to initiate movement. In the second, the energy of the moving vehicle provides the force as the stopped car absorbs the energy and jolts ahead.

CONSERVATION OF ENERGY

The law of conservation of energy states: "**Energy** can neither be created nor destroyed. It only changes from one form to another." In an auto crash, as in other trauma, identifying probable energy changes helps you assess the impacts of various collisions. Kinetic energy, possessed by a moving car and its passengers, transforms into other energy forms whenever a car stops.

If an auto slows down gradually for a stop sign, the brakes develop friction against the turning wheels, producing heat. During an auto crash, however, the energy of motion is converted at a much faster rate into different forms. This conversion of energy is manifest in the sound of impact, the deformation of the auto's structural components, the heat in the twisted steel, and the injuries to passengers as they collide with the vehicle interior. When all the kinetic energy converts to other energy forms, the auto and its passengers come to a stop.

KINETIC ENERGY

Kinetic energy is the energy of motion. It is a function of an object's **mass** and its **velocity** (Figure 13-2). (Although mass and weight—and velocity and speed—are not identical, we will consider them as such for these discussions.) Kinetic energy of an object while in motion is measured by the following formula:

$$\text{Kinetic energy} = \frac{\text{Mass (or weight)} \times \text{Velocity (or speed)}^2}{2}$$

This formula illustrates that if you double an object's weight, you double its kinetic energy. It is twice as damaging to be hit by a 2-pound baseball as to be hit by a 1-pound ball. It is three times as damaging to be hit by a 3-pound ball, and so on.

As speed (velocity) increases, there is a larger (squared) increase in kinetic energy. Being hit with a 1-pound baseball traveling at 20 miles per hour is four times as injurious as being hit with the same ball moving at 10 miles per hour. If speed increases to 30 miles per hour, trauma is nine times worse. This concept plays a key role in understanding the devastating effects of a gunshot wound in which a small bullet can do great damage (as discussed in Chapter 14, "Penetrating Trauma").

Kinetic energy is the measure of how much energy an object in motion has, not necessarily how much injury occurs. Two autos traveling at 55 miles per hour have about the same kinetic energy. The same two autos would have the same kinetic energy once they have

inertia tendency of an object to remain at rest or remain in motion unless acted upon by an external force.

motion the process of changing place; movement.

energy the capacity to do work in the strict physical sense.

kinetic energy the energy an object has while it is in motion. It is related to the object's mass and velocity.

mass a measure of the matter that an object contains; the property of a physical body that gives the body inertia.

velocity the rate of motion in a particular direction in relation to time.

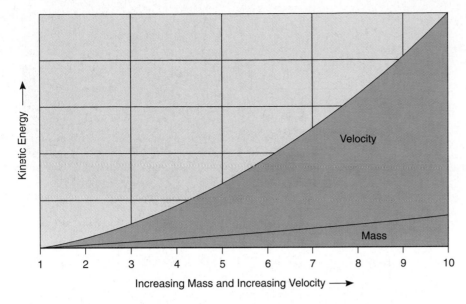

FIGURE 13-2 Increasing mass directly increases kinetic energy, whereas increasing velocity exponentially increases kinetic energy.

stopped, even if one came to rest by hitting a bridge. The difference between these two events is the rate of slowing. This rate is proportional to the crash force.

FORCE

Newton's second law of motion explains the forces at work during a collision. It is summarized by the formula below:

$$\text{Force} = \text{Mass (Weight)} \times \text{Acceleration (or Deceleration)}$$

The formula emphasizes the importance of the rate at which an object changes speed, either increasing (**acceleration**) or decreasing (**deceleration**). Slow changes in speed are usually uneventful. Normal deceleration, such as slowing for a stop sign, covers about 120 feet (from 55 miles per hour to 0 miles per hour at a braking rate of 22 feet/10 miles per hour). It therefore rarely results in injury. On the other hand, colliding with a bridge abutment and slowing from 55 miles per hour to 0 miles per hour in a matter of inches produces tremendous force and devastating injuries.

TYPES OF TRAUMA

Trauma occurs when significant kinetic energy is applied to human anatomy. Trauma is defined as a wound or injury that is externally and violently produced by some outside force. The injury may be either blunt (closed) or penetrating (open) (Figure 13-3).

Blunt trauma occurs when a body area is struck by, or strikes, an object. The transmission of energy, rather than the object, damages the tissues and organs beneath the skin as they collide with one another. An example of this is hitting your thumb with a hammer. The thumb is compressed between the hammer (which pushes the tissue) and the board (which resists the motion). Tissue injury results as flesh and bone are trapped between these two forces (acceleration and deceleration). Skin and muscle cells stretch and crush, blood vessels tear, and bone may fracture.

Blunt trauma can also induce injury deep within the body cavity. Forces of compression cause hollow organs such as the bladder or bowel to rupture, spilling their contents and hemorrhaging. In the thorax, alveoli or small airways may burst, permitting air to enter the pleural space. Solid organs, such as the spleen, liver, pancreas, and kidneys, may contuse or lacerate, leading to swelling, blood loss, or both.

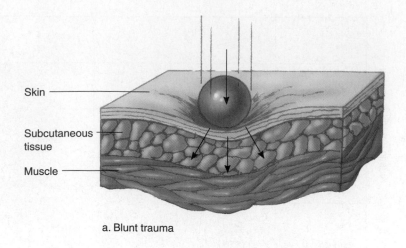

Skin

Subcutaneous tissue

Muscle

a. Blunt trauma

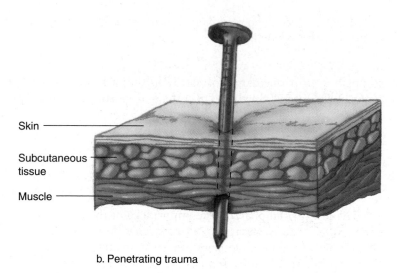

Skin

Subcutaneous tissue

Muscle

b. Penetrating trauma

FIGURE 13-3   Blunt trauma results when an object or force impacts the body and kinetic energy is transferred to the involved body tissues. Penetrating injury is produced when an object enters the body resulting in direct injury.

Other blunt trauma may result from the effects of rapid speed change on organ attachment. An example is the liver, which is suspended in the abdomen by the ligamentum teres. During severe deceleration, it may be sliced by the ligament in a way similar to cheese when cut by wire. Similarly, the aorta may be injured as the chest slows and the heart, which is suspended from the great vessels, twists on impact. Layers of the vessel are torn apart, and blood enters the injury with the force of the systolic blood pressure. The aorta balloons like a defective tire, leading to a tearing chest pain, circulatory compromise, and immediate or delayed **exsanguination** (severe blood loss).

exsanguination the draining of blood to the point at which life cannot be sustained.

Wounds that break the skin are classified as penetrating trauma. Penetrating trauma occurs when the energy source (such as a knife or bullet) progresses into the body. Energy may also be transmitted to surrounding body tissue, thus extending the trauma beyond the pathway of the object. This frequently happens with high velocity gunshot wounds.

As an EMT-I, you will encounter both blunt and penetrating trauma. The balance of this chapter deals with examples of blunt trauma. Examples of penetrating trauma are discussed in Chapter 14.

BLUNT TRAUMA

Blunt trauma most commonly results from motor-vehicle crashes (MVCs) involving auto-mobiles, motorcycles, pedestrians, or recreational vehicles (all-terrain vehicles, watercraft, snowmobiles). It can also result from explosions, falls, crush injuries, and sports injuries.

AUTOMOBILE CRASHES

Vehicular crashes account for a large proportion of EMT-I responses. Each year over 100,000 serious collisions occur on U.S. highways. Approximately 44,000 people lose their lives in these crashes, and many more are seriously injured or permanently disabled. As an EMT-I, you must be prepared to offer rapid assessment and appropriate care to victims of these crashes. To this end, you must recognize the various types of vehicular impacts, iden-tify possible mechanisms of injury, and form a reasonable index of suspicion for specific in-juries. Analysis of the types of impacts and the events associated with them help you form this index of suspicion.

Events of Impact

There are basically five types of vehicle impacts—frontal, lateral, rotational, rear-end, and rollover. Each type progresses through a series of five events (Figure 13-4). These events are:

1. *Vehicle collision.* Vehicle collision begins when the auto strikes an object. Kinetic energy converts to vehicle damage or is transferred to the object hit by the auto. The force developed in the crash depends on the stopping distance. If the auto slides into a snow bank, damage is limited. If the auto strikes a concrete retaining wall, the damage is much greater. The degree of auto deformity is a good indicator of strength and direction of forces experienced by its occupants. The auto collision slows or stops the vehicle.

2. *Body collision.* Body collision occurs when an occupant in a vehicle strikes the vehicle's interior. The vehicle and its interior have slowed dramatically during the crash, but an unrestrained occupant remains at or close to the initial speed. As the occupant contacts the interior, energy is transferred to the vehicle or is transformed into the initial tissue deformity, compression, stretching, and trauma. If the vehicle collision causes intrusion into the passenger compartment, this displacement may further injure occupants or otherwise worsen the injury process.

3. *Organ collisions.* Organ collision results when the occupant contacts the vehicle's interior and slows or stops. Tissues behind the contacting surface collide, one into another, as the occupant's body comes to a halt. This causes compression and stretching as tissues and organs violently press into each other. In the process, organs may also twist or decelerate, and tear at their attachments or at blood vessels. The result is blunt trauma.

4. *Secondary collisions.* Secondary collisions occur when objects traveling within the auto impact a vehicle occupant. During the crash, objects—such as those in the back seat, on the back window ledge, or in the back of a van—or other unrestrained passengers may continue to travel at the auto's initial speed. They then impact an occupant who has come to rest within the auto. It is important to consider the possibility of any secondary collisions and their effects on occupants when developing an index of suspicion for injuries.

5. *Additional impacts.* Additional impacts occur when a vehicle receives a second impact; for example, when it hits a vehicle, is deflected, and then hits a parked car. This second impact may induce additional patient injuries or increase the seriousness of those already received. Consider someone who sustains a femur fracture. It takes a great deal of energy to break the bone initially. Once the bone is broken, however, the energy now needed to move

Secondary collisions may cause a patient's injuries or increase their severity.

Vehicle collision

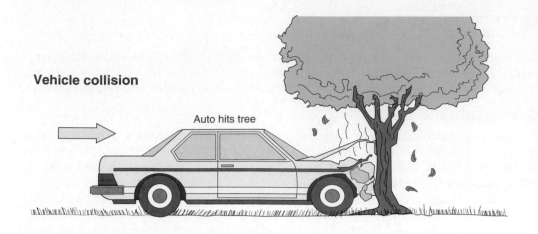

Auto hits tree

Impact points
Head vs. windshield

Body Collisions

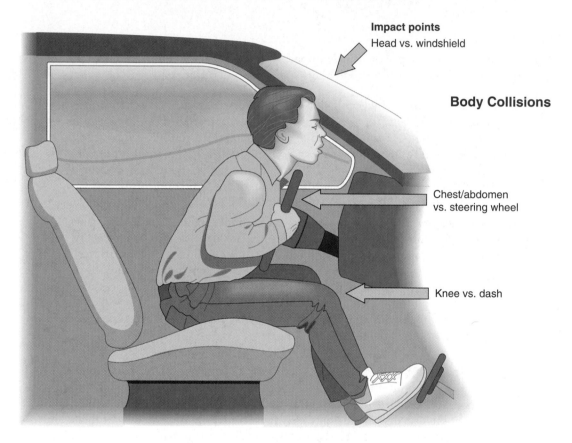

Chest/abdomen
vs. steering wheel

Knee vs. dash

FIGURE 13-4   An automobile crash generates four major collisions: the vehicle collision, the body collision, the organ collision, and secondary collisions.

those bone ends around and cause further, possibly more severe, injury to nerves and blood vessels is small. It is important to consider what effect any additional impacts may have on the initial injuries and overall patient condition.

Restraints

Restraints have had a profound effect in reducing crash-related deaths.

Restraints such as seat belts, shoulder straps, airbags, and child safety seats have a profound effect on the injuries associated with auto crashes. They have played a substantial role in reducing crash-related deaths from about 55,000 a year in the early 1970s to about 44,000 in recent years. It is important that you determine if restraints were used—and used properly— as you anticipate the possible results of an auto crash.

Organ collision

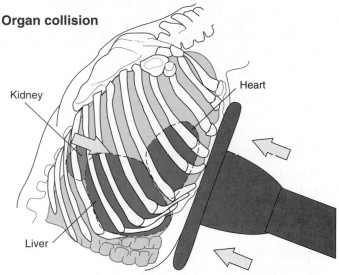

Kidney

Heart

Liver

The energy of body collision is transmitted to the interior.

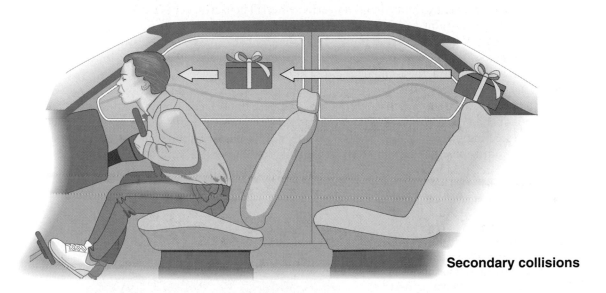

Secondary collisions

FIGURE 13-4 Continued.

EMS personnel should recognize the value of seat belts in reducing auto crash mortality and morbidity. Hence, all ambulance personnel must employ seat belts when in the patient care area of the vehicle and especially while driving. Securing the lap belt firmly provides positive positioning so drivers and other crew members are not as adversely affected by the gravitational forces (G forces) sometimes associated with emergency driving.

Seat Belts Use of seat belts and shoulder straps prevents the wearer's continuing and independent movement during a vehicle crash. The occupant slows with the auto rather than moving rapidly forward and impacting the interior suddenly. The occupant's ultimate deceleration rate is thus reduced, lessening the likelihood of serious injury from collisions within the vehicle. Seat belts and shoulder straps also lessen the chances that the wearer will be ejected from the vehicle.

Although seat belts and shoulder straps significantly reduce injury severity, they may cause some, usually much less serious, injuries. A lap belt worn alone does not restrain the torso, neck, or head from continuing forward. These body regions may impact the dash or

Seat belt use should be mandatory for all EMS personnel.

steering wheel, resulting in chest, neck, and head injuries. The sudden folding of the body at the waist during extreme impacts when only a lap belt is worn may result in intra-abdominal or lower spine injuries. If the lap belt is worn alone and too high, abdominal compression and spinal (T12 to L2) fractures may result. If worn too low, it may cause hip dislocations. If the shoulder strap is worn alone, it may cause severe neck contusions, lacerations, possible spinal injury, and even decapitation in more violent crashes. In very strong impacts, the shoulder strap may induce chest contusions and, in some cases, rib fractures. Further, the seat belt and/or shoulder strap do not protect against intrusions into the passenger compartment. In severe crashes, the dashboard may displace into the front seat, trapping or crushing the lower extremities of occupants.

Airbags Airbags, also called supplemental restraint systems (SRS), work much differently than seat belts and are extremely effective for frontal crashes. They inflate explosively upon auto impact, producing a cushion to absorb the energy exchange. Their ignition depends on several detectors sensing a very strong frontal deceleration, as can only occur with serious vehicle impact. Only after these detectors all agree does the explosive agent ignite. The ignition instantaneously fills the bag, slightly before or just as the occupant collides with it. The explosive gases escape quickly as the occupant compresses the bag, cushioning the impact similar to the inflated bags used by pole-vaulters and movie stuntmen. As with seat belts, airbags are credited with dramatically reducing vehicular death and trauma (Figure 13-5).

Airbags are positioned in the steering wheel. Their presence is indicated by an SRS (supplemental restraint system) sticker on the windshield and/or on the steering wheel itself. They may also be located in the dash for the front seat passenger. Steering wheel and dash-mounted airbags offer significant protection only in frontal impact collisions. This protection is only for the first impact and not subsequent ones.

Airbags may induce injury during their ignition and rapid inflation. As the bag inflates, especially from the steering wheel, it may impact the driver's fingers, hands, and forearms, possibly causing dislocations and fractures. In persons of small stature seated very close to the steering wheel, airbag inflation may also cause nasal fractures, minor facial lacerations, and contusions. The residue from airbag inflation may cause some irritation of the eyes; this can be relieved with gentle irrigation. Whenever an airbag has deployed, check beneath it for steering wheel deformity, which is indicative of injury to the driver.

FIGURE 13-5 Airbags cushion the driver from the forces of impact and significantly reduce mortality and morbidity in frontal impact crashes.

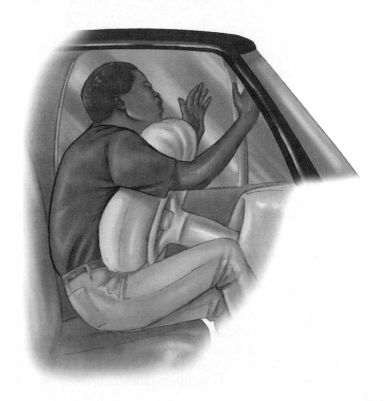

Passenger airbags have inflated in minor impacts and pushed infant and child safety carriers into seats with tremendous force. In some cases, infants and children have been severely injured or killed by inflation of the bags. For this reason, it is recommended that parents secure child safety seats in the back seat if a passenger airbag system is in an automobile.

Auto manufacturers are starting to install airbags in the seat sides, adjacent to the doors in some cars, for protection in lateral impact crashes. Some manufacturers also install airbags in the headliners above doors to provide protection for the head in such crashes. Since little experience has been gained with these types of restraints, their benefits and potential drawbacks are not well known. However, lateral impacts do account for a very high mortality rate that may be mediated with lateral-impact and head-protection airbags.

Child Safety Seats   The child's anatomy makes protection in vehicle crashes difficult. Because a child's size changes so quickly with increasing age, normal restraint systems are designed for adults only. Small children should be placed in appropriate child safety seats to ensure their relative safety during an auto impact. With infants and very small children, the child safety seat is positioned facing to the rear and held firmly to the seat with the seat belt. This positioning best distributes frontal impact forces and prevents unrestrained infant movement. As the child grows, the child carrier is turned facing forward and used as a small seat. The seat belt then crosses the child at the waistline.

Children held in an adult's lap or arms are not well protected during a crash. The holder may grasp them too tightly during impact or, more likely, will not (or cannot) hold on tightly enough. If the child is not held, he becomes an unrestrained moving object and will impact the vehicle interior suffering serious, possibly fatal, injury.

When evaluating the results of an auto impact, always be sure to examine for and ask questions about the use of restraints. Determine if seat belts and shoulder straps were used and used properly, if airbags deployed during the crash, and if child carriers were properly positioned and secured. If these restraints were properly employed, the severity of injuries to the vehicle occupants will very likely be reduced.

Types of Impact

As you have read, the five general types of auto impacts are as follows:

- Frontal
- Lateral
- Rotational
- Rear end
- Rollover

The following is a breakdown of the frequency of different types of motor-vehicle impacts (Figure 13-6). Percentages reflect an urban setting. In a more rural area, anticipate a greater percentage of frontal impacts with corresponding reductions in other categories.

Content Review

TYPES OF VEHICLE IMPACT
- Frontal
- Lateral
- Rotational
- Rear end
- Rollover

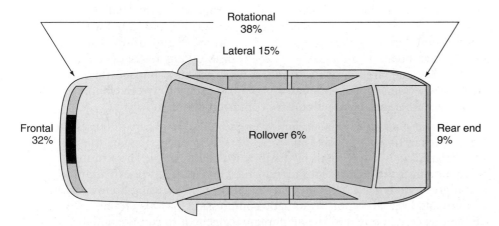

FIGURE 13-6   Incidence of motor-vehicle impacts.

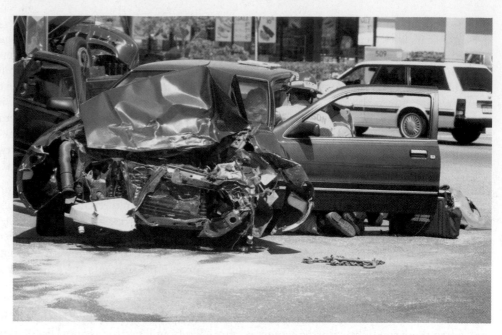

FIGURE 13-7   Frontal impact often results in a significant exchange of energy and serious injuries.

Frontal: 32%

Lateral: 15%

Rotational: 38%

Rear end: 9%

Rollover: 6%

Note that rotational impact includes four subcategories: left front, right front, left rear, and right rear.

Frontal Impact   Frontal impact is the most common type of impact (Figure 13-7) and produces three pathways of patient travel. They are:

Frontal impact is the most common type of vehicle crash.

1. *Down-and-under pathway.* In the down-and-under pathway, the occupant slides downward as the vehicle comes to a stop. The knees contact the firewall under the dash and absorb the initial impact. Knee, femur, and hip dislocations or fractures are common. Once the lower body slows, the upper body rotates forward, pivoting at the hip, and crashing against the steering wheel or dash. Chest injuries such as flail chest, myocardial contusion, and aortic tears result. If the neck contacts the steering wheel, tracheal and vascular injury may occur. An injury process frequently associated with steering wheel impact is the "paper bag" syndrome (Figure 13-8). The driver takes a deep breath in anticipation of the collision. Lung tissue (alveoli, bronchioles, and larger airways) ruptures when the chest impacts the steering wheel, much like an inflated paper bag caught between clapping hands. Pneumothorax and pulmonary contusion may result.

The up-and-over pathway accounts for over half of vehicular-crash deaths.

2. *Up-and-over pathway.* In the up-and-over pathway, the occupant tenses the legs in preparation for impact (Figure 13-9). With vehicle slowing, the unrestrained body's upper half pivots forward and upward. The steering wheel impinges the femurs, causing possible bilateral fractures. In addition, it compresses and decelerates the abdominal contents, causing hollow-organ rupture and liver laceration. Traumatic compression may also force abdominal contents against the diaphragm, causing it to rupture and allowing organs to enter the thoracic cavity. As the body continues forward,

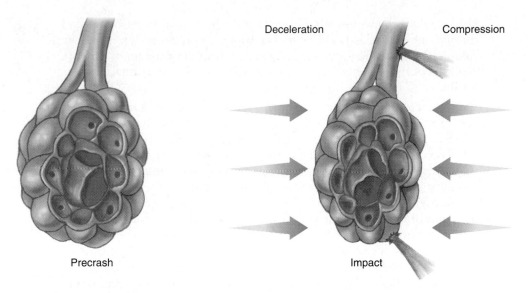

Deceleration   Compression

Precrash   Impact

FIGURE 13-8   The "paper bag" syndrome results from compression of the chest against the steering column.

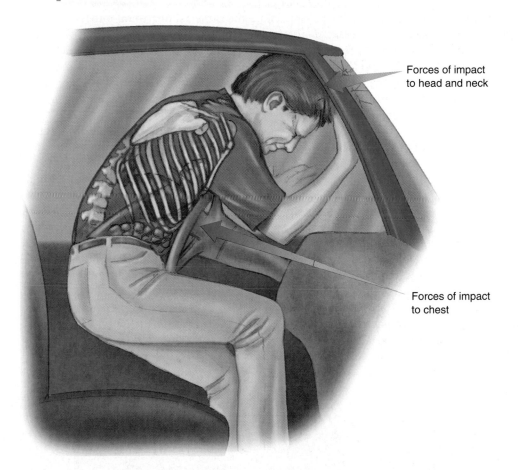

Forces of impact
to head and neck

Forces of impact
to chest

FIGURE 13-9   The up-and-over pathway is associated with frontal impact crashes.

the lower chest impacts the steering wheel and may account for the same thoracic injuries seen with the down-and-under pathway.

The same forward motion propels the head into the windshield, leading to soft tissue injury, skull or facial fractures, and internal head injury. Neck injury may result from hyperextension, hyperflexion, or the compressional forces of windshield impact. As the body is thrown upward and forward, the

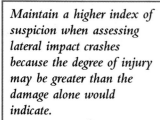

Occupants of a vehicle with no crumple zone may experience greater forces in a collision, even though damage to the vehicle itself may not appear as severe as damage to a vehicle with a crumple zone.

Maintain a higher index of suspicion when assessing lateral impact crashes because the degree of injury may be greater than the damage alone would indicate.

head contacts the windshield. The rest of the body tries to push the head through the windshield. The result is a compressional force on the cervical spine called **axial loading**. This loading may result in collapse of support elements of the vertebral column. Over half of vehicular deaths are attributed to the up-and-over pathway.

3. *Ejection.* The up-and-over pathway may lead to ejection of an unrestrained occupant. Such a victim experiences two impacts: (1) contact with the vehicle interior and windshield and (2) impact with the ground, tree, or other object. This mechanism of injury is responsible for about 27% of vehicular fatalities. Although ejection may occur with other types of impact, it is most commonly associated with frontal impact.

Recognize that a frontal impact crash interposes more vehicle between the point of impact and the vehicle occupants. Modern vehicle design techniques use this area of the vehicle (called the **crumple zone**) to absorb the impact forces and limit occupant injury (Figure 13-10). Patients in vehicle collisions such as those involving vans and lateral impacts do not benefit from these energy absorbing crumple zones. In these circumstances, the apparent vehicle damage may be less than in a frontal impact crash, even though the forces delivered to the occupants are greater.

Lateral Impact   The kinetics of lateral impact are the same as for frontal impact with two exceptions. First, occupants present a different profile (turned 90 degrees) to collision forces. Second, the amount of structural steel between the impact site and the vehicle interior is greatly reduced (Figure 13-11). Lateral impacts account for 15% of all auto collisions, yet they are responsible for 22% of vehicular fatalities. When a lateral impact occurs, the index of suspicion for serious and life-threatening internal injuries must be higher than vehicle damage alone suggests.

With lateral impacts, upper extremity injuries increase (Figure 13-12). The ribs fracture laterally on the side of impact instead of anteriorly. The clavicle, humerus, pelvis, and femur may fracture on the impact side. Cervical spine injury occurs as the body moves laterally while the head remains stationary. Vertebrae may fracture with the rapid lateral motion as may the skull as it smashes into the window. Lateral compression, affecting the body cavity, may give rise to diaphragm rupture, pulmonary contusion, splenic injury (to the driver), and much more. Aortic aneurysm may occur with this injury mechanism. The heart, which is not firmly attached in the central thorax, moves violently toward the impact as the body accelerates. This twists the aorta, tearing its inner layer, the intima. Blood seeps between the connective tissue layers and the vessel begins to delaminate. The aorta may rupture immediately or over the next few hours.

Evaluation of lateral impact collisions should take into consideration any unrestrained passenger opposite the impact site. If the driver's side is struck and such a passenger is not belted, the passenger becomes an object that will strike and injure the driver shortly after initial impact.

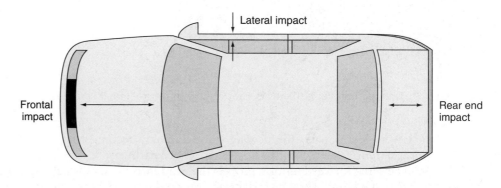

FIGURE 13-10   Crumple zones provide significant protection with both frontal and rear-end impacts but much less in cases of lateral impacts.

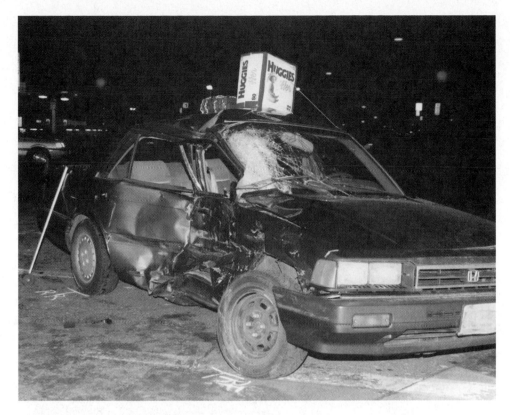

FIGURE 13-11 A lateral impact collision presents the least amount of crumple zone between the vehicle's exterior and its passenger compartment.

Rotational Impact In rotational impact, the auto is struck at an **oblique** angle and rotates as the collision forces are expended (Figure 13-13). The ensuing rotation causes injuries similar to those from frontal and lateral impacts. Acceleration (or deceleration) is greatest farther from the center of the auto and closest to impact. Autos involved are deflected from their paths rather than being stopped abruptly. Although rotational impact injuries can be serious, they are often less than vehicle damage might suggest. With the deflection of the impact, the occupant's stopping distance is much greater, deceleration is more gradual, and injuries are generally less serious.

Rear-end Impact In rear-end impact, the collision force pushes the auto forward (Figure 13-14). Within the vehicle, the seat propels the occupant forward. If the headrest is not up, the head is unsupported and remains stationary. The neck extends severely, stretching the neck muscles and ligaments while the head rotates backward. Once acceleration ceases, the head snaps forward and the neck flexes. This rapid and extreme hyperextension followed by hyperflexion may result in severe connective tissue and cervical vertebra injuries (Figure 13-15). There is also risk of injury when the auto finally ends its acceleration and an unrestrained occupant is thrown forward.

Rollover Auto rollover is normally caused by a change in elevation and/or a vehicle with a high center of gravity (Figure 13-16). As the vehicle rolls, it impacts the ground at various points. The occupant experiences an impact with each impact of the vehicle. These impacts can be especially violent due to the absence of crumple zones and internal padding at the multiple points of impact (vehicle sides and roof). The type of injuries expected with a rollover relate to the specific vehicle impacts involved. Remember, any injury occurring with the first collision is likely to be compounded with subsequent impacts. A common result of rollover is ejection or partial ejection with a limb or head trapped between the rolling vehicle and the ground. Restraints are especially effective in reducing ejection and injury during rollover.

oblique having a slanted position or direction.

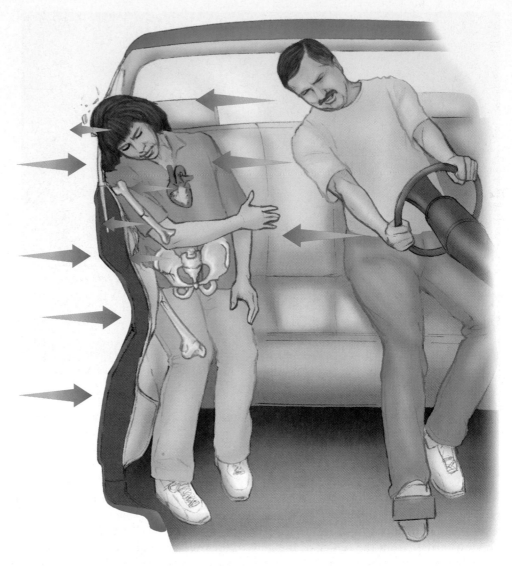

FIGURE 13-12   In a lateral impact collision, an occupant may experience lateral impact to the head, lateral bending of the neck, twisting of the heart and the aorta, plus humerus, clavicular, pelvic, and femur fractures.

Vehicle Crash Analysis

Vehicle crashes often produce hazards not only to the vehicle occupants but also to bystanders and care providers. Be alert for these hazards during the scene size-up. Such hazards may include hot engine and transmission parts, hot fluids such as radiator coolant or engine oil, caustic substances such as battery acid and automatic transmission or steering fluids, and the sharp, jagged edges of torn metal or broken glass. Also remain aware of the potential for danger from traffic moving near the crash site or from electrical power lines that may have been downed by the crash.

During the scene size-up, evaluate the vehicle to determine the direction of impact and the amount of vehicle damage. From the angle of impact, visualize the direction of forces expressed on the crash victims and the strength of those forces. Realize that the front and rear structures of modern cars are designed to crumple during impact to absorb kinetic forces. Although moderate-speed impacts may destroy the vehicle, the passengers may escape with little injury. Occupants in lateral and rollover impacts do not benefit from such crumple zones and frequently suffer injuries more directly related to the kinetic forces.

The visual examination of the crash scene can tell you a great deal about what happened to the patient(s) and what injuries should be suspected.

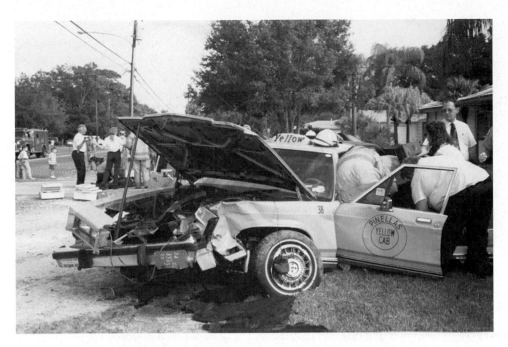

FIGURE 13-13 In rotational impacts, the energy exchange is more gradual and an occupant may have less injury than vehicle damage suggests. However, there may be multiple impacts.

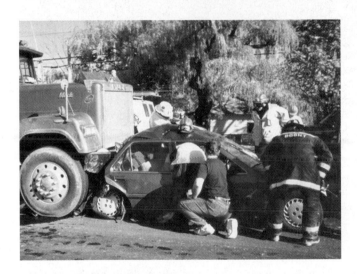

FIGURE 13-14 In rear-end impacts there is generally good protection for the body, except for the head and neck. *(Courtesy of Edward T. Dickinson, MD)*

As you evaluate the collision, consider the relative sizes of the impacting vehicles or objects. A large, heavy vehicle impacting a smaller, lighter one will experience lesser acceleration or deceleration forces than the smaller vehicle. In this case, there is likely to be more severe vehicle damage to the smaller vehicle and more serious injuries to its occupants as well. Similar considerations apply with objects impacted by vehicles. For example, a large, well-rooted tree that does not move will cause much more damage during an impact than will a telephone pole that shears off.

When evaluation of the outside of the vehicle is complete, look at the passenger compartment (Figure 13-17). Determine if there is any intrusion, which indicates the presence of forces greater than those that could be absorbed by the crumple zones. Quickly look for signs of occupant/interior impacts. A spider-web pattern on the windshield suggests a severe impact between the occupant's head and the glass. A deformed steering wheel suggests injury to the driver's chest or upper abdomen. A dented dash suggests injury to the knees or injuries transmitted to the femur or hip. Deformities of the gas, brake, or clutch pedals suggest foot injury. Deployed and deflated airbags may indicate chest, forearm, or hand injury.

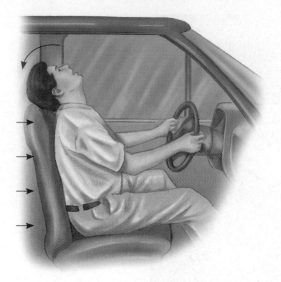

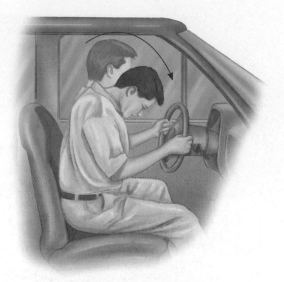

a. Victim moves ahead while head remains stationary.
Head rotates backward. Neck extends.

b. Head snaps forward. Head rotates forward. Neck flexes.

FIGURE 13-15   The effects of a rear-end collision on the occupant of a vehicle.

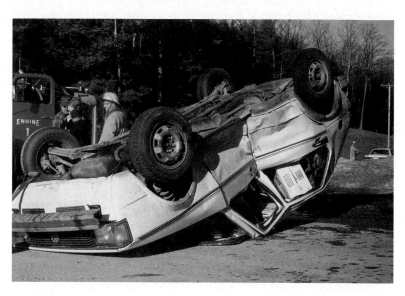

FIGURE 13-16   Rollover crashes result in multiple impacts and, possibly, multiple mechanisms of injury.

In very severe impacts, collision forces may push the dashboard and firewall into the passenger compartment, entrapping and crushing the lower extremities of occupants against the seat. In such cases, parts of the vehicle, such as the foot pedals, turn indicator arms, shift levers, and instrument panel knobs or switches may be physically imbedded in crash victims. This complicates extrication because the seat and the dash must be separated carefully to free the trapped victim. In these cases, the area should be carefully examined before and while any extrication equipment is used. Ongoing examinations should be provided frequently during extrication to ensure that the process does not result in further, unnecessary harm to the patient.

Assess whether restraints have been used or airbags deployed. Use of these devices may limit the severity of injuries in frontal impacts. Conversely, their non-use may suggest more severe injuries. Check the positions of headrests in rear-impact collisions. Their proper positioning may limit neck hyperextension and injury.

Alcohol intoxication is associated with most serious crashes.

Intoxication   Whenever you evaluate motor-vehicle trauma, consider the possibility of alcohol intoxication. Data from states requiring mandatory alcohol-level testing after fatal

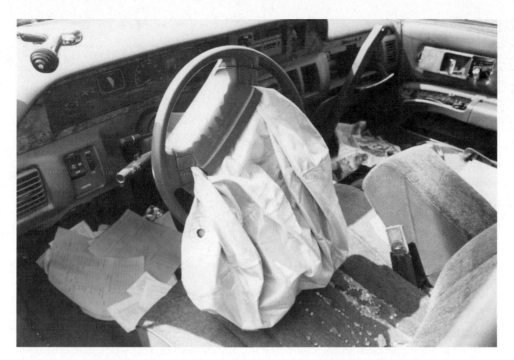

FIGURE 13-17   Study the interior of a crashed vehicle carefully to identify the strength and direction of forces expressed to the patient.

auto collisions reveal that more than 50% of the drivers were legally intoxicated. Alcohol also contributes to many recreational-vehicle collisions, boating accidents, and accidental drownings.

Whenever you suspect alcohol intoxication, your assessment must be more diligent. Remember, alcohol interferes with the patient's level of consciousness and masks signs and symptoms of injury. Intoxication may be hard to differentiate from the signs of head injury. It also anesthetizes the patient somewhat to trauma pain. These factors make the mechanism of injury analysis and the resultant index of suspicion even more important. Otherwise, significant injuries may be overlooked or brushed off as symptoms of alcohol intoxication.

Vehicular Mortality   Examination of the effects of motor-vehicle trauma on the human anatomy reveals certain areas to be especially prone to life-threatening injury. A study of the incidence of mortality and the associated location of trauma provides the findings in Table 13-1.

Trauma to the head and body cavity accounts for 85% of vehicular mortality. For this reason, the rapid trauma assessment should be directed at the head, neck, thorax, abdomen, and pelvis. Once you ensure the airway, breathing, and circulation, proceed to the rapid trauma assessment, looking at areas where your index of suspicion suggests injury. Examine the head, chest, and abdomen first to identify any evidence of life-threatening injuries.

Crash Evaluation   As an EMT-I, you must be thoroughly practiced in the assessment of trauma patients, especially because of the high incidence of serious injury associated with auto crashes. Whenever you respond to a collision, analyze the five types of collisions associated with vehicle impact. In each case, ask yourself these questions:

- How did the objects collide?
- From what direction did they come?
- At what speed were they traveling?
- Were the objects similarly sized or grossly different? (For example, did a car and a semi-truck collide?)
- Were any secondary collisions or additional transfers of energy involved?

Head and body-cavity trauma account for 85% of deaths in vehicular crashes.

Table 13-1	MOTOR-VEHICLE FATALITIES	
Incidence by Body Area		
Head		47.7%
Internal (chest/abdominal/pelvic)		37.3%
Spinal and chest fracture		8.3%
Fractures to the extremities		2.0%
All other		4.7%

In analyzing the mechanisms of injury, also consider the cause of the crash.

- Did wet pavement or poor visibility contribute to the crash?
- Was alcohol involved?
- Are skid marks absent? If so, what happened to the driver to prevent him from braking?

Examine the auto interior, which is the mass struck by the moving occupant.

- Does the windshield show evidence of impact by the victim's head?
  - Is it bloody or broken in the characteristic spider web or star-shape pattern?
  - Has it been penetrated by the patient's head or body?
- Is the steering wheel deformed or collapsed?
- Is the dash indented where the knees or head hit it?
- Has the impact damage extended into the passenger compartment (intrusion)?

Answers to such questions complement your mechanism of injury analysis and help you to develop accurate indices of suspicion.

MOTORCYCLE CRASHES

Serious trauma is likely with even low-speed motorcycle crashes because of the lack of protective vehicle structure.

In addition to auto crashes, as an EMT-I, you will respond to many motorcycle crashes. Because of the lack of protective vehicle structure, motorcycle crashes often result in serious trauma, even at low speeds. The rider, rather than the structural steel, absorbs much of the crash energy (Figure 13-18). Injuries can be severe, with an especially high incidence of head trauma. The motorcycle crash impacts differ somewhat from those of an auto crash. The four types of motorcycle impacts include frontal, angular, sliding, and ejection.

In a frontal, or head-on impact, the bike dips downward, propelling the rider upward and forward. The handlebars catch the rider's lower abdomen or pelvis, causing abdominal and/or pelvic injury. Occasionally, the rider travels through a higher trajectory. In such cases, the handlebars can trap the femurs, often resulting in bilateral fractures.

An angular impact occurs when the bike strikes an object at an oblique angle. The rider's lower extremity is trapped between the object struck and the bike. This may fracture or crush the foot, ankle, knee, and femur. Open wounds often result.

Sliding impact occurs when an experienced rider, facing an imminent crash, "lays the bike down." The rider slides the bike sideways into the object, so that the bike hits the object first, absorbing much of the energy. Laying the bike down also reduces the chances of ejection. The result is an increase in lacerations, abrasions, and minor fractures, with a decrease in more serious injuries.

Ejection during a motorcycle crash is common and usually results in serious injury. It may occur with any of the mechanisms previously described and result in the following impacts:

- Initial bike/object collision
- Rider/object impact
- Rider/ground impact

Likely injuries include skull fracture and/or head injury, spinal fractures and paralysis, internal thoracic or abdominal injury, and extremity fractures.

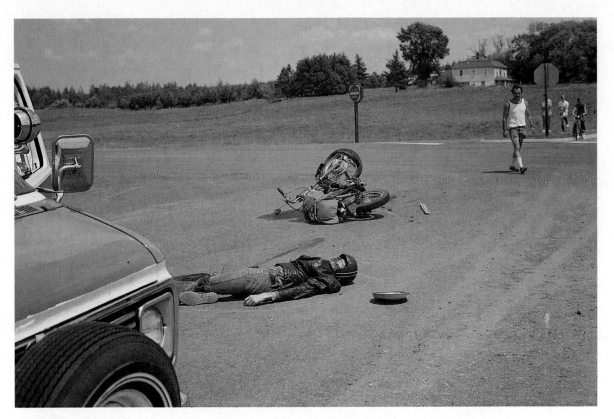

FIGURE 13-18 Motorcycle crashes result in serious trauma because the vehicle provides little protection for its rider.

In assessing a motorcycle crash, remember that protective equipment affects injury patterns. A helmet can reduce the incidence and severity of head injury from 50% to 66%. Use of a helmet, however, neither increases nor decreases the incidence of spinal trauma. Leather clothing and boots protect the rider against open soft-tissue injury, but they can also hide underlying contusions and fractures.

AUTO VS. PEDESTRIAN COLLISIONS

Some vehicular collisions involve pedestrians, who are often severely injured because of the mass and speed of the object hitting them and because of their lack of protection. Adults and children suffer different types of injuries because of differing anatomical size and differing responses to the impending accident. Recognition of these differences helps you anticipate injuries and provide the necessary treatment.

Adult pedestrians generally turn away from oncoming vehicles and present a lateral surface to impact. Anatomically, impact is low. The bumper strikes the lower leg first, fracturing the tibia and fibula. Energy transmitted to the opposing knee can lead to ligament injury. As the lower extremities are propelled forward with the car, the upper and lateral body crashes into the hood causing femur, lateral chest, or upper extremity fractures. The victim then slides into the windshield, leading to head, neck, and shoulder trauma. The adult may be further injured when thrown to the ground. This secondary collision may cause additional injury or compound those already received (Figure 13-19).

In contrast to adults, children usually turn toward an oncoming vehicle. Because of their smaller anatomy, injuries are located higher on children's bodies. The bumper impacts the femurs or pelvis, causing fracture. Children are frequently thrown in front of the vehicle because of their smaller size and lower center of gravity. They may then be run over or pushed to the side by the vehicle. If a child is thrown upward, injuries are similar to those of an adult (Figure 13-20).

When evaluating the injuries associated with auto vs. pedestrian collision, look carefully at the scene. Try to determine the speed of the vehicle at time of impact and the distance the

Helmets reduce the incidence and severity of head injuries in motorcycle crashes, but they have no effect on the incidence of spinal trauma.

In pedestrian vs. automobile crashes, adults tend to turn away from the oncoming vehicle before impact, whereas children turn toward it.

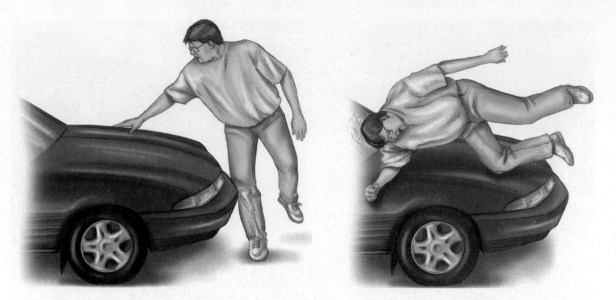

FIGURE 13-19 An adult frequently turns away from a collision with an automobile and thus impacts the vehicle first with a leg. Because of a higher center of gravity, such patients are often thrown onto the hood and into the windshield.

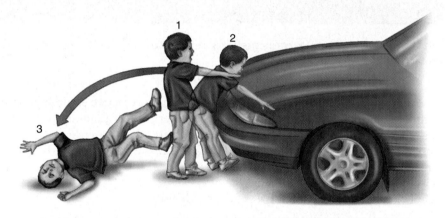

FIGURE 13-20 In collisions with autos, children often turn toward the impact and, because of their lower body heights, are frequently thrown in front of the vehicle.

pedestrian was thrown. This information may be useful to the emergency department personnel in their determination of suspected injuries.

RECREATIONAL VEHICLE CRASHES

Recreational vehicles usually lack the structure and the restraint systems that offer significant protection to automobile drivers and passengers.

Over the past years, recreational vehicle usage has increased, and with it, the incidence of related trauma. Recreational vehicle crashes often cause injuries similar to those associated with auto crashes. Drivers and passengers of recreational vehicles, however, do not have the structural protections and restraint systems found in autos. Complicating injuries is the fact that recreational vehicles travel off road, which means there is often difficulty in reaching and retrieving victims once collisions are detected. The major types of vehicles most often involved in recreational vehicle crashes are snowmobiles, watercraft, and all-terrain vehicles (ATVs).

Snowmobile crashes can be very violent because the speeds at which snowmobiles travel can approach those of cars and snowmobiles offer no crumple zones for impact absorption. These incidents commonly result in ejections, crush injuries secondary to rollover, and

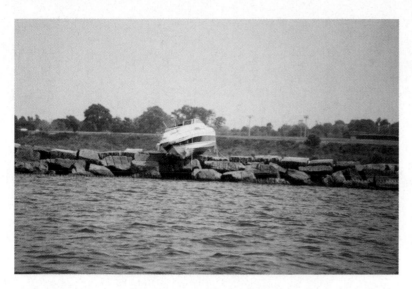

FIGURE 13-21 Watercraft accidents are common, may involve either objects on the surface or submerged, and present the risks of drowning or hypothermia.

glancing blows against obstructions in the snow. Riders also experience severe head and neck injuries from collisions with other vehicles, including autos, other snowmobiles, or with stationary objects such as trees. Snowmobile trauma may include severe neck injury when the rider runs into an unseen wire fence. The anterior neck is deeply lacerated, causing airway compromise, severe bleeding, and, in some cases, complete decapitation. Injuries to snowmobilers may be compounded by the effects of cold exposure and hypothermia.

Watercraft accidents commonly result from impact with other boats or obstructions, submerged or otherwise (Figure 13-21). These vehicles are not designed to absorb the energy of impacts nor are the occupants provided with restraint systems. As a result, watercraft crashes can cause serious injuries, even though the speeds of typical watercraft are substantially lower than those of autos. Trauma in these crashes is further complicated by the potential for drowning if the occupants are thrown into the water or the boat sinks. In northern climates, water temperatures can also rapidly induce hypothermia. Alcohol is frequently associated with watercraft incidents.

The use of personal watercraft, commonly called jet skis, for water recreation has increased greatly in recent years, as has the incidence of watercraft accidents. Jet skis are especially dangerous in the hands of inexperienced riders. The high speeds attained by these watercraft contribute to the incidence and severity of injury associated with crashes. Although the craft's propulsion unit is protected and unlikely to cause trauma, collision with other watercraft, as well as objects and people in the water, lead to blunt trauma, again complicated by the potential for drowning.

Two types of ATVs are the three- and four-wheeled versions (Figure 13-22). The three-wheeled ATV is notoriously unstable, especially when ridden by children, young adults, persons of lower body weight, or those with limited vehicle experience. The center of gravity of an ATV is relatively high, contributing to the likelihood of rollover during quick turns. As with snowmobiles, a significant incidence of frontal collision is common with both types of ATVs. The injuries expected might include upper and lower extremity fracture and head and spine injury.

BLAST INJURIES

Explosions can be caused by dust, as in a grain elevator, by fumes, such as gasoline or natural gas, or by explosive compounds (combustible and **oxidizer** mixes) such as dynamite, gunpowder, and TNT. The explosion may be the result of an accident or intentional act of terrorism or warfare. The blast magnitude may range from that of a small firecracker in the hands of a teenager to a nuclear detonation.

oxidizer an agent that enhances combustion of a fuel.

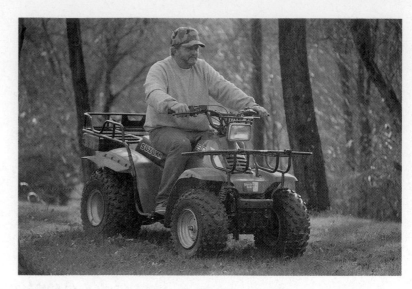

FIGURE 13-22 All-terrain vehicles (ATVs) can cause a multitude of injuries due to their speed, instability, and lack of rider protection.

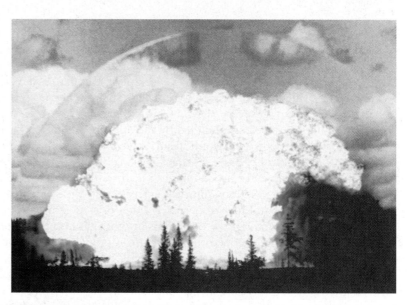

FIGURE 13-23 An explosion releases tremendous amounts of heat energy, generating a pressure wave, blast wind, and projection of debris.

Explosion

An explosion occurs when an agent or environment combusts. During a conventional (non-nuclear) explosion, the fuel and oxidizing agent combine instantaneously. Chemical bonds are broken down and reestablished, releasing tremendous energy in the form of rapidly moving molecules, known to us as heat. This heat creates a great pressure differential between the exploding agent and the surrounding air. This heat and the pressure differential produce several mechanisms of injury including a pressure wave, blast wind, projectiles, heat, and displacement of persons near the blast (Figure 13-23).

Pressure Wave

As the combustible agent ignites and burns explosively, it immediately heats the surrounding air. The molecules of heated air move very fast, increasing the pressure of the exploding cloud. The rapid increase in pressure compresses adjacent air. Adjacent air, in turn, pushes against air farther out from the point of ignition, and a **pressure wave** begins to move away from the blast epicenter. This is not a gross air movement but rather a narrow compression

Content Review

MECHANISMS ASSOCIATED WITH BLASTS

- Pressure wave
- Blast wind
- Projectiles
- Personnel displacement
- Confined spaces and structural collapses
- Burns

pressure wave area of overpressure that radiates outward from an explosion.

wave moving rapidly outward, similar to a wave through water (where the wave and not the water moves). This narrow wave, called **overpressure**, results in a drastic but brief increase, then decrease, in air pressure as it passes. The blast overpressure wave moves outward slightly faster than the speed of sound through the air or water, and its strength decreases quickly.

When the explosion involves a dust, aerosol, or gas cloud, the result is an area, not a single point, of detonation. The pressure of the exploding cloud is extremely lethal, and the area it involves can be extensive. A bomb's casing or confined spaces, such as a building interior, contain the pressure of an explosion until the structure ruptures. The ensuing rapid release of the pressure enhances the peak overpressure and the potential for injury and death.

Underwater detonation also greatly enhances the potential for injury and death associated with the pressure wave. Water is a non-compressible medium that transmits the overpressure efficiently. Any submerged portion of the victim is subject to the rapid compression and then decompression. The lethal range for an explosive charge increases threefold with an underwater detonation.

Upon striking the body, the overpressure wave instantly compresses, then decompresses, the body's air-filled spaces, causing trauma. This rapid compression/decompression may produce injury to the middle ear, sinuses, bowel, or lungs. Because overpressure intensity diminishes rapidly as the wave travels outward, most life-threatening compression injuries are usually limited to people in close proximity to the detonation, with the exceptions of gas-cloud ignitions and underwater detonations.

A victim's orientation to the blast wave is also an important factor in the production of injuries. The greater the surface a victim presents to the blast wave, the greater the impact and damage. People standing and facing directly toward or away from the blast experience the greatest pressure effect. People lying on the ground, with their heads away from or toward the blast, experience the least pressure effects. In water, the same is true, although the more deeply submerged a victim is, the greater the damaging effects of the overpressure.

Blast Wind

Following the pressure wave and traveling just behind it, is the **blast wind**. This is the actual outward movement of heated and expanding combustion gases from the explosion epicenter. The blast wind has less strength but greater duration than the pressure wave. It causes much less direct injury, although in powerful blasts it may propel debris or displace victims, which will, in turn, produce injuries.

Projectiles

If the exploding material is contained by a casing, as with military **ordnance** or a pipe bomb, or by a structure, as with a garage filled with gas fumes, the container holds the explosive force until the container breaks apart. The parts of the container then become high-speed projectiles, behaving similar to bullets and bound by the same laws of physics. Although they are not as fast as bullets and they lack good aerodynamic properties, they can cause serious injury beyond the injury zone of the blast's pressure wave itself. Some military ordnance contains special arrow-shaped missiles called **flechettes**. Their design gives the flechettes a greater following surface and aligns the missiles in flight, reducing their wind resistance and increasing their range and penetrating ability.

If the victim is in very close proximity to a strong blast, the casing and debris may move forcefully enough to tear off limbs or cause serious open wounds. The blast debris—glass fragments, building materials, or casing elements—may also impale the skin and soft tissue. Although the wounds caused by blast debris are normally small, large and heavy fragments may penetrate deeply into victims and cause serious tissue damage and hemorrhage.

Personnel Displacement

The pressure wave and blast wind may be strong enough to physically propel victims away from the center of the blast. Those victims then become projectiles and impact the ground, objects, debris, or other personnel, resulting in blunt or, in some cases, penetrating trauma. Although the effects of this mechanism of injury are limited when compared with those produced by the pressure wave, blast wind, or projectiles, significant injuries can occur.

overpressure a rapid increase then decrease in atmospheric pressure created by an explosion.

Underwater detonation increases the lethal range of an explosion threefold.

blast wind the air movement caused as the heated and pressurized products of an explosion move outward.

ordnance military weapons and munitions.

flechettes arrow-shaped projectiles found in some military ordnance.

Confined Space Explosions and Structural Collapses

The most lethal explosions are those causing structural collapses followed by those in confined spaces.

The effects of explosive devices are usually limited in range because the pressure wave and debris radiate outward in all directions from a central point. This rapidly reduces the overpressure and the concentration and, to a lesser degree, the velocity of projectiles. When an explosion occurs in a confined space, however, the pressure wave maintains its energy longer. There is also danger of structural collapse, and debris from the confining structure can increase the blast's projectile content. The blast overpressure also bounces off walls and, where pressure waves meet, the pressure greatly increases. The result can be extremely deadly overpressures. The most lethal blasts are those causing structural collapses followed by those involving confined spaces.

Structural collapses may cause severe crush-type injuries. The collapses may also make victims difficult to locate and, once found, difficult to extricate because of the weight of the material entrapping them. Damage to structures may present further hazards to rescuers and victims, including the possibility of additional collapses, electrocution, fire, or secondary explosion due to gas or fuel leaks.

Burns

An explosion can create tremendous heat. This heat may cause flash burns to those very close to the detonation. These injuries are generally superficial or partial-thickness burns and may occur with other trauma. However, victims may also be burned as the heat of the blast ignites combustibles such as clothing, debris, other munitions, or fuel. These secondary burns may be full-thickness and extensive.

incendiary an agent that combusts easily or creates combustion.

Some military and terrorist devices are designed to induce damage and injury through combustion. Napalm, for an example, is a highly **incendiary**, jellylike substance that clings to people or structures when spread by a blast. It can produce severe or fatal full-thickness burns. Other ordnance uses materials, such as phosphorus, that spontaneously combust when exposed to air.

Blast Injury Phases

The injuries produced by explosions are usually classified into three types depending on the phases of the blast that caused them: primary, secondary, and tertiary (Figure 13-24).

Content Review

BLAST INJURY PHASES
- Primary—caused by heat of explosion and overpressure wave
- Secondary—caused by blast projectiles
- Tertiary—caused by personnel displacement and structural collapse

- *Primary blast injuries.* Primary blast injuries are caused by the heat of the explosion and the overpressure wave. The pressure injuries are the most serious associated with the explosion. Burn injuries are generally limited unless caused by secondary combustion.

- *Secondary blast injuries.* Secondary blast injuries include trauma caused by projectiles. These injuries may be as or more severe than the primary blast injuries. Projectiles from an explosive blast do have the ability to extend the range of injury beyond that caused by the blast wave and wind. High concentrations of projectiles may also create multiple body penetrations and impalements over large areas of a victim's body. The resulting injuries may produce severe bleeding.

- *Tertiary blast injuries.* Tertiary blast injuries include those injuries resulting from personnel displacement and structural collapse. Blast victims may be thrown against walls, the ground, or other obstructions and suffer blunt and/or penetrating trauma. When the blast results in a structural collapse, crush injuries may also result. These injuries can be extensive and result in soft, skeletal, nervous, and vascular tissue and organ destruction.

Blast Injury Assessment

Employ disaster triage and activate the jurisdiction's disaster plan if the number of blast victims exceeds EMS system capacities.

Blast injuries produce extreme trauma in those who are close to the blast epicenter. Blasts in densely populated areas may also involve large numbers of victims. Your role as an EMT-I is to survey and size up the scene and do what you can to secure it for further EMS operations. This normally involves implementing the incident command system and ensuring overall scene management. Once command is established and operational, you will likely begin caring for patients by applying the normal assessment priorities (the ABCs of the initial assess-

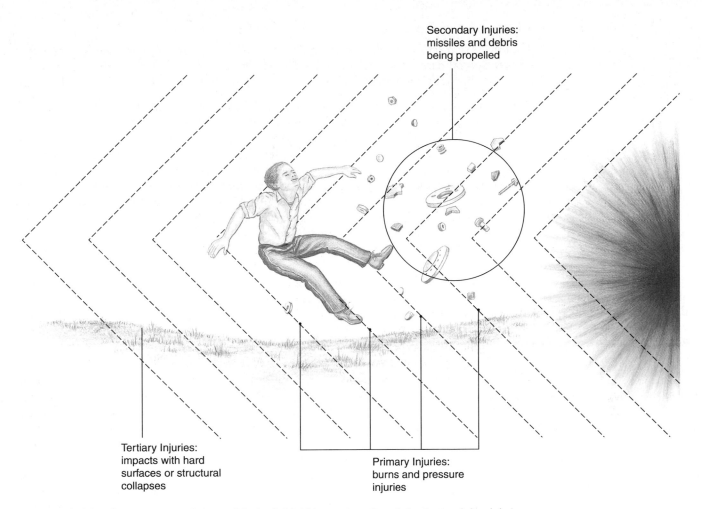

Secondary Injuries:
missiles and debris
being propelled

Tertiary Injuries:
impacts with hard
surfaces or structural
collapses

Primary Injuries:
burns and pressure
injuries

FIGURE 13-24 Blasts can cause injury with the initial blast, when the victim is struck by debris, or when the victim is thrown by the blast or injured by structural collapse.

ment) and then focusing on the seriously injured but salvageable blast victims. If the number of victims exceeds the immediate capabilities of your EMS system, employ disaster triage.

Determine, if possible, whether the blast was the result of terrorist action. If you suspect that it was, be alert to the possibility that other explosive devices may be set or the area booby-trapped to endanger rescuers. Ensure that police and bomb squad personnel sweep the area before you and your team enter it.

Carefully evaluate the scene for secondary hazards. Look for such things as gas leaks, disrupted electrical wiring, sharp debris, and the possibility of further structural collapse. During the scene size-up, determine the location of the epicenter of the blast. Note the presence of greater destruction and injury as you progress toward the epicenter. As you get closer, your index of suspicion for serious injury increases.

The most common and serious trauma associated with explosions is lung injury. Pulmonary injury may not manifest itself immediately, so anticipate it in anyone with any other significant signs or symptoms of blast trauma. Evaluate breathing and breath sounds frequently, carefully watching and listening for any dyspnea and crackles or other signs of respiratory congestion. At the first sign of breathing problems, consider high-flow, high-concentration oxygen and rapid transport.

Some blast victims may experience hearing loss due to the pressure wave. After experiencing the emotional impact of the blast itself, this injury can be extremely anxiety-producing for victims. Do your best to calm and reassure these patients. Remember that they will find it difficult to understand what others are saying and will not be able to follow spoken commands.

Pulmonary injuries are the most common and serious trauma associated with explosions.

Blast Injury Care

The effects of a serious explosion can produce injuries to the lungs, abdomen, and ears that involve special care considerations. Otherwise, care for blunt trauma, punctures/penetrations, and burns as you would for these injuries if they were produced by other mechanisms.

Lungs Pulmonary blast trauma is the most frequent and life-threatening pressure injury associated with an explosion. The blast-induced pressure wave rapidly and forcefully compresses and distorts the chest cavity, individual air passages, and the alveoli. During compression/decompression, the air pressures in these areas do not have time to equalize as they do with normal respiration. The extreme pressure damages or ruptures the thin and delicate alveolar walls, resulting in fluid accumulation, hemorrhage, and possibly even the entry of air directly into the bloodstream from the alveoli. Fluid accumulation (pulmonary edema) makes the lungs less elastic and air movement more difficult. The victim finds it more laborious and energy consuming to breathe. Alveolar wall rupture releases blood into the alveoli and may allow air to enter the capillaries. The victim may spit or cough up blood or a frothy mixture of blood and air. If the air enters the bloodstream, it may then travel through the pulmonary circulation to the heart and then to other critical organs causing small obstructions to circulation called **emboli**. These emboli may cause strokelike signs, myocardial infarction, or even death.

A patient history of exposure to a detonation should leave you suspicious of the possibility of lung injury. Since lung injury occurs more frequently with blasts than other pressure injuries and is usually more serious, assess carefully for signs and symptoms of lung injury in patients with abdominal and ear injuries. Lung injury patients may have progressively worsening crackles, difficulty breathing (**dyspnea**) and, in extreme cases, may cough up blood or blood-tinged sputum (**hemoptysis**). Patients occasionally experience a reduced level of consciousness or small, strokelike episodes. If you suspect lung injury from a blast, transport the victim immediately to the closest trauma center or other appropriate facility.

If it becomes necessary to ventilate a blast injury patient, do so with caution. The mechanism of injury may have damaged the alveolar-capillary walls and opened small blood vessels to the alveolar space. Positive pressure ventilations may push small air bubbles into the vascular system and create emboli. These emboli may quickly travel to the heart and brain, where they can cause further injury or death. The pressure of the ventilations may also induce **pneumothorax** by pushing air past blast-induced lung defects and into the pleural space. If possible, place a victim in the left lateral recumbent position with the head somewhat down. This positioning discourages emboli from traveling through the carotid arteries and toward the brain.

Despite the risks associated with ventilating blast injury patients, always provide positive pressure ventilations to any casualty with serious dyspnea. Use only the pressure needed to obtain moderate chest rise and respiratory volumes. High-flow, high-concentration oxygen, as supplied with a reservoir, is also helpful because the bloodstream absorbs small oxygen bubbles more easily than the nitrogen of room air.

Abdomen The sudden compression/decompression of the blast wave may also damage the air-filled bowel. Violent movements of the bowel wall cause hemorrhage and possible wall rupture. Rupture releases bowel contents into the abdominal cavity leading, over time, to severe infection and irritation (peritonitis).

Blast injuries to the abdomen require no special attention in the early stages of care. The impact of associated injuries—the bowel hemorrhage and spillage of bowel contents—on the patient's overall condition takes time to develop and is not usually apparent at the emergency scene. The only exceptions are when the blast is extremely powerful or the patient was very close to the detonation. In these cases, be alert for signs and symptoms of developing shock and provide rapid transport and fluid resuscitation as needed.

Ears The ears suffer greatly from blast wave forces associated with ordnance explosion, artillery fire, and even repeated small-arms fire at close range. The structure of the ears explains this. The middle ear is an air-filled cavity containing the organs of hearing (cochlea and stapes) and of positional sense (semicircular canals). The pina (the external portion of the ear) focuses and directs pressure waves (normally, sound waves) through the external

emboli undissolved solid, liquid, or gaseous matter in the bloodstream that can cause blockage of blood vessels.

dyspnea labored or difficult breathing.

hemoptysis expectoration of blood from the respiratory tract.

pneumothorax collection of air or gas in the pleural cavity between the chest wall and lung.

Provide careful positive pressure ventilations to any blast injury patient with serious dyspnea.

auditory canal to the eardrum. The eardrum (tympanic membrane) permits the passage of sound waves but excludes the movement of air into the middle ear. The eustachian tube provides a mechanism for equalizing small and gradual changes in atmospheric pressure between the middle ear and the outside atmosphere. During blast overpressure, however, the eustachian tube cannot equalize the rapid pressure changes. The pressure on the tympanic membrane becomes so great that the membrane stretches or ruptures, resulting in acute hearing loss. The pressure change may be so great as to fracture the delicate bones of hearing, also resulting in acute hearing loss. Hearing losses associated with blasts may be temporary or permanent.

Often ear injuries, even with as much as a third of the eardrum torn, will improve over time without much attention. Direct your care to supporting the victim and ensuring that the ear canal remains uncontaminated.

Penetrating Wounds Care for penetrating wounds as you would for any serious open wound. Remove as much of the contaminating material as is practical, and cover the site with a sterile dressing. If you encounter a large embedded or impaled object, stabilize the object by securing gauze pads around it or cover it with a non-Styrofoam paper cup to prevent movement during transport. Large areas of damaged tissue are prone to infection, so keep the wound as clean as possible. Care of penetrating trauma will be discussed at greater length in Chapter 14.

Burns Blasts can also cause extensive burn injuries either from the explosions themselves or from the ignition of other munitions or fuels or of debris or clothing. Care for burn injuries is discussed in detail in Chapter 16.

OTHER TYPES OF BLUNT TRAUMA

Blunt trauma can be caused by still other mechanisms. These include falls, sports injuries, and crush injuries.

Falls

In terms of physics, falls are a release of stored gravitational energy. The greater the distance a person falls, the greater the impact velocity, the greater the exchange of energy, and the greater the resultant trauma. As with auto impacts, stopping distance may be more important than the height of the fall. A person may dive pleasurably from a 12-foot platform into deep water, but a fall from a second story window to a concrete sidewalk results in serious injury. Newton's Second Law—

$$\text{Force} = \text{Mass} \times \text{Acceleration (or Deceleration)}$$

—illustrates that the more rapid the deceleration (the shorter the stopping distance), the greater the force and resultant injury. The nature of the impact surface contour may also affect the nature of the injury. An irregular surface, such as building rubble or a stairway, may focus the force of impact, increasing the seriousness of the injury.

Trauma resulting from a fall depends on the area of contact and the pathway of energy transmission. If the victim lands feet first, energy is transmitted up the skeletal structure through the calcaneus, tibia, femur, pelvis, and lumbar spine (Figure 13-25). Fractures along this skeletal pathway are common. The lumbar spine is especially prone to compression injury because it is the only skeletal component supporting the entire upper body. As the victim continues the collision, he may fall forward or backward. In forward falls, an outstretched arm may attempt to break the impact, resulting in shoulder, clavicle, and wrist fractures. Pelvic, thoracic, and head injury may result from a backward fall. In some cases, the fall will progress with the patient continuing a straight impact. The tongue may be bitten deeply as the weight of the cranium pushes the maxilla against the mandible as it impacts the sternum.

The initial impact may involve other body surfaces with kinetic energy transmitted from the contact point toward the body's center of mass. In diving injuries, the patient's head meets with the lake or pool bottom, while the rest of the body compresses the cervical spine between the head and shoulders. Axial loading crushes the vertebrae, disrupts the spinal cord, and paralyzes the patient. This may result from even a very shallow dive, as from poolside or from within the water.

The potential for injury from a fall depends on the height and stopping distance.

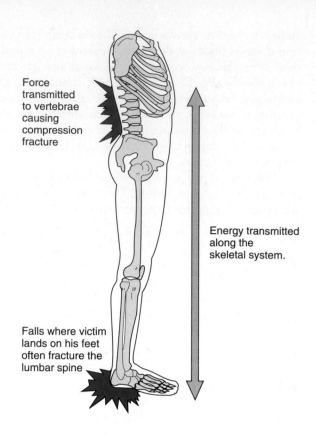

FIGURE 13-25 In falls, energy is transmitted along the skeletal system.

Force transmitted to vertebrae causing compression fracture

Energy transmitted along the skeletal system.

Falls where victim lands on his feet often fracture the lumbar spine

If the victim falls on outstretched arms, the impact energy is transmitted along the skeletal system from the hand and wrist, to the forearm, elbow, arm, and shoulder. In these cases, the clavicle often fractures because it is the smallest weight-bearing bone along the pathway of impact transmission. With collapse of the upper extremities, the head and neck may experience energy exchange and injury, as may the shoulders, upon collision with the impact surface.

In severe falls, with a person dropping more than three times his own height (20 feet for the adult, 10 feet for the small child), focus your attention on potential internal injuries. Rapid deceleration causes many organs to be compressed, displaced, and twisted. The heart, for example, is held in the center of the thorax by the aorta, the vena cavae, and the ligamentum arteriosum. When the victim contacts the ground, the heart is pulled downward with such force that it may tear from its aortic attachments, thus leading to immediate exsanguination.

In evaluating a fall, determine the point of impact, the fall height or velocity or force of impact, the impact surface, and the transmission pathway of forces along the skeleton. Then anticipate fracture sites and possible internal injuries. During your physical assessment, pay particular attention to the areas where you expect trauma for further signs of injury.

Falls are a common injury mechanism for older or geriatric patients. With increasing age come decreases in coordination, deficits in eyesight and depth perception, and weakening bones. Often, the forces required to break bones are much less in geriatric patients than in younger ones. For example, a brittle femur may actually break during ordinary activities, such as walking down a step, and result in a fall. Assess the circumstances surrounding the fall and the trauma involved, remembering that some fractures in the elderly can occur without the application of serious kinetic forces. Provide careful immobilization and gentle transport for these patients. Comfort and reassure them.

Sports Injuries

Sports medicine is a rapidly growing and extensive field, one that certainly cannot be covered completely in this chapter or text. Understanding some basic principles of sports medicine, however, may help you to better understand and care for the injured athlete.

Sports injuries are most commonly produced by extreme exertion, fatigue, or by direct trauma forces. Injuries can be secondary to acceleration, deceleration, compression, rotation, hyperextension, or hyperflexion. These forces leave behind soft-tissue damage to muscle, connective tissue injury to tendons and ligaments, skeletal trauma to long bones or the spinal column, as well as internal damage to either hollow or solid organs.

When a debilitating sports-related injury occurs, transport the athlete to an emergency department for a complete examination before further participation in the sport is allowed. Injuries that present with minimal pain may be significantly worsened by the stress of further competition. Such stress may cause complete ligament rupture or other soft-tissue injury and increase the potential for permanent disability.

In some contact sports, athletes may experience severe impacts (Figure 13-26). If collision leads to any period of unconsciousness, neurologic deficit, or lowered level of orientation, ensure that the individual is evaluated by emergency department personnel. There is often a strong desire by coaches and players alike for the athlete's return to the game. Until head and cervical spine injury can be ruled out, however, discourage such action.

Protective gear reduces the chance for and significance of injuries. Gear, however, can sometimes be a contributing factor in sports injuries. In major contact sports, for example, shoes are designed to give maximum traction, using cleats to lock the foot firmly in position. In football, a player might be struck, forcing the body to turn on an immobile foot. Ligaments in the knee may tear, resulting in severe and disabling leg injury. In other cases, protective gear may hinder your complete assessment and patient stabilization.

A newer helmet design for high-school contact sports uses an air-filled bladder to immobilize the head within the device. This fixation may be adequate to immobilize the head within the helmet in cases of suspected spinal injuries. Although it is difficult to immobilize a spherical helmet to the flat surface of a spine board, it may be preferable to attempting helmet removal. If your protocols require, attempt to immobilize the head and helmet to the long spine board, leaving the shoulder pads in place to help maintain the head and neck in a neutral position.

If a collision leads to an altered level of consciousness or neurological deficit, the athlete should be evaluated by emergency department personnel.

Crush Injuries

Crush injuries are common types of trauma. They may result from mechanisms such as structural collapse as in an explosion, an industrial or agricultural accident where a limb is caught in machinery, or when a limb is caught under a vehicle. These mechanisms direct great force to soft tissues and bones, compressing surfaces together while stretching semifluid soft tissues laterally. The result may be severe tissue disruption and serious associated hemorrhage.

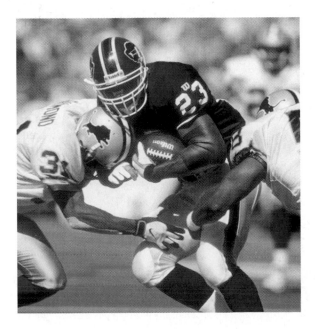

FIGURE 13-26 Contact sports may result in the exchange of great kinetic forces and produce serious injuries. *(Allsport NY)*

The injury may be further compounded if the crushing pressure remains in place for an extended period of time. The pressure can disrupt blood flow to and through the limb, causing anaerobic metabolism and some tissue death. This causes a build-up of toxins in the blood stream. If blood flow returns to the limb, the blood may carry these toxins back to the central circulation. This acidic and toxic blood may then induce cardiac dysrhythmias or seriously damage the kidneys. Another consequence of the release of the crushing pressure is severe and difficult-to-control hemorrhage. The blood vessels within the limb are severely damaged, and bleeding results from many difficult-to-identify locations. With severe and prolonged crush injury entrapment, prehospital care may include sodium bicarbonate and other medications to combat the effects of acidosis, limit damage, and improve kidney function.

SUMMARY

Blunt trauma accounts for most injury deaths and disabilities. Although vehicle crashes are the most frequent cause of blunt trauma, injuries caused by blasts, sports injuries, crush injuries, and falls also account for significant mortality and morbidity. Blunt trauma is difficult to assess accurately so you, as the care provider, must look carefully at the mechanism of injury and subtle physical signs to help anticipate serious internal injury. Careful analysis of the mechanism of injury, followed by development of indices of suspicion for injury can help guide you to recognize those patients needing rapid entry into the trauma system and those best served by on-scene care and transport to the nearest appropriate care facility.

ON THE WEB

For additional practice and review, go to the companion website at www.prenhall.com/bledsoe and click on *Intermediate Emergency Care: Principles & Practice*.

CHAPTER 14

Penetrating Trauma

Objectives

After reading this chapter, you should be able to:

1. Explain the energy exchange process between a penetrating object or projectile and the object it strikes. (pp. 625–628)

2. Determine the effects that profile, yaw, tumble, expansion, and fragmentation have on projectile energy transfer. (pp. 626–628)

3. Describe elements of the ballistic injury process including direct injury, cavitation, temporary cavity, permanent cavity, and zone of injury. (pp. 626–628, 630–633)

4. Identify the relative effects a penetrating object or projectile has when striking various body regions and tissues. (pp. 633–637)

5. Anticipate the injury types and the extent of damage associated with high-velocity/high-energy projectiles, such as rifle bullets; with medium-energy/medium-velocity projectiles

such as handgun and shotgun bullets, slugs, or pellets; and with low-energy/low-velocity penetrating objects, such as knives and arrows. (pp. 628–630)

6. Identify important elements of the scene size-up associated with shootings or stabbings. (p. 638)

7. Identify and explain any special assessment and care considerations for patients with penetrating trauma. (pp. 638–640)

8. Given several preprogrammed and moulaged penetrating trauma patients, provide the appropriate scene size-up, initial assessment, rapid trauma or focused physical exam and history, detailed exam, and ongoing assessment and provide appropriate patient care and transportation. (pp. 625–640)

CASE STUDY

An early morning traffic stop results in a gun battle between a police officer and the armed driver of a car. EMS 7 is dispatched to care for the driver, who has been shot once in the chest. The dispatch report informs the unit that officers have the patient in custody and that all weapons have been secured.

Upon arrival at the shooting scene, EMT-I Sandy O'Donnell notices several officers clustered around a male approximately 30 years old who is seated on the ground leaning back against a car. Several shell casings are on the ground near the man, and he appears to be bleeding from a small wound in his left anterior chest. The man's hands are cuffed behind his back. The man's skin color is somewhat ashen and pale, his facial expression reveals anxiety, and he appears to be breathing in an exaggerated fashion.

The arresting officer states that the man drew a weapon, a small-caliber handgun, pointed it, and fired at the officer. In response, the officer drew his weapon and fired three times, hitting the man once in the chest. The man dropped his weapon and slumped to his current position. The arresting officer took his gun, and the weapon is now in that officer's custody.

Sandy asks if the patient was searched for other weapons and the officer replies, "No." An officer performs a quick search, discovering and taking into custody a small knife. He then clears Sandy to care for the patient.

The patient seems alert and oriented to person, place, and time and does not interrupt speech to breathe. He complains of mild chest pain that increases with deep breathing. He denies any significant medical history.

Initial assessment reveals a strong pulse with a rate of about 90, respirations about 20, and full and normal chest excursion. During the rapid trauma exam, Sandy notes medium- to large-caliber bullet hole in the left anterior chest at about the fourth intercostal space along the mid-clavicular line. No air appears to be moving through the wound with respirations, and hemorrhage is very minor. Assessment of the patient's back reveals a larger wound with a more "blown-out" appearance. Again, no air seems to be moving through the wound with respirations, although hemorrhage is more significant than from the anterior wound.

Sandy quickly applies oxygen via nonrebreather mask at 15 liters per minute and listens for breath sounds. The chest sounds are reasonably clear, though there are slight crackles in the left chest near the wounds. Sandy quickly seals both anterior and posterior wounds with occlusive dressings secured on three sides while her partner takes a quick blood pressure. He reports a finding of 122/86 and a regular and strong pulse at a rate of 92. Other findings are normal, including a pulse oximeter reading of 98%.

Sandy alerts the nearby trauma center to the patient's injury mechanism and the assessment findings. They request rapid transport with one IV of normal saline run at a moderate rate. Sandy initiates the IV en route with a 14-gauge catheter, blood tubing, and a 1,000 mL bag of normal saline.

During transport to the trauma center, the ongoing assessment reveals no significant changes in the patient's condition. Upon arrival at the trauma center, Sandy provides an update on the patient's condition and vital signs to the trauma triage nurse while the patient is moved to the trauma suite for evaluation by the trauma surgical team. Moments later, he is moved to surgery.

INTRODUCTION

Modern society is experiencing a great increase in the number and severity of penetrating traumas, especially gunshot wounds. About 38,000 deaths occur each year as a result of shootings, and the number is growing. Many additional mechanisms, including knives, arrows, nails, and pieces of glass or wire, can also cause penetrating trauma. As is the case with auto crashes, physical laws govern the energy exchange process associated with penetrating trauma. Therefore, the types of weapons and projectiles involved and the characteristics of the tissue they impact all affect the severity of injury with penetrating trauma. Understanding the principles of energy exchange and projectile travel will help you to anticipate the potential for injuries, to recognize the injuries that have occurred, and, ultimately, to adequately assess and care for victims of penetrating trauma.

PHYSICS OF PENETRATING TRAUMA

The basic principles of physics that you read about in association with blunt trauma in the last chapter also apply to instances of penetrating trauma. When a projectile strikes a target, it exchanges its energy of motion, more properly called kinetic energy, with the object struck. As you recall, an object's kinetic energy is equal to its mass times the square of its velocity:

$$\text{Kinetic Energy} = \frac{\text{Mass (weight)} \times \text{Velocity (speed)}^2}{2}$$

Thus, the greater the mass of an object, the greater the energy. If you double the mass of an object, it will have twice the kinetic energy if the speed of the object remains the same. However, the speed (or velocity) of an object has a squared relationship to its kinetic energy. If you double the speed of an object, its kinetic energy increases by fourfold. If the speed triples, the energy increases by ninefold, and so on (Figure 14-1).

This relationship between mass and velocity explains why very small and relatively light bullets traveling very fast have the potential to do great harm. It also makes clear why different weights of bullets traveling at different velocities cause different amounts of damage. For example, handguns, shotguns, and low-powered rifles are considered to be medium-energy/medium velocity weapons. They deliver their bullets, slugs, and pellets much faster than low-energy/low-velocity objects like knives and arrows, but they still are slower than bullets delivered by high-energy/high-velocity weapons such as assault rifles.

Studies suggest that wounds from rifle bullets are from two to four times more lethal than wounds from handgun bullets.

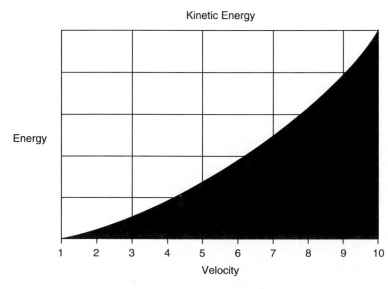

FIGURE 14-1 The extreme velocity of firearm projectiles gives them great kinetic energy and the potential to do great damage.

Thus, a handgun bullet is generally smaller and much slower (250 to 400 meters per second) than a rifle bullet. A hunting rifle, on the other hand, commonly expels a slightly heavier bullet at speeds of 600 to 1,000 meters per second. Hence, the kinetic energy of a bullet from a high-energy rifle is three to nine times greater than the bullet of a medium-energy handgun and can be expected to do significantly more damage. Experience in Northern Ireland suggests that rifle bullets are between two and four times as lethal as handgun bullets.

The Law of Conservation of Energy (energy can be neither created nor destroyed) explains why the projectile kinetic energy is transformed into damage as it slows. If a projectile such as a bullet remains within the object struck, then all its energy is transferred to the object. If the projectile passes completely through the object, then the energy transferred to the object is equal to the kinetic energy just prior to entry minus the energy remaining in the projectile as it exits.

BALLISTICS

ballistics the study of projectile motion and its interactions with the gun, the air, and the object it contacts.

trajectory the path a projectile follows.

drag the forces acting on a projectile in motion to slow its progress.

The study of the characteristics of projectiles in motion and their effects on objects they impact is called **ballistics.** The basic physics described above is the starting point for this study. One aspect of ballistics is **trajectory,** or the curved path that a bullet follows once fired from a gun. As it travels through the air, the bullet is constantly pulled downward by gravity. The faster the bullet, the flatter its curve of travel and the straighter its trajectory.

A second, more significant, aspect of projectile travel is energy dissipation. Factors that affect energy dissipation include drag, cavitation, profile, stability, expansion, and shape. As a bullet travels through the air, it experiences wind resistance, or **drag.** The faster it travels, the more drag it experiences and the greater the slowing effect. Since this represents a reduction in bullet speed, it also means, if all else is equal, that the damage caused by a bullet fired at close range will be more severe than from one fired at a distance.

Objects traveling relatively slowly, and without much kinetic energy, such as knives or arrows, will affect only the tissue they contact. High- or medium-velocity projectiles, such as rifle or handgun bullets, however, set a portion of the semi-fluid body tissue in motion, creating a shock wave and a temporary cavity in the tissue. This stage of the destruction process is known as **cavitation** and is related to the bullet's velocity and how quickly it gives up its energy. The energy exchange rate is related to the size of the projectile's contacting surface, called its profile, and to its shape.

cavitation the outward motion of tissue due to a projectile's passage, resulting in a temporary cavity and vacuum.

profile the size and shape of a projectile as it contacts a target; it is the energy exchange surface of the contact.

caliber the diameter of a bullet expressed in hundredths of an inch (.22 caliber = 0.22 inches); the inside diameter of the barrel of a handgun, shotgun, or rifle.

Profile

The **profile** is the portion of the bullet you would see if you looked at it as it traveled toward you. The larger this surface profile, the greater the energy exchange rate, the more quickly the bullet slows, and the more extensive the damage to surrounding tissue. For bullets that remain stable during their travel and do not deform, the profile is the bullet's diameter, or **caliber.** To increase the energy exchange rate, bullets are designed to become unstable as they pass from one medium to another or to deform through expansion or fragmentation.

Stability

The location of a bullet's center of mass affects its stability both during its flight and when it impacts a solid or semi-solid object. The longer the bullet, the farther the center of mass is from its leading edge. If the bullet is deflected from straight flight—for example, by the barrel exhaust or by a gust of wind—the lift created by the projectile's tip passing through air at an angle will cause the bullet to tumble. If it continues to tumble, the bullet will slow and the accuracy of the shot will be diminished. To prevent tumbling, bullets are sent spinning through the air by the gun barrel's rifling. This rotation gives a bullet gyroscopic stability similar to a spinning top. If the spinning bullet is slightly deflected, it will wobble, or **yaw,** then slowly return to straight flight.

yaw swing or wobble around the axis of a projectile's travel.

When a bullet impacts a dense substance, several things happen. If there is already a yaw, the yaw greatly increases as the bullet begins its penetration. This occurs as the bullet's mass tries to overrun the leading edge. Secondly, the gyroscopic spin designed for stability

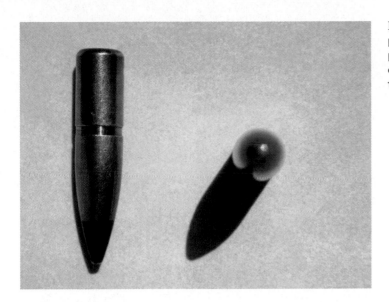

FIGURE 14-2 The presenting surface, or profile, of a bullet can change once it hits body tissue.

in air becomes insufficient. A bullet would need to spin at a rate 30 times greater in body tissue than in air to maintain the same stability. The result may be tumbling and a great increase in the bullet's presenting profile. Since a rifle bullet is generally longer than a handgun bullet and has its center of mass farther back from the leading edge, it is more likely to tumble once it hits body tissue (Figure 14-2). With increased tumbling and a larger presenting profile, the kinetic energy exchange rate of a rifle bullet increases, as does the bullet's potential for causing damage. In human tissue, a rifle bullet generally rotates 180 degrees and then continues its travel base first.

Expansion and Fragmentation

Projectiles also may increase their profile and their energy exchange rate by deforming when they strike a medium denser than air. As the bullet's nose contacts the target, it is compressed by the weight of the rest of the bullet behind it. The nose of the bullet mushrooms outward as the rear of the bullet pushes into it, increasing the projectile's diameter (Figure 14-3). In some cases, the initial impact forces are so great that the bullet separates into several pieces or fragments. This fragmentation increases the energy exchange rate of impact because the total surface area of the fragments is much greater than that of the original bullet profile (Figure 14-4). Although handgun bullets are made of relatively soft lead, their velocity, and hence their kinetic energy, is generally not sufficient to cause significant deformity. However, some bullets (dum-dums or wad-cutters) are specifically designed to mushroom and/or fragment on impact and thereby increase the damage they cause. Rifle bullets have much greater velocities than handgun bullets and much more kinetic energy. They are more prone to deform when contacting human tissue, especially bullets used for big-game hunting. Most military ammunition is fully jacketed with impact-resistant metal and seldom deforms solely with soft tissue collision.

Secondary Impacts

The energy exchange between a projectile and body tissue can also be affected by any object the projectile strikes during its travel. Branches, window glass, or articles of clothing may all deflect a bullet and induce yaw and tumble. They may also cause bullet deformity, and thereby increase the energy exchange rate once the bullet impacts the victim.

A special type of secondary impact occurs when the bullet collides with body armor. Kevlar™ and other synthetic fabrics can effectively resist the kinetic energy generated by medium-energy projectiles. This energy is absorbed by the armor and distributed to the victim in much the same way that the recoil of a gun is distributed to the shooter. The impact of the bullet may produce blunt trauma in the person hit (for example, myocardial contusion), but such injuries are generally less damaging than penetration by the bullet would have been. High-energy projectiles may pass through body armor, but in doing so

Although body armor protects against penetration, impact can result in less lethal but still serious blunt injury.

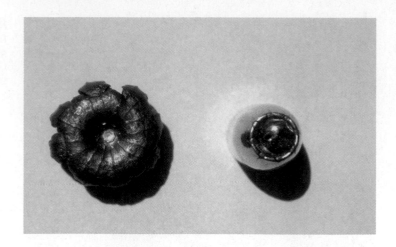

FIGURE 14-3 Some bullets are designed to mushroom on impact, thus increasing their profile, energy exchange rate, and damage potential.

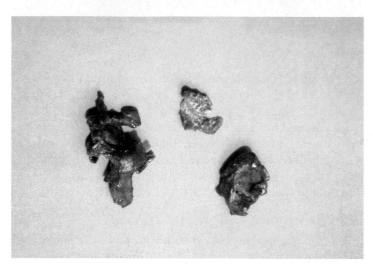

FIGURE 14-4 Some firearm projectiles break apart, or fragment, on contact, greatly increasing their profile and damage potential.

they dissipate some of their energy as blunt trauma, thereby reducing the penetrating kinetic energy as the bullet strikes body tissue. Bullet deformity may increase the rate of energy exchange, but the reduction in kinetic energy reduces the overall injury potential. Ceramic inserts for body armor will stop penetration of most rifle bullets but not without causing significant, but less lethal blunt trauma.

Shape

In addition to profile, other aspects of the shape of the bullet affect the energy exchange rate and the resulting damage. Handgun ammunition is rather blunt, is more resistant to travel through human tissue, and releases kinetic energy more quickly. Rifle bullets are more pointed and cut through the tissue more efficiently. However, if the rifle bullet tumbles, it will present a different shape and may exchange energy more rapidly both because of the shape and the increase in profile. If a bullet fragments, the irregular shape of the fragments mean that the projectile will give up its energy more rapidly and through more erratic pathways than either an intact handgun or rifle bullet.

SPECIFIC WEAPON CHARACTERISTICS

Weapons that commonly cause wounds encountered by EMT-Is include handguns, domestic rifles, assault rifles, shotguns, and knives and arrows. Each type of weapon has certain characteristics associated with the injuries it produces (Figure 14-5).

Handgun

The handgun is often a small-caliber, short-barreled, medium-velocity weapon with limited accuracy that is most effective at close range. Because a handgun does not fire a high-

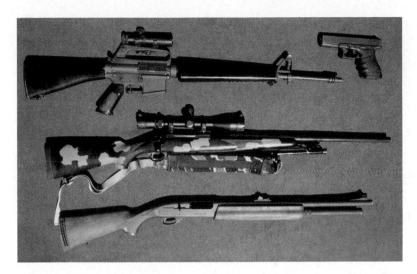

FIGURE 14-5 Firearms include (top to bottom) handguns, assault rifles, domestic rifles, and shotguns.

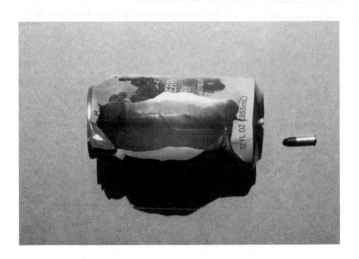

FIGURE 14-6 The energy of the handgun projectile is limited by low projectile weight and its relatively slow velocity.

velocity, high-energy projectile as a rifle does, its potential for causing damage is limited. The blunter shape of the bullet and, less frequently, its softer composition and associated mushrooming and fragmentation, may release the bullet's energy more rapidly. The damage is still, however, less than that of the higher energy rifle bullet. The severity of injury is usually related to the organs directly damaged by the bullet's passage (Figure 14-6).

Some handguns fire automatically (machine pistols). They continue to discharge bullets until the trigger is released or the magazine empties. Although the energy for each projectile remains the same, the damage potential associated with automatic weapons is increased because of the likelihood of multiple impacts or multiple victims.

Rifle

The domestic hunting rifle fires a heavier projectile than the handgun, through a much longer barrel, and with much greater muzzle velocity. It is either a manually loaded, single-shot weapon with some mechanical loading action to advance the next shell, or a semi-automatic weapon, in which the next shell is fed into the chamber by recoil or exhaust gases. However, no more than one bullet is expelled by each squeeze of the domestic hunting rifle's trigger. The high-energy rifle bullet travels much farther, with greater accuracy, and retains much more of its kinetic energy than does the handgun projectile. Because of the rifle bullet's high speed and energy, it transfers great damaging energy to the target (Figure 14-7). This results in extensive wounds with injuries that extend beyond the projectile's immediate track. Domestic hunting ammunition is especially lethal. It is often designed to expand dramatically on impact, greatly increasing the energy delivery rate and the size of both the temporary cavity and the wound pathway.

The damage caused by high-energy rifle bullets can extend well beyond the actual track of the projectile.

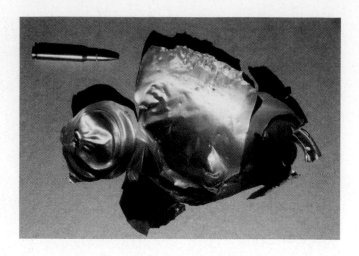

FIGURE 14-7 The energy carried by a rifle bullet is very damaging because of its heavier weight and very high velocity.

Assault Rifle

The assault rifle differs from the domestic hunting rifle in that it generally has a larger magazine capacity and will fire in both the semi-automatic and automatic mode. Examples of these weapons include the M16 and the AK47. The resulting injuries are similar to injuries produced by domestic hunting rifles, although multiple wounds and casualties can be expected. Military ammunition is fully jacketed and not designed for expansion and, though still very deadly, the energy delivery is not as severe as with domestic hunting ammunition. Assault weapons in terrorist hands, however, may be loaded with domestic hunting-type ammunition. This greatly increases their injury potential.

Shotgun

The shotgun expels a single projectile (a slug) or numerous spheres (pellets or shot) at medium velocity. The shell is loaded with a particular size of lead shot, varying from 00 (about 1/3 inch in diameter) to no. 9 shot (about the size of a pin head). The size of the projectile compartment is approximately the same with various types of loads. This means that the larger the shot, the smaller the number of projectiles. Each projectile shares a portion of the total muzzle energy and adds to the resistance as it moves through air. The shotgun is limited in range and accuracy; however, injuries sustained at close range can be very severe or lethal (Figure 14-8).

Knives and Arrows

In contrast to high- or medium-velocity projectiles such as rifle or handgun bullets, knives, arrows, and other slow-moving, penetrating objects cause low-velocity, low-energy wounds. Because low-velocity objects do not produce either a pressure shock wave or cavitation, damage is usually limited to physical injury caused by direct contact between the blade or object and the victim's tissue. The severity of a low-velocity penetrating wound, however, can often be difficult to assess because the depth and angle of the object's insertion cannot be determined from the visible wound. In addition, an attacker may move the penetrating object about inside the victim, then leave it in place or withdraw it. The penetration can result in serious internal hemorrhage or injury to individual or multiple body organs.

The hunting tips designed for arrows can be especially damaging. These feature three razor-tipped, pointed barbs that are intended to smoothly cut tissue. These tips produce severe internal hemorrhage. Also, any movement of an arrow while it is impaled in the victim increases both the tissue damage and hemorrhage rate.

DAMAGE PATHWAY

The damage pathway that a high-velocity projectile inflicts results from three specific factors. They are the direct injury, the pressure shock wave, and cavitation, or the creation of a temporary cavity. These three factors can also create a permanent cavity and a zone of injury (Figure 14-9).

The extent of damage is often difficult to assess with wounds caused by low-velocity, low-energy projectiles such as knives and arrows. Suspect internal hemorrhage and/or injury to body organs.

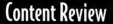

Content Review

FACTORS ASSOCIATED WITH THE DAMAGE PATHWAY OF A PROJECTILE WOUND
- Direct injury
- Pressure shock wave
- Cavitation
  - Temporary cavity
  - Permanent cavity
  - Zone of injury

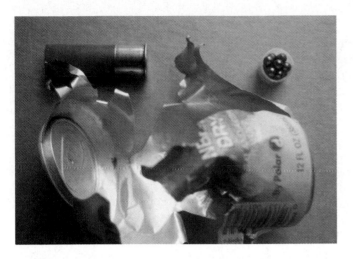

FIGURE 14-8 A shotgun propels small projectiles with limited velocity. However, because of the large number of projectiles, the weapon can be extremely damaging at close range.

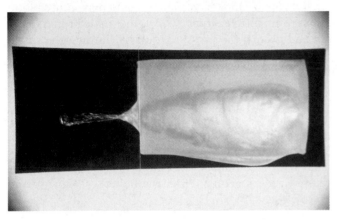

FIGURE 14-9 As a bullet passes through a gel designed to simulate human tissue, it demonstrates the wounding process.

THE PROJECTILE INJURY PROCESS

The spinning bullet smashes into a semi-fluid target, such as human tissue, with great speed and kinetic energy. The tip of the bullet impacts tissue, pushing the tissue forward and to the side along the pathway of its travel. This tissue collides with adjacent tissue, ultimately creating a shock wave of pressure moving forward and lateral to the projectile. This shock wave continues to move perpendicular to the bullet's path as it passes. The rapid compression of tissue laterally and the stretching of the tissue as it moves outward from the bullet path crushes and tears the tissue structure. The motion creates a pocket, or cavity, behind the bullet. The pressure within this cavity is reduced, creating suction. This suction draws air and debris into the cavity from the entrance wound and from the exit wound, if one is present. The body tissue's elasticity then draws the sides of the cavity back together, causing the entrance wound, exit wound, and wound pathway to close completely or remain only partially open.

The bullet's exchange of energy with the body leaves various tissues disrupted and injured. Tissue in the direct pathway of the bullet suffers most. It is severely contused and likely to have been torn from its attachments. In addition to the directly injured tissue, other debris, blood, and air are found along the bullet's pathway. The cavitational wave stretches and tears adjacent tissue, damaging cell walls and small blood vessels. The adjacent tissue is injured, but will likely regain its normal function slowly. Larger blood vessels torn by the bullet and the cavitational wave release their precious fluid in large quantities into the damage pathway. Over time, this pathway, because of the disruption in circulation and the introduction of infectious material with the drawing-in of debris, may experience severe infection, which will prolong the healing process.

Direct Injury

Direct injury is the damage done as the projectile strikes tissue, contuses and tears that tissue, and pushes the tissue out of its way. The direct injury pathway is limited to the profile of the bullet as it moves through the body or the profiles of resulting fragments as the bullet breaks apart. Except for magnum rounds (generating particularly high velocities), handgun bullet damage is usually limited to direct injury.

Pressure Shock Wave

When a high-velocity, high-energy projectile strikes human flesh, it creates a pressure shock wave (Figure 14-10). Since most human tissue is semi-fluid and elastic, the impact of the projectile transmits energy outward very quickly. The tissue cells in front of the bullet are pushed forward and to the side at great speed. They push adjacent cells forward and outward, creating a moving wave of pressure and tissue. The faster and blunter the bullet, the greater the effect. With high-velocity rifle bullets, pressures are extreme, approaching 100 times normal atmospheric pressure.

The pressure wave travels very well through fluid, such as blood, and may injure blood vessels distant from the projectile pathway. Air-filled cavities, such as the small air sacs (alveoli) of the lung, compress very easily and absorb the pressure, quickly limiting the shock wave and the resulting temporary cavity. Solid and dense organs, such as the liver and spleen, suffer greatly as the pressure wave moves through them, causing internal hemorrhage and, in extreme cases, fracture.

Temporary Cavity

The temporary cavity is a space created behind the high-energy bullet as tissue moves rapidly away from the bullet's path. The size of the cavity depends on the amount of energy transferred during the bullet's passage. With rifle bullets, the temporary cavity may be as much as twelve times larger than the projectile's profile. After the bullet's passage, tissue elasticity causes the temporary cavity to close.

Cavitation also produces a sub-atmospheric pressure within the cavity as it expands. This means that air is drawn in from the entrance wound and the exit wound, if one exists. Debris and contamination enter the cavity with the in-flowing air, adding to the risk of infection.

Permanent Cavity

The movement that creates the temporary cavity crushes, stretches, and tears the affected tissues. These processes seriously damage the area in and adjacent to the bullet's path and

> *The severity of injury in cases of bullet wounds usually depends on the organs damaged by the bullet's passage.*
>
>

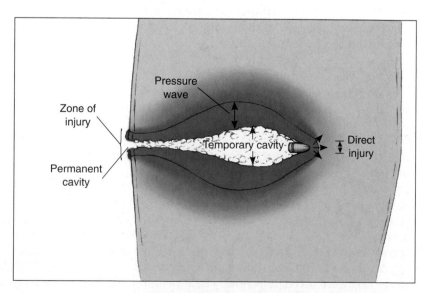

FIGURE 14-10 As a projectile passes through tissue, it creates a pressure wave and temporary cavity with results that include direct injury, a permanent cavity, and a zone of injury.

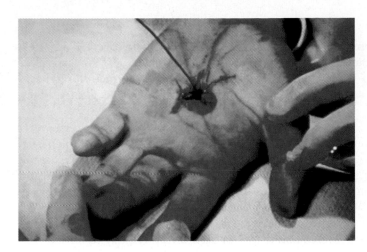

FIGURE 14-11 Damage caused by a low-velocity wounding process, such as that caused by a wire thrown by a lawnmower, is limited to the object's path of travel.

may also damage the tissue's elasticity. The tissue thus may not return to its normal orientation, resulting in a permanent cavity that in some cases may be larger than the bullet's diameter. This cavity is not a void but is filled with disrupted tissues, some air, fluid, and debris.

Zone of Injury

Associated with most projectile wounds is a zone of injury that extends beyond the permanent cavity. This zone contains contused tissue that does not function normally and may be slow to heal because of cell and tissue damage, disrupted blood flow, and infection.

LOW-VELOCITY WOUNDS

Weapons such as knives, ice picks, arrows, or flying objects such as blast debris or wires thrown by a lawn mower can cause low-velocity penetrating trauma. In these cases, the relatively slow speed of the object limits the kinetic energy exchange rate as it enters the victim's body. Consider, for example, the stabbing of a victim by a 150-pound attacker who strikes with a knife moving at about 3 meters per second. Although the mass behind the penetration of the knife blade is significantly greater than that of a rifle bullet, the velocity of the knife is vastly lower. This means that injury in such cases is usually restricted to the tissue actually contacted by the penetrating object (Figure 14-11).

Although the injury is limited to the penetrating object's pathway, that object may be twisted, moved about, or inserted at an oblique angle. As a result, the entrance wound may not reflect the depth of the object's penetration, the extent of its motion within the body, or the actual organs and tissues it contacts and injures.

Characteristics of the attacker and victim are important to keep in mind when assessing cases of low-velocity penetrating trauma. Knife-wielding males, for example, most often strike with a forward, outward, or crosswise stroke. Females usually strike with an overhand and downward stroke. Victims of these attacks initially attempt to protect themselves by using their arms. This means they often receive deep upper-extremity lacerations (commonly called defense wounds). If an attack continues, injuries are often directed to the chest, abdomen, face, neck, or back.

SPECIFIC TISSUE/ORGAN INJURIES

The extent of damage that a penetrating projectile causes within the body varies with the particular type of tissue it encounters. The density of an organ affects how efficiently the energy of the projectile is transmitted to surrounding tissues. The tissue's connective strength and elasticity, called **resiliency**, also influence how much tissue damage occurs with the kinetic energy transfer. Structures and tissues within the body that behave differently during projectile passage include connective tissue, solid organs, hollow organs, lungs, and bone.

resiliency the connective strength and elasticity of an object or fabric.

CONNECTIVE TISSUE

Muscles, the skin, and other connective tissues are dense, elastic, and held together very well. When exposed to the pressure and stretching of the cavitational wave, these types of tissue characteristically absorb energy while limiting tissue damage. The wound track closes due to the resiliency of the tissue, and serious injury is frequently limited to the projectile's pathway.

ORGANS

Another factor that has profound effects on the victim's potential for survival is the particular organ involved in a penetrating injury. Some organs, such as the heart and brain, are immediately necessary for life functions, and serious injury may cause immediate death. When large blood vessels are involved, the hemorrhage can be rapid and severe. A penetrating injury to the urinary bladder, on the other hand, may not receive surgical intervention for several hours without threatening the patient's life. When evaluating a wound's seriousness, anticipate the organs injured and the effect their injury is likely to have on the patient's condition and survivability.

Solid Organs

Be alert to the possibility of severe hemorrhage if you suspect that a projectile has damaged a solid organ.

Solid organs such as the liver, spleen, kidneys, pancreas, and brain have the density but not the resiliency of muscle and other connective tissues. When struck by the forces of bullet impact, these tissues compress and stretch, resulting in greater damage more closely associated with the size of the temporary cavity than with the bullet's profile. The tissue returns to its original location, not because of its own elasticity but because of the resiliency of surrounding tissues or the organ capsule. Hemorrhage associated with solid organ projectile damage is often severe.

Hollow Organs

pericardial tamponade filling of the pericardial sac with fluid, which in turn limits the filling and function of the heart.

Hollow organs such as the bowel, stomach, urinary bladder, and heart are muscular containers holding fluid. The fluid within is non-compressible and rapidly transmits the impact energy outward. If the container is filled and distended with fluid at the time of impact, the energy released can tear the organ apart explosively (Figure 14-12). Slower and smaller projectiles may produce small holes in an organ and permit slow leakage of its contents. If this occurs with the heart, it may produce **pericardial tamponade** (blood filling the pericardial sac, thus limiting heart function) or moderate and slowly life-threatening hemorrhage. If the container is not distended, it is more tolerant of cavitational forces. If a hollow organ, such as the bowel or stomach holds air, the air compresses with the passage of the pressure wave and somewhat limits the extent of injury. (Large blood vessels respond to projectile passage much like hollow, fluid-filled, organs.)

LUNGS

Injury to lung tissue in cases of penetrating trauma is generally less extensive than can be expected with any other body tissue.

The lungs consist of millions of small, elastic, air-filled sacs. As the bullet and its associated pressure wave pass, the air is compressed, thereby slowing and limiting the transmission of

FIGURE 14-12 If a high-velocity bullet impacts the heart during maximum cardiac filling, cardiac rupture and rapid exsanguination may occur.

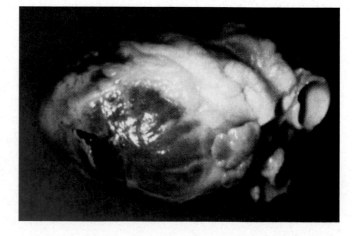

the cavitational wave. Injury to lung tissue in cases of penetrating trauma is generally less extensive than can be expected with any other body tissue.

A bullet may, however, open the chest wall or disrupt larger airways, thus permitting air to escape into the thorax (pneumothorax) or creating a valvelike defect that results in accumulating pressure within the chest (tension pneumothorax). Bullet wounds only infrequently induce an open pneumothorax (sucking chest wound) because the entrance wound diameter is usually limited to the bullet caliber. Explosive exit wounds of high-powered rifles or close-range shotgun blasts, however, may be large and cause significant disruption of the chest wall integrity. In these cases, a pneumothorax is a more likely outcome.

Suspect the possibility of pneumothorax when there has been a significant disruption of chest wall integrity.

Bone

In contrast to lung tissue, bone is the densest, most rigid, and non-elastic body tissue of all. When struck by a projectile or its associated pressure wave, bone resists displacement until it fractures, often into numerous pieces. These bone fragments then may distribute the impact energy to surrounding tissue. The projectile's contact with bone may also significantly alter the projectile's path through the body.

Content Review

Body Regions Deserving Special Attention with Penetrating Trauma

- Extremities
- Abdomen
- Thorax
- Neck
- Head

General Body Regions

Several body regions deserve special attention regarding projectile wounds. They include the extremities, abdomen, thorax, neck, and head (Figure 14-13). A projectile's passage also has a special effect on the first and last tissue contacted, the sites of the entrance and the exit wounds.

Extremities

The extremities consist of skin covering muscles and surrounding large long bones. An extremity injury may be debilitating but does not immediately threaten life unless there is severe hemorrhage associated with it. The severity of injury is limited by the resiliency of the skin and muscle, although if the bone is involved, the degree of soft tissue damage may be increased. In recent military experience, extremity injuries account for between 60% and

Approximately 90% of penetrating trauma mortality involves the head, thorax, and abdomen.

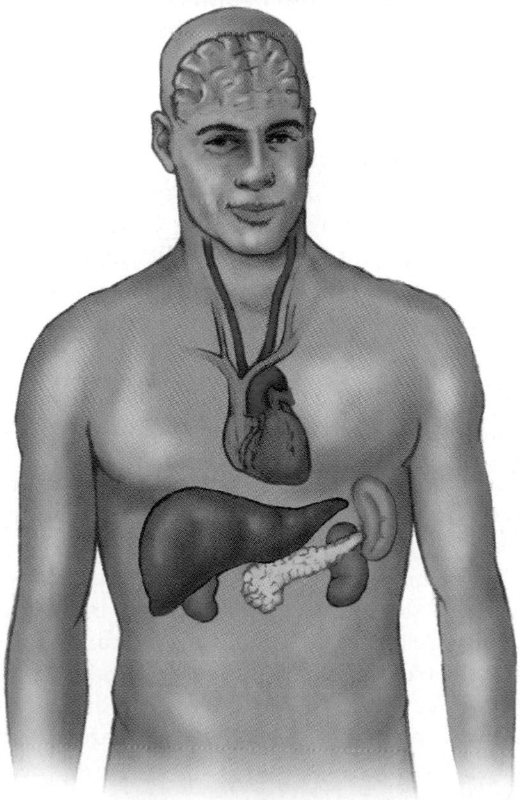

FIGURE 14-13 Critical structures in which the seriousness of a bullet's impact is increased include the brain, great vessels, heart, liver, kidneys, and pancreas.

80% of injuries yet result in less than 10% of fatalities. The remaining 20% to 40% of penetrating injuries are divided among wounds of the abdomen, thorax, and head and account for more than 90% of mortality.

Abdomen

Consider any penetrating projectile injury to the abdomen to be serious and to have the potential to cause severe internal hemorrhage.

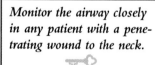

The abdomen (including the pelvic cavity) is the largest body cavity and contains most of the human organs. The area is not well protected by skeletal structures other than the upper pelvic ring, the lower rib cage border, and the lumbar vertebral column. The passage of a projectile through the abdominal cavity can produce a significant cavitational wave. The major occupant of the cavity, the bowel, is very tolerant of compression and stretching, but the liver, spleen, kidneys, and pancreas are highly susceptible to injury and hemorrhage. Since these organs occupy the upper abdominal quadrants, you should consider any penetrating projectile injury to this area to be serious and to have the potential to cause severe internal hemorrhage. Serious consequences should also be anticipated with injuries to the abdominal aorta and inferior vena cava, which are located along the spinal column in the posterior and central abdomen.

If a projectile perforates the small or large bowel, those organs may spill their contents into the abdominal cavity. This spillage results in serious peritoneal irritation due to chemical action or infection, although the signs and symptoms take some time to develop. If the injury process disrupts the blood vessels, the free blood will not result in abdominal irritation.

Thorax

Within the chest is a cavity formed by the ribs, spine, sternum, clavicles, and the diaphragm's strong muscle. This thoracic cavity houses the lungs, heart, and major blood vessels as well as the esophagus and part of the trachea. The impact of a bullet with the ribs may induce an explosive energy exchange that injures the surrounding tissue with numerous bony fragments. Lung tissue can absorb much of the cavitational energy while sustaining limited injury itself. However, the heart and great vessels, as fluid-filled containers, may suffer greatly from the energy of the bullet's passage. The damage to these structures and the associated massive hemorrhage may cause almost instant death. Because of the pressure-driven dynamics of respiration, any large chest wound may compromise breathing. Air may pass through a wound instead of the normal airway (pneumothorax) or may build up under pressure within the chest wall (tension pneumothorax).

Neck

Monitor the airway closely in any patient with a penetrating wound to the neck.

The neck is an anatomical area traversed by several critical structures. These include the larynx, the trachea, the esophagus, several major blood vessels (the carotid and vertebral arteries and the jugular veins), and the spinal cord. Penetrating trauma in this area is very likely to damage vital structures and lead to airway compromise, severe bleeding, and/or neurological dysfunction. Associated swelling and hematoma formation may compromise circulation and the airway. Additionally, any large penetrating wound may permit air to be drawn into an open external jugular vein and immediately threaten life due to the resulting pulmonary emboli.

Head

Bullet wounds to the head, particularly those that penetrate the skull, are especially lethal.

The skull is a hollow, strong, and rigid container, housing the brain's delicate semi-solid tissue. It is highly susceptible to projectile injury. If a bullet penetrates the skull, its cavitational energy is trapped within the cavity and subjects the brain to extreme pressures. If the released kinetic energy is great enough, the skull may explode outward. In some cases, a bullet may enter the skull and not have enough energy to exit; in such a case, the bullet may continue to travel along the interior of the skull, disrupting more and more brain matter. Bullet wounds to the head, particularly those that penetrate the skull, are especially lethal.

Suspect the possibility of airway compromise in patients with projectile wounds to the head and face.

The destructive forces released by a projectile wound to the head may also disrupt the airway and/or the victim's ability to control his own airway. The head and face are also areas with an extensive supply of blood vessels. Penetrating trauma may damage these vessels and result in serious and difficult-to-control hemorrhage.

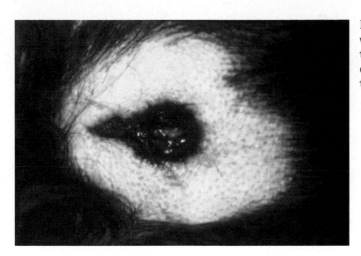

A frequent occurrence associated with suicide attempts is severe damage to the facial region. As the individual places a shotgun or rifle under the chin and pulls the trigger, the head tilts up and back. This directs the blast entirely to the facial region, but the projectile(s) may not enter the cranium or strike any immediately life-threatening structures. However, serious bleeding occurs. The bleeding and the associated damage can make the airway very hard to control. In these cases, use of an endotracheal tube to secure the airway can be difficult because many airway structures and landmarks are often obliterated by the blast.

Entrance Wound

Entrance wounds are usually the size of the bullet's profile. At this point, cavitational wave energy has not had time to develop and contribute to the wounding process (Figure 14-14). The situation is different, however, with bullets that deform or tumble during flight. With these projectiles, the initial impact can be especially violent, producing a much larger and more disrupted entry wound than the caliber of the bullet alone would suggest.

Bullet entry wounds sustained at close range, a few feet or less, display special characteristics. Such wounds may be marked by elements of the barrel exhaust and bullet passage. Tattooing from the propellant residue may form a darkened circle or an oval (if the gun is held at an angle) around the entry wound and contaminate the wound itself. At the wound site, you may notice a small (usually 1 to 2 mm) ridge of discoloration around the entrance caused by the spinning bullet. If the gun barrel is held very close or against the skin as the weapon is fired, it may push the barrel exhaust into the wound producing subcutaneous emphysema (air within the skin's tissue) and crepitus to the touch. If the barrel is held a few inches from the skin, you may notice some burns caused by the hot gases of the barrel exhaust.

Exit Wound

The exit wound is caused by the physical damage from both the passage of the bullet itself and from the cavitational wave. Since the pressure wave is moving forward and outward, the wound may have a "blown outward" appearance. The exit wound may appear as stellate, referring to the tears radiating outward in a starlike fashion (Figure 14-15). Because the cavitational wave has had time to develop, the exit wound may more accurately reflect the potential for damage caused by the bullet's passage than the entrance wound. If the bullet expends all its kinetic energy before it can exit the body, there is no exit wound and the bullet remains within the body. If the bullet does exit, the kinetic energy expended within the body is equal to the kinetic energy before impact minus the energy that remains in the bullet as it leaves the body.

An exit wound may more accurately reflect the potential damage caused by a bullet's passage through the body than an entrance wound.

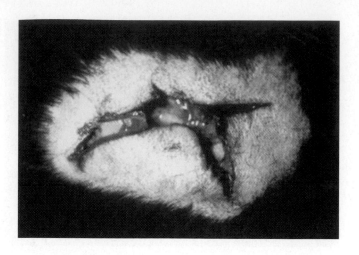

FIGURE 14-15 A bullet's exit wound often has a "blown outward" appearance, with stellate tears.

SPECIAL CONCERNS WITH PENETRATING TRAUMA

SCENE SIZE-UP

In cases involving shootings or stabbings, always be sure that police have secured the scene before you enter it.

Consider the possibility that the patient may be carrying a weapon and have the police search him if necessary.

Make every effort to preserve evidence at a crime scene, but remember that care of the patient takes priority.

The scene size-up for a shooting or stabbing raises special concerns not associated with most other emergency care situations. The very nature of these injuries should suggest the possibility of danger from further violence and potential injury to you and your crew. Do not approach a shooting or stabbing scene unless and until law-enforcement personnel arrive and secure it and direct you to enter and provide care. If law-enforcement personnel are not yet on the scene when you arrive, stage your vehicle at least a block away and out of sight of the scene. Once police or other law-enforcement personnel arrive, bring your vehicle closer to the scene, but keep the police and their vehicles between you and the shooting or stabbing site. Wait there for the police to indicate that it is safe to approach the patient (Figure 14-16).

Once you reach the patient, look carefully to determine that no weapons are within the patient's reach. Consider the possibility that the victim may be carrying a knife or other weapon. If you have any doubts, request that the police search the victim for weapons before you begin to provide care.

As you carefully size up the scene of a shooting, try to reconstruct the event. Attempt to determine the victim's original position and his or her angle to and distance from the shooter. This helps you determine the angle at which the bullet entered the patient (which may not otherwise be revealed by the entrance wound) and whether the wound was received at point-blank range or from a distance. Also try to determine the caliber of weapon and its type—handgun, rifle, or shotgun.

If the call involves a knifing injury, attempt to determine the gender and approximate weight of the attacker and the length of the blade. (You probably will not be able to determine the wound depth.) This information will help the emergency department determine the potential severity of the wound.

As you move on to your assessment of the patient, do all that you can to preserve the crime scene while providing any needed patient care. Disturb only those materials around the patient that you must move in order to render care. Cut around any bullet or knife holes in clothing and give the clothing to police for use as evidence. If you have any doubt about what to do, however, err on the side of providing patient care. If the victim is obviously dead, employ your jurisdiction's protocols for handling the body, but try to do so without disturbing evidence that may be crucial in determining what happened.

PENETRATING WOUND ASSESSMENT

When assessing the victim of penetrating trauma, try to determine the pathway of the penetrating object and the organs that may have been affected by the wound. Anticipate the impact of potential organ injury and use this determination in setting priorities for on-scene

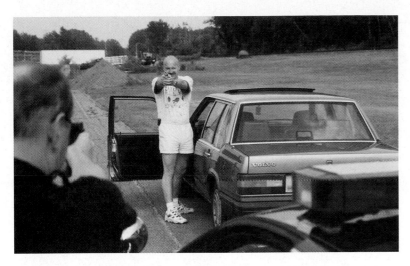

FIGURE 14-16 Ensure that any potentially violent scene is safe and secured by police before entering.

care or rapid transport of the victim. Remember, however, that a bullet may not travel in a straight line between entrance and exit wounds. Often, a very small shift in a bullet's pathway may mean the difference between tearing open a large blood vessel or missing critical organs completely. The human body is also a dynamic place. The diaphragm moves the kidneys, pancreas, liver, spleen, and heart during respirations, so whether these organs are injured may be somewhat dependent on the phase of respiration in which the injury occurs.

It is often hard to anticipate the severity of a projectile wound. Injuries to the large blood vessels, heart, and brain may be immediately or rapidly fatal. Injuries to solid organs (liver, pancreas, kidneys, or spleen) may also be deadly but take more time in working their effects. Consequently, always suspect the worst with bullet wounds that involve the head, chest, or abdomen. Provide rapid transport in these cases and treat shock aggressively.

Provide rapid transport for patients with bullet wounds to the head, chest, or abdomen and treat aggressively for shock.

PENETRATING WOUND CARE

Certain penetrating wounds need special attention. These include wounds of the face and chest and those involving impaled objects.

Facial Wounds

Some facial gunshot wounds destroy many airway landmarks (Figure 14-17). With wounds such as these, endotracheal intubation is extremely difficult. You might find it helpful to visualize the larynx with the laryngoscope while another rescuer gently presses on the chest. Look for any bubbling during the chest compression, and try to pass the endotracheal tube through the bubbling tissue. Then, very carefully assure that the endotracheal tube is properly placed in the trachea and that lung ventilation is adequate.

Chest Wounds

The chest wall is rather thick and resilient. It requires a large wound to create an opening big enough to permit free air movement through the chest wall, an open pneumothorax. Wounds caused by small-caliber handguns usually result in no air movement, whereas wounds caused by shotgun blasts and exiting high-velocity bullets more commonly cause such injuries. If frothy blood is associated with a chest wound, anticipate a developing tension pneumothorax, in which air builds up under pressure within the thorax. Remember, it takes pressure to push air through the wound and froth the blood. If you completely seal the chest wound, you may stop any outward air flow. This can increase both the speed of development of the tension pneumothorax and its severity. Cover any open chest wound with an occlusive dressing sealed on three sides (Figure 14-18). If dyspnea is significant, assess for tension pneumothorax and perform needle decompression as indicated.

Always consider the possibility of heart and great vessel damage with a penetrating chest wound. These injuries may lead rapidly to severe internal hemorrhage and death.

Anticipate a developing tension pneumothorax if your assessment reveals frothy blood in a patient with a bullet wound to the chest.

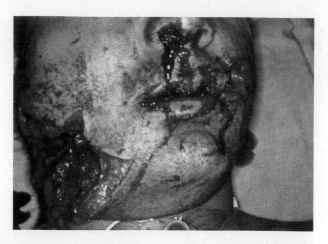

FIGURE 14-17 Facial wounds may distort or destroy airway landmarks.

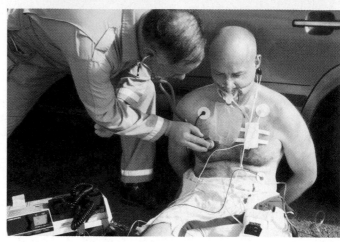

FIGURE 14-18 Seal open chest wounds and ensure adequate respirations.

Another serious complication of penetrating chest trauma is pericardial tamponade. This condition occurs when an object or projectile perforates the heart and permits blood to leak into the pericardial sac. As blood accumulates in the sac, the heart no longer fully fills with blood and circulation slows. If pericardial tamponade is uncorrected, the **prognosis** for the patient is very poor. However, a needle introduced into the pericardial space, a procedure available at the emergency department, can quickly alleviate the life threat. Therefore, if you suspect this condition, arrange for rapid transport.

prognosis the anticipated outcome of a disease or injury.

Impaled Objects

If an object that causes a low-velocity wound lodges in the body, removal of the object may be dangerous for the patient. If the object bent as it hit a bone on entry, attempts at removal may cause further injury. If the object is held firmly by soft tissue, it may obstruct blood vessels, thereby restricting blood loss; removal of the object may then increase hemorrhage.

Immobilize impaled objects in place where and as they are found and transport the patient. The only impaled objects that you should remove are those lodged in the cheek or trachea that interfere with the airway or those that you must remove to provide CPR.

Immobilize impaled objects in place. Only remove those that are lodged in the cheek or those that interfere with the airway or prevent CPR.

SUMMARY

Penetrating injuries, especially those associated with gunshot wounds are responsible for a high incidence of prehospital trauma and death. Your understanding of the mechanisms of injury that produce these wounds and an understanding of the types of injuries caused by these mechanisms (index of suspicion) can help you rapidly identify serious life threats and assure these patients receive rapid transport to a trauma center. Special prehospital care techniques such as sealing an open pneumothorax and managing a difficult airway can also help you stabilize the patient in the field and ensure that he safely reaches definitive care.

ON THE WEB

For additional practice and review, go to the companion website at www.prenhall.com/bledsoe and click on *Intermediate Emergency Care: Principles & Practice*.

CHAPTER 15

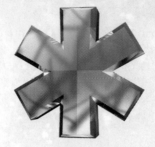

Hemorrhage and Shock

Objectives

After reading this chapter, you should be able to:

1. Describe the epidemiology, including the morbidity/mortality and prevention strategies, for shock and hemorrhage. (pp. 643–644)
2. Discuss the pathophysiology of hemorrhage and shock. (pp. 644–652, 659–662)
3. Describe the body's physiological response to changes in blood volume, blood pressure, and perfusion. (pp. 659–662)
4. Describe the effects of decreased perfusion at the capillary level. (pp. 659–661)
5. Discuss the cellular ischemic, capillary stagnation, and capillary washout phases related to hemorrhagic shock. (pp. 659–661)
6. Discuss the various types and degrees of shock and hemorrhage. (pp. 650–652, 661–662)
7. Predict shock and hemorrhage based on mechanism of injury. (pp. 652–655)
8. Identify the need for intervention and transport of the patient with hemorrhage or shock. (pp. 656–658, 665–670)
9. Discuss the assessment findings, treatment plan, and management of hemorrhage, external and internal, and shock. (pp. 662–670)
10. Differentiate between the administration rate and volume of IV fluid in patients with controlled versus uncontrolled hemorrhage. (pp. 665–667)
11. Relate pulse pressure and orthostatic vital sign changes to perfusion status. (pp. 650–656)
12. Define and differentiate between compensated and decompensated hemorrhagic shock. (pp. 661–662)
13. Discuss the pathophysiological changes, assessment findings, and management associated with compensated and decompensated shock. (pp. 661–670)
14. Identify the need for intervention and transport of patients with compensated and decompensated shock. (pp. 662–670)
15. Differentiate among normotensive, hypotensive, or profoundly hypotensive patients. (pp. 653–656, 659–662)
16. Describe differences in administration of intravenous fluid in the normotensive, hypotensive, or profoundly hypotensive patients. (pp. 665–667)
17. Discuss the physiologic changes associated with application and inflation of the pneumatic anti-shock garment (PASG). (pp. 667–668, 669)
18. Discuss the indications and contraindications for the application and inflation of the PASG. (pp. 667–668)
19. Differentiate between the management of compensated and decompensated shock. (pp. 665–667)
20. Given several preprogrammed and moulaged hemorrhage and shock patients, provide the appropriate scene size-up, initial assessment, rapid trauma or focused physical exam and history, detailed exam, and ongoing assessment and provide appropriate patient care and transportation. (pp. 644–670)

CASE STUDY

City Ambulance 1 receives a mutual aid alert. A basic life support (BLS) ambulance needs assistance in a neighboring community. A bulldozer has overturned, trapping a 39-year-old male.

Upon arrival at the scene, EMT-I Dave and his junior partner Ed take a report from the two EMT-Basics about the patient, a man named Ken. Then they assess the patient themselves and find him alert and oriented. The patient's airway and breathing appear normal as do the rate and strength of his pulse. His pelvis and lower extremities are pinned under the side of the bulldozer. The rescue team informs the EMT-I crew that it will be at least 10 minutes until they can lift and remove the bulldozer. Dave concludes the initial assessment and detects no signs of problems with airway, breathing, or circulation. The EMTs have already administered oxygen at 15 liters per minute, using a nonrebreather mask.

Next, Dave provides a rapid trauma assessment as part of the focused history and physical examination. The patient's breath sounds are good, but he cannot feel his feet. From looking at the positions of the bulldozer and the patient, Dave strongly suspects a pelvic fracture and expects increased hemorrhage to occur when the heavy machine is lifted. Ed reports vital sign findings of blood pressure 110/68, pulse 90, respirations 24, and an oxygen saturation of 99%.

Because the extrication time will be lengthy, Dave requests air medical transport to the trauma center for the patient. He then quickly establishes two IVs of normal saline, one infusing at a rapid rate. Ed prepares the pneumatic anti-shock garment (PASG) and a backboard. As the lifting equipment is readied, the EMT-Is talk with the patient, explaining the various steps in the operation. Ed rechecks vital signs every 5 minutes, and Dave documents that the vital signs and oxygen saturation remain stable.

The extrication team slowly begins to lift the bulldozer. Dave and Ed rush to position the patient on the prepared backboard and then apply and inflate the PASG. It quickly becomes apparent that the patient has suffered fractures of the pelvis, both femurs, and the left tibia. Both IVs are opened wide.

The patient reports an increase in pain, becomes restless, and attempts to get up. He then becomes lethargic. The pulse oximeter reveals that oxygen saturation has dropped to 94% and then reads erratically. The pulse rate is up to 130 very weak beats per minute. With time, the patient's level of consciousness improves, but his pulse rate remains elevated.

Dave and Ed place both IVs in pressure bags as they move the patient to the waiting helicopter. Upon arrival at the hospital, the patient's systolic blood pressure remains around 90 and the heart rate is tachycardic. The ED team starts type O-negative blood and replaces one of the field IVs. Within 20 minutes, the team transports the patient into surgery with the PASG in place.

Ken comes through the surgery well. Because of the multiple fractures, however, his rehabilitation will continue for more than a year.

INTRODUCTION

The loss of the body's most important and dynamic medium, blood, is called **hemorrhage.** Acute and continuing loss of blood robs the body of its ability to provide oxygen and nutrients to, and remove carbon dioxide and waste products from, the body's elemental building blocks, the cells. In the absence of an adequate volume of circulating blood, the cells and the organs dysfunction and, ultimately, the organism itself dies. The transition between normal function (**homeostasis**) and death is called **shock.** To recognize hemorrhage and shock and to care for them are critical skills for the EMT-I and are essential to reducing mortality and morbidity in trauma patients. This chapter provides you with an understanding of the cardiovascular system as it relates to hemorrhage and

hemorrhage an abnormal internal or external discharge of blood.

homeostasis the natural tendency of the body to maintain a steady and normal internal environment.

shock a state of inadequate tissue perfusion.

The EMT-I must be able to recognize hemorrhage and shock in trauma patients to reduce mortality and morbidity.

shock and then describes how to recognize and care for these life-threatening assaults on the human body.

HEMORRHAGE

As noted previously, hemorrhage is loss of blood from the closed vascular system because of injury to the blood vessels. Hemorrhage is usually classified based on the injured vessel from which it flows: capillary, venous, or arterial.

Capillary hemorrhage generally oozes from the wound, normally an abrasion, and clots quickly on its own. The blood is usually bright red because it is well oxygenated.

Venous hemorrhage flows more quickly, though it, too, generally stops in a few minutes. Bleeding associated with venous hemorrhage is generally dark red because the blood has already given up its oxygen as it passed though the capillary beds.

Bleeding associated with arterial hemorrhage flows very rapidly, often spurting from the wound. This blood is well oxygenated and appears bright red as it escapes from the wound. The blood volume lost can be extreme because of the pressure behind arterial bleeding. The spurting nature of arterial hemorrhage results from the variations in the blood pressure driving the blood loss.

Although it is convenient to determine the type of hemorrhage, the nature and depth of a wound may make it hard to differentiate between heavy venous and arterial bleeding. Internal hemorrhage cannot be classified by type with the diagnostic techniques available to EMT-Is providing prehospital care.

CLOTTING

clotting the body's three-step response to stop the loss of blood.

The body's response to local hemorrhage is a complex three-step process called **clotting** (Figure 15-1). As a blood vessel is torn and begins to lose blood, its smooth muscle contracts. This reduces its lumen and the volume and strength of blood flow through it. This is called the **vascular phase.**

vascular phase step in the clotting process in which smooth blood vessel muscle contracts, reducing the vessel lumen and the flow of blood through it.

At the same time, the vessel's smooth interior lining (the tunica intima) is disrupted, causing a turbulent blood flow. The disturbed blood flow causes frictional damage to the surfaces of the platelets, making them adherent. Platelets then stick to collagen, a protein fiber found in connective tissue, on the vessel's injured inner surface, and to other injured tissue in the area. The blood vessel walls also become adherent. If they are small enough, like capillaries, they may stick together, further occluding blood flow. As platelets adhere to the vessel walls, they **aggregate,** or collect, other platelets. This is the **platelet phase,** the second step of the clotting process. These events occur almost immediately after injury and effectively halt hemorrhage from capillaries and small venous and arterial vessels. Although this is a rapid method of hemorrhage control, the resulting clot is unstable.

Content Review

PHASES OF THE CLOTTING PROCESS

- Vascular phase
- Platelet phase
- Coagulation

aggregate to cluster or come together.

As time passes, the wound initiates the third and final step of the process, **coagulation.** In this phase, enzymes are released into the bloodstream, initiating a complex sequence of events. These enzymes come from the damaged blood vessel and surrounding tissue (the extrinsic pathway), from the damaged platelets (the intrinsic pathway), or from both. The release of the enzymes triggers a series of chemical reactions that result in the formation of strong protein fibers, or fibrin. These fibers entrap red blood cells and form a stronger, more durable clot. This further collection of cells halts all but the most severe hemorrhage. Coagulation normally takes from 7 to 10 minutes. Over time, the cells trapped in the clot protein matrix slowly contract, drawing the wound and the injured vessel together.

platelet phase second step in the clotting process in which platelets adhere to blood vessel walls and to each other.

The nature of the wound also affects how rapidly and well the clotting mechanisms respond to hemorrhage (Figure 15-2). If the wound lacerates the vessel cleanly in a transverse fashion, the muscles of the vessel wall contract. This retracts the vessel into the tissue, thickening the now shortened tunica media. This thickening further reduces the vessel's lumen, reduces blood flow, and assists the clotting mechanism. If the blood vessel is lacerated longitudinally rather than transversely, the smooth muscle contraction pulls the vessel open. The vessel does not withdraw and the lumen does not constrict. The result is heavy and continued bleeding. Crushing trauma often produces this type of damage. The vessels are not

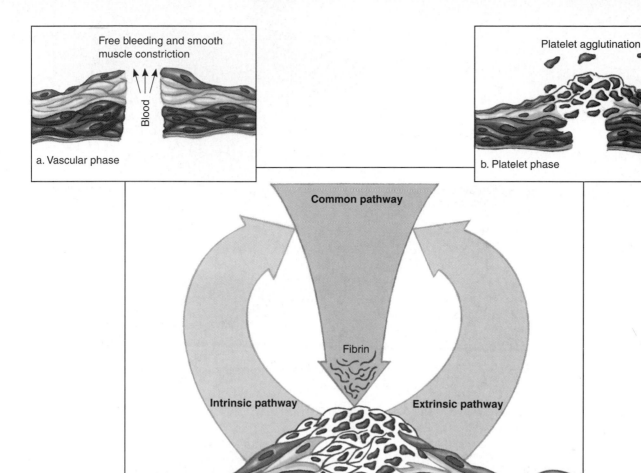

Free bleeding and smooth muscle constriction

Blood

a. Vascular phase

Platelet agglutination

b. Platelet phase

Common pathway

Fibrin

Intrinsic pathway

Extrinsic pathway

Fibrin formation

c. Coagulation phase

Figure 15-1 The three steps of the clotting process are the vascular phase, the platelet phase, and coagulation.

torn cleanly and do not withdraw. The actual hemorrhage site is lost in the disrupted tissue, resulting in severe, hard-to-control bleeding from a large wound area.

If a severe hemorrhage continues, frank hypotension reduces the blood pressure at the hemorrhage site. This limits the flow of blood and the dislodging of clots, thus improving the effectiveness of the clotting mechanism.

FACTORS AFFECTING THE CLOTTING PROCESS

The clotting process can be either helped or hindered by a variety of factors. For example, movement at or around the wound site, as in the manipulation of a fracture, may break the developing clot loose and disrupt the forming **fibrin** strands. For this reason, immediate wound immobilization (splinting) is beneficial.

Aggressive fluid therapy, which is often provided in cases of severe hemorrhage, may adversely impact the effectiveness of clotting mechanisms. Aggressive fluid resuscitation may increase blood pressure, which in turn increases the pressure pushing against the developing clots. In addition, the water and salts used in fluid therapy dilute the clotting factors, platelets, and red blood cells, further inhibiting the clotting process.

The patient's body temperature also has an effect on the clotting process. As the body temperature begins to fall, as it may in shock states, clot formation is neither as rapid nor

coagulation the third step in the clotting process; involves the formation of a protein called *fibrin*.

fibrin protein fibers that trap red blood cells as part of the clotting process.

Immediate immobilization (splinting) of the wound site aids the clotting process.

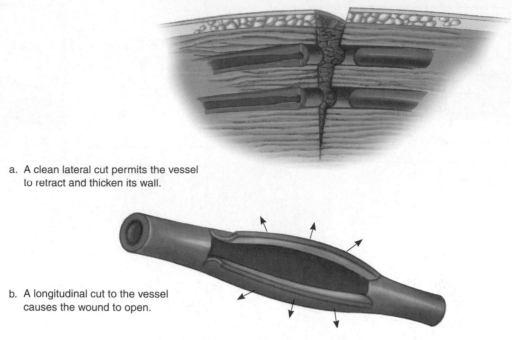

a. A clean lateral cut permits the vessel to retract and thicken its wall.

b. A longitudinal cut to the vessel causes the wound to open.

FIGURE 15-2   The type of blood vessel injury often affects the nature of the hemorrhage.

Content Review

FACTORS HINDERING THE CLOTTING PROCESS

- Movement of the wound site
- Aggressive fluid therapy
- Low body temperature
- Medications such as aspirin, heparin, or Coumadin

as effective as when the body temperature is 98.6°F (37°C). Thus it is important to keep a patient with severe hemorrhage warm.

Medications may interfere with the body's ability to form a clot and halt both internal and external hemorrhage. Aspirin modifies the enzymes on the surface of platelets that cause them to aggregate after an injury. Ibuprofen and other non-steroidal anti-inflammatory drugs (NSAIDs) may have a similar but temporary effect. Heparin and warfarin (Coumadin®) interfere with the normal generation of protein fibers that produce a stable clot. Although these drugs may prevent thrombosis and emboli in patients with heart disease, they may prolong or worsen hemorrhage when that patient is injured. Try to gather information on whether the patient uses such medications when taking the patient history.

HEMORRHAGE CONTROL

Hemorrhage is either internal or external. Though you can take steps to control external hemorrhage in the field, your care of internal hemorrhage is more limited.

External Hemorrhage

External hemorrhage is easy to identify and care for. It presents with blood oozing, flowing, or spurting from the wound. Bleeding from capillary and venous wounds is easy to halt because the pressure driving it is limited (Figure 15-3). Usually, applying **direct pressure** to the wound—or a combination of direct pressure and elevation—work quite well in stopping the bleeding. Bleeding from an arterial wound, however, is powered by the arterial blood pressure and escapes from the blood vessel with significant force. The normal control and clotting mechanisms help reduce blood loss but do not stop it if the injured vessel is large. To stop bleeding from such a wound, pressure on the bleeding site must exceed the arterial pressure. Direct digital pressure on the site of blood loss, maintained by a dressing and pressure bandage, is most effective. Elevation of the wound area and use of pressure points may also be necessary if the bandage cannot apply enough pressure directly to the hemorrhage site.

Be extremely cautious if you consider using a **tourniquet**. Employ the device only to halt persistent, life-threatening hemorrhage. If you apply the tourniquet at a pressure less than the arterial pressure, blood continues to flow into the limb, while the tourniquet restricts venous flow out. The limb's arterial and venous pressures then rise, as does the rate of hemorrhage. If the tourniquet meets its objective and halts all blood flow to the limb, blood loss stops, but so does circulation to the distal extremity. During this

direct pressure method of hemorrhage control that relies on the application of pressure to the actual site of the bleeding.

tourniquet a constrictor used on an extremity to apply circumferential pressure on all arteries to control bleeding.

Use a tourniquet only as a last resort to halt persistent, life-threatening hemorrhage.

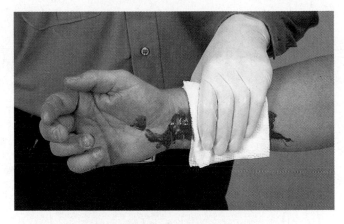

FIGURE 15-3a To control hemorrhage, apply direct pressure.

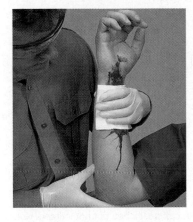

FIGURE 15-3b Elevate the extremity above the level of the heart.

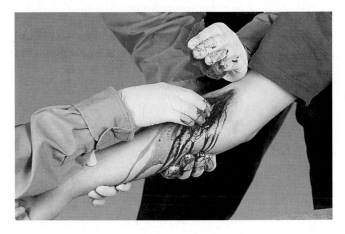

FIGURE 15-3c If bleeding does not stop, apply direct fingertip pressure.

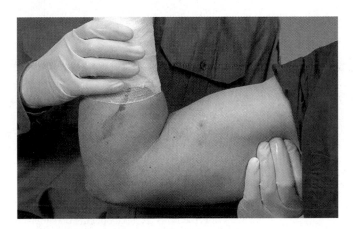

FIGURE 15-3d If bleeding continues, apply pressure to a pressure point.

absence of perfusion, **lactic acid,** potassium, and other **anaerobic** metabolites accumulate in the stagnant blood. When the tourniquet is released, the resumption of blood flow may transport these toxins into the central circulation with devastating results (Figure 15-4). Once you apply the tourniquet, therefore, leave it in place until the patient is in the emergency department or some other facility where the negative effects of re-perfusion can be addressed. If you must apply a tourniquet, use a wide cravat or belt or a blood pressure cuff. A thin or narrow constricting device may damage tissue beneath the tourniquet. Despite these hazards, the tourniquet may be essential in halting life-threatening arterial hemorrhage.

lactic acid compound produced from pyruvic acid during anaerobic glycolyis.

anaerobic able to live without oxygen.

Internal Hemorrhage

Internal hemorrhage is associated with almost all serious blunt and penetrating trauma. As with external hemorrhage, internal hemorrhage can involve capillary, venous, or arterial blood loss. The blood can accumulate in the tissue itself, forming a visible or hidden contusion, or it can be forced between **fascia** and form a pocket of blood called a **hematoma.** In most of these cases, the hemorrhage is self-limiting because the pressure within the tissue or fascia controls the blood loss. However, large contusions, massive soft tissue injuries, and large hematomas, especially those affecting large muscle masses, such as the thighs or buttocks, can account for moderate blood and body fluid loss. Fractures of the humerus and tibia/fibula may account for 500 to 750 mL of loss, whereas femur fractures may account for up to 1,500 mL of loss.

fascia a fibrous membrane that covers, supports, and separates muscles and may also unite the skin with underlying tissue.

hematoma collection of blood beneath the skin or trapped within a body compartment.

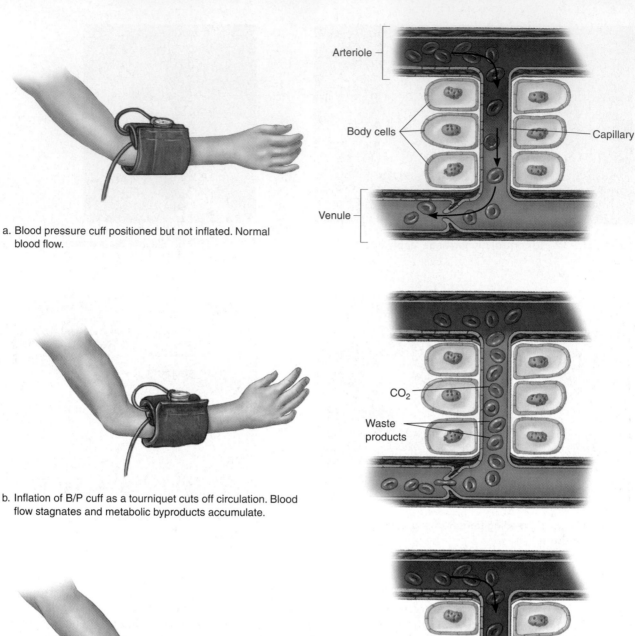

Arteriole

Body cells

Capillary

Venule

a. Blood pressure cuff positioned but not inflated. Normal blood flow.

CO_2

Waste products

b. Inflation of B/P cuff as a tourniquet cuts off circulation. Blood flow stagnates and metabolic byproducts accumulate.

CO_2

Waste products

c. Release of cuff restores circulation. Returning blood flow pushes acidic byproducts back into the central circulation.

FIGURE 15-4   Release of a tourniquet may send accumulated toxins into the central circulation with devastating results for the patient.

In body cavities such as the chest and the abdominal, pelvic, and retroperitoneal spaces, the resistance to continuing blood loss does not develop. With bleeding in these areas, loss continues unabated until the normal clotting process is effective, the blood pressure drops significantly, or surgical intervention is provided. The best indicators of significant internal hemorrhage are the mechanism of injury (MOI), local signs and symptoms of injury, and the early signs and symptoms of blood loss and shock. If a patient has sustained significant trauma to the chest, abdomen, or pelvis, anticipate significant, continuing, and uncontrolled blood loss. Such a patient requires rapid transport to a trauma center or hospital for surgical repair of any damaged vessels.

You can assist the natural internal hemorrhage control mechanisms in the extremities by providing a patient with immobilization and elevation. Continued movement of the injury site, especially if it is associated with a long bone fracture, disrupts the clotting process, causing further soft tissue, nervous, and vascular damage, and continuing the blood loss. If the patient is a victim of serious or multi-system trauma, however, do not spend time on the scene with aggressive skeletal immobilization. Instead, quickly splint the patient to a long spine board and begin transport. Provide splinting of individual limbs if time permits during transport.

Provide a patient with suspected internal bleeding with immobilization and elevation (of extremities) to aid the body's hemorrhage control mechanisms.

Internal hemorrhage is often associated with injuries to specific organs and can be related either to trauma or to pre-existing medical problems. Internal hemorrhage can also present with external signs of injury or disease in addition to the signs and symptoms of blood loss. These signs can help you identify the nature and location of the blood loss.

The nasal cavity is lined with a rich supply of capillaries to warm and help humidify incoming air. Hypertension, a strong sneeze, or direct trauma may rupture the vessels supplying these capillary beds and produce the moderate to severe hemorrhage called **epistaxis**. Prolonged epistaxis can result in hypovolemia, whereas blood flowing down the posterior nasal cavity, down the esophagus, and into the stomach may result in nausea followed by vomiting (Figure 15-5). Trauma to the oral cavity may likewise result in serious hemorrhage, followed by ingestion of blood, nausea, and then emesis.

epistaxis bleeding from the nose resulting from injury, disease, or environmental factors; a nosebleed.

There are also outward signs that indicate hemorrhage in the lungs and respiratory system. For example, degenerative diseases, such as tuberculosis or cancer, or chest trauma may rupture pulmonary vessels. This leads to the release of blood into the lower airways or alveolar space. The patient may then cough up bright red blood, a sign called hemoptysis.

Trauma, caustic ingestion, degenerative disease (for example, cancer), and rupturing **esophageal varicies** may lead to hemorrhage along the esophagus. In these pathologies, blood is likely to travel, via peristalsis, into the stomach, where it collects. Gastric hemorrhage due to ulceration or trauma may also result in the accumulation of blood in the stomach. A significant collection of blood acts as a gastric irritant, inducing vomiting. If the blood is evacuated early, it is bright red in color. If blood remains in the stomach for some time, emesis resembles coffee grounds in both color and consistency.

esophageal varicies enlarged and tortuous esophageal veins.

Hemorrhage in the small or large bowel can be associated with trauma, degenerative disease, or diverticulitis (small pouches in the walls of the bowel that collect material, become infected, and may burst). Bowel hemorrhage may present as bleeding from the rectum, or the blood may be digested before release, producing a black and tarry stool called **melena**.

melena black, tar-like feces due to gastrointestinal bleeding.

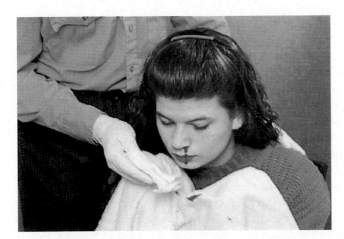

FIGURE 15-5a   To control a nosebleed, have the patient sit leaning forward.

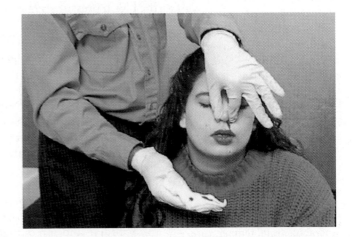

FIGURE 15-5b   Pinch the fleshy part of the patient's nostrils firmly together.

With hemorrhage patients, determine the relative severity of blood loss, the need for aggressive intervention, length of time since the incident, the current stage of hemorrhage, and how quickly the patient is moving from one stage to another.

pulse pressure difference between the systolic and diastolic blood pressures.

catecholamine a hormone, such as epinephrine or norepinephrine, that strongly affects the nervous and cardiovascular systems, metabolic rate, temperature, and smooth muscle.

Rectal injury may be caused by pelvic fracture or direct trauma. This presents with bleeding, which may be severe.

Vaginal hemorrhage may be associated with trauma, degenerative disease, menstruation, ectopic pregnancy, placenta previa, and potential or actual miscarriage. Urethral hemorrhage is generally minor and may reflect damage to the prostate or urethra. Blood in the urine reflects bladder injury.

Non-traumatic forms of hemorrhage may be either acute or chronic. Acute hemorrhage moves the victim rapidly toward shock and is quickly recognizable. Chronic hemorrhage is likely to be rather limited in volume, but it does continue over time. The resulting loss depletes the body of red blood cells and leads to **anemia.** This condition reduces the blood's oxygen-carrying capacity, and the patient experiences fatigue and lethargy. Clotting factors may likewise be depleted, which increases the rate of fluid loss and makes any secondary hemorrhage more difficult to control.

STAGES OF HEMORRHAGE

Fluid accounts for about 60% of the body's weight and is distributed among the cellular, interstitial, and vascular spaces. The cells contain about 62% of the total fluid volume, whereas the interstitial (non-vascular) space holds 26%. From 4% to 5% of body fluid is found in other spaces such as the ventricles of the brain and meninges (cerebrospinal fluid). The remaining 7% of fluid volume resides in the vascular space. This fluid, called plasma, and the blood cells account for 7% of the average adult male's body weight (about 6.5% in the female). Fluid in the vascular space is distributed among the heart, arteries, veins, and capillaries and accounts for 5 liters (10 units) of blood volume in the healthy 70-kg adult male.

The effects of hemorrhage can be categorized into four progressive stages as blood volume is lost. These stages relate to the volume of blood lost in acute hemorrhage and that result in classic signs and symptoms. Remember, however, that each individual's response to blood loss may vary as may the rate and progress of the loss. Use these categories to help determine the relative severity of the loss and the need for aggressive intervention. It is also important to identify the following: the length of time elapsed since the incident that caused the trauma, the stage of hemorrhage the victim is in when you arrive at his side, and how quickly the patient is moving from one stage to another (Table 15-1).

Stage 1 Hemorrhage

Stage 1 hemorrhage is a blood loss of up to 15% of the circulating blood volume. In the 70-kg male that is approximately 500 to 750 mL of blood, about the amount a person might give during a blood drive. The healthy human system can easily compensate for such a blood loss volume by constricting the vascular beds, especially on the venous side. In this stage, the blood pressure remains constant as do the **pulse pressure,** respiratory rate, and renal output. The central venous pressure may drop slightly, but it returns to normal quickly. The pulse rate elevates slightly, and the patient may display some signs of **catecholamine** (epinephrine and norepinephrine) release, notably nervousness and marginally cool skin with a slight pallor.

Stage 2 Hemorrhage

Stage 2 hemorrhage occurs as 15% to 25% (750 to 1,250 mL) of the blood volume is lost. The body's first-line compensatory responses can no longer maintain blood pressure, and secondary mechanisms are now employed. Tachycardia becomes very evident, and the pulse strength begins to diminish (the pulse pressure is noticeably narrowed). A strong release of catecholamines increases peripheral vascular resistance. This maintains systolic blood pressure but results in peripheral vasoconstriction and cool, clammy skin. Anxiety increases, and the patient may begin to display restlessness and thirst. Thirst is present as fluid leaves the intracellular and interstitial spaces and the osmotic pressure of the blood changes. Renal output remains normal, but the respiratory rate increases.

Table 15-1 **PATIENT SIGNS ASSOCIATED WITH STAGES OF HEMORRHAGE**

Stage	Blood Loss	Vasoconstriction	Pulse Rate	Pulse (Pressure) Strength	Blood Pressure	Respiratory Rate	Respiratory Volume
1	<15%	↑	↑	→	→	→	→
2	15–25%	↑↑	↑↑	↓	→	↑	↑
3	25–35%	↑↑↑	↑↑↑	↓↓	↓	↑↑	↓
4	>35%	↓↓	Variable	↓↓↓	↓↓↓	↓	↓↓

Stage 3 Hemorrhage

Stage 3 hemorrhage occurs when blood loss reaches between 25% to 35% of blood volume (1,250 to 1,750 mL). The body's compensatory mechanisms are unable to cope with the loss, and the classic signs of shock appear. Rapid tachycardia is present as the blood pressure begins to fall. The pulse is barely palpable as the pulse pressure remains very narrow. The patient experiences air hunger and tachypnea. Anxiety, restlessness, and thirst become more severe. The level of responsiveness decreases, and the patient becomes very pale, cool, and diaphoretic. Urinary output declines. Without rapid intervention, this patient's survival is unlikely.

Without rapid intervention, survival of a Stage 3 hemorrhage patient is unlikely.

Stage 4 Hemorrhage

Stage 4 hemorrhage occurs with a blood loss of greater than 35% of the body's total blood supply. The patient's pulse is barely palpable in the central arteries, if one can be found at all. Respirations are very rapid, shallow, and ineffective. The patient is very lethargic and confused, moving rapidly toward unresponsiveness. The skin is very cool, clammy, and extremely pale. Urinary output ceases. Even with aggressive fluid resuscitation and blood transfusions, patient survival is unlikely.

These descriptions of the stages of hemorrhage presume that the patient is a normally healthy adult. Any pre-existing condition may affect the volume of blood loss required for movement from one stage to another as well as the speed at which the patient moves through the stages. The patient's state of hydration, from dehydrated to fluid-rich, may also affect how quickly and to what degree compensation takes place.

The rate of the blood loss also has a profound effect on how quickly a patient moves from stage 1 to stage 4. If the blood loss is very rapid, the compensatory mechanisms may not work as effectively. On the other hand, a small wound bleeding uncontrollably but very slowly for days may not move the patient from stage 1 to stage 2, even with a loss much greater than 750 mL.

Certain categories of patients—pregnant women, athletes, obese patients, children, and the elderly—react differently to blood loss. The blood volume of a woman in late pregnancy is 50% greater than normal. This patient may lose rather large volumes of blood before progressing through the various stages of hemorrhage. Although the mother in this circumstance appears to be somewhat protected from the effects of serious hemorrhage, the fetus is deprived of good circulation early in the blood loss and is more susceptible to harm.

A well-conditioned athlete often has greater fluid and cardiac reserves than a typical patient. This means he or she may move more slowly through the early stages with greater percentages of loss needed to advance from one stage to another.

The obese patient, on the other hand, has a blood volume close to 7% of ideal body weight, but not actual body weight. Thus, the blood volume as a percentage of actual body weight is lower than 7%. This means that what appears to be only a small blood loss may have a more serious effect in such a patient.

In infants and young children, blood volumes approximate 8% to 9% of body weight, volumes that are proportionally about 20% greater than those of adults. However, compensatory mechanisms in infants and children are neither as well developed nor as effective

Suspect hemorrhage early in cases of child and infant trauma, and treat it aggressively.

as those in adults. These young patients may not show early signs and symptoms of compensation as clearly as adults. They may instead move quickly into the later stages of shock. Suspect hemorrhage early with child and infant trauma and treat it aggressively.

The elderly are likewise more adversely affected by blood loss. They have lower volumes of fluid reserves, and their compensatory systems are less responsive to fluid losses. These patients may also be on medications, such as beta-blockers, that further reduce the body's ability to respond to blood loss and varying blood pressures or on medications, such as aspirin, Coumadin®, and heparin, that interfere with the body's natural hemorrhage control system. Often, elderly patients do not experience the tachycardia associated with blood loss, and their blood pressures drop before those of healthy adults. Signs of blood loss and shock may be masked by reduced perceptions of pain in the elderly and by lowered levels of mental acuity due to disease. The elderly also do not tolerate periods of inadequate tissue perfusion well because of chronic cardiovascular inefficiency.

HEMORRHAGE ASSESSMENT

The assessment of various types of trauma patients is the subject of Chapters 12 to 18. Also, please refer to the patient assessment chapters, Chapters 6 to 9, for a more complete discussion of trauma assessment.

The assessment of the hemorrhage patient is directed at identifying the source of the hemorrhage and halting any serious and controllable loss. During assessment, you should also examine the circumstances of injury to approximate the volume of blood lost and the rate of past and continuing hemorrhage. This process begins with the scene size-up and continues throughout transport and care.

Scene Size-up

Remember that body substance isolation (BSI) precautions are essential during the assessment of trauma patients. A patient's blood and other body fluids may contain pathogens capable of transmitting HIV, hepatitis, and other diseases to you. Conversely, you may transmit infectious agents to the wounds of the patients you assess and care for. In fact, the risk of your transmitting disease or infection to a patient with open wounds or burns is probably much greater than the risk that he or she will transmit disease or infection to you. For these reasons, always observe BSI precautions with all trauma patients. These precautions include the use of gloves and a mask when you inspect or palpate any injured area, especially one with open wounds (Figure 15-6). If blood is spurting, as with arterial hemorrhage, if a patient is combative, or if there is airway trauma with or without bleeding, also wear eye protection and a disposable gown to protect your uniform. Be sure to wash your hands before each ambulance call and do so immediately afterward as well. Scrub vigorously when washing to remove as much of the bacterial load as possible.

If your gloves become contaminated with earth, debris, blood, or body fluids while caring for a patient, change them immediately. If you will be assessing or treating multiple patients, consider double gloving. This means that you put on two or more sets of gloves and remove a set each time you complete assessment of one patient and move on to the next. Place any contaminated gloves, clothing, dressings, or other materials in a biohazard bag and ensure proper disposal.

The handling of needles presents special problems for prehospital personnel. Once a needle is used, it carries the potential of introducing a patient's blood directly into a caregiver's or bystander's tissues. This greatly increases the likelihood of disease transmission. When dealing with needles, always ensure that they are not recapped, but rather placed in a properly marked and secure, puncture-resistant sharps container. Should you be stuck with a needle, continue your care, but document the incident immediately upon arrival at the emergency department. Wash and cover the wound, then report the incident to your service's infection control officer or other designated officer. Several prophylactic regimens are available that may protect against the transmission of some infectious diseases. Even more important, you can guard against some diseases, such as hepatitis, by obtaining immunizations before you begin your career as a care provider.

Be aware that blood loss in elderly patients may be masked by medications, bodily changes, reduced perception of pain, and effects of disease.

Assessment of the hemorrhage patient is directed at identifying the source of the hemorrhage and halting any serious and controllable blood loss.

BSI precautions protect the patient as well as the caregiver.

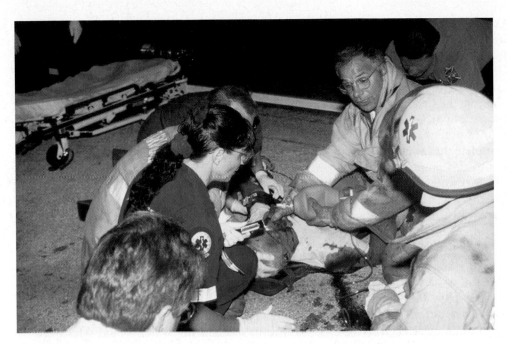

FIGURE 15-6 When caring for a hemorrhaging patient, take the appropriate body substance isolation (BSI) precautions.

Patients may see your gloves and then feel uncomfortable about being treated by someone who is "afraid to touch them." Reassure those patients. Tell them that the gloves and other precautions are for their protection as well as yours.

When appropriate BSI precautions have been taken, continue with the scene size-up. Evaluate the mechanism of injury to anticipate sites of both external and internal hemorrhage. Anticipating external hemorrhage sites focuses your subsequent assessment and care, whereas anticipating internal hemorrhage affects your decision on whether to provide rapid transport.

When evaluating the mechanism of injury (MOI), also attempt to determine the amount of time that has elapsed between the injury and your evaluation of it. Knowing the length of this time period is very important in determining the amount and rate of blood loss. For example, if you arrive on a scene 3 minutes after an accident and find a patient losing 150 mL of blood per minute, you can estimate that 450 mL of blood have been lost. You would not expect the patient to display the signs and symptoms of stage 1 hemorrhage. If, however, you arrive 10 minutes after the incident, the same patient, losing blood at the same rate, will have lost 1,500 mL of blood and is likely to have reached stage 3. In both these cases, the patient is suffering serious, life-threatening hemorrhage. Good assessment and recognition ensures provision of a proper course of care. However, the earlier you arrive at the patient's side, the harder it is to identify serious hemorrhage. For this reason, you must be aware of and appreciate the progressive effects of blood loss and use both the MOI analysis and the time since an incident to increase your suspicions of a problem. Remember, the sooner the signs of later stages of hemorrhage appear, the greater the rate and volume of blood loss.

> *The sooner the signs of the later stages of hemorrhage appear, the greater the rate and volume of blood loss.*

Initial Assessment

As you begin the initial assessment, form a general impression of the patient. Be especially alert for any signs and symptoms of internal hemorrhage. These early signs are very subtle and may go unnoticed unless you deliberately look for them. Correct any immediate life threats and provide in-line stabilization if you suspect spinal injury. Assess the patient's initial mental status to determine alertness, orientation, and responsiveness. Be alert for any signs of anxiety, confusion, or combativeness. Any central nervous system deficit may be secondary to hemorrhage, so be suspicious.

Assess both airway and breathing carefully, noting any tachypnea or air hunger. Administer oxygen via nonrebreather mask at a rate of 15 liters per minute. When assessing circulation, pay special attention to the pulse strength (the pulse pressure) and rate. Remember that the pulse pressure narrows well before the systolic pressure begins to drop. The pulse rate, too, may suggest developing shock. A fast—especially a fast, weak (thready)—pulse may be the first noticeable sign of serious internal blood loss. Note also skin color and condition. Pale or mottled skin is an early sign of shock. Cool and clammy skin is also an indicator of potential blood loss and shock.

Complete the initial assessment by establishing patient priorities. Decide, based on your findings to this point, whether the patient is to receive a rapid trauma assessment or a focused history and exam. If any indication, mechanism of injury, sign, or symptom suggests serious internal hemorrhage or uncontrolled external hemorrhage, consider the rapid trauma assessment and then immediate transport for the patient.

Focused History and Physical Exam

MOI short for mechanism of injury.

Your initial assessment findings and the evaluation of the mechanism of injury determine how you will proceed with the focused history and physical exam. For trauma patients who have a significant **MOI**, continue spinal immobilization, and perform a rapid trauma assessment. Then obtain baseline vital signs and a patient history.

For trauma patients who have no significant mechanism of injury and who have revealed no critical findings during initial assessment, perform an assessment focused on the area of injury, then obtain baseline vital signs and gather a patient history. Finally, provide care as appropriate and transport.

With both types of trauma patients, perform ongoing assessments during transport. If time and the patient's condition permit, you may also perform a detailed physical exam. However, you should never delay transport to perform the detailed examination.

Rapid Trauma Assessment For trauma patients with a significant MOI, you perform a rapid trauma assessment, inspecting and palpating the patient in an orderly fashion from head to toe. Pay particular attention to areas where critical trauma has occurred and areas where the MOI suggests forces were focused.

Carefully and quickly observe the head for serious bleeding. Internal head injury rarely accounts for the classic signs of shock. However, the scalp bleeds profusely because the vessels there are large and lack the ability to constrict as well as other peripheral vessels. If any external bleeding appears serious, halt it immediately.

Next, examine the neck. The carotid arteries and jugular veins are located close to the skin's surface. Injury to them can produce rapid and fatal exsanguination. An added danger is the aspiration of air directly into an open jugular vein. At times, venous pressure, due to deep inspiration, can be less than atmospheric pressure. Air may then be drawn into the vein, traveling to the heart and forming emboli, which then lodge in the pulmonary circulation. Quickly control any serious hemorrhage from neck wounds with sterile occlusive dressings. If spinal injury is suspected, apply a rigid cervical collar when assessment of the neck is complete, but maintain in-line manual immobilization until the patient is immobilized to a spine board.

Visually sweep the chest and abdomen for any serious external hemorrhage, though such bleeding is infrequent there. You are more likely to note signs of blunt or penetrating trauma, suggesting internal injury and hemorrhage within. Look to the abdomen for signs of soft tissue injury, contusions, abrasions, rigidity, and guarding and tenderness that suggest internal injury.

Quickly examine the pelvic and groin region. Test the integrity of the pelvic ring by pressing gently on the iliac crest. Remember that pelvic fracture can account for blood loss of more than 2,000 mL. Lacerations to the male genitalia may also account for serious external hemorrhage.

Assess the extremities and rule out fractures of the femur, tibia/fibula, or humerus. Keep in mind that femur fracture can account for up to 1,500 mL of blood loss, whereas each tibia/fibula or humerus fracture may contribute an additional 500 to 750 mL of blood loss. Hematomas and large contusions may account for up to 500 mL of blood loss in the larger

Content Review

INJURIES THAT CAN CAUSE SIGNIFICANT BLOOD LOSS

- Fractured pelvis (2,000 mL)
- Fractured femur (1,500 mL)
- Fractured tibia (750 mL)
- Fractured humerus (750 mL)
- Large contusion (500 mL)

muscle masses. Quickly check distal pulse strength and muscle tone in the extremities, comparing findings in the opposing extremities.

Finally, visually sweep the body, including the posterior, for any external hemorrhage that may have gone unnoticed in your examination to this point.

At the end of the rapid trauma assessment, assess the patient's vital signs, obtain a patient history if possible, and inventory the injuries that may contribute to shock. Provide rapid transport for any patient with a MOI or physical findings that meet trauma triage criteria (see Chapter 12, "Trauma and Trauma Systems"). Any patient with injuries likely to induce hemorrhage at the level of stage 2 or greater should likewise receive immediate transport. If travel time to the trauma center will exceed 20 minutes, consider requesting air medical transport. Be sure to record the results of your assessment carefully. Compare this information with signs and symptoms you discover during the ongoing assessment to identify trends in the patient's condition.

Perform a detailed physical exam only when all immediate life threats have been addressed. Normally, this would be when you are en route to the hospital or trauma center or when transport has been delayed for some reason.

Focused Physical Exam   Employ the focused trauma assessment for patients without a significant MOI, for example, a patient who has lacerated his or her finger with a knife. In such cases, the hemorrhage can be controlled on the scene and the MOI does not suggest additional problems. With such patients, focus your exam on the area injured, inspecting and palpating the area thoroughly, looking for additional injuries beyond the one that prompted the call. Control the hemorrhage, if you have not already done so. Obtain baseline vital signs and a patient history, and prepare and transport the patient.

In some cases, you may wish to perform a rapid trauma assessment, even though the patient does not have a significant MOI. This would be the case, for example, if you suspect the patient has more injuries than he or she has complained of or if his or her condition suddenly begins to deteriorate. With such patients, it may be necessary to perform a rapid head-to-toe examination, inspecting and palpating all body regions.

Additional Assessment Considerations   In the trauma patient with a significant MOI or the medical patient showing signs and symptoms of blood loss and shock, it is important to search for evidence of internal hemorrhage. This evidence may be in the form of blood, or material suggestive of blood, flowing from the body orifices. Bright red blood from the mouth, nose, rectum, or other orifice suggests direct bleeding. The vomiting of material that looks like coffee grounds is associated with partially digested blood in the stomach, suggestive of a long-term and slow hemorrhage. A black, tarry stool called melena suggests blood has remained in the bowel for some time. **Hematochezia** is stool with frank blood in it and reflects active bleeding in the colon or rectum.

In the patient with non-specific complaints—general ill feeling, anxiousness, restlessness—or a lowered level of responsiveness, suspect and look for other signs of internal hemorrhage. Watch for an increasing pulse rate, rising diastolic blood pressure (narrowing blood pressure), and cool and clammy skin.

Also observe for dizziness or syncope when the patient moves from a supine to a sitting or standing position. This condition is called **orthostatic hypotension** and is suggestive of a volume loss, possibly attributable to internal hemorrhage. This phenomenon is the basis of the **tilt test,** which can be employed to determine blood or fluid loss and the body's reduced ability to compensate for normal positional change. Perform this test only on patients who do not already display signs and symptoms of shock. Prepare for the test by obtaining blood pressure and pulse rates from the patient in a supine or seated position. Then have the supine patient move to a seated position or the seated patient stand up and obtain another set of blood pressure and pulse rates. If the systolic blood pressure drops more than 20 mmHg or the pulse rate rises more than 20 beats per minute, the test is considered positive, indicating hypovolemia.

Ongoing Assessment

Once you have rendered all appropriate life-saving care, perform ongoing assessments frequently—at least every 5 minutes with unstable patients and every 15 minutes with stable ones. Reevaluate your general impression, and reassess the patient's mental status, airway,

hematochezia passage of stools containing red blood.

orthostatic hypotension a decrease in blood pressure that occurs when a person moves from a supine or sitting to an upright position.

tilt test drop in the systolic blood pressure of 20 mmHg or an increase in the pulse rate of 20 beats per minute when a patient is moved from a supine to a sitting position; a finding suggestive of a relative hypovolemia.

breathing, and circulation, and obtain additional sets of vital signs. Compare each set of findings with earlier ones to determine if the patient's condition is stable, deteriorating, or improving. Pay special attention to the pulse pressure because it is a clear indicator of the body's efforts to compensate for hypovolemia. Also pay particular attention to changes in mental status, noting any increasing anxiety or restlessness.

HEMORRHAGE MANAGEMENT

The management of hemorrhage is an integral part of care for the trauma patient, one that begins during the initial assessment and is shaped by findings of the rapid trauma assessment or the focused physical exam.

First, ensure that the airway is patent, that the patient is breathing adequately, and that you have administered high-flow, high-concentration oxygen. If you have not, establish and maintain the airway and provide the necessary ventilatory support. Be prepared to provide endotracheal intubation if necessary to secure the airway.

Ensure that the patient has a pulse. If not, initiate CPR, attach a monitor-defibrillator, and employ advanced cardiac life-support measures. Rule out pericardial tamponade and tension pneumothorax as possible causes of cardiac dysfunction. Understand that cardiac arrest in trauma cases due to hypovolemia carries an extremely poor prognosis. When resources are scarce, your efforts may be better utilized caring for other salvageable patients.

During the initial assessment, care for serious hemorrhage only after any airway and breathing problems are corrected.

During the initial assessment, care for serious (arterial and heavy venous) hemorrhage only after any airway and breathing problems are corrected. Quickly apply a pressure dressing held in place by self-adherent bandage material or a firmly tied cravat. Return to provide better hemorrhage control after you complete the initial and rapid trauma assessments and set priorities for care of the hemorrhages and other trauma you discover. If the patient displays early signs of shock, consider applying a PASG and initiating fluid therapy; do not, however, delay transport to carry out these measures.

Once you have completed the focused history and physical exam stage of assessment, begin caring for injuries, including hemorrhage, as you have prioritized them. As you work down your injury priority list and come to a wound, inspect the site to identify the type and exact location of bleeding. This helps you apply pressure—either digitally or with dressings and bandages—most effectively to halt the blood flow. With cases of external hemorrhage, it is important to identify the exact source and type of bleeding and to be sure to look at the wound site.

Document your findings on the prehospital care report. If you document and convey this information clearly to the emergency department staff, you will reduce the need for others to open the wound (thus disrupting the clotting process) to determine and describe its nature.

Direct pressure usually controls all but the most persistent hemorrhage.

Direct pressure controls all but the most persistent hemorrhage (Figure 15-7). Although systolic blood pressure drives arterial hemorrhage, you can stop such a hemorrhage with simple finger pressure properly applied to the source of the bleeding. If a wound looks as

FIGURE 15-7 In most cases of moderate to severe external hemorrhage, direct pressure, maintained by a bandage and dressing, will control bleeding.

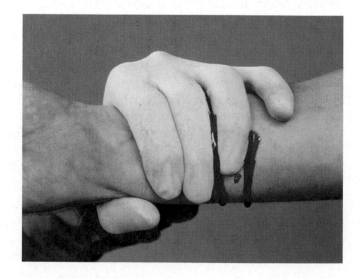

though it may pose a problem, insert a wad of dressing material over the site of the heaviest bleeding and apply a bandage over the dressing. This focuses pressure on the site and away from the surrounding area. If bleeding saturates the dressing, cover it with another dressing and apply another bandage to keep pressure on the wound. Removing the soaked bandage and dressing disrupts the clotting process and prolongs the hemorrhage. If, however, the wound continues to bleed through your layers of dressings and bandages, consider removing the dressing materials you have applied, directly visualizing the exact site of bleeding, and then re-applying a wad of dressing and firm direct pressure to the precise hemorrhage site.

If direct pressure alone does not halt the blood flow to an extremity, consider elevation. Elevation reduces the systolic blood pressure because the heart has to push the blood against gravity and up the limb. Employ elevation only when there is an isolated bleeding wound on a limb and movement will not aggravate any other injuries.

If bleeding still persists, find an arterial pulse point proximal to the wound and apply firm pressure there (Figure 15-8). This further reduces the blood pressure within the limb and should reduce the hemorrhaging.

Other techniques that can aid in hemorrhage control include limb splinting and the use of pneumatic splints. Splinting helps maintain the stability of the wound site, thus assisting the mechanisms by which clots develop. Splinting may also protect the site from injuries that might occur if the patient is jostled during extrication and transport or as you assess and care for other wounds. Pneumatic splints can also prevent movement of an injured limb.

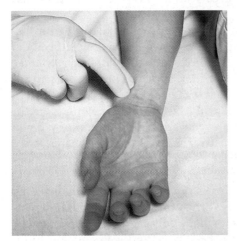

a. Radial artery for hand.

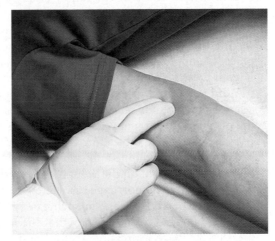

b. Brachial artery for forearm.

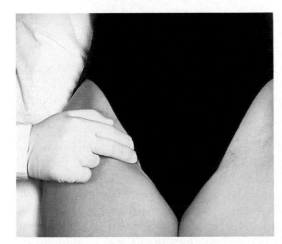

c. Femoral artery for thigh.

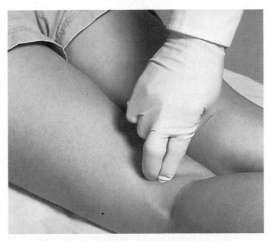

d. Popliteal artery for leg and foot.

FIGURE 15-8   Common pressure points for hemorrhage control.

They may also be helpful in holding dressings in place and in applying direct pressure to a limb circumferentially.

Consider using a tourniquet only as a last resort when hemorrhage is prolonged and persistent. As mentioned earlier, hazards are associated with tourniquet use. Apply a blood pressure cuff just proximal to the hemorrhage site and inflate it to apply a pressure about 30 mmHg greater than the systolic blood pressure. Ensure bleeding stops after you apply the tourniquet, and mark the patient's forehead with the letters "TQ" and the time of application.

Specific Wound Considerations

Several types of wounds require special attention for hemorrhage control. They include head wounds, neck wounds, large gaping wounds, and crush injuries.

Head injuries raise some special concerns regarding hemorrhage control. Head wounds may be associated with both severe hemorrhage and the loss of skull integrity (fracture). Control bleeding with such wounds very carefully, using gentle direct pressure around the wound site and against the stable skull. Fluid drainage from the ears and nose may be secondary to skull fracture. Cerebrospinal fluid, as it escapes the cranial vault, relieves building intracranial pressure. Halting the flow of fluid would end this relief mechanism and compound the increase in pressure. In addition, stopping the flow may provide a pathway for pathogens to enter the meninges and cause serious infection (meningitis). Cerebrospinal fluid quickly regenerates as the injury heals. Thus, if there is hemorrhage from either the nose or ear canal, simply cover the area with a soft, porous dressing and bandage it loosely.

Neck wounds carry the risk of air being drawn into the venous circulation with life-threatening results. Cover any open neck wound with an occlusive dressing held firmly in place. Do not employ circumferential bandages to create direct pressure with neck wounds. Digital pressure controls most, if not all, neck bleeding. It may, however, be necessary to apply and maintain this manual pressure continuously during the patient's prehospital care.

Gaping wounds often present hemorrhage control problems. With such wounds, bleeding originates from many sites and their open nature prevents application of uniform direct pressure. To manage bleeding from such a wound, create a mass of dressing material approximating the volume and shape of the wound. Place the material with the sterile, non-adherent side down on the wound and bandage it firmly in place.

Controlling hemorrhage associated with crush injuries can be particularly challenging. The source of hemorrhage in such cases is frequently difficult to determine, and the vessels are damaged in such a way that the normal hemorrhage control mechanisms may be ineffective. Place a dressing around and over the crushed tissue and a pneumatic splint over that and inflate to apply pressure and hold the dressing in place. If bleeding is heavy and persistent, consider using a tourniquet but keep in mind the precautions discussed previously.

Transport Considerations

Consider rapid transport for any patient who experiences serious external hemorrhage that you cannot control and for any patient with suspected serious internal hemorrhage. Be vigilant for any signs of compensation for blood loss and for the early signs of shock. Monitor your patient's mental status, pulse rate, and blood pressure (for narrowing pulse pressure). When in doubt, transport.

Understand that serious hemorrhage can have a significant psychological impact on patients. Stress triggers the "fight-or-flight" response, increases heart rate and blood pressure, increases the body's metabolic demands, works against the body's hemorrhage control mechanisms, and contributes to the development of shock. Do what you can to ease the anxieties of such patients. Communicate freely with them and explain what care measures you are taking and why. Be especially alert to their comfort needs and address them as appropriate. If possible, keep these patients from seeing their injuries or the serious injuries affecting friends and other accident victims.

For patients with head injury, do not attempt to stop the flow of blood or fluid from the nose or ear canal, but cover the area with porous dressing and bandage loosely.

Cover any open neck wound with an occlusive dressing held firmly in place.

Consider rapid transport for any patient with serious external hemorrhage and for any patient with suspected serious internal hemorrhage.

SHOCK

A simple medical definition of shock is "a state of inadequate tissue perfusion." Beyond that simple definition, however, shock is the transitional stage between normal life, called homeostasis, and death. It is the underlying killer of all trauma patients and often presents with only subtle signs and symptoms until the body can no longer compensate. Then the victim moves quickly, and often irreversibly, toward death. Because of this, you, as an EMT-I, must understand the process of shock and recognize its earliest signs and symptoms.

Cells are the microscopic building blocks of the human body. When cells cease to function—and if the process is not reversed—the result is cell death, which leads to tissue death, then to organ failure, and ultimately to the death of the organism. In order for cells to function, they must be continually perfused by blood, as carried through the capillaries, to receive a constant supply of oxygen and other nutrients and to eliminate waste products.

Shock is a tissue perfusion problem affecting the individual body cells. There are many causes of shock, though all are commonly manifested by signs and symptoms of cardiovascular system compensation followed by decompensation and, ultimately, collapse. The best way to understand shock and how body systems compensate for it is to look at the cell and its functions and then to examine how the body provides for the cells' metabolic needs and how this process can fail. (Cell **metabolism** is discussed in Chapter 2.)

> *Shock is the underlying killer of all trauma patients and often presents with only subtle signs and symptoms.*
>
>

metabolism the total changes that take place in an organism during physiological processes.

BODY'S RESPONSE TO BLOOD LOSS

The sympathetic nervous system and the hormones it releases begin progressive responses as hemorrhage causes blood to leave the cardiovascular system. As the draw down of the vascular volume reaches the heart, the right atrium does not completely fill. This means the atrium's output does not engorge the ventricle. Cardiac contractility therefore suffers as the ventricular myocardium does not stretch. The stroke volume drops, and there is an immediate drop in the systolic blood pressure. This reduced pressure reduces the cardiovascular system's ability to drive blood through the capillary beds. The baroreceptors in the neck recognize this decrease in blood pressure and signal to the medulla oblongata. The vasomotor center increases the peripheral vascular resistance and increases venous

---

Patho Pearls

For years the principle prehospital treatment of hypotension due to trauma was the administration of large volumes of crystalloid solutions and rapid transport. However, research is starting to show that infusing massive quantities of crystalloids, without correcting the underlying problem, may be detrimental. Consider this: if large quantities of fluid are administered without the injury being repaired, blood loss will continue and the blood will become progressively more diluted. Thus, the number of red blood cells available to carry oxygen will begin to fall. In addition, as blood becomes diluted with IV fluids, the coagulation factors are diluted and blood clotting becomes slower and less effective. Thus, some leading trauma researchers advocate limiting the amount of fluids administered prior to surgery.

Research has also started to demonstrate that hypotension (within certain parameters) following trauma may actually be protective. In fact, some are calling for "permissive hypotension" where the systolic blood pressure is maintained between 70 to 85 mmHg instead of 100 mmHg or more. The theory behind this concept is straightforward. First, several protective mechanisms appear to be activated when the blood pressure is within this range. Second, increasing the blood pressure with fluids, PASG, or similar methods might lead to a more rapid blood loss. Thus, trying to maintain normal blood pressures may actually increase the rate of blood loss and may inhibit clot formation or may cause dislodgement of a clot that formed during periods of hypotension following trauma. This concept is being aggressively studied.

The information in this box is presented to introduce you to controversies and research in the field of trauma care. Despite this information, *always follow the local protocols as established by your system and your medical director.* However, it is important to look at the ongoing research that may affect prehospital practice. EMS in the twenty-first century should be based on scientific evidence—not anecdotes or dogma.

tone, while the cardioacceleratory center increases heart rate and contractile strength. With the reduced venous capacitance and a slight increase in heart rate and peripheral vascular resistance, the blood pressure returns to normal, as does tissue perfusion. These actions normally compensate for small blood losses. If the blood loss stops, the body reconstitutes the blood from the interstitial fluid and replaces the lost red blood cells gradually, without noticeable or ill effects.

Cellular Ischemia

If blood loss continues, the venous system constricts to its limits to maintain cardiac preload. However, it becomes more and more difficult for the venous system to compensate because its limited musculature begins to tire. Peripheral vascular resistance also continues to increase to maintain the systolic blood pressure. As it does, the diastolic blood pressure rises, the pulse pressure narrows, and the pulse weakens. The constriction of arterioles means that less and less blood is directed to the non-critical organs, and those organs' supply of oxygen is reduced. The skin, the largest of the non-critical organs, receives reduced circulation and becomes cool, pale, and moist. If the hemorrhage continues, some non-critical organ cells begin to starve for oxygen. Anaerobic metabolism is their only energy source, and carbon dioxide and lactic and other acids begin to accumulate. Cellular hypoxia begins, followed by **ischemia**. The heart rate increases, but slowly, because the other compensatory mechanisms are still effectively maintaining preload.

As the blood loss increases, more and more body cells are deprived of their oxygen and nutrient supplies, and more and more waste products accumulate. The bloodstream becomes acidic, and the body's chemoreceptors stimulate an increase in depth and rate of respirations. Circulating catecholamines and increasing acidosis cause alterations in the level of orientation, and the patient becomes anxious, restless, and possibly combative. Ischemia now affects not only non-critical organs but also the arterioles. These vessels, which also require oxygen, become hypoxic and begin to fatigue. Meanwhile, the coronary arteries are providing a decreasing amount of oxygenated blood to the laboring heart.

If the blood loss stops, the blood draws fluid from within the interstitial space, at a rate of up to one liter per hour, to restore its volume, and erythropoietin accelerates the production of red blood cells. The kidneys reduce urine output to conserve water and electrolytes, and a period of thirst provides the stimulus for the patient to drink liquids and replace the lost volume on a more permanent basis. Transfusion with whole blood may be required at this point. Although some signs of circulatory compromise and fatigue are present, the patient's recovery is probable with a period of rest.

Capillary Microcirculation

If blood loss continues, sympathetic stimulation and reduced perfusion to the kidneys, pancreas, and liver cause release of hormones. Angiotensin II further increases peripheral vascular resistance and reduces the blood flow to more of the body's tissues. If the blood loss continues, circulation is further limited to only those organs most critical to life. This further decrease in circulation leads to an increase in cellular hypoxia in non-critical tissues, and more cells begin to use anaerobic metabolism for energy in a desperate attempt to survive. The build-up of lactic acid and carbon dioxide relaxes the pre-capillary sphincters. The circulating blood volume is diminished both by the continued hemorrhage and by fluid loss as the capillary beds engorge. Post-capillary sphincters remain closed, forcing fluids into the interstitial spaces by **hydrostatic pressure**. The circulatory crisis worsens as the compensatory mechanisms begin to fail. Interstitial edema reduces the ability of the capillaries to provide oxygen and nutrients to and remove carbon dioxide and other waste products from the cells. The capillary and cell membranes also begin to break down. Red blood cells begin to clump together, or agglutinate, in the hypoxic and stagnant capillaries forming columns of coagulated cells called **rouleaux.**

Capillary Washout

The building acidosis from the accumulating lactic acid and carbon dioxide (carbonic acid) finally causes relaxation of the post-capillary sphincters. With relaxation, those byproducts along with potassium (released by the cells to maintain a neutral environment in the pres-

ischemia a blockage in the delivery of oxygenated blood to the cells.

hydrostatic pressure the pressure of liquids in equilibrium; the pressure exerted by or within liquids.

rouleaux group of red blood cells that are stuck together.

Table 15-2 | STAGES OF SHOCK

Compensated Shock

Initial stage of shock in which the body progressively compensates for continuing blood loss.

- Pulse rate increases
- Pulse strength decreases
- Skin becomes cool and clammy
- Progressing anxiety, restlessness, combativeness
- Thirst, weakness, eventual air hunger

Decompensated Shock

Begins when the body's compensatory mechanisms can no longer maintain preload.

- Pulse becomes unpalpable
- Blood pressure drops precipitously
- Patient becomes unconscious
- Respirations slow or cease

Irreversible Shock

Shortly after the patient enters decompensated shock, the lack of circulation begins to have profound effects on body cells. Irreversibly damaged cells die, tissues dysfunction, organs dysfunction, and the patient dies.

---

ence of building acidosis) and the columns of coagulated red blood cells are dumped into the venous circulation. This **washout** causes profound metabolic acidosis and releases microscopic emboli. Cardiac output drops toward zero; peripheral vascular resistance drops toward zero; blood pressure drops toward zero; cellular perfusion, even to the most critical organs, drops toward zero. The body moves quickly and then irreversibly toward death.

STAGES OF SHOCK

The shock process, as described above, can be divided into three stages based on presenting signs and symptoms. The stages are progressively more serious and include compensated, decompensated, and irreversible shock (Table 15-2).

Compensated Shock

Compensated shock is the initial shock state. In this stage, the body is still capable of meeting its critical metabolic needs through a series of progressive compensating actions (Figure 15-9). These progressive compensations create a series of signs and symptoms that range from the subtle to the obvious. The compensated shock stage ends with the precipitous drop in blood pressure. Compensated shock is the shock stage in which prehospital interventions and rapid transport are most likely to meet with success.

The body's first recognizable response to serious blood loss is probably an increase in pulse rate. However, a rate increase due to blood loss may be difficult to differentiate from tachycardia due to excitement and the "fight-or-flight" response. The first sign usually attributable to shock is a narrowing pulse pressure and weakening pulse strength (weak and rapid pulse). As the condition becomes more serious, vasoconstriction causes the victim's skin to become pale, cyanotic, or ashen as blood is directed away from the skin and toward the more critical organs. The skin becomes cool and moist (clammy), and capillary refill times begin to exceed 3 seconds. As compensation becomes more acute, the victim becomes anxious, restless, or combative and complains of thirst and weakness. Near the end of the compensated shock stage, the patient may experience air hunger and tachypnea.

washout release of accumulated lactic acid, carbon dioxide (carbonic acid), potassium, and rouleaux into the venous circulation.

Content Review

STAGES OF SHOCK
- Compensated
- Decompensated
- Irreversible

compensated shock hemodynamic insult to the body in which the body responds effectively. Signs and symptoms are limited, and the human system functions normally.

At the compensated shock stage, prehospital interventions and rapid transport are most likely to meet with success.

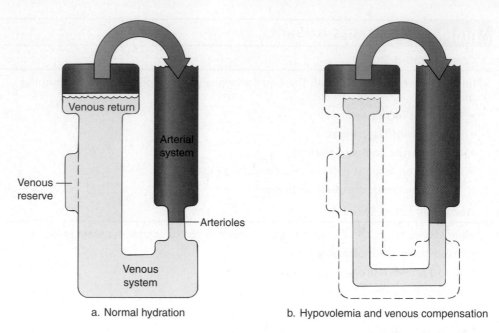

a. Normal hydration

b. Hypovolemia and venous compensation

FIGURE 15-9 In compensated shock, the body reduces venous capacitance in response to blood loss.

Decompensated Shock

decompensated shock continuing hemodynamic insult to the body in which the compensatory mechanisms break down. The signs and symptoms become very pronounced, and the patient moves rapidly toward death.

Entry into decompensated shock is indicated by a precipitous drop in systolic blood pressure.

Decompensated shock begins as the body's compensatory mechanisms can no longer respond to a continuing blood loss. Mechanisms that initially compensated for blood loss now fail, and the body moves quickly toward complete collapse. Entry into decompensated shock is indicated by a precipitous drop in systolic blood pressure. Despite all compensatory mechanisms, venous return is inadequate, and the heart no longer has enough blood volume to pump. Even extreme tachycardia produces little cardiac output. No amount of vascular resistance can maintain blood pressure and circulation. Even the most critical organs of the body are hypoperfused. The heart, already hypoxic because of poor perfusion and the increased oxygen demands created by tachycardia, begins to fail. This state may be indicated by the presence of a bradycardia. In this stage, the brain is extremely hypoxic. This means that the patient displays a rapidly dropping level of responsiveness. The brain's control over bodily functions, including respiration, ceases, and the body takes on a death-like appearance.

Irreversible Shock

irreversible shock final stage of shock in which organs and cells are so damaged that recovery is impossible.

The transition between decompensated and irreversible shock is very difficult to identify in the field.

Irreversible shock exists when the body's cells are badly injured and die in such quantities that the organs cannot carry out their normal functions. Although aggressive resuscitation may restore blood pressure and pulse, organ failure ultimately results in organism failure. The transition to irreversible shock is very difficult to identify in the field. Clearly, the longer a patient is in decompensated shock, the more likely it is that he or she has moved to irreversible shock.

SHOCK ASSESSMENT

You must be able to recognize shock as early as possible in your patient assessment and begin to provide care just as promptly. You must search for the signs and symptoms of shock in each phase of the assessment process: the scene size-up, the initial assessment, the rapid trauma assessment or focused history and physical exam, and—when appropriate—the detailed physical exam. Further, you must carefully monitor for the development or progression of shock with frequent ongoing assessments during care and transport of the trauma patient.

Scene Size-up

Anticipate shock during the scene size-up. Analyze the forces that caused the trauma and their impacts on your patient for the possibility of both external and internal injury and hemorrhage. Look especially for injury mechanisms that might result in internal chest, abdominal, or pelvic injuries or in external hemorrhage from the head, neck, and extremities. Apply trauma triage criteria as early as practical to identify the patients who are most likely to require immediate transport to the trauma center and access to air medical transport, if appropriate.

Initial Assessment

The initial assessment directs your attention to the body systems/patient priorities that present the early signs of shock. Determine the patient's level of consciousness, responsiveness, and orientation. Any mental deficit or restlessness, anxiety, or combativeness may be due to blood loss and hypovolemia. As you assess the airway and breathing, apply high-flow, high-concentration oxygen. Watch for tachypnea and air hunger, which are late signs of shock. When assessing circulation, recall that tachycardia suggests hypovolemia. Baseline rates suggestive of tachycardia are about 160 in the infant, 140 in the preschooler, 120 in the school-age child and 100 in the adult. An increase of 20 beats per minute above any of these rates suggests a significant blood loss. The weaker the pulse, the more the patient is compensating for blood loss.

During assessment, be aware that any mental deficit or restlessness, anxiety, or combativeness may be due to blood loss and hypovolemia.

Carefully observe the patient's body surface and be quick to anticipate potential shock, either as a cause of or a contributing factor to the patient's condition. Look also to the general condition of the skin. It should be warm, pink, and dry. If it is cyanotic, gray, ashen, pale, and cool and moist (clammy), suspect peripheral vasoconstriction, an early sign of shock.

Watch the pulse oximeter for the saturation value and keep it above 95%, if possible. As compensation increases and the pulse strength diminishes, the pulse oximeter readings will become more and more unreliable. If you note erratic or intermittent readings with the device, suspect increasing cardiovascular compensation and progressing shock as the reason.

Conclude the initial assessment by establishing patient priorities. If any indication, MOI, sign, or symptom suggests serious internal hemorrhage or uncontrolled external hemorrhage, consider rapid trauma assessment. If the patient has minor and isolated injuries, move to the focused history and physical exam.

Focused History and Physical Exam

As noted earlier, the order in which the steps of the focused history and physical exam are performed varies with the patient's MOI. For trauma patients who have no significant mechanism, perform an assessment focused on the area of injury, then obtain baseline vital signs and gather a patient history. For trauma patients who have a significant MOI, continue spinal immobilization and perform a rapid trauma assessment and then obtain baseline vital signs and a patient history. Remember that trauma patients with significant mechanisms of injury are the most likely to suffer from shock.

A focused physical exam is performed on a trauma patient with an expected, isolated, non-serious injury.

Rapid Trauma Assessment   When you have a trauma patient with a significant MOI, perform a rapid trauma assessment, inspecting and palpating the patient from head to toe (Figure 15-10). Immediately control any significant hemorrhage. Put a dressing and bandage over the wound and apply direct pressure. Provide more complete hemorrhage control once you attend to the other priorities.

A rapid trauma assessment is performed on a patient with a significant MOI or signs of shock or serious injury.

Be sure to examine areas of the body where you expect to find serious injury, as suggested by your scene size-up. Pay special attention to the areas most likely to produce serious, life-threatening injury: the head, neck, chest, abdomen, and pelvis. Minor reddening may be the only sign of a developing contusion and serious internal injury. Also examine the neck veins. In the supine, normovolemic patient, they should be full. If they are flat, suspect hypovolemia.

During your rapid trauma assessment, rule out the possibility of obstructive shock. Assess the chest to identify any tension pneumothorax. Look for dyspnea, a hyperinflated chest, distended jugular veins, resonant percussion, and diminished or absent breath sounds on the

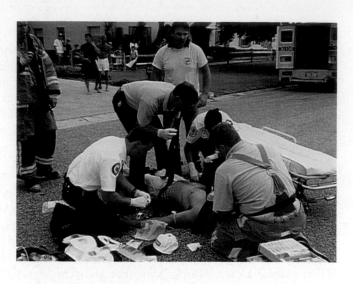

FIGURE 15-10 The rapid trauma assessment focuses on potential shock-inducing injuries to the head, neck, and torso.

affected side, lower tracheal shift to the opposite side, and any subcutaneous emphysema. Consider pleural decompression if the signs suggest tension pneumothorax (see Chapter 17, "Thoracic Trauma"). Also suspect and search for pericardial tamponade. Look for penetrating injury, distended jugular veins, muffled or distant heart tones, tachycardia, and progressive and extreme hypotension. Pericardial tamponade requires immediate and rapid transport to a trauma center. If the patient received significant anterior chest trauma, suspect myocardial contusion. Apply an electrocardiogram (ECG) monitor and analyze the cardiac rhythm.

During the assessment, be alert to the possibility that hemorrhagic shock is not the problem or is not the only problem affecting your patient. Conditions such as stroke, epilepsy, or heart attack can lead to auto crashes and other traumatic events. Be careful to rule out cardiogenic shock by questioning the patient about crushing substernal chest pain and looking for pulmonary edema, jugular vein distention, and cardiac dysrhythmias (see Chapter 20, "Cardiovascular Emergencies"). Also suspect and check for neurogenic shock (spinal trauma). Look for the presence of pink and warm skin below the point of nervous system injury, while the skin above the injury is pale, cool, and clammy. Other shock states such as anaphylactic, septic, and diabetic shock are not likely unless the patient history suggests them.

Take a quick set of vital signs, keying in on both the pulse rate and pulse pressure. If the pulse is weak, its rate is elevated, or the pulse pressure is diminished, suspect serious hemorrhage. Gauge your findings against the MOI and the time from the injury to your assessment. The shorter the time and the more pronounced the signs and symptoms, the more rapidly the patient is moving toward decompensation and then irreversible shock.

Complete this step of the assessment process by gathering a patient history. Listen to any patient complaints of weakness, thirst, or nausea, which may be further signs of shock. Be especially alert for patient complaints suggestive of a myocardial infarction. Be prepared to monitor the heart for dysrhythmias.

At the end of the rapid trauma assessment or the focused history and physical exam, inventory your findings. Set the patient's priority for transport, and set priorities for the order in which you will care for injuries. Again, if any indication, MOI, sign, or symptom suggests serious internal hemorrhage or uncontrolled external hemorrhage, consider rapid transport for the patient. Approximate the probable volume of blood lost to fractures, large contusions, and hematomas. Also note the probable locations of internal hemorrhage and attempt to approximate blood loss from them. Identify all significant injuries and assign each a priority for care. Although you may not complete care for all the injuries, setting priorities assures that you quickly address those injuries most likely to contribute to the patient's hypovolemia and shock.

During the assessment, be alert to the possibility that hemorrhagic shock may not be the only problem affecting your patient.

Detailed Physical Exam

Consider performing a detailed physical exam on a potential shock patient only after all priorities have been addressed and the patient is either en route to the trauma center or circumstances such as a prolonged extrication prevent immediate transport. If you have the time, assess the patient from head to toe and look for any additional signs of injury. Remember that your early arrival at the patient's side may mean that the ecchymosis (black-and-blue discoloration) associated with injuries has not had time to develop. So be very careful to look for reddening (erythema) and areas of local warmth, suggestive of trauma.

Ongoing Assessment

After completing the initial assessment and the rapid trauma assessment or focused history and physical exam, perform serial ongoing assessments. Reassess mental status, airway, breathing, and circulation. Reestablish patient priorities and reassess and record the vital signs. This ongoing assessment allows you to identify any trends in the patient's condition. Pay particular attention to the pulse rate and pulse pressure. If the pulse rate is increasing and the difference between the diastolic and systolic pressures is decreasing, suspect increasing compensation and worsening shock. Perform a focused assessment for any changes in symptoms the patient reports. Also, check the adequacy and effectiveness of any interventions you have performed. Provide this ongoing assessment every 5 minutes for the seriously injured patient or for any patient who displays any of the signs or symptoms of shock.

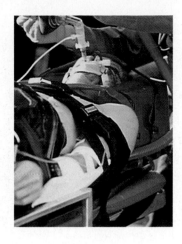

FIGURE 15-11 Make sure that the potential shock patient receives adequate ventilation, using overdrive respiration, if necessary.

SHOCK MANAGEMENT

Airway and Breathing Management

Management of the shock patient begins with corrective actions taken during the initial assessment. One of the primary principles of shock care is to ensure the best possible chance for tissue oxygenation and carbon dioxide offload. Accomplish this by ensuring or providing good ventilations with supplemental oxygen at 15 liters per minute via nonrebreather mask. If the patient is moving air ineffectively (at a breathing rate less than 12 per minute or with inadequate respiratory volume), provide positive pressure ventilations.

Positive pressure ventilation to the breathing patient—called **overdrive respiration**—is coordinated with the patient's breathing attempts if possible (Figure 15-11). However, ensure that the ventilations provide both a good respiratory volume (at least 800 mL) and an adequate respiratory rate (at least 12 to 16 per minute). Overdrive respiration may be indicated in a patient with rib fractures, flail chest, spinal injury with diaphragmatic respirations, head injury, or any condition in which the patient, because of bellows system or respiratory control failure, is not breathing adequately on his own.

If necessary, guard the airway with endotracheal intubation. If the patient is unconscious or semiconscious and unable to protect his airway, be aggressive in your care. Shock patients frequently vomit, and gastric aspiration presents a serious, possibly fatal, consequence.

If there is any sign of tension pneumothorax, confirm it and provide pleural decompression either at the second intercostal space, mid-clavicular line or at the fifth intercostal space, mid-axillary line (see Chapter 17, "Thoracic Trauma"). Continue to monitor the patient because it is common for the catheter to clog and the tension pneumothorax to reappear. Insert another needle close to the first to relieve any subsequent build-up of pressure.

Hemorrhage Control

Provide rapid control of any significant external hemorrhage. Use direct pressure, direct pressure and elevation where practical, and pressure points as needed. Apply a tourniquet to control serious and continuing hemorrhage only if it is absolutely necessary. Remember, there are serious consequences with both proper and improper use of a tourniquet.

Fluid Resuscitation

The field treatment of choice for fluid resuscitation in trauma cases is blood. Blood, however, must be refrigerated, typed, and cross-matched. (O-negative blood may be given in emergency circumstances.) Blood also has a short shelf life and is costly for field use. The most practical fluid for prehospital administration, then, is lactated Ringer's solution. Lactated Ringer's best matches the electrolyte concentration of plasma and does not produce the hyperchloremic acidosis associated with the infusion of large volumes of normal saline. However, normal saline is an acceptable second choice and has few drug and fluid incompatibility problems.

For shock care, ensure the best possible chance for tissue oxygenation and carbon dioxide offload by providing supplemental high-flow, high-concentration oxygen or positive pressure ventilation.

overdrive respiration positive pressure ventilation supplied to a breathing patient.

The most practical choice for prehospital fluid resuscitation is lactated Ringer's solution.

Some hypertonic and synthetic solutions show promise for fluid resuscitation. None of these, however, has been identified as superior to isotonic electrolyte solutions for prehospital use. Hypertonic solutions can mobilize the interstitial and cellular fluid volumes to replace lost blood volume, but they are not able to carry either the oxygen or the clotting factors essential for hemorrhage control. Synthetic agents are now available that can carry oxygen and may, in the future, assist the clotting process. These agents, however, are expensive, have short shelf lives, and pose some patient compatibility problems.

When administering fluids to a trauma patient or to any patient who may need large fluid volumes, consider the internal lumen size of both the catheter and administration set. Fluid flow is proportional to the fourth power of the internal diameter. This means that if you double the lumen's diameter, the same fluid under the same pressure will flow sixteen times more quickly. Hence, use the largest catheter you can introduce into the patient's vein and use a large-bore trauma or blood administration set (Figure 15-12).

Catheter length and fluid pressure also influence fluid flow. The longer the catheter, the greater the resistance to flow. The ideal catheter for the shock patient is relatively short, 1½ inch or shorter. An increase in pressure increases fluid flow. This means that the higher you position the bag or the greater the pressure differential between the solution and the venous system, the faster the fluid flow. If you cannot elevate the fluid bag, position it under the patient or place it in a pressure infuser or a blood-pressure cuff inflated to 100 or 200 mmHg.

Electrolyte administration is indicated for patients with the classic signs and symptoms of shock. When you have controlled external hemorrhage and there is no reason to suspect serious internal hemorrhage, employ aggressive fluid resuscitation. Moderate fluid resuscitation is also prudent for patients with blunt trauma to the chest or abdomen. Administer 1 liter of lactated Ringer's solution rapidly via IV (Figure 15-13). Use trauma or blood tubing to ensure unimpeded flow, and initiate the IV with a large-bore (14- or 16-gauge) catheter. In children, infuse 20 mL/kg of body weight rapidly when you see any signs and symptoms of shock. Administer a second fluid bolus if the vital signs do not im-

The objective of prehospital fluid resuscitation is not the return of normal vital signs but their stabilization until the patient reaches the trauma center.

FIGURE 15–12 Catheter size greatly influences fluid flow. Shown here are 22-, 18-, 14-, and 8-gauge catheters.

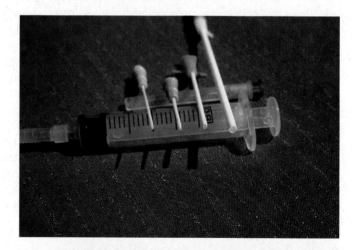

FIGURE 15–13 Supplies for initiating IV therapy.

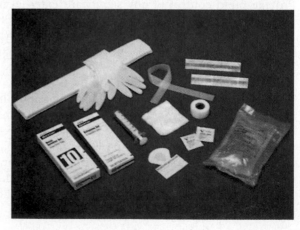

prove after the first bolus or if, at some later time, the patient again begins to deteriorate. The objective of fluid resuscitation in the field is not the return of normal vital signs but the stabilization of vital signs until the patient reaches the trauma center.

A significant drop in the patient's blood pressure (usually to below 50 mmHg) represents the shift from compensated to decompensated shock. In this circumstance, employ aggressive fluid resuscitation, up to 3 liters of normal saline, possibly the PASG, and other shock care steps to help maintain the blood pressure.

If penetrating trauma to the chest exists and/or you cannot control other hemorrhage, be more conservative with fluid administration. Cautiously control fluid volume, remembering that your goal is maintaining vital signs, not improving them. Increases in blood pressure can dislodge developing clots and disrupt the normal clotting processes. The result may be further hemorrhage with further dilution of the clotting factors and hemoglobin. Closely monitor your patient's vital signs, and administer lactated Ringer's solution to keep the patient's mental status and pulse pressure at a steady level. Maintain the blood pressure at a steady level even if it has dropped below 100 mmHg. Studies suggest that a blood pressure of 88 mmHg may be optimal for the patient with continuing internal hemorrhage. Do not, however, let the pressure drop below 50 mmHg.

Temperature Control

Trauma and blood loss seriously affect the mechanisms that normally adjust the body's core temperature. Reduced body activity reduces heat production to subnormal levels. Cutaneous vasoconstriction decreases the skin's ability to act as part of the body's temperature control system. The result is a patient highly susceptible to fluctuations in body temperature. In cases of trauma, patients commonly lose heat more rapidly than normal. At the same time, the heat-generating reflexes, such as shivering, are ineffective and, in fact, are counterproductive to the shock care process.

In all except the warmest environments, help conserve body temperature by covering the patient with a blanket and keeping the patient compartment of the ambulance very warm. If you infuse fluids, ensure that they are well above room temperature—ideally at body temperature or slightly above (no more than 104°F). Use fluid warmers or keep IV solutions in a compartment that is warmer than the rest of the ambulance. Be very sensitive to any patient complaints about being cold, and provide whatever assistance you can to ensure that heat loss is limited.

> *In all but the warmest environments, cover the hemorrhage or shock patient with a blanket and keep the patient compartment of the ambulance very warm.*

Pneumatic Anti-Shock Garment

The **pneumatic anti-shock garment (PASG),** sometimes referred to as the medical anti-shock trouser (MAST), is a device designed to apply firm circumferential pressure around the lower extremities, pelvis, and lower abdomen. The device is intended to compress the vascular space, thereby accomplishing the following four objectives:

> **pneumatic anti-shock garment (PASG)** garment designed to produce uniform pressure on the lower extremities and abdomen; used with shock and hemorrhage patients in some EMS systems.

- To increase peripheral vascular resistance by pressurizing the arteries of the lower abdomen and extremities.

- To reduce the vascular volume by compressing venous vessels.

- To increase the central circulating blood volume with blood returned from areas under the garment.

- To immobilize the lower extremities and the pelvic region.

Research has determined that the garment is responsible for a return of about 250 mL of blood to the central circulation and probably reduces the venous capacitance by the same volume. The PASG also does seem to increase the peripheral vascular resistance, although this may be detrimental to patients with uncontrolled internal hemorrhage.

Research has further revealed potential problems with PASG use. The abdominal component of the PASG pressurizes the abdominal cavity, increasing the work associated with breathing and, in some cases, reducing chest excursion. Application of the garment also increases mortality when used in cases of penetrating chest trauma. In light of this information, it is imperative that you understand the limitations of the device and comply with your local protocols and medical direction when considering use of the PASG.

The PASG is a puncture-resistant, easy to clean, three-compartment trouser attached to the patient circumferentially around the lower abdomen and extremities with Velcro® closures. The compartments can be inflated either independently or all together with a foot- or electric-powered pump. However, the abdominal segment should be inflated with the leg segments or after them, never before. A PASG may or may not come with pressure gauges, although all models should be equipped with pop-off valves to prevent inflation above 110 mmHg.

Indications for PASG use include shock patients with controlled hemorrhage, patients with pelvic fracture and instability with hypotension, patients with possible neurogenic shock, and any shock patients with uncontrolled hemorrhage below the mid-abdomen. Pulmonary edema and cardiogenic shock are contraindications to PASG application and inflation. Use the PASG with caution for patients in late pregnancy, patients with suspected diaphragmatic ruptures, and patients with objects impaled in the abdomen or with abdominal eviscerations. In these cases, do not inflate the abdominal section because doing so increases intra-abdominal pressure.

Begin application of the PASG by removing the patient's clothing, although you may leave on the undergarments for patient modesty if they are not bulky (Procedure 15-1). Assess areas of the patient's body that will lie beneath the garment, because these regions will be hidden from view and inaccessible once the PASG is applied. Then move the patient onto a spine board or other patient-carrying device with an opened garment positioned for application. One application technique calls for securing the garment's Velcro® attachments at the ends of their travel and having a caregiver at the patient's feet put one arm through each of the garment's leg sections from the foot ends. That caregiver then grasps the patient's toes while another caregiver then pulls the garment off the first caregiver's arms, onto the patient's legs, and up to the small of the patient's back. Alternatively, the device may be slid under the patient from the feet with the extra garment and the anterior abdominal segment folded between the legs. Position the PASG so that the upper portion of the abdominal segment is just below the rib margin. Secure the abdominal and leg segments with the Velcro® strips, ensuring that they hold the segments firmly around the limbs and abdomen. This reduces the air volume necessary to inflate the PASG.

Quickly take baseline vital signs and then inflate the PASG slowly. Watch for any change (improvement) in your patient's mental status, skin color, or pulse rate. If you notice such a change, stop the inflation and re-assess vital signs and level of responsiveness. The intent of using a PASG is to stabilize the patient's condition, not to return the blood pressure and circulation to normal levels. As with too-aggressive fluid resuscitation, inflation of PASG to a point where blood pressure increases can interfere with the clotting process or even increase internal hemorrhage, thus moving the patient more quickly toward decompensation and death. If vital signs and the level of responsiveness deteriorate, continue PASG inflation until you regain the level of your baseline findings. Once the pop-off valves release, stop inflation. Then inflate the garment every few minutes until the pop-off valves release to assure that the PASG maintains its maximum pressure.

Carefully monitor respirations during PASG inflation. The device may put pressure on the diaphragm, thus increasing the work of respiration as well as reducing respiratory excursion. Also listen carefully for breath sounds. The PASG may increase blood pressure and respiratory congestion as well. If you hear any crackles in the chest or if the patient complains of difficulty breathing, halt the PASG inflation.

The PASG should not be deflated in the prehospital setting. The release of circumferential pressure reduces peripheral vascular resistance, expands the size of the vascular space, and removes about 250 mL of blood from the active circulation. This could seriously harm the healthy patient and have devastating effects on one who is compensating for shock.

Pharmacological Intervention

In shock, pharmacological interventions are generally limited, especially in hypovolemic patients. The sympathetic nervous system efficiently compensates for low volume, and no agent has been shown effective in the prehospital setting, other than IV fluid and, in some cases, blood and blood products. For cardiogenic shock, fluid challenge, vasopressors such

Penetrating chest trauma, pulmonary edema, and cardiogenic shock are contraindications to PASG application and inflation.

The PASG should not be deflated in the prehospital setting.

Application of the Pneumatic Anti-Shock Garment (PASG)

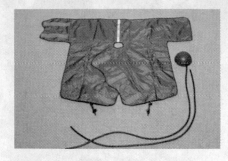

15-1a Monitor the patient before PASG application.

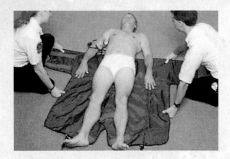

15-1b Prepare the PASG.

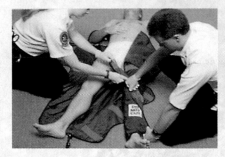

15-1c Position the patient.

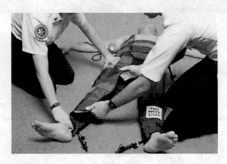

15-1d Wrap the legs, following the manufacturer's recommendations.

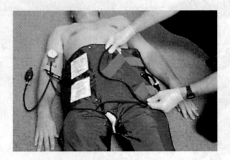

15-1e Wrap the abdomen last.

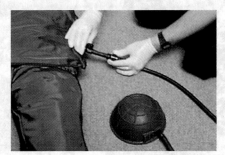

15-1f Connect the tubing.

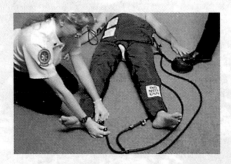

15-1g Inflate the PASG, both legs first.

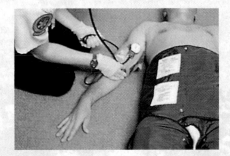

15-1h Monitor the patient.

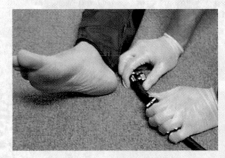

15-1i Close the stopcock valve.

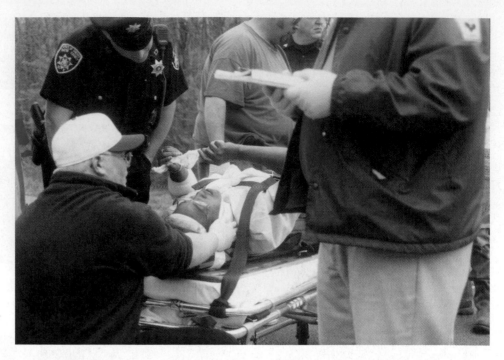

FIGURE 15-14 Emotional support for the seriously injured trauma patient is an important part of shock patient care.

as dopamine, and the other cardiac drugs are indicated (see Chapter 20, "Cardiovascular Emergencies"). For spinal and obstructive shock, consider IV fluids such as normal saline and lactated Ringer's solution. For distributive shock, consider IV fluids, dopamine, and use of the PASG.

The patient who has experienced trauma sufficient to induce hemorrhage and hypovolemia will be anxious and bewildered. As the care provider at the patient's side, it is your responsibility to be calm and reassuring, thus counteracting the natural "fight-or-flight" response (Figure 15-14). By acting in this manner, you not only help your patient deal with the event's emotional trauma but also combat some of the negative effects of sympathetic stimulation.

SUMMARY

Significant hemorrhage and its serious consequence, shock, are genuine threats to the trauma patient's life. The signs of these threats are often subtle or hidden, especially if bleeding is internal. Only through careful analysis of the mechanism of injury during the scene size-up and careful evaluation of the patient during the assessment process can you recognize and then treat these life-threatening problems. Treatment often involves rapidly bringing the patient to the services of a trauma center and, while doing so, providing aggressive care—supplemental oxygen, positive pressure ventilations, fluid resuscitation, and use of a PASG as necessary—aimed at maintaining vital signs, not necessarily improving them. With this approach, you afford your patient the best chance for survival.

ON THE WEB

For additional practice and review, go to the companion website at www.prenhall.com/bledsoe and click on *Intermediate Emergency Care: Principles & Practice.*

Chapter 16

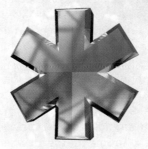

Burns

Objectives

After reading this chapter, you should be able to:

1. Describe the anatomy and physiology of the skin and remaining human anatomy as they pertain to thermal burn injuries. (see Chapter 2)

2. Describe the epidemiology, including incidence, mortality, morbidity, and risk factors for thermal burn injuries as well as strategies to prevent such injuries. (pp. 672–673)

3. Describe the local and systemic complications of a thermal burn injury. (pp. 673–676, 684–686)

4. Identify and describe the depth classifications of burn injuries, including superficial burns, partial-thickness burns, and full-thickness burns. (pp. 681–682)

5. Describe and apply the "rule of nines," and the "rule of palms" methods for determining body surface area percentage of a burn injury. (pp. 682–683)

6. Identify and describe the severity of a burn including a minor burn, a moderate burn, and a critical burn. (pp. 688–691)

7. Describe the effects age and pre-existing conditions have on burn severity and a patient's prognosis. (pp. 685, 690)

8. Discuss complications of burn injuries caused by trauma, blast injuries, airway compromise, respiratory compromise, and child abuse. (pp. 680–681, 685–686, 686–691)

9. Describe burn management including considerations for airway and ventilation, circulation,

pharmacological and non-pharmacological measures, transport decisions, and psychological support/communication strategies. (pp. 691–694)

10. Describe special considerations for a pediatric patient with a burn injury and describe the criteria for determining pediatric burn severity. (pp. 683, 685, 690)

11. Describe the specific epidemiologies, mechanisms of injury, pathophysiologies, and severity assessments for inhalation, chemical, and electrical burn injuries and for radiation exposure. (pp. 694–700)

12. Discuss special considerations that impact the assessment, management, and prognosis of patients with inhalation, chemical, and electrical burn injuries and with exposure to radiation. (pp. 694–700)

13. Differentiate between supraglottic and subglottic inhalation burn injuries. (p. 681)

14. Describe the special considerations for a chemical burn injury to the eye. (pp. 696–698)

15. Given several preprogrammed, simulated thermal, inhalation, electrical, and chemical burn injury and radiation exposure patients, provide the appropriate scene size-up, initial assessment, rapid trauma or focused physical exam and history, detailed exam, and ongoing assessment and provide appropriate patient care and transportation. (pp. 673–700)

CASE STUDY

Ben and Ronny, Fire Rescue EMT-Is, respond with trucks 23 and 56 to a working structural fire. Upon arrival, they find two fire units already deployed, with firefighters engaging a wood frame home fully engulfed in flames. As Ronny positions the vehicle, the south wall of the structure collapses onto a firefighter. Within minutes, other firefighters extinguish the burning wall and free him.

When the firefighters have secured the scene, Ben and Ronny proceed to the patient and begin their initial assessment. They approach a male who is lying supine, with his turnout gear burned and charred in places, indicating that he has received serious burns. Because the wall collapsed onto the firefighter, they provide manual in-line cervical stabilization while proceeding with the assessment. The downed firefighter's respirations appear adequate, although the patient is coughing up sooty sputum and is slightly hoarse. The firefighter, who gives his name as Karl, is conscious and alert. His airway seems clear, except for the hoarseness. The sooty sputum and hoarseness indicate the possibility of burns to the airway, making Karl a priority for rapid transport.

Ben proceeds to perform the rapid trauma assessment. Upon removal of Karl's turnout gear, Ben exposes relatively painless, dark, discolored burns to his posterior thorax and lower back as well as circumferential burns of the left upper extremity. Despite the burn severity, Karl denies much pain. Ben also finds angulation, false motion, and pain in the right forearm. Vital signs reveal normal breathing in terms of volume and rate and a strong, regular pulse at a rate of about 100. Distal pulses are also strong, and capillary refill is timed at 2 seconds. Karl is fully conscious and oriented and is joking about the incident.

The rescue crew now takes some initial care steps. Ben cuts away Karl's clothing, and then covers the burn site with a dry, sterile sheet and starts an IV line, running normal saline at a wide-open rate. Ronny applies oxygen by way of a nonrebreather mask and observes an oximetry reading of 97%. They package Karl and quickly load him into the ambulance for rapid transport. En route to the hospital, Ben checks blood pressure (120/88) and respirations (30 and shallow), noting that the patient displays increasing respiratory effort.

While Ronny is splinting the right limb, Karl begins to cough deeply and to experience severe dyspnea. Karl's dyspnea progresses, and his level of consciousness drops. Oxygen saturation falls to 86%. Ben begins to bag-valve mask Karl with supplemental oxygen, while Ronny prepares intubation equipment.

Medical direction orders the crew to intubate, and they attempt to do so during transport. The airway is edematous, and visualization of the vocal cords is difficult. After the first attempt, Ronny withdraws the tube when auscultation of breath sounds, failure to obtain chest rise, and a dropping oxygen saturation indicate esophageal placement. Ben hyperventilates Karl, and Ronny attempts another intubation. She is again unsuccessful.

As they withdraw the tube, the ambulance arrives at the emergency department. The ED physician places a large-bore catheter in the cricothyroid membrane and attempts transtracheal jet insufflation. The technique is successful. After an emergency tracheostomy, Karl begins spontaneous respirations and maintains a strong pulse. His level of consciousness does not improve, however, and the hospital staff transfer him to the burn unit for definitive care.

INTRODUCTION

The incidence of burn injuries in the United States and other developed countries has been declining for several decades. Despite the decline, an estimated 1.25 to 2 million people in the United States are treated for burns annually and 50,000 are hospitalized. Approximately

3% to 5% of these burns are considered life threatening. Persons at greatest risk for serious burns include the very young and old, the infirm, and workers, such as firefighters, metal smelters, and chemical workers. Burn injuries remain the second leading cause of death in children under 12 years of age and the fourth overall cause of trauma death.

Much of the national decline in burn mortality is attributed to improved building codes, safer construction techniques, and the use of smoke detectors. Smaller but still important effects are attributed to educational campaigns aimed primarily at school children. Other simple and inexpensive measures that have helped prevent burns include keeping cigarette lighters and matches away from children and reducing household hot-water temperatures to below scalding levels.

Burns are a specific subset of soft-tissue injuries with a specific pathologic process. The term "burn" suggests combustion, but the actual process that produces burn injuries is much different. The human body is predominantly water and does not support combustion. Instead, body tissues change chemically, evaporating water and denaturing the proteins that make up cell membranes. The result can be widespread damage to the skin, or integumentary system.

Although the skin and its functions are often taken for granted, burn injury to this organ can subject a patient to severe fluid loss, infection, hypothermia, and other injuries.

PATHOPHYSIOLOGY OF BURNS

Burns result from the disruption of proteins in the cell membranes. Burns can be caused by several different mechanisms including thermal, electrical, chemical and radiation energies. Being able to understand the mechanism of a burn and to determine the degree and area of burn helps you assess the seriousness of the burn and thus guide your care.

TYPES OF BURNS

Soft-tissue burns occur secondary to thermal (heat), electrical, chemical, or radiation insults to the body. Although the resulting burns are much the same, the damage process differs with the various mechanisms. The following sections describe each of these four types of burns.

Thermal Burns

A thermal burn causes damage by increasing the rate at which the molecules within an object move and collide with each other. The energy of this molecular motion is measured as temperature. At a temperature greater than absolute zero, the molecules of any object move about. As the object's temperature increases, so do the speed of the molecules and the incidences of their collisions with other molecules. These changes in internal energy cause many substances—for example, steel—to expand with increasing temperature. Heat energy may also cause chemical changes. As temperature increases, substances such as gasoline may combine with oxygen. The nature of matter may change as well. Water, for example, may change into ice (with decreasing heat energy) or steam (with increasing heat energy). An egg changes its nature as the proteins break down, or **denature**, in a hot frying pan. This is why cooked eggs have a rubbery consistency.

Similar changes also take place in burned tissue. As molecular speed increases, the cell components, especially membranes and proteins, begin to break down just like the egg in a frying pan. The result of exposure to extreme heat is progressive injury and cell death.

The extent of burn injury relates to the amount of heat energy transferred to the patient's skin. The amount of that heat energy in turn depends on three components of the burning agent: its temperature, the concentration of heat energy it possesses, and the length of its contact time with the patient's skin.

Obviously, the greater the temperature of an agent, the greater the potential for damage. However, it is also important to consider the amount of heat energy possessed by the object or substance. Receiving a blast of heated air from an oven at 350°F is much less damaging than contact with hot cooking oil at the same temperature. In general, water, oils, and other liquids have a fairly high heat energy content. This content is roughly related to the density of the material. In a similar fashion, solids also usually have a high heat content. Gases, on the other hand, usually have less capacity to hold heat owing to their less dense nature.

Content Review

BASIC TYPES OF BURNS
- Thermal
- Electrical
- Chemical
- Radiation

denature alter the usual substance of something.

Duration of exposure to the heat source is also obviously important in determining the severity of a burn. A patient's momentary contact with hot oil would result in less damage than if the oil were poured into his or her shoe.

A burn is a progressive process, and the greater the heat energy transmitted to the body, the deeper the wound. Initially, the burn damages the epidermis by the increase in temperature. As contact with the substance continues, heat energy penetrates further and deeper into the body tissue. Thus, a burn may involve the epidermis, dermis, and subcutaneous tissue as well as muscles, bone, and other internal tissue.

At the level of local tissues, thermal burns cause a number of effects collectively termed **Jackson's theory of thermal wounds.** This theory helps us understand the physical effects of high heat and helps explain a number of clinical effects (Figure 16-1).

With a burn, the skin nearest the heat source suffers the most profound changes. Cell membranes rupture and are destroyed, blood coagulates, and structural proteins denature. This most damaged area is the **zone of coagulation.** If the zone of coagulation penetrates the dermis, the resulting injury is termed a full-thickness or third-degree burn. Adjacent to this area is a less damaged yet still inflamed region where blood flow decreases that is called the **zone of stasis.** More distant from the burn source is a broader area where inflammation and changes in blood flow are limited. This is the **zone of hyperemia;** this zone accounts for the erythema (redness) associated with some burns.

Large burns have profound pathological effects on the body as a whole. In general, these effects are important in any burn that covers more than 15% to 20% of the patient's body surface area. To understand these effects and the resulting burn shock, you must first learn a little about the progression of burns.

The body's response to burns occurs over time and can usefully be classified into four stages: the emergent phase, the fluid shift phase, the hypermetabolic phase, and the resolution phase.

The first stage occurs immediately following the burn and is called the **emergent phase.** This is the body's initial reaction to the burn. This phase includes a pain response as well as the outpouring of catecholamines in response to the pain and the physical and emotional stress. During this stage, the patient displays tachycardia, tachypnea, mild hypertension, and mild anxiety.

The **fluid shift phase** follows the initial phase and can last for up to 18 to 24 hours. The fluid shift phase begins shortly after the burn and reaches its peak in 6 to 8 hours. You are therefore likely to see it in the prehospital setting. In this phase, damaged cells release agents that initiate an inflammatory response in the body. This increases blood flow to the capil-

Jackson's theory of thermal wounds explanation of the physical effects of thermal burns.

zone of coagulation area in a burn nearest the heat source; suffers the most damage and is characterized by clotted blood and thrombosed blood vessels.

zone of stasis area of a burn that surrounds the zone of coagulation; characterized by decreased blood flow.

zone of hyperemia area peripheral to a burn; characterized by increased blood flow.

emergent phase first stage of the burn process; characterized by a catecholamine release and pain-mediated reaction.

fluid shift phase stage of the burn process in which there is a massive shift of fluid from the intravascular to the extravascular space.

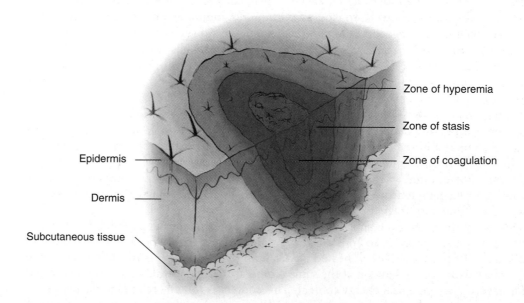

FIGURE 16-1 The zones of injury commonly caused by a thermal burn.

laries surrounding the burn and increases the permeability of the capillaries to fluid. The response results in a large shift of fluid away from the **intravascular space** into the **extravascular space** (massive edema). Note that the capillaries leak fluid (water, electrolytes, and some dissolved proteins) and not blood cells. Blood loss from burns uncomplicated by other trauma is usually minimal.

After the fluid shift phase comes the **hypermetabolic phase,** which may last for many days or weeks depending on the burn severity. This phase is characterized by a large increase in the body's demands for nutrients as it begins the long process of repairing damaged tissue. Gradually this phase evolves into the **resolution phase,** in which scar tissue is laid down and remodeled, and the burn patient begins to rehabilitate and return to normal function.

Electrical Burns

Electricity's power is the result of an electron flow from a point of high concentration to one of low concentration. The difference between the two concentrations is called the **voltage.** It is helpful to envision voltage as the "pressure" of the electric flow. The rate or the amount of flow in a given time is termed the **current** and is measured in **amperes.**

Another factor that affects the flow of electricity is **resistance.** Resistance is measured in **ohms.** Copper electrical wire has very little resistance and allows a free flow of electrons. Tungsten (the filament in a light bulb) is moderately resistant and heats, glows, and emits light as more and more current is applied to it.

The relationship between current (I), resistance (R), and voltage (V) is well known as **Ohm's law:**

$$V = IR \text{ or } I = V/R$$

Like tungsten, the internal parts of the human body are moderately resistant to the flow of electricity. The skin, on the other hand, is highly resistant to electrical flow. Moisture or sweat on the skin lowers this resistance. If the human body is subjected to voltage, the body initially resists the flow. If the voltage is strong enough, the current begins to pass into and through the body. As it does, heat energy is created. The heat produced is proportional to the square of the current flow and is related to power, P, as expressed in **Joule's law:**

$$P = I^2R$$

The highest heat occurs at the points of greatest resistance, often at the skin. This accounts for the severe entry and exit wounds sometimes seen in electrical injuries. Dry, calloused skin can have enormous resistance values, ranging from 500,000 to 1,000,000 ohms/cm. Wet skin, particularly the thin skin on the palm side of the arm or on the inner thigh can have values as low as 300 to 10,000 ohms/cm. Mucous membranes have very low resistance (100 ohms/cm) and allow even small currents to pass. This accounts for the relative ease with which household current can cause lip and oral burns in children who accidentally bite electrical cords (Figure 16-2).

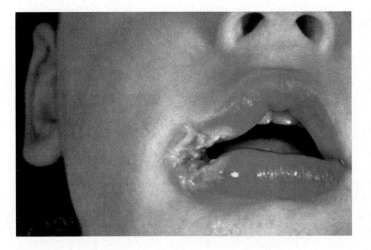

FIGURE 16-2 Electrical burns to a child's mouth caused by chewing on an electrical cord.

---

intravascular space the volume contained by all the arteries, veins, capillaries, and other components of the circulatory system.

extravascular space the volume contained by all the cells (intracellular space) and the spaces between the cells (interstitial space).

hypermetabolic phase stage of the burn process in which body metabolism increases in an attempt by the body to heal the burn.

resolution phase final stage of the burn process in which scar tissue is laid down and the healing process is completed.

voltage the difference of electric potential between two points with different concentrations of electrons.

current the rate of flow of an electric charge.

ampere basic unit for measuring the strength of an electric current.

resistance property of a conductor that opposes the passage of an electric current.

ohm basic unit for measuring the strength of electrical resistance.

Ohm's law a physical law; states that the current in an electrical circuit is directly proportional to the voltage and inversely proportional to the resistance.

Joule's law a physical law; states that the rate of heat production is directly proportional to the resistance of the circuit and to the square of the current.

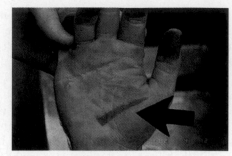
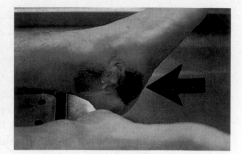

a. Entrance wound   b. Exit wound

FIGURE 16-3   Injuries due to electrical shock.

With small currents, the heat energy produced is of little consequence. But if the voltage or current is high, profound body damage can occur. The longer the duration of contact, the greater the potential for injury. Electrical burns can be particularly damaging because the burn heats the victim from the inside out, causing great damage to internal organs and structures while possibly leaving little visible damage on the surface, save for the entry and exit wounds (Figure 16-3).

Thermal injury due to electrical current occurs as energy travels from the point of contact to the point of exit. At both these points, the concentration of electricity is great, as is the degree of damage you might expect. The smaller the area of contact, the greater the concentration of current flow and the greater the injury. Between the entrance and exit points, the energy spreads out over a larger cross-sectional area and generally causes less injury. Electrical current may follow blood vessels and nerves because they offer less resistance than muscle and bone. This may lead to serious vascular and nervous injury deep within the involved limbs or body cavity.

Electrical contact also interferes with control of muscle tissue. The passage of current, especially alternating current, severely disrupts the complicated electrochemical reactions that control muscles. If contact with a current as small as 20 to 50 milliamperes (mA) is maintained for a period of time, the muscles of respiration may be immobilized. The result is prolonged respiratory arrest, anoxia, hypoxemia, and eventually death. Electrical currents greater than 50 mA may also disrupt the heart's electrical system, causing ventricular fibrillation accompanied by ineffective pumping action. Alternating electrical current such as that found in household current can also cause tetanic convulsions or uncontrolled contractions of muscles. If the victim is holding a wire at such a time, the victim may be unable to let go, thereby prolonging the exposure and increasing the severity of injury. This can occur with as little as 9 mA of current.

Electrical injury may also disrupt muscular and other tissue, leading to its degeneration. As the tissue dies, it releases materials toxic to the human body. These materials may damage the liver and kidneys, leading to failure.

At times, electrical energy may cause flash burns secondary to the heat of current passing through adjacent air. Air is very resistant to the passage of electrical current. If the current is strong enough and the space through which it passes is small, the electricity arcs, producing tremendous heat. If the patient's skin is close by, the heat may severely burn or vaporize tissue. In addition, the heat may ignite articles of clothing or other combustibles and produce thermal burns.

Chemical Burns

Chemical burns denature the biochemical makeup of cell membranes and destroy the cells. Such injuries are not transmitted through the tissue as are thermal injuries. Instead, a chemical burn must destroy the tissue before it can chemically burn any deeper. This fact generally limits the burn process unless very strong chemicals are involved (Figure 16-4). Agents that can cause chemical burns are too numerous to mention. However, the most common causes of these burns are either strong acids or bases (alkalis).

Content Review

PROCESSES OF CHEMICAL BURNS
- Acid—usually forms a thick, insoluble mass where it contacts tissue through coagulation necrosis, limiting burn damage
- Alkali—usually continues to destroy cell membranes through liquefaction necrosis, allowing it to penetrate underlying tissue and causing deeper burns

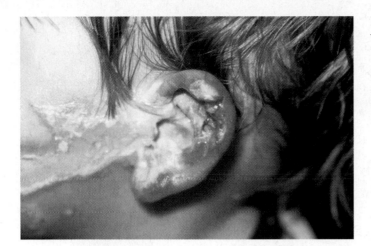

FIGURE 16-4 A chemical burn to the ear.

Both acids and alkalis burn by disrupting cell membranes and damaging tissues on contact. As they cause damage, acids usually form a thick, insoluble mass, or coagulum, at the point of contact. This process is called **coagulation necrosis** and helps limit the depth of acid burns. Alkalis, however, do not form a protective coagulum. Instead, the alkali continues to destroy cell membranes, releasing the intercellular and interstitial fluid, destroying tissue in a process called **liquefaction necrosis**. This process allows the alkali to rapidly penetrate the underlying tissue, causing progressively deeper burns. For this reason, alkali burns can be quite serious.

Radiation Injury

Nuclear radiation has bombarded Earth since long before recorded time. It is a daily, natural phenomenon. Radiation becomes a danger when people are exposed to synthetic sources that greatly increase the intensity of radiation. Medicine and industry use radioactive materials for diagnostic testing and treatment and for energy production. Deaths from exposure to radiation are extremely rare as are serious injuries because of the safety measures commonly used with the handling of nuclear materials. The risk of injury comes from accidents associated with improper handling, either in the on-site environment or during transport. In addition, the possibility of large-scale exposure to radiation from terrorist acts is considered to be increasing.

Nuclear radiation causes damage through a process known as **ionization**. A radioactive energy particle travels into a substance and changes an internal atom (Figure 16-5). In the human body, the affected cell either repairs the damage, dies, or goes on to produce damaged cells (cancer). The cells most sensitive to radiation injury are the cells that reproduce most quickly, such as those responsible for erythrocyte, leukocyte, and platelet production (bone marrow), cells lining the intestinal tract, and cells involved in human reproduction.

We commonly encounter four types of radiation. These are:

- *Alpha radiation.* The nucleus of an atom releases **alpha radiation** in the form of a small helium nucleus. Alpha radiation is a very weak energy source and can travel only inches through the air. Paper or clothing can easily stop alpha radiation. This radiation also cannot penetrate the epidermis. On the subatomic scale, however, alpha particles are massive and can cause great damage over the short distance they travel. Alpha radiation is only a significant hazard if the patient inhales or ingests contaminated material, thus bringing the source in close proximity to sensitive respiratory and digestive tract tissue.

- *Beta radiation.* A second type of radiological particle produces **beta radiation.** Its energy is greater than that of alpha radiation. However, the beta particle is relatively lightweight, with the mass of an electron. Beta radiation can travel 6 to 10 feet through air and can penetrate a few layers of clothing. Beta particles

coagulation necrosis the process in which an acid, while destroying tissue, forms an insoluble layer that limits further damage.

liquefaction necrosis the process in which an alkali dissolves and liquefies tissue.

ionization the process of changing a substance into separate charged particles (ions).

alpha radiation low level form of nuclear radiation; a weak source of energy that is stopped by clothing or the first layers of skin.

beta radiation medium-strength radiation that is stopped with light clothing or the uppermost layers of skin.

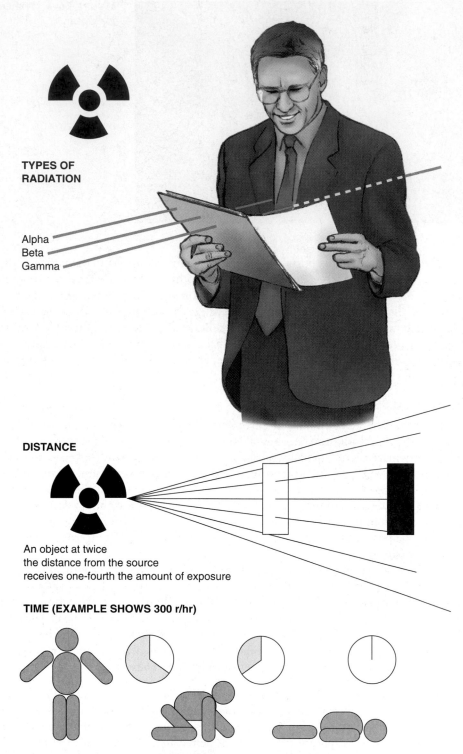

FIGURE 16-5 The injury considerations associated with nuclear radiation.

can invade the first few millimeters of skin and thus have the potential for causing external as well as internal injury.

- *Gamma radiation.* **Gamma radiation,** also known as x-rays, is the most powerful type of ionizing radiation. It has the ability to travel through the entire body or ionize any atom within. Its lack of mass or charge (it is pure electromagnetic energy) helps give it great penetrating power. Gamma radiation evokes the greatest concern for external exposure. It is the most

gamma radiation powerful electromagnetic radiation emitted by radioactive substances with penetrating properties; it is stronger than alpha and beta radiation.

dangerous and most feared type of radiation because it is difficult to protect against. Many feet of concrete or many inches of lead are needed to protect against the highest-energy gamma rays. Fortunately, exposure to high-energy gamma rays occurs only in individuals who are exposed to nuclear blasts, are near the cores of nuclear reactors, or are very close to highly radioactive materials. More modest amounts of concrete, steel, or lead can provide shielding from the more common and lower-energy x-rays and gamma rays.

- *Neutron radiation.* Neutrons are small, yet moderately massive subatomic particles with no charge. Their small size and lack of charge account for their great penetrating power. Fortunately, strong **neutron radiation** is uncommon outside of nuclear reactors and bombs.

neutron radiation powerful radiation with penetrating properties between that of beta and gamma radiation.

Exposure to radiation and the effects of ionization can occur through two mechanisms. In the first, an unshielded person is directly exposed to a strong radioactive source, for example, an unstable material such as uranium. The second mechanism of exposure is contamination by dust, debris, or fluids that contain very small particles of radioactive material. These contaminants emit weaker radiation than a direct radioactive source such as uranium. However, the close proximity of these contaminants to the body and their longer contact times with it may result in greater exposure and contamination. Note that most substances, including human tissue, do not emit radiation. The patient himself is not the danger in a radiological exposure incident. Any danger comes from the radioactive source such as the contaminated material on the patient.

Three factors are important to keep in mind whenever you are called to incidents of radiation exposure. They include the duration of exposure; the distance from the radioactive source; and the shielding between you, the patient, and the source. Knowledge of these three factors can limit your exposure and potential for injury.

- *Duration.* Radiation exposure is an accumulative danger. The longer you or the patient remain exposed to the source, the greater the potential for injury.

- *Distance.* Radiation strength diminishes quickly as you travel farther from the source. The effect is similar to that of a light bulb's intensity. At a few feet, you can easily read by it, whereas at a few hundred feet the light barely casts a shadow. Mathematically, the relationship is inverse and squared. As you double your distance from the radioactive source, its strength drops to one fourth. As you triple the distance, its strength diminishes to one ninth, and so on.

- *Shielding.* The more material between you and the source, the less radioactive exposure you experience. With alpha and beta radiation, shielding is very easy to provide and reasonably effective. With gamma and neutron sources, dense objects such as earth, concrete, metal, and lead are needed to provide any real protection.

Radiation exposure is measured with a Geiger counter. Cumulative exposure is recorded by a device called a dosimeter. They record units of radiation expressed as either the **rad** or the **Gray** (Gy), with one Gray equal to 100 rads.

rad basic unit of absorbed radiation dose.

Different tissues are sensitive to different levels of absorbed radiation. As little as 0.2 Gy can cause cataracts in exposed eyes and damage the blood–cell-producing bone marrow (also called hematopoietic) tissue. The radiation dose that is lethal to about 50% of exposed individuals is approximately 4.5 Gy.

Gray (Gy) a unit of absorbed radiation dose equal to 100 rads.

With whole body exposure, and as the radiation dose increases, the signs and symptoms of exposure appear earlier and become more severe. The first signs of serious exposure are slight nausea and fatigue, occurring between 4 and 24 hours after exposure. As the radiation dose moves into the lethal range, the severity of the nausea increases and is joined by anorexia, vomiting, diarrhea, and malaise. Erythema of the skin may be present, and fatigue becomes more intense. These signs appear within 2 to 6 hours. With exposure to even higher, fatal doses, the patient displays all the signs of radiation exposure almost immediately and soon thereafter experiences confusion, watery diarrhea, and physical collapse. Note that the signs and symptoms of radiation exposure and the injuries associated with it vary because individual sensitivity to radiation exposure varies greatly.

Prolonged exposure to even small amounts of radiation may produce long-term and delayed problems. Infertility is a potential injury, because the cells producing eggs and sperm are very susceptible to ionization damage. Cancer is another delayed and severe side effect. It may occur years or even decades after a radiation exposure.

Inhalation Injury

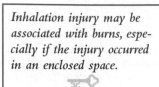
The burn environment frequently produces inhalation injury. This is especially true if the patient is in a closed space or is unconscious. A patient who is unconscious or trapped in a smoke-filled area eventually inhales gases, heated air, flames, or steam. The inhalation results in airway and respiratory injury.

You can expect to find the following inhalation conditions in a burn environment (Figure 16-6). Keep them in mind as you survey the scene and take the necessary protective measures.

Toxic Inhalation Modern residential and commercial construction uses synthetic resins and plastics that release toxic gases as they burn. Combustion of these materials can form such toxic agents as compounds of cyanide and hydrogen sulfide. If a patient inhales these gases, the gases react with the lung tissue, causing internal chemical burns, or they diffuse across the alveolar-capillary membrane and enter the bloodstream, causing systemic poisoning. The signs and symptoms of these injuries may present immediately following exposure or their onset may be delayed for an hour or two after inhalation. Toxic inhalation injury occurs more frequently than thermal inhalation burns.

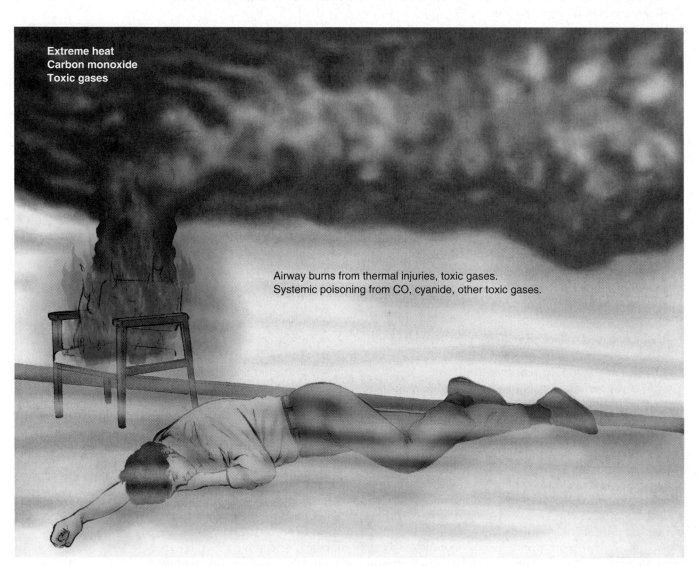

Extreme heat
Carbon monoxide
Toxic gases

Airway burns from thermal injuries, toxic gases.
Systemic poisoning from CO, cyanide, other toxic gases.

FIGURE 16-6 Hazards of fire in an enclosed environment.

Carbon Monoxide Poisoning   An additional concern associated with the burn environment is carbon monoxide (CO) poisoning. Suspect it in any patient who has been within an enclosed space during combustion. Carbon monoxide is created during incomplete combustion, similar to that which may occur with a faulty heating unit or when someone tries to heat a room with an unvented device such as a barbecue grill. Poisoning occurs because carbon monoxide has an affinity for hemoglobin more than 200 times greater than oxygen. If your patient inhales carbon monoxide, even in the smallest quantities, the carbon monoxide displaces oxygen in the hemoglobin and remains there for hours. The result is hypoxemia. Hypoxemia, which is difficult to detect, subtly compromises the delivery of oxygen to the patient's vital organs. If carbon monoxide inhalation is associated with airway burns, the respiratory compromise will be further compounded.

Airway Thermal Burn   Another, though less frequent, injury is the airway thermal burn. Very moist mucosa lines the airway and helps insulate it against heat damage. Because of this mucosa, **supraglottic,** or upper airway, structures may absorb the heat and prevent lower airway burns. High levels of thermal energy are required to evaporate the fluid and injure the cells. Inspiration of hot air or flame rarely produces enough heat to cause significant thermal burns to the lower airway.

Superheated steam has greater heat content than hot, dry air and can cause **subglottic,** or lower airway, burns. Superheated steam is created under great pressure and can have a temperature well above 212°F. A common hazard to firefighters, superheated steam develops when a stream of water strikes a hot spot and vaporizes explosively. The blast can dislodge the mask of a firefighter's self-contained breathing apparatus, exposing him or her to superheated steam inhalation. The steam contains enough heat energy to severely burn the upper airway. It also may damage the lower respiratory tract, although this happens less frequently.

Risk factors for inhalation injuries associated with burns include standing in the burn environment (hot gases rise), screaming or yelling there (the open glottis allows toxic gases to enter the lower airway), and being trapped in a closed burn environment.

With any thermal or smoke-related chemical burn injury to the respiratory tract, there is the danger of airway restriction, severe dyspnea, and possible respiratory arrest. The airway is a narrow tube, lined with extremely vascular tissue. If damaged, this tissue swells rapidly, seriously reducing the size of the airway lumen. The patient presents with minor hoarseness, followed precipitously by dyspnea. Stridor or high-pitched "crowing" sounds on inspiration are ominous signs of impending airway obstruction. Other clues leading you to suspect potential airway burns include singed facial and nasal hair, black-tinged (carbonaceous) sputum, and facial burns. The airway injury may be so extensive as to induce complete respiratory obstruction and arrest. Accurate assessment is important because 20% to 35% of patients admitted to burn centers and some 60% to 70% of burn patients who die have an associated inhalation injury.

DEPTH OF BURN

After you determine the burn source and assess the possibility of associated inhalation injury, you need to assess the burn's severity. One element in determining the severity of a burn is the depth of damage it causes. Depth of burn damage is normally classified into three categories (Figure 16-7).

Superficial Burn

The **superficial burn,** also called a first-degree burn, involves only the epidermis. It is an irritation of the living cells in this region and results in some pain, minor edema, and erythema. It normally heals without complication.

Partial-Thickness Burn

The **partial-thickness burn,** also termed a second-degree burn, penetrates slightly deeper than a superficial burn and produces blisters. Heat energy travels into the dermis, involving more of the tissue and resulting in greater destruction. The partial-thickness burn is similar to a superficial burn in that it is reddened, painful, and edematous. You can differentiate it

---

Suspect carbon monoxide poisoning in any patient who was in an enclosed space during combustion.

Superheated steam is a common cause of airway burns.

supraglottic referring to the upper airway.

subglottic referring to the lower airway.

---

superficial burn a burn that involves only the epidermis; characterized by reddening of the skin; also called a first-degree burn.

partial-thickness burn a burn in which the epidermis is burned through and the dermis is damaged; characterized by redness and blistering; also called a second-degree burn.

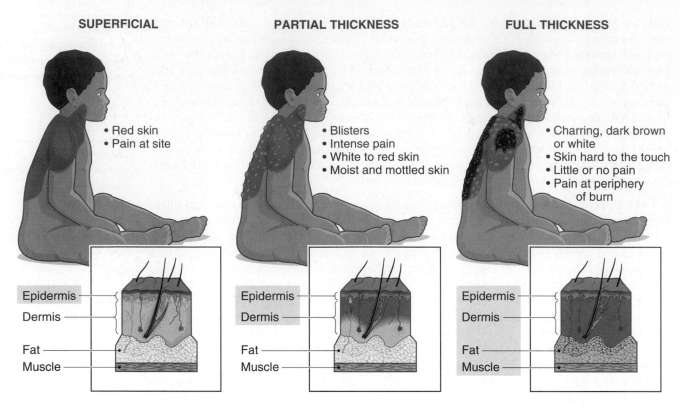

SUPERFICIAL	PARTIAL THICKNESS	FULL THICKNESS

SUPERFICIAL
- Red skin
- Pain at site

Epidermis
Dermis
Fat
Muscle

PARTIAL THICKNESS
- Blisters
- Intense pain
- White to red skin
- Moist and mottled skin

Epidermis
Dermis
Fat
Muscle

FULL THICKNESS
- Charring, dark brown or white
- Skin hard to the touch
- Little or no pain
- Pain at periphery of burn

Epidermis
Dermis
Fat
Muscle

FIGURE 16-7   Classification of burns by depth.

from the superficial burn only after blisters form. Because many nerve endings are in the dermis, both superficial and partial-thickness burns are often very painful. With both superficial and partial-thickness burns, the dermis is still intact and complete skin regeneration is very likely.

The sunburn is a common, but specialized type of burn. Ultraviolet radiation causes the burn rather than normal thermal processes. The radiation penetrates superficially and damages the uppermost layers of the dermis. Sunburn can present as either a superficial or partial-thickness burn.

Another similar type of burn occurs as someone watches an arc welder without proper protection. The lens of the eye focuses the high-intensity ultraviolet light on the retina, where it burns the tissue. This results in delayed eye pain and, possibly, transient blindness.

Full-Thickness Burn

full-thickness burn burn that damages all layers of the skin; characterized by areas that are white and dry; also called third-degree burn.

The **full-thickness,** or third-degree, burn, penetrates both the epidermis and the dermis and extends into the subcutaneous layers or even deeper, into muscles, bones, and internal organs. These burns destroy the tissue's regenerative properties and the peripheral nerve endings. The injury is painless because of the nerve destruction, but the margins of the full-thickness burn are frequently partial-thickness burns, which can be quite painful. The full-thickness burn takes on various colorations depending on the nature of the burning agent and the damaged, dying, or dead tissue. They can be white, brown, or a charred color and typically have a dry, leather-like appearance. Because the burn destroys the entire dermis, healing is difficult unless the wound is small or skin grafting is possible.

BODY SURFACE AREA

body surface area (BSA) amount of a patient's body affected by a burn.

Another factor affecting burn severity is how much of a person's **body surface area (BSA)** the burn involves. There are two approaches to estimating the BSA involved in a burn. The first, the rule of nines, is useful in estimating large burn areas. The second method, the rule of palms, is helpful in assessing smaller wounds more accurately.

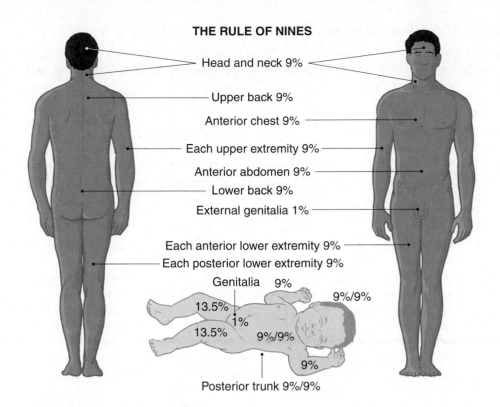

THE RULE OF NINES

Head and neck 9%

Upper back 9%

Anterior chest 9%

Each upper extremity 9%

Anterior abdomen 9%

Lower back 9%

External genitalia 1%

Each anterior lower extremity 9%

Each posterior lower extremity 9%

Genitalia 9%

13.5%

1%

13.5%

9%/9%

9%/9%

9%

Posterior trunk 9%/9%

FIGURE 16-8   The rule of nines.

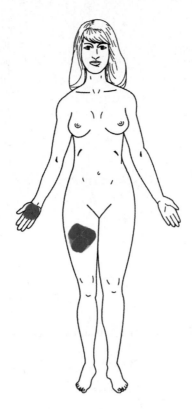

FIGURE 16-9   For the rule of palms, the surface of the patient's palm represents approximately 1% of BSA and is helpful in estimating the area of small burns.

Rule of Nines

The **rule of nines** identifies eleven topographical adult body regions, each of which approximates 9% of the patient's BSA (Figure 16-8). These regions include the entire head and neck, the anterior chest, the anterior abdomen, the posterior chest, the lower back (the posterior abdomen), the anterior surface of each lower extremity, the posterior surface of each lower extremity, and each upper extremity. The genitalia make up the remaining 1% of BSA.

Because infant and child anatomy differs significantly from that of adults, modify the rule of nines to maintain an accurate approximation of BSA. Divide the head and neck area into the anterior and posterior surface and award 9% for each. Reduce the surface area of each lower extremity by 4.5% to ensure the total body surface area remains at 100%. The rule of nines is at best an approximation of the area burned. It is, however, an expedient and useful tool to help measure the burn's extent.

> **rule of nines** method of estimating BSA burned by dividing the body into regions, each of which represents approximately 9% of total BSA (plus 1% for the genital region).

Rule of Palms

The **rule of palms,** an alternative system for approximating the extent of a burn, uses the palmar surface as a point of comparison in gauging the size of the affected body area (Figure 16-9). The patient's palm (the hand less the fingers) represents about 1% of the BSA, whether the patient is an adult, a child, or an infant. If you can visualize the palmar surface area and apply it to the burn area mentally, you can then obtain an estimate of the total BSA affected.

The rule of palms is easier to use for local burns of up to about 10% BSA, whereas the rule of nines is simpler and more appropriate for larger burns. Many other burn approximation techniques exist that are both more specific to age and, in general, more accurate. However, these techniques are more complicated and time consuming to use. Both the rule of nines and the rule of palms provide reasonable approximations of BSA when used properly in the field.

> **rule of palms** method of estimating BSA burned that sizes the area in comparison with the patient's palmar surface.

SYSTEMIC COMPLICATIONS

Burns cause several systemic complications. These can affect the overall severity of a burn. Typical complications include hypothermia, hypovolemia, eschar formation, and infection.

Hypothermia

A burn may disrupt the body's ability to regulate its core temperature. Tissue destruction reduces or eliminates the skin's ability to contain the fluid within. The burn process releases plasma and other fluids, which seep into the wound. There they evaporate and rapidly remove heat energy. If the burn is extensive, uncontrolled body heat loss induces rapid and severe hypothermia.

Hypovolemia

Hypovolemia also may complicate the severe burn. The inability of damaged blood vessels to contain plasma causes a shift of proteins, fluid, and electrolytes into the burned tissue. Additionally, the loss of plasma protein reduces the blood's ability, via osmosis, to draw fluids from the uninjured tissues. This in turn compromises the body's natural response to fluid loss and may produce a profound hypovolemia. Although this is a serious complication of the extensive burn, it takes hours to develop. Modern aggressive fluid resuscitation can effectively counteract this aspect of the burn process.

A related complication is electrolyte imbalance. With the massive shift of fluid to the interstitial space, the body's ability to regulate sodium, potassium, and other electrolytes becomes overwhelmed. In addition, large thermal and electrical burns can lead to massive tissue destruction with a resultant release of breakdown products into the bloodstream. Potassium is one such breakdown product and its oversupply, or hyperkalemia, can lead to life-threatening cardiac dysrhythmias. Careful electrocardiogram (ECG) monitoring and appropriate fluid resuscitation can help prevent hyperkalemic complications.

Eschar

eschar hard, leathery product of a deep full-thickness burn; consists of dead and denatured skin.

Skin denaturing further complicates full-thickness thermal burns. As the burn destroys the dermal cells, they become hard and leathery, producing what is known as an **eschar**. The skin as a whole constricts over the wound site, increasing the pressure of any edema beneath and restricting the flow of blood (See Figure 16-10). If the extremity burn is circumferential, the constriction may be severe enough to occlude all blood flow into the distal extremity. In the case of a thoracic burn, eschar may drastically reduce chest excursion and respiratory tidal volume.

Infection

Although infection is the most persistent killer of burn victims, its effects do not appear for several days following the acute injury. Pathogens invade the wound shortly after the burn occurs and continue to do so until the wound heals. These pathogens pose a hazard to life

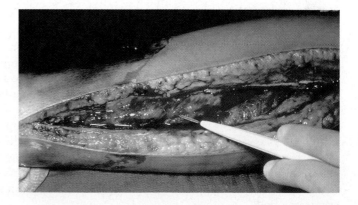

FIGURE 16-10   The constriction created by an eschar can limit chest excursion or cut off blood flow to and from a limb.

when they grow to massive numbers, a process that takes days or weeks. To reduce the patient's exposure to infectious pathogens, carefully employ body substance isolation, use sterile dressings and clean equipment, and avoid gross contamination of the burn.

Organ Failure

As previously noted, the burn process releases material from damaged or dying body cells into the bloodstream. Myoglobin from the muscles clogs the tubules of the kidneys and, with hypovolemia, may cause kidney failure. Hypovolemia and the circulating by-products of cellular destruction may also induce liver failure. In addition, the release of cellular potassium into the blood stream affects the heart's electrical system, causing dysrhythmias and possible death.

Special Factors

Certain factors involving the burn patient's overall health and age will also affect the patient's response to a burn and should influence your field decisions regarding treatment and transport. Geriatric and pediatric patients and patients who are already ill or otherwise injured have greater difficulty coping with burn injuries than do healthy individuals. The pediatric patient has a high body surface area to body weight ratio, which means the fluid reserves needed for dealing with the effects of a burn are low. Geriatric patients have reduced mechanisms for fluid retention and lower fluid reserves. They are also less able to combat infection and more apt to have underlying diseases. Ill patients are already using the energy of their bodies to fight their diseases; with burns, these patients have additional medical stresses to combat. The fluid loss that accompanies a burn also compounds the effects of blood loss in a trauma patient. This patient now must recover from two injuries.

Consider any patient with a pre-existing illness or disease or any pediatric or geriatric patient as having a more serious burn injury.

Physical Abuse

When assessing any burn, particularly in a child or an elderly and infirm adult, be alert for any signs of potential physical abuse. Look for mechanisms of injury that don't make sense, such as stove burns on an infant who cannot yet stand or walk. Certain burn patterns should also give rise to suspicion. Multiple circular burns each about a centimeter in diameter may reflect intentional cigarette burns. Infants who have been dipped in scalding hot water will have characteristic circumferential burns to their buttocks as they raise their feet and legs in an attempt to avoid the burning water (Figure 16-11). Branding is an unusual form of abuse and is sometimes seen in ritualistic or hazing ceremonies in some organizations. In all cases

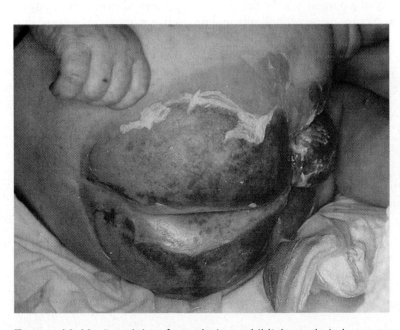

FIGURE 16-11 Burn injury from placing a child's buttocks in hot water as punishment.

of suspected abuse, document your findings objectively and accurately, report them to the person assuming patient care in the emergency department, and notify the proper authorities as state and local laws require.

ASSESSMENT OF THERMAL BURNS

Skin evaluation tells more about the body's condition than any other aspect of patient assessment. Not only is the skin the first body organ to experience the effects of burns, but it is also the first and often the only organ to display them. Therefore, assessment of the skin and the associated burns must be deliberate, careful, and complete.

Although the burn process varies, assessment is simple and well structured. Assess burn patients carefully and completely to ensure that you establish the nature and extent of each injury. This helps you to assign burns the appropriate priority for care.

The assessment of thermal burns follows established procedures for performing the scene size-up, the initial assessment, the rapid trauma assessment or focused history and physical exam, the detailed physical exam, and the ongoing assessment.

SCENE SIZE-UP

The safety of your patients, fellow rescuers, and yourself depends on a complete and thorough scene size-up. Look around carefully as you arrive at the scene to ensure there is no continuing danger to you or your patient. Examine the scene to make certain it is safe for you to enter. If there is any doubt, do not enter until the scene is made safe by appropriate emergency personnel (Figure 16-12).

On calls involving burn patients, be wary of entering enclosed spaces, such as a bedroom or a garage, if there is recent evidence of a fire. Even small fires can cause intense heat in small, enclosed spaces. This can rapidly lead to a near-explosive process (called flashover) in which the contents of a room rise in temperature to the point of rapid ignition. Flashover is frequently fatal to victims caught in the immediate area.

Another significant hazard at fire-ground scenes is the buildup of toxic gases. Carbon monoxide, cyanide, and hydrogen sulfide are common byproducts of combustion and can be produced in large quantities in some fires. Cyanide, in particular, can kill after as little as 15 seconds of exposure, a time short enough to fell any would-be rescuer without proper protection.

Never enter any potentially hazardous scene. Instead, make certain that the fire is thoroughly extinguished or that the patient is brought to you by persons skilled in working in hazardous environments who are using proper personal protective equipment. Ensure that

Be wary of entering any enclosed space associated with a fire because of the dangers of flashover and toxic gases.

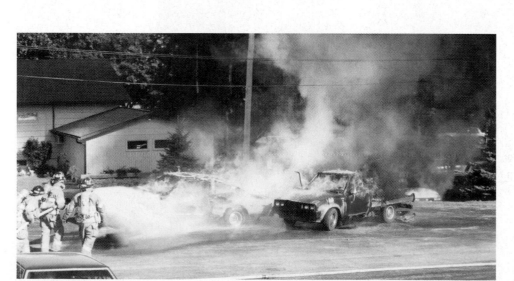

FIGURE 16-12   Never enter a fire scene until it has been safely contained by appropriately trained personnel.

the area where you will be caring for the patient is free from dangers such as structural collapse, contamination, electricity, and any other hazards.

Once at the burn patient's side, stop the burning process so it no longer threatens you or the patient. Extinguish any overt flame using copious irrigation, as water is available. As an alternative, use a heavy wool or cotton blanket (avoid most synthetics such as nylon or polyester) to smother flames.

Quickly survey the patient for other materials he or she is wearing that may continue the burn process. Remember that burn patients may be an actual hazard both to themselves and to you. Leather articles, such as shoes, belts, or watchbands, can smolder for hours and continue to induce thermal injury. Watches, rings, and other jewelry may also hold and transmit heat or may restrict swelling tissue and occlude distal circulation. Synthetics (such as a nylon windbreaker) produce great heat as they burn and leave a hot, smoldering residue once the overt flames are out. Remove materials such as those described above as soon as possible. Be careful as you check for and remove these items. They may be hot enough to burn you.

Look for and extinguish smoldering shoes, belts, or watchbands early in the assessment of burn patients.

Once the scene is safe and there are no further dangers to you or others, consider the burn mechanism. Ask yourself, "Is there any possibility that the patient was unconscious during the fire or trapped within the building?" If so, be ready to place a special emphasis on your assessment and management of the patient's airway and breathing. Watch for any signs of airway restriction and be alert to possible poisoning from carbon monoxide or other toxic gases.

Also consider and examine for other mechanisms of injury associated with the burn. Remember that the victim, in attempting to escape the flames, may have fallen down a flight of stairs or jumped from a second- or third-story window. Anticipate skeletal and internal injuries. In cases of electrical burns, consider the possibility that muscle spasms caused by contact with high voltage may also have caused skeletal fractures. Be aware that trauma injuries will increase the severity of the burn's impact on your patient.

Conclude the scene size-up by considering the need for other resources to manage the scene and treat the patient. Request additional EMS, police, and fire personnel and equipment as necessary. If you suspect serious airway involvement or carbon monoxide poisoning, consider requesting air medical service to reduce transport time to the hospital or burn/trauma center.

INITIAL ASSESSMENT

Start your initial assessment by forming a general impression of the patient. Rule out any danger of associated trauma or the possibility of head and spine injury. Evaluate the patient's level of consciousness, and, if the patient displays an altered state of consciousness, consider toxic inhalation as a cause. Protect the patient from further cervical injury if indicated by the suspected mechanism of injury or by the patient's symptoms.

Next, ensure the airway is patent. If it is not, protect it. You must give the airway of a burn patient special consideration. Look for the signs of any thermal or inhalation injury during your initial airway exam (Figure 16-13). Look carefully at the facial and nasal hairs to see if they have been singed. Examine any sputum and the areas around the mouth and nose for carbonaceous residue or any other evidence of inhalation. Listen for airway sounds, such as stridor, hoarseness, or coughing, that indicate irritation or inflammation of the mucosa. Such sounds should alert you to the possibility that the airway has been injured and that progressive swelling of the airway is likely. Stridor, in particular, is a serious finding. Consider a patient with any signs of respiratory involvement as a potential acute emergency and provide immediate care and transport.

In cases of severe airway burns, intubate early. If intubation is delayed until the patient arrives at the emergency department, the airway may be so edematous that it may be difficult or impossible to intubate.

With patients in whom respiratory involvement is suspected, provide high-flow, high-concentration oxygen and prepare the equipment for endotracheal intubation. High-concentration oxygen (at levels approaching 100%) is especially important for burn patients because they may be suffering from carbon monoxide poisoning. Very high oxygen percentages more effectively provide oxygen to body cells and may reduce the half-life of the carbon monoxide by up to two thirds.

Burn patients may progress rapidly from mild dyspnea to total respiratory arrest. Although the intubation of a respiratory burn patient may be difficult in the field, there are distinct advantages to performing it early. The edema is progressive and gradually reduces

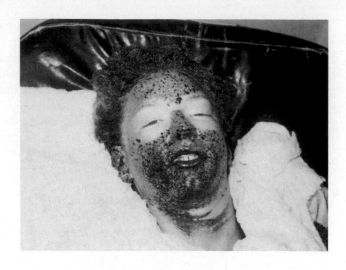

FIGURE 16–13 Facial burns or carbonaceous material around the mouth and nose suggest the potential for chemical and thermal burns to the airway.

the airway lumen. If intubation is delayed until the patient becomes extremely dyspneic or goes into respiratory arrest, the airway may be so edematous that it will be difficult, if not impossible, to intubate.

If you elect field intubation for the burn patient (and medical direction approves), perform it quickly and carefully. The airway is already narrowing, and the normal trauma associated with intubation could make matters worse. Intubation can be more complicated if the patient is conscious and fights the process. You may also find nasotracheal intubation useful. In any case, select the crew member with the most experience to ensure that intubation is completed quickly and with the least amount of associated airway trauma.

As with all intubation, it is best to maintain an airway using the largest endotracheal tube possible. Be sure, however, to have several tubes smaller than you would normally use ready, because edema may have reduced the size of the airway. Select the largest tube that you think will easily pass through the cords.

Ensure that the patient's breathing is adequate in both volume and rate. Carefully assess tidal volume if the chest has circumferential burns because the developing eschar may restrict chest excursion. Ventilate as necessary via BVM using the reservoir and high-flow, high-concentration oxygen.

FOCUSED AND RAPID TRAUMA ASSESSMENT

The focused history and physical exam for the burn patient are much the same as for any other trauma patient, beginning with a rapid trauma assessment or a focused physical exam and proceeding to the taking of baseline vital signs and a patient history. With a burn patient, however, you must also accurately approximate the area of the burn and its depth. This approximation guides your care and helps emergency department personnel prepare for patient arrival.

Except in cases of very localized burns, examine the patient's entire body surface, both anterior and posterior. Remove any clothing that was or could have been involved in the burn. If any of the clothing adheres to the burn or resists removal, cut around it as necessary.

Apply the rule of nines to determine the total BSA burned. Add 9% if the burn involves an entire rule of nines region. If it only involves a portion, add that proportion of 9%. For example, if one-third of the upper extremity is burned, the surface area approximation is 3% (⅓ of 9% = 3%). For small burns, use the rule of palms to approximate the affected BSA.

The depth of a burn injury is also an important consideration. Identify areas of painful sensation as partial-thickness burns (Figure 16-14). Consider those that present with limited or absent pain as probable full-thickness burns (Figure 16-15). This differentiation is difficult because partial-thickness injury and its associated pain commonly surround the full-thickness burn (Figure 16-16). See Table 16-1 for the characteristics of the different types of burns.

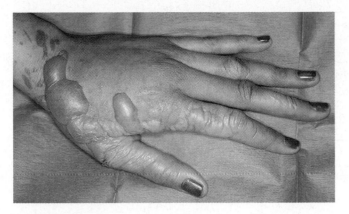

FIGURE 16-14 A partial-thickness burn.

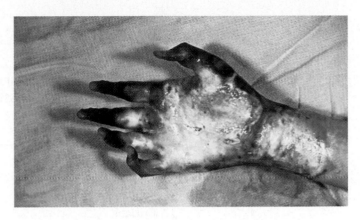

FIGURE 16-15 A deep full-thickness burn.

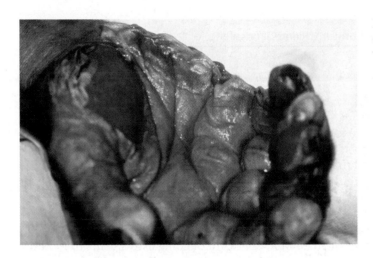

FIGURE 16-16 A hand wound displaying both partial- and full-thickness burns.

Table 16-1	CHARACTERISTICS OF VARIOUS DEPTHS OF BURNS		
	Superficial (First-Degree)	**Partial-Thickness (Second-Degree)**	**Full-Thickness (Third-Degree)**
Cause	Sun or minor flame	Hot liquids, flame	Chemicals, electricity, hot metals, flame
Skin color	Red	Mottled red	Pearly white and/or charred, translucent, and parchment-like
Skin	Dry with no blister	Blisters with weeping	Dry with thrombosed blood vessels
Sensation	Painful	Painful	Anesthetic
Healing	3–6 days	2–4 weeks	May require skin grafting

A third consideration in determining the severity of a burn is the area of the body affected. The face, hands, feet, joints, genitalia, and circumferential burns deserve particular consideration. Each presents with special problems to patients and their recovery.

You have already assessed the face for burns to eliminate respiratory involvement. But this area also needs special consideration for aesthetic reasons. Facial damage and scarring may be more socially debilitating than a joint or limb burn. Carefully assess and give a high priority to these injuries, even if you do rule out respiratory involvement.

Consider burns involving the feet or the hands as serious. These areas are critical for much of the patient's daily activities. Serious burns and the associated scar tissue make thermal hand or foot injuries very debilitating. Assess these areas and communicate the precise

Burns to the face, hands, feet, joints, genitalia, and circumferential burns are of special concern.

Table 16-2	Burn Severity
Minor	
Superficial: BSA <50% (sunburns, etc.)	
Partial thickness: BSA <15%	
Full thickness: BSA <2%	
Moderate	
Superficial: BSA >50%	
Partial thickness: BSA <30%	
Full thickness: BSA <10%	
Critical	
Partial thickness: BSA >30%	
Full thickness: BSA >10%	
Inhalation injury	
Any partial- or full-thickness burns involving hands, feet, joints, face, or genitalia	

Source: American Burn Association.

location of the injury and the degree of the burn to the receiving physician. Joint burns can likewise be debilitating for patients. Scar tissue replaces skin, leading to loss of joint flexibility and mobility. Give any burn assessed as full-thickness that involves the hands, feet, or joints a higher priority than a burn of equal surface area and depth elsewhere.

Also pay particular attention to burns that completely ring an extremity, the thorax, the abdomen, or the neck. Because of the nature of a full-thickness burn, the area underneath the burn may be drastically compressed as an eschar forms. The resulting constriction may hinder respirations, restrict distal blood flow, or cause hypoxia of the tissues beneath. Carefully assess any burn encircling a part of the body for distal circulation or other signs of vascular compromise. Once you note such an injury, perform ongoing assessments to monitor distal circulatory status.

Finally, assign a higher priority to any burns affecting pediatric or geriatric patients or patients who are ill or otherwise injured. Serious burns cause great stress for these patients. The massive fluid and heat loss as well as the infection often associated with burns challenge the ability of body systems to perform adequately. Consider a burn more serious whenever it is accompanied by any other serious patient problem.

Once you determine the depth, extent, and other factors that contribute to burn severity, categorize the patient as having either minor, moderate, or severe burns. Use the criteria in Table 16-2 as a guide.

The severity of a burn should be increased one level with pediatric and geriatric patients and patients suffering from other trauma or acute medical problems. Also consider burns as critical with a patient who shows any signs or symptoms of respiratory involvement. Such patients require immediate transport to a burn (or trauma) center, if possible (see Table 16-3).

The head-to-toe examination should continue at the scene only if significant and life-threatening burns can be ruled out.

Table 16-3	Injuries That Benefit from Burn Center Care
Partial-thickness (second-degree) burn >15% of BSA	
Full-thickness (third-degree) burn >5% BSA	
Significant burns to the face, feet, hands, or perineal area	
High-voltage electrical injuries	
Inhalation injuries	
Chemical burns causing progressive tissue destruction	
Associated significant injuries	

Source: American Burn Association.

The burn center is a hospital with a commitment to providing specialty treatment to burn patients. That commitment includes measures necessary to reduce the risk of infection presented by serious burns. The center must also have the resources to perform delicate skin grafts necessary to replace destroyed skin. Because serious burns leave scar tissue that covers joints and other important areas and affects movement, the center can provide rehabilitation programs requiring prolonged patient stays and intensive nursing care. Although immediate transport to a burn center is not as critically time dependant as transport for other seriously injured patients to a trauma center, the burn center's resources can optimize a patient's recovery prospects. Review your local protocols for criteria regarding patient transport to a burn center.

Conclude the focused history and physical exam by prioritizing the patient for transport. Rapidly transport any patient with full-thickness burns over a large portion of the BSA. Patients with associated injuries to the face, joints, hands, feet, or genitalia are also candidates for immediate transport. Other cases needing rapid transport include patients who have experienced smoke, steam, or flame inhalation, or any geriatric, pediatric, otherwise ill, or trauma patient. Direct these patients to the nearest burn center as described by your local protocols or by on-line medical direction.

ONGOING ASSESSMENT

Conduct ongoing assessments for all burn patients, every 15 minutes for minor burns and every 5 minutes for moderate or critical burns. Although the burn injury mechanism has been halted, the nature of the burn will continue to affect the patient. In addition to monitoring vital signs, watch for early signs of hypovolemia and airway problems. Also be cautious of aggressive fluid therapy. Monitor for lung sounds and respiratory effort suggestive of pulmonary edema, and slow the fluid resuscitation if any signs develop. Also carefully monitor distal circulation and sensation with any circumferential burn. Finally, monitor the ECG to identify any abnormalities, which may be caused by electrolyte imbalances secondary to fluid movement and tissue destruction.

MANAGEMENT OF THERMAL BURNS

Once you complete your burn patient assessment and correct or address any immediate life threats, you can begin certain burn management steps, either in the field or en route to the hospital. These include the prevention of shock, hypothermia, and any further wound contamination.

Thermal burn management can be divided into two categories: that for local and minor burns and that for moderate to severe burns.

LOCAL AND MINOR BURNS

Use local cooling to treat minor soft-tissue burns involving only a small proportion of the body surface area at a partial-thickness. Provide this care only for partial-thickness burns that involve less than 15% of the BSA or very small full-thickness burns (less than 2% BSA). Cooling of larger surface areas may subject the patient to the risk of hypothermia. Cold or cool water immersion has some effect in reducing pain and may limit the depth of the burning process if applied immediately (within 1 or 2 minutes) after the burn.

If you have not already done so, remove any article of clothing or jewelry from the patient that might possibly act to constrain edema. As body fluids accumulate at the injury site, the site begins to swell. If the swelling encounters any constriction, it increases pressure on other tissue and may, in effect, serve as a tourniquet. This pressure may result in the loss of pulse and circulation distal to the injury. Evaluate distal circulation and sensation frequently during care and transport.

Also provide the burn patient with comfort and support. Even rather minor burns can be very painful. Calm and reassure the patient; in severe cases, consider diazepam or morphine sulfate analgesia.

Standard in-hospital treatment for minor burns includes the application of topical (not systemic) antibiotic ointments such as silver sulfadiazine and bulky sterile dressings. Encourage the patient, as much as possible, to keep the burn elevated. Provide analgesia in either oral or parenteral form as burns can be quite painful. Full-thickness burns are open wounds, so any patient without an up-to-date tetanus immunization is given a booster of tetanus-diphtheria toxoid.

MODERATE TO SEVERE BURNS

Use dry, sterile dressings to cover partial-thickness burns that involve more than 15% BSA or full-thickness burns involving more than 5% of the BSA. Dressings keep air movement past the sensitive partial-thickness burn to a minimum, and thereby reduce pain. Bulky sterile dressings also provide padding against minor bumping and other trauma. In full-thickness burns, they provide a barrier to possible contamination.

Keep the patient warm. When burns involve large surface areas, the patient loses the ability to effectively control body temperature. If the burn begins to seep fluid, as in a full-thickness burn, evaporative heat loss can be extreme. Cover such an area with dry sterile dressings, cover the patient with a blanket, and maintain a warm environment.

When treating full-thickness burns to the fingers, toes, or other locations where burned surfaces may contact each other, place soft, non-adherent bandages between the burned skin areas (Figure 16-17). Without this precaution, the disrupted and wet wounds would stick together and cause further damage when pulled apart for care at the emergency department.

If the surface area of the burn is great, medical direction may ask you to provide aggressive fluid therapy during prehospital care. Although hypovolemia is not an early development after a burn, fluid migration into the wound later during the burn cycle eventually

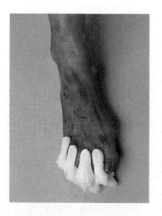
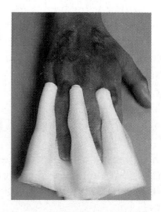
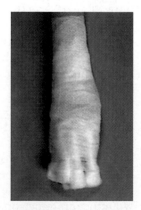

FIGURE 16-17   Separate burned toes and fingers with dry sterile gauze.

leads to serious fluid loss. Early and aggressive fluid therapy can effectively reduce the impact of this fluid loss.

If burns cover all the normal IV access sites, you may place the catheter through tissue with partial-thickness burns, proximal to any more serious injury. (Full-thickness burns usually damage the blood vessels or coagulate the blood, making IV cannulation difficult and possibly impeding effective fluid flow.) Be careful with insertion. The skin may be leathery, but the tissue underneath is very delicate.

Establish IV routes in any patient with moderate to severe burns. Introduce two large-bore catheters and hang 1,000 mL bags of either normal saline (preferred) or lactated Ringer's solution. Current fluid resuscitation formulas recommend 4 mL of fluid for every kilogram of patient weight multiplied by the percentage of body surface area burned:

$$4 \text{ mL} \times \text{Patient weight in kg} \times \text{BSA burned} = \text{Amount of fluid}$$

Thus, for a 70-kg patient with 30% BSA burned, the calculation is:

$$4 \times 70 \times 30 = 8,400 \text{ mL}$$

The patient needs half this amount of fluid in the first 8 hours after the burn. This particular fluid resuscitation protocol is known as the Parkland formula. Other variations exist and may be in use in your local area. In most prehospital situations where transport time is short (less than 1 hour), an initial fluid bolus of 0.5 mL of fluid for every kilogram of patient weight multiplied by the percentage of BSA burned is reasonable:

$$0.5 \text{ mL} \times \text{Patient weight in kg} \times \text{BSA burned} = \text{Amount of fluid}$$

Thus, for an 80-kg patient with 20% BSA burned, the calculation is:

$$0.5 \times 80 \times 20 = 800 \text{ mL}$$

You may repeat this infusion once or twice during the first hour or so of care.

Be cautious and conservative when administering fluids to the burn patient if there is any possibility of airway or lung injury. Rapid fluid administration may worsen airway swelling or the edema that accompanies toxic inhalation. Carefully monitor the airway and auscultate for breath sounds frequently whenever you administer fluid to a burn patient.

Be cautious and conservative when administering fluids to the burn patient with an inhalation injury.

Burns are quite painful, yet the pain is often paradoxical to the burn severity. Less severe superficial and partial-thickness (first- and second-degree) burns are very uncomfortable, whereas extensive full-thickness (third-degree) burns are often almost without pain. Provide patients in severe pain with narcotic analgesia. Consider morphine in 2 mg IV increments every 5 minutes until suffering is relieved. Use morphine with caution as it may depress the respiratory drive and increase any existing hypovolemia.

Infection is another classic and deadly problem associated with extensive soft-tissue burns. This life-threatening condition does not develop until well after prehospital care is concluded. However, proper field care can significantly reduce mortality and morbidity. Providing a clean environment and sterile dressings can lessen the bacterial load for the patient. Avoid prophylactic antibiotics because their early use has been shown to actually worsen outcomes for burn patients.

In dire circumstances medical direction may request you to perform an emergency escharotomy. To do this, incise the burned tissue through the eschar, perpendicular to the constriction. Be certain to incise about 1 cm deeper than the developing eschar to ensure the release of pressure. If adequate respirations or distal pulses do not return, medical direction may request you to repeat the procedure a short distance from the first incision.

Emergency department personnel will continue fluid resuscitation for serious burn patients according to the Parkland or another suitable formula. They will perform arterial blood gas evaluation to determine oxygen tension, carbon monoxide concentration, and cyanide poisoning levels. Urine output and cardiac monitoring are instituted as well. The staff will ensure adequate administration of parenteral narcotic analgesia and provide tetanus immunization if necessary. They will closely evaluate severe circumferential burns for eschar development. If the blood flow in an extremity or respirations is impaired, the physician may perform an escharotomy.

INHALATION INJURY

Early intubation can be life saving for a patient with an inhalation injury.

If you suspect thermal (or chemical) airway burns and airway compromise is imminent, intubation can be life saving. Once you ensure the patient's airway, provide high-flow, high-concentration oxygen by nonrebreather mask at 15 liters per minute. Oxygen not only counters hypoxia, but it is also therapeutic in carbon monoxide and cyanide poisoning. Consider transport to a center capable of providing hyperbaric oxygen therapy for patients with suspected carbon monoxide poisoning. The hyperbaric chamber provides oxygen under the pressure of two or more atmospheres. This pushes oxygen into the patient's blood stream, carrying it directly to the body's cells. Hyperbaric oxygenation also drives carbon monoxide from the hemoglobin, shortening the time to recovery. If hyperbaric oxygen therapy is available in your area, any smoke inhalation or suspected carbon monoxide poisoning patient should be considered for treatment at the facility.

Suspect cyanide toxicity in patients with severe symptoms such as dyspnea, chest pain, altered mental status, seizures, and unconsciousness. To be effective, antidotal treatment of serious cyanide poisoning must be started early. Vapor exposures are likely to result in severe respiratory distress or apnea in addition to unconsciousness. Rapid airway intervention with endotracheal intubation and ventilatory support with a BVM are initial priorities. However, a rapid shift to antidotal therapy is essential to save the patient.

Administration of the antidote for cyanide is a two-stage process, first using a nitrite compound, followed by a sulfur-containing compound (Figure 16-18). The nitrite acts by converting the hemoglobin (the primary oxygen-carrying protein in the blood) to methemoglobin. Methemoglobin then binds the cyanide, removing it from the cytochrome$_{a3}$ (an enzyme necessary for oxygen processing by cells). The sulfur-containing antidote then removes the cyanide by forming a nontoxic compound, excreted in the urine.

Ambulances serving industrial areas with high cyanide use may carry antidote kits containing amyl nitrite, sodium nitrite, and sodium thiosulfate. If an IV is already established, administer 300 mg sodium nitrite over 2 to 4 minutes for adults. If an IV is not yet established, crush one amyl nitrate ampule for the patient to inhale. If the patient has spontaneous respirations, place the ampule under an oxygen mask with high-flow oxygen running. In patients needing ventilatory support, place the ampule in the bag or oxygen reservoir of the BVM. Do not let the ampule fall into the patient's mouth or down the endotracheal tube. Always follow inhaled amyl nitrate with IV sodium nitrite, and do not use amyl nitrite if the patient has already received sodium nitrite.

Following administration of IV sodium nitrite, administer 12.5 gm of sodium thiosulfate for the adult. Avoid sodium thiosulfate unless the patient has received IV sodium nitrite, as it does not work well by itself. A highly effective and much safer antidote (related to vitamin B_{12}) is on the horizon, but is not yet available for general use in the United States.

FIGURE 16-18 A cyanide antidote kit.

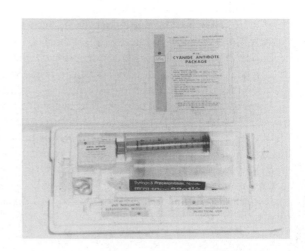

ELECTRICAL, CHEMICAL, AND RADIATION BURNS

ELECTRICAL INJURIES

Be certain that the power has been shut off before you approach the scene of a suspected electrical injury. Until it is, do not allow anyone to approach the patient or the proximity of the electrical source. Remember that an energized power line need not spark or whip around to be deadly; a power line simply lying on the ground can still present a significant danger. Note also that some utility lines have breakers that will try to re-establish power periodically. Establish a safety zone if there is any question about the status of lines that are down. Keep vehicles and personnel at a distance from downed lines or the source pole that is greater than the distance between the power poles. Also be aware that downed power lines may energize metal structures such as buildings, vehicles, or fences.

Once the scene is secure, assess the patient and prepare him or her for transport. Search for both an entrance and an exit wound. Look specifically for possible contact points with both the ground and the electrical source. In some circumstances, multiple entrance and exit wounds are present. Remember that electrical current passes through the body and therefore may result in significant internal burns, especially to blood vessels and nerves, even while the assessment reveals only minimal superficial findings. Rapidly progressive cardiovascular collapse can follow contact with an electrical source. Also, examine the patient for any fractures resulting from forceful muscle contractions caused by the current's passage.

As with thermal burns, look for smoldering shoes, belts, or other items of clothing. Such items may continue the burning process well after the current is shut off. Also remove rings, watches, and any other constrictive items from the fingers, limbs, and the neck of the patient.

Perform ECG monitoring for possible cardiac disturbances in victims of electrical burns. Electrical current may induce dysrhythmias including bradycardias, tachycardias, ventricular fibrillation, and asystole. Ensure that emergency department personnel examine any patient who has sustained a significant electrical shock. The damage the current causes may be internal and not apparent to you or your patient during assessment. Consider any significant electrical burn or exposure patient as a high priority for immediate transport.

Lightning strikes to humans occur more than 300 times each year in the United States and result in over 100 deaths. Strikes to people riding tractors, on open water, on golf courses, and under trees are most common, and men are the victims of 75% of all strikes. A lightning strike is a high-voltage (up to 100,000 volts), high-current (10,000 amperes), and high-temperature (50,000°F) event that lasts only a fraction of a second. A direct strike will impart this energy to the patient (Figure 16-19). However, the lightning will often strike a nearby object with some voltage traveling sideways (sideflash) or the voltage may radiate outward in alternate pathways from the strike point, thus diminishing the voltage (step voltage).

By the time anyone reaches the victim of a lightning strike, the electricity has long since dissipated. (There will be, however, a continued risk of further strikes as long as the storm remains nearby.) There is no danger of electrical shock from touching the victim of a lightning strike. The victim's clothing, however, may continue to smolder, so remove it as necessary. Among other serious effects, lightning can produce a sudden cessation of breathing. Despite being apneic and perhaps pulseless, these patients frequently survive with prompt prehospital intervention.

Treat visible burns (entrance and exit wounds) just as any thermal burn with cooling, if necessary, followed by the application of dry sterile dressings. Do not focus too much on the visible burns, but instead recognize that the electricity has passed through the body, possibly causing widespread internal effects.

Treat cardiac or respiratory arrest in electrical burn patients with aggressive airway, ventilatory, and circulatory management. Patients in cardiac arrest because of contact with electrical current have a high survival rate if prehospital intervention is prompt. Check immediately for ventricular fibrillation and defibrillate if necessary. Secure the airway with an endotracheal tube and begin ventilations and chest compressions. The usual resuscitative procedures for cases of cardiac arrest apply equally when the cause of the arrest is electrical injury; they might include the use of vasopressors and antidysrhythmics.

Until the power is off, no one should be allowed to approach the electrical burn patient.

Monitor the electrical burn patient for abnormalities in the ECG.

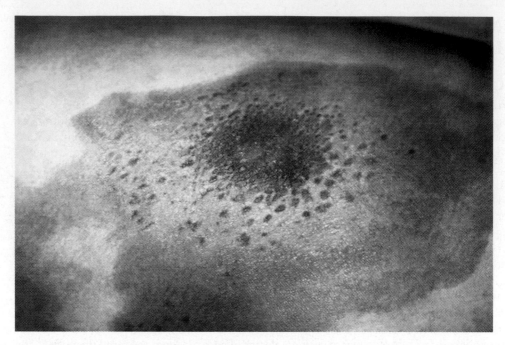

FIGURE 16-19 A typical lightning-strike injury.

For serious electrical burn injuries, initiate at least two large bore IVs and give an initial 20 mL/kg fluid bolus. If the electrical burn is severe, provide additional fluid using the Parkland or another formula. Consider use of sodium bicarbonate and mannitol, usually at the discretion of medical direction, to prevent the complications of **rhabdomyolysis** and hyperkalemia. The usual starting dose is one mEq/kg for sodium bicarbonate and 10 g for mannitol.

rhabdomyolysis acute disease that involves the destruction of skeletal muscle.

CHEMICAL BURNS

As you perform the scene size-up, identify the nature of the chemical spill/contamination and, if possible, approach from upwind. Identify the location of the chemical and ensure that it poses no hazard to you, other rescuers, or the public. Be wary of toxic fumes and cross-contamination from the patient and the surrounding environment. If necessary, have hazardous material team members evacuate and decontaminate the victim before you begin assessment and care. Seek out personnel on the scene who are familiar with the agent and consult with them regarding dangers posed by the agent and any specific medical care and patient handling procedures required with it.

During your assessment and care, always wear medical examination gloves, but never presume that they will protect you from the agent. Take appropriate protective action against airborne dust, toxic fumes, and splash exposure for both yourself and the patient (goggles and mask as needed). Wear a disposable gown if there is danger of the agent contacting your clothing. Make certain the agent is isolated and no longer a danger to the patient or others. Have any of the patient's clothing that you suspect may be contaminated removed, and isolate it from accidental contact. Save the clothing and have it disposed of properly. Identify the type of agent, its exact chemical name, the length of the patient's contact time with it, and the precise areas of the patient's body affected by it.

As you begin your initial assessment, ensure that the patient is alert and fully oriented and that airway and breathing are unaffected by the contact. If there is any airway restriction or respiratory involvement, consider early intubation. As airway tissue swells, the obstruction worsens and intubation becomes more difficult. Monitor the patient's heart rate and consider ECG monitoring, because many chemicals (for example, organophosphates) may affect the heart. If the patient is stable, begin the rapid trauma assessment.

In dealing with a chemical burn, take all precautions to ensure that no one else becomes contaminated.

Examine any chemical burn carefully to establish the depth, extent, and nature of the injury. If you suspect the involvement of phenol, dry lime, sodium or riot agents, treat as indicated below:

- *Phenol.* A gelatinous caustic called phenol is used as a powerful industrial cleaner. Phenol is very difficult to remove because it is sticky and insoluble in water. Alcohol, which dissolves it, is frequently available in places where phenol is regularly used. You can use the alcohol to remove the phenol and follow removal with irrigation using large volumes of cool water.

- *Dry lime.* Dry lime is a strong corrosive that reacts with water. It produces heat and subsequent chemical and thermal injuries. Brush dry lime off the patient gently, but as completely as possible. Then rinse the contaminated area with large volumes of cool to cold water. While the water reacts with any remaining lime, it cools the contact area and removes the rest of the chemical. By rinsing with water, you ensure the lime reacts with that water rather than with the water contained within the patient's soft tissues.

- *Sodium.* Sodium is an unstable metal that reacts destructively with many substances, including human tissue. It reacts vigorously with water, creating extreme heat, explosive hydrogen gas, and possible ignition. Sodium is normally stored submerged in oil because the metal reacts with oxygen in the air. If a patient is contaminated with sodium, decontaminate him or her quickly by gentle brushing. Then cover the wound with oil used to store the substance.

- *Riot control agents.* These agents, which include CS, CN (mace), and oleoresin capsicum (OC, pepper spray), deserve special mention because people are the targets of their intended use and because that use is frequent. These agents cause intense irritation of the eyes, mucous membranes, and respiratory tract. In general, they do not cause permanent damage when properly deployed. Patients who have been in contact with these agents typically present with eye pain, tearing, and temporary blindness. Coughing, gagging, and vomiting are not uncommon. Treatment is supportive and most patients recover spontaneously within 10 to 20 minutes of exposure to fresh air. If necessary, irrigate the patient's eyes with normal saline if you suspect that any riot agent particles remain in the eye.

If it has not been done earlier, decontaminate the patient who has come in contact with any other chemical capable of causing tissue damage. Stop the damage by irrigating the site with large volumes of water (see Figure 16-20). Water rinses away the offending material and dilutes any water-soluble agents. The water also reduces the heat and rate of the chemical reaction and, ultimately, the chemical's effects on the patient's skin. If the contamination is widespread, douse the patient with large volumes of water. Use a garden hose or low-pressure water from a fire truck. Ensure that the water is neither warm nor too cold.

Irrigation with copious amounts of cool water is indicated for burns from an unknown chemical agent.

When the patient has been thoroughly rinsed for a few minutes, remove any remaining clothing. Take care that the process does not contaminate rescuers. If the agent is dangerous, save all clothing and contain the rinse water for proper disposal at a later time. Next, gently wash the burn with a mild soap (such as ordinary dish detergent) and a gentle brush or sponge. Be careful not to cause further soft-tissue damage. After washing, gently irrigate the wound with a constant flow of water. Although the pain and the burning process may appear to subside, it is important to continue the irrigation until the patient arrives at the emergency department. If practical, transport the label from the corrosive's container or a sample of the agent (safely contained and marked) along with the patient. On arrival at the hospital, be sure to describe to emergency department personnel, and enter in your prehospital care report, any first aid given prior to your arrival.

Do not use any antidote or neutralizing agent. Neutralizing agents often react violently with the contaminants they neutralize. They may ultimately increase the heat of the reaction and induce thermal burns. In some cases, the antidote or neutralizing agent is more damaging to the skin than the contaminant.

Do not use any antidote or any neutralizing agent on chemical burns.

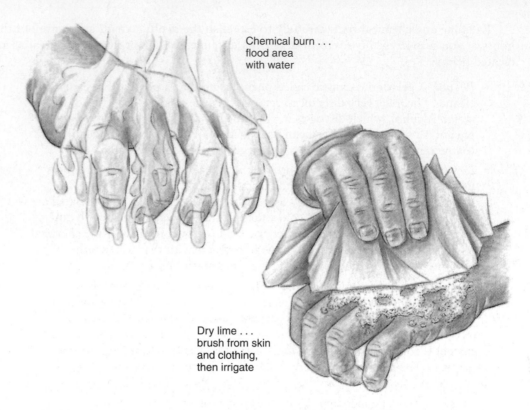

Chemical burn . . .
flood area
with water

Dry lime . . .
brush from skin
and clothing,
then irrigate

FIGURE 16-20   Chemical burns should be flushed with large quantities of water. Dry lime should be first brushed away before applying cool water.

blepharospasm twitching of the eyelids.

With chemical burns, pay particular attention to the patient's eyes. Eyes are very sensitive to chemicals and can easily be damaged, even by weak agents. Prompt treatment of chemical eye injury is critical and can reduce damage and preserve eyesight. Ask the patient about chemical contact with the eyes, eye pain, vision changes, and contact lens use. Examine the eyes for eyelid spasm (**blepharospasm**), conjunctival erythema, discoloration, tearing, and other evidence of burns or irritation.

Irrigate chemical splashes that involve the eye with large volumes of water. Alkali burns are especially damaging and with them you should flush the eye for at least 15 minutes. Irrigate acid burns for at least 5 minutes. Flush splashes of an unknown agent for up to 20 minutes. Do not, however, delay transport while irrigating.

A useful technique for irrigation is to hang a bag of normal saline (lactated Ringer's is an acceptable substitute) and use the flow regulator to control the flow of fluid into the nasal corner of the eye. Turn the patient's head to the side to facilitate drainage and avoid cross-contaminating the other eye with the waste fluid. Be alert for contact lenses in cases where chemicals are splashed into the eyes. Chemicals may become trapped under the lenses, preventing adequate irrigation. Gently remove the lenses, continuing irrigation.

RADIATION BURNS

Because radiation can be neither seen nor felt, it can endanger EMS personnel unless proper precautions are taken.

An incident involving potential radiation exposure or burns must be a concern during both dispatch and response phases of the emergency call. Because radiation can neither be seen nor felt, it can endanger EMS personnel unless the hazard has been anticipated and proper precautions taken. If you suspect radiation exposure, approach the scene very carefully (Figure 16-21). If the incident occurs at a power generation plant or in an industrial or a medical facility, seek personnel knowledgeable about the radioactive substance being used. Such persons are always on staff, and frequently on site, at these facilities. Stay a good distance from the scene and make certain that bystanders, rescuers, and patients remain remote from the source of the exposure. Remember that distance and the nature of the materials, such as concrete or earth, between you and the radiation source reduce potential exposure.

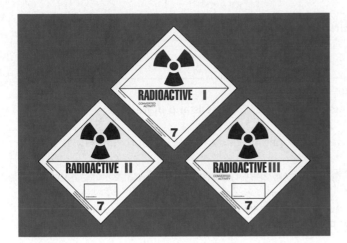

FIGURE 16-21 Warning labels indicate the presence of radioactive materials.

If the exposure may be from dust or fire, approach from and remain upwind of the radiation source.

In radiation exposure incidents, ensure that personnel trained in radiation hazards isolate the source, contain it, and test the scene for safety. If this is impossible, move the patient to a site remote from the radioactivity source where you can give care without danger either to yourself or the patient. Plan the removal carefully. Use as much shielding as possible and keep exposure times to a minimum. Remember, the dose of radiation received is related to three primary factors: duration, distance, and shielding.

If you must carry out a patient removal, use the oldest rescuers for the evacuation team. This approach is prudent because many of the effects of radiation exposure become evident many years after the exposure. If you use older rescuers, they will more likely be past their reproductive years and have fewer years of life left if and when a problem does surface. This concern is especially important with pregnant females and young adults of both sexes. Remember that radiation damages the reproductive system very easily.

If there is a risk that patients are contaminated, ensure that they are properly decontaminated before you begin assessment and care. If available for this task, use persons knowledgeable in decontamination and monitoring techniques who have the appropriate protective gear. If this is not possible, don goggles, a mask, gloves, and a disposable gown. Direct the evacuation team to place the patients in a decontamination area remote from your vehicle and other personnel and where any contamination can be contained. Have the patients disrobe or carefully disrobe them, rinse them with large volumes of water, then wash them with a soft brush and rinse again. Ordinary dish detergent is effective as a cleansing agent. Scrub, or cut off and then scrub, any areas of body hair. As in incidents of chemical contamination, save all clothing and decontamination water and dispose of them safely. Perform decontamination before moving the patients to the ambulance.

Carefully document the circumstances of the radioactive exposure. If possible, identify the source and strength of the agent. Determine the patient's proximity to the source during the exposure as well as the length of exposure.

Once decontaminated, treat a radiation exposure patient as you would any other patient. Because the human body by itself cannot be a source of ionizing radiation, the decontaminated patient poses no threat to you or your crew. Remember, however, that any contaminated material remaining on the patient or any contamination transferred to you does provide a source of radiation exposure and may contaminate you and your vehicle.

The actual assessment of a patient exposed to radiation is quite simple and usually reveals minimal signs or symptoms of injury. Only extreme exposures result in the classic presentation of nausea, vomiting, and malaise. Burns are extremely rare, although they may occur if the exposure is extremely intense. Even though a patient seems well, the delayed consequences of high-dose radiation exposure can be devastating. If you note any early patient complaints, record the findings in the patient's own words and include the time the complaint first was made. This information is helpful in determining the patient's degree of radiation exposure (Table 16-4).

Duration, distance, and shielding are important factors in determining radiation dose exposure.

Once properly decontaminated, the radiation injury patient presents no radiation danger to caregivers.

Table 16-4   DOSE-EFFECT RELATIONSHIPS TO IONIZING RADIATION

Whole Body Exposure Dose (RAD)	Effect
5–25	Asymptomatic. Blood studies are normal.
50–75	Asymptomatic. Minor depressions of white blood cells and platelets in a few patients.
75–125	May produce anorexia, nausea and vomiting, and fatigue in approximately 10% to 20% of patients within 2 days.
125–200	Possible nausea and vomiting. Diarrhea, anxiety, tachycardia. Fatal to less than 5% of patients.
200–600	Nausea and vomiting. Diarrhea in the first several hours. Weakness, fatigue. Fatal to approximately 50% of patients within 6 weeks without prompt medical attention.
600–1,000	Burning sensation within minutes. Nausea and vomiting within 10 minutes. Confusion, ataxia, and collapse within 1 hour. Watery diarrhea within 1 to 2 hours. Fatal to 100% within short time without prompt medical attention.

Localized Exposure Dose (RAD)	Effect
50	Asymptomatic
500	Asymptomatic (usually). May have risk of altered function of exposed area.
2,500	Atrophy, vascular lesion, and altered pigmentation.
5,000	Chronic ulcer, risk of carcinogenesis.
50,000	Permanent destruction of exposed tissue.

Treat the symptoms of the radiation injury patient, make the patient as comfortable as possible, and offer psychological support. Cover any burns with sterile dressing and, if general symptoms are noticeable, provide oxygen and initiate an IV. Maintain the patient's body temperature and provide transport to the emergency department.

ONGOING ASSESSMENT

Monitor patients with inhalation, chemical, and electrical burns, as well as radiation-exposure patients, for signs of increasing complications associated with their burn mechanisms. Also monitor blood pressure, pulse, and respirations and trend any changes. Perform these evaluations every 15 minutes in stable patients and every 5 minutes in unstable patients.

SUMMARY

Burn injuries may compromise the skin—the protective envelope that protects and contains the human body. Burn damage to the skin may interfere with its ability to contain water within the body and to prevent damaging agents from entering. For these reasons, assessment and care of these soft-tissue injuries are important.

Assess the burn to determine its depth and the extent of the body surface area it involves. Be sensitive to any respiratory, joint, hand, foot, or circumferential regions affected by the burn. Give special consideration to pediatric and geriatric burn patients and to burn patients who are also ill or otherwise injured. Consider all these factors in determining the overall severity of a burn. If the patient's condition warrants, institute aggressive care. Anticipate airway compromise and fluid loss. Secure the airway very early in prehospital care. Initiate IV access and begin fluid administration.

Electrical, chemical, or radiation burns require special care and assessment. An electrical burn requires careful assessment to determine the area and depth of burn involvement and should be followed by wound site dressing and cardiac monitoring. Chemical burns need rapid and effective decontamination. Radiation burns call for extreme care in removing the patient from the radiation source and in providing decontamination and supportive care.

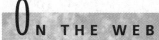

ON THE WEB

For additional practice and review, go to the companion website at www.prenhall.com/bledsoe and click on *Intermediate Emergency Care: Principles & Practice.*

Chapter 17

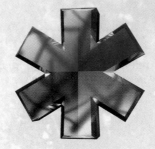

Thoracic Trauma

Objectives

CASE STUDY

Medic 101 responds to a shooting call at a Southside tavern where a man was reportedly shot during a robbery attempt. Victoria and Chris are the responding EMT-Is. They quickly size up the scene and determine it to be safe. Police are on the scene, have the assailant in custody, and have controlled the gathering crowd.

On their arrival, they find the patient supine just inside the tavern door. The tavern owner reports the man had tried to take cash from the register when he shot him with a .44 caliber handgun at close range. The initial assessment reveals a pale, ashen, weakly combative patient, who is confused. He gives his name as Conrad and his age as 34. His trachea is midline, the jugular veins are full, and there is no apparent use of accessory muscles of respiration. The EMT-Is note minimal bleeding without air leak from wounds found just below the left clavicle, left of the upper sternum, just to the right of the lower sternum, and close to the right nipple. Conrad is tachypneic with symmetrical chest rise and has slightly diminished breath sounds on the right. Radial pulses are not palpable, but weak, thready carotid pulses are present. No exit wounds are noted when the patient is log rolled and placed on a long backboard to stabilize the potential thoracolumbar spinal injury.

The patient is immediately placed on high-flow, high-concentration oxygen via nonrebreather mask, and his color improves somewhat. He is rapidly loaded into the ambulance, where bilateral antecubital large-bore IV lines are initiated and run wide open en route to Southside Hospital. Chris alerts medical direction and asks to have a trauma team standing by. As Victoria treats life threats identified during the initial assessment, she quickly reassesses the chest and notes that respirations are more labored and chest rise is no longer symmetrical. The right chest is somewhat hyperexpanded and demonstrates decreased breath sounds in comparison to the left. The patient appears more ashen, with carotid pulses now absent. His trachea appears somewhat deviated to the left with jugular venous distention also developing. Chris, suspecting tension pneumothorax, quickly re-contacts medical direction and receives an order to decompress the right chest. Victoria inserts a 14-gauge IV catheter in the right second intercostal space, along the midclavicular line and notes a significant rush of air. She observes improvement in the patient's color and better chest rise with less labored breathing. A subsequent ongoing assessment finds that the weak, thready carotid pulses have returned as the ambulance arrives at the hospital.

The emergency department physician and trauma team take over the patient's care, initiate an O-negative blood transfusion, intubate him, and place bilateral chest tubes for pneumothorax. A trauma x-ray series reveals one bullet in the area of the left scapula, another right of the thoracic spine, one in the right upper abdominal quadrant, and one in the midline upper abdomen. Continuing assessment now reveals the abdomen to be distended and that hypotension is continuing despite aggressive resuscitation with blood. The patient is rapidly transferred to the operative suite and an abdominal exploration is performed, revealing a liver laceration and partial abdominal aorta laceration. These injuries are repaired, and the patient survives.

INTRODUCTION

The thoracic cavity contains many vital structures including the heart, great vessels, esophagus, **tracheobronchial tree,** and lungs. Trauma to any one of these structures could lead to a life-threatening event. About 25% of all motor-vehicle deaths are due to thoracic trauma (about 12,000 per year in the United States). The majority of these deaths are secondary to injury to the heart and great vessels. In addition, abdominal injuries are also common in patients with traumatic chest injury and can cause significant **co-morbidity.**

tracheobronchial tree the structures of the trachea and the bronchi.

co-morbidity associated disease process.

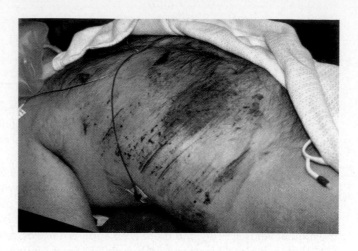

FIGURE 17-1 An example of blunt trauma to the chest. *(Courtesy of Edward T. Dickinson, MD)*

The incidence of blunt thoracic trauma has increased with the development of the modern automobile (Figure 17-1). Together with the development of a national highway system, more people are traveling greater distances, at greater speeds, and roadways are becoming more congested. This allows for an increased incidence of motor-vehicle collisions (MVCs) and thus an increase in the incidence of thoracic injuries and subsequent deaths, because most blunt thoracic trauma deaths are MVC related.

An increase in penetrating trauma has also been observed in urban areas associated with violent crime. The weapons used in violent crime in years past were likely to be of the "Saturday night special" variety, cheap small-caliber revolvers often producing just single wounds. The weapons of choice now are more likely to be large-caliber semi-automatic or automatic weapons that increase the likelihood of multiple missile injuries. With multiple wounds, there is a higher likelihood of injury to vital structures and therefore a higher mortality. Many advances in the treatment of penetrating thoracoabdominal trauma have been made in recent wars, and the incidence of mortality from these wounds has decreased from 8% to 40% in World War II to 3% to 18% today.

Prevention efforts include gun control legislation, firearm safety courses, seat belt laws, and better design of automobiles including passive restraint systems such as airbags. Statistics indicate that these efforts have already decreased the incidence of these injuries and the related morbidity and mortality.

In this chapter, you will find a discussion of thoracic trauma in relation to penetrating and blunt injury. These mechanisms have more clinical significance than simple injury categories. Certain injuries are almost exclusively associated with one type of chest trauma but unlikely with the other. For example, pericardial tamponade is almost exclusively associated with penetrating thoracic trauma whereas cardiac rupture is almost exclusively caused by blunt thoracic trauma. By considering the mechanism of injury, understanding the pathology of the various injuries, and by being aware of the patient's physical signs of injury and symptoms, you will be better able to predict, identify and treat potential life threats.

PATHOPHYSIOLOGY OF THORACIC TRAUMA

Thoracic trauma is classified into two major categories by mechanism—blunt and penetrating. It is important to examine these injury mechanisms and their effects on the organs of the thorax.

BLUNT TRAUMA

Blunt thoracic trauma is injury resulting from kinetic energy forces transmitted through the tissues. These injuries may be further subdivided by mechanism into blast, crush (compression), and deceleration injuries.

Blast injuries result from an explosive chemical reaction that creates a pressure wave traveling outward from the epicenter. This pressure wave causes tissue disruption by dramatic compression and then decompression as the wave passes. In the thorax, this action may tear blood vessels and disrupt the alveolar tissue. These injuries may lead to hemorrhage, pneumothoraces, and air embolism (air entering the disrupted pulmonary vasculature and subsequently returning to the central circulation). Other injuries associated with a blast mechanism can include disruption of the tracheobronchial tree and traumatic rupture of the diaphragm. When the blast occurs in a confined space, the pressure wave may be contained and accentuated. The result is an increase in the incidence and severity of the associated injuries.

Crush injuries occur when the body is compressed between an object and a hard surface. This leads to direct injury or disruption of the chest wall, diaphragm, heart, or tracheobronchial tree. If the victim remains pinned between two objects, significant restriction in ventilation and venous return may occur, also known as traumatic asphyxia.

Deceleration injuries occur when the body is in motion and impacts a fixed object as, for example, the chest against the steering column in a front-end collision (Figure 17-2). This impact causes a direct blunt injury to the chest wall while the internal organs of the thoracic cavity continue in motion. The organs and structures then impact with the internal surface of the thoracic cavity and may be compressed as more posterior structures collide with them. If the organ or structure has points of fixation, as with the aorta at the ligamentum arteriosum, the force of the organ moving against this point of fixation (shear force) can lead to a traumatic disruption. These sudden deceleration and shear forces can cause disruption of the myocardium, great vessel, lung, trachea, and bronchi. The rapid compression of the chest, especially against a closed glottis, may also cause alveolar and tracheobronchial rupture and pneumothorax.

The age of the blunt trauma victim may affect the trauma received and its seriousness. The cartilaginous nature of the pediatric thorax spares the infant or child from rib fractures but more easily transmits the energy of trauma to the vital organs below. The result is more minor signs of injury, few rib fractures, and a greater incidence of serious internal injury. The geriatric patient responds very differently to blunt chest trauma. That patient will suffer more frequent rib fracture than the younger adult due to calcification of the skeletal system. Though the greater incidence of rib fracture may somewhat protect the underlying organs, pre-existing disease and the progressive reduction of respiratory and cardiac reserves result in a greater morbidity and mortality from serious chest trauma.

The age of the blunt trauma victim may affect the seriousness of the trauma received.

PENETRATING TRAUMA

Penetrating thoracic trauma induces injury as an object enters the chest and causes either direct trauma or secondary injury from transmitted kinetic energy forces related to the cavitational wave of high-velocity projectiles. Penetrating chest trauma can be subdivided into three categories: low-energy, high-energy, and shotgun wounds.

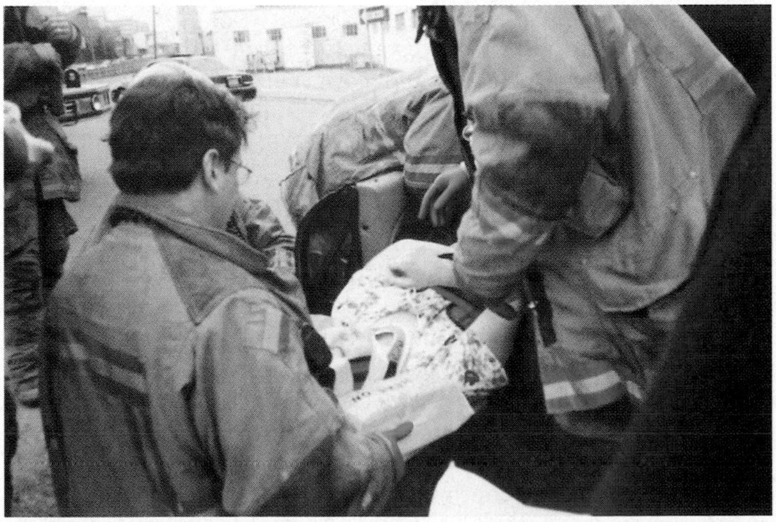

FIGURE 17-2 Frontal impact auto crashes frequently result in chest trauma.

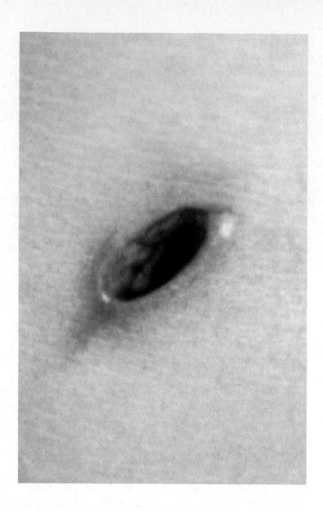

FIGURE 17-3 Penetrating (stab) wound to the chest.

Low-energy wounds are those caused by arrows, knives, handguns, and other relatively slow-moving objects (Figure 17-3). They cause injury by direct contact or very limited creation of temporary cavities. The injury that occurs from this type of wound is related to the direct path that the missile or object takes.

High-energy wounds are caused by military and hunting rifles (and some high-powered handguns at close range) that fire missiles at very high velocity. Their velocity gives the projectile very high kinetic energy. As the projectile passes through tissue, it creates a shock wave, tissue movement (including compression and stretching), and a large temporary cavity. These wounds cause extensive tissue damage perpendicular to the track of the projectile.

Shotgun wounds are classified according to the distance between the victim and the shotgun. A smaller gauge (a larger caliber) of shotgun and a larger size of shot also increase the effective range and penetrating power of the weapon and its potential to cause tissue damage. Type I injuries are those where the target is greater than 7 meters from the gun barrel at discharge. The pellets usually penetrate the skin and subcutaneous tissue but rarely penetrate the deep fascia to cause body cavity penetration. Type II injuries occur at a distance of 3 to 7 meters and often permit the pellets to penetrate the deep fascia with internal organ injury possible. Type III injuries occur at a distance of less than 3 meters and usually involve massive tissue destruction and life-threatening injury.

Penetrating thoracic trauma is often related to the structures involved. Lung tissue is very resilient when impacted by high-energy projectiles. The "spongy" nature of the air-filled alveoli absorbs the energy of cavitation and reduces the size of the temporary cavity and injury associated with the compression and stretching. The great vessels and heart (if it is distended with blood) respond much differently. The fluid transmits the kinetic energy very well and may result in cardiac or vessel rupture. With slower-moving projectiles or the heart in diastole the result may be a simple penetration. Although a projectile tends to move in a straight line, it is easily deflected by contact with a rib, clavicle, scapula, or the

Shotgun wounds within 3 meters of the discharging barrel cause serious tissue destruction and are frequently life threatening.

Table 17-1	INJURIES ASSOCIATED WITH PENETRATING THORACIC TRAUMA

Closed pneumothorax

Open pneumothorax (including sucking chest wound)

Tension pneumothorax

Pneumomediastinum

Hemothorax

Hemopneumothorax

Laceration of vascular structures, including the great vessels

Tracheobronchial tree lacerations

Esophageal lacerations

Penetrating cardiac injuries

Pericardial tamponade

Spinal cord injuries

Diaphragmatic penetration/laceration/rupture

Intra-abdominal penetration with associated organ injury

spinal column. Contact with skeletal structures may also fragment the projectile, increasing the rate of energy exchange and the seriousness of injury. Penetrating trauma frequently leads to pneumothorax, which may be bilateral, depending on the track of the missile or knife. Table 17-1 lists common injuries associated with penetrating thoracic trauma.

CHEST WALL INJURIES

Chest wall injuries are by far the most common injuries encountered in blunt chest trauma. As previously discussed, an intact and moving chest wall is necessary to develop the pressures essential for air movement into and out of the lungs (the bellows effect). Chest wall injury may disrupt this motion and result in respiratory insufficiency. Closed injuries of the chest wall include contusions, rib fractures, sternal fractures/dislocations, and flail chest. Open injuries to the chest wall are almost entirely due to penetrating trauma and are often associated with deep structure injury in addition to disruption of the changing intrathoracic pressure necessary for respiration.

Chest Wall Contusion

Chest wall contusion is the most common result of blunt injury to the thorax. The injury damages the soft tissue covering the thoracic cage and causes pain with respiratory effort. As with contusions elsewhere, contusion of the chest wall may present with erythema initially, then ecchymosis. The discoloration may outline the object that caused the trauma, may outline the ribs as the soft tissue is trapped between the ribs and the offending agent, or may outline a combination of both. The most noticeable symptom of chest wall contusion is pain, made worse with deep breathing and possibly resulting in reduced chest expansion. The area will be tender at the contusion site, and you may observe decreased chest wall movement resulting from pain. You may auscultate limited breath sounds due to decreased air movement resulting from limited chest expansion.

The pain of chest wall contusion and associated limiting of deep inspiration may lead to hypoventilation. Hypoventilation may not be apparent in a young, otherwise healthy, individual and may not pose a significant life threat due to the individual's significant pulmonary reserves. The aged patient, however, often has pre-existing medical problems, little pulmonary reserve, and does not tolerate this injury as well. Such a patient quickly becomes hypoxemic (low oxygen levels in the blood) without proper respiratory support. In a pediatric patient, the ribs are very flexible, resist fracture, and easily transmit the forces of trauma. The result may be chest wall contusion and internal injury without rib fracture.

Chest wall injuries are by far the most common injuries encountered in blunt chest trauma.

Content Review

SIGNS AND SYMPTOMS OF CHEST WALL INJURIES
- Blunt or penetrating trauma to chest
- Erythema
- Ecchymosis
- Dyspnea
- Pain on breathing
- Limited breath sounds
- Hypoventilation
- Crepitus
- Paradoxical motion of chest wall

Chest wall contusion is the most common result of blunt injury to the thorax.

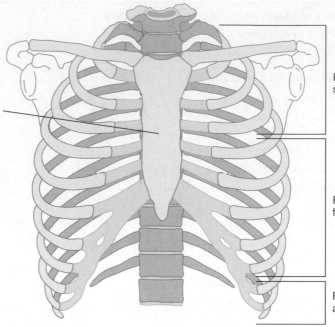

Great force is required for sternal fractures.

Ribs 1–3 are well protected by shoulder bones and muscles.

Ribs 4–8 are most frequently fractured.

Ribs 9–12 are relatively mobile and fracture less frequently.

FIGURE 17-4 Rib fractures.

Rib Fracture

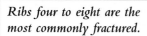

Rib fractures are found in more than 50% of cases of significant chest trauma from blunt mechanisms.

Ribs four to eight are the most commonly fractured.

In pediatric patients, more flexible ribs permit more serious internal injury before they fracture.

Rib fracture mortality increases with the number of fractures, extremes of age, and associated disease.

Rib fractures are found in more than 50% of cases of significant chest trauma from blunt mechanisms. Rib fractures are likely to occur at the point of impact or along the border of the object that impacts the chest (Figure 17-4). Fractures may also occur at a location remote from the injury site. The thoracic cage is a hollow cylinder that has some flex to it. As the compressional force of blunt trauma deforms the thorax, the ribs flex and may fracture at their weakest point—the posterior angle (along the posterior axillary line).

Ribs 4 through 8 are the most commonly fractured because they are least protected by other structures and are firmly fixed at both ends (to the spine and sternum). It takes great force to fracture the first three ribs because the shoulder, scapula, and the heavy musculature of the upper chest protect them. Their fracture is frequently associated with severe intrathoracic injuries (tracheobronchial tree injury, aortic rupture, and other vascular injuries), especially if multiple ribs are involved. Fracture of these ribs results in a mortality of up to 30% due to the associated injuries. Ribs 9 through 12 are less firmly attached to the sternum, are relatively mobile, and are thus less likely to fracture. However, they better transmit the energy of trauma to internal organs and may permit intra-abdominal injury without fracture. Fractures of ribs 9 through 12 are frequently associated with serious trauma and splenic or hepatic injury.

The incidence and significance of rib fracture varies with age. The pediatric patient has very cartilaginous ribs that bend easily. The ribs resist fracture and transmit kinetic forces to the thoracic and abdominal structures underneath. The pediatric patient hence has a decreased incidence of rib fracture and an increase in the incidence of underlying injury. The geriatric patient, on the other hand, has ribs that are calcified, less flexible, and more easily fractured. The geriatric patient is also more likely to have co-morbidity such as chronic obstructive pulmonary disease (COPD), which reduces respiratory reserves and compounds the effects of rib injury. If multiple rib fractures are noted in a young adult, they are probably associated with severe trauma and may lead to significant pain, splinting, hypoventilation, and inadequate cough. They also are likely to be associated with significant internal injuries. The mortality associated with rib fractures increases with the number of fractures, extremes of age (the very young or very old), and associated chronic respiratory or cardiac problems, especially in the elderly trauma victim.

The rib fracture is likely to be associated with an overlying chest wall contusion and presents with those signs and symptoms. The fracture site may also demonstrate a grating sensation (crepitus) as the bone ends move against each other, either during chest wall movement or during direct palpation. The pain associated with rib fracture is greater than that with chest wall contusion and will more greatly limit respiratory excursion. This reduced chest wall excursion frequently leads to hypoxia, hypoventilation, and muscle spasms at the fracture site. Hypoventilation can result in a progressive collapse of alveoli called atelectasis. This collapse reduces the lung surface available for gas exchange and contributes to hypoxia. These atelectatic segments also may become filled with blood or tissue fluid due to the injury and set the stage for secondary infection such as pneumonia. Although pneumonia does not develop in the emergency setting, it is the cause of a significant mortality in blunt chest injury patients. Serious internal injuries may also result as the jagged rib ends move about and lacerate structures beneath them. Laceration of the intercostal arteries may result in hemothorax, whereas damage to the intercostal nerves may result in a neurological deficit. Fracture and displacement of the lower ribs may injure the liver (right) or spleen (left).

Sternal Fracture and Dislocation

Sternal fractures and dislocations are usually associated with blunt anterior chest trauma. Sternal fracture results only from severe impact, as this region of the chest is well supported by the ribs and clavicles. The most likely mechanism is a direct blow, a fall against a fixed object, or the blunt force of the sternum against the steering wheel or dashboard in a motor-vehicle crash. The overall incidence of sternal fracture in thoracic trauma patients is between 5% and 8%. However, the mortality associated with it is between 25% and 45% due to underlying myocardial contusion, cardiac rupture, pericardial tamponade, and pulmonary contusion. If the surrounding ribs or costochondral joints are disrupted, the injury may result in a flail chest. The injury results in a noticeable deformity and possible crepitus with chest wall movement or palpation.

Sternal fracture is frequently associated with serious myocardial injury.

Dislocation at the sternoclavicular joint is uncommon and also requires significant force. It too may occur with blunt trauma to the anterior chest or with a lateral compression mechanism, as in side impact collisions or falls with the patient landing on the shoulder. The clavicle may dislocate from the sternum in one of two ways, anteriorly or posteriorly. The anterior dislocation creates a noticeable deformity anterior to the manubrium. The posterior dislocation displaces the head of the clavicle behind the sternum where it may compress or lacerate underlying great vessels or compress or injure the trachea and esophagus. Tracheal compression may result in stridor and voice change, though any deformity is more difficult to identify except that the shoulder may noticeably displace anteriorly and medially.

Flail Chest

Flail chest is a segment of the chest that becomes free to move with the pressure changes of respiration. The condition occurs when three or more adjacent ribs fracture in two or more places (Figure 17-5). It is one of the most serious chest wall injuries because it is often associated with severe underlying pulmonary injury (contusion) and it reduces the volume of respiration and increases the effort associated with it. This underlying injury adds to mortality in serious thoracic trauma (between 20% and 40%), as does age, head injury, shock, and other associated injuries. The most common mechanisms of injury causing flail chest are blunt traumas from falls, motor-vehicle crashes, industrial accidents, and assaults.

flail chest defect in the chest wall that allows for free movement of a segment. Breathing will cause paradoxical chest wall motion.

The flail segment created by this injury is no longer a controlled component of the chest wall and bellows system. Increasing intrathoracic pressure associated with expiration moves the flail segment outward while the rest of the chest moves inward, pushing air under the moving segment that would normally be exhaled. This reduces the change in chest volume caused by the breathing effort as well as the volume of air expired and draws the mediastinum toward the injury. During inspiration, the intrathoracic pressure falls as the respiratory muscles move the chest wall outward and the diaphragm drops caudally (tailward). The reduced pressure draws the flail segment inward. The lung beneath it moves away from the inward-moving segment, reducing the volume of air moving into the thorax and displacing the mediastinum away from the injury. In summary, the injury produces a segment of the chest wall that moves in opposition of the chest's normal respiratory effort (paradoxical movement), it reduces the volume of air moved with each breath, and it displaces

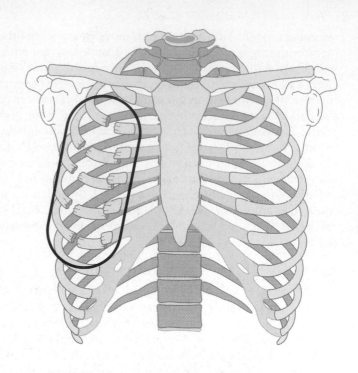

FIGURE 17-5 Flail chest occurs when three or more adjacent ribs fracture in two or more places.

the mediastinum toward and then away from the injury site with each breath (Figure 17-6). In flail chest, the patient takes more energy to move less air and the respiratory volume is further reduced as the rib fracture pain produces a natural splinting of the chest.

Over time, the muscles splinting the flail segment will fatigue and paradoxical respiration will become more evident.

It takes tremendous energy to create these six fracture sites (three or more ribs fractured in two or more places) and, accordingly, flail chest is often associated with serious internal injury. In addition, the movement of the flail segment, which is opposite to the rest of the chest wall is damaging to surrounding tissue. With each breath, the bone fracture sites move against one another causing further muscle damage, soft tissue damage, and pain. Small flail segments may go undetected as the associated intercostal muscle spasm naturally splints the segment. With time however, these muscles suffer further injury and fatigue, and the paradoxical movement of the flail segment may become more and more apparent.

Positive pressure ventilation of the patient with flail chest reverses the mechanism that causes the paradoxical chest wall movement, restores the tidal volume, and reduces the pain of chest wall movement. It accomplishes this by pushing the chest wall and the flail segment outward with positive pressure. Passive expiration then may cause both the flail segment and the rest of the chest to move inward, again, together.

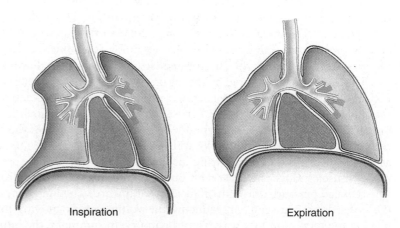

Inspiration   Expiration

FIGURE 17-6 Paradoxical movement of the chest wall seen in flail chest.

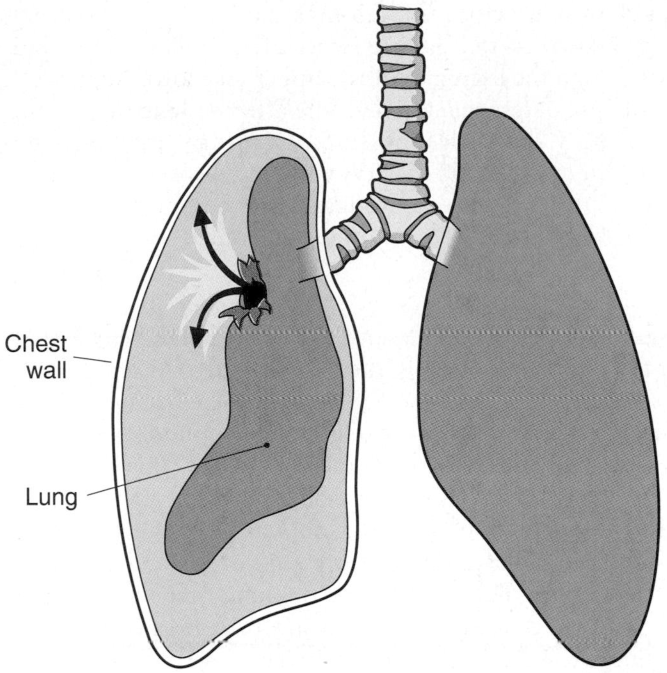

FIGURE 17-7 Simple (closed) pneumothorax.

PULMONARY INJURIES

Pulmonary injuries are injuries to lung tissue or injuries that damage the system that holds the lung to the interior of the thoracic cavity. They include the simple pneumothorax, open pneumothorax, tension pneumothorax, hemothorax, and pulmonary contusion.

Simple Pneumothorax

Simple **pneumothorax** (also known as closed pneumothorax) occurs when lung tissue is disrupted and air leaks into the pleural space (Figure 17-7). Although an external, and possibly penetrating, wound may be present, there is no communication between the pleural space and the atmosphere. The pressure within the thorax does not exceed normal expiratory pressures and there is no associated mediastinal shift. As more and more air accumulates in the pleural space, the lung collapses. With lung collapse, the alveoli collapse (atelectisis) and blood flowing past the collapsed alveoli does not exchange oxygen and carbon dioxide. As more and more of the alveoli collapse, this condition, called ventilation/perfusion mismatch becomes more pronounced and begins to lower the blood oxygen level (hypoxemia). This soon becomes life endangering, especially if there are other associated injuries or shock.

 Simple pneumothorax can occur with penetrating and blunt mechanisms. Blunt trauma may cause a pneumothorax when a rib fracture directly punctures the lung. Another mechanism may cause alveolar rupture from a sudden increase in intrathoracic pressure as the chest impacts the steering column with fully expanded lungs and a closed glottis (like a paper bag filled with air and compressed suddenly between two hands). The incidence of pneumothorax in serious thoracic trauma is between 10% and 30% and its morbidity is related to the amount of atelectisis and the degree of perfusion mismatch. Penetrating trauma to the chest is frequently associated with simple pneumothorax, or with an injury that allows air to enter the pleural space through an external wound (open pneumothorax).

 A simple pneumothorax reduces the efficiency of respiration and quickly leads to hypoxia. The hypoxia and increase in blood levels of CO_2 cause the medulla to increase the respiratory rate (tachypnea) and volume. If only a very small portion of the lung is involved, there may be no apparent signs or symptoms. A larger pneumothorax may cause mild dyspnea, or complete lung collapse may result in severe dyspnea and hypoxia. The signs, symptoms, and significance of simple pneumothorax increase with pre-existing disease.

pneumothorax air in the pleural space.

Content Review

SIGNS AND SYMPTOMS OF PNEUMOTHORAX

- Trauma to chest
- Chest pain on inspiration
- Hyperinflation of chest
- Diminished breath sounds on affected side

Pneumothorax may produce local chest pain with respiration as the pleurae become irritated (pleuritic pain). The pathology may cause the chest to hyperinflate and breath sounds to diminish on the affected side (usually in the extremes of the upper and lower lung first). A small pneumothorax involving collapse of less than 15% of the affected lung may be difficult to detect clinically and requires only supportive measures. Often the small pneumothorax will seal itself and the air in the pleural cavity will be absorbed. A larger pneumothorax is often clinically apparent and requires more aggressive therapy such as high-flow, high-concentration oxygen and chest tube placement (in the emergency department).

Open Pneumothorax

Open pneumothorax is most commonly noted in military conflicts when a high-velocity bullet creates a significant wound in the chest wall (usually the exit wound). Recently use of high-velocity assault weapons has become more common in civilian settings and thus the frequency of these injuries is on the increase. Another cause of open pneumothorax is a shotgun blast at close range with an associated large wound to the chest wall. This chest wall disruption leads to the free passage of air between the atmosphere and the pleural space (Figure 17-8). Air is drawn into the wound as the chest moves outward and the diaphragm moves downward during inspiration. The internal thoracic pressure drops and air rushes through the wound and into the chest cavity. This air replaces the lung tissue and permits its collapse and results in a large functional dead space. The inspiratory effort of the intact side of the chest draws the mediastinum toward it and away from the injury. This prevents the uninjured lung from fully inflating. On exhalation, the contracting chest wall and rising diaphragm increase the internal pressure and force air outward through the wound. This movement of air into and out of the chest through the wound is the cause of the "sucking" sound that leads to the wound's common name, "sucking chest wound."

For air movement to occur through the opening in the chest wall, the opening must be at least two-thirds the diameter of the trachea. Remember, the size of the trachea is about the size of the patient's little finger. This must be the size of the opening into the chest, not the size of the wound. The thickness and resiliency of the chest wall often closes the wound to air movement unless it is quite large. Then the remaining defect may permit the free movement of air and create an open pneumothorax.

The open pneumothorax can be recognized by the large open wound to the thorax and the characteristic air movement (or sound) it produces. Air passage through the wound and the wound's associated hemorrhage may produce frothy blood around the opening, another

Content Review

SIGNS AND SYMPTOMS OF OPEN PNEUMOTHORAX
- Penetrating chest trauma
- Sucking chest wound
- Frothy blood at wound site
- Severe dyspnea
- Hypovolemia

For air movement to occur through the opening in the chest wall, the opening must be at least two-thirds the diameter of the trachea.

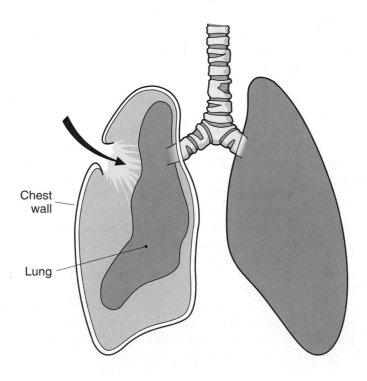

FIGURE 17-8   Open pneumothorax (sucking chest wound).

Chest wall

Lung

characteristic of the open pneumothorax. The patient is likely to experience severe dyspnea, and possibly hypovolemia from associated injury and hemorrhage. The patient's condition is further compromised because the reduced intrathoracic pressures developed during inspiration do not complement venous return to the heart as they do with the intact thorax and respiratory effort.

Tension Pneumothorax

Tension pneumothorax is an open or simple pneumothorax that generates and maintains a pressure greater than atmospheric pressure within the thorax. It may be caused by a traumatic mechanism and injury or possibly by positive pressure ventilation of a patient with chest trauma or congenital defect affecting the respiratory tree. Tension pneumothorax may also occur because an open pneumothorax is sealed and an internal injury or defect permits a build-up of pressure.

Tension pneumothorax occurs because the mechanism of injury (either the external wound, or the internal injury) forms a one-way valve. Air flows into the pleural space through the defect during inspiration as the pressure within the pleural space is less than atmospheric. With expiration, the increasing pleural pressure closes the defect and does not permit air to escape. With each breath, the volume of air and the pressure within the pleural space increase. The increasing intrapleural pressure collapses the lung on the ipsilateral (same or injury) side, causes intercostal and suprasternal bulging, and begins to exert pressure against the mediastinum. As the pressure continues to build, it displaces the mediastinum, compressing the uninjured lung and crimping the vena cava as it enters the thorax through the diaphragm or where it attaches to the heart. This reduces venous return, results in an increase in venous pressure, causes the jugular veins to distend (JVD), and narrows the pulse pressure. Tracheal shift may occur as the mediastinal structures are pushed away from the increasing pressure. This is a very late and rare finding and more commonly seen in the young trauma victim as the pediatric mediastinum is more mobile than that of the adult. Atelectasis occurs in the ipsilateral side from the initial lung collapse and on the contralateral (uninjured or opposite) side from the mediastinal shift and compression of that lung. These mechanisms lead to ventilation/perfusion mismatch, further hypoxemia, and systemic hypoxia.

Tension pneumothorax begins with the presentation of a simple or open pneumothorax (Figure 17-9). As the pressure in the pleural space begins to increase, dyspnea, ventilation/perfusion mismatch, and hypoxemia develop. The ipsilateral side of the chest becomes hyperinflated, hyperresonant to percussion, and respiratory sounds become very faint, then absent. The pressure may cause the intracostal tissues to bulge. The opposite or contralateral side of the chest becomes somewhat dull to percussion, with progressively fainter respiratory sounds as the tension pneumothorax becomes worse. Severe hypoxia results in cyanosis, diaphoresis, and an altered mental status while the increased intrathoracic pressure reduces venous return and may cause JVD and hypotension. If the condition is not quickly recognized and promptly treated, it may lead to death.

Tension pneumothorax is a serious and immediate life threat. It is corrected by relieving the intrapleural pressure by inserting a needle through the chest wall to convert the tension pneumothorax to an open pneumothorax. If a valve is added to the decompression needle, it may permit only the escape of air during respiration. If there is no continuing internal defect, this may progressively re-expand the collapsed lung and return effective respiration.

Hemothorax

Hemothorax is simply the accumulation of blood in the pleural space due to internal hemorrhage. It can be very minor and not detectable in the field or, when associated with serious or great vessel injury, may result in rapid patient deterioration. Serious hemorrhage may displace a complete lung, accumulate over 1,500 mL of blood quickly and produce a mortality rate of 75%, with most, approximately two-thirds, of those dying at the scene. Hemothorax is primarily a blood loss problem as each side of the thorax may hold up to 3,000 mL of blood (or half the total blood volume). However, the blood lost into the thorax reduces the tidal volume and efficiency of respiration in a patient who has already suffered trauma and is likely to move quickly into shock.

tension pneumothorax buildup of air under pressure within the thorax. The resulting compression of the lung severely reduces the effectiveness of respirations.

Content Review

SIGNS AND SYMPTOMS OF TENSION PNEUMOTHORAX

- Chest trauma
- Dyspnea
- Ventilation/perfusion mismatch
- Hypoxemia
- Hyperinflation of affected side of chest
- Hyperresonance of affected side of chest
- Diminished, then absent breath sounds
- Cyanosis
- Diaphoresis
- Altered mental status
- Jugular venous distention
- Hypotension
- Hypovolemia

Tension pneumothorax is a serious and immediate life threat.

hemothorax blood within the pleural space.

Content Review

SIGNS AND SYMPTOMS OF HEMOTHORAX

- Blunt or penetrating chest trauma
- Signs and symptoms of shock
- Dyspnea
- Dull percussive sounds over site of injury

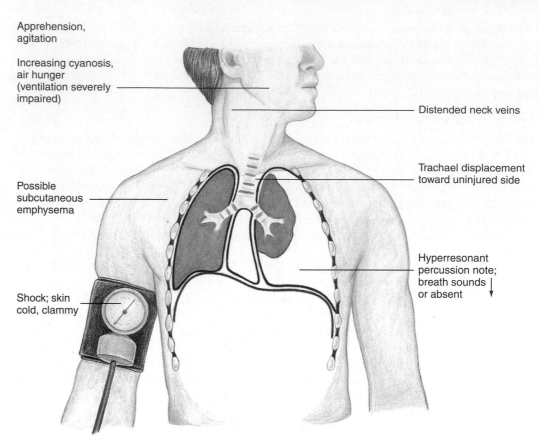

Apprehension, agitation

Increasing cyanosis, air hunger (ventilation severely impaired)

Possible subcutaneous emphysema

Shock; skin cold, clammy

Distended neck veins

Trachael displacement toward uninjured side

Hyperresonant percussion note; breath sounds ↓ or absent

FIGURE 17-9 Physical findings of tension pneumothorax.

Hemothorax is frequently associated with rib fractures and can be associated with either blunt or penetrating mechanisms. It often accompanies pneumothorax (a **hemopneumothorax**) and occurs 25% of the time with penetrating trauma. Hemorrhage into the pleural space may occur from a lung laceration (most common) or laceration of the intercostal arteries, pulmonary arteries, great vessels, or internal mammary arteries. The intercostal arteries can bleed at a rate of 50 mL/min. The bleeding into the chest is more rapid than would occur elsewhere because the pressure within the chest is often less than atmospheric pressure (Laplace's law). The blood lost into the hemothorax contributes to hypovolemia and displaces lung tissue. If the accumulation is significant, it may cause significant hypovolemia and shock, hypoxemia, respiratory distress, and respiratory failure.

The patient with hemothorax will have either a blunt or penetrating injury similar to those associated with open or simple pneumothorax. The patient may also display the signs and symptoms of shock and some respiratory distress (Figure 17-10). The blood pools in the lower chest in the seated patient or posterior chest in the supine patient. The lungs present with normal percussion and breath sounds except directly over the accumulating fluid. There the lung percussion is very dull and breath sounds are very distant, if they can be heard at all.

Pulmonary Contusion

Pulmonary contusions are simply soft tissue contusions affecting the lung. They are present in 30% to 75% of patients with significant blunt chest trauma and are frequently associated with rib fracture. Pulmonary contusions range in severity from very limited, minor, and unrecognizable injuries, to those that are extensive and quickly life threatening. They result in a mortality rate of between 14% and 20% of serious chest trauma patients.

Two specific mechanisms of injury allow the transfer of energy to the pulmonary tissue and result in pulmonary contusions. They are deceleration and the pressure wave associated with either passage of a high-velocity bullet or explosion. Deceleration injury occurs as the moving body strikes a fixed object. A common example of this mechanism is chest impact

hemopneumothorax condition in which air and blood are in the pleural space.

Content Review

SIGNS AND SYMPTOMS OF PULMONARY CONTUSION
- Blunt or penetrating chest trauma
- Increasing dyspnea
- Hypoxia
- Increasing crackles
- Diminishing breath sounds
- Hemotypsis
- Signs and symptoms of shock

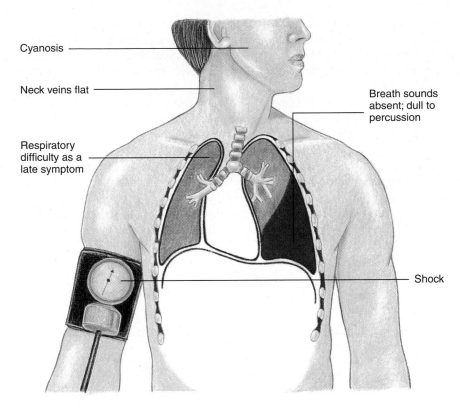

Cyanosis

Neck veins flat

Respiratory difficulty as a late symptom

Breath sounds absent; dull to percussion

Shock

FIGURE 17-10 Physical findings of massive hemothorax.

Patho Pearls

The thoracic cavity contains three general regions: the pericardial region, the pulmonary region, and the mediastinum. The pericardial region contains the heart and the origin of the great vessels. The pulmonary region contains the lungs, the airways, and the pulmonary vasculature. The mediastinum contains the esophagus, the vagus nerve, the thoracic duct, and other essential structures. Despite these, the thoracic cavity primarily involves respiratory and cardiac functions. Thus, with any thoracic injury, you would expect to see first a variation in respiratory function, cardiac function, or both. With a pneumothorax, you initially will see a subtle increase in respiratory rate and then, as the process progresses, increased respiratory effort and, finally, signs and symptoms of poor oxygenation. If this is allowed to progress untreated, cardiovascular impairment will follow. Cardiovascular impairment can result from incomplete ventricular filling due to increased intrathoracic pressure or from blood loss within the lung parenchyma.

Similarly, a penetrating injury to the heart can lead to cardiovascular collapse. With low-energy wounds, such as knife stab wounds, the pericardial sac may fill with blood thus preventing adequate ventricular filling (pericardial tamponade). This will be manifest as an initial increase in heart rate, narrowing of the pulse pressure (due to restricted ventricular filling), and distended neck veins. As cardiac efficiency declines, the pulmonary vasculature can become congested resulting in poor oxygenation. High-energy wounds that penetrate the heart are usually mortal wounds—even in the best of EMS systems and trauma centers.

Any time you have a patient with a suspected thoracic injury, first look at the respiratory or circulatory system for signs of impairment. These findings can help guide you to the exact nature of your patient's injury.

with the steering wheel during an auto crash. As the chest wall contacts the wheel and stops, the lungs continue forward, compressing and stretching the alveolar tissue or shearing it from the relatively fixed tracheobronchial tree. This causes disruption at the alveolar/capillary membrane leading to microscopic hemorrhage and edema. The second mechanism, the pressure wave of an explosion or bullet's passage, dramatically compresses and stretches the lung tissue. Due to the nature of the lung tissue (air-filled sacs surrounded by delicate and vascular membranes), the passage of this pressure is partially reflected at the gas/fluid (alveolar/capillary) interface. This leaves small, flame-shaped areas of disruption throughout the membrane leading to microhemorrhage and edema (called the Spalding effect). Pulmonary contusion is not generally associated with low-speed penetration of the chest and laceration of the lung tissues and structures.

The overall magnitude of pulmonary injury depends on the degree of deformity or stretch, and the velocity at which it occurs. Similar pulmonary contusions may result from different mechanisms. For example, an AK-47 round fired at 2,300 ft/sec striking body armor and deforming the chest wall instantaneously by 1 to 2 cm (high velocity) may cause pulmonary contusions similar to chest impact during an MVA where the chest is deformed 50% as it strikes the steering wheel at 50 ft/sec (low velocity).

Microhemorrhage into the alveolar tissue associated with pulmonary contusion may be extensive and result in up to 1,000 mL to 1,500 mL of blood loss. This hemorrhage into the tissue of the alveoli also causes irritation, initiates the inflammation process, and causes fluid to migrate into the region. The accumulation of fluid in the alveolar/capillary membrane (pulmonary edema) progressively increases its dimension and decreases the rate at which gases, and especially oxygen, can diffuse across it. The fluid accumulation also stiffens the membrane, makes the lung less compliant, and increases the work necessary to move air in and out of the affected tissue.

The thickening wall reduces the efficiency of respiration and results in hypoxemia, while the stiffening makes respiration more energy consuming. The development of edema also increases the pressure necessary to move blood through the capillary beds. This increases the pressure within the pulmonary vascular system (pulmonary hypertension) and the workload of the right heart. In combination, these effects lead to atelectasis, hypovolemia, ventilation/perfusion mismatch, hypoxemia, hypotension and, possibly, respiratory failure and shock. Although isolated pulmonary contusions can occur, they are frequently associated with chest wall injury and injuries elsewhere (87% of the time).

The patient with pulmonary contusion presents with a mechanism of injury and evidence of blunt or penetrating chest impact. Although the associated injuries may display immediate signs and symptoms (as in the pain of a rib fracture), the signs and symptoms of the pulmonary contusion take time to develop. The patient will likely complain of increasing dyspnea, demonstrate increasing respiratory effort, and show the signs of hypoxia. Oxygen saturation may gradually fall as the pathology develops. Careful auscultation of the chest may reveal increasing crackles and fainter breath sounds. Serious pulmonary contusion may cause **hemoptysis** (coughing up blood) and the signs and symptoms of shock.

CARDIOVASCULAR INJURIES

Cardiovascular injuries are the subset of thoracic trauma that leads to the most fatalities. They include myocardial contusion, pericardial tamponade, myocardial aneurysm or rupture, aortic aneurysm or rupture, and other vascular injuries.

Myocardial Contusion

Myocardial contusion is a frequent result of trauma and may occur in 76% of all serious chest trauma. It carries a high mortality rate and occurs most commonly with severe blunt anterior chest trauma. Here, the chest is struck by or strikes an object. The heart, which is relatively mobile within the chest, impacts the inside of the anterior chest wall and then may be compressed between the sternum and the thoracic spine as the thorax flexes with impact. The resulting contusion will most likely affect the right atrium and right ventricle (Figure 17-11). This is related to the heart's position in the chest, rotated somewhat counterclockwise and presenting the right atrium and ventricle surfaces toward the sternum.

The cardiac contusion is similar to a contusion in any other muscle tissue. The injury disrupts the muscle cells and microcirculation, resulting in muscle fiber tearing and damage, hemorrhage, and edema. The injury may reduce the strength of cardiac contraction and reduce cardiac output. Because of the automaticity and conductivity of the cardiac muscle, contusion may also disturb the cardiac electrical system. If the injury is serious, it may lead to hematoma, hemoperitoneum (blood in the peritoneal sac), and necrosis and may result in cardiac irritability, ectopic (irregularly occurring) beats, and conduction system defects

hemoptysis coughing up of blood that has origin in the respiratory tract.

Content Review

SIGNS AND SYMPTOMS OF CARDIAC CONTUSION
- Blunt injury to chest
- Bruising of chest wall
- Rapid heart rate—may be irregular
- Severe nagging pain not relieved with rest but may be relieved with oxygen

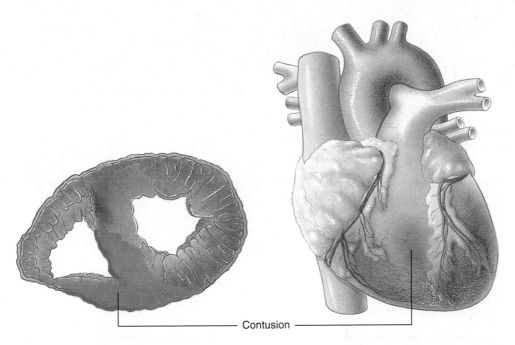

Contusion

FIGURE 17-11 Myocardial contusion most frequently affects the right atrium and ventricle as they collide with the sternum.

such as bundle branch blocks and dysrhythmias. If the injury is very extensive, it may lead to tissue necrosis (death), decreased ventricular compliance, congestive heart failure, cardiogenic shock, myocardial aneurysm, and acute or delayed myocardial rupture. In contrast to a myocardial infarction from coronary artery disease, the cellular damage from myocardial contusions heals with less scarring and there is no progression of the injury in the absence of associated coronary artery disease.

The patient experiencing myocardial contusion will have a history of significant blunt chest trauma, most likely affecting the anterior chest. The patient will likely complain of chest or retrosternal pain, very much like that of myocardial infarction and may have associated chest injuries such as anterior rib or sternal fractures. Cardiac monitoring most frequently reveals sinus tachycardia (though it may be caused by pain, hypovolemia, or hypoxia from associated chest injury). Other dysrhythmias associated with myocardial contusions are atrial flutter or fibrillation, premature atrial or ventricular contractions, tachydysrhythmias, bradydysrhythmias, bundle branch patterns, T wave inversions, and ST segment elevations. A pericardial friction rub and murmur may be auscultated over the **precordium** but is more likely to occur weeks after the injury and is associated with the development of an inflammatory pericardial effusion.

Pericardial Tamponade

Pericardial tamponade is a restriction to cardiac filling caused by blood (or other fluid) within the pericardial sac. It occurs in less than 2% of all serious chest trauma patients and is almost always related to penetrating injury. Gunshot wounds are the most frequent mechanism and carry a high overall mortality, though they often result in rapid hemorrhage through the myocardial wall and then out the defect in the pericardium. The frequency of gunshot wound mortality is probably related to the depth of injury, the degree of cardiac tissue damage caused by the cavitational wave, and a more rapid progression of the pathology.

The pathology of pericardial tamponade begins with a tear in a superficial coronary artery or penetration of the myocardium. Blood seeps into the pericardial space and accumulates (Figure 17-12). The fibrous pericardium does not stretch and the accumulating blood exerts pressure on the heart. The pressure limits cardiac filling, first affecting the right ventricle where the pressure of filling is the lowest. This restricts venous return to the heart, increases venous pressure, and causes jugular vein distention. The reduced right ventricular output limits outflow to the pulmonary arteries and then venous return to the left heart. The

precordium area of the chest wall overlying the heart.

pericardial tamponade a restriction to cardiac filling caused by blood (or other fluid) within the pericardial sac.

Content Review

SIGNS AND SYMPTOMS OF PERICARDIAL TAMPONADE
- Dyspnea and possible cyanosis
- Jugular venous distention
- Weak, thready pulse
- Decreasing blood pressure
- Shock
- Dyspnea and possible cyanosis

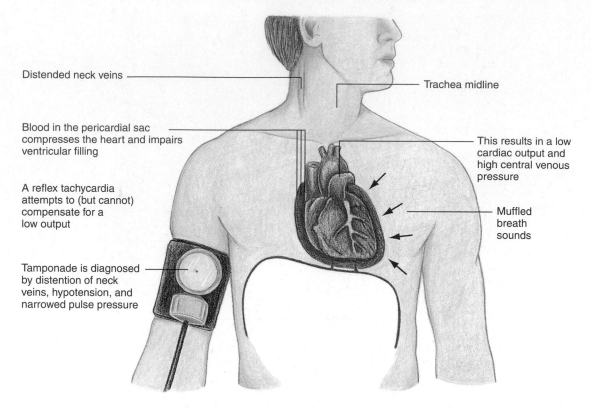

Distended neck veins

Trachea midline

Blood in the pericardial sac compresses the heart and impairs ventricular filling

This results in a low cardiac output and high central venous pressure

A reflex tachycardia attempts to (but cannot) compensate for a low output

Muffled breath sounds

Tamponade is diagnosed by distention of neck veins, hypotension, and narrowed pulse pressure

FIGURE 17-12 Physical findings of cardiac tamponade.

result is a decreasing cardiac output and systemic hypotension. The pressure exerted by the blood in the pericardium also restricts the flow of blood through the coronary arteries and to the myocardium. This may result in myocardial ischemia and infarct. It takes about 200 to 300 mL of blood to exert the pressure necessary to induce frank tamponade, while removing as little as 20 mL may provide significant relief. The progression of pericardial tamponade depends on the rate of blood flow into the pericardium. It may occur very rapidly and result in death before the arrival of emergency medical services or may gradually progress over hours.

The patient experiencing pericardial tamponade will likely have penetrating trauma to the anterior or posterior chest, though blunt trauma can also cause this problem. Although the trajectories of missiles and knife blades are difficult to predict, consider pericardial tamponade with any thoracic or upper abdominal penetrating wound, especially if it is over the precordium (central lower chest). Pericardial tamponade will diminish the strength of pulses, decrease the pulse pressure, and distend the jugular veins (JVD). The patient will likely be agitated, tachycardic, diaphoretic, and ashen in appearance. Cyanosis may be noted in the head, neck, and upper extremities. Heart tones may be muffled or distant sounding. Beck's triad (JVD, distant heart tones, and hypotension) is indicative of pericardial tamponade but may not be recognized early in the injury's progression. Another sign of pericardial tamponade is Kussmaul's sign, the decrease or absence of JVD during inspiration. As the patient inspires, the reduced intrathoracic pressure increases venous return and decreases the pressure the accumulating pericardial fluid exerts on the heart. This then translates to a better venous return and cardiac output during inspiration and the effect then seen in the jugular veins.

Other findings during pericardial tamponade may include pulsus paradoxus and electrical alternans. **Pulsus paradoxus** is a drop in systolic blood pressure of greater than 10 mmHg as the patient inspires during the normal respiratory cycle. (Normally the systolic blood pressure drops just slightly with each inspiration.) Pulsus paradoxus results because cardiac output increases with the minimal relief of the tamponade associated with the reduced intrathoracic pressure of inspiration. **Electrical alternans,** which is only rarely seen in

pulsus paradoxus drop of greater than 10 mmHg in the systolic blood pressure during the inspiratory phase of respiration that occurs in patients with pericardial tamponade.

electrical alternans alternating amplitude of the P, QRS, and T waves on the ECG rhythm strip as the heart swings in a pendulum-like fashion within the pericardial sac during tamponade.

acute pericardial tamponade, is noted on the cardiac rhythm strip as the P, QRS, and T amplitude decreasing with every other cardiac cycle. In profound pericardial tamponade, the heart displays a rhythm without producing a pulse (PEA).

Myocardial Aneurysm or Rupture

Myocardial **aneurysm** or rupture occurs almost exclusively in extreme blunt thoracic trauma as in automobile collisions. It also has been reported in cases where the blunt forces are not extreme, such as a result of CPR. The condition can affect any of the heart's chambers, the interatrial septum, the interventricular septum, or involve the valves and their supporting structures. Multiple heart chambers or structures are involved 30% of the time. Aneurysm and delayed myocardial rupture also occur secondary to necrosis from a myocardial infarction, repaired penetrating injury, or myocardial contusion. Necrosis usually develops around 2 weeks after the injury as inflammatory cells degrade the injured cells, weakening the tissue, and leading to aneurysm of the ventricular wall and/or subsequent rupture. Rupture can also occur with high velocity projectile injury as the bullet impacts the distended heart chamber.

The patient who experiences myocardial rupture will likely have suffered serious blunt or penetrating trauma to the chest and may have severe rib or sternal fracture. Specific symptoms may depend on the actual pathology. The victim may have the signs and symptoms of pericardial tamponade if the rupture is contained within the pericardial sac. If the pathology only affects the valves, the patient may present with the signs and symptoms of right or left heart failure. If there is myocardial aneurysm, rupture may be delayed. When it happens, the patient will suddenly present with the absence of vital signs or the signs and symptoms of pericardial tamponade.

Traumatic Aneurysm or Rupture of the Aorta

Aortic aneurysm and rupture are extremely life-threatening injuries resulting from either blunt or penetrating trauma. The aorta is most commonly injured by blunt trauma, carries an overall mortality of 85% to 95%, and is responsible for 15% of all thoracic trauma deaths. Aneurysm and rupture are usually associated with high-speed automobile crashes (most commonly lateral impact) and in some cases with high falls. Unlike myocardial rupture, a significant number, possibly as high as 20%, of these victims will survive the initial insult and aneurysm. Approximately 30% of these initial survivors will die within 6 hours if not treated, increasing to about 50% at 24 hours, and just under 70% by the end of the first week. It is this subset of patients who survive the initial impact and are alive at the scene that you can benefit the most by recognizing the potential injury and then by rapidly extricating, packaging, and transporting the patients to the trauma center.

The aorta is a large high-pressure vessel that provides outflow from the left ventricle for distribution to the body. It is relatively fixed at three points as it passes through the thoracic cavity and, because of this, experiences shear forces secondary to severe deceleration of the chest. The areas of fixation are the aortic annulus where the aorta joins the heart, the aortic isthmus where it is joined by the ligamentum arteriosum, and the diaphragm where it exits the chest (see Table 17-2). Traumatic dissecting aneurysm occurs infrequently to the ascending aorta and, most commonly, to the descending aorta. With severe deceleration, shear forces separate the layers of the artery, specifically the interior surface (the tunica intima) from the muscle layer (the tunica media). This allows blood to enter and, because it

> **aneurysm** a weakening or ballooning in the wall of a blood vessel.

> *Traumatic rupture of the thoracic aorta is almost always fatal.*

> *Serious lateral chest impact carries a high incidence of dissecting aortic aneurysm.*

Table 17-2	INCIDENCE AND ANATOMIC LOCATION OF TRAUMATIC AORTIC RUPTURE	
Aortic annulus		9%
Aortic isthmus		85%
Diaphragm		3%
Other		3%

is under great pressure, it begins to dissect the aortic lining like a bulging inner tube. It is likely to rupture if it is not surgically repaired.

The patient with aortic rupture will be severely hypotensive, quickly lose all vital signs, and die unless moved into surgery immediately. Dissecting aortic aneurysm progresses more slowly, though the aneurysm may rupture at any moment. The patient will probably have a history of a high fall or severe auto impact and deceleration. Lateral impact is an especially high-risk factor for aortic aneurysm. The patient may complain of severe tearing chest pain that may radiate to the back. The patient may have a pulse deficit between the left and right upper extremities and/or reduced pulse strength in the lower extremities. Blood pressure may be high (hypertension) due to stretching of sympathetic nerve fibers present in the aorta near the ligamentum arteriosum, or the pressure may be low due to leakage and hypovolemia. Auscultation may reveal a harsh systolic murmur due to turbulence as the blood exits the heart and passes the disrupted blood vessel wall.

OTHER VASCULAR INJURIES

The pulmonary arteries and vena cava are other thoracic vascular structures that can sustain injury during chest trauma. Their injury, and the resulting hemorrhage, may cause significant hemothorax, possibly leading to hypotension and respiratory insufficiency. The blood may also flow into the mediastinum and compress the great vessels, esophagus, and heart. Penetrating trauma is the primary cause of injury to the pulmonary arteries and vena cava.

The patient with pulmonary artery or vena cava injuries will likely have a penetrating wound to the central chest or elsewhere with a likelihood of central chest involvement. These injuries present with the signs and symptoms of hypovolemia and shock and result in hemothorax or hemomediastinum and then the signs and symptoms associated with those pathologies.

OTHER THORACIC INJURIES

Traumatic Rupture or Perforation of the Diaphragm

Traumatic rupture or perforation of the diaphragm can occur in both high-pressure blunt thoracoabdominal trauma as well as in penetrating trauma. Incidence is estimated from 1% to 6% of all patients with multiple trauma. It is more common in patients sustaining penetrating trauma to the lower chest, which has as much as a 30% to 40% incidence of abdominal organ and tissue involvement. Remember that during expiration the diaphragm may move superiorly to the level of the fourth intercostal space (nipple level) anteriorly and the sixth intercostal space posteriorly. Any penetrating injuries at these levels or below may penetrate the diaphragm. Diaphragmatic perforation and herniation occur most frequently on the left side because assailants are most frequently right handed and the size and solid nature of the liver protect the diaphragm on the right. The liver is also unlikely to herniate through the torn diaphragm unless the injury is sizeable.

Suspect diaphragmatic perforation with any penetrating injury to the lower thorax.

If traumatic diaphragmatic rupture occurs, the abdominal organs may herniate through the defect into the thoracic cavity causing strangulation or necrosis of the bowel, restriction of the ipsilateral lung, and displacement of the mediastinum. Mediastinal displacement occurs when the displaced abdominal contents place pressure on the lung and mediastinal structures, moving them toward the contralateral side through much the same mechanism as is seen in tension pneumothorax.

Diaphragmatic rupture presents with signs and symptoms similar to tension pneumothorax, including, dyspnea, hypoxia, hypotension, and JVD. The patient will have a history of blunt abdominal trauma or penetrating trauma to the lower thorax. The abdomen may appear hollow, and bowel sounds may be noted in one side of the thorax (most commonly the left). The patient may be hypotensive and hypoxic if the herniation is extensive. The patient may complain of upper abdominal pain, though this symptom is often overshadowed by other injuries. Diaphragmatic rupture may be recognized at the time of injury or may be missed if not extensive and present with delayed herniation months to years later.

Traumatic Esophageal Rupture

Traumatic esophageal rupture is a rare complication of blunt thoracic trauma. The incidence of it related to penetrating trauma of the thorax is somewhat higher but still only about 0.4%. Since the esophagus is rather centrally located within the chest, its injury usually coincides with other mediastinal injuries. (Esophageal rupture may also be the result of medical problems such as violent emesis, carcinoma, anatomic distortion, or gastric reflux.) Esophageal rupture carries a 30% mortality rate, even if quickly recognized, and mortality is much greater if this injury is not diagnosed promptly. The life threat from esophageal rupture is related to material entering the mediastinum as it passes down the esophagus or as emesis comes up. This results in serious infection or chemical irritation and serious damage to the mediastinal structures. Air may also enter the mediastinum through an esophageal rupture, especially during positive pressure ventilations.

The patient with espohageal rupture will probably have deep penetrating trauma to the central chest and may complain of difficult or painful swallowing, pleuritic chest pain, and pain radiating to the mid back. The patient may also display subcutaneous emphysema around the lower neck.

Tracheobronchial Injury (Disruption)

Tracheobronchial injury is a relatively rare finding in thoracic trauma with an incidence of less than 3% in patients with significant chest trauma. It may occur from either a blunt or a penetrating injury mechanism and carries a relatively high mortality similar to esophageal rupture of 30%. In contrast to patients with esophageal rupture who usually die days after injury, 50% of patients with tracheobronchial injury die within 1 hour of injury. Disruption can occur anywhere in the tracheobronchial tree but is most likely to occur within 2.5 cm of the carina.

The patient with disruption of the trachea or mainstem bronchi is generally in respiratory distress with cyanosis, hemoptysis, and, in some cases, massive subcutaneous emphysema. The patient may also experience pneumothorax and possibly, tension pneumothorax. Intermittent positive pressure ventilation drives air into the pleura or mediastinum and makes the condition worse.

Traumatic Asphyxia

Traumatic asphyxia occurs when severe compressive force is applied to the thorax and leads to backward flow of blood from the right heart into the superior vena cava and into the venous vessels of the upper extremities. (Traumatic asphyxia is not as much a respiratory problem as it is a vascular problem.) Traumatic asphyxia engorges the veins and capillaries of the head and neck with desaturated venous blood, turning the skin in this region a deep red, purple, or blue. The back flow of blood damages the microcirculation in the head and neck, producing petechiae (small hemorrhages under the skin) and stagnating blood above the point of compression. The back flow may damage cerebral circulation, resulting in numerous small strokes in the older patient whose venous vessels are not very elastic. If flow restriction continues, toxins and acids accumulate in the blood and may have a devastating effect when they return to the central circulation with the release of pressure. If the thoracic compression continues, it restricts venous return and may prevent the victim from ventilating. This results in hypotension, hypoxemia, and shock. Death may follow rapidly. Extrication of the patient may result in rapid hemorrhage from the injury site with release of the pressure. Release of the compression may likewise result in rapid patient deterioration and death.

The traumatic asphyxia patient will have suffered a severe compression force to the chest that is likely to continue until extrication. The result of the compression, the back flow of blood and restricted blood flow, will be dramatic and cause the classical discoloration of the head and neck regions. The face appears swollen, the eyes bulge, and there are numerous conjunctival hemorrhages. The patient may have severe dyspnea related to the compression and injuries associated with severe chest impact. Once the pressure is released, the patient may show the signs of hypovolemia, hypotension, and shock as well as signs related to any co-existing respiratory problems.

> *You must be ready to immediately handle the complications of traumatic asphyxia as soon as the patient is released from entrapment.*
>

ASSESSMENT OF THE THORACIC TRAUMA PATIENT

The proper assessment of the patient with a severe chest injury mechanism is critical to anticipating injury and providing the correct interventions. Although the approach to this patient follows the standard format for assessment, special considerations regarding chest trauma occur during the scene size-up, initial assessment, and especially during the rapid trauma assessment. The ongoing assessment is also critical for monitoring the thoracic trauma patient for the progression of injuries sustained during serious chest trauma.

SCENE SIZE-UP

Chest injury care, like any other serious trauma, requires BSI precautions with gloves as a minimum. Consider a face shield if you will be attending to the airway and a gown for splash protection with serious penetrating thoracic trauma. Ensure the scene is safe, including protection from the assailant, if penetrating trauma is suspected.

Examine the mechanism of injury carefully and try to determine if the central chest (heart, great vessels, trachea, and esophagus) might be in the pathway of penetrating trauma. In gunshot injuries, determine the type of weapon, caliber, distance between the gun barrel and the victim, and the probable pathway of the projectile. Determine the direction of blunt trauma impact as it may also have a bearing on which organs sustain injury. Anterior impact may rupture lung tissue and contuse the lung and heart. Lateral impact may tear the aorta as the heart displaces laterally and stresses the aorta's ligamentous attachments.

INITIAL ASSESSMENT

During the initial assessment, determine the patient's mental status and the status of the airway, breathing, and circulation. Intervene as necessary to correct life-threatening conditions. It is during the initial assessment that you will first identify the signs and symptoms of serious chest trauma. Be especially watchful for any dyspnea, asymmetrical, paradoxical, or limited chest movement, hyperinflation of the chest, or an abdomen that appears hollow. Notice any general patient color indicating hypoxia such as cyanosis or an ashen discoloration. Look for distended jugular veins, costal or suprasternal retractions, and the use of accessory muscles of respiration.

Administer ventilations with care in the patient with chest trauma.

Ensure that ventilation is adequate and administer high-flow, high-concentration oxygen by nonrebreather mask. Administer any positive pressure ventilations with care as thoracic injury may weaken the lung tissue and make the patient prone to pneumothorax or tension pneumothorax. Aggressive (or even cautious) ventilations may induce these problems. Be suspicious of internal hemorrhage and initiate at least one large-bore IV catheter and line in anticipation of hypovolemia, hypotension, and shock. With anterior blunt or penetrating trauma that may involve the heart, attach the electrocardiogram (ECG) electrodes and monitor for dysrhythmias. Attach a pulse oximeter and monitor oxygen saturation to evaluate the effectiveness of respiration. If there is any mechanism suggesting serious trauma to the chest or any physical signs of either hypoventilation or hypovolemia compensation, perform the rapid trauma assessment with a special focus on the chest and prepare for rapid patient transport to the trauma center.

RAPID TRAUMA ASSESSMENT

During the rapid trauma assessment you will examine the patient's chest in detail, carefully observing, questioning about, palpating, and auscultating the region.

Observe

Observe the chest for evidence of impact. Look for the erythema that develops early in the contusion process, especially as it outlines the ribs or forms a pattern reflecting the contours of the object the chest hit. Look carefully for penetrating trauma and try to determine the angle of entry and depth of penetration. Also look for exit wounds. Lateral chest injury is likely to involve the lungs, whereas a pathway of energy through the central chest is likely to involve the heart, great vessels, trachea, or esophagus. Injury to the mediastinal structures is also likely to result in serious hemorrhage, hypovolemia, and shock. Look for intercostal and suprasternal retractions as well as external jugular vein distention. Remember, JVD is present in supine normotensive patients and may be exaggerated in them or may continue when the patient is moved to the seated position if venous pressure is elevated.

Watch chest movement carefully during respiration. The chest should rise and the abdomen should fall smoothly with inspiration and return to position during expiration. Any limited motion, either bilaterally or unilaterally, suggests a problem. Watch for the paradoxical motion of flail chest. That movement will be limited due to muscle spasm during early care, but continued motion will further damage the surrounding soft tissue and the intracostal muscles will fatigue. This will lead to a more obvious paradoxical motion and greater respiratory embarrassment with time. Look, too, for any hyperinflation of one side of the chest and any deformity that may exist from rib fracture, sternal fracture or dislocation, or subcutaneous emphysema. Assess the volume of air effectively moved with each breath and ensure that the minute volume is greater than 6 liters. If not, consider overdrive ventilation with the bag-valve mask. Examine any open wound for air movement in or out, which is indicative of an open pneumothorax. Observe the patient's general color. If a patient's skin is dusky, ashen, or cyanotic, suspect respiratory compromise. If the head and neck are red, dark red, or blue, suspect traumatic asphyxia.

Question

Question the patient about any pain, pain on motion, pain with breathing effort (pleuritic pain), or dyspnea. Note if the pain is crushing, tearing, or is described otherwise by the patient. Have the patient describe the exact location of the pain, its severity, and any radiation of the pain. Question about other sensations and carefully monitor the patient's level of consciousness and orientation.

Palpate

Palpate the thorax carefully, feeling for any signs of injury (Figure 17-13). Feel for any swelling, deformity, crepitus, or the crackling of subcutaneous emphysema. Compress the thorax between your hands with pressure directed inward. Then apply downward pressure on the mid-sternum. Such pressure will flex the ribs and should elicit pain from any fracture site along the thorax. (Apply pressure only if you are unsure of chest injury. If you suspect rib or sternal fracture, provide appropriate care but do not aggravate the injury.) Rest your hands on the lower thorax and let the chest lift your hands with inspiration and let them fall with expiration (Figure 17-14). The motion should be smooth and equal. If not, determine the nature of any asymmetry.

You may have to rely on your palpation skills to assess chest injuries when scene noise is excessive.

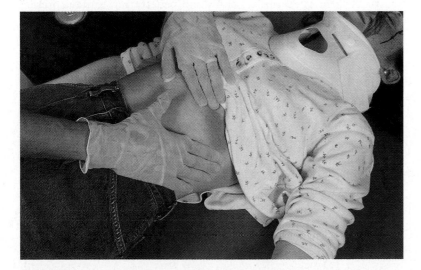

FIGURE 17-13 Carefully palpate the thorax of a patient with a suspected injury to the region.

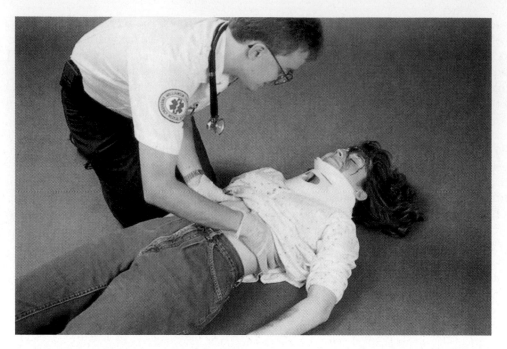

FIGURE 17-14   Place your hands on the lower thorax and let them rise and fall with respiration.

Auscultate

Auscultate all lung lobes, both anteriorly and posteriorly (Figure 17-15). Listen for both inspiratory and expiratory air movement and note any crackles, indicating edema from contusion or congestive heart failure, or any diminished breath sounds, suggesting hypoventilation. Compare one side to the other and one lobe to another. Be sensitive for distant or muffled respiratory or heart sounds.

Percuss

Percuss the chest and note the responses (Figure 17-16). Determine if the area percussed is normal, hyperresonant, or dull. A dull response suggests collecting blood or other fluid, whereas hyperresonance suggests air or air under pressure as in a pneumothorax or tension pneumothorax.

Your findings from the rapid trauma assessment may suggest an injury or multiple injuries. Identify the likely cause of the signs and symptoms you find and suspect and anticipate the worst. You are likely to note clear evidence of chest wall injury and some signs of internal injuries if they exist. As mentioned earlier, blunt and penetrating trauma present with different typical injuries.

FIGURE 17-15   Auscultate all lung lobes, both anteriorly and posteriorly.

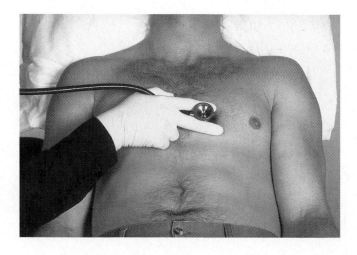

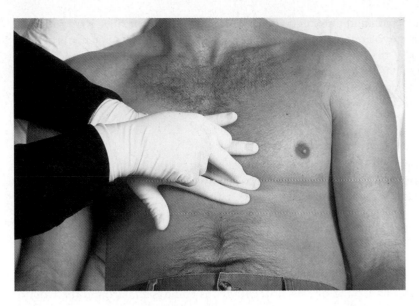

FIGURE 17-16   Percuss all lung lobes, listening for a dull response or hyperresonance.

Blunt Trauma Assessment

In blunt trauma, you commonly find slight discoloration of the surface of the chest reflective of contusions. The contusions also cause the patient pain, generally in an area or region, and somewhat limit respiration. As the impact energy increases, it may cause fractures of ribs four to nine and a greater possibility of underlying injury. If the upper ribs or ribs ten to twelve fracture, suspect serious underlying injury. Sternal fracture takes great energy and is also associated with a higher incidence of internal injury. Rib fractures generate a point-specific pain (at the fracture site) and crepitus upon deep breathing or your flexing of the patient's chest during the rapid trauma assessment. That pain may further limit chest excursion during respiration. As the energy of trauma and the seriousness of chest trauma increase, more ribs may fracture, causing a flail chest. Remember that a flail chest's paradoxical motion is initially limited by muscular splinting and grows more noticeable and causes more respiratory distress as time since the collision increases.

In blunt injury to the chest, you must anticipate and assess for additional signs suggesting internal injury. Signs specific for lung injury include increasing dyspnea, signs of hypoxemia, accessory muscle use, and intracostal and suprasternal retractions. Auscultation will help you differentiate between pulmonary contusion and pneumothorax. Contusions demonstrate progressively increasing crackles, whereas pneumothorax presents with diminished breath sounds on the ipsilateral side. Further, with pneumothorax the affected side may be hyperinflated and resonant to percussion. If the pneumothorax progresses to tension pneumothorax, you will likely note progressing dyspnea and hypoxia, use of accessory muscles, distended jugular veins, tracheal shift toward the contralateral side (a late finding), and hyperresonance of the ipsilateral chest on percussion. Subcutaneous emphysema may develop, especially if the lung defect was caused by or is associated with a rib fracture that disturbs the integrity of the parietal pleura. Hemothorax is noticeable due to the vascular loss, more so than for the respiratory component of the pathology. Suspect it if you find the signs of hypovolemia associated with blunt chest trauma. Hemothorax, when sizeable, may cause dyspnea and a lung field that is dull to percussion.

Blunt mediastinal injury will probably affect the heart, great vessels, and trachea. Heart injury may present with chest pain similar to that of the myocardial infarction and, if serious enough, with the signs of heart failure or cardiogenic shock. The ECG may reveal tachycardia, bradycardia, cardiac irritability, and, in cases of severe cardiac contusion, may demonstrate ST elevation. Cardiac rupture presents with the signs of sudden death, whereas pericardial tamponade is unlikely in blunt chest trauma. Injury to the great vessels (aneurysm) is most frequently associated with lateral impacts or feet-first high falls and may produce a tearing chest pain and pulse deficits in the extremities. If the aneurysm ruptures, rapidly progressing hypovolemia, hypotension, shock, and death ensue. Tracheobronchial injury results in rapidly developing pneumomediastinum or pneumothorax and possible subcutaneous emphysema, hemoptysis, dyspnea, and hypoxia. Positive pressure ventilations may increase the development and severity of signs. Traumatic asphyxia presents with jugular vein distention, discoloration of the head and neck, severe dyspnea, and possibly the signs of hypovolemia and shock.

Penetrating Trauma Assessment

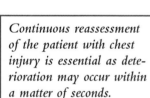

Remember, the severity of internal injury associated with penetrating trauma may be great despite seemingly minor entrance and/or exit wounds.

Penetrating injury displays a different set of signs associated with different injuries. Inspect a chest wound for frothy blood or sounds of air exchange with respirations (open pneumothorax). Remember that a wound needs to be rather large (high-velocity bullet exit wound or close-range shotgun blast) for these signs to occur. A penetrating wound, however, commonly induces a simple pneumothorax with its associated signs and symptoms. A hyperinflated chest, distended jugular veins, tracheal shift away from the injury, distant or absent breath sounds, hyperresonance to percussion, and severe dyspnea and hypotension suggest tension pneumothorax. The pressure of tension pneumothorax may push air outward through a penetrating wound or cause subcutaneous emphysema around the wound. Some degree of hemothorax is likely to be associated with penetrating chest trauma and, if extensive, may reveal diminished or absent breath sounds and a chest region that is dull to percussion. Hemothorax also causes or significantly contributes to hypovolemia and shock.

Penetrating trauma to the heart is likely to cause pericardial tamponade and present with jugular vein distention, distant heart sounds, and hypotension (Beck's triad). Pulsus paradoxus may be present and jugular filling may occur with inspiration (Kussmaul's sign), and both are indicative of pericardial tamponade. Heart sounds are distant, pulses are weak, and the patient experiences increasing hypotension and shock (Figure 17-17). Penetrating trauma to the heart may also cause myocardial rupture and associated pericardial tamponade or immediate death (Figure 17-18). The patient demonstrates vital signs that fall precipitously as the vascular volume is pumped into the mediastinum.

ONGOING ASSESSMENT

Continuous reassessment of the patient with chest injury is essential as deterioration may occur within a matter of seconds.

Although the ongoing assessment simply repeats elements of the initial assessment, the taking of vital signs, and examination of any injury signs discovered during earlier assessment, it takes on great importance for the patient with chest trauma. With any serious chest impact or any penetrating injury to the chest, observe the respiratory depth, rate, and symmetry of effort. Auscultate the lung fields for equality and crackles and monitor the distal pulses, oxygen saturation, skin color, and blood pressure for signs of progressing hypovolemia (Figure 17-19). If any signs change between assessments, search for the cause and rule out progressing chest injury. Be especially suspicious of developing tension pnuemothorax, pericardial tamponade, extensive and evolving pulmonary contusion, and hypovolemia associated with hemothorax. If any of these is found, institute the appropriate management steps.

FIGURE 17-17 Penetrating stab wound to the chest involving the heart.

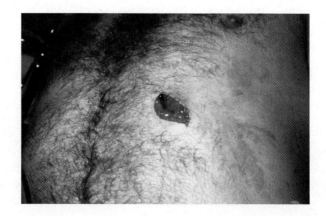

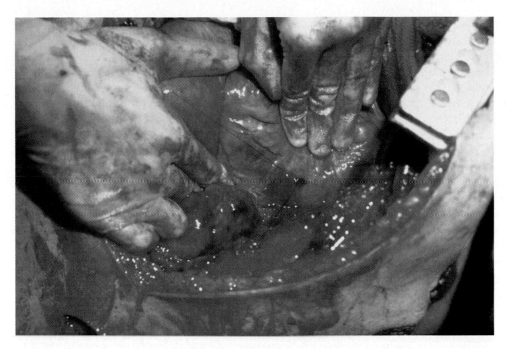

FIGURE 17-18   Stab wound that penetrated the pericardium.

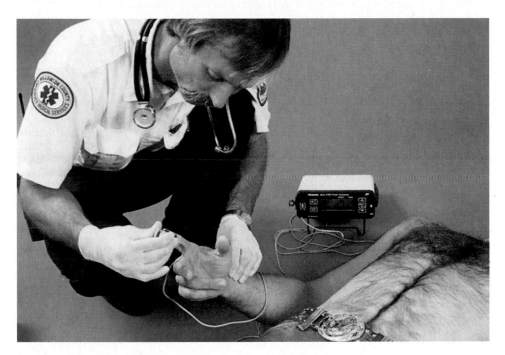

FIGURE 17-19   With pulse oximetry, you can continuously monitor the percentage of the patient's oxygen saturation.

MANAGEMENT OF THE CHEST INJURY PATIENT

The general management of the patient with significant chest injury focuses on ensuring good oxygenation and adequate respiratory volume and rate. Administer high-flow, high-concentration oxygen using the nonrebreather mask. Assure the airway is patent and consider endotracheal intubation if there is any significant loss in the level of consciousness or orientation. Consider intubation early in your care, because patients with thoracic trauma

General management of the patient with serious chest trauma requires ensurance of good oxygenation and adequate respiratory volume and rate.

are likely to get worse with time. Endotracheal intubation makes ventilation of the flail chest or pulmonary contusion patient easier.

Carefully evaluate the minute volume of the patient (breaths per minute times volume) and if it is less than 6,000 mL consider overdrive ventilation. Apply the BVM to the conscious patient with severe dyspnea at a rate of 12 to 16 full breaths per minute, trying to match the patient's respiratory rate. Closely monitor pulse oximetry, level of consciousness, and skin color. Using a BVM may also be beneficial for the patient with serious rib fractures and flail chest. The positive pressure displaces the chest outward, reducing the movement of the fracture site and moving the flail segment with the chest. It may also be beneficial to the patient who is exhausted from the increased breathing effort associated with pulmonary contusion. In this case, the ventilations help push any fluids back into the vascular system to relieve edema. Remember, however, that positive pressure ventilations change the dynamics of respiration from a less than atmospheric to a greater than atmospheric process and may exacerbate respiratory problems such as tracheobronchial injury, pneumothorax, and tension pneumothorax.

Anticipate heart and great vessel compromise with thoracic injury and be ready to stabilize the patient's cardiovascular system. Initiate at least one large-bore IV site if the patient has a serious mechanism of chest trauma and place two lines if there are any signs of hypovolemia or compensation. Be prepared to administer fluids quickly if the patient's blood pressure begins to fall. Use of the pneumatic anti-shock garment (PASG) is contraindicated for penetrating chest trauma because it may increase the rate and volume of blood loss and disrupt the clotting process. The PASG should be used only in blunt chest trauma and then only when the blood pressure drops below 60 mmHg or the pulses disappear.

IV fluid infusion for the patient with chest trauma should be conservative. Rapid fluid administration may increase the rate of hemorrhage and dilute the clotting factors, further adding to the problem. Additional fluid also increases the edema associated with pulmonary contusion, increasing the rate and extent of its development. Any time you administer fluids to the chest trauma patient, auscultate all lung fields carefully and reduce the fluid resuscitation rate whenever you hear respiratory crackles or the patient's dyspnea increases.

Care is specific for thoracic injuries including rib fractures, sternoclavicular dislocation, flail chest, open pneumothorax, tension pneumothorax, hemothorax, cardiac contusion, pericardial tamponade, aortic aneurysm, tracheobronchial injury, and traumatic asphyxia.

Remember, aggressive fluid resuscitation in the patient with chest trauma can result in hemodilution and loss of clotting factors.

RIB FRACTURES

Rib fractures, either isolated or associated with other respiratory injuries, may produce pain that significantly limits respiratory effort and leads to hypoventilation. In these patients you may consider administering analgesics to grant greater patient comfort and improve chest excursion. Ensure that the patient is hemodynamically stable, no associated abdominal or head injury is present, and that the patient is fully conscious and oriented. Consider administration of diazepam, morphine sulfate, meperidine, or nalbuphine. Note that use of nitrous oxide is contraindicated in chest trauma as the nitrogen may migrate into a pneumothorax or tension pneumothorax.

STERNOCLAVICULAR DISLOCATION

Supportive therapy with oxygen is usually all that is required for an isolated sternoclavicular dislocation. However, hemodynamic instability indicates associated injuries requiring rapid transport to the trauma center with aggressive resuscitation measures instituted en route. If you suspect posterior sternoclavicular dislocation and note the patient to be in significant respiratory distress that is not effectively treated with initial airway maneuvers and high-flow oxygen, then consider dislocation reduction. Place the patient in the supine position with a sandbag between the shoulder blades. The sandbag helps to pull the shoulders backward and moves the head of the clavicle laterally and away from the trachea. Do not perform this procedure for the multiple-trauma patient due to the probability of spine injury. An alternative reduction method is to place the patient supine and grasp the clavicle near the sternum. Pull it upward and laterally, directly perpendicular to the sternum. This distracts the clavicle forward, alleviating its impingement of the airway.

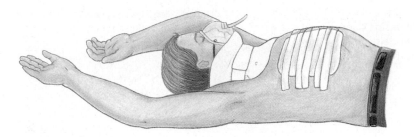

FIGURE 17-20 Flail chest should be treated with administration of oxygen and gentle splinting of the flail segment with a pillow or pad.

FLAIL CHEST

Place the patient on the side of injury if spinal immobilization is not required, or secure a large and bulky dressing with bandaging against the flail segment to stabilize it (Figure 17-20). Employ high-flow, high-concentration oxygen therapy, monitor oxygen saturation with pulse oximetry, and monitor cardiac activity with the ECG. If there is significant dyspnea, evidence of underlying pulmonary injury, or signs of respiratory compromise, these measures will not suffice. Then consider endotracheal intubation, positive pressure ventilations, and high-flow, high-concentration oxygen. Positive pressure ventilations internally splint the flail segment, expand atelectatic areas of the lung, and also treat underlying pulmonary contusion. Use of sandbags to support the flail segment is not indicated because it may diminish chest movement, adding to hypoventilation, atelectasis, and subsequent hypoxemia. Rapid transport to the trauma center is indicated as this injury, its complications, and associated injuries are life threatening.

> *Consider early intubation of the patient with flail chest, especially when oxygenation remains impaired despite the provision of high-flow, high-concentration oxygen.*

OPEN PNEUMOTHORAX

Support the patient with open pneumothorax by administering high-flow, high-concentration oxygen and monitoring oxygen saturation and respiratory effort. If you find a penetrating injury, cover it with a sterile occlusive dressing (sterile plastic wrap) taped on three sides (Figure 17-21). This process converts the open pneumothorax into a closed pneumothorax, prevents further aspiration of air, and relieves any building pressure (tension pneumothorax) through the valve-like dressing. If the dyspnea diminishes somewhat but still continues, provide positive pressure ventilations and intubate as indicated. Carefully monitor the patient when you employ intermittent positive pressure ventilation because its use may lead to a tension pneumothorax. If after the dressing has been applied, the patient has progressive breathing difficulty, appears to be hypoventilating and hypoxemic, has decreasing breath sounds on the injured side and increasing jugular distention, remove the occlusive dressing. If you hear air rush out and the patient's respirations improve, reseal the wound, monitor respiration carefully, and again remove the dressing if any respiratory signs or symptoms redevelop. If removing the dressing does not relieve the increasing signs and symptoms, suspect and treat for tension pneumothorax.

TENSION PNEUMOTHORAX

Confirm possible tension pneumothorax by auscultating the lung fields for diminished breath sounds, percussing for hyperresonnace, and observing for severe dyspnea, hyperinflation of the chest, and jugular vein distention. Successful treatment depends on rapid recognition of this condition and then pleural decompression. As you prepare to decompress the affected (ipsilateral) side, apply high-flow, high-concentration oxygen if the airway is intact and the patient is able to demonstrate adequate ventilatory effort. Provide ventilations with the BVM and supplemental oxygen and intubate if the patient is unable to maintain an airway or continues to show signs/symptoms of hypoxemia on high-flow, high-concentration oxygen. Perform needle thoracentesis by inserting a 14-gauge intravascular catheter into the second intercostal space, midclavicular line on the side of the thorax with decreased breath sounds and hyperinflation (Figure 17-22). Attach a syringe filled with sterile water or saline to the

> *Tension pneumothorax is an occasional complication of multiple trauma. Always assess for it and decompress the chest when indicated.*

On inspiration, dressing seals wound, preventing air entry

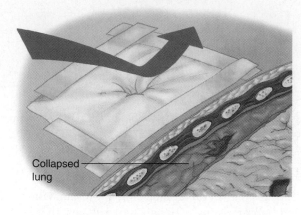

Collapsed lung

Expiration allows trapped air to escape through untaped section of dressing

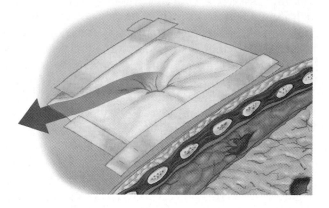

needle hub of the catheter. Then advance the catheter through the chest wall while maintaining gentle traction on the syringe plunger. Ensure you enter the thoracic cavity by passing the needle just over the rib. The intercostal artery, vein, and nerve pass just under each rib and may be injured if the needle's track is too high. As you enter the pleural space, you will feel a pop and note bubbling air through the fluid in the syringe. Advance the catheter into the chest and then withdraw the needle and syringe.

If the patient remains symptomatic, place a second or third catheter to more rapidly facilitate decompression. Secure the catheter in place with tape, being careful not to block the port or kink the catheter. Leaving the catheter open to air converts the tension pneumothorax into a simple pneumothorax and stabilizes the patient. You may create a flutter valve by cutting the finger off a latex glove, making a small perforation in its tip, and securing it to the catheter hub. Monitor the patient's respirations and breath sounds for a recurring tension pneumothorax. If signs and symptoms again appear, decompress the chest again. Frequently, the initial catheter will clog or kink and necessitate replacement by another.

Rapidly transport the patient to the trauma center for definitive treatment (usually with a chest tube). Be cautious in using IV crystalloid infusion if the patient is hemodynamically stable. An underlying pulmonary contusion may lead to edema, which is made worse with overaggressive fluid therapy. If your patient remains hypotensive after chest decompression and respirations do not become adequate, consider the possibility of internal hemorrhage and the need for (conservative) fluid resuscitation. If respirations do not dramatically improve, assess for a contralateral tension pneumothorax or pericardial tamponade as the cause.

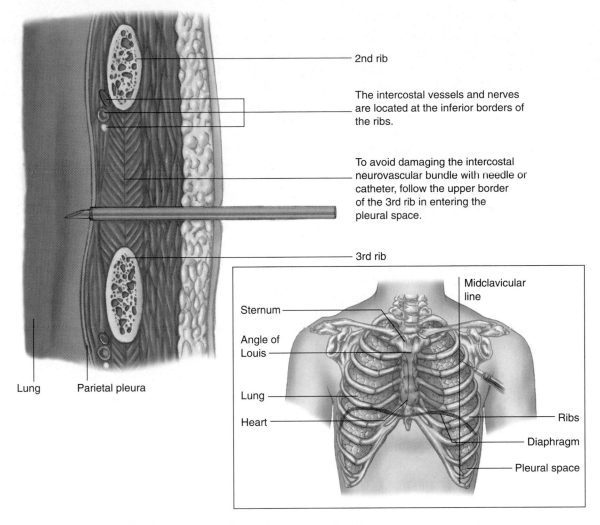

2nd rib

The intercostal vessels and nerves are located at the inferior borders of the ribs.

To avoid damaging the intercostal neurovascular bundle with needle or catheter, follow the upper border of the 3rd rib in entering the pleural space.

3rd rib

Midclavicular line

Sternum

Angle of Louis

Lung

Heart

Ribs

Diaphragm

Pleural space

Lung   Parietal pleura

FIGURE 17-22   Needle thoracentesis of a tension pneumothorax.

HEMOTHORAX

Treat the patient with suspected hemothorax with oxygen administration and respiratory support, as needed. Initiate two large-bore IV catheters, readied to infuse large volumes of fluid. Be conservative in fluid administration. Maintain blood pressure (between 90 to 100 mmHg) but do not attempt to return it to pre-injury levels. Carefully listen to breath sounds during any infusion because the increasing vascular volume may increase the edema and congestion of pulmonary contusion. It may also increase the pressure, rate, and volume of internal hemorrhage. If the pulmonary contusion is extensive and the patient cannot be adequately oxygenated by high-flow, high-concentration oxygen, positive pressure ventilations are indicated and may limit further edema that contributes to the injury.

MYOCARDIAL CONTUSION

In serious frontal impact collisions, suspect myocardial contusion and administer high-flow, high-concentration oxygen. Monitor cardiac electrical activity and watch for tachycardias, bradycardias, ectopic beats, and conduction defects. Establish an IV line in the event that antidysrhythmics (such as lidocaine) are needed, and monitor the patient for great vessel injury. Employ the pharmacological care measures recommended for advanced cardiac life support (Chapter 20, "Cardiovascular Emergencies"). Rapidly transport the patient to the trauma center for further evaluation and continued monitoring.

PERICARDIAL TAMPONADE

If pericardial tamponade is suspected, consider diverting to the closest hospital with a physician-staffed emergency department where emergency pericardiocentesis can be performed.

Maintain a high index of suspicion for pericardial tamponade in the patient with central thoracic penetrating trauma. While there is little prehospital care other than the administration of oxygen and some IV fluids to maximize venous return, definitive care is to remove some of the fluid accumulating in the pericardial sac. This action is rarely permitted in the field; hence the patient needs to be transported as rapidly as possible to the emergency department. Note that a relatively simple procedure can relieve this problem and can be adequately administered by an emergency physician. If a physician-staffed emergency department is closer to you than the trauma center, it may be the best choice for the patient with pericardial tamponade. After the pericardiocentesis is performed, the patient may then be directed to the closest trauma center.

AORTIC ANEURYSM

Care for the patient with dissecting aortic aneurysm is gentle but rapid transport to the trauma center. Any jarring during extrication, assessment, care, packaging, or transport increases the risk of rupture and rapidly fatal exsanguination. Initiate IV therapy en route, but be very conservative in fluid administration. Mild hypotension may protect the injury site. If the aneurysm ruptures, as indicated by an immediate deterioration in vital signs, provide rapid administration of fluids. Anxiety and its effect on cardiac output and blood pressure may increase the likelihood of aneurysm rupture. Place a special emphasis on calming and reassuring the patient during very gentle care and transport.

TRACHEOBRONCHIAL INJURY

Support the tracheobronchial injury patient with oxygen and clear the airway of blood and secretions. If you are unable to maintain a patent airway or adequately oxygenate the patient, then intubate the trachea and provide positive pressure ventilations. Observe the patient carefully for the development of a tension pneumothorax, which may result as a complication of positive pressure ventilations, and treat as previously prescribed. Provide rapid transport as soon as the patient can be extricated and stabilized. This is important because these patients can rapidly destabilize and then require emergency surgical intervention.

TRAUMATIC ASPHYXIA

Administer oxygen and support the airway and respiration of the traumatic asphyxia patient. This may require using positive pressure ventilations with the BVM to ensure adequate ventilation during the entrapment and possibly thereafter. Establish two large-bore IV lines for rapid infusion of crystalloid in anticipation of rapidly developing hypovolemia with chest decompression. Once the compressing force is removed, the direct effects of traumatic asphyxia spontaneously resolve; however, serious internal hemorrhage may begin. Prepare to transport immediately after release from entrapment because the patient will likely have severe coexisting injuries.

If the patient remains entrapped for a prolonged time, consider the administration of sodium bicarbonate. Prolonged stagnant blood flow and a hypoxic cellular environment may cause accumulation of metabolic acids. As the compression is released, this blood returns to the central circulation, much as it does with entrapped limbs during crush injury. Consider the administration of 1 mEq/kg of sodium bicarbonate just before or during decompression of the chest if entrapment has lasted more than 20 minutes.

SUMMARY

Thoracic trauma by either blunt or penetrating mechanisms has a great potential for posing a threat to a patient's life. In fact, 25% of all traumatic deaths are secondary to injuries in this region. In assessing these patients, the mechanism of injury, when considered along with the clinical findings, may help in differentiating among the many possible injuries. The assessment, in turn, helps guide your interventions and determines the need for rapid extrication and transport. Aggressive airway management, oxygenation, ventilation, and fluid resuscitation, when indicated, can make the difference between the patient's survival or death. Specific interventions, such as pleural decompression or stabilization of a flail segment, can also affect mortality and morbidity from chest trauma. Understanding the pathological processes affecting the chest during trauma and employing proper assessment and care measures will assure the best possible outcome for your patients.

ON THE WEB

For additional practice and review, go to the companion website at www.prenhall.com/bledsoe and click on *Intermediate Emergency Care: Principles & Practice.*

CHAPTER 18

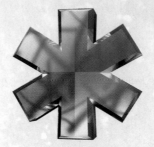

Trauma Management Skills

Objectives *(Asterisks below indicate material supplemental to the U.S. DOT curriculum.)*

After reading this chapter, you should be able to:

*1. Explain the elements of trauma assessment. (pp. 735–748)

*2. Explain the management of head, facial, and neck injury patients. (pp. 749–756)

*3. Explain the management of spinal injury patients. (pp. 756–768)

*4. Explain the management of abdominal injury patients. (pp. 768–770)

*5. Explain the management of musculoskeletal injury patients. (pp. 770–785)

*6. Explain the management of soft-tissue injury patients. (pp. 786–798)

CASE STUDY

EMT-I's Fred and Lisa are providing stand-by service at a local high school football game. Just before the end of the third quarter, they are called onto the field when a player is thrown to the ground and cannot get up.

Upon arrival at the player's side, they find a well-developed teenager who is oriented to person but not to time and place. He states that he was hit hard from the side and now has a tingling in his legs and feet. Upon further questioning, the player, Bill, complains of some localized pain just above the shoulders. Bill's medical history reveals that he has had no significant previous medical problems, has no allergies, and his tetanus vaccination is up to date.

The physical exam reveals a patient clothed in protective football gear and helmet who has no external signs of physical injury. The patient's airway is clear, and the rate, strength, and quality of his breathing and pulse are within normal limits. Physical examination of the head is limited by the helmet, but palpation of the posterior neck reveals some localized tenderness at or slightly above the first thoracic verte-bra. Respiratory excursion and diaphragm movement seem unaffected by the injury. However, there appears to be numbness to the entire chest, abdomen, lower extremities, as well as the posterior surface of the upper extremities. The patient's upper extremity grip is strong, but the strength of both feet when pushing against the EMT-I's hands appears diminished. Bill main-tains both bowel and bladder control.

Fred feels it will be very difficult to immobilize Bill with the helmet and shoulder pads in place. He has the athletic trainer hold the helmet while Lisa and he release the air pressure in the bladder and begin its removal. Lisa stabilizes Bill's head, while Fred gently and carefully ne-gotiates the helmet around Bill's face. Once the helmet is removed, Fred assumes manual stabi-lization of Bill's head, which is well above the surface of the playing field because the shoulder pads raise his shoulders more than an inch off the ground. Lisa proceeds to cut Bill's shirt and the webbing that holds the pads in place and gently removes the pads. Then, using a rope sling, Fred, Lisa, and the athletic trainer gently slide Bill with axial traction onto the spine board. After the torso is immobilized to the board, they use padding and a cervical immobilization device to im-mobilize Bill's head about 1 inch above the board to maintain neutral alignment.

Bill's blood pressure, pulse rate and strength, and respiratory rate and volume have all re-mained relatively normal during these procedures, and Fred notes no differences in skin temper-ature or capillary refill in any extremity, which makes less likely neurogenic shock from spinal cord injury. The pulse oximeter reads 98%, and the electrocardiogram (ECG) displays a normal sinus rhythm at 68. The EMT-Is load Bill into the ambulance and begin transport to the regional neu-rocenter.

Fred and Lisa learn from the local paper that Bill suffered a compression fracture of the seventh cervical vertebrae and will miss the rest of the season. The injury may limit Bill's ath-letic career but is not expected to otherwise affect his life. What the paper did not report is that, if this injury had been mishandled, Bill might have spent his life in a wheelchair.

INTRODUCTION

Trauma care provided by the EMT-I requires additional assessment and management skills for patients with soft-tissue, musculoskeletal, head, facial, neck, spinal, and abdominal trauma. This chapter addresses the assessment of the trauma patient and these individual skills.

TRAUMA ASSESSMENT

Assessment of the trauma patient is essential both to determining the priority for patient transport and identifying and prioritizing patient injuries for care. During the preceding chapters, we have discussed trauma related to body regions or systems. During these dis-cussions, we examined how the elements of assessment were applied to each system or re-gion. In this chapter, we will review the elements of assessment in a comprehensive way, much as you would when presented with a seriously injured trauma patient.

Trauma assessment progresses through the scene size-up, the initial assessment, either the rapid trauma assessment or the focused exam and history, and is then followed by serial ongoing assessments. However, your first opportunity to begin the assessment process is through a review of the dispatch information.

DISPATCH INFORMATION

The dispatch information provides critical information that you must evaluate while re-sponding to the scene. The information provides the nature of the call. Often, it specifies the mechanism of injury (such as a fall, shooting, or auto crash) or the nature of the injury (such as a broken leg, head injury, or deep laceration). This information permits you to begin preparation for patient care and to think about how to approach the scene. Occasionally, the dispatch information may suggest the scene is too dangerous to approach until it is secured by the police (such as cases of violence involving shootings, stabbings, or domestic altercations with injuries). In such cases, you should remain at a distance from the scene until police arrive and notify you that it is secure. At other times, the dispatch information may alert you to potential hazards such as a toxic gas release or downed electrical wires for which you may need to request specialized response teams to secure the scene.

Use the dispatch information to anticipate and prepare for the care of injuries. To speed your response at the scene, locate the equipment you will likely use. If appropriate, lay the equipment out on the stretcher so it can be taken immediately to the patient. (It is always easier to have a first responder or bystander return a piece of equipment to the ambulance than it is to ask them to go to the ambulance, find it, and bring it to the patient's side.) Inspect the equipment, and mentally review its application and use. If you expect severe injuries, set up an IV bag and administration set in the ambulance for later use on the patient. This saves time that would otherwise be taken from patient care to assemble the administration equipment. Finally, mentally review the assessment and care you intend to provide and, as necessary, review your protocols to ensure you are ready to respond to the emergency. These actions will help you move quickly through the required care steps and to offer the optimum patient care in the shortest span of time.

Scene Size-up

The scene size-up with trauma patients involves four major elements: determining the mechanism of injury, identifying scene hazards including the need for body substance isolation, accounting for and locating all patients, and requesting any additional resources. Initially you will don gloves because all patient contacts call for this basic form of body substance isolation. As you progress through the analysis of the mechanism of injury and anticipate injuries, you may increase your level of personal protection as indicated below. The mechanism of injury analysis is also essential to help you identify all scene hazards.

Mechanism of Injury Analysis

Analyze the mechanism of injury by re-creating the incident in your mind, and from that, anticipating the nature and severity of your patient's injuries (the index of suspicion). Take the evidence available to you as you arrive at and first view the scene (Figure 18-1), and use that evidence to determine exactly how the forces were expressed to the patient. If two autos collided, for example, determine what vehicle surfaces impacted, from which direction the vehicles were traveling, and which patient surfaces were impacted. Use the amount of vehicular damage to approximate the strength of the impact, and then determine whether restraints or other protective mechanisms were used that may have reduced the potential for injury. Frontal and rear impacts afford the vehicle occupants the most protection, especially if seatbelts are properly worn and airbags deploy. Lateral and rollover impacts are likely to cause the most serious injuries. In motorcycle, bicycle, and pedestrian vs. vehicle collisions, identify the relative speed of impact and appreciate the lack of protection afforded the victim. In other non-vehicular blunt trauma, examine the height of the fall or other indications of the energy of impact and the point of impact as well as the path of transmission of those forces through the body.

When assessing the mechanism of injury for a patient affected by penetrating trauma, look at the speed of the offending agent or projectile. Remember that an increase in mass directly increases the force's energy. An increase in speed greatly increases (a squared relationship) the impact energy and the potential for serious patient injury. With gunshot wounds, identify the nature of the weapon (handgun, shotgun, or rifle), the relative power and profile (caliber), and then the distance and angle between the gun barrel and the impact point. Visualize the pathway taken by the bullet and its destructive power as it travels through human tissue. Head, central chest, and upper abdominal injuries are most lethal. Remember, however, that the path of a bullet is frequently deflected from a straight line. In other penetrating trauma, mentally re-create the injury process and use the kinetic energy principles to analyze the nature, process, and severity of the injury. Try to determine the length of the object and the depth and angle of penetration.

Use the dispatch information to anticipate and prepare for the care of injuries.

Content Review

Scene Size-up
- Determine the mechanism of injury
- Identify scene hazards/BSI needs
- Account for and locate all patients
- Request needed additional resources

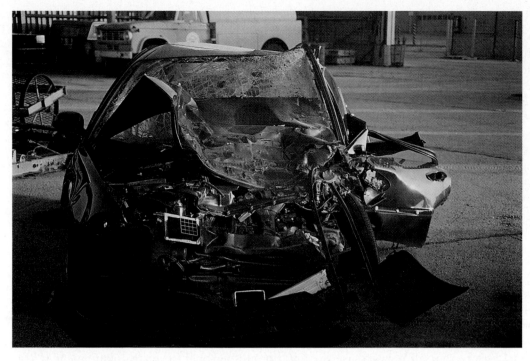

FIGURE 18-1 Analyze the mechanism of injury. Take the evidence available to you as you arrive at and first view the scene.

From your re-creation of the injury process, identify the individual organs affected and the extent of the injury to them. Approximate what significance their injury will have on the patient's condition and how it will affect him as time progresses. Assign each suspected injury a priority for both assessment and care. Finally, approximate the seriousness of your patient's overall condition and the potential need for either rapid transport with most care provided en route or on-scene care and then transport or treatment and release (as permitted by protocol). If there is more than one patient, identify the most seriously injured and order your patient assessment and care accordingly.

Hazard Identification

The mechanism of injury analysis helps you to identify many possible hazards at the scene. Search out all hazards and protect yourself, your patient, bystanders, and fellow rescuers from them. These hazards include the mechanism that injured your patient and may range from traffic associated with the auto crash to the assailant who is still holding the handgun. Search for additional sources of blunt and penetrating trauma such as the broken glass and jagged metal at an auto crash scene or moving machinery at an industrial accident site. Also search out and exclude any hazards from fire, heat, explosion, electricity, toxic chemicals, radiation, or deadly gas at each and every scene. Look for hazardous material placards. Your ambulance should carry DOT's *Hazardous Materials: The Emergency Response Guidebook*, which will help you identify the type of material and the level of risk. (However, it is ordinarily not the job of EMS to address the specific risks of hazardous materials. That responsibility lies with the hazardous material team or the fire department.)

Be aware of the presence and mood of family members, bystanders, and crowds at the emergency scene. These people may welcome your assistance or provide a serious threat to your well being.

Analyze the scene carefully to identify each of these hazards and exclude them from the scene or be prepared to deal with each before you approach the patient. Your well being and that of your patient depend on it. If you are injured at the scene you will be less able to help your patient and may, in fact, yourself become a patient rather than a caregiver.

Body Substance Isolation

A special type of hazard existing at almost every emergency scene is the presence of body fluids and substances with the potential to spread infection. Realize that the risk of infection extends to both you and your patient, especially when dealing with trauma. Although a patient's open wound releases blood that can be infectious to you, the open wound can also be a pathway through which infection enters your patient's body. The use of gloves and other body substance isolation (BSI) equipment and procedures protects both you and your patient. Ensure that all rescuers who may come into contact with the patient also employ appropriate BSI procedures as you prepare to approach the scene.

In all patient contacts, it is essential to don gloves in anticipation of contact with blood, saliva, mucus, urine, or fecal material. If the scene size-up reveals multiple patients, put on two or three sets of gloves, one over the other. Then peel gloves off as you move from one patient to another. If you prefer not to wear multiple layers of gloves, be sure to carry additional pairs of gloves and change them with each patient contact. Remember that the body fluids from one patient are potentially as infectious to another patient as they are to you and that with open wounds the risk of infection increases.

Your analysis of the mechanism of injury may also suggest airway or chest trauma or possible external arterial hemorrhage. These injuries may result in spurting blood or in blood or other fluids being propelled or coughed into the air. In such cases, wear both eye protection and splatter protection for your clothing. A mask may also be advisable. Consider wearing a mask if you have any type of respiratory infection, again to protect your patient. Ensure that all rescuers use the appropriate personal protective equipment (PPE). Once at the patient's side, your further evaluation may reveal the need for a higher level of BSI than the scene size-up suggested; for that reason, always have goggles, gowns, masks, and additional gloves handy.

Accounting for and Locating All Patients

During your scene size-up, identify the number of likely patients and their locations around the emergency scene. During a collision, patients may be thrown from the auto or trapped within a twisted wreck and completely out of sight (this often occurs with infants). A patient may also leave the vehicle and mill about the scene with bystanders or leave in an attempt to find help or simply wander from the scene in confusion. Search for evidence that suggests the number and types of patients. Consider the number of vehicles involved in a crash; the number of spider-web patterns on the windshields; purses or articles of clothing; and child seats, clothing, or toys. As you arrive at the scene, question the patients or bystanders to better determine the number and locations of any additional injured persons.

Resource Needs Determination

Once you determine the likely number of patients and their injuries, approximate the type and nature of any other emergency medical resources that will be needed at the scene. This may include additional ambulances, one for each seriously injured patient, and air medical service for patients who meet trauma triage criteria at a scene more than 20 to 30 minutes from the nearest trauma center.

Also determine the resources needed to control the hazards identified in your analysis of the scene. These resources may include the police for traffic control or for scene security (at scenes of shootings or domestic violence), the heavy rescue unit for extrication, the hazardous material team for fuel and oil spill cleanup, the power company for downed electrical lines, or the fire service for potential fire control at vehicle crashes. It is essential that you contact dispatch early so needed equipment and trained personnel are quickly en route to the scene. Waiting until later in the call delays their arrival and may hinder your ability to access and care for patients.

At the end of the scene size-up, you should have the information necessary to organize the overall response to the incident and to determine the special focus of your assessment for each patient. Take a few seconds to organize how you will address the scene and coordinate the additional resources as they arrive. Identify in your mind what you wish each respective service to accomplish and how these functions can best work together to meet your patient's needs. Then think through your initial assessment and what specific problems you might expect to find with each element of that evaluation for each patient.

INITIAL ASSESSMENT

The initial assessment is intended to identify immediate patient life threats and correct them before a more detailed assessment continues. It consists of applying spinal precautions when needed and assessing the patient's mental, airway, breathing, and circulatory status. If any serious or life-threatening problems are found, correct them immediately. As you carry out these steps, you will add to the information you gathered during the scene size-up and develop a general impression of the patient.

Spinal Precautions

Employ spinal precautions in the following circumstances: if the mechanism of injury suggests the possibility of spinal injury; if you suspect any extreme of flexion/extension, lateral bending, axial loading, distraction or rotation or that any direct penetrating or blunt force has been expressed to the neck; if the patient has a reduced level of consciousness (due to injury, intoxication, or shock); if the patient has any significant injury above the shoulders; if the patient complains of any pain along the spinal column or any limb numbness or tingling; or if, during your assessment, you notice any other distal neurological signs. If any of these conditions exists, apply manual in-line stabilization of the head and neck immediately and, after assessment of the neck (Figure 18-2), apply a cervical collar. Finally, provide complete mechanical immobilization of the entire patient to the long spine board.

General Impression

While you evaluate the patient's mental status and ABCs, develop a general impression of him or her. Combine the information you gathered during the mechanism of injury analysis, with the information gathered during the airway, breathing, and circulation check, and add to it the general appearance and mental status you observe during these first few minutes at the patient's side. The result is a general patient impression. It is your determination of the seriousness of the patient's injury and the priority for care and transport. This determination is very difficult to make early in your career; however, with experience your level of comfort in judging the severity of a patient's injuries and the need for either rapid transport or on-scene care will grow.

In some cases, your general patient impression will conflict with the seriousness of trauma suggested by the mechanism of injury or with the signs and symptoms you gather during the initial assessment. In most cases, you attend a patient very soon after an incident. In those circumstances, hemorrhage does not have the chance to accumulate and demand of the body the serious compensation that comes with time and produces the most noticeable signs and symptoms of shock. On the other hand, the mechanism of injury may not reflect the severity of the actual injuries and the patient may appear worse than expected. In all cases, base your management of the patient on the worst-case scenario. As time and further assessment continues, modify your general patient impression and the care it suggests.

Mental Status

Evaluate the patient's mental status. Begin by introducing yourself, identifying your level of training, and explaining your desire to offer care to the patient. Ask the patient what happened and what is bothering him the most. This permits the patient to consent to care, ensures that he knows who you are and that your intentions are helpful, and calls for a verbal response. Listen carefully to any responses as you continue your initial assessment.

At a minimum, identify the patient's level of consciousness using the AVPU mnemonic (*A*lert, responsive to *V*erbal stimuli, responsive to *P*ain, or *U*nresponsive). Even better, attempt to identify your patient's level of orientation. Does he know the day and time of day (orientation to time); recognize where he is (orientation to place) or know what happened (orientation to event); recognize friends and family (orientation to persons); and recognize who he is (orientation to own person)? Patients will usually lose orientation in this order.

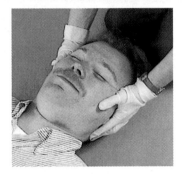

FIGURE 18-2 If spinal injury is suspected, apply manual in-line stabilization of the head and neck immediately.

Orientation is scored from 4 to 0 with the alert and completely oriented patient being oriented times 4 (A&O × 4). Some systems combine the last two—orientation to persons and orientation to own person—into a single element, resulting in a best orientation of A&O times 3. Determining a patient's level of orientation provides a baseline reading of the patient's mental status against which improvement/deterioration can be trended in ongoing assessments.

When the patient is not responsive to verbal stimuli, check for the specific response to painful stimuli. For example, if you apply a painful stimulus (usually by squeezing the fleshy region between the thumb and first finger or trapezius muscle of the shoulder), does the patient move away from the pain (purposeful); move, but not effectively, away from the pain (purposeless); or does he not move at all in response to painful stimulus? Some patients move toward a specific body position, or posture, in response to painful stimuli. With decorticate posturing, the patient's body moves toward extension with elbows flexing. With decerebrate posturing, the body and elbows extend. Determining a baseline response permits you and subsequent care providers to track patient deterioration or improvement throughout the course of care.

Airway

It is easy to evaluate the airway in the conscious patient by listening to him speak. If he can talk clearly and speak in full sentences, you know that the patient has control over an open airway, is breathing adequately, and has cerebral oxygenation enough to support conscious thought. If the speech is broken or forced, there are unusual airway sounds, or the statements are confused or unintelligible, suspect and evaluate further for airway or breathing problems.

In the unconscious patient, airway assessment requires more attention. Look, listen, and feel carefully for air movement. Watch to see if the chest rises and falls. Place your ear just in front of or over your patient's mouth, listen for the sound of air moving during respirations, and feel the volume of air escaping during exhalation. Remember that eupnea and apnea are the quietest and most difficult respirations to evaluate. If you do not hear air moving through the airway and/or you feel an insufficient volume of moving air, reposition the patient's head and jaw with the head-tilt/chin-lift or the jaw-thrust. If repositioning improves air movement, then insert a nasal or oral airway. Be cautious in using the nasal airway if the patient has any serious head trauma because a basilar skull fracture may have opened the nasal cavity to the brain. Suction as needed to remove any excessive airway fluids or if necessary, turn the patient onto his side to let gravity help drain the airway. If the patient does not have a gag reflex, consider early intubation, either now (if the airway is at immediate risk) or at the end of the initial assessment.

If you note airway sounds such as stridor, snoring, gurgling, or wheezing, presume a partial airway obstruction that will get worse during assessment and care. Trauma to soft tissue of the airway will likely cause swelling and progressive airway restriction. Expect swelling to seriously obstruct respiration and again consider early intubation.

Breathing

Apply oxygen using a nonrebreather mask with oxygen flowing at 12 to 15 liters per minute. This helps ensure inspiration of high concentration (90% to 100%) oxygen for any moderately to seriously injured trauma patient. Watch for symmetrical chest and abdominal movement with each breath. If necessary, expose the chest for a better assessment. Rule out flail chest or stabilize the flail segment and provide overdrive ventilation with a bag-valve mask (BVM) to the breathing patient. Rule out diaphragmatic breathing (associated with cervical spine injury) or provide overdrive ventilation. If the patient complains of dyspnea or if chest excursion or tidal volumes seem limited, auscultate the lung fields to identify unilateral diminished or absent breath sounds. Percuss the chest for resonance. A dull sound indicates blood in the pleural space, whereas hyperresonance indicates air in the pleural space. If you cannot rule out a building tension pneumothorax, consider pleural decompression.

If respirations are less than 12 per minute and/or the tidal volume is less than 500 mL per breath in the unconscious patient, consider the use of overdrive ventilation. If the patient is breathing rapidly but ineffectively, you should also consider overdrive ventilation. If the patient is not breathing, ventilate at 12 to 20 times per minute with full breaths (800 to 1,000 mL) with high-flow, high-concentrations of oxygen using the BVM and reservoir. Ensure good chest rise in the patient and maintain an oxygen saturation of greater than 95%.

Circulation

Quickly check the radial pulse for strength, regularity, and rate. A strong tachycardia suggests excitement, whereas a weak and thready pulse suggests shock compensation. If a radial pulse cannot be palpated, check for a carotid pulse. A rapid, weak carotid pulse suggests serious compensation for hypovolemia, the presence of severe hemorrhage (possibly internal), and the probable need for fluid resuscitation.

During the pulse check also note the patient's skin condition. Cool, clammy, ashen, or pale skin suggests shock compensation. Perform a capillary refill check. A refill that takes more than 3 seconds suggests hypovolemia and compensation. (Please note that other conditions such as smoking, low ambient temperatures, pre-existing disease, and use of medications may delay capillary refill as well.)

Make a quick visual sweep of the body, looking for any signs of serious and continuing hemorrhage. Using your analysis of the mechanism of injury, identify probable locations of bleeding and view them or, if the site is hidden from view, pass a gloved hand under the area, looking for blood loss. Also use the mechanism of injury analysis to identify likely locations of internal injury and any associated internal hemorrhage. Use this information to determine the rate of probable blood loss and the priority for rapid transport.

A critical element of the initial assessment is detecting the earliest signs of shock. Remember that internal hemorrhage is the greatest killer of patients who survive the initial impact of trauma. Look carefully at your patient for any early signs of shock. These include a decreased level of consciousness or orientation, anxiety, restlessness, or combativeness. If the patient has consumed alcohol or is otherwise affected by drugs, be especially watchful and wary.

As internal hemorrhage continues, the body employs more drastic measures to compensate for the blood loss, and signs and symptoms become more obvious with the passage of time. The sooner the signs or symptoms develop, the more rapid the internal blood loss and the more quickly the patient is moving through compensated, then uncompensated, then irreversible shock. However, do not wait for these signs and symptoms of later stages of shock to appear. At the first signs of hypovolemic compensation, prioritize the patient for immediate transport to the trauma center. If the patient demonstrates any early signs of shock or the mechanism of injury suggests serious internal injury, initiate the steps of shock care.

Concluding the Initial Assessment

As you complete the initial assessment, modify your mechanism of injury analysis based on additional evidence gained at the scene such as a bent steering wheel or intrusion into the passenger compartment. Continue to monitor the scene for safety, remaining alert to any alterations in conditions at the scene and ensuring that all providers, patients, and bystanders are protected from scene hazards (including BSI).

At the conclusion of the initial assessment for the trauma patient, you must determine whether the patient merits a rapid trauma assessment or is best served by a focused exam and history. The rapid trauma assessment aims to identify other life threats not revealed during the initial assessment, to provide appropriate rapid intervention, and to ensure that the seriously injured trauma patient receives quick transport to the trauma center. The focused exam is used for less seriously injured patients and focuses on the probable injuries and their care. With these patients, you will also make a preliminary decision about priority for transport. If the patient meets any of the trauma triage criteria, either a mechanism of injury recognized during the scene size-up or a physical condition identified during the initial assessment, consider the patient for rapid transport.

GENERAL EXAMINATION TECHNIQUES

During the rapid trauma assessment, look at the areas on the patient's body where serious life threats are most likely to occur. These include the head, neck, chest, abdomen, pelvis, extremities, and back. Also quickly study locations of injury suggested either by the mechanism

Content Review

GENERAL EXAMINATION
Conduct a rapid trauma assessment or focused physical exam using:

- Questioning
- Inspection
- Palpation
- Auscultation
- Percussion

of injury or the symptoms described by the patient. In the focused physical exam, you look specifically at areas where injury is anticipated from the mechanism of injury and patient complaints. Both the rapid trauma assessment and the focused exam use basic techniques of patient questioning, inspection, palpation, auscultation, and percussion to identify signs and symptoms of injury. Both also conclude with a quick, abbreviated patient history and the gathering of a set of baseline vital signs.

Questioning

Before you inspect or palpate a body region, question the patient about any symptoms. Symptoms may include sensations of discomfort, pain, pain on movement, tingling, a pins-and-needles sensation (paraesthesia), numbness or lack of feeling (anesthesia), weakness, inability to move, or other unusual sensations. Also note the patient's response to the complaint. Patient complaints are subjective, and different people have different levels of pain tolerance. Watch how the patient responds to the pain and how easily he is distracted from it. This gives you a good approximation of how significant the pain or sensation is to the patient. Report and record any patient complaint in the patient's own words.

Inspection

As you continue inspecting the patient, look first to the skin color. A person with a light complexion who has normal circulation will appear light pink. Note any ashen (gray or dusky), cyanotic (bluish), or pale (very light pink or white) colorations. In people of color, look at the coloration of the lips, the conjunctiva of the eyes, the palms of the hands, or soles of the feet. Any discoloration indicates a possible generalized problem like hypovolemia, hypoventilation, or hypothermia.

Use the initial coloration you observe as a baseline when you examine specific regions of the body for injury. Look at those regions for erythema, a general reddening of the skin and the first sign of injury. The discoloration of ecchymosis, the black and blue normally associated with a contusion, is delayed because it takes the erythrocytes some time to migrate into injured tissue and then lose their oxygen and turn a deeper red or blue. A portion of a limb may also change color due to problems with distal circulation. The limb may turn pale (and cold) when arterial circulation is reduced or dark red, dusky, or ashen as circulation stagnates or venous return is halted.

The second element of inspection is looking for deformities. These become most recognizable if you carefully examine and compare limb to limb or one side of the body to the other. Deformity can be either an enlargement of the dimensions of a limb or body region or an abnormal angle or position of a limb or region. Enlargement is usually due to the accumulation of fluid—blood as in a hematoma or plasma and interstitial fluid (**edema**) as in inflammation associated with a contusion—but it may also be associated with the accumulation of air associated with subcutaneous emphysema. Angulation is the unusual positioning of a limb as with a bend in a bone where a bend would not be expected. Such a condition is most likely associated with a fracture. An unusual bend in a joint, meanwhile, suggests either a fracture or dislocation. Muscle spasm or abnormal retraction of a muscle due to tendon rupture may also cause deformity. Compare any apparent deformity to the opposite limb to better determine the nature and extent of the variance from normal.

The third element of inspection is an examination for disruption of the skin (wounds). Examine for any abrasion of the skin's surface, any tearing of the skin (a laceration), or any signs of skin damage that may be associated with a burn, such as erythema, blistering or gross disruption of the skin, and discoloration. Also look for any penetrations and determine whether they are superficial or deep. Remember that deep wounds that close over encourage infection and are often more serious than more grotesque superficial open wounds.

Palpation

After inspection, palpate any area for additional signs of injury (Figure 18-3). Gently touch the entire surface of the area being evaluated, feeling for general skin and muscle tone, any unusual or warm masses, any grating sensation, or the "rice crispy" feel of subcutaneous emphysema. You should also feel for any muscle spasm (guarding) or pain on palpation

edema fluid accumulation; swelling.

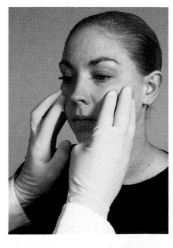

FIGURE 18-3 Palpation is an important physical examination technique—along with inspection, auscultation, and percussion.

(tenderness) that may reflect injury. Determine if that pain is pain on touch (tenderness), pain on movement, or pain on rapid release of pressure (rebound tenderness). Also palpate for relative muscle tone—normal, flaccid, or in spasm.

Auscultation

Auscultate the chest carefully to evaluate for the presence and quality of breath sounds. Note side to side, upper lobe to lower lobe, or regional differences. Crackles represent pulmonary edema most commonly related to pulmonary contusion and associated edema in trauma, whereas side-to-side inequality suggests pneumothorax or tension pneumothorax. Auscultation of the abdomen is not merited in trauma due to the time required to adequately assess for bowel sounds and their poor correlation to injury.

Percussion

Percuss each lobe of the chest for resonance. A dull response suggests fluid or blood accumulating in the pleural space. A hyperresonant response suggests air or air under pressure in the pleural space.

RAPID TRAUMA ASSESSMENT

Use the rapid trauma assessment when you suspect a patient has a serious injury to the body and are inclined to transport him or her quickly to the trauma center. Such a patient is one who meets the trauma triage criteria. During the rapid trauma assessment, quickly scan the body looking for hemorrhage or evidence of significant injury and examine the patient's head, neck, chest, abdomen, pelvis, extremities, and back (Figure 18-4). (Order your assessment to limit the movement of the patient. For example, if the patient is found lying face down, quickly assess the back before turning the patient for further assessment and care.) Check the distal function in each limb by noting distal pulse strength, skin temperature and color, capillary refill time, and—as appropriate—sensation and grip strength. If you suspect specific injuries, provide a focused evaluation of the body region using the considerations for that region as specified in the detailed physical exam, discussed later in this chapter. Conclude the rapid trauma assessment by taking a quick patient history and a set of vital signs.

FOCUSED EXAM AND HISTORY

The focused exam and history is performed on a patient who you expect has limited injuries. Direct your examination to the location of patient complaint or to any region of injury suggested by the mechanism of injury or by any signs and symptoms noted during the initial assessment. The actual focused exam uses the examination criteria for the body region as specified in the detailed exam. As with the rapid trauma assessment, it concludes with a quick patient history and vital signs.

Content Review

RAPID TRAUMA ASSESSMENT

When serious injury is suspected, conduct a rapid assessment of the

- Head
- Neck
- Chest
- Abdomen
- Pelvis
- Extremities
- Back
- Quick patient history
- Vital signs

Content Review

FOCUSED EXAM AND HISTORY

When limited injuries are expected, conduct an assessment focused on regions suggested by:

- Patient complaint
- Mechanism of injury
- Signs or symptoms noted during the initial assessment
- Also conduct a quick patient history and vital signs assessment.

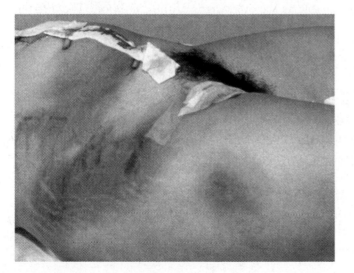

FIGURE 18-4 During the rapid trauma assessment, quickly scan the body looking for hemorrhage or evidence of significant injury.

DETAILED PHYSICAL EXAM
Used rarely, only in a
patient with:

• Altered mental status,
  and . . .
• Limited apparent minor
  injuries, and/or
• Mechanism of injury
  suggesting multiple
  injury sites

DETAILED PHYSICAL EXAM

The detailed physical exam is a comprehensive examination of the entire body to locate and identify signs of injury. It is rarely used in the prehospital setting because seriously injured patients receive attention directed at their life-threatening injuries and time becomes a premium as they are rushed to a trauma center. The patient with moderate or minor injuries receives assessment and care directed just at those injuries. The only case where a complete detailed exam may be necessary is in a patient with an altered level of consciousness, limited apparent minor injuries, and a mechanism of injury that suggests possible multiple injury sites. Only perform the detailed exam after you have concluded the initial assessment and stabilized or corrected any life-threatening conditions discovered during it.

The detailed physical exam is an organized and intensive evaluation of each body area: the head, neck, chest, abdomen, pelvis, extremities, and back. When performing the detailed exam, use the physical assessment techniques of questioning, inspection, palpation, auscultation, and percussion discussed earlier in the chapter. (Using DCAP-BTLS or some other mnemonic or system may help you remember most of the important aspects of the evaluation of a body region.)

Head

When evaluating the head, inspect and palpate its entire surface looking for any deformity, asymmetry, or hemorrhage. In addition to looking for the obvious signs of trauma, direct special attention to the eyes, the auditory canal, the nose and mouth, and the facial region.

Evaluate the eyes for pupillary response. Shade the eyes in a bright environment (or shine a light into them in a dark environment) and note their response. They should dilate (or constrict) briskly, equally, and consensually (together). Check eye movement by having the patient follow your finger as you trace an H pattern in front of him; any deficit in the patient's ability to follow your finger suggests either cranial nerve injury or orbital fracture and muscle entrapment. The auditory canal should be clear of fluid, and the tympanic membrane should be intact. The nose and mouth should be free of hemorrhage and physical obstruction. Any drainage of fluid from the mouth or nose endangers the airway and, if from the nose, suggests skull fracture and the possible leakage of cerebrospinal fluid. Notable signs of basilar skull fracture include bilateral periorbital eccymosis (raccoon's eyes), retroauricular eccymosis (Battle's sign), and eccymosis behind the tympanic membrane (hemotympanum), though the first two are late signs. Gently palpate the upper jaw and feel for any crepitus or instability indicative of a facial fracture.

Neck

Evaluate the neck for signs of injury, for the position of the trachea, and the status of the jugular veins. The trachea should be midline in the neck and not moving to one side with respiration. Displacement to one side suggests tension pneumothorax, although this is a very late sign and not as distinguishable as the other signs of the condition. The internal jugular veins should be distended in the supine, normovolemic patient and flatten as the patient's torso and head are raised to a 45-degree angle. Extremely distended jugular veins (or ones distended beyond 45 degrees) suggest tension pneumothorax, pericardial tamponade, or traumatic asphyxia. Flat jugular veins in the supine patient suggest hypovolemia. Examine the neck and head for the progressive distortion and crepitus associated with subcutaneous emphysema that may accompany tension pneumothorax. Examine for any open wounds, control any hemorrhage, and cover open wounds with occlusive dressings to prevent air embolism. Anticipate airway compromise and consider early intubation if serious neck trauma is present.

Chest

In addition to the standard elements of the physical assessment, examine the chest for intercostal or suprasternal retractions, air moving through any open wounds, and paradoxical chest wall motion. Carefully observe the surface of the chest for erythema mirroring the structure of the rib cage. When the skin is trapped between an impacting force and the ribs, it contuses and may demonstrate this sign. Auscultate all lung fields of the chest, both anteriorly and posteriorly. Also listen for heart sounds. Apply pressure to the lateral aspect of the rib cage and direct it medially to help identify any fracture site along the ribs. The pressure flexes the ribs, moves the fracture site slightly, and creates local pain. You may feel a grating sensation (crepitus) that also suggests costal fracture. Palpation may reveal a crackling sensation associated with air under the skin (subcutaneous emphysema).

Abdomen

Observe the abdomen for any asymmetry or pulsing masses. Also look for any indication of compression by the seat belt or other signs of impact. Palpate each quadrant, with one hand placing pressure on the other while you sense any unusual masses or muscle spasm (guarding). Always palpate the quadrant with the suspected injury last. Finally, inspect and palpate the flanks.

Pelvis

Evaluate the pelvis by placing firm pressure on the iliac crests directed medially and on the pubic bone directed downward. If you notice any crepitus and/or any instability of the pelvis, suspect fracture and serious internal hemorrhage. Examine the inguinal, external genitalia, and buttock areas because these locations are often sites of serious injury and hemorrhage. It is essential that you expose these areas if the mechanism of injury suggests injury there because hemorrhage is frequently hidden in jeans or other articles of clothing.

Extremities

Examine each extremity and evaluate its muscle tone, distal pulse, temperature, color, and capillary refill time. Also evaluate for motor response, sensory response, and limb strength. Compare your findings in one limb to those of the opposing limb.

Back

Examine the patient's back during your assessment or when using movement techniques such as a log roll. If spinal injury is suspected, be sure to maintain manual stabilization of the head and neck as you position the patient for examination. Examine the total surface of the back and palpate the spinal column from top to bottom. Look carefully for any slight deformities, minor reddening, very subtle pain, or tenderness; these may be the only sign or symptom indicative of spinal column injury.

Concluding the Examination

At the conclusion of the rapid trauma assessment, the focused exam, or the detailed assessment, mentally inventory all the suspected injuries you have found. Place them in descending order of priority for care and note the contribution they make to the patient's shock state. Then make your final decision as to the patient's transport status.

TRAUMA PATIENT HISTORY

Signs and Symptoms

During the rapid trauma assessment or the focused exam (or, in some cases, the detailed physical exam), conduct an abbreviated patient history. The elements of the S component of the SAMPLE history assessment, signs and symptoms, are extensively addressed as you perform the physical assessment. Gather the remaining elements of the SAMPLE history—Allergies, Medications, Past medical history, Last oral intake, and Events leading up to the incident—either while performing your physical exam or immediately after it.

Allergies

Question the patient about allergies, especially those to medications used commonly in emergency medicine. Such allergies include those to antibiotics, the -caine family of local anesthetics, analgesics, and tetanus toxoid. If any of these are noted, pass this information on to the emergency department staff.

> *Gather most of the history for the trauma patient—especially signs and symptoms—while you conduct the physical exam. Gather any remaining history information immediately after the physical exam.*

Medications

Investigate the patient's use of prescription and non-prescription medications as such use may impact response to care or suggest underlying medical problems or disease. For example, drugs, such as beta blockers, reduce the heart's ability to respond to hypovolemia with an increased rate. Be especially watchful for use of aspirin (interferes with clotting), anticoagulants such as warfarin (Coumadin®), and antibiotics.

Past Medical History

Question the patient about any significant medical history that may impact either response to shock, your care, or the medications the emergency department is likely to use during treatment. Pre-existing medical problems may limit the body's ability to compensate for shock due to trauma and may affect the presentation of signs and symptoms. For example, a heart condition may limit the ability of the heart to increase its rate in response to a reduced preload, confounding your assessment. A normally hypertensive patient may present with a normal blood pressure that, in fact, represents hypotension.

Last Oral Intake

The quantity and time since the patient's last fluid and solid oral intake should affect your index of suspicion for abdominal injury and the care a patient will receive in the emergency department. If the patient's bladder, stomach, or bowel was full and strong forces of deceleration or compression were directed to the abdomen, the risk of rupture and peritonitis is increased. Food and liquid in the stomach also pose serious risks should the patient need surgery, because the use of anesthesia may precipitate vomiting, which may result in aspiration and increase mortality and morbidity. You should also be concerned if the trauma patient has recently consumed solids or liquids because vomiting and aspiration may complicate prehospital airway care.

Events Leading Up to the Incident

The events immediately preceding the incident are very important. They may suggest that the patient's trauma was caused by a medical or other problem such as falling asleep while driving or becoming dizzy just before a fall. (Seeing no skid marks at a scene where an auto has collided with a tree is an important finding and suggests an intentional impact or some other contributing factor.)

VITAL SIGNS

Complete the physical exam by collecting a baseline set of vital signs— including pulse, blood pressure, respiration, and skin evaluations—at the scene or during transport.

Complete the rapid trauma assessment or focused exam by collecting a baseline set of vital signs. You can do this either at the scene or during transport as the patient's condition and circumstances allow. These vital signs include pulse rate and quality, blood pressure, respiration rate and quality, and skin temperature and condition. Watch for increasing pulse rate and decreasing pulse strength, increasing respiratory rate and decreasing volume, decreasing pulse pressure, and the patient's skin becoming cool and clammy. These changes all suggest increasing compensation for blood loss and shock.

TRANSPORT DECISION

The transport decision is made in a preliminary way at the end of the initial assessment and finalized at the end of the rapid trauma assessment or the focused exam and history. You will decide whether to provide rapid transport to the trauma center, treat at the scene and then transport to the nearest emergency department, or treat and release as permitted by local protocols.

Rapid Transport

If a serious mechanism of injury or physical finding is present, according to the trauma triage criteria, the patient is a candidate for rapid transport to a trauma center.

The decision to provide rapid transport to the trauma center is predicated on the trauma triage criteria. (Review Table 12-2, "Trauma Triage Criteria Indicating Need for Immediate Transport," in Chapter 12.) If any of the specified mechanisms of injury or the physical signs of injury are present, the patient is a candidate for rapid transport (Figure 18-5). If the patient demonstrates a significant mechanism of injury but the signs and symptoms and the

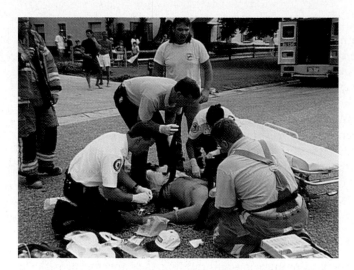

other results of your initial and rapid trauma assessment do not demonstrate the need for this level of transport, contact medical direction to possibly transport to a general hospital emergency department instead.

Revised Trauma Score

The revised trauma score is a numerical evaluation of the patient using the elements of the Glasgow Coma Scale (GCS) and the patient's respiratory rate and systolic blood pressure. Some EMS systems use this, or another trauma scoring system to predict patient outcome and help make the decision on whether the patient requires rapid transport to a trauma center. Consult your system's medical director and protocols to determine if the revised trauma score is in use in your jurisdiction and to learn what numerical score mandates rapid transport.

Treat and Transport

Provide on-scene care and then transport to the nearest emergency department for any patient who has neither a significant mechanism of injury nor physical signs of serious trauma. Manage the patient's specific injuries on the scene and transport once your care has stabilized the injuries and the patient is packaged, so movement to the ambulance and hospital will not cause further harm. If at any time during your care the patient demonstrates any signs of more serious injury or shock compensation, consider rapid transport to the trauma center.

Treat and Release

Some EMS systems permit care providers to treat patients with minor injuries and then release them to see their personal physician. Provide this service only to the patient with very minor and isolated injuries. Make certain that you carefully explain to the patient what care is needed for the injury. Describe the signs that may develop indicating that the injury requires immediate attention and advise the patient that he should call your service again if those signs appear. Finally, tell the patient that he should seek care from a family physician. If possible, provide this information in written form, approved by your system of medical direction, and have the patient acknowledge in writing the receipt of these instructions. If you have any questions about treatment or release of a patient, contact your medical direction physician.

Patient Care Refusals

Some patients with trauma will refuse assessment, care, and transport. Although this is the patient's right, the situation represents a dilemma for prehospital care providers. The patient may not understand the significance of his injuries, and the early signs of trauma may not clearly reflect its nature or seriousness.

When confronted with a patient refusing care, advise the patient that serious injury may not present with overt or painful symptoms. Try to convince him to permit you to perform an assessment and provide on-scene care. If you are not successful, attempt to have the patient talk with the physician providing on-line medical direction. Be sure the patient is an adult and is fully conscious, oriented, and able to make a rational decision. Use family members to help encourage the patient to accept your assessment and care. If your attempts to convince the patient fail, suggest that he see a personal physician at the earliest opportunity. Stress that the patient should feel free to call for EMS if additional signs or symptoms develop or existing ones worsen. Be sure to document the refusal thoroughly. Include your recommendation that the patient receive assessment, care, and transport; your warning of the dangers of refusing assessment, care, and transport; your suggestion that the patient see a family physician; and your recommendation to contact EMS again if the problem persists or worsens.

ONGOING ASSESSMENT

The ongoing assessment should be performed every 5 minutes with critically or seriously injured patients and every 15 minutes with other patients.

The ongoing assessment is important to monitoring and guiding the care you provide. It should be performed every 5 minutes with critically or seriously injured patients and every 15 minutes with other patients (Figure 18-6). Also perform an ongoing assessment whenever you note any change in the patient's condition or you institute any significant intervention.

During the ongoing assessment, perform the mental, airway, breathing, and circulation status checks of the initial assessment and recheck any significant findings of the rapid trauma assessment or focused exam. Reassess the vital signs—blood pressure; rate, regularity and strength of the pulse; respiratory rate, volume, and regularity; and skin condition. With any limb injury, re-check the distal pulse, capillary refill, muscle strength, and sensation. Pay particular attention to an increasing pulse rate, decreasing pulse strength, increasing respiratory rate, decreasing respiratory volume, increasing capillary refill time, decreasing level of consciousness or orientation, change in skin color or temperature, or increasing anxiety or restlessness. Any of these signs may indicate patient deterioration. Compare results of each ongoing assessment to baseline findings and those from previous ongoing assessments to identify any deterioration or improvement in the patient's condition. Record the results serially so that trending of the patient's signs can continue after arrival at the emergency department.

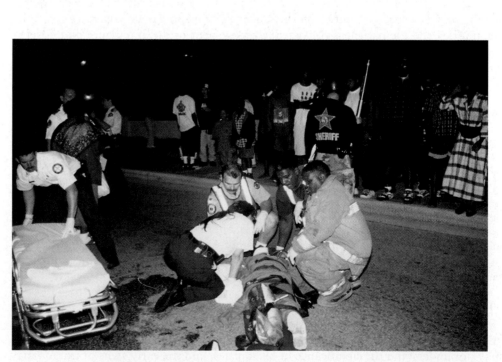

FIGURE 18-6 Repeat the ongoing assessment every 5 minutes in a seriously injured patient.

MANAGEMENT OF HEAD, FACIAL, AND NECK INJURY PATIENTS

The management priorities for the patient sustaining head, face, or neck trauma include care directed at maintaining the patient's airway and breathing, ensuring circulation through hemorrhage control, addressing or taking steps to avoid hypoxia and/or hypovolemia, and providing appropriate medications. Once these priorities have been attended to, you may dress and care for minor head, facial, and neck wounds.

AIRWAY

The airway is the most important care priority with head, face, and neck injury patients. Head, face, and neck injury can leave patients unable to control the airway either due to an altered mental status or to damaged airway structures. In addition, soft tissue trauma to the airway may cause edema that can quickly progress from restriction of the airway to its complete obstruction. Vigilant attention to the airway and aggressive airway care are the only means of ensuring that the airway of these patients remains protected and patent. Airway management techniques appropriate for such patients include patient positioning, suctioning, oral and nasal airway insertion, and endotracheal intubation. (You can review these techniques in Chapter 5, "Airway Management and Ventilation.")

Suctioning

Airway tissues are extremely vascular, bleed profusely, and swell quickly. Soft tissue injury may cause significant hemorrhage that can compromise the airway in two ways. First, the sheer volume of blood may block the airway. Note that aspiration of blood is more often responsible for hypoxia than physical obstruction of the airway, so be certain to suction as necessary to remove blood from the airway.

Secondly, blood is a gastric irritant that frequently induces emesis. If a large volume of blood is swallowed, the patient may vomit, thus further endangering the airway. In addition, vomiting is common with head injury patients because emesis is a frequent result of brain injury or increasing intracranial pressure. Vomiting often occurs without warning (without nausea) and can be projectile in nature. Vomiting is especially dangerous with head injury patients because they commonly have a depressed or absent gag reflex. Gastric contents are very acidic and will quickly damage the tissues of the lower airway if aspirated. Aspiration of gastric contents is associated with high patient mortality. Be ready to suction aggressively as needed in any patients with nasal, oral, or head trauma. Use a large-bore catheter or a suction hose without a tip to clear the airway of any blood or emesis.

Content Review

HEAD, FACE, AND NECK INJURY MANAGEMENT
- Maintain airway and breathing.
- Control hemorrhage.
- Address hypoxia and/or hypovolemia.

Vigilant attention to the airway and aggressive airway care are vital with head, facial, and neck injury patients.

Patho Pearls

Edema (swelling) is the accumulation of water in the interstitial space. It can be localized or generalized. Local swelling may appear at the site of an injury (e.g., damaged airway structures or a sprained ankle) or within a certain organ system such as the brain (cerebral edema), lungs (pulmonary edema), heart (pericardial effusion), or abdomen (ascites).

Edema not only is a sign of an underlying disease or problem, but it also causes problems. It interferes with the movement of nutrients and wastes between tissues and capillaries. It may diminish capillary blood flow, depriving tissues of oxygen. In turn, this may slow the healing of wounds, promote infection, and facilitate formation of pressure sores. Edema affecting organs such as the brain, lung, heart, or larynx may be life threatening.

Body water that is retained in the interstitial spaces is body water not available for metabolic processes in the cells. Therefore, even though the total body water is normal, edema can cause a relative condition of dehydration.

In the prehospital setting, edema can be treated through alignment of fractured or dislocated bones or joints, elevation of the affected area when possible, gentle circumferential dressings, application of cool packs, and administration of diuretics. Damage to the airway, where development of edema is life threatening, requires that the patient be intubated before the swelling develops to the point of airway obstruction.

Patient Positioning

Consider placing the patient in a position that protects the airway early in your care (during the initial assessment). The best position for the patient with suspected head injury is on the left side with the head turned slightly and facing downward, the left lateral recumbent (recovery) position. Remember, of course, that head injury patients require spinal precautions. Maintain manual stabilization until the patient is secured to a long spine board, and then be prepared to turn patient and board as a unit to facilitate airway drainage.

It is unlikely that suction alone will evacuate all emesis from the oral cavity before the unconscious or semiconscious patient attempts an inspiration. If the patient experiencing serious oral, nasal (epistaxis), or facial bleeding is conscious and alert and no serious spinal injury is suspected, have the patient sit leaning forward to promote drainage and keep fluids from flowing into the posterior airway. If the patient has sustained an isolated open neck injury with the danger of air embolism, place the patient on a spine board in the Trendelenburg position, with the lower part of the patient's body elevated about 12 inches. Otherwise, position the patient with isolated potential brain injury by elevating the head of the spine board to about 30 degrees to reduce both external hemorrhage and intracranial pressure. If in doubt, place the patient supine on a spine board and be prepared to manage the airway as needed.

Oropharyngeal and Nasopharyngeal Airways

Oropharyngeal and nasopharyngeal airways each have advantages and disadvantages when used with head, face, and neck injury patients. The nasal airway does not trigger the gag reflex as easily as the oral airway and is better tolerated by the patient. Because there is less stimulation of the gag reflex, there is also a reduction in transient increases in intracranial pressure and in the chances of increasing the severity of head injury during insertion. One hazard of nasal airway use is the possible insertion of the tube directly into the cranium through a fracture of the posterior nasal border. Always insert the nasal airway straight back, through the largest of the nares (nostrils), and use only gentle force in its introduction. If you suspect basilar skull fracture, use an oral airway or endotracheal intubation to establish and maintain the airway.

Although the oral and nasal airways help keep the respective pharynxes open, they can represent threats to the airway. The ends of the tubes sit just superior to the opening of the larynx. If a patient vomits, which frequently happens with brain injury, the vomitus is blocked from exiting the patient's mouth through the airway and remains just at the laryngeal opening. With the next breath, the patient can aspirate the gastric contents, which may have serious consequences. Whenever an oral or nasal airway is in place, monitor the patient's airway carefully and be prepared to remove the airway and evacuate any emesis.

Endotracheal Intubation

Endotracheal intubation is the most definitive method of ensuring a clear and patent airway in the head injury patient. Intubate early in the care of the unresponsive patient and consider intubation for any patient with a reduced level of consciousness. Techniques useful in caring for head injury patients include orotracheal, digital, nasotracheal, and directed intubation.

Orotracheal Intubation   Orotracheal, or oral, intubation is the most common and usually the most successful technique for placing an endotracheal tube (Figure 18-7). It does, however, pose some hazards for head, face, and neck injury patients. All patients who sustain serious injuries in these regions require spinal immobilization. Immobilization, however, limits the movement of the patient's head during intubation attempts, restricting you from manually bringing the oral opening, pharynx, and trachea in line. The result is often an inability to visualize the vocal folds and watch the endotracheal tube pass into the trachea, seriously reducing the chances of a successful oral intubation.

To improve visualization during oral intubation with spinal immobilization, employ a technique called Sellick's maneuver. Apply pressure directed posteriorly to the cricoid ring with the thumb and index finger, moving it downward toward the vertebral column. This brings the trachea more in line with the oral cavity and pharynx and compresses the esoph-

Intubate early in the care of the unresponsive patient and consider intubation for any patient with a reduced level of consciousness.

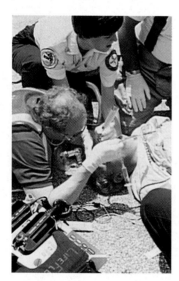

FIGURE 18-7   Oral intubation is difficult in the patient with facial trauma because landmarks may be distorted, blood may flow into the airway, and the head must remain in the neutral position.

agus, thus reducing the likelihood of vomitus entering the upper airway during intubation. Exercise caution to prevent the pressure from flexing the cervical spine. Be aware that Sellick's maneuver may not align the airway enough to permit visualized oral intubation.

Attempts at endotracheal intubation can increase the parasympathetic (vagal) tone. This, in turn, may increase intracranial pressure and lower the heart rate or increase the severity of other cardiac dysrhythmias already induced by the brain injury. Therefore, carry out the intubation rapidly. If possible, have the most experienced care provider attempt the procedure to reduce both intubation time and vagal stimulation. Also consider use of a pharmacological agent, such as a **topical anesthetic** spray, to reduce both vagal stimulation and the retching associated with stimulation of the gag reflex.

Digital Intubation   Another technique that may be effective when intubating a patient undergoing spinal precautions is digital intubation. In this procedure, the endotracheal tube is positioned without visualization; instead, the tube is directed into the trachea from the base of the tongue by the fingers of the intubator. This is a procedure best attempted by an EMT-I with long thin fingers.

A slightly smaller than usual endotracheal tube is shaped by a stylet into a J configuration. The patient's mouth is held open with a bite block while you insert the first two fingers of one hand and "walk" them back along the tongue to its base. Use these fingers to locate and lift the epiglottis. Advance the tube with your other hand along the back of the tongue and direct it with your fingers past the epiglottis and toward the tracheal opening. Continue to advance the endotracheal tube with slight anterior pressure along the posterior surface of the epiglottis for about 1½ to 2½ inches. Remove the stylet and carefully confirm tube placement in the trachea, not the esophagus. Digital intubation should only be done on unconscious patients to minimize the risk of the patient biting the EMT-I's fingers.

Nasotracheal Intubation   A third procedure for intubation of the patient with possible spinal injury is nasotracheal, or nasal, intubation. Insert the endotracheal tube into the largest of the nares. Then direct it posteriorly, curving it toward the floor of the nasal cavity. Advance the tube the length of an oral airway (the distance between the ear lobe and the corner of the mouth). At this point, slowly continue insertion while you, with your ear at the endotracheal tube opening, listen for the sounds of respirations. Gently manipulate the tube until the respiratory sounds are loudest and then advance it during inspiration. The tube should pass directly into the trachea. The technique can be made somewhat easier using an endotracheal tube with a directable tip (such as an Endotrol). With this device, a small cord connected to the end of the tube permits the user to increase or decrease the tube's curve.

The disadvantages to nasal intubation include the necessity of having a breathing patient and a quiet environment, and the danger of inserting the tube through a fractured cribiform plate and into the skull. The procedure has a lower rate of success than either oral or digital intubation. Nasal intubation also tends to raise intracranial pressure more than oral intubation because it generally takes longer and more aggressively stimulates the posterior nasal and oral pharynxes.

Directed Intubation   In some cases of serious facial or upper neck trauma, as in a shotgun blast, the landmarks of the upper airway are disrupted or destroyed. In such cases, obtaining and maintaining an airway may be extremely difficult. Use strong suction over the area and use the laryngoscope to visualize the elements of the oropharynx and laryngopharynx. If you cannot see airway landmarks themselves, look for bubbling air escaping from the trachea with expirations. If you believe you are close to the tracheal opening and can visualize the area, have an assistant compress the chest to induce bubbling. Pass the endotracheal tube along the route of bubbles and into the trachea. With this technique, it is critically important to confirm proper placement of the endotracheal tube.

Confirmation of Tube Placement   Once the endotracheal tube is inserted using one of the techniques described above, confirm its proper placement in the trachea. This is especially important when the tube has been placed blindly. Auscultate, at a minimum, the axillae and over the epigastrium. (Good breath sounds at the axillae reflect good ventilation

If possible, have the most experienced care provider attempt intubation to reduce both the length of the procedure and vagal stimulation.

topical anesthetic agent that produces partial or complete loss of sensation in the surface area to which it is applied.

Confirmation of tube placement is especially important when the tube has been placed blindly.

Endotracheal intubation
should be confirmed by the
three different methods as
described in Chapter 5.

to the distal alveoli, while sounds in the epigastrium suggest esophageal intubation.) Watch carefully for good, symmetrical chest wall excursion with each ventilation. If you hear good breath sounds bilaterally, detect no epigastric sounds, and see the chest wall move equally with each breath, the tube is most likely in the trachea. Inflate the cuff of the tube and hyperventilate the patient for a short period of time. Use an end-tidal CO_2 monitor or detection device, pulse oximetry, and observation of the patient's skin color to help confirm and monitor proper and continuing endotracheal tube placement. Remember that the endotracheal tube may dislodge from the trachea during any movement of the patient, such as from the ground to the stretcher or when the stretcher is loaded into the ambulance. Reconfirm proper tube placement frequently.

BREATHING

Ensurance of breathing is an important priority with any patient, but it becomes extremely critical with the head-injured patient. Not only is reduced air exchange a problem, but excessive air exchange and the excessive depletion of carbon dioxide can also endanger the patient. Providing supplemental oxygenation and appropriate ventilation are essential with such patients.

Oxygenation

Any patient who has
sustained a significant head
injury or who displays any
indication of lowered level of
consciousness, orientation, or
arousal is a candidate for
high-flow, high-concentration
oxygen.

Any patient who has sustained a significant head injury or who displays any indication of lowered level of consciousness, orientation, or arousal is a candidate for high-flow, high-concentration oxygen. Administer oxygen at a rate of 12 to 15 liters per minute via a nonrebreather mask with a patient who is moving an adequate respiratory volume. If the patient is not breathing adequately, supplement any positive pressure ventilations with oxygen via reservoir, again flowing at 12 to 15 liters per minute.

Ventilations

Provision of a good supply of oxygen is critical to the head injury patient, but so too is the removal of carbon dioxide. Assess the patient's respiratory status and, if the patient is not moving a normal volume of air, employ overdrive respiration. Ventilate 12 to 20 times per minute with full breaths (about 800 to 1,000 mL). Be careful not to hyperventilate the patient because doing so reduces carbon dioxide levels in the blood and significantly reduces the cerebral blood flow. Endotracheal intubation makes ventilations easier and more efficient. Be careful not to accidentally hyperventilate the head injury patient once the tube is in place. Monitor the oxygen saturation with pulse oximetry to maintain a level of 95% or greater.

CIRCULATION

Your care of the patient with head, facial, and neck injury includes both control of any serious hemorrhage and support of the body's attempts to maintain blood pressure and cerebral circulation.

Hemorrhage Control

Head and facial hemorrhage is usually easy to control because most of these injuries are to the tissues that lie over facial and cranial bones. Direct pressure is commonly an effective means of controlling such bleeding, though you should take care not to apply pressure directly on suspected skull or facial fractures. Wrap bandaging circumferentially around the head (not the neck), but be careful to keep the airway clear and give the patient the freedom to rid himself of vomitus should emesis occur. Watch the airway and be prepared to suction aggressively to limit danger from aspiration. Suctioning can also ensure that the patient does not swallow large volumes of blood, stimulating emesis. Permit the conscious and alert patient with no suspected spinal injury who is suffering epistaxis to sit leaning forward, allowing the blood to drain. This positioning keeps blood from flowing down the pharynx and entering the esophagus.

An open neck injury carries the rare but serious risk of air entering the external jugular during strong inspiration, leading to cerebral embolism with stroke-like symptoms. Seal any open neck wound with an occlusive dressing held firmly in place by bandaging and tilt the patient's body head down on a backboard or stretcher, if possible. Carefully evaluate any other open wounds for frothy blood suggestive of tracheal involvement, seal those wounds with occlusive dressings, and monitor respirations.

Blunt trauma to the neck may produce the equivalent of **compartment syndrome.** Fasciae in the region compartmentalize muscle and anatomical structures and permit pressures to rise with rapid edema or blood accumulation. Any sign of neck edema or hematoma is an indication for rapid transport. Monitor the patient's airway and level of consciousness while en route to the hospital.

Severe hemorrhage associated with open neck wounds can lead quickly to hypovolemia and shock. Control the blood loss by using a dressing and gloved fingers to apply direct pressure to the source of bleeding. You may have to maintain digital pressure throughout prehospital care because application of circumferential bandaging may restrict the airway and circulation and is contraindicated.

compartment syndrome a condition in which a structure such as a nerve or tendon is being constricted in a space.

Blood Pressure Maintenance

Another component of circulation care for the head, face, and neck injury patient is guarding against hypotension. The brain is very dependent on receiving a continuous supply of oxygenated circulation. Any interruption of the supply, such as might be caused by hypotension in response to increasing intracranial pressure, will rapidly prove fatal. Care for the patient in whom you suspect increased intracranial pressure with aggressive fluid resuscitation, even if the patient's other injuries call for different priorities. For example, the patient with penetrating chest trauma might not receive aggressive fluid resuscitation until the systolic blood pressure drops to below 60 mmHg. If that patient also has a head injury with increasing intracranial pressure, waiting for the blood pressure to drop to that level would be life threatening. Hence, provide rapid fluid (electrolyte) administration and other shock care measures well before the blood pressure reaches 60 mmHg.

Hypoxia

It is very important to monitor the patient with a head injury at all times to quickly identify and correct any hypoventilation. Hypoxia can further damage central nervous system tissue already affected by direct injury. If someone else is delivering ventilations, frequently monitor both that person's performance as well as the patient's oxygen saturation levels. Care providers often find it difficult to determine accurate ventilation rates while using a BVM during the emergency. Ensure that the patient is well oxygenated before any intubation attempt and hyperventilated for a short time after intubation. Also be watchful for interruptions in ventilations that might occur during patient movement or when changing ventilation providers.

Hypovolemia

Like hypoxia, hypovolemia and the associated hypotension reduce oxygen transport to the brain. This condition also reduces both circulation through the brain and the ability of the blood to remove the products of metabolism. Since brain tissue is especially sensitive to oxygen deprivation, with head injury patients who have already suffered some damage to brain tissue, any further circulatory loss might prove devastating. The problems of hypovolemia and hypotension are compounded if there is any increase in intracranial pressure. Such an increase further restricts cerebral blood flow, and the body's autoregulatory mechanisms cannot compensate.

Provide aggressive fluid resuscitation for any patient with significant head injury in whom you suspect brain injury and who shows signs of shock—rapid, thready pulse, slowed capillary refill, lowered level of consciousness, anxiety, or restlessness. Insert two large-bore catheters and administer lactated Ringer's solution or normal saline at a wide-open rate through non-restrictive trauma IV tubing. Administer 1,000 mL of an isotonic solution, followed by additional boluses as needed to maintain a systolic blood pressure between 90 and 100 mmHg. Consider application of a PASG and carefully monitor the vital signs to assure the blood pressure remains above 90 mmHg.

Provide aggressive fluid resuscitation for any patient with significant head injury in whom you suspect brain injury and who shows signs of shock compensation.

Cultural Considerations

Many religions and cultures have specific beliefs about blood loss and transfusions. Because of these, it is important for EMS personnel to understand and respect these beliefs. For example, large numbers of Hmong immigrated to the United States and Canada after the Vietnam conflict. The Hmong are among the oldest group of people in Asia and are often referred to as the "Hill People." They put great faith in folk medicine and sometimes will trust a shaman more than a Western medical practitioner. Many Hmong believe that the body has a limited amount of blood, and any blood loss can cause permanent problems. Furthermore, many Hmong believe that any injuries or surgical procedures sustained in life will remain with them when they enter the spirit world. Thus, many Western practices, such as surgery and autopsy, may be forbidden by members of this culture.

The Jehovah's Witnesses are a religious group that has specifically forbidden blood transfusions. This belief comes from their interpretation of a Bible verse (Acts 15:29) that states, "That ye abstain from meats offered to idols, and from blood, and from things strangled, and from fornication: from which if ye keep yourselves, ye shall do well. Fare ye well." Although some have interpreted this verse to mean the literal "eating of blood," the Jehovah's Witnesses have interpreted it to include the transfusion of blood. The beliefs will vary from individual to individual. Some Jehovah's Witnesses will allow the administration of crystalloid fluids, while others will allow the actual administration of some blood components (plasma, globulins, and platelets). However, many will refuse all blood or similar products (including IV fluids). Regardless, the EMT-I must respect this wish and change treatment plans accordingly.

MEDICATIONS

Several medications may be useful in the care of the head injury patient. These medications include oxygen, **diuretics** (mannitol, furosemide), dextrose, thiamine, and topical anesthetic sprays.

Oxygen

Oxygen is the primary first-line drug used in the care of the patient with suspected head injury. Administration of high-flow oxygen provides a high inspired oxygen level and facilitates both diffusion through the alveolar and capillary walls and the highest oxygen uptake by the hemoglobin of the red blood cells. Oxygen saturation is important for the head injury patient because the brain is acutely dependent on a good supply of oxygen. There are no contraindications nor side effects of concern for use of oxygen during prehospital emergency care. (Note, however, that hyperventilation is contraindicated in head injury patients because it reduces circulating CO_2 levels.)

Administer oxygen via a nonrebreather mask at a flow rate of between 12 and 15 liters per minute for the patient who is breathing adequately. If the patient is receiving positive pressure ventilations, supplement the ventilations with 12 to 15 liters per minute of oxygen flowing into the reservoir. Monitor oxygen administration using the pulse oximeter, and keep the saturation level above 95%. Also monitor skin color, respiratory excursion, orientation, and anxiety to ensure the patient is well oxygenated.

Diuretics

Mannitol Mannitol is a large sugar molecule that does not leave the blood stream because of its size. It is an osmolar diuretic that draws water from body tissue into the blood stream. Mannitol then is eliminated by the kidneys and, as it leaves the kidneys, takes both water and sodium with it, reducing the body's fluid load. Mannitol is especially effective in drawing fluid from the brain, thereby reducing cerebral edema and intracranial pressure. Although very effective in reducing cerebral edema, mannitol may reduce the intracranial pressure associated with intracranial hemorrhage. This may result in increased hemorrhage and, ultimately, more serious brain damage. Mannitol is contraindicated in patients with hypovolemia or hypotension because of its diuretic properties and in patients with a recent history of congestive heart failure because it transiently raises the cardiovascular fluid volume. Mannitol may be most useful in the patient with suspected isolated closed head injury who develps a dilated pupil during care or a patient who exhibits Cushing's sign (elevated blood pressure and narrowing pulse pressure).

---

diuretic agent that increases urine excretion and elimination of body water with effects including reduced blood volume and reduced intracranial pressure.

Oxygen is the primary first-line drug used in the care of the patient with suspected head injury.

Mannitol should only be used in the prehospital setting based on a consensus agreement with local neurosurgeons and the EMS system medical director.

Mannitol is usually supplied in a single-use vial with a concentration of 20%. It is given as a single slow bolus (over 5 minutes) of 1 gm/kg of the patient's weight. It is very hypertonic and forms crystals at low temperatures (below 45°F). It can be reconstituted with rewarming and gentle agitation, although it should always be administered through an in-line filter to ensure no particulate matter enters the blood stream. Flush the IV line before and after the administration of mannitol to reduce the risk of precipitation.

Furosemide Furosemide (Lasix®) is a loop diuretic that inhibits the reabsorption of sodium in the kidneys. It results in the increased secretion of water and electrolytes, including sodium, chloride, magnesium, and calcium. Furosemide also causes mild venous dilation and a reduced cardiac preload. It is often given in combination with mannitol to increase the rate of diuresis. Although it does not remove fluid from cerebral edema as well as mannitol, it does cause a more rapid fluid elimination by the kidneys. Furosemide is generally contraindicated in pregnant patients because it may cause fetal abnormalities. Since furosemide also causes diuresis, use with caution, if at all, in patients with hypotension secondary to hypovolemia.

Furosemide often comes in a pre-loaded syringe or a single-use vial and is given as a slow IV bolus or intramuscular (IM) injection. It is administered at a dose of about 0.5 to 1.0 mg/kg, frequently in doses of either 40 or 80 mg. Administer the medication very slowly, over 1 to 2 minutes.

Dextrose

In general, both hypoglycemia and hyperglycemia are detrimental to the patient with head injury. In the past, dextrose was given routinely to patients who were unresponsive with an undetermined cause. However, current practice calls for identifying the blood glucose level in all unresponsive patients, especially those with a possible history of diabetes or chronic alcoholism. If significant hypoglycemia is found, administer 25 mg of glucose and 100 mg of thiamine.

The empiric use of dextrose in the head-injured patient is contraindicated.

Dextrose is supplied in preloaded syringes containing 50 mL of a 0.5 mg/mL (50%) solution ($D_{50}W$). It is to be administered slowly through a large vein because it is a very hypertonic solution. A second dose may be administered in severe cases of hypoglycemia.

Thiamine

Thiamine, more commonly known as vitamin B1, is a substance obtained from diet and is needed for body metabolism. Thiamine is essential for the processing of glucose through Kreb's cycle, from which the body gains its life-sustaining energy. In malnourished patients (such as the chronic alcoholic), thiamine is depleted and the body tissue cannot obtain energy from glucose. The brain is especially affected since it does not store energy sources.

Thiamine is supplied in 1 mL single-use ampules, vials, and preloaded syringes containing a 100 mg/mL solution. It is administered IV bolus or IM. It should be administered before or with glucose.

Topical Anesthetic Spray

Topical sprays use an anesthetic agent, such as xylocaine or benzocaine, to anesthetize the oral and pharyngeal mucosa. This reduces the gag reflex, making endotracheal intubation easier and reducing the impact retching has on intracranial pressure. The agent is sprayed into the oral pharynx where it is rapidly absorbed by mucosal tissue. It inhibits nerve sensation, thereby reducing the gag reflex. The effects of the agent are immediate (within 15 seconds), remain local, and last for about 15 minutes. These agents are usually supplied in 2-ounce aerosol spray cannisters with long, hollow extension tubes to direct the spray down the throat. The agent is applied by directing a spray of the material into the posterior oral cavity and pharynx. Although topical anesthetic sprays permit easier intubation and reduce the associated vagal effects, they also reduce the patient's ability to remove fluids from the airway and increase the danger of aspiration.

When transporting head injury patients, limit external stimulation, such as the use of red lights and sirens, and try to provide a smooth ride.

TRANSPORT CONSIDERATIONS

Special considerations should be observed when transporting the patient with serious head injury to the hospital. Limit any external stimulation such as the use of red lights and sirens and try to achieve a smooth ride. Stimulation may further agitate the patient, increase intracranial pressure, and induce seizures.

Be cautious in considering the head injury patient as a candidate for air medical service transport. Although the time saved by helicopter transport may be very important, the head injury patient is prone to seizures, especially with the physical stimulation (noise and vibration) associated with this mode of transport. Seizures aboard any type of aircraft are very dangerous. If you elect to transport by air, ensure that the patient is firmly secured to a long spine board (including feet and hands) and that his airway is protected by endotracheal intubation.

MANAGEMENT OF SPINAL INJURY PATIENTS

Spinal precautions have one major objective: maintaining the patient in a neutral, in-line position.

Spinal injury care steps (spinal precautions) performed during the initial assessment include moving the patient to the neutral, in-line position, maintaining that position with manual immobilization until the patient is fully immobilized by mechanical means, and applying the cervical collar once the neck assessment is complete. The remaining steps in management of the spinal injury patient are related to maintaining the neutral, in-line position while moving the patient to the long spine board and then firmly securing him to the board for transport to the hospital.

These skills have but one major objective: maintaining the neutral, in-line position. Although this might seem a simple objective, it is not. Remember that the spine is a chain of thirty-three small, rather delicate bones, which is attached to other skeletal members only at the head, thorax, and pelvis. These skeletal attachments may transmit forces that attempt to flex, extend, rotate, compress, distract, and laterally bend the spine during any patient movement. The procedures and devices discussed below are intended to ensure that the patient remains in the neutral, in-line position throughout care, movement, and transport.

Constantly calm and reassure the patient with suspected spinal injury. Spinal injury can produce extreme anxiety in patients because of the severity of its effects and their potentially lifelong implications. The application of spinal precautions can compound this anxiety. The patient must endure complete immobilization on a rigid and relatively uncomfortable device, the long spine board. He will be unable to move and protect himself during the processes of immobilization, assessment, care, and transport to the hospital. To alleviate some of the anxiety, be sure to communicate frequently with the patient. Tell the patient why you are employing spinal precautions and explain, in advance, what you will be doing in each step of the process. Do what you can to make the patient comfortable and to provide assurance that you and your team are caring for his needs.

SPINAL ALIGNMENT

The first step in taking spinal precautions is to bring the patient from the position in which he is found into a neutral, in-line position adequate for assessment, airway maintenance, and spinal immobilization. This involves moving the patient to the supine position with the head facing directly forward and elevated 1 to 2 inches above the ground. Remember that the spine curves in an S shape through its length. This leaves the head displaced forward when the posterior thorax and buttocks (supporting the pelvis) rest on a firm, flat surface. Also remember that the neutral position (also known as the position of function) is generally with the joints halfway between the extremes of their motion. In spinal positioning, this means the hips and knees should be somewhat flexed for maximum comfort and minimum stress on the muscles, joints, and spine. For complete spinal immobilization, consider placement of a rolled blanket under the knees.

It is also important to ensure no distracting or compressing forces are on the spine. If the patient is seated or standing, support the head to leave only a portion of the head's weight on the spine. Be careful not to lift the entire head because this places a distracting force on the spine. Lastly, bring the spine into line by aligning the nose, navel, and toes to ensure that no rotation occurs along the length of the spine. The head must face directly forward, and the shoulders and pelvis must be in a single plane with the body. This neutral, in-line positioning allows for the greatest spacing between the cord and inner lumen of the spinal foramen. Neutral, in-line positioning both reduces pressure on the cord and increases circulation to and through it, an especially important consideration in the presence of injury. Many techniques are used for moving and immobilizing the potential spine injury patient; whichever you employ, always focus on obtaining and then maintaining neutral, in-line positioning. Doing this ensures the best opportunity to protect the vertebral column and the spinal cord of the patient during your time at his side.

The only contraindications to moving the potential spine injury patient from the position in which he is found to the neutral, in-line position are as follows: when movement causes a noticeable increase in pain, when you meet with noticeable resistance during the procedure, when you identify an increase in neurological signs as you move the head, or when the patient's spine is grossly deformed. Pain and resistance both suggest that the alignment process may be moving the injury site and thus may be causing further injury. When you meet with resistance or increased pain during any positioning of the head or spine, immobilize the patient as he lies. The same rule applies when you note an increase in the signs of neurological injury in the patient with movement of the spine. Finally, in cases of severe deformity of the spine, do not move the patient because any movement will further compromise the column and cord. Use whatever padding and immobilization devices are necessary to accommodate the patient's positioning and ensure that no further movement occurs.

Make certain that any movement of the patient during assessment or care is toward alignment. If, for example, the patient is lying twisted on the ground when you find him, assess the exposed areas, then move the patient toward alignment. If the patient is found prone, assess the patient's posterior surfaces before you log-roll him (to a long spine board) for further assessment and care. Never move a patient twice before you complete your mechanical immobilization, if possible.

Manual Cervical Stabilization

The typical trauma patient is found either seated (as in an auto) or lying on the ground. For the seated patient, initially approach from the front and carefully direct the patient not to move or turn his head. It is an almost reflexive act to turn to listen when we hear someone speak to us from behind. Such movement is dangerous in the potential spine injury patient. Ask your patient to keep his head still and explain to the patient that a caregiver is going to position himself or herself behind the patient to stabilize the spine.

Then the assigned caregiver should move behind the patient and bring his or her hands up along the patient's ears, using the little fingers to catch the mandible and the medial aspect of the heels of the hand to engage the mastoid region of the skull. Gentle pressure inward engages the head and prevents it from moving. A gentle lifting force of a few pounds helps take some of the weight of the head off the cervical spine, but care should be taken not to lift the head or apply any traction to this critical region. The patient's head should then be moved slowly and easily to a position in which the eyes face directly forward and along a line central to and perpendicular to the shoulder plane.

If there is no access to the seated patient from behind, employ the same techniques of movement and stabilization from in front with the little fingers engaging the mastoid region while the heels of the hand support the mandible. When approaching from the patient's side, place one hand under the mandible while using the other to support the occiput (Figure 18-8).

> *Move any body segment that is out of alignment toward alignment as you examine it, but if the patient feels any increase in pain or if you feel resistance to movement, immobilize the head and neck or other portion of the body in the position achieved.*

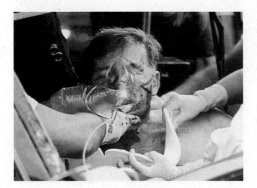

FIGURE 18-8 When you cannot access the patient from behind to apply manual stabilization, use alternative hand placement.

If the patient is supine, support the head by placing your hands along the lateral and inferior surfaces of the head. Position the little fingers and heels of the hands just lateral to the occipital region of the skull to support the head. With gentle inward pressure, hold the patient's head immobile and prevent flexion/extension, rotation, and lateral bending motion. Lift the head gently off the ground to approximate the neutral position, usually 1 to 2 inches for the adult. (If the surface on which the patient is found is not flat, adjust the height accordingly.) Position the head of a small adult or a large child at about ground level. Elevate the shoulders of infants or very small children because of their proportionally larger heads. Apply no axial pressure by either pushing or pulling the head toward or away from the body.

If a patient is found prone or on the side, position your hands according to the patient's position. If it will be some time until the patient can be moved to the supine position, place your hands so that they are comfortable during cervical stabilization. You should then reposition your hands just before the patient is moved to the final position. If the time until moving the patient to the supine position is expected to be short, place your hands so they will be properly positioned at the conclusion of the move. This may involve initially twisting your hands into a relatively uncomfortable position.

Assessment, care, and patient movement may require the caregiver holding stabilization to reposition his or her hands. To accomplish this, another caregiver supports and stabilizes the patient's head and neck by bringing his or her hands in from an alternate position. This caregiver places one hand under the patient's occiput while the other hand holds the jaw. Once the head is stable, have the original caregiver reposition his or her hands, reassume stabilization, and then have the second caregiver remove his or her hands.

Cervical Collar Application

A cervical collar by itself does not immobilize the cervical spine.

Always ensure that the cervical collar is correctly sized for the patient or choose another one.

After a potential spinal injury patient has been manually stabilized, consider the application of the cervical collar. Apply the collar as soon as the neck is fully assessed, generally during the rapid trauma assessment. The cervical collar is only an adjunct to full cervical immobilization and should never be considered to provide immobilization by itself. The collar does limit cervical spine motion and reduce the forces of compression (axial loading), but it does not completely prevent flexion/extension, rotation, or lateral bending.

To apply the cervical collar, size it to the patient according to the manufacturer's recommendations. Position the device under the chin and against the chest. Contour it over the shoulders and secure it firmly behind the neck. Be sure the Velcro® closures remain clear of sand, dirt, fabric, or the patient's hair and make a secure seal behind the neck (Figure 18-9). The collar should fit snugly around the neck but not place pressure against its anterior surface (carotid and jugular blood vessels and trachea). The collar should direct a limiting force against the jaw and occiput to restrict any flexion/extension of the head and neck. Ensure that the collar does not seriously limit the movement of the jaw, since this could prevent the patient from ridding himself of vomitus. Once the cervical collar is in place, do not release or relax manual cervical stabilization until the patient is fully im-

FIGURE 18-9 Properly place and secure the cervical collar on suspected spinal injury patients.

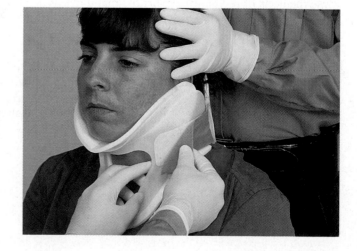

mobilized either with a vest-type immobilization device or to a long spine board with a cervical immobilization device.

Standing Takedown

Often at vehicle crash sites, you will find patients walking around when the mechanisms of injury suggest the potential for spinal injuries. These patients must receive spinal precautions, even though they are found standing. Your objective in such cases is to bring the patient to a fully supine position for further assessment, care, immobilization, and transport.

To accomplish this, employ a standing takedown procedure that maintains the spine in alignment. Have the patient remain immobile while a caregiver approaches from the rear and assumes manual cervical stabilization. Quickly assess any areas that will be covered by the cervical collar or long spine board. Apply a cervical collar and place a long spine board behind and against the patient, with the caregiver holding stabilization spreading his or her arms to accommodate the board. Position two other caregivers, one on each side of the spine board, and have each place a hand under the patient's axilla and with it grasp the closest (preferably next higher) handhold on the board. The team should then move the patient and spine board backward, tilting the patient on his heels until the patient and board are supine (Figure 18-10).

During the move, the hands in the handholds support the thorax while the caregiver holding cervical stabilization rotates his or her hands against the patient's head without either flexing or extending the head and neck as the patient moves from standing to supine. During this maneuver, the hands holding the patient's head must move from grasping the mastoid and mandible (standing) to grasping the lateral occiput (supine). This is not easy, because the head must rotate while the care-giver's hands remain in the same relative position. As with all movement procedures, the caregiver at the patient's head should be in control and direct the process.

Once the patient and board are on the ground, continue to maintain manual stabilization while assessing and caring for the patient. Then provide mechanical immobilization to the long spine board before moving the patient to the ambulance.

Helmet Removal

Helmet use in contact sports, bicycling, skateboarding, in-line skating, and motorcycling has increased over the past decade. These devices offer significant protection for the head during impact, but have not proven to reduce spine injuries. Their use also complicates spinal injury care for prehospital care providers. Many helmets are of the partial variety (such as those worn while bicycling and skateboarding) and are easy to remove at the

Helmet removal may be a tricky endeavor. You should familiarize yourself with the type of helmets used by sporting teams in your area (e.g., high school football).

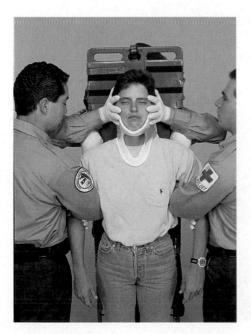

FIGURE 18-10 The standing takedown.

trauma scene. Some motorcycle and sports helmets, however, fully enclose the head and are very difficult to remove in the field. These helmets are also very difficult to secure to the spine board because of their spherical shapes. Further, most full helmets do not hold the head firmly within, so even fixing the helmet securely to the spine board does not result in effective cervical immobilization. Some newer contact sport helmets contain air bladders that expand and firmly hold the head in position within the helmet. These helmets immobilize the head well, but they are still difficult to firmly secure to a spine board. Consequently, most full-enclosure helmets must be removed to ensure adequate spinal immobilization.

The helmet must be removed if you find any of the following conditions:

- The helmet does not immobilize the patient's head within.
- You cannot securely immobilize the helmet to the long spine board.
- The helmet prevents airway care.
- The helmet prevents assessment of anticipated injuries.
- There are, or you anticipate, airway or breathing problems.
- If helmet removal will cause further injury, do not remove the helmet.

During helmet removal, have a caregiver initially stabilize the cervical spine by manually stabilizing the helmet. Remove the face mask, if present, either by unscrewing it or by cutting it off, if possible. Remove or retract any eye protection or visor and unfasten or cut away any chin strap as well. Be careful not to manipulate the helmet or otherwise transmit movement to the patient through the helmet. Then have another caregiver stabilize the head by sliding his or her hands under the helmet and placing them along the sides of the head, supporting the occiput, or by placing one hand on the jaw and the other on the occiput. This caregiver should choose the hand placement that works best for him or her and can be accommodated by the helmet. The caregiver holding the helmet should then grasp the helmet and spread it slightly to clear the ears by pulling laterally just below and anterior to the ear enclosure. That caregiver then rotates the helmet to clear the chin, counter rotates it to clear the occiput, and then rotates it to clear the nose and brow ridge (Figure 18-11). The clearance is usually very tight with a well-fitted helmet.

Execute the procedure slowly and carefully to prevent head and neck motion and to minimize patient discomfort. For helmets with air bladders, use the same procedure, but empty the bladder after someone stabilizes the head and before you begin the removal. Helmet removal is a complicated skill that you must practice frequently before you can employ it successfully in the field.

MOVING THE SPINAL INJURY PATIENT

Once you assess and provide the essential care for a patient with a potential spinal injury, plan the movement to the long spine board carefully. If any step of assessment or patient

FIGURE 18-11   Helmet removal.

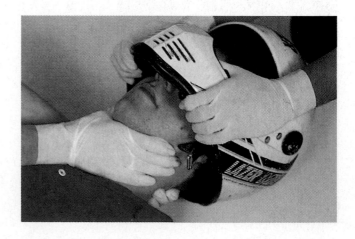

care requires patient movement, consider moving the patient onto the long spine board. Movement techniques suitable for moving the spinal injury patient to the long spine board include the log roll, straddle slide, rope-sling slide, orthopedic stretcher lift, application of a vest-type device (or short spine board), and rapid extrication. Choose a technique that affords the least spinal movement for the conditions and equipment at hand. Also select your movement technique and adjust its steps to accommodate the patient's particular injuries.

A key factor in all movement techniques for the patient with potential spinal injury is the coordination of the move. It is essential that you move the patient as a unit with his head facing forward and in a plane with the shoulders and hips. This can best be accomplished if the caregiver at the head controls and directs the move. He or she is able to see the other rescuers and has a focused and limited function (holding the head), which permits that person to evaluate what the other caregivers are doing. The caregiver at the head directs the move by counting a cadence such as, "Move on four—one, two, three, four." A four count is preferable because it gives the other caregivers a good opportunity to anticipate the actual start of movement. All moves must be slowly executed and well coordinated among caregivers.

Consider what the final positioning of the patient will be when you choose a spinal movement technique. Most spinal injury patients are best served with supine positioning on a long spine board. However, a patient with a thoracic spine injury is frequently placed in a prone position on a soft stretcher. With this patient, other positioning, such as supine on a firm spine board, puts pressure on the injury site from the body's weight and any movement is more likely to shift the site of injury and compound any damage.

Log Roll

The log roll can be used to rotate the patient 90 degrees, insert the long spine board, and then roll the patient back. It can also be used to roll the patient 180 degrees from prone to supine or vice versa.

As you begin the 90-degree roll, ensure manual spinal stabilization and apply a cervical collar. Notice that the shoulders are anatomically wider than the hips and legs. To provide a uniform roll, extend the patient's arm above his or her head. Then place a bulky blanket between the legs (with its bulkiest portion between the feet) and tie the legs together. This reduces pelvic movement and lateral bending of the lumbar spine.

Four caregivers are necessary to perform the log roll for a spinal injury patient (Figure 18-12). One caregiver holds the head, while one kneels at the patient's shoulder with the knees tight against the patient's chest. The third caregiver kneels at the patient's hip with the knees tight against the patient's hip. The last caregiver kneels at the patient's knees with the knees tight against the patient's knees.

The caregivers reach across the patient and around the opposite shoulder, hip, and knee, respectively, and grasp the patient firmly. On a count initiated by the caregiver at the head, the team, in unison, rolls the patient against their knees and up to a 90-degree angle. With a free hand, the caregiver at the knees (or an additional caregiver) slides a long spine

Choose a spinal movement technique that affords the least spinal movement.

The care giver at the head directs and controls the movement of the patient with a suspected spinal injury.

A four-count cadence is preferred because it provides a good opportunity to anticipate the start of the move.

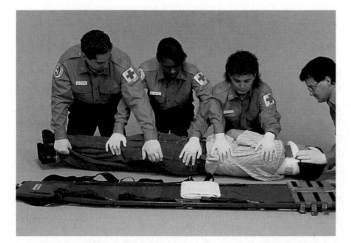

FIGURE 18-12 The four-person log roll.

board under the patient from the patient's side or the foot end. The board should be positioned tightly against the patient so that the head, torso, and pelvis will eventually rest solidly on the board. Then, at the count of the caregiver at the head, the team rolls the patient back 90 degrees onto the board.

The 180-degree log roll begins with placement of the long spine board between the caregivers and the patient, with the board resting at an angle on the caregivers' thighs. The caregivers reach across the board and grasp the patient in the same manner as for the 90-degree log roll. The caregiver at the head must be careful to anticipate the turning motion and position his or her hands so they will be comfortably positioned at the end of the roll. On the count of the caregiver at the head, the team rolls the patient past 90 degrees until he is positioned against the tilted long spine board. Then they reposition their hands against the other (lower) side of the patient and slowly back their thighs out from under the patient until the board rests on the ground.

Straddle Slide

Another technique effective for moving the patient with potential spinal injury is the straddle slide. In this procedure, three caregivers are positioned at the patient's head, shoulders, and pelvis, while a fourth prepares to insert the long spine board from either the patient's head or feet. The caregiver at the head holds cervical stabilization and guides the lift with a cadence. The second caregiver straddles the patient (facing the patient's head) and grasps the shoulders. The third caregiver straddles the patient (facing the head) and grasps the pelvis. All the caregivers keep their feet planted widely enough apart to permit the insertion of the long spine board. At the direction of the caregiver at the head, the three caregivers lift the patient just enough to permit the fourth caregiver to negotiate the long spine board underneath the patient. (**Note:** If the board is to be inserted from the patient's feet, the caregiver inserting the board lifts the patient's feet with one hand and slides the board into place with the other.) On a signal from the caregiver at the head, the team gently lowers the patient to the long spine board.

Rope-Sling Slide

A continuous ring or length of thick rope or other material can be used to help slide a supine patient, using axial traction, onto a long spine board. One caregiver holds cervical stabilization, while another places the rope across the patient's chest and under his arms. The rope is tied together (with a cravat) behind the patient's neck and brought out between the legs of the first caregiver. A long spine board is placed between the legs of the caregiver holding cervical stabilization. The second caregiver positions himself or herself at the head end of the spine board with the board resting on his thighs (this provides a small angle to more easily drag the patient onto the board). The second caregiver then pulls on the two strands of rope, guiding the patient onto the spine board as directed by the caregiver at the head. The caregiver holding cervical stabilization moves backward as the patient is moved onto the spine board. (The caregiver at the head may crouch or kneel to the patient's side to hold stabilization.) The caregiver at the head must be careful to move smoothly with the caregiver pulling axial traction. That person must ensure that the head moves with the body and does not pull against it.

Orthopedic Stretcher

The orthopedic stretcher, also known as the scoop stretcher, is a valuable device for positioning the patient on the spine board or helping to secure the patient to the long spine board. To apply the device, lengthen it to accommodate the patient's height and then separate it into its two halves. Maintain manual cervical stabilization while you gently negotiate each half of the stretcher under the patient from the sides and connect them at the top, then bottom. Be careful not to entrap the patient's skin or body parts while positioning the stretcher, especially on uneven ground. Once the device is connected, you may use the stretcher to lift the patient to the waiting spine board. Orthopedic stretchers are usually not rigid enough to use by themselves as transport devices for spinal injury patients. Rather, they are most effective in moving patients to the long spine board, where they may remain as an

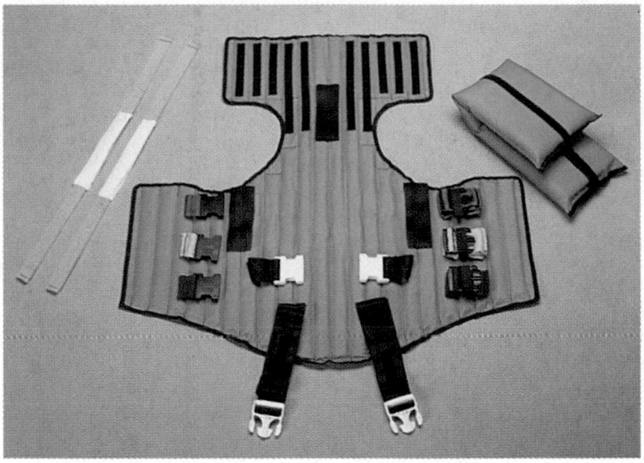

FIGURE 18-13 A vest-type immobilization device.

adjunct to full immobilization, or you may disconnect the halves, remove them, and immobilize the patient to the long spine board in the normal way.

Vest–Type Immobilization Device (and Short Spine Board)

A specialized piece of EMS equipment that may be used with some spinal injury patients is the vest-type immobilization device (Figure 18-13). This device immobilizes the patient's head, shoulders, and pelvis to a rigid board so that you can move the patient from a seated position, as in an automobile, to a fully supine position. The vest-type device is a commercially made device that usually has the needed strapping already attached. The device is usually constructed of thin, rigid wood or plastic strips embedded in a vinyl or fabric vest. It is then wrapped and secured around the patient to provide immobilization. An alternative to the vest-type device is the short spine board, a cut-out piece of rigid plywood to which you attach strapping and padding. The basic principles of application are the same with both short-board and vest-type devices.

To apply the vest-type device, manually stabilize the patient's cervical spine and apply a cervical collar while the device is being readied for application. If the patient is positioned against a soft seat (as in an automobile), gently move the patient's shoulders and head a few inches forward to permit insertion of the vest. The caregiver holding manual cervical stabilization directs and coordinates the move, while a second caregiver guides and controls shoulder motion. Negotiate the device behind the patient by either inserting the head portion under and through the arms of the caregiver providing cervical stabilization, or angling it, base first, then moving it behind the patient's back. Position the device vertically so the chest appendages fit just under the arms. This positioning permits you to fasten the straps and secure the shoulders without any upward or downward movement of the device.

First, secure the device to the chest and pelvis with strapping and ensure that the vest is immobile. Tighten the straps firmly, but be sure that they do not inhibit respiration. Secure the thigh straps because they hold the hips and thighs in the flexed position, limiting lumbar motion. Then fill the space between the occiput and the device with non-compressible padding to maintain neutral positioning. Secure both the brow ridge and chin to the device with straps, but be very careful to allow for vomiting by the patient and subsequent clearing of the airway or be prepared to cut the chin strap immediately if vomiting occurs. Tie the patient's wrists together.

The vest-type immobilization device is not meant to lift the patient but rather to facilitate rotating him on the buttocks and then to tilt the patient to the supine position for further spinal immobilization (Figure 18-14). Once the patient is positioned on the long spine board, gently and carefully release the thigh straps and slowly and gently extend the hips and knees. If after transfer to the spine board the patient's head remains firmly affixed to the vest-type device, leave the vest on the patient and secure the vest to the long spine board since doing this effectively secures both head and torso. If the head becomes loose during

The vest-type device is not meant to lift the patient but rather to facilitate rotating and tilting the patient to the supine position.

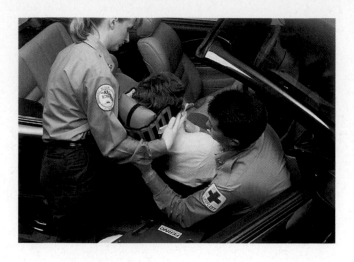

FIGURE 18-14 The vest-type immobilization device is not intended for lifting the patient but for pivoting him.

the transfer, reapply manual cervical immobilization, secure the torso with strapping, and secure the head with a cervical immobilization device.

Rapid Extrication

Applying a vest-type immobilization device is a time-consuming process. Often the circumstances of the emergency, either issues of scene safety or the need for rapid transport to the trauma center, preclude spending the time required for standard spinal immobilization. In such cases, use a rapid extrication procedure.

With whatever personnel are available, stabilize the patient's spine, shoulders, pelvis, and legs with the patient's nose, navel, and toes kept in line. Ensure that caregivers are coordinated and understand what movement is to take place. One caregiver, usually at the patient's head, should direct the move, counting a cadence to permit the crew to work together (Figure 18-15). Make certain that personnel involved in the extrication move the patient maintaining the alignment of the patient's nose, naval, and toes. Then, on the leader's count, they should move the patient from a seated or other position to a waiting spine board.

Remember the objectives of spinal movement and stabilization: keep the spine in the neutral, in-line position by keeping the patient's eyes facing directly forward and keeping the shoulders and pelvis in a plane perpendicular to that of the gaze. Be sure to prevent any flexion/extension, rotation, or lateral bending.

Although the technique of rapid extrication does not provide maximum protection for the spine, it does permit rapid movement of the patient with a spinal injury when other considerations demand it. Use the procedure only when your patient cannot afford the time it would take for normal spinal movement techniques. Rapid extrication from the confined space of a wrecked automobile is difficult at best. Plan your move carefully and execute the rapid extrication by carefully explaining the process and individual responsibilities to your team members.

During all movement of a spinal injury patient, keep the spine in the neutral, in-line position by keeping the patient's eyes facing directly forward and the shoulders, pelvis, and toes in the same plane.

Final Patient Positioning

Centering the patient on the board is essential to ensuring that the patient's spine remains in-line and he is effectively immobilized. Accomplish this by placing team members at the patient's head, shoulders, pelvis, and feet. The caregivers then place one hand on each side of the patient and prepare to move the patient toward the center of the board. On a cadence signaled by the caregiver at the head, they slide the portion of the patient that is out of alignment to an in-line position, centered on the long spine board.

Long Spine Board

The long spine board is simply a reinforced flat, firm surface designed to facilitate immobilization of a patient in a supine or prone position (Figure 18-16). Although the board may immobilize patients with multi-system trauma, pelvic and lower limb fractures, and many other types of trauma, it is primarily designed for patients with spine injuries. The board has several hand and strap holes along its lateral borders. Using nylon web strapping, you can

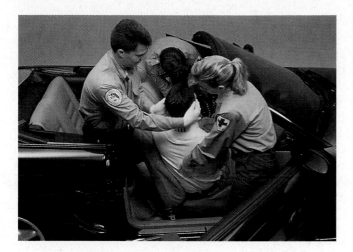

FIGURE 18-15 Rapid extrication of a patient with a spinal injury.

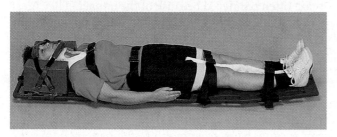

FIGURE 18-16 Immobilization of a spinal injury patient to a long spine board with a cervical immobilization device in place.

immobilize a patient with almost any combination of injuries to the board firmly enough to permit rotating the patient and board 90 degrees to clear the airway in case of vomiting.

Secure the patient to the board with the strapping, immobilizing and holding the shoulders and pelvis firmly to the board. Such strapping may cross the body and capture the shoulder and pelvic girdles. Ensure that you firmly immobilize the patient to prevent lateral motion as well as cephalad (headward) and caudad (tailward) motion. Be sure that the pressure created by strapping does not come to bear on the central abdomen. That would cause forced extension of the lumbar spine. Immobilize the lower legs and feet with strapping or cravats. Tie the legs together and place a rolled blanket under the patient's knees to immobilize them in a slightly flexed position.

Long spine board immobilization is made more effective by use of the cervical immobilization device (CID). This device is composed of two soft, padded lateral pieces that bracket the patient's head, maintaining its position, and a base plate that permits you to easily secure the device to the board. The base plate is affixed to the long spine board before the patient is moved to it. Once you position the patient on the board, fill the void between the occiput and the CID base plate with firm, non-compressible padding. Use no padding for the small adult or older child, and pad the shoulders in the young child or infant to ensure proper spinal positioning. While a caregiver maintains manual immobilization of the head, bring the lateral components of the CID against the sides of the patient's head. Use medial pressure to hold them against the head and the head in position. Then affix the lateral CID components to the Velcro® of the CID base plate.

Secure the head in position and to the long spine board using forehead and chin straps or tape. Make sure the strapping catches the brow ridge and the mandible or the upper portion of the collar. The properly secured CID must hold the patient's head in the neutral position without movement while not placing undue pressure on the neck or restricting jaw movement (in case of vomiting). Be careful that the straps do not flex, extend, or rotate the head. Bulky blanket rolls, placed on each side of the head and secured both to the head and the board will also effectively immobilize the head to the long spine board.

The long spine board does have drawbacks. Its firm surface places pressure on the skin and tissues covering the ischial tuberosities and the shoulder blades. If a patient remains immobilized to the board for more than a couple of hours, skin breakdown and ulceration injuries are likely to result.

The board also tends to encourage caregivers to immobilize the patient directly to it in a non-neutral position. In a proper neutral position, the head should be elevated about 1 to 2 inches above the board's surface and the knees should be bent at 15 to 30 degrees. This positioning relieves pressure on the cervical spine, lumbar spine, hips, and knees and increases patient comfort. You can obtain proper knee positioning by placing folded blankets under the patient's knees. Also pad under the curves of the back. Do not apply too much padding; just fill the voids at the small of the back and neck with bulky soft dressing material.

A device that is now showing merit for spinal immobilization is the full-body vacuum splint. As with the vacuum splints for the limbs, the full-body splint uses small plastic beads that maintain their position in the reduced pressure after air is evacuated from the splint. To apply the vacuum splint, place the patient on the flattened device and shape it around him. Evacuating the air causes the device to form to the contours of the patient's body and maintains immobilization.

Diving Injury Immobilization

Patients injured in shallow water dives are often paralyzed because of the impact. They must rely on others to protect their airways and remove them from the water. When carried out by untrained bystanders, however, these activities may compound any spinal injury. If you are present when such an incident occurs, be sure to carefully control any patient motion while he is still in the water. If necessary, turn him to a supine position, ensuring that the nose, navel, and toes remain in a single plane and that the eyes face directly forward. You may accomplish this by sandwiching the patient's chest between your forearms while your arms and shoulders cradle the head. Once the patient is in the supine position, water provides an almost neutral buoyancy and, if the water is calm, helps to immobilize the patient. Move the patient by pulling on the shoulders while you cradle the head, in the neutral position, with the forearms. Float a long spine board under the patient to lift and carry him from the water.

MEDICATIONS

There are several conditions in which you may use medications to treat spinal injury patients, if permitted by your system's protocols. These conditions include spinal cord injury, neurogenic shock, and the combative patient.

Medications and Spinal Cord Injury

The initial physical injury to the spinal column or cord can be further compounded by the processes of inflammation and swelling. Certain naturally occurring drugs, called **steroids,** reduce the body's response to injury and thereby reduce the associated swelling and the resulting pressure on the cord.

Methylprednisolone and Dexamethasone   Both methylprednisolone (Solu-Medrol) and dexamethasone (Decadron) are synthetic glucocorticoids with potent anti-inflammatory properties. They are similar to naturally occurring hormones and tend to reduce both capillary dilation and permeability, thus decreasing swelling. These agents have been used in the past in the treatment of various types of neurological trauma. Dexamethasone was once used routinely for closed head injuries. Methylprednisolone was recommended for the treatment of acute closed spinal cord injury. However, subsequent studies have shown that they are generally ineffective and associated with a high incidence of adverse complications.

Very high dose methylprednisolone was recommended for the treatment of acute spinal cord injury. An initial study (NINDS 2) suggested that it improved neurological function in patients who received the drug within 8 hours of their injury. However, subsequent studies failed to reproduce the findings of the initial study. Futhermore, several researchers found that the complications associated with the use of massive doses of corticosteroids (hyperglycemia, delayed wound healing, serious infections) were much higher than originally thought. Because of this, several national and international organizations have issued position and policy papers that state that high-dose methylprednisolone is *not* a standard of care or even a treatment guideline. It is only a treatment option that is supported by weak clinical evidence. EMT-Is should always defer to their local protocols and system medical directors for controversial patient care issues such as these.

Medications and Neurogenic Shock

The loss of sympathetic control leads to both a relaxation of the blood vessels (vasodilation) below the level of the lesion and the inability of the body to increase the heart rate. This expanded vascular system leads to a relative hypovolemia and lower blood pressure. The problem is further compounded because the heart, without sympathetic stimulation and in the presence of this relative hypovolemia, displays a normal or bradycardic heart rate. Frequently, the hypovolemia is treated with a fluid challenge, followed by careful use of a **vasopressor** such as dopamine. The slow heart rate is treated with atropine to reduce any parasympathetic stimulation.

The use of the PASG to combat the relative hypovolemia of neurogenic shock is controversial. The compression of the lower extremities and abdomen may counteract the vasodilation associated with the shock state, but research has not yet proven that the use of the garment contributes to a better outcome. Follow local protocols and consult with medical direction before using the device.

Fluid Challenge   The initial treatment for hypovolemia from suspected neurogenic shock is by fluid challenge. Establish an IV with a 1,000 mL bag of lactated Ringer's solution or normal saline, a non-restrictive administration set, and a large-bore IV catheter. Administer 250 mL of solution quickly, monitor the blood pressure and heart rate, and auscultate the lungs for signs of developing pulmonary edema (crackles). If the patient responds with an increasing blood pressure, a slowing heart rate, and signs of improved perfusion, consider a second bolus, or monitor the patient and administer a second bolus if the patient's signs and symptoms begin to deteriorate. If the patient does not improve with the fluid challenge, consider repeating it or changing to vasopressor therapy, as allowed by your protocols.

Dopamine   Dopamine (Intropin®) is a naturally occurring **catecholamine** that, in addition to its own actions, causes the release of norepinephrine. Dopamine increases cardiac contractility and hence cardiac output and, at higher doses, increases peripheral vascular resistance, venous constriction, cardiac preload, and blood pressure. Although there are no absolute contraindications for dopamine use in the emergency setting, its common side effects include tachydysrhythmias, hypertension, headache, nausea, and vomiting.

Dopamine is frequently packaged as either a premixed solution containing 800 or 1,600 mcg/mL or as a 5 mL vial containing 200 or 400 mg of drug. Vial contents are added to 250 mL of D_5W to yield a concentration of either 800 or 1,600 mcg/mL. Dopamine is very light sensitive and once mixed should be discarded after 24 hours. If the solution is either pink or brown, discard it. Onset of action for dopamine is about 5 minutes, and its half-life is around 2 minutes; hence, it is administered via a continuous infusion. It should be run piggyback through an already well-established IV line since infiltration can cause tissue necrosis. It is administered initially at 2.5 mcg/kg/min, then titrated to an increase in blood pressure or a maximum of 120 mcg/kg/min. (Vasoconstriction usually begins at doses above 10 mcg/kg/min.)

Atropine   Interruption of the sympathetic pathways by spinal cord injury causes unopposed parasympathetic stimulation and bradycardia (or at least prevents the compensatory tachycardia that occurs with decreased cardiac preload). The net result is a decrease in cardiac output. Atropine is administered to block the parasympathetic impulse that might contribute to slow the heart rate.

Atropine is an **anticholinergic** agent most frequently used for symptomatic bradycardia and heart blocks in the myocardial infarction patient. It is sometimes helpful in increasing the heart rate of patients with upper spinal cord injury due to unopposed vagal stimulation. It acts by inhibiting the actions of acetylcholine, the major parasympathetic neurotransmitter. Atropine has a quick onset of action and a half-life of just over 2 hours. It is available for emergency use in 5 and 10 mL preloaded syringes containing a concentration of 0.5 mg/mL. Atropine is administered rapidly in 0.5 mg (1 mL) intravenous doses every 3 to 5 minutes, up to a maximum of 2 mg. The only expected side effects in the emergency setting are dry mouth, blurred vision, and, possibly, tachycardia.

vasopressor agent causing contraction of the smooth muscle of the arteries and arterioles, thus increasing resistance to blood flow and elevating the blood pressure.

catecholamine a hormone, such as epinephrine or norepinephrine, that strongly affects the sympathetic nervous and cardiovascular systems, metabolic rate, temperature, and smooth muscle.

anticholinergic agent that blocks parasympathetic nerve impulses.

Medications and the Combative Patient

Sedatives   Frequently the patient who has sustained potentially serious spine injury has also sustained head injury, is intoxicated, or is otherwise very uncooperative or combative. In some of these cases, **sedatives** may be indicated to reduce anxiety and because the patient actively resists spinal precautions. Consider using morphine sulfate or diazepam (Valium®) to calm the patient. Sedatives should only be administered as permitted by your system's protocols and under the close and direct supervision of an on-line medical direction physician.

General Considerations

Spinal injury is a frequent consequence of serious trauma and likely to induce serious disability or death. Injury to the spinal column may occur with only minimum signs and patient symptoms. So prehospital care for any patient with a significant mechanism of injury or any trauma patient with a reduced level of consciousness must include spinal precautions. Throughout assessment and care, provide emotional support and calming reassurance to lower patient anxiety, and carefully monitor level of consciousness.

MANAGEMENT OF ABDOMINAL INJURY PATIENTS

Management of the patient with abdominal injuries is supportive, with the major emphasis on bringing the patient to surgery as quickly as possible. Prehospital care relies on rapid packaging and transport and aggressive fluid resuscitation, as needed. Specific care steps for the abdominal injury patient include proper positioning, general shock care, fluid resuscitation, possible PASG application, and care for specific injuries (open wounds and eviscerations).

The patient with minor or severe abdominal pain should be positioned for comfort (unless the positioning is contraindicated by suspicion of spinal injury). Flex the patient's knees to relax the abdominal muscles, and if the injuries permit, place the patient in the left lateral recumbent position to maintain knee flexure and the relaxed state of the abdominal muscles, and facilitate the clearing of emesis from the airway.

Ensure good ventilation and consider early administration of high-flow, high-concentration oxygen. The pain associated with peritonitis or diaphragmatic irritation may reduce respiratory excursion, adding to the potential for early shock development in these patients.

Control any moderate or serious external hemorrhage with direct pressure and bandaging. Minor bleeding or oozing may be controlled during transport, if at all.

When a serious mechanism of injury is found and the patient does not present with the signs and symptoms of shock, act in anticipation of it. Start a large-bore IV line with trauma tubing and 1,000 mL of lactated Ringer's solution or normal saline. Be prepared to run it wide open to deliver a bolus of 250 mL of fluid if any signs of shock develop. Monitor the pulse rate and blood pressure. If the pulse does not slow and the pulse pressure does not rise, consider a second bolus. Institute a second line with a non–flow-restrictive saline lock using a large-bore catheter. Use this access if the patient's blood pressure begins to drop. Do not delay transport to initiate any IV access. Start the IV access en route to the hospital if necessary. Prehospital infusion is usually limited to 3,000 mL of fluid. Titrate your administration rate to maintain a systolic blood pressure of 90 mmHg and ensure that you do not run out of fluid during field care and transport.

As with all serious trauma patients, you should communicate frequently with the patient to reduce anxiety and provide emotional support. Also watch for any changes in the patient's description of the pain or the character or intensity of the injury. Be wary of patient hypothermia, especially when providing aggressive fluid resuscitation. Provide ample blankets, keep the patient compartment of the vehicle warm, take patient complaints of being cold seriously, and warm infusion fluids when possible. Hypothermia is a special consideration with pediatric patients who have a disproportionately large body surface area to body volume and rapidly loose heat to the environment.

Cover any exposed abdominal organs (evisceration) with a dressing moistened with sterile saline. Be careful to keep the region clean and do not replace any exposed organs.

Content Review

ABDOMINAL INJURY MANAGEMENT

- Position the patient properly.
- Ensure oxygenation and ventilation.
- Control external bleeding.
- Be prepared for aggressive fluid resuscitation.
- Apply PASG if not contraindicated.

When a serious mechanism of injury is found and the patient does not present with the signs and symptoms of shock, act in anticipation of it.

Cover the wet dressing with a sterile occlusive dressing such as clear plastic wrap to keep the site as clean as possible and yet retain the moisture. If the transport is lengthy, check the dressing from time to time and remoisten as necessary.

Another wound that deserves special attention is caused by an impaled object. Do all that you can to keep the object from moving and do not remove it from the victim. Any motion causes further injury, disrupts the clotting mechanisms, and continues the hemorrhage. Removal may withdraw the object from a blood vessel, thereby permitting increased internal and uncontrollable hemorrhage. Pad around the object with bulky trauma dressings and wrap around the trunk with soft, self-adherent roller bandaging to secure it firmly. Apply direct pressure around the object if hemorrhage is anything but minor. If the object is too long to accommodate during transport or it is affixed to an immovable object, attempt to cut it. Use a saw, cutter, or torch, but be very careful to make certain that vibration, jarring, and heat are not transmitted to the patient.

Stabilize impaled objects to prevent further injury and reduce associated hemorrhage.

Carefully observe and care for penetrating wounds that may traverse both the abdominal and thoracic cavities. If the wound is large and may have penetrated the diaphragm or otherwise entered the thoracic cavity, seal the wound with an occlusive dressing taped on three sides to permit the release of the build-up of air pressure that occurs in a tension pneumothorax. Be especially watchful of respiratory excursion and effort.

The PASG is indicated for the patient with abdominal injury and the early signs of shock. However, it should not be used if a patient has concurrent penetrating trauma to the chest. The PASG applies circumferential pressure to the abdominal cavity, thereby raising intra-abdominal pressure and reducing the rate of intra-abdominal hemorrhage. Its use is generally contraindicated (inflate the leg sections only) in females in late pregnancy, abdominal evisceration patients, or patients with impaled objects. If the patient with an evisceration experiences a blood pressure below 60 mmHg, consider inflating the abdominal section of the garment because the risks associated with injury to the exposed bowel are less than those of profound hypotension. Incrementally inflate the PASG to maintain blood pressure and pulse rate, not to return them to pre-injury levels.

Inflate the PASG in increments to maintain blood pressure and pulse, not to return them to pre-injury levels.

MANAGEMENT OF THE PREGNANT PATIENT

Special care is followed for the pregnant patient because of the anatomical and physiological changes induced by pregnancy. Place the late-term mother, when possible, in the left lateral recumbent position. This ensures that the weight of the uterus does not compress the vena cava, reduce blood return to the heart, and cause hypotension. It also facilitates airway care. For the same reason, if the pregnant patient is supine on a spine board, tilt the board 20 to 30 degrees (or lift the right side about four inches). Administer high-flow, high-concentration oxygen early. (This is because the mother's respiratory reserve volume is diminished, the work necessary for her to move air is greater due to the increased intra-abdominal pressure, and the fetus is especially susceptible to hypoxia). If necessary, employ intermittent positive pressure ventilation early in your care. Also consider aggressive airway care. The pregnant mother is prone to vomiting and aspiration. If she has a significantly reduced level of consciousness, consider intubation.

Maintain a high index of suspicion for internal hemorrhage since the normal, pregnancy-induced increased blood volume of the third-term mother may permit an increased blood loss before the signs and symptoms of hypovolemia become evident. The fetus may be at risk early in the blood loss, well before the mother displays any signs. Initiate IV therapy early, but remember that pregnancy induces a relative anemia and that aggressive fluid resuscitation may further dilute the erythrocyte concentrations and lead to ineffective circulation. Consider using the PASG, inflating the leg sections first. Use of the PASG may be beneficial for the patient in early pregnancy (first term) because the pressure of the trouser is well distributed within the uterus by the amniotic fluid. However, for the late-term pregnant patient, use of the PASG's abdominal segment is contraindicated because the pressure of the garment may push the uterus more firmly against the inferior vena cava, reducing venous return to the heart, and increasing the effects of hypovolemia.

Use of the PASG's abdominal compartment is contraindicated for late-term pregnant patients.

Blunt or penetrating abdominal trauma can result in serious organ damage and life-threatening hemorrhage. Concurrently, the signs of injury are limited, non-specific, and do not reflect the seriousness of abdominal pathology. It is thus very important that your assessment carefully determine the mechanism of injury and the region of the abdomen it affects. This information must be communicated to the emergency department to ensure its personnel acknowledge the significance of your first-hand knowledge of the mechanism of injury.

Care for significant abdominal injury is rapid transport to the trauma center. Most significant abdominal injury results in serious internal bleeding or organ injury that can neither be cared for nor stabilized in the prehospital setting. Further, the definitive care for the patient with serious abdominal injury is provided via surgery. The patient must be transported to a facility capable of providing immediate surgical intervention when needed. This is a trauma center. Prehospital care is supportive of the airway and breathing, and preventive for shock.

The pregnant patient with abdominal injury deserves special attention because her vascular volume is increased and she will likely not show the signs of shock until the fetus is at risk. Careful observation while preparation for rapid transport to the trauma center is in order. If any of the slightest signs of hypoperfusion is noted, initiate aggressive fluid resuscitation.

MANAGEMENT OF MUSCULOSKELETAL INJURY PATIENTS

The objectives of musculoskeletal injury care are to reduce the possibility of any further injury during patient care and transport and to reduce the patient's discomfort. Accomplish these goals by protecting open wounds, positioning the extremity properly, immobilizing the injured extremity, and monitoring neurovascular function in the distal limb. In some cases, care involves manipulating the injury to reestablish distal circulation and sensation or simply to restore normal anatomic position for the patient expecting prolonged extrication or transport. In most cases, care for musculoskeletal injuries also includes application of a splinting device.

As you begin to care for a patient with musculoskeletal injuries, talk to him and explain what you are doing, why, and what impact it will have on the patient. Alignment and splinting will likely first cause an increase in pain followed by a significant reduction in it. By telling the patient of this in advance, you will increase confidence in both your intent to help and your ability to provide care.

PROTECTING OPEN WOUNDS

If the patient has any open wound in close proximity to the fracture or dislocation, consider the fracture or dislocation to be an open one. Carefully observe the wound and note any signs of muscle, tendon, ligament, or vascular injury and be prepared to describe the wound in your report and at the emergency department. Cover the wound with a sterile dressing held in place with bandaging or a splint. Frequently, the attempts to align a limb, the splinting process, or the application of traction will draw protruding bones back into the wound. This is an expected consequence of proper care but must be brought to the attention of the attending emergency department physician.

POSITIONING THE LIMB

Proper limb positioning is essential to ensure patient comfort, to reduce the chances of further limb injury, and to encourage venous drainage. Proper positioning is different with fractures and dislocations, although splinting with the limb in a normal anatomical position, the position of function, is beneficial for both.

Limb alignment is appropriate for any fractures of the mid-shaft femur, tibia/fibula, humerus, or radius/ulna. Alignment can be maintained by using the air splint, padded rigid splint, PASG, or traction splint. Proper alignment of a fracture enhances circulation and reduces the potential for further injury to surrounding tissue. It is also very difficult to immobilize a limb with a fracture in an unaligned, angulated position because the fracture segments are short and buried in soft tissue. Perform any limb alignment with great care so as not to damage the tissue surrounding the fracture site. During the process, the proximal limb should remain in position while you bring the distal limb to the position of alignment using gentle axial traction. Stop the process when you detect any resistance to movement or when the patient reports any significant increase in pain.

Generally, you should not attempt alignment of dislocations and serious injuries within 3 inches of a joint. Only attempt to manipulate such injury sites if the distal circulation is compromised. In such a case, try to move the joint while another care provider palpates the distal pulse. If the pulse is restored, if you meet significant resistance to movement, or if the patient complains of greatly increased pain, stop the manipulation and splint the injured limb as it is. Be sure to transport the patient quickly, because a loss of circulation can endanger the future usefulness of the limb.

If you suspect a limb will remain dislocated for an extended period, as during lengthy transports or prolonged patient entrapments, consider reducing the dislocation. Apply a firm and progressive traction to the limb, which draws the dislocated ends away from each other and moves the joint toward normal positioning. When (and if) the bone ends pop back into position, ensure there is a distal pulse and immobilize the limb in the position of function.

Proper positioning of injured limbs is important for maintaining distal circulation and sensation and increasing patient comfort. Deformities and extremes of flexion or extension put pressure on the soft tissues and may compress nerves and blood vessels. These positions also fatigue the surrounding muscles and increase the pain associated with the injury. By placing the uninjured joints of the limb halfway between flexion and extension in what is called the position of function, you place the least stress on the joint ligaments and the muscles and tendons surrounding the injury. Place the limb in the position of function whenever possible (Figure 18-17). Note, however, that some injuries and some splinting devices commonly used for musculoskeletal injuries may preclude this positioning.

When practical, elevate the injured limb. This will assist with venous drainage and reduce the edema associated with musculoskeletal injury.

IMMOBILIZING THE INJURY

The aim in immobilizing musculoskeletal injuries is to prevent further injury caused by the movement of broken bone ends and bone ends dislodged from a joint and by further stress placed on muscles, ligaments, or tendons already injured by a strain, sprain, subluxation, dislocation, or fracture. This immobilization is usually accomplished through the use of a splinting device.

Since most long bones lie buried deep within the musculature of the extremities, it is very difficult to immobilize them directly. Hence, immobilize the joint above and the joint below the injury, regardless of whether the injury occurs at a joint or mid-shaft in a long bone. This ensures that no motion is transmitted through the injury site as might occur, for example, with the rotation (supination/pronation) of the radius against the ulna at the elbow when the wrist turns.

Stop realignment attempts when you detect any resistance to movement or when the patient reports any significant increase in pain.

Do not attempt alignment of dislocations and serious injuries within 3 inches of a joint.

When possible, place injured limbs in the position of function or neutral position.

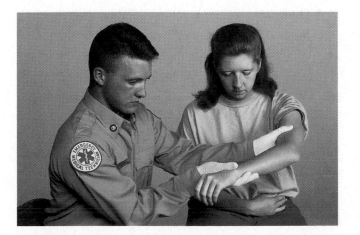

FIGURE 18-17 Gently place the limb in the position of function unless your attempts meet with resistance, there is a significant increase in pain, or the injury is within 3 inches of a joint.

Wrap any splinting device or associated bandage from a distal point to a proximal one. This ensures that the pressure of bandaging moves any blood into the systemic circulation and does not trap it in the distal limb. This method of wrapping thus assists venous drainage and reduces swelling. Apply firm pressure when wrapping, but be sure you can easily push a finger beneath the wrapping.

Checking Neurovascular Function

Always check pulses, motor function, and sensation in the distal extremity before, during, and after splinting.

It is imperative that you identify the status of the circulation, motor function, and sensation distal to the injury site before, during, and after splinting of all musculoskeletal injuries. The check before splinting identifies a baseline condition and establishes that the initial injury has not disrupted circulation. The check during splinting ensures that inadvertent limb movement or circumferential pressure does not compromise distal circulation. The check after splinting identifies any restriction caused by progressive swelling of the injured area against the splinting device. Clearly identify and document these evaluations whenever a splint is applied.

To perform this evaluation, first palpate for a pulse and ensure it is equal in strength to that of the opposing limb. If the pulse cannot be located or is weak, check capillary refill and skin temperature, color, and condition. Again compare your findings to the opposing limb. Ask the patient to describe the sensation when you rub or pinch the bottom of the foot or back of the hand and ask him to move the fingers or toes. The patient response establishes your baseline circulation, sensory, and motor findings. Reevaluate pulse, motor function, and sensation frequently during the remaining care and transport. If a care provider is holding the limb while you apply the splint, have him or her monitor both pulse and skin temperature. That care provider can then immediately note any compromise in circulation.

Splinting Devices

An essential part of managing any musculoskeletal system injury is the use of devices to immobilize a limb and permit patient transport without causing further injury. These devices, called splints, are designed to help you reduce or eliminate any movement of the injured extremity. Splints come in several forms that can assist in immobilizing common fractures and dislocations associated with musculoskeletal trauma (Figure 18-18). They include rigid, formable, soft, traction, and other splints.

Rigid Splints   Rigid splints, as the name implies, are firm and durable supports for the injured limb. They can be constructed of cardboard, metal, synthetic products, or wood. Such devices very effectively immobilize injury sites but require adequate padding to lessen patient discomfort. This padding may be built into the splint or may simply be a bulky dressing affixed to the splint with soft bandaging. Several types of commercially available rigid splints are used in prehospital care. They are usually flat and rigid devices and are about 3 inches wide and from 16 to 48 inches long. The injured limb that is in alignment is immobilized to the splint by circumferential wrapping, whereas an angulated limb may be held in position by cross-wrapping at two locations.

FIGURE 18-18   A variety of splints are available for musculoskeletal injuries.

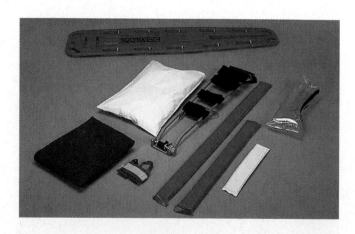

A special form of rigid splint is the preformed splint. It is usually a stamped metal or preformed plastic or fiberglass device shaped to the contours of the distal limbs. These splints are usually available for the ankles and hands.

Formable Splints   Another type of rigid splint is the formable, or malleable, splint. It consists of a material that can be easily shaped to match the angulation of a limb. Then the formed splint is affixed to the limb with circumferential bandaging. Formable splints include both the ladder splint, which is a matrix of soft metal wires soldered together, and the metal sheet splint, which is composed of thin aluminum or another easily shaped metal.

Soft Splints   Soft splints use padding or air pressure to immobilize an injured limb in place. Among the varieties of soft splints are air splints, which include the PASG, and pillow splints.

The air splint provides immobilization because air pressure fills the splint and compresses the limb. Since the splint is a formed cylinder, and may include shaping for the foot, it immobilizes the limb in an aligned position. Air splints should not be used with long bone injuries at or above the knee or elbow because they cannot prevent movement of hip or shoulder joints and are thus unable to immobilize the proximal joints of the limb. Air splints also apply a pressure that may be helpful in controlling both external and internal hemorrhage. Although these devices may limit assessment of the distal extremity, they do permit observation because they are transparent. (Note that the PASG is not often transparent, so carefully assess the patient from the rib cage to the feet before applying and inflating it.)

Monitor air splints carefully with any changes in temperature or atmospheric pressure. Increases in ambient heat or decreases in pressure, as during an ascent in a helicopter, increases the pressure within the splint. Conversely, decreases in temperature or a descent in a helicopter decreases pressure in the splint. Constantly monitor the pressure in the air splint and PASG to ensure it does not rise or fall during your care.

> *Monitor pressure within the air splint or PASG, as it may change with changes in altitude or temperature.*

The pillow splint is a comfortable splint for ankle and foot injuries. The foot is simply placed on the pillow while the outer fabric is drawn around the foot and pillow. The outer fabric is pinned together or wrapped circumferentially with bandage material around the injury site. This device applies gentle and uniform pressure to effectively immobilize the distal extremity. Using a bulky blanket or two and wrapping them firmly may also provide the same type of immobilization.

Traction Splints   The traction splint was developed during World War I and used extensively during World War II. This splint dramatically reduced both mortality and limb loss from femur fractures caused by projectile wounds, blast injuries, and other traumas. Today, the traction splint is the mainstay of prehospital care for the isolated traumatic femur fracture.

The traction splint is a frame that applies a pull (traction) on the injured extremity and against the trunk. The application of traction is useful when splinting the femur, which is surrounded by very heavy musculature. Frequently, the pain of fracture initiates muscle spasm that causes the bone ends to override each other, causing further pain and muscle spasm and aggravating the original injury. The traction splint prevents overriding of the bone ends, lessens patient pain, and may help relax any muscle spasm.

The two basic styles of traction splints are the bipolar frame device and the unipolar device (Figure 18-19). The bipolar (Hare or Thomas) traction splint has a half ring that fits up and against the ischial tuberosity of the pelvis. A distal ratchet connects to a foot harness and pulls traction from the foot and against the pelvis. The frame lifts and supports the limb, and a foot stand suspends the injured limb above the ground. This construction helps prevent motion of the limb during movement of the patient, while the elevation supplied by the stand enhances venous drainage. The unipolar (Sager) traction splint uses a single lengthening shaft to pull a foot harness against pressure applied to the pubic bone. The unipolar splint does not elevate or stabilize the extremity, so observe greater care whenever you move the patient. You can use the unipolar splint in conjunction with the PASG.

Other Splinting Aids   Vacuum splints can conform to the exact shape of a limb (Figure 18-20). An injured limb is placed on a bag of small plastic particles. The splint is shaped around the limb and then the air is withdrawn from the device. The suction locks the particles in position, immobilizing the splint to the contours of the limb. The only disadvantage

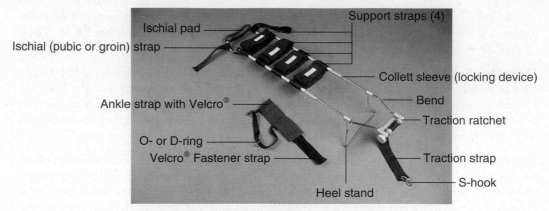

a. A bipolar frame traction splint.

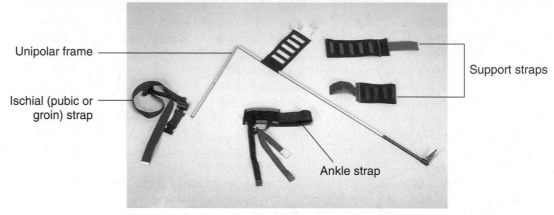

b. A unipolar frame traction splint.

FIGURE 18-19 Traction splints.

FIGURE 18-20 Suction the air out of a vacuum splint until the device is rigid. Reassess pulse, motor function, and sensation in the extremity after application.

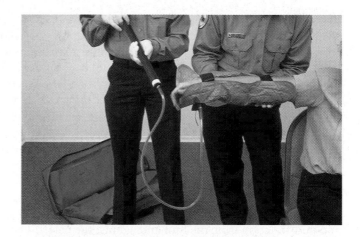

to vacuum splinting is that during air evacuation there is a small amount of shrinkage and a reduction in the splinting effect.

Cravats or Velcro® straps can augment the effectiveness of rigid splints. You can secure the lower extremities, one to the other, to help the patient control the musculoskeletal injury site or you can use a sling and swathe to help immobilize a splinted upper extremity to the chest. Fractures of the humerus are difficult to immobilize because the shoulder is such a large and mobile part of the body. A sling may hold the elbow at a fixed angle. A swathe secures the limb against the body to limit further shoulder motion. By holding a thumb in the fold of the elbow, the patient can easily reduce any motion of the limb and complement the splinting process.

In some cases of serious musculoskeletal injury, other injuries preclude the splinting of individual fractures and dislocations. In such cases, you may splint the limbs to the body with cravats or bandage material and immobilize the patient to the long spine board. Simply strap the body and limbs to the board and transport the patient as a unit. Although this is not definitive splinting, it will provide reasonable protection for musculoskeletal injuries.

FRACTURE CARE

For prehospital care purposes, consider a joint injury to be any muscular or connective tissue injury or dislocation or fracture within 3 inches of a joint. Fractures are then defined as shaft injuries at least 3 inches away from the joint. These definitions are essential because injury near the joint carries a higher incidence of blood vessel and nerve involvement and requires a different approach to positioning and splinting.

Consider any injury within 3 inches of a joint to be a joint injury.

Begin fracture care by ensuring distal pulses, sensation, and motor function. Then align the limb for splinting. Quickly recheck the circulation and motor and sensory function below the injury. If you identify any neurovascular deficit, attempt to correct the problem by gentle repositioning, even if the limb is relatively aligned. If the limb is angulated, proceed with realignment. Remember that most splinting devices are designed to immobilize aligned limbs and that alignment provides the best chance for ensuring good neurovascular function distal to the injury.

To move an injured limb from an angulated position into alignment, use gentle distal traction applied manually. Have an assisting EMT immobilize the proximal limb in the position found. Grasp the distal limb firmly and apply traction along the axis of the limb, gently moving it from the angulated to an aligned position. Should you feel any resistance to movement or notice a great increase in patient discomfort, stop the alignment attempt and splint the limb as it lies. Once you complete alignment, recheck the distal neurovascular function. If it is adequate, proceed with splinting. If function is inadequate, move the limb around slightly while another care provider monitors for a pulse. If one attempt at gentle manipulation does not reestablish a pulse, splint and transport the patient quickly.

Proceed with splinting by selecting an appropriate device and secure the limb to it in a way that ensures immobilization of both the fracture site and the adjacent joints. Have the care provider who is holding the limb apply a gentle traction to stabilize the limb (and monitor the distal pulse) during splinting. If you apply your splint properly, the device may maintain this traction and provide greater stabilization of the limb and greater patient comfort. Secure the limb to the body (upper extremity) or to the opposite limb (lower extremity) to protect it and to give the patient some control over the limb.

JOINT CARE

Joint care, too, begins with assessment for distal neurovascular function. If you find pulse, sensation, and motor function to be adequate, immobilize the joint in the position found. Use a ladder or other malleable splint, shaped to the limb's angle, or cross-wrap with a padded rigid splint to immobilize the joint in place. Ensure that splinting immobilizes the injured joint as well as the joints above and below the injury. If not, secure the limb firmly to the body to immobilize these joints.

Unless you identify a neurovascular deficit, immobilize joint injuries as you find them.

If circulation or motor or sensory function is lost below the joint injury, consider moving the limb to reestablish it. While you gently move the limb, have another care provider monitor the circulation and sensation. If you can reestablish neurovascular function quickly, splint the limb in the new position. If not, splint and provide quick transport.

With some joint injuries, you may attempt to return the displaced bone ends to their normal anatomical position. This process is called **reduction** and has both benefits and hazards. An early return to normal position reduces stress on the ligaments and basic joint structure and facilitates better distal circulation and sensation. On the other hand, the process creates the risk of trapping blood vessels or nerves when the bone ends return to their normal anatomical position. Attempt reduction of a dislocation only when you are sure the injury is a dislocation, when you expect the patient's arrival at the emergency department to be delayed (prolonged extrication or long transport time), or when there is a significant neurovascular deficit. Do not attempt a reduction if the dislocation is associated

reduction returning of displaced bone ends to their proper anatomical orientation.

with other serious patient injuries. Consult your protocols and medical direction to determine the criteria for attempting dislocation reduction used in your system.

When performing a joint reduction, you attempt to protect the articular surface while directing the bones back to their normal anatomical position. Begin the process by providing the patient with **analgesic** therapy to reduce pain associated with the injury and the reduction itself. Then have an assisting care provider hold the proximal extremity in position and provide a counter-traction during the reduction. You then apply traction to pull the bone surfaces apart, reducing the pressure between the non-articular surfaces. Slowly increase traction and direct the displaced limb toward its normal anatomical position. Successful relocation is indicated when you feel the joint pop back into position, the patient experiences a lessening of pain, and the joint becomes mobile within at least a few minutes of the procedure. Carefully evaluate the distal circulation, sensation, and motor function after the reduction. If the procedure does not meet with success within a few minutes, splint the limb as it is and provide rapid transport for the patient. If the reduction is successful, splint the limb in the position of function and transport.

analgesic agent that relieves pain.

MUSCULAR AND CONNECTIVE TISSUE CARE

Injuries to the soft tissues of the musculoskeletal system deserve special care. Although such injuries are not usually life threatening, they can be very painful, and in some cases, threaten limbs. For example, compartment syndrome can restrict capillary blood flow, venous blood return, and nerve function beyond the site of the injury. If such an injury is not discovered and relieved, it may produce severe disability. Deep contusions and especially large hematomas can also contribute to blood loss and hypovolemia. Once you care for life threats, fractures, joint injuries, and other limb problems, give injuries to muscular and connective tissues your attention.

To manage these muscle, tendon, and ligament injuries, immobilize the region surrounding them. Doing so will reduce the associated internal hemorrhage and pain. Provide gentle circumferential bandaging (loose enough to let you slide a finger underneath) to further reduce hemorrhage, edema, and pain, but be sure to monitor distal circulation and loosen the bandage further if there are any signs of neurovascular deficit. Application of local cooling will reduce both edema and patient discomfort. Be careful to wrap any cold pack or ice pack in a dressing to prevent freezing or frostbite and any consequent injury. You may apply heat to the wound after 48 hours to enhance both circulation and healing. If possible, place the limb in the position of function and elevate the extremity to ensure good venous return, limit swelling, and reduce patient discomfort. Monitor distal neurovascular function to make certain your actions do not compromise circulation, sensation, or motor function.

CARE FOR SPECIFIC FRACTURES

Pelvis

Pelvic fractures involve either the iliac crest, ischial ring, or the pelvic ring. Although iliac crest fractures may reflect serious trauma, they do not represent the life threats suggested by ring fractures. Iliac crest fractures are often isolated and stable injuries that you can care for by simple patient immobilization.

Pelvic ring fractures, on the other hand, are often serious, life-threatening events. The ring shape of the pelvis provides strength to the structure, but when it breaks, two fracture sites usually result. The kinetic forces necessary to fracture the pelvic ring are significant and are likely to produce fractures and internal injuries elsewhere. In addition, the pelvis is actively involved in blood cell production, has a rich blood supply, and its interior surface is adjacent to major blood vessels serving the lower extremities. Injury to the pelvic ring, therefore, can result in heavy hemorrhage that is likely to empty into the pelvic and retroperitoneal spaces and account for internal blood loss in excess of 2 liters. Such injury may also result in circulation loss to one or both lower extremities. Pelvic fractures may also be associated with hip dislocations and injuries to the bladder, female reproductive organs, the urethra, the prostate in the male, and the end of the alimentary canal (anus and rectum). Clearly, pelvic ring fractures are very serious injuries.

Always consider a pelvic fracture patient to be a candidate for rapid transport.

The objectives of pelvic injury care are to stabilize the fractured pelvis, support the patient hemodynamically, and provide rapid transport to a trauma center. Because of the potential for severe blood loss and the difficulty of immobilizing the broken pelvic ring, application of the PASG is standard practice with pelvic fractures (Figure 18-21). Inflate the PASG until it stabilizes the pelvis and hip joint. Start two large-bore IVs, and hang two 1,000 mL bags of lactated Ringer's solution or normal saline. Set up using trauma tubing and pressure infusion sets for rapid infusion because aggressive fluid administration may be necessary. Be prepared to run 1,000 mL of solution immediately to maintain the systolic blood pressure at between 90 and 100 mmHg. Once the initial bolus of fluid is administered, the IV lines need only run at a to-keep-open rate unless further signs of hypovolemic compensation develop or the systolic blood pressure dips below 90 mmHg. Always consider a patient who has a pelvic fracture to be a candidate for rapid transport.

FIGURE 18-21 The PASG is an effective splint for pelvic fractures and helps control internal hemorrhage.

Femur

Femur fractures may be traumatic, resulting from the application of very strong and violent forces, or atraumatic, resulting from degenerative diseases. Patients with disease-induced fractures usually are of advancing age and present with a history of a degenerative disease, a clouded or limited history of trauma, and only moderate discomfort. Care for such patients includes immobilizing them as found and then providing gentle transport. Generally, you can provide effective splinting by placing the patient on a long spine board and padding with pillows and blankets for patient comfort. Use of a traction splint is not essential because pain is not inducing the spasms that cause broken bone ends to override.

Atraumatic femur fractures may be splinted by gently placing the patient on a long spine board.

A patient who has suffered a traumatic femur fracture usually experiences extreme discomfort, often writhing in pain. In such a case, providing distal traction immobilizes both bone ends, relieves muscle spasms, and reduces the associated pain. Traction splinting is the best avenue for care of the hemodynamically stable patient with an isolated femur fracture. However, the traction splint is not indicated if the patient has concurrent serious knee, tibia, or foot injuries.

Proximal fractures (surgical neck and intertrochanteric fractures) are frequently caused by hip injuries, transmitted forces, or the degenerative effects of aging. Mid-shaft fractures often result from high-energy, lateral traumas and are associated with significant blood loss. Injuries to the distal femur (condylar and epicondylar fractures) can be extensive and are likely to involve blood vessels, nerves, and connective tissue. The energy necessary to fracture the femur may be sufficient to dislocate the hip and cause serious internal injuries elsewhere in the body.

If the femur fracture is concurrent with a severe pelvic fracture, limb immobilization and hemodynamic stability is best achieved by using the PASG alone. A traction splint may apply pressure to the fractured pelvis, thereby causing further bone displacement and hemorrhage. Also, if the early signs of shock are present or if the history suggests that the patient has sustained trauma severe enough to induce shock, the PASG may be a better choice because it effectively splints the entire region and contributes to hemodynamic stability.

You may find it difficult to differentiate between proximal fractures of the femur (hip fractures) and anterior hip dislocations. Generally, a femur fracture presents with the foot externally rotated (turned outward) and the injured limb shortened when compared with the other. This difference may be slight and may be unnoticeable if the patient's legs are not straight and parallel. An anterior dislocation presents similarly to the femur fracture, but with the head of the femur protruding in the inguinal region. When in doubt, treat as a dislocation.

If you suspect femur fracture, align the limb, determine the status of circulation and sensory and motor function, and apply the traction splint (Figure 18-22). (If you use manual traction to align the femur, maintain it until the splint is applied and continues the traction.) Adjust the length of the splint to the injured extremity, position the device against the pelvis, and secure it in position with the inguinal strap. With a bipolar splint, apply the ankle hitch, provide gentle traction, and elevate the distal limb to place the splint's ring against the ischial tuberosity. With a unipolar splint, position the T-shaped support against the pubic bone and simply apply the ankle hitch. Ensure that hitch and splint hold the foot and limb

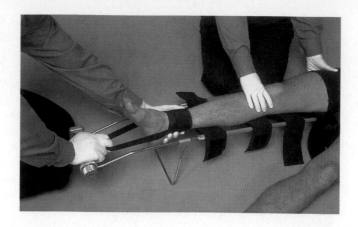

FIGURE 18-22 The traction splint effectively immobilizes femur fractures.

in an anatomical position as you apply firm traction. Position and secure the limb to the splint with straps, then gently move the patient and splint to the long spine board. Firmly secure the patient and limb for transport.

Guide your application of traction by the patient's response. Ask the patient how the limb feels as you initiate and increase the amount of traction. Stop the application of traction when the limb is immobilized and patient discomfort decreases. Remember, because the traction splint prevents the overriding of bone ends, the pain of injury decreases. This reduces the strength of muscle spasm and lets the limb return toward its initial length. This, in turn, reduces the traction provided by the splint, which means that the bone ends will no longer be as well immobilized. Check the amount of traction frequently to ensure that it does not lessen during your care. If the patient reports increasing pain, consider increasing traction gradually until some reduction in pain is noted.

When the need for rapid transport or other patient injuries preclude the use of the traction splint, consider using the long spine board for immobilizing and transporting the femur fracture patient. Use long padded rigid splints, one medial and one lateral, to quickly splint the injured limb, and then tie that limb to the uninjured one. Use an orthopedic stretcher or another device or movement technique to transfer the patient to a long spine board and secure the patient firmly on it.

Tibia/Fibula

Fibular fractures are relatively stable, whereas tibial fractures are not.

Fractures of the leg bones, the tibia and the fibula, can occur separately or together. The tibia is the most commonly fractured leg bone and may be broken by direct force, crushing injury, or twisting forces. Tibial fracture is likely to cause an open wound. Fibular fractures are often associated with damage to the knee or ankle. If the tibia is fractured and the fibula is intact, the extremity may not angulate, but it is not able to bear weight. If only the fibula is broken, the limb may be relatively stable. Injuries to either bone may result in compartment syndrome. Direct trauma suffered during an auto crash or athletic impact frequently causes these tibia and fibula injuries.

Align the injured limb, assess circulation, sensation, and motor function, and then immobilize the limb with gentle traction. A full-leg air splint (one that accommodates the foot) or lateral and medial padded rigid splints will provide effective immobilization (Figure 18-23). You may also use a cardboard splint as long as it accommodates the full limb and is rigid enough to maintain immobilization. After you splint the injured limb, secure it to the uninjured leg. This affords some protection against uncontrolled movement and may reassure the patient that he still has some control over the extremity.

Clavicle

The clavicle is the most frequently fractured bone in the human body. Fractures to it usually result from transmitted forces directed along the upper extremity that cause relatively minor skeletal injury. The clavicle, however, is located adjacent to both the upper reaches of the lung and the vasculature that serves the upper extremity and head. Hence, an injury to the clavicle has the potential to cause serious internal injury, especially if very powerful mechanisms of injury are involved. The clavicular fracture patient often presents with pain

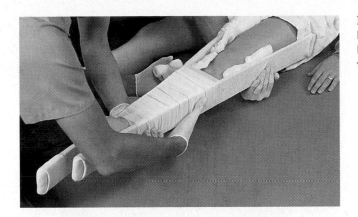

FIGURE 18-23 Placement of long padded board splints laterally and medially can effectively splint tibia/fibula fractures.

and the shoulder shifted forward with palpable deformity along the clavicle. Accomplish splinting either by immobilizing the affected limb in a sling and swathe or by wrapping a figure-eight bandage around the shoulders, drawing the shoulders back, and then securing the bandage tension. Monitor the patient carefully for any sign of internal hemorrhage or respiratory compromise, including tension pneumothorax.

Humerus

A fractured humerus is very difficult to immobilize at its proximal end. The proximal humerus is buried within the shoulder muscles, and the shoulder joint is very mobile atop the thoracic cage. The axillary artery runs through the axilla, making it difficult to apply any mechanical traction to the limb without compromising circulation. Hence, the most effective techniques for splinting this fracture are to apply a sling and swathe to immobilize the bent limb against the chest or to tie the extended and splinted limb to the body.

The preferred technique is to use the sling and swathe. Apply a short padded rigid splint to the lateral surface of the arm to distribute the pressure of the swathing and better immobilize the arm. Sling the forearm with a cravat, catching just the wrist region and not the elbow. This permits some gravitational traction in the seated patient and prevents inadvertent application of pressure by the sling, which could push the limb together. Then use several cravats to gently swathe the arm and forearm to the chest. If the patient is conscious, have him place the thumb of the uninjured extremity in the fold of the elbow to help control the injured limb's motion. This gives the patient control over the limb, decreases limb movement, and increases patient comfort.

You may also immobilize the limb by using a long padded rigid splint affixed to the extended limb. Place the splint along the medial aspect of the upper extremity and ensure that it does not apply pressure to the axilla. Such pressure disrupts axillary artery blood flow to the limb and is uncomfortable for the patient. Secure the splint firmly to the limb, wrapping from the distal end toward the proximal end. Then secure the splint to the supine patient's body, and move the patient and splint to a long spine board.

Radius/Ulna

The forearm may fracture anywhere along its length and the fracture may involve the radius, the ulna, or both. Most commonly, fracture occurs at the distal end of the radius, just above the articular surface. This is known as a Colles's fracture, and it presents with the wrist turned up at an unusual angle. Another term for this injury is the "silver fork deformity" because it is contoured like a fork and the distal limb often becomes ashen. As with most joint fractures, the major concern here is for distal circulation and innervation. If you find a neurovascular injury, use only slight adjustments to restore nervous or circulatory function because large movement in this area is likely to cause further injury.

Splint forearm fractures with a short, padded rigid splint affixed to the forearm and hand. Secure the hand in the position of function by placing a large wad of dressing material in the palm to maintain a position like that of holding a large ball. Place the rigid splint along the medial forearm surface and wrap circumferentially from the fingers to the elbow. Leave at least one digit exposed to permit checking for capillary refill. Bend the elbow across

When possible, leave a distal digit exposed to evaluate capillary refill, skin color, and temperature.

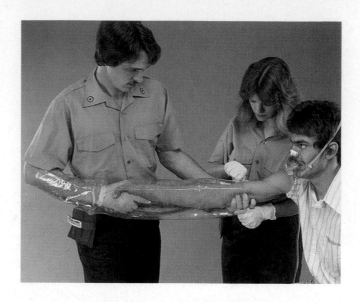

FIGURE 18-24 The full-arm air splint can effectively splint fractures of the radius and/or ulna.

the chest and use a sling and swathe to hold the limb in position. This provides relative elevation and improved venous drainage in both seated and supine patients.

The air splint or long padded rigid splint, tied firmly to the body, may also adequately immobilize forearm fractures (Figure 18-24). When using these devices, remember to place the hand in the position of function to increase patient comfort.

CARE FOR SPECIFIC JOINT INJURIES

Hip

The hip may dislocate in two directions, anteriorly and posteriorly. The anterior dislocation in uncommon and presents with the foot turned outward and the head of the femur palpable in the inguinal area. The posterior dislocation is most common and presents with the knee flexed and the foot rotated internally. The displaced head of the femur is buried in the muscle of the buttocks. Immobilize a patient with either type of dislocation on a long spine board using pillows and blankets as padding to maintain the patient's position and provide comfort. If distal circulation, sensation, or motor function is severely compromised, consider one attempt at reduction of a posterior dislocation. (Consult local protocols and medical direction to identify criteria for reduction attempts.) However, do not attempt reduction if the patient has other serious injuries, such as a pelvic fracture, associated with the hip dislocation. Anterior dislocations in general cannot be managed by reduction in the prehospital setting.

For reduction of a posterior hip dislocation, have a care provider hold the pelvis firmly against the long spine board or other firm surface by placing downward pressure on the iliac crests. Flex both the patient's hip and knee at 90 degrees and apply a firm, slowly increasing traction along the axis of the femur. Gently rotate the femur externally. It takes some time for the muscles to relax, but when they do the head of the femur will "pop" back into position. If you feel this "pop" or if the patient reports a sudden relief of pain and is able to extend the leg easily, the reduction has likely been a success. Immobilize the patient in a comfortable position, either in flexion (not to exceed 90 degrees) or fully supine with the hip and leg in full extension. Reevaluate sensation, motor function, and circulation. If the femur head does not move into the acetabulum after a few minutes of your attempted reduction, immobilize the patient as found and consider rapid transport.

Knee

Knee injuries may include fractures of the femur, the tibia, or both, patellar dislocations, or frank dislocations of the knee. Because the knee is such a large joint and bears such a great amount of weight, an injury to it is serious and threatens the patient's future ability to walk. Another concern with knee injury is possible injury to the major blood vessel traversing the area, the popliteal artery. This artery is less mobile than blood vessels in other joints, which leaves it more subject to injury and distal vascular compromise.

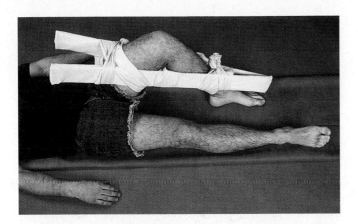

FIGURE 18-25 Angulated knee dislocations can be immobilized with two padded rigid splints.

Immobilize knee joint fractures and patellar dislocations in the position found unless distal circulation, sensation, or motor function is disrupted. If the limb is flexed, splint it with two medium rigid splints, placing one medially and one laterally (Figure 18-25). Cross-wrap with bandage material to secure the limb in position. You may also use ladder or malleable splints, conformed to the angle of the limb and placed anteriorly and posteriorly, or a vacuum splint to immobilize the knee. If the limb is extended, simply apply two padded rigid splints or a full-leg air splint.

Dislocation of the patella is more common than dislocation of the knee joint and usually leaves the knee in a flexed position with a lateral displacement of the patella. The injured knee appears significantly deformed, though patellar dislocation has a lower incidence of associated vascular injury than does knee dislocation.

Anterior dislocations of the knee produce an extended limb contour that lifts at the knee (moving from proximal to distal) whereas posterior dislocations produce a limb that drops at the knee. (Ensure that the injury is not a patellar dislocation.) If there is neurovascular compromise, have another care provider immobilize the femur. You should then grasp the limb just above the ankle and at the calf muscle and apply a firm and progressive traction, first along the axis of the tibia and then pulling the limb toward alignment with the femur. With posterior dislocations, a third care provider may provide moderate downward pressure on the distal femur and upward pressure on the proximal tibia to facilitate the reduction. As with most dislocations, success is measured by feeling the bone end pop back into place, hearing the patient report a dramatic reduction in pain, and noting a freer movement of the limb at the knee joint. Once you reduce the knee dislocation, immobilize the joint in the position of function and transport the patient. If you cannot reduce the dislocation within a few minutes of distal traction, immobilize the extremity in the position found and transport quickly. Perform a knee dislocation reduction even if the patient has good distal circulation and nervous function when the time to definitive care will exceed 2 hours.

Immobilize knee injuries in the position found unless you discover significant distal circulation, sensation, or motor deficit.

Ankle

Ankle injuries often produce a distal lower limb that is grossly deformed, either due to malleolar fracture, dislocation, or both. Sprains are also injuries of concern, although with them the limb remains in anatomical position. Splint sprains or non-displaced fractures with an air splint (shaped to accommodate the foot) or with long rigid splints positioned on either side of the limb, padded liberally, and wrapped firmly. You may also use a pillow splint, especially if the patient has any ankle deformity (Figure 18-26). Apply local cooling to ease the pain and reduce swelling.

Ankle dislocation may occur in any of three directions: anteriorly, posteriorly, and laterally. The anterior dislocation presents with a dorsiflexed (upward pointing) foot that appears shortened. The posterior dislocation appears to lengthen the plantar flexed (downward pointing) foot. The lateral dislocation is most common and presents with a foot turned outward with respect to the ankle. If distal neurovascular compromise indicates the need for reduction, have a care provider grasp the calf, hold it in position, and pull against the traction you apply. You then grasp the heel with one hand and the metatarsal arch with the other. Pull a distal traction to disengage the bone ends and protect the articular cartilage

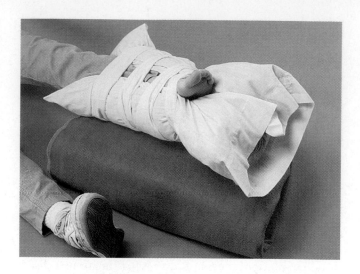

Figure 18-26 A pillow splint can be used with injuries to the ankles and feet.

during the relocation. For anterior dislocations, move the foot posteriorly with respect to the ankle; with lateral dislocations, rotate the foot medially; with posterior dislocations, pull the heel toward you and the foot toward you, then away. The joint should return to normal position with a "pop," a reduction in patient pain, and an increase in the mobility of the joint. Apply local cooling, elevate, and immobilize the limb. If the procedure does not result in joint reduction with one attempt, splint the joint as found and provide rapid transport.

Foot

Injuries to the foot include dislocations and fractures to the calcaneus (heel bone), midfoot bones, metatarsals, and phalanges. Injuries to the calcaneus generally result from falls and can cause significant pain and swelling. Injuries to the metatarsals and phalanges can result from penetrating or blunt trauma or the typical stubbing of a toe. Fatigue fractures of the metatarsal bones, or march fractures, are relatively common. These injuries are reasonably stable, even though the extremity cannot bear weight. When foot or ankle injury is suspected, anticipate both bilateral foot injuries and lumbar spinal injury.

Immobilize foot injuries in much the same way you do with ankle injuries. Use pillow, vacuum, ladder or air splints (with foot accommodation). If possible, leave some portion of the foot accessible so you can monitor distal capillary refill or, at least, skin temperature and color.

Shoulder

Fractures to the shoulder most commonly involve the proximal humerus, lateral scapula, and distal clavicle. Dislocations can include anterior, posterior, and inferior displacement of the humoral head. Anterior dislocations displace the humoral head forward, resulting in a shoulder that appears hollow or squared off, with the patient holding the arm close to the chest and forward of the midaxillary line. Posterior dislocations rotate the arm internally, and the patient presents with the elbow and forearm held away from the chest. Inferior dislocations displace the humoral head downward, with the result that the patient's arm is often locked above the head.

You should immobilize shoulder injuries, as with all joint injuries, unless pulse, sensation, or motor function distal to the injury is absent. Immobilize anterior and posterior dislocations with a sling and swathe and, if needed, place a pillow under the arm and forearm. Immobilization of any inferior dislocation (with the upper extremity fixed above the head) will call for ingenuity on your part in splinting. In such cases, immobilize the extended arm in the position found. Using cravats, tie a long, padded splint to the torso, shoulder girdle, arm, and forearm to immobilize the arm above the head. Gently move the patient to the long spine board and secure both splint and patient to the spine board.

If needed to correct neurovascular compromise, the EMT-I may attempt reduction of a shoulder dislocation. Begin reduction of anterior and posterior shoulder dislocations by placing a strap across the patient's chest, under the affected shoulder (through the axilla), and across the back. Have a care provider prepared to pull counter traction across the chest and superiorly using the strap. Meanwhile, you should flex the patient's elbow, drawing the arm somewhat away from the body (abduction) and pull firm traction along the axis of the humerus. Some slight internal and external rotation of the humerus may facilitate reduction. For reduction of inferior dislocations, have one care provider hold the thorax while you flex the elbow. Gradually apply firm traction along the axis of the humerus and gently rotate the arm externally. If the joint does not relocate in a few minutes, immobilize it as it lies and transport the patient. If reduction is successful, immobilize the upper extremity in the normal anatomical position with a sling and swathe.

Elbow

Elbow injuries display a high incidence of nervous and vascular involvement, especially in children. As in the knee, the blood vessels running through the elbow region are held firmly in place. The probability is good, therefore, that any fracture or dislocation will involve the brachial artery and the medial, ulnar, and radial nerves. Assess the distal neurovascular function and, if you detect a deficit, move the joint very carefully and minimally to restore distal circulation. Then splint the elbow with a single padded rigid splint, providing cross-strapping as necessary, or use a ladder splint bent to conform to the angle of the limb (Figure 18-27). Keeping the wrist slightly elevated above the elbow, secure the limb to the chest using a sling and swathe. This position increases venous return and reduces the swelling and pain associated with the injury.

Elbow dislocations should not be reduced in the prehospital setting.

Wrist/Hand

Fractures of the hand and wrist are commonly associated with direct trauma. They present with very noticeable deformity and significant pain reported by the patient. These fractures are of serious concern to the patient. Since the hand and wrist bones are small, any fracture is in close proximity to a joint. Exercise concern when you care for these injuries because of the possibility of vascular and neural involvement.

You can effectively immobilize musculoskeletal injuries of the forearm, wrist, hand, or fingers with a padded rigid or air splint. Place a roll of bandaging, a wad of dressing material, or some similar object in the patient's hand to maintain the position of function. Then secure the extremity to the padded board or inflate the air splint. Be sure to leave some portion of the distal extremity accessible so that you can monitor the adequacy of perfusion and sensation. Place the wrist above the elbow to assist venous return and reduce distal swelling.

Hand and wrist injuries are very common, particularly among athletes and children. A particular type of wrist fracture is the Colles's fracture in which the wrist has a silver fork appearance. Fortunately, such injuries can be managed in the prehospital setting quite easily.

When splinting the distal upper extremity, place padding in the palm of the hand to maintain the position of function.

Finger

Forces may displace the phalanges from their joints, resulting in deformity and pain. Displacement usually occurs between the phalanges or between the proximal phalanx and the metacarpal and causes the bone to be moved either anteriorly or posteriorly. (Amputations are multi-system injuries that severely damage the musculoskeletal system.)

Splint finger fractures using tongue blades or small, malleable splints designed for the purpose that you shape to the contour of the injured finger. The finger may also be taped to

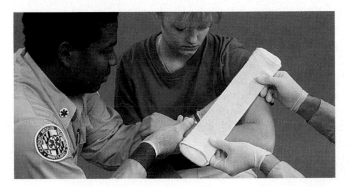

FIGURE 18-27 Use a padded board splint to immobilize angulated fractures or dislocations of the elbow.

the adjoining fingers to limit additional motion. The hand is then placed in the position of function and further immobilized.

Finger dislocations usually involve the proximal joint (and sometimes the distal joint) with the digit commonly displacing posteriorly. If reduction is indicated, grasp the distal finger and apply a firm distal traction. Then direct the digit toward the normal anatomical position by moving its proximal end. You should feel the finger pop into place, and the digit should resume its normal alignment when compared with the uninjured finger on the other hand. Splint the finger with a slight bend (10 to 15 degrees) and immobilize the hand in the position of function.

CARE FOR SOFT AND CONNECTIVE TISSUE INJURIES

Tendon, ligament, and muscle injuries are rarely life threatening.

Tendon, ligament, and muscle injuries are rarely, if ever, life threatening. Massive muscular contusions and hematomas can, however, contribute to hypovolemia. Ligament and tendon injuries can endanger the future function of a limb. Be careful about permitting the patient to put further stress on a limb, especially with higher grades of sprains. The weakened ligaments may fail completely, resulting in dislocation or complete joint instability. For the purpose of care, treat these injuries as you would dislocations and immobilize the adjacent joints. Monitor distal neurovascular function because tissue swelling within the circumferential wrapping of a splint may compress blood vessels and nerves. Care for muscular injuries with immobilization, gentle compression with snug (but not overly tight) dressings, and local cooling to suppress edema and pain using cold packs or ice wrapped in dressing material. Be watchful for signs of compartment syndrome, especially in the calf and forearm regions.

Care for muscular injuries with immobilization, gentle compression with snug dressings, and local cooling to suppress edema and pain.

Open wounds involving the muscles, tendons, and ligaments can be severe and debilitating. Carefully evaluate such wounds for signs of connective tissue involvement. Be especially watchful with deep open injuries close to the joints. With such wounds, the likelihood of tendon and ligament disruption is great and may affect the use of the joint, the muscles controlling the joint, or the muscles controlling joint movement distal to the injury. Carefully evaluate for circulation, sensation, and motor function below these injuries.

Injury to a muscle or tendon may limit its ability to either extend or flex the limb. The opposing muscle moves the limb, while the injured muscle cannot return it to the normal position. With limb injuries, note any unusual limb position, especially if the patient is unable to return the limb to a neutral position. At any sign of pain or dysfunction, splint the limb.

MEDICATIONS

Medications are frequently administered to the patient with musculoskeletal injury to relieve pain and to premedicate before the relocation of a dislocation. Medications used include nitrous oxide, diazepam, morphine, meperidine, and nalbuphine.

Sedatives/Analgesics

Nitrous Oxide   Nitrous oxide (Nitronox®) is a nitrogen and oxygen compound in a gas state. It is administered in the prehospital setting for its anesthetic properties, specifically to reduce the perception of pain in cases of musculoskeletal injuries. For prehospital care, it is administered in a 50% nitrous oxide and 50% oxygen mixture via a special regulator and a self-administration mask. Self-administration of nitrous oxide prevents over-medication because the patient will drop the mask when too heavily sedated.

Nitrous oxide is non-explosive, and its analgesic effects dissipate within 2 to 5 minutes of discontinuing administration. High concentrations of nitrous oxide may lead to hypoxia and may cause respiratory depression and vomiting. These side effects are minimized, however, because the gas is pre-mixed with oxygen by the administration set during prehospital delivery.

The chief concern with the use of nitrous oxide is that it diffuses easily into air-filled spaces in the body, increasing the pressure within them. This diffusion is especially dangerous in patients with pneumothorax or tension pneumothorax, bowel obstruction, and middle ear obstruction. Rule out chronic obstructive pulmonary disease (COPD) and these pathologies before you administer nitrous oxide in the prehospital setting.

The nitrous oxide administration device consists of two cylinders of equal size, one holding oxygen (green) and the other, nitrous oxide (blue). The gases are mixed in a special blender/regulator and distributed to the patient when his inspiration generates a less-than-atmospheric pressure. (In other countries, both gases are pre-mixed in one cylinder, reducing the weight and size of the administration device.) The patient must hold the administration mask firmly to the face to trigger administration, thus preventing administration in a patient who is heavily sedated. Nitrous oxide is a controlled substance and its use is carefully monitored for provider abuse.

Diazepam Diazepam (Valium®) is a benzodiazepine with both anti-anxiety and skeletal muscle relaxant qualities. The drug reduces the patient's perception and memory of pain. It is used with musculoskeletal injuries and to premedicate patients before painful procedures such as cardioversion and dislocation reduction. It is administered in a slow IV bolus of 5 to 15 mg, not to exceed 5 mg/minute, into a large vein. Diazepam is rather fast-acting, with IV effects occurring almost immediately and reaching peak effectiveness in 15 minutes. Its duration of effectiveness is from 15 to 60 minutes. Do not mix diazepam with any other drugs, and flush the IV line before and after administration. Administer diazepam as close to the IV catheter as possible, and do not inject it into a plastic IV bag. Diazepam is readily absorbed by plastic, which quickly reduces its concentration.

Diazepam is usually supplied in single-use vials or pre-loaded syringes containing 2 mL of a 5 mg/mL solution (10 mg). Administer 5 to 15 mg IV and repeat in 10 to 15 minutes if necessary.

The effects of diazepam may be reversed by the administration of flumazenil. Usually, 2 mL of a 0.1 mg/mL solution is given IV (over 15 seconds) with a second dose repeated at 60 seconds.

Morphine Morphine sulfate (Duramorph®, Astramorph®) is an opium alkaloid used to relieve pain (narcotic analgesic), to sedate, and to reduce anxiety. It is used with musculoskeletal injuries for its ability to reduce pain perception. Morphine may reduce vascular volume and cardiac preload by increasing venous capacitance and may thus decrease blood pressure in the hypovolemic patient. It should not be administered to a patient with hypovolemia or hypotension. Major side effects are respiratory depression, possible nausea and vomiting, hypotension, and oversedation.

Morphine is available in 10 mL single-use vials or Tubex® units of a 1 mg/mL solution or as 1 mL of a 10 mg/mL solution vial for dilution with 9 mL normal saline. Administer a 2 mg bolus slowly IV, repeating as necessary every few minutes to effect.

Naloxone hydrochloride (Narcan®) is a narcotic antagonist that can quickly reverse the effects of narcotics (morphine, meperidine, and nalbuphine) and should be available any time you use morphine sulfate. Naloxone is administered as an IV bolus of 0.4 to 2 mg, repeated every 2 to 3 minutes until effective. Naloxone is a shorter-acting drug than morphine, so repeat doses may be necessary.

Meperidine Meperidine hydrochloride (Demerol®) is a narcotic analgesic with properties similar to those of morphine, although it may produce less smooth muscle relaxation, constipation, and cough reflex suppression. As with morphine, it is used with musculoskeletal injuries for its ability to reduce the patient's perception of pain. It also may produce respiratory depression, hypotension (especially in the patient who is volume depleted), and oversedation.

Meperidine is supplied in single-dose vials and preloaded syringes and in concentrations of from 10 to 100 mg/mL. It may be administered in doses of 50 to 100 mg IM. For IV administration use a concentration of 10 mg/mL diluted in normal saline or lactated Ringer's solution and inject slowly in doses of 50 to 100 mg. Narcan® will reverse its effects.

Nalbuphine Nalbuphine hydrochloride (Nubain®) is a synthetic narcotic analgesic with properties similar to those of morphine. It is equivalent on a milligram-to-milligram basis to morphine, although it antagonizes some of the actions of that drug. Nalbuphine does not generally decrease blood pressure, although it may produce respiratory depression and bradycardia. Unlike morphine and meperidine, it is not a controlled substance. It is a rapid-acting—within 2 to 3 minutes—drug with a long duration of effectiveness—3 to 6 hours.

Nalbuphine is supplied in ampules or preloaded syringes containing 1 mL of a 10 or 20 mg/mL solution. It is administered IV in a dose of 5 mg, then 2 mg repeated as needed up to 20 mg. Narcan® will reverse its effects.

MANAGEMENT OF SOFT-TISSUE INJURY PATIENTS

The management of minor wounds is a late priority in the care of the trauma patient, unless extensive bleeding is noted.

The three objectives of bandaging are to control hemorrhage, to keep the wound clean, and to immobilize the wound site.

A combination of techniques for hemorrhage control may be effective when bleeding is resistant to direct pressure.

To halt hemorrhage, apply firm pressure to the site for at least 10 minutes.

Once you complete your patient assessment, take steps to manage the soft-tissue injury, either in the field or en route to the hospital. Control of blood loss, prevention of shock, and decontamination of affected areas take priority. The following sections describe some of the most important of these care steps.

Unless you note extensive bleeding, wound management by dressing and bandaging is a late priority in the care of trauma patients. Dress and bandage wounds whose bleeding does not represent a life threat only after you stabilize your patient by caring for higher-priority injuries.

OBJECTIVES OF WOUND DRESSING AND BANDAGING

The dressing and bandaging of a wound has three basic objectives. These are to control all hemorrhaging, to keep the wound as clean as possible, and to immobilize the wound (Procedure 18-1). The appearance of the final dressing and bandage is not as critical as achievement of these three objectives.

Hemorrhage Control

The primary method—and the most effective one—of controlling hemorrhage associated with soft-tissue injury is direct pressure. In cases of serious hemorrhage flowing from a wound with some force, place a small dressing directly over the site of the bleeding and apply pressure directly to it with a finger. When the bleeding is the more commonly encountered slow-to-moderate type, use a dressing that has been sized to cover and pad the wound. Then simply wrap the dressing with a soft, self-adherent bandage using moderate pressure to halt the blood loss. Monitor the wound frequently to ensure bleeding has stopped.

Elevation can assist in the control of hemorrhage, although it is generally not as effective as direct pressure. Elevation reduces arterial pressure in the extremity and increases venous return. Elevation can thus reduce edema and increase blood flow through the wound and injured extremity. This promotes good oxygenation and wound healing. Do not elevate a limb, however, if doing so will cause any further harm as would be the case if the patient has a suspected spinal or associated musculoskeletal injury, or if an object impaled the limb.

Use pressure points to assist with bleeding control and the clotting process when direct pressure and elevation together do not control it. Locate a pulse point immediately proximal to the wound and above a bony prominence. Apply firm pressure and maintain it for at least 10 minutes. Ensure that the hemorrhage does not continue.

Occasionally, bleeding from a soft-tissue injury can be difficult to control. If the bleeding continues despite the use of direct pressure, elevation, and pressure points, reassess the wound to be sure you have determined the exact site of blood loss. Then reapply direct digital pressure to that precise point. Too often, hemorrhage continues because the bandaging technique distributes pressure over the entire wound site rather than focusing it directly on the source of the bleeding. The force driving the hemorrhage is no greater than the patient's systolic blood pressure, and properly applied digital pressure can thus easily provide a pressure greater than this to compress the vessel and halt any blood loss.

In certain circumstances, the use of direct pressure, elevation, and a pressure point may not control hemorrhage. Crush injuries and amputations are situations in which normal bleeding control measures are often ineffective. With these traumatic injuries, several blood vessels are jaggedly torn, confounding the body's normal hemorrhage control mechanisms and making it difficult to pinpoint the source of bleeding. Even if the source of bleeding can be found, applying firm direct pressure to it may be difficult. In such cases, the application of a tourniquet may be useful. The tourniquet should be considered the last option for controlling hemorrhage. If properly applied, the tourniquet will stop the flow of blood; however, its use has serious associated risks. Keep the following precautions in mind whenever you consider using a tourniquet.

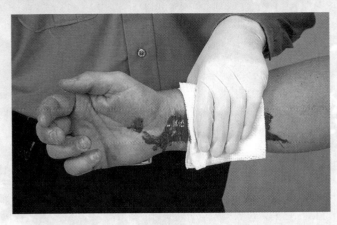

18-1a Apply direct pressure with a dressing to the site of hemorrhage.

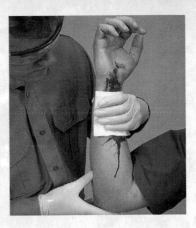

18-1b Elevate the hemorrhage site if there is no serious musculoskeletal injury.

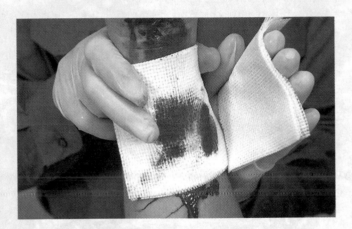

18-1c Apply additional dressings as needed.

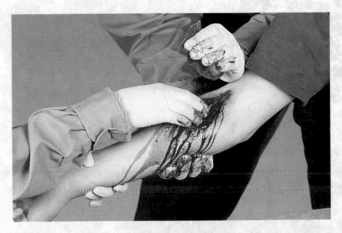

18-1d If serious hemorrhage persists, expose the wound and place digital pressure with a gloved hand on the site of bleeding.

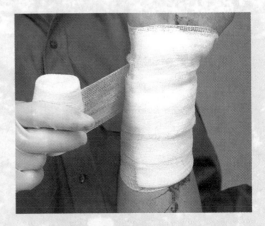

18-1e Bandage the dressing in place, maintaining pressure on the wound.

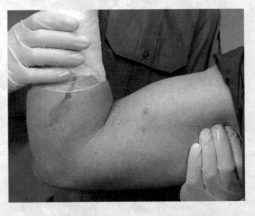

18-1f Apply digital pressure to a proximal artery if the hemorrhage persists.

1. If the pressure applied is insufficient, the tourniquet may halt venous return while permitting continued arterial blood flow into the extremity, increasing the rate and volume of blood loss.

2. When the tourniquet is applied properly, the entire limb distal to the device is without circulation. Hypoxia, ischemia, and necrosis may permanently damage the tissue distal to the tourniquet.

3. When circulation is restored, the blood flows and pools in the extremity, adding to any hypovolemia. In addition, any blood that returns to the central circulation is highly hypoxic, acidic, and toxic. This blood can cause shock, lethal dysrhythmias, renal failure, and death. The return of circulation may also restart hemorrhage and introduce emboli into the central circulation.

Do not use a tourniquet unless you cannot control bleeding by any other means.

Do not use a tourniquet unless you cannot control severe bleeding by any other means. Place it just proximal to the wound site, but stay away from the elbow or knee joints (Figure 18-28). Apply the tourniquet in a way that will not injure the tissue beneath. For example, do not use very narrow material, like rope or wire, for a tourniquet; applying great pressure to a limb with such material may cause serious injury in the compressed tissue. Instead, select a 2-inch or wider band for compression.

A readily available, effective, and easily controllable tourniquet is the sphygmomanometer (regular for the upper extremity and thigh for the lower). It is wide, simple to apply, rapid to inflate, and easy to monitor. Inflate it to a pressure 30 mmHg above the patient's systolic blood pressure and beyond the pressure at which the patient's hemorrhage ceases. Be aware, however, that blood pressure cuffs often have slow leaks that will release pressure.

Once applied, a tourniquet should be left in place until the patient arrives at the emergency department.

Once you apply a tourniquet, leave it in place until the patient arrives at the emergency department. Monitor the tourniquet during transport to ensure that it does not lose pressure, and watch for signs of renewed bleeding. If bleeding starts again, increase the tourniquet pressure. Alert the hospital staff to your use of the tourniquet during transport as well as upon arrival. Mark a piece of tape on the patient's forehead clearly with the letters TQ, and note the time the tourniquet was applied.

a. Place a bulky dressing over the distal artery.

b. Apply a pressure exceeding the systolic pressure.

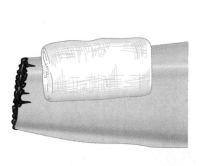

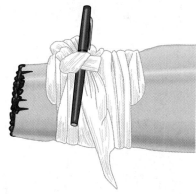

c. Secure the tourniquet and monitor the wound site for continuing hemorrhage.

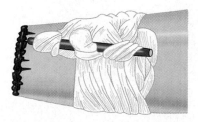

FIGURE 18-28 The steps of tourniquet application.

Do not release a tourniquet in the field except under exceptional circumstances and then only during consultation with medical direction. Be prepared to provide vigorous bleeding control, fluid resuscitation, ECG monitoring, dysrhythmia treatment, and rapid transport if a tourniquet release is attempted.

Sterility

Once you halt severe bleeding, keep the wound as clean as possible. Under field conditions, this may simply mean keeping the wound as clean as reasonably possible. With very small open wounds, like an IV start or a small laceration, you may consider the application of an antibacterial ointment to help with infection control. However, the effectiveness of such ointments on larger wounds is limited, and ointments are not generally applied to these wounds.

Under normal conditions, you need not cleanse the wound. If a wound is grossly contaminated, however, irrigate it with normal saline or lactated Ringer's solution. A 1,000 mL bag of saline, connected to a macrodrip administration set and pressurized by squeezing the bag under your arm, may allow rapid and gentle wound cleansing. Try to move any contamination from the center of the wound outward. You may also carefully remove larger particles—glass, gravel, debris, and so forth—if you can do this swiftly and without inducing further injury.

Apply a bandage to make the dressing appear as neat as time and the conditions under which you are working will allow. Often, this is as easy as covering the entire dressing with wraps of soft, self-adherent roller bandage. The neat appearance calms and reassures the patient, while the bandaging reduces contamination and the chances of post-trauma infection.

Immobilization

The last objective of bandaging is immobilization. The stability of the wound site helps the natural clotting mechanisms operate and reduces the patient's discomfort. Maintaining gentle pressure with the bandage may reduce pain and local swelling. Immobilize the limb with bandaging material to the patient's body or to a rigid surface such as a padded board or ladder splint.

When immobilizing a limb, do not use elastic bandaging material or apply the bandage too tightly. The edema that develops rapidly with an injury puts increasing pressure on underlying tissue. This pressure may quickly reduce or halt circulation.

Frequently monitor any limb that you bandage circumferentially to ensure that the distal pulse remains strong and that the distal extremity maintains good color and does not swell. If you cannot locate the distal pulse, monitor capillary refill, skin color, and temperature. If signs or symptoms suggest that the distal circulation is compromised, elevate the extremity, if possible, and check and consider loosening the bandage.

Immobilization is an important but frequently overlooked component of hemorrhage control.

PAIN AND EDEMA CONTROL

Treat painful soft-tissue injuries or those likely to cause large debilitating edema with the application of cold packs and moderate-pressure bandages. Cold reduces inflammatory response and local edema. It also dulls the pain associated with serious soft-tissue trauma. Use a commercial cold pack or ice in a plastic bag wrapped in a dry towel and apply it to the wound. Do not use a cold pack directly against the skin since it may freeze the skin. Direct application of a cold pack may also cause tissue freezing, especially in areas with reduced circulation.

Some moderate pressure over the wound area may also help reduce pain and wound edema. In cases where the patient reports severe pain, consider use of morphine sulfate or other analgesics for patient comfort. Administer morphine in 2 mg increments titrated to pain relief every 5 minutes (up to a total of 10 mg).

ANATOMICAL CONSIDERATIONS FOR BANDAGING

Each area of the body has specific anatomical characteristics. Application of bandages and dressings should take these characteristics into account to provide effective prehospital wound care (Figure 18-29).

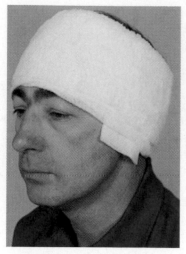

a. Head and/or ear bandage.

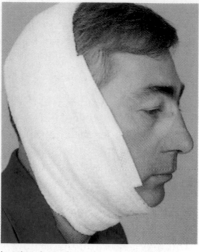

b. Cheek and ear bandage (be sure mouth will open).

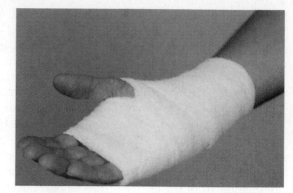

c. Hand bandage.

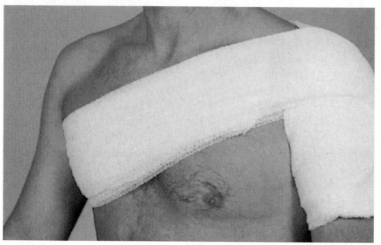

d. Shoulder bandage.

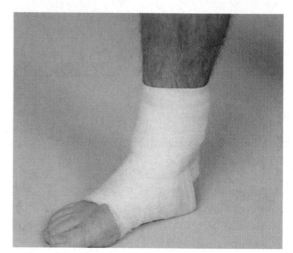

e. Foot and/or ankle bandage.

FIGURE 18-29   Good bandaging uses the natural body curves and the self-adherent characteristics of bandages to hold dressings firmly in place.

Scalp

The scalp has a rich supply of vessels that can bleed heavily when injured. It is commonly said that head wounds rarely account for shock, but scalp hemorrhage can be severe and difficult to control and can lead to the loss of moderate to large volumes of blood.

In scalp hemorrhage uncomplicated by skull fracture, direct pressure against the skull is effective in the control of bleeding. To hold a dressing in place and maintain pressure, wrap a bandage around the head, capturing the occiput or brow or, in some cases, passing the bandage under the chin (while still allowing for jaw movement).

If a head wound is complicated by fracture, be very careful in your application of pressure. Apply gentle digital pressure around the wound and attempt to locate the small scalp arteries that feed it to use as pressure points. Then simply hold a dressing on the wound without much pressure.

Face

Facial wounds are frequently gruesome and bleed heavily. Gentle direct pressure to these wounds can effectively control hemorrhage. You can maintain this pressure by wrapping a bandage around the head. Be careful to ensure a clear airway and use your bandaging to splint any facial instability.

Remember, blood is a gastric irritant and when swallowed may induce emesis. Be ready to provide suctioning in patients with oral or nasal hemorrhage because unexpected emesis may compromise the airway.

Ear or Mastoid

Wounds to the ear region can be easily bandaged by wrapping the head circumferentially. Use open gauze to collect, not stop, any bleeding or fluids flowing from the ear canal. These materials may contain cerebrospinal fluid and halting their flow may add to any increasing intracranial pressure.

Neck

Minor neck wounds may be lightly wrapped circumferentially with bandages or taped to hold dressings in place. If bleeding is moderate to severe, however, direct manual pressure may be necessary because the amount of pressure applied by circumferential wrapping may compromise both the airway and circulation to and from the head. In cases of large wounds or moderate to severe bleeding, also consider using an occlusive dressing to prevent aspiration of air into a jugular vein.

Shoulder

The shoulder is an easy area to bandage because soft, self-adherent roller bandages readily conform to body contours. Use the axilla, arm, and neck as points of fixation, but be careful not to put pressure on the anterior neck and trachea.

Trunk

For minor trunk wounds, adhesive tape may be sufficient to hold dressings in place. With larger wounds, bandaging can be more difficult because you must wrap the patient's body circumferentially to apply direct pressure to a wound. Applying a bandage in this way may require moving the patient unnecessarily and risk causing or worsening an injury. Consider instead using a ladder splint that is negotiated beneath the patient's torso, folded to the curve of the back, and then folded outward sharply at each end to serve as a bandaging fixation point. Then wrap the bandage between the ends of the ladder splint to hold the dressing in place.

Groin and Hip

The groin and the hip are easy places to affix a dressing. Bandage by following the contours of the upper thighs and waist, similar to the technique of bandaging a shoulder. Be careful here, though. Any movement of the patient is likely to affect the tightness of the bandage and the amount of pressure over the dressing. With these injuries, therefore, bandage after the patient is in final position for transport.

Elbow and Knee

Joints, especially the elbow and knee, are difficult to bandage. Bandage using circumferential wraps and then splint the area to ensure that the bandage does not loosen with movement. If possible, place the joint in a position halfway between flexion and extension. This position, called the position of function, relaxes the muscles controlling the joint and the skin tension lines, and is most comfortable for the patient during long transports or periods of immobilization.

Hand and Finger

Hand and finger injuries are easy to bandage by simple circumferential wrapping. Again, consider placing the hand or digit in the position of function, halfway between flexion and extension. Accomplish this by placing a large, bulky dressing in the palm of the patient's hand and then wrapping around it. You may use a malleable finger splint to obtain the position of function and then wrap circumferentially to splint the finger.

Ankle and Foot

Ankle and foot wounds are also easy to bandage by wrapping circumferentially and by using the natural body contours. If strong direct pressure is needed to maintain hemorrhage control, start wrapping from the toes and work proximally. This ensures that the pressure of bandaging does not form a venous tourniquet and compromise circulation to this very distal injury.

COMPLICATIONS OF BANDAGING

Bandaging can lead to some complications, although such occurrences are infrequent. If a bandage—particularly a circumferential bandage—is too tight, the area beneath it may continue to swell, increasing pressure in the area of the wound. This can lead to decreased blood flow and ischemia distal to the bandage. Pressure can build to such an extreme that the bandage acts like a tourniquet. Pain, pallor, tingling, a loss of pulses, and prolonged capillary refill time are typical signs of developing pressure and ischemia. Avoid this complication by making bandages snug but not too tight. A useful technique is to wrap a bandage only so tight that one finger can still be easily slipped beneath it.

Bandages and dressings left on too long can become soaked with blood and body fluids and then serve as incubators for infection. This problem usually takes at least 2 to 3 days to develop and is not a common concern in most prehospital settings.

The size of the dressing is an important consideration in bandaging. An unnecessarily large and bulky dressing can prevent proper inspection of a wound and hide contamination and continued serious bleeding. Too small a dressing can become lost in a wound and become, in effect, a foreign body. This is most frequently a problem with large, gaping wounds and deep wounds that penetrate the thoracic or abdominal body cavities. When dressing a wound, choose a dressing just larger than the wound yet not so small as to become lost in it.

CARE OF SPECIFIC WOUNDS

Some circumstances—amputations, impaled objects, and crush syndrome cases—deserve special attention during the patient management process. These injuries can challenge even the seasoned EMT-I to provide the most appropriate care.

Amputations

Amputations may bleed either heavily or minimally. Attempt to control hemorrhage with direct pressure by applying a large, bulky dressing to the wound. If this fails to control hemorrhage, consider using a tourniquet just above the point of severance. If a crushing wound is associated with the limb loss, apply the tourniquet just above the crushed area. Do not delay patient transport while locating or extricating the amputated body part. Transport the patient immediately, and then have other personnel transport the part once it is located or released from entrapment.

Current recommendations for managing separated body parts include dry cooling and rapid transport. Place the amputated part in a plastic bag and immerse the bag in cold water (Figure 18-30). The water may have a few ice cubes in it, but avoid direct contact between the ice and the injured part. Even if the amputated part cannot be totally reattached, skin from it may be used to cover the limb end (Figure 18-31).

Impaled Objects

When possible, immobilize all impaled objects in place (Figure 18-32). Position bulky dressings around the object to stabilize it, and tape over the dressings to hold them in place. Try to make movement of the patient to the ambulance and transport to the emergency department as smooth and nonjarring as possible. Remember that any movement of the impaled object is likely to cause continued internal bleeding and additional tissue damage.

If the impaled object is too large to transport or is affixed to something that cannot be moved, such as a reinforcing rod set in concrete, consider cutting it. Use appropriate techniques and tools depending on the circumstances of the impalement. A hand or power saw, an acetylene torch, or bolt cutters might be employed. Whatever tools and techniques are used, be sure to take steps to limit the heat, vibration, or jolting transmitted to the patient. Provide the best possible support for both the object and the patient during the cutting procedure.

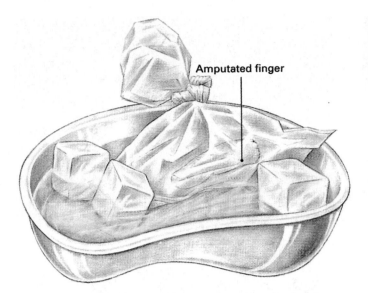

FIGURE 18–30 Amputated parts should be put in a dry bag, sealed, and placed in cool water that contains a few ice cubes.

Amputated finger

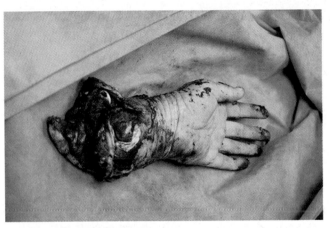

a. An amputated hand.

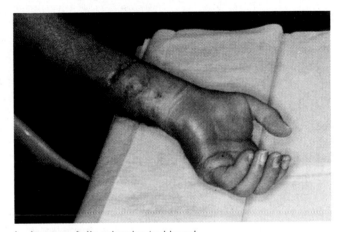

b. A successfully reimplanted hand.

FIGURE 18–31 Amputated parts should be located and transported with the patient to the hospital for possible reimplantation.

Some special circumstances occur in which you should remove an impaled object. For example, you may remove an object impaled in the cheek if the removal is necessary to maintain a patent airway (Figure 18-33). In this case, be prepared to apply direct pressure to the wound both from inside the cheek (intraorally) and externally.

Another object that would require removal is one impaled in the central chest of a patient who needs CPR. In such a circumstance, the risk associated with not performing resuscitation outweighs the risk of removing the object. Be aware, however, that a trauma patient who needs CPR has a very poor prognosis.

Another complication associated with an impaled object occurs when a patient is impaled on an object that cannot be cut or moved. In such a case, contact medical direction for advice and guidance. If the object is impaled in a limb, bleeding may be controllable. If it has entered the head, neck, chest, or abdomen, it may not be.

Only remove impaled objects that obstruct the airway or prevent CPR.

Crush Syndrome

The key to successful prehospital management of a crush syndrome patient is anticipation of the problem and prevention of its effects. Since, by definition, all crush syndrome patients are victims of prolonged entrapment, cases can be identified before extrication is complete.

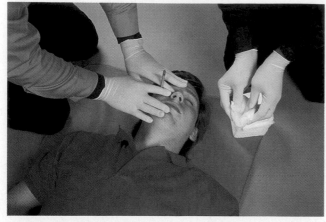

a. Manually stabilize any impaled object.

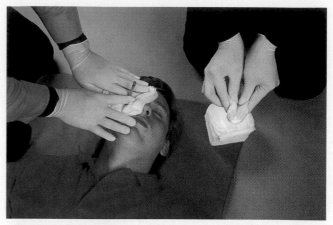

b. Use bulky padding or dressing to immobilize the object.

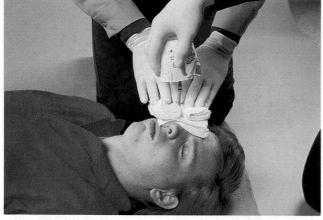

c. If the object protrudes, cover it with a paper cup.

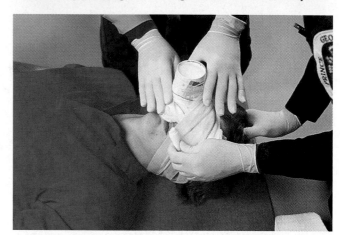

d. Bandage the cup and padding securely in place.

FIGURE 18-32   Stabilization of an impaled object.

FIGURE 18-33   Objects impaled in the cheek may be removed because the sites of hemorrhage can be controlled.

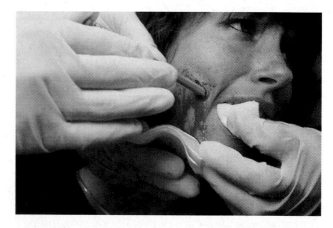

The focus of prehospital crush injury care is on rapid transport, adequate fluid resuscitation, diuresis, and, possibly, systemic alkalinization.

The prehospital approach to crush syndrome is similar to that of other trauma patients. Ensuring scene safety is particularly important in these cases. Crush syndrome victims are often buried in heavy rubble or other large debris, and access may be difficult (Figure 18-34). You may need to request the assistance of specialized personnel and their equipment—urban search and rescue teams, or trench, heavy, or confined space rescue teams. Never place yourself or other rescuers in unreasonable danger when providing care or attempting a rescue.

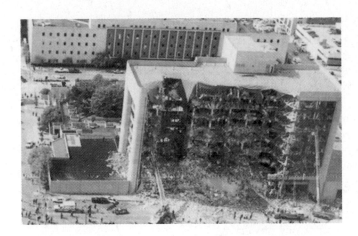

FIGURE 18-34 Explosion and structural collapse frequently produce crush injury and crush syndrome.

Once the scene is safe and you can reach the patient, conduct an initial assessment. Remove debris from around the head, neck, and thorax to minimize airway obstruction and restriction of ventilation. Control any reachable and obvious bleeding. Perform as much of the initial and rapid trauma assessment as possible, keeping in mind that portions of the patient's body will be inaccessible as a result of the entrapment. The dark, dusty, and cramped conditions of many confined space rescues may force you to improvise. Be alert for signs and symptoms of associated injuries such as dust inhalation, dehydration, and hypothermia.

Remember that the greater the body area compressed and the longer the time of entrapment, the greater the risk of crush syndrome. Initially, a trapped patient will usually complain only of entrapment symptoms: pain, lack of motor function, tingling, or loss of sensation in the affected limb. The patient may also experience flaccid paralysis and sensory loss in the limb unrelated to the normal distribution of peripheral nerve control and sensation.

As long as the body part is still trapped and the metabolic by-products of the crush injury are confined to the entrapped part, the patient will not experience the full effects of crush syndrome. With extrication, however, toxic by-products are released into the circulation, and the patient may rapidly develop shock and die. If the patient survives the initial release of the by-products, he remains at great risk of developing renal failure with serious morbidity or delayed death. Note, too, that a crush injury may also induce compartment syndrome (explained below), especially with prolonged entrapment.

Once you have ensured the patient's ABCs, turn your attention to obtaining IV access. IV fluids and selected medications are important in treating crush syndrome. Initiate two large-bore IVs if possible. Because of the entrapment, it may be necessary to consider alternative IV sites such as the external jugular vein or the veins of a lower extremity. Avoid any site distal to a crush injury.

When you encounter crush syndrome, it is unlikely that your protocols will address it. Contact the trauma center for medical direction and communicate, on-line, with the emergency physician. Expect to provide frequent vital sign and patient updates, and be prepared to administer large fluid volumes and, possibly, alkalizing agents.

Infuse 1,000 to 1,500 mL (20–30 mL/kg) of normal saline or, more ideally, 5% dextrose in ½ normal saline, even in a patient not yet showing signs of shock. Avoid lactated Ringer's or other solutions containing potassium. Then, infuse solution at a rate of 1,000 mL/hr (20 mL/kg/hr) for as long as the patient remains trapped (up to 12 liters in 24 hours). Continue this infusion rate until the patient reaches the hospital. As with all patients receiving large volumes of crystalloids, periodically query the patient for symptoms of shortness of breath and auscultate the lungs for evidence of pulmonary edema (e.g., crackles). Stop or reduce the fluid flow rate if you suspect pulmonary edema. In young, healthy adults and children, this rarely occurs at the fluid flow rates described here.

Alkalinization of the blood and urine is a consideration for preventing and treating crush syndrome. In combination with fluid resuscitation, alkalinization can correct acidosis, help prevent renal failure, and help correct hyperkalemia. Administer sodium bicarbonate 1 mEq/kg initially, followed by 0.25 mEq/kg/hr thereafter. It is preferable to add the bicarbonate to the normal saline bag rather than administering it as a bolus or IV push.

Note: The milliequivalent (mEq) is a unit of measurement for electrolytes in a standard solution and is based on the molecular weight of the electrolyte in question.

Diuretics may help keep the kidneys well perfused and more resistant to failure during crush syndrome. Mannitol, an osmotic diuretic, is the drug of choice since it draws interstitial fluid into the vascular space and eliminates it as mannitol is excreted by the kidneys. Furosemide, a loop diuretic, inhibits the reabsorption of both sodium and chloride. Its use is not advisable in hypovolemic states because it may add to the electrolyte imbalance.

Consider applying a tourniquet before the entrapping pressure is released if you have been unable to medicate the patient and provide fluid resuscitation. The tourniquet will sequester the toxins and prevent reperfusion injury. Tourniquet use, however, will continue the development of crush syndrome and worsen its effects.

In cases where the entrapping object may not be moved for many hours or days, medical direction may consider field amputation. This operation will likely be performed by a physician responding to the scene but, in dire circumstances, may be performed by an EMT-I under the on-line direction of the emergency physician.

Cardiac (ECG) monitoring is important with all crush syndrome patients. Dysrhythmias may develop at any time but are most likely to occur immediately following the release of pressure on extrication. Sudden cardiac arrest should be treated in the usual fashion with defibrillation and cardiac drugs as appropriate. Consider 500 mg calcium chloride IV push (in addition to the sodium bicarbonate) to counteract life-threatening dysrhythmias induced by hyperkalemia. Watch for the tenting, or peaking, of the T-wave, a prolonged P-R interval, and S-T segment depression. Be sure to flush the IV line between infusions or to use different lines because calcium chloride and sodium bicarbonate precipitate.

Once the patient is freed from entrapment, be prepared to treat rapidly progressing shock. Continue the normal saline infusions at 30 mL/kg/hr and provide additional boluses of sodium bicarbonate as needed. Rapidly transport the patient to an appropriate hospital (usually a trauma center) for all cases of suspected crush syndrome.

Prehospital care of the crushed limb or body parts requires no special techniques. Cover open wounds and splint fractures, keeping in mind that progressive swelling will necessitate ongoing reassessment, with monitoring of distal circulation and the tightness of bandages, straps, and splints. Handle all crushed limbs gently because the ischemic tissue is prone to injury. Elevation of severely crushed extremities is not indicated in the prehospital setting.

Care at the hospital for crush injury is aggressive and may use techniques such as debridement and hyperbaric oxygenation. During hyperbaric oxygenation, the patient is placed in a chamber with artificially high concentrations of oxygen under several atmospheres of pressure. This drives oxygen into poorly oxygenated tissue to help with the destruction of anaerobic bacteria and to increase tissue oxygenation for repair and regeneration, ultimately reducing tissue necrosis and edema. Hyperbaric oxygenation is most effective when provided early in the course of care.

Hospital care for crush injuries also includes administration of several medications as well as hemodialysis to help salvage the kidneys from the ravages of myoglobin and other toxic agents. Allopurinol, a xanthine oxidase inhibitor, interferes with the production of uric acid, a by-product of skeletal muscle destruction, and may help reperfusion of both the kidneys and the skeletal muscles. It is most effective if administered immediately before release of the compression. Amiloride hydrochloride is a potassium-sparing diuretic that inhibits the sodium/calcium exchange. Mannitol, tetanus toxoid, and prophylactic antibiotics may also be administered in the hospital to treat crush syndrome.

Compartment Syndrome

The most prominent symptom of compartment syndrome is severe pain, often out of proportion to the physical findings. Other signs are often subtle or absent, or they may be overshadowed by the original injury such as a fracture or contusion. Some people suggest using the six Ps—pain, paresthesia, paresis, pressure, passive stretching pain, pulselessness—to identify compartment syndrome, but many of these signs are not dependable or they appear very late in the course of the injury. (Passive stretching pain is pain or an increase in pain noted by a patient as a muscle is extended by a care provider.) Motor and sensory functions are usually normal with early compartment syndrome, as are distal pulses. Even capillary refill shows little change. It is important to note that compartment syndrome rarely occurs within the first 4 hours after an acute injury. It is more likely to appear 6 to 8 hours (or as much as a day or more) after the initial injury. Recognition of compartment syndrome can be challenging and requires a healthy suspicion for the problem.

The first step in prehospital treatment for compartment syndrome is care of the underlying injury. Splint and immobilize all suspected fractures, and use traction as appropriate for femur fractures. Apply cold packs to severe contusions. Elevation of the affected extremity is the single most effective prehospital treatment for compartment syndrome. This reduces edema, increases venous return, lowers compartment pressure, and helps prevent ischemia. In the hospital, compartment syndrome is treated surgically, through a procedure that incises the restrictive fascia, a fasciotomy.

Special Anatomical Sites

Several anatomical sites provide challenges to care of soft-tissue injuries. These include the face and neck, the thorax, and the abdomen.

Face and Neck   Soft-tissue injuries to the face and neck present potential challenges owing to the anatomical relationships of the airway and great vessels. Injuries to the face may result in blood and tissue debris in the airway, posing risks of airway obstruction, asphyxia, and aspiration (Figure 18-35). Pooled secretions and tissue edema may add to airway problems. Trauma to the face or neck may also distort the anatomical structures of the upper airway, leading to airway compromise, and complicating attempts at endotracheal intubation.

Emergency treatment of face and neck injuries can be challenging and may tax your skills. First, gain control of the airway. Open the airway using manual maneuvers. If you suspect the possibility of spinal injury, use the jaw-thrust maneuver in conjunction with in-line manual stabilization. Aggressively suction blood, saliva, and debris from the pharynx, but avoid stimulating the gag reflex in the patient or inducing emesis. Insert an oropharyngeal or nasopharyngeal airway as needed.

Visualized endotracheal intubation is the gold standard for securing the airway, but achieving it is fraught with complications in cases of face and neck trauma. Secretions and blood may prevent adequate visualization even with aggressive suctioning. Airway edema can distort the anatomy beyond recognition, and even prevent passage of the ET tube. In all cases, meticulous and absolute confirmation of tube placement is mandatory to avoid fatal hypoxia.

Once you have secured the airway, focus your attention on any serious facial or neck bleeding. Direct pressure is usually successful for bleeding control, but be certain to avoid compressing or occluding the airway. Pressure points and tourniquets should not be used because of the risks they present of cerebral ischemia and strangulation. Open neck wounds also carry the danger of air aspiration and emboli. Cover any open neck wound with an occlusive dressing, which should then be held or bandaged firmly in place. Because of the neck's anatomy, you may have to maintain digital pressure throughout the course of prehospital care to ensure effective bleeding control.

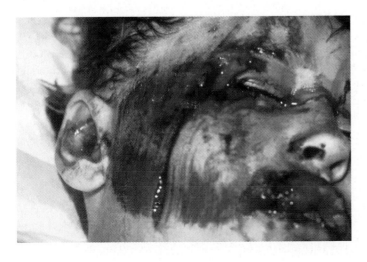

FIGURE 18-35   Severe facial soft-tissue injuries may interfere with airway control and distort landmarks used for intubation.

Thorax Superficial soft-tissue injury to the thorax may suggest more serious intrathoracic injuries. The pleural space extends superiorly to the supraclavicular fossa and inferiorly to include the entire rib cage both anteriorly and posteriorly. Trauma to this area is likely to injure both the pleura and lungs. Small lacerations may actually be deep, penetrating stab or gunshot wounds with resultant hemothorax, pneumothorax, pericardial tamponade, penetrating heart trauma, or injury to the great vessels, esophagus, bronchi, or diaphragm. A seemingly minor rib bruise may be the only visible sign of serious lung or cardiac contusions beneath.

Perform a thorough physical examination to detect any signs of internal bleeding, pulmonary edema, dysrhythmias, or shock. However, never explore a thoracic wound beyond the skin edges. Probing deeper can convert a minor wound to a pneumothorax or a bleeding disaster. Consider all thoracic wounds to be potentially life threatening until evidence proves otherwise. (See Chapter 17, "Thoracic Trauma," for detailed care procedures.)

Never explore a thoracic open wound beyond its edges. Pushing may create a pneumothorax or induce serious bleeding.

Dress all open thoracic wounds with sterile dressings in the usual fashion. Be alert, however, for the presence of air bubbling, subcutaneous emphysema, crepitus, or other hints of open pneumothorax. Be extremely cautious about making an airtight seal on any thoracic wound because doing so can rapidly lead to tension pneumothorax and death. Instead, use an occlusive dressing sealed on three sides and be prepared to assist ventilations. Auscultate the chest and monitor respirations frequently. Watch the occlusive dressing so that it does not seal with blood against the chest wall and convert a simple pneumothorax into a tension pneumothorax.

Watch any open chest wound for development of a pneumothorax or tension pneumothorax.

Abdomen The peritoneal cavity extends approximately from the symphysis pubis inferiorly to the diaphragm superiorly. Since the diaphragm rises and falls with respiration, so too does the border between the abdominal and thoracic cavities. You cannot know the exact position of the diaphragm at the time the injury occurred, so suspect associated injuries to both abdominal and thoracic organs if the soft-tissue injury involves the region between the rib margin and the fifth rib anteriorly, the seventh rib laterally, and the ninth rib posteriorly.

Blunt or penetrating trauma to the abdomen can injure both hollow and solid organs, penetrate or rupture the diaphragm, and cause serious internal bleeding. Anteriorly and just underlying the rib margin are the liver on the right and the spleen on the left. Posteriorly, the kidneys (not true abdominal organs since they lie retroperitoneally) are located in the costovertebral angle region. Hollow organs—the bowel, stomach and urinary bladder—may rupture. In addition to bleeding copiously, these organs may release their contents and inflame the peritoneum.

Consider any soft-tissue wound in the abdominal region as potentially damaging to the underlying organs. Signs and symptoms of internal damage can be subtle, particularly early on. Eviscerations and other massive injuries are obvious, but other internal injuries that are just as serious may not be apparent. Prehospital treatment is primarily supportive and includes ensuring adequate oxygenation, preventing shock, and dressing open wounds.

Wounds Requiring Transport

Transport any patient with a wound that involves a structure beneath the integument for emergency department evaluation. This includes wounds involving, or possibly involving, nerves, blood vessels, ligaments, tendons, or muscles. Also transport any patient with a significantly contaminated wound, a wound involving an impaled object, or a wound that was received in a particularly unclean environment. Also transport any patient who has a wound with likely cosmetic implications, such as facial wounds or large gaping wounds.

SUMMARY

Mastering the skills of trauma assessment and the management of specific types of trauma is critical for the EMT-I. In your basic EMT training, you learned how to assess and care for injuries to the head, face, and neck; spinal injuries, abdominal injuries, musculoskeletal injuries, and soft-tissue injuries. This chapter has reviewed the assessment and management of these types of injuries and has included information that goes beyond the basic level that you will find useful as you prepare to become an EMT-I.

ON THE WEB

For additional practice and review, go to the companion website at www.prenhall.com/bledsoe and click on *Intermediate Emergency Care: Principles & Practice*.

CHAPTER 19

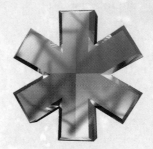

Respiratory Emergencies

Objectives

After reading this chapter, you should be able to:

1. Identify and describe the function of the structures located in the upper and lower airway. (see Chapter 2)
2. Discuss the physiology of ventilation and respiration. (pp. 802–804; and see Chapter 2)
3. Identify common pathological events that affect the pulmonary system. (pp. 804–807)
4. Discuss abnormal assessment findings and compare various airway and ventilation techniques used in the management of pulmonary diseases. (pp. 816–835)
5. Review the use of equipment utilized during the physical examination of patients with complaints associated with respiratory diseases and conditions. (pp. 812–814)
6. Identify the epidemiology, anatomy, physiology, pathophysiology, assessment findings,

   and management (including prehospital medications) for the following respiratory diseases and conditions:
   a. Bronchial asthma (pp. 819–820, 823–825)
   b. Chronic bronchitis (pp. 822–823)
   c. Emphysema (pp. 819–822)
   d. Pneumonia (pp. 827–829)
   e. Pulmonary edema (pp. 817–819)
   f. Pulmonary thromboembolism (pp. 830–832)
   g. Spontaneous pneumothorax (p. 832)
   h. Hyperventilation syndrome (p. 833)
7. Given several preprogrammed patients with non-traumatic pulmonary problems, provide the appropriate assessment, prehospital care, and transport. (pp. 802–835)

CASE STUDY

EMT-Is Tony Alvarez and Lee Smith are just finishing their barbecue lunch when they are toned out for a "medical emergency." They quickly go to the ambulance for the rest of the dispatch information. The emergency communications center dispatches them to 423 Black Champ Road where a male patient is reportedly having difficulty breathing. The dispatcher also informs the crew the First Responders from the Maypearl Fire Department are already en route. The EMT-Is are familiar with this area. It is a rural part of the county with mainly

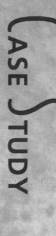

cotton farms. The response time is approximately 12 minutes. Upon arrival at the farmhouse, the EMT-Is are met by Alice Swenson, a First Responder from the Maypearl Volunteer Fire Department. Alice reports they have a 55-year-old white male who is having difficulty breathing. She further states that oxygen is already being administered.

The EMT-Is grab the drug box, monitor/defibrillator, airway kit, and stretcher. Then they enter the small farmhouse. A quick scene size-up reveals no immediate dangers. Tony and Lee find the patient seated at the kitchen table, obviously short of breath. They quickly perform an initial assessment. The airway is clear, the patient is moving little air, and has a strong pulse. Tony replaces the nasal cannula placed by the First Responders with a nonrebreather mask. Lee and Tony then complete a focused history and physical exam. The patient has diminished breath sounds, occasional rhonchi, and is using the accessory muscles of respiration. There is a hint of cyanosis around the mouth.

The team learns that, several years ago, doctors at the Veterans Administration (VA) Hospital diagnosed the patient as having emphysema. Over the last 24 hours, he has had progressive dyspnea and did not sleep at all the previous night. His wife reports that he paced the floor and repeatedly opened and closed windows. Vital signs reveal a blood pressure of 140/78 mmHg, a pulse of 96 beats per minute, and a respiratory rate of 28 breaths per minute. The monitor shows a sinus rhythm. Pulse oximetry reveals an oxygen saturation of 90% while receiving supplemental oxygen. The patient is mentally alert but slightly anxious. His current medications include an albuterol (Ventolin) metered-dose inhaler, theophylline (Slow-Bid), and amoxicillin (Amoxil). He still smokes a pack and a half of cigarettes per day and has done so for 40 years accumulating a 60 pack/year history.

The patient wants to be transported to the VA Hospital. Lee contacts medical direction and provides a brief patient report. Medical direction approves transport to the VA Hospital, since it is only 5 miles farther than the nearest hospital. The transport time will be approximately 40 minutes. Medical direction orders the placement of an IV infusion of 0.9% sodium chloride (normal saline) at a "to keep open" rate. In addition, they order a nebulizer treatment with 0.5 mL of albuterol (Ventolin) placed in 3 mL of normal saline.

Halfway through the nebulizer treatment, the patient shows marked improvement. His respiratory rate slows to 20 breaths per minute, and his oxygen saturation reading increases to 94%. Transport to the VA hospital is uneventful. He remains at the VA Hospital for two days and is discharged.

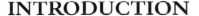

INTRODUCTION

According to one U.S. study, respiratory complaints accounted for more than 28% of all EMS calls. Over 200,000 people die each year as a result of respiratory emergencies. Several factors increase the risk of developing respiratory disease. Intrinsic risk factors are those within or influenced by the patient. The most important of these is genetic predisposition. For example, bronchial asthma, **chronic obstructive pulmonary disease (COPD)**, and lung cancer are more common in those who have family members with these diseases.

Certain respiratory conditions are increased in patients with underlying cardiac or circulatory problems. Cardiac conditions that result in ineffective pumping of blood tend to cause pulmonary edema. Cardiac and circulatory diseases may allow blood to pool in the large veins of the pelvis and lower extremities, causing pulmonary emboli. Stress may increase the severity of any respiratory complaint and can precipitate acute episodes of asthma or COPD.

Extrinsic risk factors are those that are external to the patient. The most important of these is cigarette smoking. There is a strong link between cigarette smoking and the development of pulmonary diseases such as lung carcinoma and COPD. Also, diseases such as pneumonia and pulmonary emboli are more likely in patients who smoke. Finally, cigarette smoking has been implicated as a risk factor in the development of cardiac disease. In any case, underlying lung damage caused by cigarette smoking worsens virtually all lung disorders.

The most important intrinsic factor in the development of respiratory disorders is genetic predisposition. The most important extrinsic factor is smoking.

chronic obstructive pulmonary disease (COPD) a disease characterized by a decreased ability of the lungs to perform the function of ventilation.

Another key extrinsic risk factor is environmental pollutants. The prevalence of COPD is markedly increased in areas with high environmental pollutants, as are the number and severity of acute attacks of asthma and COPD.

This chapter explores the pathophysiology of respiratory disease and how to integrate this knowledge with your assessment findings to develop a field impression and manage the patient with respiratory problems.

PHYSIOLOGICAL PROCESSES

The major function of the respiratory system is to exchange gases with the environment. Oxygen is taken in while carbon dioxide is eliminated, a process known as gas exchange.

Oxygen is vital to our bodies, allowing us to generate the energy that drives our many body functions. Oxygen from the atmosphere diffuses into the bloodstream through the lungs. Oxygen is then available for use in cellular metabolism by the body's 100 trillion cells. Waste products, including carbon dioxide, produced by cellular metabolism, must be eliminated from the body. In the lungs, carbon dioxide is exchanged for oxygen and the carbon dioxide is excreted from the lungs.

The three important processes that allow gas exchange to occur are ventilation, diffusion, and perfusion.

Content Review

PROCESSES OF GAS EXCHANGE
- Ventilation
- Diffusion
- Perfusion

VENTILATION

ventilation the mechanical process of moving air in and out of the lungs.

Ventilation is the mechanical process of moving air in and out of the lungs. In order for ventilation to occur, several body structures must be intact, including the chest wall, the nerve pathways, the diaphragm, the pleural cavity, and the brainstem.

Ventilation is divided into two phases, inspiration and expiration. During inspiration, air is drawn into the lungs. During expiration, air leaves the lungs. These phases of ventilation depend on changes in the volume of the thoracic cavity, as discussed in Chapter 2.

DIFFUSION

diffusion the movement of molecules through a membrane from an area of greater concentration to an area of lesser concentration.

Diffusion is the process by which gases move between the alveoli and the pulmonary capillaries. Remember that gases tend to flow from areas in which there is a high concentration of gas into an area of low concentration. The normal concentration of oxygen in the alveoli is 104 mmHg as opposed to a concentration of 40 mmHg in the pulmonary arterial circulation. Therefore, oxygen will move from the oxygen-rich alveoli into the oxygen-poor capillaries in response to the gradient that exists in the concentration of gases. As the red blood cells move through the pulmonary capillaries, they become enriched with oxygen. Less oxygen will pass into the blood stream as the gradient between alveolar and capillary oxygen concentration decreases.

Similarly, carbon dioxide passes out of the blood in response to a gradient that exists between the concentration of carbon dioxide in the blood in the pulmonary capillaries (45 mmHg) and in the alveoli (40 mmHg). By the time blood leaves the pulmonary capillaries, it has a dissolved concentration of oxygen of 104 mmHg and a carbon dioxide concentration of 40 mmHg.

The respiratory membrane, which normally measures 0.5 to 1.0 micrometer in thickness, must remain intact for gas exchange to occur. Any disorder that damages the alveoli or allows them to collapse will impede oxygen from entering the body and will reduce carbon dioxide elimination. Changes in the respiratory membrane or any increase in the interstitial space will also impede the process of diffusion. For example, fluid accumulation in the interstitial space as the result of pulmonary edema or pneumonia will prevent proper diffusion of gases. Finally the endothelial lining of the capillaries must be intact for exchange of oxygen and carbon dioxide to occur. Diseases that produce thickening of the endothelial lining will also interfere with the process of diffusion.

Certain measures can be taken to address problems with lung diffusion. Providing the patient with high concentrations of oxygen is one simple step that can be used. Remember

Provide oxygen to a patient with a lung diffusion problem to increase the concentration gradient that drives oxygen into the capillaries. When fluid accumulation or inflammation is present, consider administering diuretics or anti-inflammatory drugs.

that the concentration gradient provides the driving force in moving oxygen into the capillaries. Therefore, the larger the difference between the concentration of oxygen in the alveoli and the capillaries, the greater the diffusion of oxygen into the blood stream. Similarly, when fluid accumulation or inflammation is the underlying cause of the thickening of the interstitial space within the alveoli, medications such as diuretic agents or anti-inflammatory drugs (corticosteroids, antibiotics) are given to reduce fluid and inflammation.

PERFUSION

One additional process that occurs in the lungs is **perfusion**. Lung perfusion is the circulation of blood through the lungs or, more specifically, the pulmonary capillaries. Lung perfusion depends on three conditions:

- Adequate blood volume
- Intact pulmonary capillaries
- Efficient pumping of blood by the heart

For perfusion to proceed effectively, there must be an adequate volume of blood in the blood stream. Equally important is the concentration of **hemoglobin,** which is the transport protein that carries oxygen in the blood. Remember that oxygen is transported in the blood stream in one of two ways: bound to hemoglobin or dissolved in the plasma. Under normal conditions, less than 2% of all oxygen is transported dissolved in plasma (this is what is measured by the PO_2), whereas more than 98% is carried by hemoglobin.

Hemoglobin has some unique properties. It is made up four iron-containing heme molecules and a protein-containing globin portion. Oxygen molecules bind to the heme portion of the hemoglobin molecule. As oxygen binds to hemoglobin, its structure changes so that it more readily binds additional oxygen molecules. Similarly, as fully oxygen-bound hemoglobin begins to release oxygen, it more readily sheds additional oxygen. The relationship is described by the oxygen dissociation curve (Figure 19-1). You can see that with between 10 and 50 mmHg, there is a marked increase in the saturation of hemoglobin. However, as the PO_2 increases above 70 mmHg, there is only a small change in the saturation of hemoglobin which is already near 100%.

Changes in the body temperature, the blood pH, and the PCO_2 can all alter the oxygen dissociation curve. Within the tissues, as hemoglobin becomes bound with carbon dioxide, it loses its affinity for oxygen. As a result, more oxygen is released and is thus available to cells for metabolism (called the Bohr effect).

Carbon dioxide is transported from the cells to the lungs in one of three ways:

- As bicarbonate ion
- Bound to the globin portion of the hemoglobin molecule
- Dissolved in plasma (measured as PCO_2)

perfusion the circulation of blood through the capillaries.

hemoglobin the transport protein that carries oxygen in the blood.

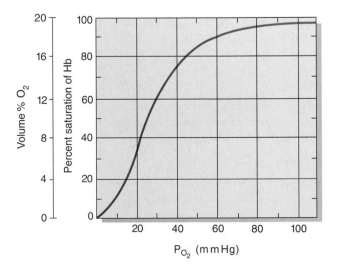

FIGURE 19-1 Oxygen dissociation curve.

The greatest portion of CO_2 produced during metabolism in cells is converted into bicarbonate ion. As the CO_2 is released into the capillaries, it enters the red blood cell where an enzyme (carbonic anhydrase) combines carbon dioxide with water to form two ions, hydrogen (H^+) and bicarbonate (HCO_3). Bicarbonate is then released from the red blood cell and transported in plasma. In the lungs, the reverse process takes place, producing water and carbon dioxide. The carbon dioxide then diffuses into the alveoli where it is eliminated during exhalation.

The carbon dioxide that is bound to hemoglobin is released in the lung because of the lower concentration of this gas in the alveoli. Additionally, as the heme portion of the hemoglobin molecule becomes saturated with oxygen, more carbon dioxide is released (called the Haldane effect). Finally, the approximately 10% of carbon dioxide that is dissolved in the plasma flows into the alveoli due to the gradient that exists between the concentration of gases (PCO_2 of 45 mmHg in pulmonary artery versus 40 mmHg in the alveoli).

For perfusion to take place, in addition to having adequate blood volume, the pulmonary capillaries must be able to transport blood through all portions of the lung tissue. These vessels must be open and not occluded, or blocked. For example, a pulmonary embolism will occlude the pulmonary artery in which it lodges, making that artery unavailable for perfusion of the portion of the lung it usually supplies with blood. Finally, the heart must pump efficiently to push blood effectively through the pulmonary capillaries to perfuse the lung tissues.

To maintain perfusion, you must ensure that the patient has an adequate circulating blood volume. In addition, take all the necessary steps to improve the pumping action of the heart. For example, in patients with acute pulmonary edema the use of diuretic agents reduces the blood return (preload) to an ineffectively pumping heart and improves cardiac efficiency.

The entire system just discussed provides for **respiration**, which is the exchange of gases between a living organism and its environment. Pulmonary respiration occurs in the lungs when the respiratory gases are exchanged between the alveoli and the red blood cells in the pulmonary capillaries through the respiratory membranes. Cellular respiration, on the other hand, occurs in the peripheral capillaries. It involves the exchange of the respiratory gases between the red blood cells and the various tissues. Many of the principles of gas exchange that occur in the lungs are reversed in the tissues, with oxygen being released to the cells and carbon dioxide accumulating in the plasma and red blood cells.

> *To maintain perfusion, make sure the patient has an adequate circulating blood volume. Also, take all necessary steps to improve the pumping action of the heart.*
>
>

respiration the exchange of gases between a living organism and its environment.

PATHOPHYSIOLOGY

Remember that many disease states affect the pulmonary system and interfere with its ability to acquire the oxygen required for normal cellular metabolism. Additionally, respiratory diseases limit the body's ability to eliminate waste products such as carbon dioxide. Your understanding of normal anatomy and physiology—ventilation, diffusion, and perfusion—will aid in understanding the mechanism of each disease process and will direct you toward the appropriate corrective actions. Ultimately, any disease process that impairs the pulmonary system will result in a derangement in ventilation, diffusion, perfusion, or a combination of these processes.

> *Your understanding of the normal processes of ventilation, diffusion, and perfusion will aid in understanding specific disease processes and direct you toward appropriate corrective actions.*
>
>

DISRUPTION IN VENTILATION

Diseases that affect ventilation will result in obstruction of the normal conducting pathways of the upper or lower respiratory tract, impairment of the normal function of the chest wall, or abnormalities involving the nervous system's control of ventilation.

Upper and Lower Respiratory Tracts

Disease states that affect the upper respiratory tract will result in obstruction of air flow to the lower structures. Upper airway trauma, for example, produces both significant hemorrhage and swelling. Infections of the upper airway structures, including epiglottitis, soft tissue infections of the neck, tonsillitis, and abscess formation within the pharynx (peritonsillar abscess and retropharyngeal abscess), can all obstruct air flow. Similarly, lower airway obstruction may be produced by trauma, foreign body aspiration, mucus accumulation (as in asthmatics), smooth muscle constriction (in asthma and COPD), and airway edema produced by infection or burns.

Chest Wall and Diaphragm

As you read earlier, the chest wall and diaphragm are mechanical components that are essential for normal ventilation. Traumatic injuries to these areas will disrupt the normal mechanics causing loss of negative pressure within the pleural space. This occurs in patients with **hemothorax** or **pneumothorax,** including open pneumothorax and tension pneumothorax. Infectious processes such as empyema (pus accumulation in the pleural space) or inflammatory conditions produce similar effects. Chest wall injuries including rib fractures or **flail chest** and diaphragmatic rupture limit the patient's ability to expand the thoracic cavity. Certain neuromuscular diseases, such as muscular dystrophy, multiple sclerosis, or amyotrophic lateral sclerosis (ALS or Lou Gehrig's Disease), impair muscular function so as to limit the ability to generate a negative pressure within the chest cavity.

hemothorax a collection of blood in the pleural space.

pneumothorax a collection of air in the pleural space, causing a loss of the negative pressure that binds the lung to the chest wall. In an *open pneumothorax,* air enters the pleural space through an injury to the chest wall. In a *closed pneumothorax,* air enters the pleural space through an opening in the pleura that covers the lung. A *tension pneumothorax* develops when air in the pleural space cannot escape, causing a build-up of pressure and collapse of the lung.

Nervous System

Finally, any disease process that impairs the nervous system's regulation of breathing may also alter ventilation. Central nervous system depressants such as alcohol, benzodiazepines, or barbiturates, alone or in combination, can alter the brain's response to important signals such as rising PCO_2. Similarly, stroke, diseases, or injuries that involve the respiratory centers within the central nervous system can change the normal ventilatory pattern. In fact, certain abnormal respiratory patterns are produced by specific brain injury (Figure 19-2):

flail chest one or more ribs fractured in two or more places, creating an unattached rib segment.

apnea absence of breathing.

- *Cheyne-Stokes respirations* describe a ventilatory pattern with progressively increasing tidal volume, followed by a declining volume, separated by periods of **apnea** at the end of expiration. This pattern is typically seen in older patients with terminal illness or brain injury.

- *Kussmaul's respirations* are deep, rapid breaths that result as a corrective measure against conditions such as diabetic ketoacidosis that produce metabolic acidosis.

- *Central neurogenic hyperventilation* also produces deep, rapid respirations that are caused by strokes or injury to the brainstem. In this case, loss of normal regulation of ventilatory controls and respiratory alkalosis is often seen.

- *Ataxic (Biot's) respirations* are characterized by repeated episodes of gasping ventilations separated by periods of apnea. This pattern is seen in patients with increased intracranial pressure.

- *Apneustic respiration* is characterized by long, deep breaths that are stopped during the inspiratory phase and separated by periods of apnea. This pattern is a result of stroke or severe central nervous system disease.

Also remember that damage to the major peripheral nerves that supply the diaphragm and intercostal muscles, the phrenic nerve, and intercostal nerves will also affect normal ventilatory mechanics. Traumatic disruption of the phrenic nerve during chest surgery, with penetrating trauma, or by neoplastic (cancerous, tumorous) invasion of the nerve can paralyze the diaphragm on the side of involvement.

DISRUPTION IN DIFFUSION

Other disease states can disrupt the diffusion of gases. Any change in the concentration of oxygen in the alveoli, such as occurs when a person ascends to high altitudes, can limit the diffusion of oxygen and produce **hypoxia.** Similarly, any disease that alters the structure or patency of the alveoli will limit diffusion. Destruction of alveoli by certain environmental pathogens such as asbestos or coal (black lung disease), in patients with COPD, or with inhalation injury reduces the capacity of the lungs to diffuse gases.

Finally, disease states that alter the thickness of the respiratory membrane will limit the diffusion of gases. The most common cause of this alteration is accumulation of fluid and inflammatory cells in the interstitial space. Fluid can accumulate in the interstitial space if

hypoxia state in which insufficient oxygen is available to meet the oxygen requirements of the cells.

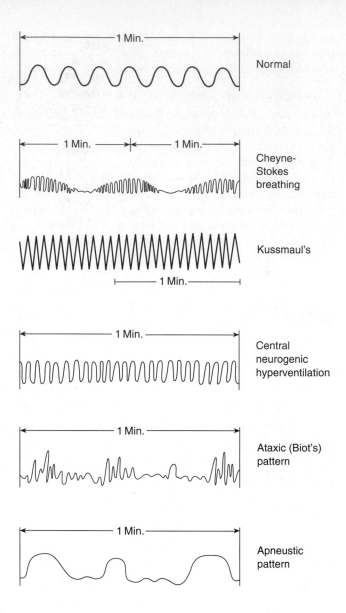

FIGURE 19-2 Abnormal respiratory patterns.

high pressure within the pulmonary capillaries forces fluid out of the circulatory system. This is seen in patients with left-sided heart failure (cardiogenic causes) and is due to increased venous pressure as a result of poor functioning of the left ventricle. Patients with pulmonary hypertension have high resting pressures in the pulmonary circulation, which ultimately leads to fluid accumulation in the interstitial space, causing right heart failure.

Similar effects can be produced by changes in the permeability (or leakiness) of the pulmonary capillaries (non-cardiogenic causes). Permeability can be affected by adult respiratory distress syndrome, asbestosis and other environmental pathogens, near-drowning, prolonged hypoxia, and inhalation injury. Also remember that disease states that alter the pulmonary capillary endothelial lining, such as advanced atherosclerosis or vascular inflammatory states, can affect diffusion.

DISRUPTION IN PERFUSION

As detailed earlier, any alteration in appropriate blood flow through the pulmonary capillaries will limit normal gas exchange in the lungs. Any disease state that reduces the normal circulating blood volume, such as trauma, hemorrhage, dehydration, shock or other causes of hypovolemia, will limit normal perfusion of the lungs. Remember that hemoglobin is the major transport protein for oxygen and plays a significant role in the elimination of carbon dioxide. Therefore, any reduction in the normal circulating hemoglobin will also affect perfusion. All causes of anemia, a condition in which the number of red blood cells or amount of hemoglobin in them is below normal, must be considered. Such causes include acute blood loss, iron or vitamin deficiency, malnutrition, and anemia from chronic disease states.

Remember that blood must be available to all of the lung segments for maximum gas exchange to occur. When an area of lung tissue is appropriately ventilated but no capillary perfusion occurs, available oxygen is not moved into the circulatory system. This is referred to as a *pulmonary shunting*. In patients with pulmonary embolism, a blockage of a division of the pulmonary artery by a clot prevents perfusion of the lung segments supplied by that branch of the artery. As a result, there may be significant shunt with return of unoxygenated blood to the pulmonary venous circulation.

ASSESSMENT OF THE RESPIRATORY SYSTEM

Assessment of the respiratory system is a vital aspect of prehospital care. You must quickly assess the airway and ventilation status during the initial assessment. If the patient's complaints suggest that the respiratory system is involved in the patient's problem, the focused history and physical examination should be directed to this aspect of the assessment.

> *If the patient's complaints suggest respiratory system involvement, direct the focused history and physical exam to this aspect.*

SCENE SIZE-UP

When you approach the scene, you should consider two major questions: (1) Is the scene safe to approach the patient? and (2) Are there visual clues that might provide information regarding the patient's medical complaint?

> *When you approach the scene, consider: (1) Is the scene safe? and (2) Are there visual cues to the patient's medical complaint?*

Remember that several hazards may result in respiratory complaints by the patient that are also potentially dangerous for emergency care providers. Certain gases and toxic products that are causing respiratory complaints from your patient may also present a significant risk to you. Carbon monoxide, for example, is a colorless and odorless gas that may be present in quantities enough to overcome unsuspecting emergency care personnel. Other toxins from incomplete combustion produced in fires or industrial processes pose a similar risk. Recent incidents involving chemical agents such as saran gas or biological agents such as anthrax highlight the need for emergency care providers to be aware of hazards to themselves as well as to their patients.

You should also be aware that in certain rescue environments the concentration of available oxygen is significantly reduced. This would include areas such as grain silos, enclosed storage containers, or any enclosed space in which there is an active fire. You must take the appropriate precautions before entering such environments, including the use of your own supplemental oxygen supply.

In any situation where you believe there is a hazard to you as a care provider, make sure that the scene is appropriately secured before you enter. If specific protective items such as hazardous materials suits, self contained breathing apparatus, or supplemental oxygen are needed, make sure they are available before you attempt to care for your patient. Similarly, if other personnel such as fire suppression units or hazardous materials teams are required, contact dispatch and have them available on scene before putting yourself at risk.

Once it is safe to enter the scene, look for clues that will provide information regarding the patient's complaints. Do you see evidence of cigarette packs or ash trays to suggest that the patient or family members are smokers? Look for any home nebulizer machines or supplemental oxygen tanks that may suggest a patient with underlying COPD or asthma. If the patient is a small child, look for small items lying around the house that could suggest potential ingested foreign bodies. Using your eyes, ears, and nose can lead you to several important clues that are useful as you begin your assessment of the patient.

INITIAL ASSESSMENT

General Impression

Take the following considerations and steps to help form your general impression of the patient's respiratory status:

- *Position.* Consider the patient's position. Patients with respiratory diseases tend to tolerate an upright posture better than lying flat. Indications of severe

> **Content Review**
>
> **GENERAL IMPRESSION OF RESPIRATORY STATUS**
> - Position
> - Color
> - Mental status
> - Ability to speak
> - Respiratory effort

FIGURE 19-3   Tripod position.

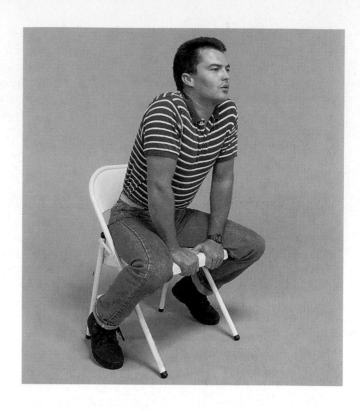

respiratory distress include a patient who is sitting upright with feet dangling over the side of the bed. In the most severe cases, the patient will assume the "tripod" position in which the patient leans forward and supports his weight with the arms extended (Figure 19-3).

pallor paleness.

diaphoresis sweatiness.

cyanosis bluish discoloration of the skin due to an increase in reduced hemoglobin in the blood. The condition is directly related to poor ventilation.

- *Color.* Patients with severe respiratory distress display **pallor** and **diaphoresis.** **Cyanosis** is a late finding and may be absent even with significant hypoxia. Peripheral cyanosis (bluish discoloration involving only the distal extremities) is not a specific finding and is also found in patients with poor circulation. Peripheral cyanosis reflects the slowing of blood flow and increased extraction of oxygen from red blood cells. Central cyanosis (involving the lips, tongue, and truncal skin) is a more ominous finding seen in hypoxia.

- *Mental status.* Briefly assess the patient's mental status. The hypoxic patient will become restless and agitated. Confusion is seen with both hypoxia (deficiency of oxygen) and hypercarbia (excess of carbon dioxide). When respiratory failure is imminent, the patient will appear severely lethargic and somnolent. The eyelids will begin to droop and the head will bob with each respiratory effort.

- *Ability to speak.* Assess the patient's ability to speak in full, coherent sentences. Determine the ease with which the patient can discuss symptoms. Patients with respiratory distress will be able to speak only one to two words before they need to pause to catch their breath. Rambling, incoherent speech indicates fear, anxiety, or hypoxia.

- *Respiratory effort.* As we have already described, normal ventilation is an active process. However, the use of accessory muscles in the neck (scalenes and sternocleidomastoids) and visible contractions of the intercostal muscles indicate significant breathing effort.

As you form your general impression, also make specific note of any of the following signs of respiratory distress:

nasal flaring excessive widening of the nares with respiration.

- **Nasal flaring**
- Intercostal muscle retraction

- Use of the accessory respiratory muscles
- Cyanosis
- Pursed lips
- **Tracheal tugging**

Your initial assessment of the patient is directed at identification of any life-threatening conditions resulting from compromise of airway, breathing, or circulation (the ABCs). Because this chapter concerns the respiratory system, it will focus on assessment of airway and breathing.

Airway

Remember that oxygen is one of the most basic necessities for life, and the respiratory system is responsible for supplying it to the body tissues. As a result, any significant abnormality in the respiratory tract must be viewed as potentially life threatening.

After quickly forming your general impression, immediately focus on the patient's airway. When assessing the airway, keep these principles in mind:

Any significant abnormality in the respiratory tract must be viewed as potentially life threatening.

- Noisy breathing nearly always means partial airway obstruction.
- Obstructed breathing is not always noisy.
- The brain can survive only a few minutes in **asphyxia.**
- Artificial respiration is useless if the airway is blocked.
- A patent airway is useless if the patient is apneic.
- If you note airway obstruction, do not waste time looking for help or equipment. Act immediately.

asphyxia a decrease in the amount of oxygen and an increase in the amount of carbon dioxide as a result of some interference with respiration.

If the airway is compromised, quickly institute basic airway management techniques. Once you have secured a patent airway, ensure that the patient has adequate ventilation. Your initial assessment of the respiratory system should be brief and directed. A more detailed examination should be conducted once you have been able to establish that an immediate threat to life does not exist.

If the airway is compromised, quickly institute basic airway management techniques. Once you have secured a patent airway, ensure that the patient has adequate ventilation.

Breathing

The following signs should suggest a possible life-threatening respiratory problem in adults. They are listed in order from most ominous to least severe:

- Alterations in mental status
- Severe central cyanosis
- Absent breath sounds
- Audible stridor
- One to two word **dyspnea** (need to breathe between every word or two)
- **Tachycardia** ≥ 130 beats per minute
- Pallor and diaphoresis
- Presence of intercostal and sternocleidomastoid retractions
- Use of accessory muscles

dyspnea difficult or labored breathing; a sensation of "shortness of breath."

tachycardia rapid heart rate.

If any of these signs are present, you should direct your efforts toward immediate resuscitation and transport of the patient to a medical facility.

FOCUSED HISTORY AND PHYSICAL EXAMINATION

History

The history and physical exam should be directed at problem areas as determined by the patient's chief complaint or primary problem. Patients with respiratory diseases will often present with a complaint of shortness of breath (dyspnea). Obtain a SAMPLE history. If the chief complaint suggests respiratory disease, ask the OPQRST questions including the

If a patient complains of dyspnea, obtain a SAMPLE history. If the chief complaint suggests respiratory disease, ask the OPQRST questions about current symptoms.

following questions about the current symptoms. The answers to these or similar questions will provide you with a pertinent patient history:

How long has the dyspnea been present?

Was the onset gradual or abrupt?

Is the dyspnea better or worse by position? Is there associated **orthopnea** or **paroxysmal nocturnal dyspnea?**

Has the patient been coughing?

    If so, is the cough productive?

    What is the character and color of the sputum?

    Is there any **hemoptysis** (coughing up of blood)?

Is there any chest pain associated with the dyspnea?

    If so, what is the location of the pain?

    Was the onset of pain sudden or slow?

    What was the duration of the pain?

    Does the pain radiate to any area?

    Does the pain increase with respiration?

Are there associated symptoms of fever or chills?

What is the patient's past medical history?

Has the patient experienced wheezing?

Is the patient or close family member a smoker?

It is also important to ask the patient if he has ever experienced similar symptoms in the past. Patients with chronic medical conditions such as COPD or asthma can usually relate the severity of their current presenting complaints to other episodes that they have experienced. Question the patient or family about prior hospitalizations for respiratory disease. In particular, you should try to determine whether the patient required care in the intensive care unit (ICU) for breathing problems. Ask if the patient has ever required endotracheal intubation and ventilatory support. Consider patients who have been previously intubated to be potentially seriously ill and approach them with great caution.

Similarly, it is important to ask the patient if he already has a known respiratory disease. The most common reason for a call to emergency care personnel is a worsening of an already present respiratory disease. This is very typical for patients with COPD, asthma, or lung cancer. If you are not familiar with the patient's diagnosis (for example, alpha-2 antitrypsin deficiency), try to determine if the disease is affecting the process of ventilation, diffusion, or perfusion.

Continue history taking by determining:

What current medications is the patient taking? (Pay particular attention to oxygen therapy, oral bronchodilators, corticosteroids, and antibiotics.)

Does the patient have any allergies?

A good history of medication use is essential and may provide useful clues to the diagnosis. If time permits, gather the patient's current medications and transport them with the patient. This is a great benefit to the Emergency Department personnel who will be evaluating the patient. Pay particular attention to any medications that suggest pulmonary disease. These would include inhaled or oral sympathomimetics such as albuterol and related agents that are used to treat diseases such as COPD or asthma. Also ask about steroid preparations, which are also used in these conditions. Other common medications used by patients with COPD or asthma include cromolyn sodium, methylxanthines such as theophylline, and antibiotic agents.

Also ask about drugs used for cardiac conditions, since cardiac patients often present with dyspnea. Nitrates, calcium channel blockers, diuretic agents, digoxin, and antidysrhythmic agents are all commonly used by patients with cardiac disease.

orthopnea dyspnea while lying supine.

paroxysmal nocturnal dyspnea short attacks of dyspnea that occur at night and interrupt sleep.

hemoptysis expectoration of blood from the respiratory tree.

Finally, inquire about medication allergies. This is important information, since it helps to avoid administering agents to which the patient is allergic. Also, it is possible that a specific medication may be the cause of an allergic reaction that has resulted in upper airway edema and respiratory complaints.

Physical Examination

First address the patient's head and neck. Look at the lips. Pursed lips indicate significant respiratory distress. This is the patient's way of maintaining positive pressure during expiration and preventing alveolar collapse. Also examine the nose, mouth, and throat for any signs of swelling or infection that might be causing upper airway obstruction.

Occasionally, the patient may also produce sputum, which can suggest an underlying cause of the patient's complaints. An increase in the amount of sputum produced suggests infection of the lungs or bronchial passages (bronchitis). Thick, green or brown sputum is characteristic of these infections. On the other hand, thin, yellow, or pale-gray sputum is more typical of inflammation or an allergic cause. Pink, frothy sputum is a sign of severe pulmonary edema. Truly bloody sputum (hemoptysis) may be seen with cancer, tuberculosis, and bronchial infection.

Assess the neck for signs of swelling or infection. Remember to look at the jugular veins for evidence of distention (Figure 19-4). This occurs when the right side of the heart is not pumping blood effectively, causing a "back-up" in the venous circulation. Such findings are often accompanied by left-sided heart failure and pulmonary edema.

Physical examination of the respiratory system should follow the standard steps of patient assessment: *inspection, palpation, percussion,* and *auscultation*:

- *Inspection.* Inspection should include an examination of the anterior-posterior dimensions and general shape of the chest. An increased anterior-posterior diameter suggests COPD. Inspect the chest for symmetrical movement. Any asymmetry may be suggestive of trauma. A paradoxical movement (moving in a fashion opposite to that expected) suggests flail chest. Note any chest scars, lesions, wounds, or deformities.

- *Palpation.* Palpate the chest, both front and back, for any abnormalities. Note any tenderness, **crepitus**, or **subcutaneous emphysema**. Palpate the anterior chest first, then the posterior. Inspect your gloved hands for blood each time

crepitus crackling sounds.

subcutaneous emphysema presence of air in the subcutaneous tissue.

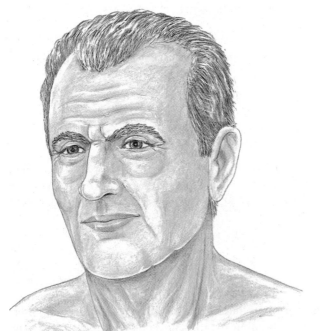

FIGURE 19-4 Jugular vein distention.

tactile fremitus vibratory tremors felt through the chest by palpation.

tracheal deviation any position of the trachea other than midline.

they are removed from behind the patient's chest. In some instances, it may be appropriate to evaluate **tactile fremitus,** the vibration felt in the chest during speaking. When evaluating tactile fremitus, compare one side of the chest with the other. Simultaneously, palpate the trachea for **tracheal deviation,** which suggests a tension pneumothorax.

- *Percussion.* If indicated, quickly percuss the chest. Limit percussion to suspected cases of pneumothorax and pulmonary edema. A hollow sound on percussion often indicates pneumothorax or emphysema. In contrast, a dull sound indicates pulmonary edema, hemothorax, or pneumonia. Remember, however, that percussion may be of little value in the noisy environment typical of most emergency scenes.

- *Auscultation.* Auscultate the chest. Begin by listening to the patient without a stethoscope and from a distance. Note any loud stridor, wheezing, or cough. If possible, the patient should be in the sitting position and the chest auscultated in a symmetrical pattern. When the patient cannot sit up, auscultate the anterior and lateral parts of the chest. Each area should be auscultated for one respiratory cycle.

Normal breath sounds heard during auscultation can be characterized according to the following descriptions:

Normal Breath Sounds

- Bronchial (or tubular)
  - Loud, high-pitched breath sounds heard over the trachea
  - Expiratory phase lasts longer than inspiratory phase
- Bronchovesicular
  - Softer, medium-pitched breath sounds heard over the mainstem bronchi (below clavicles or between scapulae)
  - Expiratory phase and inspiratory phase equal
- Vesicular
  - Soft, low-pitched breath sounds heard in the lung periphery

While the patient breathes in and out deeply with the mouth open, note any abnormal breath sounds and their location. Many terms are used to describe abnormal breath sounds. The following list includes some of the more common terms:

Abnormal Breath Sounds

- *Snoring.* Occurs when the upper airway is partially obstructed, usually by the tongue.
- *Stridor.* Harsh, high-pitched sound heard on inspiration and characteristic of an upper airway obstruction such as croup.
- *Wheezing.* Whistling sound due to narrowing of the airways by edema, bronchoconstriction, or foreign materials.
- *Rhonchi.* Rattling sounds in the larger airways associated with excessive mucus or other material.
- *Crackles* (also called *rales*). Fine, moist crackling sounds associated with fluid in the smaller airways.
- *Pleural friction rub.* Sounds like dried pieces of leather rubbing together; occurs when the pleura become inflamed, as in pleurisy.

Also examine the extremities. Look for peripheral cyanosis, which may indicate hypoxia. Examine the extremities for swelling, redness, and a hard, firm cord indicating a venous clot. This may suggest a possible cause for pulmonary embolism. Look for clubbing of the fingers (Figure 19-5), suggesting long-standing hypoxemia. This is typical of patients with COPD or cyanotic heart disease. Finally, the patient may demonstrate *carpopedal spasm* in which the fingers and toes are contracted in flexion. This is found in patients with

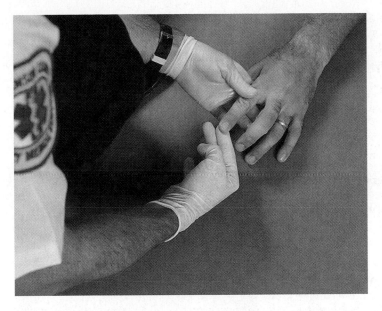
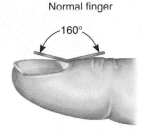
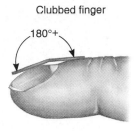

FIGURE 19-5 (a) Inspect for finger clubbing. Any clubbing may indicate chronic respiratory or cardiac disease. (b) Characteristics of finger clubbing include large fingertips and a loss of the normal angle at the nail bed.

hyperventilation and is caused by transient shifts in the blood calcium concentration caused by changes in the serum CO_2 and pH levels.

Vital Signs

The patient's vital signs may also provide information regarding the severity of the respiratory complaints. In general, tachycardia (rapid heart rate) is a very non-specific finding, seen with fear, anxiety, and fever. In patients with respiratory complaints, however, tachycardia may also indicate hypoxia. Remember that the patient may have recently used sympathomimetic drugs such as albuterol, which will accelerate the patient's heart rate. These same drugs will elevate the patient's blood pressure as well. During your assessment of the blood pressure, a patient will occasionally exhibit pulsus paradoxus, a drop in the systolic blood pressure of 10 mmHg or more with each respiratory cycle. Pulsus paradoxus is associated with COPD and cardiac tamponade. As a rule, however, you should not take the time to look for pulsus paradoxus.

A change in a patient's respiratory rate may be one of the earliest indicators of respiratory disease. The patient's respiratory rate can be influenced by several factors, including respiratory difficulty, fear, anxiety, fever, and underlying metabolic disease. Assume that an elevated respiratory rate in a patient with dyspnea is caused by hypoxia. Although fluctuations in the respiratory rate are common, a persistently slow rate indicates impending respiratory arrest.

Continually reassess the patient's respiratory rate during the time that you are caring for the patient. Trends in the respiratory rate (for example, an increasing rate) can give you an overall assessment of the effectiveness of any intervention you have made. Also assess the patient's respiratory pattern. The normal respiratory pattern (eupnea) is steady, even breaths occurring 12 to 20 times per minute with an expiratory phase that lasts between three to four times the inspiratory phase. **Tachypnea** describes a respiratory pattern with a rate that exceeds 20 breaths per minute. **Bradypnea** describes a respiratory pattern with a rate slower than 12 breaths per minute. Also, look for any abnormal respiratory patterns (e.g., Cheyne-Stokes, Kussmaul, or other) that were discussed earlier in the chapter.

Diagnostic Testing

Three diagnostic measurements of value in assessing the patient's respiratory status are pulse oximetry, peak flow, and capnometry.

Assume that an elevated respiratory rate in a patient with dyspnea is caused by hypoxia. A persistently slow rate indicates impending respiratory arrest.

Constantly reassess the patient's respiratory rate and pattern.

tachypnea rapid respiration.

bradypnea slow respiration.

Content Review

PREHOSPITAL DIAGNOSTIC TESTS
- Pulse oximetry
- Peak flow
- Capnometry

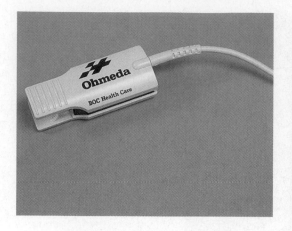

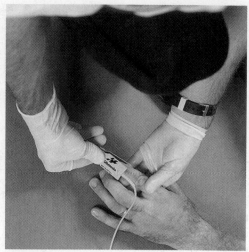

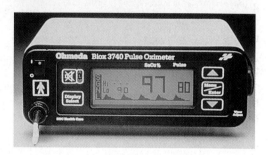

FIGURE 19-6 Sensing unit for pulse oximetry. This device transmits light through a vascular bed, such as in the finger, and can determine the oxygen saturation of red blood cells. To use the pulse oximeter, it is only necessary to turn the device on and attach the sensor to a finger. The desired graphic mode on the oximeter should be selected. The oxygen saturation and pulse rate can be continuously monitored.

Pulse Oximetry   Pulse oximetry offers a rapid and accurate means for assessing oxygen saturation. The pulse oximeter can be quickly applied to a finger or earlobe. The pulse rate and oxygen saturation can be continuously recorded. Use of the pulse oximeter, if available, is encouraged for any patient complaining of dyspnea or respiratory problems (Figure 19-6). Remember that the pulse oximetry reading may be difficult to obtain in a patient with peripheral vasoconstriction (as in sepsis or hypothermia). It may also be inaccurate under conditions in which an abnormal substance such as carbon monoxide binds to hemoglobin, since the instrument measures the saturation of hemoglobin without indicating what substance has saturated it.

The oxygen saturation measurement obtained through pulse oximetry is abbreviated as SaO_2 (oxygen saturation). When pulse oximetry first came into use, some authors abbreviated the oxygen saturation measurement as SpO_2. However, this was sometimes confused with the PaO_2 obtained during blood gas measurement. Because of this, SaO_2 has become the preferred abbreviation.

Peak Flow   Small portable hand-held devices are available for use in determining the patient's peak expiratory flow rate (PEFR). The normal expected peak flow rate is based on the patient's sex, age, and height. Remember that the measurement of the PEFR is somewhat effort dependent; you must have a cooperative patient who understands the use of the device in order to get an accurate reading.

The PEFR is obtained using a Wright Spirometer (Figure 19-7), which is inexpensive and easy to use. Place the disposable mouth piece into the meter. First have the patient take in the deepest possible inspiration. Then encourage the patient to seal his lips around the device and forcibly exhale. The peak rate of exhaled gas is recorded in liters per minute. This should be repeated twice, with the highest reading recorded as the patient's PEFR (Table 19-1).

Capnometry   Devices are now available that detect and measure exhaled carbon dioxide. The percentage of exhaled carbon dioxide is an indicator of the body's ongoing metabolic processes and the efficiency of gas exchange in the lung. For years, capnometry has been used principally to verify endotracheal tube placement. The presence of carbon dioxide is an indication that the endotracheal tube is properly placed within the trachea. Both the

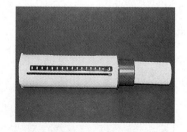

FIGURE 19-7 Wright Spirometer for determining peak expiratory flow rate (PEFR).

Table 19-1	SPIROMETRY AND PEAK FLOW VALUES FOR ADULTS		
FEV$_1$ Severity	FEV$_1$ (Liters)	FVC (%)	Peak Flow (Liters/Min)
Normal	4.0–6.0 L	80–90%	550–650 (Male) 400–500 (Female)
Mild	3.0 L	70%	300–400
Moderate	1.6 L	50%	200–300
Severe	0.6 L	40%	100

esophagus and pharynx do not contain any significant quantity of carbon dioxide. Thus, if the tube is inadvertently placed into the esophagus or pharynx, the capnometer will not register. Although use of the capnometer for detection of proper endotracheal tube placement is still a major use of the device in prehospital care, capnometry is now widely used for ongoing patient monitoring in both intubated and non-intubated patients. Information obtained from capnometry can be displayed as a wave form and can provide a great deal about the patient's underlying respiratory physiology. It can also be used to determine whether a patient with respiratory distress is deteriorating or improving, and it can help guide medical therapy and drug administration.

Although several devices are available that measure the level of carbon dioxide during the entire ventilatory cycle (as a continuous waveform called *capnography*), end-tidal CO_2 detectors focus only on the presence or absence of carbon dioxide in the sampled gas (capnometry). If the endotracheal tube becomes dislodged from its proper position, there is an almost immediate change in the readings from the end-tidal CO_2 device. This is in contrast to measurement of pulse oximetry, which may take several minutes to reflect the hypoxia produced by tube dislodgement.

Two types of devices are commonly used for capnometry. The first device gives a numerical read out or a wave form of the level of carbon dioxide detected by the device (Figure 19-8a). The other device relies on a color change produced by carbon dioxide to demonstrate the presence of the gas during exhalation (Figure 19-8b).

MANAGEMENT OF RESPIRATORY DISORDERS

The following sections will address the pathophysiology, assessment, and management of the more common respiratory disorders encountered in prehospital care. The discussion begins with a look at some general principles that can and should be applied to ALL respiratory emergencies.

MANAGEMENT PRINCIPLES

In cases of acute respiratory insufficiency, several principles should guide your actions in the prehospital setting. These include:

- Airway always has first priority. In trauma victims who may have associated cervical-spine injuries, protect and maintain the airway without extending the neck.
- Any patient with respiratory distress should receive oxygen.
- Any patient whose illness or injury suggests the possibility of hypoxia should receive oxygen.
- If there is a question whether oxygen should be given, as in COPD, administer it. *Oxygen should never be withheld from a patient suspected of suffering hypoxia.*

Keep these precautions in mind as you read through the descriptions of pathophysiology, assessment, and management of respiratory disorders frequently encountered in the field.

Principles of management for respiratory disorders include (1) giving first priority to the airway and (2) always providing oxygen to patients with respiratory distress or the possibility of hypoxia, including patients with COPD.

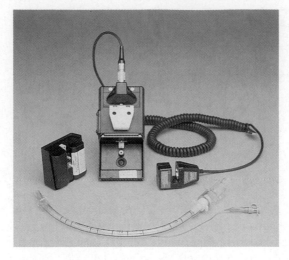

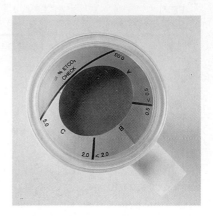

FIGURE 19-8   End-tidal CO_2 devices: (a) electronic and (b) colormetric.

SPECIFIC RESPIRATORY DISEASES

UPPER-AIRWAY OBSTRUCTION

The most common cause of upper-airway obstruction is the relaxed tongue. In an unconscious patient in the supine position, the tongue can fall into the back of the throat and obstruct the upper airway. Additionally, the upper airway can become obstructed by such common materials as food, dentures, or other foreign bodies. A typical example of upper-airway obstruction is the "cafe coronary," which tends to occur in middle-aged or elderly patients who wear dentures. These people often are unable to sense how well they have chewed their food. Thus, they accidentally inhale a large piece of food (often meat) that obstructs their airway. Concurrent alcohol consumption is often implicated in the "cafe coronary." Also, obstruction of the upper airway can be the result of facial or neck trauma, upper-airway burns, and allergic reactions. In addition, the upper airway can become blocked by an infection that causes swelling of the epiglottis (epiglottitis) or subglottic area (croup).

Assessment

Assessment of the patient with an upper-airway obstruction varies, depending on the cause of the obstruction and the history of the event. The unresponsive patient should be evaluated for snoring respirations, possibly indicating tongue or denture obstruction. If confronted by a patient suffering a "cafe coronary," determine whether the victim can speak. Speech indicates that, at present, the obstruction is incomplete. If the victim is unresponsive and has been eating, strongly suspect a food bolus lodged in the trachea. If a burn is present or suspected, assume laryngeal edema until proven otherwise.

Patients who may be having an allergic reaction to food or medications will often report an itching sensation in the palate followed by a "lump" in the throat. The situation may progress to hoarseness, inspiratory stridor, and complete obstruction. Pay particular attention to the presence of urticaria (hives). Intercostal muscle retraction and use of the strap muscles of the neck for breathing suggest attempts to ventilate against a partially closed airway.

Management

Management of the obstructed airway is based on the nature of the obstruction. Blockage by the tongue can be corrected by opening the airway, using either the head-tilt/chin-lift, the jaw-thrust, or the modified jaw-thrust maneuver. The airway can be maintained by employing either a nasopharyngeal or oropharyngeal airway. If possible, remove obstructing foreign bodies using the following basic airway maneuvers.

Conscious Adult   In an adult patient who is conscious:

1. Determine if there is a complete obstruction or poor air exchange. Ask the patient: "Are you choking?" "Can you speak?" If the patient can speak, he should be asked to produce a forceful cough to expel the foreign body.

2. If the patient has complete obstruction or poor air exchange, provide up to five abdominal thrusts in rapid succession. If the thrusts prove unsuccessful, repeat until the obstruction is relieved or the patient becomes unconscious. In very obese or pregnant patients, use chest thrusts in lieu of abdominal thrusts.

Unconscious Adult   If the patient is unconscious or loses consciousness:

1. Use the head-tilt/chin-lift, the jaw-thrust, or the modified jaw-thrust maneuver in an attempt to open the airway.

2. Pinch the patient's nostrils and attempt to give two ventilations. If the attempts to ventilate fail, reposition the head and repeat attempt. If this fails . . .

3. Straddle the patient and administer up to five abdominal thrusts in quick succession. If this fails,

4. Try the tongue-jaw lift and, if the foreign body is seen, attempt finger sweeps. If successful, resume ventilation. If unsuccessful . . .

5. Continue the abdominal thrusts and finger sweeps, while preparing the laryngoscope and the Magill forceps. Visualize the airway with the laryngoscope. If the foreign body can be seen, grasp it with the Magill forceps and remove. Once removed, begin ventilation and administer supplemental oxygen.

In cases of airway obstruction caused by laryngeal edema (e.g., anaphylactic reactions, angioedema), establish the airway by the head-tilt, chin-lift, the jaw-thrust, or triple-airway maneuver. Then administer supplemental oxygen. Attempt bag-valve-mask (BVM) ventilation. Often, air can be forced past the obstruction and the patient adequately ventilated using this technique. Next, start an IV with a crystalloid solution and administer subcutaneous epinephrine. Then administer diphenhydramine (Benadryl).

NON-CARDIOGENIC PULMONARY EDEMA/ADULT RESPIRATORY DISTRESS SYNDROME

Adult respiratory distress syndrome (ARDS) is a form of pulmonary edema that is caused by fluid accumulation in the interstitial space within the lungs. Patients with cardiogenic pulmonary edema have a poorly functioning left ventricle. This leads to increases in hydrostatic pressure and fluid accumulation in the interstitial space. In patients with ARDS, however, fluid accumulation occurs as the result of increased vascular permeability and decreased fluid removal from the lung tissue. This occurs in response to a wide variety of lung insults including:

* Sepsis, particularly with gram-negative organisms
* Aspiration
* Pneumonia or other respiratory infections
* Pulmonary injury
* Burns
* Inhalation injury
* Oxygen toxicity
* Drugs such as aspirin or opiates
* High altitude
* Hypothermia

adult respiratory distress syndrome (ARDS) form of pulmonary edema that is caused by fluid accumulation in the interstitial space within the lungs.

- Near-drowning
- Head injury
- Emboli from blood clot, fat, or amniotic fluid
- Tumor destruction
- Pancreatitis
- Procedures such as cardiopulmonary bypass or hemodialysis
- Other insults such as hypoxia, hypotension, or cardiac arrest

The mortality in patients who develop ARDS is quite high, approaching 70%. Although many patients die as the result of respiratory failure, many succumb to failure of several organ systems, including the liver and kidneys.

Pathophysiology

ARDS is a disorder of lung diffusion that results from increased fluid in the interstitial space. Each of the underlying conditions cited above results in the inability to maintain a proper fluid balance in the interstitial space. Severe hypotension, significant hypoxemia as the result of cardiac arrest, drowning, seizure activity or hypoventilation, high altitude exposure, environmental toxins and endotoxins released in septic shock—all can cause disruption of the alveolar-capillary membrane. Increases in pulmonary capillary permeability, destruction of the capillary lining, and increases in osmotic forces all act to draw fluid into the interstitial space and contribute to interstitial edema. This increases the thickness of the respiratory membrane and limits diffusion of oxygen. In advanced cases, fluid also accumulates in the alveoli, causing loss of surfactant, collapse of the alveolar sacs, and impaired gas exchange. This results in a significant amount of pulmonary shunting with unoxygenated blood returning to the circulation. The result is significant hypoxia.

Assessment

Specific clinical symptoms are related to the underlying cause of ARDS. For example, patients who develop ARDS as the result of sepsis will have symptoms related to their underlying infection. Determine if the patient has a history of prolonged hypoxia, head or chest trauma, inhalation of gases, or ascent to a high altitude without prior acclimation, all of which can suggest an underlying cause for the respiratory complaints.

Patients with ARDS experience a gradual decline in their respiratory status. In rare cases, a seemingly healthy patient has a sudden onset of respiratory failure and hypoxia. Such a presentation is characteristic of patients with high altitude pulmonary edema (HAPE).

Dyspnea, confusion, and agitation are often found in patients with non-cardiogenic pulmonary edema. Patients may also report fatigue and reduced exercise ability. Symptoms such as orthopnea, paroxysmal nocturnal dyspnea, or sputum production are not commonly reported but may be seen.

The prominent physical findings are generally those associated with the underlying lung insult. Tachypnea and tachycardia are often found in association with ARDS. Crackles (rales) are audible in both lungs. Wheezing may also be heard if there is any element of bronchospasm. Severe tachypnea, central cyanosis, and signs of imminent respiratory failure are seen in severe cases. Pulse oximetry will demonstrate low oxygen saturations in those patients with advanced disease. In those patients requiring ventilatory support, a decreased lung compliance will be noted. (It will require more operator force to deliver an adequate lung volume.)

Management

Specific management of the patient's underlying medical condition is the hallmark of treatment for this disorder. Treatment of gram negative sepsis with appropriate antibiotics, removal of the patient from any inciting toxin, or rapid descent to a lower altitude in patients with HAPE are the most important therapies for this condition. The patient will usually tolerate an upright position with the legs dangling off the cart.

Since the hypoxia seen in ARDS is the result of diffusion defects, oxygen supplementation is essential for all patients with this condition. Establish IV access, but provide fluids only if hypovolemia exists. Establish cardiac monitoring. Suctioning of lung secretions is often required to maintain airway patency.

Use positive pressure ventilation to support any ARDS patient who demonstrates signs of respiratory failure. Use BVM ventilation for initial respiratory support but note that these patients generally require endotracheal intubation and support using a mechanical ventilator for early management. **Positive end expiratory pressure (PEEP)** is often required to maintain patency of the alveoli and adequate oxygenation. Diuretics and nitrates, which are used in patients with cardiogenic pulmonary edema, are usually not helpful in patients with ARDS. Your medical director may occasionally order corticosteroids for patients with ARDS/non-cardiogenic pulmonary edema. Corticosteroids are thought to stabilize the alveolar-capillary membrane, although clinical studies have not demonstrated any benefit to their use.

Maintain cardiac monitoring and pulse oximetry throughout transport of the patient. Transport patients to a facility capable of advanced hemodynamic monitoring (including Swan-Ganz catheter) and mechanical ventilation support.

positive end expiratory pressure (PEEP) a method of holding the alveoli open by increasing expiratory pressure. Some bag-valve units used in EMS have PEEP attachments. Also EMS personnel sometimes transport patients who are on ventilators with PEEP attachments.

OBSTRUCTIVE LUNG DISEASE

Obstructive lung disease is widespread in our society. The most common obstructive lung diseases encountered in prehospital care are asthma, emphysema, and chronic bronchitis (the last two are often discussed together as COPD). Asthma afflicts 4% to 5% of the U.S. population and COPD is found in 25% of all adults. Chronic bronchitis alone affects one in five adult males. Patients with COPD have a 50% mortality rate within 10 years of the diagnosis.

Although asthma may have a genetic predisposition, COPD is known to be directly caused by cigarette smoking and environmental toxins. Other factors have been shown to precipitate symptoms in patients who already have obstructive airway disease. Intrinsic factors include stress, upper respiratory infections, and exercise. Extrinsic factors include tobacco smoke, drugs, occupational hazards (chemical fumes, dust, etc.), and allergens such as foods, animal danders, dusts, and molds.

Obstructive lung diseases all have abnormal ventilation as a common feature. This abnormal ventilation is a result of obstruction that occurs primarily in the bronchioles. Several changes occur within these air conduits. Bronchospasm (sustained smooth muscle contraction) occurs, which may be reversed by beta adrenergic receptor stimulation. Agents such as terbutaline, albuterol, and epinephrine are used to accomplish this stimulation. Increased mucus production by goblet cells that line the respiratory tree also contribute to obstruction. This effect may be worsened by the fact that in many patients, the cilia are destroyed, resulting in poor clearance of excess mucus. Finally, inflammation of the bronchial passages results in the accumulation of fluid and inflammatory cells. Depending on the underlying cause, some elements of bronchial obstruction are reversible, whereas others are not.

During inspiration, the bronchioles will naturally dilate, allowing air to be drawn into the alveoli. As the patient begins to exhale, the bronchioles constrict. When this natural constriction occurs—in addition to the underlying bronchospasm, increased mucus production,

Content Review

OBSTRUCTIVE LUNG DISEASE
- Emphysema
- Chronic bronchitis
- Asthma

Cultural Considerations

Cigarette smoking has clearly been demonstrated to be a contributing factor in the development of respiratory disease—especially chronic obstructive pulmonary disease and bronchogenic cancers. Though the use of tobacco products in the United States has declined overall, it is still more acceptable in some areas of the country than in others. For example, in some southern and eastern states where tobacco is the cash crop, there is a higher incidence of tobacco use. Smoking also is more acceptable and better tolerated in some cultures than in others. Likewise, tobacco products are more readily available. Thus, over time, one would expect the incidence of chronic obstructive pulmonary diseases and bronchogenic cancers to be higher in these groups.

and inflammation that exist in patients with obstructive airway disease—the result is significant air trapping distal to the obstruction. This is one of the hallmarks of obstructive lung disease. This section will discuss each of these disease processes—emphysema, chronic bronchitis, and asthma—detailing the pathophysiology, assessment, and treatment.

EMPHYSEMA

Emphysema results from destruction of the alveolar walls distal to the terminal bronchioles. It is more common in men than in women. The major factor contributing to emphysema in our society is cigarette smoking. Significant exposure to environmental toxins is another contributing factor.

Pathophysiology

Continued exposure to noxious substances, such as cigarette smoke, results in the gradual destruction of the walls of the alveoli. This process decreases the alveolar membrane surface area, thus lessening the area available for gas exchange. The progressive loss of the respiratory membrane results in an increased ratio of air to lung tissue. The result is diffusion defects. Additionally, the number of pulmonary capillaries in the lung is decreased, thus increasing resistance to pulmonary blood flow. This condition ultimately causes pulmonary hypertension, which in turn may lead to **cor pulmonale** and death (Figure 19-9).

> **cor pulmonale** hypertrophy of the right ventricle resulting from disorders of the lung.

Emphysema also causes weakening of the walls of the small bronchioles. When the walls of the alveoli and small bronchioles are destroyed, the lungs lose their capacity to recoil and air becomes trapped in the lungs. Thus, residual volume increases while vital capacity remains relatively normal. The destroyed lung tissue (called *blebs*) results in alveolar collapse. To counteract this effect, patients tend to breathe through pursed lips. This creates continued positive pressure similar to positive end expiratory pressure (PEEP) and prevents alveolar collapse.

> **polycythemia** an excess of red blood cells.

As the disease progresses, the PaO_2 further decreases, which may lead to increased red blood cell production and **polycythemia** (an excess of red blood cells resulting in an abnormally high hematocrit). The PaO_2 also increases and becomes chronically elevated, forcing the body to depend on hypoxic drive to control respirations. Finally, remember that emphysema is characterized by irreversible airway obstruction.

FIGURE 19-9 Long-standing chronic obstructive pulmonary disease can cause pulmonary hypertension, which in turn may lead to cor pulmonale.

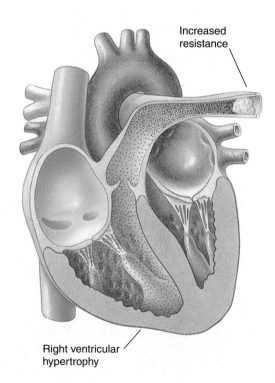

Increased resistance

Right ventricular hypertrophy

Patients with emphysema are more susceptible to acute respiratory infections, such as pneumonia, and to cardiac dysrhythmias. Chronic emphysema patients ultimately become dependent on bronchodilators, corticosteroids, and, in the final stages, supplemental oxygen.

Assessment

The patient with emphysema may report a history of recent weight loss, increased dyspnea on exertion, and progressive limitation of physical activity. Unlike chronic bronchitis, discussed in subsequent sections, emphysema is rarely associated with a cough, except in the morning. Question the patient about cigarette and tobacco usage. This is generally reported in pack/years. Ask the number of cigarette packs (20 cigarettes/pack) smoked per day and the number of years the patient has smoked. Multiply the number of packs smoked per day by the number of years. For example, a man who has smoked 2 packs per day for 15 years would have a 30 pack/year smoking history. Medical problems related to smoking, such as emphysema, chronic bronchitis, and lung cancer, usually begin after a patient surpasses a 20 pack/year history, although this can vary significantly.

Physical exam of the emphysema patient usually reveals a barrel chest evidenced by an increase in the anterior/posterior chest diameter. You may also note decreased chest excursion with a prolonged expiratory phase and a rapid resting respiratory rate. Patients with emphysema are often thin since they must use a significant amount of their caloric intake for respiration. Their skin tends to be pink due to polycythemia (excess of red blood cells), and they are referred to as "pink puffers." Emphysema patients often have hypertrophy of the accessory respiratory muscles (Figure 19-10).

The patient will often involuntarily purse his lips to create continuous positive airway pressure. Clubbing of the fingers is common. Breath sounds are usually diminished. Wheezes and rhonchi may or may not be present, depending on the amount of obstruction to air flow. The patient may exhibit signs of right-heart failure as evidenced by jugular vein distention, peripheral edema, and hepatic congestion. Signs of severe respiratory impairment in all patients with obstructive lung disease include confusion, agitation, somnolence, one to two word dyspnea, and use of accessory muscles to assist ventilation.

Emphysema is rarely associated with a cough except in the morning.

Emphysema patients usually have a barrel chest, are often thin, and have a pink skin tone ("pink puffers").

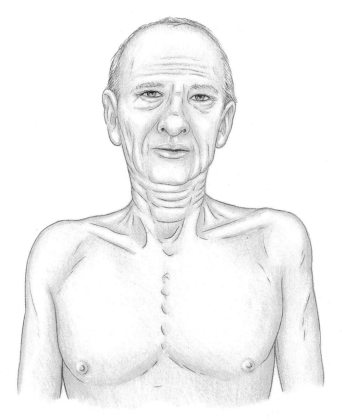

FIGURE 19-10 Typical appearance of patient with emphysema. There are well-developed accessory muscles and suprasternal retraction.

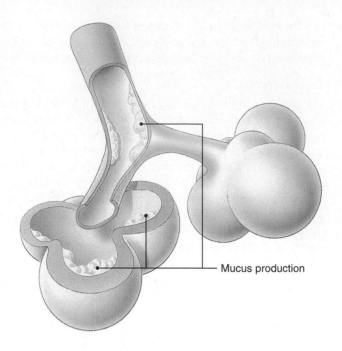

Mucus production

Management

Although emphysema differs in the disease process from chronic bronchitis, the two respiratory disorders share several of the same symptoms and pathophysiology. As a result, you will treat the two disorders in a similar manner. The discussion of management of emphysema will be taken up with chronic bronchitis. (See next section.)

CHRONIC BRONCHITIS

Chronic bronchitis results from an increase in the number of the goblet (mucus-secreting) cells in the respiratory tree (Figure 19-11). It is characterized by the production of a large quantity of sputum. This often occurs after prolonged exposure to cigarette smoke.

Pathophysiology

Unlike emphysema, in chronic bronchitis the alveoli are not severely affected and diffusion remains normal. Gas exchange is decreased because alveolar ventilation is lowered, which ultimately results in hypoxia and hypercarbia. Hypoxia may increase red blood cell production, which in turn leads to polycythemia (as occurs in emphysema). Increased $PaCO_2$ levels may lead to irritability, somnolence, decreased intellectual abilities, headaches, and personality changes. Physiologically, an increased $PaCO_2$ causes pulmonary vasoconstriction, resulting in pulmonary hypertension and, eventually, cor pulmonale. Unlike emphysema, the vital capacity is decreased, while the residual volume is normal or decreased.

Assessment

Chronic bronchitis is usually associated with a productive cough and copious sputum production.

The patient with chronic bronchitis often will have a history of heavy cigarette smoking, but the disease may also occur in nonsmokers. There may also be a history of frequent respiratory infections. In addition, these patients usually produce considerable quantities of sputum daily. Clinically, the patient is described as having a productive cough for at least three months per year for two or more consecutive years.

Chronic bronchitis patients tend to be overweight and are often cyanotic ("blue bloaters").

Patients with chronic bronchitis tend to be overweight and can be cyanotic. Because of this, they are often referred to as "blue bloaters." This can be contrasted with the "pink puffer" image of emphysema patients described above. Auscultation of the thorax often will reveal rhonchi due to occlusion of the larger airways with mucus plugs. The patient may also exhibit signs and symptoms of right-heart failure such as jugular vein distention, ankle edema, and hepatic congestion.

Management

The primary goals in the emergency management of the patient with either emphysema or chronic bronchitis are to relieve hypoxia and reverse any bronchoconstriction that may be present. However, many of these patients depend on hypoxic respiratory drive. As a result, the supplemental administration of oxygen may decrease respiratory drive and inhibit ventilation. You must continually monitor the patient and be prepared to assist ventilations if signs of respiratory depression develop.

The first step in treating a patient suffering an exacerbation of emphysema or chronic bronchitis is to establish an airway. Then place the patient in a seated or semi-seated position to assist the accessory respiratory muscles. Apply a pulse oximeter and determine the blood oxygen saturation (SaO_2). Administer supplemental oxygen at a low flow rate while maintaining an oxygen saturation above 90%. A nasal cannula can often be used, but you must constantly monitor the respiratory rate and depth as well as oxygen saturation. Alternatively, you may use a Venturi mask at a low concentration (24% to 35%). If hypoxia or respiratory failure is evident, then increase the concentration of delivered oxygen. Be prepared to support the ventilation with BVM assistance. Intubation may be required if respiratory failure is imminent.

Establish an IV line with lactated Ringer's or normal saline solution at a "to keep open" rate. More aggressive fluid administration is suggested if signs of dehydration are present. This may also aid in loosening thick mucus secretions. Then, if ordered by medical direction, administer a bronchodilator medication, such as albuterol, metaproterenol or ipratropium bromide, through a small volume nebulizer or particle inhaler (Rotohaler). Corticosteroids are also commonly used in the early management of patients with COPD.

ASTHMA

Asthma is a common respiratory illness that affects many persons. Although deaths from other respiratory diseases are steadily declining, deaths from asthma have significantly increased during the last decade. Most of the increased asthma deaths have occurred in patients who are 45 years of age or older. In addition, the death rate for black asthmatics has been twice as high as for their white counterparts. Approximately 50% of patients who die from asthma do so before reaching the hospital. Thus, EMS personnel are frequently called on to treat patients suffering an asthma attack. Prompt recognition followed by appropriate treatment can significantly improve the patient's condition and enhance his chance of survival.

Pathophysiology

Asthma is a chronic inflammatory disorder of the airways. In susceptible individuals, this inflammation causes symptoms usually associated with widespread but variable air flow obstruction. In addition to air flow obstruction, the airway becomes hyperresponsive. The air flow obstruction and hyperresponsiveness are often reversible with treatment. These conditions may also reverse spontaneously.

Asthma may be induced by one of many different factors. These factors are commonly referred to as "triggers" or "inducers" and vary from one individual to the next. In allergic individuals, environmental allergens are a major cause of inflammation. These may occur both indoors and outdoors. In addition to allergens, asthma may be triggered by cold air, exercise, foods, irritants, stress, and certain medications. Often, a specific trigger cannot be identified. Extrinsic triggers tend predominantly to affect children, whereas intrinsic factors trigger asthma in adults.

Within minutes of exposure to the offending trigger, a two-phase reaction occurs. The first phase of the reaction is characterized by the release of chemical mediators such as histamine. These mediators cause contraction of the bronchial smooth muscle and leakage of fluid from peribronchial capillaries. This results in both bronchoconstriction and bronchial edema. These two factors can significantly decrease expiratory air flow causing the typical "asthma attack."

Often, the asthma attack will resolve spontaneously in 1 to 2 hours or may be aborted by the use of inhaled bronchodilator medications such as albuterol. However, within 6 to 8 hours after exposure to the trigger, a second reaction occurs. This late phase is characterized

Administer oxygen to the COPD patient who needs it to relieve hypoxia. Since this may decrease this patient's respiratory drive, monitor him and be prepared to assist ventilations if necessary.

by inflammation of the bronchioles as cells of the immune system (eosinophils, neutrophils, and lymphocytes) invade the mucosa of the respiratory tract. This leads to additional edema and swelling of the bronchioles and a further decrease in expiratory air flow.

The second phase reaction will not typically respond to inhaled beta-agonist drugs such as metaproterenol or albuterol. Instead, anti-inflammatory agents such as corticosteroids are often required. It is important to point out that the severe inflammatory changes seen in an acute asthma attack do not develop over a few hours or even a few days. The inflammation will often begin several days or several weeks before the onset of the actual asthma attack.

Assessment

Begin the initial prehospital assessment of the asthmatic by considering immediate threats to the airway, breathing, or circulation. Then turn your attention to the focused history and physical examination.

The most common presenting symptoms of asthma are dyspnea, wheezing, and cough. Wheezing results from turbulent air flow through the inflamed and narrowed bronchioles. Many asthmatics will have a persistent cough. This is primarily due to hyperresponsiveness of the airway. It is important to point out that some asthmatics do not wheeze. Instead, their initial presentation may be a frequent and persistent cough. As asthma severity increases, the patient may exhibit hyperinflation of the chest due to trapping of air in the alveoli. In addition, tachypnea (rapid respiration) will occur. The patient may start to use accessory muscles to aid respiration.

Symptoms of a severe asthma attack include one to two word dyspnea (the inability to complete a phrase or sentence without having to stop to breathe), pulsus paradoxus (a drop of systolic blood pressure of 10 mmHg or more with inspiration), tachycardia, and decreased oxygen saturation on pulse oximetry. As hypoxia develops the patient may become agitated and anxious.

When conducting the focused history and physical examination, start by obtaining a brief patient history. Most asthmatics will report that they suffer from asthma. In addition, the patient's home medications may help confirm a history of asthma. Common asthma medications include inhaled beta-agonists (albuterol, metaproterenol), inhaled corticosteroids (betamethasone, beclomethasone), inhaled cromolyn sodium, and inhaled anticholinergics (ipratropium bromide). Often the patient will be taking oral bronchodilators such as theophylline or may be taking oral corticosteroids (prednisone).

Determine when symptoms started and what the patient has taken in an attempt to abort the attack. Also, find out whether the patient is allergic to any medications. Question the patient about hospitalizations for asthma. If the patient has been hospitalized, ask whether the patient has ever required intubation and mechanical ventilation. A prior history of intubation and mechanical ventilation should heighten your index of suspicion. Similarly, an asthmatic who is on continuous corticosteroid therapy is also a high-risk patient.

After you obtain the pertinent history, perform a brief physical examination. Place particular emphasis on the chest and neck. Examination of the chest should begin with inspection. Note any increase in the diameter of the chest that may indicate air trapping. Also, note the use of accessory muscles, including retraction of the intercostal muscles or use of the strap muscles of the neck. Following inspection, palpate the chest, noting any deformity, crepitus, or asymmetry. Next, auscultate the posterior chest. Note any abnormal breath sounds such as wheezing or rhonchi. Listen to the symmetry of breath sounds. Unilateral wheezing may indicate an aspirated foreign body or a pneumothorax.

Obtain accurate vital signs. One of the most important vital signs is the respiratory rate. An increase in the respiratory rate is one of the earliest symptoms of a respiratory problem. Many EMS personnel inaccurately measure the respiratory rate. The easiest method is to simply place your fingers on the patient's radial artery as if you were measuring the pulse rate. This will make the patient think you are obtaining the pulse rate, and he will not alter his breathing pattern. Measure the respiratory rate for at least 30 seconds. At the same time, note any alterations in the respiratory pattern. Pulse oximetry is an excellent adjunct to respiratory assessment. It will provide you with data regarding the oxygen saturation status (SaO_2) as well as an audible measure of the pulse rate.

Content Review

COMMON SIGNS OF ASTHMA

- Dyspnea
- Wheezing
- Cough

Note that some asthmatics do not wheeze; instead, they present with a frequent, persistent cough.

EMS systems should be able to measure the peak expiratory flow rate (PEFR). (Review Figure 19-7 and Table 19-1.) The PEFR is a reliable indicator of air flow. If possible, measure peak flow rates to determine the severity of an asthma attack and the degree of response to treatment. The more severe the asthma attack, the lower will be the PEFR.

Management

Treatment of asthma is designed to correct hypoxia, reverse any bronchospasm, and treat the inflammatory changes associated with the disease. Administer oxygen at a high concentration (100%). Establish IV access and place the patient on an electrocardiogram (ECG) monitor. Direct initial treatment at reversing any bronchospasm present. The most commonly used drugs are the inhaled beta-agonist preparations such as albuterol (Ventolin, Proventil) in conjunction with ipratropium bromide (Atrovent). These can be easily administered with a small volume, oxygen-powered nebulizer. Monitor the patient's response to these medications by noting improvement in PEFR and pulse oximetry readings.

Many asthmatic patients will wait before summoning EMS. The longer the time interval from the onset of the asthma attack until treatment, the less likely it will be that bronchodilator medications will work. Often, after a prolonged asthma attack, the patient may become fatigued. A fatigued patient can quickly develop respiratory failure and subsequently require intubation and mechanical ventilation. Always be prepared to provide airway and respiratory support for the asthmatic.

Content Review

MANAGEMENT GOALS FOR ASTHMA
- Correct hypoxia
- Reverse bronchospasm
- Reduce inflammation

Special Cases

Although most cases of asthma conform to the preceding descriptions, you may run into several special cases in the field. Asthma conditions that require special concern include status asthmaticus and asthmatic attacks in children.

Status Asthmaticus   Status asthmaticus is a severe, prolonged asthma attack that cannot be broken by repeated doses of bronchodilators. It is a serious medical emergency that requires prompt recognition, treatment, and transport. The patient suffering status asthmaticus frequently will have a greatly distended chest from continued air trapping. Breath sounds, and often wheezing, may be absent. The patient is usually exhausted, severely acidotic, and dehydrated. The management of status asthmaticus is basically the same as for asthma. *Recognize that respiratory arrest is imminent and be prepared for endotracheal intubation.* Transport immediately and continue aggressive treatment en route.

Asthma in Children   Asthma in children is common. The pathophysiology and treatment are essentially the same as in adults, with altered medication dosages. Several additional medications are used in the treatment of childhood asthma. (Asthma in children is discussed in greater detail in Chapter 31.)

UPPER RESPIRATORY INFECTION (URI)

Infections involving the upper airway and respiratory tract are among the most common infections for which patients seek medical attention. Although these conditions are rarely life threatening, upper respiratory infection (URI) can make many existing pulmonary diseases worse or lead to direct pulmonary infection. The best defense against the spread of URI is common practices such as good hand washing and covering the mouth during coughing and sneezing. Attention to such details is important when caring for patients with underlying pulmonary disease or those who are immunosuppressed (HIV infection, cancer) because URIs are more severe in these populations. Because of the prevalence of such infections, complete protection is impossible.

Pathophysiology

Remember that the upper airway begins at the nose and mouth, passes through the pharynx, and ends at the larynx. Other related structures are the paranasal sinuses and the eustachian tubes that connect the pharynx and the middle ear. In addition, several collections of lymphoid tissue found in the pharynx (palatine, pharyngeal, and lingual tonsils) produce antibodies and provide immune protection.

Structure	Infection	Symptoms	Signs
Nose	Rhinitis	Runny nose, congestion, sneezing	Rhinorrhea
Pharynx	Pharyngitis	Sore throat, pain on swallowing	Erythematous pharynx, tonsil enlargement, pus on tonsils, cervical lymph node enlargement
Middle ear	Otitis media	Ear pain, decreased hearing	Red, bulging eardrum, pus behind ear drum, lymph node enlargement in front of or behind ear
Larynx	Laryngitis	Sore throat, hoarseness, pain on speaking	Red pharynx, hoarse quality to voice, cervical lymph node enlargement
Epiglottis	Epiglottitis	Sore throat, drooling, ill appearing	Upright position, drooling, ill appearing
Sinuses	Sinusitis	Headache, congestion	Tenderness over the sinuses, worsening of pain with leaning forward, yellow nasal discharge

Table 19-2 · LOCATIONS AND SIGNS AND SYMPTOMS OF UPPER RESPIRATORY INFECTIONS

The vast majority of URIs are caused by viruses. A variety of bacteria may also produce infection of the upper respiratory tract. The most significant is Group A streptococcus, which is the causative organism in strep throat and accounts for up to 30% of URIs. This bacteria is also implicated in sinusitis and middle ear infections. Up to 50% of patients who have pharyngitis (inflammation of the pharynx) are not found to have a viral or bacterial cause. Fortunately, most URIs are self-limiting illnesses that resolve after several days of symptoms.

Assessment

Support the child with suspected epiglottitis in a position of comfort. Do not attempt examination of the throat, which may produce severe laryngospasm.

The major symptoms of URI depend on the portion of the upper respiratory tract that is predominantly affected (Table 19-2). Patients with URIs will often have accompanying symptoms such as fever, chills, myalgias (muscle pains), and fatigue.

Remember that any child with suspected epiglottitis (see Chapter 31) should be supported in a position of comfort. Do not attempt examination of the throat because this may produce severe laryngospasm. Adults do occasionally also develop epiglottitis, but this is generally a more benign condition.

Management

In URI, as with other medical conditions, focus attention on the patient's airway and ventilation. Give supplemental oxygen to any patient with underlying pulmonary disease.

In most cases, the diagnosis and treatment of upper respiratory conditions is based on the history and physical findings. Patients with pharyngitis are often diagnosed by obtaining a throat culture that confirms the presence of a bacterial cause of symptoms. A rapid test is also available. In patients with sinusitis and otitis media, treatment is based on a presumed bacterial cause.

As with other medical conditions, focus your attention on the patient's airway and ventilation. Generally, no intervention is required except in children with epiglottitis and in some complicated URIs where a collection of pus may occlude the airway. Give oxygen supplementation to any patient who has underlying pulmonary disease.

Most URIs are treated symptomatically. Acetaminophen or ibuprofen is prescribed for fever, headache, and myalgias. Encourage patients to drink plenty of fluids. Salt water gargles may be used for throat discomfort. Decongestants and antihistamines may be used to reduce mucus secretion. Encourage patients being treated with antibiotics for bacterial causes of URI to continue these agents.

In some patients with asthma or COPD, a URI may produce a worsening of their underlying medical condition. Use inhaled bronchodilators and corticosteroid agents according to local protocols or on advice of medical direction. Transport patients with underlying medical conditions to a health-care facility capable of continued evaluation and management of the underlying condition. Continue appropriate monitoring with pulse oximetry and ECG during transport.

PNEUMONIA

Pneumonia is an infection of the lungs and a common medical problem, especially in the aged and those infected with the human immunodeficiency virus (HIV). In fact, pneumonia is one of the leading causes of death in both groups of patients and is the fifth leading overall cause of death in the United States.

Patients with HIV infection and those on immune suppressive therapy (cancer patients) are at high risk of developing pneumonia. In addition, the very young and very old are at higher risk of acquiring pneumonia because of ineffective protective mechanisms. Other risk factors include a history of alcoholism, cigarette smoking, and exposure to cold temperatures.

Pathophysiology

Pneumonia is a collection of related respiratory diseases caused when a variety of infectious agents invade the lungs. Mucus production and the action of respiratory tract cilia play a role in protecting the body against bacterial invasion. When considering which patients are at risk, the unifying concept is that there is a defect in mucus production, ciliary action, or both.

Bacterial and viral pneumonias are the most frequent, although fungal and other forms of pneumonia do exist. More unusual forms of pneumonia are seen in those patients who are currently or recently have been hospitalized where they are exposed to a more unusual variety of microorganisms. This is referred to as hospital-acquired pneumonia. (Cases that develop in the out-of-hospital setting are described as community-acquired pneumonia.)

The infection begins in one part of the lung and often spreads to nearby alveoli. The infection may ultimately involve the entire lung. As the disease progresses, fluid and inflammatory cells collect in the alveoli, and alveolar collapse may occur. Pneumonia is primarily a ventilation disorder. Occasionally, the infection will extend beyond the lungs into the blood stream and to more distant sites in the body. This systemic spread may lead to septic shock.

Assessment

A patient with pneumonia will generally appear ill. He may report a recent history of fever and chills. These chills are commonly described as "bed shaking." There is usually a generalized weakness and malaise. The patient will tend to complain of a deep, productive cough and may expel yellow to brown sputum, often streaked with blood. Many cases involve associated **pleuritic** chest pain. Therefore, pneumonia should be considered in any patient who presents complaining of chest pain, especially if accompanied by fever and/or chills. In pneumonia involving the lower lobes of the lungs, a patient may complain of nothing more than upper abdominal pain.

Physical examination will commonly reveal fever, tachypnea, tachycardia, and a cough. Respiratory distress may be present. Auscultation of the chest usually demonstrates crackles (rales) in the involved lung segment, although wheezes or rhonchi may be heard. Usually air movement is decreased in the areas filled with infection. Percussion of the chest may reveal dullness over these areas. Egophony (a change in the spoken "E" sound to an "A" sound on auscultation) may also be noted.

In the forms of pneumonia involving viral, fungal, and rare bacterial causes, the typical symptoms described above are not seen. Instead, these patients may report a nonproductive cough with less prominent lung findings. Systemic symptoms such as headache, malaise, fatigue, muscle aches, sore throat, and abdominal complaints including nausea, vomiting, and diarrhea are more prominent. Fever and chills are not as impressive as in bacterial pneumonia.

Management

Pneumonia is generally diagnosed on the basis of physical examination, X-ray findings, and laboratory cultures. Therefore, diagnosis in the field is unlikely. The primary treatment is antibiotics to which the causative organism is susceptible. In the field, however, antibiotics are not indicated and treatment is purely supportive.

Place the patient in a comfortable position, and administer high-flow, high-concentration oxygen. Use pulse oximetry to assess the patient's oxygen requirements. In severe cases, ventilatory assistance is needed and endotracheal intubation may be required. Establish IV access and base fluid resuscitation on the patient's hydration status. Administering fluids for

> *Consider pneumonia in any patient complaining of chest pain, especially if accompanied by fever and/or chills.*

pleuritic sharp or tearing, as a description of pain.

> *Field management of suspected pneumonia is purely supportive. Place the patient in a position of comfort and administer high-flow, high-concentration oxygen.*

dehydration is appropriate, but overhydration can also worsen the respiratory condition. Medical direction may sometimes order a breathing treatment with a beta agonist, particularly if wheezing is present. Because patients with pneumonia often have some bronchospasm, these drugs will afford the patient some symptomatic relief. Give antipyretic agents such as acetaminophen or ibuprofen to reduce a high fever. Also, a cool, moistened wash cloth may soothe the patient.

Remember to be extremely careful when caring for the patient over age 65 with suspected pneumonia. These patients have high mortality and complication rates. Transport them to a facility capable of handling the significant complications associated with the disease for this population.

LUNG CANCER

Lung cancer (neoplasm) is the leading cause of cancer-related death in the United States in both men and women. Most patients with lung cancer are between the ages of 55 and 65 years. There is a high mortality rate for patients with lung cancer after only one year with the disease.

There are currently four major types of lung cancer based on the predominant cell type. About 20% of cases involve only the lung tissue. Another 35% involve spread to the lymphatic system, and 45% have distant metastases (cancer cells spreading to other tissues). In those cases where lung tissue is invaded, the primary problem is disruption of diffusion. In some larger cancers, there may also be alterations in ventilation by obstruction of the conducting bronchioles.

Cigarette smoking has long been known to be a risk factor for development of lung cancer. Environmental exposure to asbestos, hydrocarbons, radiation, and fumes from metal production have also been identified as risk factors. Finally, home exposure to radon has been implicated in the development of lung cancer. Preventive strategies include educating teenagers about the dangers of cigarette smoking and encouraging current smokers to quit. Implementing environmental safety standards that reduce the risk of exposure to such substances as asbestos will also reduce the risk of lung cancer. Finally, cancer screening of populations at risk is encouraged.

Pathophysiology

Although cancers that start elsewhere in the body can spread to the lungs, the vast majority of lung cancers are caused by carcinogens (cancer-producing substances) from cigarette smoking. A small number of lung cancers are caused by inhalation of occupational agents such as asbestos and arsenic. These substances irritate and adversely affect the various tissues of the lung, ultimately leading to the development of abnormal (cancerous) cells.

There are four major types of lung cancers depending on the type of lung tissue involved. The most common type of lung cancer is referred to as adenocarcinoma. This cancer arises from glandular-type (i.e. mucus-producing) cells found in the lungs and bronchioles. The next most frequently encountered type of lung cancer is *small cell carcinoma* (also called "oat cell" carcinoma). Small cell carcinoma arises from bronchial tissues. The third type of lung cancer is referred to as *epidermoid carcinoma*. Finally, *large cell carcinoma* is the fourth major type of lung cancer. As with small cell carcinoma, epidermoid and large cell carcinomas typically arise from the bronchial tissues. Lung cancers generally have a bad prognosis with most patients dying within a year of the diagnosis.

Assessment

In lung cancer, as with other respiratory diseases, your first priority is to address signs of respiratory distress.

As with other respiratory diseases, your first priority is to address signs of severe respiratory distress. Look for altered mental status, one to two word dyspnea, cyanosis, hemoptysis, and hypoxia as documented by pulse oximeter. Severe uncontrolled hemoptysis can be a particularly life-threatening presentation.

Patients with lung cancer will present with a variety of complaints, depending on whether they are related to direct lung involvement, invasion of local structures, or metastatic spread. Patients with localized disease will present with cough, dyspnea, hoarseness, vague chest pain, and hemoptysis. Fever, chills, and pleuritic chest pain are seen in patients who develop pneumonia. Symptoms related to local invasion include pain on swallowing (dysphagia), weakness or numbness in the arm, and shoulder pain. Metastatic symptoms are related to the area of spread and include headache, seizures, bone pain, abdominal pain, nausea, and malaise.

Physical findings are non-specific. Patients with advanced disease have profound weight loss and cachexia (general physical wasting and malnutrition). Crackles (rales), rhonchi, wheezes, and diminished breath sounds may be heard in the affected lung. Venous distention in the arms and neck may be present if the superior vena cava is occluded (called superior vena cava syndrome).

Management

Administer supplemental oxygen as needed based on the clinical status and pulse oximetry measurement. Support the patient's ventilation as needed and intubate as necessary. Be attentive, however, for any Do Not Resuscitate order or other advance directive, such as a living will, and follow your local protocol regarding these legal instruments. Consult medical direction if questions arise.

Initiate an IV of 0.9% normal saline and provide fluids if signs of dehydration are present. Follow your local protocol regarding the access of permanent indwelling catheters that many cancer victims have in place.

Out-of-hospital drug therapy consists of bronchodilator agents and corticosteroids when signs of obstructive lung disease are present. Continue any prescribed antibiotics. Transport the patient and monitor mental status, vital signs, and oxygen status, as appropriate. Be prepared to provide emotional support for both the patient and family during transport.

TOXIC INHALATION

Inhalation of toxic substances into the respiratory tract can cause pain, inflammation, or destruction of pulmonary tissues. Significant inhalations can affect the ability of the alveoli to exchange oxygen, thus resulting in hypoxemia.

Pathophysiology

The possibility of inhalation of products toxic to the respiratory system should be considered in any dyspneic patient. Causes of toxic inhalation include superheated air, toxic products of combustion, chemical irritants, and inhalation of steam. Each of these agents can result in upper airway obstruction due to edema and laryngospasm. In such cases, bronchospasm and lower-airway edema may additionally appear. In severe inhalations, disruption of the alveolar/capillary membranes may result in life-threatening pulmonary edema.

Assessment

When assessing the patient with possible toxic inhalation exposure, determine the nature of the inhalant or the combusted material. Several products can result in the formation of corrosive acids or alkalis that irritate and damage the airway. These include:

- Ammonia (ammonium hydroxide)
- Nitrogen oxide (nitric acid)
- Sulfur dioxide (sulphurous acid)
- Sulfur trioxide (sulfuric acid)
- Chlorine (hydrochloric acid)

It is also crucial to determine the duration of the exposure, whether the patient was in an enclosed area at the time of the exposure, or if he experienced a loss of consciousness. Loss of consciousness may cause the airway to become vulnerable as a result of the loss of airway protective mechanisms.

During physical examination, pay particular attention to the face, mouth, and throat. Note any burns or particulate matter. Next, auscultate the chest for the presence of any wheezes or crackles (rales). Wheezing may indicate bronchospasm. Crackles may suggest pulmonary edema.

When assessing the patient with possible toxic inhalation, determine the nature of the inhalant or combusted material.

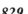

Content Review

MANAGEMENT SEQUENCE FOR TOXIC INHALATION

- Ensure safety of rescue personnel
- Remove patient from toxic environment
- Maintain an open airway
- Provide humidified, high-concentration oxygen

Management

After ensuring the safety of rescue personnel, remove the patient from the hazardous environment. Next, establish and maintain an open airway. Remember that the airway is often irritable and attempts at endotracheal intubation may result in laryngospasm, completely obstructing the airway. Laryngeal edema, as evidenced by hoarseness, brassy cough, and stridor is ominous and may require prompt endotracheal intubation. Administer humidified oxygen at high concentration. As a precaution, start an IV of a crystalloid solution to provide rapid venous access. Transport promptly.

CARBON MONOXIDE INHALATION

Carbon monoxide is an odorless, tasteless, colorless gas produced from the incomplete burning of fossil fuels and other carbon-containing compounds. Carbon monoxide can be encountered in industrial sites, such as mines and factories. It is present in the environment in various concentrations primarily because of automotive exhaust emissions. Most poisonings occur from automobile emissions and home-heating devices used in poorly ventilated areas. Carbon monoxide is often used in suicide attempts. In addition, it is a particular hazard for firefighters and rescue personnel.

Pathophysiology

Carbon monoxide exposure is potentially life threatening because it easily binds to the hemoglobin molecule. It has an affinity for hemoglobin 200 times that of oxygen. Once bound, receptor sites on the hemoglobin can no longer transport oxygen to the peripheral tissues. The result is hypoxia at the cellular level and, ultimately, metabolic acidosis. Additionally, carbon monoxide binds to iron-containing enzymes within the cells, leading to worsening cellular acidosis.

Assessment

With carbon-monoxide poisoning, determine the source of exposure, its length, and the location.

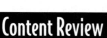

When confronted with a patient suffering possible carbon-monoxide poisoning, determine the source of exposure, its length, and the location. Less time is required to develop a significant exposure in a closed space compared with one in an area that is fairly well ventilated.

Signs and symptoms of carbon-monoxide poisoning include headache, nausea and vomiting, confusion, agitation, loss of coordination, chest pain, loss of consciousness, and even seizures. On physical examination, the skin may be cyanotic or it may be bright cherry red (a very late finding). There may be other signs of hypoxia such as peripheral cyanosis or confusion.

Management

Content Review

MANAGEMENT SEQUENCE FOR CARBON MONOXIDE INHALATION

- Ensure safety of rescue personnel
- Remove patient from exposure site
- Maintain an open airway
- Provide high-concentration oxygen

Upon detection of carbon monoxide poisoning, first ensure the safety of rescue personnel, then remove the patient from the site of exposure. Ensure and maintain the airway. Administer supplemental oxygen at the highest possible concentration. If the patient is breathing spontaneously, apply a *tight-fitting* nonrebreather mask. If respiratory depression is noted, assist respirations. If shock is present, treat. Prompt transport is essential.

Hyperbaric oxygen therapy may be used in the treatment of severe carbon monoxide poisoning. Many EMS systems have protocols established whereby patients suffering carbon monoxide poisoning are transported to hospitals with hyperbaric oxygen therapy facilities. Hyperbaric oxygen increases the PaO_2, thus promoting increased oxygen uptake and displacement of the carbon monoxide from the hemoglobin.

PULMONARY EMBOLISM

A pulmonary embolism is a blood clot (thrombus) or some other particle that lodges in a pulmonary artery, effectively blocking blood flow through that vessel. This condition is potentially life threatening because it can significantly decrease pulmonary blood flow, thus leading to hypoxemia (inadequate levels of oxygen in the blood). Pulmonary thromboembolism accounts for 50,000 deaths annually in the United States. In fact, one in five cases of sudden death are caused by pulmonary emboli. The great majority of patients with pulmonary emboli survive; only one in ten cases of documented pulmonary emboli result in death.

The incidence of pulmonary emboli is increased in certain populations. Any condition that results in immobility of the extremities can increase the risk of thromboembolism. Such conditions include recent surgery, long-bone fractures (with immobilization in casts or splints), bedridden condition, or prolonged immobilization as with long distance travel. Venous pooling that occurs during pregnancy can also lead to pulmonary emboli. Certain disease states increase the likelihood of blood clot formation. These include cancer, infections, thrombophlebitis, atrial fibrillation, and sickle cell anemia. Also, the incidence of thrombocmbolic disease is increased in patients taking oral birth control pills, particularly among smokers.

Pathophysiology

Sources of pulmonary emboli include air embolism, such as can occur during the placement of a central line; fat embolism, which can occur following a fracture; amniotic fluid embolism; and blood clots. It is also possible for a foreign body (such as part of a venous catheter) to become dislodged in the venous circulation. The vast majority of cases, however, are caused by blood clots that develop in the deep venous system of the lower extremities.

As a rule, a significant amount of blood passes through the veins of the lower extremity. During normal use of our legs, muscular contractions propel the blood through the venous system with the aid of valves that are present in the lower extremity veins. This action prevents blood from flowing backward through the venous system. When infection, venous injury, or any other condition that leads to pooling of blood in the deep veins of the lower extremity is present, clot formation occurs. If a portion of the clot becomes dislodged, it will pass through the right side of the heart and become lodged in the pulmonary vasculature.

When a pulmonary embolism occurs, the blockage of blood flow through the affected artery causes the right heart to pump against increased resistance. This results in an increase in pulmonary capillary pressure. The area of the lung supplied by the occluded pulmonary vessel can no longer effectively function in gas exchange since it receives no effective blood supply. The major derangement in patients with pulmonary emboli is a perfusion disorder. The involved lung segment is still ventilated, producing a ventilation-perfusion mismatch.

Assessment

Signs and symptoms of a patient suffering a pulmonary embolism vary, depending on the size and location of the obstruction. The patient suffering acute pulmonary embolism may report a sudden onset of severe unexplained dyspnea, which may or may not be associated with pleuritic chest pain. The patient may also report a cough that is usually not productive but may occasionally produce blood (hemoptysis). There may be a recent history of immobilization such as hip fracture, surgery, or debilitating illness.

The physical examination may reveal labored breathing, tachypnea, and tachycardia. In massive pulmonary emboli, there may be signs of right-heart failure such as jugular venous distention and, in some cases, falling blood pressure. In many cases, auscultation of the chest may reveal no significant lung findings, although rare crackles (rales) and wheezing may be noted. Occasionally, a pleural friction rub (leathery sound heard with inspiration) may be heard.

Always examine the extremities. In up to 50% of cases, findings that suggest deep venous thrombosis will be evident. These include a warm, swollen extremity with a thick cord palpated along the medial thigh and pain upon palpation or when extending the calf.

In extreme cases, the patient may present with extreme confusion as the result of hypoxia, severe cyanosis, profound hypotension, and even cardiac arrest. Physical examination may reveal petechiae (small hemorrhagic spots) on the arms and chest wall in these cases.

Management

As with all respiratory conditions, your first priorities are the airway, breathing, and circulation. Remember that a large pulmonary embolism may lead to cardiac arrest. Perform CPR if needed.

The patient with acute pulmonary embolism may have a sudden onset of severe unexplained dyspnea, with or without pleuritic chest pain.

With suspected pulmonary embolism, always examine the extremities. In up to 50% of cases, findings suggestive of deep venous thrombosis will be evident.

With pulmonary embolism, as with all respiratory conditions, your first priorities are airway, breathing, and circulation. Remember that a large pulmonary embolism may lead to cardiac arrest. Be prepared to perform CPR if needed.

If you suspect a patient is suffering a pulmonary embolism, establish and maintain an airway. Assist ventilations as required. Administer supplemental oxygen at the highest possible concentration. Endotracheal intubation may be required.

Establish an IV of lactated Ringer's or normal saline at a "to keep open" rate. The diagnosis of pulmonary embolism is often difficult and requires a high index of suspicion. Remember that patients with suspected pulmonary embolism may require a significant amount of care. This disorder has a high complication rate and a significant mortality. Carefully monitor the patient's vital signs and cardiac rhythm. Quickly transport the patient to a facility with the capabilities to care for the critical needs of the patient. Treatment in the hospital setting may include the use of various medications such as thrombolytic agents and blood thinners such as heparin.

SPONTANEOUS PNEUMOTHORAX

spontaneous pneumothorax a pneumothorax (collection of air in the pleural space) that occurs spontaneously, in the absence of blunt or penetrating trauma.

A **spontaneous pneumothorax** is defined as a pneumothorax that occurs in the absence of blunt or penetrating trauma. Spontaneous pneumothorax is a common clinical condition, with 18 cases occurring for every 100,000 population. There is also a high recurrence rate. About 50% of patients will have a recurrent episode within two years.

There is a 5:1 ratio of male to female patients with spontaneous pneumothorax. Other risk factors include a tall, thin stature and a history of cigarette smoking. This disorder tends to develop in patients between the ages of 20 and 40 years. Patients with COPD have a higher incidence of spontaneous pneumothorax, presumably because of the presence of thinned lung tissue (blebs) that may rupture.

Pathophysiology

The primary derangement is one of ventilation as the negative pressure that normally exists in the pleural space is lost. This prevents proper expansion of the lung in concert with the chest wall. A pneumothorax occupying 15% to 20% of the chest cavity is generally well tolerated by the patient unless the patient has significant underlying lung disease.

Assessment

The patient with a spontaneous pneumothorax presents with a sudden onset of sharp, pleuritic chest or shoulder pain. Often, the symptoms are precipitated by coughing or lifting. Dyspnea is commonly reported. The degree of symptoms is not strictly related to the size of the pneumothorax.

The physical examination is usually not impressive. Decreased breath sounds on the involved side may be difficult to note. They may be best heard at the lung apex. Even more subtle is hyper-resonance to percussion of the chest. Occasionally, the patient may have subcutaneous emphysema, which may be palpated as a crackling under the skin overlying the chest. Tachypnea, diaphoresis, and pallor are also seen. Cyanosis is rarely found.

Management

Use the patient's symptoms and pulse oximetry readings as guides to therapy. For most cases of spontaneous pneumothorax, supplemental oxygen is all that is required. Ventilatory support and endotracheal intubation are rarely required.

Be very careful when managing patients with a spontaneous pneumothorax who require positive pressure ventilation by mask or endotracheal tube. They are at risk for the development of a tension pneumothorax. You may note that the patient will become physically difficult to ventilate. Hypoxia, cyanosis, and hypotension may also develop. In addition to the usual signs of a pneumothorax, the patient will develop jugular vein distention and deviation of the trachea away from the pneumothorax. Needle decompression of a tension pneumothorax may be required.

Other management measures should include placing the patient in a position of comfort. Reserve IV access and ECG monitoring for patients with significant symptoms or severe underlying respiratory disease. Carefully monitor such patients during transport.

Table 19-3	CAUSES OF HYPERVENTILATION SYNDROME
Acidosis	Interstitial pneumonitis, fibrosis, edema
Beta-adrenergic agonists	Metabolic disorders
Bronchial asthma	Methyxanthine derivatives
Cardiovascular disorders	Neurologic disorders
Central nervous system infection or tumors	Pain
Congestive heart failure	Pregnancy
Drugs	Pneumonia
Fever, sepsis	Progesterone
Hepatic failure	Psychogenic or anxiety hypertension
High altitude	Pulmonary disease
Hypotension	Pulmonary emboli, vascular disease
Hypoxia	Salicylate

HYPERVENTILATION SYNDROME

Hyperventilation syndrome is characterized by rapid breathing, chest pains, numbness, and other symptoms usually associated with anxiety or a situational reaction. However, as shown in Table 19-3, many serious medical problems can cause hyperventilation. To avoid improper treatment, consider hyperventilation an indication of a serious medical problem until proven otherwise.

Consider hyperventilation an indication of a serious medical problem until proven otherwise.

Pathophysiology

Hyperventilation syndrome frequently occurs in anxious patients. The patient often senses that he cannot "catch his breath." The patient will then begin to breathe rapidly. Hyperventilation in a purely anxious patient results in the excess elimination of CO_2, causing a respiratory alkalosis. This increases the amount of bound calcium, producing a relative hypocalcemia. This results in cramping of the muscles of the feet and hands, which is called *carpopedal spasm.*

Assessment

With a hyperventilating patient, you may elicit a history of fatigue, nervousness, dizziness, dyspnea, chest pain, and numbness and tingling around the mouth, hands, and feet. The physical examination will reveal an anxious patient with tachypnea and tachycardia. As noted above, spasm of the fingers and feet may also be present. If the patient has a history of seizure disorder, the hyperventilation episode may precipitate a seizure. Other symptoms are related to the underlying cause of the hyperventilation syndrome.

Management

The primary treatment for hyperventilation syndrome is reassurance. Instruct the patient to voluntarily reduce his respiratory rate and depth of breathing. Mechanisms that will assist in increasing the PCO_2, such as breath holding or breathing into a paper bag, are discouraged in prehospital care. Hyperventilating patients require oxygen. Allowing them to rebreathe into a paper bag can be deadly. Many EMS systems permit EMT-Is to use rebreathing techniques only on physician order. It is important to exclude other medical causes before determining that a patient is hyperventilating. Check the oxygen saturation by applying a pulse oximeter. Do not withhold oxygen.

The primary treatment for hyperventilation is reassurance. Instruct the patient to reduce his respiratory rate and depth.

    The hyperventilating patient can often present a dilemma for prehospital personnel. Although anxiety is the most common cause of hyperventilation, other more serious diseases can present in exactly the same manner. For example, pulmonary embolism or acute myocardial infarction can exhibit symptoms similar to hyperventilation syndrome.

CENTRAL NERVOUS SYSTEM DYSFUNCTION

Central nervous system dysfunction, with the exception of drug overdose and massive stroke, is a relatively rare cause of respiratory emergencies. However, always consider the possibility of central nervous system dysfunction in any dyspneic patient.

Pathophysiology

Central nervous system dysfunction can be a causative factor in respiratory depression and arrest. Causes include head trauma, stroke, brain tumors, and various drugs. Several medications, such as narcotics and barbiturates, make the respiratory centers in the brain less responsive to increases in $PaCO_2$. These agents also depress areas of the brain responsible for initiating respirations.

Assessment

The assessment of patients with central nervous system dysfunction should follow the same approach as for any respiratory emergency. However, you should be alert for non-respiratory system problems such as central nervous system trauma or drug ingestion. Be careful to note any variation in the respiratory pattern, which can be an indication of central nervous system dysfunction.

Management

If central nervous system dysfunction is suspected, establish and maintain an open airway. If respiratory depression is noted or if respirations are absent, initiate mechanical ventilation. Administer supplemental oxygen, and establish an IV of normal saline at a "to keep open" rate. Direct specific therapy at the underlying problem, if it is known.

DYSFUNCTION OF THE SPINAL CORD, NERVES, OR RESPIRATORY MUSCLES

Several disease processes can affect the spinal cord, nerves, and/or respiratory muscles. Dysfunction of these structures can lead to hypoventilation and progressive hypoxemia.

Pathophysiology

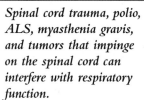

Numerous disorders can interfere with respiratory function. These include spinal cord trauma, polio, amyotrophic lateral sclerosis (ALS or Lou Gehrig's disease), and myasthenia gravis. Viral infections, in certain cases, can cause dysfunction of the nervous system. An example of this is *Guillian-Barré Syndrome (GBS)*. In GBS, the myelin covering of the nerve is damaged resulting in relative loss of nerve impulse conduction. This affects virtually every peripheral nerve. Approximately 30% of patients with GBS will require ventilatory assistance, because the nerves that stimulate respiration are impaired.

Certain tumors can impinge on the spinal cord, depressing respiratory function. These disorders result in an inability of the respiratory muscles to contract normally, thus causing hypoventilation. Tidal volume and minute volume are decreased. You should also be aware that patients with these disorders do not have the ability to generate an adequate cough reflex and as a result, are at risk of developing pneumonia.

Assessment

Patients with possible dysfunction of the spinal cord, nerves, or respiratory muscles may have a history of trauma that is not readily apparent. Always question the patient about injuries or falls. If there is any doubt about a possible injury, act accordingly and immobilize the cervical spine. Also, inquire about signs of symptoms that may suggest a problem with the peripheral nerves. These include such findings as numbness, pain, or sensory dysfunction. The assessment of patients with possible dysfunction of the spinal cord, nerves, or respiratory muscles should follow the same approach as for any respiratory emergency. However, be alert for subtle findings that may indicate a problem with the peripheral nervous system. Always be ready to protect the airway and support ventilation if the patient has symptoms of possible airway obstruction or respiratory failure.

Management

Management of spinal cord and respiratory muscle dysfunction is purely supportive. Establish an airway and provide ventilatory support. If myasthenia gravis is present and if transport time is long, the physician may request the administration of one of several agents effective in treating such patients.

Management of spinal cord and respiratory muscle dysfunction is purely supportive.

Summary

Respiratory emergencies are commonly encountered in prehospital care. It is important to recognize that all respiratory disorders may produce derangements in ventilation, perfusion, or diffusion. Recognition and treatment must be prompt. Understanding the underlying cause of the respiratory disorder can guide therapy. The primary treatment is to correct hypoxia. Necessary steps include establishing and maintaining the airway, assisting ventilations as required, and administering supplemental oxygen. Appropriate pharmacological agents may be subsequently ordered by medical direction.

On the Web

For additional practice and review, go to the companion website at www.prenhall.com/bledsoe and click on *Intermediate Emergency Care: Principles & Practice.*

CHAPTER 20

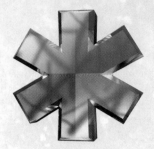

Cardiovascular Emergencies

Objectives

Part 1: Cardiovascular Anatomy and Physiology, ECG Monitoring, and Dysrhythmia Analysis (begins on page 839).

After reading Part 1 of this chapter, you should be able to:

1. Describe the incidence, morbidity, and mortality of cardiovascular disease. (pp. 838–839)
2. Review cardiovascular anatomy and physiology. (pp. 839–843, and see Chapter 2)
3. Discuss prevention strategies that may reduce morbidity and mortality of cardiovascular disease. (pp. 838–839)
4. Identify the risk factors most predisposing to coronary artery disease. (pp. 838–839)
5. Explain the purpose of ECG monitoring and its limitations. (pp. 843–855)
6. Describe how ECG wave forms are produced and correlate the electrophysiological and hemodynamic events occurring throughout the entire cardiac cycle with the various ECG

wave forms, segments, and intervals. (pp. 843–855)
7. Identify how heart rates may be determined from ECG recordings. (pp. 844–846)
8. Describe a systematic approach to the analysis and interpretation of cardiac dysrhythmias. (pp. 855–897)
9. Explain how to confirm asystole using more than one lead. (pp. 890–891)
10. List the clinical indications for defibrillation. (pp. 890–891)
11. Identify the specific mechanical, pharmacological, and electrical therapeutic interventions for patients with dysrhythmias causing compromise. (pp. 855–897)

Part 2: Assessment and Management of the Cardiovascular Patient (begins on page 897).

After reading Part 2 of this chapter, you should be able to:

1. Identify and describe the components of assessment as it relates to the patient with cardiovascular compromise (pp. 897–905)
2. List the clinical indications for an implanted defibrillation device. (p. 912)
3. Define angina pectoris and myocardial infarction (MI). (pp. 922–930)
4. List other clinical conditions that may mimic signs and symptoms of angina pectoris and myocardial infarction. (p. 923)

5. List the mechanisms by which an MI may be produced by traumatic and non-traumatic events. (pp. 923–925)
6. List and describe the assessment parameters to be evaluated in a patient with chest pain. (pp. 925–927)
7. Identify what is meant by the OPQRST of chest pain assessment. (pp. 898–899)
8. List and describe the initial assessment parameters to be evaluated in—and the anticipated presentation of—a patient with chest pain that may be myocardial in origin. (pp. 898, 923–924, 926)
9. Describe the pharmacological agents available to the EMT-Intermediate for use in the management of dysrhythmias and cardiovascular emergencies. (pp. 910, 911)
10. Develop, execute, and evaluate a treatment plan based on the field impression for the patient with chest pain that may be indicative of angina or myocardial infarction. (pp. 924, 927–930)
11. Define the terms congestive heart failure and pulmonary edema and the cardiac and non-cardiac causes and terminology associated with them. (pp. 930–931)
12. Describe the early and late signs and symptoms of pulmonary edema. (pp. 931–932)
13. Explain the clinical significance of paroxysmal nocturnal dyspnea. (pp. 931–932)
14. List and describe the pharmacological agents available to the EMT-Intermediate for use in the management of a patient with cardiac compromise. (pp. 932–933)
15. Define the term hypertensive emergency (p. 934)
16. Describe the clinical features of the patient in a hypertensive emergency. (pp. 934–935)
17. List the interventions prescribed for the patient with a hypertensive emergency. (p. 935)
18. Define the term cardiogenic shock. (p. 935)
19. Identify the clinical criteria for cardiogenic shock. (pp. 936–938)
20. Define the term cardiac arrest. (p. 938)
21. Define the term resuscitation. (p. 938)
22. Identify local protocol dictating circumstances and situations where resuscitation efforts would not be initiated or would be discontinued. (pp. 939–942)
23. Identify the critical actions necessary in caring for the patient in cardiac arrest. (pp. 938–939)
24. Synthesize patient history and assessment findings to form a field impression for the patient with chest pain and cardiac dysrhythmias that may be indicative of a cardiac emergency. (pp. 897–945)
25. Given several preprogrammed patients with cardiac complaints, provide the appropriate assessment, treatment, and transport. (pp. 897–945)

CASE STUDY

The crew of Unit 112 is called to a local nursing home to evaluate Mr. Evan Henry, an 80-year-old male with chest pain. It is Sunday afternoon, and Mr. Henry's family has been visiting from out of town. Not used to all the attention and excitement, Mr. Henry has developed substernal chest pain that radiates to his left arm. He has a history of this type of pain, but it usually resolves after one or two sublingual nitroglycerin tablets. This time, however, the nitroglycerin tablets have failed to alleviate his pain. Because of this, the nursing home staff has activated the EMS system.

Today, Unit 112 is staffed by EMT-Is David Bratcher and Bart Betik. When the crew arrives at the nursing home, the nursing home staff meets them and shows them to Mr. Henry's room. Several worried family members are nearby. The EMT-Is place Mr. Henry on a cardiac monitor, establish an IV line, and administer oxygen. They perform an initial assessment and a focused history and physical exam. While Bart is listening to Mr. Henry's chest, the patient suddenly screams and collapses. A quick check finds him to be pulseless and apneic. The monitor reveals coarse ventricular fibrillation. David charges the defibrillator and delivers a 200-joule shock. The ECG remains unchanged and David delivers a second shock, this time at 300 joules. Mr. Henry remains in ventricular

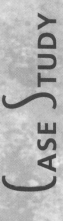
fibrillation. David again charges the defibrillator and delivers a third shock at 360 joules. Unfortunately, the patient and ECG remain the same.

An engine company arrives within 2 minutes. The crew helps to continue CPR, while Bart places an endotracheal tube. The patient is ventilated with 100% oxygen. An end-tidal carbon dioxide detector and good, equal breath sounds confirm proper placement of the endotracheal tube. David administers 1 mg of epinephrine 1:10,000 intravenously. Following this, a fourth countershock is delivered at 360 joules. This converts the patient to a slow idioventricular rhythm. This rhythm subsequently improves to a sinus tachycardia with a weak pulse. The pulse becomes stronger and cardiac compressions are stopped. Two minutes later, the blood pressure is 110 mmHg by palpation. The ECG shows a few premature ventricular contractions developing. David administers 100 milligrams of lidocaine intravenously and begins a lidocaine drip at 2 milligrams per minute. The EMT-Is and crew continue mechanical ventilation and move the patient to the ambulance.

The EMT-Is transport the patient to the hospital. En route, the patient starts to awaken and begins to breathe on his own. In the emergency department, a 12-lead ECG confirms the presence of an anterior wall myocardial infarction. The patient is transferred to the cardiac intensive care unit. Mr. Henry rapidly improves and is weaned from the ventilator. He subsequently undergoes cardiac rehabilitation. The attending physician discharges him back to the nursing home and prescribes three different medications.

INTRODUCTION

More than 60 million people in the United States have some form of cardiovascular disease.

cardiovascular disease (CVD)
disease affecting the heart, peripheral blood vessels, or both.

coronary heart disease (CHD)
a type of CVD; the single largest killer of people in the United States.

According to current estimates, more than 60 million people in the United States have some form of **cardiovascular disease (CVD). Coronary heart disease (CHD),** a type of CVD, is the single largest killer. Each year, on average, 466,000 people die of CHD. Approximately 225,000 of them, a little more than half, die before ever reaching the hospital. Another way of looking at the impact of CHD is this: An American will suffer a nonfatal heart attack every 29 seconds. About once every minute, an American will die from CHD. These deaths are usually sudden and often due to lethal cardiac rhythm disturbances that result in cardiac arrest.

Sudden death from CHD is often preventable. To decrease the chances of sudden death, the patient must recognize the signs and symptoms early and seek health care. Then, the health-care system must provide definitive care promptly, usually within the first hour after the onset of symptoms.

Public education about CHD has focused on two strategies. The first is to educate the public about the risk factors for the development of CHD. This program encourages patients to modify their lifestyle to minimize these risk factors. A variety of factors have been proven to increase the risk of cardiovascular disease. These include:

- Smoking
- Older age
- Family history of cardiac disease
- Hypertension (high blood pressure)
- Hypercholesterolemia (excessive cholesterol in the blood)
- Carbohydrate intolerance (diabetes mellitus)
- Cocaine use
- Male gender

Factors that are *thought* to increase the risk of coronary heart disease include:

- Diet
- Obesity

- Oral contraceptives (birth control pills)
- Sedentary lifestyle
- Type A personality (competitive, aggressive, hostile)
- Psychosocial tensions (stress)

The second component of public education is to teach recognition of the signs and symptoms of heart attack. Patients can only benefit from medical intervention if they recognize the signs and symptoms and promptly access the health care system. Patients are encouraged to access the EMS system early. As an EMT-I, you will treat patients who already have developed the manifestations of cardiac disease. This will be an opportunity for you to further serve your patients by teaching preventive strategies, including early recognition of symptoms, education, and alteration of lifestyle.

This chapter discusses the advanced prehospital care of cardiovascular emergencies. First, you will review the pertinent anatomy and physiology, and then that knowledge will be used to discuss assessing, recognizing, and treating cardiovascular disorders.

Part 1: Cardiovascular Anatomy and Physiology, ECG Monitoring, and Dysrhythmia Analysis

REVIEW OF CARDIOVASCULAR ANATOMY AND PHYSIOLOGY

Cardiac anatomy and physiology were discussed in detail in Chapter 2. The following is a brief review of that information.

CARDIOVASCULAR ANATOMY

The heart is located in the center of the chest in the *mediastinum*. It is a muscular organ, consisting of three tissue layers: *endocardium* (the innermost layer that lines the chambers), *myocardium* (the middle layer with its unique ability to generate and conduct electrical impulses, causing the heart to contract), and *pericardium* (the protective sac surrounding the heart).

The heart (Figure 20-1) contains four chambers—two superior, *the atria,* and two inferior, *the ventricles.* Valves control the flow of blood through the heart: the *mitral valve* between the left atrium and ventricle; the *tricuspid valve* between the right atrium and ventricle; the *aortic valve* between the left ventricle and aorta; the *pulmonary valve* between the right ventricle and pulmonary artery.

The right atrium receives deoxygenated blood from the body via the *superior* and *inferior venae cavae.* The right ventricle sends the deoxygenated blood to the lungs via the *pulmonary artery.* Oxygenated blood is returned from the lungs to the *left atrium* via the *pulmonary veins.* The left ventricle pumps the oxygenated blood to the body via the *aorta.* Oxygenated blood is pumped from the heart to the tissues via the *arteries,* and deoxygenated blood is transported from the tissues back to the heart via the *veins.* The *capillaries* connect arteries and veins. The exchange of oxygen and carbon dioxide with the body tissues takes place through the very thin capillary walls.

The heart receives its nutrients from the *coronary arteries* (Figure 20-2) that originate in the aorta and spread over the heart. The *left coronary artery* supplies the left ventricle, interventricular septum, part of the right ventricle, and the conduction system. Its two main branches are the *anterior descending artery* and *circumflex artery.* The *right coronary artery* supplies a portion of the right atrium and right ventricle and part of the conduction system. Its two major branches are the *posterior descending artery* and *marginal artery.*

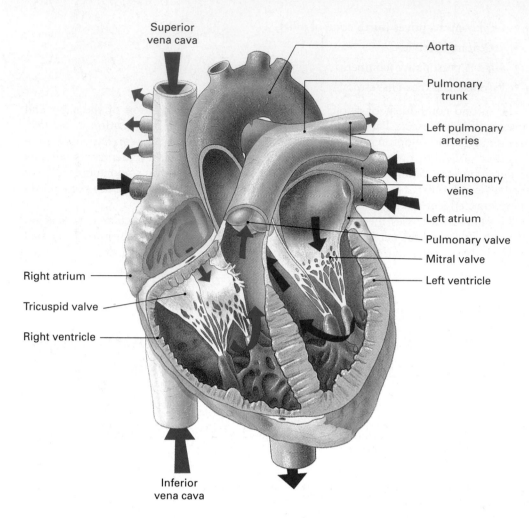

FIGURE 20-1 Blood flow through the heart.

CARDIAC PHYSIOLOGY

The *cardiac cycle* consists of *diastole,* the relaxation phase that takes place at the end of a cardiac contraction, and *systole,* the contraction phase. Normally, when the heart contracts each ventricle ejects about two-thirds of the blood it contains (the ejection fraction). The amount of blood ejected, known as the *stroke volume,* averages 70 mL. The stroke volume depends on three factors: preload, cardiac contractility, and afterload. *Preload* is the end-diastolic volume and influences the force of the next contraction because of the stretch it exerts. (*Starling's law of the heart* states that the more myocardial muscle is stretched, the greater its force of contraction will be.) *Afterload* is the resistance against which the heart muscle must pump. An increase in peripheral vascular resistance will decrease stroke volume; a decrease in resistance will increase stroke volume.

Cardiac output is calculated as stroke volume times heart rate. Since the normal heart rate is 60 to 100 beats per minute and the average stroke volume is 70 mL, the average cardiac output is about 5 liters (5,000 mL) per minute (70 mL × 70 bpm = 4,900 mL/min).

Heart function is regulated by the sympathetic and parasympathetic nervous components of the autonomic nervous system, working in opposition to one another to maintain a balance. During stress, the sympathetic system dominates to raise the heart rate and increase contractile force. During sleep, the parasympathetic system dominates to decrease heart rate and contractile force. The terms *chronotropy* (referring to heart rate), *inotropy* (referring to contractile strength), and *dromotropy* (referring to rate of nervous impulse conduction) describe autonomic control of the heart.

Cardiac function depends heavily on electrolyte balances. Electrolytes that affect cardiac function include sodium (Na^+), calcium (Ca^{++}), potassium (K^+), chloride (Cl^-), and

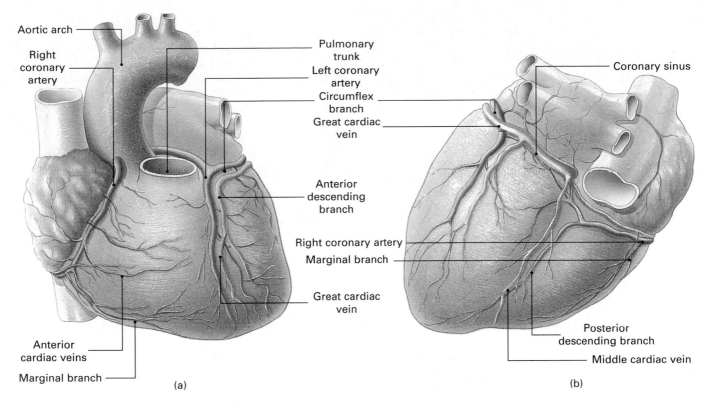

Labels for image (a):
Aortic arch
Right coronary artery
Pulmonary trunk
Left coronary artery
Circumflex branch
Great cardiac vein
Anterior descending branch
Great cardiac vein
Anterior cardiac veins
Marginal branch
(a)

Labels for image (b):
Coronary sinus
Right coronary artery
Marginal branch
Posterior descending branch
Middle cardiac vein
(b)

FIGURE 20-2   The coronary circulation: (a) anterior; (b) posterior.

magnesium (Mg^{++}). Sodium plays a major role in depolarizing the myocardium. Calcium takes part in myocardial depolarization and myocardial contraction. Potassium influences repolarization. Research is ongoing into the roles of magnesium and chloride.

ELECTROPHYSIOLOGY

Within the cardiac muscle fibers are special structures called *intercalated discs*. These discs connect cardiac muscle fibers and conduct electrical impulses quickly from one muscle fiber to the next. Thus, when one cell becomes excited, the action potential spreads rapidly across the entire group of cells, resulting in a coordinated contraction. This functional unit is a *syncytium*. The heart has two syncytia—the *atrial syncytium* and the *ventricular syncytium*. The atrial syncytium contracts from superior to inferior, so that the atria express blood to the ventricles. The ventricular syncytium contracts from inferior to superior, expelling blood from the ventricles into the aorta and pulmonary arteries. An impulse can be conducted from the atria to the ventricles only through the *atrioventricular (AV) bundle*.

Cardiac muscle functions according to an "all-or-none" principle. That is, if a single muscle fiber becomes *depolarized*, the action potential will spread through the whole syncytium. Stimulating a single atrial fiber will thus completely depolarize the atria, and stimulating a single ventricular fiber will completely depolarize the ventricles.

Cardiac Depolarization

Normally, an ionic difference exists on the two sides of a cell membrane. The cell's sodium-potassium pump expels sodium (Na$^+$) from the cell, leaving the inside of the cell more negatively charged than the outside. This difference is called the *resting potential*. When the myocardial cell is stimulated, the membrane changes to allow positively charged sodium ions to rush into the cell, giving the inside of the cell a greater positive charge than the outside. This change of membrane polarity is the *action potential*. After the influx of sodium, a slower influx of calcium ions (Ca^{++}) increases the positive charge inside the cell.

This change from the resting potential (when the inside of the cell is more negatively charged) to a relatively more positive charge inside the cell is called *cardiac depolarization*.

Once depolarization occurs in a muscle fiber, it is transmitted throughout the entire syncytium, via the intercalated discs, until the entire muscle mass is depolarized. Contraction of the muscle follows depolarization. The cell membrane remains permeable to sodium for only a fraction of a second. Thereafter, sodium influx stops and potassium escapes from inside the cell. This returns the charge inside the cell to normal (negative). In addition, sodium is actively pumped outside the cell, allowing the cell to *repolarize* and return to its normal resting state.

Understanding the process of cardiac depolarization is critical to understanding and interpreting ECGs.

Cardiac Conductive System

The cardiac conductive system stimulates the ventricles to depolarize in the proper direction. It initiates an impulse, spreads it through the atria, transmits it to the apex of the heart, and thence stimulates the ventricles to depolarize from inferior to superior. The conduction system relies on specialized conductive fibers that transmit the depolarization potential through the heart very quickly.

To accomplish their task, the cardiac conductive cells have:

- *Excitability.* The cells can respond to an electrical stimulus.
- *Conductivity.* The cells can propagate the electrical impulse from cell to cell.
- *Automaticity.* Each conductive cell can depolarize without any outside impulse (called self-excitation). Generally, the cell with the fastest rate of discharge, becomes the heart's pacemaker. Usually, this is the sinoatrial (SA) node; however, if one pacemaker cell fails to discharge, then the cell with the next fastest rate becomes the pacemaker.
- *Contractility.* The cells have the ability to contract, or constrict.

Internodal atrial pathways connect the SA node to the AV node (Figure 20-3). These internodal pathways conduct the depolarization impulse to the atrial muscle mass and through the atria to the AV junction. The AV junction (the "gatekeeper") slows the impulse and allows the ventricles time to fill. Then, the impulse passes through the AV junction into the AV node and on to the AV fibers, which conduct the impulse from the atria to the ventricles. In the ventricles the AV fibers form the *bundle of His*.

The bundle of His subsequently divides into the right and left bundle branches. The *right bundle branch* delivers the impulse to the apex of the right ventricle. From there the *Purkinje system* spreads it across the myocardium. The *left bundle branch* divides into

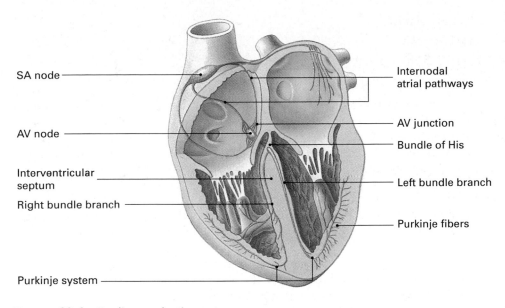

SA node		Internodal atrial pathways
AV node		AV junction
		Bundle of His
Interventricular septum		Left bundle branch
Right bundle branch		
		Purkinje fibers
Purkinje system		

FIGURE 20-3 Cardiac conductive system.

anterior and *posterior fascicles* that also ultimately terminate in the Purkinje system. At the same time that the impulse is transmitted to the right ventricle, the Purkinje system spreads it across the mass of the myocardium. Repolarization predominantly occurs in the opposite direction.

Each conductive system component has an intrinsic rate of self-excitation (SA node 60 to 100 bpm; AV node 40 to 60 bpm; Purkinje system 15 to 40 bpm).

ELECTROCARDIOGRAPHIC MONITORING

One of your most important skills as an EMT-I will be obtaining and interpreting ECG **rhythm strips.** Your patient's subsequent treatment will be based on rapid, accurate interpretation of these strips. At first, rhythm strips may seem very difficult to read, for only through classroom instruction and repeated practice can you master their interpretation. Nor will every rhythm strip you encounter be a textbook example; you must be comfortable with all possible variants. With practice and a systematic approach, however, you will soon be skilled in their interpretation. This section presents basic information about ECG monitoring, as well as recognizing and interpreting dysrhythmias.

ELECTROCARDIOGRAM

The **electrocardiogram (ECG)** is a graphic record of the heart's electrical activity. However, it tells you nothing about the heart's pumping ability, which you must evaluate by pulse and blood pressure.

The body acts as a giant conductor of electricity, and the heart is its largest generator of electrical energy. Electrodes on the skin can detect the total electrical activity within the heart at any given time. The electrical impulses on the skin surface have a very low voltage. The ECG machine amplifies these impulses and records them over time on ECG graph paper or a monitor. *Positive impulses* appear as upward deflections on the paper, and *negative impulses* as downward deflections. The absence of any electrical impulse produces an *isoelectric line,* which is flat.

Artifacts are deflections on the ECG produced by factors other than the heart's electrical activity. Common causes of artifacts include:

- Muscle tremors
- Shivering

One of your most important skills as an EMT-I will be obtaining and interpreting ECG rhythm strips.

rhythm strip
electrocardiogram printout.

electrocardiogram (ECG) the graphic recording of the heart's electrical activity, which may be displayed either on paper or on an oscilloscope.

artifact deflection on the ECG produced by factors other than the heart's electrical activity.

bipolar limb leads
electrocardiogram leads that are applied to the arms and legs and contain two electrodes of opposite (positive and negative) polarity; Leads I, II, and III.

Einthoven's triangle the triangle around the heart formed by the bipolar limb leads.

augmented limb leads another term for unipolar limb leads, reflecting the fact that the ground lead is disconnected, which increases the amplitude of deflection on the ECG tracing.

unipolar limb leads
electrocardiogram leads applied to the arms and legs, consisting of one polarized (positive) electrode and a nonpolarized reference point that is created by the ECG machine combining two additional electrodes; also called augmented limb leads; leads aVR, aVL, and aVF.

precordial (chest) leads
electrocardiogram leads applied to the chest in a pattern that permits a view of the horizontal plane of the heart; leads V_1, V_2, V_3, V_4, V_5, and V_6.

- Patient movement
- Loose electrodes
- 60 hertz interference
- Machine malfunction

It is important for ECGs to be free of artifacts. When an artifact is present, you must first try to eliminate it before recording the ECG. Loose electrodes should be replaced. Occasionally, patients may be quite diaphoretic, thus preventing the electrodes from adhering well to the skin. In these cases, you may need to wipe the skin and apply tincture of Benzoin before applying the electrode.

ECG Leads

You can obtain many views of the heart's electrical activity by monitoring the voltage change through *electrodes* placed at various places on the body surface. Each pair of electrodes is a *lead*. In the hospital, 12 leads are normally used. As a rule, most EMS systems use only three leads in the field. In fact, one lead is adequate for detecting life-threatening dysrhythmias. With the advent of thrombolytic therapy and computer interpretation, however, 12-lead ECGs are becoming more common in the field, especially in rural areas.

The three types of ECG leads are bipolar, augmented, and precordial. **Bipolar leads,** the kind most frequently used, have one positive electrode and one negative electrode. Any electrical impulse moving toward the positive electrode will cause a positive (upward) deflection on the ECG paper. Any electrical impulse moving toward the negative electrode will cause a negative (downward) deflection. The absence of a positive or negative deflection means either that there is no electrical impulse or that the impulse is moving perpendicular to the lead. Leads I, II, and III, commonly called *limb leads,* are bipolar. They are the most frequently used leads in the field. Table 20-1 lists their placement sites.

These three bipolar leads form **Einthoven's triangle,** named after Dr. Willem Einthoven, who invented the ECG machine (Figure 20-4). The direction from the negative to the positive electrode is the lead's *axis*. Each lead shows a different axis of the heart. Lead I, at the top of Einthoven's triangle, has an axis of 0°. Lead II forms the right side of the triangle and has an axis of 60°. Lead III forms the left side of the triangle and has an axis of 120°.

The bipolar leads provide only three views of the heart. **Augmented leads,** or **unipolar leads,** provide additional views that are sometimes useful. Although these leads evaluate different axes than the bipolar leads, they utilize the same electrodes. They do this by electronically combining the negative electrodes of two of the bipolar leads to obtain an axis. These augmented leads are designated aVR, aVL, and aVF. The letter *a* indicates that the lead is augmented. The letter *V* identifies it as a unipolar lead. The *R, L,* and *F* identify the extremity on which the lead is placed (*R* = right arm, *L* = left arm, and *F* = left foot).

In addition, six **precordial leads** can be placed across the surface of the chest to measure electrical cardiac activity on a horizontal axis. These leads help in viewing the left ventricle and septum. They are designated V_1 through V_6, with the letter *V* identifying them as unipolar leads.

Routine ECG Monitoring

Whether in the ambulance, emergency department, or coronary care unit, routine ECG monitoring generally uses only one lead. The most common monitoring leads are either lead II or the *modified chest lead 1* (MCL_1). Of these, Lead II is used more frequently because most of the heart's electrical current flows toward its positive axis. This gives the best view

Table 20-1 Bipolar Lead Placement Sites

Lead	Positive Electrode	Negative Electrode
I	Left arm	Right arm
II	Left leg	Right arm
III	Left leg	Left arm

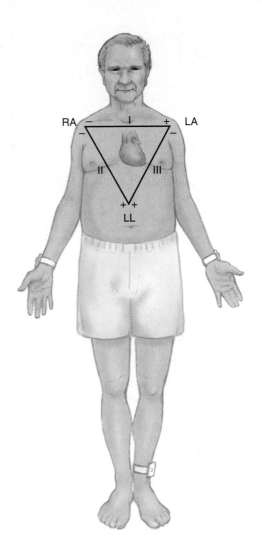

FIGURE 20-4 Einthoven's triangle as formed by Leads I, II, and III.

of the ECG waves and best depicts the conduction system's activity. MCL_1 is a special monitoring lead that some systems use selectively to help determine the origin of abnormal complexes such as premature beats. To avoid confusion, we will use Lead II as the monitor lead throughout this text.

Einthoven's triangle offers a basis for placing the leads. Usually you should place the electrodes on the chest wall instead of the extremities. This helps to reduce artifacts from arm movement. (If you use the arms, place the lead as high as possible on the extremity to decrease movement.) Make certain the skin is clean and free of hair before you place the electrodes on the chest wall. For Lead II, the positive electrode is usually placed at the apex of the heart on the chest wall (or on the left leg), the negative electrode below the right clavicle (or on the right arm). The third electrode, the ground, is placed somewhere on the left, upper chest wall (or on the left arm).

A single monitoring lead can provide considerable information, including:

- The rate of the heartbeat
- The regularity of the heartbeat
- The time it takes to conduct the impulse through the various parts of the heart

A single lead cannot provide the following information:

- The presence or location of an infarct
- Axis deviation or chamber enlargement
- Right-to-left differences in conduction or impulse formation
- The quality or presence of pumping action

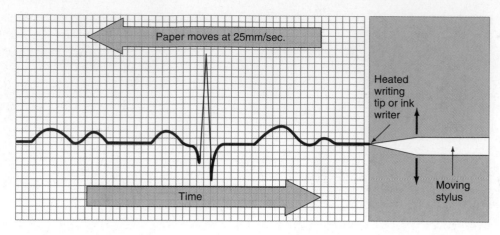

FIGURE 20-5   Recording of the ECG.

ECG Graph Paper

ECG graph paper is standardized to allow comparative analysis of ECG patterns. The paper moves across the stylus at a standard speed of 25 mm/sec (Figure 20-5). The amplitude of the ECG deflection is also standardized. When properly calibrated, the ECG stylus should deflect two large boxes when 1 millivolt (mV) is present. Most machines have calibration buttons, and a calibration curve should be placed at the beginning of the first ECG strip. Many machines do this automatically when they are first turned on.

The ECG graph is divided into a grid of light and heavy lines. The light lines are 1 mm apart, and the heavy lines are 5 mm apart. The heavy lines thus enclose large squares, each containing 25 of the smaller squares formed by the lighter lines (Figure 20-6). The following relationships apply to the horizontal axis:

1 small box = 0.04 sec

1 large box = 0.20 sec (0.04 sec × 5 = 0.20 sec)

These increments measure the duration of the ECG complexes and time intervals. The vertical axis reflects the voltage amplitude in millivolts (mV). Two large boxes equal 1.0 mV.

In addition to the grid, ECG paper has time interval markings at the top. These marks are placed at three-second intervals. Each three-second interval contains 15 large boxes (0.2 sec × 15 boxes = 3.0 sec). The time markings measure heart rate.

RELATIONSHIP OF THE ECG TO ELECTRICAL EVENTS IN THE HEART

The ECG tracing's components reflect electrical changes in the heart (Figure 20-7):

- *P wave.* The first component of the ECG, the P wave corresponds to atrial depolarization. On Lead II, it is a positive, rounded wave before the QRS complex (Figures 20-8 to 20-12).

- *QRS complex.* The QRS complex reflects ventricular depolarization. The Q wave is the first negative deflection after the P wave; the R wave is the first positive deflection after the P wave; and the S wave is the first negative deflection after the R wave. Not all three waves are always present, and the shape of the QRS complex can vary from individual to individual (Figure 20-13).

- *T wave.* The T wave reflects repolarization of the ventricles. Normally positive in Lead II, it is rounded and usually moves in the same direction as the QRS complex (Figure 20-14).

- *U wave.* Occasionally, a U wave appears. U waves follow T waves and are usually positive. U waves may be associated with electrolyte abnormalities, or they may be a normal finding.

FIGURE 20-6 ECG paper and markings.

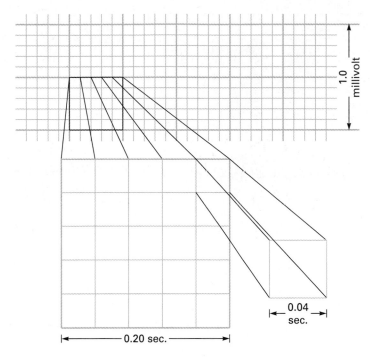

1.0 millivolt

0.04 sec.

0.20 sec.

FIGURE 20-7 Relationship of the ECG to electrical activities in the heart.

SA node

Internodal atrial conduction pathways

AV junction

Bundle of His

AV node

Bundle branches

Purkinje network

Atrial depolarization

Ventricular depolarization

Ventricular repolarization

Seconds   0   0.2   0.4   0.6

P   QRS   T

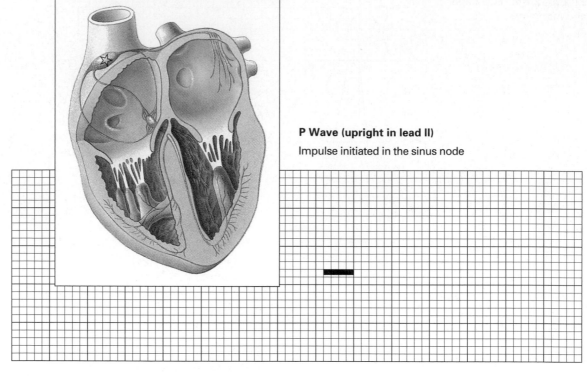

P Wave (upright in lead II)

Impulse initiated in the sinus node

FIGURE 20-8   Impulse initiation in the SA node.

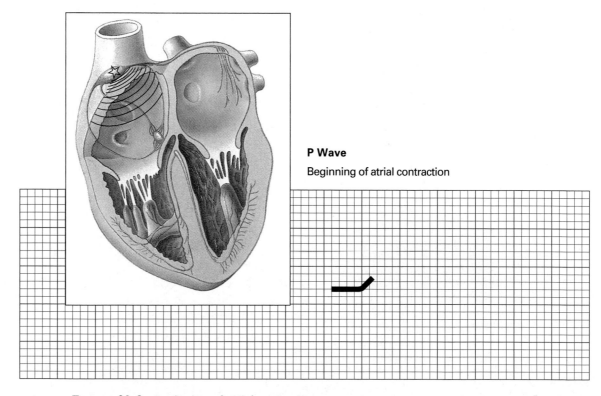

P Wave

Beginning of atrial contraction

FIGURE 20-9   Beginning of atrial contraction.

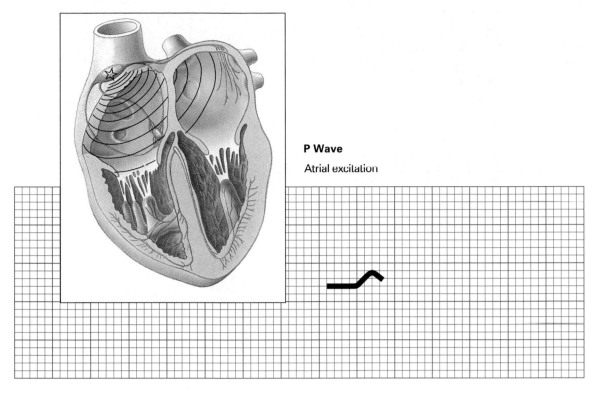

P Wave

Atrial excitation

FIGURE 20-10   Atrial excitation.

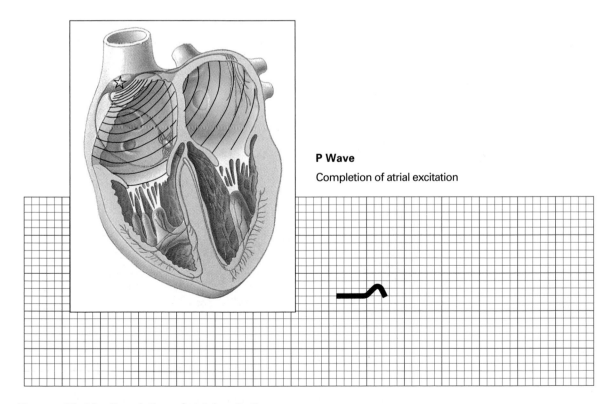

P Wave

Completion of atrial excitation

FIGURE 20-11   Completion of atrial excitation.

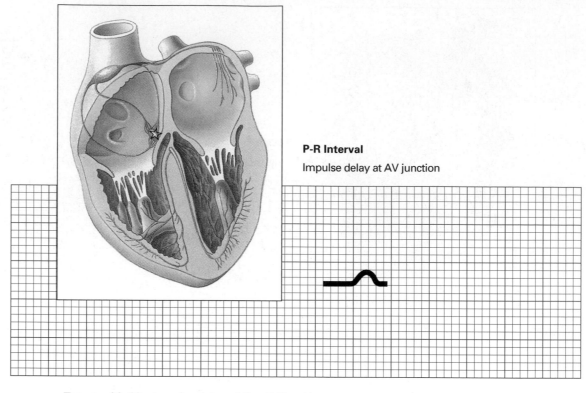

P-R Interval

Impulse delay at AV junction

FIGURE 20-12   Impulse delay at the AV junction.

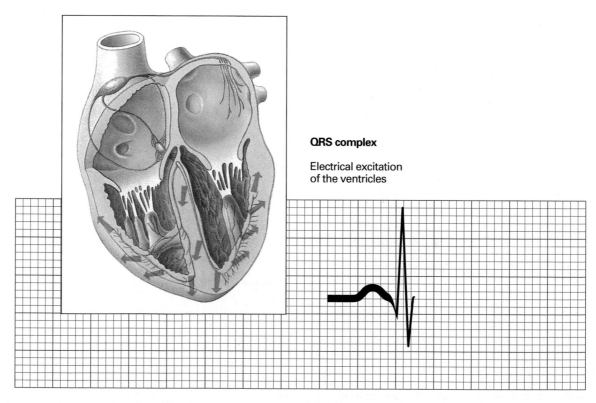

QRS complex

Electrical excitation
of the ventricles

FIGURE 20-13   Electrical excitation of the ventricles.

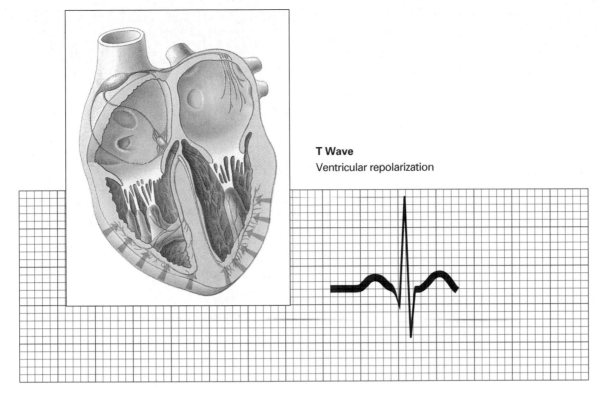

T Wave
Ventricular repolarization

FIGURE 20-14   Ventricular repolarization.

In addition to the wave forms described above, the ECG tracing reflects these important time intervals (Figure 20-15):

- *P-R interval (PRI) or P-Q interval (PQI).* The P-R interval is the distance from the beginning of the P wave to the beginning of the QRS complex. It represents the time the impulse takes to travel from the atria to the ventricles. Occasionally, the R wave is absent, in which case this interval is called the P-Q interval. The terms P-R interval and P-Q interval may be used interchangeably.

- *QRS interval.* The QRS interval is the distance from the first deflection of the QRS complex to the last. It represents the time necessary for ventricular depolarization.

- *S-T segment.* The S-T segment is the distance from the S wave to the beginning of the T wave. Usually it is an isoelectric line; however, it may be elevated or depressed in certain disease states such as ischemia.

A normal P-R interval is 0.12 to 0.20 second. A short PRI lasts less than 0.12 second; a prolonged PRI lasts longer than 0.20 second. A prolonged PRI indicates a delay in the AV node. A normal QRS complex lasts between 0.08 and 0.12 second. A value of less than 0.12 second means that the ventricles depolarized in a normal length of time.

The **QT interval** represents the total duration of ventricular depolarization. A normal QT interval is 0.33 to 0.42 second. QT intervals and heart rate have an inverse relationship: increases in heart rate usually decrease the QT interval, whereas decreases in heart rate usually prolong it. A **prolonged QT interval** is thought to be related to an increased risk of certain ventricular dysrhythmias and sudden death.

The all-or-none nature of myocardial depolarization results in an interval when the heart cannot be restimulated to depolarize. From our earlier discussion you will recall that during this time the myocardial cells have not yet repolarized and cannot be stimulated again (Figure 20-16). This **refractory period** has two parts, an **absolute refractory period** and a **relative refractory period.** During the absolute refractory period stimulation produces no depolarization whatsoever. This usually lasts from the beginning of the QRS complex to

Content Review

ECG TIME INTERVALS
- P-R interval
- QRS interval
- S-T segment

Content Review

NORMAL INTERVAL DURATIONS
- PR   0.12 to 0.20 sec
- QRS 0.08 to 0.12 sec
- QT   0.33 to 0.42 sec

QT interval period from the beginning of the QRS to the end of the T wave.

prolonged QT interval QT interval greater than 0.44 second.

refractory period the period of time when myocardial cells have not yet completely repolarized and cannot be stimulated again.

FIGURE 20-15   The ECG.

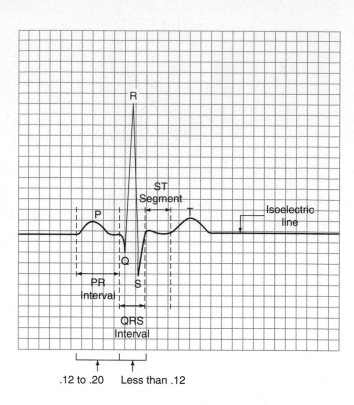

.12 to .20   Less than .12

absolute refractory period the period of the cardiac cycle when stimulation will not produce any depolarization whatever.

relative refractory period the period of the cardiac cycle when a sufficiently strong stimulus may produce depolarization.

the apex of the T wave. During the relative refractory period, a sufficiently strong stimulus may produce depolarization. This usually corresponds to the T wave's down slope.

S-T Segment Changes

The S-T segment is usually an isoelectric line. Myocardial infarctions, which are caused by lack of blood flow to a part of the heart, produce changes in this line. The affected area is then electrically dead and cannot conduct electrical impulses. Myocardial infarctions usually follow this sequence:

1. Ischemia (lack of oxygen)
2. Injury
3. Necrosis (cell death, infarction)

Each of these stages results in distinct S-T segment changes. Ischemia causes S-T segment depression or an inverted T wave. The inversion is usually symmetrical. Injury elevates the S-T segment, most often in the early phases of a myocardial infarction. As the tissue dies, a significant Q wave appears. As we noted earlier, small, insignificant Q waves may show up in normal ECG tracings. A significant Q wave is at least one small square wide, lasting 0.04 second, or is more than one-third the height of the QRS complex. Q waves may also indicate extensive transient ischemia.

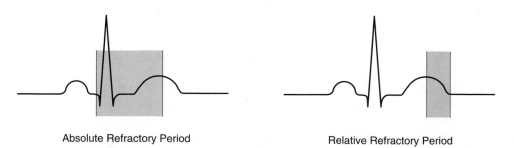

Absolute Refractory Period   Relative Refractory Period

FIGURE 20-16   Refractory periods of the cardiac cycle.

Table 20-2	OVERVIEW OF ECG LEAD GROUPINGS
Leads	**Portion of the Heart Examined**
I and aVL	Left side of the heart in a vertical plane
II, III, and aVF	Inferior (diaphragmatic) side of the heart
aVR	Right side of the heart in a vertical plane
V_1 and V_2	Right ventricle
V_3 and V_4	Intraventricular septum and the anterior wall of the left ventricle
V_5 and V_6	Anterior and lateral walls of the left ventricle

Lead Systems and Heart Surfaces

Using the various ECG leads is comparable to waiting for a train at a railroad crossing. You will want to know how long you have to wait (in other words, how long is the train), but you can only see the front of the train. If you had cameras at other viewpoints, you could see how long the train actually was. Similarly, by combining the different ECG leads you can view different parts of the heart.

Leads V_1 to V_4 view the anterior surface of the heart. Leads I and aVL view the lateral surface of the heart. The inferior surface of the heart can be visualized in leads II, III, and aVF. These leads can show ischemia, injury, and necrotic changes and can provide information about the corresponding heart surface (Table 20-2). For example, significant S–T elevation in V_1–V_4 may indicate anterior involvement, whereas elevation in II, III, and aVF may indicate inferior involvement.

Medical procedures (angioplasty) and drugs (thrombolytics) can treat acute myocardial infarction. The earlier they are initiated, the better the patient's potential outcome. Earlier identification in the field of patients with AMI will allow for earlier interventions, but the role of a 12-lead ECG in out-of-hospital care remains unresolved. Its use may not be appropriate in many EMS settings. Individual EMS medical directors will determine the application and use of the 12-lead ECG in their specific EMS settings.

Earlier field identification of patients with AMI will allow for earlier intervention.

INTERPRETATION OF RHYTHM STRIPS

The key to interpreting rhythm strips is to approach each strip logically and systematically. Attempts to nonanalytically "eyeball" the strip often lead to incorrect interpretations. Your approach to rhythm strip interpretation should include the following basic criteria:

The key to interpreting rhythm strips is to approach each strip logically and systematically.

- Always be consistent and analytical.
- Memorize the rules for each dysrhythmia.
- Analyze a given rhythm strip according to a specific format.
- Compare your analysis to the rules for each dysrhythmia.
- Identify the dysrhythmia by its similarity to established rules.

Use ECG calipers to measure ECG tracings to ensure accuracy and to avoid misinterpretation.

The health-care profession uses several standard formats for ECG analysis. We will use the following five-step procedure:

1. Analyze the rate.
2. Analyze the rhythm.
3. Analyze the P-waves.
4. Analyze the P-R interval.
5. Analyze the QRS complex.

Analyzing Rate

The first step in ECG strip interpretation is to analyze the heart rate. Usually this means the ventricular rate; however, if the atrial and ventricular rates differ, you must calculate both.

The normal heart rate is 60 to 100 beats per minute. A heart rate greater than 100 beats per minute is a **tachycardia**. A heart rate less than 60 beats per minute is a **bradycardia**. You can use any of the following methods to calculate the rate:

- *Six-second method.* Count the number of complexes in a 6-second interval. Mark off a 6-second interval by noting two 3-second marks at the top of the ECG paper. Then multiply the number of complexes within the 6-second strip by ten.
- *Heart rate calculator rulers.* Commercially available heart rate calculator rulers allow you to determine heart rates rapidly. Always use them according to the accompanying directions, since variations occur among different manufacturers. Also learn a manual method so you can still calculate rates if you forget your ruler.
- *R-R interval.* The R-R interval is related directly to heart rate. The R-R interval method is accurate only if the heart rhythm is regular. You can calculate it in the following ways:
  - Measure the duration between R waves in seconds. Divide this number into 60, giving the heart rate per minute.
    Example: $60 \div 0.65$ second = 92 (heart rate)
  - Count the number of large squares within an R-R interval, and divide the number of squares into 300.
    Example: $300 \div 3.5$ large boxes = 86 (heart rate)
  - Count the number of small squares within an R-R interval, and divide the number of squares into 1,500.
    Example: $1,500 \div 29$ small boxes = 52 (heart rate)
- *Triplicate method.* Another method, also useful only with regular rhythms, is to locate an R wave that falls on a dark line bordering a large box on the graph paper. Then assign numbers corresponding to the heart rate to the next six dark lines to the right. The order is: 300, 150, 100, 75, 60, and 50. The number corresponding to the dark line closest to the peak of the next R wave is a rough estimate of the heart rate.

Pick one of the above methods and become comfortable with it. Use it to determine the rate on all strips that you look at.

Analyzing Rhythm

The next step is to analyze the rhythm. First, measure the R-R interval across the strip. Normally, the R-R rhythm is fairly regular. Some minimal variation, associated with respirations, should be expected. If the rhythm is irregular, note whether it fits one of the following patterns:

- Occasionally irregular (only one or two R-R intervals on the strip are irregular)
- Regularly irregular (patterned irregularity or group beating)
- Irregularly irregular (no relationship among R-R intervals)

Analyzing P Waves

The P waves reflect atrial depolarization. Normally, the atria depolarize away from the SA node and toward the ventricles. In lead II, this appears as a positive, rounded P wave. When analyzing the P waves, ask yourself the following questions:

- Are P waves present?
- Are the P waves regular?
- Is there one P wave for each QRS complex?
- Are the P waves upright or inverted (compared to the QRS complex)?
- Do all the P waves look alike?

Analyzing the P-R Interval

The P-R interval represents the time needed for atrial depolarization and conduction of the impulse up to the AV node. Remember, the normal P-R interval is 0.12 to 0.20 sec (three to five small boxes). Any deviation is an abnormal finding. The P-R interval should be consistent across the strip.

Analyzing the QRS Complex

The QRS complex represents ventricular depolarization. When evaluating the QRS complex, ask yourself the following questions:

- Do all of the QRS complexes look alike?
- What is the QRS duration?

Remember, the QRS duration is usually 0.04 to 0.12 sec. Anything longer than 0.12 sec (three small boxes) is abnormal.

DYSRHYTHMIAS

On a normal ECG, the heart rate is between 60 and 100 beats per minute. The rhythm is regular (both P-P and R-R). The P waves are normal in shape, upright, and appear only before each QRS complex. The P-R interval lasts 0.12 to 0.20 sec and is constant. The QRS complex has a normal morphology, and its duration is less than 0.12 sec. All of these factors indicate a **normal sinus rhythm** (Figure 20-17a). Any deviation from the heart's normal electrical rhythm is a **dysrhythmia**. The absence of cardiac electrical activity is **arrhythmia**. The causes of dysrhythmias include:

- Myocardial ischemia, necrosis, or infarction
- Autonomic nervous system imbalance
- Distention of the chambers of the heart (especially in the atria, secondary to congestive heart failure)
- Blood gas abnormalities, including hypoxia and abnormal pH
- Electrolyte imbalances (Ca^{++}, K^{+}, Mg^{++})
- Trauma to the myocardium (cardiac contusion)
- Drug effects and drug toxicity
- Electrocution
- Hypothermia
- CNS damage
- Idiopathic events
- Normal occurrences

Dysrhythmias in the healthy heart are of little significance. No matter what the etiology or type of dysrhythmia, treat the patient and his symptoms, not the dysrhythmia. You will hear this repeated over and over: Treat the patient, not the monitor.

MECHANISM OF IMPULSE FORMATION

Several physiological mechanisms can cause cardiac dysrhythmias. The depolarization impulse is normally transmitted forward (*antegrade*) through the conductive system and the myocardium. In certain dysrhythmias, however, the depolarization impulse is conducted backward (*retrograde*).

- *Ectopic foci.* One cause of dysrhythmias is *enhanced automaticity*. This condition results when **ectopic foci** (heart cells other than the pacemaker cells) automatically depolarize, producing **ectopic** (abnormal) **beats.** Premature ventricular contractions and premature atrial contractions are examples of ectopic beats. Ectopic beats can be intermittent or sustained.

Content Review

NORMAL SINUS RHYTHM
- Rate: 60 to 100
- Rhythm: regular
- P waves: normal, upright, only before each QRS complex
- PR interval: 0.12 to 0.20 sec
  - QRS Complex:
  - Morphology: normal
  - Duration: < 0.12 sec

---

normal sinus rhythm the normal heart rhythm.

dysrhythmia any deviation from the normal electrical rhythm of the heart.

arrhythmia the absence of cardiac electrical activity; often used interchangeably with the term dysrhythmia.

Treat the patient, not the monitor.

---

ectopic focus nonpacemaker heart cell that automatically depolarizes; *plural* ectopic foci.

ectopic beat cardiac depolarization resulting from depolarization of ectopic focus.

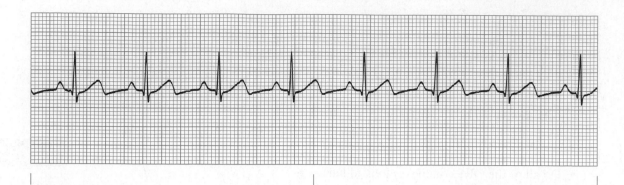

FIGURE 20-17A Normal sinus rhythm.

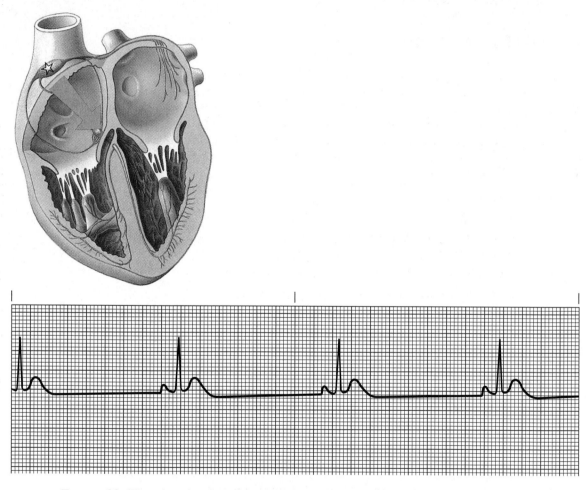

FIGURE 20-17B Sinus bradycardia.

- *Reentry.* Reentry may cause isolated premature beats, or *tachydysrhythmias.* It occurs when ischemia or another disease process alters two branches of a conduction pathway, slowing conduction in one branch and causing a unidirectional block in the other. An antegrade depolarization wave travels slowly through the branch with ischemia and is blocked in the branch with a unidirectional block. After the depolarization wave goes through the slowed branch, it enters the branch with the unidirectional block and is conducted retrograde back to the branch's origin. By now the tissue is no longer refractory and stimulation occurs again. This can result in rapid rhythms such as paroxysmal supraventricular tachycardia or atrial fibrillation.

CLASSIFICATION OF DYSRHYTHMIAS

Dysrhythmias can be classified in any number of ways. Some of the classification methods include:

- Nature of origin (changes in automaticity versus disturbances in conduction)
- Magnitude (major versus minor)
- Severity (life threatening versus non-life threatening)
- Site of origin

Classifying dysrhythmias by site of origin is closely related to basic physiology and, thus, is easy to understand. This approach divides dysrhythmias into the following categories:

- Dysrhythmias originating in the SA node
- Dysrhythmias originating in the atria
- Dysrhythmias originating within the AV junction
- Dysrhythmias sustained in or originating in the AV junction
- Dysrhythmias originating in the ventricles
- Dysrhythmias resulting from disorders of conduction

DYSRHYTHMIAS ORIGINATING IN THE SA NODE

Dysrhythmias originating in the SA node most often result from changes in autonomic tone. However, disease can exist in the SA node itself. Dysrhythmias that originate in the SA node include:

- Sinus bradycardia
- Sinus tachycardia
- Sinus dysrhythmia
- Sinus arrest

Sinus Bradycardia

Description: Sinus bradycardia results from slowing of the SA node.

Etiology: Sinus bradycardia may result from any of the following conditions:

Increased parasympathetic (vagal) tone

Intrinsic disease of the SA node

Drug effects (digitalis, propranolol, quinidine)

Normal finding in healthy, well-conditioned persons

Rules of Interpretation/Lead II Monitoring (Figure 20-17b):

Rate—less than 60

Rhythm—regular

Pacemaker site—SA node

P waves—upright and normal in morphology

P-R interval—normal (0.12 to 0.20 sec and constant)

QRS complex—normal (0.04 to 0.12 sec)

Clinical Significance: The decreased heart rate can cause decreased cardiac output, hypotension, angina, or central nervous system symptoms. This is especially true for rates slower than 50 beats per minute. The slow heart rate may also lead to atrial ectopic or ventricular ectopic rhythms. In a healthy athlete, sinus bradycardia may have no clinical significance.

Treatment: Treatment is generally unnecessary unless hypotension or ventricular irritability is present (Figure 20-18). Remember, treat your patient and not the monitor. If treatment

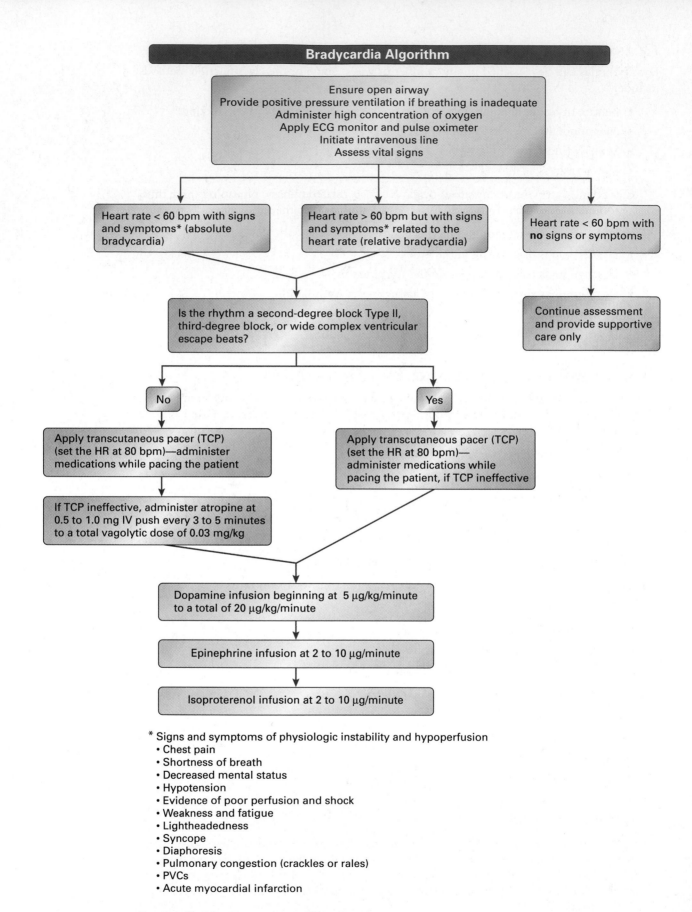

Bradycardia Algorithm

Ensure open airway
Provide positive pressure ventilation if breathing is inadequate
Administer high concentration of oxygen
Apply ECG monitor and pulse oximeter
Initiate intravenous line
Assess vital signs

Heart rate < 60 bpm with signs and symptoms* (absolute bradycardia)

Heart rate > 60 bpm but with signs and symptoms* related to the heart rate (relative bradycardia)

Heart rate < 60 bpm with **no** signs or symptoms

Is the rhythm a second-degree block Type II, third-degree block, or wide complex ventricular escape beats?

Continue assessment and provide supportive care only

No

Yes

Apply transcutaneous pacer (TCP) (set the HR at 80 bpm)—administer medications while pacing the patient

Apply transcutaneous pacer (TCP) (set the HR at 80 bpm)—administer medications while pacing the patient, if TCP ineffective

If TCP ineffective, administer atropine at 0.5 to 1.0 mg IV push every 3 to 5 minutes to a total vagolytic dose of 0.03 mg/kg

Dopamine infusion beginning at 5 μg/kg/minute to a total of 20 μg/kg/minute

Epinephrine infusion at 2 to 10 μg/minute

Isoproterenol infusion at 2 to 10 μg/minute

* Signs and symptoms of physiologic instability and hypoperfusion
- Chest pain
- Shortness of breath
- Decreased mental status
- Hypotension
- Evidence of poor perfusion and shock
- Weakness and fatigue
- Lightheadedness
- Syncope
- Diaphoresis
- Pulmonary congestion (crackles or rales)
- PVCs
- Acute myocardial infarction

FIGURE 20-18 Management of bradycardia.

is required, administer a 0.5 mg bolus of atropine sulfate. Repeat every 3 to 5 minutes until you have obtained a satisfactory rate or have given 0.04 mg/kg of the drug. If atropine fails, consider transcutaneous cardiac pacing (TCP), if available.

Sinus Tachycardia

Description: Sinus tachycardia results from an increased rate of SA node discharge.

Etiology: Sinus tachycardia may result from any of the following:

Exercise

Fever

Anxiety

Hypovolemia

Anemia

Pump failure

Increased sympathetic tone

Hypoxia

Hyperthyroidism

Rules of Interpretation/Lead II Monitoring (Figure 20-19):

Rate—greater than 100

Rhythm—regular

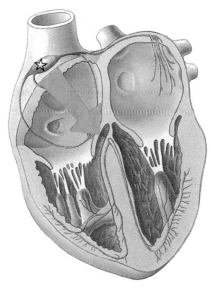

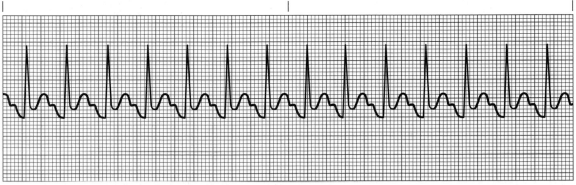

FIGURE 20-19 Sinus tachycardia.

Pacemaker site—SA node

P waves—upright and normal in morphology

P-R interval—normal

QRS complex—normal

Clinical Significance: Sinus tachycardia is often benign. In some cases, it is a compensatory mechanism for decreased stroke volume. If the rate is greater than 140 beats per minute, cardiac output may fall because ventricular filling time is inadequate. Very rapid heart rates increase myocardial oxygen demand and can precipitate ischemia or infarct in diseased hearts. Prolonged sinus tachycardia accompanying acute myocardial infarction (AMI) is often an ominous finding suggesting cardiogenic shock.

Treatment: Treatment is directed at the underlying cause. Hypovolemia, fever, hypoxia, or other causes should be corrected.

Sinus Dysrhythmia

Description: Sinus dysrhythmia often results from a variation of the R-R interval.

Etiology: Sinus dysrhythmia is often a normal finding and is sometimes related to the respiratory cycle and changes in intrathoracic pressure. Pathologically, sinus dysrhythmia can be caused by enhanced vagal tone.

Rules of Interpretation/Lead II Monitoring (Figure 20-20):

Rate—60 to 100 (varies with respirations)

Rhythm—irregular

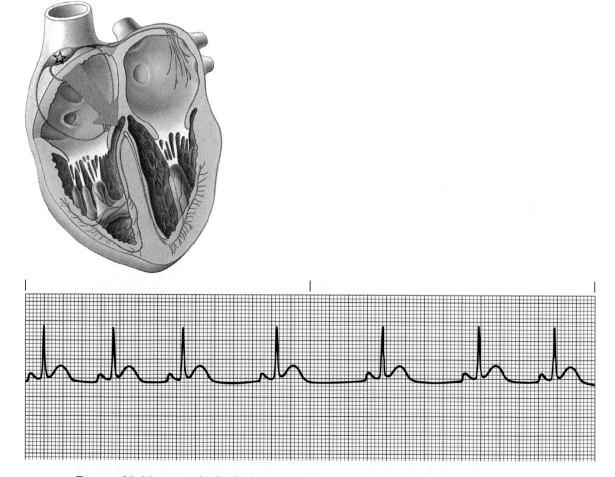

FIGURE 20-20   Sinus dysrhythmia.

Pacemaker site—SA node

P waves—upright and normal in morphology

P-R interval—normal

QRS complex—normal

Clinical Significance: Sinus dysrhythmia is a normal variant, particularly in the young and the aged.

Treatment: Typically, none required.

Sinus Arrest

Description: Sinus arrest occurs when the sinus node fails to discharge, resulting in short periods of cardiac standstill. This standstill can persist until pacemaker cells lower in the conductive system discharge (escape beats) or until the sinus node resumes discharge.

Etiology: Sinus arrest can result from any of the following conditions:

Ischemia of the SA node

Digitalis toxicity

Excessive vagal tone

Degenerative fibrotic disease

Rules of Interpretation/Lead II Monitoring (Figure 20-21):

Rate—normal to slow, depending on the frequency and duration of the arrest

Rhythm—irregular

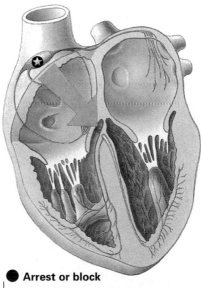

● **Arrest or block**

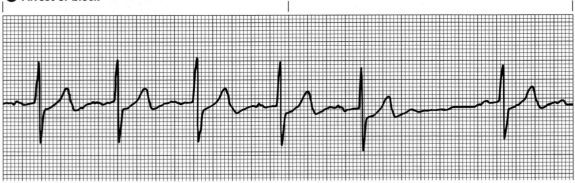

FIGURE 20-21   Sinus arrest.

Pacemaker site—SA node

P waves—upright and normal in morphology

P-R interval—normal

QRS complex—normal

Clinical Significance: Frequent or prolonged episodes may compromise cardiac output, resulting in syncope (fainting) and other problems. There is always the danger of complete cessation of SA node activity. Usually, an escape rhythm develops; however, cardiac standstill occasionally can result.

Treatment: If the patient is asymptomatic, observation is all that is required. If the patient is extremely bradycardic or symptomatic, administer a 0.5 mg bolus of atropine sulfate. Repeat every 3 to 5 minutes until you have obtained a satisfactory rate or have administered 0.04 mg/kg of the drug. If atropine fails, consider transcutaneous cardiac pacing (TCP), if available.

DYSRHYTHMIAS ORIGINATING IN THE ATRIA

Dysrhythmias can originate outside the SA node in the atrial tissue or in the internodal pathways. Ischemia, hypoxia, atrial dilation, and other factors can cause atrial dysrhythmias. Dysrhythmias originating in the atria include:

- Wandering atrial pacemaker
- Multifocal atrial tachycardia
- Premature atrial contractions
- Paroxysmal supraventricular tachycardia
- Atrial flutter
- Atrial fibrillation

Wandering Atrial Pacemaker

Description: Wandering atrial pacemaker is the passive transfer of pacemaker sites from the sinus node to other latent pacemaker sites in the atria and AV junction. Often more than one pacemaker site will be present, causing variation in R-R interval and P wave morphology.

Etiology: Wandering atrial pacemaker can result from any of the following conditions:

A variant of sinus dysrhythmia

A normal phenomenon in the very young or the aged

Ischemic heart disease

Atrial dilation

Rules of Interpretation/Lead II Monitoring (Figure 20-22):

Rate—usually normal

Rhythm—slightly irregular

Pacemaker site—varies among the SA node, atrial tissue, and the AV junction

P waves—morphology changes from beat to beat; P waves may disappear entirely

P-R interval—varies; may be less than 0.12 sec, normal, or greater than 0.20 sec

QRS Complex—normal

Clinical Significance: Wandering atrial pacemaker usually has no detrimental effects. Occasionally, it can be a precursor of other atrial dysrhythmias such as atrial fibrillation. It sometimes indicates digitalis toxicity.

Treatment: If the patient is asymptomatic, observation is all that is required. If the patient is symptomatic, consider adenosine or verapamil.

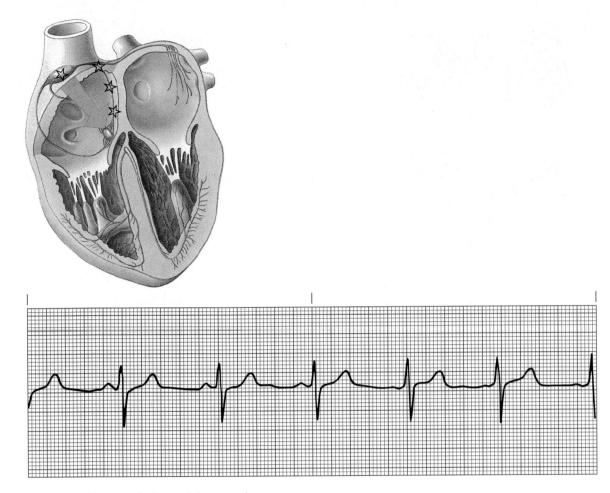

FIGURE 20-22 Wandering atrial pacemaker.

Multifocal Atrial Tachycardia

Description: Multifocal atrial tachycardia (MAT) is usually seen in acutely ill patients. Significant pulmonary disease is seen in about 60% of these patients. Certain medications used to treat lung disease (such as theophylline) may worsen the dysrhythmia. Three different P waves are noted, indicating various ectopic foci.

Etiology: Multifocal atrial tachycardia can result from any of the following conditions:

Pulmonary disease

Metabolic disorders (hypokalemia)

Ischemic heart disease

Recent surgery

Rules of Interpretation/Lead II Monitoring (Figure 20-23):

Rate—more than 100

Rhythm—irregular

Pacemaker site—ectopic sites in atria

P waves—organized, discrete nonsinus P waves with at least three different forms

P-R interval—varies

QRS complex—may be less than 0.12 sec, normal, or greater than 0.20 sec, depending on the AV node's refractory status when the impulse reaches it

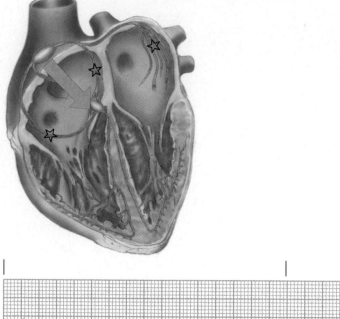

FIGURE 20-23 Multifocal atrial tachycardia.

Clinical Significance: Frequently these patients are acutely ill; this dysrhythmia may indicate a serious underlying medical illness.

Treatment: Treatment of the underlying medical disease usually resolves the dysrhythmia. Specific antidysrhythmic therapy is frequently not needed.

Premature Atrial Contractions

Description: Premature atrial contractions (PACs) result from a single electrical impulse originating in the atria outside the SA node, which in turn causes a premature depolarization of the heart before the next expected sinus beat. Because it depolarizes the atrial syncytium, this impulse also depolarizes the SA node, interrupting the normal cadence. This creates a **noncompensatory pause** in the underlying rhythm.

Etiology: A premature atrial contraction can result from any of the following conditions:

Use of caffeine, tobacco, or alcohol

Sympathomimetic drugs

Ischemic heart disease

Hypoxia

Digitalis toxicity

No apparent cause (idiopathic)

Rules of Interpretation/Lead II Monitoring (Figure 20-24):

Rate—depends on the underlying rhythm

Rhythm—depends on the underlying rhythm; usually regular except for the PAC

Pacemaker site—ectopic focus in the atrium

noncompensatory pause
pause following an ectopic beat where the SA node is depolarized and the underlying cadence of the heart is interrupted.

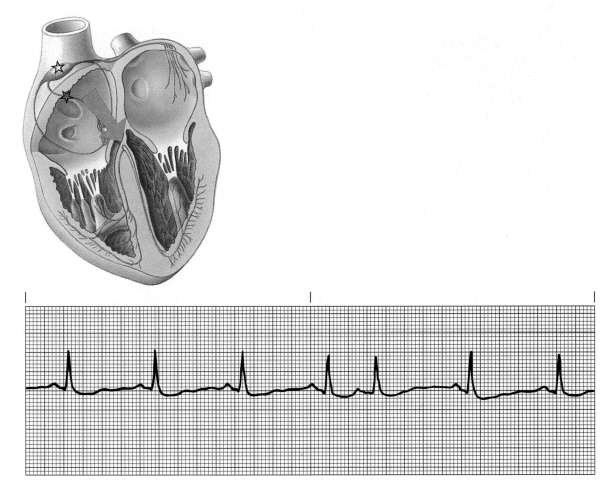

FIGURE 20-24   Premature atrial contractions.

P waves—the P wave of the PAC differs from the P wave of the underlying rhythm. It occurs earlier than the next expected P wave and may be hidden in the preceding T wave.

P-R interval—usually normal; can vary with the location of the ectopic focus. Ectopic foci near the SA node will have a P-R interval of 0.12 sec or greater, whereas ectopic foci near the AV node will have a P-R interval of 0.12 sec or less.

QRS complex—usually normal; may be greater than 0.12 sec if the PAC is abnormally conducted through partially refractory ventricles. In some cases, the ventricles are refractory and will not depolarize in response to the PAC. In these cases, the QRS complex is absent.

Clinical Significance: Isolated PACs are of minimal significance. Frequent PACs may indicate organic heart disease and may precede other atrial dysrhythmias.

Treatment: If the patient is asymptomatic, observation is all that is required in the field. If the patient is symptomatic, administer oxygen via a nonrebreather mask and start an IV line. Contact medical direction.

Paroxysmal Supraventricular Tachycardia

Description: Paroxysmal supraventricular tachycardia (PSVT) occurs when rapid atrial depolarization overrides the SA node. It often occurs in paroxysm with sudden onset, may last minutes to hours, and terminates abruptly. It may be caused by increased automaticity of a single atrial focus or by reentry phenomenon at the AV node.

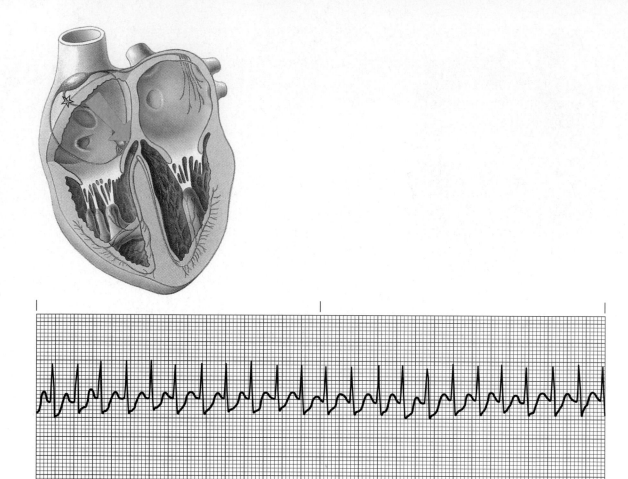

FIGURE 20-25 Paroxysmal supraventricular tachycardia.

Etiology: Paroxysmal supraventricular tachycardia may occur at any age and often is not associated with underlying heart disease. It may be precipitated by stress, overexertion, smoking, or ingestion of caffeine. It is, however, frequently associated with underlying atherosclerotic cardiovascular disease and rheumatic heart disease. PSVT is rare in patients with myocardial infarction. It can occur with accessory pathway conduction such as Wolff-Parkinson-White syndrome.

Rules of Interpretation/Lead II Monitoring (Figure 20-25):

Rate—150 to 250 per minute

Rhythm—characteristically regular, except at onset and termination

Pacemaker site—in the atria, outside the SA node

P waves—the atrial P waves differ slightly from sinus P waves. The P wave is often buried in the preceding T wave. The P wave may be impossible to see, especially if the rate is rapid. Turning up the speed of the graph paper or oscilloscope to 50 mm/sec spreads out the complex and can help identify P waves.

P-R interval—usually normal; however, it can vary with the location of the ectopic pacemaker. Ectopic pacemakers near the SA node will have P-R intervals close to 0.12 sec, whereas ectopic pacemakers near the AV node will have P-R intervals of 0.12 sec or less.

QRS complex—normal

Clinical Significance: Young patients with good cardiac reserves may tolerate PSVT well for short periods. Patients often sense PSVT as palpitations. However, rapid rates can cause a marked reduction in cardiac output because of inadequate ventricular filling time. The reduced diastolic phase of the cardiac cycle can also compromise coronary artery perfusion. PSVT can precipitate angina, hypotension, or congestive heart failure.

Treatment: If the patient is not tolerating the rapid heart rate, as evidenced by hemodynamic instability, attempt the following techniques in this order (Figure 20-26).

1. *Vagal maneuvers.* Ask the patient to perform a Valsalva maneuver. This is a forced expiration against a closed glottis, or the act of "bearing down" as if to move the bowels. This results in vagal stimulation, which may slow the heart. If this is unsuccessful, attempt carotid artery massage, if allowed and patient is eligible. Do not attempt carotid artery massage in patients with carotid **bruits** or known cerebrovascular or carotid artery disease.

2. *Pharmacological therapy.* Adenosine (Adenocard) is very safe and highly effective in terminating PSVT, especially if its etiology is reentry. Administer 6 mg of adenosine by rapid IV bolus over 1 to 3 sec through the medication port closest to the patient's heart or central circulation. (Adenosine has a very short half-life, and you must immediately follow administration with a bolus of normal saline to allow the medication to reach its site of action while it is still effective.) If the patient does not convert after 1 to 2 minutes, administer a second bolus of 12 mg over 1 to 3 sec in the medication port closest to the patient's heart or central circulation. If this fails and the patient has a normal blood pressure, then look again at the width of the cardiac QRS.

3. *Electrical therapy.* If the ventricular rate is greater than 150 beats per minute, or if the patient is hemodynamically unstable, use synchronized cardioversion (described later in the chapter). If time allows, sedate the patient with 5 to 10 mg of diazepam or 2 to 5 mg of midazolam (Versed) IV. Apply synchronized DC countershock of 100 joules. If this is unsuccessful, repeat the countershock at increased energy as ordered by medical direction. DC countershock is contraindicated if you suspect digitalis toxicity as the PSVT's cause.

bruit the sound of turbulent blood flow through a vessel; usually associated with atherosclerotic disease.

Atrial Flutter

Description: Atrial flutter results from a rapid atrial reentry circuit and an AV node that physiologically cannot conduct all impulses through to the ventricles. The AV junction may allow impulses in a 1:1 (rare), 2:1, 3:1, or 4:1 ratio or greater, resulting in a discrepancy between atrial and ventricular rates. The AV block may be consistent or variable.

Etiology: Atrial flutter may occur in normal hearts, but it is usually associated with organic disease. It rarely occurs as the direct result of an MI. Atrial dilation, which occurs with congestive heart failure, is a cause of atrial flutter.

Rules of Interpretation/Lead II Monitoring (Figure 20-27):

Rate—atrial rate is 250 to 350 per minute. Ventricular rate varies with the ratio of AV conduction.

Rhythm—atrial rhythm is regular; ventricular rhythm is usually regular, but can be irregular if the block is variable

Pacemaker site—sites in the atria outside the SA node

P waves—flutter (F) waves are present, resembling a sawtooth or picket-fence pattern. This pattern is often difficult to identify in a 2:1 flutter. However, if the ventricular rate is approximately 150, suspect 2:1 flutter.

P-R interval—usually constant but may vary

QRS complex—normal

(Continued on page 869.)

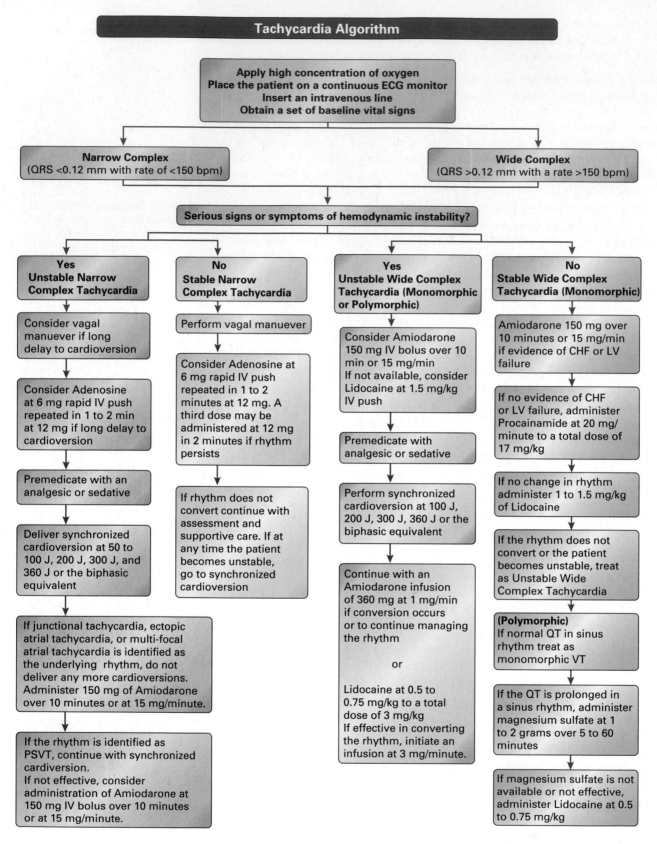

Tachycardia Algorithm

Apply high concentration of oxygen
Place the patient on a continuous ECG monitor
Insert an intravenous line
Obtain a set of baseline vital signs

Narrow Complex
(QRS <0.12 mm with rate of <150 bpm)

Wide Complex
(QRS >0.12 mm with a rate >150 bpm)

Serious signs or symptoms of hemodynamic instability?

Yes
Unstable Narrow Complex Tachycardia

Consider vagal manuever if long delay to cardioversion

Consider Adenosine at 6 mg rapid IV push repeated in 1 to 2 min at 12 mg if long delay to cardioversion

Premedicate with an analgesic or sedative

Deliver synchronized cardioversion at 50 to 100 J, 200 J, 300 J, and 360 J or the biphasic equivalent

If junctional tachycardia, ectopic atrial tachycardia, or multi-focal atrial tachycardia is identified as the underlying rhythm, do not deliver any more cardioversions. Administer 150 mg of Amiodarone over 10 minutes or at 15 mg/minute.

If the rhythm is identified as PSVT, continue with synchronized cardioversion.
If not effective, consider administration of Amiodarone at 150 mg IV bolus over 10 minutes or at 15 mg/minute.

No
Stable Narrow Complex Tachycardia

Perform vagal manuever

Consider Adenosine at 6 mg rapid IV push repeated in 1 to 2 minutes at 12 mg. A third dose may be administered at 12 mg in 2 minutes if rhythm persists

If rhythm does not convert continue with assessment and supportive care. If at any time the patient becomes unstable, go to synchronized cardioversion

Yes
Unstable Wide Complex Tachycardia (Monomorphic or Polymorphic)

Consider Amiodarone 150 mg IV bolus over 10 min or 15 mg/min
If not available, consider Lidocaine at 1.5 mg/kg IV push

Premedicate with analgesic or sedative

Perform synchronized cardioversion at 100 J, 200 J, 300 J, 360 J or the biphasic equivalent

Continue with an Amiodarone infusion of 360 mg at 1 mg/min if conversion occurs or to continue managing the rhythm

or

Lidocaine at 0.5 to 0.75 mg/kg to a total dose of 3 mg/kg
If effective in converting the rhythm, initiate an infusion at 3 mg/minute.

No
Stable Wide Complex Tachycardia (Monomorphic)

Amiodarone 150 mg over 10 minutes or 15 mg/min if evidence of CHF or LV failure

If no evidence of CHF or LV failure, administer Procainamide at 20 mg/minute to a total dose of 17 mg/kg

If no change in rhythm administer 1 to 1.5 mg/kg of Lidocaine

If the rhythm does not convert or the patient becomes unstable, treat as Unstable Wide Complex Tachycardia

(Polymorphic)
If normal QT in sinus rhythm treat as monomorphic VT

If the QT is prolonged in a sinus rhythm, administer magnesium sulfate at 1 to 2 grams over 5 to 60 minutes

If magnesium sulfate is not available or not effective, administer Lidocaine at 0.5 to 0.75 mg/kg

FIGURE 20-26   Management of tachycardia.

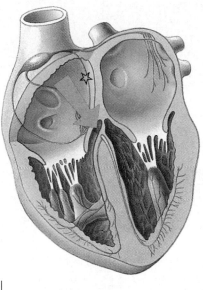

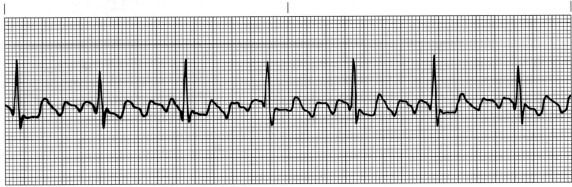

FIGURE 20-27   Atrial flutter.

Clinical Significance: Atrial flutter with normal ventricular rates is generally well tolerated. Rapid ventricular rates may compromise cardiac output and result in symptoms. Atrial flutter often occurs in conjunction with atrial fibrillation and is referred to as "atrial fib-flutter."

Treatment: Treatment is indicated only for rapid ventricular rates with hemodynamic compromise (review Figure 20-26).

1. *Electrical therapy.* Immediate cardioversion is indicated in unstable patients—those with a heart rate greater than 150 and associated chest pain, dyspnea, a decreased level of consciousness, or hypotension. If time allows, sedate the patient with 5 to 10 mg of diazepam (Valium) or 2 to 5 mg of midazolam (Versed) IV. Then apply synchronized DC countershock of 100 joules. If this is unsuccessful, repeat the countershock at increased energy as recommended by American Heart Association (AHA) guidelines.

2. *Pharmacological therapy.* Occasionally you may use pharmacological therapy in stable patients with atrial flutter, especially if the rapid heart rate is causing congestive heart failure. Several medications slow the ventricular rate. The most frequently used is diltiazem (Cardizem) although verapamil, digoxin, beta blockers, procainamide, and quinidine are also used. Procainamide and quinidine are often used to convert atrial flutter back to a sinus rhythm. Consult medical direction or refer to local protocols concerning pharmacological therapy for atrial flutter.

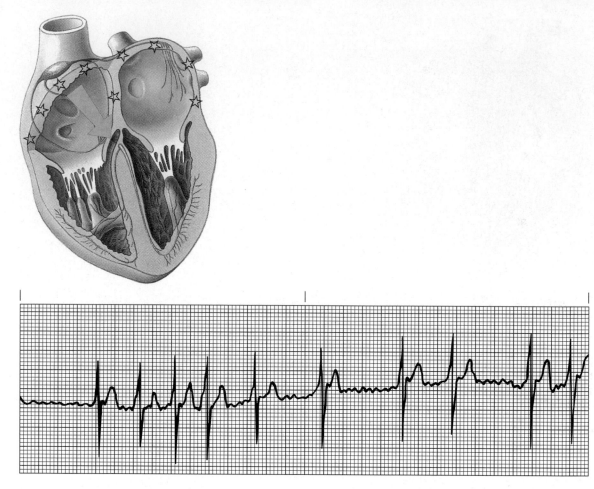

FIGURE 20-28 Atrial fibrillation.

Atrial Fibrillation

Description: Atrial fibrillation results from multiple areas of reentry within the atria or from multiple ectopic foci bombarding an AV node that physiologically cannot handle all of the incoming impulses. AV conduction is random and highly variable.

Etiology: Atrial fibrillation may be chronic and is often associated with underlying heart disease such as rheumatic heart disease, atherosclerotic heart disease, or congestive heart failure. Atrial dilation occurs with congestive heart failure and often causes atrial fibrillation.

Rules of Interpretation/Lead II Monitoring (Figure 20-28):

> Rate—atrial rate is 350 to 750 per minute (cannot be counted); ventricular rate varies greatly depending on conduction through the AV node.
>
> Rhythm—irregularly irregular
>
> Pacemaker site—numerous ectopic foci in the atria
>
> P waves—none discernible. Fibrillation (f) waves are present, indicating chaotic atrial activity.
>
> P-R interval—none
>
> QRS complex—normal

Clinical Significance: In atrial fibrillation, the atria fail to contract and the so-called atrial kick is lost, thus reducing cardiac output 20% to 25%. There is frequently a pulse deficit (a difference between the apical and peripheral pulse rates). If the rate of ventricular response is normal, as often occurs in patients on digitalis, the rhythm is usually well tolerated. If the ventricular rate is less than 60, cardiac output can fall. Suspect digitalis toxicity in patients taking digitalis with atrial fibrillation and a ventricular rate less than 60. If the ventricular response is rapid, coupled with the loss of atrial kick, cardiovascular decompensation may occur, resulting in hypotension, angina, infarct, congestive heart failure, or shock.

Treatment: Treatment is indicated only for rapid ventricular rates with hemodynamic compromise (review Figure 20-26).

1. *Electrical therapy.* Immediate cardioversion is indicated in unstable patients—those with heart rates greater than 150 and associated chest pain, dyspnea, a decreased level of consciousness, or hypotension. If time allows, sedate the patient with 5 to 10 mg of diazepam (Valium) or 2 to 5 mg of midazolam (Versed) IV. Then apply synchronized DC countershock of 100 joules. If this is unsuccessful, repeat the countershock at increased energy as ordered by medical direction.

2. *Pharmacological therapy.* Occasionally you will use pharmacological therapy in stable patients with atrial fibrillation, especially if the rapid heart rate is causing congestive heart failure. Several medications slow the ventricular rate. The most frequently used is diltiazem (Cardizem), although verapamil, digoxin, beta blockers, procainamide, and quinidine are often used. Procainamide and quinidine are used to convert atrial fibrillation to a normal sinus rhythm. Atrial fibrillation is a documented risk factor for the development of stroke. As the atria fibrillate, they dilate. This allows for stagnation of blood flow within the atria and subsequent clot development. Because of this, anticoagulants, such as heparin or warfarin (Coumadin), are administered to these patients to prevent stroke. Consult medical direction or refer to local protocols concerning pharmacological therapy of atrial fibrillation.

Patients with accessory pathways, such as in Wolff-Parkinson-White syndrome, who develop atrial flutter or atrial fibrillation, present special concerns. Usually, the electrical impulse reaches the ventricles via the accessory tract, via the AV node (normal conduction pathway), or via both. If the patient's refractory period is short in his accessory tract, more atrial impulses will be conducted down the accessory tract than through the AV node. This will result in a wide QRS complex. Rapid atrial rates occur with atrial fibrillation and flutter and can cause rapid ventricular rates. These rhythms, which have a wide complex, may resemble ventricular tachycardia. Excessive stimulation of the ventricles may actually precipitate ventricular fibrillation.

Dysrhythmias Originating within the AV Junction (AV Blocks)

Two potential problems in the AV junction (or AV node) may result in dysrhythmias. One is an atrioventricular (AV) block, in which the electrical impulse is slowed or blocked as it passes through the AV node. The other is dysrhythmias due to a malfunction of AV junctional cells themselves.

The AV junction is an important part of the conductive system, serving two important physiological purposes (Figure 20-29). First, it effectively slows the impulse between the atria and the ventricles to allow for atrial emptying and ventricular filling. Second, it serves as a back-up pacemaker if the SA node or cells higher in the conductive system fail to fire. Part of the AV tissues function as a pacemaker node and other parts serve as the junction between the atria and the ventricles.

The internodal fibers that blend to form the AV junction are called *transitional fibers*. These small fibers slow the impulse. The transitional fibers then blend into the AV junction. The lower portion of the AV node penetrates the fibrous tissue that separates the atria from the ventricles. This part of the node also slows impulse conduction. After penetrating the fibrous band, the AV node then becomes the AV bundle, which is also called the bundle of His. The bundle of His subsequently divides into the left and right bundle branches.

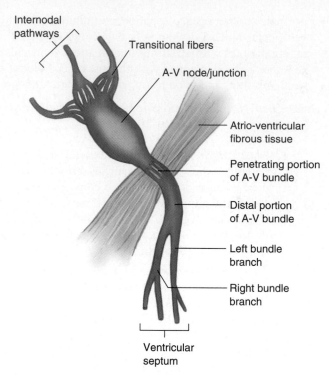

FIGURE 20-29 Organization of the AV node.

Internodal pathways

Transitional fibers

A-V node/junction

Atrio-ventricular fibrous tissue

Penetrating portion of A-V bundle

Distal portion of A-V bundle

Left bundle branch

Right bundle branch

Ventricular septum

Atrioventricular Blocks

An AV block delays or interrupts impulses between the atria and the ventricles. These dysrhythmias can be caused by pathology of the AV junctional tissue or by a physiological block, such as occurs with atrial fibrillation or flutter. Their causes include AV junctional ischemia, AV junctional necrosis, degenerative disease of the conductive system, and drug toxicity (particularly from digitalis).

AV blocks can be classified according to the site or the degree of the block. Blocks may occur at the following sites:

- At the AV node
- At the bundle of His
- Below the bifurcation of the bundle of His

Our discussion classifies AV blocks by the following degrees (traditional classification):

- First-degree AV block
- Type I second-degree AV block
- Type II second-degree AV block (Mobitz II, or Infranodal)
- Third-degree AV block

First-Degree AV Block

Description: A first-degree AV block is a delay in conduction at the level of the AV node rather than an actual block. First-degree AV block is not a rhythm in itself, but a condition superimposed on another rhythm. The underlying rhythm must also be identified (for example, sinus bradycardia with first-degree AV block).

Etiology: AV block can occur in the healthy heart. However, ischemia at the AV junction is the most common cause.

Rules of Interpretation/Lead II Monitoring (Figure 20-30):

Rate—depends on underlying rhythm

Rhythm—usually regular; can be slightly irregular

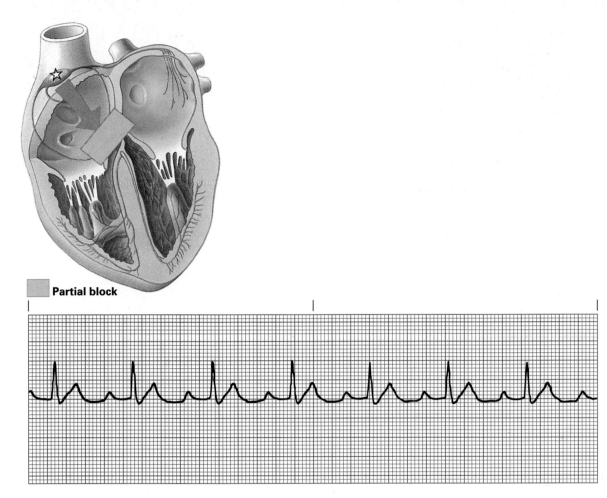

Partial block

FIGURE 20–30 First-degree AV block.

Pacemaker site—SA node or atria

P waves—normal

P-R interval—greater than 0.20 sec (diagnostic)

QRS complex—usually less than 0.12 sec; may be bizarre in shape if conductive system disease exists in the ventricles

Clinical Significance: First-degree block is usually no danger in itself. However, a newly developed first-degree block may precede a more advanced block.

Treatment: Generally, no treatment is required except observation, unless the heart rate drops significantly. If possible, avoid drugs that slow AV conduction, such as lidocaine and procainamide.

Type I Second-Degree AV Block

Description: A type I second-degree AV block (also called second-degree, Mobitz I; or Wenckebach), is an intermittent block at the level of the AV node. It produces a characteristic cyclic pattern in which the P-R intervals become progressively longer until an impulse is blocked (not conducted). The cycle is repetitive, and the P-P interval remains constant. The ratio of conduction (P waves to QRS complexes) is commonly 5:4, 4:3, 3:2, or 2:1. The pattern may be constant or variable.

Etiology: Low-grade AV blocks (first-degree and second-degree Mobitz I) can occur in the healthy heart. However, ischemia at the AV junction is the most common cause. Increased parasympathetic tone and drugs are also common etiologies.

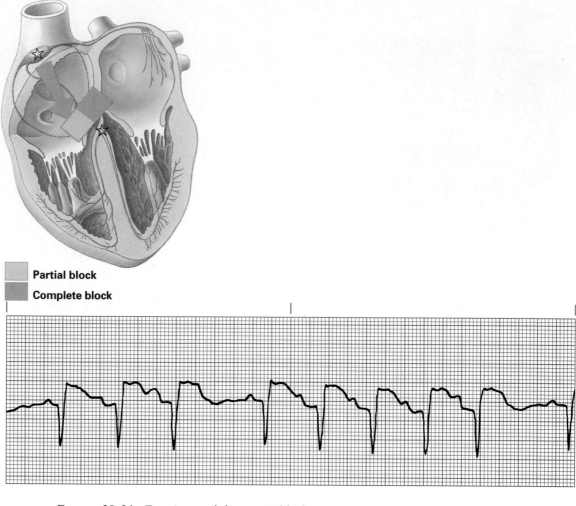

Partial block

Complete block

FIGURE 20-31   Type I second-degree AV block.

Rules of Interpretation/Lead II Monitoring (Figure 20-31):

   Rate—atrial rate is unaffected; the ventricular rate may be normal or slowed

   Rhythm—atrial rhythm is typically regular; ventricular rhythm is irregular because of the nonconducted beat

   Pacemaker site—SA node or atria

   P waves—normal; some P waves are not followed by QRS complexes

   P-R interval—becomes progressively longer until the QRS complex is dropped; the cycle then repeats

   QRS complex—usually less than 0.12 sec; may be bizarre in shape if conductive system disease exists in the ventricles

Clinical Significance: If beats are frequently dropped, second-degree block can compromise cardiac output by causing problems such as syncope and angina. This block is often a transient phenomenon that occurs immediately after an inferior wall myocardial infarction.

Treatment: Generally, no treatment other than observation is required. If possible, avoid drugs that slow AV conduction, such as lidocaine and procainamide. If the heart rate falls and the patient becomes symptomatic, administer 0.5 mg of atropine IV. Repeat every 3 to 5 minutes until you have obtained a satisfactory rate or have given 0.04 mg/kg of the drug. If atropine fails, consider transcutaneous cardiac pacing (TCP), if available.

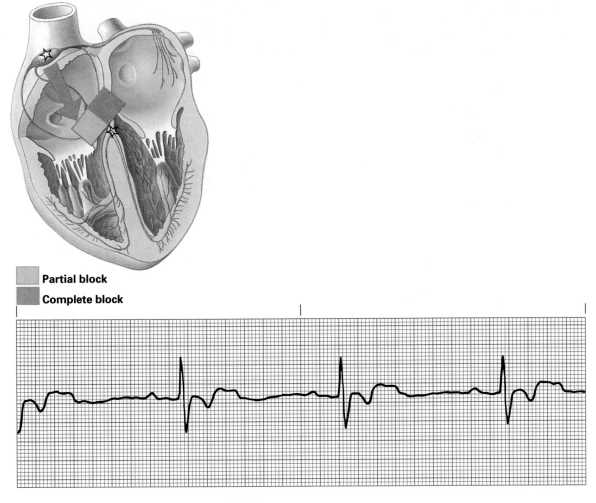

Partial block

Complete block

FIGURE 20-32   Type II second-degree AV block.

Type II Second-Degree AV Block

Description: A type II second-degree AV block (also called second-degree, Mobitz II; or infranodal) is an intermittent block characterized by P waves that are not conducted to the ventricles, but without associated lengthening of the P-R interval before the dropped beats. The ratio of conduction (P waves to QRS complexes) is commonly 4:1, 3:1, or 2:1. The ratio may be constant or may vary. A 2:1 Mobitz II block is often indistinguishable from a 2:1 Mobitz I block.

Etiology: Second-degree AV block, Mobitz II, is usually associated with acute myocardial infarction and septal necrosis.

Rules of Interpretation/Lead II Monitoring (Figure 20-32):

    Rate—atrial rate is unaffected; ventricular rate is usually bradycardic

    Rhythm—regular or irregular, depending on whether the conduction ratio is constant or varied

    Pacemaker site—SA node or atria

    P waves—normal; some P waves are not followed by QRS complexes

    P-R interval—constant for conducted beats; may be greater than 0.21 sec

    QRS complex—may be normal; however, it is often greater than 0.12 sec because of abnormal ventricular depolarization sequence

Never use lidocaine to treat third-degree heart block with ventricular escape beats.

Clinical Significance: A Mobitz II block can compromise cardiac output, causing problems such as syncope and angina if beats are frequently dropped. Since this block is often associated with cell necrosis resulting from myocardial infarction, it is considered much more serious than Mobitz I. Many Mobitz II blocks develop into full AV blocks.

Treatment: Pacemaker insertion is the definitive treatment. In the field, administer medications if stabilization is required. If the heart rate falls and the patient becomes symptomatic, administer 0.5 mg of atropine IV. Repeat every 3 to 5 minutes until you have obtained a satisfactory rate or have given 0.04 mg/kg of the drug. Use atropine with caution in patients who have high-grade blocks (second-degree Mobitz II and third-degree). The atropine may accelerate the atrial rate, but it may also worsen the AV nodal block. Consider transcutaneous cardiac pacing (TCP), if available. If the patient remains symptomatic, do not delay application of TCP while waiting for IV access or for atropine to take effect.

Third-Degree AV Block

Description: A third-degree AV block, or complete block, is the absence of conduction between the atria and the ventricles resulting from complete electrical block at or below the AV node. The atria and ventricles subsequently pace the heart independently of each other. The sinus node often functions normally, depolarizing the atrial syncytium. The escape pacemaker, located below the atria, paces the ventricular syncytium.

Etiology: Third-degree AV block can result from acute myocardial infarction, digitalis toxicity, or degeneration of the conductive system, as occurs in the elderly.

Rules of Interpretation/Lead II Monitoring (Figure 20-33):

Rate—atrial rate is unaffected. Ventricular rate is 40 to 60 if the escape pacemaker is junctional, less than 40 if the escape pacemaker is lower in the ventricles.

Rhythm—both atrial and ventricular rhythms are usually regular

Pacemaker site—SA node and AV junction or ventricle

P waves—normal. P waves show no relationship to the QRS complex, often falling within the T wave and QRS complex.

P-R interval—no relationship between P waves and R waves

QRS complex—greater than 0.12 sec if pacemaker is ventricular; less than 0.12 second if pacemaker is junctional

Clinical Significance: Third-degree block can severely compromise cardiac output because of decreased heart rate and loss of coordinated atrial kick.

Treatment: Pacemaker insertion is the definitive treatment. In the field, administer medications if stabilization is required. If the heart rate falls and the patient becomes symptomatic, administer 0.5 mg of atropine IV. You can repeat this every 3 to 5 minutes until you have obtained a satisfactory rate or have given 0.04 mg/kg of the drug. Use atropine with caution in patients with high-grade blocks (second-degree Mobitz II and third-degree). The atropine may accelerate the atrial rate, but it may also worsen the AV nodal block. Consider transcutaneous cardiac pacing (TCP), if available. If the patient remains symptomatic, do not delay application of TCP while waiting for IV access or for atropine to take effect. Never use lidocaine to treat third-degree heart block with ventricular escape beats.

DYSRHYTHMIAS SUSTAINED OR ORIGINATING IN THE AV JUNCTION

Dysrhythmias can originate within the AV node. The location of the pacemaker site will dictate the morphology of the P wave. Ischemia, hypoxia, and other factors have been identified as causes. Dysrhythmias originating in the AV junction include:

- Premature junctional contractions
- Junctional escape complexes and rhythm

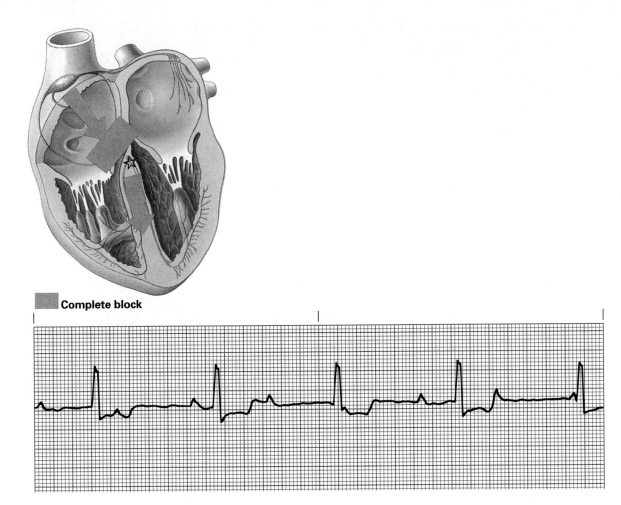

Complete block

FIGURE 20–33   Third-degree AV block.

- Accelerated junctional rhythm
- Paroxysmal junctional tachycardia

All dysrhythmias that originate in the AV junction have in common the following ECG features:

- Inverted P waves in Lead II, resulting from retrograde depolarization of the atria. The relation of the P wave to QRS depolarization depends on the relative timing of atrial and ventricular depolarization. The P wave can occur before the QRS complex, if the atria depolarize first; after the QRS, if the ventricles depolarize first; or during the QRS, if the atria and ventricles depolarize simultaneously. Depolarization of the atria during ventricular depolarization masks the P wave. Some atrial complexes that originate near the AV junction can also result in inverted P waves.
- P-R interval of less than 0.12 sec
- Normal QRS complex duration

Premature Junctional Contractions

Description: Premature junctional contractions (PJCs) result from a single electrical impulse originating in the AV node that occurs before the next expected sinus beat. A PJC can result in either a **compensatory pause** or noncompensatory pause, depending on whether the SA node is depolarized. A noncompensatory pause occurs if the premature beat depolarizes the SA node and interrupts the heart's normal cadence. A compensatory pause occurs only if the SA node discharges before the premature impulse reaches it.

compensatory pause the pause following an ectopic beat where the SA node is unaffected and the cadence of the heart is uninterrupted.

Etiology: A premature junctional contraction can result from any of the following conditions:

Use of caffeine, tobacco, or alcohol

Sympathomimetic drugs

Ischemic heart disease

Hypoxia

Digitalis toxicity

No apparent cause (idiopathic)

Rules of Interpretation/Lead II Monitoring (Figure 20-34):

Rate—depends on the underlying rhythm

Rhythm—depends on the underlying rhythm, usually regular except for the PJC

Pacemaker site—ectopic focus in the AV junction

P waves—inverted; may appear before or after the QRS complex. P waves can be masked by the QRS complex or be absent.

P-R interval—if the P wave occurs before the QRS complex, the P-R interval will be less than 0.12 sec; if the P wave occurs after the QRS complex, then technically it is an R-P interval

QRS complex—usually normal; may be greater than 0.12 sec if the PJC is abnormally conducted through partially refractory ventricles

Clinical Significance: Isolated PJCs are of minimal significance. Frequent PJCs indicate organic heart disease and may be precursors to other junctional dysrhythmias.

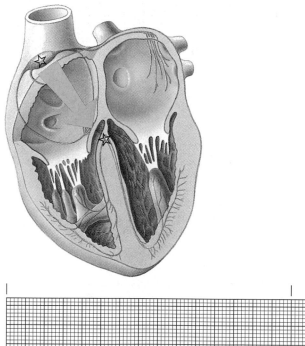

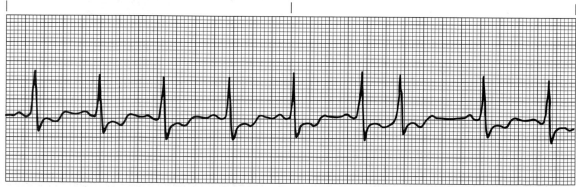

FIGURE 20-34 Premature junctional contractions.

Treatment: If the patient is asymptomatic, only observation is required in the field.

Junctional Escape Complexes and Rhythms

Description: A junctional escape beat, or junctional escape rhythm, is a dysrhythmia that results when the rate of the primary pacemaker, usually the SA node, is slower than that of the AV node. The AV node then becomes the pacemaker. The AV node usually discharges at its intrinsic rate of 40 to 60 beats per minute. This is a safety mechanism that prevents cardiac standstill.

Etiology: Junctional escape rhythm has several etiologies, including increased vagal tone, which can result in SA node slowing; pathological slow SA node discharge; or heart block.

Rules of Interpretation/Lead II Monitoring (Figure 20-35):

Rate—40 to 60 per minute

Rhythm—irregular in single junctional escape complex; regular in junctional escape rhythm

Pacemaker site—AV junction

P waves—inverted; may appear before or after the QRS complex. The P waves can be masked by the QRS or be absent.

P-R interval—if the P wave occurs before the QRS complex, the P-R interval will be less than 0.12 sec. If the P wave occurs after the QRS complex, technically it is an R-P interval.

QRS complex—usually normal; may be greater than 0.12 sec

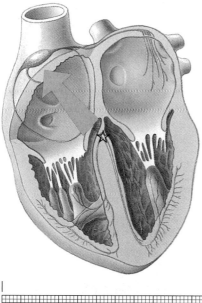

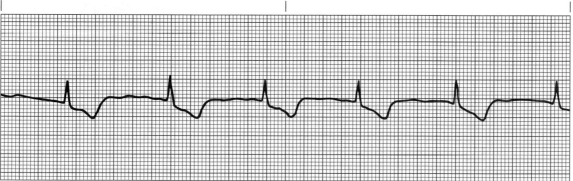

FIGURE 20-35 Junctional escape complex and rhythm.

Clinical Significance: The slow heart rate can decrease cardiac output, possibly precipitating angina and other problems. If the rate is fairly rapid, the rhythm can be well tolerated.

Treatment: If the patient is asymptomatic, only observation is required in the field. Treatment is unnecessary unless hypotension or ventricular irritability is present. If treatment is required, administer a 0.5 mg bolus of atropine sulfate. Repeat every 3 to 5 minutes until you have obtained a satisfactory rate or have given a total of 0.04 mg/kg of the drug. If atropine fails, consider transcutaneous cardiac pacing (TCP), if available.

Accelerated Junctional Rhythm

Description: An accelerated junctional rhythm results from increased automaticity in the AV junction, causing the AV junction to discharge faster than its intrinsic rate. If the rate becomes fast enough, the AV node can override the SA node. Technically, the rate associated with an accelerated junctional rhythm is not a tachycardia. However, when compared with the intrinsic rate of the AV junctional tissue (40 to 60 beats per minute), it is considered accelerated.

Etiology: Accelerated junctional rhythms often result from ischemia of the AV junction.

Rules of Interpretation/Lead II Monitoring (Figure 20-36):

    Rate—60 to 100 per minute

    Rhythm—regular

    Pacemaker site—AV junction

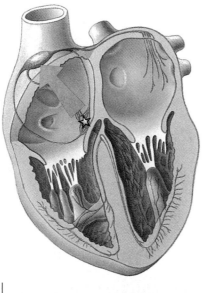

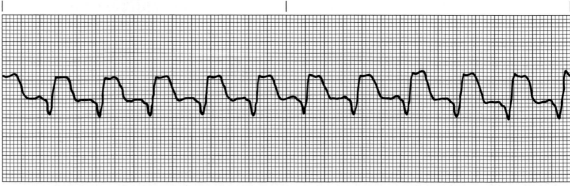

FIGURE 20-36   Accelerated junctional rhythm.

P waves—inverted; may appear before or after the QRS complex. P waves may be masked by the QRS or be absent.

P-R interval—if the P wave occurs before the QRS complex, the P-R interval will be less than 0.12 sec. If it occurs after the QRS, technically it is an R-P interval.

QRS complex—normal

Clinical Significance: An accelerated junctional rhythm is usually well tolerated. However, since ischemia is often the etiology, the patient should be monitored for other dysrhythmias.

Treatment: Prehospital treatment generally is unnecessary.

Paroxysmal Junctional Tachycardia

Description: Paroxysmal junctional tachycardia (PJT) develops when rapid AV junctional depolarization overrides the SA node. It often occurs in paroxysms (attacks with sudden onset), may last minutes or hours, and terminates abruptly. It may be caused by increased automaticity of a single AV nodal focus or by a reentry phenomenon at the AV node. Paroxysmal junctional tachycardia is often more appropriately called paroxysmal supraventricular tachycardia (PSVT), since the rapid rate may make it indistinguishable from paroxysmal atrial tachycardia.

Etiology: Paroxysmal junctional tachycardia may occur at any age and may not be associated with underlying heart disease. Stress, overexertion, smoking, or ingestion of caffeine may precipitate it. However, it is frequently associated with underlying atherosclerotic heart disease (ASHD) and rheumatic heart disease. PJT rarely occurs with myocardial infarction. It can occur with accessory pathway conduction, as in Wolff-Parkinson-White syndrome.

Rules of Interpretation/Lead II Monitoring (Figure 20-37):

Rate—100 to 180 per minute

Rhythm—characteristically regular, except at onset and termination of paroxysms

Pacemaker site—AV junction

P waves—if present, P waves are inverted. They can occur before, during, or after the QRS complex. Turning up the speed of the graph paper or oscilloscope to 50 mm/sec spreads out the complex and aids in identifying P waves.

P-R interval—if the P wave occurs before the QRS complex, the P-R interval will be less than 0.12 sec. If it occurs after the QRS complex, technically it is an R-P interval.

QRS complex—normal

Clinical Significance: Young patients with good cardiac reserve may tolerate PJT well for a short time. The patient often will sense PJT as palpitations. However, rapid rates can preclude adequate ventricular filling time and markedly reduce cardiac output. The reduced diastolic phase of the cardiac cycle can also compromise coronary artery perfusion. PJT can precipitate angina, hypotension, or congestive heart failure.

Treatment: If the patient is not tolerating the rapid heart rate, as evidenced by hemodynamic instability, attempt the following techniques in this order:

1. *Vagal maneuvers.* Ask the patient to perform a Valsalva maneuver. This is a forced expiration against a closed glottis, or "bearing down" as if to move the bowels. This results in vagal stimulation, which may slow the heart. If this is unsuccessful, attempt carotid artery massage if the patient is eligible and it is allowed in your EMS system. (Do not attempt carotid artery massage in patients with carotid bruits or known cerebrovascular or carotid artery disease.)

2. *Pharmacological therapy.* Adenosine (Adenocard) is relatively safe and highly effective in terminating PJT. This is especially true if its etiology is reentry. Administer 6 mg of adenosine by rapid IV bolus over 1 to 3 seconds

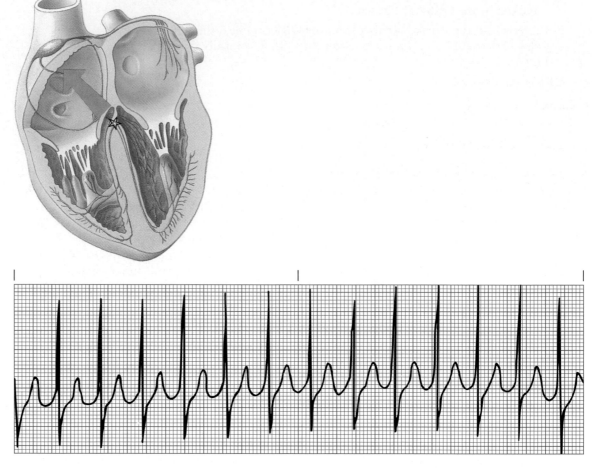

FIGURE 20-37   Paroxysmal junctional tachycardia.

through the medication port closest to the patient's heart or central circulation. If the patient does not convert after 1 to 2 minutes, administer a second bolus of 12 mg over 1 to 3 seconds in the medication port closest to the patient's heart or central circulation.

3. *Electrical therapy.* If the ventricular rate is greater than 150 beats per minute or the patient is hemodynamically unstable, use synchronized cardioversion. If time allows, sedate the patient with 5 to 10 mg of diazepam (Valium) or 2 to 5 mg of midazolam (Versed) IV. Apply synchronized DC countershock of 100 joules. If this is unsuccessful, repeat the countershock at increased energy as ordered by medical direction. DC countershock is contraindicated if you suspect digitalis toxicity as the cause of the PJT.

DYSRHYTHMIAS ORIGINATING IN THE VENTRICLES

Some dysrhythmias originate within the ventricles. The pacemaker site will dictate the morphology of the QRS complex. Many factors, including ischemia, hypoxia, and medications, have been identified as causes. Dysrhythmias originating in the ventricles include:

- Ventricular escape complexes and rhythms
- Accelerated idioventricular rhythm
- Premature ventricular contraction
- Ventricular tachycardia
- Related dysrhythmia
- Ventricular fibrillation

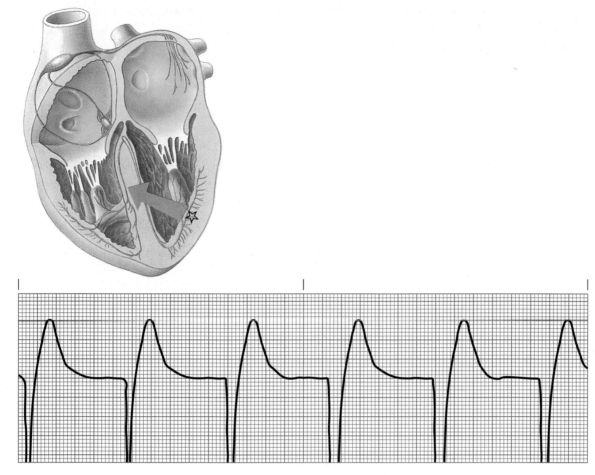

FIGURE 20-38　Ventricular escape complexes and rhythms (idioventricular rhythms).

- Asystole
- Artificial pacemaker rhythm

ECG features common to all dysrhythmias that originate in the ventricles include:

- QRS complexes of 0.12 sec or greater
- Absent P waves

Ventricular Escape Complexes and Rhythms

Description: A ventricular escape beat (ventricular escape rhythm or idioventricular rhythm) results either when impulses from higher pacemakers fail to reach the ventricles or when the discharge rate of higher pacemakers becomes less than that of the ventricles (normally 15 to 40 beats per minute). Ventricular escape rhythms serve as safety mechanisms to prevent cardiac standstill.

Etiology: Ventricular escape complexes and ventricular rhythms have several etiologies, including slowing of supraventricular pacemaker sites or high-degree AV block. They are frequently the first organized rhythms seen following successful defibrillation.

Rules of Interpretation/Lead II Monitoring (Figure 20-38):

Rate—15 to 40 per minute (occasionally less)

Rhythm—the rhythm is irregular in a single ventricular escape complex.
　　Ventricular escape rhythms are usually regular unless the pacemaker site is

low in the ventricular conductive system. Such placement makes regularity unreliable.

Pacemaker site—ventricle

P waves—none

P-R interval—none

QRS complex—greater than 0.12 sec and bizarre in morphology

Clinical Significance: The slow heart rate can significantly decrease cardiac output, possibly to life-threatening levels. The ventricular escape rhythm is a safety mechanism that you should not suppress. Escape rhythms can be perfusing or nonperfusing.

Treatment: Treatment depends on whether the escape rhythm is perfusing or nonperfusing. If it is perfusing, the object of treatment is to increase the heart rate. Administer a 0.5 mg bolus of atropine sulfate. Repeat every 3 to 5 minutes until you have obtained a satisfactory rate or have given 0.04 mg/kg of the drug. If atropine fails, consider transcutaneous cardiac pacing (TCP), if available. If the rhythm is nonperfusing, follow the pulseless electrical activity (PEA) protocol. This includes airway stabilization and CPR. Place an IV line, and administer 1 mg of epinephrine 1:10,000 IV. Direct treatment at correcting the primary problem (hypovolemia, hypoxia, cardiac tamponade, acidosis, or others). Consider a fluid challenge.

Accelerated Idioventricular Rhythm

Accelerated idioventricular rhythm is an abnormally wide ventricular dysrhythmia that usually occurs during an acute myocardial infarction. It is a subtype of ventricular escape rhythm. Typically the rate is 60 to 110 beats per minute. The patient does not require treatment unless he becomes hemodynamically unstable. If this occurs, treat the ventricular focus with atropine or overdrive pacing. The principal action should be aggressive treatment of the underlying myocardial infarction as indicated, including appropriate prehospital care.

Premature Ventricular Contractions

Description: A premature ventricular contraction (PVC, or ventricular ectopic) is a single ectopic impulse arising from an irritable focus in either ventricle that occurs earlier than the next expected beat. It may result from increased automaticity in the ectopic cell or a reentry mechanism. The altered sequence of ventricular depolarization results in a wide and bizarre QRS complex and may additionally cause the T wave to occur in the direction opposite the QRS complex.

A PVC does not usually depolarize the SA node and interrupt its rhythm. That is, it does not interrupt the heart's normal cadence. The pause following the PVC is fully compensatory. Occasionally, an **interpolated beat** occurs when a PVC falls between two sinus beats without interrupting the rhythm.

If more than one PVC occurs, each can be classified as unifocal or multifocal. Because the morphology of PVC depends on the ectopic pacemaker's location, two PVCs of different morphologies imply two different pacemaker sites (multifocal). PVCs with the same morphology imply one pacemaker site (unifocal). If the **coupling interval** (the distance between the preceding beat and the PVC) is constant, the PVCs are most likely unifocal.

PVCs often occur in patterns of group beating. These include the following terms, which can be applied to PACs and PJCs as well:

Bigeminy—every other beat is a PVC

Trigeminy—every third beat is a PVC

Quadrigeminy—every fourth beat is a PVC

Repetitive PVCs are two consecutive PVCs without a normal complex in between. They can occur in groups of two (couplets) or three (triplets). More than three consecutive PVCs are often considered ventricular tachycardia.

PVCs can trigger lethal dysrhythmias such as ventricular fibrillation if they fall within the relative refractory period (the so-called R on T phenomenon). They are often classified by their relationship to the previous normal complex.

interpolated beat a PVC that falls between two sinus beats without effectively interrupting this rhythm.

coupling interval distance between the preceding beat and the PVC.

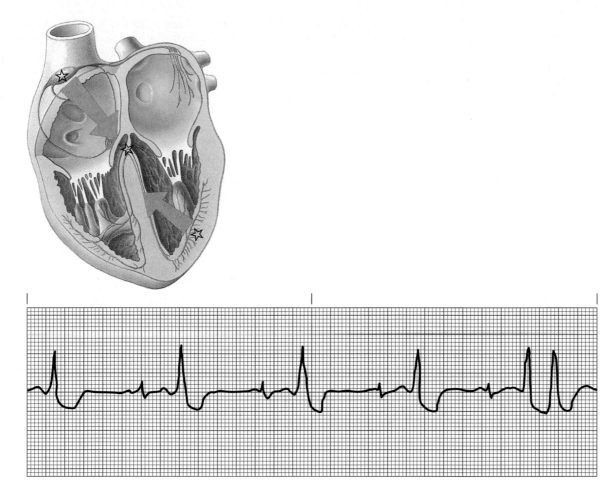

Figure 20-39   Premature ventricular contractions.

Etiologies: Etiologies for PVCs include:

   Myocardial ischemia

   Increased sympathetic tone

   Hypoxia

   Idiopathic causes

   Acid-base disturbances

   Electrolyte imbalances

   Normal variant

Rules of Interpretation/Lead II Monitoring (Figure 20-39):

   Rate—depends on underlying rhythm and rate of PVCs

   Rhythm—interrupts regularity of underlying rhythm; occasionally irregular

   Pacemaker site—ventricle

   P waves—none; however, a normal sinus P wave (interpolated P wave) sometimes
      appears before a PVC

   P-R interval—none

   QRS complex—greater than 0.12 sec and bizarre in morphology

Clinical Significance: Patients often sense PVCs as "skipped beats." In a patient without heart
   disease, PVCs may be insignificant. In patients with myocardial ischemia, PVCs may indi-

cate ventricular irritability and may trigger lethal ventricular dysrhythmias. PVCs are often classified as malignant or benign. Malignant PVCs have at least one of the following traits:

More than 6 PVCs per minute

R on T phenomenon

Couplets or runs of ventricular tachycardia

Multifocal

Associated chest pain

With most PVCs, the ventricles do not adequately fill. Because of this, you will usually not feel a pulse during the PVCs themselves. Frequent PVCs may reduce cardiac output.

PVCs can be described in terms of the Lown grading system for premature beats. The higher the grade, the more serious the ectopy:

Grade 0 = No premature beats

Grade 1 = Occasional (< 30 per hour) PVCs

Grade 2 = Frequent (> 30 per hour) PVCs

Grade 3 = Multiform (multifocal)

Grade 4 = Repetitive (couplets, salvos of 3 consecutive) PVCs

Grade 5 = R on T phenomenon

Treatment: If the patient has no history of cardiac disease and no symptoms, and if the PVCs are nonmalignant, no treatment is required. If the patient has a prior history of heart disease or symptoms, or if the PVCs are malignant, administer oxygen and place an IV line. If the patient is symptomatic, administer lidocaine at a dose of 1.0 to 1.5 mg/kg of body weight. Give an additional lidocaine bolus of 0.5 to 0.75 mg/kg every 5 to 10 minutes, if necessary, until you have given a total of 3.0 mg/kg of the drug. If the PVCs are effectively suppressed, start a lidocaine drip beginning at a rate of 2 to 4 mg/min. Reduce the dose in patients with decreased cardiac output (those with congestive heart failure or shock, for instance), in patients who are age 70 or greater, or in patients who have hepatic dysfunction. Give these patients a normal bolus dose first, followed by half the normal infusion. If the patient is allergic to lidocaine, or if you have given a maximum dose of lidocaine (3.0 mg/kg), consider procainamide or bretylium.

Ventricular Tachycardia

Description: Ventricular tachycardia (VT) consists of three or more ventricular complexes in succession at a rate of 100 beats per minute or more. This rhythm overrides the heart's normal pacemaker, and the atria and ventricles are asynchronous. Sinus P waves may occasionally be seen, dissociated from the QRS complexes. In monomorphic VT the complexes all appear the same; in polymorphic VT they have different sizes and shapes. One example of a polymorphic VT is torsade de pointes.

Etiology: As with PVCs, etiologies for ventricular tachycardia include:

Myocardial ischemia

Increased sympathetic tone

Hypoxia

Idiopathic causes

Acid-base disturbances

Electrolyte imbalances

Rules of Interpretation/Lead II Monitoring (Figure 20-40):

Rate—100 to 250 (approximately)

Rhythm—usually regular; can be slightly irregular

Pacemaker site—ventricle

P waves—if present, not associated with the QRS complexes

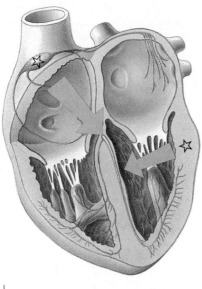

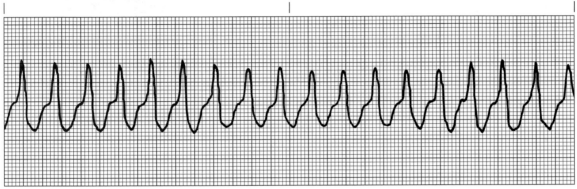

FIGURE 20-40   Ventricular tachycardia.

P-R interval—none

QRS complex—greater than 0.12 sec and bizarre in morphology

Clinical Significance: Ventricular tachycardia usually results in poor stroke volume, which, coupled with the rapid ventricular rate, may severely compromise cardiac output and coronary artery perfusion. Whether ventricular tachycardia is perfusing or nonperfusing dictates the type of treatment. Ventricular tachycardia may eventually deteriorate into ventricular fibrillation.

Treatment: If the patient is perfusing, as evidenced by the presence of a pulse, administer oxygen and place an IV line. Administer lidocaine at a dose of 1.0 to 1.5 mg/kg body weight intravenously. Administer additional doses of 0.5 to 0.75 mg/kg, until you have given a total of 3.0 mg/kg. If this treatment is unsuccessful, attempt to administer procainamide at 20 to 30 mg/minute to a maximum of 17 mg/kg. If procainamide fails, consider other second-line agents. Amiodarone (Cordarone) is becoming increasingly popular in the treatment of ventricular tachycardia. In the United States, it is primarily a second-line agent to lidocaine. In several of the Commonwealth countries, amiodarone is considered first-line treatment. The dose is 150 to 300 mg intravenously. Use synchronized cardioversion if the patient becomes unstable, as evidenced by chest pain, dyspnea, or systolic blood pressure of less than 90 mm/kg.

If the patient's condition is unstable, as evidenced by an altered level of consciousness or falling blood pressure, initiate cardioversion immediately after placing an IV line and administering oxygen. If time allows, sedate the patient first. The treatment plan is illustrated in the protocol (review Figure 20-26).

If the patient is nonperfusing, follow the protocol for ventricular fibrillation.

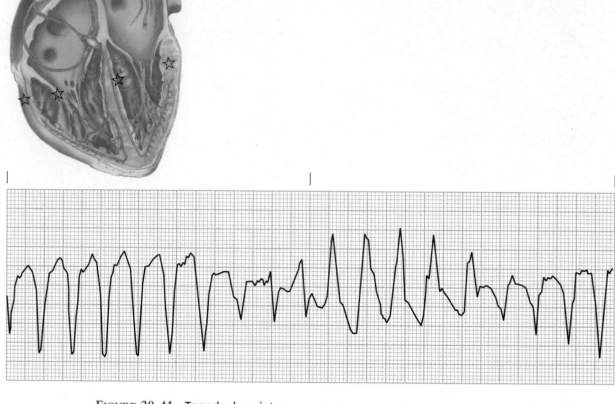

FIGURE 20–41   Torsade de pointes.

Torsade de Pointes   Torsade de pointes is a polymorphic ventricular tachycardia that differs in appearance and cause from ventricular tachycardia in general. Torsade is most commonly caused by the use of certain antidysrhythmic drugs, including quinidine (Quinidex), procainamide (Pronestyl), disopyramide (Norpace), flecanide (Tambocor), sotolol (Betapace), and amiodarone (Cordarone). These agents' effects all seem to be exacerbated by the coadministration of certain nonsedating antihistamines, most notably aztemizole (Hismanol) and terfenadine (Seldane) and, in addition, the azole antifungal agents and macrolide antibiotics; erythromycin (PCE), azithromycin, (Zithromax), and clarithramycin (Biaxin). Any of these agents increase the likelihood of the patient's developing torsade de pointes.

The morphology of the QRS varies from beat to beat (hence the term torsade de pointes, which means "twisting on a point"). In addition, the QT interval is markedly increased to 600 milliseconds or more. Torsade will usually occur in bursts that are not sustained. During the "breaks" from these bursts you should examine the rhythm strip for a prolonged Q-T interval. The QRS rate is usually between 166 and 300 beats per minute, and the R-R interval varies in an irregularly irregular pattern. The QRS complexes are wide and change in size over the span of several complexes (Figure 20-41). Attempting treatment of torsade de pointes with the antidysrhythmics usually used for the treatment of ventricular tachycardia can have disastrous consequences. Therefore, recognition of torsade de pointes as a separate dysrhythmia is essential. Treatment is 1 to 2 grams of magnesium sulfate placed in 100 mL of D_5W and administered over 1 to 2 minutes. This can be repeated every 4 hours with close monitoring of the deep tendon reflexes. Amiodarone (Cordarone) has proven effective in the treatment of torsade. Correct any underlying electrolyte problems, especially hyperkalemia.

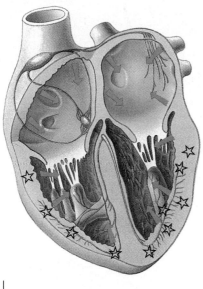

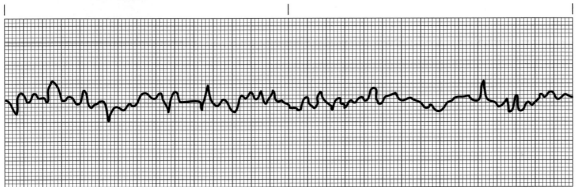

FIGURE 20-42   Ventricular fibrillation.

Ventricular Fibrillation

Description: Ventricular fibrillation is a chaotic ventricular rhythm usually resulting from the presence of many reentry circuits within the ventricles. There is no ventricular depolarization or contraction.

Etiology: A wide variety of causes have been associated with ventricular fibrillation. Most cases result from advanced coronary artery disease.

Rules of Interpretation/Lead II Monitoring (Figure 20-42):

> Rate—no organized rhythm
>
> Rhythm—no organized rhythm
>
> Pacemaker site—numerous ectopic foci throughout the ventricles
>
> P waves—usually absent
>
> P-R interval—absent
>
> QRS complex—absent

Clinical Significance: Ventricular fibrillation is a lethal dysrhythmia. The absence of cardiac output or an organized electrical pattern results in cardiac arrest.

Treatment: Ventricular fibrillation and nonperfusing ventricular tachycardia are treated identically. Initiate CPR. Follow this with DC countershock at 200 joules. If this is unsuccessful, repeat at 200 to 300 joules. If still unsuccessful, repeat at 360 joules. Subsequently, control the airway and establish an IV line. Epinephrine 1:10,000 or vasopressin are the drugs of first choice; administer every 3 to 5 minutes as required. If unsuccessful, consider second-line agents such as lidocaine, amiodarone, procainamide, or possibly magnesium sulfate.

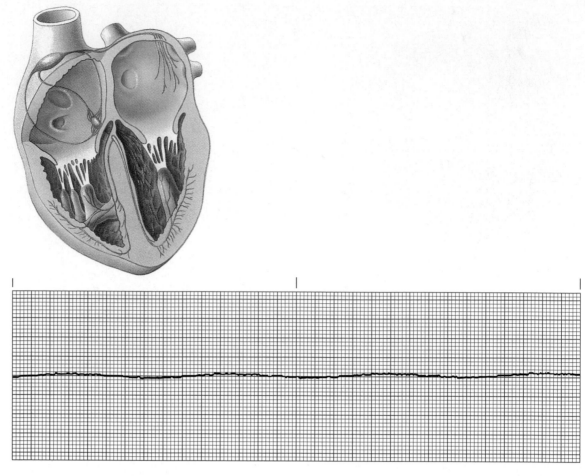

FIGURE 20-43 Asystole.

Asystole

Description: Asystole (cardiac standstill) is the absence of all cardiac electrical activity.

Etiology: Asystole may be the primary event in cardiac arrest. It is usually associated with massive myocardial infarction, ischemia, and necrosis. Resulting from heart blocks when no escape pacemaker takes over, asystole is often the final outcome of ventricular fibrillation.

Rules of Interpretation/Lead II Monitoring (Figure 20-43):

    Rate—no electrical activity

    Rhythm—no electrical activity

    Pacemaker site—no electrical activity

    P waves—absent

    P-R interval—absent

    QRS complex—absent

Clinical Significance: Asystole results in cardiac arrest. The prognosis for resuscitation is very poor.

Treatment: Treat asystole with CPR, airway management, oxygenation, and medications. If you have any doubt about the underlying rhythm, attempt defibrillation. Medications include epinephrine, and atropine (Figure 20-44).

Artificial Pacemaker Rhythm

Description: An artificial pacemaker rhythm results from regular cardiac stimulation by an electrode implanted in the heart and connected to a power source. The pacemaker lead

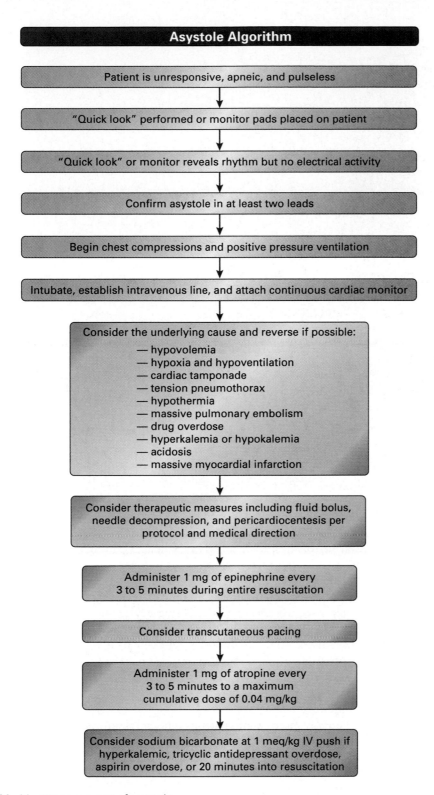

Asystole Algorithm

Patient is unresponsive, apneic, and pulseless

"Quick look" performed or monitor pads placed on patient

"Quick look" or monitor reveals rhythm but no electrical activity

Confirm asystole in at least two leads

Begin chest compressions and positive pressure ventilation

Intubate, establish intravenous line, and attach continuous cardiac monitor

Consider the underlying cause and reverse if possible:

— hypovolemia
— hypoxia and hypoventilation
— cardiac tamponade
— tension pneumothorax
— hypothermia
— massive pulmonary embolism
— drug overdose
— hyperkalemia or hypokalemia
— acidosis
— massive myocardial infarction

Consider therapeutic measures including fluid bolus, needle decompression, and pericardiocentesis per protocol and medical direction

Administer 1 mg of epinephrine every 3 to 5 minutes during entire resuscitation

Consider transcutaneous pacing

Administer 1 mg of atropine every 3 to 5 minutes to a maximum cumulative dose of 0.04 mg/kg

Consider sodium bicarbonate at 1 meq/kg IV push if hyperkalemic, tricyclic antidepressant overdose, aspirin overdose, or 20 minutes into resuscitation

FIGURE 20-44   Management of asystole.

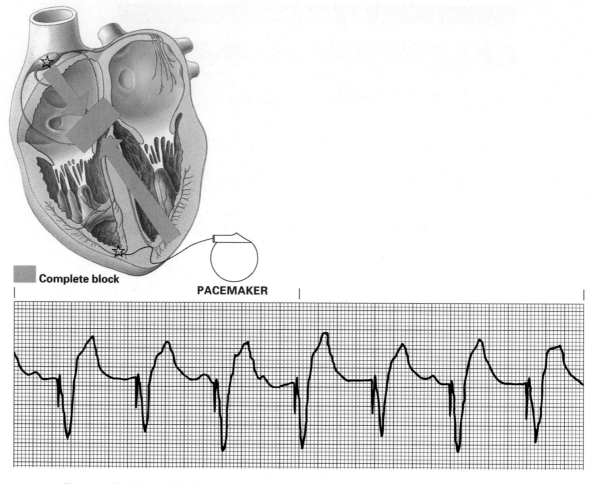

Complete block

PACEMAKER

FIGURE 20-45 Artificial pacemaker rhythm.

may be implanted in any of several locations in the heart, although it is most often placed in the right ventricle (ventricular pacemaker) or in both the right ventricle and the right atria (dual-chambered pacemaker.)

Fixed-rate pacemakers fire continuously at a preset rate, regardless of the heart's electrical activity. Demand pacemakers contain a sensing device and fire only when the natural heart rate drops below a set rate. In these cases, the pacemaker acts as an escape rhythm.

Ventricular pacemakers stimulate only the right ventricle, resulting in a rhythm that resembles an idioventricular rhythm. Dual-chambered pacemakers, commonly called AV sequential pacemakers, stimulate the atria first and then the ventricles. They are most beneficial for patients with marginal cardiac output who need the extra atrial kick to maintain cardiac output.

Pacemakers are usually inserted into patients who have chronic high-grade heart block or sick sinus syndrome or who have had episodes of severe symptomatic bradycardia.

Rules of Interpretation/Lead II Monitoring (Figure 20-45):

Rate—varies with the preset rate of the pacemaker

Rhythm—regular if pacing constantly; irregular if pacing on demand

Pacemaker site—depends on electrode placement

P waves—none produced by ventricular pacemakers. Sinus P waves may be seen but are unrelated to the paced QRS complexes. Dual-chambered pacemakers produce a P wave behind each atrial spike. A pacemaker spike is an upward or downward deflection from the baseline, which is an artifact created each time the pacemaker fires. The pacemaker spike tells you only that the pacemaker is firing. It reveals nothing about ventricular depolarization.

P-R interval—if present, varies

QRS complex—the QRS complexes associated with pacemaker rhythms are usually longer than 0.12 sec and bizarre in morphology. They often resemble ventricular escape rhythms. A QRS complex should follow each pacemaker spike. If so, the pacemaker is said to be "capturing." With demand pacemakers, some of the patient's own QRS complexes may appear. A pacemaker spike should not be associated with these complexes.

Problems with Pacemakers: Although rare, pacemakers can have problems. One cause is battery failure. Most pacemaker batteries have relatively long lives. The cardiologist can check them and usually replaces them before problems arise. If a battery fails, however, no pacing will occur and the patient's underlying rhythm, which may be bradycardic or asystolic, may return.

Occasionally, a pacemaker can run away. This condition, rarely seen with new pacemakers, results in a rapid discharge rate. Runaway pacemaker usually occurs when the battery runs low; newer models compensate for this by gradually increasing rate as their batteries run low.

Demand pacemakers can fail to shut down when the patient's intrinsic heart rate exceeds the rate set for the device. Thus the pacemaker competes with the patient's natural pacemaker. Occasionally, a paced beat can fall in the absolute or relative refractory period, precipitating ventricular fibrillation.

Finally, pacemakers can fail to capture if the leads become displaced or the battery fails. In such cases, pacemaker spikes are usually present without P waves or QRS complexes. Bradycardia often results.

Considerations for Management: Always examine any unconscious patient for a pacemaker. Battery packs are usually palpable under the skin, often in the shoulder or axillary region. Treat bradydysrhythmias, asystole, and ventricular fibrillation from pacemaker failure as in any other patient. You may use lidocaine to treat ventricular irritability without fear of suppressing ventricular response to the pacemaker. Defibrillate patients with pacemakers as usual, but do not discharge the paddles directly over the battery pack. If external cardiac pacing is available, you can use it until definitive care is available. Transport pacemaker failure patients promptly without prolonged field stabilization. Definitive care consists of battery replacement or temporary pacemaker insertion.

Use of a Magnet: Applying a magnet over the pulse generator inhibits all sensing and sets the pacemaker to a predetermined rate (usually 70). The patient should carry a card with information about his particular pacemaker, since these rates are manufacturer and model dependent. Use the magnet only for short periods to avoid the unlikely development of a serious dysrhythmia (including ventricular fibrillation). The indicator for magnet use is a runaway pacemaker.

PULSELESS ELECTRICAL ACTIVITY

Formerly termed electrical mechanical dissociation, pulseless electrical activity (PEA) essentially means that electrical complexes are present, but with no accompanying mechanical contractions of the heart. PEA is a perfect example of why you should treat the patient, not the monitor. Your monitor may show a textbook-perfect, normal sinus rhythm, but the patient may be pulseless.

Causes of PEA include:

- Hypovolemia
- Cardiac tamponade
- Tension pneumothorax
- Hypoxemia
- Acidosis
- Massive pulmonary embolism
- Ventricular wall rupture

Table 20-3 · SUGGESTED TREATMENT FOR UNDERLYING CAUSES OF PULSELESS ELECTRICAL ACTIVITY

Condition	Treatment (if allowed by local protocols)
Hypovolemia	Fluids
Cardiac tamponade	Pericardiocentesis
Tension pneumothorax	Needle thoracostomy
Hypoxemia	Intubation/oxygen

Administer epinephrine 1 mg every 3 to 5 minutes and treat the underlying cause(s). Table 20-3 shows suggested treatment for the different underlying causes. Early treatment can potentially reverse some of these conditions; therefore, prompt recognition and initiation of therapy are essential. Treatment for pulseless electrical activity is summarized in Figure 20-46.

DYSRHYTHMIAS RESULTING FROM DISORDERS OF CONDUCTION

Several dysrhythmias result from improper conduction through the heart. The three general categories of conductive disorders include:

- Atrioventricular blocks (discussed earlier in a separate section)
- Disturbances of ventricular conduction
- Pre-excitation syndromes

Disturbances of Ventricular Conduction

aberrant conduction conduction of the electrical impulse through the heart's conductive system in an abnormal fashion.

bundle branch block a kind of interventricular heart block in which conduction through either the right or left bundle branches is blocked or delayed.

Disturbances in conduction of the depolarization impulse are not limited to the AV node. Problems can arise within the ventricles as well. **Aberrant conduction** is a single supraventricular beat conducted through the ventricles in a delayed manner. **Bundle branch block** is a disorder in which all supraventricular beats are conducted through the ventricles in a delayed manner. Either the left or right bundle branch can be involved. If both branches are blocked, then a third-degree AV block exists. These complexes originate above the ventricles and should be distinguished from pure ventricular rhythms, which can have a similar QRS morphology. An incomplete bundle branch block has a normal QRS complex; a complete block has a wide QRS complex.

One of the two known causes of ventricular conduction disturbances is ischemia or necrosis of either the right or left bundle branch, rendering it incapable of conducting the impulse to the ventricle. The second is either a premature atrial contraction or a premature junctional contraction that reaches the ventricles or one of the bundle branches, usually the right, when it is still refractory. This often happens in atrial fibrillation because of the irregular rhythm's varying speed of repolarization.

The ECG features of ventricular conduction disturbances include a QRS complex longer than 0.12 sec because the blocked side of the heart is depolarized much more slowly than the unaffected side. The impulse passes much more slowly through the myocardium than through the rapid electrical conduction pathway. The QRS morphology is often bizarre. It can be notched or slurred, reflecting rapid depolarization through the normal conductive system and slow depolarization through the myocardium on the blocked side.

Ventricular conduction disturbances sometimes complicate ECG rhythm strip interpretation. In these cases, supraventricular beats can have abnormally wide QRS complexes. If you suspect a conduction system disturbance relating to supraventricular beats, then it is prudent to inspect some of the other leads to determine the problems.

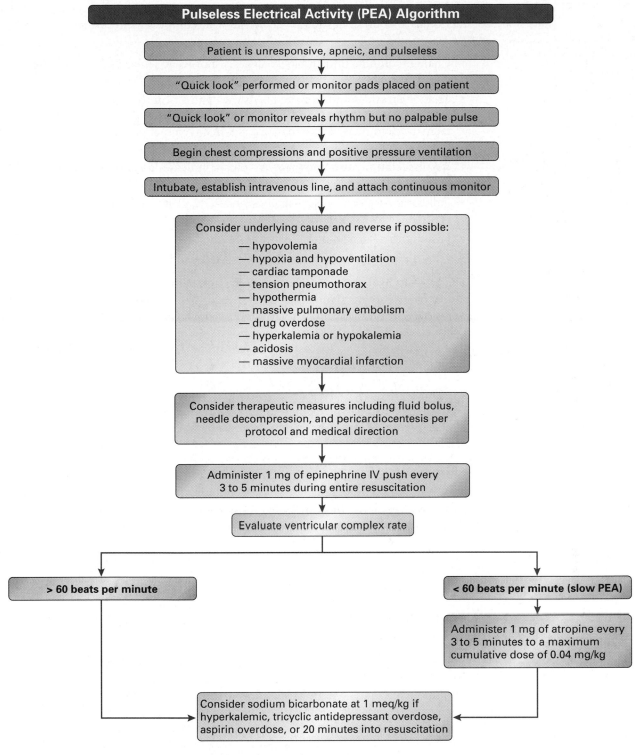

Pulseless Electrical Activity (PEA) Algorithm

Patient is unresponsive, apneic, and pulseless

"Quick look" performed or monitor pads placed on patient

"Quick look" or monitor reveals rhythm but no palpable pulse

Begin chest compressions and positive pressure ventilation

Intubate, establish intravenous line, and attach continuous monitor

Consider underlying cause and reverse if possible:

— hypovolemia
— hypoxia and hypoventilation
— cardiac tamponade
— tension pneumothorax
— hypothermia
— massive pulmonary embolism
— drug overdose
— hyperkalemia or hypokalemia
— acidosis
— massive myocardial infarction

Consider therapeutic measures including fluid bolus, needle decompression, and pericardiocentesis per protocol and medical direction

Administer 1 mg of epinephrine IV push every 3 to 5 minutes during entire resuscitation

Evaluate ventricular complex rate

> 60 beats per minute

< 60 beats per minute (slow PEA)

Administer 1 mg of atropine every 3 to 5 minutes to a maximum cumulative dose of 0.04 mg/kg

Consider sodium bicarbonate at 1 meq/kg if hyperkalemic, tricyclic antidepressant overdose, aspirin overdose, or 20 minutes into resuscitation

FIGURE 20-46 Management of pulseless electrical activity (PEA).

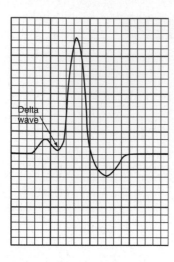

FIGURE 20-47 The delta wave of Wolf-Parkinson-White syndrome.

bundle of Kent an accessory AV conduction pathway that is thought to be responsible for the ECG findings of pre-excitation syndrome.

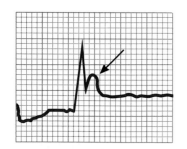

FIGURE 20-48 The Osborn (J) wave.

Although exceptions do occur, supraventricular tachycardias caused by disturbances in conduction usually differ in several ways from wide complex tachycardias originating in the ventricles:

- Changing bundle branch block suggests supraventricular tachycardia (SVT) with aberrancy.
- Trial of carotid sinus massage may slow conduction through the AV node and may terminate a reentrant SVT or slow conduction with other supraventricular tachydysrhythmias. These maneuvers will have no effect on ventricular tachycardias.
- AV dissociation, also known as AV block, indicates a ventricular origin of the dysrhythmia.
- Full compensatory pause, usually seen after a ventricular beat, indicates ventricular tachycardia.
- Fusion beats suggest ventricular tachycardia.
- QRS duration of longer than 0.14 sec usually indicates VT.

The patient's history may also help to differentiate the etiologies of wide complex tachycardias. In older patients with a history of myocardial infarction, CHF, or coronary artery disease, these dysrhythmias most likely have a ventricular origin.

When in doubt, treat the patient as if he has the more lethal dysrhythmia, ventricular tachycardia. In either case, use cardioversion if the patient is unstable; it is effective for both ventricular and supraventricular tachycardias.

Pre-Excitation Syndromes

Pre-excitation syndromes involve premature ventricular excitation by an impulse that bypasses the AV node. The most common of these is Wolff-Parkinson-White (WPW) syndrome. WPW occurs in approximately three of every 1,000 persons. It is characterized by a short P-R interval, generally less than 0.12 sec, and a long QRS duration, generally more than 0.12 sec. Additionally, the upstroke of the QRS often has a slur, called the *delta wave* (Figure 20-47). In WPW, conduction of the depolarization impulse from the atria to the ventricles is abnormal. The **bundle of Kent,** an extra conduction pathway between the atria and ventricles, effectively bypasses the AV node, shortening the P-R interval and prolonging the QRS complex. Most WPW patients are asymptomatic; however, the disorder is associated with a high incidence of tachydysrhythmias, usually through a reentry mechanism. WPW is also frequently associated with organic heart diseases such as atrial septal defects or mitral valve prolapse. Base treatment on the underlying rhythm.

ECG Changes Due to Electrolyte Abnormalities and Hypothermia

Electrolyte imbalances can cause dysrhythmias that will appear on ECG rhythm strips. Suspect hyperkalemia (excessive potassium in the blood) in patients with a history of renal failure who are on dialysis. On an ECG, tall, peaked T waves in the precordial leads are an early sign of hyperkalemia. As the levels increase further, conduction decreases and the PR and QT intervals increase. At very high potassium levels, an idioventricular rhythm may develop and eventually become a classic sine wave (a wave that rises to a maximum positive level and then drops to a maximal negative level). Prominent U waves appear with hypokalemia (deficient potassium levels in the blood). Very low levels can widen the QRS complex.

In hypothermia, the *Osborn wave,* or *J wave,* is apparent. It is a slow, positive deflection at the end of the QRS complex (Figure 20-48). Other ECG changes may include:

- T wave inversion
- PR, QRS, QT prolongation.
- Sinus bradycardia
- Atrial fibrillation or flutter

- AV block
- PVCs
- Ventricular fibrillation
- Asystole

Part 2: Assessment and Management of the Cardiovascular Patient

Part 2 of this chapter will help you build on the information about cardiovascular anatomy (in Chapter 2) and cardiac physiology, electrographic monitoring, and dysrhythmias (in Part 1 of this chapter) as you develop the skills for assessing and managing a patient suffering a cardiovascular emergency.

Part 2 begins with general principles of assessment and management of cardiovascular emergencies and concludes with discussions of a variety of specific conditions and emergencies including angina pectoris, myocardial infarction, heart failure, cardiac tamponade, hypertensive emergencies, cardiogenic shock, cardiac arrest, and cardiovascular emergencies.

ASSESSMENT OF THE CARDIOVASCULAR PATIENT

The key to providing the cardiovascular patient with the best possible medical care is to take a systematic, step-by-step approach. When you initially contact your patient, always determine the most important problems first. Airway, breathing, circulatory problems, and shock are always the most critical issues during the first minute of patient care. What may have caused any life-threatening problems does not matter at this point. In some instances such as cardiac arrest, your focus during prehospital care may never go beyond these four concerns.

Airway, breathing, and circulatory problems and shock are always the most critical issues during the first minute of patient care.

After you have managed any life-threatening problems, the focused history and physical examination will help you form your field diagnosis. Cardiovascular diseases may affect the myocardium, the electrical conductive system, the pericardium, or the blood vessels. They may also involve a combination of these problems or problems associated with other systems, such as diabetes. Diseases of the myocardium include myocardial infarction, heart failure, or cardiogenic shock. In electrical conductive illnesses, the heart rate is either too fast or too slow. Although pericardial emergencies such as pericarditis or pericardial tamponade are usually diagnosed clinically by the physical examination findings, the focused history (blunt/penetrating trauma or recent infection, for example) may help you to recognize them. Vascular problems may include coronary artery occlusion, peripheral venous or arterial occlusion, or pulmonary embolism.

In the field, therapeutic treatments are generally limited to:

- Administering nitrates, aspirin, and analgesics for symptomatic chest pain
- Treating pulmonary edema
- Giving analgesics in peripheral vascular emergencies

In your ongoing assessment, continually reevaluate your initial management. Based on the patient's needs, you will transport him in the appropriate mode to the appropriate facility. As with any patient, your management of the cardiac patient should include patient advocacy as well as communication and emotional support for the patient and his family. You must also effectively communicate the details of your assessment and management to the receiving staff. Additionally, your knowledge of nontransport criteria, education and prevention, proper documentation, and ongoing quality assurance will all contribute to providing optimum care.

Your assessment of the patient with a cardiovascular emergency should vary according to the acuity of the situation. Patients with serious illnesses should have a limited, yet focused exam. Patients who are less seriously ill should receive a more comprehensive assessment. It is important to remember that the cardiovascular system affects virtually every other body system. Signs of cardiac disease may initially be evident only in the respiratory system as dyspnea. A comprehensive exam, however, often reveals subtle findings that point to cardiovascular disease as the cause.

SCENE SIZE-UP AND INITIAL ASSESSMENT

After ascertaining that the scene is safe, begin an initial cardiovascular assessment. This allows you to identify life-threatening problems and set transport priorities. First, determine the patient's level of responsiveness. Is he speaking with you or unresponsive? Then move on to the ABCs. Make sure his airway is patent and free of debris and blood. Suction the airway if appropriate. Next, check the patient's rate and depth of breathing. Listen for the presence or absence of breath sounds. Certain breath sounds such as moist rales should heighten your suspicion of cardiovascular disease. Note the effort or work of breathing. If the patient is not breathing, initiate manual ventilation and intubate as soon as possible. Check for the rate and quality of pulses. If no pulse is present, immediately begin cardiopulmonary resuscitation. The skin can indicate the degree of perfusion present. Look for:

- Color
- Temperature
- Moisture
- Turgor
- Mobility
- Edema

Finally, check the patient's blood pressure. Is he in shock? Is this a hypertensive emergency? Treat all life-threatening conditions as you find them.

FOCUSED HISTORY

After you have completed your initial cardiovascular assessment and treated life-threatening conditions, proceed with your focused history, using the SAMPLE format (*S*ymptoms, *A*llergies, *M*edications, *P*ast medical history, *L*ast oral intake, and *E*vents preceding the incident).

Common Symptoms

Cardiac disease can manifest itself in several ways. Some common chief complaints and symptoms include:

- Chest pain or discomfort
- Dyspnea
- Cough
- Syncope
- Palpitations

Chest pain is the most common presenting symptom in cases of cardiac disease.

Not all patients who have cardiac disease will have chest pain.

Chest Pain Chest pain or discomfort that may radiate to the shoulder, neck, jaw, or back is a common symptom of cardiac disease. Always remember, however, that not all patients who have cardiac disease will have chest pain. This is especially true in diabetic patients, who may have a myocardial infarction with no pain at all. Also remember that chest pain can be benign and may have no association with cardiac disease. Differentiating between benign and life-threatening chest pain is extremely difficult; do not attempt it in the field. If a cardiac etiology is even a remote possibility, treat the patient accordingly.

Follow the OPQRST acronym to obtain the patient's description of the pain:

- *Onset.* Ask about the onset of the pain. When did it begin? What was the patient doing when it started? If the patient has had chest pain in the past, ask him to compare it to previous episodes. For instance, if he had a major heart attack in the past and tells you his present pain is the same, then strongly suspect that it is also from his heart.

- *Provocation/palliation.* What provoked the pain? Is it exertional or nonexertional? The relationship of pain to exertion is very important. During exertion, the heart muscle needs more oxygen. If it does not receive the additional oxygen, the muscle becomes ischemic and the patient has pain (angina). He may tell you that he is now walking shorter distances before the pain begins, indicating lessening blood flow to the heart. Untreated, this may lead to pain at rest and, eventually, infarction. What alleviates the pain (palliation)? Is the pain related to movement or inspiration?

- *Quality.* Ask the patient to describe the quality of the pain. Ask open-ended questions and allow the patient to characterize this symptom in his own words. Common descriptive words include sharp, tearing, pressure, and heaviness.

- *Region/radiation.* The patient may complain of pain radiating to other regions of his body, most commonly his arms, neck, jaw, and back.

- *Severity.* Ask the patient to rate the pain on a scale of 1 to 10, with 1 being very little and 10 being the worst pain he has ever felt. This can also be a useful gauge of the effectiveness of your management. Some systems will use a pain scale of 1 to 5. Regardless of the scale, it is important that the scale used is standardized in the system. It can be problematic if a EMT-I asks a patient to rate his pain on a scale of 1 to 5, but when the patient gets to the hospital, the nurse or doctor is using a scale of 1 to 10. Although seemingly trivial, this can significantly affect patient care.

- *Timing.* Check the timing of the pain. How long has the pain lasted? Always determine the time the pain began and record it. The onset and duration of pain directly affect decisions about the use of thrombolytic drugs. Is the pain constant or intermittent? Is it getting worse? better? Does it occur at rest or with activity?

Dyspnea Because of the heart's close relationship with the respiratory system, many cardiac patients have dyspnea (labored breathing). Dyspnea is often associated with myocardial infarction and in some patients may be the only symptom. Also, patients with congestive heart failure will experience increased dyspnea when lying down.

When confronted with a dyspneic patient, ask about the following:

- *Duration.* How long has it lasted? Is it continuous or intermittent?
- *Onset.* Was the onset sudden or rapid?
- *Provocation/palliation.* Does anything aggravate or relieve the dyspnea? Is it exertional or nonexertional?
- *Orthopnea.* Does sitting upright give relief?

Cough Frequently, patients who cough have chest pain. Is the cough dry or productive? Did the patient pull a chest muscle during coughing? Try to determine if the coughing results from congestive heart failure.

Other Related Signs and Symptoms Other related signs and symptoms to look for and ask about include:

- *Level of consciousness.* The level of consciousness indicates brain perfusion. An alteration in the level of consciousness can be due to problems within the cardiovascular system.

- *Diaphoresis* (perspiration). Cardiac problems significantly affect the autonomic nervous system. Stimulation of the sympathetic nervous system can result in marked diaphoresis.

- *Restlessness and anxiety.* Restlessness and anxiety are among the earliest symptoms when a patient is experiencing lowered brain perfusion, whether due to decreased oxygenation, decreased blood supply, or both.

- *Feeling of impending doom.* The significant and massive stimulation of the sympathetic nervous system associated with severe cardiovascular emergencies can cause a feeling of impending doom. This is a part of the "fight-or-flight" response. A patient with a sensation of impending doom can be experiencing a significant cardiovascular event.

- *Nausea and/or vomiting.* Nausea and vomiting are common during cardiovascular events such as myocardial ischemia. This often results from slowed peristalsis due to sympathetic stimulation.

- *Fatigue.* Fatigue is a generalized finding associated with many diseases. In patients with cardiovascular disease, it can be caused by anemia, poor oxygenation, or poor overall cardiovascular system functioning.

- *Palpitations.* Palpitations are a sensation that the heart is beating fast or skipping beats. This can result from tachycardia or simply from increased awareness of the heart's normal function.

- *Edema.* Edema is the accumulation of fluid in third (interstitial) spaces. It accompanies poor cardiac function and often indicates chronic cardiovascular disease.

  – *Extremities.* Ambulatory patients usually will develop edema in the extremities, due to the effects of gravity.

  – *Sacral.* Sacral, or presacral edema, is seen in bed-bound patients. Fluid collects in the lowest part of the patient's body, usually around the sacrum.

- *Headache.* Headache is a factor in cardiovascular disease for several reasons. First, decreased central nervous system (CNS) perfusion can result in headaches. These are often severe. Many patients with established heart disease take nitroglycerin or other nitrate drugs. Excess administration of nitrates can cause a severe headache and may indicate worsening heart disease.

- *Syncope.* Syncope is a brief loss of consciousness due to a transient decrease in cerebral blood flow. It occurs in certain cardiac dysrhythmias and in ischemic lesions where blood flow to the heart may be impaired, reducing cardiac output and interrupting CNS perfusion. Severe pain can also cause syncope as well as other forms of psychic stress.

- *Behavioral change.* A behavioral change may subtly indicate cardiovascular disease. More common in the elderly, it may point to either an acute or chronic decrease in cerebral blood flow.

- *Anguished facial expression.* The pain that accompanies myocardial ischemia can be quite severe. This, coupled with the effects of sympathetic nervous system stimulation, may cause the patient to exhibit anguished facial expressions.

- *Activity limitations.* Decreased cardiac performance can significantly limit a patient's physical activities. These limitations may develop slowly and be considered chronic or develop quickly and be considered acute.

- *Trauma.* Trauma, especially unexplained trauma, can be due to a temporary decrease in CNS perfusion. Unexplained facial injuries or bruises may indicate a cardiovascular problem.

Many of the signs and symptoms of cardiovascular disease can be subtle. Always assess for them and look for any sign or symptom patterns that point to cardiovascular disease.

Allergies

Ask about the patient's allergies. Is he allergic to any medications? Does he have an allergy to X-ray dye (IVP dye)? Try to differentiate between true medication allergies and undesirable side effects of a particular medication. For instance, the patient who tells you he breaks out in hives and stops breathing if he takes penicillin is having an allergic reaction. The patient who says he gets abdominal upset from aspirin is, most likely, experiencing a side effect. If in doubt, withhold the medication and contact medical direction.

If in doubt about a possible medication allergy, withhold the medication and contact medical direction.

Medications

The patient's current use of prescription medications is important. What medications is he currently taking? Has he recently changed any medications? The following drugs may be especially significant:

- Nitroglycerin (Nitrostat)
- Propranolol (Inderal) and other beta blockers
- Digitalis (Lanoxin)
- Diuretics (Lasix, Maxzide, Dyazide)
- Antihypertensives (Vasotec, Prinivil, Capoten)
- Antidysrhythmics (Mexitil, Quinaglute, Tambocor)
- Lipid-lowering agents (Mevacor, Lopid)

Also question the patient in detail about his compliance with his medications. Does he take his medications? Does he take the right amount? Does he take them at the right time? With the high cost of medications and limited coverage by prescription plans, more and more patients are not taking their prescriptions. Some may even borrow a friend's medication, a dangerous practice, since it may be the wrong dosage or even the wrong drug.

The patient's use of nonprescription drugs is also important. Ask if he takes any over-the-counter medications. Numerous drugs interact, and you must be aware of all medications the patient is currently taking, prescription or otherwise. Try to bring all drug containers with you to the hospital if doing so will not adversely prolong transport time. This information is very important for the hospital staff. Recreational drug use is another major problem. For example, cocaine causes vasoconstriction of the blood vessels and can lead to myocardial infarction and severe hypertension, often in the absence of coronary artery disease. These effects can last up to 2 weeks. Even though this question may make you uncomfortable, you must ask it.

Try to bring all of the patient's prescription and nonprescription drug containers to the hospital with you.

Past Medical History

Avoid spending excessive time obtaining a cardiac patient's past medical history. If the patient's condition permits, however, a past medical history may help you determine if his symptoms are attributable to a cardiac condition:

- Does the patient have a history of coronary artery disease, angina, or a previous myocardial infarction? If so, chances are good that his symptoms are cardiac in origin. Comparing his prior symptoms to his present ones is helpful. If he tells you this pain is just like his previous heart attack, then he likely is experiencing another.
- Has the patient had any prior heart problems? Ask about the following:
  - Valvular disease (rheumatic heart disease)
  - Aneurysm
  - Previous cardiac surgery
  - Congenital cardiac anomalies
  - Pericarditis or other inflammatory cardiac disease
  - Congestive heart failure
- What other medical problems does the patient have? Ask about the following:
  - Pulmonary disease/chronic obstructive pulmonary disease (COPD)

- Diabetes mellitus
- Renal (kidney) disease
- Hypertension
- Peripheral vascular disease

- Does anyone in the patient's family have cardiac disease? At what age did it first develop? Cardiac disease before the age of 50 in a close relative should heighten your concern about heart disease. If a family member had a cardiac event at a young age, especially sudden death, your patient is also at risk earlier in life. Has anyone in his family died of heart disease? At what age? Also ask if the family has a history of stroke, diabetes, or hypertension.

- Does the patient smoke? Does he know his cholesterol level? These are other modifiable risk factors for cardiac disease.

Last Oral Intake

When was the patient's last oral intake? If the patient ingested a meal high in saturated fats before the onset of symptoms, then gallbladder disease should be considered as a possible etiology. Also inquire if the patient has had an increase in caffeine intake and ask when he last drank a caffeinated beverage.

Events Preceding the Incident

What was the patient doing before the onset of symptoms? Was there emotional upset? Had he just completed a strenuous task such as mowing the yard? Has he recently started a new exercise program? Did the symptoms begin while the patient was having sex? Does the patient take Viagra? The development of chest pain during sexual intercourse is not uncommon. However, patients often will not volunteer this information. Asking about intimate events such as this may be uncomfortable, but it is necessary for optimal patient care.

PHYSICAL EXAMINATION

After addressing any life-threatening problems you find in the initial assessment, begin the physical exam. Be systematic and thorough, and remember to look (inspect), listen (auscultate), and feel (palpate) while performing your detailed examination.

Inspection

During your inspection, look for:

- *Tracheal position.* The trachea should be midline. Movement toward a side may indicate a pneumothorax. Inspect the neck veins for evidence of jugular vein distention. The internal jugular veins are major vessels. Thus, jugular vein distention often evidences an increase in central venous pressure (Figure 20-49). Pump failure or cardiac tamponade can cause back pressure in the systemic

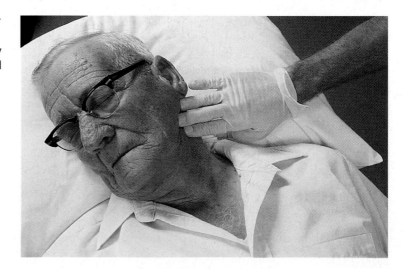

FIGURE 20-49 Look for the presence of jugular venous distension, ideally with the patient elevated at a 45-degree angle.

circulation and jugular vein engorgement. Try to have the patient seated at a 45-degree angle, not lying flat, for this examination. Remember, however, that jugular vein distention is often difficult to assess in an obese patient.

- *Thorax.* Watch the patient breathe. To do this properly, expose the patient's chest wall, maintaining patient privacy if possible. Evidence of labored breathing includes retractions and accessory muscle use. Retractions are visible depressions in the soft tissues between the ribs that occur with increased respiratory effort. Accessory muscle use involves muscles of the neck, back, and abdomen. Normally these muscles play a small role in breathing, but patients with labored breathing put them to greater use. A patient with COPD may have an increased anteroposterior (AP) diameter and may appear "barrel-chested." Examination of the thorax can provide a great deal of information about the patient, including chronic problems such as COPD. The presence of a sternotomy scar, especially in an older patient, is a significant indicator of heart disease.

- *Epigastrium.* While the chest wall is exposed, inspect the epigastrium. Look for abdominal distention and visible pulsations. This may mean the patient has an aortic aneurysm with dissection or rupture.

- *Peripheral and presacral edema.* Chronic back pressure in the systemic venous circulation causes peripheral and presacral edema. These symptoms are most obvious in dependent parts such as the ankles (Figure 20-50). Often in bedridden patients you must inspect and palpate the sacral region for edema. Edema is generally classified as either mild or pitting. To distinguish between them, press firmly on the edematous part. If the depression remains after you remove pressure, the edema is pitting; otherwise it is mild.

- *Skin.* Several changes in the skin can be associated with cardiovascular disease. Pale and diaphoretic skin indicates peripheral vasoconstriction and sympathetic stimulation. It accompanies heart disease and other problems. A mottled appearance often indicates chronic cardiac failure.

- *Subtle signs of cardiac disease.* Look for subtle indicators of cardiac disease. Observe for signs that a patient is being treated for cardiac problems. These include midsternal scars from coronary artery bypass surgeries, pacemakers, or nitroglycerin skin patches.

Auscultation

During your inspection listen for:

- *Breath sounds.* Assessing breath sounds in the cardiac patient is just as important as it is in the respiratory patient. Assess the lung fields for equality.

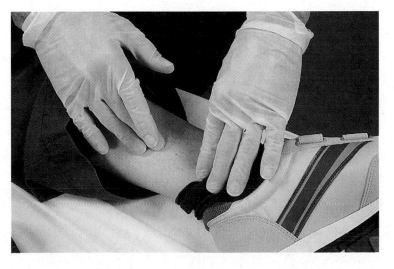

FIGURE 20-50 Check for peripheral edema.

Also listen for adventitious sounds, those that arise or occur sporadically or in unusual locations. Such sounds as crackles (rales), wheezes, or rhonchi (whistling or snoring sounds) may indicate pulmonary congestion or edema. Patients with pulmonary edema may also have foamy, blood-tinged sputum from the mouth and nose. In severe cases, this is audible from a distance as an ominous gurgling sound.

An S_3 heart sound has a cadence like "Kentucky." An S_4 heart sound has a cadence like "Tennessee."

- *Heart sounds.* Avoid spending precious time auscultating heart sounds in the field. Background noise from traffic, family members, sirens, and other sources makes it very difficult to hear heart sounds, and the information you obtain generally will not affect patient management. Nonetheless, you should be familiar with normal heart sounds and be able to distinguish abnormal from normal findings (Figure 20-51). The first heart sound (S_1) is produced by closure of the AV valves (tricuspid and mitral) during ventricular systole. The second heart sound (S_2) is produced by closure of the aortic and pulmonary valves. S_1 and S_2 are normal. Any extra heart sounds are abnormal. The third heart sound (S_3) is associated with congestive heart failure. Occasionally, the skilled listener can hear the fourth heart sound (S_4), which occurs immediately before S_1. It is associated with increased atrial contraction. Ideally, the heart should be examined from the four classic auscultatory sites: aortic, pulmonic, mitral, and tricuspid. The point on the chest wall where the heartbeat can best be heard or felt is known as the point of maximum impulse (PMI). (Find more details in Chapter 7.)

- *Carotid artery bruit.* Auscultation of the carotid arteries may reveal *bruits* (murmurs), which are a sign of turbulent blood flow through a vessel (Figure 20-52). They are audible over all major arteries, including the abdominal aorta. A bruit indicates partial blockage of the vessel, most commonly from atherosclerosis. If you detect a bruit, do not attempt carotid sinus massage. This procedure may dislodge plaque, resulting in stroke or other mishap.

Palpation

During your examination, feel for:

- *Pulse.* Determine the rate and regularity of the pulse (Figure 20-53). Also note the pulse's equality. Any pulse deficit can indicate underlying peripheral vascular disease and should be reported to medical direction.

- *Thorax.* Palpation of the thorax is extremely important because chest wall problems are quite common. These can only be elicited by palpation, which may reveal crepitus. Crepitus is a grating sensation that suggests the rubbing of

FIGURE 20-51
Auscultate the chest. Listen for heart sounds.

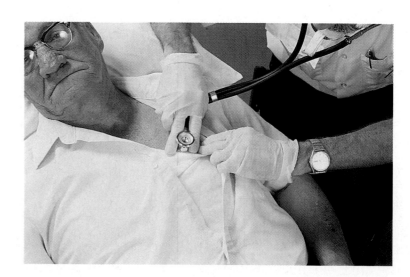

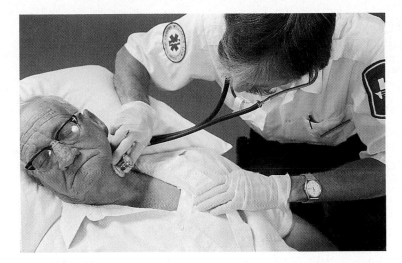

FIGURE 20-52 Listen to the carotid arteries. The presence of noisy blood flow is termed a *bruit* and may indicate underlying disease in the artery.

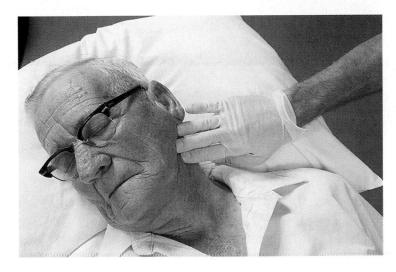

FIGURE 20-53 Check the patient's pulse for both strength and character.

broken bone ends or a "bubble wrap" crackling that suggests subcutaneous emphysema (air in the subcutaneous tissue). Palpapation may also reveal tenderness associated with a chest wall muscle strain, costochondritis (inflammation of the joint where the rib attaches to the sternum), or even rib fractures. It is important to remember that at least 15% of patients with acute myocardial infarction will have associated chest wall tenderness.

- *Epigastrium.* Also feel the abdomen for pulsations and distention, which may indicate an abdominal aortic aneurysm.

Physical examination of the chest is an essential aspect of comprehensive prehospital care. Employ the standard techniques of inspection, auscultation, palpation, and occasionally, percussion. Together these skills can provide a great deal of information about chronic problems as well as the ongoing acute episode.

MANAGEMENT OF CARDIOVASCULAR EMERGENCIES

The following section discusses management techniques frequently used in cardiac emergencies. You should also become familiar with your local protocols and procedures, since they vary from system to system.

Basic life support is the primary skill for managing serious cardiovascular problems.

BASIC LIFE SUPPORT

Basic life support is the primary skill for managing serious cardiovascular problems. These include the basic airway maneuvers as well as CPR. Review basic life support techniques frequently to keep your skills at their peak.

ADVANCED LIFE SUPPORT

Most of the procedures that EMT-Is employ to manage cardiovascular emergencies are considered advanced life support. The number of skills will vary from system to system. Advanced prehospital skills used in managing cardiovascular emergencies include:

- ECG monitoring
- Vagal maneuvers (carotid sinus massage)
- Precordial thump
- Pharmacological management
- Defibrillation
- Synchronized cardioversion
- Transcutaneous cardiac pacing

MONITORING ECG IN THE FIELD

Most systems' primary tool for ECG monitoring in the field is a combination ECG monitor/defibrillator that operates on a direct current (DC) battery source (Procedure 20-1). It has the following parts:

- Paddle electrodes
- Defibrillator controls
- Synchronizer switch
- Oscilloscope
- Paper strip recorder
- Patient cable and lead wires
- Controls for monitoring
- Special features (such as data recorders)

To monitor your patient's ECG, you will place the three limb electrodes on the chest (in left arm, right arm, and left leg positions). Some manufacturers require a fourth lead on the right leg. By placing the three principal electrodes, you can monitor any of the bipolar leads (I, II, or III). On certain machines, you can also monitor the three augmented leads (aVR, aVL, or aVF) through these three electrodes. As a rule, Lead II is usually monitored, since its axis is almost the same as that of the heart. Modified chest lead 1 (MCL_1) is used occasionally and is often better for determining the site of ectopic beats.

You can also monitor your patient through the defibrillator paddles ("quick-look"). The quick-look paddles are more frequently used in cases of cardiac arrest, when there is no time to place chest electrodes. You can also use this system when the patient cable is inoperative. Among the disadvantages of quick-look paddle electrodes are that they tend to pick up more artifacts than chest electrodes and must be held in continuous contact with the chest.

To use quick-look paddles, follow these steps:

1. Turn on oscilloscope power.
2. Apply conducting gel or other medium liberally to the paddle surface.
3. Hold the paddles firmly on the chest wall with the positive electrode on the left lower chest and the negative electrode on the right upper chest. This closely simulates Lead II.
4. Observe the monitor and obtain a tracing if desired.

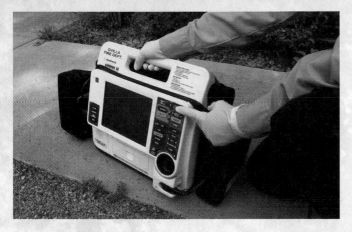

20-1a Turn on the machine.

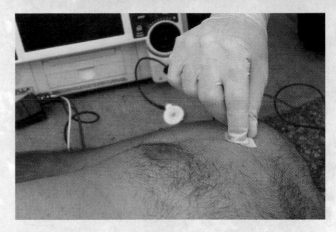

20-1b Prepare the skin.

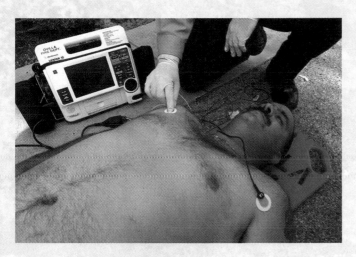

20-1c Apply the electrodes.

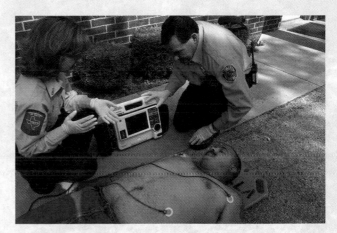

20-1d Ask the patient to relax and remain still.

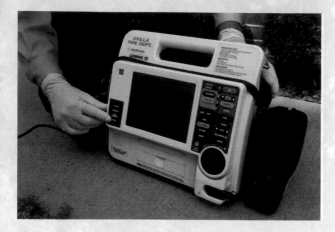

20-1e   Check the ECG.

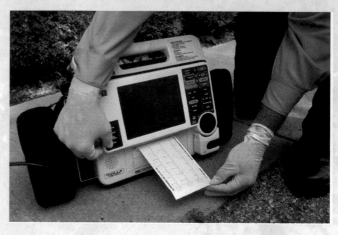

20-1f   Obtain a tracing.

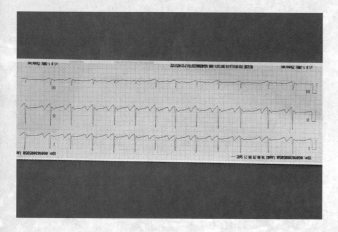

20-1g   ECG strip.

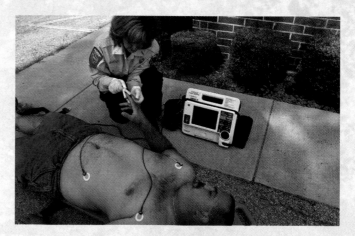

20-1h   Continue ALS care.

Chest electrodes vary from manufacturer to manufacturer. Usually to mimic Lead II, you will place the positive electrode on the patient's left lower chest and the negative electrode on his right upper chest. Placement of the ground wire varies. For MCL$_1$ place the positive electrode on the right lower chest wall and the negative electrode on the left upper chest wall. Again, placement of the ground wire varies. Place the electrodes to avoid large muscle masses, large quantities of chest hair, or anything that keeps the electrodes from resting flat on the skin. Also, avoid placing electrodes where you might have to place defibrillator paddles.

To place electrodes follow these steps:

1. Cleanse the skin with alcohol or abrasive pad. This removes dirt and body oil for better skin contact. If chest hair is thick, shave small amounts before placing the electrodes. If the patient is extremely diaphoretic, apply tincture of benzoin.
2. Apply electrodes to the skin surface.
3. Attach wires to the electrodes.
4. Plug the cable into the monitor.
5. Adjust gain or sensitivity to the proper level.
6. Adjust the QRS volume. (The continual beep of the ECG may disturb the patient.)
7. Obtain a baseline tracing.

Poor ECG signals are useless, and you should correct them. Their most common cause is faulty skin contact. Whenever you spot a poor signal, check for the following possible causes:

- Excessive hair
- Loose or dislodged electrode
- Dried conductive gel
- Poor placement
- Diaphoresis

An initially poor tracing may improve as the conductive gel breaks down skin resistance. Other causes of poor tracings include:

- Patient movement or muscle tremor
- Broken patient cable
- Broken lead wire
- Low battery
- Faulty grounding
- Faulty monitor

Obtain a paper printout from each patient you monitor. Be sure to adjust the stylus heat properly. Calibrate each strip when you begin monitoring so that 1 mV deflects the stylus 10 mm (two large boxes).

Again, treat the patient and not the monitor. Always compare the rhythm you see on the monitor with the patient's signs and symptoms. A patient may have a perfect rhythm on the monitor but have no pulse or blood pressure.

VAGAL MANEUVERS

For a stable patient with symptomatic tachycardia, vagal maneuvers sometimes help slow the heart rate. Ask the patient to perform a Valsalva maneuver (bearing down as if attempting to have a bowel movement) or to cough. If these are unsuccessful and the patient is eligible, attempt carotid artery massage. Do not attempt carotid artery massage on patients with carotid bruits or known cerebrovascular or carotid artery disease, because it may precipitate a stroke. Carotid sinus massage is discussed in more detail later in this chapter.

PRECORDIAL THUMP

The precordial thump, a blow to the midsternum with the heel of the fist, can stimulate depolarization within the heart. This is most effective when performed immediately after the onset of ventricular fibrillation or pulseless ventricular tachycardia. On occasion, the precordial thump can cause depolarization of enough ventricular cells to allow resumption of an organized rhythm. Additionally, conversions from ventricular tachycardia, complete AV block, and occasionally, ventricular fibrillation, have been reported. If no defibrillator is immediately available, you may attempt a precordial thump on a pulseless patient who has a witnessed arrest. Since the amount of energy needed to convert ventricular fibrillation increases rapidly with time, a thump is likely to succeed only if delivered early. It is not recommended in pediatric patients.

To deliver a precordial thump, strike the midsternum with the heel of your fist from a distance of 10 to 12 inches (Figure 20-54). To avoid rib fractures and other problems, keep your arm and wrist parallel to the sternum's long axis.

PHARMACOLOGICAL MANAGEMENT

The drugs that you will use to manage cardiovascular emergencies (Table 20-4) generally fall into the categories of antidysrhythmics, sympathomimetics, and drugs used specifically for myocardial ischemia (including thrombolytics), along with other prehospital medications, some of which are used only infrequently. For more detailed information on these types of drugs, see Chapter 3.

DEFIBRILLATION

defibrillation the process of passing an electrical current through a fibrillating heart to depolarize a critical mass of myocardial cells. This allows them to depolarize uniformly, resulting in an organized rhythm.

Defibrillation is the process of passing a current through a fibrillating heart to depolarize the cells and allow them to repolarize uniformly, thus restoring an organized cardiac rhythm. A critical mass of the myocardium must be depolarized to suppress all of the ectopic foci. The critical mass is related to the size of the heart, but it cannot be calculated for a given individual or situation.

The defibrillator is an electrical capacitor that stores energy for delivery to the patient at a desired time. It consists of an adjustable high-voltage power supply, energy storage capacitor, and paddles. A current-limiting inductor connects the capacitor to the paddles. Recently, different defibrillation wave forms, most commonly biphasic wave forms, have been used to decrease possible tissue damage and to increase battery life. This technology evolved with the development of the compact automated external defibrillators (AEDs).

Most defibrillators use direct current (DC). Alternating current (AC) models should not be used. DC is more effective, more portable, and causes less muscle damage. It delivers an electrical charge of several thousand volts over a very short time, generally 4 to 12 milliseconds. The shock's strength is commonly expressed in energy according to the following formula:

$$\text{energy (joules)} = \text{power (watts)} \times \text{duration (seconds)}$$

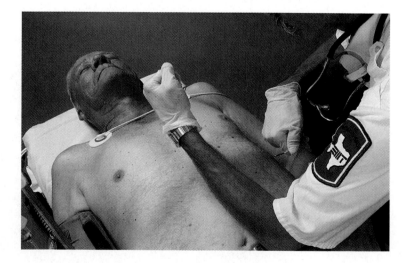

FIGURE 20-54 The precordial thump.

Table 20-4 DRUGS USED TO MANAGE CARDIOVASCULAR EMERGENCIES

Antidysrhythmics

Antidysrhythmic medications control or suppress dysrhythmias.

atropine sulfate	adenosine
lidocaine	amiodarone
procainamide	verapamil
bretylium	

Sympathomimetic agents

Sympathomimetic agents are similar to the naturally occurring hormones epinephrine and norepinephrine. They duplicate or mimic sympathetic nervous system stimulation.

dopamine	norepinephrine
dobutamine	isoproterenol
epinephrine	

Drugs used for myocardial ischemia

Drugs used to treat myocardial ischemia also act to relieve its pain.

oxygen	morphine sulfate
nitrous oxide	nalbuphine
nitroglycerin	

Thrombolytic agents

Thrombolytic agents act to break up blood clots blocking a blood vessel.

aspirin (not a thrombolytic but inhibits aggregation of platelets)	alteplase (Activase) (tPA)
	reteplase (Retavase)

Other prehospital drugs

In some situations, medical direction or local protocol may recommend the following drugs.

furosemide (diuretic)	promethazine (sedative;
diazepam (sedative-hypnotic; anticonvulsive)	antihistamine; antiemetic; anticholinergic)
	sodium nitroprusside (vasodilator)

Drugs infrequently used in the prehospital setting

The following are drugs that EMT-Intermediates who work in the emergency department may see and that many patients take on a long-term basis.

digitalis (Digoxin, Lanoxin) (cardiac 1296glycoside: increases cardiac contracile force and cardiac output)

beta blockers (propranolol) (dysrhythmia control)

calcium channel blockers (verapamil, diltiazem, nifedipine) (control supraventricular tachydysrhythmias; help manage hypertension; increase coronary artery perfusion in angina pectoris)

The chest wall offers resistance to the electrical charge, which lowers the amount of energy actually delivered to the heart. Therefore, lowering the resistance pathway between the defibrillator paddles and the chest is important. Factors that influence chest wall resistance include:

- Paddle pressure
- Paddle-skin interface

- Paddle surface area
- Number of previous countershocks
- Inspiratory vs. expiratory phase at time of countershock

The following factors influence the success of defibrillation:

- *Time until ventricular fibrillation.* When combined with effective CPR, defibrillation begun within 4 minutes after the onset of fibrillation will yield significantly improved resuscitation rates, as compared with defibrillation begun within 8 minutes.
- *Condition of the myocardium.* Converting ventricular fibrillation is more difficult in the presence of acidosis, hypoxia, hypothermia, electrolyte imbalance, or drug toxicity. Secondary ventricular fibrillation (ventricular fibrillation that results from another cause) is more difficult to treat than primary ventricular fibrillation.
- *Heart size and body weight.* The effects of heart size and body weight on defibrillation are controversial. Pediatric and adult energy requirements differ, but whether size and energy level settings are related in adults is not clear.
- *Previous countershocks.* Repeated countershocks decrease transthoracic resistance, thereby allowing the defibrillator to deliver more energy to the heart at the same energy level.
- *Paddle size.* Larger defibrillator paddles are thought to be more effective and cause less myocardial damage. The ideal size for adults, however, has not been established. Generally, the paddles should be 10 to 13 cm in diameter. In infants, 4.5 cm paddles are adequate.
- *Paddle placement.* For both adults and children in the emergency setting, place the paddles on the chest. Position one paddle to the right of the upper sternum, just below the clavicle. Place the other to the left of the left nipple in an anterior axillary line immediately over the apex of the heart. Do not place paddles over the sternum. Do not place paddles over the generator of an implanted automatic defibrillator or pacemaker, which can damage or disable the device. Place the paddles approximately 5 inches from the generator. The paddles may be marked as apex (positive electrode) and sternum (negative electrode). Although reversing polarity inverts the ECG tracing, it does not affect defibrillation.
- *Paddle-skin interface.* Paddle-skin interface should have as little electrical resistance as possible. Greater resistance decreases energy delivery to the heart and increases heat production on the skin. Many available materials decrease resistance, including gels, creams, pastes, saline-soaked pads, and prepackaged gel pads. Use only creams made specifically for defibrillation, not for ECG monitoring. When using cream, make sure that it does not run and form a bridge between paddles. Never use alcohol-soaked pads; they can ignite.
- *Paddle contact pressure.* The paddle contact pressure is important. Firm, downward pressure decreases transthoracic resistance. Do not lean on the paddles, however; they may slip.
- *Properly functioning defibrillator.* The machine should deliver the amount of energy that it indicates. Therefore, frequent inspection and testing of the machine are necessary. Change and cycle the batteries as the manufacturer directs.

To perform defibrillation, use the following steps (Procedure 20-2):

1. Confirm ventricular fibrillation or pulseless ventricular tachycardia on the cardiac monitor.
2. Place the patient in a safe environment if initially in contact with some electrically conductive material such as metal or water.

20-2a Identify rhythm on the cardiac monitor.

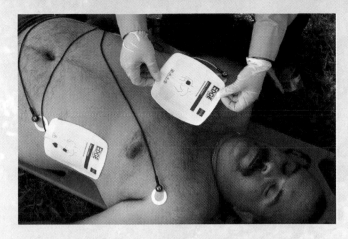

20-2b Apply electrode gel to the paddles or place commercial defibrillation pads on the patient's exposed thorax.

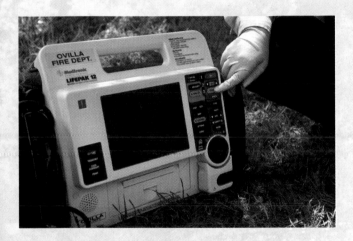

20-2c Charge the defibrillation paddles.

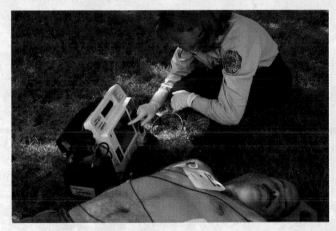

20-2d Reconfirm the rhythm on the cardiac monitor.

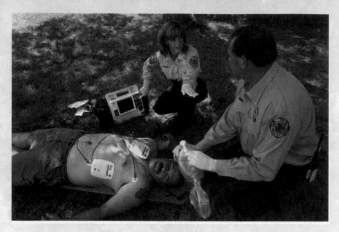

20-2e Verbally and visually clear everybody, including yourself, from the cardiac patient.

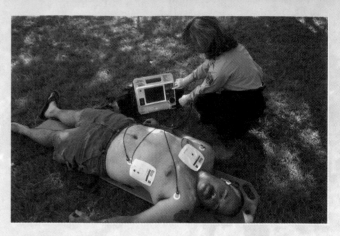

20-2f Deliver a shock by pressing both buttons simultaneously.

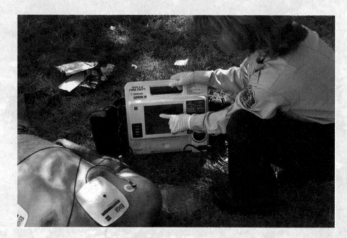

20-2g Reconfirm the rhythm on the cardiac monitor.

3. Apply electrode gel to the paddles, or place commercial defibrillation pads on the patient's exposed thorax.

4. Turn on and charge the defibrillator to 200 joules for the first shock.

5. Ensure that the electrodes are appropriately placed on the patient's thorax with proper pressure.

6. Ensure that no one else is in contact with the patient. Verbally and visually clear everybody, including yourself, before any defibrillation attempt.

7. Deliver a defibrillatory shock by depressing both red buttons simultaneously. (Depressing only one will not deliver a shock.)

8. Reconfirm the rhythm on the monitor screen; if the patient is still in ventricular fibrillation or pulseless ventricular tachycardia, recharge the defibrillator and repeat steps 5 to 7 at higher energy levels.

Keep in mind the basic energy recommendations for defibrillation. After initially attempting defibrillation at 200 joules in an adult, increase dosage to a maximum of 360 joules in one or two repeat countershocks. The pediatric dosage is generally 2 joules/kg initially, repeated at 4 joules/kg if required.

EMERGENCY SYNCHRONIZED CARDIOVERSION

Synchronized cardioversion is a controlled form of defibrillation for patients who still have organized cardiac activity with a pulse. A synchronizing circuit in the defibrillator interprets the QRS cycle and delivers the electrical discharge during the R wave of the QRS complex. This reduces the likelihood of delivering the cardioversion during the vulnerable period of the QRS cycle, which can precipitate ventricular fibrillation. Synchronizing also permits the use of lower energy levels and reduces the potential for secondary dysrhythmias. Depending on the type of dysrhythmia being treated, as little as 10 joules may be adequate, especially if the origin is atrial.

Indications for emergency synchronized cardioversion in an unstable patient include:

- Perfusing ventricular tachycardia
- Paroxysmal supraventricular tachycardia
- Rapid atrial fibrillation
- 2:1 atrial flutter

The procedure for synchronized cardioversion is the same as for defibrillation. Sedate conscious patients if at all possible. Turn on the synchronizer switch, and verify that the machine is detecting the R waves (Figure 20-55). If not, you may need to reposition the electrodes. Press and hold the discharge buttons until the machine discharges on the next R wave. Some models automatically turn off the synchronizer after a cardioversion and return to defibrillation mode. To give a second synchronized shock, you must depress the synchronizer button again. If ventricular fibrillation occurs, you must turn off the synchronizer

synchronized cardioversion the passage of an electric current through the heart during a specific part of the cardiac cycle to terminate certain kinds of dysrhythmias.

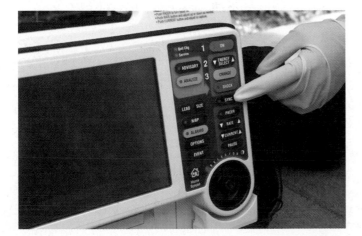

FIGURE 20-55 Activate the synchronizer.

switch and use the machine in the defibrillation mode, because the heart produces no R wave in ventricular fibrillation and the machine will not discharge. The procedure for synchronized cardioversion is summarized in Figure 20-56.

TRANSCUTANEOUS CARDIAC PACING

Many of the newer cardiac monitor/defibrillators have a built-in cardiac pacing device that enables EMT units to perform transcutaneous (external) cardiac pacing (TCP). Transcutaneous cardiac pacing allows electrical pacing of the heart through the skin via specially designed thoracic electrodes. Before the development of TCP, electrical cardiac pacing required placing an electrode through a major vein or directly into the chest. With TCP, pacing can now be provided in the prehospital setting. This is beneficial in such cases of symptomatic bradycardia as occur with high-degree AV blocks, atrial fibrillation with slow ventricular response, and other significant bradycardias (including asystole). Use transcutaneous pacing if pharmacological intervention has no effect and the patient is hypotensive or hypoperfusing.

To perform external cardiac pacing, follow these steps (Procedure 20-3):

1. Initiate IV, oxygen, and ECG monitoring.
2. Place the patient supine.
3. Confirm symptomatic bradycardia and confirm medical direction order for external cardiac pacing.
4. Apply the pacing electrodes according to the manufacturer's recommendations being sure that they interface well with the skin.
5. Connect the electrodes.
6. Set the desired heart rate on the pacemaker. This will typically range from 60 to 80 beats per minute.
7. Turn the output setting to 0.
8. Turn on the pacer.
9. Slowly increase the output until you note ventricular capture.
10. Check the pulse and blood pressure, and adjust the rate and amperage as medical direction orders.
11. Monitor the patient's response to treatment.

To manage patients in asystole, place the output on its maximum setting. Then decrease the output if capture occurs.

Occasionally, external cardiac pacing may cause patient discomfort. If this occurs, medical direction may request the administration of an analgesic.

Overdrive pacing may deter recurrent tachycardia. This involves increasing the rate above the heart's current rate to suppress ventricular ectopy. This is particularly useful in torsade de pointes. Failure of transcutaneous pacing is similar to the failure of a permanent pacemaker, as discussed earlier in the section on artificial pacemaker rhythm.

CAROTID SINUS MASSAGE

Carotid sinus massage can convert paroxysmal supraventricular tachycardia into sinus rhythm by stimulating the baroreceptors in the carotid bodies. This increases vagal tone and decreases heart rate.

To perform carotid sinus massage, have atropine sulfate readily available and use the following technique (Procedure 20-4):

1. Initiate IV, oxygen, and ECG monitoring.
2. Position patient on his back, slightly hyperextending the head.
3. Gently palpate each carotid pulse separately. Auscultate each side for carotid bruits. Do not attempt carotid sinus massage if the pulse is diminished or if carotid bruits are present.

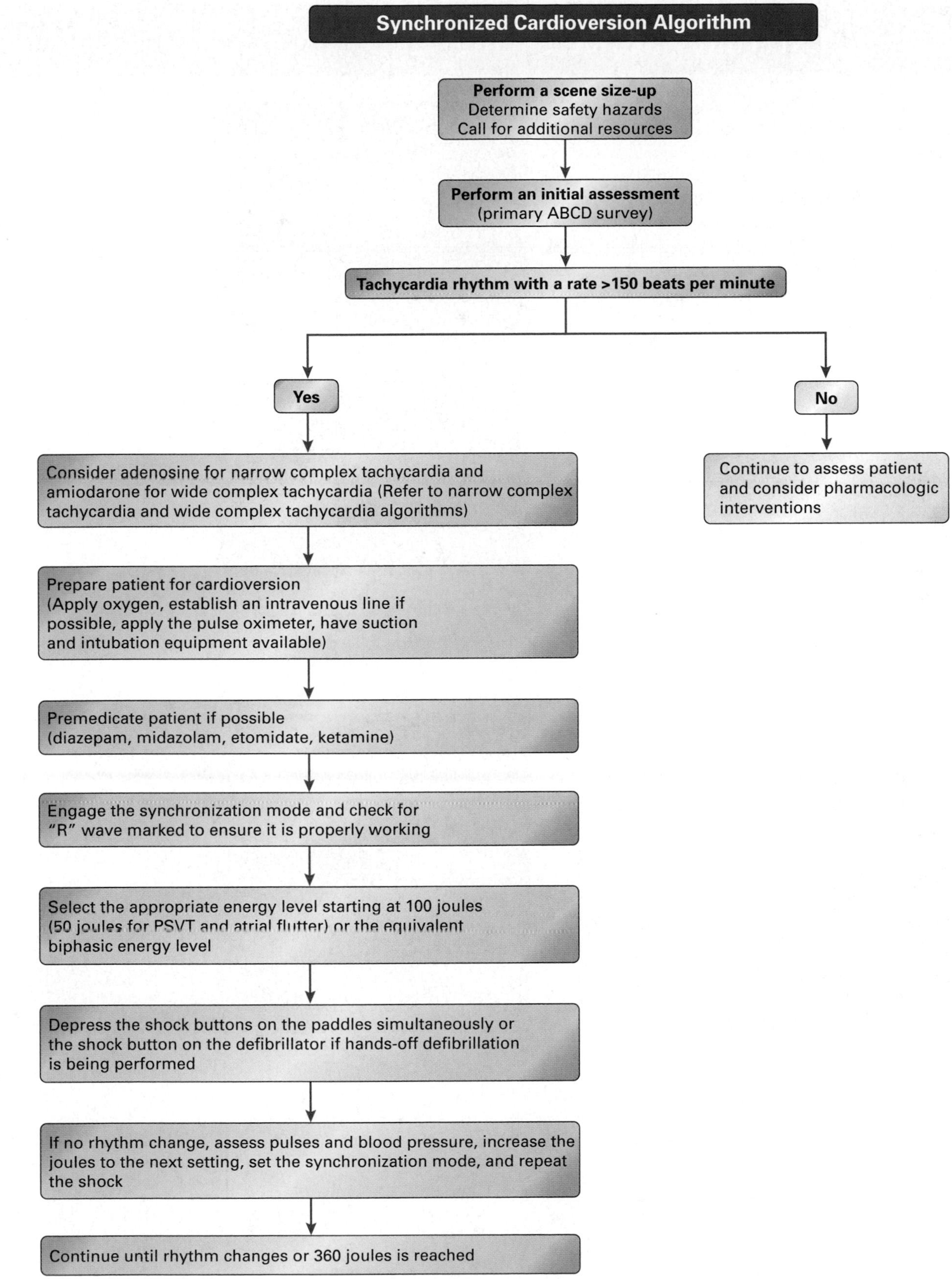

Synchronized Cardioversion Algorithm

Perform a scene size-up
Determine safety hazards
Call for additional resources

↓

Perform an initial assessment
(primary ABCD survey)

↓

Tachycardia rhythm with a rate >150 beats per minute

Yes

Consider adenosine for narrow complex tachycardia and amiodarone for wide complex tachycardia (Refer to narrow complex tachycardia and wide complex tachycardia algorithms)

↓

Prepare patient for cardioversion
(Apply oxygen, establish an intravenous line if possible, apply the pulse oximeter, have suction and intubation equipment available)

↓

Premedicate patient if possible
(diazepam, midazolam, etomidate, ketamine)

↓

Engage the synchronization mode and check for "R" wave marked to ensure it is properly working

↓

Select the appropriate energy level starting at 100 joules (50 joules for PSVT and atrial flutter) or the equivalent biphasic energy level

↓

Depress the shock buttons on the paddles simultaneously or the shock button on the defibrillator if hands-off defibrillation is being performed

↓

If no rhythm change, assess pulses and blood pressure, increase the joules to the next setting, set the synchronization mode, and repeat the shock

↓

Continue until rhythm changes or 360 joules is reached

No

Continue to assess patient and consider pharmacologic interventions

FIGURE 20–56   Electrical (synchronized) cardioversion algorithm.

External pacing is of benefit in bradycardias and heart blocks that are symptomatic. The electrodes are placed on the chest as shown. The desired heart rate is selected. The current is then adjusted until "capture" of the heart's conductive system is obtained.

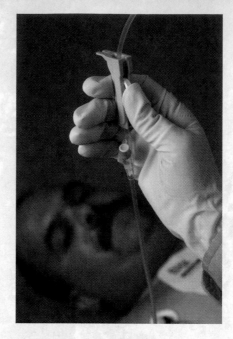

20-3a   Establish an IV line.

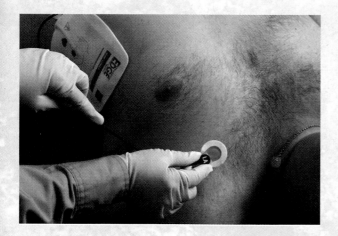

20-3b   Place ECG electrodes.

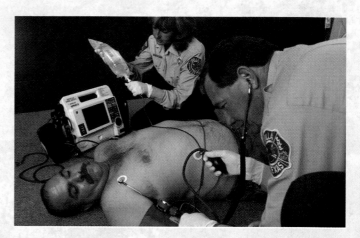

20-3c   Carefully assess vital signs and contact medical direction.

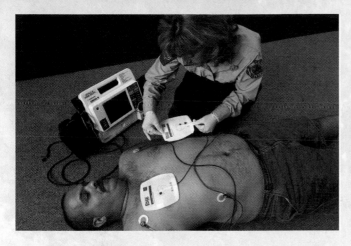

20-3d   If external pacing is ordered, apply the pacing electrodes according to the manufacturer's recommendations.

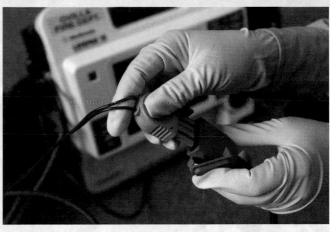

20-3e   Connect the electrodes.

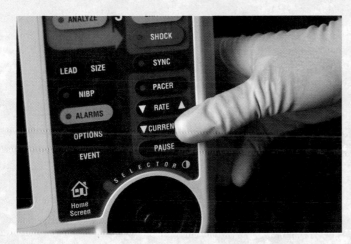

20-3f   Select the desired pacing rate and current.

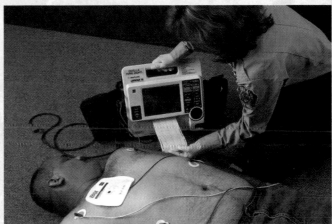

20-3g   Monitor the patient's response to treatment.

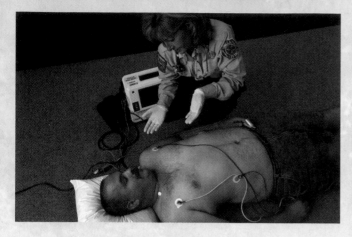

20-4a   Assess the patient.

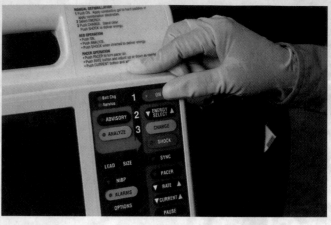

20-4b   Turn on the monitor.

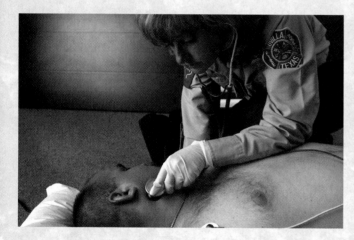

20-4c   Listen to both carotids for the presence of bruits.

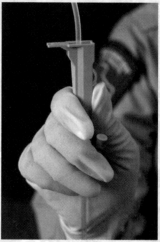

20-4d   Start an IV line.

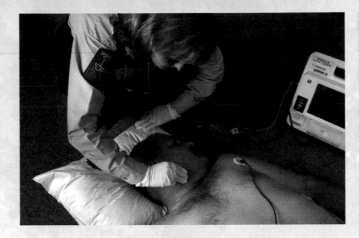

20-4e Rub either carotid. Wait.

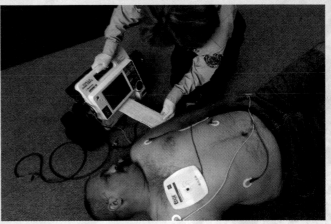

20-4f Check the rhythm.

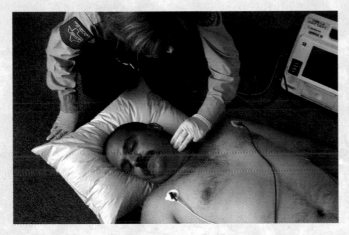

20-4g If unsuccessful, rub the other carotid.

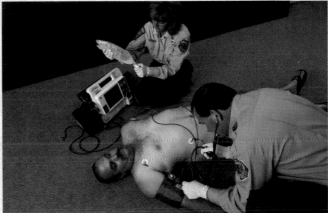

20-4h Reevalutate the patient.

4. Tilt the patient's head to either side. Place your index and middle fingers over one artery, below the angle of the jaw and as high up on the neck as possible.

5. Firmly massage the artery by pressing it against the vertebral body and rubbing.

6. Monitor the ECG and obtain a continuous readout. Terminate massage at the first sign of slowing or heart block.

7. Maintain pressure no longer than 15 to 20 seconds.

8. If the massage is ineffective, you may repeat it, preferably on the other side of the patient's neck.

Complications of carotid sinus massage include dysrhythmias such as asystole, PVCs, ventricular tachycardia, or fibrillation. In addition, this procedure can interfere with cerebral circulation, causing syncope, seizure, or stroke. Increased parasympathetic tone can cause bradycardias, nausea, or vomiting.

SUPPORT AND COMMUNICATION

As with other emergencies, appropriate support and communication are an integral part of the treatment you provide for your cardiovascular patient. Time permitting, explain your treatment to the patient and his family and offer emotional support as indicated. When rapid transport is necessary, explain why. If the patient refuses transport, you will need to clearly explain the potential consequences, and use every available means to convince him of his need for appropriate treatment. As you transfer care of your patient to the receiving facility staff, you must clearly explain your findings to the receiving nurse or physician in a formal verbal briefing. This briefing should include the patient's vital information, chief complaint and history, physical exam findings, and any treatments rendered. In cardiovascular emergencies, any ECG findings will be especially important to the receiving staff.

MANAGING SPECIFIC CARDIOVASCULAR EMERGENCIES

The following section details the pathophysiology of common cardiovascular emergencies. Each section covers epidemiology, morbidity and mortality, assessment, and management.

ANGINA PECTORIS

angina pectoris chest pain that results when the oxygen demands of the blood exceed that of the heart.

Angina pectoris literally means "pain in the chest." This condition, however, is much more complicated than simple pain. Angina occurs when the heart's blood supply is transiently exceeded by myocardial oxygen demands. In other words, during periods of increased oxygen demand, the coronary arteries cannot deliver an adequate amount of blood to the myocardium. This can cause ischemia of the myocardium and chest pain.

As a rule, the reduced blood flow through the coronary arteries results from atherosclerosis. Atherosclerotic plaques can develop throughout the coronary circulation. Some patients may have atherosclerotic lesions that are isolated to one vessel, whereas others will have diffuse disease involving several vessels. Fixed blockages in the coronary arteries decrease blood flow. Remember that blood flow through a vessel is related to its diameter. Reducing the diameter of a vessel by one-half, as can occur in atherosclerosis, drastically reduces the amount of blood that the vessel can transport.

Prinzmetal's angina variant of angina pectoris caused by vasospasm of the coronary arteries, not blockage per se; also called vasospastic angina or atypical angina.

In addition to atherosclerosis, angina can result from abnormal spasm of the coronary arteries. This disorder, commonly called **Prinzmetal's angina,** *vasospastic angina,* or *atypical angina,* can also lead to inadequate blood flow, causing pain. Approximately two-thirds of the people who have vasospastic angina also have atherosclerotic coronary artery disease. Spasm of the vessel on top of atherosclerotic blockage can cause ischemia. However, one-third of patients with vasospastic angina will have little or no coronary atherosclerosis.

Angina is generally classified as stable or unstable. *Stable angina* occurs during activity, when the heart's oxygen demands are increased. Attacks of stable angina are usually precipitated by physical or emotional stress. They are relatively brief and often respond readily to treatment. *Unstable angina,* on the other hand, occurs at rest and may not respond as readily to treatment. Because unstable angina often indicates severe atherosclerotic disease, it is also called preinfarction angina. Unstable angina usually indicates that the patient's disease process is worsening.

Angina is not a self-limiting disease. It results from underlying coronary artery disease. If it is untreated and its contributing factors are unchanged, the underlying problem remains even though the pain has resolved. Because of the nature of the episodes, angina is usually progressive (that is, it accelerates in frequency and duration). Myocardial infarction may follow a single episode of angina.

It is important to remember that there are other causes of chest pain. Although cardiac ischemia is one of its major causes, chest pain can arise from problems in the cardiovascular system, the respiratory system, the gastrointestinal system, and the musculoskeletal system. Causes of chest pain include:

- Cardiovascular causes
  - Cardiac ischemia
  - Pericarditis (viral or autoimmune)
  - Thoracic dissection of the aorta
- Respiratory causes
  - Pulmonary embolism
  - Pneumothorax
  - Pneumonia
  - Pleural irritation (Pleurisy)
- Gastrointestinal causes
  - Cholecystitis
  - Pancreatitis
  - Hiatal hernia
  - Esophageal disease
  - Gastroesophageal reflux (GERD)
  - Peptic ulcer disease
  - Dyspepsia
- Musculoskeletal causes
  - Chest wall syndrome
  - Costochondritis
  - Acromioclavicular disease
  - Herpes zoster (shingles)
  - Chest wall trauma
  - Chest wall tumors

Diagnosing the cause of a patient's chest pain can be challenging in the hospital, let alone in the prehospital setting. As frequently occurs in emergency medicine, we look for the worst and hope for the best. Always be prepared to treat patients with chest pain as if they are suffering cardiac ischemia or another major disease process. Once you have excluded these possibilities you can consider less critical causes.

Field Assessment

When you assess an angina patient, remember that weak or absent peripheral pulses indicate potential or pending shock, which you should treat immediately. Changes in skin color such as paleness or cyanosis, or changes in temperature such as cold extremities also suggest shock.

The chief complaint of a typical angina patient is a sudden onset of chest discomfort. The pain may radiate, or it may be localized to the chest. Often epigastric pain accompanies the chest pain. The patient with angina, however, often denies having chest pain, largely because he has dealt with this type of chest pain before. Although anginal episodes are common for the patient with a cardiac history, they should be considered significant when EMS is activated.

Angina usually lasts from 3 to 5 minutes, sometimes as long as 15 minutes, and is relieved with rest and/or nitroglycerin. Atypical, or Prinzmetal, angina most often occurs at rest or without a precipitating cause. Prinzmetal angina is often accompanied by S-T segment elevation on the ECG, which can indicate myocardial tissue ischemia.

Labored breathing may or may not be present. After establishing the patency of the patient's airway, auscultate the lungs for congested breath sounds, particularly in the bases. Remember, however, the lungs may be clear. The anginal patient's heart rate and rhythm may be altered. Peripheral pulses should be equal. Typically, the blood pressure will elevate during the episode and normalize afterwards.

The contributing history may indicate that this is the patient's first recognized instance of angina, that it is a recurring event, or that the episodes are increasing in frequency or duration. A recurrence of angina or an increase in its frequency or duration is often the reason an anginal patient calls EMS. Any change in typical anginal pain is significant.

ECG tracing. The most common ECG finding in the angina patient is S-T segment depression. S-T segment changes often are not specific, however, and dysrhythmias and ectopy may not be present when the tracing is obtained.

Management

The patient experiencing angina is often apprehensive. Place him at rest in a position of physical and emotional comfort to decrease myocardial oxygen demand. Administer oxygen, generally at a high-flow rate, to increase oxygen delivery to the myocardium. Establish an IV either on scene without delaying transport or en route. If possible, and again without prolonging scene time, obtain and record a 12-lead or 3-lead ECG tracing. This is important because the ECG findings may be normal once the patient is pain free. Measure any S-T segment changes and communicate them to the receiving facility. Because a single anginal episode can be a precursor to a myocardial infarction, anticipate ECG changes such as dysrhythmias and S-T segment elevation.

Administer nitroglycerin sublingually, either as a tablet or a spray. It decreases myocardial work and, to a lesser degree, dilates coronary arteries. If the patient's symptoms persist after one or two doses of nitroglycerin, assume something more serious than angina, such as myocardial infarction. Nifedipine (Procardia), or another calcium channel blocker, is now being used, in addition to nitroglycerin, to manage angina. It is a vasodilator that works through blockade of the slow calcium channels. Consider morphine sulfate for chest pain that does not respond to nitrates or calcium channel blockers.

Patients with first episodes of angina or episodes that medication does not relieve are usually admitted to the hospital for evaluation. There is often a fine line between unstable angina and early myocardial infarction. Immediate transport is indicated if the patient does not feel relief after receiving oxygen and/or nitrates. The absence of relief indicates the patient's underlying disease process may be worsening. If the event is the beginning of a myocardial infarction, reperfusion (restoring blood flow to the ischemic tissue) is crucial. Hypotension can occur, especially if the patient has taken nitroglycerin. Its presence indicates transport, because it may lead to hypoperfusion of myocardial tissue. S-T segment changes, especially S-T segment elevation, indicate rapid transport. Transport should be efficient and fast but without lights and sirens unless clinically indicated. The lights and sirens could make the patient apprehensive and increase his pain.

Sometimes, the patient experiencing anginal chest pain will call EMS and then refuse transport after his chest pain is relieved. This may be due to a number of reasons, from denial to the patient's having taken older nitrates, which take longer to work. In any case, strongly encourage immediate evaluation because of the potential serious complications such as myocardial infarction. Document patient refusal and be sure the patient signs the refusal and understands the potential risks. Encourage the patient to see his cardiologist or private care physician as soon as possible for follow-up.

Explain to the patient and family the reason and necessity for rapid transport, if indicated. Time permitting, also explain your treatment. Upon arrival at the emergency department, inform the physician of your findings—past history, vital signs, labored breathing, relief of pain, no relief of pain, and ECG findings, especially S-T segment findings.

MYOCARDIAL INFARCTION

Myocardial infarction (MI) is the death of a portion of the heart muscle from prolonged deprivation of oxygenated arterial blood. MI can also occur when the heart's oxygen demand exceeds its supply over an extended time. MI is most often associated with *atherosclerotic heart disease (ASHD)*. The precipitating event is commonly the formation of a *thrombus*, or blood clot, in a coronary artery already diseased from atherosclerosis. Atherosclerosis places many anginal patients at high risk for an MI, especially those suffering from persistent or unstable angina. MI can also result from coronary artery spasm, microemboli (as seen with the recreational use of cocaine), acute volume overload, hypotension (from any cause), or from acute respiratory failure (acute hypoxia). Trauma can also cause myocardial infarction.

The location and size of the infarction depend on the vessel involved and the site of the obstruction (Figure 20-57.) Most infarctions involve the left ventricle. Obstruction of the left coronary artery may result in anterior, lateral, or septal infarcts. Right coronary artery occlusions usually result in infarctions of the inferior wall, posterior wall, or the right ventricle. The actual infarction is often classified as either transmural or subendocardial. In a **transmural infarction,** the entire thickness of the myocardium is destroyed. This lesion is associated with Q-wave changes on the ECG and is occasionally called a pathological Q-wave infarction. A **subendocardial infarction** involves only the subendocardial layer. Because ECG Q-wave changes usually do not accompany this type of infarction, it is often called a non-Q wave infarction.

MI causes varying degrees of tissue damage. First, following occlusion of the coronary artery, the affected tissue develops ischemia. If the blockage is not relieved and collateral circulation is inadequate, the tissue will infarct and die. In trauma, the usual cause of occlusion is plaque that has broken loose. The infarcted tissue becomes necrotic and eventually forms scar tissue. A ring of ischemic tissue that surrounds the area of infarcted myocardium survives primarily because of collateral circulation. This ischemic area is the site of many dysrhythmias' origins. Cardiogenic shock can develop, typically appearing first as ischemia on the ECG (S-T depression or T-wave inversion), followed by injury (S-T elevation), and finally infarction (sometimes a pathological Q wave).

Dysrhythmias are the most common complications of MI. They are also the most common direct cause of death resulting from MI. Life-threatening dysrhythmias can occur almost

myocardial infarction (MI) death and subsequent necrosis of the heart muscle caused by inadequate blood supply; also acute myocardial infarction (AMI).

transmural infarction myocardial infarction that affects the full thickness of the myocardium and almost always results in a pathological Q wave in the affected leads.

subendocardial infarction myocardial infarction that affects only the deeper levels of the myocardium; also called non–Q-wave infarction because it typically does not result in a significant Q wave in the affected lead.

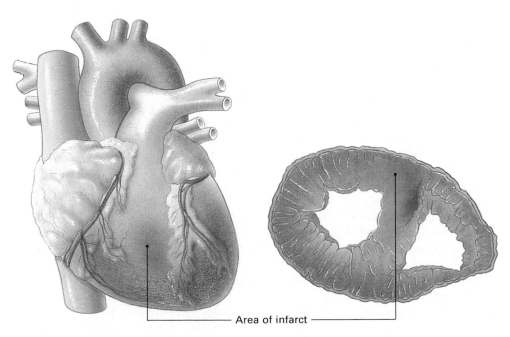

— Area of infarct —

FIGURE 20-57 Myocardial infarction.

immediately and can result in sudden death or death within 1 hour after the onset of symptoms. Ventricular fibrillation or ventricular tachycardia may present early with MI.

In addition to dysrhythmias, the destruction of a portion of the myocardial muscle mass can cause congestive heart failure. Such patients may have right heart failure, left heart failure, or both. *Heart failure* exists if the heart's pumping ability is impaired but the heart can still meet the demands of the body. That is, the heart is inefficient but adequate. If the heart cannot meet the body's oxygen demands, *inadequate tissue perfusion* results in cardiogenic shock. In cardiogenic shock, the heart is both inefficient and inadequate. Another cause of death from MI is *ventricular aneurysm* of the myocardial wall. The damaged portion of the wall weakens and in some cases bursts, resulting in sudden death. *Pump failure* resulting from extensive myocardial damage can also result in death.

The primary strategies in managing an MI are pain relief and reperfusion. For reperfusion to be effective, rapid and safe transport is paramount. Maximum efficiency on scene and in transit is the most important care you can provide for the patient suffering an MI.

Field Assessment

The patient's breathing may or may not be labored. Look for evidence of shock. Check for regularity of the peripheral pulses, which should be equal in the patient experiencing cardiac ischemia. Take the blood pressure; it usually elevates during the episode and normalizes afterward.

The chief complaint in MI is chest pain. Use the OPQRST mnemonic to determine specifics about the chest pain. Typically, the onset of the chest pain is acute, severe, constant, and unrelenting. Unlike the angina patient, the MI patient's discomfort usually lasts longer than 30 minutes. The pain can radiate to the arms (primarily left), the neck, posterior to the back, or down to the epigastric region of the abdomen. Have the patient rate his pain on a scale of 1 to 10. Patients with true myocardial ischemia can have severe pain and may rate their chest pain with high numbers such as eight, nine, ten, or above ten. Often they will confirm an acute onset of nausea and vomiting. Neither nitroglycerin nor rest offers much pain relief.

Atypically, a patient may have mild symptoms or minimize his symptoms during your assessment. This is more common in diabetics. The patient can be vague when describing chest pain and may complain of generally not feeling well. You might easily mistake this for angina. This patient generally does not complain of vomiting and may or may not have nausea. He also will rate his pain low on a scale of ten. His vague, general descriptions may arise from many pathological causes. One is that MIs generally evolve over 48 to 72 hours. If the patient is more than 24 hours into the infarction, the pain can be different than it was 12 to 24 hours after onset.

The patient experiencing chest pains tends to be very frightened, although this is not always the case. "A feeling of impending doom" describes the patient's fright and pain. This pain is so severe and intense that the patient fears death, especially if he is experiencing chest pain for the first time. Ask if this is the patient's first recognized episode of chest pain or a recurring event. A patient who has suffered infarction before or who has chronic angina may be less concerned with his current pain. If it is recurring, are the episodes increasing in frequency or duration? These patients often have angina-like pain with increasing frequency and/or duration? Denial is common among both the patient with a significant cardiac history and the first-time chest-pain sufferer.

After establishing the patient's airway, auscultate lung sounds. They may present clear or with congestion in the bases. The patient suffering an MI usually presents with pallor and diaphoresis. Temperature may vary from the norm. Cold skin or extremities indicate shock. Check the heart rate and rhythm, which may be irregular, and check the peripheral pulses for equality, which MI usually does not affect. The patient's blood pressure may be elevated, normal, or lower than normal.

Apply the ECG. First examine the underlying rhythm and potential dysrhythmias.

Cardiac dysrhythmias are the greatest threat to the patient before he arrives at the emergency department. Of the many potential dysrhythmias, the most serious are asystole (confirmed in two leads), pulseless electrical activity (PEA), ventricular fibrillation, and ventricular tachycardia. Other dysrhythmias include narrow or wide-complex tachycardia, heart block, sinus bradycardia, and sinus tachycardia with or without ectopy. Remember, life-threatening dysrhythmias are the leading cause of death among MI patients. Anticipate such dysrhythmias while caring for any patient you suspect to be having an MI.

After reviewing the patient's ECG tracing, determine if he is a likely candidate for rapid transport and reperfusion. Reperfusion uses thrombolytics such as streptokinase or tPA (Activase) to stop further injury. Used properly, thrombolytics can reperfuse all ischemic tissue and much of the injured myocardial tissue, thus reducing the total damage of an MI. They work by destroying blood clots—all clots—which, when lodged in arteries congested with plaque, are the most common cause of acute MI. The window of time in which a thrombolytic can be given and be effective is generally considered to be 6 hours from the onset of symptoms. Occasionally the window will be expanded for a particularly young patient or one who is suffering serious complications. The complications associated with giving thrombolytics include hemorrhage (which can be fatal), allergic reactions, and reperfusion dysrhythmias. Unfortunately, not all MIs are caused by blood clots. In addition, many patients have conditions that preclude them from receiving thrombolytics. These include bleeding or clotting disorders, possible blood in the stool, uncontrolled hypertension, recent trauma, recent hemorrhagic stroke, or recent surgery.

Signs of acute injury or pathological Q waves indicate rapid transport for reperfusion, if symptoms began within 6 hours. Ascertain as near as possible the exact time when the symptoms started, the locations of the ischemia and of the infarction if evidenced on the 12-lead, and any S-T segment changes occurring on the 12-lead. This will help the physician determine quickly if the patient is a candidate for reperfusion. If you are not certain the patient meets local criteria for thrombolytic therapy, assume he does.

After analyzing the patient's rhythm, prepare him for transport. Since reperfusion is the ultimate goal, time is of the utmost importance. Expediently treat any signs of acute ischemia, injury, or infarction. Carefully weigh treating the patient's pain while on scene against rapid transport. Whenever practical treat the patient suffering from an MI in transit.

Many EMS systems have a checklist similar to those that emergency departments use to determine if a patient qualifies for thrombolytic therapy. Although these checklists vary from area to area, their use has reduced the waiting time for patients who meet the clinical criteria for thrombolytic therapy. Standard information that should be relayed to the emergency department physician or staff includes the time of the pain's onset, S-T segment elevation, and the location of ischemia and infarction on a 12-lead.

If you are not certain the patient meets local criteria for thrombolytic therapy, assume he does.

Whenever practical treat the patient suffering from a myocardial infarction in transit.

Management

Prehospital Management of Acute Ischemic Chest Pain Treatment of the acute ischemic chest pain patient is summarized in Figure 20-58. Keep in mind that the patient experiencing acute ischemic chest pain is often apprehensive. Place him at rest in a position of physical and emotional comfort to decrease myocardial oxygen demand. Administer oxygen, generally at a high-flow rate, to increase oxygen delivery to the myocardium. Establish at least one IV, taking great care not to miss the vein or to have multiple misses, which could jeopardize a patient's chance of receiving thrombolytics.

Administer medications according to written protocols or upon order of medical direction. Remember, always ask the patient if he or she is allergic to any medication before giving any drug. Medications that might be indicated for the patient suspected of acute ischemic chest pain include:

- Aspirin
- Morphine sulfate
- Promethazine (Phenergan)
- Nitroglycerin
- Nitrous oxide (Nitronox)

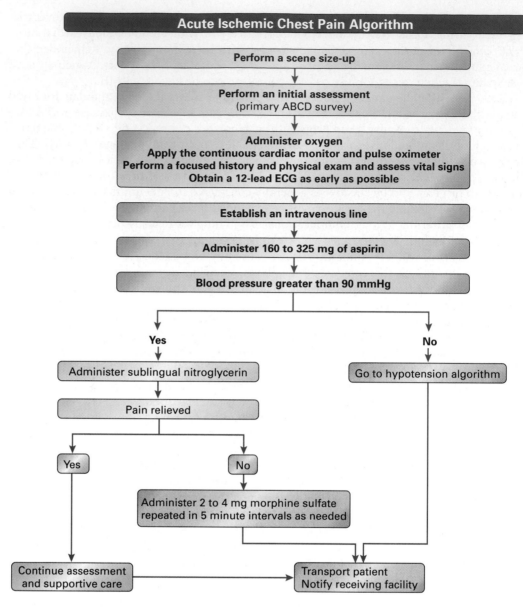

Acute Ischemic Chest Pain Algorithm

Perform a scene size-up

↓

Perform an initial assessment
(primary ABCD survey)

↓

Administer oxygen
Apply the continuous cardiac monitor and pulse oximeter
Perform a focused history and physical exam and assess vital signs
Obtain a 12-lead ECG as early as possible

↓

Establish an intravenous line

↓

Administer 160 to 325 mg of aspirin

↓

Blood pressure greater than 90 mmHg

Yes ← → **No**

Administer sublingual nitroglycerin   Go to hypotension algorithm

↓

Pain relieved

Yes   **No**

↓   ↓

                Administer 2 to 4 mg morphine sulfate
                repeated in 5 minute intervals as needed

Continue assessment   Transport patient
and supportive care   Notify receiving facility

FIGURE 20-58   Management of acute ischemic chest pain.

- Nalbuphine (Nubain)
- Atropine sulfate
- Lidocaine
- Procainamide
- Vasopressin
- Adenosine

Monitor the ECG constantly. Life-threatening dysrhythmias are possible. The patient may need rapid defibrillation or synchronized cardioversion at any moment. Plan to quickly provide defibrillation, cardioconversion, or transcutaneous pacing if needed.

Transport the patient you suspect of acute ischemic chest pain without delay. Since most such patients are very apprehensive and frightened, you should transport the normotensive patient without lights and sirens. Rapid transport is indicated if the patient exhibits S-T or Q wave anomalies, has had signs and symptoms less than 3 hours, or has no relief from medications, consider him a candidate for thrombolytic reperfusion. Hypotension indicates immediate transport, especially if the patient has taken nitroglycerin, because the potential hypoperfusion of myocardial tissue can compound the problem. Other factors that indicate rapid transport are any rhythm abnormalities and the presentation within 6 hours of the pain's onset.

If the patient is in the early stages of acute ischemic chest pain, the outcome of refusing transport is likely to be devastating, ranging from extensive, unnecessary myocardial damage to death. Avoid refusal at all cost, using every means at your disposal to convince the patient to be transported. If the patient still refuses, document the fact that the patient was repeatedly warned of the possible outcome and was also aware of the potential for severely decreased lifestyle or death. Have the patient sign to the fact that he understands the implications, and if at all possible, have a witness sign as well.

Explain to the patient and his family the reason and necessity for rapid transport, if indicated, and inform them of your treatment, time permitting. Upon arrival at the emergency department, inform the physician of your findings—past history, vital signs, labored breathing, relief of pain, no relief of pain, and ECG readings, especially S-T segment results.

In-Hospital Management of Acute Ischemic Chest Pain Your understanding of the management of the acute ischemic chest pain patient after you have delivered him to the emergency department is important. This is especially true if you belong to an EMS system whose EMT-Is also regularly staff emergency departments.

With the advent of thrombolytic therapy, many hospitals have opened specially designed chest-pain units. These facilities specialize in diagnosing and observing patients with chest pain. In addition to 12-lead ECGs, obtaining cardiac enzyme levels in chest pain patients is routine. Because dead or dying myocardial cells release cardiac enzymes, elevated levels of these enzymes indicate MI. The enzyme levels do not increase, however, until the infarction is several hours old, so intervention ideally should occur before the enzymes have a chance to rise. Commonly assayed cardiac enzymes are lactate dehydrogenase (LDH) and creatine phosphokinase (CK). Several newer markers show promise in aiding earlier identification of myocardial injury. These include troponin (I, T, and C), myoglobin, and CK-MB (a type of CK specific for cardiac muscle).

In many patients with chest pain, the diagnosis will be readily evident. In many others, however, it will remain unclear. These patients are commonly stratified according to risk. Patients with a low likelihood of cardiac ischemia may be discharged with instructions for follow-up care, which may include diagnostic tools such as stress tests. Patients with a higher likelihood of having myocardial ischemia are usually admitted to the hospital and are typically observed for 24 hours. During the patient's hospitalization, his cardiac enzyme levels are obtained several times, as is his ECG. If the tests all remain negative, the patient will usually see a cardiologist and have a stress test before going home. If the stress test is negative, the cardiologist will work up the problem as an outpatient. If the stress test is positive, additional testing is done before discharge. This testing includes nuclear medicine cardiac imaging (Cardiolyte) and, possibly, coronary angiography. Usually, cardiology immediately sees patients who have a high likelihood of cardiac ischemia but nondiagnostic ECGs and enzymes. These patients ordinarily are not observed but are taken directly to the cardiac lab for an angiogram.

Several treatment options are available. Patients with isolated coronary artery lesions may be candidates for percutaneous transluminal coronary angioplasty (PTCA). In these patients, lesions are identified during coronary angiography. A balloon catheter is then inserted into the coronary artery with the lesion. At the level of the lesion, the balloon is inflated, thus increasing the artery's diameter and reducing the relative size of the blockage. Often, the patient will have several lesions. If the arteries do not stay open following angioplasty, another alternative is to place a stent in the artery at the site of the lesion. The stent is a hollow tube that keeps the artery open. Patients with severe and diffuse coronary artery disease may not be candidates for angioplasty. The best option for these patients is

The trend in emergency cardiac care is rapid cardiac catheterization and therapeutic intervention such as PTCA.

surgical revascularization of their coronary arteries. The most common operation is the coronary artery bypass graft (CABG), in which grafts are sewn from the aorta to the coronary arteries, thus effectively bypassing the blockage. In younger patients, the surgeon may use the internal mammary artery as the source. Recently, technology has evolved to the point where some bypass grafts can be performed endoscopically. These require only small "key-hole" incisions instead of the classic sternotomy, thus markedly decreasing the pain and the recovery time. Patients whose disease is either too mild or too severe may not be candidates for surgery. These patients are managed with medication alone.

HEART FAILURE

heart failure clinical syndrome in which the heart's mechanical performance is compromised so that cardiac output cannot meet the body's needs.

Heart failure is a clinical syndrome in which the heart's mechanical performance is compromised so that cardiac output cannot meet the body's needs. Heart failure is generally divided into left ventricle or right ventricle failure. Its many etiologies include valvular, coronary, or myocardial disease. Dysrhythmias can also cause or aggravate heart failure. Many other factors can contribute to heart failure, such as excess fluid or salt intake, fever (sepsis), hypertension, pulmonary embolism, or excessive alcohol or drug use. It can manifest with exertion in the patient who has an underlying disease or as a progression of the underlying disease.

Left Ventricular Failure

Left ventricular failure occurs when the left ventricle fails as an effective forward pump, causing back pressure of blood into the pulmonary circulation, which often results in pulmonary edema. Its causes include various types of heart disease such as MI, valvular disease, chronic hypertension, and dysrhythmias. In left ventricular failure, the left ventricle cannot eject all of the blood that the right heart delivers to it via the lungs. Left atrial pressure rises and is subsequently transmitted to the pulmonary veins and capillaries. When pulmonary capillary pressure becomes too high, it forces the blood plasma into the alveoli, resulting in pulmonary edema. Progressive fluid accumulation in the alveoli decreases the lungs' oxygenation capacity and can cause death from hypoxia. Since MI is a common cause of left ventricular failure, you should consider that all patients with pulmonary edema may have had an MI.

Right Ventricular Failure

In right ventricular failure, the right ventricle fails as an effective forward pump, resulting in back pressure of blood into the systemic venous circulation and venous congestion. The most common cause of right ventricular failure is left ventricular failure. This is because MI is more common in the left ventricle than in the right and because chronic hypertension affects the left ventricle more adversely than the right. Right ventricular failure's other causes include systemic hypertension, which can affect both sides of the heart and can cause pure right ventricular failure. Pulmonary hypertension and *cor pulmonale* (heart failure due to pulmonary disease) result from the effects of COPD. These problems are related to increased pressure in the pulmonary arteries, which results in right ventricular enlargement, right atrial enlargement, and if untreated, right heart failure.

pulmonary embolism (PE) blood clot in one of the pulmonary arteries.

Pulmonary embolism (PE), a blood clot in one of the pulmonary arteries, also can cause right heart failure. If the clot is large enough to occlude a major vessel, the pressure against which the right ventricle must pump increases. This can throw the right ventricle into failure in much the same manner as pulmonary hypertension. In fact, it can be considered an acute form of pulmonary hypertension. Infarct of the right atrium or ventricle, although rare, is another cause of right ventricular failure.

Starling's law of the heart enables heart failure patients to compensate, at least for a time. Starling's law states that the more the myocardial muscle is stretched, the greater will be its force of contraction. Thus, the greater the preload (the volume of blood filling the chamber), the farther the myocardial muscle stretches and the more forceful the cardiac contraction. This has its limits, however. If myocardial muscle is stretched too far, it will not contract properly and the contraction will be weaker. Afterload (the resistance against which the ventricle must contract) also affects stroke volume. An increase in peripheral vascular resistance will decrease stroke volume. The reverse is also true: stroke volume will increase as peripheral vascular resistance decreases.

Congestive Heart Failure

In **congestive heart failure (CHF)**, the heart's reduced stroke volume causes an overload of fluid in the body's other tissues. This presents as edema, which can be pulmonary, peripheral, sacral, or ascites (peritoneal edema). CHF can manifest in an acute setting as pulmonary edema, pulmonary hypertension, or myocardial infarction. In the chronic setting, it can manifest as cardiomegaly (enlargement of the heart), left ventricular failure, or right ventricular failure. Heart failure can present in a first-time event, as in myocardial infarction, or in multiple events, as in left heart failure. CHF is one of the few diseases still on the rise in the United States. Approximately 400,000 new cases are diagnosed each year. CHF also is the most common cause of hospitalization in patients over age 65, accounting for approximately 900,000 admissions each year. Mortality is only 5 years in 50% of CHF patients. The end stage of this disease involves pulmonary edema and respiratory failure, followed by death. When the CHF patient calls EMS, one thing is clear; Starling's law is no longer allowing the patient to compensate.

Field Assessment

As in all cardiac emergencies, begin your assessment by checking the ABCs and managing any life threats. Often, patients with pulmonary edema will cough up large quantities of clear or pink-tinged sputum. Patients with profound pulmonary edema generally have labored breathing, although this may not present until the patient begins to exert himself simply by standing or walking a few steps. Look for any changes or differences in skin color on the patient's arms, face, chest, and back. In profound CHF, mottling is often present.

Focus on the patient's chief complaint. Use the OPQRST mnemonic to elicit the patient's description of symptoms. Patients with pulmonary edema will complain of progressive or acute shortness of breath and will confirm being awakened by shortness of breath (**paroxysmal nocturnal dyspnea, or PND**). If the patient's episodes of PND are becoming more frequent, the disease process usually is worsening.

Often the heart failure patient will confirm progressive accumulation of edema or weight gain over a short time. Because many heart failure patients have an underlying cardiac or prior MI history, they may complain of mild chest pain or generalized weakness. This may be due to a weakened myocardial muscle mass, myocardial ischemia, or current MI.

Determine the patient's current medications. CHF patients are generally prescribed a loop diuretic such as Lasix or Bumex and/or hypertension medication. Many are prescribed digoxin (Lanoxin), which increases the heart's contractile force; many are oxygen dependent and may be on home oxygen. Find out if the patient has been compliant in taking medications; if not, determine how long he has been off medications. Also record and report any over-the-counter medications or herbal medications that the patient is taking, as well as any prescription medications borrowed from someone else.

Unconsciousness or an altered level of consciousness indicates pending respiratory failure. If the patient shows any sign of respiratory failure, immediately assist his breathing with 100% oxygen by BVM and prepare to intubate if clinically warranted.

Next assess the patient's breathing. Often, labored breathing, dyspnea, and productive cough appear. Labored breathing is the most common symptom of CHF, and it generally worsens with activity. CHF patients frequently assume the tripod position, sitting upright with both arms supporting the upper body, and confirm PND and pillow orthopnea, the inability to recline in bed without a pillow). Ask the patient how many pillows he sleeps on at night. As a rule, the more pillows, the worse the problem.

Check the skin. CHF patients present with changes in the skin color, such as pallor, diaphoresis, mottling, or signs of cyanosis. Check the peripheral pulses for quality and rhythm. Also check for edema. Edema is usually found in the lower extremities, localized from the ankles to the mid-calf or the knees. Sometimes the edema will be so severe that it obliterates the distal pulses. Check the edematous area for pitting and record its severity on a scale from 0 to 4+. Edema may also be present in the sacral area of the back, especially in the bed-confined, or in the upper quadrants of abdominal cavity. Ascites (abdominal cavity edema or swelling) is very difficult to assess accurately without X-ray or ultrasound.

Labored breathing is the most common symptom of CHF.

Blood pressure may be elevated in the CHF patient, due to the body's attempt to compensate for decreased cardiac output, but this can change quickly. A decompensating patient can have a normal blood pressure that drops quickly.

The most serious complication of heart failure is pulmonary edema. Untreated pulmonary edema can quickly lead to respiratory failure. This is because the abundant serum fluid in a large portion of the alveoli inhibits oxygen exchange in the lungs and hypoxia ensues. Respiratory failure will quickly lead to death. Patients with severe pulmonary edema present with tachypnea and adventitious lung sounds. Pulmonary edema can present as crackles (rales) at both bases. Rhonchi, which indicates fluid in the larger airways of the lungs, is a sign of severe pulmonary edema. Wheezes in the CHF patient are a sign of the lungs' protective mechanisms, since bronchioles constrict in an attempt to keep additional fluid from entering the lungs. This wheezing in pulmonary edema and CHF is often called cardiac asthma. This term is confusing, however, and you should avoid using it. Consider wheezes in a geriatric patient to be pulmonary edema until proven otherwise.

Other complications of pulmonary edema are pulsus paradoxus and pulsus alternans. Pulsus paradoxus occurs when systolic blood pressure drops more than 10 mmHg with inspiration. This is due to compression of the great vessels or the ventricles. In pulsus alternans, the pulse alternates between weak and strong. Pulses may be thready or weak, and jugular vein distention (JVD) might be present. The apical pulse may be abnormal or difficult to auscultate because of abnormalities such as bulges in the heart, a displaced apex, or severe pulmonary edema. The patient may produce frothy sputum with coughing, and cyanosis may present in the late stages of CHF.

Management

In severe CHF with pulmonary edema, obtain pertinent medical history and complete the physical exam while initiating treatment. Reassess all life-threatening conditions and treat them accordingly. Do not have the patient exert himself in any way, including standing up or walking. Do not have the patient lie flat at any time. Seat him with his feet dangling. This will promote venous pooling, thus decreasing preload.

Administer high-flow, high-concentration oxygen. If necessary, provide positive-pressure assistance with either a demand valve if the patient can assist or a BVM unit if he is unresponsive. When possible, establish an IV at a "to keep open" (TKO) rate. Consider placing a heparin lock or saline lock. Limiting fluids is imperative; use a minidrip set to avoid accidentally infusing excessive amounts of fluid.

Place ECG electrodes. If the patient is extremely diaphoretic, apply tincture of Benzoin first. Record a baseline ECG and keep the monitor in place throughout care.

Administer medications according to written protocols or on the order of the medical director. Some left ventricular failures result from very rapid dysrhythmias. If you suspect a dysrhythmia as a cause, treat it according to established protocols. Before giving the patient any drug, ask him or his family if he is allergic to any medication. Medications frequently used in left ventricular failure and pulmonary edema include:

- Morphine sulfate
- Nitroglycerin
- Furosemide (Lasix)
- Dopamine (Intropin)
- Dobutamine (Dobutrex)
- Promethazine (Phenergan)
- Nitrous oxide (Nitronox)

Transport the heart-failure patient as a nonemergency unless clinical conditions indicate otherwise. Conditions that indicate emergency transport include hypertension or hypotension, severe respiratory distress or pending respiratory failure, or life-threatening dysrhythmias. Remember that transporting with lights and sirens can increase the conscious patient's anxiety and worsen his condition. If nonemergency transport might compromise the patient's condition, use lights and siren. Place the patient in a position of comfort, but not lying flat.

If the patient refuses transport and is indeed in the early stages of CHF, the outcome is likely to be devastating, leading to worsening signs and symptoms, unnecessary myocardial damage, severe pulmonary edema, and even death. Avoid refusal at all costs, and use every means at your disposal to convince the patient to be transported. If he still refuses, document the fact that you repeatedly warned the patient of the possible outcome.

CARDIAC TAMPONADE

In **cardiac tamponade**, excess fluid accumulates inside the pericardium. (The normal amount of fluid between the visceral pericardium and the parietal pericardium is approximately 25 cc.) This excess fluid causes an increase in intrapericardial pressure that impairs diastolic filling and drastically decreases the amount of blood the ventricles can expel with each contraction. Chest pain or dyspnea is the chief complaint; depending on the underlying cause, the chest pain may be dull or sharp and severe.

cardiac tamponade accumulation of excess fluid inside the pericardium.

Cardiac tamponade's onset may be gradual, as in pericarditis or as in a neoplasm such as benign or malignant cancer. Or it may be acute, as in MI or trauma. All forms of cardiac tamponade involve pericardial effusion of air, pus, serum, blood, or any combination of these four. Gradual onset usually results from an underlying condition, and overlooking or misdiagnosing the tamponade is easy. Renal disease and hypothyroidism can cause cardiac tamponade, though such instances are rare. Traumatic causes can include CPR and penetrating or nonpenetrating injuries. Whether onset is gradual or acute, cardiac tamponade can lead to death.

Field Assessment

Perform your initial assessment, including the patient's airway, breathing, and circulation. If you suspect cardiac tamponade, limit your history taking to determining the precipitating cause(s). Determine if the cause might be acute trauma such as penetrating or blunt trauma. Has the patient sustained recent trauma, including recent CPR? If you suspect a gradual onset, determine if the patient has recently had an infection or MI. Is he currently having an MI? Does he have a history of renal disease or hypothyroidism? Has he been ill? Use the OPQRST mnemonic to obtain information about the patient's symptoms.

Always consider the possibility of pericardial tamponade in a patient who received CPR, and then later deteriorated.

The patient generally will present with dyspnea and orthopnea. Anterior and posterior lung sounds are usually clear. Typically, the pulse is rapid and weak. In the early stages venous pressures are often elevated, as evidenced by jugular vein distention. Blood pressure readings show a decrease in systolic pressure, pulsus paradoxus, and narrowing pulse pressures. Heart sounds are normal early on but then become muffled or faint.

Do not use the ECG, whether monitor quality or 12-lead, to diagnose cardiac tamponade; rather consider it a tool to support your clinical suspicions. The ECG is generally inconclusive, but ectopy is usually a late sign of cardiac tamponade. This is because an effusion easily irritates the heart's epicardial tissue. QRS and T-wave voltages are low, and non-specific T-wave changes occur. S-T segments may elevate. Electrical alternans (weak voltage, then normal) may appear in the P, QRS, T, and S-T segments.

Management

While obtaining any pertinent medical history and completing the physical exam, initiate treatment. Management of cardiac tamponade is primarily supportive, except when you detect shock or low perfusion. Maintain a patent airway and deliver high-flow, high-concentration oxygen. If clinically indicated, secure the patient's airway with endotracheal intubation and maintain the patient's circulation with IV support, pharmacological agents, or CPR. Before administering any medication, ask the patient or family if he is allergic to any medications. Medications used in the treatment of cardiac tamponade include:

- Morphine sulfate
- Nitrous oxide (Nitronox)
- Furosemide (Lasix)
- Dopamine (Intropin)
- Dobutamine (Dobutrex)

Rapid transport is indicated for patients with cardiac tamponade. Remember to be supportive of the patient and family throughout your care. Upon arrival at the emergency department, inform the physician of your findings—past history, medications, vital signs, labored breathing, ECG readings, pulsus paradoxus, and shock. The therapy of choice is invasive pericardiocentesis, which involves aspirating fluid from the pericardium with a cardiac needle. Unless you have adequate training and local protocol permits you to do so, a physician should perform this procedure.

HYPERTENSIVE EMERGENCIES

A **hypertensive emergency** is a life-threatening elevation of blood pressure. It occurs in 1% or less of patients with hypertension, usually when the hypertension is poorly controlled or untreated. A hypertensive emergency is characterized by a rapid increase in diastolic blood pressure (usually .130 mmHg) accompanied by restlessness, confusion, blurred vision, nausea, and vomiting. It often occurs with **hypertensive encephalopathy,** a condition of acute or subacute consequence of severe hypertension characterized by severe headache, vomiting, visual disturbances (including transient blindness), paralysis, seizures, stupor, and coma. On occasion, this condition may cause left ventricular failure, pulmonary edema, or stroke.

A prior history of hypertension is the precipitating cause of most hypertensive emergencies. In many cases, the patient has not complied with his hypertensive medication or other prescribed drugs. Another cause of hypertensive crisis, toxemia of pregnancy (preeclampsia), can appear at any time between the twentieth week of pregnancy and term delivery. It occurs in 5% of pregnancies and is defined as a blood pressure of at least 140/90 mmHg. Hypertension is a sign of the toxemia, not the cause. Preeclampsia poses a high risk of abruptio placentae and generally progresses to eclampsia (coma and seizures). Left untreated, it progresses to eclampsia and death for the mother and unborn fetus.

Experts estimate that more than 50 million people in the United States are hypertensive patients. Its prevalence increases with age, and it has a higher incidence among African Americans, as well as a higher mortality and morbidity. With modern medications, hypertensive encephalopathy has become rare, yet it is still seen in the prehospital setting. Ischemic and hemorrhagic stroke are more common results of severe hypertension. Both hypertensive encephalopathy and stroke (ischemic or hemorrhagic) can have devastating consequences or lead to death if left untreated.

Field Assessment

After making your initial assessment, including airway, breathing, and circulation, conduct your focused history and physical examination. Generally, hypertensive patients have a chief complaint of headache, accompanied by nausea and/or vomiting, blurred vision, shortness of breath, epistaxis (nosebleed), and vertigo (dizziness). However any one of these symptoms might be the patient's only complaint. The patient may be semiconscious or unconscious or having a seizure. In pregnancy toxemia, the expectant mother usually has edema of the hands or face. Photosensitivity and headache are common complaints.

Determine if the patient has a history of hypertension and if he has been taking medications as prescribed. Often he has been noncompliant, taking medicines only occasionally or not at all. In some situations the patient will borrow someone else's medications or take over-the-counter medications such as herbal medications. He may be on home oxygen.

If left ventricular failure accompanies the hypertension, the lung sounds generally present with pulmonary edema; otherwise they are clear. Often the pulse is strong and at times may be bounding. By definition, hypertension is a systolic pressure greater than 160 mmHg and a diastolic pressure greater than 90 mmHg. Consider signs or symptoms of hypertensive encephalopathy associated with hypertension to be a hypertensive emergency.

The level of consciousness of a hypertensive patient may be normal or altered, or he may be unconscious. His skin may be pale, flushed, or normal, cool or warm, moist or dry. Look for edema, either pitting or nonpitting. The patient may confirm PND, orthopnea, vertigo, epistaxis, tinnitus (ringing of the ears), nausea or vomiting, or visual acuities. In addition, he may have seizures or motor/sensory deficits in parts of the body or on one side. ECG findings are generally inconclusive unless the patient has an underlying cardiac condition such as angina or MI.

Management

Place the patient in a position of comfort, unless a potential exists for airway compromise, as in stroke. Provide airway and ventilatory support, if clinically indicated. Provide oxygen and base your transport considerations on the patient's clinical presentation. Attempt supportive IV therapy on-scene time or en route. Do not prolong on-scene time to establish an IV. Place pregnant patients on their left side and transport as smoothly and quietly as possible.

In recent years, calcium channel blockers such as nifedipine (Procardia) have been widely used to treat hypertensive emergencies. Now this practice is being questioned because evidence suggests that significantly reducing the patient's blood pressure may actually be harmful. Some systems still use loop diuretics such as Lasix or nitroglycerin to reduce the patient's blood pressure by manipulating preload and afterload. These treatments' effectiveness is also being scrutinized. Follow your local protocols. In severe cases, especially if hypertensive encephalopathy is present, medical direction may order one of the following medications:

Elevated blood pressures should only be treated in the prehospital setting if these are associated with end-organ changes.

- Morphine sulfate
- Furosemide (Lasix)
- Nitroglycerin
- Sodium nitroprusside (Nipride)
- Labetalol (Trandate, Normodyne)

Explain to the patient and family the reason and necessity for rapid transport, if indicated. Advise the patient who refuses transport of the serious complications that are likely to occur without further medical attention. Stroke, seizures, pulmonary edema, and kidney damage are but a few possible outcomes. Avoid refusal at all costs. As always, use every means at your disposal to convince the patient to be transported. Document refusals as usual.

Upon arrival at the emergency department, inform the physician of your findings—vital signs, history, labored breathing, pulmonary edema, hand or facial edema, and neurological deficits.

CARDIOGENIC SHOCK

Cardiogenic shock, the most severe form of pump failure, is shock that remains after existing dysrhythmias, hypovolemia, or altered vascular tone have been corrected. It occurs when left ventricular function is so compromised that the heart cannot meet the body's metabolic demands and the compensatory mechanisms are exhausted. This usually happens after extensive MI, often involving more than 40% of the left ventricle, or with diffuse ischemia.

cardiogenic shock the inability of the heart to meet the metabolic needs of the body, resulting in inadequate tissue perfusion.

A variety of mechanisms can cause cardiogenic shock, and its onset may be acute or progressive. Among the more common mechanical causes are tension pneumothorax and cardiac tamponade. Both affect ventricular filling, or preload, and tend to manifest acutely. Interference with ventricular emptying, or afterload, as in pulmonary embolism and prosthetic valve malfunction, can also cause cardiogenic shock. Impairments in myocardial contractility, as seen in MI, myocarditis, and recreational drug use, can manifest either progressively or acutely. Trauma, too, can cause cardiogenic shock, secondary to hypovolemia or to significant underlying disease processes such as neurological, gastroenterological, renal, or metabolic disorders.

Cardiogenic shock is the most severe form of pump failure.

In cardiogenic shock, the body tries to compensate either by increasing the contractile force, by improving preload, by reducing the peripheral resistance, or by all three. In the early stages, a conscious patient presents with obvious signs of shock (cold extremities, weak pulses, and low blood pressure). As Starling's law loses effect, the patient's mental status diminishes and his radial pulses are no longer palpable. Finally, when preload, afterload, and contractility fail to meet vital organ demands, unconsciousness occurs and, if left untreated, the patient will die.

Cardiogenic shock can occur at any age, but it is most often seen as an end-stage event in the geriatric patient, with significant underlying disease(s). Mortality for cardiogenic shock is high for geriatric patients following massive MI or septic shock. This is because end-organ damage is so severe or multiple end-organ damage reaches the point that life cannot be sustained.

Cardiogenic shock has a high mortality rate.

Field Assessment

After conducting your initial assessment, including airway, breathing, and circulation, perform your focused history and physical exam. The chief complaint may range from acute onset of chest pain to shortness of breath, altered mental status or unconsciousness, or general weakness; onset may be acute or progressive. Ask about the patient's past medical history and determine if he or she has had any recent trauma. Look for evidence of a hypovolemic cause such as a gastrointestinal bleed, septic shock, and traumatic or nontraumatic internal hemorrhage. Has the patient recently suffered an MI? Cardiogenic shock is most often associated with large anterior infarction and/or loss of 40% or more of the left ventricle.

The patient's medication history may be important. Large amounts of different cardiac medications may indicate the patient has significant preexisting damage or a compromised but adequate cardiac output. Also, noncompliance with prescribed medications can further insult a preexisting weakened cardiac state, and the use of borrowed or over-the-counter medications can have unpredictable effects.

The altered mental status secondary to decreased cardiac output and unconsciousness common in cardiogenic shock may begin as restlessness and progress to confusion ending in coma. Airway findings include dyspnea, productive cough, or labored breathing. Paroxysmal nocturnal dyspnea, tripoding, adventitious lung sounds, and retractions on inspiration are also common findings. Typical ECG findings include tachycardia and atrial dysrhythmias such as atrial tachycardias. Ectopy is also common.

MI often precedes cardiogenic shock, and symptoms are initially the same as expected with MI; however, as cardiogenic shock develops and compensatory mechanisms fail, hypotension develops. The systolic blood pressure is often less than 80 mmHg. The usual heart rhythm is sinus tachycardia, a reflection of the cardiovascular system's attempts to compensate for the decreased stroke volume. If serious dysrhythmias are present, determining whether they are the cause of the hypotension or the result of the cardiogenic shock may be difficult; therefore, you must correct any major dysrhythmias.

The patient's skin is usually cool and clammy, reflecting peripheral vasoconstriction. Tachypnea is often present, since pulmonary edema is a common complication. Pitting or nonpitting peripheral edema may be present in the lower extremities or in the sacral area and may obliterate peripheral pulses.

Management

Cardiogenic shock should be aggressively treated, with rapid transport to follow.

To manage the cardiogenic shock patient, place him in a position of comfort if he is hemodynamically stable. If any pulmonary edema is present, the patient may prefer sitting upright, with both legs hanging off the stretcher. Treatment of cardiogenic shock (Figure 20-59) consists mostly of treating the underlying problem (such as MI and CHF) or treating the patient supportively. Remember to always treat the rate and rhythm first. Some medications that may be used to treat cardiogenic shock include:

- Vasopressors
  - Dopamine (Intropin)
  - Dobutamine (Dobutrex)
  - Norepinephrine (Levophed)

Other useful medications may include:

- Morphine sulfate
- Promethazine (Phenergan)
- Nitroglycerin
- Nitrous oxide (Nitronox)
- Furosemide (Lasix)
- Digitalis, digoxin (Lanoxin)

If the patient refuses transport, follow the general guidelines; however, remember that untreated cardiogenic shock has a grim outcome. No matter how well compensated the patient may appear, true cardiogenic shock will decompensate quickly into irreversible shock.

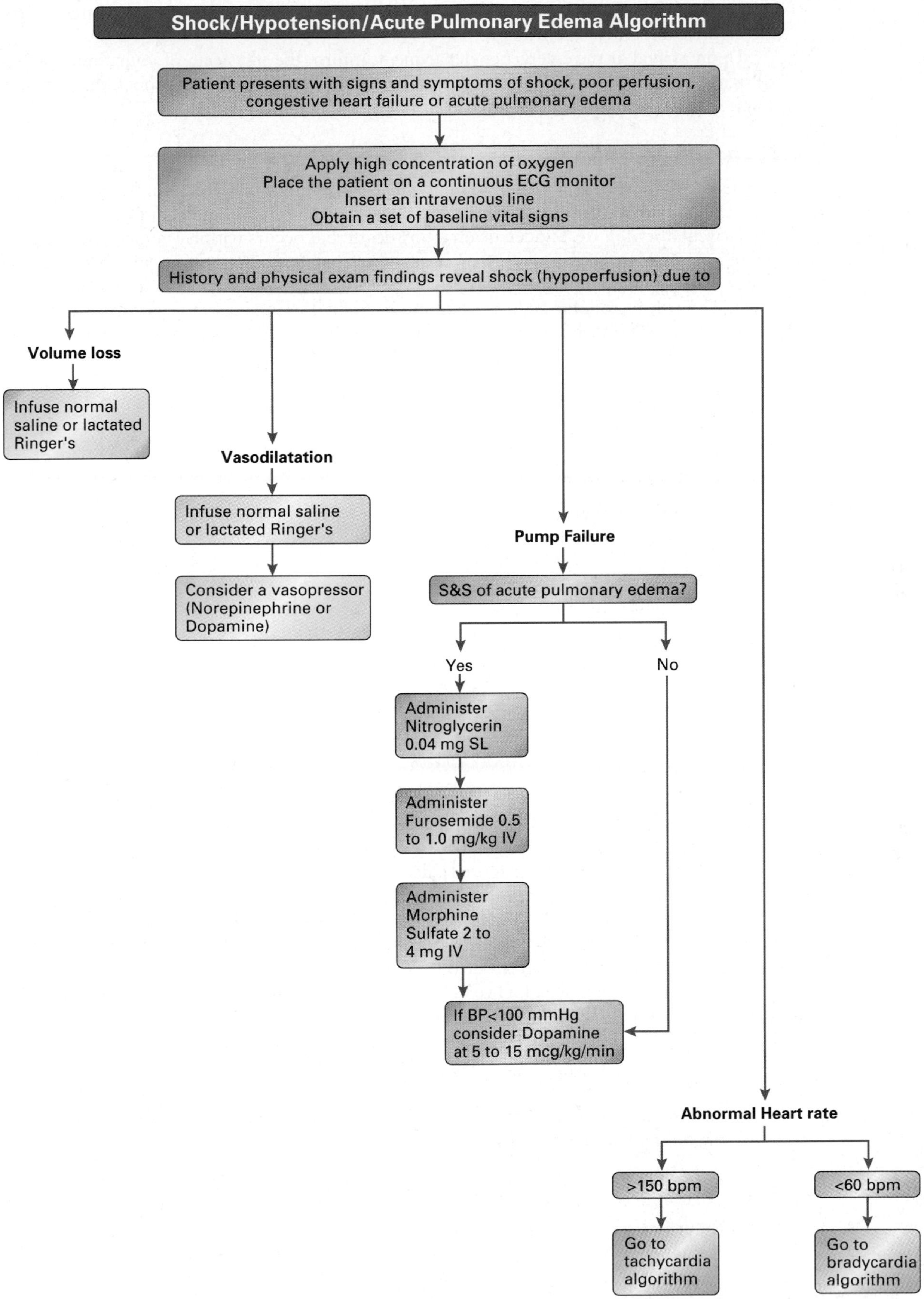

Shock/Hypotension/Acute Pulmonary Edema Algorithm

Patient presents with signs and symptoms of shock, poor perfusion, congestive heart failure or acute pulmonary edema

Apply high concentration of oxygen
Place the patient on a continuous ECG monitor
Insert an intravenous line
Obtain a set of baseline vital signs

History and physical exam findings reveal shock (hypoperfusion) due to

Volume loss

Infuse normal saline or lactated Ringer's

Vasodilatation

Infuse normal saline or lactated Ringer's

Consider a vasopressor (Norepinephrine or Dopamine)

Pump Failure

S&S of acute pulmonary edema?

Yes

No

Administer Nitroglycerin 0.04 mg SL

Administer Furosemide 0.5 to 1.0 mg/kg IV

Administer Morphine Sulfate 2 to 4 mg IV

If BP<100 mmHg consider Dopamine at 5 to 15 mcg/kg/min

Abnormal Heart rate

>150 bpm

<60 bpm

Go to tachycardia algorithm

Go to bradycardia algorithm

FIGURE 20-59   Management of shock, hypotension, and acute pulmonary edema.

Use every means at your disposal to convince the patient to be transported. If the patient still refuses, document accordingly.

Upon arrival at the emergency department, inform the physician of your findings—vital signs, labored breathing, pulmonary edema, dysrhythmias, or severe shock that remains despite your treatment.

CARDIAC ARREST

cardiac arrest the absence of ventricular contraction.

sudden death death within 1 hour after the onset of symptoms.

Cardiac arrest and sudden death accounts for 60% of all deaths from coronary artery disease. **Cardiac arrest** is the absence of ventricular contraction that immediately results in systemic circulatory failure. **Sudden death** is any death that occurs within 1 hour of the onset of symptoms. At autopsy, actual infarction often is not present. Because severe atherosclerotic disease is common, authorities usually believe that a lethal dysrhythmia is the mechanism of death. The risk factors for sudden death are basically the same as those for atherosclerotic heart disease (ASHD) and coronary artery disease (CAD). In a large number of patients, cardiac arrest is the first manifestation of heart disease. Other causes of sudden death include:

- Drowning
- Acid-base imbalance
- Electrocution
- Drug intoxication
- Electrolyte imbalance
- Hypoxia
- Hypothermia
- Pulmonary embolism
- Stroke
- Hyperkalemia (high levels of potassium)
- Trauma
- End-stage renal disease

Field Assessment

down time duration from the beginning of the cardiac arrest until effective CPR is established.

total down time duration from the beginning of the arrest until the patient's delivery to the emergency department.

A cardiac arrest patient is unresponsive, apneic, and pulseless. Peripheral pulses are absent. After initiating CPR, place ECG leads. Dysrhythmias found in the cardiac arrest patient include ventricular fibrillation, ventricular tachycardia, asystole, or PEA. If you find asystole, you should confirm it in two or more leads.

Center questions on events that occurred before the arrest. Did bystanders or EMS personnel witness the arrest? Did bystanders start CPR? How much time passed from the discovery of the arrest until CPR was initiated? From discovery until EMS was activated? These questions all focus on **down time,** the duration from the beginning of the cardiac arrest until effective CPR is established. Often physicians want to know the **total down time,** which is the time from the beginning of the arrest until you deliver the patient to the emergency department. If possible, obtain the patient's past history and medications.

Management

resuscitation provision of efforts to return a spontaneous pulse and breathing.

return of spontaneous circulation (ROSC) resuscitation results in the patient's having a spontaneous pulse.

survival when a patient is resuscitated and survives to be discharged from the hospital.

To manage the cardiac arrest patient properly, you must understand the terms resuscitation, return of spontaneous circulation, and survival.

- **Resuscitation** is the provision of efforts to return a spontaneous pulse and breathing to the patient in cardiac arrest.
- **Return of spontaneous circulation (ROSC)** occurs when resuscitation results in the patient's having a spontaneous pulse. ROSC patients may or may not have a return of breathing, and may or may not survive.
- **Survival** means that the patient is resuscitated and survives to be discharged from the hospital. Many resuscitated patients reach ROSC, but not all resuscitated patients survive.

Begin management of airway, breathing, and circulation simultaneously. When resuscitation is indicated, start CPR immediately. Remember that basic life support is the mainstay of treatment for cardiac arrest. Ventilate the patient with a BVM and 100% oxygen. Intubate or insert an alternative airway as quickly as possible. If changes in the ECG indicate defibrillation or synchronized cardioversion, perform it in conjunction with CPR, stopping CPR only to apply the pads or paddles and to deliver the shock(s). Make sure no one touches the patient when you deliver any shock. If the patient has an internal pacemaker or defibrillator, treat the arrest normally, taking care not to defibrillate over the device.

Remember, basic life support is the mainstay of prehospital cardiac care.

After establishing CPR and advanced airway management, perform IV access. The site of venipuncture should be as close to the heart as possible—for example, the antecubital area (bend of the forearm and humerus) or the external jugular vein. Follow all IV medications with a 30 to 45 second flush. After each flush, set the IV at a "to keep open" (TKO) drip rate.

Pharmacological agents that might be used in a cardiac arrest setting are:

- Atropine sulfate
- Lidocaine
- Procainamide
- Vasopressin
- Epinephrine
- Norepinephrine
- Isoproterenol
- Dopamine
- Dobutamine

Management of the successful postcardiac arrest patient generally presents an unusual situation. The patient's blood pressure can return at low, normal, or high readings because of the drugs used in resuscitation. In addition, the pulse can return at bradycardic, normal, or tachycardic rates. Ventricular ectopy is the most serious concern. If the patient presented in ventricular fibrillation or ventricular tachycardia during the arrest, or if ectopy presents in the postarrest, use an antidysrhythmic agent such as lidocaine. The blood pressure may return at low readings. The ideal range of the blood pressure is 80 to 100 mmHg in the postarrest patient. Do not be concerned if the postarrest patient does not show any signs of response. He has endured a very harsh environment, and recovery, if any, can be slow. The postarrest setting can be unnerving, with the patient's vitals and ECG changing every minute. Approach problems one at a time, and do not be fooled by a return in pulse that fades away while the monitor still has a rhythm (PEA).

Postarrest stabilization requires extreme vigilance.

Your management of all cardiac arrest patients should follow the AHA guidelines for CPR and emergency cardiac care. Figure 20-60 summarizes the treatment for ventricular fibrillation or ventricular tachycardia (VF/VT), the cardiac arrest rhythms with the best prognosis for successful resuscitation. Also review the algorithms for asystole (Figure 20-44) and pulseless electrical activity (PEA) (Figure 20-46).

Once you have established advanced life support, move the patient to the MICU as quickly as possible, while taking great care to avoid disrupting IVs, endotracheal intubation, CPR, or pharmacological treatment. Transport the patient to the nearest appropriate facility as safely and as smoothly as possible using lights and siren. Offer emotional support to the patient throughout your care. Upon arrival at the emergency department, inform the physician of your findings, especially down time, total down time, changes in rhythm, or return of pulses.

Withholding and Terminating Resuscitation

In some situations, the certainty that the patient will not survive indicates not initiating resuscitation efforts. Rigor mortis, fixed dependent lividity (pooling of the blood), decapitation, decomposition, and incineration are all situations in which you should withhold resuscitation.

In addition, withhold resuscitation efforts if the patient has an out-of-hospital advanced directive. A physician must sign and date the advanced directive, and it must state conditions that apply to the patient at the time of the arrest. For example, the directive may state that resuscitation should be withheld if the patient has an end-stage terminal illness. Each

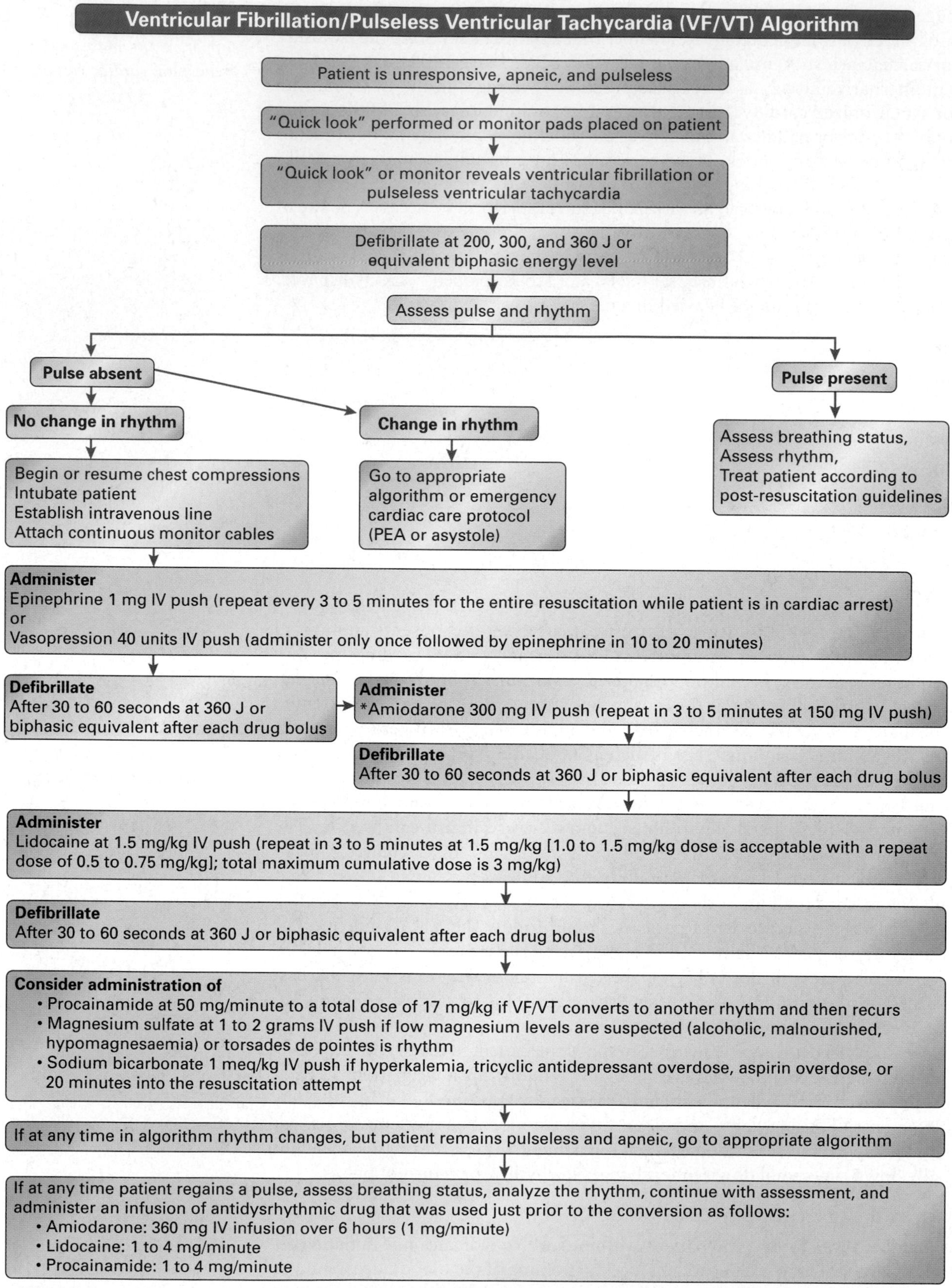

Ventricular Fibrillation/Pulseless Ventricular Tachycardia (VF/VT) Algorithm

Patient is unresponsive, apneic, and pulseless

↓

"Quick look" performed or monitor pads placed on patient

↓

"Quick look" or monitor reveals ventricular fibrillation or pulseless ventricular tachycardia

↓

Defibrillate at 200, 300, and 360 J or equivalent biphasic energy level

↓

Assess pulse and rhythm

Pulse absent → **No change in rhythm** / **Change in rhythm**

Pulse present → Assess breathing status, Assess rhythm, Treat patient according to post-resuscitation guidelines

No change in rhythm
Begin or resume chest compressions
Intubate patient
Establish intravenous line
Attach continuous monitor cables

Change in rhythm
Go to appropriate algorithm or emergency cardiac care protocol (PEA or asystole)

↓

Administer
Epinephrine 1 mg IV push (repeat every 3 to 5 minutes for the entire resuscitation while patient is in cardiac arrest)
or
Vasopression 40 units IV push (administer only once followed by epinephrine in 10 to 20 minutes)

↓

Defibrillate
After 30 to 60 seconds at 360 J or biphasic equivalent after each drug bolus

→ **Administer**
*Amiodarone 300 mg IV push (repeat in 3 to 5 minutes at 150 mg IV push)

↓

Defibrillate
After 30 to 60 seconds at 360 J or biphasic equivalent after each drug bolus

↓

Administer
Lidocaine at 1.5 mg/kg IV push (repeat in 3 to 5 minutes at 1.5 mg/kg [1.0 to 1.5 mg/kg dose is acceptable with a repeat dose of 0.5 to 0.75 mg/kg]; total maximum cumulative dose is 3 mg/kg)

↓

Defibrillate
After 30 to 60 seconds at 360 J or biphasic equivalent after each drug bolus

↓

Consider administration of
• Procainamide at 50 mg/minute to a total dose of 17 mg/kg if VF/VT converts to another rhythm and then recurs
• Magnesium sulfate at 1 to 2 grams IV push if low magnesium levels are suspected (alcoholic, malnourished, hypomagnesaemia) or torsades de pointes is rhythm
• Sodium bicarbonate 1 meq/kg IV push if hyperkalemia, tricyclic antidepressant overdose, aspirin overdose, or 20 minutes into the resuscitation attempt

↓

If at any time in algorithm rhythm changes, but patient remains pulseless and apneic, go to appropriate algorithm

↓

If at any time patient regains a pulse, assess breathing status, analyze the rhythm, continue with assessment, and administer an infusion of antidysrhythmic drug that was used just prior to the conversion as follows:
• Amiodarone: 360 mg IV infusion over 6 hours (1 mg/minute)
• Lidocaine: 1 to 4 mg/minute
• Procainamide: 1 to 4 mg/minute

*There is no evidence to suggest amiodarone has better discharge survival benefits in cardiac arrest over lidocaine; therefore, lidocaine can be used as a first-line antidysrhythmic drug prior to the administration of amiodarone.

FIGURE 20–60   Management of ventricular fibrillation and pulseless ventricular tachycardia (VF/VT).

state and many local regions treat advanced directives differently. Review local protocol and medical direction before you might have to decide whether to honor an advanced directive.

In other instances, poor prognosis and survivability of many cardiac arrest patients makes termination of resuscitation a consideration. Some of the inclusion criteria for termination of resuscitation are:

- 18 years of age or older
- Arrest is presumed cardiac in origin and not associated with a treatable cause such as hypothermia, overdose, or hypovolemia
- Successful and maintained endotracheal intubation
- ACLS standards have been applied throughout the arrest
- On-scene ALS efforts have been sustained for 25 minutes, or the patient remains in asystole through four rounds of ALS drugs
- Patient's rhythm is asystolic or agonal when the decision to terminate is made, and this rhythm persists until the resuscitation efforts are actually terminated
- Victims of blunt trauma who present in asystole or develop asystole on scene

Depending on local protocol, the exclusion criteria for termination of resuscitation may include:

- Under 18 years old
- Etiology that could benefit from in-hospital treatment (such as hypothermia)
- Persistent or recurring ventricular tachycardia or fibrillation
- Transient return of a pulse
- Signs of neurological viability
- Arrest witnessed by EMS personnel
- Family or responsible party opposed to termination

Criteria that should not be considered as either inclusionary or exclusionary:

- The patient's age if 18 or over (for example, geriatric)
- Down time before EMS arrival
- Presence of a nonofficial do-not-resuscitate (DNR) order
- Quality-of-life evaluations by EMS

Review local protocol and medical direction before attempting termination of resuscitation. Most systems use documented protocols and direct communication with an on-line medical director or physician to approve or deny termination of resuscitation. The medical director or physician may base his decision on the following information:

> *Review local protocol and medical direction before attempting termination of resuscitation.*
>

- Medical condition of the patient
- Known etiological factors
- Therapy rendered
- Family's presence and appraisal of the situation
- Communication of any resistance or uncertainty on the part of the family
- Maintain continuous documentation, including the ECG

The family should receive grief support. This requires EMS personnel or a community agency to be in place soon after termination of resuscitation. EMS personnel deal not only with the living or viable but also with the families of lost loved ones, especially when they have witnessed the death. Many systems employ assigned personnel to support the family after termination of resuscitation. In other systems, EMT-Is on the scene provide support until a predetermined person from another local agency can arrive. Although this supportive role can be uncomfortable, it will be part of your job.

Law enforcement regulations require that all local, state, or federal laws pertaining to a death be followed. These, too, may vary from region to region, but their basic principles are the same. The officer discusses the death certificate with the attending physician. He will determine if the event or patient requires assignment to a medical examiner, if the nature of the death is suspicious in any way, or if the physician is at all hesitant to sign the death certificate. The officer also may be required to assign the patient to a medical examiner if he does not have a physician. Check with local law enforcement agencies to determine their protocol.

PERIPHERAL VASCULAR AND OTHER CARDIOVASCULAR EMERGENCIES

In addition to cardiac arrest, MI, and hypertension emergencies, other common cardiovascular emergencies involve the arterial and venous systems. Such disorders are generally classified as traumatic or nontraumatic. Nontraumatic vascular emergencies typically arise from preexisting conditions or from a disease process.

Atherosclerosis

atherosclerosis a progressive, degenerative disease of the medium-sized and large arteries.

The major underlying factor in many cardiovascular emergencies is **atherosclerosis,** a progressive degenerative disease of the medium-sized and large arteries. Atherosclerosis affects the aorta and its branches, the coronary arteries, and the cerebral arteries, among others. It results from fats (lipids and cholesterol) deposited under the tunica intima (inner lining) of the involved vessels. The fat causes an injury response in the tunica intima, which subsequently damages the tunica media (middle layer) as well. Over time, calcium is deposited, causing plaques, where small hemorrhages can occur. These hemorrhages in turn lead to scarring, fibrosis, larger plaque build-up, and aneurysm. The involved arteries can become completely blocked, either by additional plaque, by a blood clot, or by an aneurysm that results from tearing in the arterial wall.

arteriosclerosis a thickening, loss of elasticity, and hardening of the walls of the arteries from calcium deposits.

The results of atherosclerosis are evident in many disease processes. First, disruption of the vessel's intimal surface destroys the vessel's elasticity. This condition, **arteriosclerosis,** can cause hypertension and other related problems. Second, atherosclerosis can reduce blood flow through the affected vessel; common manifestations include angina pectoris and intermittent **claudication.** Frequently, thrombosis will develop, totally obstructing the vessel or the tissues it supplies. MI is a classic example of this process.

claudication severe pain in the calf muscle due to inadequate blood supply. It typically occurs with exertion and subsides with rest.

Aneurysm

Aneurysm is a nonspecific term meaning dilation of a vessel. The types of aneurysm include:

aneurysm the ballooning of an arterial wall, resulting from a defect or weakness in the wall.

- Atherosclerotic
- Dissecting
- Infectious
- Congenital
- Traumatic

Most aneurysms result from atherosclerosis and involve the aorta, because the blood pressure in this area is the highest of any vessel in the body. An aneurysm occurs when blood surges into the aortic wall through a tear in the aortic tunica intima. Infectious aneurysms are most commonly associated with syphilis and are rare. Congenital aneurysms can occur with several disease states such as Marfan's syndrome, a hereditary disease that affects the connective tissue. Aortic aneurysm occurs in people with this disease because it involves the connective tissue within the vessel wall. Those affected may experience sudden death, usually from spontaneous rupture of the aorta, often at a fairly young age.

Abdominal Aortic Aneurysm Abdominal aortic aneurysm commonly results from atherosclerosis and occurs most frequently in the aorta, below the renal arteries and above the bifurcation of the common iliac arteries (Figure 20-61). It is ten times more common in men than in women and most prevalent between ages 60 and 70.

Signs and symptoms of an abdominal aneurysm include:

- Abdominal pain
- Back and flank pain
- Hypotension
- Urge to defecate, caused by the retroperitoneal leakage of blood

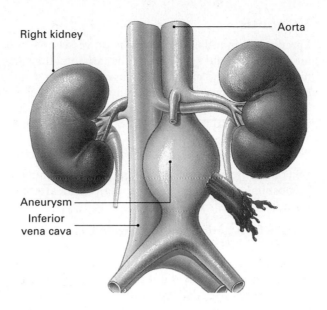

Right kidney
Aorta
Aneurysm
Inferior
vena cava

FIGURE 20-61 Rupture of an
abdominal aortic aneurysm.

Dissecting Aortic Aneurysm   Degenerative changes in the smooth muscle and elastic tissue of the aortic media cause most **dissecting aortic aneurysms.** This can result in hematoma and, subsequently, aneurysm. The original tear often results from **cystic medial necrosis,** a degenerative disease of connective tissue often associated with hypertension and to a certain extent, aging. Predisposing factors include hypertension, which is present in 75% to 85% of cases. It occurs more frequently in patients older than 40 to 50 years of age, although it can occur in younger individuals, especially pregnant women. A tendency for this disease also runs in families.

Of dissecting aortic aneurysms, 67% involve the ascending aorta. Once dissection has started, it can extend to all of the abdominal aorta as well as its branches, including the coronary arteries, aortic valve, subclavian arteries, and carotid arteries. The aneurysm can rupture at any time, usually into the pericardial or pleural cavity.

Acute Pulmonary Embolism

Acute pulmonary embolism occurs when a blood clot or other particle lodges in a pulmonary artery and blocks blood flow through that vessel. Pulmonary emboli may be composed of air, fat, amniotic fluid, or blood clots. Factors that predispose a patient to blood clots include prolonged immobilization, *thrombophlebitis* (inflammation and clots in a vein), use of certain medications, and atrial fibrillation.

When a pulmonary embolism blocks the blood flow through a vessel, the right heart must pump against increased resistance, which in turn increases pulmonary capillary pressure. The area of the lung supplied by the occluded vessel then stops functioning, and gas exchange decreases.

The signs and symptoms of pulmonary embolism depend on the size of the obstruction. The patient suffering acute pulmonary embolism may report a sudden onset of severe and unexplained dyspnea that may or may not be associated with chest pain. He may have a recent history of immobilization from a hip fracture, surgery, or other debilitating illness.

Acute Arterial Occlusion

An **acute arterial occlusion** is the sudden occlusion of arterial blood flow due to trauma, thrombosis, tumor, embolus, or idiopathic means. Emboli are probably the most common cause. They can arise from within the chamber (mural emboli), from a thrombus in the left ventricle, from an atrial thrombus secondary to atrial fibrillation, or from a thrombus caused by abdominal aortic atherosclerosis. Arterial occlusions most commonly involve vessels in the abdomen or extremities.

dissecting aortic aneurysm
aneurysm caused when blood gets between and separates the layers of the aortic wall.

cystic medial necrosis a death or degeneration of a part of the wall of an artery.

acute pulmonary embolism blockage that occurs when a blood clot or other particle lodges in a pulmonary artery.

acute arterial occlusion the sudden occlusion of arterial blood flow.

Vasculitis

Vasculitis is an inflammation of blood vessels. Most vasculitis stems from a variety of rheumatic diseases and syndromes. The inflammatory process is usually segmental, and inflammation within the media of a muscular artery tends to destroy the internal elastic lamina. Necrosis and hypertrophy (enlarging) of the vessel occur, and the vessel wall has a high likelihood of breaching, leaking fibrin and red blood cells into the surrounding tissue. This potentially can lead to partial or total vascular occlusion and subsequent necrosis.

Noncritical Peripheral Vascular Conditions

Several peripheral vascular conditions are not immediately life threatening but often require prehospital care. They include peripheral arterial atherosclerotic disease, deep venous thrombosis, and varicose veins.

peripheral arterial
atherosclerotic disease a
progressive degenerative
disease of the medium-sized
and large arteries.

Peripheral Arterial Atherosclerotic Disease Peripheral arterial atherosclerotic disease is a progressive degenerative disease of the medium-sized and large arteries. It affects the aorta and its branches, the brachial and femoral peripheral arteries, and the cerebral arteries. For reasons unknown it does not affect coronary arteries. It is a gradual, progressive disease, often associated with diabetes mellitus. In extreme cases, significant arterial insufficiency may lead to ulcers and gangrene. Occlusion of the peripheral arteries causes chronic and acute ischemia.

In the chronic setting, intermittent claudication (diminished blood flow in exercising muscle) produces pain with exertion. It occurs most commonly with the calf, but can affect any leg muscle. Rest initially relieves this pain. When the disease progresses, however, the pain presents even at rest. The extremity usually appears normal, but pulses will be reduced or absent. As the ischemia worsens, the extremity becomes painful, cold, and numb, and ulceration, gangrene, and necrosis may be present. There is no edema.

In the acute setting, arterial occlusion from an embolus, aneurysm, or thrombosis occurs. The patient experiences a sudden onset of pain, coldness, numbness, and pallor. Pulses are absent distal to the occlusion. Acute occlusion may cause severe ischemia with motor and sensory deficits. Edema is not present.

deep venous thrombosis a
blood clot in a vein.

Deep Venous Thrombosis Deep venous thrombosis is a blood clot in a vein. It most commonly occurs in the larger veins of the thigh and calf. Predisposing factors include a recent history of trauma, inactivity, pregnancy, or varicose veins.

The patient frequently complains of gradually increasing pain and calf tenderness. Often the leg and foot are swollen because of occluded venous drainage. Leg elevation may alleviate the signs and symptoms. In some cases, the patient may be asymptomatic. Gentle palpation of the calf and thigh may reveal tenderness and, on occasion, cordlike clotted veins. Dorsiflexion of the foot may cause Homan's sign, discomfort behind the knee. This is associated with deep venous thrombosis. The skin may be warm and red.

varicose veins dilated
superficial veins, usually in the
lower extremity.

Varicose Veins Varicose veins are dilated superficial veins, usually in the lower extremities. Predisposing factors include pregnancy, obesity, and genetics. Signs and symptoms include the visible distention of the leg veins, lower leg swelling and discomfort (especially at the end of the day), and skin color and texture changes in the legs and ankles. If the condition is chronic, venous stasis ulcers, a noncritical condition, can develop. Venous stasis ulcers can rupture, but direct pressure usually can control the bleeding, which occasionally is significant.

General Assessment and Management of Vascular Disorders

Occlusion of any vessel can result in ischemia, injury, and necrosis of the affected tissue. Depending on the tissue or organ involved, untreated occlusion can cause severe disability or death. In pulmonary occlusion, hypotension and cardiac collapse can ensue quickly, and death can occur rapidly. In cerebral occlusion, debilitating seizures, paralysis, or death can occur. Mesenteric occlusion can cause necrosis, giving rise to sepsis. Or it can affect vital organs, causing a slow and agonizing death. Pulmonary embolus, aortic aneurysm, and some acute arterial occlusions can produce a hypoperfusion state, and death can be rapid.

Assessment Begin your assessment by checking airway, breathing, and circulation. Breathing is usually not affected, except in pulmonary embolus and a decompensated state of shock. In decompensated shock resulting from aneurysm, arterial occlusion, or pulmonary embolus, breathing may be labored. Circulation may be compromised or absent distal to the affected area. Check circulation for the Five Ps:

- Pallor
- Pain
- Pulselessness
- Paralysis
- Paresthesia

Check the skin for pallor or mottling distal to the affected area. Skin temperature may appear normal systemically but cool or cold at the affected area, or it may be systemically cool and clammy, as occurs in decompensated shock.

Determine the patient's chief complaint. Depending on the type of vascular emergency, the patient may complain of a sudden or gradual onset of discomfort, and the pain may be localized. Use the OPQRST acronym to elicit the patient's description of symptoms and pain. Is the pain in the chest, abdomen, or extremity? Does it radiate or is it localized? Was its onset gradual or sudden? If there is claudication, is it relieved with rest?

Conduct your focused history and physical exam. Determine the contributing history. This may well be the patient's first recognized event, or it may be a recurrence. Patients with a prior vascular emergency are prone to reoccurrences. They may report an increase in the frequency or duration of events. Breath sounds may be clear to auscultation. Alterations in the heart rate and rhythm may occur with pulmonary embolus and aortic aneurysm. Unequal bilateral blood pressures may indicate a high thoracic aneurysm. Peripheral pulses may be diminished or absent in the affected extremity with arterial occlusion or peripheral arterial atherosclerotic disease. Bruits may be audible over the affected carotid artery. The skin may be cool, moist, or dry, reflecting diminished circulation to the affected area or extremity. ECG findings generally do not contribute to vascular emergency treatment. If dysrhythmias or ectopy are present, treat them accordingly.

Management Managing the patient with a vascular emergency is mostly supportive. Place the patient in a position of comfort. Give oxygen by nonrebreather mask if you suspect pulmonary embolus, aortic aneurysm, or arterial occlusion or if any hypotension or a hypoperfusion state presents.

Before administering any drug, ask the patient or his family if he is allergic to any medications. Pharmacological agents that might be used in a vascular emergency include:

- Nitrous oxide (Nitronox)
- Morphine sulfate

Transport the patient as soon as possible. Indications for rapid transport with lights and sirens include any situation in which medications do not relieve the patient's symptoms or in which you suspect pulmonary embolism, aortic aneurysm, or arterial occlusion. Also consider any presentation of hypotension or hypoperfusion to be an emergency and transport the patient rapidly. Report your findings to the emergency department staff.

If the patient refuses transport, advise him that serious complications are likely to occur without further medical attention. Vascular emergencies can reach a point where the patient permanently loses a limb or quickly decompensates into irreversible shock. Some patients will attempt to refuse transport because they have received relief from pain medications. Use every means at your disposal to convince them to be transported. Document refusals according to general guidelines.

Content Review

FIVE PS OF ACUTE ARTERIAL OCCLUSION
- Pallor
- Pain
- Pulselessness
- Paralysis
- Paresthesia

SUMMARY

Cardiovascular disease is the number one cause of death in the United States and Canada. Many deaths from heart attack occur within the first 24 hours—frequently within the first hour. With the advent of thrombolytic therapy, time is of the essence when managing the patient with suspected ischemic heart disease. EMS plays an ever-increasing role in the early recognition of patients suffering coronary ischemia. In certain areas, EMS provides definitive care by initiating thrombolytic therapy in the field. This is especially important in cases where transport times can be long. With cardiovascular disease, EMS can truly mean the difference between life and death.

ON THE WEB

For additional practice and review, go to the companion website at www.prenhall.com/bledsoe and click on *Intermediate Emergency Care: Principles & Practice*.

CHAPTER 21

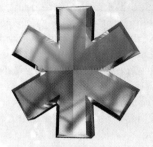

Diabetic Emergencies

Objectives

After reading this chapter, you should be able to:

1. Discuss the anatomy and physiology of the endocrine system. (pp. 948–949; and see Chapter 2)
2. Describe the pathophysiology of diabetes mellitus. (pp. 949–951)
3. Differentiate between the pathophysiology of normal glucose metabolism and diabetic glucose metabolism. (pp. 950–953)
4. Describe the mechanism of ketone body formation and its relationship to ketoacidosis. (pp. 951, 953–954)
5. Discuss the physiology of the excretion of potassium and ketone bodies by the kidneys. (pp. 951, 953–954)
6. Describe the relationship of insulin to serum glucose levels. (pp. 949–957)
7. Describe the effects of decreased levels of insulin on the body. (pp. 949–956)

8. Describe the effects of increased serum glucose levels on the body. (pp. 949–956)
9. Discuss the pathophysiology, assessment findings, and management of the following endocrine emergencies:
   a. nonketotic hyperosmolar coma (pp. 955–956)
   b. diabetic ketoacidosis (pp. 953–955)
   c. hypoglycemia (pp. 956–957)
   d. hyperglycemia (pp. 953–957)
10. Describe the actions of epinephrine as it relates to the pathophysiology of hypoglycemia. (p. 956)
11. Describe the compensatory mechanisms utilized by the body to promote homeostasis when hypoglycemia is present. (pp. 949, 956, and see Chapter 2)

CASE STUDY

Shauna White and Steve Curran leave the hospital after the Quarterly Trauma Case Conference and notify dispatch that they are in service and en route to quarters. Within minutes, they receive a dispatch call for an unknown medical emergency in a nearby residential neighborhood. The response time is less than 3 minutes. They park the unit in front of the house and don personal protective equipment. As Steve removes the

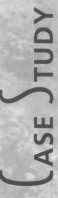

stretcher and jump kit from the back of the unit, a police cruiser pulls up to the curb. The officers intercept Steve and Shauna, explaining that they were dispatched after someone called 9-1-1 to report the sounds of a possible altercation in the home.

At that moment, a woman walks up and identifies herself as Mrs. Spencer, the 9-1-1 caller. She says that she was in her garden when she heard loud sounds suddenly coming from the McKenzie's house next door. She says she was alarmed because the noise lasted for only a short time, but it sounded like items were being thrown or broken. Moreover, she knows that Mr. McKenzie is traveling out of town. Mrs. McKenzie left the house about an hour before the noise occurred. At the moment, however, all is quiet.

The officers caution Steve, Shauna, and Mrs. Spencer to stand clear until they secure the scene. They approach the front door, identify themselves as police, and enter the house. In less than a minute, they call out "All clear," and summon the EMT-Is. Shauna and Steve quickly enter. In the living room, they see that the furniture in one corner has been overturned, and books and magazines are strewn about the floor. An officer crouches near an adolescent male who appears to be in his mid-teens. The boy is pale and diaphoretic. He looks confused as the officer speaks to him. His clothing is out of place. Mrs. Spencer looks in from the open doorway and identifies the young man as Mark McKenzie.

Shauna's initial assessment reveals a 16-year-old male without airway compromise. He is breathing rapidly, but with good depth and volume. His carotid pulse is rapid and strong. Although the patient is conscious, he responds to Shauna with incoherent muttering. Steve quickly places a nonrebreather oxygen mask over the patient's face, and then he and Shauna move him onto the stretcher. One of the police officers says he'll look around the scene for evidence of medications or illicit drugs.

Mark pulls the oxygen mask off and tries to get up and walk. Shauna replaces the mask and tries to reassure him. Finally, after he makes several more attempts to get up, Mark is gently restrained on the stretcher. Shauna begins a more detailed assessment, while Steve looks for a vein to draw blood and start an intravenous (IV) line. He notes that Mark's skin is pale, cool, and clammy. Shauna observes no obvious injuries except a small bruise forming on the right cheek. In addition, she does not smell any unusual odors, such as alcohol or paint fumes. Mark is not wearing a medical identification tag. Shauna finds that Mark's blood pressure is 130/88 mmHg, his pulse is 120 beats per minute, and his respiratory rate is 28 breaths per minute. The oxygen saturation is 99% on the nonrebreather mask.

Before starting the IV line, Steve follows protocol, filling a red-top tube with blood and obtaining a sample for immediate determination of the blood glucose level. The portable glucose detection device reports the glucose level as "LOW." As Steve gives Shauna the information, the officer returns and tells them that he found a bottle of insulin in the refrigerator with Mark's name on the label.

INTRODUCTION

hormone chemical substance released by a gland that controls or affects processes in other glands or body systems.

endocrine gland gland that secretes chemical substances directly into the blood; also called a ductless gland.

exocrine gland gland that secretes chemical substances to nearby tissues through a duct; also called a ducted gland.

The *endocrine system* is an important body system that includes eight major glands (Table 21-1). Closely linked to the nervous system, it controls numerous physiological processes. Unlike the nervous system, which exerts its control through nervous impulses, the endocrine system controls the body through specialized chemical messengers called **hormones.** The fundamental structural units of the endocrine system are the **endocrine glands.** Each endocrine gland produces one or more hormones. (An example of an endocrine gland is the pancreas.)

Endocrine glands differ from other glands in that they are ductless. Instead of releasing hormones through ducts to a local site, they secrete their hormones directly into capillaries to circulate in the blood throughout the body. In contrast, the majority of glands are **exocrine glands,** which release their chemical products through ducts and tend to have a local effect. For example, the salivary glands are a type of exocrine gland. The salivary glands are located near the pharynx and secrete digestive enzymes, such as amylase, into the pharynx.

Table 21-1	THE MAJOR ENDOCRINE GLANDS	
Hypothalamus	Thymus
Pituitary	Pancreas
Thyroid	Adrenals
Parathyroid	Gonads

Keep in mind these important points about endocrine glands:

- In contrast to the exocrine glands, whose effects tend to be localized, endocrine glands tend to have widespread effects.
- The hormones released by endocrine glands typically act on distant tissues. They exert a very specific effect on their target tissues.
- Some hormones, such as insulin, have many target organs. Other hormones have only a few target organs.
- Through the release of hormones, the endocrine system plays an important role in regulating body function.

As noted above, the principal product of an endocrine gland is a hormone. The term *hormone* comes from the Greek for "to set in motion," and hormones keep in motion, or regulate, numerous vital cell processes. For example, the hormones insulin and glucagon enable the body to maintain a stable blood glucose level, both after and between meals. This is an example of **homeostasis,** the natural tendency of the body to maintain an appropriate internal environment in the face of changing external conditions. Hormones such as growth hormone and thyroid hormone regulate **metabolism.** Metabolism encompasses all the cellular processes that produce the energy and molecules needed for growth or repair. In addition, hormones such as estrogen and testosterone regulate the sexual development of puberty and the subsequent reproductive function of adulthood.

Many people have endocrine disorders involving excessive or deficient hormone function. Some common conditions, such as hypothyroidism, are readily controlled by hormone replacement medication. Other hormonal disorders may have a more difficult course. You will find that the hormonal disorder diabetes mellitus is commonly involved in medical emergencies encountered in the prehospital setting.

DIABETIC EMERGENCIES

The most common endocrine emergencies you should expect to treat will involve complications of diabetes mellitus. This section explains the pathophysiology of diabetes and its complications, including ketoacidosis and hypoglycemia, as a basis for discussion of field management.

DIABETES MELLITUS

The disease **diabetes mellitus** is marked by inadequate insulin activity in the body. As noted earlier, insulin is critical to maintaining normal blood glucose levels. Glucose is important for all cells, but it is especially important for brain cells. In fact, glucose is the *only* substance that brain cells can readily and efficiently use as an energy source. In addition, insulin enables the body to store energy as glycogen, protein, and fat.

Diabetes mellitus, or sugar diabetes, is not only a serious disease but also a common and ancient one. Over 8 million people in the United States have been diagnosed with diabetes, and U.S. health experts believe nearly the same number of Americans may be living with undiagnosed diabetes. The disease was named in ancient times by Greek physicians who noted that affected persons produced large volumes of urine that attracted bees and other insects, hence diabetes (meaning "to siphon," or "to pass through") for excessive urine production and mellitus (meaning "honey sweet") for the presence of sugar

The effects of exocrine glands tend to be localized, whereas the effects of endocrine glands tend to be widespread.

homeostasis the natural tendency of the body to keep the internal environment and metabolism steady and normal.

metabolism the sum of cellular processes that produce the energy and molecules needed for growth and repair.

diabetes mellitus disorder of inadequate insulin activity, due to either inadequate production of insulin or to decreased responsiveness of body cells to insulin.

in the urine. If you remember that mellitus means *sweet* and insipidus means *neutral,* you will remember the common trait and the major distinctions in the presentations of untreated diabetes insipidus and diabetes mellitus.

Before presenting pathophysiology, we will examine in detail the normal body handling of glucose. The discussion of glucose metabolism will focus on events at the molecular and cellular level, whereas the discussion on regulation of blood glucose will focus on events in the blood and in major target tissues such as liver, fat cells, and kidneys.

Glucose Metabolism

You learned in the chapter introduction that metabolism is the sum of the processes that produce the energy and molecules needed for cell growth or repair. The word *metabolism* comes from the Greek for "to change." Two kinds of change take place within a cell. One kind builds complex molecules from simpler ones. The synthesis of glycogen from glucose is an example. The other kind breaks down complex molecules into simpler ones. The breakdown of glucose into carbon dioxide, water, and energy in the form of adenosine triphosphate, or ATP, is an example.

The building processes within a cell are collectively called **anabolism.** The prefix *ana-* comes from the Greek for "up," and anabolic pathways build molecules of higher complexity. Breakdown processes are collectively called **catabolism.** The prefix *cata-* comes from the Greek for "down," and catabolic pathways produce molecules of lower complexity. Anabolic pathways usually require energy to drive them, and catabolic pathways often release energy as part of the process. In other words, anabolic activity uses energy whereas catabolic activity produces energy.

Look at the summary of effects of insulin and glucagon in Table 21-2. When materials are abundant after meals and blood glucose is high, insulin enables cells to use glucose directly and to store energy as glycogen, protein, and fat. Insulin stimulates anabolic pathways. In contrast, glucagon is the dominant hormone during periods of low blood glucose. It stimulates catabolic pathways to produce usable energy from the body's stores.

In order for anabolic pathways to proceed, insulin must first exert its stimulatory effects. Insulin acts by binding to receptors in the outer cell membrane. These receptors are proteins whose structure reacts specifically with insulin. When insulin is bound to a receptor, it changes the permeability of the membrane such that glucose enters the cell far more readily. The rate at which glucose can be transported into cells can be increased tenfold or more by the action of insulin. Without insulin activity, the amount of glucose that can enter cells is far too small to meet average body energy demands. Note the two requirements for insulin effectiveness:

- Sufficient insulin must be circulating in the bloodstream to satisfy cellular needs.
- Insulin must be able to bind to body cells in such a way that adequate levels of stimulation occur.

The importance of these two requirements will become clear when you learn about the two types of diabetes mellitus.

anabolism the constructive or "building up" phase of metabolism.

catabolism the destructive or "breaking down" phase of metabolism.

Table 21-2	SUMMARY OF GLUCOSE METABOLISM
Hormonal Effects of Insulin and Glucagon	
Insulin	**Glucagon**
Dominant hormone when blood glucose level is high	Dominant hormone when blood glucose level is low
Major Effects on Target Tissues	**Major Effects on Target Tissues**
All cells: ↑ uptake glucose	
Liver: ↑ production of glycogen, protein, fat	Liver: ↑ glycogenolysis → glucose
Liver, fat: ↑ production of fats	Liver: ↑ gluconeogenesis (protein, fat → glucose)

Sometimes the body cannot use glucose as a primary energy source. In diabetes, this occurs when insufficient insulin activity exists for blood glucose to be taken in and used by cells. Other conditions, such as a high-fat, low-carbohydrate diet or starvation (which can occur in conjunction with some eating disorders) cause depletion of body stores of carbohydrate. Under any of these conditions, the body slowly switches from glucose to fat as the primary energy source. Adipose cells break down fats into their component free fatty acids, and the blood concentration of fatty acids rises considerably.

Most of the fatty acid is used directly by body cells as an energy source. Some is taken in by liver cells. In the liver, catabolism of fatty acids produces acetoacetic acid. When more acetoacetic acid is released from the liver than can be used by body cells, it accumulates in the blood along with two closely related substances, acetone and β-hydroxybutyric acid. These three substances are collectively called **ketone bodies,** and their presence in biologically significant quantity in the blood is called **ketosis.** This catabolic state is significant in the context of the emergency condition called diabetic ketoacidosis, or diabetic coma.

Regulation of Blood Glucose

Homeostasis of blood glucose is remarkably effective. If you draw venous blood samples from a group of healthy persons, you'll find that fasting blood glucose (generally done after an overnight fast) is usually between 80 to 90 mg glucose/dL blood. In the first hour or so after a meal, blood glucose may increase to about 120 to 140 mg/dL before falling toward the fasting, or baseline, level. The principal tissues involved in homeostasis are the alpha and beta tissues of the islets of Langerhans (producing glucagon and insulin, respectively) and the liver, as shown in Table 21-2. Liver disease, even in the presence of normal pancreatic function, can cause significant disturbances in glucose homeostasis.

A blood glucose level lower than baseline (often defined as less than 80 mg/dL) reflects **hypoglycemia,** or low blood sugar. Similarly, a blood glucose level higher than that expected shortly after a meal (often defined as greater than 140 mg/dL when drawn in a setting other than directly following a meal) reflects **hyperglycemia,** or high blood sugar. Both terms indicate the blood glucose level only, not the cause of the abnormality.

The last factor to consider in discussing regulation of blood glucose is the role of the kidneys. When blood is filtered through the glomeruli of the kidneys, glucose, along with water and many other small molecules, passes from the blood into the proximal tubule. Water, glucose, and other useful materials are then reabsorbed, while waste products that are not reabsorbed become part of the urine, which will be excreted from the body. The amount of glucose that is reabsorbed depends on the blood level of glucose that already exists. Reabsorption of glucose is essentially complete at blood glucose levels up to about 180 mg/dL. Above that level, glucose begins to be lost in urine.

Glucose loss in urine can lead to dehydration, which has its physiological basis in osmosis. Osmosis is the tendency of water molecules to migrate across a semipermeable membrane such that the concentrations of particles approach equivalence on both sides. Our example is the cell membranes that form the boundaries between the tubules of the kidney and the capillaries that surround them.

When glucose spills into urine, the osmotic pressure, or concentration of particulates, rises inside the kidney tubule to a level higher than that of the blood. Water follows glucose into urine to cause a marked water loss termed **osmotic diuresis,** which is the basis of the excessive urination characteristic of untreated diabetes. The term **diuresis** alone refers to increased formation and secretion of urine. The presence of glucose in urine, **glycosuria,** creates the sweet urine that added *mellitus* to *diabetes.*

Last, you should note that whenever the flow rate of fluid inside the kidney tubules rises, as in osmotic diuresis, an increase in excretion of potassium occurs. This leads to the potential for significant hypokalemia and its effects, including cardiac dysrhythmias.

Type I Diabetes Mellitus

When we discussed the elements essential to normal insulin activity, the first was the presence of adequate amounts of insulin in the body. *Type I diabetes mellitus* is characterized by very low production of insulin by the pancreas. In many cases, no insulin is produced at all. Type I diabetes is commonly called juvenile-onset diabetes because of the average age

ketone bodies compounds produced during the catabolism of fatty acids, including acetoacetic acid, β-hydroxybutyric acid, and acetone.

ketosis the presence of significant quantities of ketone bodies in the blood.

hypoglycemia deficiency of blood glucose. Sometimes called insulin shock. Hypoglycemia is a medical emergency.

hyperglycemia excessive blood glucose.

osmotic diuresis greatly increased urination and dehydration that results when high levels of glucose cannot be reabsorbed into the blood from the kidney tubules and the osmotic pressure of the glucose in the tubules also prevents water reabsorption.

diuresis formation and secretion of large amounts of urine.

glycosuria glucose in urine, which occurs when blood glucose levels exceed the kidney's ability to reabsorb glucose.

at diagnosis. The term *insulin-dependent diabetes mellitus (IDDM)* is also used because patients require regular insulin injections to maintain glucose homeostasis. This type of diabetes is less common than is Type II diabetes, but it is more serious. Diabetes is regularly among the ten leading causes of death in the United States, and Type I diabetes accounts for most diabetes-related deaths.

Heredity is an important factor in determining which persons will be predisposed to development of Type I diabetes. The cause of Type I diabetes is often unclear. However, viral infection, production of autoantibodies directed against beta cells, and genetically determined early deterioration of beta cells are all possible. The immediate cause of the disease is destruction of beta cells.

In untreated Type I diabetes, blood glucose levels rise because, without adequate insulin, cells cannot take up the circulating sugar. Hyperglycemia in the range of 300 to 500 mg/dL is not uncommon. As glucose spills into urine, large amounts of water are lost, too, through osmotic diuresis. Catabolism of fat becomes significant as the body switches to fatty acids as the primary energy source. Overall, this pathophysiology accounts for the constant thirst (*polydipsia*), excessive urination (*polyuria*), ravenous appetite (*polyphagia*), weakness, and weight loss associated with untreated Type I diabetes. Ketosis can occur as the result of fat catabolism, and it may proceed to frank diabetic ketoacidosis, a medical emergency that you will encounter in the field and that will be discussed later in this chapter.

Type II Diabetes Mellitus

The second requirement for proper insulin activity is insulin binding such that adequate stimulation of cells occurs. Type II diabetes mellitus is associated with a moderate decline in insulin production accompanied by a markedly deficient response to the insulin that is present in the body. Type II diabetes is also called adult-onset diabetes or *non–insulin-dependent diabetes mellitus (NIDDM)*.

Heredity may play a role in predisposition. In addition, obese persons are more likely to develop Type II diabetes, and obesity probably plays a role in development of the disease. Increased weight (and increased size of fat cells) causes a relative deficiency in the number of insulin receptors per cell, which makes fat cells less responsive to insulin. This type of diabetes is far more common than is type I diabetes, accounting for about 90% of cases of diabetes mellitus. It is also less serious.

Content Review

SYMPTOMS OF UNTREATED DIABETES MELLITUS

- Polydipsia
- Polyuria
- Polyphagia
- Weakness
- Weight loss

Untreated Type II diabetes typically presents with a lower level of hyperglycemia and fewer major signs of metabolic disruption. For instance, glucose use is usually sufficient to keep the body from switching to fats as the primary energy source. Thus, diabetic ketoacidosis is uncommon in these patients. However, a complication called hyperglycemic hyperosmolar nonketotic coma can occur, and you may see it as a medical emergency. It is discussed later in this chapter.

Medical treatment of Type II diabetes is less intensive than that required for Type I diabetes. Initial therapy often consists of dietary change and increased exercise in an attempt to improve body weight. If nonpharmacological therapy is insufficient to bring blood glucose levels down to the normal range, oral hypoglycemic agents may be prescribed. These drugs stimulate insulin secretion by beta cells and promote an increase in the number of insulin receptors per cell. In some cases, however, control may eventually require use of insulin.

DIABETIC KETOACIDOSIS (DIABETIC COMA)

Diabetic ketoacidosis is a serious, potentially life-threatening complication associated with Type I diabetes. It occurs when profound insulin deficiency is coupled with increased glucagon activity. It may occur as the initial presentation of severe diabetes, as a result of patient noncompliance with insulin injections, or as the result of physiological stress such as surgery or serious infection. Some of the major characteristics of diabetic ketoacidosis are listed in Tables 21-3 and 21-4.

diabetic ketoacidosis complication of Type I diabetes due to decreased insulin intake. Marked by high blood glucose, metabolic acidosis, and, in advanced stages, coma. Ketoacidosis is often called diabetic coma.

Pathophysiology

Reread the discussion of ketosis in the prior section on "Glucose Metabolism." Diabetic ketoacidosis reflects amplification of the same physiological mechanisms as ketosis.

Table 21-3 DIABETIC EMERGENCIES

Diabetic Ketoacidosis	Hyperglycemic Hyperosmolar Nonketotic (HHNK) Acidosis	Hypoglycemia
Common Causes	**Common Causes**	**Common Causes**
Cessation of insulin injections	Physiological stress (such as infection or stroke) producing hyperglycemia and a noncompensated diuresis, modulated by both insulin and glucagon activity	Excessive administration of insulin
Physiological stress (such as infection or surgery) that causes release of catecholamines, potentiating glucagon effects and blocking insulin effects		Excess insulin for dietary intake
		Overexertion, resulting in lowered blood glucose level
Signs and Symptoms	**Signs and Symptoms**	**Signs and Symptoms**
Polyuria, polydipsia, polyphagia	Polyuria, polydipsia, polyphagia	Weak, rapid pulse
Warm, dry skin and mucous membranes	Warm, dry skin and mucous membranes	Cold, clammy skin
Nausea/vomiting	Orthostatic hypotension	Weakness, uncoordination
Abdominal pain	Tachycardia	Headache
Tachycardia	Decreased mental function or frank coma	Irritable, agitated behavior
Deep, rapid respirations (Kussmaul's respirations)		Decreased mental function or bizarre behavior
Fruity odor on breath		Coma (severe cases)
Fever (if associated with infection)		
Decreased mental function or frank coma		
Management	**Management**	**Management**
Fluids, insulin as directed	Fluids, insulin as directed	Dextrose

Table 21-4 DIAGNOSTIC SIGNS BY SYSTEM FOR DIABETIC EMERGENCIES

	Diabetic Ketoacidosis	Hyperglycemic Hyperosmolar Nonketotic (HHNK) Coma	Hypoglycemia
Cardiovascular System			
Pulse	Rapid	Rapid	Normal
Blood pressure	Low	Normal to Low (may be affected by position, or orthostatic)	Normal
Respiratory System			
Respiration rate	Exaggerated air hunger	Normal, unlabored	Normal or shallow
Breath odor	Acetone (sweet fruity)	None	None
Nervous System			
Headache	Absent	None	Present
Mental state	Restlessness/ unconsciousness	Lethargy/unconsciousness	Apathy, irritability/ unconsciousness
Tremors	Absent	Absent	Present
Convulsions	None	Possible	In late stages
Gastrointestinal System			
Mouth	Dry	Dry	Drooling
Thirst	Intense	Excessive	Absent
Vomiting	Common	Common	Uncommon
Abdominal pain	Frequent	Common	Absent
Ocular System			
Vision	Dim	Normal	Double vision (diplopia)

In the initial phase of diabetic ketoacidosis, profound hyperglycemia exists because of lack of insulin. Body cells cannot take in glucose. The compensatory mechanism for low glucose levels within cells, gluconeogenesis, only contributes more blood glucose. The consequent loss of glucose in the urine, accompanied by loss of water through osmotic diuresis, produces significant dehydration.

As the body switches to fat-based metabolism, the blood level of ketones rises. The ketone load accounts for the observed acidosis. By the time the characteristic decrease in pH from about 7.4 to about 6.9 has occurred, the patient is hours from death if left untreated.

Signs and Symptoms

The onset of clinically obvious diabetic ketoacidosis is slow, lasting from 12 to 24 hours. In the initial phase, signs of diuresis appear, including increased urine production and dry, warm skin and mucous membranes. The individual often has excessive hunger and thirst, coupled with a progressive sense of general malaise. Volume depletion induces tachycardia and feelings of physical weakness.

The presence of a sweet, fruity odor on the patient's breath is a hallmark of diabetic ketoacidosis.

As ketoacidosis develops, a major compensatory mechanism for acidosis appears: the rapid, deep breathing pattern termed *Kussmaul's respirations,* which helps expel carbon dioxide, CO_2, from the body (Figure 21-1). The breath itself may have a fruity or acetone-like smell since some blood acetone is expelled through the lungs. The blood profile not only includes hyperglycemia and acidic pH, but also electrolyte abnormalities. Low bicarbonate levels reflect loss of acid-base buffer via Kussmaul's respirations. Low potassium levels may be found secondary to diuresis, with marked hypokalemia increasing the risk for cardiac dysrhythmias or death. Over time, mental function declines and frank coma may occur. A fever is not characteristic of ketoacidosis. If present, it is a signal of infection.

Type of respiration	Diagram	Discussion
Normal	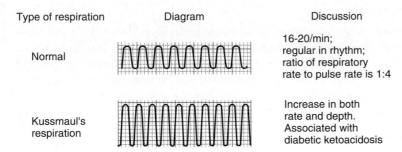	16-20/min; regular in rhythm; ratio of respiratory rate to pulse rate is 1:4
Kussmaul's respiration		Increase in both rate and depth. Associated with diabetic ketoacidosis

FIGURE 21-1 Kussmaul's respirations.

Assessment and Management

The approach used with the patient suffering from diabetic ketoacidosis is essentially the same as with any other patient who has mental impairment or is unconscious. First, complete your initial assessment of airway, breathing, and circulation. Then complete a focused history and physical exam. Look for a medical identification device, such as a Medic-Alert bracelet, and/or insulin in the refrigerator. Obtain a history from any bystanders. The sweet, fruity odor of ketones occasionally can be detected in the breath. If possible, complete the rapid test for blood glucose level. It is not uncommon for patients with ketoacidosis to have blood glucose levels well in excess of 300 mg/dL.

Focus field management on maintenance of the ABCs and fluid resuscitation to counteract dehydration. In such cases, draw a red top tube (or the tube specified by local protocols) of blood. Following blood sampling, administer 1 to 2 liters of normal saline per protocol. If transport time is lengthy, the medical direction physician may request intravenous or subcutaneous administration of regular insulin.

If the blood glucose level cannot be quickly determined, draw a red top tube of blood for analysis and start an IV of normal saline. Following this, administer 50 mL (25 grams) of 50% dextrose solution. The additional glucose load will not adversely affect the ketoacidotic patient because it is negligible compared with the quantity present in the body. If the patient were hypoglycemic, however, the additional glucose might be sufficient to protect brain cells from damage. If the patient is a known alcoholic, consider administering 100 mg of thiamine.

Expedite transport to an appropriate facility for definitive therapy.

HYPERGLYCEMIC HYPEROSMOLAR NONKETOTIC (HHNK) COMA

Hyperglycemic hyperosmolar nonketotic (HHNK) coma is a serious complication associated with Type II diabetes. Typically, both insulin and glucagon activity are present. HHNK coma develops when two conditions occur: Sustained hyperglycemia causes osmotic diuresis sufficient to produce marked dehydration, and water intake is inadequate to replace lost fluids. Dialysis, high-osmolarity feeding supplements, infection, and certain drugs can also be associated with development of HHNK coma. Some characteristics of HHNK coma are listed in Tables 21-3 and 21-4.

hyperglycemic hyperosmolar nonketotic (HHNK) coma complication of Type II diabetes due to inadequate insulin activity. Marked by high blood glucose, marked dehydration, and decreased mental function. Often mistaken for ketoacidosis.

Pathophysiology

As sustained hyperglycemia develops, glucose spills into the urine, causing osmotic diuresis and resultant dehydration. The level of hyperglycemia is often much higher than the levels seen in ketoacidosis (up to 1,000 mg/dL). However, insulin activity in patients with HHNK coma prevents significant production of ketone bodies. Inadequate fluid replacement results in characteristic signs and symptoms.

The mortality rate for HHNK coma is higher than that for ketoacidosis, ranging from 40% to 70%. The higher mortality rate may be due to the lack of early signs and symptoms that bring patients with ketoacidosis to the attention of family or health-care professionals. The mortality rate of HHNK is also high because it primarily affects the elderly.

Signs and Symptoms

The onset of HHNK coma is even slower than that of ketoacidosis, with development often occurring over several days. Early signs include increased urination and increased thirst. Subsequent volume depletion can result in orthostatic hypotension when the patient gets out of bed, along with other signs such as dry skin and mucous membranes as well as tachycardia. The patient may become lethargic, confused, or enter frank coma. Kussmaul's respirations are rarely seen because of the lack of acidosis.

Assessment and Management

The approach used with the patient suffering from HHNK coma is essentially the same as with any other patient who has mental impairment or is unconscious. It is often difficult in the field to distinguish diabetic ketoacidosis from HHNK coma. Therefore, the prehospital treatment of both emergencies is identical (see earlier discussion of management of ketoacidosis) and transportation should be expedited.

HYPOGLYCEMIA (INSULIN SHOCK)

Hypoglycemia, or low blood glucose, is a medical emergency. It can occur when a patient takes too much insulin, eats too little to match an insulin dose, or overexerts and uses almost all available blood glucose. As the period of hypoglycemia lengthens, the risk rises that brain cells will be permanently damaged or killed due to lack of glucose. You have learned that brain cells can adapt to use fats as an energy source. Note, however, that this adaptation requires hours to develop, and the switch to fat-based metabolism cannot correct any damage already incurred. This is why every second counts in treating hypoglycemia.

Pathophysiology

Hypoglycemia, or insulin shock, reflects high insulin and low blood glucose. Regardless of the reason for low blood sugar, insulin causes almost all remaining blood glucose to be taken up by cells. Because of the high level of insulin, glucagon may be ineffective in raising blood glucose levels. In prolonged fasts, almost half the glucose normally produced through gluconeogenesis is of renal origin. This activity is stimulated by epinephrine. Diabetic patients with kidney failure may be predisposed to hypoglycemia because of lack of renal gluconeogenesis.

Signs and Symptoms

The signs and symptoms of hypoglycemia are many and varied. Altered mental status is the most important. In the earliest stages of hypoglycemia, the patient may appear restless or impatient or complain of hunger. As blood glucose falls lower, he may display inappropriate anger (even rage) or display a bizarre behavior. Sometimes the patient may be placed in police custody for such behavior or be involved in an automobile accident.

Physical signs may include diaphoresis and tachycardia. If blood glucose falls to a critically low level, the patient may have a **hypoglycemic seizure** or become comatose.

In contrast to diabetic ketoacidosis, hypoglycemia can develop quickly. A clear change in mental status can occur without warning. Always consider hypoglycemia when encountering a patient with bizarre behavior. Review Tables 21-3 and 21-4 for additional information.

Assessment and Management

In suspected cases of hypoglycemia, perform the initial assessment quickly. Look for a medical identification device, such as a Medic-Alert bracelet. If possible, determine the blood glucose level. Because of the urgency of this emergency, most EMT-I units need to have the capability to perform this task or to rush a blood sample along with the patient.

If the blood glucose level is less than 60 mg/dL, draw a red top tube of blood and start an IV of normal saline. Next, administer 50 to 100 mL (25 to 50 grams) of 50% dextrose intravenously. If the patient is conscious and able to swallow, complete glucose administration with orange juice, sugared sodas, or commercially available glucose pastes.

---

hypoglycemia deficiency of blood glucose.

Hypoglycemia is a true medical emergency that requires prompt intervention to prevent permanent brain injury.

Hypoglycemia virtually never occurs outside the setting of diabetes mellitus.

hypoglycemic seizure seizure that occurs when brain cells are not functioning normally due to low blood glucose.

All ALS vehicles must have the capability of rapidly determining a patient's blood glucose level.

If blood glucose cannot be obtained and the patient is unconscious, start an IV of normal saline and administer 50 to 100 mL (25 to 50 grams) of 50% dextrose. Expedite transport to a medical facility. If you suspect alcoholism, also administer 100 mg of thiamine.

When an IV cannot be started, hypoglycemic patients may improve following the administration of glucagon. This is a much slower process and will only work if adequate stores of glycogen are available. Glucagon must be reconstituted immediately prior to administration. A dose of 0.5 to 1.0 mg intramuscularly is usually adequate.

Summary

In conjunction with the nervous system, the endocrine system regulates body functions. The vast majority of endocrine emergencies involve complications of diabetes mellitus such as hypoglycemia or ketoacidosis. Other endocrine emergencies tend to be rare and will more likely be part of the history rather than the emergency. In the field, you should always suspect diabetes when patients present with unexplained changes in mental status. Hypoglycemia, the most urgent diabetic emergency, must be quickly treated to prevent serious nervous system damage. When the exact type of diabetic emergency is undetermined, treat for hypoglycemia. Treatment of diabetic ketoacidosis is primarily a hospital procedure.

On the Web

For additional practice and review, go to the companion website at www.prenhall.com/bledsoe and click on *Intermediate Emergency Care: Principles & Practice*.

CHAPTER 22

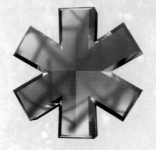

Allergic Reactions

Objectives

After reading this chapter, you should be able to:

1. Discuss the pathophysiology of allergy and anaphylaxis. (pp. 960–963)
2. Describe the common routes of substance entry into the body. (pp. 962–963)
3. Define allergic reaction, anaphylaxis, antibody, antigen, natural and acquired immunity, and allergen. (pp. 959–962)
4. List common antigens most frequently associated with anaphylaxis. (pp. 959–962)
5. Describe the physical manifestations of anaphylaxis. (pp. 963–965, 967)
6. Identify and differentiate between the signs and symptoms of an allergic reaction and anaphylaxis. (pp. 963–965, 967–968)
7. Explain the various treatment and pharmacological interventions used in the management of allergic reactions and anaphylaxis. (pp. 965–968)
8. Correlate abnormal findings in assessment with the clinical significance in the patient with an allergic reaction or anaphylaxis. (pp. 963–965, 967–968)
9. Given several pre-programmed and moulaged patients, provide the appropriate assessment, care, and transport for the allergic reaction and anaphylaxis patient. (pp. 960–968)

CASE STUDY

Cherokee Nation EMS is dispatched to a clinic on the outskirts of town for a medical emergency. Upon arrival at the scene, EMT-Is are met by clinic staff who direct them to a treatment room. The nurse practitioner reports that a 39-year-old male had received an immunization injection approximately 15 minutes earlier. Immediately after the injection, the man developed a red rash and generalized itching. This quickly progressed to obvious hives, wheezing, and associated dyspnea. As the reaction worsened, the patient became hoarse, more dyspneic, and hypotensive. A nurse was now administering supplemental oxygen while another clinic employee was setting up an intravenous infusion.

Initial assessment reveals an alert 39-year-old Native-American male in marked distress. His airway is open, but there is marked stridor and audible wheezing. The carotid pulse is rapid and weak. The EMT-Is quickly remove the nasal cannula placed by the clinic staff and replace it with a nonrebreather oxygen mask. The airway kit is opened in case endotracheal intubation is required.

Steve Williams, the lead EMT-I, begins a more detailed assessment while his partner, Beth White Cloud, begins to search for a vein to catheterize. The patient is diaphoretic and has urticarial lesions on the trunk and extremities. In addition, he is tachypneic with a weak and thready pulse. Blood pressure is 88/50 mmHg, pulse is 120 beats per minute, respirations are 32 breaths per minute, and oxygen saturation is 100% on the nonrebreather.

While Beth places the IV, Steve administers 0.4 milligrams of epinephrine 1:1,000 subcutaneously per system standing orders. Within approximately two minutes, the patient's stridor begins to improve and respirations slow. Beth completes placement of the IV and secures it with tape and tincture of benzoin because of the patient's marked diaphoresis. Beth administers 50 milligrams of diphenhydramine (Benadryl) intravenously. Steve prepares a pre-fill of epinephrine 1:10,000 for intravenous administration in case the patient does not improve.

Within five minutes, significant improvement is noted. In fact, it appears that most of the urticarial lesions have cleared. The patient's respiratory rate is down to 22 breaths per minute, but the patient's heart rate is up to 136 beats per minute, which the EMT-Is attribute to the epinephrine. A repeat blood pressure is 100/74 mmHg. Steve opens the IV infusion and administers a 500 mL fluid bolus.

The patient continues to improve and is moved to the ambulance for transport to the emergency department. Upon arrival, the patient is assessed by Stephen Johnston, M.D. Dr. Johnston orders the administration of an intravenous corticosteroid and additional IV fluids. The patient is observed for two hours and discharged symptom-free. A phone call to the clinic reveals that the patient received a tetanus immunization. In reviewing the case, Dr. Johnston learns from the patient that he had a similar reaction with a prior tetanus immunization but failed to relay this information to the clinic staff.

INTRODUCTION

An **allergic reaction** is an exaggerated response by the immune system to a foreign substance. Allergic reactions can range from mild skin rashes to severe, life-threatening reactions that involve virtually every body system. The most severe type of allergic reaction is called **anaphylaxis.** Anaphylaxis is a life-threatening emergency that requires prompt recognition and specific treatment by EMT-Is. The emergency treatment of anaphylaxis is one area of prehospital care where advanced life-support measures often mean the difference between life and death. Anaphylaxis can develop within seconds and cause death just minutes after exposure to the offending agent. Fortunately, several emergency medications are available that can reverse the adverse effects of anaphylaxis.

The first complete description of anaphylaxis was reported in 1902 by Portier and Richet. Portier and Richet were French immunologists who were attempting to immunize dogs against the toxin of the deadly sea anemone (sea flower). They were injecting small, non-lethal quantities of the toxin into the animals in hopes of stimulating immunity to the toxin. However, when the animals received secondary injections of sub-lethal quantities of the toxin, at a time when it might be expected that they would be immune, the dogs developed shock and died. Richet called this dramatic and unexpected phenomenon *anaphylaxis*, which means the opposite of "phylaxis" or protection.

Anaphylaxis results from exposure to a particular substance that sets off a biochemical chain of events that can ultimately lead to shock and death. The exact incidence of anaphylaxis is unknown. However, an estimated 400 to 800 deaths annually in the United States are attributed to anaphylaxis. Injected penicillin and bee and wasp (*Hymenoptera*)

Anaphylaxis is the most severe form of allergic reaction and is often life threatening.

allergic reaction an exaggerated response by the immune system to a foreign substance.

anaphylaxis an unusual or exaggerated allergic reaction to a foreign protein or other substance.

Hymenoptera any of an order of highly specialized insects such as bees and wasps.

immune system the body
system responsible for
combating infection.

stings are the two most common causes of fatal anaphylaxis. Approximately 100 to 500
deaths per year are attributed to the parenteral administration of penicillin. Approximately
25 to 40 persons die each year from *hymenoptera* stings. Fortunately, the incidence of anaphylaxis appears to be declining. This is presumably due to better recognition and treatment, as well as the availability of numerous potent antihistamines.

PATHOPHYSIOLOGY

The immune system is the principal body system involved in allergic reactions. However,
other body systems are also affected by an allergic reaction. These include the cardiovascular system, the respiratory system, the nervous system, and the gastrointestinal system,
among others. To fully appreciate the complexity of allergic and anaphylactic reactions, it
is first necessary to review the anatomy and physiology of the immune system as it relates
to the immune response.

IMMUNE SYSTEM

immune response events
within the body that work
toward the destruction or
inactivation of pathogens,
abnormal cells, or foreign
molecules.

pathogen a disease-producing
agent or invading substance.

toxin any poisonous chemical
secreted by bacteria or
released following destruction
of the bacteria.

cellular immunity immunity
resulting from a direct attack
of a foreign substance by
specialized cells of the immune
system.

humoral immunity immunity
resulting from attack of an
invading substance by
antibodies.

antibody principal agent of a
chemical attack of an invading
substance.

immunoglobulin (Ig)
alternative term for antibody.

antigen any substance that is
capable, under appropriate
conditions, of inducing a
specific immune response.

The **immune system** is a complicated body system responsible for combating infection.
Components of the immune system can be found in the blood, the bone marrow, and the
lymphatic system.

The **immune response** is a complex cascade of events that occurs following activation
by an invading substance, or **pathogen**. The goal of the immune response is the destruction
or inactivation of pathogens, abnormal cells, or foreign molecules such as **toxins**. The body
can accomplish this through two mechanisms, cellular immunity and humoral immunity.
Cellular immunity involves a direct attack of the foreign substance by specialized cells of the
immune system. These cells physically engulf and deactivate or destroy the offending agent.
Humoral immunity, on the other hand, is much more complicated. Humoral immunity is
basically a chemical attack of the invading substance. The principal chemical agents of this
attack are **antibodies,** also called **immunoglobulins (Igs).** Antibodies are a unique class of
chemicals that are manufactured by specialized cells of the immune system called *B cells.*
The five different classes of antibodies are IgA, IgD, IgE, IgG, and IgM.

The humoral immune response begins with exposure of the body to an antigen. An
antigen is defined as any substance capable of inducing an immune response (Table 22-1).
Most antigens are proteins. Following exposure to an antigen, antibodies are released from
cells of the immune system. These antibodies attach themselves to the invading substance to
facilitate removal of that substance from the body by other cells of the immune system.

If the body has never been exposed to a particular antigen, the response of the immune
system is different than if it has been previously exposed to the particular antigen. The ini-

Table 22-1	AGENTS THAT MAY CAUSE ANAPHYLAXIS

Antibiotics and other drugs

Foreign proteins (e.g., horse serum, streptokinase)

Foods (nuts, eggs, shrimp)

Allergen extracts (allergy shots)

Hymenoptera stings (bees, wasps)

Hormones (Insulin)

Blood products

Aspirin

Non-steroidal anti-inflammatory drugs (NSAIDs)

Preservatives (sulfiting agents)

X-ray contrast media

Dextran

tial response to an antigen is called the **primary response.** Following exposure to a new antigen, several days are required before both the cellular and humoral components of the immune system respond. Generalized antibodies (IgG and IgM) are first released to help fight the antigen.

At the same time, other components of the immune system begin to develop antibodies specific for the antigen. These cells also develop a *memory* of the particular antigen. If the body is exposed to the same antigen again, the immune system responds much faster. This is called the **secondary response.** As a part of the secondary response, antibodies specific for the offending antigen are released. Antigen-specific antibodies are much more effective in facilitating removal of the offending antigen than the generalized antibodies released during the primary response.

Immunity may be either natural or acquired. **Natural immunity,** also called *innate immunity,* is genetically predetermined. It is present at birth and has no relation to previous exposure to a particular antigen. All humans are born with some innate immunity.

Acquired immunity develops over time and results from exposure to an antigen. Following exposure to a particular antigen, the immune system will produce antibodies specific for the antigen. This protects the organism as subsequent exposure to the same antigen will result in a vigorous immune response. **Naturally acquired immunity** normally begins to develop after birth and is continually enhanced by exposure to new pathogens and antigens throughout life. For example, a child contracts chicken pox (varicella) at age 18 months. Following the infection, the child's immune system creates antibodies specific for the varicella virus. Repeated exposure to the varicella virus usually will not result in another infection. In fact, it is not unusual for a patient exposed to varicella to develop lifelong immunity to the infection.

Induced active immunity, also called *artificially acquired immunity,* is designed to provide protection from exposure to an antigen at some time in the future. This is achieved through vaccination and provides relative protection against serious infectious agents. In vaccination, an antigen is injected into the body so as to generate an immune response. This results in the development of antibodies specific for the antigen and provides protection against future infection. Most vaccines contain antigenic proteins from a particular virus or bacterium. Later, when the individual is actually exposed to the pathogen, the immune response will be vigorous and will often be enough to prevent the infection from developing.

An example of a vaccine commonly used is the diphtheria/pertussis/tetanus (DPT) vaccine. This vaccine contains antigenic proteins from the bacteria that cause diphtheria, whooping cough, and tetanus. The vaccine is administered at several intervals during the first 5 years of life. It provides protection against infection from these bacteria. Some vaccinations will impart lifelong immunity whereas others must be periodically followed with a booster dose to ensure continued protection.

Acquired immunity can be either active or passive. **Active immunity** occurs following exposure to an antigen and results in the production of antibodies specific for the antigen. Most vaccinations result in the development of active immunity. However, it takes some time for a patient to develop specific antibodies. In certain cases, it is necessary to administer antibodies to provide protection until the active immunity can kick in. The administration of antibodies is referred to as **passive immunity.** There are two types of passive immunity. *Natural passive immunity* occurs when antibodies cross the placental barrier from the mother to the infant so as to provide protection against embryonic or fetal infections. *Induced passive immunity* is the administration of antibodies to an individual to help fight infection or prevent diseases. An example of the clinical use of both active and passive immunity is the regimen used for the prevention of tetanus.

Most persons who are from developed countries have typically received some form of tetanus vaccination during their life. These persons typically have some antibodies to tetanus and often need nothing more than a tetanus booster. However, some persons have never received any sort of tetanus vaccination. When these persons seek treatment for a tetanus-prone wound, they must receive prophylaxis for tetanus in addition to care for their wound. This is best achieved by the provision of both passive and active immunity. To provide immediate protection, the patient is administered antibodies specific for tetanus (tetanus immune globulin [TIG] Hypertet®). Then, they are administered a tetanus vaccination (Td or

primary response initial, generalized response to an antigen.

secondary response response by the immune system that takes place if the body is exposed to an antigen a second time; in secondary response, antibodies specific for the offending antigen are released.

natural immunity genetically predetermined immunity that is present at birth; also called innate immunity.

acquired immunity immunity that develops over time and results from exposure to an antigen.

naturally acquired immunity immunity that begins to develop after birth and is continually enhanced by exposure to new pathogens and antigens throughout life.

induced active immunity immunity achieved through vaccination given to generate an immune response that results in the development of antibodies specific for the injected antigen; also called artificially acquired immunity.

active immunity acquired immunity that occurs following exposure to an antigen and results in the production of antibodies specific for the antigen.

passive immunity acquired immunity that results from administration of antibodies either from mother to infant across the placental barrier (natural passive immunity) or through vaccination (induced passive immunity).

Dt). The tetanus immune globulin (TIG) provides passive immunity until such time as the body's immune system can respond to the tetanus vaccination with the development of antibodies specific for tetanus. This should be followed by periodic tetanus boosters until such time as the patient's immunization program is complete.

ALLERGIES

The initial exposure of an individual to an antigen is referred to as **sensitization.** Sensitization results in an immune response. Subsequent exposure induces a much stronger secondary response. Some individuals can become hypersensitive (overly sensitive) to a particular antigen. **Hypersensitivity** is an unexpected and exaggerated reaction to a particular antigen. In many instances, hypersensitivity is used synonymously with the term **allergy.** Two types of hypersensitivity reactions are: delayed and immediate.

Delayed and Immediate Hypersensitivity

Delayed hypersensitivity is a result of *cellular immunity* and therefore does not involve antibodies. Delayed hypersensitivity usually occurs in the hours and days following exposure and is the sort of allergy that occurs in normal people. Delayed hypersensitivity most commonly results in a skin rash and is often due to exposure to certain drugs and chemicals. The rash associated with poison ivy is an example of delayed hypersensitivity.

When people use the term *allergy* they are usually referring to **immediate hypersensitivity** reactions. Examples of immediate hypersensitivity reactions include hay fever, drug allergies, food allergies, eczema, and asthma. Some persons have an allergic tendency. This allergic tendency is usually genetic, meaning it is passed from parent to child and is characterized by the presence of large quantities of IgE antibodies. An antigen that causes release of the IgE antibodies is referred to as an **allergen.** Common allergens include:

- Drugs
- Foods and food additives
- Animals
- Insects (*Hymenoptera* stings) and insect parts
- Fungi and molds
- Radiology contrast materials

Patho Pearls

The allergic response to an antigen is designed to rapidly eliminate the offending antigen from the body. In most people, this response is mild. However, in those previously sensitized to the antigen, the response can be massive, even life threatening. The cascade of events following exposure to the antigen serves to remove the antigens from the body and to prevent additional ones from entering it. For example, shortly after exposure, in patients previously sensitized to the antigen, patients will develop bronchospasm and, in some cases, coughing. The bronchospasm serves to prevent additional antigens from entering the respiratory tract, whereas the cough and increased sputum production help to remove any antigens there. Likewise, following exposure, histamine is released from mast cells and basophiles. Histamine, in addition to causing bronchospasm, causes the capillaries to become leaky, allowing fluid to leave the intravascular space and enter the interstitial space. This can cause the antigen to be taken from the blood, where it is causing problems, and moved to the interstitial space where it can be eventually removed by the lymphatic system and its components. Likewise, vomiting and diarrhea are common with severe allergic reactions. These serve to help remove any offending pathogens from the gastrointestinal tract.

Unfortunately, when the allergic response becomes severe, it can lead to cardiovascular collapse, massive bronchospasm, and fluid shifts. Because of this, EMT-Is may have to intervene with drugs such as epinephrine and diphenhydramine (Benadryl), which will help counter some of the untoward effects described here.

Allergens can enter the body through various routes. These include oral ingestion, inhalation, topically, and through injection or envenomation. The vast majority of anaphylactic reactions result from injection or envenomation.

Parenteral penicillin injections are the most common cause of fatal anaphylactic reactions. Insect stings are the second most frequent cause of fatal anaphylactic reactions. Insects in the order *Hymenoptera* are the most frequent offending insects. There are three families in this order: fire ants (*Formicoidea*); wasps, yellow jackets, and hornets (*Vespidae*); and the honey bees (*Apoidea*). All produce a unique venom, although there are similar components in each. Honey bees often will leave their stinger embedded in the victim following a sting.

Following exposure to a particular allergen, large quantities of IgE antibodies are released. These antibodies attach to the membranes of **basophils** and **mast cells**—specialized cells of the immune system that contain chemicals which assist in the immune response. When the allergen binds to IgE attached to the basophils and mast cells, these cells release histamine, heparin, and other substances into the surrounding tissues. Histamine and other substances are stored in *granules* found within the basophils and mast cells. In fact, because of this feature, basophils and mast cells are often called *granulocytes*. The process of releasing these substances from the cells is called *degranulation*. This release results in what people call an allergic reaction, which can be very mild or very severe.

The principal chemical mediator of an allergic reaction is histamine. **Histamine** is a potent substance that causes bronchoconstriction, increased intestinal motility, vasodilation, and increased vascular permeability. Increased vascular permeability causes the leakage of fluid from the circulatory system into the surrounding tissues. A common manifestation of severe allergic reactions and anaphylaxis is angioneurotic edema. **Angioneurotic edema,** also called *angioedema,* is marked edema of the skin and usually involves the head, neck, face, and upper airway. Histamine acts by activating specialized histamine receptors present throughout the body.

There are two classes of histamine receptors. H1 receptors, when stimulated, cause bronchoconstriction and contraction of the intestines. H2 receptors cause peripheral vasodilation and secretion of gastric acids. The goal of histamine release is to minimize the body's exposure to the antigen. Bronchoconstriction decreases the possibility of the antigen entering through the respiratory tract. Increased gastric acid production helps destroy an ingested antigen. Increased intestinal motility serves to move the antigen quickly though the gastrointestinal system with minimal absorption of the antigen into the body. Vasodilation and capillary permeability help remove the allergen from the circulation where it has the potential to do the most harm.

ANAPHYLAXIS

Anaphylaxis usually occurs when a specific allergen is injected directly into the circulation. This is the reason anaphylaxis is more common following injections of drugs and diagnostic agents and following bee stings. When the allergen enters the circulation, it is distributed widely throughout the body. The allergen interacts with both basophils and mast cells, resulting in the massive dumping of histamine and other substances associated with anaphylaxis. The principal body systems affected by anaphylaxis are the cardiovascular system, the respiratory system, the gastrointestinal system, and the skin. Histamine causes widespread peripheral vasodilation as well as increased permeability of the capillaries. Increased capillary permeability results in marked loss of plasma from the circulation. People sustaining anaphylaxis can actually die from circulatory shock.

Also released from the basophils and mast cells is a substance called **slow-reacting substance of anaphylaxis (SRS-A).** This causes spasm of the bronchial smooth muscle, resulting in an asthma-like attack and occasionally asphyxia. SRS-A potentiates the effects of histamine, especially on the respiratory system.

ASSESSMENT FINDINGS IN ANAPHYLAXIS

The signs and symptoms of anaphylaxis begin within 30 to 60 seconds following exposure to the offending allergen. In a small percentage of patients the onset of signs and symptoms may be delayed over an hour. The signs and symptoms of anaphylaxis can vary significantly.

basophil type of white blood cell that participates in allergic responses.

mast cell specialized cell of the immune system which contains chemicals that assist in the immune response.

histamine a product of mast cells and basophils that causes vasodilation, capillary permeability, bronchoconstriction, and contraction of the gut.

angioneurotic edema marked edema of the skin that usually involves the head, neck, face, and upper airway; a common manifestation of severe allergic reactions and anaphylaxis.

slow-reacting substance of anaphylaxis (SRS-A) substance released from basophils and mast cells that causes spasm of the bronchiole smooth muscle, resulting in an asthma-like attack and occasionally asphyxia.

The severity of the reaction is often related to the speed of onset. Reactions that develop very quickly tend to be much more severe.

A rapid and focused assessment is crucial to the early detection and treatment of anaphylaxis. Patients having an anaphylactic reaction often have a sense of impending doom. This sense of impending doom is often followed by development of additional signs and symptoms.

If the patient's condition permits, a brief history should be gathered, including previous allergen exposures and reactions. If possible, try to determine how quickly symptoms started and how severe they were.

Next, quickly evaluate the patient's level of consciousness. Upper airway problems, including laryngeal edema, may result in the patient being unable to speak. As the emergency progresses, the patient will become restless. As cardiovascular collapse continues, the patient will exhibit a decreased level of consciousness. If untreated, this may continue to unresponsiveness.

As noted earlier, a common manifestation of anaphylaxis is angioneurotic edema, involving the face and neck. Laryngeal edema is also a frequent complication and can threaten the airway. Initially, laryngeal edema will cause a hoarse voice. As the edema worsens, the patient may develop stridor. Finally, this all may lead to complete airway obstruction from either massive laryngeal edema, laryngospasm, or pharyngeal edema, or a combination of any of these.

The respiratory system is significantly involved in an anaphylactic reaction. Initially, the patient will become tachypneic. Later, as lower airway edema and bronchospasm develop, respirations will become labored as evidenced by retractions, accessory muscle usage, and prolonged expirations. Wheezing, resulting from bronchospasm and edema of the smaller airways, is a common manifestation and may be so pronounced that it can be heard without the aid of a stethoscope. Ultimately, anaphylaxis can result in markedly diminished lung sounds, which reflect decreased air movement and hypoventilation.

The skin is typically involved early in severe allergic reactions and anaphylaxis. Generally, a fine red rash will appear diffusely on the body. As histamine is released, fluid will diffuse from leaky capillaries, resulting in urticaria. **Urticaria,** also called "hives," is a wheal and flare reaction characterized by red raised bumps, which may appear and disappear across the body (Figure 22-1). As cardiovascular collapse and dyspnea progresses, the patient will become diaphoretic. This may, if untreated, progress to cyanosis and pallor.

The effect of histamine on the gastrointestinal system is pronounced. Initially, the patient may note a rumbling sensation in the abdomen as gastrointestinal motility increases. On physical examination, this may be evident as hyperactive bowel sounds. Later, nausea, vomiting, and diarrhea develop as the body tries to rid itself of the offending allergen.

The vital signs will vary depending on the severity and stage of the severe allergic or anaphylactic reaction. Initially both the heart and respiratory rate will increase. As airway edema and dyspnea occurs, the respiratory rate can fall—an ominous finding. The blood pressure will fall when significant capillary leakage and peripheral vasodilation occurs. This will often result in a reflex tachycardia as the body attempts to compensate for the fall in

urticaria the raised areas, or wheals, that occur on the skin, associated with vasodilation due to histamine release; commonly called "hives."

FIGURE 22-1 Hives are red, itchy blotches, sometimes raised, that often accompany an allergic reaction.

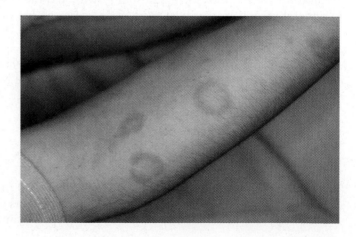

blood pressure. Very late in anaphylaxis the heart rate will fall. This too should be considered a very ominous sign.

State-of-the-art advanced prehospital care of anaphylaxis includes use of all available monitoring devices. These include the cardiac monitor, the pulse oximeter, and, if the patient is intubated, an end-tidal carbon dioxide detector. As anaphylaxis progresses, the end-tidal carbon dioxide level may climb due to the development of both respiratory and metabolic acidosis, which results in increased carbon dioxide elimination.

MANAGEMENT OF ANAPHYLAXIS

When responding to a patient with an anaphylactic reaction, first ensure that the scene is safe to approach. The presence of chemicals or patrolling bees can pose a risk to EMS personnel as well as to the patient and bystanders. If the patient is still in contact with the agent causing the reaction, he should be moved a safe distance away. Honey bees often leave their stinger behind during a sting. If present, the stinger should be removed by scraping the skin with a fingernail or scalpel blade.

Always consider the possibility of trauma in anaphylaxis. If there is any suspicion of co-incidental trauma, stabilize the cervical spine. It is not uncommon for people to fall or otherwise injure themselves as they try to escape from wasps and bees. Signs and symptoms of trauma may be masked by those of anaphylaxis.

PROTECT THE AIRWAY

Position the patient and protect the airway. Administer oxygen via a nonrebreather mask. If the patient is hypoventilating or apneic, initiate ventilatory assistance. If an airway problem is detected, first apply basic airway maneuvers such as head positioning or the modified jaw-thrust maneuver. Use oropharyngeal and nasopharyngeal airways with caution because they can cause laryngospasm. If the patient is having severe airway problems, consider early endotracheal intubation to prevent complete occlusion of the airway. It is important to remember that the glottic opening may be smaller than expected due to laryngeal edema. Also, the larynx will be very irritable, and any manipulation of the airway may lead to laryngospasm. Ideally, the most experienced member of the crew should perform endotracheal intubation, since only one attempt may be possible.

Establish an IV as soon as possible with a crystalloid solution such as lactated Ringer's or normal saline. Remember that patients suffering anaphylaxis are volume depleted due to histamine-mediated third spacing of fluid. If the patient is hypotensive, administer fluids wide open. If time allows, place a second IV line.

ADMINISTER MEDICATIONS

The primary treatment for anaphylaxis is pharmacological. If the necessary drugs cannot be administered in the field, then the patient should be transported to the emergency department immediately. Emergency medications used in the treatment of anaphylaxis include oxygen, epinephrine, antihistamines, corticosteroids, and vasopressors. Occasionally, inhaled beta agonists, such as albuterol, may be required.

Oxygen

Oxygen is always the first drug to administer to a patient with an anaphylactic reaction. Administer high-flow, high-concentration oxygen with a nonrebreather mask or similar device. If mechanical ventilation is required, attach supplemental oxygen to ensure as high an oxygen delivery as possible.

Epinephrine

The primary drug for use in treatment of severe allergic reactions and anaphylaxis is epinephrine. Epinephrine is a sympathetic agonist. It causes an increase in heart rate, an increase in the strength of the cardiac contractile force, and peripheral vasoconstriction. It can also reverse some of the bronchospasm associated with anaphylaxis. Epinephrine also reverses

Epinephrine is the primary drug for management of anaphylaxis.

much of the capillary permeability caused by histamine. It acts within minutes of administration. In severe anaphylaxis, characterized by hypotension and/or severe airway obstruction, administer epinephrine 1:10,000 intravenously. Epinephrine 1:10,000 contains one milligram of epinephrine in 10 milliliters of solvent. The standard adult dose is 0.3 to 0.5 mg; child dose is 0.01 mg/kg. The effects of intravenous epinephrine wear off in 3 to 5 minutes, so repeat boluses may be required. In severe cases of sustained anaphylaxis, medical direction may order the preparation and administration of an epinephrine drip.

Antihistamines

Antihistamines are second-line agents in the treatment of anaphylaxis. They should only be given following the administration of epinephrine. Antihistamines block the effects of histamine by blocking histamine receptors. They do not displace histamine from the receptors. They only block additional histamine from binding. They also help reduce histamine release from mast cells and basophils. Most antihistamines are non-selective and block both H_1 and H_2 receptors. Others are more selective for either H_1 or H_2 receptors.

Diphenhydramine (Benadryl) is probably the most frequently used antihistamine in the treatment of allergic reactions and anaphylaxis. It is non-selective and acts on both H_1 and H_2 receptors. The standard dose of diphenhydramine is 25 to 50 milligrams intravenously or intramuscularly. It should be administered slowly when given intravenously. The pediatric dose of diphenhydramine is 1 to 2 milligrams per kilogram of body weight. Other non-selective antihistamines frequently used are hydroxyzine (Atarax, Vistaril) and promethazine (Phenergan). Hydroxyzine is a potent antihistamine, but it can only be administered intramuscularly. Promethazine can be administered intravenously or intramuscularly, but does not appear to be as potent as diphenhydramine.

Selective histamine blockers are primarily H_2 blockers used to treat ulcer disease. Blockage of the H_2 receptors decreases gastric acid secretion. However, H_2 receptors are also present in the peripheral blood vessels. Administration of H_2 blockers conceivably will reverse some of the vasodilation associated with anaphylaxis. The two most frequently used H_2 blockers are cimetidine (Tagamet) and ranitidine (Zantac). Typically, 300 milligrams of cimetidine or 50 milligrams of ranitidine are administered by slow IV push (over 3 to 5 minutes). Some recent studies have questioned the effectiveness of H_2 blockers in the treatment of allergic reactions. Also, these agents are more expensive than the non-selective antihistamines.

Corticosteroids

Corticosteroids are important in the treatment and prevention of anaphylaxis. Although they are of little benefit in the initial stages of treatment they help suppress the inflammatory response associated with these emergencies. Commonly used corticosteroids include methylprednisolone (Solu-Medrol), hydrocortisone (Solu-Cortef), and dexamethasone (Decadron).

Vasopressors

Severe and prolonged anaphylactic reactions may require the use of potent vasopressors to support blood pressure. Use these medications in conjunction with first line therapy and adequate fluid resuscitation. Commonly used agents include dopamine, norepinephrine, and epinephrine. These medications are prepared as infusions and are continuously administered to support blood pressure and cardiac output.

Beta Agonists

Many patients with severe allergic reactions and anaphylaxis will develop bronchospasm, laryngeal edema, or both. In these cases, an inhaled beta agonist can be useful. The most frequently used beta agonist in prehospital care is albuterol (Ventolin, Proventil). Although usually used in the treatment of asthma, these agents will help reverse some of the bronchospasm and laryngeal edema associated with anaphylaxis. Give the adult patient 0.5 mL of albuterol in 3 mL of normal saline via a hand-held nebulizer. Children should receive 0.2 to 0.5 mL of albuterol based on their weight. Other beta agonists, such as metaproterenol (Alupent) and isoetharine (Bronkosol) may be used instead of albuterol.

Other Agents

Other drugs occasionally used in the treatment of anaphylaxis include aminophylline and cromolyn sodium. Aminophylline is a bronchodilator unrelated to the beta agonists. It can be administered by slow intravenous infusion to treat the bronchospasm associated with anaphylaxis. Although cromolyn sodium (Intal) is not used in the treatment of allergic reactions and anaphylaxis, it is used in their prevention. Cromolyn sodium helps to stabilize the membranes of the mast cells, thus reducing the amount of histamine and other mediators released when these cells are stimulated.

OFFER PSYCHOLOGICAL SUPPORT

A severe allergic or anaphylactic reaction is a harrowing experience for the patient. Although it is essential to work fast, prehospital crews should provide the patient emotional support and explain the treatment regimen. Caution patients about the potential side effects of administered medications. For example, epinephrine will often cause a rapid heart rate, anxiety, and tremulousness. Likewise, the antihistamines may cause a dry mouth, thirst, and sedation. Careful explanation and emotional support will help allay patient anxiety and apprehension.

ASSESSMENT FINDINGS IN ALLERGIC REACTION

Many patients you will be called to treat will be suffering from forms of allergic reaction less severe than anaphylaxis. An allergic reaction, as contrasted with an anaphylactic reaction, will have a more gradual onset with milder signs and symptoms and the patient will have a normal mental status (Table 22-2).

MANAGEMENT OF ALLERGIC REACTIONS

Common manifestations of mild (non-anaphylactic) allergic reactions include itching, rash, and urticaria. Patients with simple itching and non-urticarial rashes may be treated with antihistamines alone. In addition to antihistamines, epinephrine is often necessary for the treatment of urticaria.

Table 22-2	SIGNS AND SYMPTOMS OF ALLERGIC AND ANAPHYLACTIC REACTIONS	
	Mild Allergic Reaction	**Severe Allergic Reaction or Anaphylaxis**
Onset	Gradual	Sudden (30-60 seconds but can be more than an hour after exposure)
Skin/vascular system	Mild flushing, rash, or hives	Severe flushing, rash, or hives; angioneurotic edema to the face and neck
Respiration	Mild bronchoconstriction	Severe bronchoconstriction (wheezing), laryngospasm (stridor), breathing difficulty
GI system	Mild cramps, diarrhea	Severe cramps, abdominal rumbling, diarrhea, vomiting
Vital signs	Normal to slightly abnormal	Increased pulse early, may fall in late/severe case; increased respiratory rate early, falling respiratory rate late; falling blood pressure late
Mental status	Normal	Anxiety, sense of impending doom, may decrease to confusion and to unconsciousness
Other clues		Symptoms occur shortly after exposure to parenteral penicillin, *Hymenoptera* sting (fire ant, wasp, yellow-jacket, hornet, bee), or ingestion of foods to which patient is allergic such as nuts or shellfish
Ominous signs		Respiratory distress, signs of shock, falling respiratory rate, falling pulse rate, falling blood pressure

Note: Not all signs and symptoms will be present in every case.

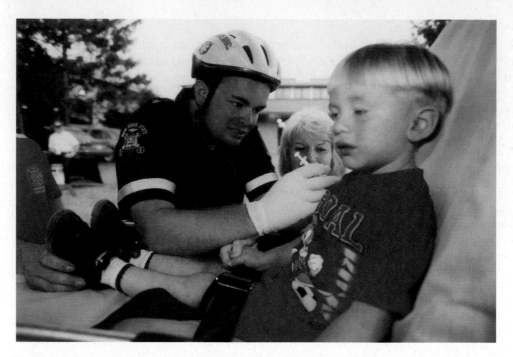

FIGURE 22-2   Epinephrine being administered to a pediatric patient.

Any patient having an allergic reaction who exhibits dyspnea or wheezing should receive supplemental oxygen. This should be followed by subcutaneous epinephrine 1:1,000. Lesser allergic reactions that are not accompanied by hypotension or airway problems can be adequately treated with epinephrine 1:1,000 administered subcutaneously (Figure 22-2). Epinephrine 1:1,000 contains one milligram of epinephrine in one milliliter of solvent. When administered into the subcutaneous tissue, the drug is absorbed more slowly and the effect prolonged. The subcutaneous dose is the same as the intravenous dose (0.3 to 0.5 milligram). The subcutaneous route should not be used in severe anaphylaxis. Many physicians prefer to give epinephrine 1:1,000 intramuscularly, because this has a faster rate of onset although a shorter duration of action.

SUMMARY

Fortunately, severe allergies and anaphylaxis are uncommon. However, when they do occur, they can progress quickly and result in death in minutes. The central physiological action in anaphylaxis is the massive release of histamine and other mediators. Histamine causes bronchospasm, airway edema, peripheral vasodilation, and increased capillary permeability. The prehospital treatment of anaphylaxis is intended to reverse the effects of these agents.

The primary, and most important, drug used in the treatment of anaphylaxis is epinephrine. Epinephrine helps reverse the effects of histamine. It also supports the blood pressure and reverses detrimental capillary leakage. Following the administration of epinephrine, potent antihistamines should be used to block the adverse effects of the massive histamine release. Inhaled beta agonists are useful in cases of severe bronchospasm and airway involvement. IV fluid replacement is crucial in preventing hypovolemia and hypotension.

The key to successful prehospital management of anaphylaxis is prompt recognition and treatment.

ON THE WEB

For additional practice and review, go to the companion website at www.prenhall.com/bledsoe and click on *Intermediate Emergency Care: Principles & Practice*.

CHAPTER 23

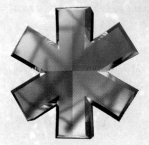

Poisoning and Overdose Emergencies

Objectives

After reading this chapter, you should be able to:

1. Identify appropriate personal protective equipment and scene safety awareness concerns and situations in which additional non-EMS resources need to be contacted in dealing with toxicologic emergencies. (p. 973)
2. Describe the routes of entry of toxic substances into the body. (pp. 971–972)
3. Discuss the role of Poison Control Centers in the United States. (p. 971)
4. Discuss the pathophysiology, assessment findings, need for rapid intervention and transport, and management of toxic emergencies. (pp. 970–1006)
5. Differentiate among the most common poisonings, pathophysiology, assessment findings, and management of poisoning by ingestion, inhalation, absorption, injection, and overdose. (pp. 971–1006)
6. Define substance abuse and drug overdose and differentiate among the most common drugs of abuse, including alcohol, and their assessment and management. (pp. 999–1006)
7. Discuss common causative agents or offending organisms, pharmacology, assessment findings, and management for a patient with food poisoning, a bite, or a sting. (pp. 992–999)
8. Given several scenarios of poisoning or overdose, provide the appropriate assessment, treatment, and transport. (pp. 970–1006)

CASE STUDY

Rescue 190 is staffed by EMT-Is Kevin Lucia, Charles Wright, and David Schrodt. Dispatch reports an unconscious person at 1301 North Seventh Street. As the EMT-Is turn the corner and approach the residence, they immediately remember this location. They have been called here many times in the past to attend to a chronically

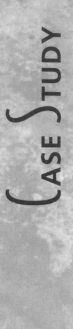
depressed young woman who has trouble coping with stressful situations. David reports that the crew from another shift was there 4 days ago.

Inside they find the young woman unresponsive and lying on the floor beside the sofa. She was found like this by her boyfriend, who states that she called him at work 2 hours ago crying that "she just couldn't take it anymore." On the floor beside her is an empty bottle of acetaminophen (Tylenol) and an empty bottle of nortriptyline (Pamelor), a tricyclic antidepressant. A pharmacy receipt on the floor shows that the bottles were just purchased today. Because of this, the EMT-Is have to assume that the bottles were full. The smell of alcohol pervades the air. A quick look around the scene reveals several empty bottles of an expensive wine on the sofa table.

Initial assessment shows that the young woman is unresponsive but alive. Respirations are slow and shallow. She is tachycardic with weak pulses. The EMT-Is intubate her and begin mechanical ventilation. They then establish an IV access and place the various monitors. A focused history from the patient's boyfriend provides no additional information. The police arrive and start to interrogate the boyfriend in an adjacent room. Kevin and Charles complete a rapid medical assessment. The only noteworthy findings are multiple shallow scars across both wrists.

The EMT-Is quickly transport the patient to the hospital, remembering to bring all bottles of medicines (full and empty) found at the scene. The patient does not seem to improve while en route. Shortly after arrival at the emergency department, the patient has a grand mal seizure that requires intravenous diazepam for treatment. The patient continues to deteriorate despite aggressive medical intervention. She does not regain consciousness and is eventually transferred to the ICU. She dies in ICU 48 hours later from cardiac dysrhythmias and hepatic failure. Her physicians hope to learn the cause of death from an autopsy performed by the hospital's pathologist. Results should be known in several weeks.

INTRODUCTION

toxicology study of the detection, chemistry, pharmacological actions, and antidotes of toxic substances.

toxin any chemical (drug, poison, or other) that causes adverse effects on an organism that is exposed to it.

Toxicology is the study of **toxins** (drugs and poisons) and antidotes and their effects on living organisms. Toxicological emergencies result from the ingestion, inhalation, surface absorption, or injection of toxic substances that then exert their adverse effects on the body's tissues and metabolic mechanisms. Theoretically, all toxicological emergencies can be classified as poisoning. However, in this discussion, the term *poisoning* will be used to describe exposure to non-pharmacological substances. The term *overdose* will be used to describe exposure to pharmacological substances, whether the overdose is accidental or intentional. Substance abuse, although technically a form of poisoning, will be addressed separately.

In this chapter we will discuss various aspects of toxicological emergencies as they apply to prehospital care. We will establish general treatment guidelines for each type of toxic exposure, then address the specific issues surrounding some of the more common substances involved. Because the field of toxicology is rapidly changing, it is virtually impossible for an EMT-I to remain up to date on treatment guidelines for each type of toxic exposure. Specific treatment should be supervised by medical direction in association with a Poison Control Center. This plan ensures that the patient receives the most current level of care available.

EPIDEMIOLOGY

Over the years, the occurrence of toxicological emergencies has continued to increase in number and severity. The following statistics reveal the high potential for toxic substance involvement on an EMS call:

- The American Association of Poison Control Centers estimates over 4 million poisonings occur annually.

- 10% of all emergency department visits and EMS responses involve toxic exposures.
- 70% of accidental poisonings occur in children under the age of 6 years.
- A child who has experienced an accidental ingestion has a 25% chance of another, similar ingestion within 1 year.
- 80% of all attempted suicides involve a drug overdose.

Although over half of all poisonings occur in children age 1 to 5, they are generally accidental and relatively mild, accounting for only 10% of hospital admissions for poisoning and only 5% of the fatalities. EMS personnel must be aware that more serious poisonings, especially in children older than 5, may represent intentional poisoning by parents or caretakers. Unfortunately, poisoning due to drug experimentation and suicide attempts are also becoming a common consideration in older children.

Adult poisonings and overdoses, although less frequent, account for 90% of hospital admissions for toxic substance exposure. They also account for 95% of the fatalities in this category. Most adult poisonings and overdoses are intentional. Intentional poisonings and overdoses can be due to illicit drug use, alcohol abuse, attempted suicide, and "suicidal gesturing" in which the patient is making a cry for help but may miscalculate and take a type or amount of toxin that does actually cause injury. More rarely, intentional poisoning can result from attempted homicide or chemical warfare. Accidental poisonings are increasingly caused by exposure to chemicals and toxins on the farm or in the industrial workplace. More often they are the result of idiosyncratic (individual hypersensitivity) reactions or dosage errors when taking prescribed medications, but these usually do not require medical attention.

POISON CONTROL CENTERS

Poison Control Centers have been set up across the United States and Canada to assist in the treatment of poison victims and to provide information on new products and new treatment recommendations. They are usually based in major medical centers and teaching hospitals and serve a large population. Almost all Poison Control Centers now have computer systems to rapidly access information.

Poison Control Centers are usually staffed by physicians, toxicologists, pharmacists, nurses, or EMT-Is with special training in toxicology. These experts provide information to callers 24 hours a day, 7 days a week. They update information regularly and offer the most current treatment guidelines.

Memorize the number of the nearest Poison Control Center and access it routinely. There are several advantages to this. First, the Poison Control Center can help you immediately determine potential toxicity based on the type of agent, amount and time of exposure, and physical condition of the patient. Second, the most current, definitive treatment can sometimes be started in the field. Finally, the Poison Control Center can notify the receiving hospital of current treatment and recommendations even before arrival of the patient.

ROUTES OF TOXIC EXPOSURE

Poisons must gain entrance into the body to have a destructive effect. The four portals of entry are ingestion, inhalation, surface absorption, and injection. It is important to note that, regardless of the portal of entry, toxic substances have both immediate and delayed effects.

INGESTION

Ingestion is the most common route of entry for toxic exposure. Frequently ingested poisons include:

- Household products
- Petroleum-based agents (gasoline, paint)
- Cleaning agents (alkalis and soaps)

Memorize the number of the nearest Poison Control Center and access it routinely for information regarding a poisoning or overdose.

Content Review

ROUTES OF TOXIC EXPOSURE

- Ingestion
- Inhalation
- Surface absorption
- Injection

It is important to remember that toxic substances have both immediate and delayed effects.

ingestion entry of a substance into the body through the gastrointestinal tract.

- Cosmetics
- Drugs (prescription, non-prescription, illicit)
- Plants
- Foods

Immediate toxic effects of ingestion of corrosive substances, such as strong acids or alkalis, can involve burns to the lips, tongue, throat, and esophagus. Delayed effects result from absorption of the poison from the gastrointestinal tract. Most absorption occurs in the small intestine, with only a small amount being absorbed from the stomach. Some poisons may remain in the stomach for up to several hours, because the intake of a large bolus of poison can retard absorption. Aspirin ingestion is a classic example of this. When a patient ingests a large number of aspirin tablets, the tablets can bind together to form a large bolus that is difficult to remove or break down.

INHALATION

inhalation entry of a substance into the body through the respiratory tract.

Inhalation of a poison results in rapid absorption of the toxic agent through the alveolar-capillary membrane in the lungs. Inhaled toxins can irritate pulmonary passages, causing extensive edema and destroying tissue. When these toxins are absorbed, wider systemic effects can occur. Causative agents can appear as gases, vapors, fumes, or aerosols. Common inhaled poisons include:

- Toxic gases
- Carbon monoxide
- Ammonia
- Chlorine
- Freon
- Toxic vapors, fumes, or aerosols
- Carbon tetrachloride
- Methyl chloride
- Tear gas
- Mustard gas
- Nitrous oxide

SURFACE ABSORPTION

surface absorption entry of a substance into the body directly through the skin or mucous membrane.

Surface absorption is the entry of a toxic substance through the skin or mucous membranes. This most frequently occurs from contact with poisonous plants such as poison ivy, poison sumac, and poison oak. Many toxic chemicals may also be absorbed through the skin. **Organophosphates,** often used as pesticides, are easily absorbed through dermal contact.

organophosphates phosphorus-containing organic chemicals.

INJECTION

injection entry of a substance into the body through a break in the skin.

Injection of a toxic agent under the skin, into muscle, or into a blood vessel results in both immediate and delayed effects. The immediate reaction is usually localized to the site of the injection and appears as red, irritated, edematous skin. An allergic or anaphylactic reaction can also appear (see Chapter 22). Later, because the toxin is distributed throughout the body by the circulatory system, delayed systemic reactions can occur.

Other than intentional injection of illicit drugs, most poisonings by injection result from the bites and stings of insects and animals. Most insects that can sting and bite belong to the class *Hymenoptera,* which includes honeybees, hornets, yellow jackets, wasps, and fire ants. Only the females in this group can sting. In addition, spiders, ticks, and other arachnids, such as scorpions, are notorious for causing poisonings by injection. Higher animals that bite and sting include snakes and certain marine animals. Marine animals with venomous stings include jellyfish (especially the Portuguese man-of-war), stingrays, anemones, coral, hydras, and certain spiny fish.

GENERAL PRINCIPLES OF TOXICOLOGIC ASSESSMENT AND MANAGEMENT

Although specific protocols for managing toxicological emergencies may vary, certain basic principles apply to most situations. Keep in mind the importance of recognizing the poisoning promptly. Have a high index of suspicion if circumstances suggest involvement of a toxin in the emergency.

SCENE SIZE-UP

Always begin assessment with a thorough evaluation of the scene. Take note of where you are and who is around you. Be alert for any potential danger to you, the rescuer. Remember, despite your natural urge to immediately assess and treat the patient, if you are incapacitated you will not be able to help anyone and you will become a patient yourself. In toxicological emergencies keep in mind the following specific hazards:

- Patients who are suicidal may have the potential for violence. They are often intoxicated, may act irrationally, and will not always be cooperative or happy to see you. Therefore, look for signs of overdose such as empty pill bottles and used needles or other drug paraphernalia. Never put your hand blindly into a patient's pocket because it may contain used needles.
- Chemical spills and hazardous material emergencies can quickly incapacitate any individuals who are nearby. Make sure you have the proper clothing and equipment needed for the particular emergency. Distribute this gear to rescuers who have been trained in their use.

Call for specially trained rescue teams and other resources as needed.

INITIAL ASSESSMENT

After the scene size-up, perform the standard initial assessment. Form a general impression and quickly assess mental status. Assessment of the ABCs is critical in toxicological emergencies because airway and respiratory compromise are common complications. This can be due to direct airway injury, pulmonary injury, profuse secretions, or decreased respiratory effort secondary to altered mental status. After assessing the patient's ABCs, set a transport priority.

HISTORY, PHYSICAL EXAM, AND ONGOING ASSESSMENT

For responsive patients, start by obtaining a history. It is important to find out not only what toxin the patient was exposed to but also when the exposure took place, since toxic effects develop over time. Then proceed to a focused physical exam with full vital signs. With unresponsive patients, start with a rapid head-to-toe exam. Be alert for signs of trauma inconsistent with the suspected intoxication. Then proceed to obtain a history from relatives or other bystanders. Relay this information to the local Poison Control Center. They will advise you on the most current protocol for treatment. Be aware of your local policy, which will outline whether you can initiate this protocol or whether you must first contact on-line medical direction. Never delay supportive measures or immediate transport to the hospital based on a delay in contacting or obtaining information from the Poison Control Center.

A detailed physical exam can be performed en route if time and the patient's condition permit. Ongoing assessment is essential for these patients. Poisoned patients can deteriorate suddenly and quickly. Repeat the initial assessment and vital signs and re-evaluate every 5 minutes for critical/unstable patients and every 15 minutes for stable patients.

TREATMENT

Decontamination

Once you have initiated supportive treatment (airway control, breathing assistance, and IV fluids), proceed to a mode of treatment that is specific to toxicological emergencies:

decontamination. **Decontamination** is the process of minimizing toxicity by reducing the amount of toxin absorbed into the body. There are three steps to decontamination:

1. *Reduce intake of the toxin.* This means that you must remove a person from an environment where they are inhaling toxic fumes, or you must properly remove a stinger and sac from someone stung by a bee. A classic example involves a person who has had organophosphates spilled on him. The patient's clothes must be removed and the skin cleaned with soap and water to reduce absorption of the toxins.

2. *Reduce absorption of the toxin once it is in the body.* This usually applies to ingested toxins, which wait in the stomach and intestines while the body absorbs them into the blood stream.

   In the past, syrup of ipecac was used to induce vomiting in order to empty the stomach. *Use of syrup of ipecac is no longer acceptable.* Studies consistently show that the use of syrup of ipecac to induce emesis reduces absorption by only 30%. This still leaves 70% of the toxin to be absorbed and cause injury. Vomiting also limits the use of other oral agents that are more effective for decontamination (e.g., activated charcoal) or oral antidotes (e.g., N-Acetylcysteine). There is also an increased risk of aspiration with vomiting, which makes induction of vomiting a procedure with minimal usefulness and high risk. Although ipecac may have some minor role in home management of some pediatric poisonings, it has generally become an obsolete treatment.

   Gastric lavage ("pumping the stomach") has also been found to be of limited use. This process involves passing a tube into the stomach and repeatedly filling and emptying the stomach with water or saline in hopes of removing the ingested poison. Most studies have shown that gastric lavage removes almost no poisons from the stomach unless it is initiated within one hour of the ingestion. Possible complications, such as aspiration or perforation, make this procedure a risk without much benefit. Except in limited situations with ingestions of highly toxic substances that do not bind to charcoal and for which there is no antidote, gastric lavage has become an uncommon decontamination procedure.

   The most effective and widely used method of reducing absorption of toxins is **activated charcoal**. Because of its extremely large surface area, it can adsorb, or bind, molecules from the offending toxin and prevent their absorption into the bloodstream.

3. *Enhance elimination of the toxin.* Cathartics, such as sorbitol (often mixed with activated charcoal), increase gastric motility, thereby shortening the amount of time toxins stay in the gastrointestinal tract to be absorbed. Cathartics must be used cautiously, since there is controversy regarding their effectiveness. Cathartics should not be used in pediatric patients because of the potential to cause severe electrolyte derangements.

   Whole bowel irrigation is another method of enhancing elimination. Using a gastric tube, polyethylene glycol electrolyte solution is administered continuously at 1 to 2 liters per hour until the rectal effluent is clear or objects recovered. This technique seems effective with few complications and is therefore gaining popularity. Its availability, however, is limited to a few centers.

Antidotes

Finally, if indicated, the appropriate antidote should be administered. An **antidote** is a substance that will neutralize a specific toxin or counteract its effect on the body. There are not many antidotes (Table 23-1), and they will rarely be 100% effective. Most poisonings will not require the administration of an antidote.

Table 23-1 — ANTIDOTES FOR TOXICOLOGICAL EMERGENCIES

Toxin	Antidote	Adult Dosage (Pediatric Dosage)
Acetaminophen	N-Acetylcysteine	Initial: 140 mg/kg
Arsenic	see Mercury, arsenic, gold	
Atropine	Physostigmine	Initial: 0.5–2 mg IV
Benzodiazepines	Flumazenil	Initial: 0.2 mg q 1 min to total of 1–3 mg
Carbon monoxide	Oxygen	
Cyanide	Amyl nitrite	Inhale crushed pearl for 30 seconds, then oxygen for 30 seconds
	then sodium nitrite	10 mL of 3% solution over 3 min IV (Pediatric: 0.33 mL/kg)
	then sodium thiosulfate	50 mL of 25% solution over 10 min IV (Pediatric: 1.65 mL/kg)
Ethylene glycol	Fomepizole (or as methyl alcohol)	Initial: 15 mg/kg IV
Gold	see Mercury, arsenic, gold	
Iron	Defroxamine	Initial: 10–15 mg/kg/hr IV
Lead	Edetate calcium disodium or dimercaptosuccinic acid (DMSA)	1 amp/250 mL D₅W over 1 hr; 250 mg PO
Mercury, arsenic, gold	BAL (British anti-Lewisite) DMSA	5 mg/kg IM; 250 mg PO
Methyl alcohol	Ethyl alcohol +/− dialysis	1 mL/kg of 100% ethanol IV
Nitrates	Methylene blue	0.2 mL/kg of 1% solution IV over 5 min
Opiates	Naloxone	0.4–2.0 mg IV
Organophosphates	Atropine Pralidoxime (protopam)	Initial: 2–5 mg IV; Initial: 1 g IV

The specific actions you take when dealing with toxicological emergencies will be dictated by consultation with medical direction, by protocols obtained from the Poison Control Center, and by your local policy and procedures on initiating these protocols.

SUICIDAL PATIENTS AND PROTECTIVE CUSTODY

Before leaving a suicidal patient who claims to have been "just kidding," consider the legal ramifications. You may be charged later with patient abandonment. At the same time, be aware of protective custody laws in your state. Always involve law enforcement personnel in these cases and involve them early. Only law enforcement personnel can place a patient in protective custody and ultimately consent to treatment.

Involve law enforcement early in any possible suicide case.

INGESTED TOXINS

Poisoning by ingestion is the most common route of poisoning you will encounter in prehospital care. It is essential to initiate the following principles of assessment and treatment promptly.

Assessment

It takes time for an ingested toxin to make its way from the gastrointestinal system into the circulatory system. Therefore, you need to find out not only what was ingested but also when it was ingested. Following are some general guidelines for managing patients who have ingested toxins as well as information about specific substances.

History   Begin your history by trying to find out the type of toxin ingested, the quantity of the toxin, the time elapsed since ingestion, and whether the patient took any alcohol or other potentiating substance. Also ask the patient about drug habituation or abuse and underlying medical illnesses and allergies. Remember that in cases of poisoning, inaccuracies

In cases of poisoning, histories are often unreliable due to drug-induced confusion, patient misinformation, or deliberate deception.

creep into nearly one-half of the histories because of drug-induced confusion, patient misinformation, or deliberate patient attempts at deception.

The following questions will help you to develop a relevant history:

- What did you ingest? (Obtain pill containers and any remaining contents, samples of the ingested substance, or samples of vomitus. Bring them with the patient to the emergency department.)
- When did you ingest the substance? (Time is critical for decisions regarding lab tests and the use of gastric lavage and/or antidotes.)
- How much did you ingest?
- Did you drink any alcohol?
- Have you attempted to treat yourself (including inducing vomiting)?
- Have you been under psychiatric care? If so, why? (Answers may indicate a potential for suicide.)
- What is your weight?

Physical Examination   Because the history can be unreliable, the physical examination is extremely important. It has two purposes: (1) to provide physical evidence of intoxication and (2) to find any underlying illnesses that may account for the patient's symptoms or that may affect the outcome of the poisoning. As you complete the initial assessment and rapid physical exam, pay attention to the following patient features:

- *Skin.* Is there evidence of cyanosis, pallor, wasting, or needle marks? Flushing of the skin may indicate poisoning with an anticholinergic substance. Staining of the skin may occur from chronic exposure to mercuric chloride, bromine, or similar chemicals.
- *Eyes.* Constriction or dilation of the pupils can occur with various types of poisons (e.g., marijuana, methamphetamines, narcotics). Ask about impaired vision, blurring of vision, or coloration of vision.
- *Mouth.* Look for signs of caustic ingestion, presence of the gag reflex, the amount of salivation, any breath odor, or the presence of vomitus.
- *Chest.* Breath sounds may reveal evidence of aspiration, atelectasis, or excessive pulmonary secretions.
- *Circulation.* Cardiac examination may give clues as to the type of toxin ingested. For example, the presence of tachydysrhythmias (e.g., from methamphetamine) or bradydysrhythmias (e.g., from organophosphates) may suggest specific toxins.
- *Abdomen.* Abdominal pain may result from poisoning by salicylates, methyl alcohol, caustics, or botulism toxin.

You can expect to frequently encounter patients who have ingested more than one toxin. This may be the result of a suicide attempt or of experimentation with illicit drugs. Such multiple ingestions present a diagnostic and therapeutic dilemma. Signs and symptoms may be inconsistent with a single diagnosis, and attempted treatment may produce unexpected results. A common example of this is the "speedball" (heroin mixed with cocaine). If the narcotic overdose is treated, the rescuer is often presented with a patient who is now in a cocaine-induced catecholamine crisis (tachycardia, hypertension, seizures). In such cases, or if you cannot identify what the patient has ingested, consult medical direction and/or the Poison Control Center according to your local protocols.

Maintaining airway, breathing, and circulation is top priority in treating a poisoned patient. Preventing aspiration must be a major objective.

Management

Prevent Aspiration   As previously discussed, initiation of supportive measures (maintaining the ABCs) is top priority in the treatment of the poisoned patient. Aspiration is a frequent complication of poisoning, resulting from an altered level of consciousness and a decreased gag reflex. Preventing aspiration must be one of your major objectives.

Administer Fluids and Drugs   Once you have ensured the ABCs, establish intravenous access. An IV of lactated Ringer's or normal saline at a "to-keep-open" rate is recommended for all potentially dangerous ingestions. In addition to volume replacement with a crystalloid solution, conduct cardiac monitoring and repeat assessments, including frequent monitoring of vital signs.

Many EMS systems still utilize an empiric therapeutic regimen for comatose patients consisting of $D_{50}W$, naloxone (Narcan), and thiamine (Vitamin B_1). This so-called "coma cocktail" should not be used. Instead, treatment should be guided by objective patient information obtained on scene. If immediate determination of blood glucose levels is available (glucometer and chemstrips), withhold the administration of $D_{50}W$ until determination of hypoglycemia is made. If indicated, use 25 to 50 grams of $D_{50}W$ IV push. If narcotic intoxication is suspected (respiratory depression or pinpoint pupils), give 1 to 2 mg of naloxone IV push. Naloxone reverses the effects of narcotic intoxication. If chronic alcoholism is suspected, consider administration of 100 mg of thiamine IV to address possible encephalopathy. *Do not give these medications empirically.*

Follow these supportive measures with the decontamination procedures outlined earlier. Often, decontamination is performed in the emergency department rather than on scene or during transport. This also applies to the use of most antidotes. There are exceptions, of course, and each case needs to be treated individually. Consult the Poison Control Center and medical direction according to your local protocols.

Do Not Induce Vomiting   As mentioned earlier, induction of vomiting is no longer an accepted routine intervention for patients who have ingested toxins. It is still important to contact the Poison Control Center about this, since, in rare cases of pediatric ingestion, induction of vomiting may play some role. However, for the overwhelming majority of cases, inducement of vomiting is not required and may even be contraindicated.

INHALED TOXINS

Toxic inhalations can be self-induced or the result of accidental exposure from such sources as house fires or industrial accidents. Commonly abused inhaled toxins include paint (and other hydrocarbons), freon, propellants, glue, amyl nitrite, butyl nitrite, and nitrous oxide. The general guidelines for assessment and management of toxicological emergencies apply to inhaled toxins, but the following provides some specifics.

Assessment

Inhaled toxic substances produce signs and symptoms primarily in the respiratory system. These symptoms are particularly severe in patients who have inhaled chemicals and propellants concentrated in paper or plastic bags. Patients who inhale paint or propellants are often referred to as "huffers." Look for the presence of paint on the upper or lower lip. Huffers often prefer gold paint because they believe it is more potent. The presence of paint on the upper or lower lips should alert you to the possibility of inhalant abuse. The sniffing of paint, propellants, or hydrocarbons has become an epidemic problem in many developing countries. This is particularly true in the lower socioeconomic groups, most notably the legions of street children in Latin and South America. "Huffing" can lead to serious, irreversible brain damage. As the toxins are inhaled, oxygen is gradually displaced from the respiratory system, producing a relative hypoxia. Signs and symptoms of aerosol inhalation include:

- *Central nervous system:* dizziness, headache, confusion, seizures, hallucinations, coma
- *Respiratory:* tachypnea, cough, hoarseness, stridor, dyspnea, retractions, wheezing, chest pain or tightness, rales or rhonchi
- *Cardiac:* dysrhythmias

Management

Your first priority in the case of toxin inhalation is to remove the patient from the source as soon as it is safe to do so. Then follow these guidelines:

Your first priority in any inhalation emergency is personal safety and then removal of the patient from the toxic environment.

- Safely remove the patient from the poisonous environment. In doing so, take the following essential precautions:
  - Wear protective clothing.
  - Use appropriate respiratory protection.
  - Remove the patient's contaminated clothing.
- Perform the initial assessment, history, and physical exam.
- Initiate supportive measures.
- Contact the Poison Control Center and medical direction according to your local protocols.

SURFACE-ABSORBED TOXINS

Many poisons, including organophosphates, cyanide, and other toxins, can be absorbed through the skin and mucous membranes.

Assessment and Management

Your first priority in any surface-absorbed poisoning emergency is personal safety and then removal of the patient from the toxic environment.

Signs and symptoms of absorbed poisons can vary depending on the toxin involved. See the discussion of specific toxins in the sections that follow. Whenever you suspect absorption of a toxin (especially cyanide or organophosphates), take the following steps:

- Safely remove the patient from the poisonous environment. It is essential that you follow these guidelines:
  - Wear protective clothing.
  - Use appropriate respiratory protection.
  - Remove the patient's contaminated clothing.
  - Perform the initial assessment, history, and physical exam.
  - Initiate supportive measures.
  - Contact the Poison Control Center and medical direction according to your local protocols.

SPECIFIC TOXINS

toxidrome a toxic syndrome; a group of typical signs and symptoms consistently associated with exposure to a particular type of toxin.

To recognize and implement the proper procedure in a given poisoning, you must be familiar with the signs and symptoms that a particular toxin will trigger. Often, you may not be able to identify the exact toxin a patient has been exposed to, but usually a group of toxins will have very similar manifestations and effects and will require similar interventions. Similar toxins with similar signs and symptoms are organized into **toxidromes** (toxic syndromes), which make remembering the details of their effects much simpler. Study the toxidromes listed in Table 23-2.

The following sections address specific toxins commonly encountered. Although the standard toxicological emergency procedures discussed earlier apply to all of these toxins, pay close attention to variations in treatment. Variations include specific procedures you must perform in a particular case or a poisoning in which an antidote is available or immediately necessary. Management of injected toxins, drug overdose, and substance abuse will be covered later in the chapter.

CYANIDE

Cyanide can enter the body by a variety of routes. It is present in many commercial and household items that can be either ingested or absorbed—rodenticides, silver polish, and fruit pits and seeds (apricots, cherries, pears, and so on). It also can be inhaled, especially in fires that release cyanide from products containing nitrogen. A room full of burning plastics, silks, or synthetic carpeting can also be a roomful of cyanide-filled smoke. Cyanide also forms in patients on long-term sodium nitroprusside therapy. Suicidal patients have been known to take cyanide salt. Regardless of the entry route, cyanide is an extremely fast-acting

Table 23-2 TOXIC SYNDROMES

Toxidromes	Toxin			Signs and Symptoms
Anticholinergic	Belladonna alkaloids			Dry skin and mucous membranes
	Atropine (hyoscyamine)			Thirst
	Belladonna alkaloid mixtures: belladonna			Dysphagia
	leaf, fluid extract, tincture			Vision blurred for near objects
	Homatropine			Fixed dilated pupils
	Methscopolamine			Tachycardia
	Methylatropine nitrate			Sometimes hypertension
	Plants: *Atropa belladonna, Datura stramonium,*			Rash, similar to scarlet fever
	Hyoscyamus niger, Amanita muscaria			Hyperthermia, flushing
	or *pantherina*			Urinary urgency and retention
	Scopolamine (l-hyoscine)			Lethargy
	Synthetic anticholinergics			Confusion to restlessness, excitement
	Adiphenine	Isopropamide	Pipenzolate	Delirium, hallucinations
	Anisotropine	Mepenzolate	Piperiodolate	Ataxia
	Cyclopentolate	Methantheline	Poldine	Seizures
	Dicyclomine	Methixene	Propantheline	Respiratory failure
	Diphemanil	Oxyphencyclimine	Thiphenamil	Cardiovascular collapse
	Eucatropine	Oxyphenonium	Tridihexethyl	
	Glycopyrrolate	Pentapiperide	Tropicamide	
	Hexocyclium			
	Incidential anticholinergics			
	Antihistamines	Benactyzine	Phenothiazines	
	Tricyclic antidepressants			
Acetylcholinesterase inhibition	Organophosphates			Sweating, constricted pupils, lacrimation, excessive salivation, wheezing, cramps, vomiting, diarrhea, tenesmus, bradycardia or tachycardia, hypotension or hypertension, blurred vision, urinary incontinence
	TEPP			
	OMPA			
	Dipterex			
	Chlorthion			
	Di-Syston			
	Co-ral			
	Phosdrin			Striated muscle: cramps, weakness, twitching, paralysis, respiratory failure, cyanosis, arrest
	Parathion			
	Methylparathion			
	Malathion			
	Systox			Sympathetic ganglia: tachycardia, elevated blood pressure
	EPN			
	Diazinon			
	Guthion			CNS effects: anxiety, restlessness ataxia, seizures, insomnia, coma, absent reflexes, Cheyne-Stokes respirations, respiratory and circulation depression
	Trithion			
Cholinergic	Acetylcholine	Carbachol	Pilocarpine	Sweating, constricted pupils, lacrimation, excessive salivation, wheezing, cramps, vomiting, diarrhea, tenesmus, bradycardia or tachycardia, hypotension or hypertension, blurred vision, urinary incontinence
	Area catechu	*Clitocybe dealbata*	*Pilocarpus species*	
	Betel nut	Methacholine		
	Bethanechol	Muscarine		

Continued

Table 23-2 TOXIC SYNDROMES (CONTINUED)

Toxidromes	Toxin			Signs and Symptoms
Extrapyramidal	Acetophenazine Butaperazine Carphenazine Chlorpromazine Haloperidol	Mesoridazine Perphenazine Piperacetaxine Promazine Thioridazine	Thiothixene Trifluoperazine Triflupromazine	Parkinsonian Dysphagia, eye muscle spasm, rigidity, tremor, neck spasm, shrieking, jaw spasm, laryngospasm
Hemoglobinopathies	Carbon monoxide Methemoglobin			Headache, nausea, vomiting, dizziness, dyspnea, seizures, coma, death Cutaneous blisters, gastroenteritis Epidemic occurrence with carbon monoxide Cyanosis, chocolate blood with non-functional hemoglobin
Metal fume fever	Fumes of oxides of: Brass Cadmium Copper Iron	Magnesium Mercury Nickel Titanium	Tungsten Zinc	Chills, fever, nausea, vomiting, muscular pain, throat dryness, headache, fatigue, weakness, leukocytosis, respiratory disease
Narcotic	Alphaprodine Anileridine Codeine Cyclazocine Dextromethorphan Dextromoramide Diacetylmorphine Dihydrocodeine Dihydrocodeinone Dipipanone Diphenoxylate (Lomotil)	Ethoheptazine (meperidene metabolite) Ethylmorphine Fentanyl Heroin Hydromorphone Levorphanol Meperidine Methadone Metopon Morphine	Normeperidene Opium Oxycodone Oxymorphone Pentazocine Phenazocine Piminodine Propoxyphene Racemorphan	CNS depression Pinpoint pupils Slowed respirations Hypotension Response to naloxone: pupils may be dilated and excitement may predominate Normeperidine: tremor, CNS excitation, seizures
Sympathomimetic	Aminophylline Amphetamines Caffeine Catha edulus (Khat) Cocaehylene Cocaine Dopamine	Ephedrine Epinephrine Fenfluramine Levarterenol Metaraminol Methamphetamine Methcathinone	Methylphenidate (Ritalin) Pemoline Phencyclidine Phenmetrazine Phentermine	CNS excitation Seizures Hypertension Hypotension with caffeine Tachycardia
Withdrawal	Alcohol Barbiturates Benzodiazepines Chloral hydrate	Cocaine Ethchlorvynol Glutethimide Meprobamate	Methaqualone Methyprylon Opiods Paraldehyde	Diarrhea, large pupils, piloerection, hypertension, tachycardia, insomnia, lacrimation, muscle cramps, restlessness, yawning, hallucinations Depression with cocaine

Source: Adapted from Done AK. *Poisoning—A Systematic Approach for the Emergency Department Physician.* Presented at Snowmass Village, Colo. Symposium sponsored by Rocky Mountain Poison Center. Used by permission.

toxin. Once cyanide enters the body, it acts as a *cellular asphyxiant*. It inflicts its damage by inhibiting an enzyme vital to cellular use of oxygen.

Signs and Symptoms

Signs and symptoms of cyanide poisoning include:

- A burning sensation in the mouth and throat
- Headache, confusion, combative behavior
- Hypertension and tachycardia followed by hypotension and further dysrhythmias
- Seizures and coma
- Pulmonary edema

Management

First, safely remove the patient from the source of exposure. To prevent inhalation, always wear breathing equipment when entering the scene of a fire. Initiate supportive measures immediately. Follow this with the cyanide antidote kit (Figure 23-1). This kit contains amyl nitrite ampules, a sodium nitrite, and a sodium thiosulfate solution. Adding nitrites to blood converts some hemoglobin to methemoglobin, which allows cyanide to bind to it. Thiosulfate then binds with the cyanide to form thiocyanate, a nontoxic substance readily excreted renally. Because cyanide is rapidly toxic, you must administer the cyanide antidote kit without delay. If your unit carries this kit, familiarize yourself with its contents and use.

CARBON MONOXIDE

Carbon monoxide (CO) is an odorless, tasteless gas that is often the by-product of incomplete combustion. Because of its chemical structure, it has more than 200 times the affinity of oxygen to bind with the red blood cell's hemoglobin (producing carboxyhemoglobin). Once this molecule has bound with hemoglobin, it is very resistant to removal and causes an effective hypoxia. Because of the variability of the signs and symptoms, people usually ignore CO poisoning until very toxic levels occur. Common circumstances for CO poisoning include improperly vented heating systems or the use of a small barbecue to heat a house or camper. Symptoms of early poisoning are very similar to those of influenza. Be alert for

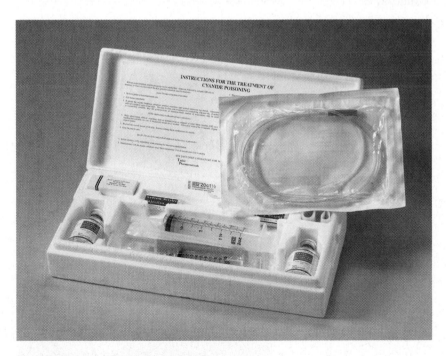

FIGURE 23-1 Cyanide antidote kit.

CO poisoning in multiple patients living together in a poorly heated and vented space, having flu-like symptoms.

Signs and Symptoms

Signs and symptoms of CO poisoning include:

- Headache
- Nausea, vomiting
- Confusion or other altered mental status
- Tachypnea

Management

Because of the difficulty in removing CO from hemoglobin, definitive treatment is often performed in a hyperbaric chamber (Figure 23-2). In this specially designed environment, oxygen under several atmospheres of pressure surrounds the body. This increases oxygenation of available hemoglobin. In field settings, take the following supportive steps:

- Ensure safety of rescue personnel.
- Remove the patient from the contaminated area.
- Begin immediate ventilation of the area.
- Initiate supportive measures. High-flow, high-concentration oxygen by nonrebreather mask is critical in this setting.

CARDIAC MEDICATIONS

The list of cardiac medications grows almost daily. Many classes of these drugs exist, including antidysrythmics, beta blockers, calcium channel blockers, glycosides, ACE inhibitors, and so on. Generally these medications regulate heart function by decreasing heart rate, suppressing automaticity, and/or reducing vascular tone. Overdoses of these drugs can be intentional but are more often due to errors in dosage.

Signs and Symptoms

In overdose quantities, signs and symptoms of cardiac medication poisoning include:

- Nausea and vomiting
- Headache, dizziness, confusion
- Profound hypotension
- Cardiac dysrhythmias (usually bradycardia)

FIGURE 23-2 Hyperbaric chamber.

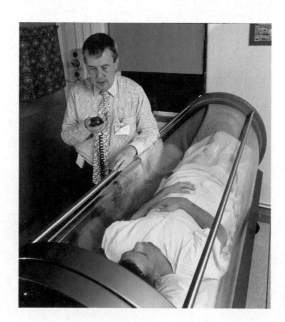

- Heart conduction blocks
- Bronchospasm and pulmonary edema (especially beta blockers)

Management

Initiate standard toxicological emergency assessment and treatment immediately. Be aware that severe bradycardia may not respond well to atropine; therefore, you may need to use an external pacing device. Some cardiac medications do have antidotes that may help with severe adverse effects. These include calcium for calcium channel blockers, glucagon for beta blockers, and Digoxin-specific Fab (Digibind) for digoxin. Contact medical direction before giving these antidotes.

CAUSTIC SUBSTANCES

Caustic substances are either **acids** or **alkalis** (bases) that are found in both the home and the industrial workplace. Approximately 12,000 exposures occur annually with 150 major complications or deaths. Strong caustics can produce severe burns at the site of contact and, if ingested, cause tissue destruction at the lips, mouth, esophagus, and other areas of the gastrointestinal tract.

Strong *acids* have a pH less than 2. They are found in plumbing liquids such as drain openers and bathroom cleaners. Contact with strong acids usually produces immediate and severe pain. This is a result of tissue coagulation and necrosis. Often this type of contact injury will produce *eschar* at the burn site, which will act like a shield and prevent further penetration or damage to deeper tissues. If ingested, acids will cause local burns to the mouth and throat. Because of the rapid transit through the esophagus, the esophagus is not usually damaged. More likely, the stomach lining will be injured. Immediate or delayed hemorrhage can occur and may be associated with perforation. Pain is severe and usually due to direct injury and spasm from irritation. Absorption of acids into the vascular system will occur quite readily, causing a significant acidemia, which will need to be managed along with the direct local effects.

Strong *alkaline* agents typically have a pH greater than 12.5. They can be in solid or liquid form (such as in Drano or Liquid Plumber) and are routinely found around the house. These agents cause injury by inducing liquefaction necrosis. Pain is often delayed, which allows for longer tissue contact and deeper tissue injury before the exposure is even recognized. Solid alkaline agents can stick to the oropharynx or esophagus. This can cause perforation, bleeding, and inflammation of central chest structures. Liquid alkalis are more likely to injure the stomach because they pass quickly through the esophagus. Within 2 to 3 days of exposure, complete loss of the protective mucosal tissue can occur, followed by either gradual healing and recovery or further bleeding, necrosis, and stricture formation.

acid a substance that liberates hydrogen ions (H^+) when in solution.

alkali a substance that liberates hydroxyl ions (OH^-) when in solution; a strong base.

Signs and Symptoms

Signs and symptoms of caustic injury include:

- Facial burns
- Pain in the lips, tongue, throat, or gums
- Drooling, trouble swallowing
- Hoarseness, stridor, or shortness of breath
- Shock from bleeding, vomiting

Management

Assessment and intervention must be aggressive and rapid to minimize morbidity and mortality. Take precautions to prevent injury to rescuers. Initiate standard toxicological emergency assessment and treatment, but pay particular attention to establishing an airway. Since caustics will not adsorb to activated charcoal, there is no indication to administer it. In the past, rescuers often gave water or milk to dilute any ingested caustics but there is controversy as to whether this is beneficial. Rapid transport to the emergency department is essential.

HYDROFLUORIC ACID

Hydrofluoric (HF) acid deserves special attention because it is extremely toxic and can be lethal despite the appearance of only moderate burns on skin contact. HF acid penetrates deeply into tissues and is inactivated only when it comes in contact with *cations* such as calcium. Calcium fluoride is formed by this inactivation and settles in the tissue as a salt. The removal of calcium from cells causes a total disruption of cell functioning and can even cause bone destruction since calcium leeches out of the bones. Death has been reported from exposure of less than 2.5% body surface area to a highly concentrated solution.

Signs and Symptoms

Signs and symptoms of HF acid exposure include:

- Burning at site of contact
- Trouble breathing
- Confusion
- Palpitations
- Muscle cramps

Management

Management includes:

- Ensure the safety of rescue personnel.
- Initiate supportive measures.
- Remove exposed clothing.
- Irrigate the affected area with water thoroughly.
- Immerse the affected limb in iced water with magnesium sulfate, calcium salts, or benzethonium chloride.
- Transport immediately for definitive care.

ALCOHOL

See the section on "Alcohol Abuse" later in this chapter.

HYDROCARBONS

Hydrocarbons are organic compounds composed of mostly carbon and hydrogen. They include such common recognizable names as kerosene, naphtha, turpentine, mineral oil, chloroform, toluene, and benzene. These chemicals are found in common household products such as lighter fluid, paint, glue, lubricants, solvents, and aerosol propellants. Toxicity from hydrocarbons can occur through any route, including ingestion, inhalation, or surface absorption.

Signs and Symptoms

Signs and symptoms of hydrocarbon poisoning will vary with the type and route of exposure but may include:

- Burns due to local contact
- Wheezing, dyspnea, hypoxia, and pneumonitis from aspiration/inhalation
- Headache, dizziness, slurred speech, ataxia (irregular and difficult-to-control movements), and obtundation (dulled reflexes)
- Foot and wrist drop with numbness and tingling
- Cardiac dysrhythmias

Management

Recent studies have shown that very few poisonings with hydrocarbons are serious, and less than 1% require physician intervention. If you know the exact chemical that the patient has been exposed to and the patient is asymptomatic, medical direction may suggest that the patient can be left at home. On the other hand, a few hydrocarbon poisonings can be very serious. Any patient who is symptomatic, does not know what he has taken, or who has taken a hydrocarbon that requires gastrointestinal decontamination (halogenated or aromatic hydrocarbons) must be treated using standard toxicological emergency procedures. Since charcoal will not bind hydrocarbons, this may be one of the few cases in which gastric lavage can be useful.

TRICYCLIC ANTIDEPRESSANTS

Tricyclic antidepressants were once commonly used to treat depression. Close monitoring was required because these medications have a narrow **therapeutic index,** meaning that a relatively small increase in dose can quickly lead to toxic effects. The very nature of their use, treating depression, presents a dilemma because the patients most seriously in need of treatment may also be the most likely to attempt to take an overdose. Deaths due to antidepressant overdose have dropped significantly in recent years since the development and rapid acceptance of safer agents unrelated to tricyclics. However, tricyclic antidepressants are still used for various clinical problems such as chronic pain or migraine prophylaxis and may still be responsible for more deaths due to intentional overdose than any other medication. Common agents include amitriptyline (Elavil), amoxapine, clomipramine, doxepin, imipramine, and nortriptyline.

therapeutic index the maximum tolerated dose divided by the minimum curative dose of a drug; the range between curative and toxic dosages; also called therapeutic window.

Signs and Symptoms

Signs and symptoms of tricyclic antidepressant toxicity include:

- Dry mouth
- Blurred vision
- Urinary retention
- Constipation

Late into an overdose, more severe toxicity may produce:

- Confusion, hallucinations
- Hyperthermia
- Respiratory depression
- Seizures
- Tachycardia and hypotension
- Cardiac dysrhythmias (heart block, wide QRS, torsades de pointes)

Management

Toxicity from tricyclic antidepressants requires immediate initiation of standard toxicological emergency procedures. Cardiac monitoring is critical since dysrhythmias are the most common cause of death. If you suspect a mixed overdose with benzodiazepines, do not use Flumazenil, since it may precipitate seizures. If significant cardiac toxicity occurs, sodium bicarbonate can be used as an additional therapy. Contact medical direction as necessary.

If you suspect a mixed overdose with benzodiazepines, do not use Flumazenil, since it may precipitate seizures.

MAO INHIBITORS

Monoamine oxidase inhibitors (MAOIs) have been used, although rarely, to treat depression. Recently they have been used, on a limited basis, to treat obsessive-compulsive disorders. They are relatively unpopular because of a narrow therapeutic index, multiple-drug interactions, serious interactions with foods containing *tyramine* (for example, red wine and cheese), and high morbidity and mortality when taken in overdose. These drugs inhibit the breakdown of neurotransmitters such as norepinephrine and dopamine while increasing the availability of the components needed to make even more neurotransmitters. When taken in overdose, MAOIs can be extremely dangerous, although symptoms may not appear for up to 6 hours.

Signs and Symptoms

Signs and symptoms of MAOI overdose include:

- Headache, agitation, restlessness, tremor
- Nausea
- Palpitations
- Tachycardia
- Severe hypertension
- Hyperthermia
- Eventually bradycardia, hypotension, coma, and death occur

New MAOIs have recently entered the marketplace. These next-generation drugs are reversible, less toxic, and do not have the same reactions with food as the older MAOIs. Data is not yet available on the outcome of patients overdosing with these newer agents.

Management

No antidote exists for MAOI overdose because the inhibition is not reversible except with newer drugs. Therefore, institute standard toxicological emergency procedures as soon as possible. If necessary, give symptomatic support for seizures and hyperthermia using benzodiazepines. If vasopressors are needed, use norepinephrine.

NEWER ANTIDEPRESSANTS

In recent years, several new agents have been developed to treat depression. Because of their high safety profile in therapeutic and overdose amounts, these drugs have been widely accepted and have virtually replaced tricyclic antidepressants.

Recently introduced drugs include trazodone (Desyrel), bupropion (Wellbutrin), and the large group of very popular *selective serotonin re-uptake inhibitors* (SSRIs) (Prozac, Luvox, Paxil, Zoloft). SSRIs prevent the re-uptake of serotonin in the brain, theoretically making it more available for brain functions. The true mechanism by which these drugs treat depression is unclear.

Signs and Symptoms

When these drugs are taken in overdose, usually the signs and symptoms are mild. Occasionally trazodone and buprorion will cause CNS depression and seizures, but deaths are very rare and have only been reported in mixed overdoses with multiple ingestions. More commonly, signs and symptoms of overdose with the newer antidepressant agents include:

- Drowsiness
- Tremor
- Nausea and vomiting
- Sinus tachycardia

SSRIs are now also associated with *serotonin syndrome*. This syndrome is caused by increased serotonin levels and is often triggered by increasing the dose of SSRI or adding a second drug such as Demerol, codeine, dextromethorphan (cough syrup), or other antidepressants. Signs and symptoms of serotonin syndrome include:

- Agitation, anxiety, confusion, insomnia
- Headache, drowsiness, coma
- Nausea, salivation, diarrhea, abdominal cramps
- Cutaneous piloerection, flushed skin
- Hyperthermia, tachycardia
- Rigidity, shivering, incoordination, myoclonic jerks

Management

Overdose with these new antidepressants is not as life threatening as with previous agents unless other drugs or alcohol are taken simultaneously. Consequently, treat overdoses with the standard toxicological emergency procedures. Also have the patient discontinue all serotonergic drugs and implement supportive measures. Benzodiazepines or beta blockers occasionally are used to improve patient comfort, but these are rarely given in the field.

LITHIUM

In the treatment of bipolar (manic-depressive) disorder, no other drug has been proven to be more effective than lithium. It is unclear how lithium exerts its therapeutic effect. However, as with tricyclic antidepressants, lithium has a narrow therapeutic index, which results in toxicity during normal use and in overdose situations.

Signs and Symptoms

Signs and symptoms of lithium toxicity include:

- Thirst, dry mouth
- Tremor, muscle twitching, increased reflexes
- Confusion, stupor, seizures, coma
- Nausea, vomiting, diarrhea
- Bradycardia, dysrhythmias

Management

Treat lithium overdose with mostly supportive measures. Use the standard toxicological emergency procedures, but remember that activated charcoal will not bind lithium and need not be given. Alkalinizing the urine with sodium bicarbonate and osmotic diuresis using mannitol may increase elimination of lithium, but severe toxic cases require hemodialysis.

SALICYLATES

Salicylates are some of the more common drugs taken in overdose, largely because they are readily available over the counter. The most recognizable forms are aspirin, oil of wintergreen, and some prescription combination medications.

Aspirin in large doses can cause serious consequences. About 300 mg/kg is required to cause toxicity. In such amounts, salicylates inhibit normal energy production and acid buffering in the body. This results in a metabolic acidosis, which further injures other organ systems.

Signs and Symptoms

Signs and symptoms of salicylate overdose include:

- Rapid respirations
- Hyperthermia
- Confusion, lethargy, coma
- Cardiac failure, dysrhythmias
- Abdominal pain, vomiting
- Pulmonary edema, adult respiratory distress syndrome (ARDS)

Chronic overdose symptoms are somewhat less severe and do not tend to include abdominal complaints. It is difficult to distinguish chronic overdose from very early acute overdose or early overdose that has progressed past the abdominal irritation stage.

Management

In all cases, salicylate poisoning should be treated using standard toxicological emergency procedures. Activated charcoal definitely reduces drug absorption and should be used. If possible, find out the time of ingestion, since blood levels measured at the right time can indicate the expected degree of injury. Most symptomatic patients will require generous IV fluids and may need urine alkalinization with sodium bicarbonate. Severe cases may require dialysis.

ACETAMINOPHEN

Due to its few side effects in normal dosages, acetaminophen (e.g., paracetamol, Tylenol) is one of the most common drugs in use today. It is used to treat fever and/or pain and is a common ingredient in hundreds of over-the-counter preparations. It can be also obtained by prescription in combination with various other drugs.

In large doses, however, acetaminophen can be a very dangerous pharmaceutical. A dose of 150 mg/kg is considered toxic and may result in death due to injury to the liver. A highly reactive by-product of acetaminophen metabolism is responsible for most adverse effects, but this is usually avoided by the body's detoxification system. When large amounts of acetaminophen enter the system, the detoxification system is overwhelmed and gradually depleted, leaving the toxic metabolite in the circulation to cause hepatic necrosis.

Signs and Symptoms

Signs and symptoms of acetaminophen toxicity appear in four stages:

Stage 1	½ hour to 24 hours	Nausea, vomiting, weakness, fatigue
Stage 2	24 to 48 hours	Abdominal pain, decreased urine, elevated liver enzymes
Stage 3	72 to 96 hours	Liver function disruption
Stage 4	4 to 14 days	Gradual recovery or progressive liver failure

Management

Treat acetaminophen overdose with standard toxicological emergency procedures. Find out the time of ingestion since blood levels taken at the right time can predict the potential for injury. An antidote called N-acetylcysteine (NAC, Mucomyst) is available and highly effective. However, NAC is usually administered based on clinical and laboratory studies and is rarely given in the prehospital setting.

OTHER NON-PRESCRIPTION PAIN MEDICATIONS

Non-steroidal anti-inflammatory drugs (NSAIDs) are another group of medications that are readily available and are often overdosed. Common examples include naproxen sodium, indomethacin, ibuprofen, and ketorolac (Toradol).

Signs and Symptoms

The presentation of toxicity caused by NSAIDs varies greatly but can include:

- Headache
- Ringing in the ears (tinnitus)
- Nausea, vomiting, abdominal pain
- Swelling of the extremities
- Mild drowsiness
- Dyspnea, wheezing, pulmonary edema
- Rash, itching

Management

There is no specific antidote for NSAID toxicity. Use general overdose procedures, including supportive care as soon as possible and transport to the emergency department for observation and any necessary symptomatic treatment.

Theophylline

Theophylline belongs to a group of medications called xanthines. It is usually used for patients with asthma or chronic obstructive pulmonary disease (COPD) because of its moderate bronchodilation and mild anti-inflammatory effects. As with other drugs with a narrow therapeutic index and high toxicity, theophylline has become less popular recently and therefore is not implicated in as many overdose injuries as in the past.

Signs and Symptoms

Symptoms of theophylline toxicity include:

- Agitation
- Tremors
- Seizures
- Cardiac dysrhythmias
- Nausea and vomiting

Management

Theophylline can cause significant morbidity and mortality. In overdose situations, it is essential that you institute toxicological emergency procedures immediately. In fact, theophylline is on the small list of drugs that have significant *entero-hepatic circulation*. This means that multiple doses of activated charcoal over time will continuously remove more and more of the drug from the body. Treat any dysrhythmias according to ACLS procedures.

Metals

With the exception of iron, overdose of heavy metals is a rare occurrence. Other possible involved metals include lead, arsenic, and mercury. All metals affect numerous enzyme systems within the body and therefore present with a variety of symptoms. Some also have direct local effects when ingested and when accumulated in various organs.

Iron

The body only requires small amounts of iron on a daily basis to maintain a sufficient store for enzyme and hemoglobin production. Excess amounts are easily obtained from nonprescription supplements and multi-vitamins. Children have a tendency to accidentally overdose on iron by taking too many candy-flavored chewable vitamins containing iron. To determine the amount of iron ingested, you must calculate the amount of elemental iron present in the type of pill ingested. Symptoms occur when more than 20 mg/kg of elemental iron are ingested.

Signs and Symptoms   Excess iron will cause gastrointestinal injury and possible shock from hemorrhage, especially if it forms *concretions* (lumps of iron formed when tablets fuse together after being swallowed). Patients with significant iron ingestions will often have visible tablets or concretions in the stomach or small intestine when an x-ray is taken. Other signs and symptoms of iron ingestion include:

- Vomiting (often hematemesis), diarrhea
- Abdominal pain, shock
- Liver failure
- Metabolic acidosis with tachypnea
- Eventual bowel scarring and possible obstruction

Management   It is essential to initiate standard toxicological emergency procedures immediately. Since iron tends to inhibit gastrointestinal motility, pills sit longer in the stomach and may possibly be easier to remove through gastric lavage. Because activated charcoal will not bind iron (or any metals), it should not be used. Deferoxamine, a chelating agent, may be used in iron overdose as an antidote since it binds to iron so that less is moved into cells and tissues to cause damage.

Lead and Mercury

Both lead and mercury are heavy metals found in varying amounts in the environment. Lead was often used in glazes and paints before the toxic potential of such exposure became apparent. Mercury is a contaminant from industrial processing but is also found in thermometers and temperature-control switches in most homes. Chronic and acute exposures are possible with both metals.

Signs and Symptoms   Signs and symptoms of heavy metal toxicity include:

- Headache, irritability, confusion, coma
- Memory disturbance
- Tremor, weakness, agitation
- Abdominal pain

Management   Chronic poisoning can cause permanent neurological injury, which makes it imperative that the proper agencies monitor heavy metal levels in the environment of a patient who has presented with toxicity. Learn to recognize the signs of heavy metal toxicity and institute standard toxicology emergency procedures as needed. Activated charcoal will not bind heavy metals but various chelating agents (DMSA, BAL, CDE) are available and may be used in definitive management in the hospital.

CONTAMINATED FOOD

Food poisoning is caused by a spectrum of different factors. For example, bacteria, viruses, and toxic chemicals notoriously produce varying levels of gastrointestinal distress. The patient may present with nausea, vomiting, diarrhea, and diffuse abdominal pain.

Bacterial food poisonings range in severity. Bacterial **exotoxins** (secreted by bacteria) or **enterotoxins** (exotoxins associated with gastrointestinal diseases, including food poisoning) cause the adverse gastrointestinal complaints noted previously. Food contaminated with other bacteria such as *Shigella, Salmonella,* or *E. coli* can produce even more severe gastrointestinal reactions, often leading to electrolyte imbalance and hypovolemia. *Clostridium botulinum,* the world's most toxic poison, presents as severe respiratory distress or arrest. The incubation of this toxin can range from 4 hours to 8 days. Fortunately, botulism rarely occurs, except in cases of improper food storage methods such as canning.

A variety of seafood poisonings are a result of specific toxins found in dinoflagellate contaminated shellfish such as clams, mussels, oysters, and scallops and can produce a syndrome referred to as *paralytic shellfish poisoning.* This condition can lead to respiratory arrest in addition to standard gastrointestinal symptoms.

Increased fish consumption by North Americans has also increased the number of cases of poisonings from toxins found in many commonly eaten fish. *Ciguatera (bony fish) poisoning* most frequently turns up in fish caught in the Pacific Ocean or along the tropical reefs of Florida and the West Indies. Ciguatera normally takes 2 to 6 hours to incubate and may produce myalgia and paresthesia. *Scombroid (histamine) poisoning* results from bacterial contamination of mackerel, tuna, bonitos, and albacore. Both types of poisoning cause the common gastrointestinal symptoms. Scombroid poisoning will present with an immediate facial flushing as histamines cause vasodilation.

Signs and Symptoms

As mentioned above, signs and symptoms of food poisoning may include:

- Nausea, vomiting, diarrhea, abdominal pain
- Facial flushing, respiratory distress (with some seafood poisonings)

Management

Except for botulism, food poisoning is rarely life threatening. Treatment, therefore, is largely supportive. In suspected cases of food poisoning, contact poison control and medical direction, and take the following steps:

---

exotoxin a soluble poisonous substance secreted during growth of a bacterium.

enterotoxin an exotoxin that produces gastrointestinal symptoms and diseases such as food poisoning.

- Perform the necessary assessment.
- Collect samples of the suspected contaminated food source.
- Perform the following management actions:
  - Establish and maintain the airway.
  - Administer high-flow, high-concentration oxygen.
  - Intubate and assist ventilations, if appropriate.
  - Establish venous access.
- Consider the administration of antihistamines (especially in seafood poisonings) and antiemetics.

POISONOUS PLANTS AND MUSHROOMS

Plants, trees, and mushrooms contribute heavily to the number of accidental toxic ingestions. Although the vast majority of plants are nontoxic, many of the popular decorative houseplants can present a danger to children, who frequently ingest non-food items. Most Poison Control Centers distribute pamphlets that identify toxic household plants. (These pamphlets will help "poison proof" the home.)

It is impossible to cover all the toxic plants and mushrooms. Few rescuers are trained as botanists, and they find it difficult to identify the offending material. Mushrooms are particularly difficult to identify from small pieces. Additionally, most people recognize mushrooms and other plants by common names rather than by the nomenclature of scientific species. A general approach is to obtain a sample of the plant, if possible. Try to find a full leaf, stem, and any flowers.

Since many ornamental plants contain irritating chemicals or crystals, examine the patient's mouth and throat for redness, blistering, or edema. Identify other abnormal signs during the focused physical exam.

Mushroom poisonings generally fall into two categories: people seeking edible mushrooms and accidental ingestions by children. Fortunately, few of the many mushroom species possess extremely dangerous toxins. Toxic mushrooms fall into seven classes. *Amanita* and *Galerina* belong to the deadly *cyclopeptide* group (Figure 23-3). (*Amanita* accounts for over 90% of all deaths.) These mushrooms produce a poison that is extremely toxic to the liver, with a mortality rate of about 50%.

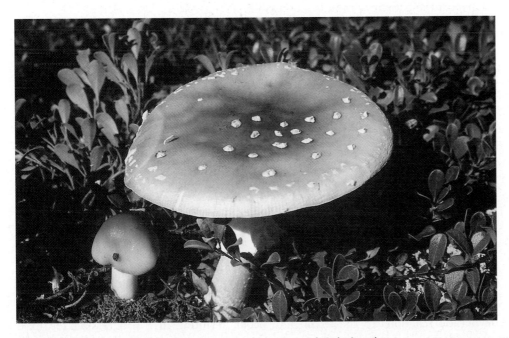

FIGURE 23-3 Poisonous mushrooms from *Amanita* and *Galerina* class.

Signs and Symptoms

Signs and symptoms of poisonous plant ingestion include:

- Excessive salivation, lacrimation (secretion of tears), diaphoresis
- Abdominal cramps, nausea, vomiting, diarrhea
- Decreasing levels of consciousness, eventually progressing to coma

Management

For guidance on the treatment of plant poisonings, call the Poison Control Center. If contact cannot be made, use the procedures outlined under treatment of food poisoning earlier.

INJECTED TOXINS

Although we generally think of intentional or accidental drug overdoses as sources of injected poisons, the most common source for these poisonings is the animal kingdom. Bites and stings from a variety of insects, reptiles, and animals are among the most common injuries sustained by humans. Further injury can result from bacterial contamination or from a reaction produced by an injected substance.

GENERAL PRINCIPLES OF MANAGEMENT

In case of a bite or sting, remember to protect rescue personnel. The offending organism may still be around.

The general principles of field management for bites and stings include:

- Protect rescue personnel—the offending organism may still be around.
- Remove the patient from danger of repeated injection, especially in the case of yellow jackets, wasps, or hornets.
- If possible, identify the insect, reptile, or animal that caused the injury and bring it to the emergency department along with the patient (if it can be done safely).
- Perform an initial assessment and rapid physical exam.
- Prevent or delay further absorption of the poison.
- Initiate supportive measures as indicated.
- Watch for anaphylactic reaction (see Chapter 5).
- Transport the patient as rapidly as possible.
- Contact the Poison Control Center and medical direction according to your local protocols.

INSECT BITES AND STINGS

Insect Stings

Many people die from allergic reactions to the stings from an order of insects known as *Hymenoptera*. As mentioned earlier, Hymenoptera includes wasps, bees, hornets, and ants. Only the common honeybee leaves a stinger. Wasps, yellow jackets, hornets, and fire ants sting repeatedly until removal from contact.

In most cases of insect bite, local treatment is all that is necessary. Unless an allergic reaction occurs, most patients will tolerate the isolated *Hymenoptera* sting.

Signs and Symptoms   Signs and symptoms include:

- Localized pain
- Redness
- Swelling
- Skin wheal

Idiosyncratic reactions to the toxin may occur, resulting in a progressing localized swelling and edema. This is not an allergic reaction, however, if it responds well to an antihistamine such as diphenhydramine hydrochloride. The major problem resulting from a

Hymenoptera sting is an allergic reaction or anaphylaxis. Signs and symptoms of allergic reaction include the following:

- Localized pain, redness, swelling, and a skin wheal
- Itching or flushing of the skin, rash
- Tachycardia, hypotension, bronchospasm, or laryngeal edema
- Facial edema, uvular swelling

Management For *Hymenoptera* stings, take the following supportive measures:

- Wash the area.
- Gently remove the stinger, if present, by scraping without squeezing the venom sac.
- Apply cool compresses to the injection site.
- Observe for and treat allergic reactions and/or anaphylaxis. (See Chapter 22.)

Brown Recluse Spider Bite

The brown recluse spider lives in the southern and midwestern states. It is found in large numbers in Tennessee, Arkansas, Oklahoma, and Texas. It has also been reported in Hawaii and California.

The brown recluse spider is about 15 mm in length. It generally lives in dark, dry locations and can often be found in and around the house. There is a characteristic violin-shaped marking on the back, giving the spider its nickname, "fiddleback spider" (Figure 23-4). Another identifying feature is the presence of six eyes (three pairs in a semicircle), instead of the eight eyes common to most spiders.

Signs and Symptoms Brown recluse spider bites are usually painless. Not uncommonly, bites occur at night while the patient sleeps. Most victims are unaware they have been bitten until the local reaction starts. Initially a small erythematous macule surrounded by a white ring forms at the site (Figure 23-5). This usually appears within a few minutes of the bite. Over the next 8 hours localized pain, redness, and swelling develop. Tissue necrosis at the site occurs over days to weeks (Figure 23-6). Other symptoms include chills, fever, nausea and vomiting, joint pain and in severe situations, bleeding disorders (disseminated intravascular coagulation).

Management Treatment is mostly supportive. Since there is no antivenin, the emergency department treatment consists of antihistamines to reduce systemic reactions and possible surgical excision of necrotic tissue.

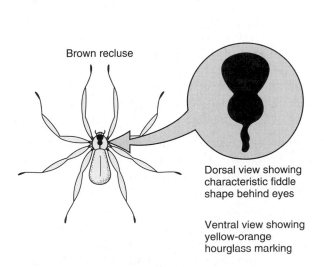

Brown recluse

Dorsal view showing characteristic fiddle shape behind eyes

Ventral view showing yellow-orange hourglass marking

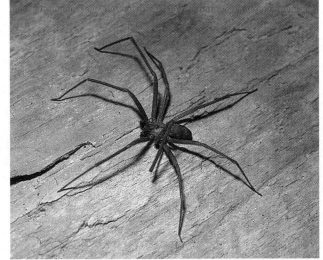

FIGURE 23-4 Brown recluse spider.

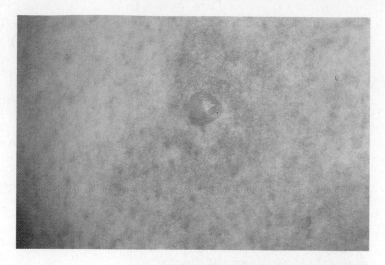

FIGURE 23-5 Brown recluse spider bite 24 hours after bite. Note the bleb and surrounding white halo. (Courtesy of Scott and White Hospital and Clinic)

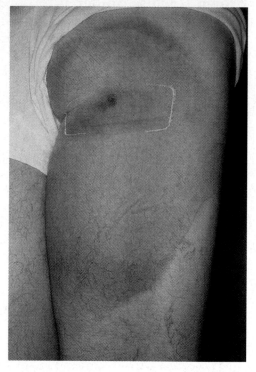

FIGURE 23-6 Brown recluse spider bite 4 days after the bite. Note the spread of erythema and early necrosis. (Courtesy of Scott and White Hospital and Clinic)

Black Widow Spider Bites

Black widow spiders live in all parts of the continental United States. They are usually found in woodpiles or brush. The female spider is responsible for bites and can be easily identified by the characteristic orange hourglass marking on her black abdomen (Figure 23-7). The venom of the black widow is very potent, causing excessive neurotransmitter release at the synaptic junctions.

Signs and Symptoms   Signs and symptoms of black widow spider bites start as immediate localized pain, redness, and swelling. Progressive muscle spasms of all large muscle groups can occur and are usually associated with severe pain. Other systemic symptoms include nausea, vomiting, sweating, seizures, paralysis, and decreased level of consciousness.

Management   Prehospital treatment is mostly supportive. It is important to reassure the patient. IV muscle relaxants may be necessary for severe spasms. With physician order you may use diazepam (2.5 to 10 mg IV) or calcium gluconate (0.1 to 0.2/kg of 10% solution IV). Note that calcium chloride is not effective and should not be used. Since hypertensive crisis is possible, monitor blood pressure carefully. Antivenin is available, so transfer the patient to the emergency department as soon as possible.

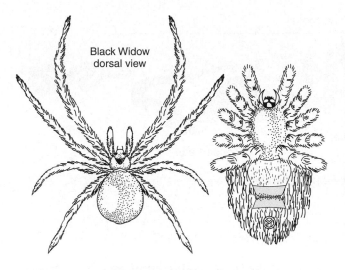

Black Widow
dorsal view

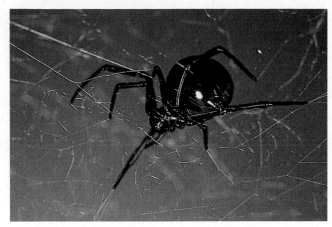

FIGURE 23-7   Black widow spider.

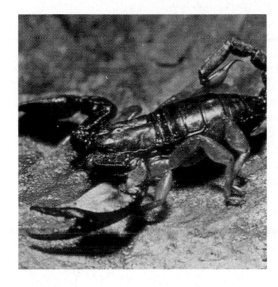

FIGURE 23-8   Scorpion.

Scorpion Stings

Many species of scorpion are found in the United States (Figure 23-8). All can sting, causing localized pain, but only one, the bark scorpion, has caused fatalities. These arthropods live mostly in Arizona and adjacent areas of California, Nevada, New Mexico, and Texas. There have been no deaths in Arizona from scorpion stings since 1970.

Scorpions move mostly at night, hiding in the day under debris and buildings. The venom they inject is stored in a bulb at the end of the tail. If provoked the scorpion will sting with its tail, injecting only a small amount of poison.

Signs and Symptoms   The bark scorpion's venom acts on the nervous system, producing a burning and tingling effect without much evidence of injury initially. Gradually this progresses to numbness. Systemic effects are more pronounced with slurred speech, restlessness (hyperactivity in 80% of children), muscle twitching, salivation, abdominal cramping, nausea and vomiting, and seizures.

Management   Begin treatment by reassuring the patient. Apply a constricting band above the wound site no tighter than a watchband to occlude lymphatic flow only. Avoid the use of analgesics, which may increase toxicity and potentiate the venom's effect on airway control. Transport the patient to the emergency department if systemic symptoms develop. Antivenin is available but is an unlicensed goat–serum–derived product found in Arizona only. It can produce allergic or anaphylactic reactions and should be used only in severe cases.

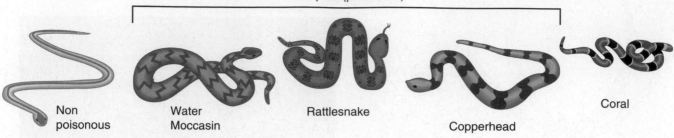

Non poisonous   Water Moccasin   Rattlesnake   Copperhead   Coral

FIGURE 23-9   Venomous snakes in the United States.

SNAKEBITES

Several thousand snakebites occur each year in the United States. Fortunately, these bites result in very few deaths. The signs and symptoms of snakebite depend upon the snake, the location of the bite, and the type and amount of venom injected.

There are two families of poisonous snakes native to the United States (Figure 23-9). One family (*Crotalidae*) includes the pit vipers. Common pit vipers are cottonmouths (water moccasins), rattlesnakes, and copperheads. Pit vipers are so named because of the distinctive pit between the eye and the nostril on each side of the head. These snakes have elliptical pupils, two well-developed fangs, and a triangular-shaped head. Only the rattlesnake, the most common pit viper, has rattles on the end of its tail.

The second family of poisonous snakes is the *Elapidae,* or coral snake, which is a distant relative of the cobra. Several varieties of coral snakes are found in the United States, primarily in the southwest. Because it is a small snake and has small fangs, the coral snake cannot readily attach itself to a large surface, such as an arm or leg. The coral snake has round eyes, a narrow head, and no pit. It has characteristic yellow-banded red and black rings around its body. Several nonpoisonous snakes, such as the King Snake, mimic this coloration pattern. Keep in mind a helpful mnemonic: "red touch yellow, kill a fellow; red touch black, venom lack." This rhyme indicates the distinctive pattern of the coral snake—a pattern that signals danger.

Pit Viper Bites

Pit viper venom contains hydrolytic enzymes that are capable of destroying proteins and most other tissue components. These enzymes may produce destruction of red blood cells and other tissue components and may affect the body's blood clotting system within the blood vessels. This will produce infarction and tissue necrosis, especially at the site of the bite.

A severe pit-viper bite can result in death from shock within 30 minutes. However, most deaths from pit-viper bites occur from 6 to 30 hours after the bite, with 90% occurring within the first 48 hours.

Signs and Symptoms   Signs and symptoms of pit viper bite include:

- Fang marks (often little more than a scratch mark or abrasion)
- Swelling and pain at the wound site
- Continued oozing at the wound site
- Weakness, dizziness, or faintness
- Sweating and/or chills
- Thirst
- Nausea and vomiting
- Diarrhea
- Tachycardia and hypotension
- Bloody urine and gastrointestinal hemorrhage (late)

- Ecchymosis
- Necrosis
- Shallow respirations progressing to respiratory failure
- Numbness and tingling around face and head (classic)

Management In treating a person who has been bitten by a pit viper, the primary goal is to slow absorption of the venom. Remember, about 25% of all rattlesnake bites are "dry" and no venom is injected. The amount of venom a pit viper injects varies significantly. It is helpful to try to classify the degree of envenomation:

Degree of Envenomation	Signs and Symptoms
None	None (either local or systemic)
Minimal	Swelling
	Pain
	No systemic symptoms
Moderate	Progressive swelling
	Mild systemic symptoms
	– paresthesias
	– nausea and vomiting
	– unusual tastes
	– mild hypotension
	– mild tachycardia
	– tachypnea
Severe	Swelling (spreading rapidly)
	Severe pain
	Systemic symptoms
	– altered mental status
	– nausea and vomiting
	– hypotension (systolic, 80)
	– severe tachycardia
	– severe respiratory distress
	Blood oozes freely from puncture wounds

Antivenin is available for the various common pit vipers found in the United States. However, antivenin should only be considered for severe cases where there is marked envenomation as evidenced by severe systemic symptoms. In some cases, people become more ill from the antivenin than they do from the snakebite itself. Routine emergency treatment of pit viper bites includes the following steps:

- Keep the patient supine.
- Immobilize the limb with a splint.
- Maintain the extremity in a neutral position. Do not apply constricting bands.

Initiate supportive care using the following guidelines:

- Apply high-flow, high-concentration oxygen.
- Start IV with crystalloid fluid.
- Transport the patient to the emergency department for management, which may include the administration of antivenin.

- DO NOT apply ice, cold pack, or freon spray to the wound.
- DO NOT apply an arterial tourniquet.
- DO NOT apply electrical stimulation from any device in an attempt to retard or reverse venom spread.

Coral Snake Bites

The venom of the coral snake contains some of the enzymes found in pit viper venom. However, because of the presence of neurotoxin, coral snake venom primarily affects nervous tissue. The classic, severe coral snake bite will result in respiratory and skeletal muscle paralysis.

Signs and Symptoms   After the bite of a coral snake, there may be no local manifestations or even any systemic effects for as long as 12 to 24 hours. Signs and symptoms of a coral snake bite include:

- Localized numbness, weakness, and drowsiness
- Ataxia
- Slurred speech and excessive salivation
- Paralysis of the tongue and larynx (produces difficulty breathing and swallowing)
- Drooping of eyelids, double vision, dilated pupils
- Abdominal pain
- Nausea and vomiting
- Loss of consciousness
- Seizures
- Respiratory failure
- Hypotension

Management   Treatment in cases of suspected coral snake bites includes the following steps:

- Wash the wound with copious amounts of water.
- Apply a compression bandage and keep the extremity at the level of the heart.
- Immobilize the limb with a splint.
- Start an IV using crystalloid fluid.
- Transport the patient to the emergency department for administration of antivenin.
- DO NOT apply ice, cold pack, or freon sprays to the wound.
- DO NOT incise the wound.
- DO NOT apply electrical stimulation from any device in an attempt to retard or reverse venom spread.

MARINE ANIMAL INJECTION

Although most dangerous marine life prefer warm, tropical waters, some can be found in more northern waters. With the large number of people who flock to beaches and coastal recreation areas every year, the number of injuries from marine life has increased moderately. The most common encounters occur while the person is walking on the beach but can also happen while wading in shallow waters or scuba diving in deeper waters. Injection of toxins from marine life can result from stings of jellyfish and corals or from punctures by the bony spines of animals such as sea urchins and stingrays (Figure 23-10). All venoms of marine animals contain substances that produce pain out of proportion to the size of the injury. These poisonous toxins are unstable and heat sensitive. Heat will relieve pain and inactivate the venom.

Both fresh water and salt water contain considerable bacterial and viral pollution. Therefore, secondary infection is always a possibility in injuries from marine animals. Particularly severe and life-threatening infections can be inflicted by a number of organisms. In all cases of marine-acquired infections, *Vibrio* species must be considered.

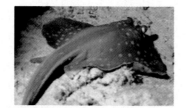

FIGURE 23-10   Stingray.

Signs and Symptoms Signs and symptoms of marine animal injection include:

- Intense local pain and swelling
- Weakness
- Nausea and vomiting
- Dyspnea
- Tachycardia
- Hypotension or shock (severe cases)

Management In suspected cases of marine animal injection, take the following steps:

- Establish and maintain the airway.
- Apply a constricting band between the wound and the heart no tighter than a watchband to occlude lymphatic flow only.
- Apply heat or hot water (110°F to 113°F).
- Inactivate or remove any stingers.

SUBSTANCE ABUSE AND OVERDOSE

Substance abuse, the use of a pharmacological substance for purposes other than medically defined reasons, is a very serious problem in our nation. Drugs are abused because they stimulate a feeling of euphoria in the abuser. Eventually, abusers begin to crave the feeling the drug gives them and therefore develop a *dependence* on the drug, also called **addiction.** An addiction exists when a person repeatedly uses and feels an overwhelming need to obtain and continue using a particular drug. Becoming accustomed to the use of the drug is called *habituation*. *Physiological dependence* is the resulting condition if removal of the drug causes adverse physical reactions. There can also be *psychological dependence*, in which use of the drug is required to prevent or relieve tension or emotional stress. With continued use, **tolerance** develops, which means that the abuser must use increasingly larger doses to get the same effect.

Attempts to stop the drug can trigger a psychological or physical reaction known as **withdrawal.** Withdrawal reactions can be quite unpleasant and severe. In some cases (especially with alcohol), withdrawal can be severe enough to cause death. These reactions further strengthen the victim's dependence on the drug. At this point the abuser may begin to withdraw from regular activities. He may have conflicts with family, friends, and coworkers as his

substance abuse use of a pharmacological substance for purposes other than medically defined reasons.

addiction compulsive and overwhelming dependence on a drug; may be physiological dependence, a psychological dependence, or both.

tolerance the need to progressively increase the dose of a drug to reproduce the effect originally achieved by smaller doses.

withdrawal referring to alcohol or drug withdrawal in which the patient's body reacts severely when deprived of the abused substance.

Patho Pearls

Prolonged exposure to many different drugs can result in addiction to and tolerance of the drug in question. Addiction is the continued use of the drug despite the fact that it may be harmful and serves no medical purpose. Tolerance describes the need for an increased amount of the drug to obtain effects previously obtained from a lower dose of the same drug. Addiction can be psychological, physical, or both. With addiction, patients will often use larger and larger quantities of the drug to get the euphoria they seek. As they become physically addicted, they will begin to suffer physical manifestations as the drug levels fall. This phenomenon is referred to as "withdrawal." Most drug withdrawals are very uncomfortable for the patient, but rarely life threatening. However, with alcohol and the benzodiapzepines, withdrawal can be potentially fatal and complicated by seizures and similar problems.

The symptoms of drug withdrawal vary depending on the drug involved. But, as a rule, withdrawal symptoms are usually the physiological opposite of those caused by the drug. For example, alcohol is a CNS depressant. Withdrawal from alcohol is characterized by CNS stimulation including anxiety, tremulousness, difficulty sleeping, hallucinations, and possibly seizures. Patients addicted to amphetamines, a CNS stimulant, experience a loss of energy, excessive sleepiness, slowed mentation, and similar symptoms. Thus, it is not necessary to memorize the various withdrawal syndromes—simply remember the physiological effects of the particular drug in question. Patients suffering physical withdrawal from those drugs often manifest symptoms exactly opposite of those caused by the drugs.

personality and priorities change. Often the abuser will be involved in criminal activities to support the habit. The abuser has formed an addiction at the point when the substance abuse begins to affect some part of his life. This includes affecting the abuser's health, work, or relationships. Also, the abuser begins to act in a manner so as to seek out the drug he abuses.

The National Institute on Drug Abuse performed a survey to estimate national use and exposure to illicit drugs. The results were astounding:

- 28 million people used illicit drugs at least once.
- 14.5 million use illicit drugs regularly.
- 20 million have tried cocaine.
- 860,000 people use cocaine weekly.
- 11.6 million use marijuana regularly.
- 770,000 use hallucinogens such as PCP or LSD regularly.
- 2.5 million have used heroin.

The use of illicit drugs has fluctuated in recent years. Most recently, heroin has regained popularity, especially among middle to upper class teenagers and young adults. Beyond hurting themselves, substance abusers are eighteen times more likely to be involved in criminal activities. These include violent crimes as well as theft to support drug habits. (The Secretary of Health and Human Services has estimated that cocaine is a $65 billion per year industry.)

> **drug overdose** poisoning from a pharmacological substance in excess of that usually prescribed or that the body can tolerate.

In general terms, **drug overdose** refers to poisoning from a pharmacological substance, either legal or illegal. This can occur by accident, miscalculation, changes in the strength of a drug, suicide, polydrug use, or recreational drug usage. Many overdose emergencies seen in the field occur in the habitual drug abuser. It is most difficult to obtain a good history in these cases. However, if the EMT-I is familiar with street-drug slang, a more accurate history may be obtained. It is imperative that the EMT-I maintain a nonjudgmental attitude in these cases, even though this may be difficult.

The presentation of the drug overdose will vary based on the substance used. Management should be the same as for any ingested, inhaled, or injected poison. Poison control should be contacted for additional direction.

DRUGS OF ABUSE

Drugs Commonly Abused

Drugs of abuse are both common and dangerous. These drugs all have various signs and symptoms and require supportive treatment and general toxicological emergency management. Refer to Table 23-3 for further details on what you may find on assessment and the interventions required.

Remember these specific guidelines for patients who have taken the following drugs:

- *Alcohol*—May require thiamine and $D_{50}W$ for hypoglycemia.
- *Cocaine*—Benzodiazepines (diazepam) may be needed for sedation and to treat seizures. Beta blockers are absolutely contraindicated because unopposed alpha receptor stimulation can cause cardiac ischemia, hypertension, and hyperthermia.
- *Narcotics/Opiates*—Naloxone is effective in reversing respiratory depression and sedation, but be careful, since it may trigger a withdrawal reaction in chronic opiate abusers.
- *Amphetamines*—Use benzodiazepines (diazepam) for seizures and in combination with haloperidol for hyperactivity.
- *Hallucinogens*—Use benzodiazepines for seizures and in combination with haloperidol for hyperactivity.
- *Benzodiazepines*—Use flumazenil to counteract adverse effects. Be careful not to trigger a withdrawal syndrome with seizures.
- *Barbiturates*—Forced diuresis and alkalinization of the urine improve elimination of barbiturates from the body.

Table 23-3 COMMON DRUGS OF ABUSE

Drug	Signs and Symptoms	Routes	Prehospital Management
Alcohol			
beer whiskey gin vodka wine tequila	CNS depression Slurred speech Disordered thought Impaired judgment Diuresis Stumbling gait Stupor Coma	Oral	ABCs Respiratory support Oxygenate Establish IV access Administer 100 mg thiamine IV ECG monitor Check glucose level Administer $D_{50}W$, if hypoglycemic
Barbiturates			
thiopental phenobarbital primidone	Lethargy Emotional lability Incoordination Slurred speech Nystagmus Coma Hypotension Respiratory depression	Oral IV	ABCs Respiratory support Oxygenate Establish IV access ECG monitor Contact Poison Control—may order bicarbonate
Cocaine			
crack rock	Euphoria Hyperactivity Dilated pupils Psychosis Twitching Anxiety Hypertension Tachycardia Dysrhythmias Seizures Chest pain	Snorting Injection Smoking (freebasing)	ABCs Respiratory support Oxygenate ECG monitor Establish IV access Treat life-threatening dysrhythmias Seizure precautions: diazepam 5–10 mg
Narcotics			
heroin codeine meperidine morphine hydromorphone pentazocine Darvon Darvocet methadone	CNS depression Constricted pupils Respiratory depression Hypotension Bradycardia Pulmonary edema Coma Death	Oral Injection	ABCs Respiratory support Oxygenate Establish IV access Administer 1–2 mg naloxone IV or endotracheally as ordered by medical direction until respirations improve* Larger than average doses (2–5 mg) have been used in the management of Darvon overdose and alcoholic coma ECG monitor

*With the advent of the opiate antagonist naloxone, narcotic overdosage became easier to manage. It is possible to titrate this effective medication to increase respirations to normal levels without fully awakening the patient. In the case of narcotics addicts, this prevents hostile and confrontational episodes.

Continued

| Table 23-3 | COMMON DRUGS OF ABUSE (CONTINUED) |

Drug	Signs and Symptoms	Routes	Prehospital Management
Marijuana			
grass	Euphoria	Smoked	ABCs
weed	Dry mouth	Oral	Reassure the patient
hashish	Dilated pupils		Speak in a quiet voice
	Altered sensation		ECG monitor if indicated
Amphetamines			
Benzedrine	Exhilaration	Oral	ABCs
Dexedrine	Hyperactivity	Injection	Oxygenate
Ritalin	Dilated pupils		ECG monitor
"speed"	Hypertension		Establish IV access
	Psychosis		Treat life-threatening dysrhythmias
	Tremors		Seizure precautions: diazepam 5–10 mg
	Seizures		
Hallucinogens			
LSD	Psychosis	Oral	ABCs
STP	Nausea	Smoked	Reassure the patient
mescaline	Dilated pupils		"Talk down" the "high" patient
psilocybin	Rambling speech		Protect the patient from injury
PCP†	Headache		Provide a dark, quiet environment
	Dizziness		Speak in a soft, quiet voice
	Suggestibility		Seizure precautions: diazepam 5–10 mg
	Distortion of sensory perceptions		
	Hallucinations		
Sedatives			
Seconal	Altered mental status	Oral	ABCs
Valium	Hypotension		Respiratory support
Librium	Slurred speech		Oxygenate
Xanax	Respiratory depression		Establish IV access
Halcion	Shock		ECG monitor
Restoril	Bradycardia		Medical direction may order naloxone
Dalmane	Seizures		
Phenobarbital			
Benzodiazepines‡			
Valium	Altered mental status	Oral	ABCs
Librium	Slurred speech		Respiratory support
Xanax	Dysrhythmias		Oxygenate
Halcion	Coma		Activated charcoal as ordered by medical direction
Restoril			Establish IV access
Dalmane			ECG monitor
Centrax			Contact Poison Control Center
Ativan			
Serax			

†Although PCP was originally an animal tranquilizer, it manifests hallucinogenic properties when used by humans. In addition to bizarre delusions, it can cause violent and dangerous outbursts of aggressive behavior. The rescuer is advised to remain safe when attempting to treat this type of overdose. PCP patients have been known to have almost superhuman strength and high pain tolerance.

‡Deaths due to pure benzodiazepine are rare. Minor toxicity ranges are 500–1,500 mg. A benzodiazepine antagonist (Romazicon) is available (IV dosage 1–10 mg or infusion 0.5 mg/hr). It may cause seizures in a benzodiazepine-dependent patient.

Drugs Used for Sexual Purposes

A number of drugs deserve mention as a separate category. These drugs are used to stimulate and enhance the sexual experience, but without medically approved indications for such use. *Ecstasy,* also called MDMA, is one such drug. Ecstasy is a modified form of methamphetamines and has similar, although milder effects. It is very popular in today's university and nightclub environments.

Use of Ecstasy initially causes anxiety, nausea, tachycardia, and elevated blood pressure, followed by relaxation, euphoria, and feelings of enhanced emotional insight. No definitive data exists as to whether the experience of sexual intercourse is improved. Studies show that prolonged use may cause brain damage. Some deaths from MDMA ingestion have been reported. These cases present with confusion, agitation, tremor, high temperature, and diarrhea. No specific treatment exists. Standard supportive measures should be initiated.

Rohypnol (flunitrazepam) is another drug abused for sexual purposes. Illegal in the United States, it is commonly called the "date rape drug," since it can be secretly slipped into a woman's drink. This drug is a strong benzodiazepine similar to diazepam, lorazepan, and midazolam. The resulting sedation and amnesia allows the perpetrator to rape the victim. Treatment is the same as for any benzodiazepine, but consequences of the sexual assault require attention as well.

ALCOHOL ABUSE

Alcohol is the most common substance of abuse in the United States and most of the world. Almost 75% of people in the United States have at least one drink per year, with the average person consuming 2.5 gallons of pure ethanol every year. Alcohol has been linked to 5% of deaths in the United States. Alcoholism costs over $100 billion per year due to lost work time and medical costs to treat complications and injuries. Alcoholism progresses in much the same way as drug dependence, discussed earlier.

PHYSIOLOGICAL EFFECTS

Alcohol (ethyl alcohol, or ethanol) depresses the central nervous system, potentially to the point of stupor, coma, and death. In patients with severe liver disease, metabolism of alcohol may become impaired, which increases the course and severity of intoxication. At low doses, alcohol has excitatory and stimulating effects, thus depressing inhibitions. At higher doses alcohol's depressive effect is more obvious. Alcohol abuse and dependence is called *alcoholism.* It is a major problem, contributing to highway traffic fatalities, drownings, burns, trauma, and drug overdoses.

Alcohol is completely absorbed from the stomach and intestinal tract in approximately 30 to 120 minutes after ingestion. Once absorbed, alcohol is distributed to all body tissues and fluids, with concentrations of alcohol in the brain rapidly approaching the alcohol level in the blood.

Some alcoholics will drink methanol (wood alcohol) or ethylene glycol (a component of antifreeze) if ethanol is unavailable. Ingestion of these chemicals can cause blindness or death.

In addition, alcohol causes a peripheral vasodilator effect on the cardiovascular system, resulting in flushing and a feeling of warmth. In cold conditions, alcohol's dilation of the blood vessels results in an increased loss of body heat. The diuretic effect seen when large amounts of alcohol are ingested is due to the inhibition of *vasopressin,* which is the hormone responsible for the conservation of body fluids. Without vasopressin, an increase in urine flow occurs. The "dry mouth syndrome" experienced after alcohol consumption may be the result of alcohol-induced cellular dehydration.

In addition, methanol will also cause visual disturbances, abdominal pain, and nausea and vomiting even at low doses. In fact, death has been reported after ingestion of only 15 mL of a 40% solution. Occasionally patients will complain of headache or dizziness and may even present with seizures and obtundation. Ethylene glycol ingestion has similar symptoms, but the central nervous system effects such as hallucinations, coma, and seizures are more pronounced in the early stages.

GENERAL ALCOHOLIC PROFILE

The classic alcoholic portrayed in movies is an unkempt, continually intoxicated street person who is completely non-functional. Although alcoholics of this type exist, it would be a grave error to consider this the typical picture of someone dependent on alcohol. More commonly, alcoholism is characterized by impaired control over drinking, preoccupation with the drug ethanol, use of ethanol despite adverse consequences, and distortions in thinking, such as denial. This is the definition used by the National Council on Alcoholism and Drug Dependence. Obviously, this definition applies to many people, including many functional people at all levels of society who have masked their addiction well. Take note of these warning signs, which may indicate alcohol abuse:

- Drinks early in the day
- Prone to drink alone and secretly
- Periodic binges (may last for several days)
- Partial or total loss of memory ("blackouts") during period of drinking
- Unexplained history of gastrointestinal problems (especially bleeding)
- "Green tongue syndrome" (using chlorophyll-containing substances to disguise the odor of alcohol on the breath)
- Cigarette burns on clothing
- Chronically flushed face and palms
- Tremulousness
- Odor of alcohol on breath under inappropriate conditions

CONSEQUENCES OF CHRONIC ALCOHOL INGESTION

Alcohol has many deleterious effects on the body. Chronic abuse can be devastating, effecting every organ system as shown in Figure 23-11. Some of the more common effects include:

- Poor nutrition
- Alcohol hepatitis
- Liver cirrhosis with subsequent esophageal varices
- Loss of sensation in hands and feet
- Loss of cerebellar function (balance and coordination)
- Pancreatitis
- Upper gastrointestinal hemorrhage (often fatal)
- Hypoglycemia
- Subdural hematoma (due to falls)
- Rib and extremity fractures (due to falls)

Conditions such as subdural hematomas, sepsis, diabetic ketoacidosis, and others may mimic signs and symptoms of alcohol intoxication.

Keep in mind that conditions such as subdural hematomas, sepsis, and other life-threatening disease processes may mimic the signs and symptoms of alcohol intoxication. For example, diabetic ketoacidosis produces a breath odor that can easily be confused with the odor of alcohol.

Withdrawal Syndrome

delirium tremens (DTs) disorder found in habitual and excessive users of alcoholic beverages after cessation of drinking for 48 to 72 hours. Patients experience visual, tactile, and auditory disturbances. Death may result in severe cases.

The alcoholic may suffer a withdrawal reaction from either abrupt discontinuation of ingestion after prolonged use or from a rapid fall in blood-alcohol level after acute intoxication. Alcohol withdrawal can be potentially fatal. Withdrawal symptoms can occur several hours after sudden abstinence and can last up to 5 to 7 days. Seizures (sometimes called "rum fits") may occur within the first 24 to 36 hours of abstinence. **Delirium tremens (DTs)** usually develops on the second or third day of the withdrawal. Delirium tremens is characterized by a decreased level of consciousness during which the patient hallucinates and misinterprets

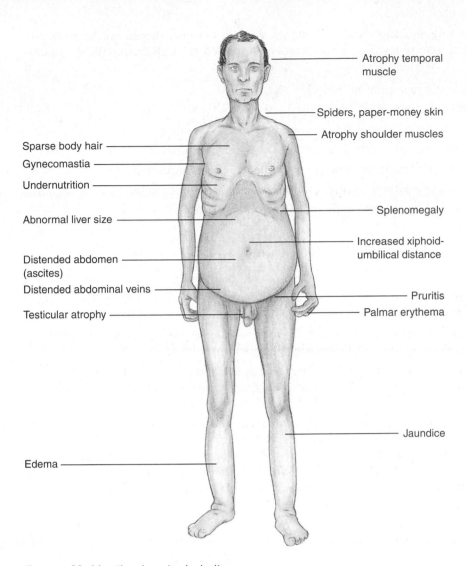

Atrophy temporal muscle

Spiders, paper-money skin

Atrophy shoulder muscles

Sparse body hair

Gynecomastia

Undernutrition

Abnormal liver size

Distended abdomen (ascites)

Distended abdominal veins

Testicular atrophy

Splenomegaly

Increased xiphoid-umbilical distance

Pruritis

Palmar erythema

Jaundice

Edema

FIGURE 23-11   The chronic alcoholic.

nearby events. Seizures and delirium tremens are ominous signs. There is a significant mortality from delirium tremens. Medical direction may order diazepam in severe cases.

Signs and Symptoms   Signs and symptoms of withdrawal syndrome include:

- Coarse tremor of hands, tongue, and eyelids
- Nausea and vomiting
- General weakness
- Increased sympathetic tone
- Tachycardia
- Sweating
- Hypertension
- Orthostatic hypotension
- Anxiety
- Irritability or a depressed mood
- Hallucinations
- Poor sleep

Management Alcohol intoxication, whether acute or chronic, should not be underestimated as a toxic emergency problem. In cases of suspected alcohol abuse, take the following steps:

- Establish and maintain the airway.
- Determine if other drugs are involved.
- Start an IV using lactated Ringer's solution or normal saline.
- Chemstrip and administer 25 grams of $D_{50}W$ if hypoglycemic.
- Administer 100 mg of thiamine intravenously or intramuscularly.
- Maintain a sympathetic attitude and reassure the patient of help.
- Transport to the emergency department for further care.

SUMMARY

Clearly, there is much to remember when dealing with toxicological emergencies. To effectively manage these situations you must focus on three things:

- Recognize the poisoning promptly. In other words, you must have a high index of suspicion when circumstances suggest a toxin may be involved.

- Be thorough in your initial assessment and evaluation of the patient. This will facilitate your efforts to identify the toxin and the measures needed to control the situation.

- Initiate the standard treatment procedures required for all toxicological emergencies. Beyond the usual concern for rescuer safety and rapid implementation of ABCs and supportive measures, consider the methods needed to minimize any further exposure to the toxin, decontaminate the patient from the toxins already involved, and finally administer any useful antidote if one exists for the particular toxin.

If you remember these three steps, you will be equipped to handle most toxicological emergencies promptly and efficiently.

ON THE WEB

For additional practice and review, go to the companion website at www.prenhall.com/bledsoe and click on *Intermediate Emergency Care: Principles & Practice.*

CHAPTER 24

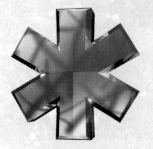

Neurological Emergencies

Objectives

After reading this chapter, you should be able to:

1. Define and discuss the epidemiology (including the morbidity/mortality and preventative strategies), pathophysiology, assessment findings, and management for the following neurologic problems:
   a. Coma and altered mental status (pp. 1018–1019)
   b. Seizures (pp. 1025–1029)
   c. Syncope (pp. 1029–1031)
   d. Headache (pp. 1030–1031)
   e. Weakness/dizziness (pp. 1031–1032)
   f. Stroke (pp. 1020–1025)
   g. Intracranial hemorrhage (p. 1021)
   h. Transient ischemic attack (pp. 1023–1025)
2. Describe and differentiate the major types of seizures. (pp. 1025–1027)

3. Describe the phases of a generalized seizure. (pp. 1025–1026)
4. Define and discuss the pathophysiology, assessment findings, and management for nontraumatic spinal injury, including:
   a. Low back pain (p. 1032)
   b. Herniated intervertebral disk (pp. 1032–1033)
   c. Spinal-cord tumors (p. 1033)
5. Differentiate between neurologic emergencies based on assessment findings. (pp. 1010–1017)
6. Given several preprogrammed nontraumatic neurological emergency patients, provide the appropriate assessment, management, and transport. (pp. 1010–1034)

CASE STUDY

A call is received by Engine Company 201 and Ambulance 68 for a "possible stroke patient." Dispatch reports that the patient is a male in his 60s with reported right-sided weakness and inability to speak. He is being assisted by bystanders in the lobby of a local bank. The response time is approximately 3 minutes. Upon arrival, the bank manager leads EMT-Is Jack Tory and Linda Alvarez to a corner area of the lobby where they see an elderly male sitting in a chair and being held upright by bystanders.

Jack and Linda quickly perform an initial assessment. Although unable to speak, the patient appears to be alert and cooperative. His airway is patent. His respiratory rate is 18 breaths per minute and regular. His pulse is 88 beats per minute and strong. The blood pressure is 160/90 mmHg taken in the left arm (because of the weakness in his right arm). The patient's skin is warm and dry, yet pale. The blood glucose level is 80 mg/dL. He has marked right-sided weakness but otherwise appears to be well nourished and in good overall health.

Jack quickly administers oxygen via nonrebreather mask while Linda obtains a more detailed medical history from the patient's family. Linda places a saline lock in the patient's left forearm while Jack places the electrocardiogram (ECG) leads and turns on the monitor. The patient exhibits atrial fibrillation with a rate of 90. Linda applies the pulse oximeter. The patient appears to be well oxygenated with an SpO$_2$ of 99% on the nonrebreather mask. Jack and Linda move the patient to a stretcher, being careful to protect the paralyzed extremity. They load the patient into the ambulance and transport him to the nearest emergency department with a "brain attack team."

Upon arrival at the emergency department, the patient's condition remains unchanged. His airway remains patent and his symptoms persist. A routine laboratory profile is normal. Because the patient has a hemiparesis and is unable to speak, the emergency physician orders a computed tomography (CT) scan of the brain. A neuroradiologist reads the CT scan and reports no evidence of hemorrhage in the brain. The brain attack team is consulted. They feel that thrombolytic therapy is indicated and tPA is started in the emergency department by the consulting neurologist. The patient is then admitted to the neurologic intensive care unit.

Following thrombolytic therapy, the patient recovers his speech, and most of his right-sided weakness is alleviated. Several days later, the patient is discharged to the rehabilitation unit.

INTRODUCTION

Nervous system conditions and diseases affect millions of lives in the United States. Strokes attack a half million people every year, of whom 150,000 die. Epilepsy affects 2.5 million people, or approximately 1% of the United States population. An additional 50,000 people in the United States are diagnosed with Parkinson's disease each year. These are only a few examples of the impact of nervous system disorders.

Many conditions, diseases, and injuries can cause nervous system disorders. Such disorders may be caused by internal or external factors. Modern advances and clinical studies continue to yield new medications and treatments for many conditions. EMT-Is should maintain a solid knowledge of the nervous system and remain familiar with current trends and advancements in treating the neurological patient.

This chapter provides an overview of the common neurological conditions that may be encountered in the prehospital setting. It discusses the relevant pathophysiology of the nervous system, assessment techniques, and the recommended prehospital management. Figure 24–1 provides an overview of the central and peripheral nervous systems.

PATHOPHYSIOLOGY

A firm grasp of the pathophysiology of nontraumatic neurologic emergencies is essential in order for the EMT-I to provide appropriate and timely emergency care.

ALTERATION IN COGNITIVE SYSTEMS

Consciousness is a condition in which an individual is fully responsive to stimuli and demonstrates awareness of the environment. The ability to respond to stimuli depends on

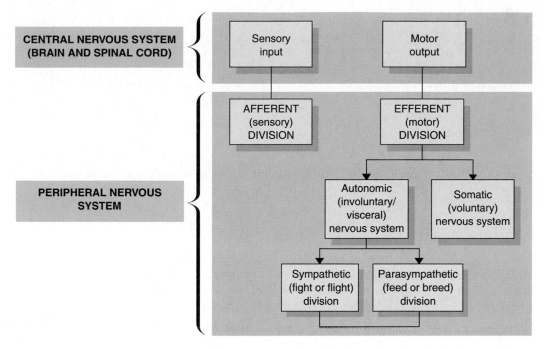

FIGURE 24-1 Overview of the nervous system.

an intact reticular activating system (RAS). Cognition and the ability to respond to the environment rely on an intact cerebral cortex. Therefore, altered forms of consciousness can result from dysfunction or interruption of the central nervous system.

CENTRAL NERVOUS SYSTEM DISORDERS

An alteration in mental status is the hallmark sign of CNS injury or illness. Any alteration in mental status is abnormal and warrants further examination. Alterations may vary from minor thought disturbances to unconsciousness. Unconsciousness, also called **coma,** is a state in which the patient cannot be aroused, even by powerful external stimuli. Generally, two mechanisms are capable of producing alterations in mental status:

- *Structural lesions.* Structural lesions (e.g., tumors, contusions) depress consciousness by destroying or encroaching on the substance of the brain. Examples of causes of structural lesions include brain tumor (neoplasm), degenerative disease, intracranial hemorrhage, parasites, and trauma.

- *Toxic-metabolic states.* Toxic-metabolic states involve either the presence of circulating toxins or metabolites or the lack of metabolic substrates (oxygen, glucose, or thiamine). These states produce diffuse depression of both sides (hemispheres) of the cerebrum, with or without depression within the brainstem. Various causes of toxic-metabolic states include anoxia (lack of oxygen), diabetic ketoacidosis, hepatic failure, hypoglycemia, renal failure, thiamine deficiency, and toxic exposure (e.g., cyanide, organophosphates).

Within the two general mechanisms (structural lesions and toxic metabolic states), there are many difficult-to-classify causes of altered mental status. Some of the more common causes are listed in the following four general categories:

- Drugs
  - Depressants (including alcohol)
  - Hallucinogens
  - Narcotics
- Cardiovascular
  - Anaphylaxis
  - Cardiac arrest

An alteration in mental status is the hallmark sign of central nervous system (CNS) injury or illness.

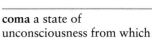

coma a state of unconsciousness from which the patient cannot be aroused.

- Stroke
- Dysrhythmias
- Hypertensive encephalopathy
- Shock
- Respiratory
  - Chronic obstructive pulmonary disease (COPD)
  - Inhalation of toxic gas
  - Hypoxia
- Infectious
  - Acquired immunodeficiency syndrome (AIDS)
  - Encephalitis
  - Meningitis

CEREBRAL HOMEOSTASIS

The autonomic nervous system (ANS) maintains cerebral homeostasis (internal balance) and regulates and coordinates the body's vital functions, such as blood pressure, temperature regulation, respiration, and metabolism. It can be strongly affected by emotional influences, resulting in blushing, palpitations, clammy hands, and dry mouth.

GENERAL ASSESSMENT FINDINGS

SCENE SIZE-UP AND INITIAL ASSESSMENT

A great deal of crucial information can be obtained while approaching the patient. Size up the scene and the surroundings as well as the patient to form a general impression. Is there evidence of toxic exposure or trauma? Look for clues that can indicate a patient's condition, such as:

- *General appearance.* Is the patient conscious? Alert? Confused? Sitting upright?
- *Speech.* Can the patient speak? Clearly and coherently? In full sentences? Is the speech slurred?
- *Skin.* Color (pink, pale, cyanotic?) Temperature (warm, hot, cool?) Moisture (diaphoretic, clammy?)
- *Face.* Is facial drooping present?
- *Posture/gait.* Upright? Leaning? Staggered? Steady gait?

Next, quickly check the patient's mental status using the "AVPU" method:

A—*Alert and aware of his surroundings.* A patient alert and orientated to time, place, person, and one's own person, is said to be "alert and oriented times four." Remember, no patient is "oriented" unless he has answered the questions that the EMT-I has to ask.

V—*Responds to verbal stimuli.* The patient responds when talked to, perhaps in a loud voice. Note if the patient delivers the answers normally or sluggishly. Also observe whether the patient has purposeful or uncoordinated movements.

P—*Responds to painful stimuli.* The patient responds when tactile stimulation is used, such as a sternal rub, a squeeze of the trapezius muscle, or pinching the thenar (thumb) web space.

U—*Unresponsive.* The patient is not alert and does not respond to verbal or painful stimuli.

Assessment of cerebral functioning also includes assessing the patient's emotional status. If the patient is conscious, you can detect changes in the following:

- *Mood.* Is the patient's affect natural or is the patient irritable, anxious, or apathetic? Does the patient appear depressed? manic? happy? solemn? reserved?

- *Thought.* What is the patient's thought pattern? Is it logical? appropriate? scattered?

- *Perception.* How does the patient perceive his surroundings? Are his interactions appropriate?

- *Judgment.* Is the patient using reasonable and sound judgment? Is he logical?

- *Memory and attention.* Is short-term memory present? long-term memory? Question family members or caregivers to obtain this information. Does the patient maintain conversation? Pay attention? Repeatedly ask or answer questions?

Any alteration from the patient's normal mental status or mood should be considered significant and warrants additional assessment.

Once a patient's level of consciousness is determined, place the greatest emphasis on maintenance of the airway. If the patient is unconscious, assume that a cervical spine injury exists and treat it appropriately. Use the modified jaw-thrust maneuver to open the airway. Once opened, insert the appropriate airway adjunct. In unresponsive patients, the tongue may be occluding the airway. In such cases, you may need only to place an oropharyngeal or nasopharyngeal airway to maintain the airway. If the patient tolerates an oropharyngeal airway, consider intubation.

Vigilantly monitor the airway in any patient with CNS injury. It is essential to observe for respiratory arrest that can result from increased intracranial pressure. Remain alert for an absent gag reflex and vomiting. In addition, blood from facial injuries and possible aspiration of gastric contents further threaten the patient's airway.

Observe the patient for any signs and symptoms of inadequate or impaired breathing or the presence of any abnormal respiratory patterns. Remember, the body's breathing center is located in the brain. Certain neurological conditions can cause these areas to malfunction and limit the patient's ability to breathe.

Complete assessment of the body's circulatory status is also a crucial part of the initial assessment. Evaluation of the heart rate, rhythm, and ECG pattern can shed light on the body's overall state of perfusion. Observe the patient's skin color, temperature, and moisture for abnormal findings such as cyanosis and moisture. A healthy adult's skin is usually warm, dry, and pink.

FOCUSED HISTORY AND PHYSICAL EXAM

Following completion of the initial assessment and correction of any immediate threats to the patient's life, turn your attention to the focused history and physical exam. This assessment should include an accurate history and a physical exam, including vital signs. Remember that any indications of nervous system dysfunction should cause you to place particular emphasis on neurological evaluation. Neurological evaluation will be detailed under "Nervous System Status" later in this chapter.

History

A thorough, accurate history of a patient is crucial in determining the current problem and subsequent treatment of a patient. One of the first steps in obtaining a thorough history involves attempting to determine whether the neurological problem is traumatic or medical. Clarification will help determine the plan for subsequent prehospital treatment. The initial history may not be easy to obtain because of the patient's altered mental status. In these cases, it is critical for you to obtain information from family, friends, or other bystanders, if available.

If the neurological emergency is due to trauma, ask the following questions:

- When did the incident occur?
- How did the incident occur, or what is the mechanism of injury?

- Was there any loss of consciousness?
- Was there evidence of incontinence? (Incontinence suggests loss of consciousness.)
- What is the patient's chief complaint?
- Has there been any change in symptoms?
- Are there any complicating factors?

If there is no evidence of a traumatic cause of the neurological emergency, ask the following questions to determine the nature of illness:

- What is the chief complaint?
- What are the details of the present illness, or the nature of the illness?
- Is there a pertinent underlying medical problem, such as cardiac disease, chronic seizures, diabetes, hypertension?
- Have these symptoms occurred before?
- Are there any environmental clues? These may include evidence of current medications, medical identification tag, alcohol bottles or drug paraphernalia, chemicals, hazardous materials.

Physical Examination

The physical examination of a patient with a neurological emergency should include the standard head-to-toe examination and a more detailed neurological assessment. Pay particular attention to the pupils, respiratory status, and spinal evaluation.

Face A patient's ability to smile, frown, and wrinkle his forehead indicates an intact facial nerve (cranial nerve VII). If the patient is conscious, test these abilities. Note any drooping or facial paralysis.

Eyes The pupils are controlled by the oculomotor nerve (cranial nerve III). This nerve follows a long course through the skull and is easily compressed by brain swelling. While slight pupillary inequality is normal, abnormal pupils can be an early indicator of increasing intracranial pressure. If both pupils are dilated and do not react to light, the patient probably has a brainstem injury or has suffered serious brain anoxia. If the pupils are dilated but still react to light, the injury may be reversible. However, the patient must be transported quickly to an emergency facility capable of treating CNS injuries. A unilaterally dilated pupil that remains reactive to light may be the earliest sign of increasing intracranial pressure. The patient with altered mental status who presents with or develops a unilaterally dilated pupil is in the "immediate transport" category. Constricted, or pinpoint, pupils suggest a toxic etiology for the altered mental status.

A common method of assessing extraocular movement is to have the patient follow finger movements. For example, ask the patient to follow your finger to the extreme left, then up, then down. Repeat the same motions to the extreme right. These positions are referred to as the cardinal positions of gaze. Because extraocular movements are controlled by cranial nerves III (oculomotor), IV (trochlear), and VI (abducens), inability to look in all directions with both eyes can be an early indication of a CNS problem. This is particularly important in the indication of facial trauma.

When examining a patient's pupils, it is important to check for contact lenses. Contact lenses, if present, should be removed and placed into their container or a saline solution and transported with the patient.

Nose/Mouth In the presence of facial paralysis, drooping of the patient's mouth may occur. Pay particular attention to any of these changes that may potentially compromise the patient's airway. A common way to assess for mouth droop is to ask the patient to smile. Also, ask the patient to "show your teeth." Both maneuvers will help determine whether there is any degree of facial drooping.

Respiratory Status Respiratory derangement can occur with CNS illness or injury. Any of five abnormal respiratory patterns may commonly be observed (Figure 24-2):

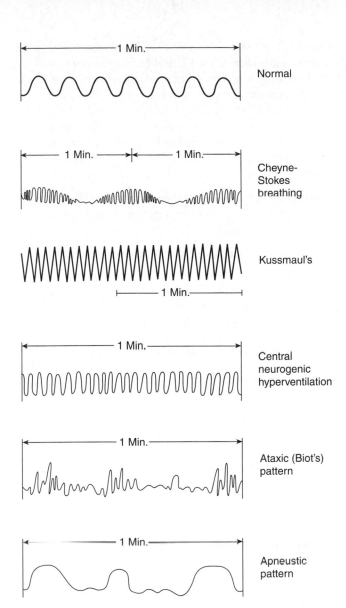

Figure 24-2 Respiratory patterns seen with CNS dysfunction.

- Normal
- Cheyne-Stokes breathing
- Kussmaul's
- Central neurogenic hyperventilation
- Ataxic (Biot's) pattern
- Apneustic pattern

- **Cheyne-Stokes respiration.** A breathing pattern characterized by a period of apnea lasting 10 to 60 seconds, followed by gradually increasing depth and frequency of respirations.
- **Kussmaul's respiration.** Rapid, deep respirations caused by severe metabolic and CNS problems.
- **Central neurogenic hyperventilation.** Hyperventilation caused by a lesion in the central nervous system, often characterized by rapid, deep, noisy respirations.
- **Ataxic respirations.** Poor respirations due to CNS damage, causing ineffective thoracic muscular coordination.
- **Apneustic respirations.** Breathing characterized by prolonged inspiration unrelieved by expiration attempts. This is seen in patients with damage to the upper part of the pons.

Several other respiratory patterns are also possible, depending on the injury. A patient's respirations can be affected by so many factors—fear, hysteria, chest injuries, spinal-cord injuries, or diabetes—that they are not as useful as other signs in monitoring the course of CNS problems. Just before death, the patient may present with central neurogenic hyperventilation.

Cheyne-Stokes respiration a breathing pattern characterized by a period of apnea lasting 10 to 60 seconds, followed by gradually increasing depth and frequency of respirations.

Kussmaul's respiration rapid deep respirations caused by severe metabolic and CNS problems.

central neurogenic hyperventilation hyperventilation caused by a lesion in the central nervous system, often characterized by rapid, deep, noisy respirations.

ataxic respiration poor respirations due to CNS damage, causing ineffective thoracic muscular coordination.

apneustic respiration breathing characterized by a prolonged inspiration unrelieved by expiration attempts, seen in patients with damage to the upper part of the pons.

It is important to remember that the level of carbon dioxide ($PaCO_2$) in the blood has a critical effect on cerebral vessels. The normal blood $PaCO_2$ is 40 mmHg. Increasing the $PaCO_2$ causes cerebral vasodilatation, whereas decreasing it results in cerebral vasoconstriction. If the patient is poorly ventilated, the $PaCO_2$ will increase, causing even further vasodilatation with a subsequent increase in intracranial pressure. Hyperventilation can decrease the $PaCO_2$ effectively causing vasoconstriction of the cerebral vessels. This will assist in minimizing brain swelling. Therefore, hyperventilate any patient who is suspected of having increased intracranial pressure at a rate of 20 breaths per minute. It is important to avoid excessively hyperventilating a patient so as to prevent decreasing $PaCO_2$ levels to dangerously low levels.

Cardiovascular Status   Patients suffering from a neurological event are also likely to suffer changes to the cardiovascular system. Vigilant assessment of a patient's vital signs is necessary to observe these changes. Look for these changes:

- *Heart rate.* A heart rate that is too fast (tachycardia), too slow (bradycardia), or irregular (dysrhythmias).
- *ECG/rhythm.* Development of any changes to the ECG rhythm, including S-T segment changes, the onset of bradycardia, tachycardia, or potentially lethal dysrhythmias, such as ventricular fibrillation or ventricular tachycardia.
- *Bruits.* The sound of turbulent blood flow through the carotid arteries, known as a bruit, may indicate atherosclerotic disease and decreased blood flow to the brain.
- *Jugular venous distention (JVD).* Increased jugular venous pressure, known as jugular venous distention, may be present, indicating that the heart is not pumping effectively.

Nervous System Status   To evaluate nervous system status, take into account sensorimotor status, motor system status, and the status of the cranial nerves.

Sensorimotor Evaluation   The purpose of sensorimotor evaluation is to document loss of sensation and/or motor function. To initially assess the patient with a possible spinal injury, perform these steps:

1. If the patient is unconscious, determine the response to voice, gentle tactile stimulation, and then, if necessary, pain.
2. Evaluate the spine for pain and tenderness.
3. Observe for bruises on the spine.
4. Observe for deformity of the spine.
5. Note any incontinence.
6. Check for circulation, motor function, and sensation in each extremity. Does the patient have feeling in his hands and feet? Ask the patient to wiggle his toes and push them against resistance. Compare both sides. Check bilateral grip strength. If the patient is unconscious, pain response should be observed. If the unconscious patient withdraws or localizes to the pinching of fingers and toes, there is intact sensation and motor function. This is a sign of normal or only minimally impaired cortical function.

A patient with a suspected spinal-cord injury will require full spinal immobilization on a long spine board.

Both **decorticate posturing** (arms flexed, legs extended) and **decerebrate posturing** (arms and legs extended) are ominous signs of deep cerebral or upper brainstem injury (Figures 24-3 and 24-4). Flaccid paralysis usually indicates spinal-cord injury.

Motor System Status   A thorough examination of the motor system of the body includes an assessment of muscle tone, strength, flexion, extension, coordination, and balance. Assess the patient for the following:

- *Muscle tone.* Are the patient's muscles firm? Or, is atrophy present?
- *Strength.* Does the patient have adequate muscle strength? Or is weakness present? Does the patient have strong and equal grip strength?

decorticate posturing
characteristic posture associated with a lesion at or above the upper brainstem. The patient presents with the arms flexed, fists clenched, and legs extended.

decerebrate posturing
sustained contraction of extensor muscles of the extremities resulting from a lesion in the brainstem. The patient presents with stiff and extended extremities and retracted head.

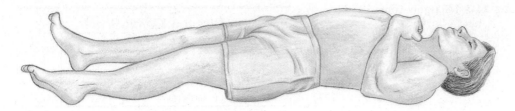

FIGURE 24-3 Patient with decorticate posturing.

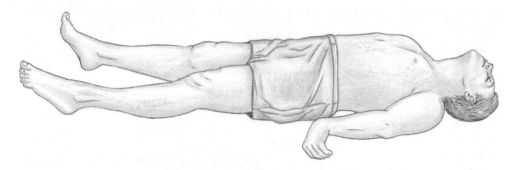

FIGURE 24-4 Patient with decerebrate posturing.

- *Flexion/extension.* Can the patient flex, extend, and move extremities adequately?
- *Coordination.* Are the patient's gait and movements steady and smooth? Can the patient touch finger to nose?
- *Balance.* Can the patient stand or sit upright without becoming dizzy?

Cranial Nerves Status   As you learned earlier, twelve pairs of cranial nerves extend from the lower surface of the brain. Each pair is designated by a Roman numeral from I to XII. Proper and intact functioning of these nerves may be assessed during a complete neurological examination as detailed in, Chapter 7, "Techniques of Physical Examination." Review Figure 2-72 in Chapter 2, which outlines the cranial nerves and their functions.

Further Mental Status Assessment   For patients with an altered mental status or those who are unresponsive, the **Glasgow Coma Scale (GCS)** is a simple tool that can be used to evaluate and monitor the patient's condition. Although it is used most commonly in trauma situations, the scale can also be a valuable tool for monitoring a medical patient's status.

The scale includes three components: eye opening, verbal response, and motor response (Figure 24-5). A number is applied to each of the components based on the patient's condition. The total score can serve as an indicator of survival. The lowest GCS score possible is 3; the highest possible score is 15. The GCS can also be used as a predictor of long-term morbidity and mortality. The following are examples of the predictive value of the GCS system:

Patient with a total score of:	Has an estimated:
8 or better	94% favorable outcome
5, 6, 7	50% favorable (adult), 90% (children)
3.4	10% favorable outcome
5, 6, 7 who drops a grade	0% favorable outcome
5, 6, 7 who improves to more than 7	80% favorable outcome

Glasgow Coma Scale (GCS) tool used in evaluating and quantifying the degree of coma by determining the best motor, verbal, and eye-opening response to standardized stimuli.

Vital Signs

Vital signs are crucial in following the course of neurological problems. Such signs can indicate changes in intracranial pressure. Increased intracranial pressure is characterized by the following changes in vital signs, sometimes collectively referred to as **Cushing's reflex:**

- Increased blood pressure
- Decreased pulse

Cushing's reflex a collective change in vital signs (increased blood pressure and temperature and decreased pulse and respirations) associated with increasing intracranial pressure.

FIGURE 24-5 Glasgow Coma Scale.

Glasgow Coma Scale

Eye Opening	Spontaneous	4	
	To Voice	3	
	To Pain	2	
	None	1	
Verbal Response	Oriented	5	
	Confused	4	
	Inappropriate Words	3	
	Incomprehensible Words	2	
	None	1	
Motor Response	Obeys Commands	6	
	Locailzes Pain	5	
	Withdraw (Pain)	4	
	Flexion (Pain)	3	
	Extension (Pain)	2	
	None	1	
Glasgow Coma Score Total			

TOTAL GLASGOW
COMA SCALE POINTS

13 – 15 = 5

9 – 12 = 4

6 – 8 = 3

4 – 5 = 1

Conversion =
Approximately
One - Third
Total Value

Neurologic Assessment	

- Decreased respirations
- Increased temperature

A patient in the early stages of increased intracranial pressure usually exhibits a decrease in pulse rate and an increase in blood pressure and temperature. Later, if the intracranial pressure continues to rise without correction, the pulse will increase, the blood pressure will fall, and the body temperature will remain elevated. Dysrhythmias may be seen with increased intracranial pressure. Continuous ECG monitoring and pulse oximetry, if available, should be utilized to spot early signs of CNS lesions. Table 24-1 compares vital signs of a patient in shock with those of a patient with head injury and increased intracranial pressure. Remember, if you suspect that a patient has a CNS injury, take and record vital signs every 5 minutes.

Additional Assessment Tools

Additional technological tools may be useful in assessing and monitoring the neurological patient. Such tools should be used as adjuncts to a complete patient assessment, and they should not be relied on as sole indicators of a patient's condition. EMT-Is should continue to base their clinical decisions on a patient's entire presentation. Use such instruments as the end-tidal CO_2 detector, pulse oximeter, and blood glucometer to gain further insight into a patient's condition.

Capnography The capnometer (end-tidal CO_2 detector) monitors the amount of carbon dioxide being exhaled by a patient while being ventilated. This device works on the premise that during exhalation CO_2 should be detected. In the apneic patient with a suspected neurological injury, the device can be used to monitor the effectiveness of the assisted ven-

Table 24-1	COMPARISON OF VITAL SIGNS IN SHOCK AND INCREASED INTRACRANIAL PRESSURE (ICP)	
Vital Signs	Shock	Increased ICP
Blood pressure	Decreased	Increased
Pulse	Increased	Decreased
Respirations	Increased	Decreased
Level of Consciousness	Decreased	Decreased

tilations. Monitoring the levels of CO_2 can ensure that ventilation rate and quality are appropriate for decreasing the increased intracranial pressure.

Pulse Oximeter   The pulse oximeter is an effective tool for monitoring a patient's general state of perfusion. Any patient with a pulse oximetry reading of less than 90% is likely to be hypoxic. In a patient who has suffered a stroke, altered mental status, or syncope, the oximeter can be a useful adjunct in monitoring a patient's condition. It can also monitor the effectiveness of airway management techniques.

Blood Glucometer   A common cause of an altered mental status or focal neurological deficits is hypoglycemia. Determining the blood glucose level is often a crucial step in caring for the neurological patient. Use the glucometer to obtain an accurate blood glucose level. See Chapter 21 for a discussion of this procedure. Documented hypoglycemia should be treated with a bolus of 50% dextrose.

Geriatric Considerations in Neurological Assessment

The neurological system of the geriatric patient is susceptible to systemic illness and is often affected by other body disorders. In addition, certain neurological changes such as pupil sluggishness, loss of overall body strength, and muscle atrophy occur naturally with the aging process. Slowing of nerve conduction is another characteristic often seen in the geriatric patient. Such slowing may indicate that a little more time is necessary to obtain a complete neurological history.

The level of consciousness and overall mental status of a geriatric patient is evaluated by assessing judgment, memory, affect, mood, orientation, speech, and grooming. Interviewing family members about the patient's normal state may reveal any change in mental status. Common neurological problems of the older patient include headache, low back pain, dizziness, weakness, loss of balance, disorders such as Parkinson's disease, and vascular emergencies such as stroke.

ONGOING ASSESSMENT

Any patient suffering from a neurological emergency should be reassessed every 5 minutes during your care and during transportation. Constantly re-evaluate and monitor the patient's airway and neurological system.

MANAGEMENT OF SPECIFIC NERVOUS SYSTEM EMERGENCIES

The primary treatment for nervous system emergencies in the field is supportive.

The major concerns in any CNS emergency are always the airway, breathing, circulation, and, if indicated, C-spine control.

The primary treatment for nervous system emergencies in the field is supportive. Most conditions will not be "cured" in the prehospital setting but symptoms may be reduced or controlled. Make a strong effort to make the patient comfortable and to reduce any of the existing symptoms. Follow these steps:

- *Airway and breathing.* Properly position any patient who you suspect has a neurological emergency and protect the airway. If there is known or possible trauma, maintain C-spine immobilization. Administer oxygen via a nonrebreather mask. If the patient is breathing inadequately or is apneic, initiate ventilatory assistance. If an airway problem is detected, first apply basic airway maneuvers such as head positioning or the modified jaw-thrust maneuver. Intubate, if indicated.

- *Circulatory support.* Establish an IV with a crystalloid solution such as lactated Ringer's or normal saline. Alternatively, consider placing a heparin or saline lock. It is important to have an accessible route for medications. Generally, running an IV at a keep-open rate will be sufficient.

- *Pharmacological interventions.* Medications are available to alleviate signs and symptoms in patients with neurological emergencies. Medications include dextrose, thiamine, naloxone, and diazepam.

- *Psychological support.* Patients suffering from a nervous system emergency, acute or chronic, are likely also to suffer anxiety. Neurological deficits of any kind are frightening experiences. Provide the patient with emotional support and explain the treatment regimen. In most cases, it is appropriate to explain to the patient what is occurring and why. Careful explanation and emotional support will help allay anxiety and apprehension.

- *Transport considerations.* Assess, provide emergency care, and package the patient as quickly and safely as possible. Rapidly transport any patient with a neurological deficit or altered mental status to an appropriate emergency department, equipped with a computerized tomography (CT) or magnetic resonance imaging (MRI) scanner and facilities capable of managing strokes with thrombolytic therapy. Modern medicine has seen the development of new advances in pharmacological and surgical interventions that are only available in the hospital setting.

There are numerous causes of nervous system emergencies. The more common non-traumatic nervous emergencies encountered in the prehospital setting include altered mental status, seizures, stroke, transient ischemic attacks (TIA), and headache. The following discussion details the assessment and management of these frequently encountered non-traumatic nervous system emergencies.

ALTERED MENTAL STATUS

When evaluating a patient, you may find mnemonic devices useful as assessment aids. A mnemonic that may help you remember some of the common causes of altered mental status is "AEIOU-TIPS":

A — Acidosis, alcohol

E — Epilepsy

I — Infection

O — Overdose

U — Uremia (kidney failure)

T — Trauma, tumor, toxin

I — Insulin (hypoglycemia or diabetic ketoacidosis)

P — Psychosis, poison

S — Stroke, seizure

Make an effort through history taking and patient assessment to determine the underlying cause of the altered level of consciousness. Oftentimes, however, a clear cause will not be evident and cannot be determined in the prehospital setting.

Assessment

Using the AVPU method discussed earlier, determine the patient's level of consciousness. Unresponsive patients require vigilant monitoring and protection of the airway. Use information from family, friends, or other bystanders to try to determine the underlying cause of unconsciousness. Perform a physical exam to uncover any hidden injuries, signs, or symptoms.

Management

Your initial priority is to ensure that the patient's airway is open and cervical spine is immobilized (in cases of suspected head/neck injury). Simultaneously secure the patient's airway and administer supplemental oxygen. If the patient is breathing inadequately, support respirations. An unresponsive patient requires an appropriate airway adjunct. Then assess the patient's circulatory status. Evaluate the patient's heart rate, blood pressure, and monitor the cardiac rhythm.

After the above are completed, perform the following steps:

- Establish an IV of normal saline or lactated Ringer's solution at a keep-open rate or place a heparin or saline lock.

- Determine the blood glucose level using a reagent strip or glucometer. A serum glucose determination will assist in determining if the altered mental status is due to hypoglycemia.

- If the blood glucose level is low, administer 50% dextrose. This will mediate hypoglycemia, which may be the cause of the altered mental status. Even if the patient is an uncontrolled diabetic whose body is not producing enough insulin, hyperglycemia produced by administration of glucose will do limited harm in the short time before arrival at the hospital. If, however, the patient is hypoglycemic, for example from too much insulin or missing a meal, the administration of glucose can be life saving, and the patient may respond immediately. For the alcoholic patient who is hypoglycemic, the glucose may be life saving as well. For more information or diabetic emergencies, see Chapter 21.

- Administer naloxone if the patient is suspected of having a narcotic overdose. Naloxone, a narcotic antagonist, has proven effective in the management and reversal of overdose caused by narcotics or synthetic narcotic agents. For more information, see Chapter 23.

- If the patient is a suspected alcoholic, consider the administration of 100 mg of thiamine (vitamin B$_1$). It is required for the conversion of pyruvic acid to acetyl-coenzyme-A (an important step in normal metabolism). Without this conversion, a significant amount of energy available in glucose cannot be obtained. The brain is extremely sensitive to thiamine deficiency.

Chronic Alcoholism Chronic alcoholism interferes with the intake, absorption, and use of thiamine. A significant percentage of alcoholics have thiamine deficiency that can cause Wernicke's syndrome or Korsakoff's psychosis. **Wernicke's syndrome** is an acute but reversible encephalopathy (brain disease) characterized by ataxia, eye muscle weakness, and mental derangement. Of even greater concern is **Korsakoff's psychosis,** characterized by memory disorder. Once established, Korsakoff's psychosis may be irreversible. EMT-Is should follow local protocols. If ordered by medical direction, administer 100 mg of thiamine intravenously or intramuscularly.

Increased Intracranial Pressure If an increase in intracranial pressure is likely, as occurs in a closed head injury, hyperventilate the patient at 20 breaths per minute. Decreasing the carbon dioxide level will cause cerebral vasoconstriction and will help minimize brain swelling. Use caution not to over-hyperventilate, which could decrease CO$_2$ levels to dangerously low levels. Medical direction may order administration of the osmotic diuretic mannitol (Osmotrol). Mannitol causes diuresis, eliminating fluid from the intravascular space through the kidneys. Many authorities feel that its oncotic effect also causes a fluid shift from the substance of the brain to the circulation, thus reducing brain edema. As with all drugs, follow local protocols.

Wernicke's syndrome condition characterized by loss of memory and disorientation, associated with chronic alcohol intake and a diet deficient in thiamine.

Korsakoff's psychosis psychosis characterized by disorientation, muttering delirium, insomnia, delusions, and hallucinations. Symptoms include painful extremities, bilateral wrist drop (rarely), bilateral foot drop (frequently), and pain on pressure over the long nerves.

STROKE AND INTRACRANIAL HEMORRHAGE

stroke caused by either ischemic or hemorrhagic lesions to a portion of the brain, resulting in damage or destruction of brain tissue. Commonly also called a cerebrovascular accident or "brain attack."

Stroke, also called a "brain attack," is a general term that describes injury or death of brain tissue usually due to interruption of cerebral blood flow. The term *brain attack* is used because it compares the physiology of a stroke with that of a heart attack. In both cases, oxygen deprivation causes damage to the affected tissue.

"Brain attack" also reflects recent trends in the treatment of a stroke, which in many cases now parallels the treatment available for heart attack. Before 1995, prehospital care of the stroke patient was considered primarily supportive. Since then, modern medicine has discovered new therapies and has realized the importance of early intervention. Now, early recognition and rapid transport to the hospital are identified as crucial to improving the outcome for stroke patients. The National Institute of Neurological Disorders and Stroke (NINDS) suggests transport to an emergency facility with the capability to respond to a stroke patient quickly, such as a facility equipped with computed tomography (CT) and neurological services.

The use of *tissue plasminogen activator (tPA)* and other thrombolytic agents used in the treatment of heart attack is under increasing scrutiny, as additional studies were not able to replicate the NINDS study findings. Most major emergency medicine organizations have issued position statements that thrombolytics for acute ischemic stroke are *not* the standard of care.

Prompt identification and transport are critical in cases of stroke. Patients who need thrombolytic therapy must reach definitive treatment within 3 hours of onset.

Stroke patients who may be candidates for the thrombolytic therapy must receive definitive treatment within 3 hours of onset. Because of the possibility of intervention with thrombolytics, it is crucial to determine the exact time of the onset of symptoms as accurately as possible. In addition, it is essential that the public be aware of the signs and symptoms of stroke so that EMS can be notified. Therefore, extensive public education is necessary in achieving early recognition of symptoms and appropriate intervention and treatment. Transportation to an emergency facility is crucial in achieving the best possible outcome for these patients.

Strokes are the third most common cause of death and, in middle-aged and older patients, are a frequent cause of disability. Therefore the public, particularly those with a history of atherosclerosis (hardening of the arteries), heart disease, or hypertension, should be educated on the signs and symptoms of stroke as well as the need to contact EMS at the outset of symptoms. Likewise, EMT-Is must understand stroke as a serious, potentially life-threatening condition that warrants rapid recognition and prompt transport.

Strokes can be divided into two broad categories: those caused by occlusion (blockage) of an artery and those caused by hemorrhage from a ruptured cerebral artery (Figure 24-6).

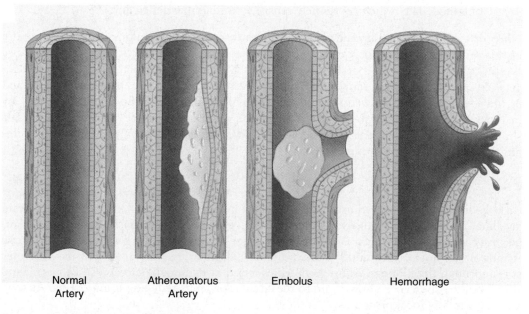

| Normal | Atheromatorus | Embolus | Hemorrhage |
| Artery | Artery | | |

FIGURE 24-6 Etiologies of stroke.

Occlusive Strokes

An occlusive stroke occurs when a cerebral artery is blocked by a clot or other foreign matter. This results in ischemia, an inadequate blood supply to the brain tissue, and progresses to infarction, the death of tissues as a result of cessation of blood supply. In infarction, the tissue that has died will swell, causing further damage to nearby tissues, which only have a marginal blood supply. If swelling is severe, herniation (protrusion of brain tissue from the skull through the foramen magnum, the narrow opening at the base of the skull) may result. Occlusive strokes are classified as either embolic or thrombotic, depending on the cause:

- *Embolic stroke.* An embolus is a solid, liquid, or gaseous mass carried to a blood vessel from a remote site. The most common emboli are clots (thromboemboli) that usually arise from diseased blood vessels in the neck (carotid) or from abnormally contracting chambers in the heart. Atrial fibrillation often results in atrial dilation, a precursor to the formation of clots. Other types of emboli that may cause occlusion in cerebral blood vessels are air, tumor tissue, and fat. Embolic strokes occur suddenly and may be characterized by severe headaches.

- *Thrombotic stroke.* A cerebral thrombus is a blood clot that gradually develops in and obstructs a cerebral artery. As a person ages, atheromatous plaque deposits can form on the inner walls of arteries. The buildup causes a narrowing of the arteries and reduces the amount of blood that can flow through them. This process is known as atherosclerosis. Once the arteries are narrowed, platelets adhere to the roughened surface and can create a blood clot that blocks the blood flow through the cerebral artery. This ultimately results in brain tissue death. Unlike the embolic stroke, the signs and symptoms of thrombotic stroke develop gradually. This type of stroke often occurs at night and is characterized by a patient awakening with altered mental status and/or loss of speech, sensory, or motor function.

Hemorrhagic Strokes

Hemorrhagic strokes are usually categorized as being within the brain (intracerebral) (Figure 24-7a) or in the space around the outer surface of the brain (subarachnoid) (Figure 24-7b). Onset is often sudden and marked by a severe headache. Most intracranial hemorrhages occur in the hypertensive patient when a small vessel deep within the brain tissue ruptures. Subarachnoid hemorrhages most often result from congenital blood vessel abnormalities or from head trauma. Congenital abnormalities include aneurysms (weakened vessels) and arteriovenous malformations (collections of abnormal blood vessels). Aneurysms tend to be on the surface and may hemorrhage into the brain tissue or the subarachnoid space. Arteriovenous malformations may be within the brain, in the subarachnoid space, or both. Hemorrhage inside the brain often tears and separates normal brain tissue. The release of blood into the cavities within the brain that contain cerebrospinal fluid may paralyze vital centers. If blood in the subarachnoid space impairs drainage of cerebrospinal fluid, it may cause a rise in the intracranial pressure. Herniation of brain tissue may then occur.

Assessment

Signs and symptoms of a stroke will depend on the type of stroke and the area of the brain damaged. Areas commonly affected are the motor, speech, and sensory centers. The onset of symptoms will be acute, and the patient may experience unconsciousness. The patient may have stertorous breathing (laborious breathing accompanied by snoring) due to paralysis of a portion of the soft palate. Respiratory expiration may be puffs of air out of the cheeks and mouth. The patient's pupils may be unequal, with the larger pupil on the side of the hemorrhage. Paralysis will usually involve one side of the face, one arm, and one leg. The eyes often will be turned away from the side of the body paralysis. The patient's skin may be cool and clammy. Speech disturbances, or aphasia, may also be noted.

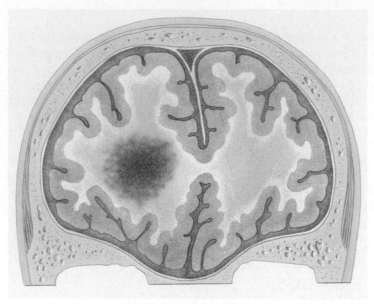

(a)

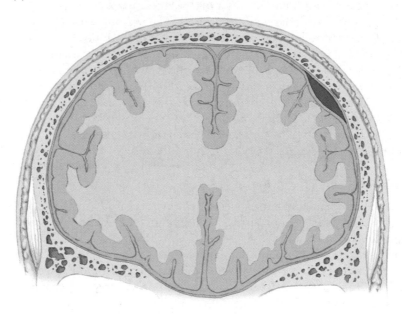

(b)

FIGURE 24-7   (a) Intracerebral hemorrhage, and (b) subarachnoid hemorrhage.

Signs and symptoms of a stroke include:

- Facial drooping
- Headache
- Confusion and agitation
- Dysphasia (difficulty in speaking)
- Aphasia (inability to speak)
- Dysarthria (impairment of the tongue and muscles essential to speech)
- Vision problems such as monocular blindness (blindness in one eye) or double vision
- Hemiparesis (weakness on one side)
- Hemiplegia (paralysis on one side)

- Paresthesia (numbness or tingling)
- Inability to recognize by touch
- Gait disturbances or uncoordinated fine motor movements
- Dizziness
- Incontinence
- Coma

Predisposing factors that may contribute to the stroke include hypertension, diabetes, abnormal blood lipid levels, oral contraceptives, sickle cell disease, and some cardiac dysrhythmias (e.g., atrial fibrillation).

Distinguishing Transient Ischemic Attacks (TIAs) Some patients may have transient strokelike symptoms known as **TIAs, or transient ischemic attacks.** These indicate temporary interference with the blood supply to the brain, producing symptoms of neurological deficit. These symptoms may last for a few minutes or for several hours but usually resolve within 24 hours. After the attack, the patient will show no evidence of residual brain or neurological damage. The patient who experiences a TIA may, however, be a candidate for an eventual stroke. In fact, one-third of TIA patients have a stroke soon thereafter.

The onset of a transient ischemic attack is usually abrupt. The specific signs and symptoms depend on the area of the brain affected. Any one or a combination of stroke symptoms may be present. In fact, it is virtually impossible to determine whether such a neurological event is due to a stroke or to a TIA in the prehospital setting.

The most common cause of a TIA is carotid artery disease. Other causes can be a small embolus, decreased cardiac output, hypotension, overmedication with antihypertensive agents, or cerebrovascular spasm.

While obtaining the history of the patient suspected of sustaining a TIA, you should try to collect information on or take note of the following factors:

- Previous neurological symptoms
- Initial symptoms and their progression
- Changes in mental status
- Precipitating factors
- Dizziness
- Palpitations
- History of hypertension, cardiac disease, sickle cell disease, or previous TIA or stroke

transient ischemic attack (TIA) temporary interruption of blood supply to the brain.

Management

Care for the stroke or TIA patient emphasizes early recognition, supportive measures, rapid transport, and notification of the emergency department (Figure 24-8). Aggressive airway

Patho Pearls

Despite the great strides in medicine, there is still very little that can be provided to help minimize the effects of a stroke. Stroke therapy usually involves medically stabilizing the patient after the stroke and then getting him into a physical rehabilitation program where he can regain as much motor function as possible.

The use of thrombolytic therapy for stroke initially showed great promise. However, the scientific studies that demonstrated thrombolytic therapy for stroke to be beneficial have not been duplicated. In addition, more recent studies have questioned the use of thrombolytics for stroke and several medical organizations have issued position statements that declare thrombolytic therapy for stroke is *not* a standard of care.

It is clear that thrombolytic therapy can help a limited number of stroke patients. Additional studies will help to clarify when and how to administer it. However, at present, the best treatment for stroke is prevention. And, this should begin at an early age with prudent lifestyle changes that modify the risk factors for later developing a stroke.

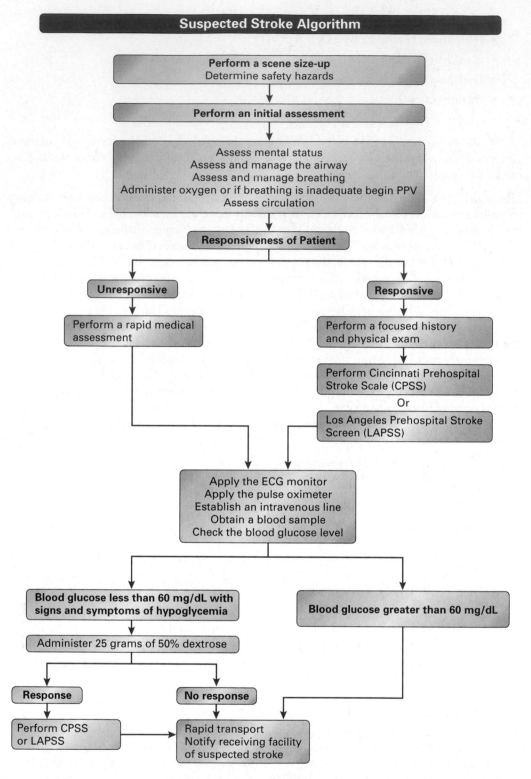

Suspected Stroke Algorithm

Perform a scene size-up
Determine safety hazards

Perform an initial assessment

Assess mental status
Assess and manage the airway
Assess and manage breathing
Administer oxygen or if breathing is inadequate begin PPV
Assess circulation

Responsiveness of Patient

Unresponsive

Perform a rapid medical assessment

Responsive

Perform a focused history and physical exam

Perform Cincinnati Prehospital Stroke Scale (CPSS)

Or

Los Angeles Prehospital Stroke Screen (LAPSS)

Apply the ECG monitor
Apply the pulse oximeter
Establish an intravenous line
Obtain a blood sample
Check the blood glucose level

Blood glucose less than 60 mg/dL with signs and symptoms of hypoglycemia

Blood glucose greater than 60 mg/dL

Administer 25 grams of 50% dextrose

Response

Perform CPSS or LAPSS

No response

Rapid transport
Notify receiving facility of suspected stroke

FIGURE 24-8   Management of suspected stroke.

management is a priority in caring for these patients. Field management of the stroke patient generally includes the following procedures:

- Ensure scene safety, including body substance isolation.
- Establish and maintain an adequate airway. Have suction equipment readily available. Control of the patient's airway is a priority. Brain damage can affect a patient's ability to swallow and maintain an open airway.

- If patient is apneic or if breathing is inadequate, provide positive pressure ventilations at a rate of 20 per minute. Hyperventilation of the stroke patient will eliminate excessive CO_2 levels. Avoid overzealous hyperventilation that may lower CO_2 levels to detrimentally low levels causing profound cerebral vasoconstriction.
- If breathing is adequate, administer oxygen via a nonrebreather mask at 15 liters per minute.
- Complete a detailed patient history.
- Keep the patient supine or in the recovery position. If the patient has congestive heart failure, he could be maintained in a semi upright position, if necessary.
- If an altered mental status is present or there is potential for airway compromise, place the patient in the left lateral recumbent, or recovery position.
- Determine the blood glucose level.
- Start an IV of normal saline or lactated Ringer's solution at a keep-open rate or place a heparin or saline lock. (Avoid dextrose solutions that may increase intracranial pressure due to increased osmotic effects.) If hypoglycemia is present, consider the administration of 50% dextrose by IV push.
- Monitor the cardiac rhythm.
- Protect the paralyzed extremities.
- Give the patient reassurance—all procedures should be explained. The patient may be unable to speak but still may be able to hear and understand.
- Rapidly transport without excessive movement or noise to an appropriate medical facility.

SEIZURES AND EPILEPSY

A **seizure** is a temporary alteration in behavior due to the massive electrical discharge of one or more groups of neurons in the brain. Seizures in any individual may be caused by stresses to the body, such as hypoxia, or a rapid lowering of blood sugar. Febrile seizures can occur in young children with sudden elevations in body temperature. Structural diseases of the brain such as tumors, head trauma, toxic eclampsia, and vascular disorders also cause seizures. The most common cause is idiopathic epilepsy. The term *idiopathic* means "without a known cause." The term *epilepsy* or *epileptic* indicate nothing more than the potential to develop seizures in circumstances that would not induce them in most individuals. Seizures can provoke a great deal of anxiety in both yourself and bystanders.

To assess seizures quickly under such conditions, you need to be thoroughly familiar with their various forms.

Types of Seizures

Seizures can be clinically classified as generalized or partial. **Generalized seizures** begin as an electrical discharge in a small area of the brain but spread to involve the entire cerebral cortex, causing widespread malfunction. **Partial seizures** may remain confined to a limited portion of the brain, causing localized malfunction, or may spread and become generalized.

Generalized Seizures Generalized seizures include tonic-clonic and absence seizures. Another type, pseudoseizures, may mimic generalized seizures.

A **tonic-clonic seizure**, also known as a *grand mal seizure*, is a generalized motor seizure, producing a loss of consciousness. It typically includes a **tonic** (increased tone) **phase,** characterized by tensed, contracted muscles, and a **clonic phase,** characterized by rhythmic jerking movements of the extremities. During the seizure episode, a patient's intercostal muscles and diaphragm become temporarily paralyzed, interrupting respirations and producing cyanosis. The patient's neck, head, face, and eye muscles may also jerk. Once respirations resume, copious amounts of oral secretions (frothing) may be present. Incontinence is also

seizure a temporary alteration in behavior due to the massive electrical discharge of one or more groups of neurons in the brain. Seizures can be clinically classified as generalized or partial.

generalized seizures seizures that begin as an electrical discharge in a small area of the brain but spread to involve the entire cerebral cortex, causing widespread malfunction.

partial seizures seizures that remain confined to a limited portion of the brain, causing localized malfunction. Partial seizures may spread and become generalized.

Content Review

TYPES OF SEIZURES
- Generalized Seizures
  - Tonic-clonic
  - Absence
- Partial Seizures
  - Simple partial seizures
  - Complex partial seizures

tonic-clonic seizure type of generalized seizure characterized by rapid loss of consciousness and motor coordination, muscle spasms, and jerking motions.

tonic phase phase of a seizure characterized by tension or contraction of muscles.

clonic phase phase of a seizure characterized by alternating contraction and relaxation of muscles.

PHASES OF A GENERALIZED SEIZURE
- Aura
- Loss of consciousness
- Tonic phase
- Hypertonic phase
- Clonic phase
- Post-seizure
- Postictal

common during a seizure. Agitation or confusion, drowsiness, or coma may also follow the seizure.

Tonic-clonic seizures have a specific progression of events. It is descriptively convenient to refer to this progression as ranging from warning phase to period of recovery. However, not all seizure patients experience all of these events:

- *Aura.* An aura is a subjective sensation preceding seizure activity. The aura may precede the attack by several hours or by only a few seconds. An aura may be of a psychic or a sensory nature, with olfactory, visual, auditory, or taste hallucinations. Some common types include hearing noise or music, seeing floating lights, smelling unpleasant odors, feeling an unpleasant sensation in the stomach, or experiencing tingling or twitching in a specific body area. Not all seizures are preceded by an aura.

- *Loss of consciousness.* The patient will become unconscious at some point after the aura sensations, if any.

- *Tonic phase.* This is a phase of continuous muscle tension, characterized by contraction of the patient's muscles.

- *Hypertonic phase.* The patient experiences extreme muscular rigidity, including hyperextension of the back.

- *Clonic phase.* The patient experiences muscle spasms marked by rhythmic movements, The patient's jaw usually remains clenched, making airway management difficult.

- *Post seizure.* The patient remains in a coma.

- *Postictal.* The patient may awaken confused and fatigued. He may complain of a headache and may experience some neurological deficit. In many cases, patients will be in this postictal state upon the arrival of EMT-I crews. There may be evidence of incontinence, which supports the likelihood that seizure activity has taken place.

An **absence seizure,** also called a *petit mal seizure,* is a brief, generalized seizure that usually presents with a 10 to 30-second loss of consciousness or awareness, eye or muscle fluttering, and an occasional loss of muscle tone. Loss of consciousness may be so brief that the patient or observers may be unaware of the episode. Absence seizures are idiopathic disorders of early childhood and rarely occur after age 20. Children who suffer frequent absence seizures are often accused of day dreaming or inattentiveness. Absence seizures may not respond to normal treatment modalities.

Pseudoseizures, also called "hysterical seizures," stem from psychological disorders. The patient presents with sharp and bizarre movements that can often be interrupted with a terse command, such as "stop it!" The seizure is usually witnessed, and there will not be a postictal period. Very rarely do patients experiencing a pseudoseizure injure themselves.

Partial Seizures   Partial Seizures may be either simple or complex. **Simple partial seizures,** also sometimes called focal motor, focal sensory, or Jacksonian seizures, are characterized by chaotic movement or dysfunction of one area of the body. When an abnormal electrical discharge occurs from a specific portion of the brain, only those functions served by that area will have dysfunction. Simple partial seizures involve no loss of consciousness and begin as localized tonic/clonic movements. They frequently spread and can progress to generalized tonic-clonic seizures. Therefore, it is crucial that you document how such seizures begin and the course that they subsequently take.

Complex partial seizures, sometimes called temporal lobe or psychomotor seizures, are characterized by distinctive auras. They include unusual smells, tastes, sounds, or the tendency of objects to look either very large and near or small and distant. Sometimes a seizure patient may visualize scenes that look very familiar (*deja vu*) or very strange. A metallic taste in the mouth is a common psychomotor seizure aura. These are focal seizures, lasting approximately 1 to 2 minutes. The patient experiences a loss of contact with his surroundings. Additionally, the patient may act confused, stagger, perform purposeless movement, or make unintelligible sounds. He may not understand what is said. The patient may even re-

---

absence seizure type of generalized seizure with sudden onset, characterized by a brief loss of awareness and rapid recovery.

simple partial seizure type of partial seizure that involves local motor, sensory, or autonomic dysfunction of one area of the body. There is no loss of consciousness.

complex partial seizure type of partial seizure usually originating in the temporal lobe characterized by an aura and focal findings such as alterations in mental status or mood.

fuse medical aid. Some patients develop automatic behavior or show a sudden change in personality, such as abrupt explosions of rage.

Assessment

Your initial contact with the patient and bystanders will offer a unique opportunity to obtain a history that may influence your plan of management. What an untrained observer calls a seizure may be a simple fainting spell. Therefore, you need to ascertain exactly what the patient may recall or what bystanders witnessed.

Many other problems can mimic or suggest a seizure. These include migraine headaches, cardiac dysrhythmias, hypoglycemia after exercise or drug ingestion, and the tendency to faint when rising from a supine or sitting position (orthostatic hypotension). Hyperventilation, meningitis, intracranial hemorrhage, or certain tranquilizers can cause stiffness of the extremities. Decerebrate movements, if present, may be caused by increased intracranial pressure. If you are unsure whether the patient has had a seizure, it may be more harmful than beneficial to administer an anticonvulsant medication.

It is also important to try to distinguish between syncope and true seizure (Table 24-2). Syncope patients sometimes have a short initial period of seizurelike activity (usually less than 1 minute), but this is not followed by a postictal state. The most common cause of fainting is vasovagal syncope associated with fatigue, emotional stress, or cardiac disease. Syncope will be discussed in greater detail later in this chapter.

When obtaining a history, remember to include the following points:

- History of seizures. This data should include length of any past seizure; whether it was generalized or focal; presence of auras, incontinence, or trauma to the tongue.
- Recent history of head trauma.
- Any alcohol and/or drug abuse.
- Recent history of fever, headache, or stiff neck.
- History of diabetes, heart disease, or stroke.
- Current medications. Most chronic seizure patients take anticonvulsant medication on a regular basis. Common anticonvulsant medications include phenytoin (Dilantin), phenobarbital, carbamazepine (Tegretol), and valproic acid (Depakote).

The physical examination of the seizure patient should include the following steps:

- Note any signs of head trauma or injury to the tongue.
- Note any evidence of alcohol and/or drug abuse.
- Document dysrhythmias.

Management

Remember that seizures tend to provoke anxiety in patients, families, and EMT-Is. From a medical standpoint, however, most of these situations only require managing the airway and preventing the patient from injuring himself. Because the patient may become hypothermic

A good history will be important in distinguishing a seizure from other conditions.

The prime concerns in seizure management are control of the airway and prevention of injury.

Table 24-2 DIFFERENTIATION BETWEEN SYNCOPE AND GENERALIZED TONIC-CLONIC SEIZURE

Syncope	Seizure
Usually begins in a standing position	May begin in any position
Patient will usually remember a warning of fainting (feeling of weakness or dizziness)	May begin without warning or may be preceded by an aura
Jerking motions usually not present	Jerking motions present during unconsciousness
Patient regains consciousness almost immediately on becoming supine	Patient remains unconscious during seizure, remains drowsy during postictal period

or hyperthermic if exposed, protecting body temperature is also crucial. Field management of the seizure patient generally includes the following procedures:

- Ensure scene safety.
- Maintain the airway. Do not force objects between the patient's teeth—this includes padded tongue blades. Pushing objects into the patient's mouth may cause him to vomit or to aspirate. It can also cause laryngospasm.
- Administer high-flow, high-concentration oxygen.
- Establish IV access. Initiate normal saline or lactated Ringer's solution at a keep-open rate. Do not use dextrose solutions; emergency department personnel may later administer phenytoin (Dilantin), which is incompatible with dextrose solutions.
- Determine the blood glucose level. If hypoglycemic, administer 50% dextrose.
- Never attempt to restrain the patient. This may injure him. However, protect the patient from hitting objects in the environment (Figure 24-9). (Note: If there is evidence of head trauma, C-spine immobilization must be considered as in any other head injury.)
- Maintain body temperature.
- Position the patient on his left side after the clonic-tonic phase (Figure 24-10).
- Suction, if required.
- Monitor cardiac rhythm.
- If seizure is prolonged (less than 5 minutes), consider an anticonvulsant.
- Provide a quiet, reassuring atmosphere.
- Transport the patient in the supine or lateral recumbent position.

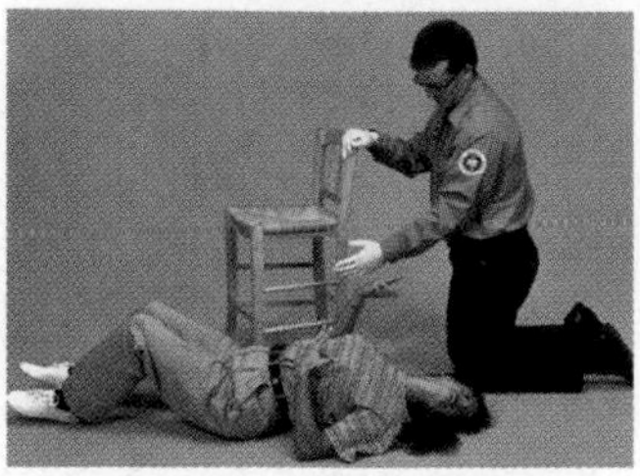

FIGURE 24-9 Protection of a patient having a seizure.

Status Epilepticus

Status epilepticus is a series of two or more generalized motor seizures without an intervening return of consciousness. The most common cause in adults is failure to take prescribed anticonvulsant medications. Status epilepticus is a major emergency since it involves a prolonged period of apnea, which in turn can cause hypoxia of vital brain tissues. These seizures may result in respiratory arrest, severe metabolic and respiratory acidosis, extreme hypertension, increased intracranial pressure, serious elevations in body temperature, fractures of the long bones and spine, necrosis of the cardiac muscle, and severe dehydration.

The most valuable intervention is to protect the patient from airway obstruction and deliver 100% oxygen. Preferably this should be accomplished by bag-valve-mask assistance, since the normal ventilatory mechanisms of the patient are seriously impaired and air ex-

status epilepticus series of two or more generalized motor seizures without any intervening periods of consciousness.

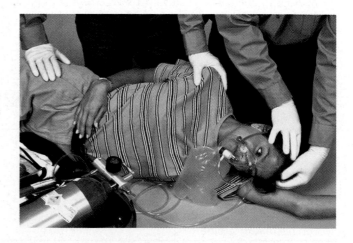

FIGURE 24-10 Place a seizing patient with no suspected spine injury on her left side.

change is generally ineffective. Once the airway is maintained and ventilations are being assisted, take the following steps:

- Start an IV of normal saline at a keep-open rate.
- Monitor cardiac rhythm.
- Administer 25 gms of 50% dextrose IV push, if hypoglycemia is present.
- Administer 5 to 10 mg diazepam IV push for an adult. (Diazepam is a sedative and anticonvulsant that depresses the spread of seizure activity across the motor cortex of the brain.)
- Continue to monitor the airway. Some patients may require large doses of diazepam. Always have flumazenil (Romazicon) available in case it is needed to reverse any significant respiratory depression caused by diazepam. Remember, administration of flumazenil may result in the return of seizures. It should only be used when absolutely necessary.

SYNCOPE

As discussed earlier, **syncope** (fainting) is a neurological condition characterized by the sudden, temporary loss of consciousness caused by insufficient blood flow to the brain, with recovery of consciousness almost immediately upon becoming supine. Nearly 50% of all the people in the United States will experience at least one episode of syncope during their lifetimes. According to the National Institutes of Health, syncope accounts for 3% of all emergency department visits.

syncope transient loss of consciousness due to inadequate flow of blood to the brain with rapid recovery of consciousness upon becoming supine; fainting.

Assessment

Focus on what caused the patient to faint, or lose consciousness. The causes of syncope can be classified into these three general categories:

- *Cardiovascular* conditions, such as dysrhythmias or mechanical problems—A heart rate that is too fast or too slow, or an abnormally functioning heart valve may trigger hypoxia in the brain and subsequent fainting.
- *Non-cardiovascular* disease, such as metabolic, neurological, or psychiatric conditions—Hypoglycemia, a transient ischemic attack, or an anxiety attack can all be causes of syncope.
- *Idiopathic,* or unknown, cause—Oftentimes, the cause of a patient's syncope remains unknown despite careful assessment and diagnostic tests.

Syncope can occur in all ages from the very young to the very old. Symptoms may include feeling faint, dizziness, lightheadedness, or a loss of consciousness without warning. Keep in mind, however, that the definition of syncope includes rapid recovery of consciousness (usually less than a minute). If a patient does not spontaneously regain consciousness within a few moments, it is NOT syncope—it is something more serious.

Syncope involves rapid recovery of consciousness. If a patient does not regain consciousness within a few moments, it is NOT syncope, but something more serious.

Management

When caring for someone who has fainted, it is important to attempt to identify the underlying cause and treat it. If no cause can be identified, anyone who loses consciousness should be transported to an appropriate emergency department and evaluated. Field management of the syncopal patient generally includes the following procedures:

- Ensure scene safety.
- Establish and maintain an adequate airway.
- Administer high-flow, high-concentration oxygen and assist ventilations when required.
- Check circulatory status (heart rate, blood pressure, cardiac rhythm).
- Check and continuously monitor mental status.

- Start an IV of normal saline or lactated Ringer's solution at a keep-open rate.
- Determine the blood glucose level.
- Monitor the cardiac rhythm.
- Reassure the patient.
- Transport the patient to an emergency department.

HEADACHE

Headache can seriously disrupt a person's life. Nearly 45 million people in the United States suffer from chronic headaches. Of these, approximately 17 million have migraine headaches. An estimated 4 billion dollars is spent annually on over-the-counter pain relievers for headache.

Headache pain can be acute (sudden onset) or chronic (constant or recurring), generalized (all over) or localized (in one specific area) and can range from mild to severe. In some cases the cause is known. In others it is not. The most common types of headache can be classified into three categories:

- *Vascular.* Vascular headaches include migraines and cluster headaches. Migraines can last from several minutes to several days. They can be characterized by an intense or throbbing pain, photosensitivity (sensitivity to light), nausea, vomiting, and sweats. Migraines are frequently unilateral (on one side of the head) and may be preceded by an aura. Cluster headaches usually occur as a series of one-sided headaches that are sudden, intense, and may continue for 15 minutes to 4 hours. Symptoms may include nasal congestion, drooping eyelid, and an irritated or watery eye. Migraines occur more commonly in women, whereas cluster headaches generally occur in men.

- *Tension.* A significant percentage of headaches are tension headaches. Most personnel in the emergency medical field have, at one time or another, suffered from a tension headache. Sometimes such headaches occur on a daily basis. Sufferers often awake in the morning with a mild headache that gets worse during the course of the day. The tension headache produces a dull, achy pain that feels like a forceful pressure is being applied to the neck and/or head.

- *Organic.* A third, less common category includes organically caused headaches. They occur in individuals suffering from tumors, infection, or other diseases of the brain, eye, or other body system.

A continuous throbbing headache (often predominantly over the occiput) with fever, confusion, and nuchal rigidity (stiffness of the neck) are classic signs and symptoms of meningitis. Be alert for these features while assessing patients complaining of headache, particularly those who have also been complaining of nausea, vomiting, or rash.

Assessment

When assessing a patient complaining of headache, ascertain any associated signs and symptoms, such as nausea, vomiting, blurred vision, dizziness, weakness, or watery eyes.

In addition to pain, those suffering from a headache of any type may also complain of nausea, vomiting, blurred vision, dizziness, weakness, or watery eyes. A complete and thorough history of the patient's headache is crucial to its treatment. Determine as much as you can about the pain, including:

- What was the patient doing during the onset of pain?
- Does anything provoke, or worsen, the pain (light, sound, or movement)?
- What is the quality of the pain? (Is it throbbing? crushing? tension?)
- Does the pain radiate to the neck, arm, back, or jaw?
- What is the severity of the pain (On a scale of 1 to 10, how does the patient rate the pain?)
- How long has the headache been present? (acute vs. chronic?)

Headache of acute onset or of a changing pattern demands immediate attention. A sudden onset of pain, description of the pain as "the worst headache in my life," or changes in the pattern of pain should all be considered characteristics of potential serious conditions, such as intracranial hemorrhage.

Management

Treatment for a victim of headache is supportive. Field management of the headache patient generally includes the following:

- Ensure scene safety.
- Establish and maintain an adequate airway.
- Place the patient in a position of comfort. Patients will often place themselves in a position that best alleviates the symptoms, such as lying flat in a dark room.
- Administer high-flow, high-concentration oxygen and assist ventilations when required.
- Start an IV of normal saline or lactated Ringer's solution at a keep-open rate.
- Determine the blood glucose level.
- Monitor the cardiac rhythm.
- Reassure the patient.
- Consider antiemetics or pain control measures. Migraine headaches typically are accompanied by nausea and vomiting. Antiemetic medications, such as prochlorperazine (Compazine), have proven extremely effective in terminating migraine headaches as well as the accompanying nausea and vomiting. The current pharmacological approach to migraines first includes abortive agents such as sumatriptan (Imitrix) and prochlorperazine (Compazine). If these agents fail, then small doses of analgesics should be considered.
- Ensure a calm, quiet environment. Dimming the interior ambulance lights will help comfort the headache patient with photosensitivity.
- Transport the patient to an emergency department.

"WEAK AND DIZZY"

A frequent problem that EMT-Intermediates encounter is the patient who is "weak and dizzy" or "weak all over." Generalized weakness and dizziness, although vague, can be symptoms of many diseases. Furthermore, the feeling of being weak or the feeling of being dizzy can be quite disconcerting, especially to the elderly.

Assessment

Obtain a more detailed history of the illness. Has the patient ever had symptoms such as this before? Has he had vomiting and/or diarrhea? Has there been a change in his medication regimen recently or has he taken a new medication in the past 72 hours?

Patients with weakness and/or dizziness should receive a focused assessment including a neurological examination. Be alert for the presence of nystagmus (a constant, involuntary, cyclical motion of the eyeball), which can indicate a CNS or inner ear problem. Assess the various muscle groups to try and determine whether the weakness reported by the patient is localized or diffuse. Be alert for potential causes. These can be neurological, respiratory, cardiovascular, endocrine, or infectious. Many viral illnesses will cause a feeling of malaise in the early stages. Inner ear infections (labyrinthitis) often will cause dizziness, especially with sudden movements of the head. Mild volume depletion (dehydration) can cause both weakness and dizziness. Sometimes the dizzy patient will become nauseated or may actually vomit.

Management

While assessing the patient, provide supportive care. This includes:

- Ensure scene safety.
- Establish and maintain an adequate airway.
- Place the patient in a position of comfort, generally with head elevated. Avoid sudden or exaggerated movement of the head because it can exacerbate symptoms.

- Administer high-flow, high-concentration oxygen.
- Start an IV of normal saline or lactated Ringer's solution at a keep-open rate. Consider a fluid bolus if the patient appears dehydrated.
- Check the blood glucose level.
- Monitor the cardiac rhythm.
- Consider the administration of an antiemetic. Often, antiemetics such as dimenhydrinate (Dramamine, Gravol) are helpful in treating dizziness and nausea. If the patient is nauseated or vomiting, consider promethezine (Phenergan) or prochlorperazine (Compazine).
- Ensure a calm, quiet environment.
- Reassure the patient.
- Transport the patient to an emergency department.

BACK PAIN AND NONTRAUMATIC SPINAL DISORDERS

Low Back Pain

Back pain can be felt anywhere along the spinal column. However, low back pain (LBP) is the most common back-pain complaint. It is a common, yet debilitating condition. Low back pain is defined as back pain felt between the lower rib cage and the gluteal muscles, often radiating to the thighs.

Both chronic and new-onset low back pain are increasingly common. This complaint of low back pain is the cause of great amount of lost work time in the United States. Between 60% and 90% of the population experience some form of low back pain at some time in their life. Men and women are equally affected, although women over 60 years of age report low back pain symptoms more often, most likely as a result of post-menopausal osteoporosis. Occupations that involve exposure to vibrations from vehicles or machinery and those that require repetitious lifting are often implicated in low back pain. As an EMT-I, you are particularly at risk for back problems.

About one percent of acute low back pain results from sciatica, which causes severe pain along the path of the sciatic nerve, down the back of the thigh and inner leg. This is sometimes accompanied by motor and sensory deficits such as muscle weakness. Sciatica may be caused by compression or trauma to the sciatic nerve or its roots, often resulting from a herniated intervertebral disk or osteoarthrosis of the lumbosacral vertebrae. It may also be caused by inflammation of the sciatic nerve from metabolic, toxic, or infectious causes.

Pain occurring at the level of L-3, L-4, L-5, and S-1 may be due to inflammation of the interspinous bursae. Low back pain may also result from inflammation or sprains or strains of the muscles and ligaments that attach to the spine or from vertebral fractures. Additional causes of back pain include tumors, inflammation of the synovial sacs, rising venous pressure, degenerative joint disease, abnormal bone pressure, problems with spinal mobility, and inflammation caused by infection (osteomyelitis).

In fact, however, most low back pain is idiopathic. That is, the cause may be difficult or impossible to diagnose, even by a physician or in a hospital setting. This makes treatment of many cases of low back pain frustrating and sometimes unsuccessful.

Causes of Nontraumatic Spinal Disorders and Back Pain

Spinal problems may be caused by trauma, but many spinal disorders have nontraumatic causes. Nontraumatic spinal injuries most often result from three causes:

- Degeneration or rupture of the disks that separate the vertebrae
- Degeneration or fracture of the vertebrae
- Cyst or tumor that impinges on the spine

Type and degree of pain that results from these conditions differs from person to person.

Disk Injury   The cartilaginous disks that separate the vertebrae may rupture as a result of injury or may rupture or degenerate as part of the process of aging. Degeneration may cause a narrowing of the disk that compromises spinal stability. Degenerative disk disease is more common in patients over 50 years of age.

A herniated disk occurs when the gelatinous center of the disk (the nucleus pulposa) extrudes through a tear in the tough outer capsule (the anulus fibrosa). The pain that results from these conditions usually results from pressure on the spinal cord or muscle spasm at the site. The intervetebral disks themselves have no innervation. Herniation may be caused by degenerative disk disease, by trauma, or by improper lifting. Improper lifting is the most common cause. Men aged 30 to 50 years are more prone to disk herniation than women. Herniation most commonly affects the disks at L-4, L-5, and S-1 but may also occur in C-5, C-6, and C-7.

Vertebral Injury   The vertebrae themselves may break down (vertebral spondylolysis), especially the lamina or vertebral arch between the articulating facets (the areas where adjoining vertebrae contact one another). Heredity is thought to be a significant factor in the development of spondylolysis. Rotational fractures are common at these sites. Spinal fractures are frequently associated with osteoporosis (brittle bones), which tends to develop in many elderly persons.

Cysts and Tumors   A cyst or tumor along the spine or intruding into the spinal canal may cause pain by pressing on the spinal cord, by causing degenerative changes in the bone, or by interrupting blood supply. The specific manifestations depend on the location and the type of the cyst or tumor.

Other Medical Causes   Back pain can also be caused by medical conditions associated with neither traumatic nor non-traumatic spinal injury. For example, back pain may manifest as referred pain from disorders such as diabetic neuropathy, renal calculus, abdominal aortic aneurysm, and many other conditions such as those discussed in this chapter. It would be a mistake to assume that all back complaints are related to the spinal cord, the vertebrae, the intervetebral disks, or the muscles and ligaments surrounding the vertebrae.

Assessment

Assessment of back pain is based on the patient's chief complaint, the history, and the physical exam. When the complaint is low back pain, a precise diagnosis is likely to be difficult. Preliminary diagnosis may be based on a history of risk factors, such as an occupation requiring repetitive lifting, exposure to vibrations from vehicles or industrial machinery, or a known history of osteoporosis.

The complaint of low back pain often involves radiation of the pain from the gluteus to the thigh, leg, and foot. Usually there is history of slow onset over several weeks to months and the patient has called for your help secondary to an increase in pain and the lack of relief from warm compresses or over-the-counter analgesics. The patient may or may not recall a particular incident that has caused this "low back pain;" direct trauma is very rarely a contributing factor in this type of pain.

Just because low back pain is a common complaint that can be hard to diagnose, do not dismiss this type of complaint as "not real pain." A complete history and physical exam by a physician are necessary to determine the cause of any back pain. Diagnosis will often depend on the results of a CT or MRI scan, electromyelography, or other in-hospital testing.

In the prehospital setting, the important task is to determine if the patient's pain is caused by a life-threatening or a non–life-threatening condition. A good patient history will help in this determination. A history of work or play involving lifting or twisting and a sudden onset of pain, often associated with straining, coughing, or sneezing, may point to a mechanical type of muscle or ligament injury. A gradual onset of pain may point instead to a chronic condition such as degenerative disk disease or tumor development. The presence of associated neurological deficit may also point to a more serious underlying cause. When the complaint is back pain, be sure to inquire about prior back surgery, physical therapy, and time lost from work.

Location of the injury may be revealed by a limited range of motion in the lumbar spine, tenderness on palpation at the location of the injury, alterations in sensation, pain, and temperature at the site, pain or paresthesia below the injury (in the upper extremities with cervical injury, symptoms increasing with neck motion, with possible slight motor weakness in the biceps and triceps; similar symptoms in the lower extremities with injury to the thoracic or lumbar spine).

Keep in mind that you are very unlikely to be able to determine the cause of your patient's back pain in the field. Primarily, you need to gather information from the history and physical exam that you will report to the receiving physician and that will help you determine what degree of immobilization, if any, will be necessary during transport.

Management

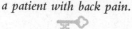

Prehospital care of back pain is aimed at decreasing pain and discomfort. Follow local protocols regarding immobilization of a patient with back pain.

Prehospital management of back pain is primarily aimed at decreasing any pain or discomfort caused by moving the patient and keeping a watchful eye for signs and symptoms of any serious underlying disorder.

Should C-spine precautions be taken with the patient complaining of back pain? Should this patient be immobilized to a long backboard or a vacuum-type stretcher? These questions are best answered, "It depends." First you must consider trauma as a possible cause of the patient's pain. If there is no recent mechanism of injury, consider whether the patient has a possible history of osteoporosis or another disease that might lead to spinal fracture. In these cases, consider immobilizing the patient.

If trauma and possible fracture are ruled out, you may still undertake C-spine precautions and immobilization, because the less movement a patient is put through the more comfortable he will feel. Long-board or vacuum-stretcher immobilization may be the best mode of transportation. If in doubt, immobilize, remembering the injunction to "do no harm."

Some patients with back pain and back spasms may require parenteral analgesics and parenteral diazepam before they can even lie on the stretcher. Contact medical direction regarding analgesic and muscle relaxant therapy.

Conduct ongoing assessment en route with special attention to the airway, breathing, vital signs, and the possible presence or development of motor and sensory deficits that may indicate a critical condition and that can adversely affect the patient's breathing effort.

Summary

Nervous system emergencies include a complex variety of illnesses and injuries. A thorough patient assessment and medical history will help guide your care and will prove invaluable for subsequent hospital management.

Initial field management is directed at ensuring an adequate airway and ventilation. The brain requires a constant supply of oxygen, glucose, and vitamins. After 10 to 20 seconds without blood flow, the patient becomes unconscious. Significant loss of oxygen (anoxia) or low blood sugar (hypoglycemia) can cause coma or seizures. Supply high-flow, high-concentration oxygen to patients with neurological disorders. Administer dextrose to any neurological patient with hypoglycemia.

Neurological injuries and illnesses often require treatment as soon as possible to prevent progressive damage. Patients suffering from an altered level of consciousness, stroke (brain attack), transient ischemic attack, seizures, and syncope require early intervention and transportation to the closest appropriate facility.

You will also be called to care for patients suffering from a headache or a complaint of back pain. These conditions may be relatively minor or indicate a much more serious underlying condition. They too require a complete patient assessment, medical history, and supportive care.

Care for the neurological patient may simply be supportive. In other cases, you should provide drug therapy or other interventions to limit or reduce the presenting symptoms. Airway management remains a priority in caring for any patient with an alteration in neurological function.

On the Web

For additional practice and review, go to the companion website at www.prenhall.com/bledsoe and click on *Intermediate Emergency Care: Principles & Practice.*

CHAPTER 25

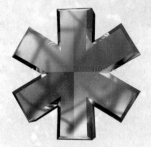

Non-Traumatic Abdominal Emergencies

Objectives

After reading this chapter, you should be able to:

1. Discuss the pathophysiology of non-traumatic abdominal emergencies. (pp. 1036–1037)
2. Discuss the signs and symptoms of non-traumatic acute abdominal pain. (pp. 1037–1050)
3. Describe the technique for performing a comprehensive physical examination on a patient with non-traumatic abdominal pain. (pp. 1050–1052)
4. Describe the management of the patient with non-traumatic abdominal pain. (p. 1052)
5. Given several preprogrammed patients with non-traumatic abdominal pain and symptoms, provide the appropriate assessment, treatment, and transport. (pp. 1036–1052)

CASE STUDY

Shortly after midnight, Rachel Gutierrez and Jack White receive a call that a man has fallen in his bathroom and cannot get up. When they arrive at the house, they are met by a young woman who identifies herself as Amy Jackson, the patient's wife and the person who called 9-1-1 for help. She says she woke up hearing her husband, David, yelling from the bathroom that he needed help. As the three go up the steps, they can hear a man calling, "Hurry up. This pain is awful."

Rachel and Jack see an athletic-looking man in pajamas lying in the bathroom and moaning. He is pale, sweating profusely, and restlessly moving over the floor. When Rachel asks about the pain, he says "It's in my lower back. On the right. I can't move, it's so bad. And I have to pee. Help me." Rachel gets a urine bottle, while Jack introduces himself quietly to David and begins the assessment. Jack helps David to void and then checks the bottle. The urine is reddish yellow. Jack looks for a vein to start an IV line, and Rachel asks David

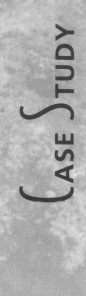
about the pain. He answers that the same spot in his back hurt a bit after dinner, but he was in a lot of pain when he woke up and tried to go to the bathroom. David says his brother had a kidney stone last year. "Could this be one? Am I going to die?" Rachel answers that it might be a kidney stone and that they will take care of him and get him to a hospital. Then she asks more questions quietly, trying to find out if his urination pattern had been normal before he got up, and whether he has ever had bloody urine or been told he had any kind of urinary system trouble before.

Jack completes the physical exam, and Rachel reports vital signs of blood pressure 140/90, pulse 150, and respirations 36/min. After an IV line is established and an oxygen mask is in place, Rachel and Jack help the patient onto the stretcher and out to the ambulance.

David stays in the emergency department for almost 24 hours, medicated with meperidine to relieve pain and with an IV drip to keep him well hydrated and move fluid through his kidneys. An intravenous pyelogram (IVP) shows complete obstruction midway down the right ureter with what appears to be a radiopaque stone. His urine is intermittently bloody, and all samples are screened for stones. Finally David passes a visible stone, and with his pain easing to an ache, he sleeps a bit before going home.

INTRODUCTION

Non-traumatic abdominal pain is a common reason people seek EMS care. Although most non-traumatic abdominal emergencies are not life-threatening, some are. There are numerous causes of non-traumatic abdominal pain, but it is not within the scope of this text to discuss them all. Instead, this chapter focuses on those problems that are potentially life threatening.

The most threatening non-traumatic abdominal emergency is referred to as an **acute abdomen.** An acute abdomen is generally defined as acute abdominal pain in which emergency surgical intervention must be considered. In addition to abdominal pain, other signs and symptoms, such as nausea, vomiting, or diarrhea, may be present. Conditions that can cause an acute abdomen include, but are not limited to, appendicitis, small bowel obstruction, cholecystitis, ischemic bowel, and pelvic inflammatory disease.

GENERAL PATHOPHYSIOLOGY

Non-traumatic abdominal emergencies usually result from an underlying pathologic process that can be predicted by evaluating numerous risk factors. These risk factors are commonly known to physicians; most are self-induced by patients. They include excessive alcohol consumption, excessive smoking, increased stress, ingestion of caustic substances, and poor bowel habits. The wide variety of risk factors and potential causes requires the emergency care provider to complete a thorough focused history and physical examination before making a field diagnosis, along with assessing the seriousness of the emergency and the need for any prevention strategy to minimize organ damage.

Pain is the hallmark of the acute abdominal emergency. The three main classifications of abdominal pain are visceral, somatic, and referred. **Visceral pain** originates in the walls of hollow organs such as the gallbladder or appendix, in the capsules of solid organs such as the kidney or liver, or in the visceral peritoneum. Three separate mechanisms that can produce this pain are inflammation, distention (being stretched out or inflated), and ischemia (inadequate blood flow). Because these processes progress at varying rates, they likewise can cause varying intensities, characteristics, and locations of pain.

Inflammation, distention, and ischemia all transmit a pain signal from visceral afferent neural fibers back to the spinal column. Because the nerves enter the spinal column at various levels, visceral pain usually is not localized to any one specific area. Instead, it is often described as very vague or poorly localized, dull, or crampy. The body most often responds

---

acute abdomen abnormal condition of the abdomen in which there is a sudden, abrupt onset of severe pain; emergency surgical intervention must be considered.

Non-traumatic abdominal emergencies require a thorough focused history and physical exam before making a field diagnosis.

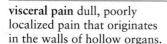

visceral pain dull, poorly localized pain that originates in the walls of hollow organs.

Content Review

ABDOMINAL PAIN
- Visceral
- Somatic
- Referred

to this vague pain with sympathetic stimulation that causes nausea and vomiting, diaphoresis, and tachycardia.

Organs that consist of hollow viscera can frequently cause visceral pain, e.g., the gallbladder (cholecystitis) and the small and large intestines. Many hollow organs first cause visceral pain when they become distended and then cause a different, more specific type of pain (somatic pain, described below) when they rupture or tear. For example, appendicitis initially presents with vague periumbilical abdominal pain that is classified as visceral. If the appendix ruptures, it can spill its contents into the peritoneal cavity, causing bacterial **peritonitis** and generating somatic pain. Various microbes associated with pelvic inflammatory diseases can also cause bacterial peritonitis.

peritonitis inflammation of the peritoneum, which lines the abdominal cavity.

Somatic pain, as contrasted to visceral pain, is a sharp type of pain that travels along definite neural routes (determined by the dermatomes, or tissue blocks, present during embryonic development) to the spinal column. Because these routes are clearly defined, the pain can be localized to a particular region or area. As previously noted, bacterial and chemical irritations of the abdomen commonly cause somatic pain. Bacterial irritation can originate from a perforated or ruptured appendix or gallbladder. Chemical irritation of the abdomen can result from leakage of acidic juices from a perforated ulcer or from an inflamed pancreas. Whether the cause is bacterial or chemical, the resulting peritonitis can lead to sepsis and even death. The degree of pain is initially proportional to the spread of the irritant through the abdominal cavity. Somatic pain allows the examiner to locate the specific area of irritation, providing valuable information.

somatic pain sharp, localized pain that originates in walls of the body such as skeletal muscles.

The third type of pain, **referred pain,** is not a true pain-producing mechanism. As its name implies, referred pain originates in a region other than where it is felt. Many neural pathways from various organs pass through or over regions where the organ was formed during embryonic development. For example, the afferent neural pathways that originate in the diaphragm enter the spinal column at the cervical enlargement at the fourth cervical vertebra. Therefore, patients who have an inflammation or injury of the diaphragm often feel pain in their necks or shoulders. One of the most significant hemorrhagic emergencies, the dissecting abdominal aortic artery, produces referred pain felt between the shoulder blades. Some common non-hemorrhagic emergencies are associated with referred-pain patterns, too. Appendicitis often presents with periumbilical pain, whereas pneumonia can cause pain below the lower margin of the rib cage.

referred pain pain that originates in a region other than where it is felt.

COMMON CAUSES OF NON-TRAUMATIC ABDOMINAL PAIN

There are numerous causes of non-traumatic abdominal pain, but it is difficult to determine the exact one in the prehospital setting. Common causes—some more common than others—include: appendicitis, cholecystitis, pancreatitis, peptic ulcers, bowel obstruction, acute renal failure, chronic renal failure, kidney stones, and urinary tract infection.

APPENDICITIS

Appendicitis is an inflammation of the vermiform appendix, located at the junction of the large and small intestines (the ileocecal junction). Appendicitis occurs in approximately 10% to 20% of the population in the United States, and it is most common in young adults. Acute appendicitis is the most common surgical emergency you will encounter in the field, mostly in older children and young adults. There are no particular risk factors.

appendicitis inflammation of the vermiform appendix at the juncture of the large and small intestines.

The appendix has no known anatomical or physiological function; most of its tissue is lymphoid in type. It lies just inferior to the ileocecal valve and the first section of the ascending colon. Depending on the individual patient, it may be in the retroperitoneal, pelvic, or abdominal cavity. The appendix can become inflamed, and if left untreated, it can rupture, spilling its contents into the peritoneal cavity and contributing to peritonitis.

Appendicitis is evaluated in the ED and eventually treated in the OR more frequently than any other abdominal emergency.

The pathogenesis of appendicitis is most often due to obstruction of the appendiceal lumen by fecal material. The shape and location of the appendix make it particularly vulnerable to obstruction by feces or other material such as food particles or tumor. This inflames the lymphoid tissue and often leads to bacterial or viral infection that ulcerates the mucosa.

The inflammation also causes the appendix's internal diameter to expand, which can block the appendicular artery and cause thrombosis. With its blood supply cut off, the appendix becomes ischemic, and infarction and necrosis of tissue follows. At this point the vessel walls often weaken to the point of rupture, spilling the appendiceal contents into the peritoneal cavity.

Appendicitis is frequently misdiagnosed due to the wide variety of signs and symptoms that can accompany it. Mild or early appendicitis causes diffuse, **colicky** pain often associated with nausea and vomiting and sometimes a low-grade fever. Often the pain is initially located in the periumbilical region. Due to appendiceal blockage, the patient usually loses his appetite. As the appendix continues to dilate the pain will localize in the right lower quadrant. A common site of pain is **McBurney's point,** 1½ to 2 inches above the anterior iliac crest along a direct line from the anterior crest to the umbilicus (Figure 25-1). Once the appendix ruptures the pain becomes diffuse due to development of peritonitis.

Physical assessment will find a patient who appears to be in discomfort. The abdominal exam will reveal tenderness or guarding around the umbilicus or right lower quadrant. Do not repeatedly palpate for rebound tenderness. The pressure that this procedure exerts can cause an inflamed appendix to rupture.

Prehospital care for appendicitis includes placing the patient in a position of comfort, giving psychological support, diligently managing his airway to prevent aspiration, establishing IV access, and transporting him. In most cases the appendix will not have ruptured, and the patient will remain hemodynamically stable. Monitor as you would for bowel obstruction, and treat any complications such as tachycardia or other signs of shock as they arise.

CHOLECYSTITIS

Cholecystitis is an inflammation of the gallbladder. Cholelithiasis (the formation of gallstones), which causes 90% of cholecystitis cases, occurs in approximately 15% of the adult population in the United States, with over one million new cases diagnosed annually. The two types of gallstones are cholesterol-based and bilirubin-based. Cholesterol-based stones are far more common and are associated with a specific risk profile: obese, middle-aged women with more than one biological child.

Definitive treatment of acute cholecystitis includes antibiotic therapy, laparoscopic surgery, lithotripsy (ultrasound treatment to break up the stones), and surgery if the other, less invasive, therapies fail. With the advent of laparoscopic surgery, mortality has fallen to less then 1%, with an overall morbidity of approximately 6%.

Cholecystitis caused by gallstones can be chronic or acute. The liver produces bile, the primary vehicle for removing cholesterol from the body. The bile travels down the common bile duct to empty into the small intestine at the sphincter of Oddi. The sphincter of Oddi opens when chyme exits the stomach through the cardiac sphincter. When the sphincter of Oddi closes, the flow of bile backs up into the gallbladder via the cystic duct. The bile remains in the gallbladder until the sphincter of Oddi opens again.

The bile can become supersaturated. Calculi, which are stone-like masses based on bilirubin, cholesterol, or both, then form. These calculi travel down the cystic duct, fre-

colic acute pain associated with cramping or spasms in the abdominal organs.

McBurney's point common site of pain from appendicitis, 1 to 2 inches above the anterior iliac crest in a direct line with the umbilicus.

cholecystitis inflammation of the gallbladder.

FIGURE 25-1 McBurney's point is a common site of pain in appendicitis.

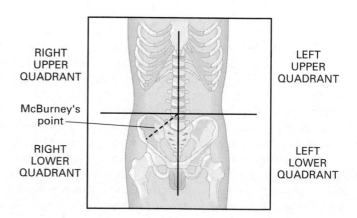

RIGHT UPPER QUADRANT

LEFT UPPER QUADRANT

McBurney's point

RIGHT LOWER QUADRANT

LEFT LOWER QUADRANT

quently lodging in the common bile duct. When they obstruct the flow of bile, gallbladder inflammation and irritation result. The bile salts subsequently attack the mucosal membrane lining the gallbladder, leaving the underlying epithelial tissue without protection. Prostaglandins are also released, further irritating the epithelial wall. As irritation continues, the inflammation grows, increasing intraluminal pressure and ultimately reducing blood flow to the epithelium.

Other causes of cholecystitis include acalculus cholecystitis (cholecystitis without associated stones) and chronic inflammation caused by bacterial infection. Acalculus cholecystitis usually results from burns, sepsis, diabetes, and multiple organ failure. Chronic cholecystitis resulting from a bacterial infection (*Escherichia coli* and enterococci) presents with an inflammatory process similar to cholelithiasis.

An inflamed gallbladder usually causes an acute attack of right upper quadrant abdominal pain. The inflammation can cause an irritation of the diaphragm with referred pain in the right shoulder. If the gallstones are lodged in the cystic duct, the pain may be colicky, due to expansion and contraction of the duct. Often the pain occurs after a meal that is high in fat content because of the secondary release of bile from the gallbladder. The right subcostal region may be tender because of abdominal muscle spasms. Patients may experience extreme pain as the epithelium in the gallbladder erodes away. Sympathetic stimulation because of the pain may cause pale, cool, clammy skin. If peritonitis occurs, the skin may be warm due to increased blood flow to the inflamed peritoneum. Nausea and vomiting are common, due to cystic duct spasm.

Visual inspection may reveal scars from previous gallstone surgeries, but distention and ecchymosis are rarely seen. Palpation may reveal either diffuse right-sided tenderness or point tenderness under the right costal margin, a positive **Murphy's sign.**

Prehospital treatment of the patient with acute cholecystitis is mainly palliative. Place the patient in the position of comfort, maintain his ABCs, ensuring adequate oxygenation, and finally establish intravenous access. Pain medications commonly used include meperidine (Demerol) and butorphanol (Stadol). Morphine is contraindicated because it is believed to cause spasms of the cystic duct.

PANCREATITIS

Pancreatitis is an inflammation of the pancreas. Its four main categories, based on cause, are metabolic, mechanical, vascular, and infectious. Metabolic causes, specifically alcoholism, account for approximately 80% of all cases; consequently, pancreatitis is widespread in the United States, due to the high incidence of alcoholism. Mechanical obstructions caused by gallstones or elevated serum lipids account for another 9%. Vascular injuries caused by thromboembolism or shock, along with infectious diseases, account for the remaining 11%. Overall mortality in acute pancreatitis is relatively high, approximately 30% to 40%, mainly due to accompanying sepsis and shock, which lead to multisystem organ failure. In acute pancreatitis, the rate of serious morbidity and mortality has been found to be 14% in patients with fewer than three positive findings. The mortality rate exceeded 95% when there were three or more positive findings.

The vast bulk of the pancreas's tissue is arranged in glandular structures called *acini* (singular, *acinus*). These cells produce digestive enzymes that empty into the duodenum at the ampulla of Vater, near the junction with the stomach. The other function of the pancreas is endocrine: A small amount of tissue located in isolated islets of tissue secretes the hormones insulin and glucagon. Frequently, gallstones leaving the common bile duct become lodged at the ampulla of Vater and obstruct the pancreatic duct. These obstructions back up pancreatic digestive enzymes into the pancreatic duct and the pancreas itself. The digestive enzymes inflame the pancreas and cause edema, which reduces blood flow, as in the pathogenesis of acute appendicitis. In turn, the decreased blood flow causes ischemia and, finally, acinar destruction. This is often called acute pancreatitis based on rapidity of onset.

Acinar tissue destruction causes a second form of pancreatitis, chronic pancreatitis. Acinar tissue destruction commonly occurs due to chronic alcohol intake, drug toxicity, ischemia, or infectious diseases. Alcohol ingestion results in the deposit of platelet plugs in the acinar tissue. The plugs disrupt the enzymes' flow from the pancreas. When digestive juices back up into the pancreas from the ampulla of Vater, the digestive enzymes can become

Murphy's sign pain caused when an inflamed gallbladder is palpated by pressing under the right costal margin.

pancreatitis inflammation of the pancreas.

activated and begin to digest the pancreas itself. Morphologically this autodigestion appears as lesions and fatty tissue changes on the pancreas.

As tissue digestion continues, the lesion can erode and begin to hemorrhage. This acute exacerbation of pancreatitis causes intense abdominal pain. Its intensity reflects the number of lesions affected or the degree of acinar tissue death. The pain can be localized to the left upper quadrant or may radiate to the back or the epigastric region. Most patients experience nausea followed by uncontrolled vomiting and retching that can further aggravate the hemorrhage. Visual inspection may reveal previous surgical scars for lesion removal; ecchymosis and swelling of the left upper quadrant may also be present due to hemorrhage or significant organ edema. The patient will appear acutely ill with diaphoresis, tachycardia, and possible hypotension if massive hemorrhaging is involved.

Prehospital treatment is supportive and aimed at maintaining the ABCs by providing high-flow, high-concentration oxygen and establishing IV access. Fluid resuscitation with crystalloid may be warranted if the patient appears hemodynamically unstable. Definitive treatment involves gastric intubation and suctioning for emesis control, diagnostic peritoneal lavage, antibiotic therapy, fluid resuscitation, and surgery to remove the blockage.

PEPTIC ULCERS

peptic ulcer erosion caused by gastric acid.

Peptic ulcers are erosions caused by gastric acid (Figure 25-2). They can occur anywhere in the gastrointestinal (GI) tract; terminology is based on the portion of the GI tract affected. Duodenal ulcers most frequently occur in the proximal portion of the duodenum; gastric ulcers occur exclusively in the stomach. Overall, peptic ulcers occur in males four times more frequently than in females, and duodenal ulcers occur from two to three times more frequently than do gastric ulcers. Current statistics place the number of peptic ulcers at 4 to 5

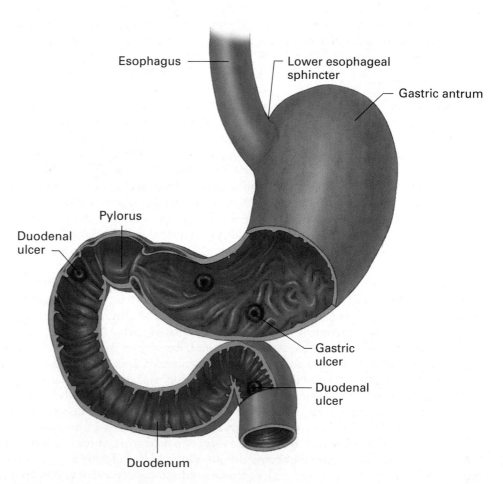

FIGURE 25-2 Peptic ulcer.

million, with approximately 500,000 new cases diagnosed yearly. Those patients who are more likely to have gastric ulcers are over 50 years old and work in jobs requiring physical activity. Their pain usually increases after eating or with a full stomach and they usually have no pain at night. Duodenal ulcers are more common in patients from 25 to 50 years old who are executives or leaders under high stress. There is also some familial tendency toward duodenal ulcer, suggesting genetic predisposition. Patients with duodenal ulcers commonly have pain at night or whenever their stomach is empty. Thus, it is important in taking the focused history to get family history and a reliable estimate of the patient's last oral intake. Measurement of hematocrit may substantiate any suspicions of chronic or acute hemorrhage.

Nonsteroidal anti-inflammatory medications (aspirin, Motrin, Advil, Naprosyn), acid-stimulating products (alcohol, nicotine), or *Helicobacter pylori* bacteria are the most common causes of peptic ulcers. To help break down food boluses, the stomach secretes hydrochloric acid. One of the enzymes that control this secretion is pepsinogen. The hydrochloric acid helps to convert pepsinogen into its active form, pepsin. Between them, the pepsin and the hydrochloric acid can make the digestive enzymes very irritating to the mucosal lining of the GI tract. Ordinarily, mucous gland secretions protect the stomach's mucosal barrier from these irritants. But when nonsteroidal anti-inflammatory medications, acid stimulators, or *H. pylori* damage the barrier, the mucosa is exposed to the highly acidic fluid, and peptic ulcers result. Prostaglandin, an important locally acting hormone, decreases the stimulation for blood flow through the gastric mucosa, thus allowing its further destruction. Treatment strategies in the prehospital setting focus on antacid treatment and support of any complications such as hemorrhage.

The recent discovery that *H. pylori* bacteria appear in over 80% of gastric and duodenal ulcers has enabled physicians to treat the disease by eliminating its cause with antacids and antibiotics, rather than merely treating its symptoms. Definitive treatment includes tamponade of any bleed, possibly by surgical resection, and antibiotic therapy along with histamine blockers and antacids. If medical therapy fails and the problem persists, it may require surgical resection of the vagus nerve (vagotomy) to reduce the stimulation for acid secretion.

A blocked pancreatic duct can also contribute to duodenal ulcers. As chyme passes through the pyloric sphincter from the stomach into the duodenum, the pancreas secretes an alkalotic solution laden with bicarbonate ions that neutralize the acidic hydrogen ions in the chyme. If the pancreatic duct is blocked, however, the acidic chyme can cause ulcerations throughout the intestine. One other cause of duodenal ulcers is **Zollinger-Ellison syndrome,** in which an acid-secreting tumor provokes the ulcerations.

Zollinger-Ellison syndrome condition that causes the stomach to secrete excessive amounts of hydrochloric acid and pepsin.

Findings on clinical examination of a patient with peptic ulcer can vary. Chronic ulcers can cause a slow bleed with resulting anemia. Visual inspection of the abdomen is usually helpful only if significant hemorrhage has occurred, in which case the same signs of ecchymosis and distention are found as in other causes of upper GI bleeding. On palpation, pain may be localized or diffuse. These patients often have relief of pain after eating or coating their GI tract with a liquid such as milk.

Acute, severe pain is probably due to a rupture of the ulcer into the peritoneal cavity causing hemorrhage. Depending on the ulcer's location, the patient may have **hematemesis** or may have **melena**-colored stool. Bouts of nausea and vomiting due to the irritation of the mucosa are common. If the ulcer has eroded through a highly vascular area, massive hemorrhage can occur. Along with the signs of hemorrhage on visual inspection, these patients will appear very ill and have signs of hemodynamic instability such as pale, cool, and clammy skin, tachycardia, decreased blood pressure, and possibly, altered mental status. Most patients will lie still to decrease the pain. They may have surgical scars from previous ulcer repair. Bowel sounds will usually be absent.

hematemesis bloody vomitus.

melena dark, tarry, foul smelling stool indicating presence of partially digested blood.

Treatment for peptic ulcers depends on the severity of the patient's pain. Those who have abdominal pain or hemodynamic instability may require comfortable positioning and psychological support, high-flow, high-concentration oxygen, IV access for fluid resuscitation and pharmacological administration, and rapid transport. Common medications to reduce the mucosal irritation include histamine blockers such as Zantac and Pepcid and antacids such as Carafate.

BOWEL OBSTRUCTION

An obstructed bowel segment can be catastrophic if not rapidly diagnosed and treated.

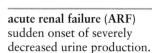

Bowel obstructions are blockages of the hollow space, or lumen, within the small and large intestines. Obstructions can be either partial or complete. An obstructed bowel segment can be catastrophic if not rapidly diagnosed and treated. Of this malady's many different causes, **hernias, intussusception, volvulus,** and **adhesions** are the four most frequent, accounting for over 70% of all reported cases (Figure 25-3). Other common causes are foreign bodies, gallstones, tumors, adhesions from previous abdominal surgery, and bowel **infarction.** The most common location for obstructions is the small intestine, due to its smaller diameter and its greater length, flexibility, and mobility.

The obstruction may be chronic, as with tumor growth or adhesion progression, or its onset may be sudden and acute, as with obstruction by a foreign body. Chronic obstruction usually results in a decreased appetite, fever, malaise, nausea and vomiting, weight loss, or if rupture occurs, peritonitis. Acute-onset pain may follow ingestion of a foreign body. Pain might also be due to a strangulated hernia, one that has rotated through the muscle wall of the abdomen such that blood flow is suddenly cut off (the herniated tissue has been "strangulated") and ischemia, or even infarction, of tissue occurs. Patients with bowel obstruction will frequently vomit, with the vomitus often containing a significant amount of bile. Severe bowel obstructions may result in the patient's vomiting material that looks and smells like feces. All of these findings suggest a bowel obstruction.

These patients present with diffuse visceral pain, usually poorly localized to any one specific location. They may be hemodynamically unstable due to necrosis within an organ, and you may see signs and symptoms of shock (pale, cool, clammy skin, tachycardia, alterations in level of consciousness, and hypotension). Visual inspection may reveal distention, peritonitis, or free air within the abdomen secondary to rupture of a strangulated segment of intestine. Look for scars left from previous surgery, as well as for the ecchymosis indicating that significant hemorrhage has occurred into the abdominal cavity. In the earliest phase of acute obstruction, bowel sounds may be present as a high-pitched obstruction sound. In most cases, however, bowel sounds will be greatly reduced or absent. Palpation will reveal tenderness. Be careful to palpate very lightly if you suspect obstruction, because additional pressure may bring about rupture of the obstructed segment.

The treatment for a patient with an obstructed bowel is based on physiological and psychological support during expedited transport to an appropriate facility. Measures include airway management, oxygenation via a nonrebreather mask at 15 Lpm, position of comfort or shock position, and fluid resuscitation to prevent shock.

ACUTE RENAL FAILURE

Acute renal failure (ARF) is a sudden (often over a period of days) drop in urine output to less than 400 to 500 mL per day, a condition called **oliguria.** Output may literally fall to zero, a condition called **anuria.** ARF is not uncommon among severely ill, hospitalized patients. It is less common in the field. Noting ARF in the prehospital setting is vital because the condition may be reversible, depending on the cause and extent of damage associated with the disorder. Overall mortality is roughly 50%, in part because the condition usually appears in significantly injured or ill persons.

Normally, the kidneys receive about 20% to 25% of cardiac output. This high level of perfusion is essential to sustaining a glomerular filtration rate (GFR) sufficient to maintain blood volume and composition and to clear wastes such as urea and creatinine from the bloodstream. As GFR drops, less urine forms, and the bloodstream retains water, electrolytes, and wastes such as urea and creatinine. Because the retained electrolytes include H^+ and K^+, metabolic acidosis and hyperkalemia may appear.

The focused history will often provide clues to the severity and duration of ARF. For instance, if the patient complains of inability to void for a number of hours associated with a feeling of painful bladder fullness, the cause may simply be acute obstruction at the bladder neck or urethra. In contrast, a patient with poor mentation may be unable to give a coherent history, and a family member will tell you that the patient has felt increasingly ill for several days and has not urinated at all within the past 12 hours or so. Questions likely to provide useful information include the following:

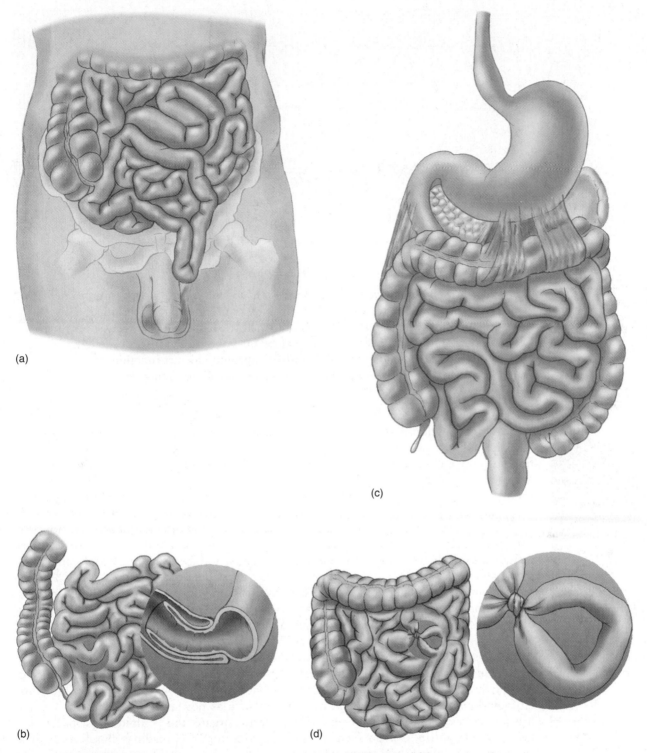

(a)

(c)

(b)

(d)

FIGURE 25-3 The most common causes of bowel obstruction: (a) hernia, (b) intussusception, (c) adhesion, and (d) volvulus.

- *When was the decrease or absence of urine first noticed, and has there been any observed change in output since the problem was first noted? What was the patient's previous output?* The last question may be useful because patients with chronic renal failure due to inadequate renal function can develop ARF as a complication.

- *Has the patient noted development of edema (swelling) in the face, hands, feet, or torso? What about feelings of heart palpitations or irregular rhythm? Has a*

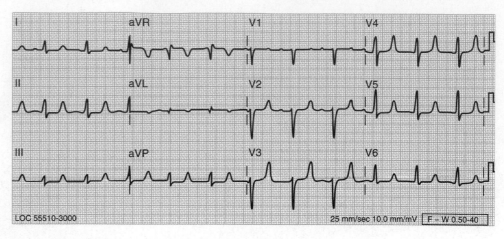

FIGURE 25-4 ECG with signs of hyperkalemia.

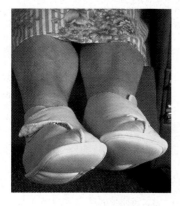

FIGURE 25-5 Edema of the feet consistent with fluid retention in acute renal failure.

chronic renal failure (CRF) permanently inadequate renal function due to nephron loss.

family member or friend noticed decreased mental function, lethargy, or overt coma? If the patient continued to consume fluids after ARF developed, retention of water and Na$^+$ can lead to visible edema in a relatively short time. Retention of K$^+$ can lead to hyperkalemia, a condition that can be lethal, especially in a person with previously compromised heart function. Increasingly poor mentation can be a sign of metabolic acidosis.

The focused physical examination may be helpful in assessing the degree of ARF present, the antecedent condition, and any immediate threats to life. Impaired mentation or clear decreases in consciousness in a person with previously good mental function suggest severe ARF and a potential threat to life. In a patient without evidence of shock, cardiovascular findings may include hypertension due to fluid retention, tachycardia, and electrocardiogram (ECG) evidence of hyperkalemia (Figure 25-4). If shock triggered the ARF or has developed more recently, profound hypotension may be present, accompanied by tachycardia and hyperkalemia.

General visual inspection will usually show pale, cool, moist skin; if shock is not present, these findings may still represent homeostatic shunting of blood to the internal organs, including the kidneys. Look for edema in face, hands, and feet (Figure 25-5). Examination of the abdomen will reveal very different findings dependent on the cause of ARF. As with any abdominal complaint, look for scars, ecchymosis, and distention. If the abdomen is distended, note whether the swelling is symmetrical. Palpate for pulsing masses, which may indicate an abdominal aortic aneurysm. Auscultation is rarely helpful in renal and urological emergencies, and bowel sounds may be muffled if ascites (fluid within the abdomen) is present. Percussion and palpation findings will depend on the trigger condition.

Because ARF can lead to life-threatening metabolic derangements, monitoring and supporting the ABCs is vital. Use high-flow, high-concentration oxygen to maximize breathing efficiency; couple this with circulatory supports such as positioning with head down and legs up to assist blood flow to the brain and internal organs and IV fluid resuscitation (bolus followed by drip) if hypovolemia is present. Monitor ECG readings closely and adjust supports per local protocol or discussion with medical direction. During transportation, be sure to talk quietly to the patient, both to calm him and to keep him informed of time until arrival or other pertinent matters. As always, your actions should reflect caring competence. Even if the patient is confused or comatose, you should still address him respectfully as you perform procedures and avoid saying anything you do not want him to hear.

CHRONIC RENAL FAILURE

Chronic renal failure (CRF) is inadequate kidney function due to permanent loss of nephrons. Usually, at least 70% of the nephrons (healthy norm, one million per kidney) must be lost before significant clinical problems develop and the diagnosis is made. Metabolic instability does not occur until about 80% or more of nephrons are destroyed. When this point of dysfunction is reached, an individual is said to have developed end-stage renal failure and must have either dialysis or a kidney transplant to survive. Anuria is not necessarily present in either CRF or end-stage renal failure.

Together, diabetes mellitus and hypertension cause more than 50% of all cases of end-stage renal failure. The death toll from CRF is high. More than 250,000 people in the United States have end-stage renal failure, and more than 50,000 die yearly from kidney disease. Roughly 30,000 new cases of CRF are diagnosed each year. The number of donor kidneys available in recent years has been sufficient for only about one-third of the persons on the waiting list to receive a kidney.

During the focused history and physical exam, you will probably find many characteristics of uremia in patients with CRF and end-stage disease. Table 25-1 lists some of these signs and symptoms, which affect nearly every organ system. Many of the listed problems can precipitate shock or other major physiologic instability; this is one reason you must always be alert when dealing with patients with CRF or end-stage disease, even when they initially appear stable. In addition, this list is by no means exhaustive. Kidney failure affects almost every organ and major function in the body.

Always stay alert for shock or other major physiologic instability when dealing with CRF or end-stage disease, even when the patient initially appears to be stable.

Table 25-1 COMMON ELEMENTS OF UREMIC SYNDROME

System	Pathophysiology	Clinical Signs/Symptoms
Fluid/electrolyte	Water/Na$^+$ retention	Edema, arterial hypertension*
	K$^+$ retention	Hyperkalemia*
	H$^+$ retention	Metabolic acidosis
	PaO$_2$ retention	Hyperphosphatemia/hypocalcemia*
Cardiovascular/pulmonary	Fluid volume overload	Ascites, pulmonary edema
	Arterial hypertension	Congestive heart failure, accelerated atherosclerosis
	Dysfunctional fat metabolism; retention urea, other wastes	Pericarditis
Neuromuscular		
Central nervous system	Retention urea, other wastes	Headache, sleep disorders, impaired mentation, lethargy, coma, seizures
Skeletal muscle	Retention urea, other wastes; hypocalcemia	Muscular irritability and cramps, muscle twitching
Gastrointestinal (GI)	Retention urea, other wastes	Anorexia, nausea, vomiting
	Impaired hemostasis	Peptic ulcer, GI bleeding
Endocrine/metabolic	Low vitamin D, other factors	Osteodystrophy
	Cellular resistance to insulin	Glucose intolerance
	Mechanisms unclear	Poor growth and development, delayed sexual maturation†
Dermatologic	Chronic anemia	Pallor skin, mucous membranes
	Retention urea, pigments	Jaundice, uremic frost
	Clotting disorders	Ecchymoses, easy bleeding
	Secondary hyperparathyroidism	Pruritus, scratches
Hematologic	Lack of renal erythropoeitin	Chronic anemia
	Impaired platelet function and prothrombin consumption	Impaired hemostasis, with easy bleeding, bruising; splenomegaly
Immunologic	Lymphopenia, general leukopenia	Vulnerability to infection

*Although relatively uncommon, fluctuations to the other extreme (example, hypokalemia) may occur if oral intake is poor over prolonged period or during or after dialysis treatment.

†Primarily seen in children, adolescents, and young adults.

The focused history will typically show GI symptoms such as anorexia and nausea, sometimes with vomiting. The patient's mentation as he speaks is an important clue to central nervous system impairment. Signs may be as subtle as anxiety or mood swings or as immediately serious as seizures or coma.

Your general impression before the focused physical exam is likely to note marked abnormalities. Skin will typically be pale, moist, and cool. Scratches and ecchymoses are common skin changes associated with CRF. Mucous membranes may also be very pale, depending on the degree of anemia. Jaundice may be present, depending on the degree of retention of urea and other pigmented metabolic wastes. A skin condition called uremic frost appears when excessive amounts of urea are eliminated through sweat. As the sweat dries, a white "frosty" dust of urea may appear on the skin.

The major organ systems often show significant abnormalities on direct examination (Table 25-1). Because of the failure of vital urinary system functions, cardiovascular stress can be enormous. Either hypertension or hypotension may occur, depending on the degree of fluid retention (retention detectable as peripheral edema or pulmonary edema) and the level of cardiac function; tachycardia is common with both presentations. ECG findings may include a dysrhythmia secondary to hyperkalemia. Metabolic acidosis, when present, compounds the effects of hyperkalemia. Pericarditis is also common, and a rub may be heard on chest auscultation. Neuromuscular abnormalities, in addition to impaired mentation, include muscle cramps and "restless legs syndrome," as well as muscle twitching or tonic-clonic or other forms of seizure.

In CRF emergencies, the challenge is to separate chronic findings from those of recent onset or aggravated by the emergency.

Your abdominal exam will reveal many abnormalities. The challenge is to begin separating (by exam and history) chronic findings from those of recent onset or aggravated by the emergency that led to your call. For instance, you know that ecchymoses on the abdomen or flank may suggest acute hemorrhage. You may find a patient with ecchymoses scattered over the body surface. Look for evidence of new abdominal ecchymoses versus older bruises or a clear history of recent onset as signs of a current problem. Be sure to note abdominal contour, including the presence of symmetric distention or localized bulges, scars, and ecchymoses before the exam and to clearly document the pre-exam appearance. Findings on auscultation, percussion, and palpation will depend on the presenting problem.

As with ARF, CRF can lead to life-threatening complications, so monitoring and supporting the ABCs is vital. Use high-flow, high-concentration oxygen to maximize breathing efficiency. Couple this with circulatory supports such as positioning with the head down and the legs up to support blood flow to the brain and internal organs. Consider a small IV bolus for fluid resuscitation if hypovolemia is evident. Monitor the ECG readings closely and adjust supports according to your local protocol or discussion with medical direction. Expedite transportation to an appropriate facility in the same manner appropriate for patients with ARF. Be sure to talk quietly to the patient, both to calm him and to keep him informed of the time until arrival or other pertinent matters. If the patient is confused, ask short orientation questions periodically to assess lucidity and level of consciousness.

KIDNEY STONES

Kidney stones occur more frequently in summer and autumn.

Kidney stones, or *renal calculi* (singular, *calculus*), represent crystal aggregation in the kidney's collecting system (Figure 25-6). This condition is also called *nephrolithiasis* (from Greek *lithos*, stone). Kidney stones affect about 500,000 persons each year. Brief hospitalization is common due to the severity of pain as a stone travels from the renal pelvis, through the ureter, to the bladder, and is eliminated in urine. If necessary, additional in-patient treatment may include shock-wave lithotripsy, a procedure that uses sound waves to break large stones into smaller ones. Overall morbidity and mortality are low, unless a complication such as hemorrhage or urinary-tract obstruction results. Stones form more commonly in men than women, although the ratio varies for types of stones with different compositions. Certain stones also occur in familial patterns, suggesting hereditary factors. Another risk factor for calculus formation is immobilization due to surgery or injury, with the latter including immobilization secondary to paraplegia or other paralysis syndromes that involve the absence of motor impulses, sensation, or both. Last, the use of certain medications, including anesthetics, opiates, and psychotropic drugs, increases the risk for stones.

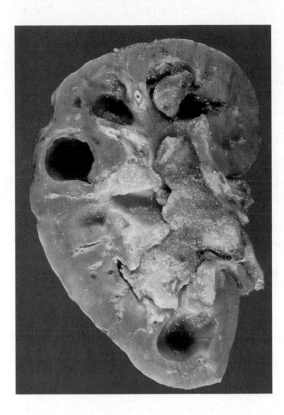

FIGURE 25-6 Sectioned kidney with kidney stones.

Stones may form in metabolic disorders such as gout or primary hyperparathyroidism, which produce excessive amounts of uric acid and calcium, respectively. More often, they occur when the general balance between water conservation and dissolution of relatively insoluble substances such as mineral ions and uric acid is lost and excessive amounts of the insolubles aggregate into stones. The problem boils down to "too much insoluble stuff" and urine "too concentrated," a situation that may more likely arise with change in diet, climate, or physical activity.

Stones consisting of calcium salts (namely, calcium oxalate and calcium phosphate) are by far the most common. These compounds are found in from 75% to 85% of all stones. Calcium stones are two to three times more common in men than in women, and the average age at onset is between 20 and 30 years. Their formation frequently runs in families, and anyone who has had a calcium stone is at fairly high risk to form another within 2 to 3 years.

The focused history almost always centers on pain. (Kidney stones are generally conceded to be among the most painful of medical conditions.) Typically, the patient first notes discomfort as a vague, visceral pain in one flank. Within 30 to 60 minutes it progresses to an extremely sharp pain that may remain in the flank or migrate downward and anteriorly toward the groin. Migrating pain indicates that the stone has passed into the lowest third of the ureter. Stones that lodge in the lowest part of the ureter, within the bladder wall, often cause characteristic bladder symptoms such as frequency during the day or during the night (nocturia), urgency, and painful urination. Because the latter three symptoms more frequently suggest bladder infection, making the probable diagnosis may be difficult, particularly in women. Visible hematuria is not uncommon in urine specimens taken during passage of a stone. Fever, however, is not typical unless infection is present. Whenever kidney stones are suspected, be sure to get the patient's personal medical history and family history, because both will often provide useful information.

The physical exam will almost always reveal someone who is very uncomfortable. The patient may be agitated or physically restless; walking sometimes reduces the pain. Vital signs will vary with level of discomfort, with highest blood pressure and heart rate associated with greatest pain. Skin will typically be pale, cool, and clammy. Abdominal examination may be difficult, depending on the patient's ability to remain still. First inspect the abdomen for contour and symmetry. Auscultation and percussion are generally useful only in ruling out GI conditions. Palpation results will vary and may depend, in part, on whether

Whenever kidney stones are suspected, be sure to get the patient's personal medical history and family history.

pain is so great that muscle guarding is present, making palpation of underlying structures impossible.

Parenteral narcotic analgesics or ketorolac (Toradol) should be considered for the patient with renal colic.

As always, management begins with the ABCs. Positioning should center on comfort, but be prepared for vomiting due to the severe pain, especially if the patient's last meal occurred within several hours. Consider analgesia en route to the hospital, according to your local protocol and your perception of the patient's condition. Use narcotics cautiously if a GI condition is at all possible or if mentation is impaired. If the pain is in the initial, intermittent, colicky phase, consider coaching pain management through breathing techniques similar to those used for women in labor. An IV line is useful for volume replacement or drug administration. The usual prevention strategy, if kidney function is adequate, is IV fluid to promote urine formation and movement through the system. Transport is the same as that for other abdominal conditions, i.e., position of comfort and supportive care.

URINARY TRACT INFECTION

urinary tract infection (UTI) usually a bacterial infection, which can occur at any site in the urinary tract.

Urinary tract infection (UTI) affects the urethra, bladder, or kidney, as well as the prostate gland in men. UTIs are extremely common, accounting for over six million office visits yearly. Almost all UTIs start with pathogenic colonization of the bladder by bacteria that enter through the urethra. Thus, females in general are at higher risk because of their relatively short urethra. Other groups at risk for UTI are paraplegic patients or patients with nerve disruption to the bladder, including some diabetic persons. Any condition that promotes **urinary stasis** (incomplete urination with urine remaining in the bladder that may serve as nutrition for pathogens) places a person at higher risk. Pregnant women often have urinary stasis due to pressure from the gravid uterus. People with neurological impairment (some patients with spina bifida or with diabetic neuropathy, for example) also tend to have urinary stasis, which predisposes them to infection. The use of instrumentation in patients who require bladder catheterization places them at even higher risk of UTIs.

urinary stasis condition in which the bladder empties incompletely during urination.

Morbidities such as scarring, abscesses, or eventual development of CRF are most likely in persons with anatomical abnormalities of the urinary system or chronic calculi (the latter acting as a focus for continuing infection and inflammation), those who are immunocompromised, or those who have renal disease due to diabetes mellitus or another condition.

UTIs are generally divided into those of the lower urinary tract, namely, urethritis (urethra), cystitis (bladder), and prostatitis (prostate gland), and those of the upper urinary tract, pyelonephritis (kidney).

Lower UTIs are far more common than upper UTIs, for two reasons. First, seeding of infection via the bloodstream is rare. Second, asymptomatic bacterial colonization of the urethra, especially in females, is very common, and can predispose a person to infection by other, pathogenic bacteria.

In females, infection may begin when gram-negative bacteria normally found in the bowel (that is, the enteric flora) colonize the urethra and bladder. Symptomatic **urethritis,** inflammation secondary to urethral infection, is very uncommon. More often you will see joint symptomatic infection of the urethra and bladder (urethritis and **cystitis,** respectively). Sexually active females are at higher risk, which may be attributed to use of contraceptive devices or agents, to the introduction of enteric flora during intercourse, or both. Recently, homosexually active men who engage in anal sex have also been found to be at higher risk for bacterial cystitis, possibly due to introduction of enteric bacterial flora during intercourse. In any case, sexually active persons who suffer from urinary stasis are at even higher risk for infection. Persons who urinate after intercourse might lower their risk because voiding eliminates some bacteria. The pathophysiology for persons using bladder catheterization probably differs only in that pathogenic bacteria are introduced directly into the bladder via the catheter. In general, the likelihood that active cystitis will develop, that antibiotic treatment will clear such infections, and that reinfection will occur are all determined by the interplay of the pathogen's virulence, the size of its colony, its sensitivity to antibiotic treatment, and the strength of the host's local and systemic immune functions.

Prostatitis, inflammation of the prostate gland, in our context, denotes inflammation secondary to bacterial infection, as well as any general inflammatory condition. Men with acute bacterial prostatitis, the closest parallel to acute cystitis in women, also tend to show evidence of joint urethritis, and the same bowel flora tend to be involved. The major difference between acute bacterial prostatitis and acute cystitis is the much lower incidence of prostatitis among men who do not require bladder catheterization.

Upper UTIs usually evolve from infection that spreads upward into the kidney. **Pyelonephritis** is an infectious inflammation of the renal parenchyma: nephrons, interstitial tissue, or both. Acute pyelonephritis is ten times more common in women than in men. Its incidence is highest in pregnancy and during periods of sexual activity, reflecting the epidemiology of lower UTIs. If the infection of pyelonephritis persists, intrarenal or perinephric abscesses may occur, but these complications are uncommon. **Intrarenal abscesses** form within the renal parenchyma. If they rupture and spill their contents into the adjacent fatty tissue, **perinephric abscesses** may result. From 20% to 60% of patients who develop perinephric abscesses have a clear predisposing factor such as renal calculi, anatomical abnormalities of the kidney, history of urological surgery or injury, or diabetic renal disease.

The focused history of lower UTI typically centers on three symptoms: painful urination, frequent urge to urinate, and difficulty in beginning and continuing to void. Pain often begins as visceral discomfort that progresses to severe, burning pain, particularly during and just after urination. The evolution of pain corresponds roughly to the degree of epithelial damage caused by the pathogen. In both men and women, pain is often localized to the pelvis and perceived as in the bladder (in women) or bladder and prostate (in men). The patient may complain of a strong or foul odor in the urine. Many women will give a history of similar episodes, which may or may not have been diagnosed or treated. Patients with pyelonephritis are more likely to feel generally ill or feverish. They typically complain of constant, moderately severe or severe pain in a flank or lower back (just under the rib cage). Pain may be referred to the shoulder or neck. The triad of urgency, pain, and difficulty may or may not be present or included in the past history.

On physical exam, patients with UTI appear restless and uncomfortable. Typically, patients with pyelonephritis appear more ill and are far more likely to have a fever. Skin will often be pale, cool, and moist (in lower UTI) or warm and dry (in febrile upper UTI). Vital signs will vary with the degree of illness and pain, but in an otherwise healthy individual they should not be far from the norms. Inspect and auscultate the abdomen to document findings, but neither procedure is likely to be very useful, because visible appearance and bowel sounds are usually within normal limits. Percussion and palpation will probably reveal painful tenderness over the pubis in lower UTI and at the flank in upper UTI. Lloyd's sign, tenderness to percussion of the lower back at the costovertebral angle (CVA), indicates pyelonephritis.

UTI management should center on the ABCs and circulatory support. If pain is severe, help the patient to a comfortable position, but consider the risk of aspiration during vomiting.

urethritis an infection and inflammation of the urethra.

cystitis an infection and inflammation of the urinary bladder.

prostatitis an infection and inflammation of the prostate gland.

pyelonephritis an infection and inflammation of the kidney.

intrarenal abscess a pocket of infection within kidney tissue.

perinephric abscess a pocket of infection in the layer of fat surrounding the kidney.

With acute pyelonephritis, the patient will usually appear quite ill. With cystitis, the patient will be uncomfortable but will not appear toxic.

Analgesics should be considered as with renal calculi; they will probably be needed only for severely painful cases of pyelonephritis. Consider nonpharmacological pain management with breathing and relaxation techniques. The best prevention technique is hydration to increase blood flow through the kidneys and to produce a more dilute urine. In many cases, this is better accomplished by IV administration, which eliminates the risk of vomiting and satisfies the guidelines for possible surgical cases. Expedite transport to an appropriate facility.

GENERAL ASSESSMENT

Your assessment of a patient who complains of abdominal discomfort or whom you suspect of having an abdominal pathology is similar to a trauma assessment with an expanded history. Do not approach the patient until you and your partner have determined the scene to be free and clear of any apparent dangers. Always take appropriate body substance isolation measures, including gloves, eyewear, mask, and disposable body gown to prevent contamination. As you approach the patient, survey the scene for potential evidence of your patient's problem. Medication bottles, alcohol containers, ashtrays, and buckets with emesis or sputum, for instance, can provide valuable information.

SCENE SIZE-UP AND INITIAL ASSESSMENT

As you approach, look for mechanisms of injury to help determine whether the call is medical or trauma. If you suspect trauma, always immobilize the cervical spine as you assess the adequacy of the patient's airway and his level of responsiveness. In the vast majority of medical patients you can check responsiveness and airway patency by asking the patient his name and chief complaint (why he called the ambulance today) and noting the answers. You can further evaluate the rate, depth, and quality of the patient's respirations fairly rapidly and without great difficulty. As you evaluate the respiratory functions, quickly palpate a pulse and check skin color, temperature, and circulation, including signs of bleeding and capillary refill. If you discover a life-threatening condition during the initial assessment, treat it and then rapidly continue the assessment to identify any other life threats.

HISTORY AND PHYSICAL EXAM

Once you have completed the initial assessment and dealt with any life threats, conduct the focused history and physical examination. Your ability to obtain a history from the patient will depend on his level of responsiveness. In some cases, you may detect deterioration of the patient's mental status over time as you take the history.

History

The history of the present illness and past medical history will be especially helpful in piecing together a clear picture of the underlying pathophysiology.

An accurate and thorough history can provide invaluable information. After you conduct the SAMPLE history (*Symptoms, Allergies, Medications, Past medical history, Last oral intake, and Events leading up to the emergency), you can take a more thorough, focused history, exploring the chief complaint, the history of the present illness, the past medical history, and the current health status. The history of the present illness and the past medical history will be especially helpful in sorting the multitude of signs and symptoms and piecing together a clear picture of the underlying pathophysiology.

History of the Present Illness Your OPQRST-ASPN history for gastrointestinal patients should address the following specific concerns:

   O—*Onset.* When did the pain first start? Was the onset very sudden or gradual? Sudden onsets of abdominal pain are generally caused by perforations of abdominal organs or capsules. Gradual onset of pain usually is associated with the blockage of hollow organs.

   P—*Provocation/palliation.* What makes the pain worse? What makes the pain better? If the pain lessens when the patient draws his legs up to his chest or lies on his side, it usually indicates peritoneal inflammation, which is often of

GI origin. If walking relieves the pain, the cause may be in the GI or urinary systems—perhaps an obstruction of the gallbladder or a stone caught in the renal pelvis or ureter.

Q—_Quality._ How would you describe the pain: dull, sharp, constant, intermittent? Localized, tearing pain is usually associated with the rupture of an organ. Dull, steadily increasing pain may indicate a bowel obstruction. Sharp pain, particularly in the flank, may indicate a kidney stone.

R—_Region/radiation._ Does the pain travel to any other part of your body? Radiated pain, or pain that seems to change location, is common because it involves the same neural routes as referred pain. Pain referred to the shoulder or neck is usually associated with an irritation of the diaphragm, such as happens with cholecystitis.

S—_Severity._ On a scale of 1 to 10, with 10 representing the worst pain possible, how would you rate the pain you are feeling now? The severity of pain usually worsens as the pathology (ischemia, inflammation, or stretching) of the organ advances.

T—_Time._ When did the pain first start? Estimation of the pain's time of onset is important to determine its possible causes. Any abdominal pain lasting over 6 hours is considered a surgical emergency and needs to be evaluated in the emergency department.

AS—_Associated symptoms._ Have you experienced any associated nausea and or vomiting with the discomfort? If yes, try to determine the content, color, and smell of the vomitus. Ask if the vomitus contained any bright red blood, "coffee grounds," or clots. Determining if your patient has an active GI bleed is imperative.

Have you experienced any changes in bowel habits—constipation or diarrhea—associated with this discomfort/pain? Question the patient further to determine if there have been any changes in feces such as a tarry, foul-smelling stool. Changes in bowel morphology, color, or smell can be the only indication of such conditions as a lower GI hemorrhage, gastritis, or bleeding diverticula.

Have you had an associated loss of appetite or weight loss? Patients who have an acute abdomen usually have an associated loss of appetite.

PN—_Pertinent negatives._ The absence of symptoms associated with GI function or the presence of symptoms related to urinary function may mean the problem originates in the urinary system. Pain in the lowest part of the abdomen, the pelvis, can be due to problems in the reproductive system. Last, remember that an inferior myocardial infarction (MI) can irritate the diaphragm and generate its referred-pain pattern. Be sure to check for cardiovascular history when this pain pattern (pain in shoulder and/or neck area) is present.

Keep in mind the information that your SAMPLE history gave you about your patient's last oral intake. It can help you to differentiate the possible causes of your patient's pain if the problem is in the GI system.

Not all abdominal emergencies result in abdominal pain. Some may cause chest pain. This, typically, is referred pain. Common gastrointestinal emergencies that can cause chest pain include: gastroesophageal reflux, gastric ulcers, duodenal ulcers, and, in some cases, gall bladder disease. When confronted by a patient with chest pain, always consider the gastrointestinal system as a possible cause.

Past Medical History Have you ever experienced this same type of pain or discomfort before? If the patient answers yes, then investigate whether he saw a physician for the problem and how it was diagnosed. Commonly, patients have been treated for the complaint in the past and the pain is a flare-up of an old problem.

Physical Examination

While you are conducting the history you can also begin the physical examination. Your patient's general appearance and posture strongly suggest his apparent state of health and the severity of his complaint. Usually patients with severe abdominal pathology lie as still as possible, often in the fetal position. They do not writhe around on the floor or cry out, because doing so increases the pain. You also should continually monitor the patient's level of consciousness for any subtle changes that indicate early signs of shock.

Take a complete set of vital signs to establish a baseline for further evaluation and treatment. These include pulse, respiratory rate, blood pressure, and pulse oximetry. You can also ascertain additional important information such as body temperature.

Visually inspect the abdomen before palpating it, auscultating it, or moving the patient. Remove the patient's clothing as necessary to freely visualize the entire abdomen. Distention of the abdomen may be an ominous sign. It can be caused by a build-up of free air due to an obstruction of the bowel. If the distention is caused by hemorrhage, the patient has lost a large amount of his circulating volume, for the abdomen can hold from four to six liters of fluid before any noticeable change in abdominal girth occurs. Other signs of fluid loss include periumbilical ecchymosis (**Cullen's sign**) and ecchymosis in the flank (**Grey-Turner's sign**).

Auscultating the abdomen usually provides little helpful information because bowel sounds are heard throughout this area. If you auscultate the abdomen, you must do so before palpating it. Listen for at least two minutes in each quadrant, beginning with the quadrant farthest from the affected area and auscultating the affected area last. Like auscultation, percussion requires a quiet environment and an experienced clinician. It too provides little or no useful information and, therefore, is not routinely performed in the field.

Palpating the abdomen, on the other hand, can give you a plethora of information. It can define the area of pain and identify the associated organs. Before palpating, ask the patient to point to where he is experiencing the most discomfort. Then work in reverse order, palpating that area last. Palpate the abdomen with a gentle pressure, feeling for muscle tension or its absence, as well as for masses, pulsations, and tenderness beneath the muscle. If you identify a pulsating mass, stop palpating at once; the increase in pressure may cause the affected blood vessel or organ to rupture.

GENERAL TREATMENT

Once you have completed the initial assessment and the focused history and physical examination, you can address treatment and transport. Your highest priority when treating a patient with abdominal pain is to secure and maintain his airway, breathing, and circulation. Be prepared to suction the airway of vomitus and blood. High-flow, high-concentration oxygenation and aggressive airway management may be indicated, depending on your patient's status. Monitor circulation by placing the patient on a cardiac monitor and frequently assessing his blood pressure. Measurement of the hematocrit will give an indirect measure of blood loss.

Establish a large-bore IV line in patients who complain of abdominal discomfort for use if emergency blood transfusion becomes necessary. You can use the IV for pharmacological intervention or to replace volume lost to hemorrhage or dehydration. In general, the need to avoid masking any abdominal pain for further evaluation will limit your pharmacological interventions to palliative agents such as antiemetics. Place the patient in a comfortable position and provide emotional reassurance based on your field assessment, any conversation with hospital staff or family, and knowledge of estimated transport time. Keep your voice and actions quiet and collected. Calm, as well as anxiety, are transmitted easily to patients and family. How you transport the patient will depend on his physiological status. Normally, gentle but rapid transport is sufficient. Remember that persistent abdominal pain lasting longer than 6 hours is classified as a surgical emergency and always requires transport. In all cases, be sure to maintain monitoring of mental status and vital signs and to give nothing by mouth. Bring vomitus to the emergency department for evaluation.

Usually, patients with severe abdominal pathology lie as still as possible, often in the fetal position.

Cullen's sign ecchymosis in the periumbilical area.

Grey-Turner's sign ecchymosis in the flank.

Distention of the abdomen may be an ominous sign.

If you auscultate the abdomen, you must do so before palpating it.

Your highest priority for a patient with abdominal pain is to secure and maintain his airway, breathing, and circulation.
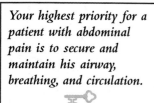

Persistent abdominal pain lasting longer than 6 hours always requires transport.

SUMMARY

Abdominal pain can originate from a wide variety of causes, either from the abdominal organs or from areas outside of the abdominal cavity. The prehospital management priorities for the abdominal patient are to establish and maintain his airway, breathing, and circulation. The differential diagnosis can include a multitude of causes that usually cannot be identified without laboratory and radiographic analysis. Airway management is of paramount importance, since patients frequently suffer from severe bouts of nausea and vomiting. Be prepared to turn the patient onto his side if necessary to clear large amounts of vomitus from the airway. Oxygenation usually can be adequately stabilized by placing the patient on high-flow, high-concentration oxygen via a nonrebreather mask. Fluid loss, hemorrhage, or sepsis may compromise the circulatory status. You should initiate fluid resuscitation for the hemodynamically unstable patient in the field, but never delay transport. Patients who have abdominal pain lasting more than 6 hours should always be evaluated by a physician.

ON THE WEB

For additional practice and review, go to the companion website at www.prenhall.com/bledsoe and click on *Intermediate Emergency Care: Principles & Practice*.

CHAPTER 26

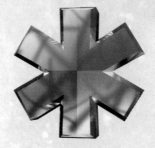

Environmental Emergencies

Objectives

After reading this chapter, you should be able to:

1. Define environmental emergency. (pp. 1055–1056)

2. Identify risk factors most predisposing to environmental emergencies. (pp. 1055–1056)

3. Identify environmental factors that may cause illness, exacerbate a preexisting illness, or complicate treatment or transport decisions. (pp. 1055–1056)

4. Identify normal, critically high, and critically low body temperatures. (pp. 1058-1060)

5. Describe several methods of temperature monitoring. (p. 1060)

6. Describe the body's compensatory processes for over-heating and for excess heat loss. (pp. 1056–1060, 1065)

7. List the common forms of heat and cold disorders. (pp. 1060–1072)

8. Define heat illness and hyperthermia, and list their common predisposing factors and preventive measures. (pp. 1060–1061)

9. Identify the signs, symptoms, and treatment for heat cramps, heat exhaustion, and heat-stroke. (pp. 1061–1063)

10. Discuss the role of dehydration and the role of fluid therapy in heat disorders. (p. 1064)

11. Discuss how to differentiate fever from heat-stroke and treatment for fever. (p. 1064)

12. Define hypothermia and list its common predisposing factors and preventive measures. (pp. 1065–1066)

13. Identify differences between mild, severe, chronic, and acute hypothermia. (p. 1066)

14. Identify the signs, symptoms, and treatment for hypothermia. (pp. 1066–1071)

15. Discuss the impact of severe hypothermia on standard BCLS and ACLS algorithms and transport considerations. (pp. 1069, 1070–1071)

16. Define frostbite and trench foot, and discuss the degrees of frostbite and the treatment for frostbite and trench foot. (pp. 1071–1072)

17. Define near-drowning, list its signs and symptoms, and discuss its treatment. (pp. 1072–1075)

18. Discuss the complications and protective role of hypothermia in the context of near-drowning. (pp. 1072–1074)

19. Discuss the pathophysiology, signs and symptoms, and management of diving emergencies. (pp. 1075–1081)

20. Discuss the pathophysiology, signs and symptoms, and management of high altitude illness. (pp. 1081–1084)

21. Discuss the pathophysiology, signs and symptoms, and management of radiation injuries. (pp. 1084–1088)

22. Given several pre-programmed simulated environmental emergency patients, provide the appropriate assessment, management, and transportation. (pp. 1056–1088)

CASE STUDY

Today is Sunday, you and your partner are staffing Medic 7. Because of the bad weather, you pick up your partner from his home in your four-wheel drive sport utility vehicle and ride together to work at the Thunder Bay station. It is another bitterly cold January day, so you warm up with a mug of hot chocolate, awaiting what the day will bring. Suddenly, central dispatch calls in a "priority A" situation at 1050 Ventura Road, a downtown office building in the bar and nightclub district. Apparently, someone on the way to work found an unconscious man lying in the snow. You and your partner depart immediately.

Upon arrival you find an approximately 20-year-old male huddled and shivering on the ice-covered ground. His breathing is shallow and irregular. He is quite stuporous and confused but manages to tell you that he had been out celebrating his twenty-first birthday last night and early this morning. He thinks he passed out here a couple of hours ago but really is not sure.

Your assessment reveals that the patient is bradycardic and mildly hypotensive. His core temperature is 86°F (30°C). While you are speaking with the patient, he stops shivering and his speech becomes unintelligible. You and your partner gently and slowly put him in the ambulance, remove his wet clothing, apply cardiac and core temperature monitors, and then place warm water bottles at his head, neck, chest, and groin. Your partner notes his core temperature has dropped to 85°F (29.4°C).

En route to Foothills General Hospital, your vehicle passes through a bumpy area of road construction, jostling your patient considerably. The alarms go off, and ventricular fibrillation appears on the monitor. Vital signs are absent after checking for two minutes. Your partner administers 200J, 300J, and 360J shocks, without success. You intubate the patient, ventilate with warmed oxygen, and begin chest compressions. You give no medications through the IV.

In the emergency department, the patient is gradually rewarmed, using active techniques. Once the core temperature is above 86°F (30°C), the usual ACLS protocols are initiated. The patient is converted from ventricular fibrillation and slowly regains vital signs and eventually is admitted to the ICU. Following admission, he does well and is discharged five days later. The day before his discharge you and your partner stop by to check his progress. He reports that he is doing very well but does not remember the prehospital care or the ambulance ride. The patient is adamant about one thing, however. He vows never to drink alcohol again.

INTRODUCTION

The term *environment* can be defined as all of the surrounding external factors that affect the development and functioning of a living organism. Human beings obviously depend on the environment for life. But they also must be protected from its extremes. When factors such as temperature, weather, terrain, and atmospheric pressure act on the body, they can create stresses that the body is unable to compensate for. A medical condition caused or exacerbated by such environmental factors is known as an **environmental emergency.**

Environmental emergencies include a variety of conditions such as heatstroke, hypothermia, drowning or near-drowning, altitude sickness, nuclear radiation, and diving accidents or barotraumas, among others. Such emergencies often call for special rescue resources.

Although environmental emergencies can affect anyone, several risk factors predispose certain individuals to developing environmental illnesses. These factors include:

- Age—very young children and older adults do not tolerate environmental extremes very well.

environmental emergency medical condition caused or exacerbated by weather, terrain, atmospheric pressure, or other local factors.

- Poor general health
- Fatigue
- Predisposing medical conditions
- Certain medications—either prescription or over-the-counter

Environmental factors must also be considered when determining the risk for environmental emergencies. For example, climate in a particular place may vary greatly from moment to moment. Areas where change in temperature can be drastic over the course of the day may catch unwary individuals off guard. For example, desert areas can have temperatures of 105°F during the day but drop below freezing at night, placing unprepared travelers in a difficult situation. Temperatures in parts of southern Alberta can change drastically when the Chinook winds kick up. Other considerations include the season, local weather patterns, atmospheric pressures (high altitude or underwater), and the type of terrain, which can cause injury or hinder rescue efforts.

As an EMT-I, you will frequently be called upon to treat medical emergencies related to environmental conditions. It is critical that you understand the particular conditions that prevail in your region. If you live in a mountain area, near large caves, in an area with swift moving water, or in a resort area where diving is prominent, you need to be familiar with the specialized rescue resources these situations may require and the particular environmental emergencies they may cause. Understanding their causes and underlying pathophysiologies can help you recognize these emergencies promptly and manage them effectively.

Although many environmental factors can result in medical emergencies, this chapter will focus primarily on problems related to temperature extremes, drowning or near-drowning, diving emergencies, high altitude illness, and nuclear radiation.

HOMEOSTASIS

homeostasis the natural tendency of the body to maintain a steady and normal internal environment.

In order for the human body to function properly, it must interact with the environment to obtain oxygen, nutrients, and other necessities, but it must also avoid being damaged by extreme external environmental conditions. The process of maintaining constant suitable conditions within the body is called **homeostasis.** Various body systems respond in an effort to maintain the correct core and peripheral temperature, oxygen level, and energy supply to maintain life.

The following sections address how the body attempts to maintain these normal settings and what happens when certain environmental conditions exceed the ability of the body to compensate.

PATHOPHYSIOLOGY OF HEAT AND COLD DISORDERS

MECHANISMS OF HEAT GAIN AND LOSS

The body gains and loses heat in two ways, from within the body itself and by contact with the external environment.

thermal gradient the difference in temperature between the environment and the body.

The body receives heat from or loses it to the environment via the **thermal gradient.** The thermal gradient is the difference in temperature between the environment (the ambient temperature) and the body. The ambient temperature is usually different from body temperature. If the environment is warmer than the body, heat flows from the environment to the body. If the body is warmer than the environment, heat flows from the body to the environment. Other environmental factors, including wind and relative humidity (the percentage of water vapor in the air), also affect heat gain and loss.

The mechanisms by which heat is generated within the body and by which heat is gained or lost to the environment are discussed in more detail in the following sections.

THERMOGENESIS (HEAT GENERATION)

The amount of heat in the body continually fluctuates as a result of the heat generated or gained and the heat lost. The body gains heat from both external and internal sources. In addition to the heat the body absorbs from the environment, the body also generates heat through energy-producing chemical reactions (metabolism).

The creation of heat is called **thermogenesis.** There are several types of thermogenesis. One is *work-induced thermogenesis* that results from exercise. Our muscles need to create heat because warm muscles work more effectively than cold ones. One way muscles can produce heat is by shivering. Another type, *thermoregulatory thermogenesis,* is controlled by the endocrine system. The hormones norepinephrine and epinephrine can cause an immediate increase in the rate of cellular metabolism, which in turn increases heat production. The last type, metabolic thermogenesis, or *diet-induced thermogenesis,* is caused by the processing of food and nutrients. When a meal is eaten, digested, absorbed, and metabolized, heat is produced as a by-product of these activities.

thermogenesis the production of heat, especially within the body.

THERMOLYSIS (HEAT LOSS)

The heat generated by the body is constantly lost to the environment. This occurs because the body is usually warmer than the surrounding environment. The transfer of heat into the environment occurs through the following mechanisms (Figure 26-1):

thermolysis loss of heat from the body.

- **Conduction.** Direct contact of the body's surface to another, cooler object causes the body to lose heat by conduction. Heat flows from higher temperature matter to lower temperature matter.

conduction moving electrons, ions, heat, or sound waves through a conductor or conducting medium.

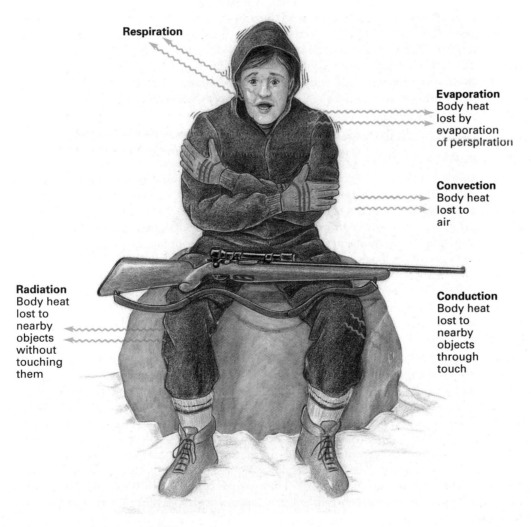

Respiration

Evaporation
Body heat lost by evaporation of perspiration

Convection
Body heat lost to air

Radiation
Body heat lost to nearby objects without touching them

Conduction
Body heat lost to nearby objects through touch

FIGURE 26-1   Heat loss by the body.

convection transfer of heat via currents in liquids or gases.

radiation transfer of energy through space or matter.

evaporation change from liquid to a gaseous state.

respiration the exchange of gases between a living organism and its environment.

thermoregulation the maintenance or regulation of a particular temperature of the body.

core temperature the body temperature of the deep tissues, which usually does not vary more than a degree or so from its normal 98.6°F (37°C).

Content Review

COMPARATIVE BODY TEMPERATURES

Celsius	Fahrenheit
40.6°	105°
37.8°	100°
37°	98.6°
35°	95°
32°	89.6°
30°	86°
20°	68°

Content Review

MECHANISMS OF HEAT DISSIPATION/CONSERVATION

Dissipation
- Sweating
- Vasodilation

Conservation
- Shivering
- Vasoconstriction

hypothalamus portion of the diencephalon that produces neurosecretions important in the control of certain metabolic activities, including body temperature regulation.

- **Convection.** Heat loss to air currents passing over the body is called convection. Heat, however, must first be conducted to the air before being carried away by convection currents.

- **Radiation.** An unclothed person will lose approximately 60% of total body heat by radiation at normal room temperature. This heat loss is in the form of infrared rays. All objects not at absolute zero temperature will radiate heat into the atmosphere.

- **Evaporation.** Evaporation is the change of a liquid to vapor. Evaporative heat loss occurs as water evaporates from the skin. Additionally, a great deal of heat loss occurs through evaporation of fluids in the lungs. Water evaporates from the skin and lungs at approximately 600 mL/day.

- **Respiration.** Respiration combines the mechanisms of convection, radiation, and evaporation. It accounts for a large proportion of the body's heat loss. Heat is transferred from the lungs to inspired air by convection and radiation. Evaporation in the lungs humidifies the inspired air (adds water vapor to it). During expiration this warm, humidified air is released into the environment, creating heat loss.

THERMOREGULATION

Thermoregulation is the maintenance or regulation of temperature. The body temperature of the deep tissues, commonly called the **core temperature,** usually does not vary more than a degree or so from its normal 98.6°F (37°C). A naked person can be exposed to an external environment ranging anywhere from 55°F to 144°F and still maintain a fairly constant internal body temperature. This characteristic of warm-blooded animals is called steady-state metabolism. The various biochemical reactions occurring within the cell are most efficient when the body temperature is within this narrow temperature range.

Evaluation of peripheral body temperature can be measured by touch or by taking the temperature by oral or axillary means. Core body temperatures can be measured using tympanic or rectal thermometers.

The body maintains a balance between the production and loss of heat almost entirely through the nervous system and negative feedback mechanisms. The **hypothalamus,** located at the base of the brain, is responsible for temperature regulation. It functions as a thermostat, controlling temperature through the release of neurosecretions (secretions produced by nerve cells). When the hypothalamus senses an increased body temperature, it shuts off the mechanisms designed to create heat (for example, shivering). When it senses a decrease in body temperature, the hypothalamus shuts off mechanisms designed to cool the body (for example, sweating). Because the action involved requires stopping, or negating, a process, it is called a **negative feedback** system.

When the heat-regulating function of the hypothalamus is disrupted, the result can be an abnormally high or low body temperature. At the extremes, such abnormal temperatures can result in death (Figure 26-2).

Thermoreceptors

Although the hypothalamus plays a key role in body temperature regulation, temperature receptors in other parts of the body also help to moderate temperatures. There are thermoreceptors in the skin and certain mucous membranes (peripheral thermoreceptors) as well as in certain deep tissues of the body (central thermoreceptors). The skin has both cold and warm receptors. Because cold receptors outnumber warm receptors, peripheral detection of temperature consists mainly of detecting cold rather than warmth. Deep body temperature receptors lie mostly in the spinal cord, abdominal viscera, and in or around the great veins. These receptors are exposed to the body's core temperature rather than the peripheral temperature. They also respond mainly to cold rather than warmth. Both peripheral and central thermoreceptors act to prevent lowering of the body temperature.

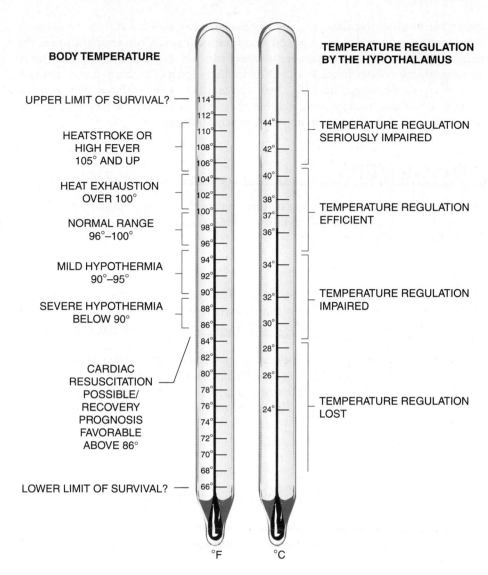

BODY TEMPERATURE

TEMPERATURE REGULATION BY THE HYPOTHALAMUS

UPPER LIMIT OF SURVIVAL? — 114°

112°

HEATSTROKE OR HIGH FEVER 105° AND UP — 110° 108° 106°

TEMPERATURE REGULATION SERIOUSLY IMPAIRED — 44° 42°

HEAT EXHAUSTION OVER 100° — 104° 102° 100°

TEMPERATURE REGULATION EFFICIENT — 40° 38° 37°

NORMAL RANGE 96°–100° — 98° 96° — 36°

MILD HYPOTHERMIA 90°–95° — 94° 92° 90° — 34°

TEMPERATURE REGULATION IMPAIRED — 32°

SEVERE HYPOTHERMIA BELOW 90° — 88° 86° — 30°

84° 82° — 28°

CARDIAC RESUSCITATION POSSIBLE/ RECOVERY PROGNOSIS FAVORABLE ABOVE 86° — 80° 78° 76° 74° — 26° 24°

TEMPERATURE REGULATION LOST

72° 70° 68°

LOWER LIMIT OF SURVIVAL? — 66°

°F   °C

FIGURE 26-2 Temperature regulation by the hypothalamus.

Metabolic Rate

The **basal metabolic rate (BMR)** is the metabolism that occurs when the body is completely at rest. It is the rate at which the body consumes energy just to maintain itself—the rate of metabolism that maintains brain function, circulation, and cell stability. Any additional activity that the body performs demands energy consumption beyond that supported by the basal rate, metabolizing more nutrients and releasing more calories (units of heat). The rate of metabolism that supports this additional activity is called an **exertional metabolic rate.**

The body continually adjusts the metabolic rate in order to maintain the temperature of the core (where the crucial structures such as the heart and brain are located). The body also achieves temperature maintenance by dilating some blood vessels and constricting others so that the blood carries the excess heat from the core to the periphery where it is close to the skin. This allows heat to dissipate through the skin into the environment.

Conversely, when the environment is too cold, counter-current heat exchange is used to shunt warm blood away from the superficial veins near the skin and back into the deep veins near the core to keep vital structures warm. Another body response that counters a cold environment is shivering, a physical activity that increases metabolism and generates heat.

negative feedback homeostatic mechanism in which a change in a variable (here, core temperature) ultimately inhibits the process that led to the shift.

basal metabolic rate (BMR) rate at which the body consumes energy just to maintain stability; the basic metabolic rate (measured by the rate of oxygen consumption) of an awake, relaxed person 12–14 hours after eating and at a comfortable temperature.

exertional metabolic rate rate at which the body consumes energy during activity. It is faster than the basic metabolic rate.

It is important to note that these various mechanisms can create a difference between the core body temperature and the peripheral body temperature. Core temperature is the crucial measurement since, as noted, the core is where the major organs are located. Therefore, it is important in any heat-related or cold-related emergency to obtain a core temperature reading such as from the rectum. Oral and axillary temperatures may provide convenient approximations in some situations but may lead to incorrect interventions if relied on for treatment of the patient with an environmental illness.

HEAT DISORDERS

heat illness increased core body temperature due to inadequate thermolysis.

hyperthermia unusually high core body temperature.

Disruption of the body's normal thermoregulatory mechanisms can produce a number of heat illnesses, such as hyperthermia and fever. **Heat illness** is increased *core body temperature (CBT)* due to inadequate thermolysis.

HYPERTHERMIA

Hyperthermia is a state of unusually high body temperature, specifically the core body temperature. Hyperthermia is usually caused by heat transfer from the external environment for which the body cannot compensate. Occasionally it is caused by excessive generation of heat within the body.

As the body attempts to eliminate this excessive heat, you will see the general signs of thermolysis (heat loss). These signs are caused by the body's two chief methods of heat dissipation, sweating (which leads to evaporative heat loss) and vasodilation (which allows the blood to carry heat to the periphery for dissipation through the skin). These include:

- Diaphoresis (sweating)
- Increased skin temperature
- Flushing

As heat illness progresses, you will also note signs of thermolytic inadequacy (the failure of the body's thermoregulatory mechanisms to compensate adequately): altered mentation and altered level of consciousness.

Hyperthermia can manifest as heat cramps, heat exhaustion, or heatstroke, which will be discussed in following sections.

PREDISPOSING FACTORS

Age, general health, and medications are predisposing factors in hyperthermia. Factors that may contribute to a susceptibility to hyperthermia include:

autonomic neuropathy condition that damages the autonomic nervous system, which usually senses changes in core temperature and controls vasodilation and perspiration to dissipate heat.

- *Age of the patient.* Pediatric and geriatric populations can tolerate less variation in temperature and their heat-regulating mechanisms are not as responsive as those of young adult and adult populations.
- *Health of the patient.* Diabetics can become hyperthermic more easily because they develop **autonomic neuropathy.** This condition damages the autonomic nervous system, which may interfere with thermoregulatory input and with vasodilation and perspiration, which normally dissipate heat.
- *Medications.* Various medications can affect body temperature in the following ways. Diuretics predispose to dehydration, which worsens hyperthermia. Beta blockers interfere with vasodilation and reduce the capacity to increase heart rate in response to volume loss and may also interfere with thermoregulatory input. Psychotropics and antihistamines, such as antipsychotics and phenothiazines, interfere with central thermoregulation.

acclimatization the reversible changes in body structure and function by which the body becomes adjusted to a change in environment.

- *Level of acclimatization.* **Acclimatization** is the process of becoming adjusted to a change in environment. In response to an environmental change, reversible changes in body structure and function take place that help to maintain homeostasis.

- *Length of exposure*
- *Intensity of exposure*
- *Environmental factors* such as humidity and wind

PREVENTIVE MEASURES

Ideally, prevention of heat disorders is preferable to treating an illness already in progress. Measures to prevent hyperthermia include the following:

- Maintain adequate fluid intake, remembering that thirst is an inadequate indicator of dehydration.
- Allow time for gradual acclimatization to being out in the heat. Acclimatization results in more perspiration with lower salt concentration and increases body-fluid volume.
- Limit exposure to hot environments.

SPECIFIC HEAT DISORDERS

Inevitably, you will be required to respond to heat-related emergencies such as heat cramps, heat exhaustion, or heatstroke. Heat cramps and heat exhaustion result from dehydration and depletion of sodium and other electrolytes. Heatstroke, a far more serious and potentially life-threatening condition, occurs when the thermoregulatory mechanisms of the body fail.

Signs and symptoms and emergency care procedures for heat cramps, heat exhaustion, and heatstroke are discussed in the following sections.

Heat (Muscle) Cramps

Heat cramps are muscle cramps caused by overexertion and dehydration in the presence of high atmospheric temperatures. Sweating occurs as sodium (salt) is transported to the skin. Because "water follows sodium," water is deposited on the skin surface where evaporation occurs, aiding in the cooling process. Since sweating involves not only the loss of water but also the loss of electrolytes (such as sodium), intermittent cramping of skeletal muscles may occur. Heat cramps are painful but are not considered to be an actual heat illness.

heat cramps acute painful spasms of the voluntary muscles following strenuous activity in a hot environment without adequate fluid or salt intake.

Signs and Symptoms   The patient with heat cramps will present with cramps in the fingers, arms, legs, or abdominal muscles. He will generally be mentally alert with a feeling of weakness. He may feel dizzy or faint. Vital signs will be stable. Body temperature may be normal or slightly elevated. The skin is likely to be moist and warm.

Treatment   Treatment of the patient with heat cramps is usually easily accomplished. First, remove the patient from the environment. Place him in a cool environment such as a shaded area or the air conditioned back of the ambulance. In the case of severe cramps, administer an oral saline solution (approximately four teaspoons of salt to one gallon of water) or a sports drink. Do NOT administer salt tablets, which are not absorbed as readily and may cause stomach irritation and ulceration or **hypernatremia**. If the patient is unable to take fluids orally, an IV of normal saline may be needed.

hypernatremia excess of sodium in the blood.

Some EMS systems recommend massaging the painful muscles. Application of moist towels to the patient's forehead and over the cramped muscles may also be helpful.

Heat Exhaustion

Heat exhaustion, which is considered to be a mild heat illness, is an acute reaction to heat exposure. It is the most common heat-related illness seen by prehospital personnel. An individual performing work in a hot environment will lose one to two liters of water per hour. Each liter lost contains 20 to 50 milliequivalents of sodium. The resulting loss of water and sodium, combined with general vasodilation, leads to a decreased circulating blood volume, venous pooling, and reduced cardiac output.

heat exhaustion a mild heat illness; an acute reaction to heat exposure.

Dehydration and sodium loss due to sweating account for the presenting symptoms. However, these signs and symptoms are not exclusive to heat exhaustion. Instead, they mimic those of an individual suffering from fluid and sodium loss from any of a number of other causes. A history of exposure to high environmental temperatures is needed to obtain an accurate assessment.

If not treated, heat exhaustion may progress to heatstroke.

Signs and Symptoms Signs and symptoms that you may encounter include increased body temperature (over 100°F or 37.8°C), skin that is cool and clammy with heavy perspiration, breathing that is rapid and shallow, and a weak pulse. The patient may have signs of active thermolysis such as diarrhea and muscle cramps. The patient will feel weak and, in some cases, may lose consciousness. There may be central nervous system (CNS) symptoms such as headache, anxiety, paresthesia, and impaired judgment or even psychosis.

Treatment Prehospital management of the patient with heat exhaustion is aimed at immediate cooling and fluid replacement. Steps include:

1. Remove the patient from the environment. Place the patient in a cool environment such as a shaded area or the air-conditioned ambulance.
2. Place the patient in a supine position.
3. Administer an oral saline solution (approximately four teaspoons of salt to one gallon of water) or a sports drink. Do NOT administer salt tablets, which are not absorbed as readily and may cause stomach irritation and ulceration or hypernatremia. If the patient is unable to take fluids orally, an IV of normal saline may be needed.
4. Remove some clothing and fan the patient. Remove enough clothing to cool the patient without chilling him. Fanning increases evaporation and cooling. Again, be careful not to cool the patient to the point of chilling. If the patient begins to shiver, stop fanning and perhaps cover the patient lightly.
5. Treat for shock, if shock is suspected. However, be careful not to cover the patient to the point of overheating him.

Symptoms should resolve with fluids, rest, and supine posturing with knees elevated. If they do not, consider that the symptoms may be due to an increased core body temperature, which is predictive of impending heatstroke and should be treated aggressively, as outlined in the following section.

Heatstroke

heatstroke acute, dangerous reaction to heat exposure, characterized by a body temperature usually above 105°F (40.6°C) and central nervous system disturbances. The body usually ceases to perspire.

Heatstroke is a true environmental emergency.

Heatstroke is a true environmental emergency that occurs when the body's hypothalamic temperature regulation is lost, causing uncompensated hyperthermia. This in turn causes cell death and damage to the brain, liver, and kidneys. There is no arbitrary core temperature at which heatstroke begins. However, heatstroke is generally characterized by a body temperature of at least 105°F (40.6°C), central nervous system disturbances, and usually the cessation of sweating.

Signs and Symptoms Sweating is thought to stop due to destruction of the sweat glands or when sensory overload causes them to temporarily dysfunction. However, the patient's skin may be either dry or covered with sweat that is still present on the skin from earlier exertion. In either case, the skin will be hot.

The patient may present with the following signs and symptoms:

- Cessation of sweating
- Hot skin that is dry or moist
- Very high core temperature
- Deep respirations that become shallow, rapid at first but may later slow
- Rapid, full pulse, may slow later
- Hypotension with low or absent diastolic reading
- Confusion or disorientation or unconsciousness
- Possible seizures

Classic heatstroke commonly presents in those with chronic illnesses, with the increased core body temperature due to deficient thermoregulatory function. Predisposing conditions include age, diabetes, and other medical conditions. Hot, red, dry skin is common in this type of heatstroke.

Exertional heatstroke commonly presents in those who are in good general health, with the increased core body temperature due to overwhelming heat stress. There is excessive ambient temperature as well as excessive exertion with prolonged exposure and poor acclimatization. In this type of heatstroke you will find that, although sweating has ceased and the skin is hot, moisture from prior sweating may still be present.

If the patient develops heatstroke due to exertion, he may go into severe metabolic acidosis caused by lactic acid accumulation. Hyperkalemia (excessive potassium in blood) may also develop because of the release of potassium from injured muscle cells, renal failure, or metabolic acidosis.

Treatment Prehospital management of the heatstroke patient is aimed at immediate cooling and replacement of fluids. Steps include the following:

> *The heatstroke patient should be cooled immediately and given fluids.*

1. Remove the patient from the environment. This first step is essential. If you do not remove the patient from the hot environment, any other measures will be only minimally useful. Move the patient to a cool environment, such as the air-conditioned ambulance.

2. Initiate rapid active cooling. Body temperature must be lowered to 102°F (39°C). A target of 102°F (39°C) is used to avoid an overcorrection. This can be accomplished en route to the hospital. Remove the patient's clothing and cover the patient with sheets soaked in tepid water. Fanning and misting may also be used if necessary. Refrain from overcooling, because it may cause reflex hypothermia (low body temperature). This results in shivering, which can raise the core temperature again. Tepid water is used because ice packs and cold-water immersion may affect peripheral thermoreceptors, producing reflex vasoconstriction and shivering.

3. Administer high-flow, high-concentration oxygen by nonrebreather mask. If respirations are shallow, assist with a bag-valve-mask unit supplied with 100% oxygen. Utilize pulse oximetry, if available.

4. Administer fluid therapy if the patient is alert and able to swallow.
   - *Oral fluids.* In many cases oral fluid therapy will be all that is needed. Some salt additive is beneficial, but salt tablets should be avoided because they may cause gastrointestinal irritation and ulceration or hypernatremia. There is a very limited need for other electrolytes in oral rehydration.
   - *Intravenous fluids.* Begin one to two IVs, using normal saline. Initially infuse them wide open.

5. Monitor the ECG. Cardiac dysrhythmias may occur at any time. S-T segment depression, non-specific T-wave changes with occasional PVCs, and supraventricular tachycardias are common.

6. Avoid vasopressors and anticholinergic drugs. These agents may potentiate heatstroke by inhibiting sweating. They can also produce a hypermetabolic state in the presence of high environmental temperatures and relatively high humidity.

7. Monitor body temperature. EMS systems operating in extremely warm climates should carry some device to record the body temperature, whether a simple rectal thermometer or a sophisticated electronic device. Simple glass thermometers generally do not measure above 106°F (41°C) or below 95°F (35°C). This may become significant during long transport when it is essential to detect changes in the patient's condition.

ROLE OF DEHYDRATION IN HEAT DISORDERS

Dehydration often goes hand in hand with heat disorders because it inhibits vasodilation and therefore thermolysis. Dehydration leads to orthostatic hypotension (increased pulse and decreased blood pressure on rising from a supine position) and the following symptoms, which may occur along with the signs and symptoms of heatstroke:

- Nausea, vomiting, and abdominal distress
- Vision disturbances
- Decreased urine output
- Poor skin turgor
- Signs of hypovolemic shock

When these signs and symptoms are present, rehydration of the patient is critical. Oral fluids may be administered if the patient is alert and not nauseated. Administration of IV fluids may be necessary, especially if the patient has an altered mental status or is nauseated. It is not uncommon for the adult patient with moderate to severe dehydration to require 2 to 3 liters of IV fluids (occasionally more!).

FEVER (PYREXIA)

pyrexia fever, or above-normal body temperature.

A fever (**pyrexia**) is the elevation of the body temperature above the normal temperature for that person. (An individual person's normal temperature may be one or two degrees above or below 98.6°F or 37°C.) The body develops a fever when pathogens enter and cause infection, which in turn stimulates the production of pyrogens.

pyrogen any substance causing a fever, such as viruses and bacteria or substances produced within the body in response to infection or inflammation.

Pyrogens are any substances that cause fever, such as viruses and bacteria or substances produced within the body in response to infection or inflammation. They reset the hypothalamic thermostat to a higher level. Metabolism is increased, which produces the elevation of temperature. The increased body temperature fights infection by making the body a less hospitable environment for the invading organism. The hypothalamic thermostat will reset to normal when pyrogen production stops or when pathogens end their attack on the body.

Fever is sometimes difficult to differentiate from heatstroke, and neurological symptoms may present with either, but usually there is a history of infection or illness with a fever. Although the heatstroke patient usually has a history of exertion and exposure to high ambient temperatures, this is not always the case. In some cases, heatstroke can be caused by impaired functioning of the hypothalamus without exertion or exposure to ambient heat. Treat for heatstroke if you are unsure which it is.

Although fever may be beneficial, it can be disconcerting to the parents of children with fever. In addition, fever can be uncomfortable for the patient. If the patient is uncomfortable, measures should be taken to treat the fever. Also, if a child has a history of febrile seizures, the fever should be treated. Parents will often have their febrile children wrapped in several layers of clothing or blankets because the child is "cold." These should be removed, leaving only the diaper or underclothes, exposing the child to the ambient air. This will allow a controlled cooling.

Do not use sponge baths to cool febrile children.

Sponge baths and cool-water immersion should not be used. These cause a rapid drop in the body core temperature and result in shivering. This again elevates the core temperature, which complicates the process. Several medications are good antipyretics (that is, they lower body temperature in fever). These include acetaminophen (Tylenol) and ibuprofen (Motrin). Many EMS systems will utilize an antipyretic in the treatment of fever, particularly in pediatric patients. Liquid acetaminophen and ibuprofen are easy to administer and effective. Acetaminophen is also available in a suppository form for patients with active vomiting. These antipyretics are typically dosed based on the patient's weight:

Consider administering an antipyretic, primarily for patient comfort. This is especially important in services with long transportation times.

- *Acetaminophen*—15 mg/kg for pediatric patients; adult dose is typically 650 mg
- *Ibuprofen*—10 mg/kg for pediatric patients; adult dose is typically 600 to 800 mg

These liquid medications should be dosed with syringes because teaspoons are inaccurate measuring devices. EMS services with prolonged transport times should consider the use of antipyretics for patient comfort as well as for the prevention of febrile seizures.

COLD DISORDERS

Disruption of the body's normal thermoregulation may produce cold-related disorders such as hypothermia, frostbite, and trench foot.

HYPOTHERMIA

Hypothermia is a state of low body temperature, specifically low core temperature. When the core temperature of the body drops below 95°F (35°C), an individual is considered to be hypothermic. Hypothermia can be attributed to inadequate thermogenesis, excessive cold stress, or a combination of both.

MECHANISMS OF HEAT CONSERVATION AND LOSS

Exposure to cold normally triggers compensatory mechanisms designed to conserve and generate heat in order to maintain a normal body temperature. One such mechanism is piloerection (hair standing on end, or "goose bumps") to impede air flow across the skin. Shivering and increased muscle tone occur, resulting in increased metabolism. There is peripheral vasoconstriction with an increase in cardiac output and respiratory rate. When these mechanisms can no longer adequately compensate for heat lost from the body surface, the body temperature falls. As the body temperature falls, so do the metabolic rate and cardiac output.

As discussed, major mechanisms of body heat loss are conduction, convection, radiation, evaporation, and respiration. Heat loss can be increased by the removal of clothing (decreased insulation, increased radiation), the wetting of clothing by rain or snow (increased conduction and evaporation), air movement around the body (increased convection), or contact with a cold surface or cold-water immersion (increased conduction).

PREDISPOSING FACTORS

Several factors can contribute to the risk of developing hypothermia. They also contribute to the severity of damage if cold injury occurs. Risk factors that increase the danger of developing hypothermia include:

- *Age of the patient.* Pediatric or geriatric patients cannot tolerate cold environments and have less responsive heat-generating mechanisms to combat cold exposure. Elderly persons often become hypothermic in environments that seem only mildly cool to others.

- *Health of the patient.* Hypothyroidism suppresses metabolism, preventing patients from responding appropriately to cold stress. Malnutrition, hypoglycemia, Parkinson's disease, fatigue, and other medical conditions can interfere with the body's ability to combat cold exposure.

- *Medications.* Some drugs interfere with proper heat-generating mechanisms. These include narcotics, alcohol, phenothiazines, barbiturates, antiseizure medications, antihistamines and other allergy medications, antipsychotics, sedatives, antidepressants, and various pain medications such as aspirin, acetaminophen, and NSAIDs.

- *Prolonged or intense exposure.* The length and severity of cold exposure have a direct effect on morbidity and mortality.

- *Coexisting weather conditions.* High humidity, brisk winds, or accompanying rain can all magnify the effect of cold exposure on the human body by accelerating the loss of heat from skin surfaces.

PREVENTIVE MEASURES

Certain precautions can decrease the risk of morbidity related to cold injury:

- Dress warmly.
- Get plenty of rest to maximize the ability of heat-generating mechanisms to replenish energy supplies.

Content Review

COLD DISORDERS
- Hypothermia
- Frostbite
- Trench foot

hypothermia state of low body temperature, particularly low core body temperature.

- Eat appropriately and at regular intervals to support metabolism.
- Limit exposure to cold environments.

DEGREES OF HYPOTHERMIA

Hypothermia can be classified as mild or severe, as follows:

- *Mild*—a core temperature greater than 90°F (32°C) with signs and symptoms of hypothermia
- *Severe*—a core temperature less than 90°F (32°C) with signs and symptoms of hypothermia

Initially some patients may exhibit compensated hypothermia. In this case, signs and symptoms of hypothermia will be present but with a normal core body temperature, temporarily maintained by thermogenesis. As energy stores from the liver and muscle glycogen are exhausted, the core body temperature will drop.

The onset of symptoms may be *acute,* as occurs when a person suddenly falls through ice into frigid water. *Subacute* exposure can occur in situations such as when mountain climbers are trapped in a snowy, cold environment. Finally, *chronic* exposure to cold is a growing problem in our inner cities where homeless people endure frequent and prolonged cold stress without shelter.

In some cases cold exposure is the primary cause of hypothermia, but in others, hypothermia may develop secondary to other problems, such as medical problems. For example, hypothyroidism depresses the body's heat-producing mechanisms. Brain tumors or head trauma can depress the hypothalamic temperature control center, causing hypothermia. Other conditions such as myocardial infarction, diabetes, hypoglycemia, drugs, poor nutrition, sepsis, or old age can also contribute to metabolic and circulatory disorders that predispose to hypothermia. Any patient thought to have hypothermia, but with no history of exposure to a cold environment, should be assessed for any predisposing factors. Evaluate the patient for level of consciousness, cool skin, and shivering. Also, evaluate the rectal temperature. A rectal temperature of less than 95°F (35°C) indicates hypothermia. Key findings at different degrees of hypothermia are summarized in Table 26-1.

Patients who experience body temperatures above 86°F (30°C) will usually have a favorable prognosis. Those with temperatures below 86°F (30°C) show a significant increase in mortality rate. Remember that most thermometers used in medicine do not register below 95°F (35°C). EMS systems in colder areas should carry special thermometers for recording subnormal temperature readings because there is no reliable correlation between signs and symptoms and actual core body temperature.

Signs and Symptoms

Signs and symptoms of hypothermia are summarized in Table 26-2. Patients experiencing mild hypothermia (core temperature >90°F or 32°C) will generally exhibit shivering. The patient may be lethargic and somewhat dulled mentally. (In some cases, however, the patient may be fully oriented.) Muscles may be stiff and uncoordinated, causing the patient to walk with a stumbling, staggering gait.

Patients experiencing severe hypothermia (core temperature < 90°F or 32°C) may be disoriented and confused. As their temperatures continue to fall, they will proceed into stupor and complete coma. Shivering will usually stop, and physical activity will become uncoordinated. Muscles may be stiff and rigid. Continuous cardiac monitoring is indicated for anyone experiencing hypothermia. The ECG will frequently show pathognomonic (indicative of a disease) **J waves,** also called Osborn waves, associated with the QRS complexes (Figure 26-3), but these are not useful diagnostically. Atrial fibrillation is the most common presenting dysrhythmia seen in hypothermia. As the body cools, however, the myocardium becomes progressively more irritable and may develop a variety of dysrhythmias. In severe hypothermia, bradycardia is inevitable.

Ventricular fibrillation becomes more probable as the body's core temperature falls below 86°F (30°C). The severely hypothermic patient requires assessment of pulse and respirations for at least 30 seconds every one to two minutes.

Services operating in colder environments should carry specialized hypothermia thermometers for cold exposure patients.

J wave ECG deflection found at the junction of the QRS complex and the ST segment. It is associated with hypothermia and seen at core temperatures below 32°C, most commonly in leads II and V₆; also called an Osborn wave.

Table 26-1 KEY FINDINGS AT DIFFERENT DEGREES OF HYPOTHERMIA

°C	°F	Clinical Findings
37.6°	99.6°	Normal rectal temperature
37°	98.6°	Normal oral temperature
36°	96.8°	Metabolic rate increased
35°	95°	Maximum shivering seen, impaired judgment
34°	93.2°	Amnesia, slurred speech
33°	91.4°	Severe clouding of consciousness/apathy, uncoordinated movement
32°	89.6°	Most shivering ceases, pupils dilate
31°	87.8°	Blood pressure may no longer be obtainable
30°	86°	Atrial fibrillation/other dysrhythmias develop, pulse and cardiac output decreased by 33%
29°	84.2°	Progressive decrease in pulse and breathing, progressive decrease in level of consciousness
28°	82.4°	Pulse and oxygen consumption decreased by 50%, severe slowing of respiration, increased muscle rigidity, loss of consciousness, high risk of ventricular fibrillation
27°	80.6°	Loss of reflexes and voluntary movement, patients appear clinically dead
26°	78.8°	No reflexes or response to painful stimuli
25°	77°	Cerebral blood flow decreased by 66%
24°	75.2°	Marked hypotension
22°	71.6°	Maximum risk for ventricular fibrillation
19°	66.2°	Flat electroencephalogram (EEG)
18°	64.4°	Asystole
16°	60.8°	Lowest reported adult survival from accidental exposure
15.2°	59.2°	Lowest reported infant survival from accidental exposure
10°	50°	Oxygen consumption 8% of normal
9°	48.2°	Lowest reported survivor from therapeutic exposure

Table 26-2 HYPOTHERMIA: SIGNS AND SYMPTOMS

Mild	Severe
Lethargy	No shivering
Shivering	Dysrhythmias, asystole
Lack of coordination	Loss of voluntary muscle control
Pale, cold, dry skin	Hypotension
Early rise in blood pressure, heart, and respiratory rates	Undetectable pulse and respirations

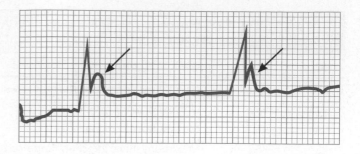

FIGURE 26-3 ECG tracing showing J wave following the QRS complex as seen in hypothermia.

Treatment for Hypothermia

All victims of hypothermia should have the following care (see also Figure 26-4):

1. Remove wet garments.
2. Protect against further heat loss and wind chill. Use passive external warming methods such as application of blankets, insulating materials, and moisture barriers.
3. Maintain the patient in a horizontal position.
4. Avoid rough handling, which can trigger dysrhythmias.
5. Monitor the core temperature.
6. Monitor the cardiac rhythm.

Rewarming is not the opposite of the cooling process.

Active Rewarming   Victims of mild hypothermia may also be rewarmed, using *active external methods*. This includes the use of warmed blankets and/or heat packs placed over areas of high heat transfer with the core: the base of the neck, the axilla, and the groin. Be sure to insulate between the heat packs and the skin to prevent burning. IV fluid heaters (i.e., Hot I.V.) can be used to warm the IV fluid from 95°F to 100°F (35° to 38°C). Warmed IV fluids are helpful in treating mild to moderate hypothermia. Heat guns and lights may also be used, but this will most likely take place in the emergency department. Warm water immersion in water between 102°F and 104°F (39°C to 40°C) may be used but can induce rewarming shock (see below), so this method also has little application in an out-of-hospital setting.

Active rewarming of the severely hypothermic patient is best carried out in the hospital using a prearranged protocol. Most patients who die during rewarming do so from ventricular fibrillation, the risk of which is related to both the depth and the duration of hypothermia. Rough handling of the hypothermic patient may also induce ventricular fibrillation. Active rewarming should not be attempted in the field unless travel to the emergency department will take more than 15 minutes.

Defer active rewarming of the severely hypothermic patient until the patient is at the hospital unless transport time is long and rewarming is ordered by medical direction.

If such is the case, active internal means may also be used, including the use of warmed—102°F to 104°F (38°C to 40°C)—humidified oxygen, and administration of IV fluids also warmed from 102°F to 104°F (38°C to 40°C). This is crucial to prevent further heat loss, but actual heat transferred is minimal, so there is limited contribution to the rewarming effort.

Rewarming Shock   Although application of warmed blankets is a safe and effective means of rewarming the hypothermic patient, application of external heat, as with heat packs, is usually not recommended in the prehospital setting. For effective rewarming, more heat transference is generally required than is possible with out-of-hospital methods. Additionally, application of external heat may result in *rewarming shock* by causing reflex peripheral vasodilatation. This reflex vasodilation causes the return of cool blood and acids from the extremities to the core. This may cause a paradoxical "afterdrop" core temperature decrease and further worsen core hypothermia. This, in turn, may cause the blood pressure to fall, especially when there is also volume depletion.

If active rewarming is necessary in the prehospital setting, for example when transport is delayed, administration of warmed IV fluids during rewarming can prevent the onset of rewarming shock.

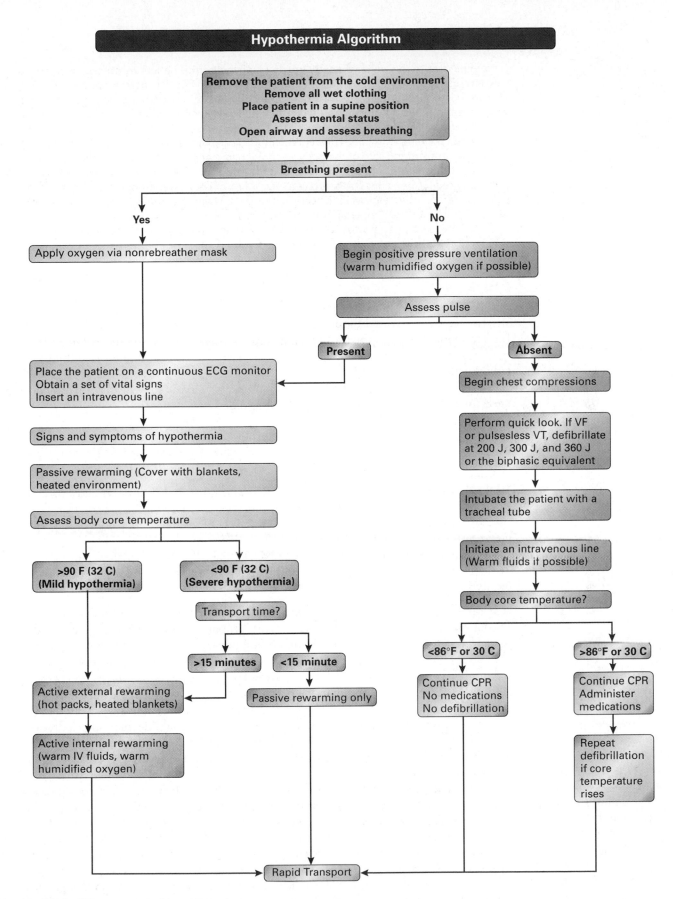

FIGURE 26-4 Management of hypothermia.

Cold Diuresis Volume depletion can occur as a result of *cold diuresis*. Core vasoconstriction causes increased blood volume and blood pressure, so the kidneys remove excess fluid to reduce the pressure, thus causing diuresis. A warmed IV volume expander (e.g., normal saline) should be used both to prevent rewarming shock and to replace fluid lost from cold diuresis.

The conscious patient who is able to manage his airway may be given warmed, sweetened fluids. Alcohol and caffeine should be avoided.

Resuscitation

There are certain resuscitation considerations when handling cardiac arrest victims with core temperatures below 86°F (30°C).

Basic Cardiac Life Support BLS providers should start cardiopulmonary resuscitation (CPR) immediately, although pulse and respirations may need to be checked for longer periods to detect minimal cardiopulmonary efforts. Use normal chest compression and ventilation rates and ventilate with warmed, humidified oxygen. If an AED is available and ventricular fibrillation is detected, three shocks may be given. Further shocks should be avoided until after rewarming to above 86°F. CPR, rewarming, and rapid transport should immediately follow the three defibrillation attempts.

Advanced Cardiac Life Support Since there is no increased risk of inducing ventricular fibrillation from orotracheal or nasotracheal intubation, ALS providers may intubate the patient and ventilate with warmed, humidified oxygen. Drug metabolism is reduced however, so administered medications, such as epinephrine, lidocaine, and procainamide may accumulate to toxic levels if used repeatedly in the severely hypothermic victim. In addition, administered drugs may remain in the peripheral circulation. When the patient is rewarmed and perfusion resumes, large, toxic boluses of these medications may be delivered to the central circulation and target tissues. Lidocaine and procainamide may also paradoxically lower the fibrillatory threshold in a hypothermic heart and increase resistance to defibrillation. Bretylium and magnesium sulfate, however, may be effective even in hypothermic hearts.

The American Heart Association recommends that, if the patient fails to respond to initial defibrillation attempts or initial drug therapy, subsequent defibrillations or boluses of medication should be avoided until the core temperature is about 86°F (30°C). This is because it is generally impossible to electrically defibrillate a heart that is colder than 86°F. Active core rewarming techniques are the primary modality in hypothermia victims who are either in cardiac arrest or unconscious with a slow heart rate.

Techniques that may be used include the administration of heated, humidified oxygen and warmed IV fluids, preferably normal saline, infused centrally at rates of 150 to 200 mL per hour to avoid overhydration. Peritoneal lavage with warmed potassium-free fluid adminis-

If the hypothermic cardiac arrest patient fails to respond to initial defibrillation or drug therapy, avoid subsequent defibrillations or medication until the core temperature is about 86°F (30°C). It is generally impossible to defibrillate a heart that is colder than 86°F.

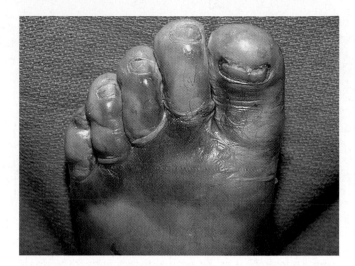

FIGURE 26-5 Frostbite.

tered two liters at a time may be used, as may extracorporeal blood warming with partial cardiac bypass. Obviously some of these techniques may only be carried out in a hospital setting.

Transportation

When transporting a hypothermic patient, remember that gentle transportation is necessary due to myocardial irritability and that the patient should be kept level or slightly inclined with head down. Contact the receiving hospital for general rewarming options. When determining your destination, consider the availability of cardiac bypass rewarming.

FROSTBITE

Frostbite is environmentally induced freezing of body tissues (Figure 26-5). As the tissues freeze, ice crystals form within and water is drawn out of the cells into the extracellular space. These ice crystals expand, causing the destruction of cells. During this process, intracellular electrolyte concentrations increase, further destroying cells. Damage to blood vessels from ice crystal formation causes loss of vascular integrity, resulting in tissue swelling and loss of distal nutritional flow.

Superficial and Deep Frostbite

Generally, there are two types of frostbite: superficial and deep. **Superficial frostbite** (frostnip) exhibits some freezing of epidermal tissue, resulting in initial redness, followed by blanching. There will also be diminished sensation. **Deep frostbite** affects the epidermal and subcutaneous layers. There is a white appearance and the area feels hard (frozen) to palpation. There is also a loss of sensation in deep frostbite.

Frostbite mainly occurs in the extremities and in areas of the head and face exposed to the environment. Subfreezing temperatures are required for frostbite to occur, although they are not necessary to produce hypothermia. Many patients who have frostbite will also have hypothermia.

There can be tremendous variation in how an individual can present with frostbite. For example, some patients feel little pain at onset. Others will report severe pain. A certain degree of compliance may be felt beneath the frozen layer in superficial frostbite, but in deep frostbite, the frozen part will be hard and noncompliant.

Treatment for Frostbite

In treating frostbite, take the following recommended steps:

- Do not thaw the affected area if there is any possibility of refreezing.
- Do not massage the frozen area or rub with snow. Rubbing the affected area may cause ice crystals within the tissues to damage the already injured tissues more seriously.
- Administer analgesia prior to thawing.

frostbite environmentally induced freezing of body tissues causing destruction of cells.

superficial frostbite freezing involving only epidermal tissues resulting in redness followed by blanching and diminished sensation; also called frostnip.

deep frostbite freezing involving epidermal and subcutaneous tissues resulting in a white appearance, hard (frozen) feeling on palpation, and loss of sensation.

Do not thaw frozen flesh if there is any possibility of refreezing. Do not massage the frozen area or rub it with snow.

- Transport to the hospital for rewarming by immersion. If transport will be delayed, thaw the frozen part by immersion in a 102°F to 104°F (39°C to 40°C) water bath. Water temperature will fall rapidly, requiring additions of warm water throughout the process.
- Cover the thawed part with loosely applied dry, sterile dressings.
- Elevate and immobilize the thawed part.
- Do not puncture or drain blisters.
- Do not rewarm frozen feet if they are required for walking out of a hazardous situation.

TRENCH FOOT

Trench foot (immersion foot) is similar to frostbite, but it occurs at temperatures above freezing. It is rarely seen in the civilian population. It received its name in World War I, when troops confined to trenches with standing cold water developed progressive symptoms over days. Symptoms are similar to frostbite, but there may be pain. Blisters may form upon spontaneous rewarming.

Treatment of Trench Foot

Treatment of trench foot requires early recognition of developing symptoms and immediate steps to warm, dry, aerate, and elevate the feet. Measures to prevent trench foot are most effective, such as avoiding prolonged exposure to standing water, changing wet socks frequently, and never sleeping in wet boots or socks.

DROWNING AND NEAR-DROWNING

Drowning is asphyxiation resulting from submersion in liquid. There has been an attempt made to differentiate between the terms drowning and near-drowning. The term *drowning* means that death occurred within 24 hours of submersion, whereas the term **near-drowning** indicates that death either did not occur or occurred more than 24 hours after submersion.

It is estimated that in the United States, approximately 4,500 persons die annually due to drowning. Many more sustain serious injury due to near-drowning. This makes drowning the third most common cause of accidental death in the United States. Approximately 40% of these deaths are in children under five years of age. A second peak incidence occurs in teenagers and a final third peak in the elderly as a result of accidental bathtub drownings. Approximately 85% of near-drowning victims are male, and two-thirds of these do not know how to swim. Most commonly, these situations are due to fresh-water submersion, especially in swimming pools. Unfortunately, alcohol use by the victim or the supervising adult is frequently associated with this type of accident.

It is important to note that other emergency conditions are often associated with near-drowning. If the cause of the submersion is unknown, you must consider the possibility of trauma and treat the patient accordingly.

Frequently the submersion occurs in cold water, causing hypothermia. Hypothermia slows the body's metabolic processes thereby decreasing the need for oxygen. This can have a protective effect on organs and tissues that become hypoxic (low in oxygen) in submersion situations. However, it is important to treat the hypoxia first, once you have initiated rescue.

PATHOPHYSIOLOGY OF DROWNING AND NEAR-DROWNING

As an EMT-I, you need to understand the sequence of events in drowning or near-drowning. Following submersion, if the victim is conscious, he will undergo a period of complete apnea for up to three minutes. This apnea is an involuntary reflex as the victim strives to keep his head above water. During this time, blood is shunted to the heart and brain because of the mammalian diving reflex, which is described later in this chapter.

When the victim is apneic, the $PaCO_2$ in the blood rises to greater than 50 mmHg. Meanwhile, the PaO_2 of the blood falls below 50 mmHg. The stimulus from the hypoxia ultimately overrides the sedative effects of the hypercarbia, resulting in CNS stimulation.

Dry vs. Wet Drowning

Until unconscious, the victim experiences a great deal of panic. During this stage the victim makes violent inspiratory and swallowing efforts. At this point, copious amounts of water enter the mouth, posterior oropharynx, and stomach, stimulating severe laryngospasm (airway obstruction due to aspirated water) and bronchospasm. In approximately 10% of drowning victims, and in a much greater percentage of near-drowning victims, this laryngospasm prevents the influx of water into the lungs. If a significant amount of water does not enter the lungs, it is referred to as a *dry drowning*. Conversely, if a laryngospasm does not occur, and a significant quantity of water does enter the lungs, it is referred to as a *wet drowning*.

The laryngospasm further aggravates the hypoxia, with coma ultimately ensuing. Persistent anoxia (absence of oxygen) results in a deeper coma. Following unconsciousness, reflex swallowing continues, resulting in gastric distention and increased risk of vomiting and aspiration. If untreated, hypotension, bradycardia, and death result in a short period.

Drowning and near-drowning are primarily due to asphyxia from airway obstruction in the lung secondary to the aspirated water or the laryngospasm. If, in a near-drowning episode, this process does not end in death, any fluid that has entered the lungs may cause lower-airway disease.

Fresh-Water vs. Saltwater Drowning

You should expect different physiological reactions in cases of fresh-water and saltwater drownings or near-drownings. However, these mechanistic differences do not make any difference in the end metabolic result or in the prehospital management.

Fresh-Water Drowning In fresh-water drowning or near-drowning, the large surface area of the alveoli and small airways allow a massive amount of hypotonic water to diffuse across the alveolar/capillary membrane and into the vascular space. This results in hemodilution, an expansion in blood plasma volume and relative reduction in red blood cell concentration. Hemodilution produces a thickening of the alveolar walls with inflammatory cells, hemorrhagic pneumonitis (bleeding lung inflammation), and destruction of surfactant.

Surfactant is a substance in the alveoli responsible for keeping the alveoli open. In drowning, some surfactant is lost when the capillaries of the alveoli are damaged. Plasma proteins then leak back into the alveoli, resulting in the accumulation of fluid in the small airways. This in turn leads to multiple areas of atelectasis—areas of alveolar collapse. Atelectasis causes shunting, which is the return of unoxygenated blood from the damaged alveoli to the bloodstream. In other words, blood is traveling through the lungs without being oxygenated. The result is hypoxemia (inadequate oxygenation of the blood) (Figure 26-6).

Saltwater Drowning In saltwater drowning or near-drowning, the hypertonic nature of sea water, which is three to four times more hypertonic than plasma, draws water from the bloodstream into the alveoli (Figure 26-6). This produces pulmonary edema, leading to profound shunting. The result is failure of oxygenation, producing hypoxemia. Additionally, respiratory and metabolic acidosis develop due to the retention of CO_2 and developing anaerobic (without-oxygen) metabolism.

Factors Affecting Survival

A number of factors have an impact on drowning and near-drowning survival rates. These include the cleanliness of the water, the length of time submerged, and the age and general health of the victim. Children have a longer survival time and a greater probability of a successful resuscitation. Even more significant is the water temperature. The concept of developing brain death after 4 to 6 minutes without oxygen is not applicable in cases of near-drowning in cold water. Some patients in cold water (below 68°F) can be resuscitated after 30 minutes or more in cardiac arrest. However, persons under water 60 minutes or longer usually cannot be resuscitated.

A possible contribution to survival may be the **mammalian diving reflex.** When a person dives into cold water, he reacts to the submersion of the face. Breathing is inhibited, the heart rate becomes bradycardic, and vasoconstriction develops in tissues relatively resistant to asphyxia. Meanwhile cerebral and cardiac blood flow is maintained. In this way, oxygen

Although the pathophysiology of fresh-water and saltwater drownings differs, there is no difference in the end result or in prehospital management.

surfactant secreted by cells in the lungs, regulates the surface tension of the fluid that lines the alveoli; important in keeping the alveoli open for gas exchange.

mammalian diving reflex resulting from submersion of the face and nose in water, a complex cardiovascular reflex that constricts blood flow everywhere except to the brain.

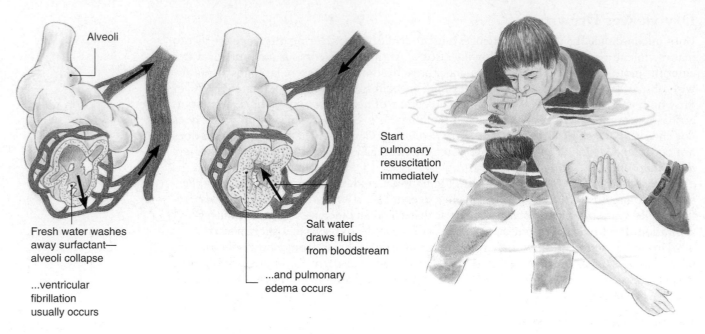

Alveoli

Fresh water washes
away surfactant—
alveoli collapse

...ventricular
fibrillation
usually occurs

Salt water
draws fluids
from bloodstream

...and pulmonary
edema occurs

Start
pulmonary
resuscitation
immediately

FIGURE 26-6 Pathophysiological effects of drowning.

is sent and used only where it is immediately needed to sustain life. The colder the water, the more oxygen is diverted to the heart and brain.

A common saying in emergency medicine states: "The cold-water drowning victim is not dead until he is warm and dead." In other words, a person who has been submerged in cold water may only seem to be dead, but due to the continued supply of oxygen to the heart and brain may indeed still be alive.

TREATMENT FOR NEAR-DROWNING

Since fresh-water and saltwater near-drownings both involve factors that disrupt normal pulmonary function, initial field treatment must be directed toward correcting the profound hypoxia. Take the following steps:

- Remove the patient from the water as soon as possible. This should be done by a trained rescue swimmer.
- Initiate ventilation while the patient is still in the water. Rescue personnel should wear protective clothing if water temperature is less than 70°F. In addition, attach a safety line to the rescue swimmer. In fast water, it is essential to use personnel specifically trained for this type of rescue.
- Suspect head and neck injury if the patient experienced a fall or was diving. Rapidly place the victim on a long backboard and remove him from the water. Use C-spine precautions throughout care.
- Protect the patient from heat loss. Avoid laying the patient on a cold surface. Remove wet clothing and cover the body to the extent possible.
- Examine the patient for airway patency, breathing, and pulse. If indicated, begin CPR and defibrillation.
- Manage the airway using proper suctioning and airway adjuncts.
- Administer oxygen at a 100% concentration.
- Use respiratory rewarming, if available, and if transport time is longer than 15 minutes. (In the past, prophylactic abdominal thrusts were used to clear the airway, but there are conflicting recommendations regarding the practice since no definitive scientific data supports this maneuver.)
- Establish an IV of lactated Ringer's solution or normal saline for venous access and run at 75 mL/hr. If indicated, carry out defibrillation.

The cold-water drowning victim is not dead until he is warm and dead.

Never attempt to rescue a drowning victim unless you have been trained to do so and have the necessary safety equipment.

- Follow ACLS protocols if the patient is normothermic. If the patient is hypothermic, treat him according to the hypothermia protocol presented earlier in the chapter.

Resuscitation is not indicated if immersion has been extremely prolonged (unless hypothermia is present) or if there is evidence of putrefaction (decomposition).

Adult Respiratory Distress Syndrome

More than 90% of near-drowning patients survive without *sequelae* (after effects). However, all near-drowning patients should be admitted to the hospital for observation since complications may not appear for 24 hours.

Adult respiratory distress syndrome (ARDS) is one of the more severe post-resuscitation complications, with a high rate of mortality. The physiological stress of near-drowning causes the lungs to leak fluid into the alveoli. This fluid is loaded with various chemical factors that cause severe inflammation of the tissues and failure of the respiratory system. In addition, some of these patients have problems with pulmonary parenchymal injury, destruction of surfactant, aspiration pneumonitis, or pneumothorax. A number require an extended hospital stay due to renal failure, hypoxia, hypercarbia, and mixed metabolic and respiratory acidosis. The effects of cerebral hypoxia occasionally require treatment throughout hospitalization and beyond.

All near-drowning patients should be admitted to the hospital for observation since complications may not appear for 24 hours.

DIVING EMERGENCIES

Scuba diving has become an extremely popular recreational sport. Divers wear portable equipment containing compressed air, which allows the diver to breathe underwater. Although scuba diving accidents are fairly uncommon, inexperienced divers have a higher rate of injury. Scuba diving emergencies can occur on the surface, in three feet of water, or at any depth. The more serious emergencies usually occur following a dive. To better assess and care for diving injuries, you need to understand a few principles of pressure.

scuba abbreviation for self-contained underwater breathing apparatus; portable apparatus that contains compressed air, which allows the diver to breathe underwater.

EFFECTS OF AIR PRESSURE ON GASES

Water is an incompressible liquid. Fresh water has a density, or weight per unit of volume, of 62.4 pounds per cubic foot. Saltwater has a density of 64.0 pounds per cubic foot. This density can be equated to pressure, which is defined as the weight or force acting upon a unit area. Thus, a cubic foot of fresh water exerts a pressure ("weight") of 62.4 pounds over an area of one square foot. This measurement is typically stated in *pounds per square inch (psi)*.

Air at sea level exerts a pressure of 14.7 psi (760 mmHg). This pressure, however, may vary within the environment. For example, ascending to an altitude of one mile will decrease the atmospheric pressure by 17% to approximately 12.2 pounds.

To understand how air pressure affects diving accidents, you need to look at three physical laws: Boyle's Law, Dalton's Law, and Henry's Law.

Boyle's Law

Boyle's Law states that the volume of a gas is inversely proportional to its pressure if the temperature is kept constant. As you increase pressure, the gas is compressed into a smaller space. For example, doubling the pressure of a gas mixture will decrease its volume by one-half. The pressure of air at sea level is 14.7 psi, or 760 mmHg. This pressure is called one "atmosphere absolute" or one ata. Two ata occur at a depth of 33 feet of water, three ata occur at a depth of 66 feet of water, and so on. Therefore, one liter of air at the surface is compressed to 500 mL at 33 feet. At 66 feet, one liter of air would be compressed to 250 mL.

Dalton's Law

Dalton's Law states that the total pressure of a mixture of gases is equal to the sum of the partial pressures of the individual gases. The air we breathe is a mixture of nitrogen (about 78%), oxygen (about 21%), and carbon dioxide plus traces of argon, helium, and other rare gases (about 1%). Since the pressure of air at sea level is 760 mmHg, the pressure of nitrogen is about 593 mmHg, the pressure of oxygen is about 160 mmHg, and the pressure of carbon dioxide is somewhat less than 4 mmHg—each gas exerting its proportion of the total pressure of the mixture.

At different altitudes above sea level or depths below sea level, the pressure of air will change (less at higher altitudes, more at greater depths), but the component gases will still account for the same proportion of whatever the total pressure is at that level: nitrogen 78%, oxygen 21%, and carbon dioxide less than 1%.

Henry's Law

Henry's Law states that the amount of gas dissolved in a given volume of fluid is proportional to the pressure of the gas above it. When we descend below sea level, and the pressure bearing down on us increases, the gases that make up the air we breathe tend to dissolve in the liquids (mainly blood plasma) and tissues of the body.

Compare what happens to the two chief components of the air—oxygen and nitrogen—when a person descends to greater and greater depths below sea level. Much of the oxygen is used up in the normal metabolism of the cells, leaving only a small amount to be dissolved in the blood and tissues. Nitrogen, however, is an inert gas and, as such, is not used by the body. Therefore, a far greater quantity of nitrogen is available to dissolve in the blood and tissues as a person descends below sea level. In brief, at depths below sea level, oxygen metabolizes but nitrogen dissolves.

When the person ascends toward sea level again, the gases that are dissolved in the blood and tissues, being under less and less pressure, come out of the blood and tissues and, if the ascent is too rapid, form bubbles. To understand this phenomenon, compare the human body to a bottled carbonated soft drink—that is, a liquid in which carbon dioxide gas is dissolved. The gas is kept dissolved in the liquid by the cap on the bottle and a high-pressure gas under the cap, on top of the liquid. When the cap is removed and the pressure is released, the gas bubbles out of the liquid, causing a fizz that will sometimes rise completely out of the bottle.

The following sections offer a discussion on how the phenomena of gases and pressure can cause serious problems for divers.

PATHOPHYSIOLOGY OF DIVING EMERGENCIES

As noted above, gases are dissolved in the diver's blood and tissues under pressure. As the diver goes deeper into the water, pressure increases, causing more gas to dissolve in the blood (Henry's Law). According to Boyle's Law, these gases will have a smaller volume due to the increased ambient pressure. During controlled ascent, with decreasing pressure, dissolved gases come out of the blood and tissues slowly, escaping gradually through respiration.

If ascent is too rapid, however, the dissolved gases, mostly nitrogen, come out of solution and expand quickly, forming bubbles in the blood, brain, spinal cord, skin, inner ear, muscles, and joints. Once bubbles of nitrogen have formed in various tissues, it is difficult for the body to remove them. The ascending diver who comes to the surface too rapidly, not adhering to safety measures, is at risk of becoming a veritable living bottle of soda.

CLASSIFICATION OF DIVING INJURIES

Scuba diving injuries are due to barotrauma, pulmonary over-pressure, arterial gas embolism, decompression illness, cold, panic, or a combination of these. Accidents generally occur at one of the following four stages of a dive: on the surface, during descent, on the bottom, and during ascent.

Injuries on the Surface

Surface injuries can involve any of several factors. One such factor can be entanglement of lines or entanglement in kelp fields while swimming to the area of the dive. Divers in these situations may panic, become fatigued, even drown. Another factor may be cold water that produces shivering and blackout. Boats in the area are another potential source of injury to the diver. To prevent such accidents, divers will usually mark the area of their dive with a flag. Maritime rules require boat operators to stay clear of a flagged area.

Injuries during Descent

Barotrauma means injuries caused by changes in pressure. Barotrauma during descent is commonly called "the squeeze." It can occur if the diver cannot equilibrate the pressure between the nasopharynx and the middle ear through the eustachian tube. The diver can experience middle ear pain, ringing in the ears, dizziness, and hearing loss. In severe cases, rupture of the eardrum can occur. A diver who has an upper respiratory infection, and who therefore cannot clear the middle ear through the eustachian tube, should not dive. A similar lack of equilibration can occur in the sinuses, producing severe frontal headaches or pain beneath the eye in the maxillary sinuses.

Injuries on the Bottom

Major diving emergencies while at the bottom of the dive often involve **nitrogen narcosis** (a state of stupor), commonly called "raptures of the deep." This is due to nitrogen's effect on cerebral function. The diver may appear to be intoxicated and may take unnecessary risks. Other emergencies occur when a diver runs low on or out of air. The diver who panics will exacerbate this situation by consuming even more oxygen and producing even more carbon dioxide.

Injuries during Ascent

Serious and life-threatening emergencies, many involving barotrauma, can occur during the ascent. For example, as during descent, an ascending diver may be unable to equilibrate inner ear and nasopharyngeal pressure.

Dives below 40 feet require staged ascent to prevent **decompression illness,** also called "the bends." This condition develops in divers subjected to rapid reduction of air pressure while ascending to the surface following exposure to compressed air, with formation of nitrogen bubbles causing severe pain, especially in the abdomen and the joints.

The most serious barotrauma that occurs during ascent is injury to the lung from **pulmonary over-pressure.** This can occur with a deep dive, or it can occur with a dive of as little as three feet below the surface. The injury results from the diver holding his breath during the ascent. As the diver ascends, the air in the lung, which has been compressed, expands. If it is not exhaled, the alveoli may rupture. If this occurs, the result will be structural damage to the lung and, possibly, **arterial gas embolism (AGE),** an air bubble, or air embolism, that enters the circulatory system from the damaged lung. Another result may be **pneumomediastinum,** the release of gas (air) through the visceral pleura into the mediastinum and pericardial sac around the heart as well as into the tissues of the neck. **Pneumothorax** is possible if the alveoli rupture into the pleural cavity. Air embolism can occur if the air ruptures into the pulmonary veins or arteries and returns to the left atrium and finally into the left ventricle and out into the systemic circulation.

GENERAL ASSESSMENT OF DIVING EMERGENCIES

In the early assessment of diving accidents, all symptoms of air embolism and decompression illness are considered together. Early assessment and treatment of a diving injury is of more importance than trying to distinguish the exact problem. One of your most important tasks in a diving-related injury is elicitation of a diving history or profile. Several essential factors to consider include:

- Time at which the signs and symptoms occurred
- Type of breathing apparatus utilized
- Type of hypothermia protective garment worn
- Parameters of the dive:
  - Depth of dive(s)
  - Number of dive(s)
  - Duration of dive(s)

barotrauma injuries caused by changes in pressure. When it occurs from increasing pressure during a diving descent, it is commonly called "the squeeze."

nitrogen narcosis a state of stupor that develops during deep dives due to nitrogen's effect on cerebral function; also called "raptures of the deep."

decompression illness development of nitrogen bubbles within the tissues due to a rapid reduction of air pressure when a diver returns to the surface; also called "the bends."

pulmonary over-pressure expansion of air held in the lungs during ascent. If not exhaled, the expanded air may cause injury to the lungs and surrounding structures.

arterial gas embolism (AGE) an air bubble, or air embolism, that enters the circulatory system from a damaged lung.

pneumomediastinum the presence of air in the mediastinum.

pneumothorax a collection of air in the pleural space. Air may enter the pleural space through an injury to the chest wall or to the lungs. In a tension pneumothorax, pressure builds because there is no way for the air to escape, causing lung collapse.

In a diving emergency, consider all symptoms of air embolism and decompression illness together. Early assessment and treatment are more important than identifying the exact problem.

- Aircraft travel following a dive (in a pressurized cabin?)
- Rate of ascent
- Associated panic forcing rapid ascent
- Experience of the diver (for example, student, inexperienced, or professional)
- Properly functioning depth gauge
- Previous medical diseases
- Old injuries
- Previous episodes of decompression illness
- Use of medications
- Use of alcohol

From a quick assessment of the patient's diving profile, you can rapidly determine if the diver is a likely candidate for a pressure disorder.

PRESSURE DISORDERS

Injuries caused by pressure, as noted earlier, are known as barotrauma. In the case of diving accidents, most barotrauma results from a pressure imbalance between the external environment and gases within the body. The following sections describe some of the most common forms of barotrauma involved in diving accidents.

Decompression Illness

Decompression illness develops in divers subjected to rapid reduction of air pressure after ascending to the surface following exposure to compressed air. A number of general and individual factors can contribute to the development of decompression illness, or the bends (Table 26-3). Decompression illness results as nitrogen bubbles come out of solution in the blood and tissues, causing increased pressure in various body structures and occluding circulation in the small blood vessels. This occurs in joints, tendons, the spinal cord, skin, brain, and inner ear. Symptoms develop when a diver rapidly ascends after being exposed to a depth of 33 feet or more for a time sufficient to allow the body's tissues to be saturated with nitrogen.

Signs and Symptoms   The principal signs and symptoms of decompression illnesses are joint and abdominal pain, fatigue, paresthesias, and CNS disturbances. The nitrogen bubbles produced by rapid decompression are thought to produce obstruction of blood flow and lead to local ischemia, subjecting tissues to anoxic stress. In some cases, this stress may lead to tissue damage.

Table 26-3 | FACTORS RELATED TO THE DEVELOPMENT OF DECOMPRESSION ILLNESS

General Factors	Individual Factors
Cold water dives	Age—older individuals
Diving in rough water	Obesity
Strenuous diving conditions	Fatigue—lack of sleep prior to dive
History of previous decompression dive incident	Alcohol—consumption before or after dive
Overstaying time at given dive depth	History of medical problems
Dive at 80 feet or greater	
Rapid ascent—panic, inexperience, unfamiliarity with equipment	
Heavy exercise before or after dive to the point of muscle soreness	
Flying after diving (24-hour wait is recommended)	
Driving to high altitude after dive	

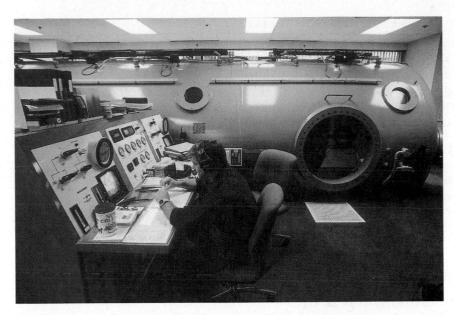

FIGURE 26-7 Hyperbaric oxygen chamber used in the treatment of decompression illness.

Treatment Patients with decompression illness usually seek medical treatment within 12 hours of ascent from a dive. Some patients may not seek treatment for as long as 24 hours after the last dive. It is generally safe to assume that signs or symptoms developing more than 36 hours after a dive cannot reasonably be attributed to decompression illness.

Decompression illness may require urgent definitive care through **recompression**. This can be accomplished by placing the patient in a **hyperbaric oxygen chamber** (Figure 26-7). There the patient is subjected to oxygen under greater-than-atmospheric pressure to force the nitrogen in the body to re-dissolve, then gradually decompressed to allow the nitrogen to escape without forming bubbles. However, prompt stabilization at the nearest emergency department should be accomplished before transportation to a recompression chamber.

Early oxygen therapy may reduce symptoms of decompression illness substantially. Divers who are administered high concentrations of oxygen have a considerably better treatment outcome. The following list outlines some of the steps in the prehospital management of decompression illnesses:

- Assess the patient's ABCs.
- Administer CPR, if required.
- Administer oxygen at 100% concentration with a nonrebreather mask. An unconscious diver should be intubated.
- Keep the patient in the supine position.
- Protect the patient from excessive heat, cold, wetness, or noxious fumes.
- Give the conscious, alert patient nonalcoholic liquids such as fruit juices or oral balanced salt solutions.
- Evaluate and stabilize the patient at the nearest emergency department prior to transport to a recompression chamber. Begin IV fluid replacement with electrolyte solutions for unconscious or seriously injured patients. You may use lactated Ringer's solution or normal saline. Do not use 5% dextrose in water.
- If there is evidence of CNS involvement, administer dexamethasone, heparin, or Valium as ordered by medical direction.
- If air evacuation is used, do not expose the patient to decreased barometric pressure. Cabin pressure must be maintained at sea level, or fly at the lowest possible safe altitude.
- Send the patient's diving equipment with the patient for examination. If that is impossible, arrange for local examination and gas analysis.

recompression resubmission of a person to a greater pressure so that gradual decompression can be achieved; often used in the treatment of diving emergencies.

hyperbaric oxygen chamber recompression chamber used to treat patients suffering from barotrauma.

Pulmonary Over-Pressure Accidents

Lung overinflation due to rapid ascent is the common cause of a number of emergencies, particularly at shallow depths of less than 6 feet. Air can become trapped in the lungs by mucous plugs, bronchospasm, or simple breath holding. With rapid ascent, ambient pressure drops quickly, causing the trapped air to expand. Air expansion can rupture the alveolar membranes. This can result in hemorrhage, reduced oxygen and carbon dioxide transport, and capillary and alveolar inflammation. Air can also escape from the lung into other nearby tissues and cause pneumothorax and tension pneumothorax, subcutaneous emphysema, or pneumomediastinum.

Signs and Symptoms   Divers with this type of condition will complain of substernal chest pain. Respiratory distress and diminished breath sounds are common findings on examination.

Treatment   Treatment for this condition is the same as for pneumothorax caused by any other mechanism (see Chapter 27). Rest and supplemental oxygen are important but hyperbaric oxygen is not usually necessary.

Arterial Gas Embolism (AGE)

As described above, a pressure buildup in the lung can damage and rupture alveoli. This can allow air in the form of a large bubble to escape into the circulation. This air embolism, or arterial gas embolism, can travel to the left atrium and ventricle of the heart and out into various parts of the body where it may lodge and obstruct blood flow, causing ischemia and possibly infarct. Such obstruction of blood flow can have devastating effects triggered by cardiac, pulmonary, and cerebral compromise.

Signs and Symptoms   Signs and symptoms of air embolism include onset within 2 to 10 minutes of ascent, a rapid and dramatic onset of sharp, tearing pain, and other symptoms related to the organ system affected by blocked blood flow. The most common presentation mimics a stroke with confusion, vertigo, visual disturbances, and loss of consciousness. Although rare, you may also encounter paralysis on one side of the body (hemiplegia), as well as cardiac and pulmonary collapse. If any person using scuba equipment presents with neurological deficits during or immediately after ascent, an air embolism should be suspected. Because death or serious disability can result, prompt medical treatment is crucial.

Treatment   Management of air embolism includes the following steps:

- Assess the patient's ABCs.
- Administer oxygen by nonrebreather mask at 100%.
- Place the patient in a supine position.
- Monitor vital signs frequently.
- Administer IV fluids at a TKO rate.
- Administer a corticosteroid agent, if ordered by medical direction.
- Transport to a recompression chamber as rapidly as possible. If air transport is utilized, it is very important to use a pressurized aircraft or to fly at a low altitude.

Pneumomediastinum

As noted earlier, a pneumomediastinum is the release of gas (air) through the visceral pleura into the mediastinum and pericardial sac around the heart. It can result from a pulmonary over-pressure accident during rapid ascent from a dive.

Signs and Symptoms   Signs and symptoms of a pneumomediastinum include substernal chest pain, irregular pulse, abnormal heart sounds, reduced blood pressure and narrow pulse pressure, and a change in voice. Evidence of cyanosis may or may not be present.

Treatment   The field management of pneumomediastinum includes:

- Administer high-flow, high-concentration oxygen via nonrebreather mask.
- Start an IV lactated Ringer's solution or normal saline per medical direction.
- Transport to the emergency department.

Treatment generally ranges from observation to recompression for relief of acute symptoms. The patient should be observed for 24 hours for any other signs of lung overpressure. He should not be recompressed unless air embolism or decompression illness is also present.

Nitrogen Narcosis

Nitrogen narcosis develops during deep dives and contributes to major diving emergencies while the diver is at the bottom. With an elevated partial pressure, more nitrogen dissolves in the bloodstream. With higher concentrations of nitrogen in the body, including the brain, the result is intoxication and altered levels of consciousness very similar to the effects of alcohol or narcotic use. Between 70 and 100 feet these effects become apparent in most divers, but at 200 feet most divers become so impaired that they cannot do any useful work. At 300 to 350 feet unconsciousness occurs. The main concern with nitrogen narcosis is the same as with any person who is intoxicated while in a situation requiring alertness and common sense. Impaired judgment can cause accidents and unnecessary risk taking.

Signs and Symptoms   Altered levels of consciousness and impaired judgment.

Treatment   Treatment simply requires return to a shallow depth since this condition is self-resolving on ascent. To avoid this problem altogether in deep dives, oxygen mixed with helium is used, since helium does not have the anesthetic effect of nitrogen.

OTHER DIVING-RELATED ILLNESSES

Less frequent problems can occur as a result of scuba diving. For example, oxygen toxicity caused by prolonged exposure to high partial pressures of oxygen can cause lung damage or even convulsions. Hyperventilation due to excitement or panic may lead to a decreased level of consciousness or muscle cramps and spasm. This will impair the diver's ability to function properly, possibly leading to injury. Inadequate breathing or faulty equipment may lead to increased CO_2 levels, or *hypercapnia*. This also may cause unconsciousness. Finally, poorly prepared air tanks may be contaminated with other gases, which can increase the risk of hypoxia, narcosis, and accidental injury.

DIVERS ALERT NETWORK (DAN)

Clearly, scuba diving has a unique set of potential problems. With the popularity of this activity rising so dramatically, it is important for EMS personnel in popular diving areas to become familiar with recognition and treatment of these problems. If assistance is needed, the Divers Alert Network (DAN) operates a non-profit consultation and referral service in affiliation with Duke University Medical Center. In an emergency, contact (919) 684-8111. For non-emergency situations call (919) 684-2948 or see the DAN website at http://www.diversalertnetwork.org.

HIGH ALTITUDE ILLNESS

In contrast to illnesses related to diving and high atmospheric pressure, high altitude illnesses are caused by a decrease in ambient pressure. Essentially, high altitude is a low-oxygen environment. As noted in the discussion of Dalton's law, earlier, oxygen concentration in the atmosphere remains constant at 21%. Therefore, as you go higher and barometric pressure decreases, the partial pressure of oxygen also decreases (is 21% of a lower total pressure). Oxygen becomes less available, triggering a number of related illnesses as well as aggravating pre-existing conditions such as angina, congestive heart failure, chronic obstructive pulmonary disease, and hypertension.

High altitude illnesses start to become manifest at altitudes greater than 8,000 feet.

Even in healthy individuals, ascent to high altitude, especially if it is very rapid, can cause illness. It is difficult to predict who will be affected and to what degree. The only predictor is the hypoxic ventilatory response.

Every year millions of visitors to mountains expose themselves to altitudes greater than 2,400 meters (8,000 feet) the altitude at which high altitude illnesses start to become manifest. For reference purposes, Denver is at 1,610 meters where there is 17% less oxygen than at sea level. Aspen at 2,438 meters has 26% less oxygen, and at the top of Mount Everest (8,848 meters or 29,028 feet) there is 66% less oxygen than at sea level. At *high altitude* (4,900 to 11,500 feet) the hypoxic environment causes decreased exercise performance, although without major disruption of normal oxygen transport in the body. However, if ascent is very rapid, altitude illness will commonly occur at 8,000 feet and beyond. *Very high altitude* (11,500 to 18,000 feet) will result in extreme hypoxia during exercise or sleep. It is important to ascend to these altitudes slowly, allowing for acclimatization to the environment. *Extreme altitude* beyond 18,000 feet will cause severe illness in almost everyone.

Some of the signs and symptoms of altitude illness are malaise, anorexia, headache, sleep disturbances, and respiratory distress that increases with exertion.

PREVENTION

Acclimatization, exertion, sleep, diet, and medication are key considerations in preventing or limiting high altitude medical emergencies. A description of each follows.

Gradual Ascent

To avoid developing high altitude medical problems, it is important to allow a period of acclimatization. Slow, gradual ascent over days to weeks gives the body a chance to adjust to the hypoxic state caused by high altitudes. A person who would normally become short of breath, dizzy, and confused by a rapid drop in oxygen can function quite well if the oxygen level is decreased to the same level gradually over a long period of time. Acclimatization occurs through several mechanisms. They are:

- *Ventilatory changes.* The hypoxic ventilatory response (HVR) is triggered by decreased oxygen. When oxygen is decreased, ventilation increases. This hyperventilation causes a decrease in CO_2, but the kidneys compensate by eliminating more bicarbonate from the body. In essence, the body resets its normal ventilation and operating level of CO_2. The process takes 4 to 7 days at a given altitude.

- *Cardiovascular changes.* The heart rate increases at high altitude, allowing more oxygen to be delivered to the tissues. In addition, peripheral veins constrict, increasing the central blood volume. In response, the central receptors, which sense blood volume, induce a diuresis, which causes concentration of the blood. Unfortunately, pulmonary circulation also constricts in a hypoxic environment. This causes or exacerbates pre-existing hypertension and predisposes to developing high altitude pulmonary edema.

- *Blood changes.* Within 2 hours of ascent to high altitude the body begins making more red blood cells to carry oxygen. Over time, this mechanism will significantly compensate for the hypoxic environment. It is this mechanism that fostered the idea of "blood-doping" during athletic competition, especially at high altitudes. Athletes donate their own blood long in advance of a competition at high altitude. This allows them time to rebuild their red blood cells. Just before the competition they receive a transfusion of their own blood to increase their oxygen-carrying capacity. This practice is frowned upon by most athletic governing bodies.

Limited Exertion

Clearly, one of the easiest ways to avoid some effects of high altitude is to limit the amount of exertion. By limiting the body's need for oxygen, the effect of oxygen deprivation will be minimized.

Sleeping Altitude

Sleep is often disrupted by high altitude. Hypoxia causes abnormal breathing patterns and frequent awakenings in the middle of the night. Descending to a lower altitude for sleep improves rest and allows the body to recover from hypoxia. This practice will, however, interfere with the process of acclimatization.

High Carbohydrate Diet

Carbohydrates are converted by the body into glucose and rapidly released into the blood stream, providing quick energy. The theory that this is helpful in acclimatizing to high altitude is controversial.

Medications

Two medications will limit or prevent the development of medical conditions related to high altitude. They are:

- *Acetazolamide.* Acetazolamide (Diamox) acts as a diuretic. It forces bicarbonate out of the body, which greatly enhances the process of acclimatization as discussed above. The hypoxic ventilatory response reaches a new set point more quickly. This improves ventilation and oxygen transport with less alkalosis. In addition, the periodic breathing that occurs at high altitude is resolved, thereby preventing sudden drops in oxygen.
- *Nifedipine.* Nifedipine (Procardia, Adalat) is a medication usually used to treat high blood pressure. It causes blood vessels to dilate, preventing the increase in pulmonary pressure that often causes pulmonary edema.

Other treatments are currently under evaluation. Phenytoin (Dilantin), for example, is being studied because of its membrane stabilization effects. Steroids are commonly used but their efficacy is still controversial.

TYPES OF HIGH ALTITUDE ILLNESS

A variety of symptoms occur when the average person ascends rapidly to high altitude. These may range from fatigue and decreased exercise tolerance to headache, sleep disturbance, and respiratory distress. The following section will deal with some of the specific syndromes that will occur.

Acute Mountain Sickness (AMS)

Acute mountain sickness usually manifests in an unacclimatized person who ascends rapidly to an altitude of 2,000 meters (6,600 feet) or greater.

Signs and Symptoms   The mild form of acute mountain sickness presents with the following symptoms:

- Lightheadedness
- Breathlessness
- Weakness
- Headache
- Nausea and vomiting

These symptoms can develop from 6 to 24 hours after ascent. More severe cases can develop especially if the person continues to ascend to higher altitudes. These symptoms include:

- Weakness (requiring assistance to eat and dress)
- Severe vomiting
- Decreased urine output
- Shortness of breath
- Altered level of consciousness

Mild AMS is self-limiting and will often improve within 1 to 2 days if no further ascent occurs.

Treatment Treatment of AMS consists of halting ascent, possibly lowering altitude, using acetazolamide (Diamox), and anti-nauseants such as prochlorperazine (Compazine) as necessary. It is not usually necessary to descend to sea level. Supplemental oxygen will relieve symptoms but is usually used only in severe cases. In severe cases oxygen, if available, will help. In addition, immediate descent is the definitive treatment. For very severe cases, hyperbaric oxygen may be necessary.

High Altitude Pulmonary Edema (HAPE)

HAPE develops as a result of increased pulmonary pressure and hypertension caused by changes in blood flow at high altitude. Children are most susceptible, and men are more susceptible than women.

Signs and Symptoms Initially symptoms include dry cough, mild shortness of breath on exertion, and slight crackles in the lungs. As the condition progresses, so will the symptoms. Dyspnea can become quite severe and cause cyanosis. Coughing may be productive of frothy sputum, and weakness may progress to coma and death.

Treatment In the early stages, HAPE is completely and easily reversible with descent and the administration of oxygen. It is therefore critical to recognize the illness early and initiate appropriate treatment. If immediate descent is not possible, supplemental oxygen can completely reverse HAPE but requires 36 to 72 hours. Such a supply of oxygen is rarely available to mountain climbers. In this situation the portable hyperbaric bag can be very useful. This is a sealed bag that can be inflated to 2 psi, which simulates a descent of approximately 5,000 feet. Acetazolamide can be used to decrease symptoms. Medications such as morphine, nifedipine (Procardia), and furosemide (Lasix) have been used with some success, but complications such as hypotension and dehydration can result, so they should be used with caution.

High Altitude Cerebral Edema (HACE)

The exact cause of high altitude cerebral edema is not known. It usually manifests as progressive neurological deterioration in a patient with AMS or HAPE. The increased fluid in the brain tissue causes a rise in intracranial pressure.

Signs and Symptoms The symptoms of high altitude cerebral edema include:

- Altered mental status
- Ataxia (poor coordination)
- Decreased level of consciousness
- Coma

Headache, nausea, and vomiting are less common. Occasionally actual focal neurological changes may occur.

Treatment As in all altitude illnesses, definitive treatment is descent to lower altitude. Oxygen and steroids may also help to improve recovery. If descent is not possible, the use of oxygen with steroids and a hyperbaric bag may be sufficient, although often unavailable. If coma develops, it may persist for days after descent to sea level but usually resolves, although sometimes leaving residual disability.

NUCLEAR RADIATION

Injury due to exposure to ionizing radiation occurs infrequently. However, the incidence of radiation emergencies has increased in recent years due to the expansion of nuclear medicine procedures and commercial nuclear facilities.

Keep in mind that radiation emergencies should be handled only by those with proper protective equipment and adequate training.

BASIC NUCLEAR PHYSICS

Radiation is a general term applied to the transmission of electromagnetic or particle energy. This energy can include nuclear energy, ultraviolet light, visible light, infrared, and x-ray. A radioactive substance emits ionizing radiation. Such a substance is referred to as a *radionuclide* or *radioisotope*.

To understand nuclear radiation, you might begin by taking a look at the structure of an atom and by becoming familiar with some of the basic terms associated with nuclear physics. The atom consists of various subatomic particles. These include:

- *Protons.* Positively charged particles that form the nucleus of hydrogen and are present in the nuclei of all elements. The atomic number of the element indicates the number of protons present.
- *Neutrons.* Subatomic particles that are approximately equal in mass to a proton, but lack an electrical charge. As a free particle, a neutron has an average life of less than 17 minutes.
- *Electrons.* Minute particles with negative electrical charges that revolve around the nucleus of an atom. When emitted from radioactive substances, electrons are called beta particles.

You should also be familiar with two basic terms associated with nuclear medicine:

- *Isotopes* (radioisotope). Atoms in which the nuclear composition is unstable. That is, they give off **ionizing radiation.**
- *Half-life.* The time required for half the nuclei of a radioactive substance to lose its activity due to radioactive decay is called **half-life.**

A radioactive substance is one that emits ionizing radiation. The four types of ionizing radiation are:

- *Alpha particles.* Alpha particles are slow-moving, low-energy particles that usually can be stopped by such things as clothing and paper. When they contact the skin, they only penetrate a few cells deep. Because they can be absorbed (stopped) by a layer of clothing, a few inches of air, or the outer layer of skin, alpha particles usually constitute a minor hazard. However, they can produce serious effects if taken internally by ingestion or inhalation.
- *Beta particles.* Smaller than alpha particles, beta particles are higher in energy. Although beta particles can penetrate air, they can be stopped by aluminum and similar materials. Beta particles generally cause less local damage than alpha particles, but they can be harmful if inhaled or ingested.
- *Gamma rays.* Gamma rays are more highly energized and penetrating than alpha and beta particles. The origin of gamma rays is related to that of x-rays. Gamma radiation is extremely dangerous, carrying high levels of energy capable of penetrating thick shielding. Gamma rays easily pass through clothing and the entire body, inflicting extensive cell damage. They also create indirect damage by causing internal tissue to emit alpha and beta particles. Lead shielding can provide protection from gamma radiation.
- *Neutrons.* Neutrons are more penetrating than the other types of radiation. The penetrating power of neutrons is estimated to be three to ten times greater than gamma rays, but less than the internal hazard associated with ingestion of alpha and beta particles. Exposure to neutrons causes direct tissue damage. However, in nuclear accidents, neutron exposure is not normally a problem for EMT-Is because neutrons tend to be present only near a reactor core.

EFFECTS OF RADIATION ON THE BODY

Ionizing radiation cannot be seen, felt, or heard. Therefore, a detection instrument is required to measure the radiation given off by the radiation source. The most commonly used

ionizing radiation electromagnetic radiation (e.g., x-ray) or particulate radiation (e.g., alpha particles, beta particles, and neutrons) that, by direct or secondary processes, ionizes materials that absorb the radiation. Ionizing radiation can penetrate the cells of living organisms, depositing an electrical charge within them. When sufficiently intense, this form of energy kills cells.

half-life time required for half of the nuclei of a radioactive substance to lose activity by undergoing radioactive decay. In biology and pharmacology, the time required by the body to metabolize and inactivate half the amount of a substance taken in.

device is the Geiger counter. The rate of radiation is measured in roentgens per hour (R/hr) or milliroentgens per hour (mR/hr) (1,000 mR = 1R).

The unit of local tissue energy deposition is called *radiation absorbed dose (RAD)*. *Roentgen equivalent in man (REM)* provides a gauge of the likely injury to the irradiated part of an organism. For all practical purposes, RAD and REM are equal in clinical value. When neutrons or other high-energy radiation sources are used, a *quality factor (QF)* is applied to determine the equivalent dose.

Simply stated, ionizing radiation causes alterations in the body's cell, primarily the genetic material (DNA). Depending on the dosage received, the changes can be in cell division, cell structure, and cellular biochemical activities. Cell damage due to ionizing radiation is cumulative over a lifetime. If a person is exposed to ionizing radiation long enough, the number of white blood cells decreases. Additionally, there may be defects in offspring, an increased incidence of cancer, and various degrees of bone marrow damage.

Detection of the first biological effects of exposure to ionizing radiation occurs at varying times (Table 26-4). Biological effects include:

- *Acute*. Effects appearing in a matter of minutes or weeks.
- *Long-term*. Effects appearing years or decades later.

PRINCIPLES OF SAFETY

Three basic principles allow rescue personnel and patients to limit exposure to ionizing radiation. These are *time*, *distance*, and *shielding*. Determining exposure, absorption, and damage done by radiation requires specialized training. The amount of radiation received by a person depends on the source of radiation, the length of time exposed, the distance from the source, and the shielding between the exposed person and the source. For example, the amount of radiation at the patient's initial location may be 300 R/hr. If exposure is for 20 minutes, this is the same radiation equivalent as working for one hour at a 100 R/hr scene.

Limiting radiation exposure is based on three principles: time, distance, and shielding.

Content Review

CLEAN RADIATION ACCIDENTS

Patient is exposed to radiation but not contaminated by radioactive particles, liquids, gases, or smoke.

DIRTY RADIATION ACCIDENTS

Patient is contaminated by radioactive particles, liquids, gases, or smoke.

Table 26-4 DOSE-EFFECT RELATIONSHIPS TO IONIZING RADIATION

Whole Body Exposure

Dose (RAD)	Effect
5–25	Asymptomatic. Blood studies are normal.
50–75	Asymptomatic. Minor depressions of white blood cells and platelets in a few patients.
75–125	May produce anorexia, nausea, and vomiting, and fatigue in approximately 10%–20% of patients within 2 days.
125–200	Possible nausea and vomiting. Diarrhea, anxiety, and tachycardia. Fatal to fewer than 5% of patients.
200–600	Nausea and vomiting, diarrhea in the first several hours, weakness, fatigue. Fatal to approximately 50% of patients within 6 weeks without prompt medical attention.
600–1,000	Severe nausea and vomiting, diarrhea in the first several hours. Fatal to 100% of patients within 2 weeks without prompt medical attention.
1,000 or more	"Burning sensation" within minutes, nausea and vomiting within 10 minutes, confusion ataxia, and prostration within 1 hour, watery diarrhea within 1–2 hrs. Fatal to 100% within short time without prompt medical attention.

Localized Exposure

Dose (RAD)	Effect
50	Asymptomatic.
500	Asymptomatic (usually). May have risk of altered function of exposed area.
2,500	Atrophy, vascular lesion, and altered pigmentation.
5,000	Chronic ulcer, risk of carcinogenesis.
50,000	Permanent destruction of exposed tissue.

The amount of radiation may drop off rapidly as the patient is decontaminated and moved away from the exposure. The distance from an ionizing radiation source is crucial since exposure is determined by the inverse square relationship. Doubling the distance away from a radiation source reduces the exposure by a factor of four. Conversely, halving the distance to a radiation source increases exposure by a factor of four.

There are basically two types of ionizing radiation accidents, clean and dirty. In a *clean accident,* the patient is exposed to radiation but is not contaminated by the radioactive substance, particles of radioactive dust, or radioactive liquids, gases, or smoke. If he is properly decontaminated before arrival of rescue personnel, there will be little danger, provided the source of the radiation is no longer exposed at the scene. After exposure to ionizing radiation, the patient is not radioactive. Therefore, he poses no hazard to rescue personnel.

In contrast, the *dirty accident,* often associated with fire at the scene of a radiation accident, exposes the patient to radiation and contaminates him with radioactive particles or liquids. The scene may be highly contaminated, although the primary source of radiation is shielded when rescue personnel arrive. Unless you are properly trained in dealing with this type of emergency, you may have to delay rescue procedures until properly trained technical assistance arrives.

MANAGEMENT

If you find yourself involved in a radioactive emergency, take the following precautionary steps:

- Park the rescue vehicle upwind to minimize contamination.
- Look for signs of radiation exposure. Radioactive packages are marked by clearly identifiable color-coded labels (Figure 26-8).
- Use portable instruments to measure the level of radioactivity. If dose estimates are significant, rotate rescue personnel.
- Normal principles of emergency care should be applied, for example, ABCs, shock management, and trauma care.
- Externally radiated patients pose little danger to rescue personnel. Initiate normal care procedures for injuries other than radiation.
- Internally contaminated patients (who have ingested or inhaled radioactive particles) pose little danger to rescue personnel. Normal care procedures should be undertaken. Collect body wastes. If assisted ventilation is required, use a BVM unit or demand valve. If radioactive particles are inhaled, swab the nasal passages and save the swabs.
- Externally contaminated patients (liquids, dirt, smoke) require decontamination. Following decontamination, initiate normal emergency care

In a radiation accident, externally radiated and internally contaminated patients pose little danger to rescue personnel. Provide normal emergency care.

Externally contaminated patients must be decontaminated before normal emergency care is initiated. EMS personnel and equipment must be decontaminated after the call.

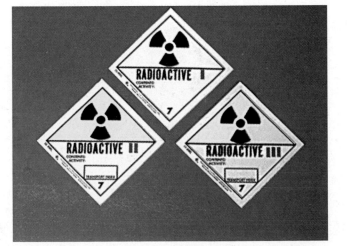

FIGURE 26-8 Radioactive warning labels.

procedures. Decontamination of EMS personnel and equipment is required after the call is completed.

- Patients with open, contaminated wounds require normal emergency care procedures. Avoid cross-contamination of wounds.

SUMMARY

Our environment provides us with all that we need to survive and prosper. The extremes of our environment, however, can have significant impact on human metabolism. Our bodies will, of course, compensate for these extremes, but sometimes it is not enough. Sometimes the heat gain or loss is too much. Sometimes the pressure change is too much. As a result, medical illnesses and emergencies arise. These can range from abnormal core body temperatures to decompensation, shock, and even death.

Basic knowledge of common environmental, recreational, and exposure emergencies is necessary in order for you to administer prompt and proper treatment in the prehospital setting. It is not easy to remember this type of information since these problems are not usually encountered on a daily basis. Remember the general principles involved. Remove the environmental influence causing the problem. Support the patient's own attempt to compensate. Finally, select a definitive care location and transport the patient as rapidly as possible.

In every case, remember that you must maintain your own safety. There are too many cases in which EMT-Is have lost their lives as a result of attempting a rescue for which they were not properly trained. Rapid action is always necessary when performing an environmental rescue. However, common sense must prevail.

ON THE WEB

For additional practice and review, go to the companion website at www.prenhall.com/bledsoe and click on *Intermediate Emergency Care: Principles & Practice*.

CHAPTER 27

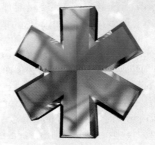

Behavioral Emergencies

Objectives

After reading this chapter, you should be able to:

1. Distinguish between normal and abnormal behavior. (p. 1090)
2. Discuss the pathophysiology of behavioral and psychiatric disorders. (pp. 1091–1092)
3. Describe the medical legal considerations for management of emotionally disturbed patients. (p. 1107)
4. Describe the overt behaviors associated with specific behavioral and psychiatric disorders. (pp. 1095–1105)
5. List the appropriate measures to ensure the safety of the EMT-Intermediate, the patient, and others. (pp. 1092–1094, 1107–1110)
6. Describe the circumstances when relatives, bystanders, and others should be removed from the scene. (p. 1093)
7. Describe techniques to systematically gather information from the disturbed patient. (pp. 1093–1094, 1106–1107)

8. Identify techniques for physical assessment in a patient with behavioral problems. (pp. 1093–1094)
9. List situations in which you are expected to transport a patient forcibly and against his will. (p. 1107)
10. Describe restraint methods necessary in managing the emotionally disturbed patient. (pp. 1107–1110)
11. List the risk factors and behaviors that indicate a patient is at risk for suicide. (pp. 1103–1104)
12. Given several preprogrammed behavioral emergency patients, provide the appropriate scene size-up, initial assessment, focused assessment, and detailed assessment, then provide the appropriate care and patient transport. (pp. 1090–1110)

CASE STUDY

On a hot August night, EMT-I ambulance crew Kelly Underwood and Charles Bear have been dispatched to a possible psychiatric emergency at a local supermarket. They carefully approach the scene and observe a man standing in front of the store with his back to them. The manager approaches the ambulance and tells Kelly and

Charles that the man came to the store and announced that the produce was poisonous. The manager also warns them that the man's behavior is somewhat bizarre. The man turns and begins shouting loudly, "Don't come in here! They're selling poison. They're trying to kill us all!" Charles radios for police assistance. He and Kelly remain in the ambulance and observe the patient until police arrive.

When the police arrive, Kelly quickly briefs them on the situation and the patient's status. The officers recognize the man as a psychiatric patient with whom they have recently had contact at a local motel. The man begins yelling and says he is working for the government. He yells at the top of his voice, "We'll close this place down!" The police ask Kelly and Charles to prepare the stretcher and restraints as a precaution. As the police approach the man, he calls them "poisoners." His agitation continues to escalate despite the efforts of the crew and officers to calm him. It becomes obvious that restraint is needed.

The police officers make the initial approach and control the patient's arms. Kelly is able to safely control the man's legs, while Charles moves the stretcher into place. After moving the patient to the stretcher, they place him face-up and restrain his arms and legs using wide roller bandages. Kelly performs an assessment to rule out medical or traumatic causes of the patient's altered mental status. He monitors the man carefully en route to the emergency department. From there, the patient is eventually transferred to the psychiatric center.

INTRODUCTION

A significant difference between behavioral and psychiatric conditions and other types of medical emergencies is that most of your assessment and care will depend on your people skills. You can evaluate a bradycardia with a cardiac monitor and treat it with atropine or a pacing unit. You evaluate the psychiatric patient, on the other hand, by observing his behavior, by gathering information from his family and bystanders, and by interviewing him. Your care, which includes support, calming reassurance, and occasionally restraint, requires interpersonal skills more than diagnostic equipment.

BEHAVIORAL EMERGENCIES

behavior a person's observable conduct and activity.

behavioral emergency situation in which a patient's behavior becomes so unusual that it alarms the patient or another person and requires intervention.

Behavior is a person's observable conduct and activity. A **behavioral emergency** is a situation in which a patient's behavior becomes so unusual, bizarre, threatening, or dangerous that it alarms the patient or another person such as a family member or bystander and requires the intervention of emergency service and/or mental health personnel.

Notice that the definition of behavioral emergency does not use the word *abnormal*. The differentiation between normal and abnormal is largely subjective. What is normal varies based on culture, ethnic group, socioeconomic class, and personal interpretation and opinion. What one person considers normal, another might consider highly abnormal. Generally, however, normal behavior can be defined as behavior that is readily acceptable in a society.

Indications of a behavioral or psychological condition include actions that:

- Interfere with core life functions (eating, sleeping, ability to maintain housing, interpersonal or sexual relations)
- Pose a threat to the life or well-being of the patient or others
- Significantly deviate from society's expectations or norms

PATHOPHYSIOLOGY OF PSYCHIATRIC DISORDERS

Experts estimate that up to 20% of the population has some type of mental health problem and that as many as one person in seven will actually require treatment for an emotional disturbance. These problems may be severely disabling and require inpatient care, or the patient may quietly tolerate them with no outward symptoms. A misconception is that all people with psychiatric conditions exhibit bizarre or unusual behavior. The small percentage of patients with psychiatric disorders who publicly exhibit bizarre behavior tends to create this misconception among lay people. In reality, most patients who suffer from disorders such as anxiety, depression, eating disorders, or mild personality disorders function normally on a daily basis, going unnoticed in society. Nonetheless, behavioral and psychiatric disorders incapacitate more people than all other health problems combined. Most patients with mental illness are cared for in outpatient settings such as public mental health centers. Only those with severe psychiatric illnesses remain institutionalized. Because of this, EMS providers are increasingly being called to care for patients with behavioral complaints. A common reason for EMS intervention in psychiatric illness is patient failure to take psychiatric medications. When mental health patients such as schizophrenics begin to deteriorate and develop bizarre behavior, they most likely have not been adhering to their psychiatric medication regimen.

Another common misconception is that all mental patients are unstable and dangerous and that their conditions are incurable. This is simply not true. Research in psychiatry, as with other areas in medicine, has made great strides in determining causes and treatments for many psychiatric conditions. Having a mental disorder is not reason for embarrassment or shame, although society often stigmatizes these patients unfairly. The general causes of behavioral emergencies are biological (or organic), psychosocial, and sociocultural. Each of these three possible causes should guide your questioning during the patient interview. Keep in mind, however, that a patient's condition may result from more than one pathological process.

BIOLOGICAL

For many years, medical practitioners have used the terms **biological** and **organic** interchangeably when discussing certain types of psychiatric disorders whose causes are physical rather than purely psychological. They result from disease processes such as infections and tumors or from structural changes in the brain such as those brought on by the abuse of alcohol or drugs (over-the-counter and prescription medications). It could be argued, however, that even purely psychological conditions originate in the brain and for that very reason are organic. Indeed, many psychiatric conditions do originate from alterations in brain chemistry.

Behavioral emergencies frequently involve biological conditions. Never assume a patient with an altered mental status or unusual behavior is suffering from a purely psychological condition or disease until you have completely ruled out medical conditions and substance abuse.

Content Review

GENERAL CAUSES OF BEHAVIORAL EMERGENCIES
- Biological (organic)
- Psychosocial (personal)
- Social (situational)

biological/organic related to disease processes or structural changes.

Never assume a patient with an altered mental status or unusual behavior is suffering from a purely psychological condition or disease until you have completely ruled out medical conditions and substance abuse.

Patho Pearls

Although you may encounter a patient with a bonafide psychiatric problem, it is important to remember that drug and alcohol use cause a significant amount of aberrant and violent behavior problems. Any time you encounter a violent patient or a patient with acute psychosis, first try to identify a medical or toxicological cause for the behavior. Many medical conditions, such as diabetes mellitus, can cause behavioral changes. Likewise, many medications and recreational drugs can cause behavior that is similar to that of mental illness. Always consider the possibility of drugs and alcohol in any patient with a behavioral emergency.

PSYCHOSOCIAL

Psychosocial (personal) conditions are related to a patient's personality style, dynamics of unresolved conflict, or crisis management methods. These disorders are not attributable to substance abuse or medical conditions.

Environment plays a large part in psychosocial development. Traumatic childhood incidents may affect a person throughout life. Parents or other persons in positions of authority can have a tremendous impact on a child's development. Dysfunctional families, abusive parents, alcohol or drug abuse by parents, or neglect can cause behavioral problems from childhood through adulthood. Such conditions, in addition to—or in combination with genetic predisposition and brain chemistry—form the basis for psychosocial conditions.

SOCIOCULTURAL

Sociocultural (situational) causes of behavioral disorders are related to the patient's actions and interactions within society and to factors such as socioeconomic status, social habits, social skills, and values. These problems are usually attributable to events that change the patient's social space (relationships, support systems), social isolation, or otherwise have an impact on socialization.

Some events in the lives of children and adults that may cause a profound psychological change are rape, assault, witnessing the victimization of another, death of a loved one, and acts of violence such as war or riots. Events that occur over time may also have an impact on the individual. These include the loss of a job, economic problems such as poverty, and ongoing prejudice or discrimination. Sometimes simply doing anything outside the norms of society can lead to stress and psychological changes.

ASSESSMENT OF BEHAVIORAL EMERGENCY PATIENTS

The assessment and care of behavioral emergency patients is similar to that for other medical conditions. The order of assessment (scene size-up, initial assessment, focused history and physical examination) remains unchanged. Potential medical conditions that mimic behavioral emergencies require you to perform a thorough medical assessment.

Among the differences between your assessment and care of a patient with a medical condition and one with a behavioral emergency is that, as already noted, you actually begin your care at the same time you begin your assessment by developing a rapport with the patient. Interpersonal skills are important for all patients, but perhaps never more than for one who is experiencing a behavioral emergency. Additionally, the focused history and physical exam for a behavioral emergency includes a mental status examination.

SCENE SIZE-UP

Approach every patient cautiously to protect yourself and your crew from injury.

As with any call, determining scene safety is of the utmost importance. Approach the scene carefully. If a patient is experiencing a behavioral emergency that is significant enough to warrant EMS, it is most likely significant enough to have law enforcement authorities respond. Most patients experiencing behavioral emergencies or crises will not attack you; however, those who are behaving unusually, experiencing hallucinations or delusions, or are under the effect of a substance may become violent. Approach every patient cautiously to protect yourself and your crew from injury (Figure 27-1).

The scene size-up also includes making observations that relate to patient care. Look for evidence of substance use or abuse, for therapeutic medications that may indicate an underlying medical condition (or abuse of that medication), and for signs of violence or destruction of property. Examine the general environmental condition and, when possible, observe the patient from a distance to note any visible behavior patterns or violent behavior.

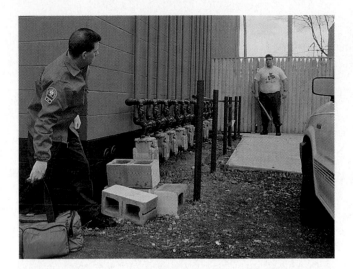

FIGURE 27-1 Approach every patient cautiously. If you determine a potential for violence, request police assistance.

INITIAL ASSESSMENT

Because many behavioral emergencies are caused by or concurrent with medical conditions, you should be acutely suspicious of life-threatening emergencies. As with any other injury or condition, assess the ABCs and intervene when necessary. Continue to observe the patient for any clues to his underlying condition. Be cautious of any overt behavior such as **posture** or hand gestures. Note any emotional response such as rage, **fear,** anxiety, **confusion,** or anger. Early in the evaluation try to determine the patient's **mental status,** the state of his cerebral functioning. Continue assessing mental status throughout the patient encounter by evaluating his awareness, orientation, cognitive abilities, and **affect** (visible indicators of mood).

Control the scene as soon as possible. Remove anyone who agitates the patient or adds confusion to the scene. Generally, a limited number of people around the patient is best. At times, performing an effective assessment and care may necessitate totally clearing a room or moving the patient to a quiet area. Finally, observe the patient's affect in greater detail. To avoid being grabbed or struck by the patient, stay alert for signs of aggression.

FOCUSED HISTORY AND PHYSICAL EXAMINATION

Your examination of a patient experiencing a behavioral emergency is largely conversational. This makes your interpersonal technique very important. Just as starting an IV access with poor technique most likely will not establish a patent IV line, interviewing with poor interpersonal skills most likely will not obtain significant information. Remove the patient from the crisis area and limit interruptions. Focus your questioning and assessment on the immediate problem and follow these guidelines:

- *Listen.* Ask open-ended questions (those that require more than a yes-or-no response). These will encourage your patient to respond in detail and share important information. Listen to the answer. Pay attention. No one likes being ignored. When you need information from a patient, listen.

- *Spend time.* Rushing the patient's answers, cutting him off, or appearing hurried will cause him to "shut down" and stop answering questions.

- *Be assured.* Communicate self-confidence, honesty, and professionalism.

- *Do not threaten.* Avoid rapid or sudden movements or questions that the patient might interpret as threats. Approach him slowly and confidently.

- *Do not fear silence.* Silence can be appropriate. Encourage the patient to tell his or her story, but do not be forceful or antagonizing.

- *Place yourself at the patient's level.* Standing over the patient may be intimidating. Unless you are intentionally attempting to gain a position of

posture position, attitude, or bearing of the body.

fear feeling of alarm and discontentment in the expectation of danger.

confusion state of being unclear or unable to make a decision easily.

mental status the state of the patient's cerebral functioning.

affect visible indicators of mood.

Stay alert for signs of aggression.

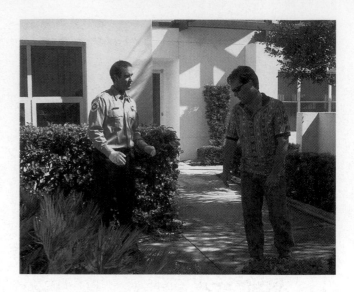

FIGURE 27-2 Avoid invading the patient's personal space, the area within about three feet of the patient.

authority, crouch, kneel, or sit near the patient. Do not position yourself where you cannot respond appropriately to danger or attack.

- *Keep a safe and proper distance.* The surest way to make a behavioral emergency patient violent is to invade his personal space (Figure 27-2). This is an area within an approximately three-foot radius around a person; encroaching upon it causes anxiety. If appropriate, however, you may touch the patient's shoulder or use another consoling touch when he allows.

- *Appear comfortable.* Do not appear uncomfortable—even if you are. Talking to patients about suicide, self-mutilation, or other psychological conditions is difficult. If the patient sees that you are uncomfortable, however, he is unlikely to open up to you. Would you expect a patient to tell you his reasons for attempting suicide when you appear uncomfortable even saying the word? To help, use terms the patient has used. If he says he wanted to "end it all," begin with that. Caregivers sometimes hesitate to use the word suicide because it might give the patient ideas of suicide. If you are there to care for a suicidal or potentially suicidal patient, however, he has already had those thoughts.

- *Avoid appearing judgmental.* Patients who are experiencing behavioral emergencies may feel strong emotions toward their caregivers. The patient should believe that you are interested in his condition and welfare. Be supportive and empathetic, and avoid judgments, pity, anger, or any other emotions that may damage your relationship with the patient.

- *Never lie to the patient.* Honesty is the best policy. Do not reinforce false beliefs or hallucinations or mislead the patient in any way.

MENTAL STATUS EXAMINATION

As part of the focused history and physical examination for behavioral emergencies, do not overlook any physical or medical complaint. In addition to the medical evaluation, which is covered in depth throughout this and the other volumes of this program, your examination of the patient with psychiatric or behavioral disorders should include a psychological evaluation, also known as a **mental status examination (MSE).** The components of the MSE include:

- *General appearance.* The patient's appearance can provide important information when looking at his "big picture." Observe hygiene, clothing, and overall appearance.

- *Behavioral observations.* Observe verbal or nonverbal behavior, strange or threatening appearance, or facial expressions. Note tone of voice, rate, volume, and quality.

mental status examination (MSE) a structured exam designed to quickly evaluate a patient's level of mental functioning.

- *Orientation.* Does the patient know who he is and who others are? Is he oriented to current events? Can he concentrate on simple questions and answer them?
- *Memory.* Is the patient's memory intact for recent and long-term events?
- *Sensorium.* Is the patient focused? Paying attention? What is his level of awareness?
- *Perceptual processes.* Are the patient's thought patterns ordered? Does he appear to have any hallucinations, delusions, or phobias?
- *Mood and affect.* Observe for indicators of the patient's mood. Is it appropriate? What is his prevailing emotion? Depression, elation, anxiety, or agitation? Other?
- *Intelligence.* Evaluate the patient's speech. What is his level of vocabulary? His ability to formulate an idea?
- *Thought processes.* What is the patient's apparent form of thought? Are his thoughts logical and coherent?
- *Insight.* Does the patient have insight into his own problem? Does he recognize that a problem exists? Does he deny or blame others for his problem?
- *Judgment.* Does the patient base his life decisions on sound, reasonable judgments? Does he approach problems thoughtfully, carefully, and rationally?
- *Psychomotor.* Does the patient exhibit an unusual posture or is he making unusual movements? Patients with hallucinations may react to them. For example, a patient who believes he is covered with insects may be picking at his skin to remove the "bugs."

PSYCHIATRIC MEDICATIONS

Many patients who suffer from psychiatric or behavioral disorders are under the care of a mental health professional and may be taking prescription medications. During the interview and history-taking process, determine whether the patient is taking medications and, if so, what type. The patient's use of such medications can provide clues to his underlying condition. Additionally, if a patient is not taking a medication as directed, his condition may deteriorate. Some schizophrenic patients may receive periodic injections of extremely long-acting antipsychotics (for example, haloperidol deconoate) because of poor compliance. They will often carry an identification card or may report that they "go to the clinic every three weeks for a shot." Types of psychiatric medications are discussed in Chapter 3, "Emergency Pharmacology."

SPECIFIC PSYCHIATRIC DISORDERS

Almost all psychiatric disorders have two diagnostic elements: symptoms of the disease or disorder and indications that the disease or disorder has impaired major life functions resulting in loss of relationships, a job, or housing or in another significant social problem. To define specific conditions, mental health professionals use the *Diagnostic and Statistical Manual of Mental Disorders,* fourth edition (DSM-IV). Published by the American Psychiatric Association (APA), the DSM-IV details diagnostic criteria for all currently defined psychiatric disorders, which are grouped according to the patient's signs and symptoms. The recognized types of behavioral and psychiatric disorders include:

- Cognitive disorders
- Schizophrenia
- Anxiety disorders
- Mood disorders
- Substance-related disorders
- Somatoform disorders

- Factitious disorders
- Dissociative disorders
- Eating disorders
- Personality disorders
- Impulse control disorders

The following summaries of the major criteria for these illnesses do not imply that you should diagnose behavioral disorders. Even for skilled psychologists and psychiatrists, diagnosis is complicated by the considerable overlap in symptoms from one disease to another. A patient may actually fit into several categories. You should use the information here only as a guide to better understanding the science of psychiatry and the criteria applied to patients with behavioral emergencies. Knowledge of these terms and conditions will also allow you to communicate better with psychiatric care providers.

COGNITIVE DISORDERS

Psychiatric disorders with organic causes such as brain injury or disease are known as *cognitive disorders*. This family of disorders includes conditions caused by metabolic disease, infections, neoplasm, endocrine disease, degenerative neurological disease, and cardiovascular disease. They might also be caused by physical or chemical injuries due to trauma, drug abuse, or reactions to prescribed drugs. The specific brain pathology will differ based on the type of disease. Two types of cognitive disorders are delirium and dementia.

Delirium

Delirium is characterized by a relatively rapid onset of widespread disorganized thought. These patients suffer from inattention, memory impairment, disorientation, and a general clouding of consciousness. In some cases, individuals may experience vivid visual hallucinations. Delirium is characterized by a fairly acute onset (hours or days) and may be reversible. Delirium may be due to a medical condition, substance intoxication, substance withdrawal, or multiple etiologies. Confusion is a hallmark of delirium.

Dementia

Dementia may be due to several medical problems. Included among the more common causes of dementia are Alzheimer's disease (both early and late onset), vascular problems, AIDS, head trauma, Parkinson's disease, substance abuse, and other chronic problems. Regardless of its cause, dementia involves memory impairment, cognitive disturbance, and pervasive impairment of abstract thinking and judgment. Unlike delirium, dementia usually develops over months and, in many cases, is irreversible.

Dementia involves cognitive deficits manifested by both memory impairment (diminished ability to learn new information or to recall previously learned information) and one or more of the following cognitive disturbances:

- *Aphasia.* Impaired ability to communicate.
- *Apraxia.* Impaired ability to carry out motor activities despite intact sensory function.
- *Agnosia.* Failure to recognize objects or stimuli despite intact sensory function.
- *Disturbance in executive functioning.* Impaired ability to plan, organize, or sequence.

These conditions must significantly impair social or occupational functioning and represent a significant decline from a previous level of functioning. Your approach to patients with either of these conditions should be supportive. Assess and manage any medical complaints or conditions and transport to an appropriate medical facility.

SCHIZOPHRENIA

Schizophrenia is a common mental health problem, affecting an estimated one percent of the United States population. Its hallmark is a significant change in behavior and a

---

Content Review

COGNITIVE DISORDERS
- Delirium
- Dementia

---

delirium condition characterized by relatively rapid onset of widespread disorganized thought.

dementia condition involving gradual development of memory impairment and cognitive disturbance.

schizophrenia common disorder involving significant change in behavior often including hallucinations, delusions, and depression.

loss of contact with reality. Signs and symptoms often include hallucinations, delusions, and depression. The schizophrenic patient may live in his own world and be preoccupied with inner fantasies. Although several biological and psychosocial theories attempt to explain the condition and its manifestations, its definitive cause is unknown.

The symptoms of schizophrenia include:

- **Delusions.** Fixed, false beliefs that are not widely held within the context of the individual's cultural or religious group.
- **Hallucinations.** Sensory perceptions with no basis in reality. These are often auditory (hearing voices).
- Disorganized speech, marked by frequent derailment or incoherence.
- Grossly disorganized or **catatonic** behavior.
- Negative symptoms (**flat affect**).

A diagnosis of schizophrenia requires that two or more symptoms must each be present for a significant portion of each month over the course of six months. The symptoms must cause a social or occupational dysfunction (decline in social relations or work from the predisease state). Most schizophrenics are diagnosed in early adulthood.

The DSM-IV defines several major types of schizophrenia:

- *Paranoid.* The patient is preoccupied with a feeling of persecution and may have delusions or auditory hallucinations.
- *Disorganized.* The patient often displays disorganized behavior, dress, or speech.
- *Catatonic.* The patient exhibits catatonic rigidity, immobility, stupor, or peculiar voluntary movements. Catatonic schizophrenia is exceedingly rare.
- *Undifferentiated.* The patient does not readily fit into one of the categories above.

Your approach to the schizophrenic patient should be supportive and nonjudgmental. Do not reinforce the patient's hallucinations, but understand that he considers them real. Speak openly and honestly with him. Be encouraging yet realistic. Remain alert for aggressive behavior, and restrain the patient if he becomes violent or presents a danger to you, to himself, or to others.

ANXIETY AND RELATED DISORDERS

The group of illnesses known as **anxiety disorders** is characterized by dominating apprehension and fear. These disorders affect approximately 2% to 4% of the population. Broadly defined, **anxiety** is a state of uneasiness, discomfort, apprehension, and restlessness. More specifically, anxiety disorders fall into three categories: panic disorder, phobia, and post-traumatic stress syndrome.

Panic Attack

The DSM-IV does not list **panic attacks** in themselves as a disease. Characterized by recurrent, extreme periods of anxiety resulting in great emotional distress, they are symptoms of disease and are included among the criteria for other disorders (panic disorder, agoraphobia). Panic attacks differ from generalized feelings of anxiety in their acute nature. They are usually unprovoked, peaking within 10 minutes of their onset and dissipating in less than one hour.

The presentation of panic and anxiety may resemble a cardiac or respiratory condition. This presents a dilemma for EMS personnel. Ruling out those conditions is difficult in the prehospital setting; psychiatrists usually diagnose anxiety or panic disorders by excluding known medical conditions. Keys to identifying panic or anxiety in the field are the patient's having a history of the condition and being outside the expected age range for certain cardiac or respiratory illnesses. This, of course, is not to say that young people cannot have myocardial infarction. Many symptoms of panic resemble those of hyperventilation, and some

---

delusions fixed, false beliefs not widely held within the individual's cultural or religious group.

hallucinations sensory perceptions with no basis in reality.

catatonia condition characterized by immobility and stupor; often a sign of schizophrenia.

flat affect appearance of being disinterested, often lacking facial expression.

Content Review

MAJOR TYPES OF SCHIZOPHRENIA

- Paranoid
- Disorganized
- Catatonic
- Undifferentiated

Content Review

ANXIETY-RELATED DISORDERS

- Panic attack
- Phobia
- Post-traumatic stress syndrome

anxiety disorder condition characterized by dominating apprehension and fear.

anxiety state of uneasiness, discomfort, apprehension, and restlessness.

panic attack extreme period of anxiety resulting in great emotional distress.

do appear to be correlated, such as the paresthesia from panic being due largely to hyperventilation.

The diagnostic criteria for a panic attack require a discrete period of intense fear or discomfort, during which four or more of the following symptoms develop abruptly and reach a peak within 10 minutes:

- Palpitations, pounding heart, or accelerated heart rate
- Sweating
- Trembling or shaking
- Sensations of shortness of breath or smothering
- Feeling of choking
- Chest pain or discomfort
- Nausea or abdominal distress
- Feeling dizzy, unsteady, lightheaded, or faint
- Derealization (feelings of unreality) or depersonalization (being detached from oneself)
- Fear of losing control or going crazy
- Fear of dying
- Paresthesia (numbness or tingling sensations)
- Chills or hot flashes

Management for anxiety disorders is generally simple and supportive. Show empathy. Assess any medical complaints and manage them appropriately. If the patient experiences hyperventilation, calm and reassure him in order to decrease his respiratory rate to normal. Patients with severe or incapacitating symptoms may benefit from the administration of a sedative. Benzodiazepines, such as diazepam (Valium) and lorazepam (Ativan) can be administered in the prehospital setting. In addition, antihistamines, such as hydroxyzine (Vistaril) and diphenhydramine (Benadryl), have sedative effects and are useful in treating patients with significant anxiety. Consult medical direction in accordance with local protocol and transport to an appropriate medical facility.

Phobias

phobia excessive fear that interferes with functioning.

Everyone has some source of fear or anxiety that they consciously avoid. When this fear becomes excessive and interferes with functioning, it is a **phobia**. A phobia, generally considered an intense, irrational fear, may be due to animals, the sight of blood (or injection or injury), situational factors (elevators, enclosed spaces), or environmental conditions (heights or water). Exposure to the situation or item will induce anxiety or a panic attack. Some patients experience extreme phobias that prevent or limit their normal daily activities. For example, a patient suffering from agoraphobia (fear of crowds) may confine himself to his home and avoid ever venturing outdoors. In most patients, however, the phobia is less severe; the patient realizes that his fear is unreasonable, and the anxiety dissipates.

Management for a patient with a phobia is supportive. Understand that the patient's fear is very real. Do not force him to do anything that he opposes. Manage any underlying problems and transport for evaluation.

Post-traumatic Stress Syndrome

post-traumatic stress syndrome reaction to an extreme stressor.

EMS providers often are particularly interested in **post-traumatic stress syndrome** because their responsibilities may make them susceptible to it. Originally recognized on the battlefields of war, post-traumatic stress syndrome is a reaction to an extreme, usually lifethreatening stressor such as a natural disaster, victimization (rape, for instance), or other emotionally taxing situation. It is characterized by a desire to avoid similar situations, recurrent intrusive thoughts, depression, sleep disturbances, nightmares, and persistent symptoms of increased arousal. The patient may feel guilty for having survived the incident, and substance abuse may frequently complicate his condition.

Treat any post-traumatic stress syndrome patient with respect, empathy, and support, and transport him to an appropriate facility for evaluation.

MOOD DISORDERS

The DSM-IV defines mood as "a pervasive and sustained emotion that colors a person's perception of the world." Common examples of mood alterations include depression, elation, **anger,** and anxiety. The main **mood disorders** are depression and bipolar disorder.

Depression

Depression is characterized by a profound sadness or feeling of melancholy. It is common in everyday life and is to be expected following the break-up of a relationship or the loss of a loved one. Most of us have experienced some sort of depression, at least in its mildest form. It is one of the most prevalent psychiatric conditions, affecting from 10% to 15% of the population. When depression becomes prolonged or severe, however, it is diagnosed as a *major depressive episode*.

The symptoms of major depressive disorder include:

- Depressed mood most of the day, nearly every day, as indicated by subjective report or observation by others.
- Markedly diminished interest in pleasure in all, or almost all, activities most of the day nearly every day.
- Significant weight loss (without dieting) or weight gain. A 5% change in body weight is considered significant.
- Insomnia or hypersomnia nearly every day.
- Psychomotor agitation or retardation every day (observable by others, not just the subjective feeling of the patient).
- Feelings of worthlessness or excessive inappropriate guilt (may be delusional) nearly every day.
- Diminished ability to think or concentrate, or indecisiveness nearly every day.
- Recurrent thoughts of death (not just fear of dying), recurrent suicidal ideation without a specific plan, or a suicide attempt or a specific plan for committing suicide. (Depression greatly increases the risk of suicide.)

The diagnostic criteria for major depressive disorder require that five or more of the symptoms have been present during the same two-week period and represent a change from previous functioning; at least one of the symptoms must be either a depressed mood or loss of interest in pleasure. The condition must cause clinically significant distress or impairment in social, occupational, or other important functions. Further, it must not meet the criteria for a mixed episode (mixtures of mania and depression); it must not be due to the direct physiological effects of a substance such as drug abuse or a medication, or to a general medical condition such as hypothyroidism; finally, it must not be better accounted for by **bereavement.** The acronym *In SAD CAGES* provides a screening mnemonic for major depression: *In*terest, *S*leep, *A*ppetite, *D*epressed mood, *C*oncentration, *A*ctivity, *G*uilt, *E*nergy, *S*uicide.

Depression may occur as an isolated condition, but it is often accompanied by other disorders such as substance abuse, anxiety disorders, and schizophrenia. Depression can also affect a patient without meeting all of the identified clinical criteria. It can affect different people in different ways and is often atypical. Bereavement is one of the situations in which depression is expected. If the depression lasts longer than two months or is accompanied by suicidal ideation or marked functional impairment, it could be classified as a major depressive episode. Depression is more prevalent in females and is spread evenly throughout the life span.

Bipolar Disorder

Bipolar disorder is characterized by one or more **manic** episodes (periods of elation), with or without subsequent or alternating periods of depression. In the past, the term manic-depressive

Content Review

MOOD DISORDERS
- Depression
- Bipolar disorder

anger hostility or rage to compensate for an underlying feeling of anxiety.

mood disorder pervasive and sustained emotion that colors a person's perception of the world.

depression profound sadness or feeling of melancholy.

bereavement death of a loved one.

bipolar disorder condition characterized by one or more manic episodes, with or without periods of depression.

manic characterized by excessive excitement or activity (mania).

was used to describe this condition. Bipolar disorder is not particularly common, affecting approximately less than one percent of the population.

Manic-depressive episodes are not the "Jeckyl and Hyde" transformations that television and the movies often portray. However, they often begin suddenly and escalate rapidly over a few days. In contrast to major depressive disorders, bipolar disorders usually develop in adolescence or early adulthood and occur as often in males as in females. Some patients with major depressive episodes will eventually develop a bipolar disorder and experience manic episodes. Commonly patients have several depressive episodes before having a manic episode.

The diagnostic criteria for a manic episode require a distinct period of abnormally and persistently elevated, expansive, or irritable mood lasting for at least one week (or for any duration when hospitalization is necessary). Three or more (four or more if the mood is only irritable) of the following symptoms must have been present to a certain degree and must have persisted during that time:

- Inflated self-esteem or grandiosity
- Decreased need for sleep
- More talkative than usual or pressure to keep talking
- Flight of ideas or subjective experience that thoughts are racing
- Distractibility
- Increase in goal-directed activity (socially, at work or school, or sexually) or psychomotor agitation
- Excessive involvement in pleasurable activities that have a high potential for painful consequences (buying sprees, sexual indiscretions, foolish business investments)
- Delusional thoughts (grandiose ideas or unrealistic plans)

The symptoms must not meet the criteria for a mixed episode. The mood disturbance must be severe enough to markedly impair occupational or social functioning, to require hospitalizing the patient to prevent harm to himself or others, or present with psychotic features. As with depression, the symptoms must not be due to the direct physiological effects of a substance or a general medical condition. Patients with bipolar illness are often prescribed lithium (Lithobid, Eskalith) for treatment.

Management of these patients includes maintaining a calm, protective environment. Avoid confronting the manic patient. Never leave a depressed or suicidal patient alone. Assess and manage any other coexisting medical problems, and transport to an appropriate medical facility. Bipolar patients in an extreme manic phase may be overtly psychotic. In these cases, medication with an antipsychotic medication such as haloperidol may be indicated. Always contact medical direction for treatment options.

Many patients with bipolar disorder are treated with lithium. Lithium has a very narrow therapeutic index, making lithium toxicity a significant complicating factor.

SUBSTANCE-RELATED DISORDERS

Substance abuse is a common disorder. Any patient exhibiting symptoms of a psychiatric or behavioral disorder should be screened for substance use and/or abuse. Substance abuse patients may present as being depressed, psychotic, or delirious, and their signs and symptoms may mimic those of many behavioral disorders. The DSM-IV lists substance abuse as a psychiatric disorder; you should consider it a serious condition. Any mood-altering chemical has the potential for abuse. Alcohol is a common part of our culture, but can be abused. The user of a substance may be intoxicated from the effects of the chemical or may be ill from addiction or withdrawal of the chemical. Intoxication, in and of itself, may cause behavioral problems.

Repetitive use of a mood-altering chemical may lead to dependence or addiction. Dependence on a substance is characterized by repeated use of the substance. Dependence may be either psychological, physical, or both. Psychological dependence is a compelling desire to use the substance, inability to reduce or stop use, and repeated efforts to quit. Physical dependence is characterized by the need for increased amounts of the chemical to obtain the desired effect. Also, the presence of withdrawal symptoms when the substance is reduced or stopped is characteristic of physical dependence. All drugs have the potential to cause psychological dependence; many have the potential to cause physical dependence as well.

SOMATOFORM DISORDERS

Somatoform disorders are characterized by physical symptoms that have no apparent physiological cause. They are believed to be attributable to psychological factors. People who suffer from somatoform disorders believe their symptoms are serious and real. The major types of somatoform disorder are:

- *Somatization disorder.* The patient is preoccupied with physical symptoms.
- *Conversion disorder.* The patient sustains a loss of function, usually involving the nervous system (for instance, blindness or paralysis), unexplained by any medical illness.
- *Hypochondriasis.* Exaggerated interpretation of physical symptoms as a serious illness.
- *Body dysmorphic disorder.* A person believes he or she has a defect in physical appearance.
- *Pain disorder.* The patient suffers from pain, usually severe, that is unexplained by a physical ailment.

Somatoform disorders are often difficult to identify and diagnose. They can mimic and be confused with various bona fide physical conditions. Never attribute physical symptoms to a behavioral disorder until medical conditions have been ruled out.

FACTITIOUS DISORDERS

Factitious disorders are sometimes confused with somatoform disorders. They are characterized by the following three criteria:

- Intentional production of physical or psychological signs or symptoms.
- Motivation for the behavior is to assume the "sick role."
- External incentives for the behavior (e.g., economic gain, avoiding work, avoiding police) are absent.

Although patients suffering from factitious disorders essentially feign their illnesses, that does not preclude the possibility of true physical or psychological symptoms. The disorder is apparently more common in males than in females. In severe cases, patients will go to great length to obtain medical or psychological treatment. Patients with factitious disorders often will voluntarily produce symptoms and will present with a very plausible history. They often have an extensive knowledge of medical terminology and can be very demanding and disruptive. In severe cases (Munchausen syndrome), patients will undergo multiple surgical operations and other painful procedures.

DISSOCIATIVE DISORDERS

Like somatoform disorders, **dissociative disorders** are attempts to avoid stressful situations while still gratifying needs. In a manner, they permit the person to deny personal responsibility for unacceptable behavior. The individual avoids stress by dissociating from his core personality. These behavior patterns can be complex but are quite rare. The disorders include:

- **Psychogenic amnesia.** While amnesia is a partial or total inability to recall or identify past events, psychogenic amnesia is a failure to recall. The "forgotten" material is present but "hidden" beneath the level of consciousness.
- **Fugue state.** An amnesic individual may withdraw even further by retreating in what is known as a fugue state. A patient in a fugue state actually flees as a defense mechanism and may travel hundreds of miles from home.
- **Multiple personality disorder.** In multiple personality disorder the patient reacts to an identifiable stress by manifesting two or more complete systems of

- **Depersonalization.** Depersonalization is a relatively more frequent dissociative disorder that occurs predominantly in young adults. Patients experience a loss of the sense of one's self. Such individuals suddenly feel "different"—that they are someone else or that their body has taken on a different form. The disorder is often precipitated by acute stress.

depersonalization feeling detached from oneself.

EATING DISORDERS

The two classifications of eating disorders are anorexia nervosa and bulimia nervosa. Both generally occur between adolescence and the age of 25. The condition afflicts women more than men at a rate of 20:1.

Anorexia is the loss of appetite. **Anorexia nervosa** is a disorder marked by excessive fasting. Individuals with this disorder have an intense fear of obesity and often complain of being fat even though their body weight is low. They suffer from weight loss (25% of body weight or more), refusal to maintain body weight, and often a cessation of menstruation from severe malnutrition.

Recurrent episodes of seemingly uncontrollable binge eating with compensatory self-induced vomiting or diarrhea, excessive exercise, or dieting and with a full awareness of the behavior's abnormality characterize **bulimia nervosa**. Individuals often display personality traits of perfectionism, low self-esteem, and social withdrawal.

The weight loss and body changes experienced by anorexic and bulimic patients can lead to serious physical problems. Starvation and attempts to purge can have drastic consequences such as anemia, dehydration, vitamin deficiencies, hypoglycemia, and cardiovascular problems. In addition to psychological support, prehospital care is likely to include treatment for dehydration and physical problems. Both disorders have a high potential morbidity and mortality.

PERSONALITY DISORDERS

Most adult personalities are attuned to social demands. Some individuals, however, often seem ill-equipped to function adequately in society. These people might be suffering from a **personality disorder.** Stemming largely from immature and distorted personality development, these personality, or character, disorders result in persistently maladaptive ways of perceiving, thinking, and relating to the world.

The broad category of personality disorder includes problems that vary greatly in form and severity. Although others might describe them as eccentric or troublesome, some patients with personality disorders function adequately. In extreme cases, patients act out against or attempt to manipulate society.

Personality Disorder Clusters

The DSM-IV groups similar personality disorders into three broad types, Cluster A, Cluster B, and Cluster C.

Cluster A   These individuals often act oddly or eccentricly. Their unusual behavior can take drastically different forms. This cluster includes the following:

- *Paranoid personality disorder.* Pattern of distrust and suspiciousness.
- *Schizoid personality disorder.* Pattern of detachment from social relationships.
- *Schizotypal personality disorder.* Pattern of acute discomfort in close relationships, cognitive distortions, and eccentric behavior.

Cluster B   These individuals often appear dramatic, emotional, or fearful. This cluster includes the following:

- *Antisocial personality disorder.* Pattern of disregard for the rights of others.
- *Borderline personality disorder.* Pattern of instability in interpersonal relationships, self-image, and impulsivity.

Content Review

EATING DISORDERS
- Anorexia nervosa
- Bulimia nervosa

anorexia nervosa psychological disorder characterized by voluntary refusal to eat.

bulimia nervosa recurrent episodes of binge eating.

Content Review

PERSONALITY DISORDER CLUSTERS

Cluster A personality disorders
- Paranoid
- Schizoid
- Schizotypal

Cluster B personality disorders
- Antisocial
- Borderline
- Histrionic
- Narcissistic

Cluster C personality disorders
- Avoidant
- Dependent
- Obsessive-compulsive

personality disorder condition that results in persistently maladaptive behavior.

- *Histrionic personality disorder.* Pattern of excessive emotions and attention seeking.
- *Narcissistic personality disorder.* Pattern of grandiosity, need for admiration, and lack of empathy.

Cluster C   These individuals often appear anxious or fearful. This cluster includes:

- *Avoidant personality disorder.* Pattern of social inhibition, feelings of inadequacy, and hypersensitivity to criticism.
- *Dependent personality disorder.* Pattern of submissive and clinging behavior related to an excessive need to be cared for.
- *Obsessive-compulsive disorder.* Pattern of preoccupation with orderliness, perfectionism, and control.

Diagnosing a personality disorder requires evaluating the individual's long-term functioning and behavior. In many cases, the individual suffers from multiple disorders. A complete interview, history, and assessment will assist you in determining your approach. Your prehospital care will vary based on the patient's chief complaint and overall presentation.

IMPULSE CONTROL DISORDERS

Related to the personality disorders are the **impulse control disorders**. Recurrent impulses and the patient's failure to control them characterize these disorders. Examples of impulse control disorders include:

impulse control disorder condition characterized by the patient's failure to control recurrent impulses.

- *Kleptomania.* A recurrent failure to resist impulses to steal objects not for immediate use or for their monetary value
- *Pyromania.* A recurrent failure to resist impulses to set fires
- *Pathological gambling.* A chronic and progressive preoccupation with gambling and the urge to gamble
- *Trichotillomania.* A recurrent impulse to pull out one's own hair
- *Intermittent explosive disorder.* Recurrent and paroxysmal episodes of significant loss of control of aggressive responses

Disorders of impulse control may be harmful to the patient and others. Prior to committing the act the patient will have an increasing sense of tension. After the act, he will either have pleasure gratification or release.

SUICIDE

Suicide, simply stated, is when a person intentionally takes his or her own life. In the year 2000, the Centers for Disease Control reported that 29,350 people in the United States took their own lives (10.7 deaths per 100,000 population), making suicide the eleventh leading cause of death among all groups. However, in the 10–24 age group, suicide was the third leading cause of death. The incidence of suicide deaths among the elderly remains higher than the rate for the population as a whole. Women attempt suicide more frequently than men, but men are more likely to succeed. The most common methods of suicide (2000) are:

1. Firearms (57%)
2. Hanging, strangulation, suffocation (19%)
3. Solid and liquid poisons (12%)
4. Gas poisons (5%)
5. Jump from high places (2.1%)
6. Other methods (5.5%)

Assessing Potentially Suicidal Patients

In cases of attempted suicide, many focus on whether the patient really wanted to kill himself. Indeed this question will be at the heart of the patient's future psychiatric care, and information from the EMT-I will be crucial to making that determination. But never lose sight of patient care while probing the psychological nature of attempted suicide.

Perform an appropriate focused history and physical exam concurrently with providing sound psychological care. Mental health professionals are rarely on the scene. It is up to you to document observations at the scene, especially any detailed suicide plans, any suicide notes, and any statements of the patient and bystanders. This information may not be available after the event when the patient receives psychiatric screening at the hospital. Such care and observations at the scene, combined with detailed documentation, are critical to the patient's long-term psychological care.

Risk Factors for Suicide

The risk factors for suicide are numerous. When assessing a patient who has indicated suicidal intentions, screen for any of these risk factors:

- Previous attempts (Of those who successfully commit suicide, 80% have made a previous attempt.)
- Depression (Suicide is 500 times more common among patients who are severely depressed than those who are not.)
- Age (Incidence is high between 15 and 24 and over the age of 40.)
- Alcohol or drug abuse
- Divorced or widowed (The rate is five times higher than among other groups.)
- Giving away personal belongings, especially cherished possessions
- Living alone or in increased isolation
- Presence of **psychosis** with depression (for example, suicidal or destructive thoughts or hallucinations about killing or death)
- Homosexuality (especially homosexuals who are depressed, aging, alcoholic, or HIV-infected)
- Major separation trauma (mate, loved one, job, money)
- Major physical stresses (surgery, childbirth, sleep deprivation)
- Loss of independence (disabling illness)
- Lack of goals and plans for the future
- Suicide of same-sex parent
- Expression of a plan for committing suicide
- Possession of the mechanism for suicide (gun, pills, rope)

Patients who have attempted suicide must be evaluated in a hospital or psychiatric facility. Many people assume that "they were just looking for attention." Applied to the wrong patient, that conjecture may contribute to his death.

AGE-RELATED CONDITIONS

Some behavioral disorders are particularly common among patients at the ends of the age spectrum—the young and the elderly. Your awareness of age-related conditions will help you to assess and interact with these patients.

Crisis in the Geriatric Patient

Common physical problems among the elderly include dementia, chronic illness, and diminished eyesight and hearing. The elderly also experience depression that is often mistaken for dementia. When confronted with an elderly person in a crisis, take the following steps:

- Assess the patient's ability to communicate.
- Provide continual reassurance.
- Compensate for the patient's loss of sight and hearing with reassuring physical contact.

Document observations at the scene of an attempted suicide, especially any detailed suicide plans, suicide notes, and statements by the patient and bystanders.

psychosis extreme response to stress characterized by impaired ability to deal with reality.

- Treat the patient with respect. Call the patient by name and title, such as "Mrs. Jones." Avoid such terms as "dear," "honey," and "babe."
- Avoid administering medication.
- Describe what you are going to do before you do it.
- Take your time. Do not convey the impression that you are in a hurry.
- Allow family members and friends to remain with the patient if possible.

Crisis in the Pediatric Patient

Behavioral emergencies are not limited to adults. Children also have behavioral crises. Although the child's developmental stage will affect his or her behavior, these general guidelines will assist you when confronting an emotionally distraught or disruptive child:

- Avoid separating a young child from his parent.
- Attempt to prevent the child from seeing things that will increase his distress.
- Make all explanations brief and simple, and repeat them often.
- Be calm and speak slowly.
- Identify yourself by giving both your name and your function.
- Be truthful with the child. Telling the truth will develop trust.
- Encourage the child to help with his care.
- Reassure the child by carrying out all interventions gently.
- Do not discourage the child from crying or showing emotion.
- If you must be separated from the child, introduce the person who will assume responsibility for his care.
- Allow the child to keep a favorite blanket or toy.
- Do not leave the child alone, even for a short period.

Always be mindful of every young or elderly patient's uniqueness. Treat him equally and fairly, as you would any other patient.

MANAGEMENT OF BEHAVIORAL EMERGENCIES

Patients who are experiencing behavioral emergencies require both medical and psychological care. In general, take the following measures when you treat a patient who is experiencing a behavioral emergency:

1. Ensure scene safety and body substance isolation (BSI) precautions.
2. Provide a supportive and calm environment.
3. Treat any existing medical conditions.
4. Do not allow the suicidal patient to be alone.
5. Do not confront or argue with the patient.
6. Provide realistic reassurance.
7. Respond to the patient in a direct, simple manner.
8. Transport to an appropriate receiving facility.

Remember to treat the whole patient. Never overlook any serious, or potentially serious, medical complaints while focusing on the psychiatric assessment.

Never overlook any serious, or potentially serious, medical complaints while focusing on the psychiatric assessment.

MEDICAL

Patients who are experiencing apparent behavioral emergencies often have concurrent medical conditions—some of which may be responsible for the behavioral problem. Current literature indicates that medical conditions and/or substance abuse cause a much higher proportion of behavioral emergencies than previously believed. Medical care may include treatment for overdose, lacerations, toxic inhalation, hypoxia, or metabolic conditions. Many patients with chronic psychiatric conditions take medications for their illnesses; when abused, those medications have extremely toxic side effects. (See Chapter 3, "Emergency Pharmacology.") Additionally these patients often live in conditions ranging from substandard housing to the street. This existence may predispose them to other medical problems such as exposure, infections, and untreated illnesses.

PSYCHOLOGICAL

Patients who present with an apparent behavioral emergency also require psychological care. The time you spend developing a rapport with the patient—before, during, and after assessment—is actually a part of the care you provide. In effect, when you begin an assessment you are also beginning your care, and you will continue to perform psychological assessment and care concurrently with medical assessment and care. Be calm and reassuring while you interview your patient.

Since much of your care will be aimed at the psychological problem, you should steer your conversation and actions in that direction. Visualize your patients on a continuum ranging from agitated and out-of-control to introverted and depressed (Figure 27-3). As an EMT-I, you will need to defuse the agitated patient and attempt to communicate with the withdrawn patient. These situations especially will require the interviewing skills you learned earlier in this chapter.

As you approach the patient, introduce yourself and state that you want to help, since this might not be intuitively clear to a person with distorted perceptions. As you begin to converse, note how the patient reacts to you. Generally, if he responds appropriately to your actions, you should continue what you are doing. If the patient becomes more agitated or further withdrawn, rethink. Perhaps you are getting too close, talking too fast, or addressing difficult topics too early. Be sure your exit path is not blocked.

Your approach to these patients requires excellent people skills—especially listening and observing. If you do not use these skills, or if you rush or seem disinterested, your care

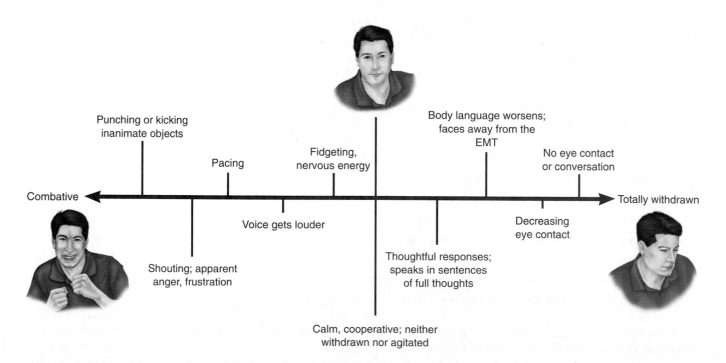

FIGURE 27-3 Continuum of patient responses during behavioral emergency. Whether dealing with an agitated or withdrawn patient, you will use your interpersonal skills to bring him to the calm, cooperative state in the middle of the continuum.

will likely fail. Therapeutic communication, as this interaction has been called, is an art. "Talking down" the behavioral emergency patient requires effort and skill. Some patients, however, will not react favorably even to the best people skills. Extremely withdrawn patients or those with severe psychotic symptoms may never fully respond during the time you spend with them out of the hospital. These patients still deserve quality care and compassion, even when they are uncommunicative or restrained.

Just as we must observe the patient, the patient observes us. Patients may actually be able to read us as accurately (or more accurately) than we read them. Perform your assessment and care confidently and competently. If patients sense uneasiness or indecision, they are more likely to act out. Never play along with a patient's hallucinations or delusions. It may seem to be the easiest route, but ultimately it may be harmful. Often the patient will recognize that you are patronizing him. Or the patient may talk of hallucinations or appear delusional, but not fully believe what he says. If you play along, you will lose credibility.

VIOLENT PATIENTS AND RESTRAINT

The role of providing medical care in the prehospital environment often places EMTs in harm's way. Agitation or confusion can result from a variety of the patient's medical or traumatic conditions. Likewise, various psychiatric and behavioral disorders can result in violent patients who pose a risk to EMT-Is, themselves, and others. The restraint of violent patients at an emergency scene is a controversial aspect of modern EMS. In fact, as a result of several prehospital deaths related to patient restraint, the practice has come under increasing scrutiny.

In 2002, the National Association of EMS Physicians (NAEMSP) adopted a position paper entitled, "Patient Restraint in Emergency Medical Services Systems." The purpose of this document is to provide guidelines that will help to minimize the possibility of injury to patients and EMS personnel. It is important to remember that many medical and trauma conditions can result in agitation and combativeness. Because of this, EMT-Is must be knowledgeable about these conditions and their appropriate treatment. All EMS systems should have protocols in place for the restraint and management of agitated and combative patients.

It is important to remember that many medical and trauma conditions can result in agitation and combativeness.

MEDICAL/LEGAL ISSUES

EMS systems and medical directors must be aware of the laws of their state. Local legislation related to an individual's rights, processes for involuntarily restraining or holding patients with mental health disorders, an individual's right to refuse treatment, and other related laws must be considered when developing a patient restraint protocol.

In general, legislation attempts to ensure the safety of individuals who are an immediate threat to themselves or others. It may be necessary to involve law enforcement or a mental health official to restrain a competent individual against his or her will. When possible, EMS systems should make certain that patients are accompanied by personnel of the same gender as the patient during treatment and transportation. This is of particular importance when pharmacologic agents are used for chemical restraint.

The application of physical and chemical restraints to a patient must be performed with the understanding that overstepping the boundaries of restraint may be perceived as battery, assault, or even false imprisonment. Restraint of an individual could even lead to serious allegations of civil rights violations. For this reason, the EMS service should always review patient restraint policies with appropriate legal counsel.

METHODS OF RESTRAINT

EMT-Is should always be alert for unexpectedly agitated patients or for those with escalating emotions. Because the safety of EMS personnel is paramount, it is appropriate for EMT-Is to withdraw from a violent situation until law enforcement or additional resources arrive.

The safety of EMS personnel is always paramount.

If a patient is known to be violent, make sure that law enforcement has secured the scene before you enter it.

Anticipate the potential for exposure to blood and body fluids during patient restraint, where you can be exposed to blood, saliva, urine, or feces. Based on the situation, appropriate BSI precautions should be taken during patient restraint activities.

The methods of restraint include *verbal deescalation, physical restraint,* and *chemical restraint.* The chosen method of restraint should always be the least restrictive method that ensures the safety of the patient and EMS personnel. These methods of restraint may be applied in a step-by-step fashion in many cases, but in extremely violent individuals, immediate physical restraint may be indicated to ensure the safety of the patient, bystanders, and EMS personnel.

VERBAL DEESCALATION

The use of verbal techniques to calm the patient is usually the first method that EMT-Is should employ. Verbal deescalation is safest because it does not require any physical contact with the patient. The conversation must be honest and straightforward with a friendly tone. Avoid direct eye contact and encroachment on the patient's "personal space," because this may induce added stress and anxiety. Always attempt to have equally open escape routes for both yourself and the patient should it become necessary. Always assess the patient for suicidal and/or homicidal ideation. Verbal intervention sometimes can diffuse the situation, prevent further escalation, and may avoid the need for further restraint tactics.

PHYSICAL RESTRAINT

When physically restraining a patient, EMT-Is must make every effort to avoid injuring the patient.

When physically restraining a patient, EMT-Is must make every effort to avoid injuring the patient (Figures 27-4 and 27-5). Because of this, patient restraint policies must recommend restraint devices that are associated with the least chance of injury. Physical restraint is accomplished with materials and techniques that allow for the restriction of movement of a person who is considered a danger to himself or others. Examples include soft restraints (sheets, wristlets, and chest Posey) and hard restraints (plastic ties, handcuffs, and leathers).

In general, EMS personnel should avoid the use of hard restraints. If a system chooses to use hard restraints, all personnel should be proficient in their use, and the patient's extremities should be evaluated frequently for injury or possible neurovascular compromise.

Ideally, five people should be present to safely apply physical restraint to a violent patient, which will allow for control of the head and each limb. This requirement may be difficult for some EMS systems due to a limited number of available personnel. Before beginning physical restraint, there should be a plan and a team leader who directs the restraining process.

A restrained patient should never be transported in a prone position.

Four-point restraints (restraints for both arms and both legs) are preferred over two-point restraints. It is often helpful to tether the hips, thighs, and chest. Tethering the thighs, just above the knees, often prevents kicking, more than restraint of the ankles does. Restrained patients should *not* be transported in a prone position. This has been associated

FIGURE 27-4 Never try to physically restrain a patient until you have sufficient help and an appropriate plan. If necessary, retreat to a safe area and await law enforcement.

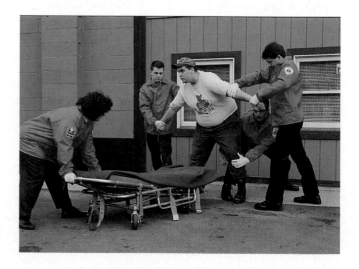

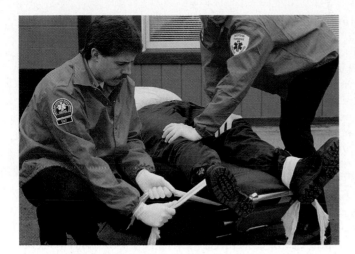

FIGURE 27-5 Place the patient supine on the ambulance stretcher and apply soft four-point restraints to the extremities.

with **positional asphyxia**. In addition, nothing should be placed over the face, head, or neck of the patient. A surgical mask placed loosely on the patient may prevent spitting. A hard cervical collar may limit the mobility of the patient's neck and may decrease the patient's range of motion in any attempt to bite.

While gaining initial control of the patient during restraint, it may be acceptable to temporarily restrain the patient in a prone position or sandwich the patient with a mattress, but personnel must be extremely vigilant for respiratory compromise. Gaining initial control of the patient in the prone position limits the patient's visual awareness of the environment and decreases the range of motion of the extremities. As soon as the team has control of the patient's movement, the team should work to move the patient into a supine four-point restrained position.

A patient should never be hobbled or "hog-tied" with the arms and legs tied together behind the back. During transport, a patient should never be restrained to a stretcher in the prone position or sandwiched between backboards or mattresses.

Once the patient has been restrained, he should never be left unattended. If a patient vomits, it may be necessary to immediately position him or suction him to protect the airway. Also, EMT-Is should perform and document frequent neurovascular assessments of the extremities that are restrained to ensure adequate circulation.

A patient who has undergone physical restraint should not be allowed to continue to struggle against the restraints. This may lead to severe acidosis and fatal dysrhythmia. In general, for the safety of EMS personnel, physical restraints applied in the field should not be removed until the patient is reevaluated upon arrival at the receiving facility.

Weapons used by law enforcement officers—including but not limited to pepper spray, mace defensive spray, stun guns, air tasers, stun batons, and telescoping steel batons—are not appropriate choices for patient restraint by EMS. They should be avoided since they may exacerbate the patient's agitation and increase the risk of injury or death. Although appropriately trained law enforcement officers may use these weapons, the use of weapons should be excluded from routine EMS protocols.

CHEMICAL RESTRAINT

Chemical restraint is defined as the addition of specific pharmacological agents to decrease agitation and increase the cooperation of patients who require medical care and transportation. EMS systems may use a variety of agents for chemical restraint of the agitated or combative patient. The goal of chemical restraint is to subdue excessive agitation and struggling against physical restraints. Ideally, this pharmacologic sedation will change the patient's behavior without reaching the point of amnesia or altering the patient's level of consciousness.

Butyrophenones (haloperidol, droperidol) and/or benzodiazepines (diazepam, midazolam, lorazepam) are the most commonly used medications for chemical restraint in emergency departments and in prehospital care. Some other historical, but less advisable,

positional asphyxia death from positioning that prevents sufficient intake of oxygen.

Law enforcement weapons should not be used as a part of EMS patient restraint.

medications include the barbiturates (pentothal), opioids (morphine), and phenothiazines (chlorpromazine).

Chemical restraint protocols often include a butyrophenone, a benzodiazepine, or a combination of both. Diazepam (Valium), lorazepam (Ativan) and midazolam (Versed) are the benzodiazepines that are most commonly used for patent restraint. Droperidol (Inapsine) and haloperidol (Haldol) are the butyrophenones that are commonly used. All five of these medications can be given intramuscularly or intravenously. Although several limited prehospital studies support the effectiveness of droperidol in decreasing the agitation of combative patients in the prehospital setting, the FDA has issued a warning of possible dysrhythmias associated with droperidol administration. It has been associated with problems in patients who have a prolonged QT interval on their ECG. However, haloperidol and benzodiazepines have been shown to be effective in the emergency department setting, and these are probably also effective in the prehospital environment.

Neuromuscular-blocking medications with endotracheal intubation are never indicated to paralyze a patient solely for the purpose of restraining violent behavior. Only patients who have coexisting medical conditions, for example, severe head injury or respiratory failure, may benefit from paralysis and intubation. Regardless, the decision to paralyze a patient should be based on medical indications beyond violent or combative behavior.

When considering the use of chemical restraint, EMT-Is must weigh the risks of struggling while physically restrained against the side effect profile of the medications that are considered for sedation of agitated patients. At present, there is no consensus on the best medication or dosage for chemical restraint, and this decision is best deferred to the individual EMS system and its medical director.

> *Neuromuscular-blocking medications with endotracheal intubation are never indicated to paralyze a patient solely for the purpose of restraining violent behavior.*
>

SUMMARY

Calls involving psychiatric and behavioral emergencies will challenge your skills as an EMT-I. Differentiating physiological and psychological conditions will try your diagnostic skills, and developing the interview abilities that form the basis of psychiatric assessment and care will test your people skills. Ultimately, you will be called on to help patients in a time of great need—a time of crisis. Once you determine that the patient is experiencing a purely behavioral emergency, your compassion and communication skills, rather than medications and procedures, will, benefit him most.

EMS providers routinely encounter patients who are violent or combative due to a behavioral illness or a medical condition. Verbal, physical, and chemical restraint techniques provide effective ways of restraining patients who are a threat to themselves or require medical assessment and treatment for a condition associated with combative or agitated behavior. Life-threatening adverse events have occurred in restrained individuals, and adherence to the principles of restraint presented here will minimize the occurrence of these adverse events. EMS personnel and their medical directors should ensure that their systems are prepared to appropriately treat violent or combative patients by providing training, policies, and protocols to deal with these situations.

Situations involving crisis can drain your emotions. Observing a suicide or attempted suicide or struggling with or restraining a patient can take its toll. Take care of yourself before, during, and after these calls.

ON THE WEB

For additional practice and review, go to the companion website at www.prenhall.com/bledsoe and click on *Intermediate Emergency Care: Principles & Practice.*

CHAPTER 28

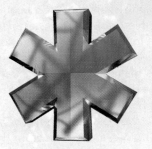

Gynecological Emergencies

Objectives

After reading this chapter, you should be able to:

1. Review the anatomic structures and physiology of the female reproductive system. (see Chapter 2)
2. Describe how to assess a patient with a gynecological complaint. (pp. 1113–1115)
3. Explain how to recognize a gynecological emergency. (pp. 1113–1115)
4. Describe the general care for any patient experiencing a gynecological emergency. (p. 1115)
5. Describe the pathophysiology, assessment, and management of specific gynecological emergencies, including:
   a. Pelvic inflammatory disease (pp. 1115–1116)

    b. Ruptured ovarian cyst (p. 1116)
    c. Cystitis (p. 1116)
    d. Ectopic pregnancy (p. 1117)
    e. Vaginal bleeding (pp. 1117–1118)
6. Describe the assessment, care, and emotional support of the sexual assault patient. (pp. 1118–1120)
7. Given several preprogrammed gynecological patients, provide the appropriate assessment, management, and transportation. (pp. 1113–1120)

CASE STUDY

It is near dusk on a warm summer evening when you and Sam Rusk, your partner, are dispatched from quarters to a nearby community park for an "assault." Within 4 minutes, you are pulling up to the park access gate near the security office, where you are met by a police officer and the park security supervisor. The police officer tells you that a 28-year-old female was found wandering in the park by a security officer just as the park was closing. He tells you that the Crime Scene Unit is en route. The supervisor reports that the officer who found her is sitting with her in the office.

You enter the security office as Sam gets the stretcher and jump kit from the back of the medic unit. The patient is seated on a cot facing away from the door. The security officer is sitting on a chair next to the cot, talking quietly to her. The patient has a white cotton blanket, provided by the officer, wrapped tightly over her shoulders and around her body. You observe that her hair is in disarray, tangled and matted with leaves and small twigs. As you approach her, you identify and introduce yourself and Sam as EMT-Is who are there to help her. She turns her tear-stained, battered face toward you and nods, saying "I know" so quietly that you can barely hear her. The park officer stands and tells you that your patient's name is Stephanie. He then excuses himself, telling her that she's in good hands and that he'll be right outside.

You pull up the chair that had been used by the officer and position it in front of Stephanie to complete your initial assessment. Although your priority is the assessment of her ABCs, you cannot ignore her obvious injuries. She has dried blood on her nose and mouth and her left eye is bruised and nearly swollen shut. You tell her that you need to perform some simple procedures to make sure that she's okay and ask her permission to do so. Again she nods, her eyes never leaving your face. In a soft hoarse voice, she says quietly, "He raped me, even though I begged him not to."

Stephanie's airway is open and her breathing is regular in rate and depth. You ask her if you can check her pulse, and she unwraps the blanket just enough to let her right forearm extend toward you. You find that her pulse is strong but rapid and her skin is cool and dry. You notice an abrasion around her wrist that makes you wonder if she had been tied down. You also observe that she has several broken nails on the trembling hand she extends toward you. Again with her permission you gently unwrap the blanket to reveal a torn, dirty T-shirt that is splattered with blood. She is wearing nothing else. Her inner thighs are covered with dried blood, as well as dirt and bits of leaves. You limit your rapid trauma assessment to merely a search for life-threatening injuries, since Stephanie will undergo a thorough exam by the sexual assault nurse examiner (SANE). Stephanie's blood pressure is 108/70. Her pulse is strong and regular at 110 beats per minute. Her breathing is quiet and non-labored at a rate of 24 breaths per minute with a pulse oximeter reading of 99% on room air.

Explaining exactly what you're going to do and asking her permission to do so, you and Sam help her stand and then pivot her onto the stretcher, leaving her wrapped in the blanket in which you found her. You move her to the medic unit. As you get her settled, and before beginning the short drive to the hospital, Sam contacts medical direction and requests that the SANE meet you at the hospital.

En route you complete Stephanie's SAMPLE history. She denies allergies and reports that the only medication she takes is a multivitamin tablet daily. Stephanie denies any significant past medical history. She ate a chef's salad for lunch about mid-afternoon. Stephanie says that she was grabbed from behind while she was jogging and that she was dragged off the path and into the woods. You reassure her that she is safe now and no one will hurt her. Within minutes you arrive at the hospital.

Emma Cannise, RN, the SANE coordinator, meets you at the emergency entrance to the hospital. You introduce Stephanie to Emma, who then accompanies you to the evaluation unit located behind the main emergency department. You give her a brief report, and she signs off on your patient care report.

Returning to quarters, you and Sam discuss how ironic it was that this month's continuing medical education (CME) program was a presentation by Emma Cannise on caring for victims of sexual assault.

---

gynecology the branch of medicine that deals with the health maintenance and the diseases of women, primarily of the reproductive organs.

obstetrics the branch of medicine that deals with the care of women throughout pregnancy.

INTRODUCTION

The term **gynecology** is derived from Greek, *gynaik*, meaning "woman." Gynecology is the branch of medicine that deals with the health maintenance and the diseases of women and primarily of their reproductive organs. **Obstetrics** is the branch of medicine that deals with the care of women throughout pregnancy. This chapter focuses on the assessment and care of non-pregnant patients with problems of the reproductive system. The assessment and care of the obstetrical patient is the subject of the next chapter.

ASSESSMENT OF THE GYNECOLOGICAL PATIENT

Beyond labor and delivery, the most common emergency complaints of women in the child-bearing years are abdominal pain and vaginal bleeding. Abdominal pain is often due to problems of the reproductive organs. In addition to the usual history and physical assessment activities, you will need to ask specific questions pertinent to reproductive function and dysfunction. However, don't allow yourself to get distracted from getting complete medical histories including chronic medical problems, medications, and allergies.

You may feel uncomfortable asking a patient about her reproductive history, but remember that you are a health-care professional who is trying to obtain pertinent information in order to provide the best possible care for your patient. If you conduct yourself in this manner, it should not be uncomfortable for you or your patient. Assess your patient's emotional state. If she is reluctant to discuss her complaint in detail, respect her wishes and transport her to the emergency department where a more thorough assessment can be done.

HISTORY

Use the SAMPLE approach for obtaining additional information about the history of the present illness. If the chief complaint is pain, then use the mnemonic OPQRST to gather more information. Is the patient's pain abdominal or in the pelvic region? Is it localized in a specific quadrant of the pelvis? Is she having her menstrual period? If so, how does the pain she is having now compare with how she usually feels? Some women have severe discomfort during their menstrual periods. This is called **dysmenorrhea.** Others may experience **dyspareunia,** painful sexual intercourse. Does walking or defecation aggravate her pain? What, if anything, alleviates her pain? Does positioning herself on her back or side with her knees bent relieve her discomfort?

You need to determine if there are any associated signs or symptoms that will be helpful in determining what is wrong with your patient. For instance, does your patient report a fever or chills? Is she reporting signs of gastrointestinal problems, such as nausea, vomiting, diarrhea, or constipation? Or perhaps she's complaining of urinary problems, such as frequency, painful urination, or "colicky" urinary cramping. Does she report a vaginal discharge or bleeding? If so, you should obtain information about the color, amount, frequency, or odors associated with either vaginal bleeding or discharge. If she reports vaginal bleeding, how does the amount compare with the volume of her usual menstrual period? Does she report dizziness with changes in position (orthostatic hypotension), syncope, or diaphoresis?

You will need to obtain specific information about her obstetric history. Has she ever been pregnant? *Gravida (G)* is the term used to describe the number of times a woman has been pregnant, including this one if she is pregnant. How many of those pregnancies ended in the delivery of a viable infant? *Para or parity (P)* refers to the number of deliveries. *Abortion (Ab)* refers to any pregnancy that ends before 20 weeks of gestation, regardless of cause. You may see this information recorded in shorthand, for example, $G_3 P_2 Ab_1$, or gravida 3, para 2, ab 1. This means that she has been pregnant three times and had two prior deliveries and one pregnancy that ended before 20 weeks gestation. These terms refer to the number of pregnancies and deliveries, not the number of infants delivered, so even twins or triplets counts only as one pregnancy and one delivery.

You will also need to obtain a gynecological history. Question the patient about previous ectopic pregnancies, infections, cesarean sections, pelvic surgeries such as tubal ligation, abortions (either elective or therapeutic), and dilation and curettage (D&C) procedures. Also ask the patient about any prior history of trauma to the reproductive tract. It is often helpful to find out whether the patient, if sexually active, has had pain or bleeding during or after sexual intercourse.

It is important to document the date of the patient's last menstrual period, commonly abbreviated LMP (or LNMP, last normal menstrual period). Ask whether the period was of a normal length and whether the flow was heavier or lighter than usual. An easy way for women to estimate menstrual flow is by the number of pads or tampons used. She can easily compare

dysmenorrhea painful menstruation.

dyspareunia painful sexual intercourse.

this number to her routine usage. It is also important to inquire how regular the patient's periods tend to be. Ask her what form of birth control, if any, she uses. Also, find out if she uses it regularly. Direct questions such as "Could you be pregnant?" are generally unlikely to get an accurate response. Indirect questioning is often more helpful in determining the likelihood of pregnancy, such as "When did your last menstrual period start?" If you suspect pregnancy, inquire about other signs, including a late or missed period, breast tenderness, bloating, urinary frequency, or nausea and vomiting. Until proven otherwise, you should assume that any missed or late period is due to pregnancy even though your patient may deny it.

Contraception, or the prevention of pregnancy, takes many forms. Remember that many contraceptives are medications, so don't forget to ask about their use. With the exception of oral contraceptives ("the pill") and intrauterine devices (IUDs), side effects caused by contraceptives are relatively rare. Oral contraceptives have been associated with hypertension, rare incidents of stroke and heart attack, and possibly pulmonary embolism. IUDs can cause perforation of the uterus, uterine infection, or irregular uterine bleeding. This is especially true for IUDs that have remained in place longer than the time recommended by the manufacturer, which rarely exceeds two years.

PHYSICAL EXAM

Physical examination of the gynecological patient is limited in the field. More than at any other time, the patient's comfort level should guide your actions. Respect your patient's modesty and maintain her privacy. This may mean that you need to exclude parents from the room when assessing adolescent patients or that you need to exclude spouses of married patients. Recognizing that most people are not comfortable discussing matters related to sexuality or reproductive organs, take your cues from the patient. Maintain a professional demeanor. Explain all procedures thoroughly so that your patient can understand them before initiating any care. Some women may feel more comfortable if they can be cared for by a female EMT-I.

As always, the level of consciousness is the best indicator of your patient's status. Assess your patient's general appearance, paying particular attention to the color of her skin and mucous membranes. Cyanosis and pallor may indicate shock or a gas-exchange problem, whereas a flushed appearance is more indicative of fever.

Remember that vital signs are useful clues to the nature of your patient's problem. Pain and fever tend to cause an increase in pulse and respiratory rates along with a slight increase in blood pressure. Significant bleeding will cause increased pulse and respiratory rates as well as narrowing pulse pressures (the difference between systolic and diastolic pressures). Perform a tilt test to assess for orthostatic changes in her vital signs (a decrease in blood pressure and an increase in pulse rate when the patient rises from a supine or seated position), which again points to significant blood loss.

Assess your patient for evidence of vaginal bleeding or discharge. If possible estimate blood loss. The use of more than two sanitary pads per hour is considered significant bleeding. If serious bleeding is reported or evident, it may be necessary to inspect the patient's perineum. Document the color and character of the discharge, as well as the amount, and the presence or absence of clots. *Do not perform an internal vaginal exam in the field.*

Legal Notes

Fortunately, EMT-Is seldom have to examine a woman's genitalia. Even when necessary, all that is required is a brief look at the external structures for injury and for any evidence of hemorrhage. Always have a chaperone when examining the genitalia of any person (of the opposite sex or even the same sex). This will protect you from possible allegations of sexual assault or inappropriate touching. Always explain to the patient what you are planning to do and talk to her throughout the examination. With the exception of emergent treatment for a breech birth (to maintain the infant's airway) or for a prolapsed cord (to keep the baby's head off the cord), there is no reason to perform an internal vaginal examination in the field. Even significant vaginal bleeding (unless due to a tear in the labia or introitus) cannot be controlled with packing. These patients require immediate transport, treatment for shock, and rapid gynecological examination.

Pay particular attention to the abdominal examination. Auscultate the abdomen and note whether bowel sounds are absent or hyperactive. Gently palpate the abdomen. Document and report any masses, distention, guarding, localized tenderness, or rebound tenderness. In thin patients, a palpable mass in the lower abdomen may be an intrauterine pregnancy. At three months, the uterus is barely palpable above the symphysis pubis. At four months, the uterus is palpable midway between the umbilicus and the symphysis pubis. At five months (approximately 20 weeks), it is palpable at the level of the umbilicus.

MANAGEMENT OF GYNECOLOGICAL EMERGENCIES

In general, the management of the patient experiencing a gynecological emergency is focused on supportive care. Rely on your initial assessment to guide your decision making about the need for oxygen therapy or intravenous access. If your patient's status warrants it, administer oxygen or assist ventilation as necessary. As a rule, IV access and fluid replacement is usually not indicated. However, if your patient has excessive bleeding or demonstrates signs of shock, then establish at least one large-bore IV and administer normal saline at a rate indicated by the patient's presentation. You may also want to initiate cardiac monitoring if your patient is unstable.

General management of gynecological emergencies is focused on supportive care.

Continue to monitor and evaluate serious bleeding. *Do not pack dressings in the vagina.* Discourage the use of tampons to absorb blood flow. If your patient is bleeding heavily, count and document the number of sanitary pads used. If your patient demonstrates signs of impending shock, you may elect to place her in the Trendelenburg position (head lower than feet). The use of a pneumatic anti-shock garment in this situation should be governed by your local protocol. If shock is not a consideration, then position your patient for comfort in the left lateral recumbent position or supine with her knees bent, since this decreases tension on the peritoneum. Analgesics (pain-control medications) are not usually given in the field for gynecological complaints because these drugs tend to mask signs and symptoms of a deteriorating condition and make assessment and diagnosis difficult.

Do not pack dressings in the vagina.

Since it is not appropriate to perform an internal vaginal exam in the field, most patients with gynecological complaints will be transported to be evaluated by a physician. Some problems may require surgical intervention, so you should consider emergency transport to the appropriate facility based on your local protocols.

Psychological support is particularly important when caring for patients with gynecological complaints. Keep calm. Maintain your patient's modesty and privacy. Remember that this is likely to be a very stressful situation for your patient, and she will appreciate your gentle, considerate care.

SPECIFIC GYNECOLOGICAL EMERGENCIES

Generally, gynecological emergencies can be divided into two categories, medical and traumatic.

MEDICAL GYNECOLOGICAL EMERGENCIES

Gynecological emergencies of a medical nature are often hard to diagnose in the field. The most common symptoms of a medical gynecological emergency are abdominal pain and/or vaginal bleeding.

Gynecological Abdominal Pain

Pelvic Inflammatory Disease Probably the most common cause of non-traumatic abdominal pain is pelvic inflammatory disease (PID). **Pelvic inflammatory disease (PID)** is an infection of the female reproductive tract that can be caused by a bacterium, virus, or fungus. The organs most commonly involved are the uterus, fallopian tubes, and ovaries. Occasionally the adjoining structures, such as the peritoneum and intestines, also become

pelvic inflammatory disease (PID) an acute infection of the reproductive organs that can be caused by a bacteria, virus, or fungus.

involved. PID is the most common cause of abdominal pain in women in the childbearing years, occurring in 1% of that population. The highest rate of infection occurs in sexually active women ages 15 to 24. The most common causes of PID are gonorrhea (*Neisseria gonorrhoeae*) or chlamydia (*Chlamydia trachomatis*), although rarely streptococcus or staphylococcus bacteria may cause it. Commonly, gonorrhea or chlamydia progresses undetected in a female until frank PID develops.

Predisposing factors include multiple sexual partners, prior history of PID, recent gynecological procedure, or an IUD. Post-infection damage to the fallopian tubes is a common cause for infertility. PID may be either acute or chronic. If it is allowed to progress untreated, sepsis may develop. Additionally, PID may cause adhesions, in which the pelvic organs "stick together." Adhesions are a common cause of chronic pelvic pain and increase the frequency of infertility and ectopic pregnancies.

Although it is possible for a patient with PID to be asymptomatic, most PID patients complain of abdominal pain. It is often diffuse and located in the lower abdomen. It may be moderate to severe, which occasionally makes it difficult to distinguish it from appendicitis. Pain may intensify either before or after the menstrual period. It may also worsen during sexual intercourse, as movement of the cervix tends to cause increased discomfort. Patients with PID tend to walk with a shuffling gait, since walking often intensifies their pain. In severe cases, fever, chills, nausea, vomiting, or even sepsis may accompany PID. Occasionally, patients have a foul-smelling vaginal discharge, often yellow in color, as well as irregular menses. It is common also to have mid-cycle bleeding.

Generally, on physical examination, the patient with PID appears acutely ill or toxic. The blood pressure is normal, although the pulse rate may be slightly increased. Fever may or may not be present. Palpation of the lower abdomen generally elicits moderate to severe pain. Occasionally, in severe cases, the abdomen will be tense with obvious rebound tenderness. Such cases may be impossible to distinguish from appendicitis in the prehospital setting.

The primary treatment for PID is antibiotics, often administered intravenously over an extended period. Once the causative organism is determined, the sexual partner may also require treatment. In the field, the primary goal is to make the patient as comfortable as possible. Place the patient on the ambulance stretcher in the position in which she is most comfortable. She may wish to draw her knees up toward her chest, because this decreases tension on the peritoneum. *Do not perform a vaginal examination.* If your patient has signs of sepsis, administer oxygen and establish IV access.

Ruptured Ovarian Cyst *Cysts* are fluid-filled pockets. When they develop in the ovary, they can rupture and be a source of abdominal pain. When an egg is released from the ovary, a cyst, known as a corpus luteum cyst, is often left in its place. Occasionally, cysts develop independent of ovulation. When the cysts rupture, a small amount of blood is spilled into the abdomen. Because blood irritates the peritoneum, it can cause abdominal pain and rebound tenderness. Ovarian cysts may be found during a routine pelvic examination. However, in the field setting, your patient is likely to complain of moderate to severe unilateral abdominal pain, which may radiate to her back. She may also report a history of dyspareunia, irregular bleeding, or a delayed menstrual period. It is not uncommon for patients to rupture ovarian cysts during intercourse or physical activity. This often results in immediate, severe abdominal pain causing the patient to immediately stop intercourse or other physical activity. Ruptured ovarian cysts may be associated with vaginal bleeding.

cystitis infection of the urinary bladder.

Cystitis Urinary bladder infection, or **cystitis**, is a common cause of abdominal pain. Bacteria usually enter the urinary tract via the urethra, ascending into the bladder and ureters. The bladder lies anterior to the reproductive organs and, when inflamed, causes pain, generally immediately above the symphysis pubis. If untreated, the infection can progress to the kidneys. In addition to abdominal pain, your patient may report urinary frequency, pain or burning with urination (**dysuria**), and a low-grade fever. Occasionally the urine may be blood tinged.

dysuria painful urination often associated with cystitis.

mittelschmerz abdominal pain associated with ovulation.

Mittelschmerz Occasionally, ovulation is accompanied by mid-cycle abdominal pain known as **mittelschmerz**. It is thought that the pain is related to peritoneal irritation due to follicle rupture or bleeding at the time of ovulation. The unilateral lower quadrant pain is usually self-limited and may be accompanied by mid-cycle spotting. Although some women may report a low-grade fever, it should be noted that body temperature normally increases at the time of ovulation and remains elevated until the day before the onset of the menstrual period. Treatment is symptomatic.

Endometritis   An infection of the uterine lining called **endometritis** is an occasional complication of **miscarriage,** childbirth, or gynecological procedures such as dilatation and curettage (D&C). Commonly reported signs and symptoms include mild to severe lower abdominal pain, a bloody, foul-smelling discharge, and fever (101°F to 104°F). The onset of symptoms is usually 48 to 72 hours after the gynecological procedure or miscarriage. These infections often mimic the presentation of PID and can be quite serious if not quickly treated with the appropriate antibiotics. Complications of endometritis may include sterility, sepsis, or even death.

Endometriosis   **Endometriosis** is a condition in which endometrial tissue is found outside of the uterus. Most commonly it is found in the abdomen and pelvis, although it has been found virtually everywhere in the body, including the central nervous system and lungs. Regardless of its site, the tissue responds to the hormonal changes associated with the menstrual cycle and thus bleeds in a cyclic manner. This bleeding causes inflammation, scarring of adjacent tissues, and the subsequent development of adhesions, particularly in the pelvic cavity.

   Endometriosis is usually seen in women between the ages of 30 to 40 and is rarely seen in postmenopausal women. The exact cause is unknown. The most common symptom is dull, cramping pelvic pain that is usually related to menstruation. Dyspareunia and abnormal uterine bleeding is also commonly reported. Painful bowel movements have also been reported when the endometrial tissue has invaded the gastrointestinal tract. It is not uncommon for endometriosis to be diagnosed when the patient is being evaluated for infertility. Definitive treatment may include medical management with hormones, analgesics, and anti-inflammatory drugs, and/or surgery to remove the excessive endometrial tissue or adhesions from other organs.

Ectopic Pregnancy   An **ectopic pregnancy** is the implantation of a fetus outside of the uterus. The most common site is within the fallopian tubes. This is a surgical emergency, because the tube can rupture, triggering a massive hemorrhage. Patients with ectopic pregnancy often have severe unilateral abdominal pain which may radiate to the shoulder on the affected side, a late or missed menstrual period, and, occasionally, vaginal bleeding. Additional discussion of ectopic pregnancy is presented in the next chapter.

Management of Gynecological Abdominal Pain

Any woman with significant abdominal pain should be treated and transported to the hospital for evaluation. Administer oxygen and establish IV access if indicated. Refer to the earlier section on management of gynecological emergencies for additional information.

Non-Traumatic Vaginal Bleeding

Non-traumatic vaginal bleeding is rarely seen in the field unless it is severe. Refer to the earlier section in this chapter on completing a patient history. You should not presume that vaginal bleeding is due to normal menstruation. Occasionally a woman will experience **menorrhagia,** or excessive menstrual flow, but rarely is it the cause for a 9-1-1 call. Hemorrhage, regardless of cause, is always potentially life threatening, so be alert for signs of impending shock.

   The most common cause of non-traumatic vaginal bleeding is a spontaneous abortion (miscarriage). If it has been more than 60 days since your patient's last menstrual period, you should assume that this is the cause. Vaginal bleeding due to miscarriage is often associated with cramping abdominal pain and the passage of clots and tissue. The loss of a pregnancy, even at a very early phase, is a significant emotional event for your patient, so your kind and considerate care is important. Spontaneous abortion and other causes of bleeding in the obstetric patient will be discussed further in the next chapter. Other potential causes of vaginal bleeding include cancerous lesions, PID, or the onset of labor.

Management of Non-Traumatic Vaginal Bleeding

Your field management of patients suffering non-traumatic vaginal bleeding will depend on the severity of the situation and your assessment of the patient's status. Absorb the blood flow. *Do not pack the vagina.* If your patient is passing clots or tissue, save these for evaluation by a physician. Transport your patient in a position of comfort. The initiation of oxygen therapy and IV access should be guided by the patient's condition.

TRAUMATIC GYNECOLOGICAL EMERGENCIES

Most cases of vaginal bleeding result from obstetrical problems or are related to the menstrual period. However, trauma to the vagina and perineum can also cause bleeding and abdominal pain.

Causes of Gynecological Trauma

The incidence of genital trauma is increasing, with vaginal injury occurring far more commonly than male genital injury. Gynecological trauma may occur at any age. Blunt trauma occurs more frequently than penetrating trauma. Straddle injury (such as may occur with riding a bicycle) is the most common form of blunt trauma. Vaginal injuries are most often lacerations due to sexual assault. Other causes of gynecological trauma include blunt force to the lower abdomen due to assault or seat-belt injuries, direct blows to the perineal area, foreign bodies inserted into the vagina, self-attempts at abortion, and lacerations following childbirth.

Management of Gynecological Trauma

Injuries to the external genitalia should be managed by direct pressure over the laceration or a chemical cold pack applied to a hematoma. In most cases of vaginal bleeding, the source is not readily apparent. If bleeding is severe or your patient demonstrates signs of shock, establish IV access to maintain intravascular volume and monitor vital signs closely. Blunt force may cause organ rupture leading to the development of peritonitis or sepsis. *Never pack the vagina with any material or dressing,* regardless of the severity of the bleeding. Expedite transport to the emergency department since surgical intervention is often required.

Sexual Assault

Sexual assault continues to represent the most rapidly growing violent crime in the United States. Over 700,000 women are sexually assaulted annually. Unfortunately, it is estimated that more than 60% of all sexual assaults are never reported to authorities. Male victims represent 5% of reported sexual assaults. Sexual abuse of children is reported even less frequently. It is estimated that the incidence of sexual abuse in children ranges from 50,000 to 350,000/year. There is no typical victim of sexual assault. No one—from small children to aged adults—is immune.

Most victims of sexual assault know their assailants. Friends, acquaintances, intimates, and family members commit the vast majority (80%) of sexual assaults against women. Acquaintance rape is particularly common among adolescent victims. Sexual assault is a crime of violence, not passion, that is motivated by aggression and a need to control, humiliate, or inflict pain. There are very few predictors of who is capable of committing sexual assault, since age, economic status, and ethnic origins vary widely. Common behavioral characteristics found among rapists include poor impulse control, the need to achieve sexual satisfaction within the context of violence, and immaturity.

The definition of sexual assault varies from state to state. The common element of any definition is sexual contact without consent. Generally, rape is defined as penetration of the vagina or rectum of an unwilling female or the rectum in an unwilling male. In most states, penetration must occur for an act to be classified as rape. Sexual assault also includes oral-genital sex. Regardless of the legal definition, sexual assault is a crime of violence with serious physical and psychological implications.

Assessment The victim of sexual assault is a unique patient with unique needs. Your patient needs emergency medical treatment and psychological support. Your patient also needs to have legal evidence gathered. Your objectivity is essential, because your attitude may affect long-term psychological recovery. As a rule, victims of sexual abuse *should not* be questioned about the incident in the field. Do not ask questions about specific details of the assault. It is not important, from the standpoint of prehospital care, to determine whether penetration took place. Do not inquire about the patient's sexual practices. Confine your questions to the physical injuries the patient received. Even well-intentioned questions may lead to guilt feelings in the patient. Do not ask questions, such as why did you go with him or get in his car.

The psychological response of sexual assault victims is widely variable. The victim of sexual assault may be withdrawn or hysterical. Some use denial, anger, or fear as defense mechanisms. Approach the patient calmly and professionally. Allay the patient's fear and anxiety. Respond to the patient's feelings but be aware of your own. If the patient is incompletely dressed, a cover should be offered. Respect the patient's modesty. Explain all procedures and obtain the patient's permission before beginning them. Avoid touching the patient other than to take vital signs or examine other physical injuries. *Do not examine the genitalia* unless there is life-threatening hemorrhage.

Management In most situations, psychological and emotional support is the most important help you can offer. Maintain a nonjudgmental attitude and assure the patient of confidentiality. If the patient is female, allow her to be cared for by a female EMT-I (if available). If the patient desires, have a female accompany her to the hospital (Figure 28-1). Provide a safe environment, such as the back of a well-lit ambulance. Respond to the patient's feelings and respect the patient's wishes. Unless your patient is unconscious, do not touch the patient unless given permission. Even when your patient appears to have an altered level of consciousness, explain what's going to be done before initiating any treatment.

Preservation of physical evidence is important. When the patient arrives at the hospital, a physician or sexual assault nurse examiner will complete a sexual assault examination to gather physical evidence. To protect this evidence, it is important that you adhere to the following guidelines:

- Consider the patient a crime scene and protect that scene.
- Handle clothing as little as possible, if at all.
- If you must remove clothing, bag separately each item that must be bagged.
- Do not cut through any tears or holes in the clothing.
- Place bloody articles in brown paper bags.
- Do not examine the perineal area.
- If the assault took place within the hour or the patient is bleeding, put an absorbent underpad (e.g., Chux) under the patient's hips to collect that evidence.
- If you cover the patient with a sheet or blanket, turn that over to the hospital as evidence.
- Do not allow patients to change their clothes, bathe, or douche (if female) before the medical examination.

Do not ask about specific details of a sexual assault.

Do not examine the external genitalia of a sexual assault victim unless there is life-threatening hemorrhage.

Psychological and emotional support are the most important elements of care for the sexual assault patient.

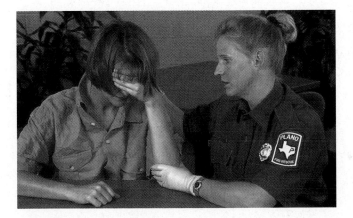

FIGURE 28-1 If possible, have a female EMT accompany the sexual assault patient to the hospital.

- Do not allow patients to comb their hair, brush their teeth, or clean their fingernails.
- Do not clean wounds, if at all possible.
- If you must initiate care on scene, avoid disruption of the crime scene.

Documentation When completing your patient care report, keep the following documentation guidelines in mind:

- State patient remarks accurately.
- Objectively state your observations of the patient's physical condition, environment, or torn clothing.
- Document any evidence (e.g., clothing, sheets) turned over to the hospital staff and the name of the individual to whom you gave it.
- Do NOT include your opinions as to whether rape occurred.

SUMMARY

Most gynecological emergency patients have either abdominal pain or vaginal bleeding. The patient with abdominal pain should be made comfortable and transported to the emergency department. The management of vaginal bleeding depends on the severity. Minor bleeding should be monitored. Severe bleeding should be treated with IV fluids, if indicated.

In the case of sexual assault, you should first determine if any life-threatening physical injuries exist. Second, respect the patient's wishes and offer emotional support. Third, in treating victims of sexual assault, make every effort to preserve physical evidence. As with any type of emergency care, the primary concern is the patient.

ON THE WEB

For additional practice and review, go to the companion website at www.prenhall.com/bledsoe and click on *Intermediate Emergency Care: Principles & Practice.*

CHAPTER 29

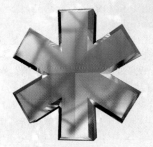

Obstetrical Emergencies

Objectives

After reading this chapter, you should be able to:

1. Describe the anatomical structures and physiology of the reproductive system during pregnancy. (pp.1122–1126)
2. Identify the normal events of pregnancy. (p. 1126)
3. Describe how to assess an obstetrical patient. (pp. 1128–1130)
4. Identify the stages of labor and the EMT-Intermediate's role in each stage. (pp. 1140–1141)
5. Differentiate between normal and abnormal delivery. (pp. 1147–1151)
6. Identify and describe complications associated with pregnancy and delivery. (pp. 1131–1140, 1147–1153)
7. Identify predelivery emergencies. (pp. 1131–1140)
8. State indications of an imminent delivery. (p. 1141)
9. Differentiate the management of a patient with predelivery emergencies from a normal delivery. (pp. 1131–1140)
10. State the steps in the predelivery preparation of the mother. (pp. 1141, 1144)
11. State the steps to assist in the delivery of a newborn, including cutting the umbilical cord and delivery of the placenta. (pp. 1141–1145)
12. Describe how to care for the newborn, including routine care and neonatal resuscitation. (pp. 1145–1147)
13. Describe the management of the mother post-delivery. (pp. 1151–1153)
14. Describe the procedures for handling abnormal deliveries, complications of pregnancy, and maternal complications of labor. (pp. 1131–1140, 1147–1153)
15. Describe special considerations when meconium is present in amniotic fluid or during delivery. (p. 1151)
16. Describe special considerations of a premature baby. (pp. 1126, 1139–1140)
17. Given several simulated delivery situations, provide the appropriate assessment, management, and transport for the mother and child. (pp. 1122–1153)

CASE STUDY

The crew members of Fire Station 32 are relaxing in the television room when, suddenly, they hear an automobile screech to a halt at the station door. The captain rushes to it and finds an old station wagon with a man standing beside it yelling, "Help! My wife needs help!"

The whole crew spills out the door. In the back seat of the station wagon, they see a pregnant female. She keeps saying, "The baby is coming. The baby is coming." The ambulance normally based at Station 32 has gone out for gas. The captain notifies fire dispatch, which orders the ambulance to return. Meanwhile, the EMT-Is assigned to the engine learn that the patient is 29 years old and that this is her sixth pregnancy. She exclaims that she feels as if she has to move her bowels.

Now the patient begins to scream. "I've got to push. I've got to push," she yells. The crew dons gloves and goggles, and the senior EMT-I checks for crowning. He easily spots the top of the baby's head during a contraction. One member of the crew retrieves an obstetrical (OB) kit and an oxygen bottle from the medic box on the fire engine. Shortly thereafter, the patient gives birth to a baby girl in the back of the station wagon.

At the time of delivery, the ambulance crew arrives. They assist the engine crew in cutting the cord, then dry and wrap the baby in a warming blanket. APGAR scores are 8 at one minute and 9 at five minutes. The mother receives fundal massage, oxygen, and an IV solution of normal saline. The EMT-Is then transport both mother and daughter to the hospital without incident. The father follows in the station wagon.

The next morning, as the Station 32 crew members are walking to their cars, they see a stork artfully painted on the window of the car belonging to the EMT-I who delivered the baby.

INTRODUCTION

Pregnancy, childbirth, and the potential complications of each are the focus of this chapter. Pregnancy is a normal, natural process of life that results from ovulation and fertilization. Complications of pregnancy are uncommon, but when they do occur, you must be prepared to recognize them quickly and manage them. Childbirth occurs daily, usually requiring only the most basic assistance. This chapter will prepare you to assess and care for the female patient throughout her pregnancy and delivery of her child.

PRENATAL PERIOD

The *prenatal period* (literally "prebirth period") is the time from conception until delivery of the fetus. During this period, fetal development takes place. In addition, significant physiological changes occur in the mother.

ANATOMY AND PHYSIOLOGY OF THE OBSTETRIC PATIENT

ovulation the release of an egg from the ovary.

As you learned in the previous chapter, the first 2 weeks of the menstrual cycle are dominated by the hormone estrogen, which causes the endometrium (the inner lining of the uterus) to thicken and become engorged with blood. In response to a surge of luteinizing hormone (LH) and follicle stimulating hormone (FSH), **ovulation,** or release of an egg (ovum) from the ovary, takes place. The egg travels down the fallopian tube to the uterus. If the egg has been fertilized, it becomes implanted in the uterus and pregnancy begins. If the egg has not been fertilized, menstruation (discharge of blood, mucus, and cellular debris from the endometrium) takes place 14 days after ovulation. (The time from ovulation to menstruation is always exactly 14 days. However, the time from menstruation to the next ovulation may vary by several days from the average of 14 days, which is why it can be difficult for couples to find the optimum time of the month to conceive, or to avoid conceiving, a baby.)

If the woman has had intercourse within 24 to 48 hours before ovulation, fertilization may occur. The male's seminal fluid carrying numerous spermatozoa, or male sex cells, enters the vagina and uterus and travels toward the fallopian tubes. Fertilization, which usually takes place in the distal third of the fallopian tube, occurs when a male spermatozoon fuses with the female ovum (Figure 29-1). After fertilization, the ovum begins cellular divi-

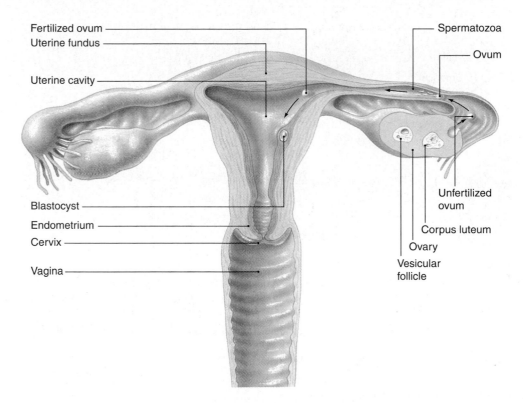

FIGURE 29-1 Fertilization and implantation of the ovum.

Labels in figure:
- Fertilized ovum
- Uterine fundus
- Uterine cavity
- Blastocyst
- Endometrium
- Cervix
- Vagina
- Spermatozoa
- Ovum
- Unfertilized ovum
- Corpus luteum
- Ovary
- Vesicular follicle

sion immediately, which continues as it moves through the fallopian tube to the uterus. The ovum then becomes a *blastocyst* (a hollow ball of cells). The blastocyst normally implants in the thickened uterine lining, which has been prepared for implantation by the hormone progesterone, where the fetus and placenta subsequently develop.

Approximately 3 weeks after fertilization, the placenta develops on the uterine wall at the site where the blastocyst attached (Figure 29-2). The **placenta**, known as the "organ of pregnancy," is a temporary, blood-rich structure that serves as the lifeline for the developing fetus. It transfers heat while exchanging oxygen and carbon dioxide, delivering nutrients such as glucose, potassium, sodium, and chloride, and carrying away wastes such as urea, uric acid, and creatinine. The placenta also serves as an endocrine gland throughout pregnancy, secreting hormones necessary for fetal survival as well as the estrogen and progesterone required to maintain the pregnancy. Additionally, the placenta serves as a protective barrier against harmful substances. (However, some drugs such as narcotics, steroids, and some antibiotics, are able to cross the placental membrane from the mother to the fetus.) When expelled from the uterus following birth of the child, the placenta and accompanying membranes are called the **afterbirth**.

The placenta is connected to the fetus by the **umbilical cord**, a flexible, rope-like structure about 2 feet long and three-quarters of an inch in diameter. Normally, the cord contains two arteries and one vein. The umbilical vein transports oxygenated blood to the fetus, while the umbilical arteries return relatively deoxygenated blood to the placenta.

The fetus develops within the **amniotic sac**, sometimes called the "bag of waters" (BOW). This thin-walled membranous covering holds the **amniotic fluid** that surrounds and protects the fetus during intrauterine development. The amniotic fluid increases in volume throughout the course of the pregnancy. After 20 weeks of gestation, the volume varies from 500 to 1,000 cc. The presence of amniotic fluid allows for fetal movement within the uterus and serves to cushion and protect the fetus from trauma. The volume changes constantly as amniotic fluid moves back and forth across the placental membrane. During the latter part of the pregnancy, the fetus contributes to the volume by secretions from the lungs and urination. Although it may rupture earlier, the amniotic sac usually breaks during labor, and the amniotic fluid flows out of the vagina. This is called *rupture of the membranes (ROM)*. It is what has happened when the pregnant woman says, "My water has broken."

placenta the organ that serves as a lifeline for the developing fetus. It is attached to the wall of the uterus and to the umbilical cord.

afterbirth the placenta and accompanying membranes that are expelled from the uterus after the birth of a child.

umbilical cord structure containing two arteries and one vein that connects the placenta and the fetus.

amniotic sac the membranes that surround and protect the fetus throughout the period of intrauterine development.

amniotic fluid clear, watery fluid that surrounds and protects the developing fetus.

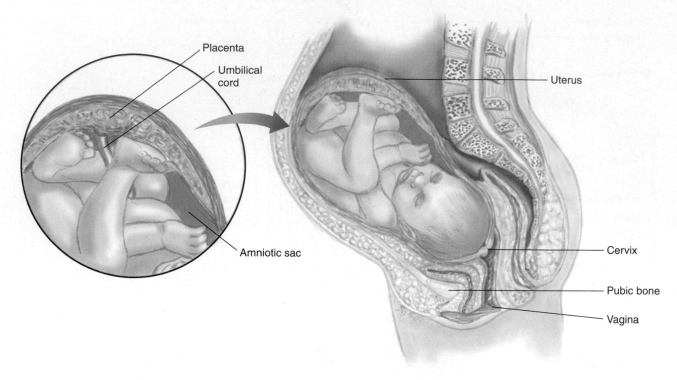

Labels: Placenta, Umbilical cord, Amniotic sac, Uterus, Cervix, Pubic bone, Vagina

FIGURE 29-2   Anatomy of the placenta.

Physiologic Changes of Pregnancy

The physiologic changes associated with pregnancy are due to an altered hormonal state, the mechanical effects of the enlarging uterus and its significant vascularity, and the increasing metabolic demands on the maternal system. It is important for you to understand the physiologic changes associated with pregnancy so that you can better assess your pregnant patients.

Reproductive System   It is understandable that the most significant pregnancy-related changes occur in the uterus. In its non-pregnant state, the uterus is a small pear-shaped organ weighing about 60 grams (two ounces) with a capacity of approximately 10 cc. By the end of pregnancy, its weight has increased to 1,000 grams (slightly more than two pounds) while its capacity is now approximately 5,000 mL (Figure 29-3). Another notable change is that during pregnancy the vascular system of the uterus contains about one-sixth (16%) of the mother's total blood volume.

   Other changes include the formation of a mucous plug in the cervix that protects the developing fetus and helps to prevent infection. This plug will be expelled when cervical dilatation begins prior to delivery. Estrogen causes the vaginal mucosa to thicken, vaginal secretions to increase, and the connective tissue to loosen to allow for delivery. The breasts enlarge and become more nodular as the mammary glands increase in number and size in preparation for lactation.

Respiratory System   As maternal oxygen demands increase, progesterone causes a decrease in airway resistance. This results in a 20% increase in oxygen consumption and a 40% increase in tidal volume. There is only a slight increase in respiratory rate. The diaphragm is pushed up by the enlarging uterus, resulting in flaring of the rib margins to maintain intrathoracic volume.

Cardiovascular System   Various changes take place in the cardiovascular system during pregnancy. Cardiac output increases throughout pregnancy, peaking at 6 to 7 liters per minute by the time the fetus is fully developed. The maternal blood volume increases by 45% and, although both red blood cells and plasma increase, there is slightly more plasma, resulting in a relative anemia. To combat this anemia, pregnant women receive supplemental iron to increase the oxygen-carrying capacity of their red blood cells. Due to the in-

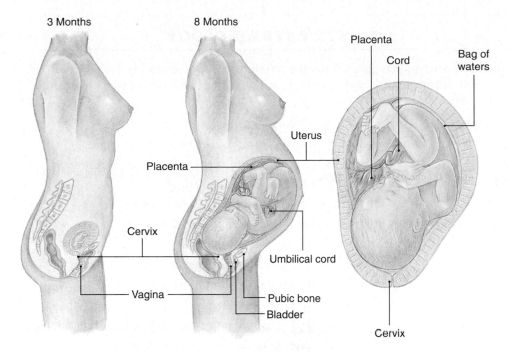

FIGURE 29-3   Uterine changes associated with pregnancy.

crease in blood volume, the pregnant female may have a blood loss of 30% to 35% without a significant change in vital signs. The maternal heart rate increases by 10 to 15 beats per minute. Blood pressure decreases slightly during the first two trimesters, then rises to near non-pregnant levels during the third trimester.

Supine hypotensive syndrome occurs when the gravid uterus compresses the inferior vena cava when the mother lies in a supine position, causing decreased venous return to the right atrium, which lowers blood pressure. Current research suggests that the abdominal aorta may also be compressed. The enlarging uterus also may press on the pelvic and femoral vessels, causing impaired venous return from the legs and venous stasis. This may lead to the development of varicose veins, dependent edema, and postural hypotension. Some patients are predisposed to this problem because of an overall decrease in circulating blood volume or because of anemia. Assessment and management of supine hypotensive syndrome will be discussed later in this chapter.

Gastrointestinal System   Nausea and vomiting are common in the first trimester as a result of hormone levels and changed carbohydrate needs. Peristalsis is slowed, so delayed gastric emptying is likely and bloating or constipation is common. As the uterus enlarges, abdominal organs are compressed, and the resulting compartmentalization of abdominal organs makes assessment difficult.

Urinary System   Renal blood flow increases during pregnancy. The glomerular filtration rate increases by nearly 50% in the second trimester and remains elevated throughout the remainder of the pregnancy. As a result, the renal tubular absorption also increases. Occasionally glucosuria (large amounts of sugar in the urine) may result from the kidney's inability to reabsorb all of the glucose being filtered. Glucosuria may be normal or may indicate the development of gestational diabetes. The urinary bladder gets displaced anteriorly and superiorly increasing the potential for rupture. As a result, urinary frequency is common, particularly in the first and third trimesters.

Musculoskeletal System   Loosened pelvic joints caused by hormonal influences account for the waddling gait that is often associated with pregnancy. As the uterus enlarges and the mother's center of gravity changes, postural changes take place to compensate for anterior growth, causing low back pain.

OBSTETRIC TERMINOLOGY

The field of obstetrics has its own unique terminology. You should be familiar with it, since patient documentation and communications with other health care personnel, including physicians, often require it.

antepartum	time interval prior to delivery of the fetus
postpartum	time interval after delivery of the fetus
prenatal	time interval prior to birth, synonymous with *antepartum*
natal	relating to birth or the date of birth
gravidity[*]	the number of times a woman has been pregnant
parity[*]	number of pregnancies carried to full term
primigravida	woman who is pregnant for the first time
primipara	woman who has given birth to her first child
multigravida	woman who has been pregnant more than once
nulligravida	woman who has not been pregnant
multipara	woman who has delivered more than one baby
nullipara	woman who has yet to deliver her first child
grand multiparity	woman who has delivered at least seven babies
gestation	period of time for intrauterine fetal development

[*] The gravidity and parity of a woman is expressed in the following shorthand: G4P2. *G* refers to the gravidity, and *P* refers to the parity. The woman in this example would have had four pregnancies and two births.

FETAL DEVELOPMENT

Fetal development begins immediately after fertilization and is quite complex. The time at which fertilization occurs is called conception. Since conception occurs approximately 14 days after the first day of the last menstrual period, it is possible to calculate, with fair accuracy, the approximate date the baby should be born. This estimate is usually made during the mother's first prenatal visit. The normal duration of pregnancy is 40 weeks from the first day of the mother's last menstrual period. This is equal to 280 days, which is ten lunar months or, roughly, nine calendar months. This estimated birth date is commonly called the due date. Medically, it is known as the **estimated date of confinement (EDC)**. Generally, pregnancy is divided into *trimesters*. The length of each trimester is approximately 13 weeks, or three calendar months.

> **estimated date of confinement (EDC)** the approximate day the infant will be born. This date is usually set at 40 weeks after the date of the mother's last menstrual period (LMP).

Several different terms are used to describe the stages of development. The *pre-embryonic stage* covers the first 14 days following conception. The embryonic stage begins at day 15 and ends at approximately 8 weeks. The period from 8 weeks until delivery is known as the *fetal stage*. As an EMT-I, you should be familiar with some of the significant developmental milestones that occur during these three periods (Table 29-1). During normal fetal development, the sex of the infant can usually be determined by 16 weeks gestation. By 20 weeks, *fetal heart tones (FHTs)* can be detected by stethoscope. The mother also has generally felt fetal movement. By 24 weeks, the baby may be able to survive if born prematurely. Fetuses born after 28 weeks have an excellent chance of survival. By 38 weeks, the baby is considered *term,* or fully developed.

Most of the fetus's organ systems develop during the first trimester. Therefore, this is when the fetus is most vulnerable to the development of birth defects.

FETAL CIRCULATION

The fetus receives its oxygen and nutrients from its mother through the placenta. Thus, while in the uterus, the fetus does not need to use its respiratory system or its gastrointestinal tract. Because of this, the fetal circulation shunts blood around the lungs and gastrointestinal tract.

Table 29-1 SIGNIFICANT FETAL DEVELOPMENTAL MILESTONES

	Pre-embryonic Stage
2 weeks	Rapid cellular multiplication and differentiation
	Embryonic Stage
4 weeks	Fetal heart begins to beat
8 weeks	All body systems and external structures are formed Size: approximately 3 cm (1.2 in)
	Fetal Stage
8–12 weeks	Fetal heart tones audible with Doppler Kidneys begin to produce urine Size: 8 cm (3.2 in), weight about 1.6 oz Fetus most vulnerable to toxins
16 weeks	Sex can be determined visually Swallowing amniotic fluid and producing meconium Looks like a baby, although thin
20 weeks	Fetal heart tones audible with stethoscope Mother able to feel fetal movement Baby develops schedule of sucking, kicking, and sleeping Hair, eyebrows, and eyelashes present Size: 19 cm (8 in), weight approximately 16 oz
24 weeks	Increased activity Begins respiratory movement Size: 28 cm (11.2 in), weight 1 lb 10 oz
28 weeks	Surfactant necessary for lung function is formed Eyes begin to open and close Weighs 2 to 3 lbs
32 weeks	Bones are fully developed but soft and flexible Subcutaneous fat being deposited Fingernails and toenails present
38–40 weeks	Considered to be full-term Baby fills uterine cavity Baby receives maternal antibodies

The infant receives its blood from the placenta by means of the umbilical vein (Figure 29-4). The umbilical vein connects directly to the inferior vena cava by a specialized structure called the *ductus venosus.* Blood then travels through the inferior vena cava to the heart. The blood enters the right atrium and passes through the tricuspid valve into the right ventricle. It then exits the right ventricle, through the pulmonic valve, into the pulmonary artery. The fetus's heart has a hole between the right and left atria, termed the *foramen ovale,* which allows mixing of the oxygenated blood in the right atrium with that leaving the left ventricle bound for the aorta.

At this time, the blood is still oxygenated. Once in the pulmonary artery, the blood enters the *ductus arteriosus,* which connects the pulmonary artery with the aorta. The ductus arteriosus causes blood to bypass the uninflated lungs. Once in the aorta, blood flow is basically the same as in extrauterine life. Deoxygenated blood containing waste products exits the fetus, after passage through the liver, via the umbilical arteries.

The fetal circulation changes immediately at birth. As soon as the baby takes his first breath, the lungs inflate, greatly decreasing pulmonary vascular resistance to blood flow. Also, the ductus arteriosus closes, diverting blood to the lungs. In addition, the ductus venosus closes, stopping blood flow from the placenta. The foramen ovale also closes as a result of pressure changes in the heart, which stops blood flow from the right to left atrium.

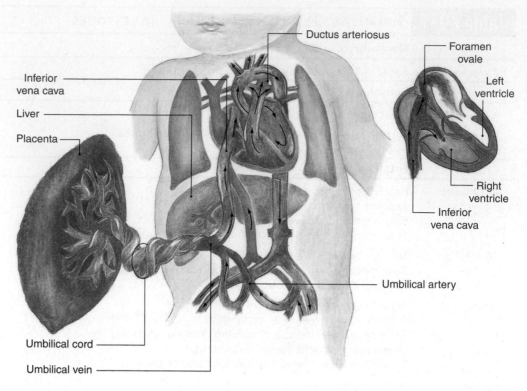

FIGURE 29-4 The maternal-fetal circulation.

GENERAL ASSESSMENT OF THE OBSTETRIC PATIENT

INITIAL ASSESSMENT

The initial approach to the obstetrical patient should be the same as for the non-obstetrical patient, with special attention paid to the developing fetus. Complete initial assessment quickly. Next, obtain essential obstetric information.

HISTORY

The SAMPLE history will allow you to gain specific information about the mother's situation as well as her pertinent medical history.

General Information

You will want to obtain information about the pregnancy, such as the mother's gravidity and parity, the length of gestation, and the estimated date of confinement (EDC), if known. In addition, you should determine whether the patient has had any cesarean sections or any gynecological or obstetrical complications in the past. It is also important to ascertain whether the patient has had any prenatal care. Determine what type of health-care professional (physician or nurse midwife) is providing her care and when she was last evaluated. Ask the patient whether a sonogram examination was done. A sonogram reveals the age of the fetus, the presence of more than one fetus, abnormal presentations, and certain birth defects. A general overview of the patient's current state of health is important. Pay particular attention to current medications and drug and/or medication allergies.

Pre-existing or Aggravated Medical Conditions

Pregnancy aggravates many pre-existing medical conditions and may trigger new ones.

Diabetes   Previously diagnosed diabetes can become unstable during pregnancy due to altered insulin requirements. Diabetics are at increased risk of developing preeclampsia and

Obtain information about the pregnancy. Ask about gravidity, parity, length of gestation, and EDC. Ask about past gynecological or obstetrical complications and prenatal care. Determine current medications and any drug allergies.

Pregnancy can aggravate pre-existing medical conditions such as diabetes, heart disease, hypertension, seizure disorders, and neuromuscular disorders, and may trigger new ones. (However, a remission of neurological disorder symptoms during pregnancy is not unusual.)

hypertension (discussed later in this chapter). Pregnancy may also accelerate the progression of vascular disease complications of diabetes. It is not uncommon for pregnant diabetics to have problems with fluctuating blood sugar levels, causing hypoglycemic or hyperglycemic episodes. Also, many patients develop diabetes during pregnancy (*gestational diabetes*). Pregnant diabetics cannot be managed with oral hypoglycemic agents because these drugs tend to cross the placenta and affect the fetus. Therefore, all pregnant diabetics are placed on insulin, if their blood sugar levels cannot be controlled by diet alone. It has been shown that maintaining careful control of the mother's blood sugar between 70 and 120 mg/dL reduces risks to mother and fetus.

Diabetes also affects the infant. Infants of diabetic mothers, especially those with poorly controlled blood sugar levels, tend to be large. This complicates delivery. Such infants also may have trouble maintaining body temperature after birth and may be subject to hypoglycemia. Babies born to diabetic mothers are also at increased risk of congenital anomalies (birth defects).

Heart Disease   During pregnancy, cardiac output increases up to 30%. Patients who have serious pre-existing heart disease may develop congestive heart failure in pregnancy. When confronted by a pregnant patient in obvious or suspected heart failure, inquire about pre-existing heart disease or murmurs. It is important to be aware, however, that most patients develop a quiet systolic flow murmur during pregnancy. This is caused by increased cardiac output and is rarely a source of concern.

Hypertension   Hypertension is also aggravated by pregnancy. Generally, blood pressure is lower in pregnancy than in the non-pregnant state. However, women who were borderline hypertensive before becoming pregnant may become dangerously hypertensive when pregnant. Also, many common blood pressure medications cannot be used during pregnancy. In addition, preeclampsia (discussed later in this chapter) may contribute to maternal hypertension. Persistent hypertension may adversely affect the placenta, thus compromising the fetus as well as placing the mother at increased risk for stroke, seizure, or renal failure.

Seizure Disorders   Most women with a history of seizure disorders controlled by medication have uneventful pregnancies and deliver healthy babies. However, women who have poorly controlled seizure disorders are likely to have increased seizure activity during pregnancy. Medications to control seizures are commonly administered throughout the pregnancy.

Neuromuscular Disorders   Disabilities associated with neuromuscular disorders, such as multiple sclerosis, may be aggravated by pregnancy. However, it is more common that pregnant women enjoy remission of symptoms during pregnancy and a slight increase in relapse rate during the postpartum period. The strength of uterine contractions is not diminished in these patients. Also, their subjective sensation of pain is often less than seen in other patients.

Pain

If the patient is in pain, try to determine when the pain started and whether its onset was sudden or slow. Also, attempt to define the character of the pain—its duration, location, and radiation, if any. It is especially important to determine whether the pain is occurring on a regular basis.

Vaginal Bleeding

The presence of vaginal bleeding or spotting is a major concern in an obstetrical patient. Ask about events immediately prior to the start of bleeding. You also need to gain information about the color, amount, and duration. To assess the amount of bleeding, count the number of sanitary pads used. If your patient is passing clots or tissue, save this material for evaluation. In addition, question the patient about the presence of other vaginal discharges, as well as the color, amount, and duration.

Active Labor

When confronted with a patient in active labor, assess whether the mother feels the need to push or has the urge to move her bowels. Determine whether the patient thinks her membranes have ruptured. Patients often sense this as a dribbling of water or, in some cases, a true gush of water.

PHYSICAL EXAMINATION

Physical examination of the obstetric patient is essentially the same as for any emergency patient. However, you should be particularly careful to protect the patient's modesty as well as to maintain her dignity and privacy.

When examining a pregnant patient, first estimate the date of the pregnancy by measuring the *fundal height*. The fundal height is the distance from the symphysis pubis to the top of the uterine fundus. Each centimeter of fundal height roughly corresponds to a week of gestation. For example, a woman with a fundal height of 24 centimeters has a gestational age of approximately 24 weeks. If the fundus is just palpable above the symphysis pubis, the pregnancy is about 12 to 16 weeks gestation. When the uterine fundus reaches the umbilicus, the pregnancy is about 20 weeks. As pregnancy reaches term, the fundus is palpable near the xiphoid process. If fetal movement is felt when the abdomen is palpated, the pregnancy is at least 20 weeks. Fetal heart tones can be heard by stethoscope at approximately 18 to 20 weeks. The normal fetal heart rate ranges from 140 to 160 beats per minute.

Generally, vital signs in the pregnant patient should be taken with the patient lying on her left side. As noted earlier, as pregnancy progresses, the uterus increases in size. Ultimately, when the patient is supine, the weight of the uterus compresses the inferior vena cava, severely compromising venous blood return from the lower extremities. Turning the patient to her left side alleviates this problem. Occasionally, it may be helpful to perform orthostatic vital signs. First, obtain the blood pressure and pulse rate after the patient has rested for 5 minutes in the left lateral recumbent position. Then repeat the vital signs with the patient sitting up or standing. A drop in the blood pressure level of 15 mmHg or more, or an increase in the pulse rate of 20 beats per minute or more, is considered significant and should be reported and documented. When performing this maneuver, it is always important to be alert for syncope. This procedure should not be performed if the patient is in obvious shock.

You may need to examine the genitals to evaluate any vaginal discharge, the progression of labor, or the presence of a *prolapsed cord*, an umbilical cord that comes out of the uterus ahead of the fetus. This can be accomplished simply by looking at the perineum. If, during the physical examination, the patient reports that she feels the need to push, or if she feels as though she must move her bowels, examine her for crowning. Crowning is the bulging of the fetal head past the opening of the vagina during a contraction. **Crowning** is an indication of impending delivery. Examine for crowning only during a contraction. *Do not perform an internal vaginal examination in the field.*

GENERAL MANAGEMENT OF THE OBSTETRIC PATIENT

The first consideration for managing emergencies in obstetric patients is to remember that you are in fact caring for two patients, the mother and the fetus. Fetal well-being is dependent on maternal well-being. Also keep in mind that your calm, professional demeanor and caring attitude will go a long way in reducing the emotional stress during any obstetric emergency. Remember to protect your patient's privacy and maintain her modesty.

The physiologic priorities for obstetric emergencies are identical to those for any other emergency situation. Focus your efforts on maintaining the airway, breathing, and circulation (ABC). Administer high-flow, high-concentration oxygen as needed based on the patient's condition. Initiate IV access by using a large bore catheter in a large vein and consider fluid resuscitation based on your local protocols. If your patient is bleeding or showing signs of shock, establish two IV lines. Cardiac monitoring is also appropriate. Place your patient in a position of comfort, but remember that left lateral recumbent is preferred after 24 weeks.

If pain is the primary complaint, administer analgesics such as morphine. However, analgesics should be used with caution since they can alter your ability to assess a deteriorating condition as well as other changes in patient status and may negatively affect the fetus. Nitrous oxide is the preferred analgesic in pregnancy, but narcotics are acceptable.

When transport is indicated, transport immediately to a hospital that is capable of managing emergency obstetric and neonatal care. Report the situation to the receiving hospital before your arrival, because emergency department personnel may want to summon obstetrics department staff to assist with patient care.

Always remember that you are caring for two patients, the mother and the fetus.

Focus on airway, breathing, and circulation. Monitor for shock. As needed, administer oxygen, initiate IV access, consider fluid resuscitation, and monitor the heart. Place the patient in a position of comfort. The left lateral recumbent position is preferred after the 24th weeks.

COMPLICATIONS OF PREGNANCY

Pregnancy is a normal process. However, women who are pregnant are not immune from injury or other health problems. There may also be complications associated with the pregnancy itself.

TRAUMA

EMT-Is frequently receive calls to help a pregnant woman who has been in a motor vehicle collision or who has sustained a fall. In pregnancy, syncope occurs frequently. The syncope of pregnancy often results from compression of the inferior vena cava, as described earlier, or from normal changes in the cardiovascular system associated with pregnancy. Also, the weight of the gravid uterus alters the patient's balance, making her more susceptible to falls.

Pregnant victims of major trauma are more susceptible to life-threatening injury than are non-pregnant victims because of the increased vascularity of the gravid uterus. Trauma is the most frequent, non-obstetric cause of death in pregnant women. Some form of trauma, usually a motor vehicle crash or a fall but sometimes physical abuse, occurs in 6% to 7% of all pregnancies. Since the primary cause for fetal mortality is maternal mortality, the pregnant trauma patient presents a unique challenge. The later in the pregnancy, the larger the uterus and the greater the likelihood of injury. All patients at 20 weeks (or more) gestation with a history of direct or indirect injury should be transported for evaluation by a physician.

EMT-Is should *anticipate* the development of shock based on the mechanism of injury rather than waiting for overt signs and symptoms. Due to the cardiovascular changes of pregnancy, overt signs of shock are late and inconsistent. Trauma significant enough to cause maternal shock is associated with a 70% to 80% fetal mortality. In the face of acute blood loss, significant vasoconstriction will occur in response to catecholamine release, resulting in maintenance of a normotensive state for the mother. However, this causes significant uterine hypoperfusion (20% to 30% decrease in cardiac output) and fetal bradycardia.

Generally, the amniotic fluid cushions the fetus from blunt trauma fairly well. However, in direct abdominal trauma, the pregnant patient may suffer premature separation of the placenta from the uterine wall, premature labor, abortion, uterine rupture, and possibly fetal

Transport all trauma patients at 20 weeks or more gestation. Anticipate the development of shock.

 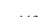

death. The presence of vaginal bleeding or a tender abdomen in a pregnant patient should increase your suspicion of serious injury. Fetal death may result from death of the mother, separation of the placenta from the uterine wall, maternal shock, uterine rupture, or fetal head injury. Any pregnant patient who has suffered trauma should be immediately transported to the emergency department and evaluated by a physician. Trauma management essentials include the following:

- Apply a C-collar to provide cervical stabilization and immobilize on a long backboard.
- Administer high-flow, high-concentration oxygen.
- Initiate two large bore IVs for crystalloid administration per protocol.
- Transport tilted to the left to minimize supine hypotension.
- Reassess frequently.
- Monitor the fetus.

MEDICAL CONDITIONS

The pregnant patient is subject to all of the medical problems that occur in the non-pregnant state. Abdominal pain is a common complaint. It is often caused by the stretching of the ligaments that support the uterus. However, appendicitis and cholecystitis can also occur. Pregnant women are at increased risk of developing gallstones as a result of hormonal influences that delay emptying of the gallbladder. In pregnancy, the abdominal organs are displaced because of the increased mass of the gravid uterus in the abdomen, which makes assessment more difficult. The pregnant patient with appendicitis may complain of right upper quadrant pain or even back pain. The symptoms of acute cholecystitis may also differ from those in non-pregnant patients. Any pregnant patient with abdominal pain should be evaluated by a physician.

BLEEDING IN PREGNANCY

Vaginal bleeding may occur at any time during pregnancy. Bleeding is usually due to abortion, ectopic pregnancy, placenta previa, or abruptio placentae. Generally, the exact etiology of vaginal bleeding during pregnancy cannot be determined in the field. Refer to the earlier discussion in this chapter and your own local protocols for management of obstetric emergencies. Vaginal bleeding is associated with potential fetal loss. Keep in mind that this is a very emotionally stressful situation for your patient, so a professional, caring demeanor is imperative.

Abortion

Abortion, the expulsion of the fetus prior to 20 weeks gestation, is the most common cause of bleeding in the first and second trimesters of pregnancy. The terms *abortion* and *miscarriage* can be used interchangeably. Generally, the lay public thinks of abortion as termination of pregnancy at maternal request and of miscarriage as an accident of nature. Medically, the term abortion applies to both kinds of fetal loss. Spontaneous abortion, the naturally occurring termination of pregnancy that is often called miscarriage, is most commonly seen between 12 and 14 weeks of gestation. It is estimated that 10% to 20% of all pregnancies end in spontaneous abortion. If the pregnancy has not yet been confirmed, the mother often assumes she is merely having a period with unusually heavy flow.

About half of all abortions are due to fetal chromosomal anomalies. Other causes include maternal reproductive system abnormalities, maternal use of drugs, placental defects, or maternal infections. Although many people believe that trauma and psychological stress can cause abortion, research does not support that belief.

Assessment   The patient experiencing an abortion is likely to report cramping abdominal pain and a backache. She is also likely to report vaginal bleeding, which is often accompanied by the passage of clots and tissue. If the abortion was not recent, then frank signs and symptoms of infection may be present. In addition to your routine emergency assessments, assess for orthostatic vital sign changes and ascertain the amount of vaginal bleeding.

abortion termination of pregnancy before 20 weeks of gestation. The term *abortion* refers to both miscarriage and induced abortion. Commonly, abortion is used for elective termination of pregnancy and miscarriage for the loss of a fetus by natural means. A miscarriage is sometimes called a spontaneous abortion.

Management   Place the patient who is experiencing an abortion in a position of comfort. Treat for shock with oxygen therapy and IV access for fluid resuscitation. As mentioned earlier, any tissue or large clots should be retained and given to emergency department personnel. If the abortion occurs during the late first trimester or later, a fetus may be passed. Often, the placenta does not detach, and the fetus is suspended by the umbilical cord. In such a case, place the umbilical clamps from the OB kit on the cord and cut it. Carefully wrap the fetus in linen or other suitable material and transport it to the hospital with the mother.

> *Treat the patient suffering an abortion as you would any patient at risk for hypovolemic shock.*

An abortion is generally a very sad occurrence. Provide emotional support to the parents. This can be a devastating psychological experience for the mother, so avoid saying trite but inaccurate phrases meant to provide comfort. Inappropriate remarks include "You can always get pregnant again" or "This is nature's way of dealing with a defective fetus." Parents who wish to view the fetus should be allowed to do so. Occasionally, Roman Catholic parents may request baptism of the fetus. You can perform this by making the sign of a cross and stating, "I baptize you in the name of the Father and of the Son and of the Holy Spirit. Amen."

> *Provide emotional support to the parents.*

Ectopic Pregnancy

As you learned earlier, the fertilized egg normally is implanted in the endometrial lining of the uterine wall. The term *ectopic pregnancy* refers to the abnormal implantation of the fertilized egg outside of the uterus. Approximately 95% are implanted in the fallopian tube. Occasionally (< 1%), the egg is implanted in the abdominal cavity. Current research indicates that the incidence of ectopic pregnancy is one for every forty-four live births. Improved diagnostic technology is credited with an increased incidence, as most are detected between the second and twelfth week. Ectopic pregnancy accounts for approximately 10% of maternal mortality.

Predisposing factors in the development of ectopic pregnancy include scarring of the fallopian tubes due to pelvic inflammatory disease (PID), a previous ectopic pregnancy, or previous pelvic or tubal surgery, such as a tubal ligation. Other factors include endometriosis or use of an intrauterine device (IUD) for birth control.

Assessment   Ectopic pregnancy most often presents as abdominal pain, which starts out as diffuse tenderness and then localizes as a sharp pain in the lower abdominal quadrant on the affected side. This pain is due to rupture of the fallopian tube when the fetus outgrows the available space. The woman often reports that she missed a period or that her last menstrual period (LMP) occurred 4 to 6 weeks ago, but with decreased menstrual flow that was brownish in color and of shorter duration than usual. As the intra-abdominal bleeding continues, the abdomen becomes rigid and the pain intensifies and is often referred to the shoulder on the affected side. The pain is often accompanied by syncope, vaginal bleeding, and shock.

Assume that any female of childbearing age with lower abdominal pain is experiencing an ectopic pregnancy.

> *Assume that any female of childbearing age with lower abdominal pain is experiencing an ectopic pregnancy.*

Management   Ectopic pregnancy poses a significant life threat to the mother. Transport this patient immediately, since surgery is often required to resolve the situation. Interim care measures should include oxygen therapy and IV access for fluid resuscitation. Trendelenburg position or the use of a pneumatic anti-shock garment may be indicated by your local protocols.

> *Ectopic pregnancy is life-threatening. Transport the patient immediately.*

Placenta Previa

Placenta previa occurs as a result of abnormal implantation of the placenta on the lower half of the uterine wall, resulting in partial or complete coverage of the cervical opening (Figure 29-5). Vaginal bleeding, which may initially be intermittent, occurs after the seventh month of the pregnancy as the lower uterus begins to contract and dilate in preparation for the onset of labor. This process pulls the placenta away from the uterine wall, causing bright red vaginal bleeding. Placenta previa occurs in about 1 of every 250 live births. It is classified as complete, partial, or marginal, depending on whether the placenta covers all or part of the cervical opening or is merely in close proximity to the opening.

Although the exact cause of placenta previa is unknown, certain predisposing factors are commonly seen. These factors include a previous history of placenta previa, multiparity,

> *Third-trimester bleeding should be attributed to either placenta previa or abruptio placentae until proven otherwise. Placenta previa usually presents with painless bleeding. Abruptio placentae usually presents with sharp pain, with or without bleeding.*

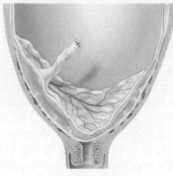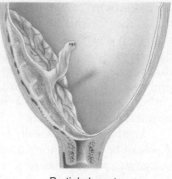

Total placenta previa   Partial placenta previa

FIGURE 29-5   Placenta previa (abnormal implantation).

or increased maternal age. Other factors include the presence of uterine scars from cesarean sections, a large placenta, or defective development of blood vessels in the uterine wall.

Assessment   The patient with placenta previa is usually a multigravida in her third trimester of pregnancy. She may have a history of prior placenta previa or of bleeding early in the current pregnancy. She may report a recent episode of sexual intercourse or vaginal examination just before vaginal bleeding began, or she may not bleed until the onset of labor. The onset of painless bright red vaginal bleeding, which may occur as spotting or recurrent hemorrhage, is the hallmark of placenta previa. In fact, any painless bleeding in pregnancy is considered placenta previa until proven otherwise. The bleeding may or may not be associated with uterine contractions. The uterus is usually soft, and the fetus may be in an unusual presentation. *Vaginal examination should never be attempted, because an examining finger can puncture the placenta, causing fatal hemorrhage.*

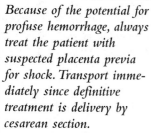

Never attempt vaginal examination since an examining finger can puncture the placenta and cause fatal hemorrhage.

The presence of placenta previa may already have been diagnosed with an ultrasound during prenatal care, in which case the mother is anticipating the onset of symptoms. The prognosis for the fetus depends on the extent of the previa. Obviously, in profuse hemorrhage the fetus is at risk of severe hypoxia and the viability of the placenta is compromised. You should perform your assessment and physical exam as discussed earlier in this chapter.

Because of the potential for profuse hemorrhage, always treat the patient with suspected placenta previa for shock. Transport immediately since definitive treatment is delivery by cesarean section.

Management   If the placenta previa was previously diagnosed, your patient may already have been managed by placing her on bed rest. Because of the potential for profuse hemorrhage, you should treat for shock. Administer oxygen and initiate IV access. Additionally, continue to monitor the maternal vital signs and fetal heart tones. Since the definitive treatment is delivery of the fetus by cesarean section, it is imperative to transport the patient to a hospital with obstetric surgical capability.

Abruptio Placentae

Abruptio placentae, or the premature separation (abruption) of a normally implanted placenta from the uterine wall, poses a potential life threat for both mother and fetus (Figure 29-6). The incidence of abruptio placentae is one in 120 live births. It is associated with 20% to 30% fetal mortality, which rises to 100% in cases where the majority of the placenta has separated. Maternal mortality is relatively uncommon, although it rises markedly if shock is inadequately treated. Abruptio placentae is classified as marginal (or partial), central (severe), or complete, as explained below.

Although the cause of abruptio placentae is unknown, predisposing factors include multiparity, maternal hypertension, trauma, cocaine use, increasing maternal age, and history of abruption in previous pregnancy.

Assessment   The presenting signs and symptoms of abruptio placentae vary depending on the extent and character of the abruption. Partial abruptions can be marginal or central. Marginal abruptio is characterized by vaginal bleeding but no increase in pain. In central abruptio, the placenta separates centrally and the bleeding is trapped between the placenta

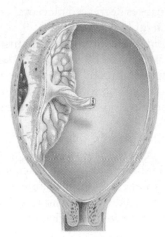
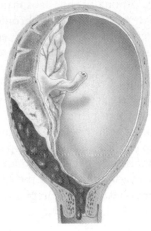
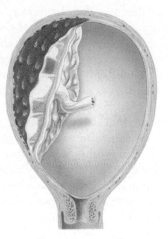

Partial separation
(concealed hemorrhage)

Partial separation
(apparent hemorrhage)

Complete separation
(concealed hemorrhage)

FIGURE 29-6 Abruptio placentae (premature separation).

and the uterine wall, or concealed, so there is no vaginal bleeding. However, there is a sudden sharp, tearing pain and development of a stiff, board-like abdomen. In complete abruptio placentae there is massive vaginal bleeding and profound maternal hypotension. If the patient is in labor at the time of the abruptio, separation of the placenta from the uterine wall will progress rapidly, with fetal distress versus fetal demise dependent on percentage of separation.

Management Abruptio placentae is a life-threatening obstetrical emergency. Immediate intervention to maintain maternal oxygenation and perfusion is imperative. Immediately place two large-bore IV lines and begin fluid resuscitation. Position your patient in the left lateral recumbent position. Transport immediately to a hospital with available surgical obstetric and high-risk neonatal care.

MEDICAL COMPLICATIONS OF PREGNANCY

As discussed earlier, pregnancy can exacerbate pre-existing medical conditions such as diabetes, heart disease, hypertension, and seizure or neuromuscular disorder.

Hypertensive Disorders

The American College of Obstetricians and Gynecologists has identified four classifications of *hypertensive disorders of pregnancy* (formerly called "toxemia of pregnancy"). They include preeclampsia and eclampsia, chronic hypertension, chronic hypertension superimposed with preeclampsia, and transient hypertension.

    Preeclampsia and Eclampsia Pregnancy-induced hypertension (PIH), which includes *preeclampsia* and *eclampsia,* occurs in approximately 5% of all pregnancies. Preeclampsia is the most common hypertensive disorder seen in pregnancy. A higher incidence is found among primigravidas, particularly if they are teenagers or over the age of 35. Others at increased risk are diabetics, women with a history of preeclampsia, and those who are carrying multiple fetuses.

    Preeclampsia is a progressive disorder that is usually categorized as mild or severe. Seizures (or coma) develop in its most severe form, known as eclampsia. Preeclampsia is defined as an increase in systolic blood pressure by 30 mmHg and/or a diastolic increase of 15 mmHg over baseline on at least two occasions at least six hours apart. Remember that maternal blood pressure normally drops during pregnancy, so a woman may be hypertensive at 120/80 if her baseline in early pregnancy was 90/66. If there is no baseline blood pressure available, then a reading ≥140/90 is considered to be hypertensive.

    Preeclampsia is most commonly seen in the last 10 weeks of gestation, during labor, or in the first 48 hours postpartum. The exact cause of preeclampsia is unknown. It is thought to be caused by abnormal vasospasm, which results in increased maternal blood pressure

Signs and symptoms of abruptio placentae vary. With a marginal abruption, there will be bleeding but no pain. With a central abruption, there will be sharp, tearing pain and a stiff, boardlike abdomen. Complete abruption will result in massive hemorrhage.

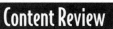

Abruptio placentae is a life-threatening emergency. Treat for shock, including fluid resuscitation, and transport immediately in the left lateral recumbent position.

Content Review

MEDICAL COMPLICATIONS OF PREGNANCY
- Hypertensive disorders
- Supine hypotensive syndrome
- Gestational diabetes

and other associated symptoms. Additionally, the vasospasm causes decreased placental perfusion, contributing to fetal growth retardation and chronic fetal hypoxia.

Mild preeclampsia is characterized by hypertension, edema, and protein in the urine. Severe preeclampsia progresses rapidly with maternal blood pressures reaching 160/110 or higher, while the edema becomes generalized and the amount of protein in the urine increases significantly. Other commonly seen signs and symptoms in the severe state include headache, visual disturbances, hyperactive reflexes, and the development of pulmonary edema, along with a dramatic decrease in urine output.

Patients who are preeclamptic have intravascular volume depletion, since a great deal of their body fluid is in the third space. Those who develop severe preeclampsia and eclampsia are at increased risk for cerebral hemorrhage, pulmonary embolism, abruptio placentae, disseminated intravascular coagulopathy (DIC), and the development of renal failure.

Eclampsia, the most serious manifestation of pregnancy-induced hypertension, is characterized by grand mal (major motor) seizure activity. Eclampsia is often preceded by visual disturbances, such as flashing lights or spots before the eyes. Also, the development of epigastric pain or pain in the right upper abdominal quadrant often indicates impending seizure. Eclampsia can often be distinguished from epilepsy by the history and physical appearance of the patient. Patients who become eclamptic are usually grossly edematous and have markedly elevated blood pressure, whereas epileptics usually have a prior history of seizures and are usually taking anticonvulsant medications. If eclampsia develops, death of the mother and fetus frequently results. The risk of fetal mortality increases by 10% with each maternal seizure.

Chronic Hypertension　Hypertension is considered chronic when the blood pressure is ≥140/90 before pregnancy or before 20 weeks of gestation, or if it persists for more than 42 days postpartum. As a general rule, if the diastolic pressure exceeds 80 mmHg during the second trimester, chronic hypertension is likely. The cause of chronic hypertension is unknown. The goal of management is to prevent the development of preeclampsia.

Chronic Hypertension Superimposed with Preeclampsia　It is not uncommon for the chronic hypertensive who develops preeclampsia to progress rapidly to eclampsia even before 30 weeks of gestation. The same diagnostic criteria for preeclampsia are used (systolic blood pressure increases >30 mmHg over baseline, edema, and protein in the urine).

Transient Hypertension　Transient hypertension is defined as a temporary rise in blood pressure that occurs during labor or early in postpartum and which normalizes within 10 days.

Assessment　Obtaining an accurate history is extremely important whenever you suspect one of the hypertensive disorders of pregnancy. Question the patient about excessive weight gain, headaches, visual problems, epigastric or right upper quadrant abdominal pain, apprehension, or seizures. On physical exam, patients with PIH or preeclampsia are usually markedly edematous. They are often pale and apprehensive. The reflexes are hyperactive. The blood pressure, which is usually elevated, should be taken after the patient has rested for 5 minutes in the left lateral recumbent position.

Management　Definitive treatment of the hypertensive disorders of pregnancy is delivery of the fetus. However, in the field, use the following management tactics to prevent dangerously high blood pressures or seizure activity:

- *Hypertension.* Closely monitor the patient who is pregnant and has elevated blood pressure without edema or other signs of preeclampsia. Record the fetal heart tones and the mother's blood pressure level.

- *Preeclampsia.* The patient who is hypertensive and shows other signs and symptoms of preeclampsia, such as edema, headaches, and visual disturbances, should be treated quickly. Keep the patient calm and dim the lights. Place the patient in the left lateral recumbent position and quickly carry out the initial assessment. Begin an IV of normal saline. Transport the patient rapidly, without lights or sirens. If the blood pressure is dangerously high (diastolic >110), medical direction may request the administration of hydralazine (Apresoline) or similar antihypertensives that are safe for use in pregnancy. If

With suspected hypertensive disorder, it is critical to obtain an accurate history, including weight gain, headaches, visual problems, epigastric or right upper quadrant abdominal pain, apprehension, or seizures.

Preeclampsia and eclampsia are life-threatening. Keep the patient calm. Dim the lights. Place patient in left lateral recumbent position and transport quickly without lights or sirens. Administer magnesium sulfate to control seizures if they occur. Medical direction may request administration of antihypertensive or sedative drugs.

the transport time is long, the administration of magnesium sulfate may also be ordered.

- *Eclampsia.* If the patient has already suffered a seizure or a seizure appears to be imminent, then, in addition to the above measures, administer oxygen and manage the airway appropriately. Administer a bolus dose of magnesium sulfate (2 to 5 grams diluted in 50 to 100 mL slow IV push) to control the seizures. If you are unable to control the seizures with magnesium sulfate, you may consider diazepam (Valium) or other sedative. It is important to keep calcium gluconate available for use as an antidote to magnesium sulfate. Also monitor your patient closely for signs (vaginal bleeding or abdominal rigidity) of abruptio placentae or developing pulmonary edema. Transport immediately to a hospital with surgical obstetric and neonatal care availability.

Supine-Hypotensive Syndrome

Supine-hypotensive syndrome usually occurs in the third trimester of pregnancy. Also known as vena caval syndrome, supine hypotensive syndrome occurs when the gravid uterus compresses the inferior vena cava when the mother lies in a supine position (Figure 29-7).

Assessment Supine-hypotensive syndrome usually occurs in a patient late in her pregnancy who has been supine for a period of time. The patient may complain of dizziness, which results from the decrease in venous return to the right atrium and consequent lowering of the patient's blood pressure. Question the patient about prior episodes of a similar nature and about any recent hemorrhage or fluid loss. Direct the physical examination at determining whether the patient is volume depleted.

Management If there are no indications of volume depletion, such as decreased skin turgor or thirst, place the patient in the left lateral recumbent position or elevate her right hip. Monitor the fetal heart tones and maternal vital signs frequently. If there is clinical evidence of volume depletion, administer oxygen and start an IV of normal saline. Check for orthostatic changes (a decrease in blood pressure and increase in heart rate when rising from the

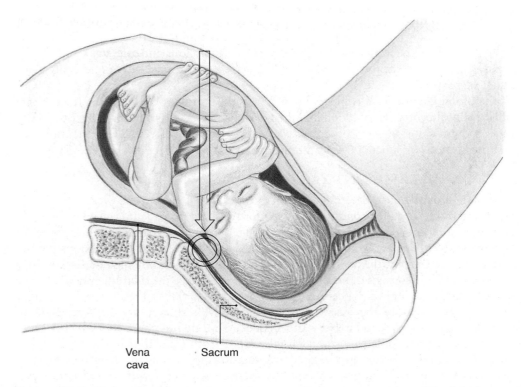

Vena cava   Sacrum

FIGURE 29-7 The supine-hypotensive syndrome results from compression of the inferior vena cava by the gravid uterus.

supine position) and place electrodes for cardiac monitoring. Transport the patient promptly in the left lateral recumbent position

Gestational Diabetes

Diabetes mellitus occurs in approximately 4% of all pregnancies. Hormonal influences cause an increase in insulin production as well as an increased tissue response to insulin during the first 20 weeks of gestation. However, during the last 20 weeks placental hormones cause an increased resistance to insulin and a decreased glucose tolerance. This causes catabolism (the "breaking down" phase of metabolism) between meals and during the night. At these times, ketones may be present in the urine because fats are metabolized more rapidly. Further, maternal glucose stores are used up, because they are the sole source of glucose to meet the energy needs of the growing fetus. This is known as the *diabetogenic* (diabetes-causing) effect of pregnancy. Gestational diabetes usually subsides after pregnancy.

Routine prenatal care includes screening to detect diabetes throughout the pregnancy. Women who are considered to be at high risk for developing gestational diabetes are given a glucose tolerance test at their first prenatal visit. High risk is associated with maternal age (over 35), obesity, hypertension, family history of diabetes, and history of prior stillbirth.

Management of gestational diabetes requires good prenatal care. The mother will be instructed on diabetic management and the importance of balancing diet and exercise as well as how to monitor her glucose levels and administer insulin. Fetal development will be monitored on an ongoing basis throughout the pregnancy.

Assessment   When you encounter a pregnant patient with an altered mental status, consider hypoglycemia as a likely cause. Remember that the clinical signs and symptoms of hypoglycemia are many and varied. An abnormal mental status is the most important. Physical signs may include diaphoresis and tachycardia. If the blood sugar falls to a critically low level, she may sustain a hypoglycemic seizure or become comatose, which poses a potential life threat to the mother and fetus. Obtaining an accurate history of associated signs and symptoms, such as nausea, vomiting, abdominal pain, increased urination, or a recent infection, will allow you to ascertain whether diabetic ketoacidosis might be the cause of your patient's altered mental status. Determine the blood glucose level in addition to obtaining baseline vital signs and fetal heart tones.

Management   If the blood glucose level is noted to be less that 60 mg/dL, draw a red-top tube of blood and start an IV of normal saline. Next, administer 50 to 100 mL (25 to 50 grams) of 50% dextrose intravenously. If the patient is conscious and able to swallow, complete glucose administration with orange juice, sugared soft drinks, or commercially available glucose pastes.

If the blood glucose level is in excess of 200 mg/dL, draw a red-top tube (or the tube specified by local protocols) of blood and then establish IV access to administer 1 to 2 liters of 0.9% sodium chloride per protocol. If transport time is lengthy, medical direction may request intravenous or subcutaneous administration of regular insulin.

BRAXTON-HICKS CONTRACTIONS

It is occasionally difficult to determine the onset of labor. As early as 13 weeks, the uterus contracts intermittently, thus conditioning itself for the birth process. It is also believed that these contractions enhance placental circulation. These painless, irregular contractions are known as Braxton-Hicks contractions. As the EDC approaches, these contractions become more frequent. Ultimately, the contractions become stronger and more regular, signaling the onset of labor. Labor consists of uterine contractions that cause the dilation and **effacement** (thinning and shortening) of the cervix. The contractions of labor are firm, fairly regular, and quite painful. Before the onset of labor, Braxton-Hicks contractions—occasionally called *false labor*—increase in intensity and frequency but do not cause cervical changes.

It is virtually impossible to distinguish false labor from true labor in the field. Distinguishing the two requires repeated vaginal examinations, over time, to determine whether the cervix is effacing and dilating. *Remember: Internal vaginal exams should not be performed in the field.* Therefore, all patients with uterine contractions should be transported to the hospital for additional evaluation.

effacement the thinning and shortening of the cervix during labor.

Braxton-Hicks contractions do not require treatment by the EMT-I aside from reassurance of the patient and, if necessary, transport for evaluation by a physician.

PRETERM LABOR

As you have already learned, normal gestation is 40 weeks and, in terms of fetal development, the fetus is not considered to be full term until 38 weeks of gestation. True labor that begins before 38 weeks is called preterm labor and frequently requires medical intervention. A variety of maternal, fetal, or placental factors may cause this potentially life-threatening situation for the mother and fetus:

- Maternal factors
  - Cardiovascular disease
  - Renal disease
  - Pregnancy-induced hypertension (PIH)
  - Diabetes
  - Abdominal surgery during gestation
  - Uterine and cervical abnormalities
  - Maternal infection
  - Trauma, particularly blows to the abdomen
  - Contributory factors: history of preterm birth, smoking, and cocaine abuse
- Placental factors
  - Placenta previa
  - Abruptio placentae
- Fetal factors
  - Multiple gestation
  - Excessive amniotic fluid
  - Fetal infection

In many cases, physicians attempt to stop preterm labor to give the fetus additional time to develop in the uterus. Prematurity is the primary neonatal health problem in the nation and occurs in 7% to 10% of all live births. All of the preterm infant's organ systems are immature to some degree, but lung development is of greatest concern. Although technological advances in the care of preterm infants have improved the prognosis dramatically, the consequences of a preterm birth can last a lifetime.

Assessment When confronted by a patient with uterine contractions, first determine the approximate gestational age of the fetus. If it is less than 38 weeks, then suspect preterm labor. If gestational age is greater than 38 weeks, treat the patient as a term patient, as described later in this chapter.

After determining gestational age, obtain a brief obstetrical history. Then question the mother about the urge to push or the need to move her bowels or urinate. Also ask if her membranes have ruptured. Any sensation of fluid leakage or "gushing" from the vagina should be interpreted as ruptured membranes until proven otherwise. Next, palpate the contractions by placing your hand on the patient's abdomen. Note the intensity and length of the contractions, as well as the interval between contractions.

Commonly reported signs and symptoms of preterm labor include contractions that occur every 10 minutes or less, low abdominal cramping that is similar to menstrual cramps, or a sensation of pelvic pressure. Other complaints such as low backache, changes in vaginal discharge, and abdominal cramping with or without diarrhea may also be reported. Rupture of the membranes is confirmatory for preterm labor.

Management Preterm labor, especially if quite early in the pregnancy, should be stopped if possible. The process of stopping labor, or **tocolysis,** is frequently practiced in obstetrics. However, it is infrequently done in the field.

There are three general approaches to tocolysis. The first is to sedate the patient, often with narcotics or barbiturates, thus allowing her to rest. Often, after a period of rest, the contractions stop on their own. The second approach is to administer a fluid bolus intravenously. The administration of approximately one liter of fluid intravenously increases the intravascular

tocolysis the process of stopping labor.

> *The patient with suspected preterm labor should be transported immediately.*

fluid volume, thus inhibiting ADH secretion from the posterior pituitary. Since oxytocin and ADH are secreted from the same area of the pituitary gland, the inhibition of ADH secretion also inhibits oxytocin release, often causing cessation of uterine contractions. Ultimately, if the above methods fail, a beta agonist, such as terbutaline or ritodrine, or magnesium sulfate may be administered to stop labor by inhibiting uterine smooth muscle contraction. Current research in tocolysis includes the administration of calcium channel blockers, such as nifedipine, and prostaglandin inhibitors, such as indomethacin. You may also find that a patient with preterm labor has been given corticosteroids to accelerate fetal lung maturity.

As a rule, tocolysis in the field is limited to sedation and hydration, especially if transport time is long. EMT-Is may, however, transport a patient from one medical facility to another with beta agonist administration underway. You should therefore be familiar with its use. Commonly associated side effects include being jittery, tachycardia usually described by the patient as palpitations, and occasionally abdominal pain. Transport your patient to the nearest facility that has neonatal intensive care capabilities. Careful and frequent monitoring of maternal vital signs and fetal heart tones is imperative during tocolysis.

PUERPERIUM

The **puerperium** is the time period surrounding birth of the fetus. Childbirth generally occurs in a hospital or similar facility with appropriate equipment. Occasionally, prehospital personnel may be called on to attend a delivery in the field. Therefore, you should be familiar with the birth process and some of the complications that may be associated with it.

LABOR

Childbirth, or the delivery of the fetus, is the culmination of pregnancy. The process by which delivery occurs is called **labor,** the physiologic and mechanical process in which the baby, placenta, and amniotic sac are expelled through the birth canal. The duration of labor is widely variable.

Before the onset of true labor, the head of the fetus descends into the bony pelvis area. The frequency and intensity of the Braxton-Hicks contractions increase in preparation for true labor. Increased vaginal secretions and softening of the cervix occur. Bloody show, pink-tinged secretions, is generally considered a sign of imminent labor as the mucous plug is expelled from the cervix. Labor then usually begins within 24 to 48 hours. Many people also consider the rupture of the membranes as a sign of impending labor. If labor does not begin spontaneously within 12 to 24 hours after rupture, labor will likely require induction because of the risk of infection.

Pressure exerted by the fetus on the cervix causes changes that lead to the subsequent expulsion of the fetus. Muscular uterine contractions increase in frequency, strength, and duration. You can assess the frequency and duration of contractions by placing one hand on the fundus of the uterus. Time contractions from the beginning of one contraction until the beginning of the next. It is important to note whether the uterus relaxes completely between contractions. It is also desirable to monitor fetal heart tones during and between contractions. Occasional fetal bradycardia occurs during contractions, but the heart rate should increase to a normal rate (120 to 160) after the contraction ends. Failure of the heart rate to return to normal between contractions is a sign of fetal distress.

Labor is generally divided into three stages: dilatation, expulsion, and placental.

Stage One (Dilatation Stage)

The first stage of labor begins with the onset of true labor contractions and ends with the complete dilatation and effacement of the cervix. Early in pregnancy the cervix is quite thick and long, but after complete *effacement* it is short and paper thin. Effacement usually begins several days before active labor ensues. *Dilatation* is the progressive stretching of the cervical opening. The cervix dilates from its closed position to 10 centimeters, which is considered complete dilation. This stage lasts approximately 8 to 10 hours for the woman in her first labor, the nullipara, and about 5 to 7 hours in the woman who has given birth previously, the multipara. Early in this stage the contractions are usually mild, lasting for 15 to 20

Content Review

STAGES OF LABOR
1. Dilatation
2. Expulsion
3. Placental

seconds with a frequency of 10 to 20 minutes. As labor progresses, the contractions increase in intensity and occur approximately every 2 to 3 minutes with duration of 60 seconds.

Stage Two (Expulsion Stage)

The second stage of labor begins with the complete dilatation of the cervix and ends with the delivery of the fetus. In the nullipara, this stage lasts 50 to 60 minutes. It takes about half that amount of time for the multipara. The contractions are very strong, occurring every 2 minutes and lasting for 60 to 75 seconds. Often, the patient feels pain in her lower back as the fetus descends into the pelvis. The urge to push or bear down usually begins in the second stage. The membranes usually rupture at this time, if they have not ruptured previously. Crowning during contractions is evident as the delivery of the fetus nears. Crowning occurs when the head (or other presenting part of the fetus) is visible at the vaginal opening during a contraction and is the definitive sign that birth is imminent. The most common presentation is for the infant to be delivered headfirst, face down (vertex position).

Stage Three (Placental Stage)

The third and final stage of labor begins immediately after the birth of the infant and ends with the delivery of the placenta. The placenta generally delivers within 5 to 20 minutes. There is no need to delay transport to wait for its delivery. Classic signs of placental separation include a gush of blood from the vagina; a change in size, shape, or consistency of the uterus; lengthening of the umbilical cord protruding from the vagina; and the mother's report that she has the urge to push.

MANAGEMENT OF A PATIENT IN LABOR

Probably one of the most important decisions you must make with a patient in labor is whether to attempt to deliver the infant at the scene or to transport the patient to the hospital. It is generally preferable to transport the mother unless delivery is imminent. You should take several factors into consideration when making this decision. They include the patient's number of previous pregnancies, the length of labor during the previous pregnancies, the frequency of contractions, the maternal urge to push, and the presence of crowning. Some women have rapid labors and may be completely dilated in a short period of time. Also, as mentioned above, multiparas generally have shorter labors than nulliparas. The maternal urge to push or the presence of crowning indicates that delivery is imminent. In such cases, the infant should be delivered at the scene or in the ambulance.

Transport the patient in labor unless delivery is imminent. Maternal urge to push or the presence of crowning indicates imminent delivery. Delivery at the scene or in the ambulance will be necessary.

Traditionally, a woman who had previously delivered by a cesarean section was advised to deliver all subsequent infants by cesarean sections. However, current thinking encourages women to attempt vaginal birth after cesarean (VBAC). If your patient has had prenatal care during this pregnancy she has probably already discussed this with her health-care provider. The only absolute contraindication for VBAC is a classic vertical uterine incision. However, most cesarean sections done today are done using a low transverse uterine incision. (Note that a horizontal skin incision does not ensure that the uterine incision is horizontal.) A patient in labor who is opting for VBAC requires no more special care than any other labor patient does.

However, certain factors should prompt immediate transport, despite the threat of delivery. These include prolonged rupture of membranes (>24 hours), since prolonged time between rupture and delivery often leads to fetal infection; abnormal presentation, such as breech or transverse; prolapsed cord; or fetal distress, as evidenced by fetal bradycardia or meconium staining (the presence of meconium, the first fetal stools, in the amniotic fluid). The presence of multiple fetuses may also contribute to your decision to transport. You will read more about these conditions later in this chapter.

FIELD DELIVERY

If delivery is imminent, you can assist the mother to deliver the baby in the field (Procedure 29-1 and Figures 29-8 through 29-16). Equipment and facilities must be quickly prepared. Set up a delivery area. This should be out of public view, such as in a bedroom or the back of the ambulance. Administer oxygen to the mother via nasal cannula or nonrebreather mask. If time permits, establish IV access and administer normal saline at a keep-open rate. Place the patient on her back with knees and hips flexed and buttocks slightly elevated. It

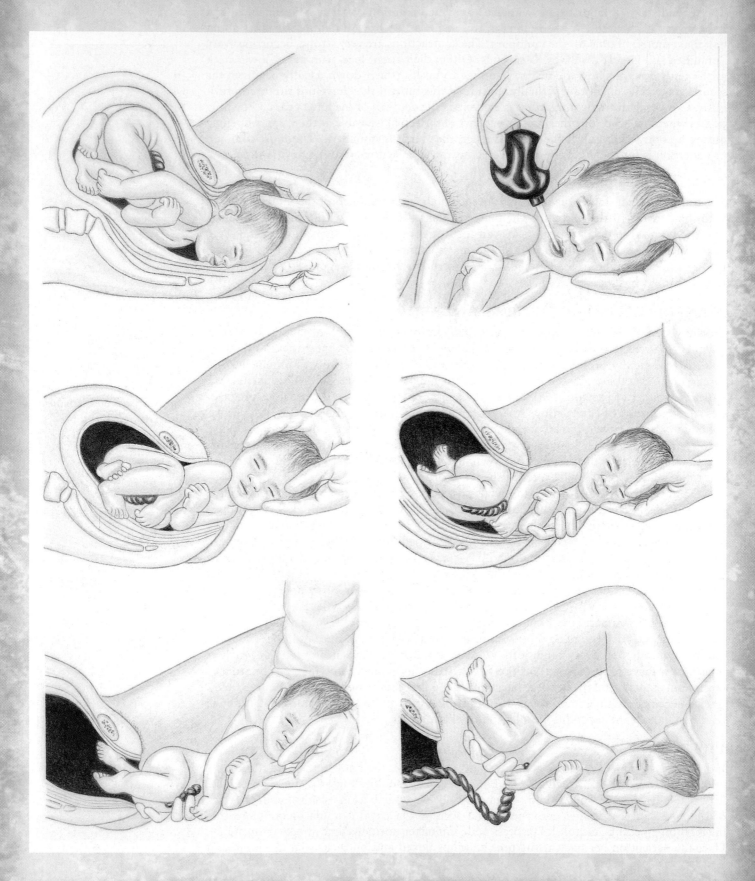

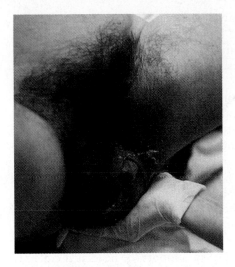

FIGURE 29-8   Crowning.

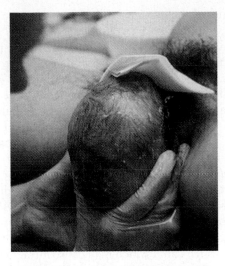

FIGURE 29-9   Delivery of the head.

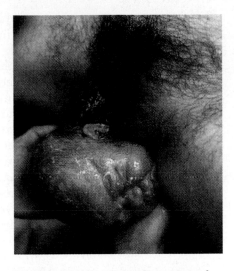

FIGURE 29-10   External rotation of the head.

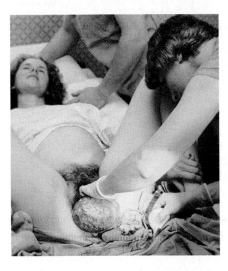

FIGURE 29-11   As soon as possible, suction the mouth and then the nose.

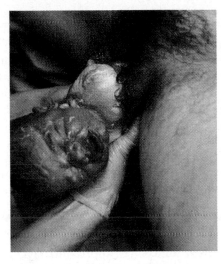

FIGURE 29-12   Delivery of the anterior shoulder.

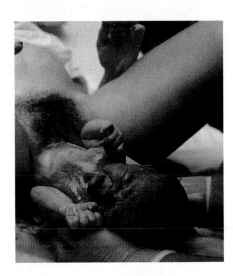

FIGURE 29-13   Complete delivery of the infant.

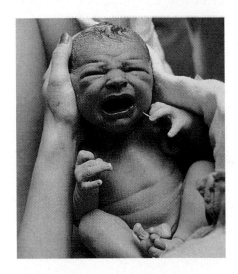

FIGURE 29-14   Dry the infant.

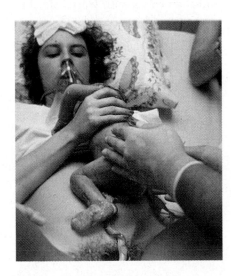

FIGURE 29-15   Place the infant on the mother's stomach.

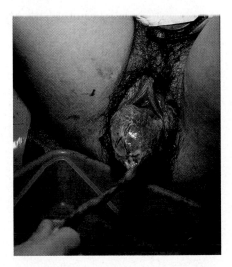

FIGURE 29-16   Deliver the placenta and save for transport with the mother and infant.

should be noted that this position is easier on you than the mother. She may prefer to squat or lie in a semi-Fowler's position with her knees and hips flexed. Either of these positions enables gravity to facilitate the delivery. If time permits, drape the mother with toweling from the OB kit. Place one towel under the buttocks, another below the vaginal opening, and another across the lower abdomen.

Until delivery, the fetal heart rate should be monitored frequently. A drop in the fetal heart rate to less than 90 beats per minute indicates fetal distress and should prompt immediate transport with the mother in the left lateral recumbent position. Coach the mother to breathe deeply between contractions and to push with contractions. If the baby does not deliver after 20 minutes of contractions every 2 to 3 minutes, *transport immediately.*

Prepare the OB equipment and don sterile gloves, gown, and goggles. If time permits, wash your hands and forearms before gloving. As the head crowns, control it with gentle pressure. Providing support to the head and perineum decreases the likelihood of vaginal and perineal tearing and decreases the potential for rapid expulsion of the baby's skull through the birth canal which may cause intracranial injury. Support the head as it emerges from the vagina and begins to turn. If it is still enclosed in the amniotic sac, tear the sac open to permit escape of the amniotic fluid and enable the baby to breathe.

Gently slide your finger along the head and neck to ensure that the umbilical cord is not wrapped around the baby's neck. If it is, try to gently slip it over the shoulder and head. If this cannot be done and it is wrapped so tightly as to inhibit labor, carefully place two umbilical cord clamps approximately 2 inches apart and cut the cord between the clamps. As soon as the infant's head is clear of the vagina, instruct the mother to stop pushing. While supporting the head, suction the baby's mouth, then nose, using a bulb syringe. If meconium-stained fluid is noted, suction the mouth, nares, and pharynx with mechanical suction to prevent aspiration. Then tell the mother to resume pushing, while you support the infant's head as it rotates.

Gently guide the baby's head downward to allow delivery of the upper shoulder. Do not pull! Gently guide the baby's body upward to allow delivery of the lower shoulder. Once the head and shoulders have been delivered, the rest of the body will follow rapidly. Be prepared to support the infant's body as it emerges. Remember to keep the baby at the level of the vagina to prevent over- or under-transfusion of blood from the cord. Never "milk" the cord. Clamp and cut the cord as follows (Figure 29-17). Supporting the baby's body, place the first umbilical clamp approximately 10 centimeters from the baby. Place the second clamp approximately 5 centimeters above the first. Then carefully cut the umbilical cord between the clamps. Wipe the baby's face clean of blood and mucus and repeat suctioning of the mouth and nose until the airway is clear. Dry the infant thoroughly and then cover with warm, dry blankets or towels, and position on his side. Record the time of birth.

Figure 29-17 Clamp and cut the cord.

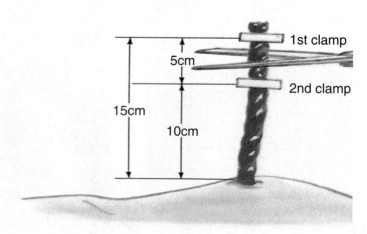

Usual maternal blood loss with delivery is 1 pint (about 500 cc). Following delivery, if the uterus is contracting normally, the fundus should be at the level of the umbilicus and have the size and consistency of a grapefruit. After birth, the mother's vagina should continue to ooze blood. Do not pull on the umbilical cord. Eventually, the cord will appear to lengthen, which indicates separation of the placenta. The placenta should be delivered and transported with the mother to the hospital. If it does deliver, place it in a plastic biohazard bag and bring it to the hospital for evaluation. Retained placenta may cause maternal hemorrhage or become a source of infection. However, there is no need to delay transport for delivery of the placenta. At this time, massage the uterine fundus by placing one hand immediately above the symphysis pubis and the other on the uterine fundus. Cup the uterus between the two hands and support it. Massage until the uterus assumes a woody hardness. Avoid overmassage. Putting the baby to the mother's breast also stimulates uterine contractions, which will further decrease bleeding.

Following delivery, inspect the mother's perineum for tears. If any tears are present, apply direct pressure. Continuously monitor vital signs. Note the presence of continued hemorrhage and report it to medical direction. In some systems, EMT-Is may administer oxytocin (Pitocin) to facilitate uterine contraction in the control of postpartum hemorrhage. Oxytocin should only be administered after delivery of the placenta has been confirmed. Following stabilization, transport the mother and infant to the hospital.

NEONATAL CARE

Care of the **neonate** will be discussed in detail in Chapter 30. Initial care of the neonate has been described in the preceding section. Several additional important considerations regarding routine care of the neonate, APGAR scoring, and neonatal resuscitation are briefly discussed in the following sections.

> **neonate** newborn infant.

Routine Care of the Neonate

Newborns are slippery and will require both hands to support the head and torso. Position yourself so that you can work close to the surface where you have placed the infant.

Maintain warmth! Cold infants rapidly become distressed infants. Quickly dry the infant with towels, discarding each as it becomes wet. Then cover the infant with a dry receiving blanket or use a commercial warming blanket made of a material such as Thinsulate™.

Repeat suctioning of the mouth and nose as needed until the infant's airway is clear. Generally, suctioning and drying the baby will stimulate respirations, crying, and activity. This should cause the infant to "pink up." (Do not be alarmed if the extremities remain dusky. This is known as acrocyanosis and is very common in the first hours of life.) If this is not effective, you may try flicking your finger against the soles of the feet or rubbing gently in a circular motion in the middle of the back (Figure 29-18).

Assess the neonate as soon as possible after birth. The normal neonatal respiratory rate should average 30 to 60 breaths per minute whereas the heart rate should be between 100 to 180 beats per minute. If resuscitation is not indicated, assign APGAR scores. Do not, however, delay resuscitative efforts and transport in order to complete APGAR scoring.

Support the infant's head and torso, using both hands. Maintain warmth, repeat suctioning of the mouth and nose as needed, and assess using APGAR scoring.

APGAR Scoring

Named for Dr. Virginia Apgar, who developed the assessment tool, the APGAR scoring system is a means of evaluating the status of a newborn's vital functions at one minute and five minutes after delivery. There are five parameters and each is given a score from a low value of 0 to a normal value of 2. APGAR is an acronym for the names of the five parameters, which are *A*ppearance (skin color), *P*ulse rate, *G*rimace (irritability), *A*ctivity (muscle tone), and *R*espiratory effort (Table 29-2).

The majority of infants are healthy and active and have total scores between 7 and 10, requiring only routine care. Infants scoring between 4 and 6 are moderately depressed and require oxygen and stimulation to breathe. Infants scoring 0 to 3 are severely depressed and require immediate ventilatory and circulatory assistance. By repeating the

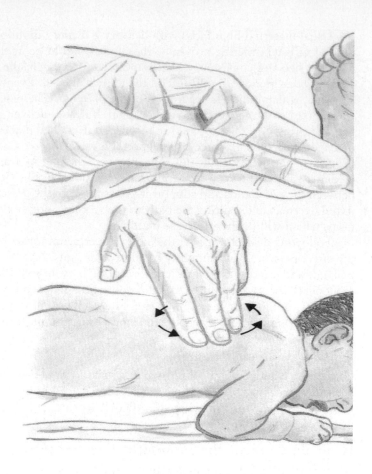

FIGURE 29-18 Stimulate the infant as required.

Table 29-2 THE APGAR SCORE

Element	0	1	2	Score
Appearance (skin color)	Body and extremities blue, pale	Body pink, extremities blue	Completely pink	
Pulse rate	Absent	Below 100/min	100/min or above	
Grimace (Irritability)	No response	Grimace	Cough, sneeze, cry	
Activity (Muscle tone)	Limp	Some flexion of extremities	Active motion	
Respiratory effort	Absent	Slow and irregular	Strong cry	
				TOTAL SCORE =

score at one and five minutes, it is possible to determine whether intervention has caused a change in infant status.

Neonatal Resuscitation

It is estimated that approximately 6% of all neonates born in a hospital require resuscitation. It is likely that this percentage is higher for out-of-hospital deliveries, although the exact numbers are not available. Factors that contribute to the need for resuscitation include prematurity, pregnancy and delivery complications, maternal health problems, or inadequate prenatal care.

If tactile stimulation does not increase the neonate's respiratory rate, immediately assist ventilations using a pediatric bag-valve-mask device attached to high-flow, high-concentration oxygen. Reassess after 15 to 30 seconds. If the respiratory rate is now within normal limits, assess the heart rate. If not, continue ventilations.

Assess the heart rate using a stethoscope to auscultate the apical pulse, by feeling the pulse at the base of the umbilical cord, or by palpating the brachial or femoral artery. The heart rate should normally be between 100 and 180 beats per minute with a range of 140 to 160 beats per minute being optimal. If the pulse is 100 or greater with spontaneous respirations, continue assessment. If less than 100, continue positive pressure ventilations. If less than 80 and not responding to ventilations, initiate chest compressions. Continue to reassess respiratory status and heart rate frequently.

Make every effort to expedite transport to a facility capable of providing neonatal intensive care while you continue resuscitative efforts. If you have a long transport time, it may be necessary to initiate vascular access in order to administer medications or fluid resuscitation. The most logical (and easiest) access is the umbilical vein. If this is not feasible, consider peripheral veins or an intraosseous access. Although many medications (epinephrine, atropine, lidocaine, and naloxone) can be administered via the endotracheal route, this route is not suitable for fluid resuscitation. During transport, continue to maintain warmth while supporting ventilations, oxygenation, and circulation. Refer to Chapter 30 for more information on neonatal resuscitation.

ABNORMAL DELIVERY SITUATIONS

Breech Presentation

Most infants present head first and face down, which is called the vertex position. Breech presentation is the term used to describe the situation in which either the buttocks or both feet present first. This occurs in approximately 4% of all live births. In such presentations, there is an increased risk for delivery trauma to the mother, as well as an increased potential for cord prolapse, cord compression, or anoxic insult for the infant. Although the cause is unknown, breech presentations are most commonly associated with preterm birth, placenta previa, multiple gestation, and uterine and fetal anomalies.

Management   Because cesarean section is often required, delivery of the breech presentation is best accomplished at the hospital. However, if field delivery is unavoidable, the following maneuvers are recommended. First, position the mother with her buttocks at the edge of a firm bed. Ask her to hold her legs in a flexed position. She will often require assistance in doing this. As the infant delivers, do not pull on the infant's legs. Simply support them. Allow the entire body to be delivered with contractions while you merely continue to support the infant's body (Figure 29-19).

As the head passes the pubis, apply gentle upward traction until the mouth appears over the perineum. If the head does not deliver, and the baby begins to breathe spontaneously with its face pressed against the vaginal wall, place a gloved hand in the vagina with the palm toward the infant's face. Form a V with the index and middle fingers on either side of the infant's nose, and push the vaginal wall away from the infant's face to allow unrestricted respiration (Figure 29-20). If necessary, continue during transport.

Alternatively, you may find that the shoulders, not the head, are the most difficult part to deliver. In that case, allow the body to deliver to the level of the umbilicus. Support the infant's body in your palm while gently extracting approximately 4 to 6 inches of umbilical cord. Be very careful that you do not compress the cord during this extraction. Gently rotate the infant's body so that the shoulders are now in an anterior-posterior position. Apply gentle traction to the body until the axilla become visible. Guide the infant's body upward to deliver the posterior shoulder. Then, guide the neonate downward to facilitate delivery of the anterior shoulder. Now gently ease the head through the birth canal. Continue your care of the mother and infant as you would with a normal delivery.

If the infant's respirations are below 30 per minute and tactile stimulation does not increase the rate to a normal range, immediately assist ventilations using a pediatric bag-valve-mask with high-flow oxygen. If the heart rate is below 80 and does not respond to ventilations, initiate chest compressions. Transport to a facility with neonatal intensive care capabilities.

Content Review

ABNORMAL DELIVERIES

- Breech presentation
- Prolapsed cord
- Limb presentation
- Occiput posterior

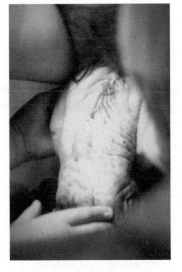

FIGURE 29-19 Breech delivery.

If the infant starts to breathe with face pressed against the vaginal wall, form a V with the index and middle fingers on either side of the infant's nose and push the vaginal wall away from the face. If necessary, continue during transport.

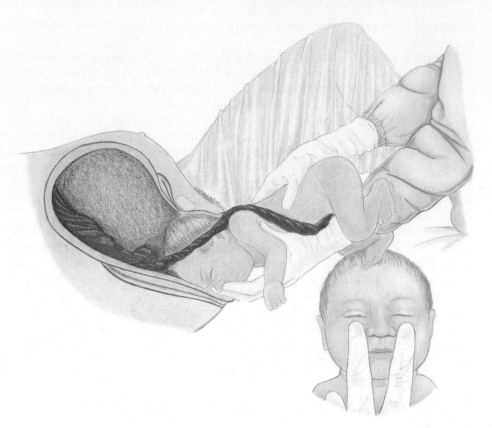

FIGURE 29-20   Placement of the fingers to maintain the airway in a breech birth.

Prolapsed Cord

A *prolapsed cord* occurs when the umbilical cord precedes the fetal presenting part. This causes the cord to be compressed between the fetus and the bony pelvis, shutting off fetal circulation (Figure 29-21). A prolapsed cord occurs once in every 250 deliveries. Predisposing factors include prematurity, multiple births, and premature rupture of the membranes before the head is fully engaged. It is a serious emergency, and fetal death will occur quickly without prompt intervention.

Management   If the umbilical cord is seen in the vagina, insert two fingers of a gloved hand to raise the presenting part of the fetus off the cord. At the same time, gently check the cord for pulsations, but take great care to ensure that you do not compress the cord. Place the mother in a Trendelenburg or knee-chest position (Figure 29-22). Administer high-flow, high-concentration oxygen to the mother and transport her immediately, with the fingers continuing to hold the presenting part off the umbilical cord. If assistance is available, apply a dressing moistened with sterile saline to the exposed cord. *Do not attempt delivery, do not pull on the cord,* and *do not attempt to push the cord back into the vagina!*

Limb Presentation

Sometimes, if the baby is in a transverse lie across the uterus, an arm or leg is the presenting part protruding from the vagina. This is seen in less than 1% of births and is more commonly associated with preterm birth and multiple gestation.

Management   When examination of the perineum reveals a single arm or leg protruding from the birth canal, a cesarean section is necessary. Under no circumstance should you attempt a field delivery. Do not touch the extremity, as to do so may stimulate the infant to gasp, risking inhalation and aspiration of amniotic fluid. *Do not pull on the extremity or attempt to push it back into vagina!*

If the umbilical cord is seen in the vagina, insert two gloved fingers to raise the fetus off the cord. Place the mother in Trendelenburg or knee-chest position, administer oxygen, and transport immediately. Do not attempt delivery.

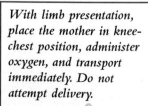

With limb presentation, place the mother in knee-chest position, administer oxygen, and transport immediately. Do not attempt delivery.

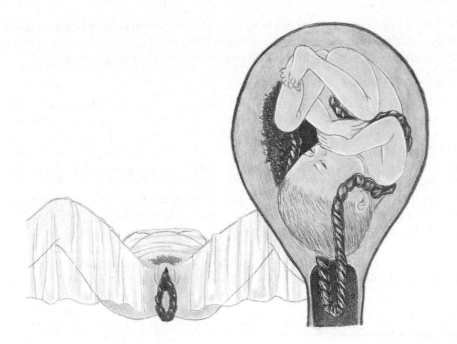

FIGURE 29-21 Prolapsed cord.

- Elevate hips, administer oxygen and keep warm
- Keep baby's head away from cord
- Do not attempt to push cord back
- Wrap cord in sterile moist towel
- Transport mother to hospital, continuing pressure on baby's head

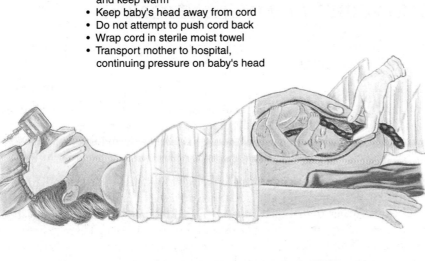

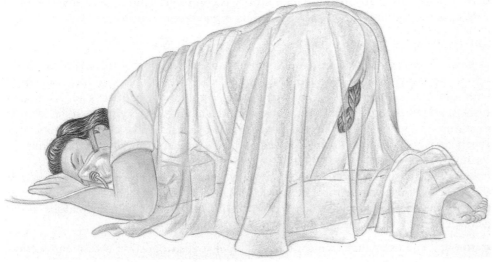

FIGURE 29-22 Patient positioning for prolapsed cord.

Assist the mother into a knee-chest position as is also done when there is a prolapsed cord and administer oxygen via nonrebreather mask. Provide reassurance to the mother. Transport immediately (still in knee-chest position) for emergency cesarean section.

Other Abnormal Presentations

Other abnormal presentations can complicate delivery. One of the most common is the *occiput posterior position*. Normally, as the infant descends into the pelvis, its face is turned posteriorly. This is important, as extension of the head assists delivery. However, if the infant descends facing forward, or occiput posterior, its passage through the pelvis is delayed. This presentation occurs most frequently in primigravidas. In multigravidas it usually resolves spontaneously.

The presenting part may also be the face or brow, rather than the crown of the head. Occasionally, during these presentations, the face or brow can be seen high in the pelvis during a contraction. Usually, vaginal delivery is impossible in these cases.

As described earlier for a limb presentation, the fetus can lie transversely in the uterus. In such a case, the fetus cannot enter the pelvis for delivery. If the membranes rupture, the umbilical cord can prolapse, or an arm or leg can enter the vagina. Vaginal delivery is impossible.

Management Early recognition of an abnormal presentation is important. If one is suspected, the mother should be reassured, placed on oxygen, and transported immediately, since forceps or cesarean delivery is often required.

OTHER DELIVERY COMPLICATIONS

Although most deliveries proceed without incident, complications can arise. Therefore, you should be prepared to deal with them.

Multiple Births

Multiple births are fairly rare, with twins occurring approximately once in every 90 deliveries, about 40% of those being preterm. Usually, the mother knows or at least suspects the presence of more than one fetus. Multiple births should also be suspected if the mother's abdomen remains large after delivery of one baby and labor continues.

Management Manage this situation with the normal delivery guidelines, recognizing that you will need additional personnel and equipment to manage a multiple birth. In twin births, labor often begins earlier than expected, and the infants are generally smaller than babies born singly. Usually, one twin presents vertex and the other breech. There may be one shared placenta or two placentas. After delivery of the first baby, clamp and cut the cord. Then deliver the second baby. Because prematurity is common in multiple births, low birth weight is common and prevention of hypothermia is even more crucial.

Cephalopelvic Disproportion

Cephalopelvic disproportion occurs when the infant's head is too big to pass through the maternal pelvis easily. This may be caused by an oversized fetus. Large fetuses are associated with diabetes, multiparity, or post-maturity. Fetal abnormalities such as hydrocephalus, conjoined twins, or fetal tumors may make vaginal delivery impossible. Women of short stature or women with contracted pelvises are at increased risk for this problem. If cephalopelvic disproportion is not recognized and managed appropriately, fetal demise or uterine rupture may occur.

Cephalopelvic disproportion tends to develop most frequently in the primigravida. Strong contractions may occur for an extended period of time. On physical examination, the fetus may feel large. Also, labor generally does not progress. The fetus may be in distress, as evidenced by fetal bradycardia or meconium staining.

Management The usual management of cephalopelvic disproportion is cesarean section. Administer oxygen to the mother and establish IV access. Transport should be immediate and rapid.

Whenever an abnormal presentation or position of the fetus makes normal delivery impossible, reassure the mother, administer oxygen, and transport immediately. Do not attempt field delivery in these circumstances.

Content Review

OTHER DELIVERY COMPLICATIONS

- Multiple births
- Cephalopelvic disproportion
- Precipitous delivery
- Shoulder dystocia
- Meconium staining

Precipitous Delivery

A precipitous delivery is a delivery that occurs after less than 3 hours of labor. This type of delivery occurs most frequently in the grand multipara and is associated with a higher-than-normal incidence of fetal trauma, tearing of the umbilical cord, or maternal lacerations.

Management   The best way to handle precipitous delivery is to be prepared. Do not turn your attention from the mother. Be ready for a rapid delivery, and attempt to control the infant's head. Once delivered, the baby may have some difficulty with temperature regulation and must be kept warm.

Shoulder Dystocia

A *shoulder dystocia* occurs when the infant's shoulders are larger than its head. This occurs most frequently with diabetic and obese mothers and in post-term pregnancies. In shoulder dystocia, labor progresses normally and the head is delivered routinely. However, immediately after the head is delivered, it retracts back into the perineum because the shoulders are trapped between the symphysis pubis and the sacrum ("turtle sign").

Management   If a shoulder dystocia occurs, do not pull on the infant's head. Administer oxygen to the mother and have her drop her buttocks off the end of the bed. Then flex her thighs upward to facilitate delivery and apply firm pressure with an open hand immediately above the symphysis pubis. If delivery does not occur, transport the patient immediately.

Meconium Staining

Meconium staining occurs when the fetus passes feces into the amniotic fluid. Between 10% and 30% of all deliveries have meconium-stained fluid. It always indicates fetal hypoxic incident. Hypoxia causes an increase in fetal peristalsis along with relaxation of the anal sphincter, causing meconium to pass into the amniotic fluid. In addition to the stress that caused the incident, there is a risk of aspiration of the meconium-stained fluid.

Meconium staining is often associated with prolonged labor but may be seen in term, post-term, and low birth weight infants. The incident may occur a few days before delivery or during labor. Some meconium staining is virtually always associated with breech deliveries. This is due to vagal stimulation, which occurs as a result of the pressure of the contracting uterus on the fetus's head.

Evidence of meconium staining is readily observable. Normally the amniotic fluid is clear or possibly light straw-colored. When meconium is present, the color varies from a light yellowish-green to light green or worst case, dark green, which is sometimes described as "pea soup." As a rule, the thicker and darker the color, the higher the risk of fetal morbidity.

Management   As noted earlier, once the head of the newborn is out of the birth canal you should suction the mouth and nose on the perineum. If the meconium is thin and light colored no further treatment is required, and you should continue with the delivery and routine care. However, if the meconium is thick, visualize the glottis and suction the hypopharynx and trachea using an endotracheal tube until you have cleared all of the meconium from the newborn's airway. Failure to do so will cause the meconium to be pushed farther into the airway and down into the lungs during the delivery process.

If meconium is thick, visualize the infant's glottis and suction the hypopharynx and trachea using an endotracheal tube until all meconium has been cleared from the airway.

MATERNAL COMPLICATIONS OF LABOR AND DELIVERY

Several maternal problems can arise during and after delivery. These include postpartum hemorrhage, uterine rupture, uterine inversion, and pulmonary embolism.

Postpartum Hemorrhage

Postpartum hemorrhage is the loss of more than 500 cc of blood immediately following delivery. It occurs in approximately 5% of deliveries. The most common cause of postpartum hemorrhage is *uterine atony*, or lack of uterine muscle tone. This tends to occur most frequently in the multigravida and is most common following multiple births or births of large infants.

Content Review

MATERNAL COMPLICATIONS
- Postpartum hemorrhage
- Uterine rupture
- Uterine inversion
- Pulmonary embolism

Uterine atony also occurs after precipitous deliveries and prolonged labors. In addition to uterine atony, postpartum hemorrhage can be caused by placenta previa, abruptio placentae, retained placental parts, clotting disorders in the mother, or vaginal and cervical tears. Occasionally, the uterus fails to return to its normal size during the postpartum period, and postpartum hemorrhage occurs long after the birth, potentially as much as 2 weeks postpartum.

Assessment of the patient with postpartum hemorrhage should focus on the history and the predisposing factors described above. You must rely heavily on the clinical appearance of the patient and her vital signs. Often, the uterus will feel boggy and soft on physical examination. Vaginal bleeding is usually obvious as a steady, free flow of blood. Counting the number of sanitary pads used is a good way to monitor the bleeding. When postpartum bleeding occurs in the hospital setting the pads are often weighed, since 500 cc of blood weighs approximately 1 pound. You should also examine the perineum for evidence of traumatic injury, which may be the source of the bleeding.

Management   When confronted by a patient with postpartum hemorrhage, complete the initial assessment immediately. Administer oxygen and begin fundal massage. Establish at least one, preferably two, large-bore IVs of normal saline. If shock is evident, apply anti-shock trousers according to your local protocols. Never attempt to force delivery of the placenta or pack the vagina with dressings. In severe cases, medical direction may request the administration of oxytocin (Pitocin). The usual dose is 10 to 20 USP units (20 mg) oxytocin in one liter of normal saline to run at 125 cc per hour titrated to response. If IV access cannot be obtained, an alternative therapy is to administer 10 USP units intramuscularly.

Uterine Rupture

Uterine rupture is the actual tearing, or rupture, of the uterus. It usually occurs with the onset of labor. However, it can also occur before labor as a result of blunt abdominal trauma. During labor, it often results from prolonged uterine contractions or a surgically scarred uterus, such as occurs from previous cesarean sections, especially in those with the classic vertical incision. It can also occur following a prolonged or obstructed labor, as in the case of cephalopelvic disproportion or in conjunction with abnormal presentations. Although it is a rare occurrence, it carries with it an extremely high maternal and fetal mortality rate.

The patient with uterine rupture will complain of excruciating abdominal pain and will often be in shock. Uterine rupture is virtually always associated with the cessation of labor contractions. If the rupture is complete, the pain usually subsides. On physical examination, there is often profound shock without evidence of external hemorrhage, although it is sometimes associated with vaginal bleeding. Fetal heart tones are absent. The abdomen is often tender and rigid and may exhibit rebound tenderness. It is often possible to palpate the uterus as a separate hard mass found next to the fetus.

Management   Management is the same as for any patient in shock. Administer oxygen at high concentration. Next, establish two large-bore IVs with normal saline and begin fluid resuscitation. Monitor vital signs and fetal heart tones continuously. Transport the patient rapidly. If the fetus is still viable, the definitive treatment is cesarean section with subsequent repair or removal of the uterus.

Uterine Inversion

Uterine inversion is a rare emergency occurring only once in every 2,500 live births. It occurs when the uterus turns inside out after delivery and extends through the cervix. When uterine inversion occurs, the supporting ligaments and blood vessels supplying blood to the uterus are torn, usually causing profound shock. The average blood loss associated with uterine inversion ranges from 800 to 1,800 cc. Uterine inversion usually results from pulling on the umbilical cord while awaiting delivery of the placenta or from attempts to express the placenta when the uterus is relaxed.

Management   If uterine inversion occurs, you must act quickly. First, place the patient in a supine position and begin oxygen administration. Do *not* attempt to detach the placenta or pull on the cord. Initiate two large-bore IVs of normal saline and begin fluid resuscitation. Make one attempt to replace the uterus, using the following technique. With the palm of the hand, push the fundus of the inverted uterus toward the vagina. If this single attempt is unsuccessful, cover the uterus with towels moistened with saline and transport the patient immediately.

Pulmonary Embolism

Pulmonary embolism is the presence of a blood clot in the pulmonary vascular system (see Chapter 19). It can occur after pregnancy, usually as a result of venous thromboembolism. It is one of the most common causes of maternal death and appears to occur more frequently following cesarean section than vaginal delivery. Pulmonary embolism may occur at any time during pregnancy. There is usually a sudden onset of severe dyspnea accompanied by sharp chest pain. Some patients also report a sense of impending doom. On physical examination, the patient may show tachycardia, tachypnea, jugular vein distention, and, in severe cases, hypotension.

Management   Management of pulmonary embolism consists of administration of high-flow, high-concentration oxygen and ventilatory support as needed. Also establish an IV of normal saline at a keep-open rate. Initiate cardiac monitoring and carefully monitor the patient's vital signs and oxygen saturation while transporting her immediately.

> *In the rare occurrence of uterine inversion, begin fluid resuscitation, then make one attempt to replace the uterus. If this fails, cover the uterus with towels moistened with saline and transport immediately.*
>

> *Pulmonary embolism usually presents with sudden severe dyspnea and sharp chest pain. Administer high-flow, high concentration oxygen and support ventilations as needed. Establish an IV of normal saline. Transport immediately, monitoring the heart, vital signs, and oxygen saturation.*
>

SUMMARY

Childbirth is a normal process and obstetrical emergencies are fairly uncommon. However, all pregnant patients are at risk for developing complications, and it is impossible to predict which ones will actually occur. It is therefore important to recognize these complications and act accordingly. Keep in mind that you are caring for two patients, and as long as you remember the priorities of patient care, the situation should go smoothly. Relax and enjoy the opportunity to help bring a new life into the world.

ON THE WEB

For additional practice and review, go to the companion website at www.prenhall.com/bledsoe and click on *Intermediate Emergency Care: Principles & Practice.*

CHAPTER 30

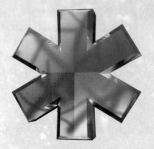

Neonatal Resuscitation

Objectives

After reading this chapter, you should be able to:

1. Define newborn and neonate. (p. 1155)
2. Identify important antepartum factors that can affect childbirth and determine high-risk newborns. (p. 1156)
3. Identify the primary signs utilized for evaluating a newborn during resuscitation. (p. 1158)
4. Identify the appropriate use of the APGAR scale and calculate the APGAR score given various newborn situations. (pp. 1158–1159, also see Chapter 29)
5. Formulate an appropriate treatment plan for providing initial care to a newborn. (p. 1159)
6. Discuss the initial steps in resuscitation of a newborn. (pp. 1162–1170)
7. Describe the indications, equipment needed, application, and evaluation of effectiveness for the following management techniques for the newborn in distress:
   a. Blow-by oxygen (pp. 1167–1168)
   b. Ventilatory assistance (p. 1168)
   c. Chest compressions (pp. 1168–1169)
8. Discuss appropriate transport guidelines for a newborn. (p. 1172)
9. Describe the epidemiology, including the incidence, morbidity/mortality, risk factors and prevention strategies, pathophysiology, assessment findings, and management for the following neonatal problems:
   a. Meconium aspiration (pp. 1159, 1164–1165, 1172–1173)
   b. Bradycardia (pp. 1174–1175)
   c. Respiratory distress/cyanosis (p. 1176)
   d. Hypothermia (p. 1178)
   e. Cardiac arrest (p. 1181)
10. Given several neonatal emergencies, provide the appropriate procedures for assessment, management, and transport. (pp. 1155–1181)

CASE STUDY

A storm rages outside, making travel dangerous. Around midnight, you receive a call from the dispatcher. A woman has just gone into labor. She lives about 20 minutes from the hospital, but her husband is worried about weather conditions and requests help from your EMS unit.

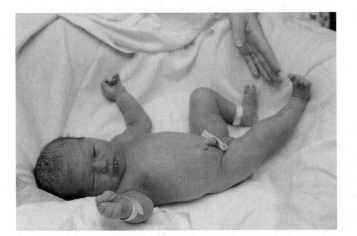
Upon arrival, you find a 24-year-old female who is about to deliver her second baby. You quickly determine that there is not enough time to transport the patient to the hospital. You and your partner begin to prepare the equipment needed for a field delivery.

The delivery goes beautifully, and you announce the arrival of the couple's new daughter. Following the birth, however, the baby remains blue and limp—even after you suction the airway. You quickly dry the baby and then wrap her in a dry blanket. You stimulate the baby by rubbing her back and flicking the soles of her feet gently. Once again, you suction the baby, first the mouth and then the nose.

When the baby stays blue and limp, you push aside a very normal urge to panic and deliver blow-by oxygen. When her heart rate remains less than 100, you grab the bag-valve-mask unit and apply artificial ventilation. The baby "pinks up" almost immediately and begins to cry.

Using the pulse oximeter, you determine that the oxygen saturation is 95% and increasing. You prepare the baby for transport, making sure her head is covered. You ask the mother to hold her new daughter and then load both of your patients into the ambulance.

En route to the hospital, you continue to administer blow-by oxygen and assign a five-minute APGAR score of 9. The trip is uneventful. The baby leaves the hospital only one day after the mother. The parents later pay a surprise visit to your EMS unit. They proudly introduce a healthy baby daughter, who is named after you.

INTRODUCTION

Babies pass through stages of physical and emotional development. This chapter concerns itself with babies one month old and under. Babies less than one month old are called neonates. Recently born **neonates**—those in the first few hours of their lives—may also be called **newborns** or newly born infants (Figure 30-1).

After an unscheduled delivery in the field, you have two patients to manage—the mother and the baby. You can review information on care of the mother in Chapter 29. The present chapter describes the initial care of newborns, focusing on the special needs of distressed and premature newborns.

neonate an infant from the time of birth to one month of age.

newborn a baby in the first few hours of his life; also called a newly born infant.

After an unscheduled delivery in the field, you have two patients to manage—the mother and the baby.

GENERAL PATHOPHYSIOLOGY, ASSESSMENT, AND MANAGEMENT

The care of newborns follows the same priorities as for all patients. You should complete the initial assessment first. Correct any problems detected during the initial assessment before proceeding to the next step. The vast majority of newborns require no resuscitation beyond suctioning the airway, mild stimulation, and maintenance of body temperature.

FIGURE 30-1 Term newborn.

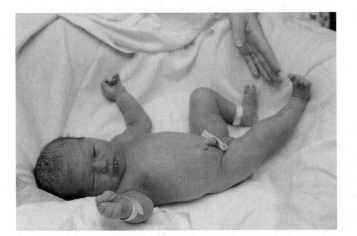

Table 30-1	RISK FACTORS INDICATING POSSIBLE COMPLICATIONS IN NEWBORNS	
Antepartum Factors	**Intrapartum Factors**	
Multiple gestation	Premature labor	
Inadequate prenatal care	Meconium-stained amniotic fluid	
Mother's age (<16 or >35)	Rupture of membranes more than 24 hours before delivery	
History of perinatal morbidity or mortality	Use of narcotics within 4 hours of delivery	
Post-term gestation	Abnormal presentation	
Drugs/medications	Prolonged labor or precipitous delivery	
Toxemia, hypertension, diabetes	Prolapsed cord or bleeding	

For newborns who require additional care, your quick actions can make the difference between life and death.

antepartum before the onset of labor.

intrapartum occurring during childbirth.

Your success in treating at-risk newborns increases with training, ongoing practice, and proper stocking of equipment on board the ambulance.

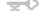

extrauterine outside the uterus.

ductus arteriosus channel between the main pulmonary artery and the aorta of the fetus.

The time of a newborn's first breath is unrelated to the cutting of the umbilical cord.

However, for newborns who require additional care, your quick actions can make the difference between life and death.

EPIDEMIOLOGY

Approximately 6% of field deliveries require life support. The incidence of complications increases as the birth weight decreases. About 80% of newborns weighing less than 1,500 grams (3 pounds, 5 ounces) at birth require resuscitation. Determine at-risk newborns by considering the **antepartum** and **intrapartum** factors that may indicate complications at the time of delivery (Table 30-1).

Your success in resuscitating these at-risk infants increases with training, ongoing practice, and proper stocking of equipment on board the ambulance. Make sure your ambulance carries a basic obstetrical (OB) kit and resuscitation equipment for newborns of various sizes. (See the list under "Resuscitation," later in this chapter.)

Plan transport in advance. Know the type of facilities available in your locality and local protocols governing use of these facilities. A nearby neonatal intensive care unit (NICU) makes the best choice for at-risk newborns. However, if you must transport to a distant NICU, determine whether it might be in the best interests of the infant to transport him or her to the nearest facility for stabilization. Follow local protocols and consult medical direction as needed.

PATHOPHYSIOLOGY

Upon birth, dramatic changes occur within the newborn to prepare him for **extrauterine** life. The respiratory system, which is essentially nonfunctional when the fetus is in the uterus, must suddenly initiate and maintain respirations. While in the uterus, fetal lung fluid fills the fetal lungs. The capillaries and arterioles of the lungs are closed. Most blood pumped by the heart bypasses the nonfunctional respiratory system by flowing through the **ductus arteriosus.**

Approximately one-third of fetal lung fluid is removed through compression of the chest during vaginal delivery. Under normal conditions, the newborn takes his first breath within the first few seconds after delivery. The timing of the first breath is unrelated to the cutting of the umbilical cord. Factors that stimulate the baby's first breath include:

- Mild acidosis
- Initiation of stretch reflexes in the lungs
- Hypoxia
- Hypothermia

With the first breaths, the lungs rapidly fill with air, which displaces the remaining fetal fluid. The pulmonary arterioles and capillaries open, decreasing pulmonary vascular resistance. At this point, the resistance to blood flow in the lungs is now less than the resistance of the ductus arteriosus. Because of this pressure difference, blood flow is diverted from the ductus arteriosus to the lungs, where it picks up oxygen for transport to the peripheral tissues (Figure 30-2).

Soon, there is no need for the ductus arteriosus, and it eventually closes. However, if hypoxia or severe acidosis occurs, the pulmonary vascular bed may constrict again and the

FIGURE 30-2 Hemodynamic
changes in the newborn at birth.

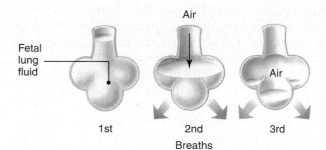

Air

Fetal
lung
fluid

Air

1st   2nd   3rd
Breaths

Following birth, the lungs
expand as they are filled with air.
The fetal lung fluid gradually
leaves the alveoli.

Arterioles dilate and blood flow increases

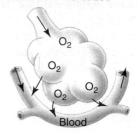

O_2
O_2
O_2
O_2
O_2
Blood

At the same time as the lungs
are expanding and the fetal lung
fluid is clearing, the arterioles in
the lung begin to open, allowing
a considerable increase in the
amount of blood flowing through
the lungs.

Pulmonary blood flow increases

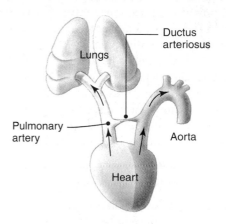

Ductus
arteriosus
Lungs

Pulmonary
artery
Aorta

Heart

Blood previously diverted
through the ductus arteriosus
flows through the lungs where it
picks up oxygen to transport to
tissues throughout the body.
Soon there is no need for the
ductus and it eventually closes.

ductus may reopen. This will retrigger fetal circulation with its attendant shunting and ongoing hypoxia. (This condition is called **persistent fetal circulation.**) To help the newborn make his transition to extrauterine life, it is very important for the EMT-I to facilitate the first few breaths and to prevent ongoing hypoxia and acidosis.

Remain alert at all times to signs of respiratory distress. Infants are susceptible to hypoxemia, which can lead to permanent brain damage. After initial hypoxia, the infant rapidly gasps for breath. If the asphyxia continues, respiratory movements cease altogether, the heart rate begins to fall, and neuromuscular tone gradually diminishes. The infant then enters a period of apnea known as *primary apnea*. In most cases, simple stimulation and exposure to oxygen will reverse bradycardia and assist in the development of pulmonary perfusion.

With ongoing asphyxia, however, the infant will enter a period known as *secondary apnea*. During secondary apnea, the infant takes several last, deep gasping respirations. The heart rate, blood pressure, and oxygen saturation in the blood continue to fall. The infant becomes unresponsive to stimulation and will not spontaneously resume respiration on his own. Death will occur unless you promptly initiate resuscitation. For this reason, always assume that apnea in the newborn is secondary apnea and rapidly treat with ventilatory assistance including oxygen and, when appropriate, chest compressions.

Congenital Anomalies

Approximately 2% of infants are born with some sort of congenital problem. Congenital problems typically arise from a problem in fetal development. Most fetal development

persistent fetal circulation
condition in which blood
continues to bypass the fetal
respiratory system, resulting in
ongoing hypoxia.

*Always assume that apnea
in the newborn is secondary
apnea and rapidly treat
with ventilatory assistance.*

occurs during the first trimester of pregnancy. It is during this time that the developing fetus is most sensitive to environmental factors and substances that can affect normal development.

There are many types of congenital anomalies. These may affect a single organ or structure or may affect many organs or structures. Several recognized patterns, called *syndromes,* can occur. It is not within the scope of this text to discuss all the various congenital anomalies. However, a few congenital anomalies can make resuscitation more difficult. For example, some children may be born with a defect in the diaphragm that allows some of the abdominal contents to enter the chest. This abnormality is referred to as a **diaphragmatic hernia.** If you suspect a diaphragmatic hernia, do not treat the infant with BVM ventilation. This procedure will distend the stomach, which protrudes into the chest cavity, thus decreasing ventilatory capacity. Instead, immediately intubate the infant. (Diaphragmatic hernia will be discussed in more detail later in this chapter.)

Some infants are born with a defect in their spinal cords. In some cases, the spinal cord and associated structures may be exposed. This abnormality is called a **meningomyelocele.** Infants born with a meningomyelocele should not be placed on their backs. Instead, place them on their stomachs or sides and conduct resuscitation in this position, if possible. Cover the spinal defect with sterile gauze pads soaked in warm sterile saline and inserted in a plastic covering.

A newborn may exhibit a defect in the area of the umbilicus. In some cases, the abdominal contents will fill this defect, resulting in an **omphalocele.** If you encounter a newborn with an omphalocele, cover the defect with an occlusive plastic covering to decrease water and heat loss.

Since newborns are obligate nose breathers, **choanal atresia** can cause upper airway obstruction and respiratory distress. Choanal atresia is the most common birth defect involving the nose and is due to the presence of a bony or membranous septum between the nasal cavity and the pharynx. Suspect this condition if you are unable to pass a catheter through either nare into the oropharynx. An oral airway will usually bypass the obstruction.

A fairly common congenital anomaly is cleft lip and cleft palate. During fetal development, the lip and palate come together in the middle forming the oral cavity. Failure of the palate to completely close during fetal development can result in a defect known as **cleft palate.** Cleft palate may also be associated with failure of the upper lip to close. This condition, referred to as **cleft lip,** can make it difficult to obtain an adequate seal for effective mask ventilation. If a child with a cleft lip or cleft palate will require more than brief mechanical ventilation, you should place an endotracheal tube.

Pierre Robin Syndrome is a congenital condition characterized by a small jaw and large tongue in conjunction with a cleft palate. In this condition, the tongue is likely to obstruct the upper airway. A nasal or oral airway usually bypasses the obstruction. If the obstruction cannot be bypassed with a simple airway, then intubation will be necessary, although it can be very difficult to carry out on newborns with this condition.

ASSESSMENT

Assess the newborn immediately after birth. (Ideally, if two EMT-Is are available, one EMT-I attends the mother, while the other attends the newborn.) Make a mental note of the time of birth and then quickly obtain vital signs. Remember that newborns are slippery and will require both hands to support the head and torso. Position yourself so that you can work close to the surface where you have placed the infant.

The newborn's respiratory rate should average 40 to 60 breaths per minute. If respirations are not adequate or if the newborn is gasping, immediately start positive-pressure ventilation.

Expect a normal heart rate of 150 to 180 beats per minute at birth, slowing to 130 to 140 beats per minute thereafter. A pulse rate of less than 100 beats per minute indicates distress and requires emergency intervention.

Evaluate the skin color as well. Some cyanosis of the extremities is common immediately after birth. However, cyanosis of the central part of the body is abnormal, as is persistent peripheral cyanosis. In such cases, administer 100% oxygen until the cause is determined or the condition is corrected.

APGAR SCALE

As discussed in Chapter 29, as soon as possible, assign the newborn an **APGAR score.** (See Table 29-2 in Chapter 29.) Ideally, try to do this at one and five minutes after birth. How-

---

diaphragmatic hernia protrusion of abdominal contents into the thoracic cavity through an opening in the diaphragm.

meningomyelocele herniation of the spinal cord and membranes through a defect in the spinal column.

omphalocele congenital hernia of the umbilicus.

choanal atresia congenital closure of the passage between the nose and pharynx by a bony or membranous structure.

cleft palate congenital fissure in the roof of the mouth, forming a passageway between oral and nasal cavities.

cleft lip congenital vertical fissure in the upper lip.

Pierre Robin Syndrome unusually small jaw, combined with a cleft palate, downward displacement of the tongue, and an absent gag reflex.

APGAR scoring a numerical system of rating the condition of a newborn.

Content Review

APGAR
- Appearance
- Pulse rate
- Grimace
- Activity
- Respiratory effort

ever, if the newborn is not breathing, DO NOT withhold resuscitation to determine the AP-GAR score. The APGAR scoring system helps distinguish between newborns who need only routine care and those who need greater assistance. The system also predicts long-term survival. A score of 0, 1, or 2 is given for each of the above parameters. The minimum total score is 0 and the maximum is 10. A score of 7 to 10 indicates an active and vigorous newborn who requires only routine care. A score of 4 to 6 indicates a moderately distressed newborn who requires oxygenation and stimulation. Severely distressed newborns, those with APGAR scores of less than 4, require immediate resuscitation.

TREATMENT

Treatment starts before delivery. Begin care by preparing the environment and assembling the equipment needed for delivery and immediate care of the newborn. The initial care of a newborn follows the same priorities as for all patients. Complete the initial assessment first. Correct any problems detected during the initial assessment before proceeding to the next step. The vast majority of term newborns—approximately 80%—require no resuscitation beyond suctioning of the airway, mild stimulation, and maintenance of body temperature by drying and warming with blankets.

Establishing the Airway

Airway management is one of the most critical steps in caring for the newborn. During delivery, fluid is forced out of the baby's lungs, into the oropharynx, and out through the nose and mouth. Fluid drainage occurs independently of gravity. As soon as you deliver the newborn's head, suction the mouth and then the nose, using a bulb suction. Always suction the mouth first so that there is nothing for the infant to aspirate if he or she gasps when the nose is suctioned.

Immediately following delivery, maintain the newborn at the same level as the mother's vagina, with the head approximately 15 degrees below the torso. This facilitates the drainage of secretions and helps to prevent aspiration. If there appears to be a large amount of secretions, attach a **DeLee suction trap** to a suction source. As previously explained, suction the mouth first and then the nose (Figure 30-3a). Repeat these steps until the airway is clear. If you detect **meconium,** prepare intubation equipment and a meconium aspirator (Figure 30-3b). (Meconium staining will be discussed in more detail in several later sections of this chapter.)

Drying and suctioning produce enough stimulation to initiate respirations in most newborns. If the newborn does not immediately cry, stimulate him by flicking the soles of his feet or gently rubbing his back (Figure 30-4). DO NOT spank or vigorously rub a newborn baby.

Prevention of Heat Loss

Heat loss can be a life-threatening condition in newborns. Cold infants quickly become distressed infants. Heat loss occurs through evaporation, convection, conduction, and radiation. Most heat loss in newborns results from evaporation. The newborn comes into the world wet, and the amniotic fluid quickly evaporates. Immediately after birth, the newborn's core temperature can drop 1°C (1.8°F) or more from his birth temperature of 38°C (100.4°F).

Loss of heat can also occur through convection, depending on the temperature of the room and the movement of the air around the newborn. The newborn can lose additional heat through contact with surrounding surfaces (convection) or by radiating heat to colder objects nearby.

To prevent heat loss, take these steps:

- Dry the newborn immediately to prevent evaporative cooling (Figure 30-5).
- Maintain the ambient temperature—the temperature in the delivery room or ambulance—at a *minimum* of 23°C to 24°C (74°F to 76°F).
- Close all windows and doors.

FIGURE 30-3A Suctioning of the mouth using flexible suction catheter.

When head is delivered

As soon as the baby's head is delivered (prior to delivery of the shoulders) *the mouth, oropharynx, and hypopharynx should be thoroughly suctioned,* using a 10 Fr. DeLee suction catheter or other flexible suction catheter. Any catheter used should be no smaller than a 10 Fr.

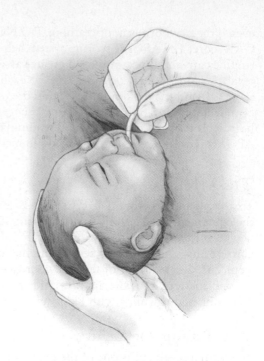

FIGURE 30-3B Intubation for removal of residual meconium.

Following delivery

After delivery of the infant, if a great deal of meconium is present, the trachea should be intubated and any residual meconium removed from the lower airway.

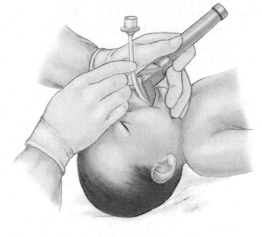

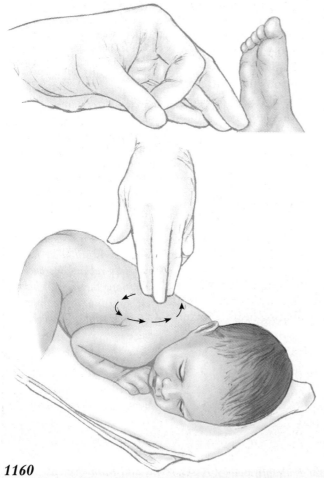

FIGURE 30-4 Stimulate the newborn as required.

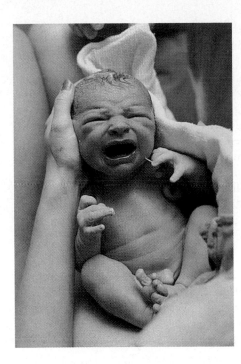

FIGURE 30-5 Dry the infant to prevent loss of evaporative heat.

- Discard the towel used to dry the newborn and swaddle the infant in a warm, dry receiving blanket or other suitable material. Cover the head.
- In colder areas, place well-insulated water bottles or rubber gloves filled with warm water (40°C or 104°F) around the newborn to help maintain a warm body temperature. To avoid burns, do not place these items against the skin. Be sure the newborn is wrapped in a blanket, and place the water bottle or rubber glove against the blanket.

Cutting the Umbilical Cord

After you have stabilized the newborn's airway and minimized heat loss, clamp and cut the umbilical cord. You can prevent over- and under-transfusion of blood by maintaining the baby at the same level as the vagina, as previously described. Do not "milk" or strip the umbilical cord, since this increases blood viscosity, or **polycythemia**. Polycythemia can cause cardiopulmonary problems. It can also contribute to excessive red blood cell destruction, which may in turn lead to **hyperbilirubinemia**—an increased level of bilirubin in the blood that causes jaundice.

Apply the umbilical clamps within 30 to 45 seconds after birth. Place the first clamp approximately 10 centimeters (four inches) from the newborn. Place the second clamp about five centimeters (two inches) farther away than the first. Then cut the cord between the two clamps. (See Figure 29-17 in Chapter 29.) After the cord is cut, inspect it periodically to make sure there is no additional bleeding.

THE DISTRESSED NEWBORN

The distressed newborn can be either full term or premature. (See "Premature Infants" later in this chapter.) The presence of fetal meconium at birth indicates that fetal distress has occurred at some point during pregnancy. If the newborn is simply meconium stained, then distress may have occurred at a remote time. If you see *particulate* meconium, however, distress may have occurred recently and the newborn should be managed accordingly.

Aspiration of meconium can cause significant respiratory problems and should be prevented. Whenever you spot meconium during delivery, do not induce respiratory effort until you have removed the meconium from the trachea by suctioning under direct

Do not "milk" or strip the umbilical cord.

polycythemia an excess of red blood cells. In a newborn, the condition may reflect hypovolemia or prolonged intrauterine hypoxia.

hyperbilirubinemia an excessive amount of bilirubin—the orange-colored pigment associated with bile—in the blood. In newborns, the condition appears as jaundice. Precipitating factors include maternal Rh or ABO incompatibility, neonatal septis, anoxia, hypoglycemia, and congenital liver or gastrointestinal defects.

visualization with the laryngoscope. (This will be discussed in more detail under "Meconium Stained Amniotic Fluid.") Be sure to report the presence of meconium to the medical direction physician.

The most common problems experienced by newborns during the first minutes of life involve the airway. For this reason, resuscitation usually consists of ventilation and oxygenation. Except in special situations, the use of IV fluids, drugs, or cardiac equipment is usually not indicated. (See "Inverted Pyramid for Resuscitation" below.) The most important procedures include suctioning, drying, and stimulating the distressed newborn.

Of the vital signs, fetal heart rate is the most important indicator of neonatal distress. The newborn has a relatively fixed stroke volume. Thus, cardiac output depends more on heart rate. Bradycardia, as caused by hypoxia, results in decreased cardiac output and, ultimately, poor perfusion. A pulse rate of less than 60 beats per minute in a distressed newborn should be treated with chest compressions. In distressed newborns, monitor the heart rate manually. Do not depend on external electronic monitors.

Of the vital signs, fetal heart rate is the most important indicator of neonatal distress.

RESUSCITATION

The vast majority of newborns do not require resuscitation beyond stimulation, maintenance of the airway, and maintenance of body temperature. Unfortunately, it is difficult to predict which newborns ultimately will require resuscitation. Each EMS unit, therefore, should contain a neonatal resuscitation kit with the following items:

- Neonatal BVM unit
- Bulb syringe
- DeLee suction trap
- Meconium aspirator
- Laryngoscope with size 0 and 1 blades
- Uncuffed endotracheal tubes (2.5, 3.0, 3.5, 4.0) with appropriate suction catheters
- Endotracheal tube stylet
- Tape or device to secure endotracheal tube
- Umbilical catheter and 10 mL syringe
- Three-way stopcock
- 20 mL syringe and 8 French feeding tube for gastric suction
- Glucometer
- Assorted syringes and needles
- Towels (sterile)
- Medications:
  - Epinephrine 1:10,000 and 1:1,000
  - Neonatal naloxone (Narcon)
  - Volume expander (lactated Ringer's solution or saline)

INVERTED PYRAMID FOR RESUSCITATION

Resuscitation of the newborn follows an inverted pyramid (Figure 30-6). As this pyramid indicates, most distressed newborns respond to relatively simple maneuvers. Few require CPR or advanced life support measures.

The following are steps for the initial care of the newborn. Also see the resuscitation steps illustrated in Procedure 30-1 and Figure 30-7.

Step 1: Drying, Warming, Positioning, Suctioning, and Tactile Stimulation

Resuscitation begins with drying, warming, positioning, suctioning, and stimulating the newborn. Immediately upon delivery, minimize heat loss by drying the newborn. Next, place the newborn in a warm, dry blanket. Make sure the environment is warm and free of drafts.

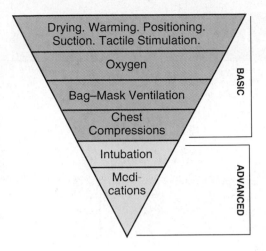

FIGURE 30-6 The inverted pyramid of neonatal resuscitation, showing approximate relative frequencies of neonatal care and resuscitative efforts. Note that a majority of infants respond to the simple measures noted at the top (wide part) of the pyramid.

NORMAL NEWBORN ASSESSMENT AND SUPPORT

Temperature: Dry, warm
Airway: Position, suction
Breathing: Gentle stimulation to cry
Circulation: Pulse rate, color

ASSISTANCE SOME NEWBORNS MAY REQUIRE

(Note: Moving down the list, progressively fewer patients will require the listed interventions.)

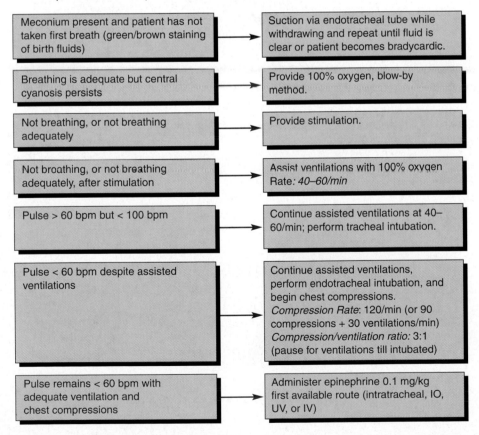

Meconium present and patient has not taken first breath (green/brown staining of birth fluids)	Suction via endotracheal tube while withdrawing and repeat until fluid is clear or patient becomes bradycardic.
Breathing is adequate but central cyanosis persists	Provide 100% oxygen, blow-by method.
Not breathing, or not breathing adequately	Provide stimulation.
Not breathing, or not breathing adequately, after stimulation	Assist ventilations with 100% oxygen Rate: *40–60/min*
Pulse > 60 bpm but < 100 bpm	Continue assisted ventilations at 40–60/min; perform tracheal intubation.
Pulse < 60 bpm despite assisted ventilations	Continue assisted ventilations, perform endotracheal intubation, and begin chest compressions. *Compression Rate*: 120/min (or 90 compressions + 30 ventilations/min) *Compression/ventilation ratio:* 3:1 (pause for ventilations till intubated)
Pulse remains < 60 bpm with adequate ventilation and chest compressions	Administer epinephrine 0.1 mg/kg first available route (intratracheal, IO, UV, or IV)

FIGURE 30-7 Resuscitation of the newborn. *(Adapted from David S. Markenson,* Pediatric Prehospital Care, *Prentice Hall, 2002)*

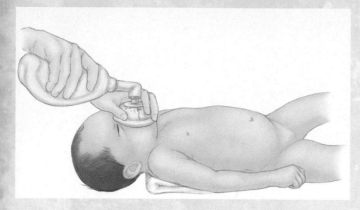

30-1a Ventilate with 100% oxygen for 15 to 30 seconds.

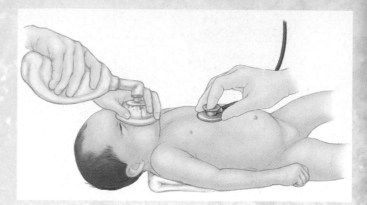

30-1b Evaluate heart rate.

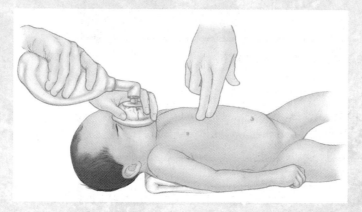

30-1c Initiate chest compressions if: heart rate less than 60, or between 60 and 80 and **not** increasing.

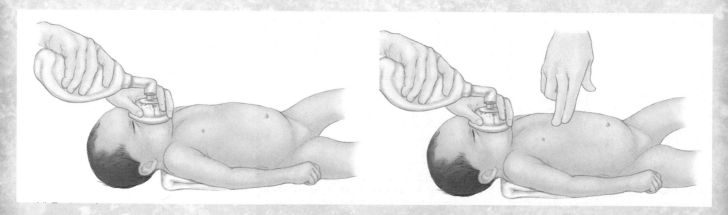

30-1d Evaluate heart rate: below 80—continue chest compressions; 80 or above—discontinue chest compressions.

CORRECT

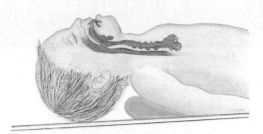

Neck slightly extended

Care should be taken to prevent hyperextension or underextension of the neck since either may decrease air entry.

INCORRECT

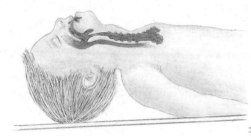

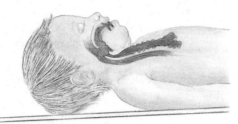

Neck hyperextended   Neck underextended

FIGURE 30-8   Positioning the newborn to open the airway.

Table 30-2	GUIDELINES FOR TRACHEAL TUBE SIZES AND DEPTH OF INSERTION IN THE NEWBORN		
Tube Size (mm) ID	**Depth of Insertion from Upper Lip (cm)**	**Weight (g)**	**Gestation (wk)**
2.5	6.5–7	<1,000	<28
3.0	7–8	1,000–2,000	28–34
3.5	8–9	2,000–3,000	34–38
3.5–4.0	>9	>3,000	>38

After you have dried the newborn, place the infant on his back with his head slightly below his body and his neck slightly extended (Figure 30-8). This facilitates drainage of secretions and fluids from the lungs. Place a small blanket, folded to a 2 centimeter (¾ inch) thickness, under the newborn's shoulders to help maintain this position.

Next, suction the newborn again, using a bulb syringe or DeLee suction trap. Deep suctioning can cause a **vagal response**, resulting in bradycardia. Because of this, suctioning should last no longer than 10 seconds. If meconium is present, avoid stimulating the infant and visualize the airway with a laryngoscope. Suction the meconium, preferably with a DeLee suction trap. If there is a great deal of meconium, place an appropriately sized endotracheal tube (Table 30-2) and suction the meconium directly through the tube. Remove the tube and discard. Do not use the same tube for mechanical ventilation. (See Procedure 30-2.) Following adequate tracheal suctioning, stimulate the newborn by flicking the soles of his feet or rubbing his back.

Suctioning of a newborn should last no longer than 10 seconds.

vagal response stimulation of the vagus nerve causing a parasympathetic response.

Endotracheal Intubation and Tracheal Suctioning in the Newborn

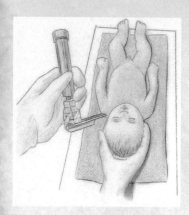

30-2a   Position the infant.

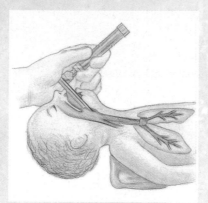

30-2b   Insert the laryngoscope.

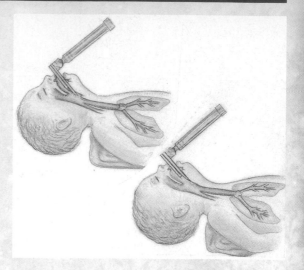

30-2c   Elevate the epiglottis by lifting.

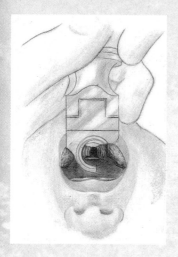

30-2d   Visualize the cords.

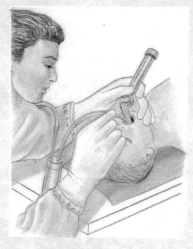

30-2e   Suction any meconium present.

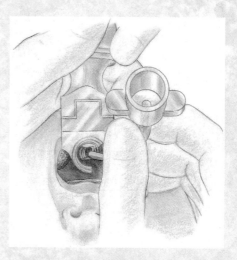

30-2f   Insert a fresh tube for ventilation.

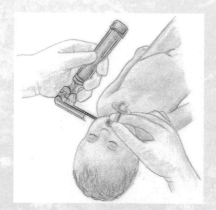

30-2g   Remove the laryngoscope.

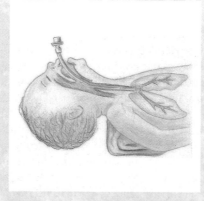

30-2h   Check proper tube placement.

After carrying out the preceding procedures, assess the newborn as noted below.

Newborn Assessment Parameters

- *Respiratory effort.* The rate and depth of the newborn's breathing should increase immediately with tactile stimulation. If the respiratory response is adequate, evaluate the heart rate next. If the respiratory rate is inadequate, begin positive-pressure ventilation (see Step 3).

- *Heart rate.* As noted earlier, heart rate is critical in the newborn. Check the heart rate by listening to the apical area of the heart with a stethoscope, feeling the pulse by lightly grasping the umbilical cord, or feeling either the brachial or femoral pulse. If the heart rate is greater than 100 and spontaneous respirations are present, continue the assessment. If the heart rate is less than 100, immediately begin positive-pressure ventilation (see Step 3).

- *Color.* A newborn may be cyanotic despite a heart rate greater than 100 and spontaneous respirations. If you note central cyanosis, or cyanosis of the chest and abdomen, in a newborn with adequate ventilation and a pulse rate greater than 100, administer supplemental oxygen (see Step 2). Newborns with peripheral cyanosis do not usually need supplemental oxygen UNLESS the cyanosis is prolonged.

- *APGAR score.* Unless resuscitation is required, obtain one-minute and five-minute APGAR scores.

Step 2: Supplemental Oxygen

If central cyanosis is present or the adequacy of ventilation is uncertain, administer supplemental oxygen by blowing oxygen across the newborn's face (Figure 30-9). If possible, the oxygen should be warmed and humidified. Continue oxygen administration until the newborn's color has improved. Although oxygen toxicity is a concern, this condition usually results from prolonged usage over several days. Administration of blow-by oxygen in the

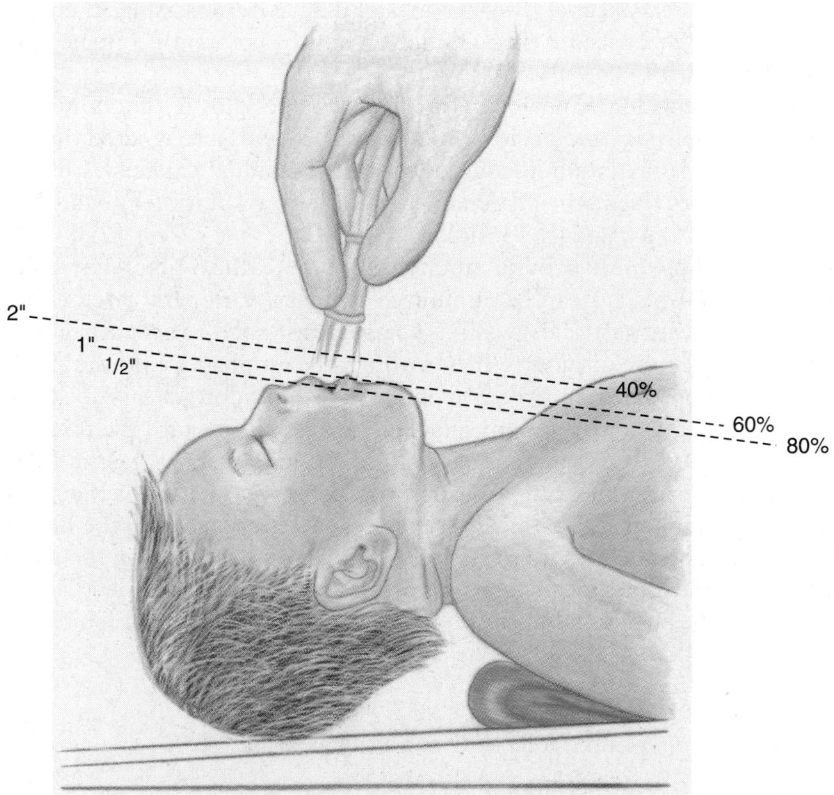

Content Review

NEWBORN ASSESSMENT PARAMETERS
- Respiratory effort
- Heart rate
- Color
- APGAR score

Content Review

NORMAL NEWBORN VITAL SIGNS
- Respirations 30–60
- Heart rate 100–180
- Blood pressure 60–90 systolic
- Temperature 36.7°C to 37.8°C (98°F to 100°F)

FIGURE 30-9 Guidelines for estimating oxygen concentration. Based on oxygen flow rate of 5 liters per minute.

prehospital setting will not cause problems. NEVER DEPRIVE A NEWBORN OF OXYGEN IN THE PREHOSPITAL SETTING FOR FEAR OF OXYGEN TOXICITY.

Step 3: Ventilation

Begin positive-pressure ventilation if any of the following conditions is present:

- Heart rate less than 100 beats per minute
- Apnea
- Persistence of central cyanosis after administration of supplemental oxygen

A ventilatory rate of 40 to 60 breaths per minute is usually adequate. A BVM unit is the device of choice. A self-inflating bag of an appropriate size (450 mL is optimal) should be used. Many self-inflating bags have a pressure-limiting pop-off valve that is preset at 30 to 45 cm/H_2O. However, since the initial pressures required to ventilate a newborn may be as high as 60 cm/H_2O, you may have to depress the pop-off valve to deactivate it and ensure adequate ventilation. If prolonged ventilation is required, it may be necessary to disable the pop-off valve.

Face masks in various sizes must be available. The most effective ones are designed to fit the contours of the newborn's face and have a low dead space volume (less than 5 mL). When a mask is correctly sized and positioned, it covers the newborn's nose and mouth, but not the eyes.

Endotracheal intubation of a newborn should be carried out in the following situations:

- BVM unit does not work.
- Tracheal suctioning is required (such as in cases of thick meconium).
- Prolonged ventilation will be required.
- Diaphragmatic hernia is suspected.
- Inadequate respiratory effort is found.

Because of the narrowness of the neonatal airway at the level of the cricoid cartilage, always use an *uncuffed* endotracheal tube. (Review Table 30-2.) After inserting it, ensure proper placement by noting symmetrical chest wall motion and equal breath sounds. (Review Procedure 30-2.)

glottic function opening and closing of the glottic space.

PEEP positive end-expiratory pressure.

Intubation has several effects in the newborn. First, it bypasses **glottic function**. Second, it eliminates **PEEP**—the physiologic positive end-expiratory pressure created during normal coughing and crying. To maintain adequate functional residual capacity, a PEEP of 2 to 4 cm/H_2O should be provided when mechanical ventilation is initiated by adding a magnetic-disk PEEP valve to the bag-valve outlet.

Gastric distention, caused by a leak around an uncuffed endotracheal tube, may compromise ventilation of a newborn. This can be minimized by using a properly sized endotracheal tube. If there is significant gastric distension, a **nasogastric tube** or **orogastric tube** should be inserted (through the nose or mouth, then through the esophagus into the stomach) as soon as the airway is controlled. It is recommended that the endotracheal tube be in place before the gastric tube is placed to avoid misplacing the gastric tube into the trachea.

nasogastric tube/orogastric tube a tube that runs through the nose or mouth and esophagus into the stomach, used for administering liquid nutrients or medications or for removing air or liquids from the stomach.

Make sure the newborn is well oxygenated before attempting to insert a gastric tube. To determine the depth of insertion, measure a nasogastric tube from the tip of the nose, around the ear, to below the xiphoid process. Measure an orogastric tube from the lips to below the xiphoid process. Lubricate the end of the tube and pass it gently along the nasal floor or the mouth and into the esophagus. Confirm that the tube is in the stomach by injecting 10 cc of air into the tube and auscultating a bubbling sound, or sound of rushing air, over the epigastrium.

Step 4: Chest Compressions

Initiate chest compressions if *either* of the following conditions exists:

- Heart rate is less than 60 beats per minute.
- Heart rate is between 60 and 80, *but does not increase* with 30 seconds of positive-pressure ventilation and supplemental oxygenation.

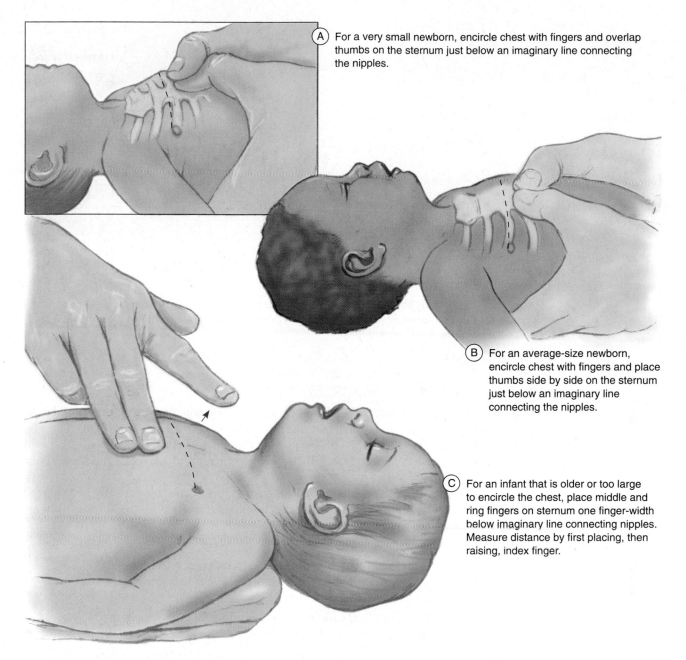

A) For a very small newborn, encircle chest with fingers and overlap thumbs on the sternum just below an imaginary line connecting the nipples.

B) For an average-size newborn, encircle chest with fingers and place thumbs side by side on the sternum just below an imaginary line connecting the nipples.

C) For an infant that is older or too large to encircle the chest, place middle and ring fingers on sternum one finger-width below imaginary line connecting nipples. Measure distance by first placing, then raising, index finger.

FIGURE 30–10 Position fingers for chest compressions according to the size of the infant.

Perform chest compressions by following these steps:

- Encircle the newborn's chest, placing both of your thumbs on the lower one-third of the sternum. If the newborn is very small, you may need to overlap your thumbs. If the newborn is very large, you may need to place the ring and middle fingers of one hand just below the nipple line and perform two-finger compression (Figure 30-10).

- Compress the sternum 1.5 to 2.0 centimeters (½ to ⅓ inch) at a rate of 120 times per minute. Accompany compressions with positive-pressure ventilation. Maintain a ratio of three compressions to one ventilation.

- Reassess the newborn after 20 cycles of compressions and ventilations, or at approximately one-minute intervals.

- Discontinue compressions if the spontaneous heart rate exceeds 80.

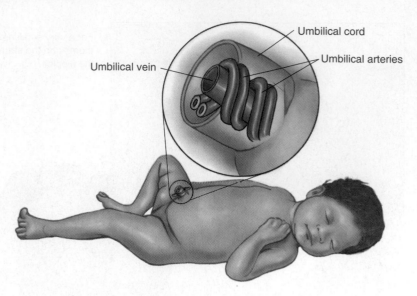

Umbilical cord

Umbilical arteries

Umbilical vein

FIGURE 30-11 The umbilical cord contains two arteries and one vein. The umbilical vein can be accessed for vascular administration of fluids and drugs. The vein is larger than the arteries and has a thinner wall.

Step 5: Medications and Fluids

Most cardiopulmonary arrests in newborns result from hypoxia. Because of this, initial therapy consists of ventilation and oxygenation. However, when these measures fail, fluid and medications should be administered. They may also be necessary in cases of persistent bradycardia, hypovolemia, respiratory depression secondary to narcotics, and metabolic acidosis.

Vascular access for the administration of fluids and drugs can most readily be managed by using the umbilical vein. The umbilical cord contains three vessels—two arteries and one vein. The vein is larger than the arteries and has a thinner wall (Figure 30-11). To establish venous access, follow these procedures:

Vascular access for the administration of fluids and drugs can most readily be managed by using the umbilical vein.

- Trim the umbilical cord with a scalpel blade to one centimeter above the abdomen. Be sure to save enough of the umbilical cord stump in case neonatal personnel have to place additional lines.

- Insert a 5 French umbilical catheter into the umbilical vein. Connect the catheter to a three-way stopcock and fill it with saline.

- Insert the catheter until the tip is just below the skin and you note the free flow of blood. (If the catheter is inserted too far, it may become wedged against the liver, and it will not function.)

- After the catheter is in place, secure it with umbilical tape.

If an umbilical vein catheter cannot be placed, some medications can be given via the endotracheal tube. They include atropine, epinephrine, lidocaine, and naloxone. Other options for vascular access are peripheral vein cannulation and intraosseous cannulation. Table 30-3 lists recommended medications and doses for the newborn. Fluid therapy should consist of 10 mL/kg of saline or lactated Ringer's solution given by syringe as a slow IV push.

MATERNAL NARCOTIC USE

Maternal abuse of narcotics—either illegal or prescribed—can complicate field deliveries. Maternal narcotic use has been shown to produce low-birth-weight infants. Such infants may demonstrate withdrawal symptoms such as tremors, startles, and decreased alertness. They also face a serious risk of respiratory depression at birth.

Naloxone (Narcan), which is extremely safe even at high doses, is the treatment of choice for respiratory depression secondary to maternal narcotic use *within four hours of delivery.*

Table 30-3 Neonatal Resuscitation Drugs

Medication	Concentration to Administer	Preparation	Dosage/Route*	Total Dose/Infant		Rate/Precautions
Epinephrine	1:10,000	10 mL	0.1–0.3 mL/kg IV or IT	weight 1 kg 2 kg 3 kg 4 kg	total mLs 0.1–0.3 mL 0.2–0.6 mL 0.3–0.9 mL 0.4–1.2 mL	Give rapidly
Volume Expanders	Whole blood 5% Albumin Normal saline Lactated Ringer's solution	40 mL	10 mL/kg IV	weight 1 kg 2 kg 3 kg 4 kg	total mLs 10 mL 20 mL 30 mL 40 mL	Give over 5–10 min
Narcan Neonatal	1.0 mg/mL or 0.4 mg/mL (dilute 1.0 mg in 9mL of saline)	2 mL	0.1 mg/kg IV, IM, SQ, IT	weight 1 kg 2 kg 3 kg 4 kg	total mLs (0.1 mg/mL) 1.0 mL 2.0 mL 3.0 mL 4.0 mL	Give rapidly
Dopamine	$6 \times \dfrac{\text{weight (kg)} \times \text{desired dose (mcg/kg/min)}}{\text{desired fluid (mL/hr)}} = \text{mg of dopamine per 100 mL of solution}$		Begin at 5 mcg/kg/min (may increase to 20 mcg/kg/min if necessary) IV	weight 1 kg 2 kg 3 kg 4 kg	total mcg/min 5–20 mcg/min 10–40 mcg/min 15–60 mcg/min 20–80 mcg/min	Give as continuous infusion using an infusion pump. Monitor heart rate and blood pressure closely. Seek consultation.

Source: From Textbook of Neonatal Resuscitation, © 2001, copyright American Heart Association.

*IM = Intramuscular, IT = Intratracheal, IV = Intravenous, SQ = Subcutaneous

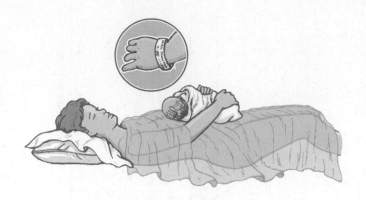

FIGURE 30-12 A healthy newborn can be placed on the mother's abdomen. Write the mother's last name and time of delivery on a tape and place it around the infant's wrist. (Do not allow adhesive to contact the infant's skin.)

Ventilatory support must be provided before administration of naloxone. Because the duration of the narcotics may exceed that of the naloxone, repeat administration as necessary.

Keep in mind, however, that the naloxone may induce a withdrawal reaction in an infant born to a *narcotic-addicted* mother. Medical direction may advise that naloxone NOT be administered if the mother is drug addicted, advising that prolonged ventilatory support be provided instead.

The dosage of naloxone is 0.1 mg/kg. The initial dose may be repeated every two to three minutes as needed. Naloxone may be given by intravenous, intraosseous, endotracheal, subcutaneous, or intramuscular routes.

As with other newborns, continue all resuscitative measures until the newborn is resuscitated or until the emergency staff assumes care.

Keep in mind that naloxone may induce a withdrawal reaction with an infant born to a narcotic-addicted mother.

NEONATAL TRANSPORT

Healthy newborns should be allowed to begin the bonding process with the mother as soon as possible (Figure 30-12). Distressed newborns, however, must be positioned on their side to prevent aspiration and rapidly transported.

In addition to field deliveries, EMT-Is are frequently called upon to transport a high-risk newborn from a facility where stabilization has occurred to a neonatal intensive care unit (NICU). The trip may be across the street or across the state. Usually, a pediatric nurse, respiratory therapist, and, often, a physician accompany the newborn. During transport, an EMT-I crew will help maintain a newborn's body temperature, control oxygen administration, and maintain ventilatory support. Often, a transport **isolette** with its own heat, light, and oxygen source is available. In such cases, IV medications are usually infused through the umbilical vein. The umbilical artery is catheterized as well.

If a self-contained isolette is not available for transport, it is important to keep the ambulance warm. Wrap the newborn in several blankets, keep the infant's head covered, and place hot-water bottles containing water heated to no more than 40°C (104°F) near, but not touching, the newborn. Do not use chemical packs to keep the newborn warm. These can generate excessive heat and may burn the infant.

isolette a clear plastic-enclosed bassinet used to keep prematurely born infants warm. The temperature of an isolette can be adjusted regardless of the room temperature. Some isolettes also provide humidity control.

SPECIFIC NEONATAL SITUATIONS

Rapid assessment and treatment of a distressed newborn is the key to the infant's survival. The following information will help you to formulate treatment plans for specific emergencies involving newborns. Remember that, unless otherwise directed, it will be necessary to transport these infants to a facility that is able to handle high-risk neonates. A reference card should be available in the ambulance and in the dispatch office that tracks the availability of neonatal unit beds. Whenever possible, keep the parents advised of what is happening and the reason for any treatments being given to the infant. However, do not discuss "chances of survival" with the family or caregivers.

Do not discuss "chances of survival" with a newborn's family or caregivers.

MECONIUM-STAINED AMNIOTIC FLUID

Meconium-stained amniotic fluid occurs in approximately 10% to 15% of deliveries, mostly in post-term or in small-for-gestational-age (SGA) newborns. The mortality rate for meconium-stained infants is considerably higher than the mortality rate for non-stained infants, and meconium aspiration accounts for a significant proportion of neonatal deaths.

Fetal distress and hypoxia can cause the passage of meconium into the amniotic fluid. Meconium is a dark green substance found in the digestive tract of full-term newborns. It arises from secretions of the various digestive glands and amniotic fluid. Either *in utero,* or more often with the first breath, thick meconium is aspirated into the lungs, resulting in small-airway obstruction and aspiration pneumonia. This may produce respiratory distress within the first hours, or even minutes, of life as evidenced by tachypnea, retraction, grunting, and cyanosis in severely affected newborns.

The partial obstruction of some airways may lead to pneumothorax. A pneumothorax may occur in an infant, cause no distress, and require no active treatment. If, however, the infant has significant respiratory distress, then the pneumothorax must be evacuated. If tension pneumothorax has occurred, needle decompression may be required.

An infant born through thin meconium may not require treatment, but depressed infants born through thick, particulate (pea-soup) meconium-stained fluid should be intubated immediately, before the first ventilation (Figure 30-13). Aspiration of meconium by a newborn can result in either partial or complete airway obstruction. Complete airway obstruction causes atelectasis (collapsed or airless lungs). In addition, some aspects of fetal blood flow resume a right-to-left shunt of blood across the foramen ovale (the opening between the atria of the fetal heart). This results from increased pulmonary pressures. Incomplete obstruction can act as a ball-valve in the smaller airways, thus preventing exhalation. Also, the newborn is at increased risk of developing a pneumothorax.

Before stimulating the infant to breathe, apply suction with a meconium aspirator attached to an endotracheal tube. Connect to suction at 100 cm/H_2O or less to remove meconium from the airway. Withdraw the endotracheal tube as suction is applied.

Repeat intubation and suction until the meconium clears, usually not more than two times. Once the airway is clear and the infant is able to breathe on his own, ventilate with 100% oxygen. If the infant is found to be hypotensive, consider a fluid challenge. Remember to warm the infant to prevent hypothermia. The parents will probably question the treatment being performed on the infant. Explain what you are doing and why, without discussing chances of survival. Stress the need for rapid transport to a facility able to handle high-risk infants.

APNEA

Apnea is a common finding in pre-term infants, infants weighing under 1,500 grams (3 pounds, 5 ounces), infants exposed to drugs, or infants born after prolonged or difficult labor and delivery. Typically, the infant fails to breathe spontaneously after stimulation, or the infant experiences respiratory pauses of greater than 20 seconds.

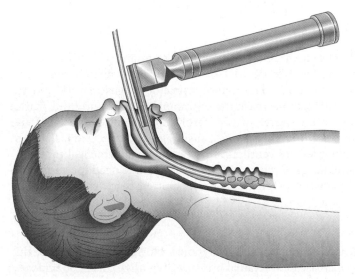

FIGURE 30-13 Intubate the infant born through particulate, thick meconium immediately—before the first ventilation.

Although apnea is usually due to hypoxia or hypothermia, there may be other causative factors. These include:

- Narcotic or central nervous depressants
- Weakness of the respiratory muscles
- Septicemia
- Metabolic disorders
- Central nervous system disorders

Begin management of apnea with tactile stimulation. Flick the soles of the infant's feet or gently rub his back. If necessary, ventilate using a BVM with the pop-off valve disabled. If the infant still does not breathe on his own, or if he has a heart rate of less than 60 with adequate ventilation and chest compressions, perform tracheal intubation with direct visualization. Gain circulatory access, and monitor the heart rate continuously. If the apnea is due to narcotics administered within the previous four hours, consider naloxone. As noted earlier, however, the use of narcotic antagonists is generally contraindicated if the mother is a drug abuser.

Early and aggressive treatment of apnea usually results in a good outcome. Throughout treatment, keep the infant warm to prevent hypothermia. Also explain procedures to parents and the need for rapid transport.

DIAPHRAGMATIC HERNIA

Diaphragmatic hernias rarely occur. They are seen in approximately one out of every 2,200 live births. When they do appear, the **herniation** takes place most often in the posterolateral segments of the diaphragm, and most commonly (90%) on the left side. The defect is caused by the failure of the pleurperitoneal canal (foramen of Bochdalek) to close completely. The survival rate for infants who require mechanical ventilation in the first 18 to 24 hours is approximately 50%. However, if there is no respiratory distress in the first 24 hours of life, the survival rate approaches 100%.

herniation protrusion or projection of an organ or part of an organ through the wall of the cavity that normally contains it.

Protrusion of abdominal viscera through the hernia into the thoracic cavity occurs in varying degrees. In severe cases, the stomach and a large part of the intestines and the spleen, liver, and kidneys displace the lungs and heart to the opposite side. The lung on the affected side is compressed, causing diminished total lung volume. In at least one-third of patients, pulmonary hypertension is present. With a patent ductus arteriosus, there may be severe right-to-left shunting, further aggravating tissue hypoxia.

Assessment findings may include:

- Little to severe distress present from birth
- Dyspnea and cyanosis unresponsive to ventilations
- Small, flat (scaphoid) abdomen
- Bowel sounds in the chest
- Heart sounds displaced to the right

As soon as you suspect a diaphragmatic hernia, position the infant with his head and thorax higher than the abdomen and feet (Figure 30-14). This will help facilitate the downward displacement of the abdominal organs. Place a nasogastric or orogastric tube and apply low, intermittent suctioning. This will decrease the entrapment of air and fluid within the herniated viscera and will lessen the degree of ventilatory compromise. DO NOT use BVM ventilation, which can worsen this condition by causing gastric distention. If necessary, cautiously administer positive-pressure ventilation through an endotracheal tube.

This condition usually requires surgical repair. Explain the possible need for surgery to parents, assuring them that their newborn child will be transported quickly to the facility best able to handle this procedure.

BRADYCARDIA

Bradycardia in the newborn is most commonly caused by hypoxia. However, it may also be due to several other factors, including increased intracranial pressure, hypothyroidism, or acidosis.

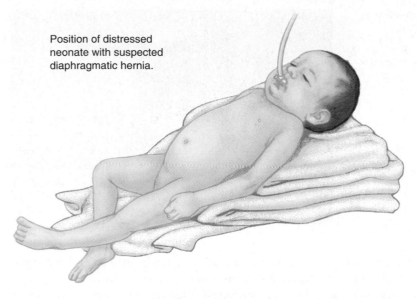

Position of distressed neonate with suspected diaphragmatic hernia.

FIGURE 30-14 If a diaphragmatic hernia is suspected, position the infant with his head and thorax higher than the abdomen and feet to facilitate downward displacement of abdominal organs.

In cases of hypoxia, the infant experiences minimal risk if the hypoxia is corrected quickly. In providing treatment, follow the procedures in the inverted pyramid, as discussed earlier. Check for secretions in the airway, check tongue and soft tissue positioning, and check for possible foreign body obstruction. Resist the inclination to treat the bradycardia with pharmacological measures alone. Although epinephrine may be necessary, in all likelihood you will be able to correct the problem with suctioning, positioning, administration of oxygen (blow-by or BVM), or tracheal intubation. Throughout treatment, keep the newborn warm and transport to the nearest facility.

> *Resist the temptation to treat bradycardia in a newborn with pharmacological measures alone.*
>
>

PREMATURE INFANTS

A premature newborn is an infant born before 37 weeks of gestation or with weight ranging from 0.6 to 2.2 kg (1 pound, 5 ounces to 4 pounds, 13 ounces). Healthy premature infants weighing more than 1,700 grams (3 pounds, 12 ounces) have a survivability and outcome approximately that of full-term infants. The mortality rate decreases weekly as the gestational age surpasses the age of fetal viability. With the technology currently available, fetal viability is considered to be 23 to 24 weeks of gestation.

Premature newborns are at greater risk of respiratory suppression, head or brain injury caused by hypoxemia, changes in blood pressure, intraventricular hemorrhage, and fluctuations in serum osmolarity. They are also more susceptible to hypothermia than full-term newborns. Reasons premature newborns lose heat more readily include:

- Premature newborns have a relatively large body surface area and comparatively small weight.
- Premature newborns have not sufficiently developed the various control mechanisms needed to regulate body temperature.
- Premature newborns have smaller subcutaneous stores of insulating fat.
- Newborns cannot shiver and must maintain body temperature through other mechanisms.

The degree of immaturity determines the physical characteristics of a premature newborn (Figure 30-15). Premature newborns often appear to have a larger head relative to body size. They may have large trunks and short extremities, transparent skin, and few wrinkles.

Prematurity should not be a factor in short-term treatment. Resuscitation should be attempted if there is any sign of life, and the measures of resuscitation should be the same as

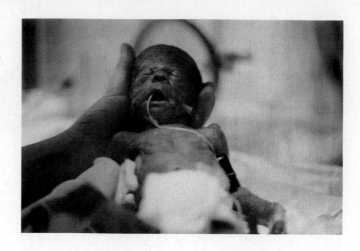

FIGURE 30-15 The premature newborn.

those for newborns of normal weight and maturity. Maintain a patent airway and avoid potential aspiration of gastric contents. Medical direction may advise administration of epinephrine. Throughout treatment, maintain the newborn's body temperature and transport to a facility with special services for low-birth-weight newborns.

RESPIRATORY DISTRESS/CYANOSIS

Prematurity is the single most common factor causing respiratory distress and cyanosis in the newborn. The problem occurs most frequently in infants less than 1,200 grams (2 pounds, 10 ounces) and 30 weeks of gestation. Premature infants have an immature central respiratory control center and are easily affected by environmental or metabolic changes. Multiple gestations or prenatal maternal complications may also increase the risk of respiratory distress and cyanosis.

The severely ill newborn with respiratory distress and cyanosis presents a difficult diagnostic challenge. There may be many contributing factors, including lung or heart disease, central nervous system disorders, meconium aspiration, metabolic problems, obstruction of the nasal passages, shock and sepsis, diaphragmatic hernia, and more. Assessment findings include:

- Tachypnea
- Paradoxical breathing
- Intercostal retractions
- Nasal flaring
- Expiratory grunt

Follow the inverted pyramid of treatment, paying particular attention to airway and ventilation. Suction as needed and provide a high concentration of oxygen. Ventilate, as needed, with a BVM. If prolonged ventilation will be required, consider placing an endotracheal tube. Perform chest compressions, if indicated. Consider dextrose ($D_{10}W$ or $D_{25}W$) solution if the newborn is hypoglycemic. Maintain body temperature and transport. Be sure to keep the parents informed and provide needed psychological support.

HYPOVOLEMIA

Hypovolemia is the leading cause of shock in newborns. It may result from dehydration, hemorrhage, or third-spacing of fluids. Dehydration is by far the most common cause. Signs of hypovolemia include:

- Pale color
- Cool skin
- Diminished peripheral pulses
- Delayed capillary refill, despite normal ambient temperature

Prematurity should not be a factor in short-term treatment. Resuscitation should be attempted if there is any sign of life.

- Mental status changes
- Diminished urination (oliguria)

When you observe these signs, administer a fluid bolus and assess the infant's response. If signs of shock continue, administer a second bolus. Additional boluses should be infused as indicated by repeated assessments. A hypovolemic infant may often need 40 to 60 mL/kg of fluid during the first hour of resuscitation.

Fluid bolus resuscitation consists of 10 mL/kg of an isotonic crystalloid solution, such as Ringer's lactate or normal saline. Administer the bolus over 5 to 10 minutes as soon as intravascular or intraosseous access is obtained. Do not use solutions containing dextrose, as they can produce hypokalemia or worsen ischemic brain injury.

In treating hypovolemia in a newborn, do not use solutions containing dextrose, as they can produce hypokalemia or worsen ischemic brain injury.

SEIZURES

Although seizures occur in a very small percentage of all newborns, they usually indicate a serious underlying abnormality and represent a medical emergency. Prolonged and frequent multiple seizures may result in metabolic changes and cardiopulmonary difficulties.

Neonatal seizures differ from seizures in a child or an adult, because generalized tonic-clonic convulsions normally do not occur during the first month of life. Seizures in neonates include:

- *Subtle seizures.* These seizures consist of chewing motions, excessive salivation, blinking, sucking, swimming movements of the arms, pedaling movements of the legs, apnea, and changes in color.
- *Tonic seizures.* These seizures are characterized by rigid posturing of the extremities and trunk. They are sometimes associated with fixed deviation of the eyes. They occur more commonly in premature infants, especially those with an intraventricular hemorrhage.
- *Focal clonic seizures.* These seizures consist of rhythmic twitching of muscle groups, particularly the extremities and face. They may occur in both full-term and premature infants.
- *Multifocal seizures.* These seizures are similar to focal clonic seizures, except that multiple muscle groups are involved. Clonic activity randomly migrates. These seizures occur primarily in full-term newborns.
- *Myoclonic seizures.* These seizures involve brief focal or generalized jerks of the extremities or parts of the body that tend to involve distal muscle groups. They may occur singly or in a series of repetitive jerks.

Causes of neonatal seizures include sepsis, fever, hypoglycemia, hypoxic-ischemic encephalopathy, metabolic disturbances, meningitis, developmental abnormalities, or drug withdrawal. Assessment findings include a decreased level of consciousness and seizure activities such as those described above. Treatment focuses on airway management and oxygen saturation. With medical direction, consider administration of an anti-convulsant. You might also administer a benzodiazepine (usually lorazepam) for status epilepticus or dextrose ($D_{10}W$ or $D_{25}W$) for hypoglycemia. As with all distressed newborns, maintain body temperature and transport rapidly.

FEVER

Average normal temperature in a newborn is 37.5°C (99.5°F). A rectal temperature of 38.0°C (100.4°F) or higher is considered fever. Neonates do not develop fever as readily as older children. Thus, any fever in a neonate requires extensive evaluation, because it may be caused by life-threatening conditions such as pneumonia, sepsis, or meningitis. Fever may be the only sign of meningitis in a neonate. Because of their immature development, they do not develop the classic symptoms such as a stiff neck. Thus, any neonate with a fever should be considered to have meningitis until proven otherwise.

Any neonate with fever should be considered to have meningitis until proven otherwise.

In assessing a neonate with fever, remember that infants have a limited ability to control their body temperature. As a result, fever can be a serious problem. Assessment findings will probably include the following:

- Mental status changes (irritability/somnolence)
- Decreased feeding
- Skin warm to the touch
- Rashes or *petechia* (small, purplish, hemorrhagic spots on the skin)

Term infants may produce beads of sweat on their brow, but not on the rest of their body. Premature infants will have no visible sweat at all.

Treatment of a neonate with fever will, for the most part, be limited to ensuring a patent airway and adequate ventilation. Do not use cold packs, which may drop the temperature too quickly and may also cause seizures. If the newborn becomes bradycardic, provide chest compressions. In the prehospital setting, administration of an antipyretic agent to a neonate is of questionable benefit and should be avoided. Select the appropriate treatment facility, and explain the need for transport to the parents or caregivers.

HYPOTHERMIA

As previously noted, hypothermia presents a common and life-threatening condition for newborns. Adults sometimes fail to realize that a newborn may die because of exposure to temperatures that adults find comfortable. The increased surface-to-volume relationship in newborns makes them extremely sensitive to environmental temperatures, especially right after delivery when they are wet. As a result, it is important to control the four methods of heat loss—evaporation, conduction, convection, and radiation.

In treating hypothermia—a body temperature below 35°C (95°F)—keep in mind that it can also be an indicator of sepsis in the newborn. Regardless of the cause, the increased metabolic demands created by hypothermia can produce a variety of related conditions including metabolic acidosis, pulmonary hypertension, and hypoxemia.

In assessing a hypothermic newborn, remember that they do not shiver. Instead, expect these findings:

- Pale color
- Skin cool to the touch, particularly in the extremities
- **Acrocyanosis**
- Respiratory distress
- Possible apnea
- Bradycardia
- Central cyanosis
- Initial irritability
- Lethargy in later stages

acrocyanosis cyanosis of the extremities.

Management focuses on ensuring adequate ventilations and oxygenation. Chest compressions may be performed, if necessary. With medical direction, you might administer warm fluids through an IV fluid heater. Do not microwave fluids, because there can be a great variation in fluid temperature. Dextrose ($D_{10}W$ or $D_{25}W$) may also be given if the newborn is hypoglycemic. Above all, the newborn must be kept warm. Set the ambulance temperature at 24°C to 26°C (75.2°F to 78.8°F). Also remember to warm your hands before touching the newborn. Select the appropriate receiving facility and transport rapidly.

HYPOGLYCEMIA

Newborns are the only age group that can develop severe hypoglycemia and not have diabetes mellitus. Hypoglycemia may be due to inadequate glucose intake or increased glucose utilization. Stress and other factors can also cause the blood sugar to fall, sometimes to a critical level.

Hypoglycemia is more common in premature or small-for-gestational-age (SGA) infants, the smaller twin, and newborns of a diabetic mother, because these infants often have decreased glycogen stores. Hypoglycemia can also develop due to increased glucose utilization. Causes include respiratory illnesses, hypothermia, toxemia, CNS hemorrhage, asphyxia, meningitis, and sepsis. In an older infant, hypoglycemia may be due to an inadequate glucose intake or increased utilization of glucose. Infants receiving glucose infusions can develop hypoglycemia if the infusion is suddenly stopped.

Infants with hypoglycemia may be asymptomatic or they may exhibit symptoms such as apnea, color changes, respiratory distress, lethargy, seizures, acidosis, and poor myocardial contractility.

Persistent hypoglycemia can have catastrophic effects on the brain. The normal newborn's glycogen stores are sufficient to meet glucose requirements for only 8 to 12 hours. This time frame is diminished in infants with decreased glycogen stores or the presence of other problems where glucose utilization increases. As a result, you should determine the blood glucose on all sick infants. A blood glucose screening test of less than 45 mg/dL indicates hypoglycemia.

In response to hypoglycemia, the newborn's body will release counter-regulatory hormones such as glucagon, epinephrine, cortisol, and growth hormone. These hormones help raise the blood glucose level by mobilizing glucose stores. In fact, this hormone response may cause transient symptoms of hyperglycemia that may last for several hours. However, when the infant's glucose stores are depleted, the glucose level will again fall.

In assessing hypoglycemic newborns, expect these findings:

- Twitching or seizures
- Limpness
- Lethargy
- Eye-rolling
- High-pitched cry
- Apnea
- Irregular respirations
- Possible cyanosis

Treatment begins with management of the airway and ventilations. Ensure adequate oxygenation. Perform chest compressions, if indicated. With medical direction, administer dextrose ($D_{10}W$ or $D_{25}W$). Maintain a normal body temperature in the newborn and transport to the appropriate facility.

VOMITING

Vomiting in a neonate may result from a variety of causes and rarely presents as an isolated symptom. Vomiting (a forceful ejection of stomach contents) is uncommon during the first weeks of life and may be confused with regurgitation (a simple backflow of stomach contents into the mouth, or "spitting up"). Vomiting in the neonate usually occurs because of an anatomical abnormality such as a tracheoesophageal fistula or upper gastrointestinal obstruction. More often, it may be a symptom of some disease such as increased intracranial pressure or an infection. Vomitus containing dark blood often signals a life-threatening illness. Keep in mind, however, that vomiting of mucus—which may occasionally be blood streaked—in the first few hours after birth is not uncommon.

Assessment findings may include a distended stomach, signs of infection, increased intracranial pressure, or drug withdrawal. Because vomitus can be aspirated, management considerations focus on ensuring a patent airway. If you detect respiratory difficulties or obstruction of the airway, suction or clear vomitus from the airway and assure adequate oxygenation. Fluid administration may be needed to prevent dehydration. Also remember that, as with older patients, vagal stimulation may cause bradycardia in the neonate.

After you have protected the airway, place the infant on his side and transport to an appropriate facility. As with all other situations involving distressed neonates, advise parents or caregivers of steps taken and why.

Because hypoglycemia can have a catastrophic effect on a neonate's brain, you should determine blood glucose in all sick infants.

DIARRHEA

Diarrhea in a neonate can cause severe dehydration and electrolyte imbalances. Although diarrhea may be harder to assess in neonates than in other patients, consider five to six stools per day as normal, especially in breast-fed infants.

Causes of diarrhea in a neonate include:

- Bacterial or viral infection
- Gastroenteritis
- Lactose intolerance
- **Photorapy**
- **Neonatal abstinence syndrome (NAS)**
- **Thyrotoxicosis**
- Cystic fibrosis

In treating neonates with diarrhea, remember to take appropriate body substance isolation precautions, just as you would do in any situation involving body fluids. Expect to find loose stools, decreased urinary output, and other signs of dehydration such as prolonged capillary refill time, cool extremities, and listlessness or lethargy. It is often difficult for the parents to estimate the number of stools. In such cases, it might be better to inquire about the number of diapers the baby is using.

Management consists of maintenance of airway and ventilations, adequate oxygenation, and chest compressions, if indicated. With medical direction, you might also consider fluid therapy. Explain all treatments to parents or caregivers, and transport the neonate to a facility able to handle high-risk infants.

COMMON BIRTH INJURIES

A **birth injury** occurs in an estimated 2 to 7 of every 1,000 live births in the United States. About 5 to 8 of every 100,000 infants die of birth trauma and 25 of every 100,000 die of anoxic injuries. Such injuries account for 2% to 3% of infant deaths. Risk factors for birth injury include:

- Prematurity
- Postmaturity
- Cephalopelvic disproportion
- Prolonged labor
- Breech presentation
- Explosive delivery
- Diabetic mother

Birth injuries take various forms. Cranial injuries may include molding of the head and overriding of the parietal bones, erythema (reddening of the skin), abrasions, ecchymosis (black-and-blue discoloration) and subcutaneous fat necrosis, subconjunctival and retinal hemorrhage, subperiosteal hemorrhage, and fracture of the skull. Intracranial hemorrhage may result from trauma or asphyxia. Often the infant will develop a large scalp hematoma during the birth process. This injury, called *caput succedaneum,* will usually resolve over a week's time. There may be damage to the spine and spinal cord from strong traction exerted when the spine is hyperextended or there is a lateral pull. Other birth injuries include peripheral nerve injury, injury to the liver, rupture of the spleen, adrenal hemorrhage, fractures of the clavicle or extremities, and, of course, hypoxia-ischemia.

Assessment findings may include:

- Diffuse, sometimes ecchymotic, edematous swelling of soft tissues around the scalp
- Paralysis below the level of the spinal cord injury
- Paralysis of the upper arm with or without paralysis of the forearm

---

photorapy exposure to sunlight or artificial light for therapeutic purposes. In newborns, light is used to treat hyperbilirubinemia or jaundice.

neonatal abstinence syndrome (NAS) a generalized disorder presenting a clinical picture of CNS hyperirritability, gastrointestinal dysfunction, respiratory distress, and vague autonomic symptoms. It may be due to intrauterine exposure to heroin, methadone, or other less potent opiates. Non-opiate central nervous system depressants may also cause NAS.

thyrotoxicosis toxic condition characterized by tachycardia, nervous symptoms, and rapid metabolism due to hyperactivity of the thyroid gland.

In treating a neonate with diarrhea, remember to take appropriate body substance isolation precautions.

birth injury avoidable and unavoidable mechanical and anoxic trauma incurred by the newborn during labor and delivery.

- Diaphragmatic paralysis
- Movement on only one side of the face when crying
- Inability to move the arm freely on the side of the fractured clavicle
- Lack of spontaneous movement of the affected extremity
- Hypoxia
- Shock

Management of a newborn or newborn with birth injuries usually centers on protection of the airway, provision of adequate ventilation and oxygen, and, if needed, chest compressions. With medical direction, you may administer medications or take other non-pharmacological steps to support the specific injury. Newborns with birth injuries usually require treatment at specialized facilities. As in the management of other neonatal emergencies, provide professional and compassionate communication to parents or caregivers.

In treating distressed neonates with birth injuries or other critical conditions, provide professional and compassionate communication with parents or caregivers.

CARDIAC RESUSCITATION, POST RESUSCITATION, AND STABILIZATION

The incidence of neonatal cardiac arrest is related primarily to hypoxia. As previously explained, the outcome will be poor unless you immediately initiate appropriate interventions. As you might expect, cases involving cardiac arrest have an increased chance of brain and organ damage. Risk factors for cardiac arrest in newborns include:

- Bradycardia
- Intrauterine asphyxia
- Prematurity
- Drugs administered to or taken by the mother
- Congenital neuromuscular diseases
- Congenital malformations
- Intrapartum hypoxemia

Cardiac arrest can be caused by primary or secondary apnea, bradycardia, persistent fetal circulation, or pulmonary hypertension. Assessment findings may include peripheral cyanosis, inadequate respiratory effort, and ineffective or absent heart rate.

In managing neonatal cardiac arrest, follow the inverted pyramid for resuscitation. Administer drugs or fluids according to medical direction. Maintain normal body temperature while you transport the distressed newborn to the appropriate facility. This situation will require delicate handling of the parents or caregivers. Explain what is being done for the infant, without entering into the possibilities of survival.

Content Review

CAUSES OF NEONATAL CARDIAC ARREST
- Primary or secondary apnea
- Bradycardia
- Persistent fetal circulation
- Pulmonary hypertension

Cultural Considerations

Occasionally, prehospital childbirth may result in the delivery of a stillborn infant. The reasons for the infant's demise may be obvious or the infant may appear otherwise normal. Some Christian families may request that the infant be baptized as soon as possible after birth. In fact, in some faiths, failure to baptize the infant might "deny a child the priceless grace of becoming a child of God." Infant baptism is primarily a practice of the Roman Catholic church, although similar religions (Episcopalian, Anglican) often practice the rite. If you are asked to baptize an infant, remember, despite your own personal religious beliefs, this is very important to the parents and they have put a great deal of trust in you. According to the Catechism of the Catholic Church, dip your finger into a bowl of water and make a sign of the cross on the infant's forehead. Then say, "I baptize you in the name of the Father and of the Son and of the Holy Spirit. Amen." Even if you are not baptized, in an emergency you may baptize an infant if that is the parents' wish, provided you act in the spirit of church teaching. Most parents will appreciate the act. Sometimes, even in this era of sophisticated medical technology, there is little we can do other than provide support to the survivors.

SUMMARY

After a woman gives birth, you must care for two patients, the mother and her newborn child. The newborn has several special needs, the most important of which are protection of the airway and support of ventilations. The newborn must be kept warm at all times. If assessment reveals a distressed newborn, you should initiate ventilatory support, stimulation, and, if required, CPR. If possible, newborns should be transported to a facility with an NICU. Maintain communications with family members or caregivers, explaining all procedures performed on the newborn.

ON THE WEB

For additional practice and review, go to the companion website at www.prenhall.com/bledsoe and click on *Intermediate Emergency Care: Principles & Practice.*

CHAPTER 31

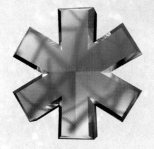

Pediatric Emergencies

Objectives

After reading this chapter, you should be able to:

1. Identify methods/mechanisms that prevent injuries to infants and children. (p. 1186)
2. Identify the common family responses to acute illness and injury of an infant or child. (pp. 1187–1188)
3. Describe techniques for successful interaction with families of acutely ill or injured infants and children. (pp. 1187–1188)
4. Identify key anatomical, physiological, growth, and developmental characteristics of infants and children and their implications. (pp. 1188–1191)
5. Outline differences in adult and childhood anatomy, physiology, and "normal" age-group-related vital signs. (pp. 1191–1194)
6. Describe techniques for successful assessment of infants and children. (pp. 1195–1204)
7. Discuss normal age-group vital signs and the appropriate equipment used to obtain pediatric vital signs. (pp. 1203–1204)
8. Determine appropriate airway adjuncts, ventilation devices, and endotracheal intubation equipment; their proper use; and complications of use for infants and children. (pp. 1204–1213)
9. List the indications and methods of gastric decompression for infants and children. (pp. 1213, 1214)

10. Define pediatric respiratory distress, failure, and arrest. (pp. 1220–1221)
11. Differentiate between upper airway obstruction and lower airway disease. (pp. 1221–1227)
12. Describe the general approach to the treatment of children with respiratory distress, failure, or arrest from upper airway obstruction or lower airway disease. (pp. 1221–1227)
13. Describe the pathophysiology, assessment, and treatment of infants and children with:
    a. Croup (p. 1222)
    b. Epiglottitis (pp. 1222–1224)
    c. Foreign body aspiration (pp. 1224–1225)
    d. Asthma (pp. 1225–1226)
    e. Bronchiolitis (pp. 1226–1227)
    f. Pneumonia (p. 1227)
    g. Foreign body lower airway obstruction (p. 1227)
    h. Shock (hypoperfusion) (pp. 1227–1231)
    i. Dysrhythmias, including tachydysrhythmias, bradydysrhythmias, and arrest (pp. 1232–1234)
    j. Seizures (pp. 1236–1237)

Continued

k. Hypoglycemia and hyperglycemia (pp. 1238–1240)

l. Trauma emergencies, including injuries to the head, neck, chest, abdomen, and extremities and burns (pp. 1242–1250)

m. Abuse or neglect (pp. 1251–1254)

n. Sudden infant death syndrome (SIDS), including parent/caregiver responses (pp. 1250–1251)

o. Children with special needs, including children dependent on various technological devices (pp. 1255–1258)

14. Discuss the primary etiologies of cardiopulmonary arrest in infants and children. (pp. 1196, 1209–1221)

15. Discuss basic cardiac life support (CPR) guidelines for infants and children. (pp. 1204–1209)

16. Discuss age-appropriate sites, equipment, techniques, and complications of vascular access and fluid therapy for infants and children. (pp. 1215–1216)

17. Identify common lethal mechanisms of injury in infants and children. (pp. 1243–1245)

18. Discuss anatomical features of children that predispose or protect them from certain injuries. (pp. 1248–1250)

19. Describe aspects of infant and child airway management that are affected by potential cervical spine injury. (pp. 1245–1246)

20. Identify infant and child trauma patients who require spinal immobilization. (pp. 1217–1218)

21. Given several pre-programmed simulated pediatric patients, provide the appropriate assessment, treatment, and transport. (pp. 1185–1258)

CASE STUDY

Three tones sound on the EMS radios in the ED. A message crackles: "LA 54, I need you to be 10-8." The crew of LA 54 transfers care of the patient in bed no. 6 to the hospital staff. Within 60 seconds, they depart from the hospital parking lot. En route to the emergency, they review information provided by the dispatcher. They will be treating a 5-month-old female who is described as "not breathing" by the father.

The response time is 4 minutes. Upon arrival, the parents lead the EMT-Is into the patient's bedroom. The little girl is lying in a crib. Immediately, EMT-Is note that she has pale, cool, and clammy skin. Her anterior fontanelle is noticeably sunken. The respiratory rate and quality is 20 and shallow. Upon mild painful stimuli, the infant cries vigorously, increasing her tidal rate and volume. However, no tears appear. After taking appropriate BSI precautions, the EMT-Is check the diaper and find that it is dry. "She hasn't kept any food down for 3 days," explains the mother. "She hasn't wet her diaper in hours."

The crew places the patient on 15 liters/minute supplemental oxygen via a nonrebreather mask. The infant responds to the mask by crying, but she makes no effort to remove it. Capillary refill is borderline (2.5 seconds). The EMT-Is prepare to transport the infant to the ED, informing the parents of all the steps that will be taken to help their daughter.

En route to the hospital, the crew establishes an IV access and administers a fluid bolus of 20 mL/kg of normal saline. By the time they pull up to the ambulance ramp at the ED, the patient's color and respiratory rate have improved greatly. Capillary refill time and pulse rate move toward normal limits. The ED staff evaluates the patient and admits her for 24-hour observation and IV fluid therapy. She returns home the following day. The EMT-Is later learn that she had contracted a viral gastroenteritis that was going around her day care center. Within 48 hours, she was back to her usual playful self.

INTRODUCTION

The ill or injured child presents special concerns for prehospital personnel. Current research indicates that more than 20,000 pediatric deaths occur each year in the United States. The leading causes of death are age specific. They include motor-vehicle collisions, burns, drownings, suicides, and homicides. These alarming facts become even more troublesome when experts theorize that many of them could have been prevented by early intervention. Tragedies involving children—neonates to adolescents—account for some of the most stressful incidents that you will encounter in EMS practice.

Treatment of pediatric patients presents a number of challenges for the EMT-I. Children, especially young ones, often cannot describe what is bothering them or what has happened to them. In addition to the child patient, you must deal with the parents or caregivers. Finally, a child's size often makes routine procedures more difficult. Keep in mind that children are not simply small adults. They have special considerations and needs. This chapter will present the topic of pediatric emergencies as it applies to advanced prehospital care.

ROLE OF EMT-INTERMEDIATES IN PEDIATRIC CARE

When considering the reduction of pediatric morbidity and mortality, your role as an EMT-I centers around two key concepts. First, you must realize that pediatric injuries have become a major health concern. Second, you should remember that children are at a higher risk of injury than adults and that they are more likely to be adversely affected by the injuries that they suffer.

Numerous factors account for the high pediatric injury rates. Some factors, such as geography and weather, cannot be altered. However, other factors, particularly dangers within the home and community, can be eliminated or minimized. All health-care professionals must get involved in identifying and implementing methods and mechanisms that prevent injuries to infants and children. Those of us who deliver prehospital care must do more than simply enter the picture after an injury has taken place.

In addition to pediatric injuries, EMT-Is are often responsible for treating the ill child. Many aspects of disease and disease processes are unique to children. It is important that the EMT-I be familiar with these, since early intervention is often the key to reduced morbidity and mortality.

CONTINUING EDUCATION AND TRAINING

Your role in improving the health care offered to pediatric patients begins with your own training. Because you will encounter pediatric patients less frequently than adult patients, you have a professional responsibility to maintain and improve your pediatric knowledge, particularly your clinical skills. Continuing education programs include:

- Pediatric Advanced Life Support (PALS)
- Pediatric Basic Trauma Life Support (PBTLS)
- Advanced Pediatric Life Support (APLS)
- Prehospital Pediatric Care (PPC)

In addition to these programs, you can also attend regional conferences and seminars designed to increase your knowledge of pediatric care. These are often conducted by regional children's hospitals. You can further enhance your clinical skills by spending time in pediatric emergency departments, pediatric hospitals, or pediatric departments in local hospitals. You might also visit the offices of pediatricians or talk with Pediatric Nurse Practitioners—registered nurses who provide primary health care to children.

For self-study, you can choose among many excellent pediatric textbooks currently available or read articles on pediatric care in the various EMS journals. Many good pediatric educational sites are available on the Internet. A particularly useful source of information is the Center for Pediatric Medicine (CPEM), established in 1985 at the New York

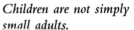

Content Review

TOP CAUSES OF PEDIATRIC DEATHS
- Motor-vehicle collisions
- Burns
- Drownings
- Suicides
- Homicides

Tragedies involving children account for some of the most stressful incidents that you will encounter in EMS practice.

Children are not simply small adults.

You have a professional responsibility to maintain and improve your pediatric knowledge, particularly your clinical skills.

University Medical Center and Bellevue Hospital. This federally funded center promotes education, research, and development of systems aimed at improving emergency medical services for children in the United States. CPEM has made available the *Teaching Resource for Instructors in Prehospital Pediatrics* (TRIPP), a progressive and comprehensive resource for instructors of prehospital providers. This resource contains a thorough review of prehospital pediatric emergencies.

IMPROVED HEALTH CARE AND INJURY PREVENTION

Emergency Medical Services for Children (EMSC) federally funded program aimed at improving the health of pediatric patients who suffer from life-threatening illnesses and injuries.

Funding for CPEM comes largely from a group known as the **Emergency Medical Services for Children (EMSC)**. This federally funded program falls under the management of the Maternal and Child Health Bureau, an agency of the U.S. Department of Health and Human Services. The EMSC was formed for the express purpose of improving the health of pediatric patients who suffer potentially life-threatening illnesses or injuries. This nationally coordinated effort has identified a number of pediatric health-care concerns, including:

- Community education
- Data collection
- Quality improvement
- Injury prevention
- Access
- Prehospital care
- Emergency care
- Definitive care
- Finance
- Rehabilitation
- A systems approach to pediatric care
- Ongoing health care from birth to young adulthood

As an EMT-I, you can take part in this national effort by actively participating in programs that promote injury prevention. Prehospital care providers see the consequences of pediatric trauma all too often. You can help reduce the rate of injury by taking advantage of opportunities to share "teaching points" in your daily life, both personally and professionally. Take part in, or offer to organize, school or community programs in injury prevention or health care. Engage student interest in the EMS profession by volunteering to speak on career days, emphasizing those aspects of your job that relate to young people. Use non-urgent ambulance calls as a chance to educate family members or caregivers on the importance of "child-proofing" a home or neighborhood. Work with appropriate agencies in initiating or conducting safety inspections, block watches, and more.

There has been an increased effort to identify the severity and nature of prehospital pediatric emergencies. Many regions now have both pediatric and trauma registries. These, in addition to standard epidemiological research conducted by local health departments, depend on quality prehospital documentation. If your area is participating in a registry program or research study, be sure to obtain and record all required data. Information gained from these registries will help identify the need for more or specialized resources.

GENERAL APPROACH TO PEDIATRIC EMERGENCIES

The approach to the pediatric patient varies with the age of the patient and with the problem being treated. Foremost in approaching any pediatric emergency is consideration of the patient's emotional and physiological development. Care also involves the family members or caregivers responsible for the child. They will demand information, express fears, and, ultimately, give or refuse consent for treatment and/or transport.

COMMUNICATION AND PSYCHOLOGICAL SUPPORT

Treatment of an infant, child, or teenager begins with communication and psychological support. Interaction with pediatric patients and related adults continues throughout assessment and management. When obtaining the medical history of the pediatric patient, you should gather information as quickly and as accurately as possible. The parents and caregivers are often the primary source of information, especially in the case of infants. However, as children become older, they can also be a good source of information. Older children, for example, can often give accurate descriptions of symptoms or other details. Treat pediatric patients with respect, allowing them to express opinions and ask questions. Your listening skills will play an important role in alleviating the fears of child patients. You can even communicate a calm and caring attitude to infants, who respond to touch and voice just like any other human being.

> *Treatment of an infant, child, or teenager begins with communication and psychological support.*

Responding to Patient Needs

As previously mentioned, a child's response to an emergency will vary, depending on the age and emotional maturity of the child. The child's most common response to illness or injury is fear. Common fears of children include:

- Fear of being separated from the parents or caregivers
- Fear of being removed from a family place, such as home, and never returning
- Fear of being hurt
- Fear of being mutilated or disfigured
- Fear of the unknown

These fears may be intensified if the child detects fear or anxiety from the parents or caregivers. The general chaos and panic that often surround pediatric emergency situations may further distress the child.

Remember that children have the right to know what is being done to them. You should be as honest as possible with them. If a procedure such as an IV needle stick will hurt, tell them so. Tell them immediately before performing a procedure. Do not say that a procedure will be painful and then take 5 minutes to prepare the equipment, allowing time for the child's anticipation of pain to build.

> *Remember that children have the right to know what is being done to them. Be as honest as possible.*

Always use language that is appropriate for the age of the child. Medical and anatomical terms that EMTs routinely use may be completely foreign to children. Telling a child that you are going to "apply a cervical collar" means nothing. Instead, tell the child: "I'm going to put this collar around your neck to keep it from moving." "Try to hold your head still." "Tell me if it is too tight." This will involve children in their own care and reduce their feelings of helplessness.

Responding to Parents or Caregivers

As you might expect, the reaction of parents or caregivers to a pediatric emergency will vary. Initial reactions might include shock, grief, denial, anger, guilt, fear, or complete loss of control. Their behavior may change during the course of the emergency. Communication is the key. Preferably only one EMT-I will speak with adults at the scene. This will avoid any chance of conflicting information and allow a second EMT-I to focus on the child. If parents or caregivers sense your confidence and professionalism, they will regain control and trust your suggestions for care. As with the child, most parents and caregivers feel overwhelmed by fear. They often express their fears in questions such as the following:

"Is my child going to die?"

"Did my child suffer brain damage?"

"Is my child going to be all right?"

"What are you doing to my child?"

"Will my child be able to walk?"

It may be difficult to answer these questions in the prehospital setting. However, the following actions may help allay parents' fears:

- Tell them your name and qualifications.
- Acknowledge their fears and concerns.
- Reassure them that it is all right to feel the way they do.
- Redirect their energies toward helping you care for the child.
- Remain calm and appear in control of the emergency.
- Keep the parents or caregivers informed as to what you are doing.
- Don't "talk down" to them.
- Assure them that everything possible is being done for their child.

If conditions permit, you should allow one of the parents or caregivers to remain with the child at all times. Some family members may be extremely emotional in emergency situations. The child will react more positively to a family member who appears calm and reassuring. If a parent or caregiver is out of control, have another person take him or her away from the immediate area to settle down. Maintain a reasonable level of suspicion if a child shows a pattern of injuries, some old and some new. In such cases, the parent or caregiver may try to cover up what may be an abusive situation. They may also try to block examination and treatment. (There will be more on potential abuse or neglect later in this chapter.)

GROWTH AND DEVELOPMENT

Children progress through developmental stages on their way to adulthood. You should tailor your approach to the developmental level of your pediatric patient.

Newborns (First Hours after Birth)

Although the terms *newborn* and *neonate* are often used interchangeably, *newborn* refers to a baby in the first hours of extrauterine life. The term *neonate* describes infants from birth to 1 month of age. The method most frequently used to assess newborns is the APGAR scoring system, which was described in Chapter 29. Resuscitation of the newborn generally follows the inverted pyramid described in Chapter 30 and the guidelines established in the Neonatal Advanced Life Support (NALS) curriculum.

Neonates (Ages Birth to 1 Month)

The neonate, as noted above (and described in Chapter 30), is an infant up to 1 month of age. This is a major stage of development. Soon after birth, the neonate typically loses up to 10% of his birth weight as he adjusts to extrauterine life. This lost weight, however, is ordinarily recovered within 10 days. Gestational age affects early growth. Children born at term (40 weeks) should follow accepted developmental guidelines. Infants born prematurely will not be as developed, either neurologically or physically, as their term counterparts.

The neonatal stage of development centers on reflexes. The neonate's personality also begins to form. The infant is close to the mother and may stare at faces and smile. The mother, and occasionally the father, can comfort and quiet the child. Obviously, the history must be obtained from the parents or caregivers. However, it is also important to observe the child. Common illnesses in this age group include jaundice, vomiting, and respiratory distress. Serious illnesses, such as meningitis, are difficult to distinguish from minor illnesses in neonates. Often, fever is the only sign, although the majority of neonates with fever have minor illnesses (96% to 97%). The few who are seriously ill can be easily missed. For this reason, any fever in a neonate requires extensive evaluation.

The approach to this age group should include several factors. First, the child should always be kept warm. Observe skin color, tone, and respiratory activity. The absence of tears when crying may indicate dehydration. The lungs should be auscultated early during the exam, while the infant is quiet. You might find it helpful to have the child suck on a pacifier during the examination. Allowing the infant to remain in a parent's or caregiver's lap may help keep the child calm.

Infants (Ages 1 to 5 Months)

Infants should have doubled their birth weight by 5 to 6 months of age. They should be able to follow the movements of others with their eyes. Muscle control develops in a cephalocaudal progression. This means, literally, that development of muscular control begins at the head (*cephalo*) and moves toward the tail (*caudal*). Muscular control also spreads from the trunk toward the extremities during this period. The infant's personality at this stage still centers closely on the parents or caregivers. The history must be obtained from these individuals, with close attention to possible illnesses and accidents, including sudden infant death syndrome (SIDS), vomiting, dehydration, meningitis, child abuse, and household accidents.

Concentrate on keeping these patients warm and comfortable. Allow the infant to remain in the parent's or caregiver's lap. A pacifier or bottle can be used to help keep the baby quiet during the examination.

Infants (Ages 6 to 12 Months)

Infants in this age group may stand or even walk with assistance. They are quite active and enjoy exploring the world with their mouths. In this stage of development, the risk of **foreign body airway obstruction (FBAO)** becomes a serious concern.

Infants 6 months and older have more fully formed personalities and express themselves more readily. They have considerable anxiety toward strangers. They do not like lying on their backs. Children in this age group tend to cling to the mother, though the father "will do" in many cases. Common illnesses and accidents include febrile seizures, vomiting, diarrhea, dehydration, bronchiolitis, car accidents, croup, child abuse, poisonings, falls, airway obstructions, and meningitis.

These children should be examined while sitting in the lap of the parent or caregiver (Figure 31-1). The exam should progress in a toe-to-head order, since starting at the face may upset the child. If time and conditions permit, allow the child to become familiar with you before beginning the examination.

Toddlers (Ages 1 to 3 Years)

Great strides occur in gross motor development during this stage. Children tend to run underneath or stand on almost everything. They seem to always be on the move. As they grow older, toddlers become braver and more curious or stubborn. They begin to stray away from the parents or caregivers more frequently. Yet these remain the only people who can comfort them quickly, and most children will cling to a parent or caregiver if frightened.

At ages 1 to 3 years, language development begins. Often children can understand better than they can speak. Therefore, the majority of the medical history will still come from the parents or caregivers. Remember, however, that you can ask toddlers simple and specific questions.

Accidents of all types are the leading cause of injury deaths in pediatric patients ages 1 to 15 years. Common accidents in this age group include motor-vehicle collisions, homicides, burn injuries, drownings, and pedestrian accidents. Common illnesses and injuries in the toddler age group include vomiting, diarrhea, febrile seizures, poisonings, falls, child abuse, croup, and meningitis. Keep in mind that FBAO is still a high risk for toddlers.

Be cautious when treating toddlers. Approach toddlers slowly and try to gain their confidence. Conduct the exam in a toe-to-head order. The child may be difficult to examine and may resist being touched. Speak quietly and use only simple words. Avoid asking questions that allow the child to say "no." If the situation permits, allow toddlers to hold transitional objects such as a favorite blanket or toy. Be sure to tell the child if something will hurt. If at all possible, avoid procedures on the dominant arm/hand, which the child will try to pull away.

Preschoolers (Ages 3 to 5 Years)

Children in this age group show a tremendous increase in fine and gross motor development. Language skills increase greatly. Children in this age group know how to talk. However, if frightened, they often refuse to speak, especially to strangers. They often have vivid imaginations and may see monsters as part of their world. Preschoolers may have tempers and will express them. During this stage of development, children fear mutilation and may feel threatened by treatment. Avoid frightening or misleading comments.

foreign body airway obstruction (FBAO) blockage or obstruction of the airway by an object that impairs respiration; in the case of pediatric patients, tongues, abundant secretions, and deciduous (baby) teeth are more likely to block airways.

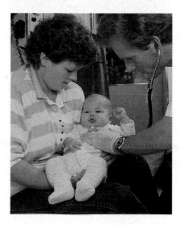

FIGURE 31-1 Infants and young children should be allowed to remain in their mother's arms.

Examine infants and toddlers in a toe-to-head order.

Preschoolers often run to a particular parent or caregiver, depending on the occasion. They stick up for the people they love and are openly affectionate. They still seek support and comfort from within the home.

When evaluating children in this age group, question the child first, keeping in mind that imagination may interfere with the facts. The child often has a distorted sense of time, and thus you must rely on the parents or caregivers to fill in the gaps. Common illnesses and accidents in this age group include croup, asthma, poisonings, auto accidents, burns, child abuse, ingestion of foreign bodies, drownings, epiglottitis, febrile seizures, and meningitis.

Treatment of preschoolers requires tact. Avoid baby talk. If time and situation permit, give the child health-care choices. Often the use of a doll or stuffed animal will assist in the examination. Allow the child to hold a piece of equipment, such as a stethoscope, and to use it. Let the child sit on your lap. Start the examination with the chest and evaluate the head last. Avoid misleading comments. Do not trick or lie to the child, and always explain what you are going to do.

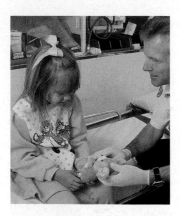

FIGURE 31-2 A small toy may calm a child in the 6 to 10 year age range.

School-Age Children (Ages 6 to 12 Years)

Children in this age group are active and carefree. Growth spurts sometimes lead to clumsiness. The personality continues to develop. School-age children are protective and proud of their parents or caregivers and seek their attention. They value peers, but also need home support.

When examining school-age children, give them the responsibility of providing the history. However, remember that children may be reluctant to provide information if they sustained an injury while doing something forbidden. The parents or caregivers can fill in the pertinent details. When assessing children in this age group, it is important to respect their modesty. Be honest and tell the child what is wrong. A small toy may help to calm the child (Figure 31-2). Common illnesses and injuries for this age group include drownings, auto collisions, bicycle accidents, falls, fractures, sports injuries, child abuse, and burns.

Adolescents (Ages 13 to 18)

Adolescence covers the period from the end of childhood to the start of adulthood (age 18). It begins with puberty, roughly age 13 for male children and age 11 for female children. (For this reason, adolescence is often defined as including ages 11 to 18, rather than 13 to 18.) Puberty is highly child specific and can begin at various ages. A female child, for example, may experience her first menstrual period as early as age 7 or 8.

Adolescents vary significantly in their development. Those over age 15 are physically nearer to adults in terms of their vital signs but emotionally may still be children. Regardless of physical maturity, remember that teenagers as a group are "body conscious." They worry about their physical image more than any other pediatric age group. You should tactfully address their stated concerns about body integrity or disfigurement. The slightest possibility of a lasting scar may be a tremendous issue to the adolescent patient.

Although patients in this age are not yet legally adults, most consider themselves to be grown up. They take offense at the use of the word "child." They have a strong desire to be liked by their peers and to be included. Relationships with parents and caregivers may at times be strained as the adolescent demands greater independence. They value the opinions of other adolescents, especially members of the opposite sex. Generally, these patients make good historians. Do not be surprised, however, if their perception of events differs from that of their parents or caregivers.

Common illnesses and injuries in this age group include mononucleosis, asthma, auto collisions, sports injuries, drug and alcohol problems, suicide gestures, and sexual abuse. Remember that pregnancy is also possible in female adolescents. When assessing teenagers, remember that vital signs will approach those of adults. In gathering a history, be factual and address the patient's questions. It may be wise to interview the patient away from the parents or caregivers. Listen to what the teenager is saying, as well as what he or she is not saying. If you suspect substance abuse or endangerment of the patient or others, approach the subject with tact and compassion. If you must perform a detailed physical exam, respect the teenager's sense of privacy. If the patient exhibits modesty or bodily shame, have an

Table 31-1 ANATOMIC AND PHYSIOLOGIC CHARACTERISTICS OF INFANTS AND CHILDREN

Differences in Infants and Children as Compared to Adults	Potential Effects That May Impact Assessment and Care
Tongue proportionately larger	More likely to block airway
Smaller airway structures	More easily blocked
Abundant secretions	Can block the airway
Deciduous (baby) teeth	Easily dislodged; can block the airway
Flat nose and face	Difficult to obtain good face mask seal
Head heavier relative to body and less-developed neck structures and muscles	Head may be propelled more forcefully than body producing a higher incidence of head injury in trauma
Fontanelle and open sutures (soft spots) palpable on top of young infant's head	Bulging fontanelle can be a sign of increased intracranial pressure (but may be normal if infant is crying); shrunken fontanelle may indicate dehydration
Thinner, softer brain tissue	Susceptible to serious brain injury
Head larger in proportion to body	Tips forward when supine; possible flexion of neck, which makes neutral alignment of airway difficult
Shorter, narrower, more elastic (flexible) trachea	Can close off trachea with hyperextension of neck
Short neck	Difficult to stabilize or immobilize
Abdominal breathers	Difficult to evaluate breathing
Faster respiratory rate	Muscles easily fatigue, causing respiratory distress
Newborns breathe primarily through the nose (obligate nose breathers)	May not automatically open mouth to breathe if nose is blocked; airway more easily blocked
Larger body surface relative to body mass	Prone to hypothermia
Softer bones	More flexible, less easily fractured; traumatic forces may be transmitted to internal organs, causing injury without fracturing the ribs; lungs easily damaged with trauma
Spleen and liver more exposed	Organ injury likely with significant force to abdomen

EMT-I of the same sex as the teenager conduct the examination, if possible. Regardless of the situation, provide psychological support and reassurance.

ANATOMY AND PHYSIOLOGY

The differences between the anatomy and physiology of infants and children and that of adults form the basis for the differences in the emergency medical care offered to the two groups (Table 31-1). As previously mentioned, children are not simply small adults. They possess bodies well suited to growth. As a rule, they have healthier organs, a greater ability to compensate for most illnesses, and softer, more flexible tissues. Because you will probably have infrequent contact with pediatric patients, you need to regularly review the physical characteristics that distinguish them from the adult patients that you encounter more often.

Head

The pediatric patient's head is proportionally larger than an adult's and the occipital region is significantly larger. In comparison with their head size, most pediatric patients have small faces and flat noses, which makes it difficult to obtain a good face mask seal.

With infants, pay special attention to the fontanelles—areas of the skull that have not yet fused. The fontanelles allow for compression of the head during childbirth and for rapid growth of the brain during early life. The posterior fontanelle generally closes by 4 months

In assessing infants, pay special attention to the fontanelles, especially the anterior fontanelle.

of age. The anterior fontanelle diminishes after 6 months of age and usually closes between 9 and 18 months.

During assessment, always inspect the anterior fontanelle. Normally, it should be level with the surface of the skull or slightly sunken. It also may pulsate. With increased intracranial pressure, as with meningitis or head trauma, the fontanelle may become tight and bulging and pulsations may diminish or disappear. In the presence of dehydration, the anterior fontanelle often falls below the level of the skull and appears sunken.

The heavy head relative to body size places an infant or child at risk of blunt head trauma. In accidents, the head may be propelled more forcefully than the body, resulting in a higher incidence of brain injury. Head size also affects the airway positioning techniques you should use in treating pediatric patients. In general, follow these guidelines:

- In treating seriously injured patients less than 3 years of age, place a thin layer of padding under their back to obtain a neutral position. This will prevent the head from tipping forward when supine, causing flexion of the neck (Figure 31-3).
- In treating medically ill children over 3 years of age, place a folded sheet or towel under the occiput to obtain a sniffing position (neck flexed slightly forward, head extended slightly backward to align pharynx and trachea).

Airway

In managing the airway of an infant or child, keep in mind these anatomical and physiological considerations:

- Pediatric patients have narrower airways at all levels and these are more easily blocked by secretions or obstructions.
- Infants are obligate nose breathers. If their noses are blocked by secretions, for example, they may not automatically open their mouths to breathe.
- The tongue takes up more space proportionately in a child's mouth and can more easily obstruct breathing in an unconscious patient.
- The trachea is softer and more flexible in a child and can collapse if the neck and head are hyperextended.
- A child's larynx is higher (C-3 to C-4) and extends into the pharynx.
- In young children, the cricoid ring is the narrowest part of the airway.
- Infants have an omega-shaped (horseshoe-shaped) epiglottis that extends at a 45-degree angle into the airway. Because epiglottic folds in pediatric patients have softer cartilage than in adults, they can be more floppy, especially in infants.

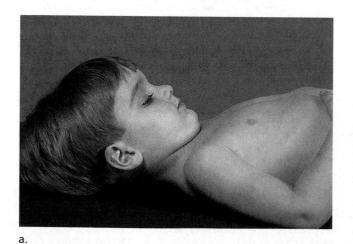
a.

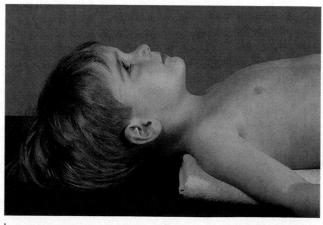
b.

FIGURE 31-3 In the supine position, an infant's or child's larger head tips forward, causing airway obstruction (a). Placing padding under the patient's back and shoulders will bring the airway to a neutral or slightly extended position (b).

Take these anatomical and physiological differences into account by following these general procedures: Always keep the nares clear in infants less than 6 months of age. Do not overextend the neck, which may collapse the trachea. Open the airway gently to avoid soft-tissue injury. Because any device placed in the infant's or child's airway further narrows the passage's diameter and may result in localized swelling, consider use of an oral or a nasal airway only after other manual maneuvers have failed to keep the airway open. (There will be more information on pediatric airway management later in this chapter.)

Consider use of an oral or nasal airway in a pediatric patient only after other manual maneuvers have failed to keep the airway open.

Chest and Lungs

In evaluating the chest and lungs of an infant or child, remember that tissues and muscles are more immature than in adults. Chest muscles tire easily, and lung tissues are more fragile. The soft, pliable ribs offer less protection to organs. Expect the ribs to be positioned horizontally and the mediastinum to be more mobile.

Take into account the following anatomical and physiological considerations when assessing the chest and lungs of a pediatric patient:

- Infants and children are diaphragmatic breathers.
- Pediatric patients, especially young infants, are prone to gastric distention.
- Although rib fractures occur less frequently in children, they are not uncommon in cases of child abuse.
- Because of the softness of a child's ribs, greater energy can be transmitted to underlying organs following trauma. As a result, significant internal injury can be present without external signs.
- Pulmonary contusions are more common in pediatric patients who have been subjected to major trauma.
- An infant's or child's lungs are more prone to pneumothorax following barotrauma.
- The mediastinum of a child or infant will shift more with tension pneumothorax than in an adult.
- Thin chest walls in infants and children allow for easily transmitted breath sounds. This may result in perception of breath sounds from elsewhere in the chest, which may cause you to miss a pneumothorax or misplaced intubation.

Abdomen

Note that the liver and spleen, both very vascular organs, are proportionally larger in the pediatric patient than in the adult patient. Abdominal organs lie closer together. Because of the immature abdominal muscles in an infant or child, expect to find more frequent damage to the liver and spleen and more multiple organ injuries than in an adult.

Extremities

Until pediatric patients reach adolescence, they have softer and more porous bones than adults. Therefore, you should treat sprains and strains as fractures and immobilize them accordingly.

During early stages of development, injuries to the **growth plate** may also disrupt bone growth. Keep this in mind when inserting an intraosseous needle, which could mistakenly pierce the plate. (Intraosseous infusion is discussed later in this chapter.)

growth plate the area just below the head of a long bone in which growth in bone length occurs; the epiphyseal plate.

Skin and Body Surface Area (BSA)

There are three distinguishing features of the pediatric patient's skin and BSA. First, the skin of an infant or child is thinner than that of an adult. Second, infants and children generally have less subcutaneous fat. Finally, they have a larger BSA-to-weight ratio.

As a result of these features, children risk greater injury from extremes in temperature or thermal exposure. They lose fluids and heat more quickly than adults and have a greater likelihood of dehydration and hypothermia. They also burn more easily and deeply than adults, explaining why burns account for one of the leading causes of death among pediatric trauma patients.

During the early stages of development, injuries to the growth plate by an intraosseous needle may disrupt bone growth.

Respiratory System

Although infants and children have a tidal volume proportionately similar to that of adolescents and adults, they require double the metabolic oxygen. They also have proportionately smaller oxygen reserves. The combination of increased oxygen requirements and decreased oxygen reserves makes infants and children especially susceptible to hypoxia.

Cardiovascular System

Infants and children increase their cardiac output by increasing their heart rate. They have a very limited capacity to increase their stroke volume.

Cardiac output is rate dependent in infants and small children. They possess vigorous, but limited, cardiovascular reserves. Although infants and children have a circulating blood volume proportionately larger than adults, their absolute blood volume is smaller. As a result, they can maintain blood pressure longer than an adult but still be at risk of shock (hypoperfusion). In assessing a pediatric patient for shock, keep in mind the following points:

- Smaller absolute volume of fluid/blood loss is needed to cause shock in infants and children.

- Larger proportional volume of fluid/blood loss is needed to cause shock in these same patients.

- As with all categories of patients, hypotension is a late sign of shock. In pediatric patients, it is an ominous sign of imminent cardiopulmonary arrest.

- The child may be in shock despite a normal blood pressure.

- Shock assessment in children and infants is based on clinical signs of tissue perfusion. (See the later discussion of circulation assessment.)

- Suspect shock if tachycardia is present.

- Monitor the pediatric patient carefully for the development of hypotension.

Bleeding that would not be dangerous in an adult may be life-threatening in an infant or child.

Once again, remember that children are not small adults. Bleeding that would not be dangerous in an adult may be a serious and life-threatening condition in an infant or child. Shock can develop in the small child who has a laceration to the scalp (with its many blood vessels), or in the 3-year-old who loses as little as a cup of blood. (Management of shock in pediatric patients will be discussed in detail later in the chapter.)

Nervous System

The nervous system develops continually throughout childhood. Even so, the neural tissue remains more fragile than in adults. The skull and spinal column, which are softer and more pliable than in adults, offer less protection of the brain and spinal cord. Therefore, greater force can be transmitted to a child's neural tissue with more devastating consequences. These injuries can occur without injury to the skull or to the spinal column. (Treatment of head and neck trauma will be discussed later in the chapter.)

Metabolic Differences

You may have noticed the repeated emphasis on the need to keep neonatal and pediatric patients warm during treatment and transport. The emphasis on warming techniques is based on the following metabolic considerations:

- Infants and children have a limited store of glycogen and glucose.

- Pediatric patients are prone to hypothermia because of their greater BSA-to-weight ratio.

- Significant volume loss can result from vomiting and diarrhea.

- Newborns and neonates lack the ability to shiver.

To prevent heat loss, always cover the patient's head and maintain adequate temperature controls in the ambulance. Ensure that the ambulance is always stocked with an adequate supply of blankets and, if you live in a cold area, hot water bottles.

GENERAL APPROACH TO PEDIATRIC ASSESSMENT

Priorities in the management of the pediatric patient, as with all patients, are established on a threat-to-life basis. If life-threatening problems are not present, you will complete each of the general steps discussed in the following sections.

BASIC CONSIDERATIONS

Many of the components of the initial patient assessment can be done during a visual examination of the scene. (This is sometimes called the "assessment from the doorway," during which you quickly note signs of an ill child such as lethargy.) Whenever possible, involve the parent or caregiver in efforts to calm or comfort the child. Depending on the situation, you may decide to allow the parent or caregiver to remain with the child during treatment and transport. As previously mentioned, the developmental stage of the patient and the coping skills of the parents or guardians will be key factors in making this decision.

When interacting with parents or other responsible adults, keep in mind the communication techniques suggested earlier. Pay attention to the way in which parents or caregivers interact with the child. Are the interactions appropriate to the emergency? Are family members concerned? Are they angry? Are they overly emotional or entirely indifferent?

From the time of dispatch, you will continually acquire information relative to the patient's condition. As with all patients, personal safety must be your first priority. In treating pediatric patients, follow the same guidelines in approaching the scene as you would with any other patient. Observe for potentially hazardous situations, and make sure you take appropriate BSI precautions. Remember that infants and young children are at especially high risk of an infectious process.

Remember to take appropriate BSI precautions when treating infants and children.

SCENE SIZE-UP

Upon arrival, conduct a quick scene size-up. Dispatch information received en route, as well as your own observations, can provide critical indicators of scene safety. Be aware of the increased anxiety and stress in any situation involving an infant or child. Try to set aside thoughts of your own children and adopt the professional, systematic approach to assessment necessary for scene safety and effective patient management. If you find yourself getting angry or upset, temporarily turn over care to another EMT-I until you compose yourself.

As you survey the scene, look for clues to the mechanism of injury (MOI) or the nature of the illness (NOI). These clues will help guide your assessment and determine appropriate interventions. Note the presence of dangerous substances, such as medicine bottles, household chemicals, or poisonous plants, that the child may have ingested. Spot environmental hazards such as unprotected stairwells, kerosene heaters, and so on. Identify possible causes of trauma, especially in motor-vehicle collisions. Remain alert for evidence of child abuse, particularly in cases in which the injury and history do not coincide. As already mentioned, pay attention to the way parents or caregivers respond to the child and the way the child responds to them.

Keep the child in mind while conducting your scene size-up. Pace your approach to give the child time to adjust to your presence. Speak in a soft voice, using simple words. As soon as you reach the child, position yourself at eye level with the patient and make every effort to win his trust. If the child bonds more readily with one member of the team than another, allow that person to remain with the child and, if possible, to conduct most of the physical exam.

INITIAL ASSESSMENT

The patient's condition determines the course of your initial assessment. An active and alert child will allow for a more comfortable approach, with more time spent on communication with the child and appropriate adults. A critically ill or injured child, however, may require quick intervention and rapid transport. Your choice of action depends on your general impression of the patient.

General Impression

The major points in forming your general impression are outlined in an assessment tool called the pediatric assessment triangle. Many experts recommend this assessment tool as a way of quickly evaluating the level of severity and the need for immediate intervention. It is a rapid "eyes-open, hands-on" approach that allows you to detect a life-threatening situation without the use of a stethoscope, blood pressure cuff, pulse oximeter, or other medical device. The triangle's three components are:

- *Appearance*—focuses on the child's mental status and muscle tone
- *Breathing*—directs attention to respiratory rate and respiratory effort
- *Circulation*—uses skin signs and color as well as capillary refill as indicators of the patient's circulatory status

Vital Functions

After quickly applying the pediatric assessment triangle to form a general impression, you will evaluate vital functions—mental status (level of consciousness) and the ABCs—as they apply to infants and children. Although assessment steps are basically the same as for adults, certain modifications must be made to collect accurate data.

Never shake an infant or child.

Level of Consciousness Employ the AVPU method (*A*lert, responds to *V*erbal stimuli, responds to *P*ainful stimuli, *U*nresponsive) to evaluate the pediatric patient's level of consciousness. Adjust the techniques for the child's age. With an infant, you may need to shout to elicit a response (perhaps crying) to verbal stimulus. An infant should withdraw from a noxious stimulus. *Never shake an infant or child.*

Airway and respiratory problems are the most common cause of cardiac arrest in infants and young children.

Airway Assess the airway using the techniques shown in Figures 31-4 to 31-7. If at any point the patient shows little or no movement of air, intervene immediately. Keep this fact in mind: *Airway and respiratory problems are the most common cause of cardiac arrest in infants and young children.*

As you inspect the airway, ask yourself the following questions:

- Is the airway patent?
- Is the airway maintainable with head positioning, suctioning, or airway adjuncts?
- Is the airway not maintainable? If so, what action is required? (Airway management techniques are discussed later in this chapter.)

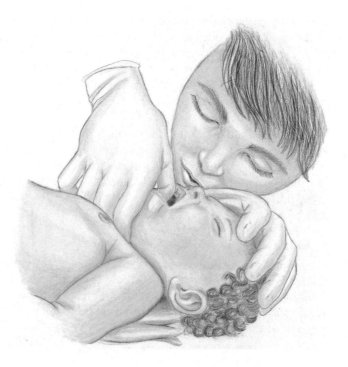

FIGURE 31-4 Opening the airway in a child.

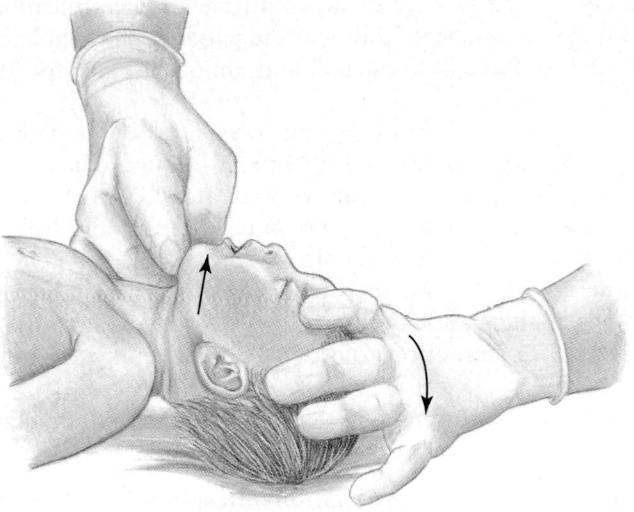

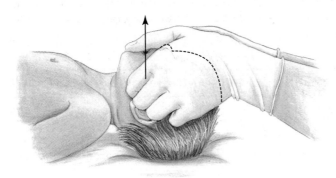

FIGURE 31-5   Head-tilt/chin-lift maneuver.

FIGURE 31-6   Jaw-thrust maneuver.

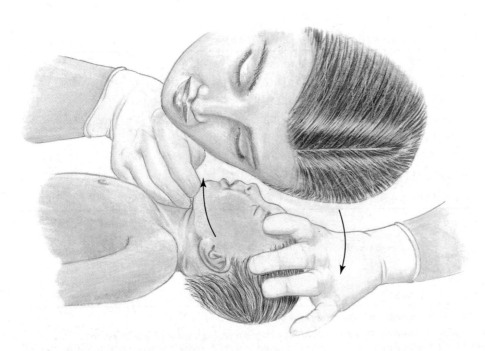

FIGURE 31-7   Assessing breathing.

Breathing   In assessing the breathing of a pediatric patient, recall the CPR certification courses in which you learned to "look, listen, and feel." *Look* at the patient's chest and abdomen for movement. *Listen* for breath sounds, both normal and abnormal. *Feel* for air movement at the patient's mouth.

Keep in mind that pediatric patients have small chests. For this reason, place the stethoscope near each of the armpits in order to minimize transmitted breath sounds. When considering the respiratory rate, remember that pain or fear can increase a child's respiratory efforts. Tachypnea, an abnormally rapid rate of breathing, may indicate fear, pain, inadequate oxygenation, or, in the case of neonates, exposure to cold.

If you suspect trauma, check the infant or child for life-threatening chest injuries. Keep in mind that even a minor injury to the chest can interfere with a child's breathing efforts. A chest injury can also interfere with your effort to provide adequate oxygenation or ventilation.

Your goal is to identify any evidence of compromised breathing. Evaluation of breathing includes assessment of the following conditions:

- *Respiratory rate.* Tachypnea is often the first manifestation of respiratory distress in infants. Regardless of the cause, an infant breathing at a rapid rate will eventually tire. Keep in mind that a decreasing respiratory rate may be a result of tiring and is not necessarily a sign of improvement. A slow respiratory rate in an acutely ill infant or child is an ominous sign. (Normal respiratory rates are listed in Table 31-2.) In short, be alert for a respiratory rate that is either abnormally fast or abnormally slow.

Table 31-2   NORMAL VITAL SIGNS: INFANTS AND CHILDREN*

Normal Pulse Rates (Beats per Minute, at Rest)

Newborn	100 to 180
Infant (0–5 mo)	100 to 160
Infant (6–12 mo)	100 to 160
Toddler (1–3 yrs)	80 to 110
Preschooler (3–5 yrs)	70 to 110
School age (6–10 yrs)	65 to 110
Early adolescence (11–14 yrs)	60 to 90

Normal Respiration Rates (Breaths per Minute, at Rest)

Newborn	30 to 60
Infant (0–5 mo)	30 to 60
Infant (6–12 mo)	30 to 60
Toddler (1–3 yrs)	24 to 40
Preschooler (3–5 yrs)	22 to 34
School Age (6–10 yrs)	18 to 30
Early Adolescence (11–14 yrs)	12 to 26

Normal Blood Pressure Ranges (mmHg, at Rest)

	Systolic Approx. 90 plus 2 × age	Diastolic Approx. ⅔ systolic
Preschooler (3–5 yrs)	average 98 (78 to 116)	average 65
School age (6–10 yrs)	average 105 (80 to 122)	average 69
Early adolescence (11–14 yrs)	average 114 (88 to 140)	average 76

*Adolescents ages 15 to 18 approach the vital signs of adults.

Note: A high pulse in an infant or child is not as great a concern as a low pulse. A low pulse may indicate imminent cardiac arrest. Blood pressure is usually not taken in a child under 3 years of age. In cases of blood loss or shock, a child's blood pressure will remain within normal limits until near the end, then fall swiftly.

- *Respiratory effort.* The quality of air entry can be assessed by observing for chest rise, breath sounds, stridor, or wheezing. An increased respiratory effort in the infant or child is also evidenced by nasal flaring and the use of accessory respiratory muscles. (Signs of increased respiratory effort are listed in Table 31-3.)
- *Color.* Cyanosis is a fairly late sign of respiratory failure and is most frequently seen in the mucous membranes of the mouth and the nail beds. Cyanosis of the extremities alone is more likely due to circulatory failure (shock) than to respiratory failure.

Circulation   As mentioned earlier, you should assess a pediatric patient's circulation by first checking the child's color. Keep in mind that the pediatric patient tends to become hypothermic; therefore, you should check the capillary refill time in an area of central circulation, such as the sternum or forehead. (Note that capillary refill time, as discussed later in this chapter, is considered reliable as a sign of perfusion primarily in children less than 6 years of age.) In general, evaluate the following conditions when assessing circulation during the initial assessment:

- *Heart rate.* As previously mentioned, infants develop sinus tachycardia in response to stress. Thus any tachycardia in an infant or child requires further evaluation to determine the cause. Bradycardia in a distressed infant or child may indicate hypoxia and is an ominous sign of cardiac arrest. (Normal heart rates are listed in Table 31-2.)
- *Peripheral circulation.* The presence of peripheral pulses is a good indicator of the adequacy of end-organ perfusion. Loss of central pulses is an ominous sign.
- *End-organ perfusion.* End-organ perfusion is most evident in the skin, kidneys, and brain. Decreased perfusion of the skin is an early sign of shock. A capillary refill time of greater than 2 seconds is indicative of low cardiac output. Impairment of brain perfusion is usually evidenced by a change in mental status. The child may become confused or lethargic. Seizures may occur. Failure of the child to recognize the parents' faces is often an ominous sign. Urine output directly relates to kidney perfusion. Normal urine output is 1 to 2 mL/kg/hr. Urine flow of less than 1 mL/kg/hr is an indicator of poor renal perfusion.

Remember that evaluation of mental status and ABCs during the initial assessment is rapid and not detailed—aimed at discovering and correcting immediate life-threatening conditions. More thorough measurements will be performed during the focused history and physical exam.

Table 31-3	SIGNS OF INCREASED RESPIRATORY EFFORT
Retraction	Visible sinking of the skin and soft tissues of the chest around and below the ribs and above the collarbone
Nasal flaring	Widening of the nostrils; seen primarily on inspiration
Head bobbing	Observed when the head lifts and tilts back as the child inhales and then moves forward as the child exhales
Grunting	Sound heard when an infant attempts to keep the alveoli open by building back pressure during expiration
Wheezing	Passage of air over mucous secretions in bronchi; heard more commonly upon expiration; a low- or high-pitched sound
Gurgling	Coarse, abnormal bubbling sound heard in the airway during inspiration or expiration; may indicate an open chest wound
Stridor	Abnormal, musical, high-pitched sound, more commonly heard on inspiration

Anticipating Cardiopulmonary Arrest

At each stage of evaluating vital functions, ask yourself, "Does this child have pulmonary or circulatory failure that may lead to cardiopulmonary arrest?"

Your initial assessment, and the repeated assessments that follow, help you to recognize and prevent cardiopulmonary arrest. At each stage of evaluating vital functions, ask yourself this question: *"Does this child have pulmonary or circulatory failure that may lead to cardiopulmonary arrest?"* Early recognition of the physiologically unstable child is one of the main goals of pediatric advanced life support (PALS). Conditions that place a pediatric patient at risk of cardiopulmonary arrest include:

- Respiratory rate greater than 60
- Heart rate greater than 180 or less than 80 (under 5 years)
- Heart rate greater than 180 or less than 60 (over 5 years)
- Respiratory distress
- Trauma
- Burns
- Cyanosis
- Altered level of consciousness
- Seizures
- Fever with petechiae (small purple spots resulting from skin hemorrhages)

Evaluate the patient for these conditions throughout assessment and transport. Cardiopulmonary arrest in infants and children is usually not a sudden event. Instead, it is the end result of progressive deterioration in respiratory and cardiac function. Therefore, you need to determine whether the patient's condition is deteriorating or improving. Any decompensation or change in the patient's status will prompt you to perform basic or advanced life support measures, as appropriate.

Transport Priority

Based on your initial assessment, you will assign the patient one of the following transport priorities:

- *Urgent*—Proceed with the rapid trauma assessment, if trauma is suspected, then transport immediately with further assessment and treatment performed en route.
- *Non-urgent*—Complete the focused history and physical exam at the scene, then transport.

Transitional Phase

The way in which the pediatric patient is transferred to EMS care depends entirely on the seriousness of the patient's condition. A transitional phase is intended for the conscious, non-acutely ill child. This phase of assessment allows the infant or child to become familiar with you and the equipment that you will be using. When dealing with the unconscious or acutely ill patient, however, you will skip this phase and proceed directly to the treatment and transport phases of assessment. In essence, you assign the patient an "urgent" status.

FOCUSED HISTORY AND PHYSICAL EXAM

After you have prioritized patient care at the end of the initial assessment, you will obtain a history and perform a physical exam. If the patient has a medical illness, the history will precede the physical exam. If the patient is suffering from trauma, the physical exam will take precedence. If partners are working together, the history and physical exam may be performed simultaneously.

History

Whenever a patient is identified as a priority patient, then the focused history will occur en route to the hospital, after essential treatments or interventions for life-threatening conditions have been performed.

To obtain a history for a pediatric patient, you will probably need to involve a family member or caregiver. Remember, however, that school-age children and adolescents like to take part in their own care. As previously mentioned, you can elicit valuable information from even very young patients. As a general precaution, question older adolescent patients in private, especially about issues such as sexual activity, pregnancy, or illicit drug and alcohol use. If you question adolescents about these subjects in the presence of an adult, they will probably be more reticent for fear of later repercussions.

As with any patient, you will use the history to uncover additional pertinent injuries or medical conditions. The history should center on the chief complaint and past medical history.

To evaluate the nature of the chief complaint, determine each of the following:

- Nature of the illness/injury
- Length of time the patient has been sick/injured
- Presence of fever
- Effects of the illness/injury on patient behavior
- Bowel/urine habits
- Presence of vomiting/diarrhea
- Frequency of urination

The past medical history identifies chronic illnesses, use of medications, and allergies. Be sure to inquire whether the infant or child is currently under a doctor's care. If so, obtain the name of the physician and present it at the receiving hospital. In the case of trauma patients, reconsider the mechanism of injury and the results of your on-scene physical examination (which, as noted earlier, will precede the history in the case of trauma).

Physical Exam

Focused Exam Carry out the physical exam after all life-threatening conditions have been identified and addressed. If there is a significant mechanism of injury or if the patient is unresponsive, perform a complete rapid trauma assessment or rapid medical assessment. Use the toe-to-head approach with the younger child (or begin with the chest and examine the head last) and the head-to-toe approach in the older child. If the injury is minor or if the ill patient is responsive, perform a physical exam that is focused on the affected areas and systems.

Perform the physical exam. Depending on the particular situation, some or all of the following assessment techniques may be appropriate to include in the exam:

- *Pupils.* Inspect the patient's pupils for equality and reaction to light.
- *Capillary refill.* As noted earlier, this technique is valuable for pediatric patients less than 6 years of age. Blanch the nail bed, base of the thumb, or sole of one of the feet. Remember that normal capillary refill is 2 seconds or less. Recall that this technique is less reliable in cold environments.
- *Hydration.* Note skin turgor, presence of tears and saliva and, with infants, the condition of the fontanelles.
- *Pulse oximetry.* Use this mechanical device on moderately injured or ill infants and children. Readings will give you immediate information regarding peripheral oxygen saturation and allow you to follow trends in the patient's pulse rate and oxygenation status. Keep in mind, however, that hypothermia or shock can affect readings.

Content Review

ELEMENTS OF THE GLASGOW COMA SCALE
- Verbal responses
- Motor functions
- Eye movements

To use the Glasgow coma scale with pediatric patients, remember: the younger the patient, the more adjustments you will need to make.

Glasgow Coma Scale In cases of trauma, you may need to apply the Glasgow coma scale (GCS)—a scoring system for monitoring the neurological status of patients with possible head injuries. The GCS assigns scores based on verbal responses, motor functions, and eye movements.

In using the GCS with pediatric patients, you will have to make certain modifications. The younger the patient, the more adjustments you will need to make. Verbal responses, for example, will not be possible for neonates and infants. However, motor function may be assessed in very young children by observing voluntary movement. Infants under 4 months of age should have a grasp reflex when an object is placed on the palmar surface of their hand. The grasp should be immediate. Children over 3 years of age will follow directions, when encouraged. Sensory function can be observed by the withdrawal reaction from tickling the patient. (See Table 31-4 for a modified GCS for infants.)

After you score the GCS for the patient, prioritize the patient according to severity. Guidelines are:

- *Mild*—GCS 13 to 15
- *Moderate*—GCS 9 to 12
- *Severe*—GCS less than or equal to 8

Table 31-4 GLASGOW COMA SCALE MODIFICATIONS FOR INFANTS

Category	Response	Score
Verbal	Happy, coos, babbles, or cries spontaneously	5
	Irritable crying, but consolable	4
	Cries to pain, weak cry	3
	Moans to pain	2
	None	1
Motor	Spontaneous movement	6
	Withdraws to touch	5
	Withdraws to pain	4
	Abnormal flexion	3
	Abnormal extension	2
	None	1
Eye opening (same as adult)	Spontaneous	4
	To speech	3
	To pain	2
	None	1

Source: Adapted from James, H.E., (1986): "Neurological evaluation and support in the child with acute brain insult," *Pediatric Annals*, 15(1):17.

Vital Signs   Remember that poorly taken vital signs are of less value than no vital signs at all. The following guidelines will help you obtain accurate pediatric readings. (Review Table 31-2 for normal pediatric vital signs.)

- Take vital signs with the patient in as close to a resting state as possible. If necessary, allow the child to calm down before attempting vital signs. Vital signs in the field should include pulse, respiration, blood pressure, and temperature.

- Take vital signs with the patient in as close to a resting state as possible. If necessary, allow the child to calm down before attempting vital signs. Vital signs in the field should include pulse, respiration, blood pressure, and temperature.

- Obtain blood pressure with an appropriate-sized cuff. The cuff should be two-thirds the width of the upper arm. Note that the pulse pressure (the difference between the systolic and diastolic blood pressure) narrows as shock develops. *Note that hypotension is a late and often sudden sign of cardiovascular decompensation.* Even mild hypotension should be taken seriously and treated quickly and vigorously, since cardiopulmonary arrest is probably imminent.

- Feel for peripheral, brachial, or femoral pulses. There is often a significant variation in pulse rate in children due to varied respirations. Therefore, it is important to monitor the pulse for at least 30 seconds, a full minute if possible.

- It is generally not possible to weigh the child. However, if medications are required, make a good estimate of the child's weight. Often the parents or caregivers can provide a fairly reliable weight from a recent visit to the doctor.

- Observe respiratory rate before beginning the examination. After the examination is started, the child will often begin to cry. It will then be impossible to determine respiratory rate. For an estimate of the upper limit of respiratory rate, subtract the child's age from 40. It is also important to identify respiratory pattern, as well as retractions, nasal flaring, or paradoxical chest movement.

- Measure temperature early in the patient encounter and repeat toward the end. IV fluid and exposure to the environment can cause a drop in core temperature.

- Continue to observe the child for level of consciousness. There may be a wide variety in levels of consciousness and activity during treatment.

Noninvasive Monitoring   Modern noninvasive monitoring devices all have their application in pediatric emergency care (Figure 31-8). These may include the pulse oximeter, automated blood pressure devices, self-registering thermometers, and electrocardiograms (ECGs). To promote the goal of early recognition of cardiopulmonary arrest, every seriously ill or injured child should receive continuous pulse oximetry. This will provide you with essential information regarding the patient's heart rate and peripheral O_2 saturation. It will also help you to monitor the effects of any medications administered. ECG and automated blood pressure/pulse monitor should also be considered. However, these devices may

Poorly taken vital signs are of less value than no vital signs at all.

Even mild hypotension should be taken seriously in infants and young children.

Every seriously ill or injured child should receive continuous ECG monitoring.

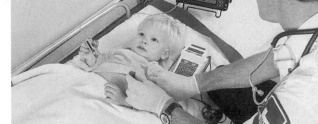

FIGURE 31-8   If available, noninvasive monitoring, including pulse oximetry and temperature measurement, should be used in prehospital pediatric care.

frighten the child. Before applying any monitoring device, explain what you are going to do. Demonstrate the display or lights. If the monitoring device makes noise, allow the child to hear the noise before you apply it. Reassure the child that the device will not hurt him.

ONGOING ASSESSMENT

Because a pediatric patient's condition can rapidly change for the better or the worse, it is necessary to repeat relevant portions of the assessment. (For this reason, ongoing assessment is sometimes called "reassessment.") You should continually monitor the patient's respiratory effort, skin color, mental status, temperature, and pulse oximetry. Retake vital signs and compare them with baseline vitals. In general, reassess stable patients every 15 minutes, critical patients every 5 minutes.

GENERAL MANAGEMENT OF PEDIATRIC PATIENTS

The same ABCs that guide the management of adult patients apply to pediatric patients: Your top priorities in treating an infant or child are airway, breathing, and circulation. However, because of the special anatomical and physiological considerations that influence the management of pediatric patients, you need to practice these skills on an ongoing and regular basis.

BASIC AIRWAY MANAGEMENT

In treating the pediatric patient, basic life support (BLS) should be applied according to current standards and protocols. BLS should include maintenance of the airway, artificial ventilation, and if required, chest compressions. (See Table 31-5.) As with all patients, your priority is to ensure an open airway. The following modifications of BLS airway skills will ensure that you take into account the clinical implications of the pediatric airway.

Manual Positioning

Allow the pediatric patient to assume a position of comfort, if possible. When placing the patient in a supine position, avoid hyperextension of the neck. As previously mentioned, infants and small children risk collapsed tracheas from hyperextension of the neck. For

Table 31-5 SUMMARY OF BLS MANEUVERS IN INFANTS AND CHILDREN		
Target of Maneuver	Infant (<1 year)	Child (1 to 8 years)
Airway		
Open airway	Head-tilt/chin-lift (unless trauma present)	Head-tilt/chin-lift (unless trauma present)
	Jaw-thrust	Jaw-thrust
Clear foreign body obstruction	Back blows/chest thrusts	Heimlich maneuver
Breathing		
Initial	2 breaths at 1 to 1½ sec/breath	2 breaths at 1 to 1½ sec/breath
Subsequent	20 breaths/min	20 breaths/min
Circulation		
Pulse check	Brachial/femoral	Carotid
Compression area	Lower third of sternum	Lower third of sternum
Compression width	2 or 3 fingers	Heel of 1 hand
Depth	Approximately ½ to 1 in (newborn ½ to ¾ in)	Approximately 1 to 1½ in
Rate	At least 100/min (newborn 120/min)	100/min
Compression-ventilation ratio	5:1 (Newborn 3:1)	5:1

trauma patients less than 3 years old, place support under the torso. For supine medical patients 3 years old and older, provide occipital elevation.

Foreign Body Airway Obstruction (FBAO)

Before administering treatment, determine if an airway obstruction is partial or complete. Infants or children with a partial airway obstruction will have a cough, hoarse voice or cry, stridor, or some other evidence that at least some air is passing through the airway. Avoid any maneuvers that will turn a partial obstruction into a complete obstruction. Instead, place the patient in a position of comfort and transport immediately.

In the case of complete airway obstruction, take one of the following age-specific maneuvers:

- *Children.* For children older than 1 year of age, perform a series of abdominal thrusts.
- *Infants.* For infants less than 1 year old, deliver a series of five back blows followed by five chests thrusts. Inspect the infant's mouth on completion of each series.

As you recall from the basic CPR courses, never check a pediatric patient's mouth with blind finger sweeps.

Never use blind finger sweeps in a pediatric patient.

Suctioning

Apply suctioning whenever you detect heavy secretions in the nose or mouth of a pediatric patient, especially if the patient has a diminished level of consciousness. You can use a bulb syringe, flexible suction catheter, or rigid-tip suction catheter, depending on the patient's age or size (Figure 31-9). Make sure that flexible catheters are correctly sized (Table 31-6).

Although pediatric suctioning techniques vary very little from adult suctioning techniques, keep the following modifications in mind:

- Decrease suction pressure to less than 100 mmHg in infants.
- Avoid excessive suctioning time (suction less than 10 seconds) in order to decrease the possibility of hypoxia.

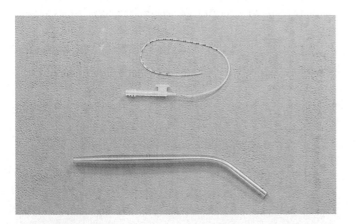

FIGURE 31-9 Pediatric-size suction catheters. Top: soft suction catheter. Bottom: rigid or hard suction catheter.

Table 31-6	SUCTION CATHETER SIZES FOR INFANTS AND CHILDREN

Age	Suction Catheter Size (French)
Up to 1 year	8
2 to 6 years	10
7 to 15 years	12
16 years	12 to 14

- Avoid stimulation of the vagus nerve, which may produce bradycardia. As a general rule, suction no deeper than you can see and for no more than 15 seconds per attempt.
- Frequently check the patient's pulse. If bradycardia occurs, stop suctioning immediately and oxygenate.

Oxygenation

Adequate oxygenation is the hallmark of pediatric patient management. Methods of oxygen delivery include blow-by techniques (especially for neonates) and pediatric-sized nonrebreather masks. Although nonrebreather masks provide the highest concentration of supplemental oxygen, children may resist their use. Try to overcome their fear by demonstrating the use of the mask on yourself (Figure 31-10). Better yet, enlist the support of a parent or caregiver, and ask them to demonstrate the mask. As an alternative, you might place the mask over the face of a stuffed animal.

If the child refuses to accept the nonrebreather mask, resort to high-flow, blow-by oxygen. Some units place oxygen tubing through the bottom of a colorful paper cup and use it to deliver the blow-by supplemental oxygen. Children often find a familiar object less frightening than complicated medical equipment.

Airway Adjuncts

As a general rule, use airway adjuncts in pediatric patients only if prolonged artificial ventilations are required. There are two reasons for this. First, infants and children often improve quickly through the administration of 100% oxygen. Second, airway adjuncts may create greater complications in children than in adults. Pediatric patients risk soft-tissue damage, vomiting, and stimulation of the vagus nerve.

Oropharyngeal Airways Oropharyngeal airways should be used only in pediatric patients who lack a gag reflex. (Patients with a gag reflex risk vomiting and bradycardia.) Size the airway by measuring from the corner of the mouth to the front of the earlobe. Remember: Oropharyngeal airways that are too small can obstruct breathing; ones that are too large can both block the airway and cause trauma. (For general sizing suggestions, see Table 31-7.)

In placing an oropharyngeal airway, use a tongue blade to depress the tongue and jaw (Figure 31-11). If you detect a gag reflex, continue to maintain an open airway with a manual maneuver (jaw-thrust or head tilt/chin lift) and consider the use of a nasal airway. Remember that with a pediatric patient, the oral airway is inserted with the tip pointing toward the tongue and pharynx.

Nasopharyngeal Airways Use nasopharyngeal airways for those children who possess a gag reflex and who require prolonged artificial ventilations. DO NOT use them on any child

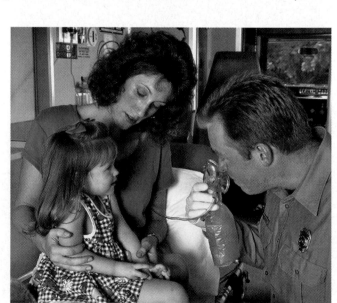

FIGURE 31-10 To overcome the child's fear of the nonrebreather mask, try it on yourself or have the parent try it on before attempting to place it on the child.

Table 31-7   EQUIPMENT GUIDELINES ACCORDING TO AGE AND WEIGHT

Equipment	Age (50th Percentile Weight)					
	Premature (1–2.5 kg)	Neonate (2.5–4.0 kg)	6 Mo (7.0 kg)	1–2 Yrs (10–12 kg)	5 Yrs (16–18 kg)	5–10 Yrs (24–30 kg)
Airway Oral	infant (00)	infant (small) (0)	small (1)	small (2)	medium (3)	medium large (4.5)
Breathing Self-inflating bag	infant	infant	child	child	child	child/adult
O$_2$ ventilation mask	premature	newborn	infant/child	child	child	small adult
Endotracheal tube	2.5–3.0 (uncuffed)	3.0–3.5 (uncuffed)	3.5–4.0 (uncuffed)	4.0–4.5 (uncuffed)	5.0–5.5 (uncuffed)	5.5–6.5 (uncuffed)
Laryngoscope blade	0 (straight)	1 (straight)	1 (straight)	1–2 (straight)	2 (straight or curved)	2–3 (straight or curved)
Suction/stylet (F)	6–8/6	8/6	8–10/6	10/6	14/14	14/14
Circulation BP cuff	newborn	newborn	infant	child	child	child/adult
Venous access Angiocath	22–24	22–24	22–24	20–22	18–20	16–20
Butterfly needle	25	23–25	23–25	23	20–23	18–21
Intracath	—	—	19	19	16	14
Arm board	6 in	6 in	6–8 in	8 in	8–15 in	15 in
Orogastric tube (F)	5	5–8	8	10	10–12	14–18
Chest tube (F)	10–14	12–18	14–20	14–24	20–32	28–38

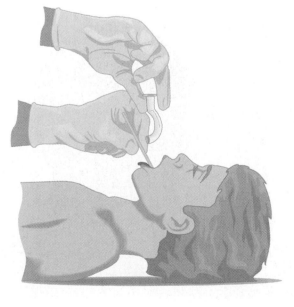

FIGURE 31-11 Inserting an oropharyngeal airway device in a child with the use of a tongue blade.

with midface or head trauma. You might mistakenly pass the airway through a fracture into the sinuses or the brain.

Size a nasal airway in the same fashion as for adult patients. (Use the outside diameter of the patient's little finger as a measure.) Although nasopharyngeal airways come in a variety of sizes, they are not readily available for infants less than 1 year old. Equipment required for insertion of a nasal airway includes: appropriately sized soft, flexible latex tubing; and a water-based lubricant.

When inserting the nasal airway, follow the same basic method as you would in an adult patient. It is important to remember that younger children often have enlarged adenoids (lymphatic tissues in the nasopharynx), which can be easily lacerated when inserting a nasopharyngeal airway. Because of this, always use care when inserting a nasopharyngeal airway in a younger child. If resistance is met, do not force the airway because significant bleeding can result.

Ventilation

Adequate tidal volume and ventilatory rate provide more than just a high oxygen saturation for your patient. Ventilation is a two-way physiological street: Maintenance of appropriate oxygen levels results in appropriate carbon dioxide levels as well. However, you will achieve neither of these clinically important events without tailoring the ventilatory device and technique to your pediatric patient. Important points to remember include:

- Avoid excessive bag pressure and volume. Ventilate at an age-appropriate rate, using only enough ventilation to make the chest rise.
- Use a properly sized mask to ensure a good fit. In general, the mask should fit on the bridge of the nose and the cleft of the chin (Figure 31-12).
- Obtain a chest rise with each breath.
- Allow adequate time for exhalation.
- Assess BVM ventilation. (Provide 100% oxygen by using a reservoir attached to the BVM.)
- Remember that flow-restricted, oxygen-powered ventilation devices are contraindicated in pediatric resuscitation.
- Do not use BVMs with pop-off valves unless they can be readily occluded, if necessary. (Ventilatory pressures required during pediatric CPR may exceed the limit of the pop-off valve.)
- Apply cricoid pressure through application of the Sellick maneuver to minimize gastric inflation and passive regurgitation (Figure 31-13).
- Ensure correct positioning to avoid hyperextension of the neck.

FIGURE 31-12 A mask should fit on the bridge of the child's nose and on the cleft of the chin.

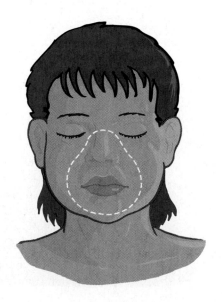

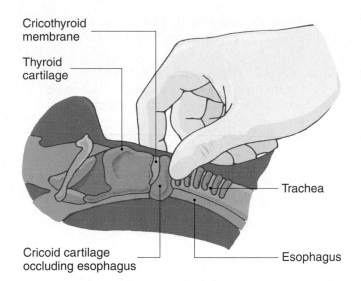

Cricothyroid membrane

Thyroid cartilage

Trachea

Cricoid cartilage occluding esophagus

Esophagus

FIGURE 31-13 In the Sellick maneuver, pressure is placed on the cricoid cartilage, compressing the esophagus. This reduces regurgitation and helps bring the vocal cords into view, which is useful if intubation is to be performed.

ADVANCED AIRWAY AND VENTILATORY MANAGEMENT

As an EMT-I, you will be expected to master the advanced life support (ALS) procedures that make you a leader in the EMS system. Your clinical skills will help save the lives of pediatric patients whose respiratory systems have failed so severely that BLS measures are insufficient. When signs of impending cardiopulmonary arrest have been identified (as discussed earlier), you may be called on to implement the following pediatric advanced life support (PALS) techniques, either in your own unit or in a transfer of care from a BLS unit. The success of these techniques requires knowledge of the procedures that set pediatric skills apart from the ALS skills used on adults. (Review the advanced airway skills for adults discussed in Chapter 5.)

Foreign Body Airway Obstruction

One advantage of being able to perform endotracheal intubation is that it gives you another treatment modality for children with FBAOs. If a child's airway cannot be cleared by basic airway procedures, visualize the airway with the laryngoscope. Often, the obstructing foreign body can be seen. Once visualized, grasp the foreign body with the Magill forceps and remove it. If you cannot remove the foreign body with Magill forceps, try to intubate around the obstruction. This often requires using an endotracheal tube smaller than you would normally choose. However, this will provide an adequate airway until the foreign body can be removed at the hospital.

Endotracheal Intubation

Endotracheal intubation allows direct visualization of the lower airway through the trachea, bypassing the entire upper airway. It is the most effective method of controlling a patient's airway, whether the patient is an adult or a child. However, endotracheal intubation is not without complications. It is an invasive technique with little room for error. A tube that is mistakenly sized or misplaced, especially in an apneic patient, can quickly lead to hypoxia and death.

Anatomical and Physiological Concerns   Although endotracheal intubation of a child and an adult follow the same basic procedures, the special features of the pediatric airway complicate placement of any orotracheal tube. In fact, variations in the airway size of children discourage the use of certain airways, including esophageal obturator airways (EOA), pharyngeotracheal lumen airways (PtL), and esophageal-tracheal combitubes (ETC). In using an endotracheal tube, keep in mind these points:

- In infants and small children, it is often more difficult to create a single clear visual plane from the mouth, through the pharynx, and into the glottis. A straight-blade laryngoscope is preferred, since it provides greater displacement

An endotracheal tube that is mistakenly sized or misplaced—especially in the apneic patient—can quickly lead to hypoxia and death.

Alternative airways (EOA, PtL, ETC) cannot be used in children.

Remember that LMAs do not protect the airway from aspiration.

of the tongue and better visualization of the relatively cephalad and anterior glottis. For larger children, a curved blade may sometimes be used. (Review Table 31-7.)

- Variations in the sizes of pediatric airways, coupled with the fact that the narrowest portion of the airway is at the level of the cricoid ring, makes proper sizing of the endotracheal tube crucial. To determine correct size, apply any of the following methods:
  - Use a resuscitation tape, such as the Broselow/™ tape, to estimate tube size based on height.
  - Estimate the correct tube size by using the diameter of the patient's little finger or the diameter of the nasal opening.
  - Calculate the correct tube size by using this simple numerical formula:

$$\text{(Patient's age in years} + 16) \div 4 = \text{tube size}$$

- Depth of insertion can be estimated based on age (Table 31-8). However, the best method of determining depth is direct visualization. Due to the distance between the mouth and the trachea, a stylet is rarely needed to position the tube properly. When a stylet is used, select a malleable yet rigid style.
- Because the pediatric airway narrows at the level of the cricoid cartilage, uncuffed tubes should be used in children younger than 8 years old. The tubes should display a vocal cord marker to ensure correct placement.
- Infants and small children may have greater vagal response than adults. Therefore, laryngoscopy and passage of an endotracheal tube are likely to cause a vagal response, dramatically slowing the child's heart rate and decreasing the cardiac output and blood pressure. As a result, pediatric intubations must be carried out swiftly, accurately, and with continuous monitoring.

Indications   The indications for endotracheal intubation in a pediatric patient are the same as those for an adult. They include:

- Need for prolonged artificial ventilations
- Inadequate ventilatory support with a BVM
- Cardiac or respiratory arrest
- Control of an airway in a patient without a cough or gag reflex
- Necessary for providing a route for drug administration
- Need to gain access to the airway for suctioning

Additionally, if local protocols allow it, endotracheal intubation may be used in a child who has croup or epiglottitis and an increasingly compromised airway.

Techniques for Pediatric Intubation   To perform endotracheal intubation on a pediatric patient, follow the basic steps in Procedure 31-1. Detailed steps include:

Pediatric intubation must be carried out swiftly, accurately, and with continuous monitoring.

1. While maintaining ventilatory support, hyperventilate the patient with 100% oxygen. If time allows, hyperventilate for a full 2 minutes.

Table 31-8 INFANT/CHILD ENDOTRACHEAL TUBES	
Age of Patient	**Measurement of the Endotracheal Tube at the Teeth**
6 mo to 1 yr	12 cm—teeth to mid-trachea
2 yrs	14 cm—teeth to mid-trachea
4 to 6 yrs	16 cm—teeth to mid-trachea
6 to 10 yrs	18 cm—teeth to mid-trachea
10 to 12 yrs	20 cm—teeth to mid-trachea

Endotracheal Intubation in the Child

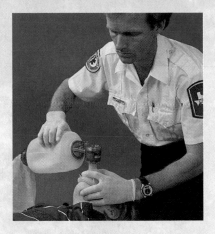

31-1a Hyperventilate the child.

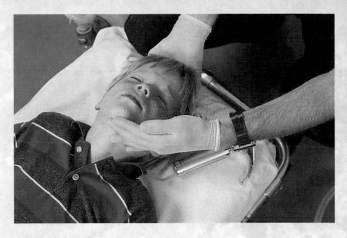

31-1b Position the head.

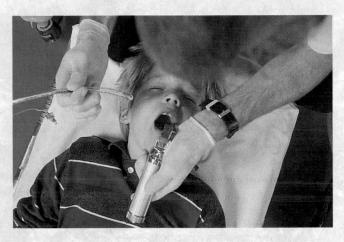

31-1c Insert the laryngoscope and visualize the airway.

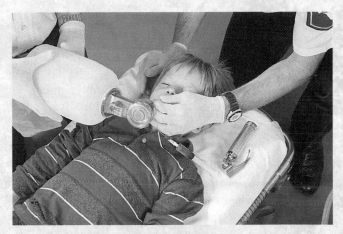

31-1d Insert the tube and ventilate the child.

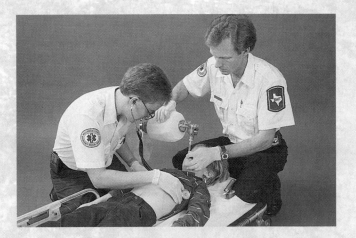

31-1e Confirm tube placement.

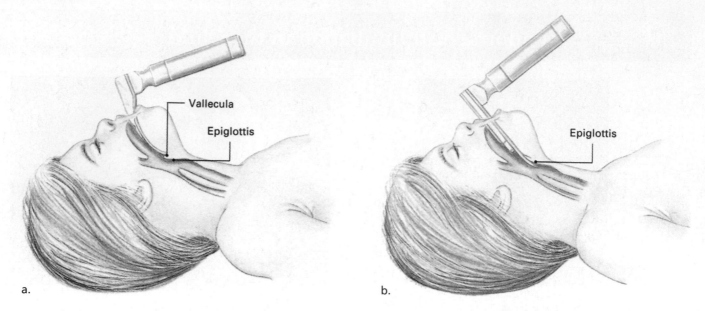

Vallecula

Epiglottis

Epiglottis

a.

b.

FIGURE 31-14   Placement of the laryngoscope: (a) MacIntosh (curved) blade and (b) Miller (straight) blade.

2. Assemble and check your equipment. As stated earlier, a straight-blade laryngoscope is preferred. Assorted sizes of endotracheal tubes, both cuffed and uncuffed, should be stocked in the pediatric kit aboard your ambulance.

3. Place the patient's head and neck into an appropriate position. With a pediatric patient, the head should be maintained in a sniffing position.

4. Hold the laryngoscope in your left hand.

5. Insert your laryngoscope blade into the right side of the patient's mouth. With a sweeping action, displace the tongue to the left.

6. Move the blade slightly toward the midline, and then advance it until the distal end is positioned at the base of the tongue (Figure 31-14).

7. Look for the tip of the epiglottis and place the laryngoscope blade into its proper position. Keep in mind that a child, particularly an infant, has a shorter airway and a higher glottis than an adult. Because of this, you will see the cords much sooner than you may expect.

8. With your left wrist straight, use your shoulder and arm to lift the mandible and tongue at a 45-degree angle to the floor until the glottis is exposed. Use the little finger of your left hand to apply gentle downward pressure to the cricoid cartilage. This will permit easier visualization of the cords.

9. Grasp the endotracheal tube in your right hand. To pass the tube into your patient's mouth, it may be helpful to hold it so that its curve is in a horizontal plane (bevel sideways). Insert the tube through the right corner of the child's mouth.

10. Under direct observation, insert the endotracheal tube into the glottic opening and pass it through until its distal cuff disappears past the vocal cords, approximately 5 to 10 centimeters. As a tube is advanced, it should be rotated into the proper plane. In some cases, it will be difficult to advance an endotracheal tube at the level of the cricoid. DO NOT force the tube through this region, because it may cause laryngeal edema.

11. Hold the tube in place with your left hand. Attach an infant- or child-size bag-valve device to the 15/22 mm adapter and deliver several breaths.

12. Check for proper tube placement. Watch for chest rise and fall with each ventilation and listen for equal, bilateral breath sounds. There should also be

DO NOT force an endotracheal tube through the cricoid region, because it may cause laryngeal edema.

an absence of sounds over the epigastrium with ventilations. Confirm placement with an ETCO$_2$ detector.

13. If the tube has a distal cuff, inflate it with the recommended amount of air.

14. Recheck for proper placement of the tube and hyperventilate the patient with 100% oxygen.

15. Secure the endotracheal tube with umbilical tape while maintaining ventilatory support.

16. Continue supporting the tube manually while maintaining ventilations. Check periodically to ensure proper tube position. As with adults, allow no more than 30 seconds to pass without ventilating your patient.

Nasogastric Intubation

If gastric distention is present in a pediatric patient, you may consider placing a nasogastric (NG) tube. In infants and children, gastric distention may result from overly aggressive artificial ventilations or from air swallowing. Placement of an NG tube will allow you to decompress the stomach and proximal bowel of air. An NG tube can also be used to empty the stomach of blood or other substances. Indications for use of a nasogastric intubation include:

- Inability to achieve adequate tidal volumes during ventilation due to gastric distention
- Presence of gastric distention in an unresponsive patient

As with nasopharyngeal airways, an NG tube is contraindicated in pediatric patients who have sustained head or facial trauma. Because the NG tube might migrate into the cranial sinuses, consider the use of an orogastric tube instead. Other contraindications include possible soft-tissue damage in the nose and inducement of vomiting.

Equipment for placing an NG tube includes:

- Age-appropriate NG tubes
- 20 mL syringe
- Water-soluble lubricant
- Emesis basin
- Tape
- Suctioning equipment
- Stethoscope

In sizing the NG tube, keep in mind the following recommended guidelines:

- Newborn/infant: no. 8.0 French
- Toddler/preschooler: no. 10 French
- School-age children: no. 12 French
- Adolescents: no. 14 to 16 French

In determining the correct length, measure the tube from the top of the nose, over the ear, to the tip of the xiphoid process. The steps for inserting the tube can be followed in Procedure 31-2. Keep in mind as you examine these steps that many experts believe that an NG tube should only be inserted when an endotracheal tube is in place. This precaution will prevent misplacement of the tube into the trachea instead of the esophagus. Consult protocols in your area on the use of NG tubes.

NG tube insertion is safest when the airway is protected with an ET tube.

CIRCULATION

As mentioned earlier, the respiratory and cardiovascular systems are interdependent. In pediatrics, you are encouraged to look at the total child. You should assess the child by assessing the various body systems. For example, instead of simply checking a pulse, you should look for end-organ changes that indicate the effectiveness of respiratory and cardiovascular function. These include such things as mental status, skin color, skin temperature,

Two problems lead to cardiopulmonary arrest in children: shock and respiratory failure.

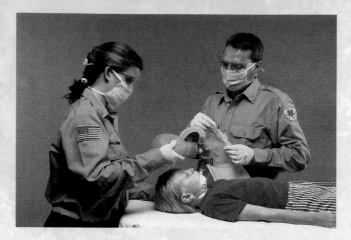

31-2a   Oxygenate and continue to ventilate, if possible.

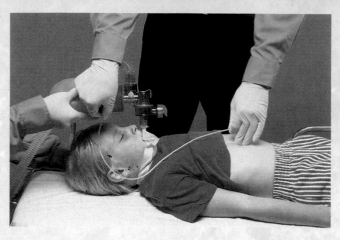

31-2b   Measure the nasogastric tube from the tip of the nose, over the ear, to the tip of the xiphoid process.

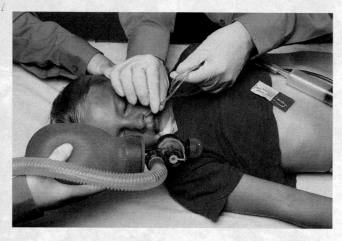

31-2c   Lubricate the end of the tube. Then pass it gently downward along the nasal floor to the stomach.

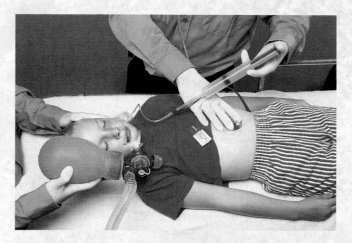

31-2d   Auscultate over the epigastrium to confirm correct placement. Listen for bubbling while injecting 10 to 20 cc of air into the tube.

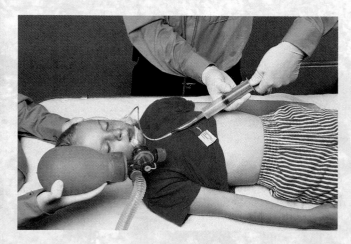

31-2e   Use suction to aspirate stomach contents.

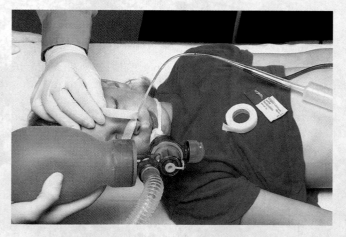

31-2f   Secure the tube in place.

urine output, and others. Two problems lead to cardiopulmonary arrest in children: shock and respiratory failure. Both must be identified and corrected early. The following section will address assessment of the cardiovascular system. Particular emphasis is placed on venous access and fluid resuscitation, because these are essential skills for prehospital ALS personnel who treat pediatric patients.

Vascular Access

Intravenous techniques for children are basically the same as for adults. (See Chapter 4.) However, additional veins may be accessed in the infant. These include veins of the neck and scalp, as well as of the arms, hands, and feet. The external jugular vein, however, should only be used for life-threatening situations.

Intraosseous Infusion

The use of intraosseous (IO) infusion has become popular in the pediatric patient. (See Figure 31-15a.) This is especially true when large volumes of fluid must be administered, as occurs in hypovolemic shock, and when other means of venous access are unavailable. Certain drugs can be administered intraosseously, including epinephrine, atropine, dopamine, lidocaine, sodium bicarbonate, and dobutamine. Indications for IO infusion include:

- Children less than 6 years old
- Existence of shock or cardiac arrest
- An unresponsive patient
- Unsuccessful attempts at peripheral IV insertion

The primary contraindications for IO infusion include:

- Presence of a fracture in the bone chosen for infusion
- Fracture of the pelvis or extremity fracture in the bone proximal to the chosen site

In performing IO perfusion, you can use a standard 16- or 18-gauge needle (either hypodermic or spinal). However, an intraosseous needle is preferred and significantly better (Figure 31-15b). The anterior surface of the leg below the knee should be prepped with antiseptic solution such as povidone iodine. The needle is then inserted, in a twisting fashion, 1 to 3 centimeters below the tuberosity. Insertion should be slightly inferior in direction (to avoid the growth plate) and perpendicular to the skin (Figure 31-16). Placement of the needle into the marrow cavity can be determined by noting a lack of resistance as the needle passes through the bony cortex. Other indications include the needle standing upright without support, the

Content Review

DRUGS ADMINISTERED BY INTRAOSSEOUS ROUTE
- Epinephrine
- Atropine
- Dopamine
- Lidocaine
- Sodium bicarbonate
- Dobutamine

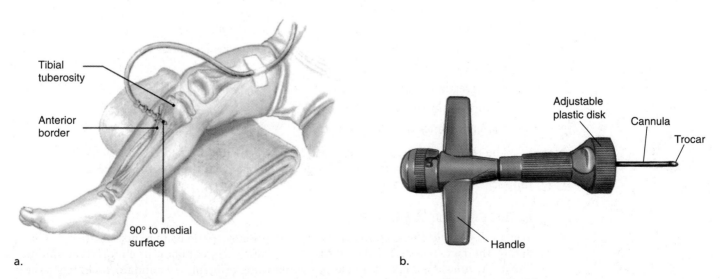

a.   b.

FIGURE 31-15   Intraosseous administration in the pediatric patient (a). An intraosseous needle (b).

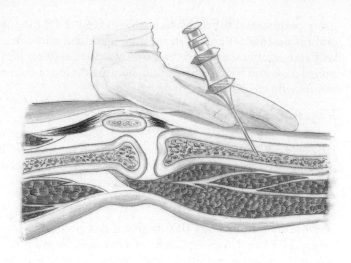

FIGURE 31-16 Correct needle placement for intraosseous administration. Note that the needle tip is in the marrow cavity.

ability to aspirate bone marrow into a syringe, or free flow of the infusion without infiltration into the subcutaneous tissues. (See also the discussion of IO infusion in Chapter 4.)

Fluid Therapy

In children, too much fluid can result in heart failure and pulmonary edema. Too little fluid can be ineffective.

The accurate dosing of fluids in children is crucial. Too much fluid can result in heart failure and pulmonary edema. Too little fluid can be ineffective. The initial dosage of fluid in hypovolemic shock should be 20 mL/kg of an isotonic solution such as lactated Ringer's or normal saline, as soon as IV access is obtained. After the infusion, the child should be reassessed. If perfusion is still diminished, then a second bolus of 20 mL/kg should be administered. A child with hypovolemic shock may require 40 to 60 mL/kg, whereas a child with septic shock may require at least 60 to 80 mL/kg. Fluid therapy should be guided by the child's clinical response.

DO NOT allow a full liter bag of fluid to be directly connected to a small child or infant without having a flow limiter attached.

Intravenous infusions in children should be closely monitored with frequent patient reassessment. Minidrip administration sets, flow limiters, or infusion pumps should be routinely used in pediatric cases.

Medications

Cardiopulmonary arrest in infants and children is almost always due to a primary respiratory problem, such as drowning, choking, or smoke inhalation. The major aim in pediatric resuscitation is airway management and ventilation, as well as replacement of intravascular volume, if indicated. In certain cases, medications may be required. The objectives of medication therapy in pediatric patients include:

- Correction of hypoxemia
- Increased perfusion pressure during chest compressions
- Stimulation of spontaneous or more forceful cardiac contractions
- Acceleration of the heart rate
- Correction of metabolic acidosis
- Suppression of ventricular ectopy
- Maintenance of renal perfusion

The dosages of medications must be modified for the pediatric patient. Table 31-9 and Table 31-10 illustrate recommended pediatric drug dosage in advanced cardiac life support.

ELECTRICAL THERAPY

You are less likely to use electrical therapy on pediatric patients than adult patients. This is due to the fact that ventricular fibrillation is much less common in children than adults. However, you should review and keep the following principles in mind for times when these emergencies arise:

Table 31-9 DRUGS USED IN PEDIATRIC ADVANCED LIFE SUPPORT*

Drug	Dose	Remarks
Adenosine	0.1 to 0.2 mg/kg Maximum strength dose 12 mg	Rapid IV bolus
Amiodarone	5 mg/kg IV/IO	Rapid IV bolus
Atropine sulfate	0.02 mg/kg per dose	Minimum dose 0.1 mg Maximum single dose: 0.5 mg in child; 1.0 mg in adolescent
Calcium chloride 10%	20 mg/kg per dose	Give slowly
Dopamine hydrochloride	2–10 mcg/kg per min	Adrenergic action dominates at ≥ 15–20 mcg/kg per min
Epinephrine *for bradycardia*	IV/IO 0.01 mg/kg (1:10,000) ET: 0.1 mg/kg (1:1,000)	Be aware of effective dose of preservatives administered (if preservatives are present in epinephrine preparation) when high doses are used
for asystolic or pulseless arrest	*First dose:* IV/IO: 0.01 mg/kg (1: 10,000) ET: 0.1 mg/kg (1:1,000) Doses as high as 0.2 mg/kg may be effective *Subsequent doses:* IV/IO/ET: 0.1 mg/kg (1:1,000) Doses as high as 0.2 mg/kg may be effective	Be aware of effective dose of preservatives administered (if preservatives are present in epinephrine preparation) when high doses are used
Epinephrine infusion	Initial at 0.1 mcg/kg per min Higher infusion dose used if asystole present	Titrate to desired effect (0.1–1.0 mcg/kg per minute)
Lidocaine	1 mg/kg per dose	Rapid bolus
Lidocaine infusion	20–50 mcg/kg per min	
Sodium bicarbonate	1 mEq/kg per dose or 0.3 × kg × base deficit	Infuse slowly and only if ventilation is adequate

*IV, intravenous; IO, intraosseous; ET, endotracheal.

- Administer an initial dosage of 2 joules per kilogram of body weight.
- If this is unsuccessful, increase the dosage to 4 joules per kilogram.
- If this is unsuccessful, focus your attention on correcting hypoxia and acidosis.
- Transport to a pediatric critical care unit, if possible.

C-SPINE IMMOBILIZATION

Spinal injuries in children are not as common as in adults. However, because of a child's disproportionately larger and heavier head, the cervical spine (C-spine) is vulnerable to injury. Any time an infant or child sustains a significant head injury, assume that a neck injury may also be present. Children can suffer a spinal cord injury with no noticeable damage to the vertebral column as seen on cervical spine X-rays. Thus, negative cervical spine X-rays do not necessarily ensure that a spinal cord injury does not exist. Because of this, children should remain immobilized until a spinal cord injury has been excluded by hospital personnel. As previously noted, even children secured in a car safety seat can suffer neck injuries if the heads are propelled forward during an accident or sudden stop.

Any time an infant or child sustains a head injury, assume that a neck injury is also present.

Table 31-10 PREPARATION OF INFUSIONS

Drug	Preparation*	Dose
Epinephrine	0.6 × body weight (kg) equals milligrams added to diluent† to make 100 mL	Then 1 mL/h delivers 0.1 mcg/kg per min; titrate to effect
Dopamine/ dobutamine	0.6 × body weight (kg) equals milligrams added to diluent† to make 100 mL	Then 1 mL/h delivers 0.3 mcg/kg per min; titrate to effect
Lidocaine	120 mg of 40 mg/mL solution added to 97 mL of 5% dextrose in water, yielding 1,200 mcg/mL solution	Then 1 mL/kg per h delivers 20 mcg/kg per min

*Standard concentration may be used to provide more dilute or more concentrated drug solution, but then individual dose must be calculated for each patient and each infusion rate:

$$\text{Infusion rate (mL/h)} = \frac{\text{Weight (kg)} \times \text{Dose (mcg/kg/min)} \times 60 \text{ min/h}}{\text{Concentration (mcg/mL)}}$$

†Diluent may be 5% dextrose in water, 5% dextrose in half-normal, normal saline, or Ringer's lactate solution.

Always make sure that you use the appropriate-sized pediatric immobilization equipment. These supplies may include rigid cervical collars, towel or blanket rolls, foam head blocks, commercial pediatric immobilization devices, vest-type or short wooden backboards, and long boards with the appropriate padding. For pediatric patients found in car seats, you can also use the seat for immobilization. The Kendrick Extrication Device (KED) can be quickly modified to immobilize a pediatric patient. Because of the significant variations in the size of children, you must be creative in devising a plan for pediatric immobilization.

In securing the pediatric patient to the backboard, use appropriate amounts of padding to secure infants, toddlers, and preschoolers in a supine, neutral position. Never use sandbags when immobilizing a pediatric patient's head. If you must tip the board to manage vomiting, the weight of the sand bag may worsen the head injury.

Any time you immobilize a pediatric patient, remember that many children, especially those under age 5, will protest or fight restraint. Try to minimize the emotional stress by having a parent or caretaker stand near or touch the child. Often the child will quit struggling when secured totally in an immobilization device. Ideally, a rescuer or family member should remain with the child at all times to reassure and calm the child, if possible.

TRANSPORT GUIDELINES

In managing a pediatric patient, never delay transport to perform a procedure that can be done en route to the hospital.

In managing a pediatric patient, never delay transport to perform a procedure that can be done en route to the hospital. After deciding on necessary interventions—first BLS, then ALS—determine the appropriate receiving facility. In reaching your decision, consider three factors:

- Time of transport
- Specialized facilities
- Specialized personnel

If you live in an area with specialized prehospital crews such as Critical Care Crews and Neonatal Nurses, their availability should weigh in your decision as well. Consider whether the patient would benefit by transfer by one of these crews. If so, request support. If not, determine the closest definitive care facility for the infant or child placed in your care. If time allows, continue to reduce the fear involved in transition of care from the family to the hospital. If you have won the trust of the child, and conditions permit, you might allow the patient to sit on your lap en route to the hospital (Figure 31-17). Think of what you would do or say to calm your own child or the child of a close relative or friend.

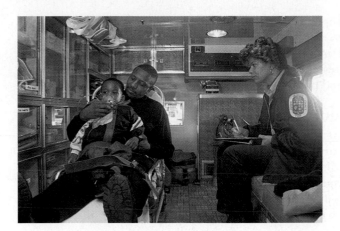

FIGURE 31-17 Emotional support of the infant or child continues during transport.

SPECIFIC MEDICAL EMERGENCIES

As you already realize from your earlier training and experience, a variety of pediatric medical problems can activate the EMS system. Although the majority of childhood medical emergencies involve the respiratory system, other body systems can be involved as well. To help you recognize and treat pediatric medical emergencies, the following sections cover some of the specific conditions you may encounter.

INFECTIONS

Childhood is a time of frequent illnesses because of the relative immaturity of the pediatric immune system. Infectious diseases may be caused by the infection or infestation of the body by an infectious agent such as a virus, bacterium, fungus, or parasite. Most infections are minor and self-limiting. However, several infections can be life-threatening. These include meningitis, pneumonia, and septicemia (a systemic infection, usually bacterial, in the bloodstream).

The impact of an infection on physiological processes depends on the type of infectious agent and the extent of the infection. Signs and symptoms also vary, depending on the type of infection and the time since exposure. Any of the following conditions may indicate the presence of an infection: fever, chills, tachycardia, cough, sore throat, nasal congestion, malaise, tachypnea, cool or clammy skin, petechiae, respiratory distress, poor appetite, vomiting, diarrhea, dehydration, hypoperfusion (especially with septicemia), purpura (purple blotches resulting from hemorrhages into the skin that do not disappear under pressure), seizures, severe headache, irritability, stiff neck, or bulging fontanelle (infants).

The management of infections depends on the body system or systems affected. Treatment of some of the most common and serious infections will be found in the sections that follow. As a general rule, you should adhere to these guidelines when treating an infectious illness:

- Take all BSI precautions, due to the unknown cause of the infection.
- Become familiar with the common pediatric infections encountered in your area.
- If possible, try to determine which, if any, pediatric infections you have not been exposed to or vaccinated for. For example, if you did not have chicken pox (varicella) or measles (rubeola) as a child, and were not vaccinated for them, then you should consider receiving vaccination for these illnesses. If you encounter a child suspected of having an infectious disease to which you may be susceptible, consider allowing another rescuer to be the primary person to care for the child.

RESPIRATORY EMERGENCIES

Respiratory emergencies constitute the most common reason EMS is summoned to care for a pediatric patient. Respiratory illnesses can cause respiratory compromise due to their affect on the alveolar/capillary interface. Some illnesses are quite minor, causing only mild

Infectious diseases account for the majority of pediatric illnesses.

Prompt recognition of a respiratory emergency in an infant or child can literally mean the difference between life and death.

symptoms, whereas others can be rapidly fatal. Your approach to the child with a respiratory emergency will depend on the severity of respiratory compromise. If the child is alert and talking, then you can take a more relaxed approach. However, if the child is ill-appearing and exhibiting marked respiratory difficulty, then you must immediately intervene to prevent respiratory arrest and possible cardiopulmonary arrest.

Severity of Respiratory Compromise

The severity of respiratory compromise can be quickly classified into the following categories: respiratory distress, respiratory failure, and respiratory arrest.

Respiratory emergencies in pediatric patients may quickly progress from respiratory distress to respiratory failure to respiratory arrest. You must learn to recognize the phase your patient is in and take the appropriate interventions. Prompt recognition and treatment can literally mean the difference between life and death for an infant or child suffering from respiratory compromise.

Respiratory Distress   The mildest form of respiratory impairment is classified as respiratory distress. The most noticeable finding is an increased work of breathing. One of the earliest indicators of respiratory distress is an increase in respiratory rate. Unfortunately, respiratory rate is one of the vital signs that is most often estimated. As mentioned previously, it is essential to obtain an accurate respiratory rate in children. Ideally, the respiratory rate should be measured for an entire minute. If time does not allow it, or if the child is deteriorating, then the respiratory rate should be measured for at least 30 seconds and multiplied by two to obtain the respiratory rate.

In addition to an increased work of breathing, the child in respiratory distress will initially have a slight decrease in the arterial carbon dioxide tension as the respiratory rate increases. However, as respiratory distress increases, the carbon dioxide tension will gradually increase.

The signs and symptoms of respiratory distress include:

- Normal mental status deteriorating to irritability or anxiety
- Tachypnea
- Retractions
- Nasal flaring (in infants)
- Good muscle tone
- Tachycardia
- Head bobbing
- Grunting
- Cyanosis that improves with supplemental oxygen

If not corrected immediately, respiratory distress will lead to respiratory failure.

Respiratory Failure   Respiratory failure occurs when the respiratory system is not able to meet the demands of the body for oxygen intake and for carbon dioxide removal. It is characterized by inadequate ventilation and oxygenation. During respiratory failure, the carbon dioxide level begins to rise as the body is not able to remove carbon dioxide. This ultimately leads to respiratory acidosis.

The signs and symptoms of respiratory failure include:

- Irritability or anxiety deteriorating to lethargy
- Marked tachypnea later deteriorating to bradypnea
- Marked retractions later deteriorating to agonal respirations
- Poor muscle tone
- Marked tachycardia later deteriorating to bradycardia
- Central cyanosis

Respiratory failure is a very ominous sign. If immediate intervention is not provided, the child will deteriorate to full respiratory arrest.

Respiratory Arrest   The end result of respiratory impairment, if untreated, is respiratory arrest. The cessation of breathing typically follows a period of bradypnea and agonal respirations.

Signs and symptoms of respiratory arrest include:

- Unresponsivenes deteriorating to coma
- Bradypnea deteriorating to apnea
- Absent chest wall motion
- Bradycardia deteriorating to asystole
- Profound cyanosis

Respiratory arrest will quickly deteriorate to full cardiopulmonary arrest if appropriate interventions are not made. The child's chances of survival markedly decrease when cardiopulmonary arrest occurs.

Management of Respiratory Compromise

The management of respiratory compromise should be based on the severity of the problem. The goals of management include increasing ventilation and increasing oxygenation. You should try to identify the signs and symptoms of respiratory distress early so that you can intervene before the child deteriorates.

Your initial attention should be directed at the airway. Is it patent? Is it maintainable with simple positioning? Is endotracheal intubation required?

After assessing the airway, ensure continued maintenance of the airway by positioning, placement of an airway adjunct (oropharyngeal or nasopharyngeal airway), or endotracheal intubation.

For children in respiratory distress or early respiratory failure, administer oxygen at high flow. Some children will tolerate a nonrebreather mask. Others may not and may require that someone (perhaps a parent) hold blow-by oxygen for them to breathe. If the child fails to improve with supplemental oxygen administration, the patient should be treated more aggressively. Often, it is necessary to separate the parents from the child so that you can provide the necessary care without interruption or distraction.

Pediatric patients with late respiratory failure or respiratory arrest require aggressive treatment. This includes:

- Establishment of an airway
- High-flow supplemental oxygen administration
- Mechanical ventilation with a BVM device attached to a reservoir delivering 100% oxygen
- Endotracheal intubation if mechanical ventilation does not rapidly improve the patient's condition
- Consideration of gastric decompression with an orogastric or nasogastric tube if abdominal distension is impeding ventilation
- Consideration of needle decompression of the chest if a tension pneumothorax is thought to be present

In addition to the above, you should obtain venous access. The child should be promptly transported to a facility staffed and equipped to handle critically ill children. While en route, continue to reassess the child. Signs of improvement include an improvement in skin color and temperature. As end-organ perfusion improves, the child will exhibit an increase in pulse rate, an increase in oxygen saturation, and an improvement in mental status. Provide emotional and psychological support to the parents and keep them abreast of the results of your care.

SPECIFIC RESPIRATORY EMERGENCIES

Respiratory problems typically arise from obstruction of a part of the respiratory tract or impairment of the mechanics of respiration. The following discussion will present the common pediatric respiratory emergencies based on the part of the airway they most affect.

COMMON CAUSES
OF UPPER AIRWAY
OBSTRUCTION
- Croup
- Epiglottitis
- Bacterial tracheitis
- Foreign body aspiration

Whenever you find an infant, toddler, or young child in respiratory or cardiac arrest, assume complete upper airway obstruction until proven otherwise.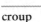

croup laryngotracheobronchitis; a common viral infection of young children, resulting in edema of the subglottic tissues; characterized by barking cough and inspiratory stridor.

epiglottitis bacterial infection of the epiglottis, usually occurring in children older than age 4; a serious medical emergency.

Upper Airway Obstruction

Obstruction of the upper airway can be caused by many factors. As previously mentioned, upper airway obstruction may be partial or complete. It can be caused by inflamed or swollen tissues caused by infection or by an aspirated foreign body. Appropriate care depends on prompt and immediate identification of the disorder and its severity. Whenever you find an infant, toddler, or young child in respiratory or cardiac arrest, assume complete upper airway obstruction until proven otherwise.

Croup Croup, medically referred to as *laryngotracheobronchitis*, is a viral infection of the upper airway. It most commonly occurs in children 6 months to 4 years of age and is prevalent in the fall and winter. Croup causes an inflammation of the upper respiratory tract involving the subglottic region. The infection leads to edema beneath the glottis and larynx, thus narrowing the lumen of the airway. Severe cases of croup can lead to complete airway obstruction. Another form of croup called spasmodic croup occurs mostly in the middle of the night without any prior upper respiratory infection.

Assessment The history for croup is fairly classic. Often, the child will have a mild cold or other infection and be doing fairly well until evening. After dark, however, a harsh, barking or brassy cough develops. The attack may subside in a few hours but can persist for several nights.

The physical exam will often reveal inspiratory stridor. There may be associated nasal flaring, tracheal tugging, or retraction. You should never examine the oropharynx. Often, in the prehospital setting, it is difficult to distinguish croup from epiglottitis. (See Table 31-11 and Figure 31-18.) If epiglottitis is present, examination of the oropharynx may result in laryngospasm and complete airway obstruction. If the attack of croup is severe and progressive, the child may develop restlessness, tachycardia, and cyanosis. Although croup can result in complete airway obstruction and respiratory arrest, this is a rare event.

Management Management of croup consists of appropriate airway maintenance. Place the child in a position of comfort and administer cool mist oxygen at 4 to 6 L/minute. Oxygen can be delivered by face mask or blow-by method. If the attack is severe, the medical direction physician may order the administration of racemic epinephrine or albuterol. Some physicians also advocate the use of steroids, because they feel these drugs will shorten the course of the illness.

In preparing the patient for transport, remember that the journey from the house to the ambulance will often allow the child to breathe cool air. Because cool air causes a decrease in subglottic edema, the child may be clinically improved by the time you reach the ambulance. If appropriate, keep the parent or caregiver with the infant or child. Do not agitate the patient, which could worsen the croup, by administering nonessential measures such as IVs or blood pressure readings.

Epiglottitis Epiglottitis is an acute infection and inflammation of the epiglottis and is potentially life-threatening. (Recall that the epiglottis is a flap of cartilage that protects the airway during swallowing.) Epiglottitis, unlike croup, is caused by a bacterial infection, usually *Haemophilus influenzae* type B. Due to the availability of the H. flu vaccine, epiglottitis has become an uncommon occurrence. When it does occur, it tends to strike preschool and school-age children ages 3 to 7 years.

Table 31-11 SYMPTOMS OF CROUP AND EPIGLOTTITIS

Croup	Epiglottitis
Slow onset	Rapid onset
Generally wants to sit up	Prefers to sit up
Barking cough	No barking cough
No drooling	Drooling; painful to swallow
Fever approx. 100°F to 101°F	Fever approx. 102°F to 104°F
	Occasional stridor

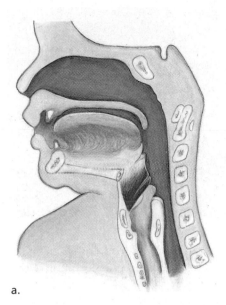 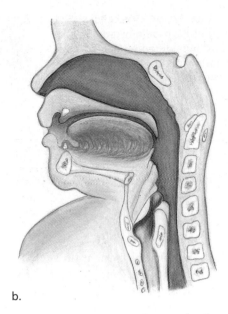

a.   b.

FIGURE 31-18 Epiglottitis is characterized by inflammation of the epiglottis and supraglottic tissues (a). Croup is characterized by subglottic edema (b).

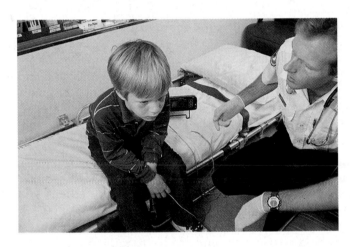

FIGURE 31-19 Posturing of the child with epiglottitis. Often, there will be excessive drooling.

Assessment Epiglottitis presents similarly to croup. Often the child will go to bed feeling relatively well, usually with what parents or caregivers consider to be a mild infection of the respiratory tract. Later, the child awakens with a high temperature and a brassy cough. The progression of symptoms can be dramatic. There is often pain on swallowing, sore throat, high fever, shallow breathing, dyspnea, inspiratory stridor, and drooling (Figure 31-19).

On physical examination, the child will appear acutely ill and agitated. *Never attempt to visualize the airway.* If the child is crying, the tip of the epiglottis can be seen posterior to the base of the tongue. In epiglottitis, the epiglottis is cherry red and swollen. As airway obstruction develops, the child will exhibit retractions, nasal flaring, and pulmonary hyperexpansion. As the epiglottis swells, he may not be able to swallow his saliva and will begin to drool. Often the child will want to remain seated. Patients will often assume the tripod position to help maximize their airway. If they lean backward or lie flat, the epiglottis can fall back and completely obstruct the airway.

Management Management of epiglottitis consists of appropriate airway maintenance and oxygen administration by face mask (Figure 31-20) or the blow-by technique. Ideally, the oxygen should be humidified to minimize drying of the epiglottis and airway. To reduce the child's anxiety, you might ask the parent or caregiver to administer the oxygen. If the airway becomes obstructed, two-rescuer ventilation with BVM is almost always effective.

Never attempt to visualize the airway in patients with epiglottitis.

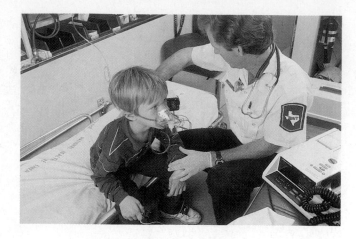

FIGURE 31-20 The child with epiglottitis should be administered humidified oxygen and transported in a comfortable position.

Make sure that all intubation equipment is available, including an appropriate-sized endotracheal tube. Remember, however, that intubation is contraindicated unless complete obstruction has occurred.

Also, do not intubate in settings with short transport times. If endotracheal intubation is required, it may be necessary to use a smaller endotracheal tube because of narrowing of the glottic opening. If you perform chest compression on glottic visualization during intubation, a bubble at the tracheal opening may form. This may help to establish upper airway landmarks that are distorted by the disease.

Pediatric patients with epiglottitis require immediate transport. Handle the child gently, since stress could lead to total airway obstruction from spasms of the larynx and swelling tissues. Avoid IV sticks, do not take a blood pressure, and do not attempt to look into the mouth. During transport, allow the child to sit on the lap of the parent or caregiver, if appropriate. Constantly monitor the child, and notify the hospital of any changes in status. Remember, if the patient is maintaining his airway, *do not put anything in the child's mouth,* including a thermometer. At all times, consider epiglottitis a critical condition.

Bacterial Tracheitis Bacterial tracheitis is a bacterial infection of the airway, subglottic region. Although the condition is very uncommon, it is most likely to appear following episodes of viral croup. It afflicts mainly infants and toddlers 1 to 5 years of age.

Assessment In assessing this condition, parents or caregivers will typically report that the child has experienced an episode of croup in the preceding few days. They will also indicate the presence of a high-grade fever accompanied by coughing up of pus and/or mucus. The patient may exhibit a hoarse voice and, if able to talk, the child may complain of a sore throat. A physical examination may reveal inspiratory or expiratory stridor.

Management As with all respiratory emergencies, the child must be carefully monitored since respiratory failure or arrest may be an end result. Carefully manage airway and breathing, providing oxygenation by face mask or blow-by technique. Keep in mind that ventilations may require high pressure to adequately ventilate the patient. This may require depressing the pop-off valve of the pediatric BVM device, if the valve is present. Consider intubation only in cases of complete airway obstruction. Transport guidelines are similar to those for cases of epiglottitis.

Foreign Body Aspiration Children—especially toddlers and preschoolers ages 1 to 4—like to put objects into their mouths. As a result, these children are at increased risk of aspirating foreign bodies, especially when they run or fall. In fact, foreign body aspiration is the number one cause of in-home accidental deaths in children under 6 years of age. In addition, many children choke on, or aspirate, food given to them by their parents or other well-meaning adults. Young children have not yet developed coordinated chewing motions in their mouth and pharynx and cannot adequately chew food. Common foods associated with aspiration and airway obstruction in children include hard candy, nuts, seeds, hot dogs, sausages, and grapes. Non-food items include coins, balloons, and other small objects.

Do not put anything in the mouth of an epiglottitis patient, including a thermometer.

At all times, consider epiglottitis a critical condition.

bacterial tracheitis bacterial infection of the airway, subglottic region; in children, most likely to appear after episodes of croup.

Assessment   The child with a suspected aspirated foreign body may present in one of two ways. If the obstruction is complete, the child will have minimal or no air movement. If the obstruction is partial, the child may exhibit inspiratory stridor, a muffled or hoarse voice, drooling, pain in the throat, retractions, and cyanosis.

Management   Whenever you suspect that a child has aspirated a foreign body, immediately assess the patient's respiratory efforts. If the obstruction is partial, make the child as comfortable as possible and administer humidified oxygen. If old enough, place the child in a sitting position. Do not attempt to look in the mouth. Intubation equipment should be readily available since complete airway obstruction can occur. Transport the child to a hospital, where the foreign body can be removed by hospital personnel in a controlled environment.

If the obstruction is complete, clear the airway with accepted BLS techniques. Sweep visible obstructions with your gloved finger. Do not perform blind finger sweeps, as this can push a foreign body deeper into the airway. Following BLS foreign body removal procedures, attempt ventilation with a BVM. If unsuccessful, visualize the airway with a laryngoscope. If the foreign body is seen and readily accessible, try to remove it with Magill forceps. Intubate if possible. Continue BLS foreign body removal procedures. Transport following appropriate guidelines, avoiding further agitation of the child.

Lower Airway Distress

As already discussed, suspect lower airway distress when the following conditions exist: an absence of stridor, presence of wheezing during exhalation, and increased work of breathing. Common causes of lower airway distress include respiratory diseases such as asthma, bronchiolitis, and pneumonia. Although infrequent, you may also encounter cases of foreign body lower airway aspiration, especially in toddlers and preschoolers.

Asthma   Asthma is a chronic inflammatory disorder of the lower respiratory tract. The disease affects more than 6 million people in the United States. It occurs before age 10 in approximately 50% of the cases, and before age 30 in another 33% of cases. The disease tends to run in families. It is also commonly associated with atopic conditions, such as eczema and allergies. Although deaths from other respiratory conditions have been steadily declining, asthmatic deaths have risen significantly in recent decades. Hospitalization of children for treatment of asthma has increased by more than 200% over the past 20 years. Because children can readily succumb to asthma, prompt prehospital recognition and treatment are essential.

Pathophysiology   Asthma is a chronic inflammatory disorder of the airways, characterized by bronchospasm and excessive mucus production. In susceptible children, this inflammation causes widespread, but variable, airflow obstruction. In addition to airflow obstruction, the airways become hyperresponsive.

Asthma may be induced by one of many different factors, commonly called "triggers." The triggers vary from one child to the next. Common triggers include environmental allergens, cold air, exercise, foods, irritants, emotional stress, and certain medications.

Within minutes of exposure to the trigger, a two-phase reaction occurs. The first phase of the reaction is characterized by the release of chemical mediators such as histamine. These cause bronchoconstriction and bronchial edema that effectively decreases expiratory airflow, causing the classic "asthmatic attack." If treated early, asthma may respond to inhaled bronchodilators. If the attack is not aborted, or does not resolve spontaneously, a second phase may occur. The second phase is characterized by inflammation of the bronchioles as cells of the immune system invade the respiratory tract. This causes additional edema and further decreases expiratory airflow. The second phase is typically unresponsive to inhaled bronchodilators. Instead, antiinflammatory agents, such as corticosteroids, are often required.

As the attack continues, and swelling of the mucous membranes lining the bronchioles worsens, the bronchi may become plugged by thick mucus. This further obstructs airflow. As a result, there is an increase in sputum production. In addition, the lungs become progressively hyperinflated, since airflow is more restricted in exhalation. This effectively reduces vital capacity and results in decreased gas exchange by the alveoli, resulting in hypoxemia. If allowed to progress untreated, hypoxemia will worsen, and unconsciousness and death may ensue.

If an asthma attack is allowed to progress untreated, hypoxemia will worsen and unconsciousness and death may result.

In severe asthma attacks, the patient may not wheeze at all. This is an ominous finding.

Subcutaneous epinephrine or terbutaline may be used when inhaled medications are poorly tolerated or are unavailable.

Status asthmaticus requires immediate transport with aggressive treatment administered en route.

bronchiolitis viral infection of the medium-sized airways, occurring most frequently during the first year of life.

Assessment   Asthma can often be differentiated from other pediatric respiratory illnesses by the history. In many cases, there is a prior history of asthma or reactive airway disease. The child's medications may also be an indicator. Children with asthma often have an inhaler or take a theophylline or oral beta agonist preparation.

On physical examination, the child is usually sitting up, leaning forward, and tachypneic. Often, there is an associated unproductive cough. Accessory respiratory muscle usage is usually evident. Wheezing may be heard. However, in a severe attack, the patient may not wheeze at all. This is an ominous finding. Some children will not wheeze, but will cough, often continuously. Generally, there is associated tachycardia, which should be monitored, since virtually all medications used to treat asthma increase the heart rate.

Management   The primary therapeutic goals in the asthmatic are to correct hypoxia, reverse bronchospasm, and decrease inflammation. First, it is imperative that you establish an airway. Next, administer supplemental, humidified oxygen as necessary. Initial pharmacological therapy is the administration of an inhaled beta agonist (Figure 31-21). All EMT-I units should have the capability of administering nebulized bronchodilator medications, such as albuterol, metaproterenol, or isoetharine. Alternatively, a metered-dose inhaler (MDI) may be used. If transport time is prolonged, the medical direction physician may also request administration of a steroid preparation.

Status Asthmaticus   Status asthmaticus is defined as a severe, prolonged asthma attack that cannot be broken by aggressive pharmacological management. This is a serious medical emergency and prompt recognition, treatment, and transport are required. Often, the child suffering status asthmaticus will have a greatly distended chest from continued air trapping. Breath sounds, and often wheezing, may be absent. The patient is usually exhausted, severely acidotic, and often dehydrated. The management of status asthmaticus is basically the same as for asthma. However, you should recognize that respiratory arrest is imminent and remain prepared for endotracheal intubation. Transport should be immediate, with aggressive treatment continued en route.

Bronchiolitis   Bronchiolitis is a respiratory infection of the medium-sized airways, the bronchioles, that occurs in early childhood. It should not be confused with bronchitis, which is an infection of the larger bronchi. Bronchiolitis is caused by a viral infection, most commonly *respiratory syncytial virus (RSV)*, which affects the lining of the bronchioles.

Bronchiolitis is characterized by prominent expiratory wheezing and clinically resembles asthma. It most commonly occurs in winter in children less than 2 years of age. Bronchiolitis often spreads quickly through day care and preschool facilities. Most children will develop life-long immunity to RSV following infection. The exception is the very young infant who has an immature immune system.

Assessment   A history is necessary to distinguish bronchiolitis from asthma. Often, with bronchiolitis, there is a family history of asthma or allergies although neither is yet present in the child. In addition, the child often has a low-grade fever. A major distinguishing factor is age. Asthma rarely occurs before the age of 1 year, where bronchiolitis is more frequent in this age group.

FIGURE 31-21   The young asthma patient may be making use of a prescribed inhaler to relieve symptoms. *(The Stock Market Photo Agency)*

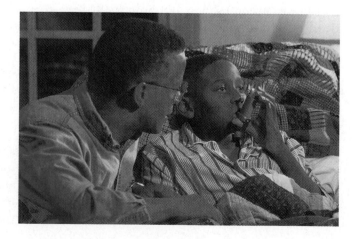

Your physical examination should be systematic. Pay particular attention to the presence of crackles or wheezes. Also, note any evidence of infection or respiratory distress.

Management Prehospital management of suspected bronchiolitis is much the same as with asthma. Place the child in a semi-sitting position, if old enough, and administer humidified oxygen by mask or blow-by method. Ventilations should be supported as necessary. Equipment for intubation should be readily available. If respiratory distress is present, consider administration of a bronchodilator such as albuterol (Ventolin, Proventil) by small-volume nebulizer. The cardiac rhythm should be constantly monitored. Pulse oximetry, if available, should be used continuously.

Pneumonia Pneumonia is an infection of the lower airway and lungs. It may be caused by either a bacterium or a virus. Pneumonia can occur at any age, but in pediatric patients, it most commonly appears in infants, toddlers, and preschoolers ages 1 to 5 years. Most cases of pneumonia in children are viral and self-limited. As children get older, they can contract bacterial pneumonias like adults. A pneumonia vaccine is available. However, its use is reserved for patients with an immune system problem or who are asplenic.

Assessment Persons with pneumonia often have a history of a respiratory infection, such as a severe cold or bronchitis. Signs and symptoms include a low-grade fever, decreased breath sounds, crackles, rhonchi, and pain in the chest area. Conduct a systematic assessment of a patient with suspected pneumonia, paying particular attention to evidence of respiratory distress.

Management Prehospital management of pneumonia is supportive. Place the patient in a position of comfort. Ensure a patent airway and administer supplemental oxygen via a nonrebreather device. If respiratory failure is present, support ventilations with a BVM device. If prolonged ventilation will be required, perform endotracheal intubation. Transport the patient in a position of comfort. Provide emotional and psychological support to the parents.

Foreign Body Lower Airway Obstruction The same pediatric patients that are at risk from upper airway obstruction are at risk for lower airway obstruction. A foreign body can enter the lower airway if it is too small to lodge in the upper airway. The object is often food (nuts, seeds, candy), small toys, or parts of toys. The child will take a deep breath or will fall and accidentally aspirate the foreign body. The foreign body will fall into the lower airway until it reaches the airway that is smaller than the foreign body. Depending on positioning, the foreign body can act as a one-way valve either trapping air in distal lung tissues or preventing aeration of distal lung tissues, causing a ventilation/perfusion mismatch.

Assessment There will often be a history of the child having a foreign body in the mouth and then it is gone. The parents may be unsure whether the child swallowed it, aspirated it, or simply lost the object. If the object is fairly large and aspirated, then respiratory distress may be present. There is often considerable, often intractable, coughing. The child will be anxious and may have diminished breath sounds in the part of the chest affected by the foreign body. There may be crackles or rhonchi, usually unilateral. In some cases, there may be unilateral wheezing where some air is getting past the object. Unilateral wheezing should be considered to be due to an aspirated foreign body until proven otherwise.

Management The management of an aspirated foreign body is supportive. Place the child in a position of comfort and avoid agitation. Provide supplemental oxygen. Transport the child to a facility that has the capability of performing pediatric fiber-optic bronchoscopy. The bronchoscope can be used to visualize the airway and remove any foreign objects detected.

SHOCK (HYPOPERFUSION)

The second major cause of pediatric cardiopulmonary arrest—after respiratory impairment—is shock. Shock can most simply be defined as inadequate perfusion of the tissues with oxygen and other essential nutrients and inadequate removal of metabolic waste products. This ultimately results in tissue hypoxia and metabolic acidosis. Ultimately, if untreated, cellular death will occur.

When compared with the incidence of shock in adults, shock is an unusual occurrence in children because their blood vessels constrict so efficiently. However, when blood pressure does drop, it drops so far and so fast that the child may quickly develop cardiopulmonary arrest. A number of factors place infants and young children at risk of shock. As mentioned in Chapter 30, newborns and neonates can develop shock as a result of a loss of body heat. Other

Content Review

PREDISPOSING FACTORS OF PEDIATRIC SHOCK
- Hypothermia
- Dehydration (vomiting, diarrhea)
- Infection
- Trauma
- Blood loss
- Allergic reactions
- Poisoning
- Cardiac events (rare)

causes include dehydration (from vomiting and/or diarrhea), infection (particularly septicemia), trauma (especially from abdominal injuries), and blood loss. Less common causes of shock in infants and children include allergic reactions, poisoning, and cardiac events (rare).

The definitive care of shock takes place in the emergency department of a hospital. Because shock is a life-threatening condition in pediatric patients, it is important to recognize early signs and symptoms—or even the possibility of shock in a situation where signs and symptoms have not yet developed. In a situation in which you suspect a possibility of shock, provide oxygen to boost tissue perfusion and transport as quickly as possible. Also, keep the patient in a supine position and take steps to protect the child from hypothermia and agitation that might worsen the condition.

Severity of Shock

Shock is classified by degrees of severity as compensated, decompensated, and irreversible. The child responds to decreased perfusion by increasing heart rate and by increasing peripheral vascular resistance. The child has very little capacity to increase stroke volume. The key to early identification of shock is detecting the subtle signs that result from the body's various compensatory mechanisms.

Compensated Shock   Early shock is known as compensated shock because the body is able to compensate for decreased tissue perfusion through various physiological mechanisms. In compensated shock, the patient exhibits a normal blood pressure. The signs and symptoms of compensated shock include:

- Irritability or anxiety
- Tachycardia
- Tachypnea
- Weak peripheral pulses, full central pulses
- Delayed capillary refill (more than 2 seconds in children less than 6 years of age)
- Cool, pale extremities
- Systolic blood pressure within normal limits
- Decreased urinary output

Compensated shock is generally reversible if appropriate treatment measures are instituted. Again, the key to a good outcome is prompt detection of the early signs and symptoms and initiation of therapy based on this. Management is directed at correcting the underlying problem. High-flow oxygen should be administered and venous access obtained. If the patient is hypovolemic, then fluid replacement should be initiated. If the cause is cardiogenic, then medications should be administered to support cardiac output and increase peripheral vascular resistance. Sometimes definitive care of shock is surgical. However, in these cases, fluid therapy and oxygen administration will help buy time until the patient can be taken to surgery.

Decompensated Shock   Decompensated shock develops when the body can no longer compensate for decreased tissue perfusion. The hallmark of decompensated shock is a fall in blood pressure (an ominous sign in children). This results in hypoperfusion and inadequate end-organ perfusion. It is important to remember that a child's compensatory mechanisms are quite efficient. Thus, when a child develops decompensated shock, there has been a significant loss of fluid or a significant impairment of cardiac output. The signs and symptoms of decompensated shock (Figure 31-22) include:

- Lethargy or coma
- Marked tachycardia or bradycardia
- Absent peripheral pulses, weak central pulses
- Markedly delayed capillary refill
- Cool, pale, dusky, mottled extremities
- Hypotension

The definitive care of shock takes place in the ED. However, early detection makes sure the patient gets to the hospital.

A slight increase in the heart rate is one of the earliest signs of shock.

The hallmark of decompensated shock is a fall in blood pressure (an ominous sign in children).

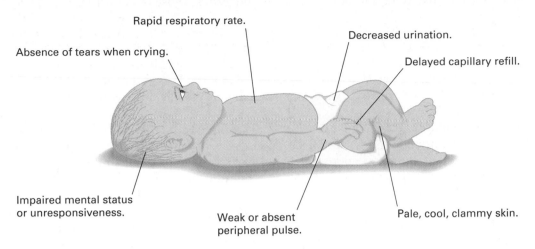

Rapid respiratory rate.

Absence of tears when crying.

Decreased urination.

Delayed capillary refill.

Impaired mental status or unresponsiveness.

Weak or absent peripheral pulse.

Pale, cool, clammy skin.

FIGURE 31-22   Signs and symptoms of shock (hypoperfusion) in a child.

- Markedly decreased urinary output
- Absence of tears

Decompensated shock can become irreversible if aggressive treatment measures are not undertaken. In some cases, it may be irreversible despite the fact that aggressive treatment measures have been provided. Management is directed at treatment of the underlying cause. You should have a low threshold for initiating mechanical ventilation with a BVM device and 100% oxygen. Consider intubating the patient if mechanical ventilation will be prolonged.

Irreversible Shock   Irreversible shock occurs when treatment measures are inadequate or too late to prevent significant tissue damage and death. Sometimes, blood pressure and pulse can be restored. However, the patient later succumbs due to organ failure. The best treatment for irreversible shock is prevention.

Categories of Shock

There are a number of ways of categorizing shock. Shock can be categorized as *cardiogenic* (caused by impaired pumping power of the heart), *hypovolemic* (caused by decreased blood or water volume), *obstructive* (caused by an obstruction that interferes with return of blood to the heart, such as a pulmonary embolism, cardiac tamponade, or tension pneumothorax), and *distributive* (caused by abnormal distribution and return of blood resulting from vasodilation, vasopermeability, or both, as in septic, anaphylactic, or neurogenic shock).

Often, shock is classified into two general categories, cardiogenic and noncardiogenic. As noted above, **cardiogenic shock** results from an inability of the heart to maintain an adequate cardiac output to the circulatory system and tissues. Cardiogenic shock in a pediatric patient is ominous and often fatal. **Noncardiogenic shock** includes types of shock that result from causes other than inadequate cardiac output. Causes may include hemorrhage, abdominal trauma, systemic bacterial infection, spinal cord injury, and others.

Noncardiogenic Shock

Noncardiogenic shock is more frequently encountered in prehospital pediatric care than cardiogenic shock. (Recall that children have a much lower incidence of cardiac problems than adults.) The forms that you will most commonly assess and manage are hypovolemic and distributive shock. (See also the discussion of metabolic problems in children later in the chapter.)

Hypovolemic Shock   **Hypovolemic shock** results from loss of intravascular fluids. In pediatric patients, the most common causes include severe dehydration from vomiting and/or

The child in decompensated shock is critically ill and will rapidly die without aggressive intervention.

cardiogenic shock the inability of the heart to meet the metabolic needs of the body, resulting in inadequate tissue perfusion.

noncardiogenic shock types of shock that result from causes other than inadequate cardiac output.

hypovolemic shock decreased amount of intravascular fluid in the body; often due to trauma that causes blood loss into a body cavity or frank external hemorrhage; in children, can be the result of vomiting and diarrhea.

diarrhea and blood loss, usually as a result of trauma. Trauma may include blood loss into a body cavity (particularly the abdomen) or frank external hemorrhage. Children are also at risk of fluid loss as a result of burns, the second leading cause of pediatric deaths in the United States.

Treatment of hypovolemic shock involves administration of supplemental oxygen and establishment of IV access. This should be followed by a 20 mL/kg bolus of lactated Ringer's solution or normal saline. Following the bolus, the child should be reassessed. If signs and symptoms of compensated shock still exist, then administer a second bolus. Some children may require 80 to 100 mL/kg of fluid, depending on the volume of fluid lost.

Distributive Shock   **Distributive shock** presents with a marked decrease in peripheral vascular resistance, usually due to a loss of vasomotor tone. In pediatric patients, causes include septicemia from bacterial infection, anaphylactic reaction, and damage to the brain and/or spinal cord. Cardiac output and fluid volume are adequate.

Septic Shock   This condition is caused by sepsis, an infection of the bloodstream by some pathogen, usually bacterial. Sepsis commonly occurs as a complication of an infection at some other site such as pneumonia, an ear infection, or a urinary tract infection. Meningitis is frequently associated with sepsis. The etiology can be varied, as can be the signs and symptoms.

The septic child is critically ill. Septic shock may develop when the pathogen causing the infection releases deadly toxins. These toxins cause peripheral vasodilatation, leading to a drop in blood pressure and decreased tissue perfusion. Sepsis can be rapidly fatal if not promptly identified and treated.

Signs of sepsis include:

- Ill appearance
- Irritability or altered mental status
- Fever
- Vomiting and diarrhea
- Cyanosis, pallor, or mottled skin
- Nonspecific respiratory distress
- Poor feeding

Signs and symptoms of septic shock include:

- Very ill appearance
- Altered mental status
- Tachycardia
- Capillary refill time greater than 2 seconds
- Hyperventilation, leading to respiratory failure
- Cool and clammy skin
- Inability of child to recognize parents

Your goal in treating sepsis is to prevent the development of septic shock. Supplemental oxygen should be administered and IV access obtained. Administer a 20 mL/kg bolus of lactated Ringer's solution or normal saline. Consider initiating pressor therapy with dopamine. Begin at 2 mcg/kg/minute and gradually increase the dose until the blood pressure improves or there is evidence of improved end-organ perfusion. Definitive treatment includes antibiotics and other therapy. Transport should be rapid with care provided en route.

Anaphylactic Shock   Anaphylactic shock results from exposure to an antigen to which the patient has been previously exposed. Milder cases may simply result in an allergic reaction. More severe reactions can impair tissue perfusion. This primarily occurs as a result of the release of histamine and other similar chemicals. Histamine causes peripheral vasodilation and leakage of fluid from the intravascular space into the interstitial space. Anaphylactic shock can be differentiated from a severe allergic reaction by the presence of signs and symptoms of impaired end-organ perfusion. These include:

---

distributive shock marked decrease in peripheral vascular resistance with resultant hypotension; examples include septic shock, neurogenic shock, and anaphylactic shock.

Septic shock kills!

Your goal in treating sepsis is to prevent the development of septic shock.

The child in septic shock may require pressor therapy (dopamine or epinephrine).

- Tachycardia
- Tachypnea
- Wheezing
- Urticaria (hives)
- Anxiousness
- Edema
- Hypotension

Treatment of a severe allergic reaction includes administration of subcutaneous epinephrine 1:1,000 and an antihistamine. Treatment of anaphylactic shock includes supplemental oxygen administration and IV access. If the patient is exhibiting decompensated shock, administer epinephrine 1:10,000 intravenously and diphenhydramine (Benadryl) intravenously. Patients not exhibiting hypotension may be given an initial dose of epinephrine subcutaneously. If this does not rapidly improve the situation, then an IV dose of epinephrine should be considered. Contact medical direction for additional assistance. EMS systems with long transport times may be asked to administer an initial dose of a corticosteroid such as methylprednisolone (Solu-Medrol).

Neurogenic Shock   Neurogenic shock is due to sudden peripheral vasodilation resulting from interruption of nervous control of the peripheral vascular system. The most common cause is injury to the spinal cord. Cardiac output and intravascular fluid volume are usually adequate.

Treatment is directed at increasing peripheral vascular resistance. This is primarily through administration of a pressor agent such as dopamine. Care should also include stabilization of the injury and administration of supplemental oxygen.

Cardiogenic Shock

Cardiogenic shock results from inadequate cardiac output. In children, cardiogenic shock usually results from a secondary cause such as near-drowning or a toxic ingestion. Children, unlike adults, rarely have primary cardiac disease. The exceptions are congenital heart disease and cardiomyopathy.

Congenital heart disease is an abnormality or defect in the heart that is present at birth. Many congenital cardiac problems are detected at birth. However, some may not be detected until later in life. Cardiomyopathy causes a decrease in cardiac output due to impairment of cardiac muscle contraction. Dysrhythmias, although rare in children, can cause a decrease in cardiac output. Rapid dysrhythmias may impair ventricular filling and thus cause a decrease in cardiac output. Likewise, slow dysrhythmias may cause decreased cardiac output simply due to their slow rate.

The following sections provide more detail on congenital heart disease, cardiomyopathy, and dysrhythmias which, as noted, are primary causes of pediatric cardiogenic shock. Remember, however, cardiogenic shock in children most often results from secondary causes.

Congenital Heart Disease

Congenital heart disease is the primary cause of heart disease in children. As noted above, although most congenital heart problems are detected at birth, some problems may not be discovered until later in childhood. A common symptom of congenital heart disease is cyanosis. This occurs when blood going to the lungs for oxygenation mixes with blood bound for other parts of the body. This may result from holes in the internal walls of the heart or from abnormalities of the great vessels.

The child with congenital heart disease may develop respiratory distress, congestive heart failure, or a "cyanotic spell." Cyanotic spells occur when oxygen demand exceeds that provided by the blood. They begin as irritability, inconsolable crying, or altered mental status, and progressive cyanosis with severe dyspnea. In severe and prolonged cases, seizures, coma, or cardiac arrest may result. Non-cyanotic problems associated with congenital heart disease include respiratory distress, tachycardia, decreased end-organ perfusion, drowsiness, fatigue, and pallor.

Allergic reactions can usually be managed with subcutaneous epinephrine 1:1000, whereas severe allergic reactions require intravenous epinephrine 1:10,000.

congenital present at birth.

Tetralogy of Fallot, a type of congenital heart disease with a right-to-left shunt, is often characterized by cyanotic episodes ("tet" spells) that are relieved by the child squatting.

Treatment includes the standard primary assessment. Administer oxygen at a high concentration. If necessary, provide ventilatory support. If the patient is having a cyanotic spell, place the child in the knee-chest position facing downward. This will help increase the cardiac return. Apply the ECG monitor, and start an IV line at a keep-open rate. Transport immediately.

Cardiomyopathy

Cardiomyopathy is a disease or dysfunction of the cardiac muscle. Although fairly rare, cardiomyopathy can result from congenital heart disease or infection. A frequent cause of infectious cardiomyopathy is Coxsackie virus. Cardiomyopathy causes mechanical pump failure, which is usually biventricular. It often develops slowly and is not detectable until heart failure develops.

The signs and symptoms of cardiomyopathy include early fatigue, crackles, jugular venous distension, engorgement of the liver, and peripheral edema. Later, as the disease progresses, the signs and symptoms of shock can develop.

The prehospital treatment of cardiomyopathy is supportive. Supplemental oxygen should be administered via a nonrebreather mask. Fluids should be restricted. If possible, IV access should be obtained. Severe cases resulting in the development of severe dyspnea should be treated with furosemide and pressor agents (dobutamine, dopamine). The child should be transported to a facility capable of managing critically ill children. Most cases of cardiomyopathy are managed with medication. Definitive care in severe cases may include cardiac transplantation.

Dysrhythmias

Dysrhythmias in children are uncommon. When dysrhythmias occur, bradydysrhythmias are the most common. Supraventricular tachydysrhythmias are uncommon and ventricular tachydysrhythmias are very uncommon. Dysrhythmias can cause pump failure ultimately leading to cardiogenic shock. Children have a very limited capacity to increase stroke volume. The primary mechanism through which they increase cardiac output is through changes in the heart rate. The treatment of dysrhythmias is specific for the dysrhythmia in question.

Tachydysrhythmias   Tachydysrhythmias are dysrhythmias in which the rate is greater than the estimated maximum normal heart rate for the child. These can result from primary cardiac disease or from secondary causes. Tachydysrhythmias from any cause are relatively uncommon in children.

Supraventricular Tachycardia   True supraventricular tachycardia is a narrow complex tachycardia with a heart rate of 220 per minute or greater. Supraventricular tachycardia is typically due to a problem in the cardiac conductive system. Rarely, it can be due to a secondary cause such as drug ingestion. It is occasionally seen in infants with no prior history. The cause is uncertain but may be due to immaturity of the cardiac conductive system. Rapid heart rates often do not allow time for adequate cardiac filling, eventually causing congestive heart failure and cardiogenic shock.

The signs and symptoms of supraventricular tachycardia include irritability, poor feeding, jugular venous distension, hepatomegaly (enlarged liver), and hypotension. The ECG will show a narrow complex (supraventricular) tachycardia with a rate greater than 220 per minute. Children can often tolerate the rapid rate well.

Prehospital treatment of supraventricular tachycardia depends on the clinical findings. Children who are tolerating the heart rate (normal blood pressure) and are stable should receive supplemental oxygen and transport. Adenosine should be considered if the child is stable. If the child is exhibiting signs of decompensation (hypotension, mental status change, poor skin color) then synchronized cardioversion should be attempted at initial dose of 0.5 to 1.0 Joules/kg of body weight. This can be increased to 2 Joules/kg if the initial shock is unsuccessful. The child should be transported to the appropriate facility.

Ventricular Tachycardia with a Pulse   Ventricular tachycardia and ventricular fibrillation are exceedingly rare in children. They are occasionally seen following drowning or following a prolonged resuscitation attempt. Unlike adults, where ventricular tachydysrhythmias result from primary heart disease, ventricular tachydysrhythmias in children are almost always due to a secondary cause. The exception is structural, congenital heart disease.

The signs and symptoms of ventricular tachycardia with a pulse include poor feeding, irritability, and a rapid, wide complex tachycardia. Children are unable to tolerate this dysrhythmia very long. They soon develop signs of shock.

The prehospital management of ventricular tachycardia with a pulse includes supplemental oxygen and IV access. Stable patients who are not hypotensive should be transported. Unstable patients (hypotension) should be aggressively treated. Initially, amiodarone, procainamide, or lidocaine should be administered. However, ventricular tachycardia due to structural heart disease often does not respond to antidysrhythmic drugs. If the patient is unstable or deteriorating, administer synchronized cardioversion at 0.5 to 1.0 Joules/kg. This can be increased to 2 Joules/kg if needed. Transport emergently and provide care en route.

Bradydysrhythmias   Bradydysrhythmias are the most common type of pediatric dysrhythmia. They most frequently result from hypoxia. Although rare, they can also result from vagal stimulation from such causes as marked gastric distension.

The signs and symptoms of bradycardia include a slow, narrow complex rhythm. The child may be lethargic or exhibiting early signs of congestive heart failure.

Stable children with bradydysrhythmias should receive supportive care. Unstable children should be ventilated with a BVM unit and 100% oxygen. If the heart rate does not readily increase, consider endotracheal intubation. Perform chest compressions if oxygenation and ventilation do not increase the heart rate. Consider administering epinephrine or atropine down the endotracheal tube until IV access can be obtained. Transport emergently with care provided en route. (See the algorithm for treatment of pediatric bradycardia, Figure 31-23.)

Absent Rhythm   The absence of a cardiac rhythm is an ominous finding. Most cases are asystole. However, some cases may be a very fine ventricular fibrillation. If necessary, turn up the gain on the ECG to distinguish between the two.

Asystole   Asystole is the absence of a rhythm and may be the initial rhythm seen in cardiopulmonary arrest. (Remember, children rarely develop ventricular fibrillation, which is often the precursor to arrest in adults.) Bradycardias can degenerate to asystole if appropriate intervention is not provided. The mortality rate associated with asystole in children is very high.

The child with asystole is pulseless and apneic. The cardiac rhythm is a straight line that should be confirmed in two leads. Treatment is often futile. However, CPR should be initiated. The patient should be intubated and ventilated with 100% oxygen. Chest compressions should be continued. Emergency resuscitative drugs (epinephrine, atropine) should be administered through the endotracheal tube until IV access can be obtained. (See the algorithm for pediatric asystole and cardiac arrest, Figure 31-24.)

Ventricular Fibrillation/Pulseless Ventricular Tachycardia   Ventricular fibrillation and pulseless ventricular tachycardia are functionally the same rhythm. They are exceedingly rare in children. Causes include electrocution and drug overdoses. The mortality rate is very high.

The child with ventricular fibrillation/pulseless ventricular tachycardia will be pulseless and apneic. The ECG will exhibit a wide complex tachycardia or fibrillation. In unmonitored patients, provide CPR. If the patient was monitored at the time of the arrest, then defibrillate three times (2 Joules/kg, then 4 Joules/kg, then repeat at 4 Joules/kg). Ventilate the patient with 100% oxygen and intubate. Continue chest compressions. Resuscitative medications (epinephrine, lidocaine, amiodarone) can be administered down the endotracheal tube until IV access can be obtained. Transport as soon as possible.

Pulseless Electrical Activity   Pulseless electrical activity (PEA) is the presence of a cardiac rhythm without an associated pulse. This is due to noncardiogenic causes such as hypoxia, pericardial tamponade, tension pneumothorax, trauma, acidosis, hypothermia, hypoglycemia, and others.

The patient with PEA is pulseless and apneic. Resuscitation should be directed toward correcting the underlying cause. The patient should receive CPR, be intubated and ventilated,

Wide-complex tachycardia should be treated with amiodarone, procainamide, or lidocaine, if stable. If unstable, go directly to synchronized cardioversion.

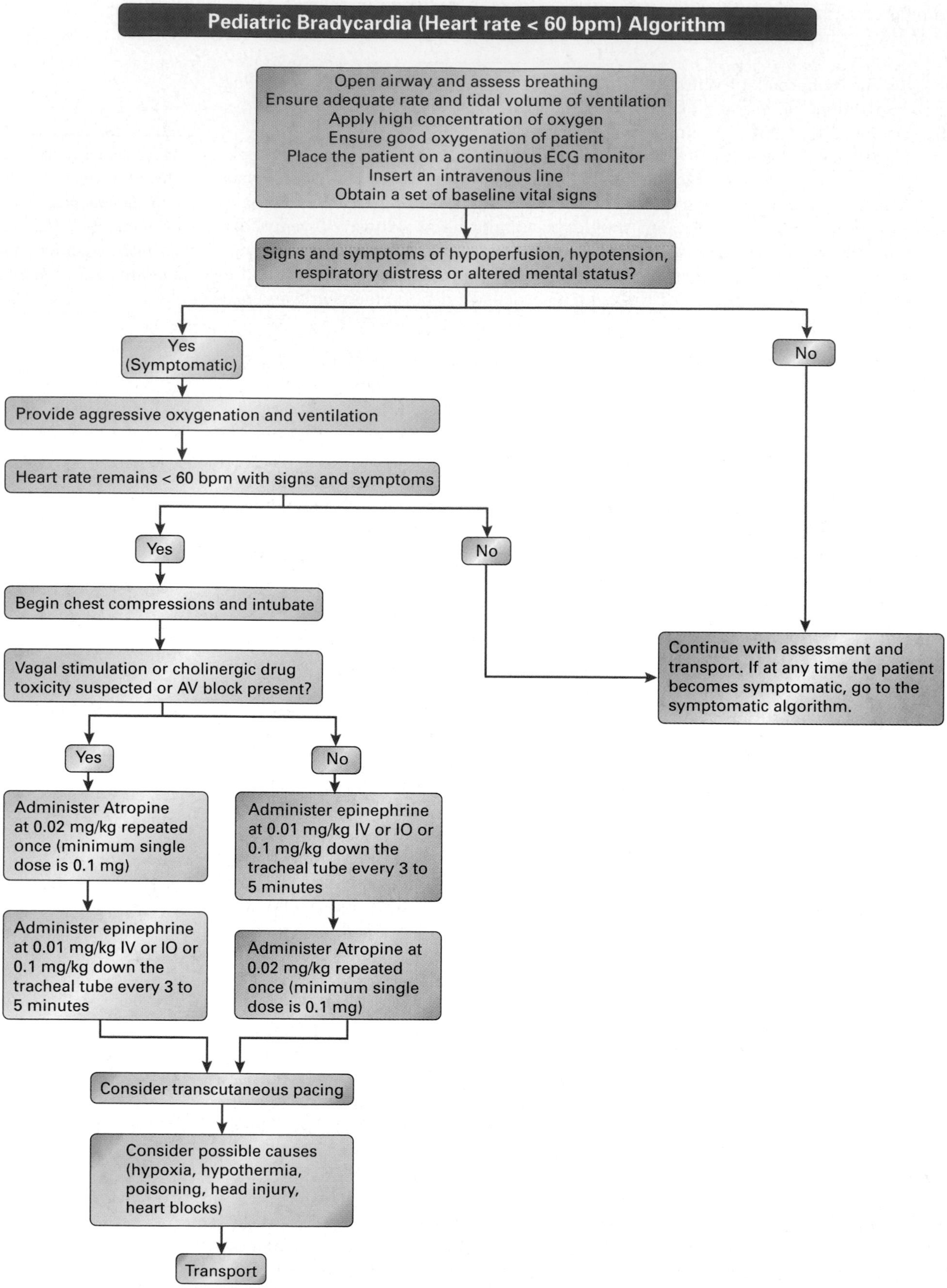

Pediatric Bradycardia (Heart rate < 60 bpm) Algorithm

Open airway and assess breathing
Ensure adequate rate and tidal volume of ventilation
Apply high concentration of oxygen
Ensure good oxygenation of patient
Place the patient on a continuous ECG monitor
Insert an intravenous line
Obtain a set of baseline vital signs

Signs and symptoms of hypoperfusion, hypotension, respiratory distress or altered mental status?

Yes (Symptomatic)

No

Provide aggressive oxygenation and ventilation

Heart rate remains < 60 bpm with signs and symptoms

Yes

No

Begin chest compressions and intubate

Continue with assessment and transport. If at any time the patient becomes symptomatic, go to the symptomatic algorithm.

Vagal stimulation or cholinergic drug toxicity suspected or AV block present?

Yes

No

Administer Atropine at 0.02 mg/kg repeated once (minimum single dose is 0.1 mg)

Administer epinephrine at 0.01 mg/kg IV or IO or 0.1 mg/kg down the tracheal tube every 3 to 5 minutes

Administer epinephrine at 0.01 mg/kg IV or IO or 0.1 mg/kg down the tracheal tube every 3 to 5 minutes

Administer Atropine at 0.02 mg/kg repeated once (minimum single dose is 0.1 mg)

Consider transcutaneous pacing

Consider possible causes (hypoxia, hypothermia, poisoning, head injury, heart blocks)

Transport

FIGURE 31–23   Pediatric bradycardia treatment algorithm.

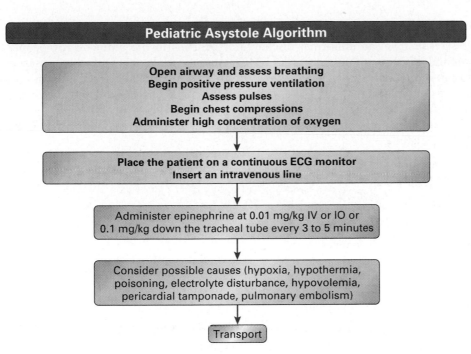

Pediatric Asystole Algorithm

> Open airway and assess breathing
> Begin positive pressure ventilation
> Assess pulses
> Begin chest compressions
> Administer high concentration of oxygen

> Place the patient on a continuous ECG monitor
> Insert an intravenous line

> Administer epinephrine at 0.01 mg/kg IV or IO or
> 0.1 mg/kg down the tracheal tube every 3 to 5 minutes

> Consider possible causes (hypoxia, hypothermia,
> poisoning, electrolyte disturbance, hypovolemia,
> pericardial tamponade, pulmonary embolism)

> Transport

FIGURE 31-24 Pediatric asystole treatment algorithm.

and given the standard resuscitative medications (epinephrine). Transport should be prompt with care provided en route.

NEUROLOGICAL EMERGENCIES

Neurological emergencies in childhood are fairly uncommon. However, seizures can and do occur in children. In fact, they are a frequent reason for summoning EMS. In addition to seizures, meningitis tends to show up more often in children than in adults. Although your chances of encountering either of these two conditions are small, both are life threatening and should be promptly identified and treated.

Seizures

Seizures result from an abnormal discharge of neurons in the brain. Many people have seizures and it is a common reason why EMS is summoned. People with chronic seizure disorders can often control their seizures with medications. However, a seizure can be an exceptionally scary event for both the parents and the child. This is especially true if the child has never had a seizure before.

Although the etiology for seizures is often unknown, several risk factors have been identified. They include:

- Fever
- Hypoxia
- Infections
- Idiopathic epilepsy (epilepsy of unknown origin)
- Electrolyte disturbances
- Head trauma
- Hypoglycemia
- Toxic ingestions or exposure
- Tumor
- Central nervous system (CNS) malformations

Seizures in pediatric patients may be either partial or generalized. (Recall that generalized seizures normally do not occur during the first month of life.) Simple partial seizures, sometimes called focal motor seizures, involve sudden jerking of a particular part of the body, such as an arm or a leg. Other characteristics include lip smacking, eye blinking, staring, confusion, and lethargy. There is usually no loss of consciousness. Generalized seizures involve sudden jerking of both sides of the body, followed by tenseness and relaxation of the body. In a generalized seizure, patients typically experience a loss of consciousness.

Keep in mind that children can have **status epilepticus**—a series of one or more generalized seizures without any intervening periods of consciousness. Status epilepticus is a serious medical emergency because it involves a prolonged period of apnea, which in turn can cause hypoxia of vital brain tissues. (For more on seizures and status epilepticus, see Chapter 24.)

Most of the pediatric seizures that you will probably encounter are febrile seizures. **Febrile seizures** are those seizures that occur as a result of a sudden increase in body temperature. They occur most commonly between the ages of 6 months and 6 years. Febrile seizures seem related to the rate at which the body temperature increases, not to the degree of fever. Often, the parents or caregivers will report the recent onset of fever or cold symptoms. The diagnosis of febrile seizure should not be made in the field. All pediatric patients having a seizure must be transported to the hospital so that other etiologies can be excluded.

Assessment   The history is a major factor in determining seizure type. Febrile seizure should be suspected if the temperature is above 103°F (39.2°C). The history of a previous seizure may suggest idiopathic epilepsy or another CNS problem. However, there is also a tendency for recurrence of febrile seizures in children.

When confronted with a seizing child, determine whether there is a history of seizures or seizures with fever. Has the child had a recent illness? Also, determine how many seizures occurred during the incident. If the child is not seizing upon arrival, elicit a description of the seizure activity. Note the condition and position of the child when found. Question parents, caregivers, or bystanders about the possibility of head injury. A history of irritability or lethargy prior to the seizure may indicate CNS infection. If possible, find out whether the child suffers from diabetes or has recently complained of a headache or a stiff neck. Note any current medications, as well as possible ingestions.

The physical examination should be systematic. Pay particular attention to the adequacy of respirations, the level of consciousness, neurological evaluation, and signs of injury. Also inspect the child for signs of dehydration. Dehydration may be evidenced by the absence of tears or, in an infant, by the presence of a sunken fontanelle.

status epilepticus prolonged seizure or multiple seizures with no regaining of consciousness between them.

Status epilepticus is a serious medical emergency because it involves a prolonged period of apnea, which in turn can cause hypoxia of vital brain tissues.

febrile seizures seizures that occur as a result of a sudden increase in body temperature; occur most commonly between ages 6 months and 6 years.

The diagnosis of febrile seizure should not be made in the field.

Management   Management of pediatric seizures is essentially the same as for seizing adults. Place patients on the floor or on the bed. Be sure to lay them on their side, away from the furniture. Do not restrain patients, but take steps to protect them from injury. Maintain the airway, but do not force anything, such as a bite stick, between the teeth. Administer supplemental oxygen. Then take and record all vital signs. If the patient is febrile, remove excess layers of clothing, while avoiding extreme cooling. If status epilepticus is present, institute the following steps:

Some medical directors prefer lorazepam (Ativan) as the anticonvulsant of choice for pediatric patients.

- Start an IV of normal saline or lactated Ringer's solution and perform a glucometer evaluation.
- Administer diazepam as follows:
  - Children who are 1 month to 5 years old: 0.2 to 0.5 mg slowly IV push every 2 to 5 minutes up to a maximum of 2.5 mg.
  - Children who are 5 years and older: 1 mg slowly IV push every 2 to 5 minutes to a maximum of 5 mg.
- Contact medical direction for additional dosing. Diazepam can be administered rectally if an IV cannot be established.
- If the seizure appears to be due to fever and a long transport time is anticipated, medical direction may request the administration of acetaminophen to lower the fever. Acetaminophen is supplied as an elixir or as suppositories. The dose should be 15 mg/kg body weight.

As mentioned previously, all pediatric patients should be transported. Reassure and support the parents or caregivers, since this is a very stressful and frightening situation for them.

Meningitis

Meningitis is an infection of the meninges, the lining of the brain and spinal cord. Meningitis can result from both bacteria and viruses. Viral meningitis is frequently called *aseptic meningitis,* since an organism cannot be routinely cultured from cerebrospinal fluid. Aseptic meningitis is generally less severe than bacterial meningitis and self-limiting. Bacterial meningitis most commonly results from *Streptococcus pneumoniae, Haemophilus influenzae,* and *Neisseria meningitides.* These infections can be rapidly fatal if they are not promptly recognized and treated appropriately.

Assessment   Meningitis is more common in children than in adults. Findings in the history that may suggest meningitis include a child who has been ill for one day to several days, recent ear or respiratory tract infection, high fever, lethargy or irritability, a severe headache, or a stiff neck. Infants generally do not develop a stiff neck. They will generally become lethargic and will not feed well. Some babies may simply develop a fever.

On physical examination, the child with meningitis will appear very ill. With an infant, the fontanelle may be bulging or full unless accompanied by dehydration. Extreme discomfort with movement may be present due to irritability of the meninges.

Be alert for rapid cardiopulmonary collapse in the child with fulminant meningitis, or severe meningitis with a rapid onset.

Management   Prehospital care of the pediatric patient with meningitis is supportive. Rapidly complete the primary assessment and transport the child to the emergency department. If shock is present, treat the child with IV fluids (20 mL/kg) and oxygen.

GASTROINTESTINAL EMERGENCIES

Childhood gastrointestinal problems almost always present with nausea and vomiting as a chief complaint. As a child gets older, other gastrointestinal system emergencies, such as appendicitis, become more common.

Nausea and Vomiting

Nausea and vomiting are not diseases themselves, but are symptoms of other disease processes. Virtually any medical problem can cause these conditions in an infant or child. The most common causes include fever, ear infections, and respiratory infections. In addition, many viruses and certain bacteria can infect the gastrointestinal system. These infections—collectively known as *gastroenteritis*—readily cause vomiting, diarrhea, or both.

Table 31-12	SIGNS AND SYMPTOMS OF DEHYDRATION		
Signs/Symptoms	Mild	Moderate	Severe
Vital signs			
Pulse	Normal	Increased	Markedly increased
Respirations	Normal	Increased	Tachypneic
Blood pressure	Normal	Normal	Hypotensive
Capillary refill	Normal	2–3 sec	>2 sec
Mental status	Alert	Irritable	Lethargic
Skin	Normal	Dry and ashen	Dry, cool, mottled
Mucous membranes	Dry	Very dry	Very dry/no tears

Vomiting and diarrhea carry the potential for dehydration and electrolyte abnormalities, serious conditions in the pediatric patient.

The biggest risks associated with nausea and vomiting in children are dehydration and electrolyte abnormalities. Infants and toddlers can quickly become dehydrated from bouts of vomiting. If diarrhea or fever is also present, fluid loss is further accelerated, worsening the situation. Dehydration in infants and toddlers is more difficult to detect than in older children. (See Table 31-12 for a description of the signs and symptoms of dehydration.)

Treatment of pediatric nausea and vomiting is primarily supportive. If the child is dehydrated and unable to keep oral fluids down, IV fluid therapy may be indicated. Severe dehydration, as evidenced by prolonged capillary refill time, should be treated by 20 mL/kg fluid boluses of lactated Ringer's solution or 0.9% sodium chloride solution (normal saline).

Diarrhea

Diarrhea is a common occurrence in childhood. Often, what parents call diarrhea is actually loose bowel movements. Generally, ten or more stools per day is considered diarrhea. As with nausea and vomiting, the main concern associated with diarrhea is dehydration. Most diarrhea is due to viral infections of the gastrointestinal system or secondary to infections elsewhere in the body. However, certain bacterial infections can cause significant, even life-threatening, diarrhea.

Treatment of the child suffering from diarrhea is primarily supportive. If dehydration is evident, administer fluids. Severe dehydration should be treated with 20 mL/kg boluses of IV fluids (lactated Ringer's solution or normal saline).

METABOLIC EMERGENCIES

Metabolic problems are uncommon in children. However, diabetes can occur in very young children. It is rarely diagnosed until the child comes to the hospital in diabetic ketoacidosis. Diabetic children can have great swings in their blood glucose levels due to diet, growth, and physical activity. Because of this, hypoglycemia and hyperglycemia are possible. It is important to remember that very young children, unlike adults, can develop hypoglycemia without having diabetes. This can occur with severe illnesses such as meningitis and pneumonia. The following section will present the prehospital treatment of pediatric hypoglycemia and hyperglycemia.

Hypoglycemia

hypoglycemia abnormally low concentration of glucose in the blood.

Hypoglycemia is an abnormally low concentration of sugar (glucose) in the blood. It is a true medical emergency that must be treated immediately. Without treatment, a low blood sugar may progress to unconsciousness and convulsions.

Hypoglycemia is a true medical emergency that must be treated immediately.

In the prehospital setting, hypoglycemia in pediatric patients usually occurs in newborn infants and children with Type I diabetes. Diabetic children increase their risk of hypoglycemia through overly strenuous exercise, too much insulin, and dehydration from illness. Non-diabetic children can develop hypoglycemia from physical activity, diet changes, illness, and growth.

In known diabetics or hypoglycemics, preventive steps include:

- Taking extra snacks for extra activity
- Eating immediately after taking insulin if the blood sugar is less than 100 mg/dL
- Eating regular meals
- Regularly monitoring blood sugar
- Eating an extra snack of carbohydrate and protein if the blood sugar is less than 120 mg/dL at bedtime
- Replacing carbohydrates in the meal plan with regular soda pop or regular popsicles on days when the child is sick

Assessment Suspect hypoglycemia when the patient exhibits signs and symptoms such as weakness, dizziness, tachypnea, tachycardia, pallor, sweating, tremors, vomiting, or altered mental status. Measure blood glucose with a glucometer, and elicit a history of conditions known to cause hypoglycemia in infants and children. Treatment should be initiated whenever you have a high index of suspicion and/or blood sugar drops below 70 mg/dL.

Management As with all patients, continually monitor the ABCs. Be sure to find out if parents or caregivers have given the patient any glucose tablets, gels, foods (cake icing, honey, maple syrup, sugar, raisins), or drinks (juice, regular soda pop, milk) to correct the situation. If so, find out what was given, how much was given, and when it was given. Take a blood glucose test, if possible.

In the conscious, alert patient, administer oral fluids with sugar or oral glucose. (Amounts are age and/or weight specific, so check with medical direction.) If there is no response, or if the patient exhibits an altered mental status, transport immediately. Consult your medical direction physician on orders for the administration of dextrose or IM glucagon. A 25% dextrose solution ($D_{25}W$) can be prepared by diluting 50% dextrose solution 1:1 with sterile water or saline. It is easier to dose children with this concentration and does not cause as much discomfort as with IV administration. Repeat blood glucose tests within 10 to 15 minutes of infusion or the administration of glucose.

In treating diabetic pediatric patients, remember that most children have been taught about their condition and can participate, in varying degrees, in their care. Most understand how glucometers work, for example, and can hand you a test strip (Figure 31-25). Also, they may be sensitive to their condition. So avoid labeling any tests as "good" or "bad."

Hyperglycemia

Hyperglycemia is an abnormally high concentration of blood sugar. For patients with type I diabetes, hyperglycemia may lead to dehydration and **diabetic ketoacidosis,** a very serious medical emergency. Left untreated, the condition will deteriorate to coma. Hyperglycemia and diabetic ketoacidosis are the most common findings in new-onset diabetics.

hyperglycemia abnormally high concentration of glucose in the blood.

diabetic ketoacidosis complication of diabetes due to decreased insulin secretion or intake; characterized by high levels of blood glucose, metabolic acidosis, and, in advanced stages, coma; often referred to as diabetic coma.

Diabetic ketoacidosis is a very serious medical emergency, which may quickly deteriorate into coma.

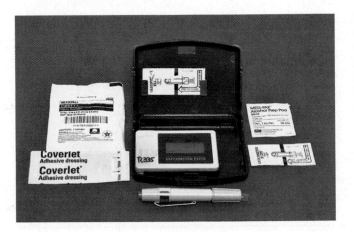

FIGURE 31-25 Many diabetic children have home glucometers to test their blood glucose levels. Older children know what the readings mean and will be curious about any glucose testing device that you may use.

In the prehospital setting, pediatric hyperglycemia is commonly associated with Type I diabetes. Causes include:

- Eating too much food relative to injected insulin
- Missing an insulin injection
- Defective insulin pump, blockage of tubing, or disconnection of insulin pump infusion set
- Illness or stress

Hyperglycemia can occur with other severe illnesses and not necessarily mean that the child is developing diabetes mellitus.

Assessment In cases of hyperglycemia, glucose is spilled into the urine, taking water with it through osmotic diuresis. This can result in a significant fluid loss with resultant dehydration.

Keep in mind that acidosis results from the accumulation of ketones, a by-product of fat metabolism. A continual increase in the ketones eventually leads to metabolic acidosis, which produces the fruity breath odor commonly associated with hyperglycemia. For other signs and symptoms, see Table 31-13.

As with hypoglycemia, elicit a history to determine causes linked with hyperglycemia. If possible, confirm your suspicions with blood glucose test. A blood sugar reading of greater than 200 mg/dl typically indicates hyperglycemia.

Management Carefully monitor the ABCs and vital signs. If you cannot confirm the presence of hyperglycemia with a blood glucose test, consider administering oral fluids with sugar or oral glucose in case the patient is hypoglycemic. If IV access is possible, consider initiating an IV of either normal saline or lactated Ringer's solution. Administer an IV bolus of 20 mL/kg, and repeat the bolus if the patient's vital signs do not change. Monitor the patient's mental status and be prepared to intubate if the respirations continue to decrease.

Remember this is a potentially life-threatening situation. Consult with medical direction on all actions taken and transport immediately.

POISONING AND TOXIC EXPOSURE

Accidental poisoning or toxic exposure is a common reason for summoning EMS. Pediatric patients account for the majority of poisonings treated by EMS. Most poisonings result from accidental ingestion of a toxic substance, usually by a young child. Toddlers and preschoolers like to taste things, especially colorful objects and substances that look like food or beverages. They also mimic their parents or caregivers, swallowing pills or drinking alcohol

Table 31-13	SIGNS AND SYMPTOMS OF HYPERGLYCEMIA	
Early	**Late**	**Ketoacidosis**
Increased thirst	Weakness	Continued decreased level of consciousness progressing to coma
Increased urination	Abdominal pain	
Weight loss	Generalized aches	
	Loss of appetite	Kussmaul respirations (deep and slow)
	Nausea	Signs of dehydration
	Vomiting	
	Signs of dehydration, except increased urinary output	
	Fruity breath odor	
	Tachypnea	
	Hyperventilation	
	Tachycardia	

"just like Mommy and Daddy." Teenagers on antidepressants are also at risk of misusing or abusing their prescriptions, especially if given a one- or two-month supply of a medication.

Poisonings are the leading cause of preventable death in children under age 5. Because of their immature respiratory and cardiovascular systems, even a single pill can poison or, in some cases, kill a child. Iron-containing supplements are the leading cause of poisonings, especially in toddlers and preschoolers.

The most dangerous rooms in a house in terms of poisons are the kitchen, where household cleaners are stored, and the bathroom, where many people keep their over-the-counter and prescription medications. Garages and utility rooms also contain toxic substances, made more attractive to children when they are poured into everyday containers such as coffee cans, soda bottles, or plastic cups. Living rooms may have poisonous plants and liquor bottles.

The best way to prevent pediatric poisonings is by helping the families in your communities learn how to "poison-proof" their homes. You can obtain guidelines from the Food and Drug Administration in Rockville, Maryland. Poisoning prevention should be a major goal of EMS prevention and community education programs.

Assessment   Common substances involved in pediatric poisonings include:

- Alcohol, barbiturates, sedatives
- Amphetamines, cocaine, hallucinogens
- Anticholinergic agents (jimson weed, belladonna products)
- Aspirin, acetaminophen
- Lead
- Vitamins and iron-containing supplements
- Corrosives
- Digitalis and beta blockers
- Hydrocarbons
- Narcotics
- Organic solvents (inhaled)
- Organophosphates (insecticides)

Poisoning can cause many different signs and symptoms (Figure 31-26). Narcotics and some of the hydrocarbons can cause respiratory system depression. Digitalis, beta blockers, and many of the antihypertensive agents can cause circulatory depression or collapse. The central nervous system can be impaired by many agents, including alcohol, barbiturates, narcotics, cocaine, and others. Thought and behavior can be affected by virtually any substance. Common agents include the anticholinergics, alcohol, narcotics, hydrocarbons, and many others. Aspirin, corrosives, and hydrocarbons can irritate or destroy the gastrointestinal system. Acetaminophen can cause liver necrosis and liver failure.

Management   Although scenarios vary, take these general steps in managing a pediatric poisoning patient:

Responsive Poisoning Patient

- Administer oxygen.
- Contact medical direction and/or the poison control center.
- Consider the need for activated charcoal.
- Transport. (Be sure to take all pills, substances, and containers to the hospital.)
- Monitor the patient continuously in case the child suddenly becomes unresponsive.

Unresponsive Poisoning Patient

- Ensure a patent airway. Apply suctioning, if necessary.
- Administer oxygen.

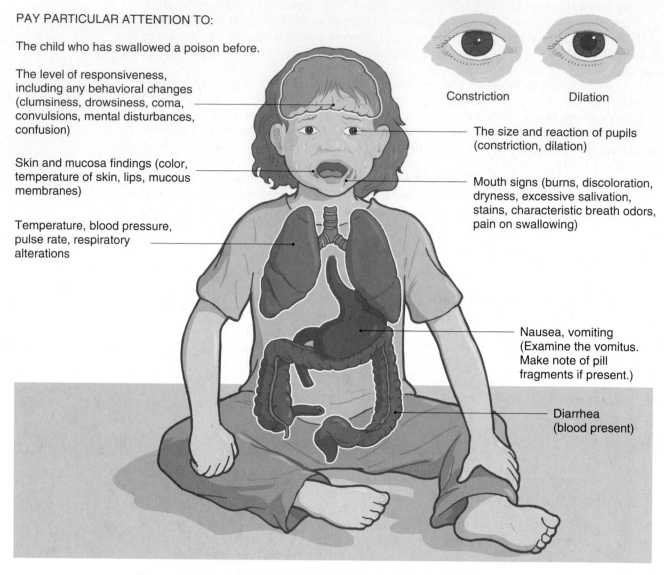

PAY PARTICULAR ATTENTION TO:

The child who has swallowed a poison before.

The level of responsiveness, including any behavioral changes (clumsiness, drowsiness, coma, convulsions, mental disturbances, confusion)

Skin and mucosa findings (color, temperature of skin, lips, mucous membranes)

Temperature, blood pressure, pulse rate, respiratory alterations

Constriction   Dilation

The size and reaction of pupils (constriction, dilation)

Mouth signs (burns, discoloration, dryness, excessive salivation, stains, characteristic breath odors, pain on swallowing)

Nausea, vomiting (Examine the vomitus. Make note of pill fragments if present.)

Diarrhea (blood present)

FIGURE 31-26 Possible indicators of ingested poisoning in children.

- Be prepared to provide artificial ventilations if respiratory failure or cardiac arrest is present.
- Contact medical direction and/or the poison control center.
- Transport.
- Monitor the patient continuously, and rule out trauma as a cause of altered mental status.

For more on poisonings and toxic exposure, see Chapter 23.

TRAUMA EMERGENCIES

Trauma is the number one cause of death in infants and children. Most pediatric injuries result from blunt trauma. As previously mentioned, children have thinner body walls that allow forces to be more readily transmitted to body contents, increasing the possibility of injury to internal tissues and organs. If you serve in an urban area, you can expect to see a higher incidence of penetrating trauma, mostly intentional and mostly from gunfire or knife

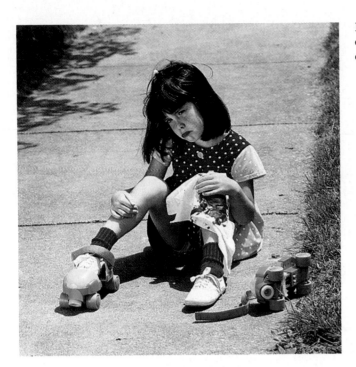

wounds. There is also a significant incidence of penetrating trauma outside the cities, mostly unintentional from hunting and agricultural accidents.

MECHANISMS OF INJURY

Children tend to be more susceptible to certain types of injuries than adults. The following categories describe the most common mechanisms of injury among infants and children.

Falls

Falls are the single most common cause of injury in children (Figure 31-27). Fortunately, serious injury or death from accidental falls is relatively uncommon unless from a significant height. Falls from bicycles account for a significant number of injuries. The incidence of head injuries is declining, primarily because of bicycle safety helmets.

Motor-Vehicle Collisions

Approximately 25,000 children in the United States die annually from trauma. Approximately one-third of these die from motor-vehicle collisions, making motor-vehicle collisions the leading cause of traumatic death in children. In addition, motor-vehicle collisions are the leading cause of permanent brain injury and the new onset of epilepsy. Improperly seated children are at increased risk of sustaining injury or death from automobile air bags when they deploy (Figure 31-28). This is an area where EMS prevention strategies can make a difference. Public education programs on drunk driving, safe driving, air bags, and proper use of children's car seats can be a major focus of EMS personnel. Some states have given EMT-Is the ability to issue citations for persons who do not correctly buckle their children or place them in child safety seats.

Car vs. Pedestrian Injuries

Car vs. child pedestrian injuries are more common in cities where children play close to the street. These types of injuries are a particularly lethal form of trauma in children, because their short stature tends to push them down under the car. There are two phases of injury in car vs. pedestrian incidents. The first group of injuries occur when the auto contacts the child. Because of the energy present, the child may be propelled away from the car or pushed down underneath the car. It is at this point that the second group of injuries occur as the child contacts the ground or other objects. Head and spinal injuries often occur with the secondary impact. The best treatment for car vs. child pedestrian

Content Review

MOST COMMON MECHANISMS OF PEDIATRIC INJURY
- Falls
- Motor-vehicle collisions
- Car vs. pedestrian collisions
- Drownings and near-drownings
- Penetrating injuries
- Burns
- Physical abuse

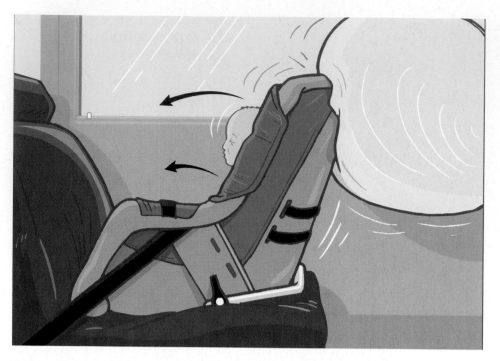

FIGURE 31-28   A deploying airbag can propel a child safety seat back into the vehicle's seat, seriously injuring the child secured in it.

injuries is prevention. This too can be a major area of emphasis for prehospital prevention programs.

Drownings and Near-Drownings

Drowning is the third leading cause of death in children between birth and 4 years of age, with approximately 2,000 deaths occurring in the United States annually. The term drowning is used to describe deaths that occur within 24 hours of the accident. *Near-drowning* refers to injuries where the child did not die or where the death occurred more than 24 hours after the injury. Many children who do not die from drowning suffer severe and irreversible brain injuries as a result of anoxia. Approximately 20% to 25% of near-drowning survivors exhibit severe neurological deficits. The outcomes are better when the water is cold, because the body's protective mechanisms protect against brain injury.

Again, as with the other injury processes, the best treatment is prevention. EMS systems, in conjunction with local building inspectors, can inspect pools for safety. A pool should be fenced off with a gate that closes automatically. Essential rescue equipment (pole, life saver) should be immediately available and the local emergency number posted. The best time for drowning prevention is late spring and early summer. Encourage parents to enroll their children in water safety classes as soon as possible.

Penetrating Injuries

Until 20 years ago, penetrating injuries in children were fairly uncommon. Since then, an increase in violent crime (although violent crime rates have both risen and fallen within that period) has resulted in an increasing number of children sustaining penetrating trauma. Stab wounds and firearm injuries account for approximately 10% to 15% of all pediatric trauma admissions. The risk of death increases with age. Children are usually innocent victims of crimes perpetrated against adults. However, children are sometimes the intended victims of gunfire and stabbings, as in the shootings that have taken place in schools.

It is important to remember that visual inspection of external injuries does not provide adequate evaluation of internal injuries. This is especially true with high-energy, high-velocity weapons that can cause massive internal injury with only minimal external trauma.

EMT-Is can play a major role in preventing pediatric shootings. During public education and community service programs, it is prudent to talk about gun safety, including such measures as using trigger locks or locking weapons in places where children cannot reach them. You might emphasize the fact that children have an uncanny ability to find and gain access to weapons that adults think they have hidden and secured. As with many other pediatric emergencies, the best treatment is prevention.

Burns

Burn injuries are the leading cause of accidental death in the home for children under 14 years of age. Children can sustain both burn injuries and smoke inhalation in house fires. Unsupervised children with matches or cigarette lighters are responsible for many fires that result in pediatric injury.

Fire prevention programs are a major area of emphasis for fire departments. The importance of smoke detectors cannot be overemphasized. Citizens should be encouraged to change the batteries in their smoke detectors when the clock is moved backward or forward for daylight savings time. Many fire departments and EMS systems replace smoke detector batteries as a part of their fire prevention program. Part of the fire prevention program should be specifically directed at children. It is especially important to teach children how to exit their house in case fire erupts.

Physical Abuse

Unfortunately, children are at risk for physical abuse by adults and older children. Factors leading to child abuse are known to include social phenomena such as poverty, domestic disturbances, younger-aged parents, substance abuse, and community violence. EMT-Is are often the first members of the health-care team to come into contact with the abused child. It is very important to not accuse the parents or to confront a suspected abuser. Instead, document all pertinent findings, treatments, and interventions and report these to the proper authorities. (Child abuse is discussed in more detail later in this chapter.)

SPECIAL CONSIDERATIONS

As mentioned previously, children are not small adults. You should keep this in mind and modify treatment accordingly. Specific items to consider include the following:

Airway Control

Special considerations are related to characteristics of the child's airway. These include the following:

- Maintain in-line stabilization in neutral instead of the sniffing position to prevent possible pinching of the trachea (Figure 31-29).
- Administer 100% oxygen to all trauma patients.
- Maintain a patent airway with suctioning and the jaw-thrust maneuver.
- Be prepared to assist ineffective respirations. Remember that airway pressures can be high in children and it may be necessary to depress the pop-off valve to ventilate the child adequately.
- Intubate the child when the airway cannot be maintained, while simultaneously maintaining cervical-spine stabilization (Figure 31-30).
- A gastric tube should be placed following intubation to decompress the stomach.

Immobilization

Use appropriate-sized pediatric immobilization equipment including:

- Rigid cervical collar
- Towel or blanket roll
- Child safety seat
- Pediatric immobilization device

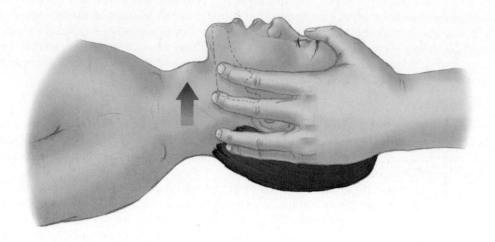

FIGURE 31-29 In the pediatric trauma patient, use the combination of jaw-thrust/spine-stabilization to open the airway.

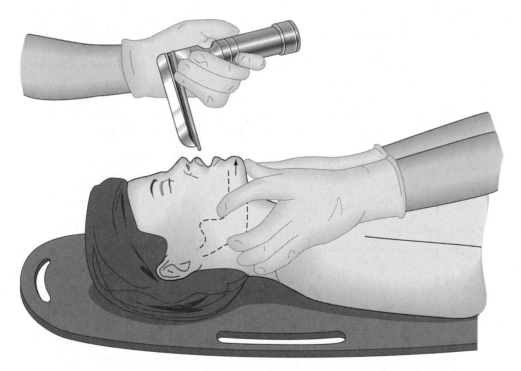

FIGURE 31-30 Simultaneous cervical-spine stabilization and intubation in a pediatric patient.

- Vest-type device (such as the Kendrick Extrication Device)
- Short wooden backboard
- Straps and cravats
- Tape
- Padding

Keep infants, toddlers, and preschoolers supine with the cervical spine in a neutral in-line position by placing padding from the shoulders to the hips. (Review the discussion of pediatric immobilization earlier in this chapter.)

Fluid Management

Management of the airway and breathing takes priority over management of circulation, because circulatory compromise is less common in children than in adults. When obtaining vascular access, remember the following:

- If possible, insert a large-bore IV catheter into a peripheral vein.
- Do not delay transport to gain venous access.
- Intraosseous access in children less than 6 years of age is an alternative when a peripheral IV cannot be obtained.
- Administer an initial fluid bolus of 20 mL/kg of lactated Ringer's solution or normal saline.
- Reassess the vital signs and re-bolus with another 20 mL/kg if there is no improvement.
- If improvement does not occur after the second bolus, there is likely to be a significant blood loss that may require surgical intervention. Rapid transport is essential.

Pediatric Analgesia and Sedation

An often overlooked aspect of prehospital pediatric care is pain control. Many pediatric injuries are painful and analgesics are indicated. These include burns, long bone fractures, dislocations, and others. Unless there is a contraindication, pediatric patients should receive analgesics. Commonly used analgesics include meperidene, morphine, and fentanyl. It is best to avoid using the synthetic analgesics (e.g., butorphanol [Stadol], nalbuphine [Nubain]) because their effects on children are unpredictable. Also, certain pediatric emergencies may benefit from sedation. These include such problems as penetrating eye injuries, prolonged rescue from entrapment in machinery, cardioversion, and other painful procedures. Always consult medical direction if you feel pediatric analgesia or sedation may be indicated.

Traumatic Brain Injury

Children, because of the relatively large size of their head and weak neck muscles, are at increased risk for traumatic brain injury. These injuries can be devastating and are often fatal. Early recognition and aggressive management can reduce both morbidity and mortality. Pediatric head injuries can be classified as follows:

- *Mild:* Glasgow coma score is 13 to 15.
- *Moderate:* Glasgow coma score is 9 to 12.
- *Severe:* Glasgow coma score is less than or equal to 8.

Traumatic head injuries can cause intracranial bleeding or swelling. This ultimately results in an increase in intracranial pressure. The signs of increased intracranial pressure can be subtle. They include:

- Elevated blood pressure
- Bradycardia
- Rapid, deep respirations progressing to slow, deep respirations
- Bulging fontanelle in infants

Increased intracranial pressure will eventually lead to herniation of a portion of the brain through the foramen magnum. This is an ominous development that is often associated with irreversible injury. Signs and symptoms of herniation include:

- Asymmetrical pupils
- Decorticate posturing
- Decerebrate posturing

Specific management of traumatic head injuries in children is similar to that for adults. As a rule, follow these steps:

- Administer a high concentration of oxygen for mild to moderate head injuries.
- Intubate children with a Glasgow coma score of less than or equal to 8 (severe head injury) and ventilate at a normal rate with 100% oxygen.
- Consider using intravenous or tracheal lidocaine prior to intubation to blunt the rise in intracranial pressure that often occurs in association with this procedure.

Consider hyperventilation if the child's condition deteriorates as evidenced by asymmetrical pupils, active seizures, or neurological posturing. Children with traumatic head injuries do best at facilities that treat a great number of children and who have pediatric neurosurgeons on staff. Consider diverting to a pediatric trauma facility if a moderate or severe traumatic head injury is present.

SPECIFIC INJURIES

As previously mentioned, more pediatric patients die of trauma than of any other cause. Statistics reveal that nearly 50% of these deaths occur within the first hour of injury. The quick arrival of EMS at the scene can literally mean the difference between life and death for a child. Although management of trauma is basically the same for children as adults, anatomical and physiological differences cause pediatric patients to have different patterns of injury.

Head, Face, and Neck

The majority of children who sustain multiple trauma will suffer associated head and/or neck injuries. As previously mentioned, the larger relative mass of the head and lack of neck muscle strength provide for increased momentum in acceleration-deceleration injuries and a greater stress on the cervical spine. The fulcrum of cervical mobility in the younger child is at the C2–C3 level. As a result, nearly 60% to 70% of pediatric fractures occur in C1–C2.

Injuries to the head are the most common cause of death in pediatric trauma victims. School-age children tend to sustain head injuries from bicycle accidents, falls from trees, or auto-pedestrian accidents. Older children most commonly suffer head injuries from sporting events. Heads injuries in all age groups may result from abuse.

In treating head injuries, remember that diffuse injuries are common in children, whereas focal injuries are rare. Because the skull is softer and more compliant in children than in adults, brain injuries occur more readily in infants and young children. Because of open fontanelles and sutures, infants up to an average age of 16 months may be more tolerant to an increase in intracranial pressure and can have delayed signs. (Keep this fact in mind when taking the history of children in the 1-month to 2-year age range.)

Children also frequently injure their faces. The most common facial injuries are lacerations secondary to falls. Young children are very clumsy when they first start walking. A fall onto a sharp object, such as the corner of a coffee table, can result in a laceration. Older children sustain dental injuries in falls from bicycles, skateboard accidents, fights, and sports activities.

Spinal injuries in children are not as common as in adults. However, as noted earlier, a child's proportionally larger and heavier head makes the cervical spine vulnerable to injury. Any time a child sustains a severe head injury, always assume that a neck injury may also be present.

Chest and Abdomen

Most injuries to the chest and abdomen result from blunt trauma. As noted earlier, infants and young children lack the rigid rib cages of adults. Therefore, they suffer fewer rib fractures and more intrathoracic injuries. Likewise, their relatively undeveloped abdominal musculature affords minimal protection to the viscera.

Because of the high mortality associated with blunt trauma, children with significant blunt abdominal or chest trauma should be transported immediately to a pediatric trauma center with appropriate care provided en route.

Injuries to the Chest   Chest injuries are the second most common cause of pediatric trauma deaths. Because of the compliance of the chest wall, severe intrathoracic injury can be present without signs of external injury. Pneumothorax and hemothorax can occur in the pediatric patient, especially if the mechanism of injury was a motor-vehicle collision. Tension pneumothorax can also occur in children. The condition is poorly tolerated by pediatric patients and a needle thoracostomy may be lifesaving. Tension pneumothorax presents with the following signs and symptoms:

> *Children tend to develop pulmonary contusions, sometimes massive, following blunt trauma to the chest.*
>

- Diminished breath sounds over the affected lung
- Shift of the trachea to the opposite side
- Progressive decrease in ventilatory compliance

Keep in mind that children with cardiac tamponade may have no physical signs of tamponade other than hypotension. Also remember that flail chest is an uncommon injury in children. When noted without a significant mechanism of injury, suspect child abuse.

Injuries to the Abdomen   Significant blunt trauma to the abdomen can result in injury to the spleen or liver. In fact, the spleen is the most commonly injured organ in children. Signs and symptoms of a splenic injury include tenderness in the left upper quadrant of the abdomen, abrasions on the abdomen, and hematoma of the abdominal wall. Symptoms of liver injury include right upper quadrant abdominal pain and/or right lower chest pain. Both splenic and hepatic injuries can cause life-threatening internal hemorrhage.

In treating blunt abdominal trauma, keep in mind the small size of the pediatric abdomen. Be certain to palpate only one quadrant at a time. In cases of both chest and abdominal trauma, treat for shock with positioning, fluids, and maintenance of body temperature.

Extremities

Extremity injuries in children are typically limited to fractures and lacerations. Children rarely sustain amputations and other serious extremity injuries. An exception includes farm children who are vulnerable to becoming entangled in agricultural equipment.

The most common injuries are fractures, usually resulting from falls. Because children have more flexible bones than adults, they tend to have incomplete fractures such as **bend fractures, buckle fractures,** and **greenstick fractures.** In younger children, the bone growth plates have not yet closed. Some types of growth plate fractures can lead to permanent disability if not managed correctly.

bend fractures fractures characterized by angulation and deformity in the bone without an obvious break.

Whenever indicated, perform splinting in order to decrease pain and prevent further injury and/or blood loss. In rare cases, the pneumatic anti-shock garment may be useful in unstable pelvic fractures with hypotension.

buckle fractures fractures characterized by a raised or bulging projection at the fracture site.

Burns

Burns are the second leading cause of death in children. They are the leading cause of accidental death in the home for children under 14. Burns may be chemical, thermal, or electrical. The most common type of burn injury encountered by EMS personnel is scalding. Children can scald themselves by pulling hot liquids off tables or stoves. In cases of abuse, they can be scalded by immersion in hot water.

greenstick fractures fractures characterized by an incomplete break in the bone.

Estimation of the burn surface area is slightly different for children than for adults (Figure 31-31). In adults, the "rule of nines" assigns 9% of the body surface area (BSA) to each of eleven body regions: the entire head and neck, the anterior chest, the anterior abdomen, the posterior chest, the lower back (posterior abdomen), the anterior surface of each lower extremity, the posterior surface of each lower extremity, and the entirety of each upper extremity. The remaining 1% is assigned to the genitalia.

In a child, the head accounts for a larger percentage of BSA, while the legs make up a smaller percentage. So for children the rule of nines is modified to take away 8% from the lower extremities (2% from the front and 2% from the back of each leg) plus the 1% assigned to the adult genitalia. This 9% that is taken from the lower part of the body is reassigned to the head. So whereas the adult's entire head and neck are counted as 9%, in the child the anterior head and neck count as 9% and the posterior head and neck count as another 9%.

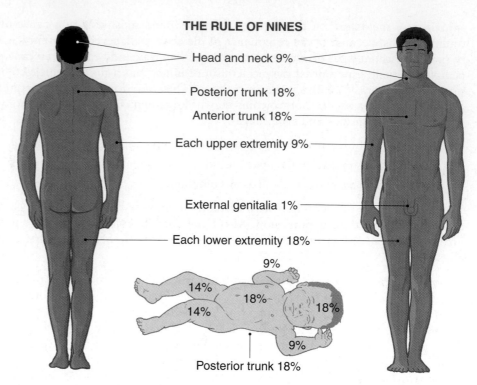

THE RULE OF NINES

Head and neck 9%

Posterior trunk 18%

Anterior trunk 18%

Each upper extremity 9%

External genitalia 1%

Each lower extremity 18%

9%

14%

18%

18%

14%

9%

Posterior trunk 18%

FIGURE 31-31   The rule of nines helps to estimate the extent of a burn in adults and children. Note the modifications for the child.

You can also use the child's palm as a guide (the "rule of palm"). The palm equals about 1% of the body surface area. You can calculate a burn area by estimating how many palm areas it equals. Usually, the rule of nines works best for more extensive burns. The rule of palm works best for less extensive ones.

Management considerations for pediatric burn patients include the following:

- Provide prompt management of the airway, since swelling can develop rapidly.

- If intubation is required, you may need to use an endotracheal tube up to two sizes smaller than normal.

- Thermally burned children are very susceptible to hypothermia. Be sure to maintain body heat.

- When treating serious electrical burn patients, suspect musculoskeletal injuries and perform spinal immobilization.

SUDDEN INFANT DEATH SYNDROME (SIDS)

sudden infant death syndrome (SIDS) illness of unknown etiology that occurs during the first year of life, with the peak at ages 2 to 4 months.

Sudden infant death syndrome (SIDS) is defined as the sudden death of an infant during the first year of life from an illness of unknown etiology. The incidence of SIDS in the United States is approximately two deaths per 1,000 births. SIDS is the leading cause of death between the ages of 2 weeks and 1 year. It is responsible for a significant number of deaths between the ages of 1 and 6 months, with peak incidence occurring at 2 to 4 months old.

SIDS occurs most frequently in the fall and winter months. It tends to be more common in males than in females. It is more prevalent in premature and low birth-weight infants, in infants of young mothers, and in infants whose mothers did not receive prenatal care. Infants of mothers who used cocaine, methadone, or heroin during pregnancy are at greater risk. Occasionally, a mild upper respiratory infection will be reported prior to death. SIDS is not caused by external suffocation from blankets or pillows. Neither is it related to allergies to cow's milk or regurgitation and aspiration of stomach contents. It is not thought to be hereditary.

Current theories vary about the etiology of SIDS. Some authorities feel it may result from an immature respiratory center in the brain that leads the child to simply stop breathing. Others think there may be an airway obstruction in the posterior pharynx as a result of pharyngeal relaxation during sleep, a hypermobile mandible, or an enlarged tongue. Studies strongly link SIDS to a prone sleeping position. Soft bedding, waterbed mattresses, smoking in the home, and/or an overheated environment are other potential associations. A small percentage of SIDS may be abuse related.

Although research into SIDS continues, the American Academy of Pediatrics suggests that infants be placed supine unless medical conditions prevent this. In addition, the academy urges parents or caregivers to avoid placing infants in overheated environments, overwrapping them with too many clothes or blankets, smoking before and after pregnancy, and filling the crib with soft bedding.

Assessment   Physical findings are similar among infants suffering SIDS. From an external standpoint, there is a normal state of nutrition and hydration. The skin may be mottled. There are often frothy, occasionally blood-tinged, fluids in and around the mouth and nostrils. Vomitus may be present. Occasionally, the infant may be in an unusual position as a result of muscle spasm or high activity at the time of death. Common findings noted at autopsy include intrathoracic petechiae (small hemorrhages) in 90% of cases. There is often associated pulmonary congestion and edema. Sometimes, stomach contents are found in the trachea. Microscopic examination of the trachea often reveals the presence of inflammatory changes.

Management   The immediate needs of the family with a SIDS baby are many. Unless the infant is obviously dead, undertake active and aggressive care of the infant to assure the family that everything possible is being done. A first responder or other personnel should be assigned to assist the parents and to explain the procedures. At all points, use the baby's name.

After arrival at the hospital, direct management at the parents or caregivers, since nothing can be done for the child. Allow the family to see the dead child. Expect a normal grief reaction. Initially, there may be shock, disbelief, and denial. Other times, the parents or caregivers may express anger, rage, hostility, blame, or guilt. Often, there is a feeling of inadequacy as well as helplessness, confusion, and fear. The grief process is likely to last for years. SIDS has major long-term effects on family relations. It may also affect you, the on-scene EMT-I. If so, do not be reluctant to request a Critical Incident Stress Debriefing.

> *In SIDS, active and aggressive care of the infant should continue until delivery to the ED unless the infant is obviously dead.*
>
>

> *At all times in a SIDS case, use the baby's name when speaking with parents or caregivers.*
>
>

CHILD ABUSE AND NEGLECT

A tragic truth is that some people cause physical and psychological harm to children, either through intentional abuse or through intentional or unintentional neglect. In fact, child abuse is the second leading cause of death in infants less than 6 months of age. An estimated 2,000 to 5,000 children die each year as a result of abuse or neglect.

Several characteristics are common to abused children. Often, the child is seen as "special" and different from others. Premature infants and twins stand a higher risk of abuse than other children. Many abused children are less than 5 years of age. Physically and mentally handicapped children as well as those with other special needs are at greater risk. So are uncommunicative (autistic) children. Boys are more often abused than girls. A child who is not what the parents wanted (e.g., the "wrong" gender) is at increased risk of abuse, too.

PERPETRATORS OF ABUSE OR NEGLECT

Abuse or neglect may be instigated by a parent, a legal guardian, or a foster parent. It can be carried out by a person, an institution, or an agency or program entrusted with custody. Abuse or neglect can also result from the actions of a caretaker, such as a baby-sitter or a nanny.

The person who abuses or neglects a child can come from any geographical, religious, ethnic, racial, occupational, educational, or socioeconomic background. Despite their diversity, people who abuse children tend to share certain traits. The abuser is usually a parent or a full-time caregiver. When the mother spends the majority of the time with the child, she is the parent most frequently identified as the abuser. Most abusers were abused themselves as children.

Three conditions can alert you to the potential for abuse. They include:

- Parent or adult who seems capable of abuse, especially one who exhibits evasive or hostile behavior
- Child in one of the high-risk categories
- Presence of a crisis, particularly financial stress, marital or relationship stress, or physical illness in a parent or child

TYPES OF ABUSE

Child abuse can take several forms. These forms include:

- Psychological abuse
- Physical abuse
- Sexual abuse
- Neglect (either physical or emotional)

Abused children suffer every imaginable kind of mistreatment. They are battered with fists, belts, broom handles, hair brushes, baseball bats, electric cords, and any other objects that can be used as weapons (Figure 31-32). They are locked in closets, denied food, or deprived of access to a toilet. They are intentionally burned or scalded with anything from hot water to cigarette butts to open flames (Figure 31-33). They are severely shaken, thrown into cribs, pushed down stairs, or shoved into walls. Some are shot, stabbed, or suffocated.

FIGURE 31–32 An abused child. Note the marks on the legs are associated with beatings with an electric wire. The burns on the buttocks are from submersion in hot water. *(Courtesy of Scott and White Hospital and Clinic)*

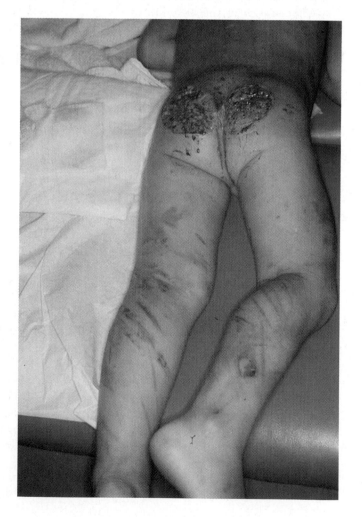

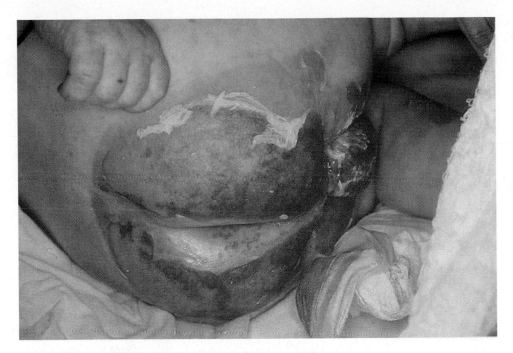

FIGURE 31-33 Burn injury from placing a child's buttocks in hot water as a punishment. *(Courtesy of Scott and White Hospital and Clinic)*

Sexual abuse ranges from adults exposing themselves to children to overt sexual acts to sexual torture. Sexual abuse can occur at any age, and the victims may be either male or female. Generally, the sexual abuser is someone the child knows and, perhaps, trusts. Stepchildren or adopted children face a greater risk for sexual abuse than biological children. Cases in which sexual abuse causes physical harm may get reported. Other cases, especially those with emotional and minor physical injury, may go undetected.

ASSESSMENT OF THE POTENTIALLY ABUSED OR NEGLECTED CHILD

Signs of abuse or neglect can be startling (Figure 31-34). As a guide, the following findings should trigger a high index of suspicion:

- Any obvious or suspected fractures in a child under 2 years of age
- Multiple injuries in various stages of healing, especially burns and bruises (Figure 31-35)
- More injuries than usually seen in children of the same age or size
- Injuries scattered on many areas of the body
- Bruises or burns in patterns that suggest intentional infliction
- Increased intracranial pressure in an infant
- Suspected intra-abdominal trauma in a young child
- Any injury that does not fit with the description of the cause given

Information in the medical history may also raise the index of suspicion. Examples include:

- History that does not match the nature or severity of the injury
- Vague parental accounts or accounts that change during the interview
- Accusations that the child injured himself intentionally
- Delay in seeking help
- Child dressed inappropriately for the situation
- Revealing comments by bystanders, especially siblings

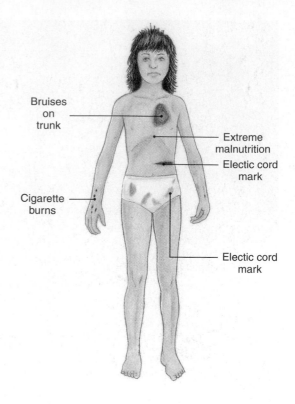

FIGURE 31-34 The stigmata of child abuse.

Bruises on trunk

Cigarette burns

Extreme malnutrition

Electic cord mark

Electic cord mark

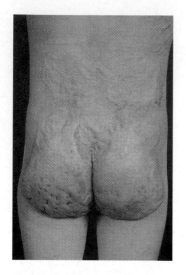

FIGURE 31-35 The effects of child abuse, both physical and mental, can last a lifetime. *(Courtesy of Scott and White Hospital and Clinic)*

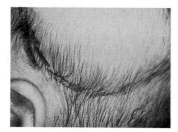

FIGURE 31-36 Child neglect from a lack of appropriate medical care.

Never leave transport of an abused child to an alleged abuser.

In many states, prehospital personnel are required by law to report suspected child abuse or neglect to the appropriate authorities.

Suspect child neglect if you spot any of the following conditions:

- Extreme malnutrition
- Multiple insect bites
- Long-standing skin infections
- Extreme lack of cleanliness
- Verbal or social skills far below those you would expect for a child of similar age and background
- Lack of appropriate medical care (Figure 31-36)

MANAGEMENT OF THE POTENTIALLY ABUSED OR NEGLECTED CHILD

In cases of child abuse or neglect, the goals of management include appropriate treatment of injuries, protection of the child from further abuse, and notification of proper authorities. You should obtain as much information as possible, in a nonjudgmental manner. Document all findings or statements in the patient report. Don't cross-examine the parents—this job belongs to the police or other authorities. Try to be supportive toward the parents, especially if it helps you to transport the child to the hospital. Remember: Never leave transport to the alleged abuser.

Upon arrival at the emergency department, report your suspicions to the appropriate personnel. Complete the patient report and all available documentation at this time, since delay may inhibit accurate recall of data.

Child abuse and neglect are particularly stressful aspects of EMS. You must recognize and deal with your feelings. Don't hesitate to seek out a mental-health professional to help you.

RESOURCES FOR ABUSE AND NEGLECT

You can contact your local child protection agency for additional information on child abuse. Consider taking a course in the recognition of child abuse and neglect. These are often offered by children's hospitals. The Internet has several sites that provide up-to-date information on child abuse.

INFANTS AND CHILDREN WITH SPECIAL NEEDS

Historically, infants and children with devastating congenital conditions or diseases either died or remained confined to a hospital. In recent decades, however, medical technology has lowered infant mortality rates and allowed a greater number of children with special needs to live at home. Some of these infants and children include:

- Premature babies
- Infants and children with lung disease, heart disease, or neurological disorders
- Infants and children with chronic diseases, such as cystic fibrosis, asthma, childhood cancers, cerebral palsy, and others
- Infants and children with altered functions from birth (Examples include cerebral palsy, spina bifida, and other congenital birth defects.)

In caring for these children, family members receive education relative to the special equipment required by the infant or child. Even so, they may feel a great deal of apprehension when care moves from the hospital to the home. As a result, they may summon EMS at the first indication of trouble. This is especially true in the initial weeks following discharge.

COMMON HOME-CARE DEVICES

Devices you might commonly find in the home include tracheostomy tubes, apnea monitors, home artificial ventilators, central IV lines, gastric feeding tubes, gastrostomy tubes, and shunts. In treating children with special needs, remember that the parents and caregivers are often very knowledgeable about their children and the devices that sustain their lives. Listen to them. They know their children better than anybody else.

Tracheostomy Tubes

Patients who are on prolonged home ventilators or who have chronic respiratory problems may have surgically placed tubes in the inferior trachea (Figure 31-37). A **tracheostomy** (trach) tube may be used as a temporary or a permanent device. Although there are various types of tubes, you might expect some common complications. They include:

- Obstruction, usually by a mucous plug
- Site bleeding, either from the tube or around the tube
- An air leakage

tracheostomy a surgical incision in the neck held open by a metal or plastic tube.

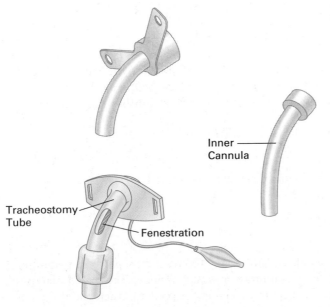

FIGURE 31-37 Tracheostomy tubes. Top: plastic tube. Bottom: metal tube with inner cannula.

Inner Cannula

Tracheostomy Tube

Fenestration

- A dislodged tube
- Infection—a condition that will worsen an already impaired breathing ability

Management steps for a patient with a tracheostomy include:

- Maintaining an open airway
- Suctioning the tube, as needed
- Allowing the patient to remain in a position of comfort, if possible
- Administering oxygen in cases of respiratory distress
- Assisting ventilations in cases of respiratory failure/arrest by:
  - Intubating orally in the absence of an upper airway obstruction
  - Intubating via the **stoma** if the upper airway is obstructed
- Transporting the patient to the hospital

stoma a permanent surgical opening in the neck through which the patient breathes.

Apnea Monitors

Apnea monitors are used to alert parents or caregivers to the cessation of breathing in an infant, especially a premature infant. Some types of monitors signal changes in heart rate, such as bradycardia or tachycardia. They operate via pads attached to the baby's chest and connected to the monitor by wires. If the device does not detect a breath within a specific time frame or if the infant's heart rate is too slow or too fast, an alarm will sound.

Most parents who have infants on apnea monitors have received training in pediatric CPR.

When an apnea monitor is placed in a home, the parents are typically instructed on what to do if the alarm sounds (stimulate the child, provide artificial respirations, and so on). If these fail, EMS may be summoned. Also, nervous parents who have just brought a baby home on an apnea monitor may panic the first couple of times the alarm sounds and call 9-1-1. Be patient and kind while instructing them on what to do when the alarm sounds.

Home Artificial Ventilators

Various configurations exist for home ventilators. Demand ventilators sense rate and quality of a patient's respiration as well as several other parameters, including pulse oximetry. They typically respond to pre-set limits. Other devices provide a constant positive end-expiratory pressure (PEEP) and a set oxygen concentration for the patient.

Two complications commonly result in EMS calls: (1) a device's mechanical failure and (2) shortages of energy during an electrical failure. Treatment typically includes:

- Maintaining an open airway
- Administering artificial ventilations via an appropriately sized BVM with oxygen
- Transporting the patient to a hospital until the home ventilator is working

Central Intravenous Lines

Children who require long-term IV therapy will often have central lines placed into the superior vena cava near the heart. In cases where IV therapy is necessary for only several weeks, percutaneous intravenous catheter (PIC) lines may be placed in the arm and threaded into the superior vena cava. Otherwise the lines are placed through subclavian venipuncture. **Central IV lines** are commonly used to administer nutrition. antibiotics, or chemotherapy for cancer.

central IV line intravenous line placed into the superior vena cava for the administration of long-term fluid therapy.

Possible complications for central IV lines include:

- Cracked line
- Infection, either at the site or at more distal aspects of the line
- Loss of patency, such as clotting
- Hemorrhage, which can be considerable
- Air embolism

Emergency medical care steps include control of any bleeding through direct pressure. If a large amount of air is in the line, try to withdraw it with a syringe. If this fails, clamp the line and transport. In cases of a cracked line, place a clamp between the crack and the patient.

If the patient exhibits an altered mental status following the cracked line, position the child on the left side with head down. Transport the child to the hospital as quickly as possible.

Gastric Feeding Tubes and Gastrostomy Tubes

Children who are not capable of swallowing or eating receive nutrition through either a gastric feeding tube or a gastrostomy tube. (A gastric feeding tube is placed through the nostrils into the stomach. A gastrostomy tube is placed through the abdominal wall directly into the stomach.) These special devices are commonly used in disorders of the digestive system or in situations in which the developmental ability of the patient hinders feeding. Food consists of nutritious liquids.

Possible emergency complications include:

- Bleeding at the site
- Dislodged tube
- Respiratory distress, particularly if a tube feeding backs up into the esophagus and is aspirated into the trachea and lungs
- In the case of diabetics, altered mental status due to missed feedings

Emergency medical care involves supporting the ABCs, including possible suctioning and administration of supplemental oxygen. Patients should be transported to a definitive care facility, either in a sitting position or lying on the right side with the head elevated. The goal is to reduce the risk of aspiration, a serious condition.

Shunts

A **shunt** is a surgical connection that runs from the brain to the abdomen. It removes excess cerebrospinal fluid from the brain through drainage. A subcutaneous reservoir is usually palpable on one side of the patient's head. A pathological rise in intracranial pressure, secondary to a blocked shunt, is a primary complication. Shunt failure may also result when the shunt's connections separate, usually because of a child's growth.

Cases of shunt failure present as altered mental status. The patient may exhibit drowsiness, respiratory distress, or the classic signs of pupil dysfunction or posturing. Be aware that an altered mental status may be caused by infection, a distinction to be made in a hospital setting.

Care steps involve maintenance of an open airway, administration of ventilations as needed, and immediate transport. Shunt failures require correction in the operating room, where the cerebrospinal fluid can be drained or, in rare cases, an infection identified and treated.

shunt surgical connection that runs from the brain to the abdomen for the purpose of draining excess cerebrospinal fluid, thus preventing increased intracranial pressure.

GENERAL ASSESSMENT AND MANAGEMENT PRACTICES

Remember that pediatric patients with special needs require the same assessment as other patients. Always evaluate the airway, breathing, and circulation. (Recall that in the initial assessment, "disability" refers to patient's neurological status, not to the child's special need.) If you discover life-threatening conditions in the initial assessment, begin appropriate interventions. Keep in mind that the child's special need is often an ongoing process. In most cases, you should concentrate on the acute problem.

During the assessment, ask pertinent questions of the patient, parent, or caregiver such as: "What unusual situation caused you to call for an ambulance?" As already mentioned, the parent or caregiver is usually very knowledgeable about the patient's condition.

In most cases, the physical examination is essentially the same as with other patients. It is important to explain everything that is being done, even if the patient does not seem to understand. Do not be distracted by the special equipment. Be aware of the help that the patient, parent, or caregiver may be able to provide in handling home-care devices.

In managing patients with special needs, try to keep several thoughts in mind:

- Avoid using the term *disability* (in reference to the child's special need). Instead, think of the patient's many abilities.
- Never assume that the patient cannot understand what you are saying.

Remember that pediatric patients with special needs require the same assessment as other patients.

In most cases, concentrate on the acute problem rather than the ongoing special need.

- Involve the parents, caregivers, or the patient, if appropriate, in treatment. They manage the illness or congenital condition on a daily basis.
- Treat the patient with a special need with the same respect as any other patient.

SUMMARY

Pediatric emergencies can be stressful for both you and the adults responsible for the child's well-being. Most pediatric emergencies result from trauma, respiratory distress, ingestion of poisons, or febrile seizure activity. In addition, you must always be on the lookout for signs and symptoms of child abuse or neglect. The approach and management of pediatric emergencies must be modified for the age and size of the child. Certain skills generally considered routine, such as IV administration, become difficult in the pediatric patient because of size and other factors. It is important to remember that children are not small adults. They have special considerations—both physical and emotional—that must be managed accordingly.

ON THE WEB

For additional practice and review, go to the companion website at www.prenhall.com/bledsoe and click on *Intermediate Emergency Care: Principles & Practice*.

Chapter 32

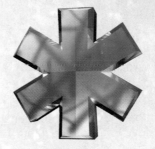

Geriatric Emergencies

Objectives

After reading this chapter, you should be able to:

1. Discuss dependent and independent living environments of elderly patients. (pp. 1262–1263)
2. Discuss common emotional and psychological reactions to aging, including causes and manifestations. (pp. 1261–1263, 1299–1301)
3. Discuss pathophysiology changes associated with the elderly in regard to drug distribution, metabolism, and elimination—including polypharmacy, dosing errors, increased drug sensitivity, and medication non-compliance. (pp. 1264–1265)
4. Discuss the use and effects of commonly prescribed drugs for the elderly patient. (pp. 1264–1265, 1296–1298)
5. Discuss the problem of mobility in the elderly and develop strategies to prevent falls. (pp. 1265–1266)
6. Discuss age-related changes in sensations in the elderly and describe the implications of these changes for communication and patient assessment. (pp. 1266, 1269–1270)
7. Discuss the problems with continence and elimination in the elderly patient. (pp. 1266–1267)
8. Discuss factors that may complicate the assessment of the elderly patient. (pp. 1267–1272)
9. Discuss common complaints of elderly patients. (pp. 1278–1301)

10. Discuss the normal and abnormal changes of age in relation to the following systems:
    a. Pulmonary system (p. 1273)
    b. Cardiovascular system (pp. 1273–1275)
    c. Nervous system (pp. 1275–1276)
    d. Endocrine system (p. 1276)
    e. Gastrointestinal system (p. 1276)
    f. Thermoregulatory system (pp. 1276–1277)
    g. Integumentary system (p. 1277)
    h. Musculoskeletal system (p. 1277)
    i. Renal system (p. 1277)
    j. Genitourinary system (pp. 1277–1278)
    k. Immune system (p. 1278)
    l. Hematology system (p. 1278)
11. Discuss the assessment and management of the elderly patient with complaints related to the following body systems:
    a. Respiratory system (pp. 1278–1281)
    b. Cardiovascular system (pp. 1281–1285)
    c. Nervous system (pp. 1285–1289)
    d. Endocrine system (pp. 1289–1290)
    e. Gastrointestinal system (pp. 1290–1291)
    f. Integumentary system (pp. 1291–1292)
    g. Musculoskeletal system (pp. 1293–1294)
    h. Renal and Urinary system (pp. 1294–1295)
12. Describe the assessment and management of the elderly patient with an environmental emergency. (pp. 1295–1296)

Continued

13. Describe the assessment and management of the elderly patient with a toxicological or substance abuse problem. (pp. 1296–1299)
14. Describe the assessment and management of the elderly patient with a behavioral or psychological problem. (pp. 1299–1301)
15. Describe the incidence, morbidity/mortality, risk factors, prevention strategies, pathophysiology, assessment, need for intervention and transport, and management of the elderly trauma patient. (pp. 1301–1303)

16. Describe the assessment and management of the elderly patient with
    a. Orthopedic injuries (pp. 1304–1305)
    b. Burns (pp. 1305–1306)
    c. Head and spinal injuries (p. 1306)
17. Given several preprogrammed simulated geriatric patients with various complaints, provide the appropriate assessment, management, and transport. (pp. 1261–1306)

CASE STUDY

"Turnpike Rescue, respond Priority One to 957 Homestead Road for a 79-year-old female with abdominal pain."

You've just arrived on duty when this call comes into the station. "The day is starting early," you say to a coworker. Oh well, you think. It's a good chance to teach the EMT-I student intern assigned to your crew about elderly patients. "Hey Andy," you call out to the student. "What are the causes of abdominal pain in an elderly patient?"

Andy tells you that the pain could be related to any number of bowel complaints—from obstruction to simple constipation. He also mentions problems such as ulcers, urinary infections, and even trauma. He ends with a quip: "Probably isn't related to too many beers and a taco, huh?"

You've just pulled up to the house, so you let Andy's remark slide for now. A man standing in the doorway calls out: "Come quickly. I think my mother may be dying."

You and your partner allow Andy to conduct a complete scene size-up. You concur with his decision that the scene is safe at the present time and enter what appears to be a well-kept home. "Does your mother live alone?" you ask.

The son, who identifies himself as Michael, replies: "Yes, Mom lives alone. She's extremely independent. She drives everywhere, even at night. She does volunteer work and still likes to travel. This past summer, she took a cruise to the Bahamas all by herself." Michael then adds, "That's why I'm so worried. I stopped in to visit, and there was Mom still in bed, crying out in pain."

Upon entering the patient's bedroom, you see a well-nourished elderly woman, tossing and turning on her bed. "My stomach hurts so much," she sobs. Between cries of anguish, she manages to tell you that the pain woke her up early this morning. She has not gotten out of bed since. When you ask if she has fallen recently, she says, "No."

You notice that Andy has instructed your partner to set up high-flow, high-concentration O_2. You nod approval and ask him to begin the initial assessment. Meanwhile, you obtain a history from the son.

Michael explains that his mom, Mrs. Hildegaard, has been very healthy. She has hypertension, but is compliant with her medication of lisinopril-hydochlorthiazide. When you ask about allergies, Michael mentions aspirin. He knows of no changes in his mom's diet, and her appetite has been good. In fact, she and his brother, Allen, went out to dinner last night. Michael explains that Mrs. Hildegaard was clinically depressed after the death of her husband 7 years ago, but bounced back after therapy. She's taken no antidepressants for more than 5 years.

After performing an initial assessment, Andy reports: "Airway is open and clear. Breathing is slightly fast at 22 per minute, but is interspersed with crying. Lungs are clear. Skin is cool, but dry. No overt bleeding. Pupils equal and reactive, with no neuro deficits noted." He then states the vital signs as BP 154/90, pulse 110 and irregular, respirations 22 and non-labored. Upon examination of the patient's abdomen, Andy found no evidence of guarding and no specific area of tenderness. Mrs. Hildegaard told him: "My stomach hurts all over, everywhere you touch."

Andy has started oxygen at 10 liters by nonrebreather mask, per protocols. Your partner has also established an IV line of normal saline and placed the patient on the cardiac monitor. The monitor shows atrial fibrillation with an average rate of 110 bpm.

The patient is packaged and transported to the emergency department. En route, you contact medical direction.

In the emergency department, the attending physician orders blood work, chest film, and an abdominal CT. Following an exploratory laparotomy, the physician admits Mrs. Hildegaard to the surgical intensive care unit. The diagnosis is an infarcted bowel. The patient's prognosis is poor.

Back at the station, you take time to address Andy's quip about the "beers and a taco." You say: "You probably know that as people age they often lose life-long support systems, like a job or a spouse. But did you realize that the elderly sometimes turn to alcohol to relieve the pain, just like people our own age?"

You then offer some pointers for providing quality EMS care to the elderly. "The most important thing to remember about the elderly patient is that while many changes occur as a result of aging, you must avoid jumping to conclusions. Give proper attention to assessment, and think about normal changes of aging versus changes as a result of disease. Provide prompt treatment as the elderly patient has less physiologic reserve than a younger patient. Once the elderly patient starts to deteriorate, the process is difficult to stop. Always remember that when complaints of abdominal pain are out of proportion to your exam, you should suspect a serious medical condition—in this case, bowel infarct."

As you walk away, you say: "So Andy, do you want to talk about what went right with this call and what we could have done better while we restock the ambulance?"

"You bet," he replies.

INTRODUCTION

Aging—the gradual decline of biological functions—varies widely from one individual to another. Most people reach their biological peak in the years before age 30. For practical purposes, however, the aging process does not affect their daily lives until later years. Many of the decrements commonly ascribed to aging are caused by other factors, such as lifestyle, diet, behavior, or environment. The aging process becomes even more complicated if we remember that age-related changes in organ functions also occur at different rates. For example, a person's kidneys may decline rapidly with age, while the heart remains strong or vice versa.

As people age, they actually become less alike, both physiologically and psychologically. Although some functional losses in old age are due to normal age-related changes, many others result from abnormal changes, particularly disease. In assessing and treating older patients, it is important to distinguish, when possible, normal age-related changes from abnormal changes. The purpose of this chapter is to present some of the most common physiological changes associated with aging and the implications of these changes to the quality of EMS care provided to the elderly—one of the fastest-growing segments of our population.

> Many of the decrements commonly ascribed to aging are caused by other factors, such as lifestyle, diet, behavior, or environment.

elderly a person age 65 or older.

EPIDEMIOLOGY AND DEMOGRAPHICS

The twentieth century, with its tremendous medical and technological advances, was a period of both a reduction in infant mortality rates and an increase in life expectancies. The cumulative effect was a population boom worldwide, with the greatest gains seen among people age 65 or older. During the 1900s, the population of the United States increased threefold, while the number of elderly increased tenfold. The growing number of elderly patients presents a challenge to all health-care services, including EMS, not only in terms of resources, but in the enormous impact that aging has on our society.

POPULATION CHARACTERISTICS

The population in the United States is getting older. Between 1960 and 1990, the number of elderly people nearly doubled. By late 1998, the total reached more than 34 million, with nearly 400,000 people ages 95 and older. As the 2000s began, demographers talked about the "graying of America," a process in which the number of elderly people is pushing up the average age of the U.S. population as a whole. Reasons for this trend include:

- Mean survival rate of older persons is increasing.
- Birth rate is declining.
- There has been an absence of major wars and other catastrophes.
- Health care and standards of living have improved significantly since World War II.

In 2030, when the post-World War II baby boomers enter their 80s, more than 70 million people will be age 65 or older. By 2040, the elderly will represent roughly 20% of the population. In other words, one in five people in the United States will be age 65 or older.

Not only will the elderly population increase in size, its members will live longer, which in turn will swell the number of the **old-old**. By 2040, the number of people age 85 and over is expected to rise by 17%. Whether longer life spans mean longer years of active living or longer years of disease and disability is unknown.

old-old an elderly person age 80 or older.

Gerontology, the study of the effects of aging on humans, is a relatively new science. (The Gerontological Society of America [GSA] was formed in 1945.) Gerontologists still do not fully understand the underlying causes of aging. However, most believe that some form of cellular damage or loss, particularly of nerve cells (neurons), is involved. The result is a general decline in the body's efficiency, such as a reduction in the size and function of most internal organs.

gerontology scientific study of the effects of aging and of age-related diseases on humans.

To treat age-related changes, physicians and other health-care workers have increasingly specialized in the care of the elderly. This aspect of medicine, known as **geriatrics**, is essential in caring for our aging population.

geriatrics the study and treatment of diseases of the aged.

The demographic changes will also affect your EMS career. Today nearly 36% of all EMS calls involve the elderly. The percentage is expected to grow. Therefore, you will need to be familiar with the fundamental principles of geriatrics, especially those related to advanced prehospital care. You will also need to be aware of the social issues that can affect the health and mental well-being of the elderly patients that you will be treating.

SOCIETAL ISSUES

For a typical working person, the post-retirement years can be up to one-third of an average life span. The years include a series of transitions, such as reduced income, relocation, and loss of friends, family members, spouse, or partner.

Emotional, physical, and/or financial difficulties can help create a context in which illnesses occur. An understanding of those difficulties is involved in successful medical treatment of elderly patients.

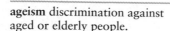

After years of working and/or raising a family, an elderly person must not only find new roles to fulfill, but also, in many cases, overcome the societal label of "old person." A lot of elderly people disprove **ageism**—and all the stereotypes it engenders—by living happy, productive, and active lives (Figure 32-1). Others, however, feel a sense of social isolation or uselessness. Physical and financial difficulties reinforce these feelings and help create an emotional context in which illnesses can occur. Therefore, successful medical treatment of elderly patients involves an understanding of the broader social situation in which they live.

ageism discrimination against aged or elderly people.

The elderly live in both independent and dependent living environments. Many continue to live alone or with their partner well into their 80s or 90s. The oldest old are the most likely to live alone, and, in fact, nearly half of those age 85 and over live by themselves. The great majority of these people, an estimated 78%, are women. This is because married

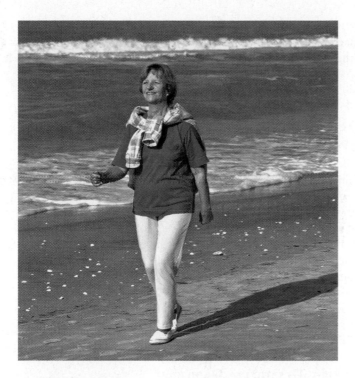

FIGURE 32-1 Many older adults live active lives, participating in sports and exercises popular among people of all ages. *(The Stock Market Photo Agency)*

Table 32-1	PREVENTION STRATEGIES FOR THE OLDER PERSON
Issues	**Strategies**
Lifestyle	
Exercise	Weight-bearing and cardiovascular exercise (walking) for 20–30 min at least three times a week
Nutrition	Varies, but generally low fat, adequate fiber (complex carbohydrates), reduced sugar (simple carbohydrates), moderate protein; adequate calcium, especially for women*
Alcohol/tobacco	Moderate alcohol, if any; abstinence from tobacco
Sleep	Generally 7–8 hours a night
Accidents	Maintain good physical condition; add safety features to home (handrails, nonskid surfaces, lights, etc.); modify potentially dangerous driving practices (driving at night with impaired night vision, traveling in hazardous weather, etc.)
Medical health	
Disease/Illness	Routine screening for hearing, vision, blood pressure, hemoglobin, cholesterol, etc.; regular physical examinations; immunizations (tetanus booster, influenza vaccine, once-in-a-lifetime pneumococcal vaccine)
Pharmacological	Regular review of prescriptive and over-the-counter medications, focusing on potential interactions and side effects
Dental	Regular dental checkups and good oral hygiene (important for nutrition and general well-being)
Mental/emotional	Observe for evidence of depression, disrupted sleep patterns, psychosocial stress; ensure effective support networks and availability of psychotherapy; compliance with prescribed antidepressants

*Vitamin supplements may be required, but should be taken only after other medications are reviewed and in correct dosages. Excessive doses of vitamin A or D, for example, can be toxic.

men tend to die before their wives, and widowed men tend to remarry more often than widowed women.

PREVENTION AND SELF-HELP

In treating the elderly, remember that the best intervention is prevention (Table 32-1). The goal of any health-care service, including EMS, should be to help keep people from becoming sick or injured in the first place. As previously mentioned, disease and disability in later life are often linked to unhealthy or unsafe behavior. As an EMT-I, you can reduce morbidity among the elderly by taking part in community education programs and by cooperating with agencies or organizations that support the elderly. Some possible resources are described in the following sections.

GENERAL PATHOPHYSIOLOGY, ASSESSMENT, AND MANAGEMENT

In treating elderly patients, it is important to recall several facts. First, medical disorders in the elderly often present as **functional impairment** and should be treated as an early warning of a possibly undetected medical problem. Second, signs and symptoms do not necessarily point to the underlying cause of the problem or illness. For example, although confusion often indicates a brain disease in younger patients, this may not be the case in an elderly patient. The confused patient may be suffering from a wide range of disorders, including drug toxicity, malnutrition, or accidental hypothermia.

A thorough evaluation must always be done to detect possible causes of an impairment. If identified early, an environmental- or disease-generated impairment can often be reversed. Your success depends on a knowledge of age-related changes and the implications of these changes for patient assessment and management.

PATHOPHYSIOLOGY OF THE ELDERLY PATIENT

As mentioned, patients become less alike as they enter their elderly years, Even so, certain generalizations can be made about age-related changes and the disease process in the elderly.

Multiple-System Failure

There is no escaping the fact that the body becomes less efficient with age, increasing the likelihood of malfunction. The body is susceptible to all the disorders of young people, but its maintenance, defense, and repair processes are weaker. As a result, the elderly often suffer from more than one illness or disease at a time. On average, six medical disorders may coexist in an elderly person and perhaps even more in the old-old. Neither the patient nor the patient's doctor may be aware of all of these problems. Furthermore, disease in one organ system may result in the deterioration of other systems, compounding existing acute and/or chronic conditions.

Because of concomitant diseases (**comorbidity**) in the elderly, complaints may not be specific to any one disorder. Common complaints of the elderly include: fatigue and weakness, dizziness/vertigo/syncope, falls, headaches, insomnia, **dysphagia,** loss of appetite, inability to void, and/or constipation/diarrhea.

Elderly patients often accept medical problems as a part of aging and fail to monitor changes in their condition. In some cases, such as a silent myocardial infarction, pain may be diminished or absent. In others, an important complaint may seem trivial, such as constipation.

Although many medical problems in the young and middle-aged populations present with a standard set of signs and symptoms, the changes involved in aging lead to different presentations. In pneumonia, for example, the classic symptom of fever is often absent in the elderly. Chest pain and a cough are also less common. Finally, many cases of pneumonia among the elderly are due to aspiration, not infection. The presentation of pneumonia and other diseases commonly found in the elderly will be covered later in the chapter.

Pharmacology in the Elderly

The existence of multiple chronic diseases in the elderly leads to the use of multiple medications. Persons age 65 and older use one-third of all prescriptive drugs in the United States, taking an average of 4.5 medications per day. This does not include over-the-counter medications, vitamin supplements, or herbal remedies.

If medications are not correctly monitored, **polypharmacy** can lead to a number of problems among the elderly. In general, a person's sensitivity to drugs increases with age.

---

functional impairment decreased ability to meet daily needs on an independent basis.

comorbidity having more than one disease at a time.

dysphagia inability to swallow or difficulty swallowing.

The existence of multiple chronic diseases in the elderly often leads to the use of multiple medications.

polypharmacy multiple drug therapies in which there is a concurrent use of a number of drugs.

When compared with younger patients, the elderly experience more adverse drug reactions, more drug-drug interactions, and more drug-disease interactions. Because of age-related pharmacokinetic changes such as a loss of body fluid and atrophy of organs, drugs concentrate more readily in the plasma and tissues of elderly patients. As a result, drug dosages often must be adjusted to prevent toxicity. (The problem of toxicity will be discussed in more detail later in the chapter.)

In taking a medical history of an elderly patient, remember to ask questions to determine if a patient is taking a prescribed medication as directed. Noncompliance with drug therapy, usually underadherence, is common among the elderly. Up to 40% do not take medications as prescribed. Factors that can decrease compliance in the elderly include:

- Limited income
- Memory loss due to decreased or diseased neural activity
- Limited mobility
- Sensory impairment (cannot hear/read/understand directions)
- Multiple or complicated drug therapies
- Fear of toxicity
- Child-proof containers (especially with arthritic patients)
- Duration of drug therapy (The longer the therapy, the less likely a patient will stick with it.)

Factors that can increase compliance among the elderly include:

- Good patient-physician communication
- Belief that a disease or illness is serious
- Drug calendars or reminder cards
- Compliance counseling
- Blister-pack packaging or other easy-to-open packaging
- Multi-compartment pill boxes
- Transportation services to pharmacy
- Clear, simple directions written in large type
- Ability to read

Problems with Mobility and Falls

Regular exercise and a good diet are two of the most effective preventive measures for ensuring mobility among the elderly. However, not all elderly take these measures. They may suffer from a severe medical problem, such as crippling arthritis. They may fear for their personal safety, either from accidental injury or intentional injury, such as robbery. Certain medications also may increase their lethargy. Whatever the cause, a lack of mobility can have detrimental physical and emotional effects. Some of these include:

- Poor nutrition
- Difficulty with elimination
- Poor skin integrity
- A greater predisposition for falls
- Loss of independence and/or confidence
- Depression from "feeling old"
- Isolation and lack of a social network

Fall-related injuries represent the leading cause of accidental death among the elderly. Intrinsic factors include a history of repeated falls, dizziness, a sense of weakness, impaired vision, an altered gait, central nervous system (CNS) problems, decreased mental status, or use of certain medications. Extrinsic factors include environmental hazards such as slippery floors, a lack of handrails, or loose throw rugs.

In taking a medical history of an elderly patient, remember to ask if the patient is taking a prescribed medication as directed.

In assessing an elderly patient who has fallen, remember that a fall often has multiple causes. An over-medicated patient, for example, trips over a throw rug. A fall may also be a presenting sign of an acute illness, such as a myocardial infarction, or a sign that a chronic illness has worsened. Bear in mind the possibility of physical abuse, especially if the injury does not match the story.

Communication Difficulties

Most elderly patients suffer from some form of age-related sensory changes. Normal physiological changes may include impaired vision or blindness, impaired or loss of hearing, an altered sense of taste or smell, and/or a lower sensitivity to pain (touch). Any of these conditions can affect your ability to communicate with the patient. For communication strategies, see Table 32-2. (A discussion on the implications of sensory impairment on patient assessment appears later in the chapter.)

Problems with Continence and Elimination

The elderly often find it embarrassing to talk about problems with continence and elimination. They may feel stigmatized, isolated, and/or helpless. When confronted with these problems, DO NOT make a big deal out of them. Respect the patient's dignity, and assure the person that, in many cases, the problem is treatable.

incontinence inability to retain urine or feces because of loss of sphincter control or cerebral or spinal lesions.

Incontinence The problem of **incontinence** can affect nearly any age group, but is most commonly associated with the elderly. Incontinence may be either urinary or fecal. An estimated 15% of the elderly who live at home experience some form of urinary incontinence. Nearly 30% of the hospitalized elderly and 50% of those living in nursing homes suffer from the same condition. Although fecal, or bowel, incontinence is less common, it seriously impairs activity and may lead to dependent care. Between 16% and 60% of the institutionalized elderly have some kind of fecal incontinence.

Incontinence can lead to a variety of conditions such as rashes, skin infections, skin breakdown (ulcers), urinary tract infections, sepsis, and falls or fractures. As mentioned, the condition takes a high emotional toll on both the patient and the caregiver. Management of incontinence costs billions of dollars each year.

In general, effective continence requires several physical conditions. These include:

- An anatomically correct gastrointestinal/gastrourinary tract
- Competent sphincter mechanism
- Adequate cognition and mobility

Table 32-2 | AGE-RELATED SENSORY CHANGES AND IMPLICATIONS FOR COMMUNICATION

Sensory Change	Result	Communication Strategy
Clouding and thickening of lens in eye	Cataracts; poor vision, especially peripheral vision	Position yourself in front of patient where you can be seen; put hand on arm of blind patient to let patient know where you are; locate a patient's glasses, if necessary.
Shrinkage of structure in ear	Decreased hearing, especially ability to hear high frequency sounds; diminished sense of balance	Speak clearly; check hearing aids as necessary; write notes if necessary; allow the patient to put on the stethoscope, while you speak into it like a microphone.
Deterioration of teeth and gums	Patient needs dentures, but they may inflict pain on sensitive gums, so patient doesn't always wear them	If patient's speech is unintelligible, ask patient to put in dentures, if possible.
Lowered sensitivity to pain and altered sense of taste and smell	Patient underestimates the severity of the problem or is unable to provide a complete pertinent history	Probe for significant symptoms, asking questions aimed at functional impairment.

Although incontinence is not necessarily caused by aging, several factors predispose older patients to this condition. As mentioned, the elderly tend to have several medical disorders, each of which may require drug therapy. These disorders and/or the drugs used to treat them may compromise the integrity of either the urinary or bowel tracts. In addition, bladder capacity, urinary flow rate, and the ability to postpone voiding appear to decline with age. Certain diseases, such as diabetes and autonomic neuropathy, may also cause sphincter dysfunction. Diarrhea, or lack of physical sensation, may produce bowel incontinence as well.

Management of incontinence depends on the cause, which cannot be easily diagnosed in the field. Some cases of incontinence can be managed surgically. In most cases, however, patients use some type of absorptive devices, such as leak-proof underwear or panty liners. Indwelling catheters are less common and may cause infections when used, particularly if not properly managed. Of critical importance is respect for the patient's modesty and dignity.

Elimination Difficulty with elimination can be a sign of a serious underlying condition (Table 32-3). It can also lead to other complications. Straining to eliminate may have serious effects on the cerebral, coronary, and peripheral arterial circulations. In elderly people with cerebrovascular disease or impaired baroreceptor reflexes, efforts to force a bowel movement can lead to a **transient ischemic attack (TIA)** or syncope. In the case of prolonged constipation, the elderly may experience colonic ulceration, intestinal obstruction, and urinary retention.

In assessing a patient with difficulty eliminating, remember to inquire about their medications. Any of the following drugs can cause constipation:

- Opioids
- Anticholinergics (e.g., antidepressants, antihistamines, muscle relaxants, antiparkinsonian drugs)
- Cation-containing agents (e.g., antacids, calcium supplements, iron supplements)
- Neurally active agents (e.g., opiates, anticonvulsants)
- Diuretics

ASSESSMENT CONSIDERATIONS

As with all patients, be sure to take appropriate body substance isolation (BSI) precautions when assessing an elderly patient. Because of the increased risk of tuberculosis in patients who are in nursing homes, consider wearing a HEPA or N-95 respirator. Remain alert to the environment, particularly the temperature of the surroundings and evidence of prescription medications.

In general, assessment of the elderly patient follows the same basic approach used with any patient. However, you need to keep in mind several factors that will improve the quality of your evaluation and make subsequent treatment more successful.

General Health Assessment

As already mentioned, you need to set a context for illness when assessing an elderly patient. When performing a general health assessment, take into account the patient's living situation, level of activity, network of social support, level of independence, medication history (both prescription and non-prescriptive), and sleep patterns.

In treating incontinence, remember to respect the patient's modesty and dignity.

Difficulty with elimination can be a sign of a serious underlying condition.

transient ischemic attacks (TIA) reversible interruptions of blood flow to the brain; often seen as a precursor to a stroke.

Because of the increased risk of tuberculosis in nursing home patients, consider using a HEPA or N-95 respirator.

Content Review

FACTORS IN PERFORMING A GENERAL ASSESSMENT
- Living situation
- Level of activity
- Network of social support
- Level of independence
- Medication history
- Sleep patterns

Table 32-3	POSSIBLE CAUSES OF ELIMINATION PROBLEMS
Difficulty in Urination	**Difficulty with Bowel Movements**
Enlarged prostate in men	Diverticular disease
Urinary tract infection	Constipation*
Acute or chronic renal failure	Colorectal cancer

*Constipation may be related to dietary, medical, or surgical conditions. It could also be the result of a malignancy, intestinal obstruction, or hypothyroidism. Treat constipation as a serious medical problem.

Unfortunately, many elderly are economically disadvantaged. In fact, many elderly patients, especially elderly females, live at or below the poverty line. The reasons for this are many. Most importantly, they live on a fixed income—either from retirement pensions or social security benefits. While this income remains fixed, the cost of living continues to increase. Thus, some elderly must make decisions as to what they can and cannot afford. Some will forgo certain medications. Others will try to live with reduced heating or cooling to save energy costs. And, unfortunately, others will forgo food to maintain their independence.

When called to assess a geriatric patient, try to get an idea as to how well they are living. Is the house unusually hot or cold? Are they forgoing certain medications that they consider are too expensive? Is the house safe and clean? Are they eating well? Are they able to prepare meals for themselves? And, most importantly, do family members or friends periodically check in on them? If you have any concerns, you should notify the proper authorities or the hospital staff so that social services can provide an evaluation to ensure that they can live safely in their present setting.

Pay particularly close attention to the patient's nutrition. Elderly patients often have a decreased sense of smell and taste, which decreases their pleasure in eating. They also may be less aware of internal cues of hunger and thirst. Although caloric requirements generally decrease with age, an elderly patient may still suffer from malnutrition. Conditions that may complicate or discourage eating among the elderly include:

- Breathing or respiratory problems
- Abdominal pain
- Nausea/vomiting, sometimes a drug-induced condition as with antibodies or aspirin
- Poor dental care
- Medical problems, such as hyperthyroidism, hypercalcemia, and chronic infections (e.g., cancer or tuberculosis)
- Medications (e.g., digoxin, vitamin A, fluoxetine)
- Alcohol or drug abuse
- Psychological disorders, including depression and **anorexia nervosa**
- Poverty
- Problems with shopping or cooking

As with any person, nutrition greatly affects a patient's overall health. Because of reasons cited above, patients may suffer from a number of by-products of malnutrition, including vitamin deficiencies, dehydration, and hypoglycemia. Also remember that when a malnourished elderly person is fed, the food may produce yet other side effects, including electrolyte abnormalities, hyperglycemia, aspiration pneumonia, and a significant drop in blood pressure.

Pathophysiology and Assessment

Assessment of the elderly reflects the pathophysiology of this age group. As already mentioned, the chief complaint of the elderly may seem trivial or vague at first. Also, the patient may fail to report important symptoms. Therefore, you should try to distinguish the patient's chief complaint from the patient's primary problem. A patient may report nausea, which is the chief complaint. The primary problem, however, may be the rectal bleeding that the patient neglected to mention.

The presence of multiple diseases also complicates the assessment process. The presence of chronic problems may make it more difficult to assess an acute problem. It is easy to confuse symptoms from a chronic illness with those of an acute condition. When confronted with an elderly patient who has chest pain, for example, it is difficult to determine whether the presence of frequent premature ventricular contractions is acute or chronic.

anorexia nervosa eating disorder marked by excessive fasting.

Content Review

BY-PRODUCTS OF MALNUTRITION

- Vitamin deficiencies
- Dehydration
- Hypoglycemia

Try to distinguish the patient's chief complaint from the primary problems.

Lacking access to the patient's medical record, you should treat the patient on a threat-to-life basis.

Other complications stem from age-related changes in an elderly patient's response to illness and injury. Pain may be diminished, causing both you and the patient to underestimate the severity of the primary problem. In addition, the temperature-regulating mechanism may be altered or depressed. This can result in the absence of fever, or a minimal fever, even in the presence of a severe infection. Alterations in the temperature-regulating mechanism, coupled with changes in the sweat glands, also makes the elderly more prone to environmental thermal problems.

Because of the complexity of factors that can affect assessment, you must probe for significant symptoms, and ultimately, the primary problem. Patience, respect, and kindness will elicit the answers needed for a pertinent medical history.

History

You should be prepared to spend more time obtaining histories from elderly patients. You may need to split the interview into sessions. For example, you might need to allow patients time to rest, if they become fatigued during the interview, or you might take a break to talk with caregivers.

When gathering the history, keep in mind the complications that arise from multiple diseases and multiple medications. Medications can be an especially important indicator of the patient's diseases. Therefore, you should find the patient's medications and take them to the hospital with the patient. Try to determine which of the medications, including over-the-counter medications, are currently being taken. In cases of multiple medications, there is an increased incidence of medication errors, drug interactions, and noncompliance.

Communication Challenges As previously mentioned, communications may be more difficult when dealing with the aged. **Cataracts** (Figure 32-2) and **glaucoma** can diminish sight. Blindness, often resulting from diabetes and stroke, is more common in the elderly. The level of anxiety increases when a patient is unable to see his or her surroundings clearly. As a result, you should talk calmly to the visually impaired patient. Yelling does not help. Instead, position yourself so the patient can see or touch you.

Alterations in the temperature-regulating mechanism, coupled with changes in the sweat glands, make the elderly more prone to environmental thermal problems.

Be prepared to spend more time obtaining a history from an elderly patient.

cataracts medical condition in which the lens of the eye loses its clearness.

glaucoma medical condition where the pressure within the eye increases.

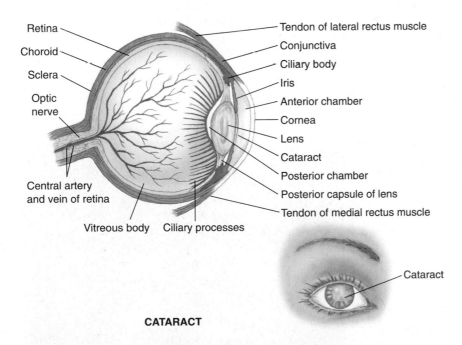

CATARACT

FIGURE 32-2 Cataracts, which cloud the lens, can diminish eyesight in the elderly.

tinnitus subjective ringing or tingling sound in the ear.

Meniere's disease a disease of the inner ear characterized by vertigo, nerve deafness, and a roar or buzzing in the ear.

Age also affects hearing. Overall hearing decreases and patients may have auditory disorders such as **tinnitus** or **Meniere's disease**. Diminished hearing or deafness can make it virtually impossible to obtain a history. In such cases, try to determine the history from a friend or family member. DO NOT shout at the patient. This will not help if the patient is deaf, and it may distort sounds and make it difficult for the patient who still has some hearing to understand you. Write notes if necessary. If the patient can lip-read, speak slowly and directly toward the patient. Whenever possible, verify the history with a reliable source. Also, because loss of hearing may result from other causes (such as a build up of earwax), confirm whether deafness is a pre-existing condition.

Patients may also have trouble with speech. They find it difficult to retrieve words. They will often speak slowly and exhibit changes in voice quality, which may be a normal age-related change. If a patient has forgotten to put in dentures, politely ask the person to do so.

To improve your skill at communicating with the elderly, keep these techniques in mind:

- Always introduce yourself.
- Speak slowly, distinctly, and respectfully.
- Speak to the patient first, rather than family members, caregivers, or bystanders.
- Speak face to face, at eye level with eye contact (Figure 32-3).
- Locate the patient's hearing aid or eyeglasses, if needed.
- Allow the patient to put on the stethoscope, while you speak into it like a microphone (Figure 32-4).
- Turn on the room lights.
- Display verbal and nonverbal signs of concern and empathy.
- Remain polite at all times.
- Preserve the patient's dignity.
- Always explain what you are doing and why.
- Use your power of observation to recognize anxiety—tempo of speech, eye contact, tone of voice—during the telling of the history.

Altered Mental Status and Confusion   Remember that age sometimes diminishes mental status. The patient can be confused and unable to remember details. In addition, the noise of radios, electrocardiogram (ECG) equipment, and strange voices may add to the confusion. Both senility and organic brain syndrome may manifest themselves similarly. Common symptoms include:

- Delirium
- Confusion

FIGURE 32-3   If possible, talk to the elderly patient rather than talking about the patient to others.

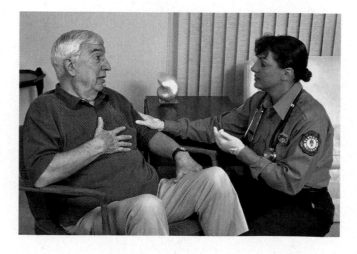

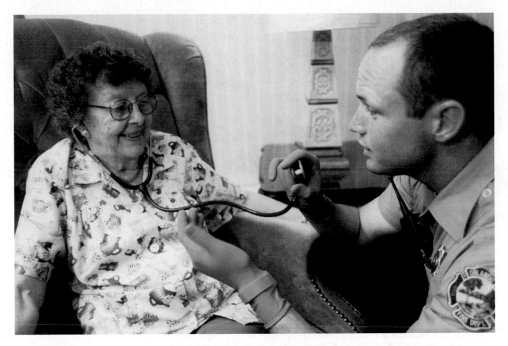

FIGURE 32-4 Allow the elderly patient with hearing difficulties to put on the stethoscope while you speak into it like a microphone.

- Distractibility
- Restlessness
- Excitability
- Hostility

When confronted with a confused patient, try to determine whether the patient's mental status represents a significant change from normal. DO NOT assume that a confused, disoriented patient is "just senile," thus failing to assess for a serious underlying problem (Figure 32-5). Alcoholism, for example, is more common in the elderly than was once recognized. It can further complicate taking the history.

Another complication results from depression, which can be mistaken for many other disorders. It can often mimic senility and organic brain syndrome. Depression may also inhibit patient cooperation. The depressed patient may be malnourished, dehydrated, overdosed, contemplating suicide, or simply imagining physical ailments for attention. If you suspect depression, question the patient regarding drug ingestion or suicidal ideation. It is important to remember that suicide is now the fourth-leading cause of death among the elderly in the United States.

Concluding the History   After obtaining the history, and if time allows, try to verify the patient's history with a credible source. This will often be less offensive to the patient if done out of his or her presence. While at the scene, it is important to observe the surroundings for indications of the patient's self-sufficiency. Look for evidence of drug or alcohol ingestion or for medical identification devices such as Medic Alert or Vial-of-Life items. It is also important to spot signs of abuse or neglect, particularly in dependent living arrangements.

Physical Examination

Certain considerations must be kept in mind when examining the elderly patient. Remember that some patients are often easily fatigued and cannot tolerate a long examination. Also, because of the problems with temperature regulation, the patient may be wearing several layers of clothing, which can make examination difficult. Be sure to explain all actions clearly before initiating the examination, especially to patients with impaired vision. Be aware that the patient may minimize or deny symptoms because of a fear of becoming institutionalized or loss of self-sufficiency.

DO NOT assume that a confused, disoriented patient is "just senile" and fail to assess for a serious underlying problem.

Treat depression as a warning sign of substance abuse and/or suicide ideation—both more common among the elderly than previously understood.

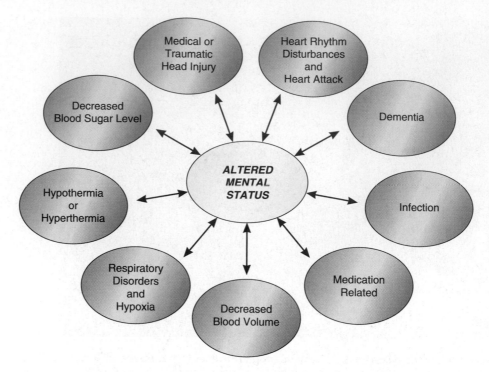

FIGURE 32-5 DO NOT assume that an altered mental status is a normal age-related change. A number of serious underlying problems may be responsible for changes in consciousness.

Try to distinguish signs of chronic disease from an acute problem. Peripheral pulses may be difficult to evaluate, because of peripheral vascular disease and arthritis. The elderly may also have non-pathological crackles (rales) upon lung auscultation. In addition, the elderly often exhibit an increase in mouth breathing and a loss of skin elasticity, which may be easily confused with dehydration. Dependent edema may be caused by inactivity, not congestive heart failure. Only experience and practice will allow you to distinguish acute from chronic physical findings.

MANAGEMENT CONSIDERATIONS

As you have read, people become less alike as they age. Therefore, each elderly patient presents a unique challenge in terms of assessment and management. You will need to tailor your management plan to fit a patient's illness, injury, and overall general health. Because of the potential for rapid deterioration among the elderly, you must quickly spot conditions requiring rapid transport. As with any other patient, your first concern is airway, breathing, and circulation. Remain alert at all times for changes in an elderly patient's neurological status, vital signs, and general cardiac status. (Management of specific disorders is covered in other sections of this chapter.)

In general, remember that transport to a hospital is often more stressful to the elderly than to any other age group except for the very young. Avoid lights and sirens in all but the most serious cases, such as when you suspect a pulmonary embolism or bowel infarction. A calm, smooth transport helps to reduce patient anxiety and the resulting strain on an elderly patient's heart.

Provide emotional support at every phase of the call. Nearly any serious illness or injury in the elderly can provoke a sense of impending doom. Death is a very real possibility to this age group. To help reduce patient fears, keep these guidelines in mind:

- Encourage patients to express their feelings.
- DO NOT trivialize their fears.
- Acknowledge nonverbal messages.
- Avoid questions that are judgmental.

- Confirm what the patient says.
- Recall all you have learned about communicating with the elderly, thus avoiding communication breakdowns.
- Assure patients that you understand that they are adults on an equal footing with their care providers, including you.

SYSTEM PATHOPHYSIOLOGY IN THE ELDERLY

Although aging begins at the cellular level, it eventually affects virtually every system in the body. Age-related changes in the structure and function of organs increase the probability of disease, modify the threshold at which signs and symptoms appear, and affect assessment and treatment of the elderly patient (Table 32-4). You should be familiar with normal systemic changes related to aging so that you can more easily identify the abnormal changes that may point to a serious underlying problem.

RESPIRATORY SYSTEM

The effects of aging on the respiratory system begin as early as age 30. Age-related changes in the respiratory system include:

- Decreased chest wall compliance
- Loss of lung elasticity
- Increased air trapping due to collapse of the smaller airways
- Reduced strength and endurance of the respiratory muscles

Functionally, by the time a person reaches age 65, vital capacity may be reduced by as much as 50%. In addition, the maximum breathing capacity may decrease by as much as 60%, while the maximum oxygen uptake may decrease by as much as 70%. These changes ultimately result in decreased ventilation and progressive hypoxemia. Any presence of underlying pulmonary diseases, such as emphysema and chronic bronchitis, further reduces respiratory function.

In addition, there is a decrease in an effective cough reflex and the activity of the cilia—the small hairlike fibers that trap particles and infectious agents. The decline of these two defense mechanisms leaves the lungs more susceptible to recurring infection.

Other factors that may affect pulmonary function in the elderly include:

- **Kyphosis**
- Chronic exposure to pollutants
- Long-term cigarette smoking

kyphosis exaggeration of the normal posterior curvature of the spine.

The management of respiratory distress in elderly patients is essentially the same as for all age groups. Position the patient for adequate breathing, usually upright or sitting. Teach breathing patterns that assist in exhalation, such as pursed-lip breathing. (Tell patients to pretend they are blowing out a candle with each exhalation.) Use bronchodilators as needed, and provide high-flow, high-concentration supplemental oxygen.

At all points, remain attentive for possible complications, such as **anoxic hypoxemia.** Monitor ventilations closely as an elderly patient can become easily fatigued from any increase in the work of breathing. Remember that many elderly patients with respiratory disease have underlying cardiac disease. With this in mind, drugs such as theophylline and the beta agonists should be used with extreme caution. Monitor cardiovascular status, and administer IV fluids judiciously. DO NOT FLUID OVERLOAD. When infusing fluids, frequently reassess lung sounds to check for the pressure of pulmonary edema.

anoxic hypoxemia an oxygen deficiency due to disordered pulmonary mechanisms of oxygenation.

In treating respiratory disorders in the elderly patient, DO NOT FLUID OVERLOAD.

CARDIOVASCULAR SYSTEM

A number of variables unrelated to aging influence cardiovascular function. They include diet, smoking and alcohol use, education, socioeconomic status, and even personality traits.

Table 32-4 COMMON AGE-RELATED SYSTEMIC CHANGES

Body System	Changes with Age	Clinical Importance
Respiratory	Loss of strength and coordination in respiratory muscles	Increased likelihood of respiratory failure
	Cough and gag reflex reduced	
Cardiovascular	Loss of elasticity and hardening of arteries	Hypertension common
	Changes in heart rate, rhythm, efficiency	Greater likelihood of strokes, heart attacks
		Great likelihood of bleeding from minor trauma
Neurological	Brain tissue shrinks	Delay in appearance of symptoms with head injury
	Loss of memory	
	Clinical depression common	Difficulty in patient assessment
	Altered mental status common	Increased likelihood of falls
	Impaired balance	
Endocrine	Lowered estrogen production (women)	Increased likelihood of fractures (bone loss) and heart disease
	Decline in insulin sensitivity	
	Increase in insulin resistance	Diabetes mellitus common with greater possibility of hyperglycemia
Gastrointestinal	Diminished digestive functions	Constipation common
		Greater likelihood of malnutrition
Thermoregulatory	Reduced sweating	Environmental emergencies more common
	Decreased shivering	
Integumentary (skin)	Thins and becomes more fragile	More subject to tears and sores
		Bruising more common
		Heals more slowly
Musculoskeletal	Loss of bone strength (osteoporosis)	Greater likelihood of fractures
	Loss of joint flexibility and strength (osteoarthritis)	Slower healing
		Increased likelihood of falls
Renal	Loss of kidney size and function	Increased problems with drug toxicity
Genitourinary	Loss of bladder function	Increased urination/incontinence
		Increased urinary tract infection
Immune	Diminished immune response	More susceptible to infections
		Impaired immune response to vaccines
Hematological	Decrease in blood volume and/or red blood cells	Slower recuperation from illness/injury
		Greater risk of trauma-related complications

Of particular importance is the level of physical activity. Even though maximum exercise capacity and maximum oxygen consumption decline with age, a well-trained elderly person can match, or even exceed, the aerobic capacity of an unconditioned younger person.

This said, the cardiovascular system still experiences, in varying degrees, age-related deterioration. The wall of the left ventricle may thicken and enlarge (**hypertrophy**), often by as much as 25%. This is even more pronounced if there is associated hypertension. In addition, **fibrosis** develops in the heart and peripheral vascular system, resulting in hypertension, arteriosclerosis, and decreased cardiac function.

The aorta also becomes stiff and lengthens. This results from deposits of calcium and changes in the connective tissue. These changes predispose the aorta to partial tearing, resulting in dissection (thoracic) or aneurysm (abdominal).

hypertrophy an increase in the size or bulk of an organ.

fibrosis the formation of fiber-like connective tissue, also called scar tissue in an organ.

As a person ages, the pattern of ventricular filling changes. Less blood enters the left ventricle during early diastole when the mitral valve is open. Therefore, filling and stretch (preload) depend on atrial contraction. Loss of the atrial kick (as will occur with atrial fibrillation) is not well tolerated in the elderly.

Over time, the conductive system of the heart degenerates, often causing dysrhythmias and varying degrees of heart block. Ultimately, the stroke volume declines and the heart rate slows, leading to decreased cardiac output. Because of this, the heart's ability to respond to stress diminishes. In such situations, expect exercise intolerance, which is an inability of the heart to meet an exercising muscle's need for oxygen.

To adequately manage complaints related to the cardiovascular system, ask the patient to stop all activity. This reduces the myocardial oxygen demand. DO NOT walk a patient with a cardiovascular complaint to your rig. Take the following basic steps per local protocols:

DO NOT walk a patient with a cardiovascular disorder to your rig.

- Provide high-flow, high-concentration supplemental oxygen.
- Start an IV for medication administration. Medications will vary with the complaint, but may include:
  - Antianginal agents
  - Aspirin
  - Diuretics
  - Antidysrhythmics
- Inquire about age-related dosages.
- Monitor vital signs and rhythm.
- Remain calm, professional, and empathetic. A heart attack is one of the most fearful situations for the elderly.

NERVOUS SYSTEM

Unlike cells in other organ systems, cells in the central nervous system cannot reproduce. The brain can lose as much as 45% of its cells in certain areas of the cortex. Overall, there is an average 10% reduction in brain weight from age 20 to age 90. Keep in mind that reductions in brain weight and ventricular size are not well correlated with intelligence, and elderly people may still be capable of highly creative and productive thought. Once again, DO NOT assume that an elderly person possesses less cognitive skill than a younger person. Slight changes that may be expected include:

- Difficulty with recent memory
- Psychomotor slowing
- Forgetfulness
- Decreased reaction times

Although brain size may not have clinical implications in terms in intelligence, it does have implications for trauma. A reduction in brain size leaves room for increased bleeding following a blow to the head, making the elderly more prone to subdural hematomas. In cases of altered mental status, maintain a suspicion of trauma, especially when an accident has been reported.

Whenever you assess an elderly patient for mental status, determine a baseline. Presume your patient to have been mentally sharp unless proven otherwise. (Talk with partners, caregivers, family members, and so on.) Focus on the patient's perceptions, thinking processes, and communication. In questioning an elderly patient, provide an environment with minimal distractions. As already mentioned, ask clear and unhurried questions.

In assessing an elderly patient with altered mental status, presume the patient to have been mentally sharp unless proven otherwise.

In forming a patient plan, observe for weakness, chronic fatigue, changes in sleep patterns, and syncope or near syncope. If you suspect a stroke, think "brain attack" and assign the patient a priority status. (Additional material on strokes will appear later in the chapter.) Consider blood pressure control per local protocol, but remember that perfusion of the brain tissue depends on an adequate blood pressure. DO NOT plan to reduce the blood pressure to an average of 120/80 as cerebral blood flow may be diminished. Consider the causes of changes in mental status, keeping in mind the possibility of trauma. Apply oxygen, and monitor ventilations. Depending upon the situation, you may be called on to administer dextrose, thiamine, and naloxone.

ENDOCRINE SYSTEM

Early diagnosis of disorders in the endocrine system offers some of the greatest opportunities to prevent disabilities through appropriate hormonal therapy and/or lifestyle changes. Diabetes mellitus, for example, is extremely common among the elderly. However, normalization of glucose levels—through diet, exercise, and/or drug therapy—can reduce some of the devastating vascular and neurological complications.

In women, menopause—a normal age-related hormonal deficiency—can be similarly treated in a variety of ways, including hormone replacement therapy (HRT). By taking preventive measures, women can reduce and/or delay the incidence of heart disease, bone loss, and possibly Alzheimer's disease.

Thyroid disorders are "clinical masqueraders," especially in the elderly. Common signs and symptoms may be absent or diminished. When signs and symptoms are present, they may be attributed to aging or tied to other diseases, such as cardiovascular, gastrointestinal, or neuromuscular disorders. However, it has been shown that thyroid disorders, especially hypothyroidism and thyroid nodules, increase with age. (For more on thyroid disorders, see "Metabolic and Endocrine Disorders" later in the chapter.)

With the exception of glucose disorders, most endocrine disorders cannot be easily determined in the field. Many endocrine emergencies will present as altered mental status, especially with insulin-related diseases. Monitor for cardiovascular effects of endocrine changes such as aortic aneurysm in a patient with **Marfan's syndrome,** a disorder resulting in abnormal growth of distal tissues and a dilatation of the root of the aorta. Also remain alert to blood pressure swings in thyroid disorders such as hyperthyroidism and hypothyroidism.

GASTROINTESTINAL SYSTEM

Age affects the gastrointestinal system in various ways. The volume of saliva may decrease by as much as 33%, leading to complaints of dry mouth, nutritional deficiencies, and a predisposition to choking. Gastric secretions may decrease to as little as 20% of the quantity present in younger people. Esophageal and intestinal motility also decrease, making swallowing more difficult and delaying digestive processes. The production of hydrochloric acid also declines, further disrupting digestion and, in some adults, contributing to nutritional anemia. Gums atrophy and the number of taste buds decrease, reducing even further the desire to eat.

Other conditions may also develop. **Hiatal hernias** are not age-related per se, but can have serious consequences for the elderly. They may incarcerate, strangulate, or, in the most severe cases, result in massive gastrointestinal hemorrhage. A diminished liver function, which is associated with aging, can delay or impede detoxification. A common drug toxicity problem for EMS personnel is the use of lidocaine for ventricular arrythmias. (See "Toxicological Emergencies" later in the chapter.) A diminished liver function can also reduce the production of clotting proteins, which in turn leads to bleeding abnormalities.

Complications in the gastrointestinal system can be life-threatening. Use shock protocols as necessary and remember that not all fluid loss occurs outside the body.

THERMOREGULATORY SYSTEM

The elderly and infants are highly susceptible to variations in environmental temperatures. This occurs in the elderly because of altered or impaired thermoregulatory mechanisms. Aging seems to reduce the effectiveness of sweating in cooling the body. Older persons tend to sweat at higher core temperatures and have less sweat output per gland than younger people. As people age, they also experience deterioration of the autonomic nervous system, including a decrease in shivering and lower resting peripheral blood flow. In addition, the elderly may have a diminished perception of the cold. Drugs and disease can further affect an elderly patient's response to temperature extremes, resulting in hyperthermia or accidental hypothermia.

Many endocrine emergencies encountered in the field present as altered mental status, especially with insulin-related disorders.

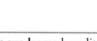

Marfan's syndrome hereditary condition of connective tissue, bones, muscles, ligaments, and skeletal structures characterized by irregular and unsteady gait, tall lean body type with long extremities, flat feet, stooped shoulders. The aorta is usually dilated and may become weakened enough to allow an aneurysm to develop.

hiatal hernia protrusion of the stomach upward into the mediastinal cavity through the esophageal hiatus of the diaphragm.

A diminished liver function, which is associated with aging, can delay or impede detoxification. A common drug toxicity problem for EMS personnel is the use of lidocaine for ventricular arrythmias.

Environmental emergencies are common causes of EMS calls, especially among the elderly living alone or in poverty. For more on these emergencies, see the discussion of heatstroke, hypothermia, and hyperthermia later in the chapter.

INTEGUMENTARY SYSTEM

As people age, the skin loses collagen, a connective tissue that gives elasticity and support to the skin. Without this support, the skin is subject to a greater number of injuries from bumping or tearing. The lack of support also makes it more difficult to start an IV because the veins "roll away." Furthermore, the assessment of tenting skin becomes an inaccurate indicator of fluid status in the elderly. Without elasticity, the skin often will remain tented regardless of water balance.

As the skin thins, cells reproduce more slowly. Injury to skin is often more severe than in younger patients and healing time is increased. As a rule, the elderly are at a higher risk of secondary infection, skin tumors, drug-induced eruptions, and fungal or viral infections. Decades of exposure to the sun also make the elderly vulnerable to melanoma and other sun-related carcinomas (e.g., basal cell carcinoma, squamous cell carcinoma).

MUSCULOSKELETAL SYSTEM

An aging person may lose as much as 2 to 3 inches of height from narrowing of the intervertebral discs and **osteoporosis.** Osteoporosis is the loss of mineral from the bone, resulting in softening of the bones. This is especially evident in the vertebral bodies, thus causing a change in posture. The posture of the aged individual often reveals an increase in the curvature of the thoracic spine, commonly called kyphosis, and slight flexion of the knee and hip joints. The demineralization of bone makes the patient much more susceptible to hip and other fractures. Some fractures may even occur from simple actions such as sneezing.

In addition to skeletal changes, a decrease in skeletal muscle weight commonly occurs with age, especially with sedentary individuals. To compensate, elderly women develop a narrow, short gait, whereas older men develop a wide gait. These changes make the elderly more susceptible to falls and, consequently, a possible loss of independence.

Because of the changes in the musculoskeletal system, simple trauma in the elderly can lead to complex injuries. In treating musculoskeletal disorders, supply supplemental oxygen, initiate an IV line, and consider pain control. Many extremity injuries should be splinted as found because of changes in the bone and joint structure of the elderly. To determine the cause of any injury, be sure to look beyond the obvious. Keep in mind the possibility of underlying medical conditions, drug complications, abuse or neglect, and ingestion of alcohol or drugs.

> **osteoporosis** softening of bone tissue due to the loss of essential minerals, principally calcium.

> *Many extremity injuries should be splinted as found because of changes in the bone and joint structure in the elderly.*
>
>

RENAL SYSTEM

Aging affects the renal system through a reduction in the number of functioning **nephrons,** which may be decreased by 30% to 40%. Renal blood flow may also be reduced by up to 45%, increasing the waste products in the blood and upsetting the fluid and electrolyte balance. Because the kidneys are responsible for the production of erythropoietin (which stimulates the production of red blood cells in the bone marrow) and renin (which stimulates vasoconstriction), a decrease in renal function may result in anemia or hypertension in the older patient.

Prehospital treatment of complaints involving the renal and urinary systems is directed toward adequate oxygenation, fluid status, monitoring output, and pain control. Pay attention to the airway, as nausea and vomiting are complications of pain secondary to renal obstruction. Also monitor vital signs to detect changes in blood pressure and pulse.

> **nephrons** the functional units of the kidneys.

GENITOURINARY SYSTEM

As people age, they experience a progressive loss of bladder sensation and tone. The bladder does not empty completely and consequently the patient may sense a frequent need to urinate. This urge increases the risk of falls, especially during the middle of the night when lighting is dim or the patient is sleepy. Furthermore, the lack of emptying increases the likelihood of urinary tract infection and perhaps sepsis. In the male, the prostate often becomes enlarged (benign prostatic hypertrophy), causing difficulty in urination or urinary retention. As already mentioned, the elderly also commonly develop, in varying degrees, problems with incontinence.

Treatment for a complaint in the genitourinary system is described in the preceding section on the renal system and in the earlier discussion of incontinence.

IMMUNE SYSTEM

As a person ages, the function of T cells declines, making them less able to notify the immune system of invasion by antigens. A diminished immune response, sometimes called **immune senescence,** increases the susceptibility of the elderly to infections. It also increases the duration and severity of an infection.

Unless contraindicated, the elderly should receive vaccinations suggested by the health department. However, keep in mind that aging impairs the immune response to vaccines. The best prevention is adequate nutrition, infection control measures (e.g., washing hands), and exercise. Recognition and treatment of diseases such as diabetes mellitus, heart failure, thyroid disease, and occult malignancy also reduce the risk and severity of infections. As an EMT-I, you should treat alterations in immune status as life-threatening and seek to prevent exposure of patients to infectious agents. DO NOT transmit an illness—even a mild cold— to an elderly patient.

HEMATOLOGY SYSTEM

The hematology system is affected by a failure of the renal system to stimulate the production of red blood cells. Nutritional abnormalities may also produce abnormal red blood cells. Since there is less body water present in the elderly, blood volume similarly decreases. This makes it difficult for an elderly patient to recuperate from an illness or injury. Intervention must be started early in order to make a lasting difference.

In addition to providing supplemental oxygen, you should prepare for increases in bleeding time. Monitor the elderly patient closely as deterioration is difficult to stop.

COMMON MEDICAL PROBLEMS IN THE ELDERLY

In general, the elderly suffer from the same kinds of medical emergencies as younger patients. However, illnesses may be more severe, complications more likely, and classic signs and symptoms absent or altered. In addition, the elderly are more likely to react adversely to stress and deteriorate much more quickly than young or middle-aged adults. The following are some of the medical disorders that you may encounter.

PULMONARY/RESPIRATORY DISORDERS

Respiratory emergencies are some of the most common reasons elderly persons summon EMS or seek emergency care. Most elderly patients with a respiratory disorder present with a chief complaint of dyspnea. However, coughing, congestion, and wheezing are also common chief complaints.

Many factors can trigger respiratory distress among the elderly (Figure 32-6). Descriptions of the most common ones follow.

Pneumonia

Pneumonia is an infection of the lung. It is usually caused by a bacterium or virus. However, aspiration pneumonia may also develop as a result of difficulty swallowing.

Pneumonia is a serious disease for the elderly. It is the fourth leading cause of death in people age 65 and older. Its incidence increases with age at a rate of 10% for each decade beyond age 20. It is found in up to 60% of the autopsies performed on the elderly. Reasons the elderly develop pneumonia more frequently than younger patients include:

- Decreased immune response
- Reduced pulmonary function

immune senescence diminished vigor of the immune response to the challenge and rechallenge of pathogens.

DO NOT transmit an illness—even a mild cold—to an elderly patient.

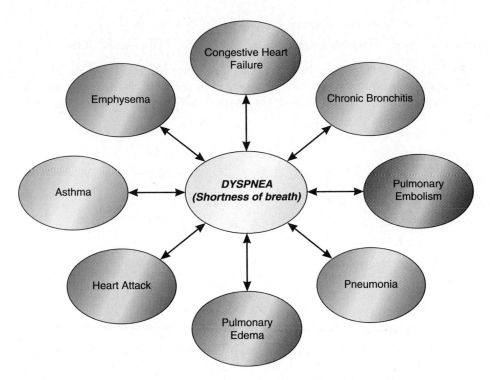

FIGURE 32-6 Dyspnea can be caused by a number of respiratory and cardiac problems in the elderly.

- Increased colonization of the pharynx by gram-negative bacteria
- Abnormal or ineffective cough reflex
- Decreased effectiveness of mucociliary cells of the upper respiratory system

The elderly who are at greatest risk for contracting pneumonia include frail adults and those with chronic, multiple diseases or compromised immunity. Institutionalized patients, either in hospitals or nursing homes, are especially vulnerable because of increased exposure to microorganisms and limited mobility. A patient in an institutional setting is up to fifty times more likely to contract pneumonia than an elderly patient receiving home care.

Common signs and symptoms of pneumonia include increasing dyspnea, congestion, fever, chills, tachypnea, sputum production, and altered mental status. Occasionally, abdominal pain may be the only symptom. Because of thermoregulatory changes, a fever may be absent in an elderly patient.

Prevention strategies include prophylactic treatment with antibiotics. Efforts should also be taken to reduce exposure to infectious patients and to promote patient mobility.

In treating an elderly patient with pneumonia, manage all life threats. Maintain adequate oxygenation. Transport the patient to the hospital for diagnosis, keeping in mind that patients with respiratory disease often have other underlying problems.

Chronic Obstructive Pulmonary Disease

Chronic obstructive pulmonary disease (COPD) is really a collection of diseases, characterized by chronic airflow obstruction with reversible and/or irreversible components. Although each COPD has its own distinct features, elderly patients commonly have two or more types at the same time. COPD usually refers to some combination of emphysema, chronic bronchitis, and, to a lesser degree, asthma. Pneumonia, as well as other respiratory disorders, can further complicate COPD in the elderly.

In the United States, COPD is among the ten leading causes of death. Its prevalence has been increasing over the past 20 years. Several factors combine to produce the damage of COPD. They include:

- Genetic disposition
- Exposure to environmental pollutants

- Existence of a childhood respiratory disease
- Cigarette smoking, a contributing factor in up to 80% of all cases of COPD

The physiology of COPD varies, but may include inflammation of the air passages with increased mucous production or actual destruction of the alveoli. The outcome is decreased airflow in the alveoli, resulting in reduced oxygen exchange. Usual signs and symptoms include:

- Cough
- Increased sputum production
- Dyspnea
- Accessory muscle use
- Pursed-lip breathing
- Tripod positioning
- Exercise intolerance
- Wheezing
- Pleuritic chest pain
- Tachypnea

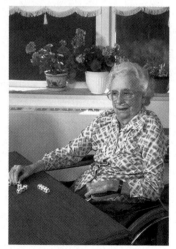

FIGURE 32-7 The COPD patient may use a nasal cannula with a home oxygen unit.

COPD is progressive and debilitating (Figure 32-7). The patient can often keep the signs and symptoms under control until the body is stressed. When the condition becomes disabling, it is called exacerbation of COPD. This condition can lead rapidly to patient death because hypoxia and hypercapnia alter acid-base balance and deprive the tissues of the oxygen needed for efficient energy production.

The most effective prevention involves elimination of tobacco products and reduced exposure to cigarette smoke (in non-smokers). Recent legislation has sought to keep public places smoke free and to discourage cigarette smoking in the young. Once the disease is present, patients are taught to identify stresses that exacerbate the condition. Appropriate self-care includes exercise, avoidance of infections, appropriate use of drugs, and, when necessary, calling EMS.

When confronted with an elderly patient with COPD, treatment is essentially the same as for all age groups. Supply supplemental oxygen and possibly drug therapy, usually for reducing dyspnea.

Pulmonary Embolism

Pulmonary embolism (PE) should always be considered as a possible cause of respiratory distress in the elderly. Although statistics for the elderly are unavailable, approximately 650,000 cases occur annually in the United States alone. Of this number, a pulmonary embolism is the primary cause of death in 100,000 people and a contributing factor in another 100,000 deaths. Nearly 11% of pulmonary embolism deaths take place in the first hour and 38% in the second hour.

Blood clots are the most frequent cause of pulmonary embolism. However, the condition may also be caused by fat, air, bone marrow, tumor cells, or foreign bodies. Risk factors for developing pulmonary embolism include:

- Deep venous thrombosis
- Prolonged immobility, common among the elderly
- Malignancy (tumors)
- Paralysis
- Fractures of the pelvis, hip, or leg
- Obesity
- Trauma to the leg vessels
- Major surgery
- Presence of a venous catheter

- Use of estrogen (in women)
- Atrial fibrillation

Pulmonary emboli usually originate in the deep veins of the thigh and calf. The condition should be suspected in any patient with the acute onset of dyspnea. Often, it is accompanied by pleuritic chest pain and right heart failure. If the pulmonary embolus is massive, you can expect severe dyspnea, cardiac dysrhythmias, and, ultimately, cardiovascular collapse.

Definitive diagnosis of a pulmonary embolism takes place in a hospital setting. The goals of field treatment are to manage and minimize complications of the condition. General treatment considerations include delivery of high-flow, high-concentration oxygen via mask, maintaining oxygen levels above an SaO_2 of 90%. Establishment of an IV for possible administration of medications is appropriate, but vigorous fluid therapy should be avoided, if possible.

Prehospital pharmacological therapy for pulmonary embolism is limited. Upon advice from medical direction, you may administer small doses of morphine sulfate to reduce patient anxiety. After confirming the absence of gastrointestinal bleeding, medical direction may also prescribe anticoagulants to prevent clot formation and/or to speed clot dissolution. If the administration of a vasopressor is indicated by low blood pressure, then dopamine may be prescribed. In such cases, remember to titrate the dopamine to a desirable blood pressure.

The risk of death from pulmonary embolism is greatest in the first few hours. As a result, rapid transport is essential. Position the patient in an upright position and avoid lifting the patient by the legs or knees, which may dislodge thrombi in the lower extremities. During transport, continue to monitor changes in skin color, pulse oximetry, and changes in breathing rate and rhythm. Your field assessment and interventions can save the patient's life and guide the hospital physician in a direction that will result in an accurate diagnosis and rapid treatment.

> *The risk of death from pulmonary embolism is greatest in the first few hours. As a result, rapid transport is essential.*
>
>

Pulmonary Edema

Pulmonary edema is an effusion or escape of serous fluids into the alveoli and interstitial tissues of the lungs. Acute pulmonary edema can develop rapidly in the elderly. Although most commonly associated with acute myocardial infarction, it can also occur due to other factors including pulmonary infections, inhaled toxins, narcotic overdose, pulmonary embolism, and decreased atmospheric pressure.

Pulmonary edema causes severe dyspnea associated with congestion. Other signs and symptoms include rapid labored breathing, cough with blood-stained sputum, cyanosis, and cold extremities. Physical examination usually reveals the presence of moist crackles and accessory muscle use. Severe cases will exhibit rhonchi.

Treatment is directed toward altering the cause of the condition. The existence of pulmonary edema can be life-threatening and is often the symptom of a fatal cardiovascular disease.

> *The existence of pulmonary edema can be life-threatening and is often the symptom of a fatal cardiovascular disease.*
>
>

Lung Cancer

North America has the highest incidence of lung cancer in the world. The incidence increases with age, with about 65% of all lung cancer deaths occurring among people age 65 and older. The leading cause of lung cancer is cigarette smoking.

Often, progressive dyspnea will be the first presentation of a cancerous lesion. Hemoptysis (bloody sputum), chronic cough, and weight loss are also common symptoms.

Treatment of lung cancer occurs in a hospital setting. However, you may be called to assist in the follow-up home care or, in terminal stages, a hospice.

CARDIOVASCULAR DISORDERS

The leading cause of death in the elderly is cardiovascular disease. Assessment and treatment of cardiovascular disease in the elderly patient is often complicated by non–age-related factors and disease processes in other organ systems. In conducting your history, determine the patient's level of cardiovascular fitness, changes in exercise tolerance, recent diet history, use of medications, and use of cigarettes and/or alcohol. Ask questions about breathing difficulty, especially at night, and evidence of palpitations, flutter, or skipped beats.

In performing the physical exam, look for hypertension and orthostatic hypotension (a decrease in blood pressure and an increase in heart rate when rising from a seated or supine position). Watch for dehydration or dependent edema. When taking an elderly patient's blood pressure, consider checking both arms. Routinely determine pulses in all the extremities. In auscultating the patient, remember that a bruit or noise in the neck, abdomen, or groin indicates a high probability of carotid, aortorenal, or peripheral vascular disease. Keep in mind, too, that heart sounds are generally softer in the elderly, probably because of a thickening of lung tissue between the heart and chest wall.

In evaluating the problem, recall the cardiovascular disorders commonly found in elderly patients. They include angina pectoris, myocardial infarction, heart failure, dysrhythmias, aortic dissection, aneurysm, hypertension, and syncope.

Angina Pectoris

The likelihood of developing angina increases dramatically with age. This is especially true of women, who are estrogen protected until after menopause. Angina is usually triggered by physical activity, especially after a meal, and by exposure to very cold weather. Attacks vary in frequency, from several a day to occasional episodes separated by weeks or months.

Angina pectoris literally means "pain in the chest." However, the pain of angina is actually felt in only about 10% to 20% of elderly patients. The changes in sensory nerves, combined with the myocardial changes of aging, make dyspnea a more likely symptom of angina than pain.

Angina develops when narrowing of coronary vessels due to plaque or vasospasm lead to an inability to meet the oxygen demands of the heart muscle. The heart muscle usually responds by sending out pain signals, which represent a build-up of lactic acid. In an elderly patient, exercise intolerance is a key symptom of angina. In obtaining a history, you should ask the patient about sudden changes in routine. In addition, inquire about any increased stresses on the heart, such as anemia, infection, dysrhythmias, and thyroid changes.

General prevention strategies in the elderly are similar to those in young patients. Blood pressure control, combined with diet, exercise, and smoking modifications reduces the risk in all groups.

Myocardial Infarction

A myocardial infarction (MI) involves actual death of muscle tissue due to a partial or complete occlusion of one or more of the coronary arteries. The greatest number of patients hospitalized for acute MI are older than 65. The elderly patient with MI is less likely to present with classic symptoms such as chest pain than a younger counterpart. Atypical presentations that may be seen in the elderly include:

- Absence of pain
- Exercise intolerance
- Confusion/dizziness
- Syncope
- Dyspnea—common in patients over age 85
- Neck, dental, and/or epigastric pain
- Fatigue/weakness

The mortality rate associated with MI and/or resulting complications doubles after age 70. Unlike younger patients, the elderly are more likely to suffer a **silent myocardial infarction.** They also tend to have larger MIs. The majority of deaths that occur in the first few hours following an MI are due to dysrhythmias.

In auscultating a patient, remember that a bruit in the neck, abdomen, or groin indicates a high probability of carotid, aortorenal, or peripheral vascular disease.

Generally, heart sounds in the elderly are softer, probably because of thickening lung tissues between the heart and chest wall.

In an elderly patient, exercise intolerance is a key symptom of angina.

The elderly patient with myocardial infarction is less likely to present with classic symptoms.

silent myocardial infarction a myocardial infarction that occurs without exhibiting obvious signs and symptoms.

An MI is most commonly triggered by some form of physical exertion or a preexisting heart disease. Because of the high mortality associated with MIs in the elderly, early detection and emergency management are critical.

Heart Failure

Heart failure takes place when cardiac output cannot meet the body's metabolic demands. The incidence rises exponentially after age 60. The condition is widespread among the elderly and is the most common diagnosis in hospitalized patients over age 65. The causes of heart failure fall in one of four categories: impairment to flow, inadequate cardiac filling, volume overload, and myocardial failure.

Typical age-related factors, such as prolonged myocardial contractions, make the elderly vulnerable to heart failure. Other factors that place them at risk include:

- Noncompliance with drug therapy
- Anemia
- Ischemia
- Thermoregulatory disorders (hypothermia/hyperthermia)
- Hypoxia
- Infection
- Use of non-steroidal anti-inflammatory drugs

Signs and symptoms of heart failure vary. In most patients, regardless of age, some form of edema exists. However, edema in the elderly can indicate a range of problems, including musculoskeletal injury. Assessment findings specific to the elderly include:

- Fatigue (left failure)
- **Two-pillow orthopnea**
- Dyspnea on exertion
- Dry, hacking cough progressing to productive cough
- Dependent edema (right failure)
- **Nocturia**
- Anorexia, **hepatomegaly,** ascites

Nonpharmacologic management of heart failure includes modifications in diet (e.g., less fat and cholesterol), exercise, and reduction in weight, if necessary. Pharmacologic management may include treatment with diuretics, vasodilators, antihypertensive agents, or inotropic agents. Check to see if the patient is already on any of these medications and if the patient is compliant with scheduled doses.

Dysrhythmias

Many cardiac dysrhythmias develop with age. Atrial fibrillation is the most common dysrhythmia encountered.

Dysrhythmias occur primarily as a result of degeneration of the patient's conductive system. Anything that decreases myocardial blood flood can produce a dysrhythmia. They may also be caused by electrolyte abnormalities.

To complicate matters further, the elderly do not tolerate extremes in heart rate as well as a younger person would. For example, a heart rate of 140 in an older patient may cause syncope, whereas a younger patient can often tolerate a heart rate greater than 180. In addition, dysrhythmias can lead to falls from cerebral hypoperfusion. They can also result in congestive heart failure (CHF) or a transient ischemic attack (TIA).

Treatment considerations depend on the type of dysrhythmia. Patients may already have a pacemaker in place. In such cases, keep in mind that pacemakers have a low but significant rate of complications such as a failed battery, fibrosis around the catheter site, lead fracture, or electrode dislodgment. In a number of situations, drug therapy may be indicated. Whenever you discover a dysrhythmia, remember that an abnormal or disordered

two-pillow orthopnea the number of pillows—in this case, two—needed to ease the difficulty of breathing while lying down; a significant factor in assessing the level of respiratory distress.

nocturia excessive urination during the night.

hepatomegaly enlarged liver.

Content Review

POSSIBLE PACEMAKER COMPLICATIONS

- Failed battery
- Fibrosis around the catheter site
- Lead fracture
- Electrode dislodgment

Abnormal or disordered heart rhythm may be the only clinical finding in an elderly patient suffering acute myocardial infarction.

heart rhythm may be the only clinical finding in an elderly patient suffering acute myocardial infarction.

Aortic Dissection/Aneurysms

Aortic dissection is a degeneration of the wall of the aorta, either in the thoracic or abdominal cavity. It can result in an **aneurysm** or in a rupture of the vessel.

Approximately 80% of thoracic aneurysms are due to atherosclerosis combined with hypertension. The remaining cases occur secondary to other factors, including Marfan's syndrome or blunt trauma to the chest. Patients with dissections will often present with tearing chest pain radiating through to the back or, if rupture occurs, cardiac arrest.

The distal portion of the aorta is the most common site for abdominal aneurysms. Approximately 1 in 250 people over age 50 die from a ruptured abdominal aneurysm. The aneurysm may appear as a pulsatile mass in a patient with a normal girth, but lack of an identifiable mass does not eliminate this condition. Patients may present with tearing abdominal pain or unexplained low back pain. Pulses in the legs are diminished or absent and the lower extremities feel cold to the touch. There may be sensory abnormalities such as numbness, tingling, or pain in the legs. The patient may fall when attempting to stand.

Treatment of an aneurysm depends on its size, location, and the severity of the condition. In the case of thoracic aortic dissection, continuous IV infusion and/or administration of drug therapy to lower the arterial pressure and to diminish the velocity of left ventricle contraction may be indicated. Rapid transport is essential, especially for the older patient who most commonly requires care and observation in an intensive care unit.

Hypertension

Hypertension appears to be a product of industrial society. In developed nations, such as the United States, the systolic and diastolic pressures have a tendency to rise until age 60. Systolic pressure may continue to rise after that time, but diastolic pressure stabilizes. Since this rise in blood pressure is not seen in less developed nations, experts believe that hypertension is not a normal age-related change.

Today more than 50% of the people in the United States over age 65 have clinically diagnosed hypertension, defined as blood pressure greater than 140/90 mmHg. Prolonged elevated blood pressure will eventually damage the heart, brain, or kidneys. As a result of hypertension, elderly patients are at greater risk for heart failure, stroke, blindness, renal failure, coronary heart disease, and peripheral vascular disease. In men with blood pressure greater than 160/95 mmHg, the risk of mortality nearly doubles.

Hypertension increases with atherosclerosis, which is more common with the elderly than other age groups. Other contributing factors include obesity and diabetes. The condition can be prevented or controlled through diet (sodium reduction), exercise, cessation of smoking, and compliance with medications.

Hypertension is often a silent disease that produces no clinically obvious signs or symptoms. It may be associated with nonspecific complaints such as headache, tinnitus, **epistaxis**, slow tremors, or nausea and vomiting. An acute onset of high blood pressure without any kidney involvement is often a telltale indicator of thyroid disease.

Management of hypertension depends on its severity and the existence of other conditions. For example, hypertension is often treated with beta-blockers—medications that are contraindicated in patients with chronic obstructive lung disease, asthma, or heart block greater than first degree. Diuretics, another common drug used in treating hypertension, should be prescribed with care for patients on digitalis. Keep in mind that centrally acting agents are more likely to produce negative side effects in the elderly. Unlike younger patients, the elderly may experience depression, forgetfulness, sleep problems, or vivid dreams and/or hallucinations.

Syncope

Syncope is a common presenting complaint among the elderly. The condition results when blood flow to the brain is temporarily interrupted or decreased. It is most often caused by problems with either the nervous system or the cardiovascular system. In general, syncope has a higher incidence of death in elderly patients than in younger individuals. The following are some of the common presentations that you may encounter:

aortic dissection a degeneration of the wall of the aorta.

aneurysm abnormal dilation of a blood vessel, usually an artery, due to a congenital defect or a weakness in the wall of the vessel.

Most abdominal aortic aneurysms occur below the renal arteries.

Content Review

HYPERTENSION PREVENTION STRATEGIES
• Modified diet (low sodium)
• Exercise
• Cessation of smoking
• Compliance with medications

epistaxis nosebleed.

- *Vasodepressor syncope.* Vasodepressor syncope is the common faint. It may occur following emotional distress; pain; prolonged bed rest; mild blood loss; prolonged standing in warm, crowded rooms; anemia; or fever.

- *Orthostatic syncope.* Orthostatic syncope occurs when a person rises from a seated or supine position. There are several possible causes. First, there may be a disproportion between blood volume and vascular capacity. That is, a pooling of blood in the legs reduces blood flow to the brain. Causes of this include hypovolemia, venous **varicosities**, prolonged bed rest, and **autonomic dysfunction.** Many drugs, especially blood pressure medicines, can cause drug-induced orthostatic syncope due to the effects of the medications on the capacitance vessels.

- *Vasovagal syncope.* Vasovagal syncope occurs as a result of a **valsalva maneuver,** which happens during defecation, coughing, or similar maneuvers. This effectively slows the heart rate and cardiac output, thus decreasing blood flow to the brain.

- *Cardiac syncope.* Cardiac syncope results from transient reduction in cerebral blood flow due to a sudden decrease in cardiac output. It can result from several mechanisms. Syncope can be the primary symptom of silent MI. In addition, many dysrhythmias can cause syncope. Dysrhythmias that have been shown to cause syncope include bradycardias, **Stokes-Adams syndrome,** heart block, tachydysrhythmia, and **sick sinus syndrome.**

- *Seizures.* Syncope may result from a seizure disorder or syncope (prolonged) may cause seizure activity. Syncope due to seizures tends to occur without warning. It is associated with muscular jerking or convulsions, incontinence, and tongue-biting. Postictal confusion may follow.

- *Transient ischemic attacks.* TIAs occur more frequently in the elderly. They may cause syncope.

NEUROLOGICAL DISORDERS

Elderly patients are at risk for several neurological emergencies. Often, the exact cause is not initially known and may require probing at the hospital.

Many of the neurological disorders that you will encounter in the field will exhibit an alteration in mental status. You may discover a range of underlying causes from stroke to degenerative brain disease. Some of the most common causes of altered mental status include:

- Cerebrovascular disease (stroke or transient ischemic attack)
- Myocardial infarction
- Seizures
- Medication-related problems (drug interactions, drug underdose, and drug overdose)
- Infection
- Fluid and electrolyte abnormalities (dehydration)
- Lack of nutrients (hypoglycemia)
- Temperature changes (hypothermia, hyperthermia)
- Structural changes (dementia, subdural hematoma)

As mentioned, it is often impossible in the field to distinguish the cause of an altered mental status. Even so, you should carry out a thorough assessment. Administer supplemental oxygen. As soon as practical, obtain a blood glucose level to exclude hypoglycemia as a possible cause. Overall, the approach to the elderly patient with altered mental status is the same as with any other patient presenting with similar symptoms.

Cerebrovascular Disease (Stroke/Brain Attack)

Stroke is the third leading cause of death in the United States. Annually, about 500,000 people suffer strokes and about 150,000 die. Incidence of stroke and the likelihood of dying

varicosities an abnormal dilation of a vein or group of veins.

autonomic dysfunction an abnormality of the involuntary aspect of the nervous system.

valsalva maneuver forced exhalation against a closed glottis, such as with coughing. This maneuver stimulates the parasympathetic nervous system via the vagus nerve, which in turn slows the heart rate.

Stokes-Adams syndrome a series of symptoms resulting from heart block, most commonly syncope. The symptoms result from decreased blood flow to the brain caused by the sudden decrease in cardiac output.

sick sinus syndrome a group of disorders characterized by dysfunction of the sinoatrial node in the heart.

As soon as practical, obtain a blood glucose level to exclude hypoglycemia as a possible cause of altered mental status in an elderly patient.

stroke injury to or death of brain tissue resulting from interruption of cerebral blood flow and oxygenation.

from a stroke increase with age. Occlusive stroke is statistically more common in the elderly and relatively uncommon in younger individuals. Older patients are at higher risk of stroke because of atherosclerosis, hypertension, immobility, limb paralysis, congestive heart failure, and atrial fibrillation. TIAs are also more common in older patients. More than one-third of patients suffering TIAs will develop a major, permanent stroke. As previously mentioned, TIAs are a frequent cause of syncope in the elderly.

Strokes usually fall in one of two major categories. **Brain ischemia**—injury to brain tissue caused by an inadequate supply of oxygen and nutrients—accounts for about 80% of all strokes. Brain hemorrhage, the second major category, may be either **subarachnoid hemorrhage** or **intracerebral hemorrhage**. These different patterns of bleeding have different presentations, causes, and treatments. However, together they account for a high percentage of all stroke deaths.

Because of the various kinds of strokes, signs and symptoms can present in many ways—altered mental status, coma, paralysis, slurred speech, a change in mood, and seizures. Stroke should be highly suspect in any elderly patient with a sudden change in mental status.

Whenever you suspect a stroke, it is essential that you complete the Prehospital Stroke Score or a similar objective assessment tool for later comparison in the emergency department. Thrombolytic agents administered to a patient suffering an occlusive (ischemic) stroke can decrease the severity of damage if administered within 3 hours of onset. Rapid transport is essential for avoiding brain damage or limiting its extent. In the case of stroke, "time is brain tissue."

By far the most preferred treatment is prevention of strokes in the first place. Strategies include:

- Control of hypertension
- Treatment of cardiac disorders, including dysrhythmias and coronary artery disease
- Treatment of blood disorders, such as anemia and **polycythemia**
- Cessation of smoking
- Cessation of recreational drugs
- Moderate use of alcohol
- Regular exercise
- Good eating habits

Seizures

Seizures may be easily mistaken for stroke in the elderly. Also, a first-time seizure may occur due to damage from a previous stroke. Not all seizures experienced by the elderly are of the major motor type. Some are more subtle. Many causes of seizure activity in the elderly have been identified. Common causes include:

- Seizure disorder (epilepsy)
- Syncope
- Recent or past head trauma
- Mass lesion (tumor or bleed)
- Alcohol withdrawal
- Hypoglycemia
- Stroke

Often the cause of the seizure cannot be determined in the field. As a result, treat the condition as a life-threatening emergency and transport as quickly as possible to eliminate the possibility of stroke. If the patient has fallen during a seizure, check for evidence of trauma and treat accordingly.

Dizziness/Vertigo

Dizziness is a frightening experience and a frequent complaint of the elderly. The complaint of dizziness may actually mean that the patient has suffered syncope, pre-syncope, light-

brain ischemia injury to brain tissues caused by an inadequate supply of oxygen and nutrients.

subarachnoid hemorrhage bleeding that occurs between the arachnoid and dura mater of the brain.

intracerebral hemorrhage bleeding directly into the brain.

When you suspect stroke, complete the Prehospital Stroke Score or a similar objective assessment tool for later comparison in the emergency department.

polycythemia an excess of red blood cells.

Treat seizures in the elderly as a life-threatening condition and transport as quickly as possible to eliminate the possibility of stroke.

headedness, or true **vertigo.** Vertigo is a specific sensation of motion perceived by the patient as spinning or whirling. Many patients will report that they feel as though they are spinning. Vertigo is often accompanied with sweating, pallor, nausea, and vomiting. Meniere's disease can cause severe, **intractable** vertigo. It is often, however, associated with a constant roaring sound in the ears, as well as pressure in the ear.

Vertigo results from so many factors that it is often hard, even for the physician, to determine the actual cause. Any factor that impairs visual input, inner-ear function, peripheral sensory input, or the central nervous system can cause dizziness. In addition, alcohol and many prescription drugs can cause dizziness. So can hypoglycemia in its early stages. It is virtually impossible to distinguish dizziness, syncope, and pre-syncope in the prehospital setting.

Delirium, Dementia, Alzheimer's Disease

Approximately 15% of all people in the United States over age 65 have some degree of dementia or delirium. **Dementia** is a chronic global cognitive impairment, often progressive or irreversible. The best-known form of dementia is **Alzheimer's disease,** a condition that affects 4 million in the United States. **Delirium** is a global mental impairment of sudden onset and self-limited duration. (For differences between dementia and delirium, see Table 32-5.)

Delirium Many conditions can cause delirium. The cause may be either organic brain disease or disorders that occur elsewhere in the body. Delirium in the elderly is a serious condition. According to some estimates, about 18% of hospitalized elderly patients with delirium die. Possible etiologies or causes include:

- Subdural hematoma
- Tumors and other mass lesions
- Drug-induced changes or alcohol intoxication
- CNS infections
- Electrolyte abnormalities
- Cardiac failure
- Fever
- Metabolic disorders, including hypoglycemia
- Chronic endocrine abnormalities, including hypothyroidism and hyperthyroidism
- Postconcussion syndrome

The presentation of delirium varies greatly and can change rapidly during assessment. Common signs and symptoms include the acute onset of anxiety, an inability to focus, disordered thinking, irritability, inappropriate behavior, fearfulness, excessive energy, or psychotic behavior such as hallucinations or paranoia. Aphasic or speaking errors and/or prominent slurring may be present. Normal patterns of eating and sleeping are almost always disrupted.

vertigo the sensation of faintness or dizziness; may cause a loss of balance.

intractable resistant to cure, relief, or control.

dementia a deterioration of mental status that is usually associated with structural neurological disease. It is often progressive and irreversible.

Alzheimer's disease a progressive, degenerative disease that attacks the brain and results in impaired memory, thinking, and behavior.

delirium an acute alteration in mental functioning that is often reversible.

Table 32-5 DISTINGUISHING DEMENTIA AND DELIRIUM*

Dementia	Delirium
Chronic, slowly progressive development	Rapid in onset, fluctuating course
Irreversible disorder	May be reversed, especially if treated early
Greatly impairs memory	Greatly impairs attention
Global cognitive deficits	Focal cognitive deficits
Most commonly caused by Alzheimer's disease	Most commonly caused by systemic disease, drug toxicity, or metabolic changes
Does not require immediate treatment	Requires immediate treatment

*These are general characteristics that apply to most, but not all cases. For example, some forms of dementia, such as those caused by hypothyroidism, may be reversed.

In distinguishing between delirium and dementia, err on the side of delirium. The condition is often caused by life-threatening, but reversible, conditions. Causes of delirium such as infections, drug toxicity, and electrolyte imbalances generally have a good prognosis if identified quickly and managed promptly.

Dementia   Dementia is more prevalent in the elderly than delirium. Over 50% of all nursing home patients have some form of dementia. It is usually due to an underlying neurological disease. This mental deterioration is often called organic brain syndrome, **senile dementia,** or senility. It is important to find out whether an alteration in mental status is acute or chronic. Causes of dementia include:

- Small strokes
- Atherosclerosis
- Age-related neurological changes
- Neurological diseases
- Certain hereditary diseases (e.g., Huntington's disease)
- Alzheimer's disease

Signs and symptoms of dementia include progressive disorientation, shortened attention span, **aphasia** or nonsense talking, and hallucinations. Dementia often hampers treatment through the patient's inability to communicate and exhausts caregivers. In moderate to severe cases, you will need to rely on the caregiver for information. (Remain alert to signs of abuse or neglect, which occurs in a disproportionate number of elderly suffering from dementia.)

Alzheimer's Disease   Alzheimer's disease is a particular type of dementia. It is a chronic degenerative disorder that attacks the brain and results in impaired memory, thinking, and behavior. It accounts for more than half of all forms of dementia in the elderly.

Alzheimer's disease generally occurs in stages, each with different signs and symptoms. These stages include:

- *Early stage.* Characterized by loss of recent memory, inability to learn new material, mood swings, and personality changes. Patients may believe someone is plotting against them when they lose items or forget things. Aggression or hostility is common. Poor judgment is evident.
- *Intermediate stage.* Characterized by a complete inability to learn new material; wandering, particularly at night; increased falls; loss of ability for self-care, including bathing and use of the toilet.
- *Terminal stage.* Characterized by an inability to walk and regression to infant stage, including the loss of bowel and bladder function. Eventually the patient loses the ability to eat and swallow.

Families caring for an Alzheimer's patient at home also have signs of stress. Remember to treat both the Alzheimer patient and the family and/or caregivers with respect and compassion. Evaluate the needs of the family and make an appropriate report at your facility. Support groups are available to assist families.

Parkinson's Disease

Parkinson's disease is a degenerative disorder characterized by changes in muscle response, including tremors, loss of facial expression, and gait disturbances. It mainly appears in people over age 50 and peaks at age 70. The disease affects about 1 million people in the United States, with 50,000 new cases diagnosed each year. It is the fourth most common neurodegenerative disease among the elderly.

The cause of primary Parkinson's disease remains unknown. However, it affects the basal ganglia in the brain, an area that deciphers messages going to muscles. Secondary Parkinson's disease is distinguished from primary Parkinson's disease by having a known cause. Some of the most common causes include:

- Viral encephalitis
- Atherosclerosis of cerebral vessels

- Reaction to certain drugs or toxins, such as antipsychotics or carbon monoxide
- Metabolic disorders, such as anoxia
- Tumors
- Head trauma
- Degenerative disorders, such as **Shy-Drager syndrome**

It is impossible in a field setting to distinguish primary and secondary Parkinson's disease. The most common initial sign of a Parkinson's disorder is a resting tremor combined with a **pill-rolling motion.** As the disease progresses, muscles become more rigid and movements become slower and/or more jerky. In some cases, patients may find their movements halted while carrying out some routine task. Their feet may feel "frozen to the ground." Gaits become shuffled with short steps and unexpected bursts of speed, often to avoid falling. Kyphotic deformity is a hallmark of the disease.

Patients with Parkinson's disease commonly develop mask-like faces devoid of all expression. They speak in slow, monotone voices. Difficulties in communication, coupled with a loss of mobility, often lead to anxiety and depression.

There is no known cure for Parkinson's disease, with the exception of drug-induced secondary Parkinson's disorders. Exercise may help maintain physical activity or teach the patient adaptive strategies. In calls involving a Parkinson's patient, observe for conditions that may have involved the EMS system, such as a fall or the inability to move. Manage treatable conditions and transport as needed.

METABOLIC AND ENDOCRINE DISORDERS

As previously mentioned, the endocrine system undergoes a number of age-related changes, which affect hormone levels. The most common endocrine disorders include diabetes mellitus and problems related to the thyroid gland. Of the two, you will more often treat diabetic-related emergencies, particularly hypoglycemia.

Diabetes Mellitus

An estimated 20% of older adults have diabetes mellitus, primarily Type II diabetes. Almost 40% have some type of glucose intolerance. Reasons that the elderly develop these disorders include:

- Poor diet
- Decreased physical activity
- Loss of lean body mass
- Impaired insulin production
- Resistance by body cells to the actions of insulin

Diagnosis of Type II diabetes usually occurs during routine screening in a physical exam. In some cases, urine tests may register negative because of an increased renal glucose threshold in the elderly. The condition may present, in its early stages, with such vague constitutional symptoms as fatigue or weakness. Allowed to progress, diabetes can result in neuropathy and visual impairment. These manifestations often lead to more aggressive blood testing, which in most cases will reveal elevated glucose levels.

The treatment of diabetes involves diet, exercise, the use of sulfonylurea agents, and/or insulin. Many diabetics use self-monitoring devices to test glucose levels. Unfortunately, the cost of these devices and the accompanying test strips, sometimes discourages the elderly from using them. Elderly patients on insulin also risk hypoglycemia, especially if they accidentally take too much insulin or do not eat enough food following injection. The lack of good nutrition can be particularly troublesome to elderly diabetics. They often find it difficult to prepare meals, fail to enjoy food because of altered taste perceptions, have trouble chewing food, or are unable to purchase adequate and/or the correct food because of limited income.

Management of diabetic and hypoglycemic emergencies for the elderly is generally the same as for any other patient. DO NOT rule out alcohol as a complicating factor, especially in cases of hypoglycemia. In addition, remember that diabetes places the elderly at increased

Shy-Drager syndrome chronic orthostatic hypotension caused by a primary autonomic nervous system deficiency.

pill-rolling motion an involuntary tremor, usually in one hand or sometimes in both, in which fingers move as if they were rolling a pill back and forth.

DO NOT rule out alcohol as a complicating factor in cases of hypoglycemia.

retinopathy any disorder of the retina.

risk of other complications, including atherosclerosis, delayed healing, **retinopathy**, blindness, altered renal function, and severe peripheral vascular disease, leading to foot ulcers and even amputations.

Thyroid Disorders

With normal aging the thyroid gland undergoes moderate atrophy and changes in hormone production. An estimated 2% to 5% of people over age 65 experience hypothyroidism, a condition resulting from inadequate levels of thyroid hormones. It affects women in greater numbers than men, and the prevalence rises with age.

Less than 33% of the elderly present with typical signs and symptoms of hypothyroidism. When they do, their complaints are often attributed to aging. Common nonspecific complaints in the elderly include mental confusion, anorexia, falls, incontinence, and decreased mobility. Some patients also experience an increase in muscle or joint pain. Treatment involves thyroid hormone replacement.

Hyperthyroidism is less common among the elderly but may result from medication errors such as an overdose of thyroid hormone replacement. The typical symptom of heat intolerance is often present. Otherwise, hyperthyroidism presents atypically in the elderly. Common nonspecific features or complaints include atrial fibrillation, failure to thrive (weight loss and apathy combined), abdominal distress, diarrhea, exhaustion, and depression.

Diagnosis and treatment of thyroid disorders do not take place in the field. Elderly patients with known thyroid problems should be encouraged to go to the hospital for medical evaluation.

GASTROINTESTINAL DISORDERS

Gastrointestinal emergencies are common among the elderly. The most frequent emergency is gastrointestinal bleeding. However, older people will also describe a variety of other gastrointestinal complaints—nausea, poor appetite, diarrhea, and constipation, to name a few. Remember, that like other presenting complaints, these conditions may be symptomatic of more serious diseases. Bowel problems, for example, may point to cancer of the colon or other abdominal organs.

Regardless of the complaint, remember that prompt management of a gastrointestinal emergency is essential for young and old alike. For the elderly, there is a significant risk of hemorrhage and shock. There is a tendency to take gastrointestinal patients less seriously than those suffering moderate or severe external hemorrhage. This is a serious mistake. Patients with gastrointestinal complaints should be aggressively managed, especially the elderly. Keep in mind that older patients are far more intolerant of hypotension and anoxia than younger patients. Treatment should include:

- Airway management
- Support of breathing and circulation
- High-flow, high-concentration oxygen therapy
- IV fluid replacement with a crystalloid solution
- Pneumatic anti-shock garment (PASG) placement, if indicated
- Rapid transport

Some of the most critical gastrointestinal problems that you may encounter in the field will involve internal hemorrhage and bowel obstruction. You may also be called on to treat **mesenteric infarct,** a serious and life-threatening condition in an elderly patient. The following will help you to recognize each of these gastrointestinal disorders.

Gastrointestinal Hemorrhage

Gastrointestinal bleeding falls into two general categories: upper GI bleed and lower GI bleed.

Upper GI Bleed   This form of gastrointestinal bleeding includes:

- *Peptic ulcer disease.* Injury to the mucous lining of the upper part of the gastrointestinal tract due to stomach acids, digestive enzymes, and other agents, such as anti-inflammatory drugs.

Patients with gastrointestinal complaints should be aggressively managed, especially the elderly.

mesenteric infarct death of tissue in the peritoneal fold (mesentery) that encircles the small intestine; a life-threatening condition.

- *Gastritis.* An inflammation of the lining of the stomach.
- *Esophageal varices.* An abnormal dilation of veins in the lower esophagus; a common complication of cirrhosis of the liver.
- *Mallory-Weiss tear.* A tear in the lower esophagus that is often caused by severe and prolonged retching.

Lower GI Bleed   Conditions categorized as lower gastrointestinal bleeding include:

- *Diverticulosis.* The presence of small pouches on the colon that tends to develop with age causes 70% of life-threatening lower gastrointestinal bleeds.
- *Tumors.* Tumors of the colon can cause bleeding when the tumor erodes into blood vessels within the intestine or surrounding organs.
- *Ischemic colitis.* An inflammation of the colon due to impaired or decreased blood supply.
- *Arteriovenous malformations.* An abnormal link between an artery and a vein.

Signs of significant gastrointestinal blood loss include the presence of "coffee ground" emesis, black tar-like stools (**melena**), obvious blood in the emesis or stool, orthostatic hypotension, pulse greater than 100 (unless on beta blockers), and confusion. Gastrointestinal bleeding in the elderly may result in such complications as a recent increase in angina symptoms, congestive heart failure, weakness, or dyspnea.

melena a dark, tarry stool caused by the presence of digested free blood.

Bowel Obstruction

Bowel obstruction in the elderly typically involves the small bowel. Causes include tumors, prior abdominal surgery, use of certain medications, and occasionally the presence of vertebral compression fractures. The patient will typically complain of diffuse abdominal pain, bloating, nausea, and vomiting. The abdomen may feel distended when palpated. Bowel sounds may be hypoactive or absent. If the obstruction has been present for a prolonged period of time, the patient may have fever, weakness, shock, and various electrolyte disturbances.

Mesenteric Infarct

Vessels arising from the superior or inferior mesenteric arteries generally serve the bowel. An infarct occurs when a portion of the bowel does not receive enough blood to survive. Certain age-related changes make the elderly more vulnerable to this condition. First, as a person ages, changes in the heart (such as atrial fibrillation) or the vessels (atherosclerosis) predispose the patient to a clot lodging in one of the branches serving the bowel. Second, changes in the bowel itself can promote swelling that effectively cuts off blood flow.

The primary symptom of a bowel infarct is pain out of proportion to the physical exam. Signs include:

- Bloody diarrhea, but usually not a massive hemorrhage
- Some tachycardia, although there may be a vagal effect masking the sign
- Abdominal distention

The patient is at great risk for shock because the dead bowel attracts interstitial and intravascular fluids, thus removing them from use. Necrotic products are released to the peritoneal cavity, leading to a massive infection. The prognosis, in part, is poor due to decreased physiological reserves on the part of the older patient.

SKIN DISORDERS

Younger and older adults experience common skin disorders at about the same rates. However, age-related changes in the immune system make the elderly more prone to certain chronic skin diseases and infections. They are also more likely to develop **pressure ulcers** (bed sores) than any other age group.

Content Review

SIGNS AND SYMPTOMS OF BOWEL OBSTRUCTION

- Diffuse abdominal pain
- Bloating
- Nausea
- Vomiting
- Distended abdomen
- Hypoactive/absent bowel sounds

---

pressure ulcer ischemic damage and subsequent necrosis affecting the skin, subcutaneous tissue, and often the muscle; result of intense pressure over a short time or low pressure over a long time; also known as pressure sore or bed sore.

Skin Diseases

Elderly patients commonly complain about **pruritus,** or itching. This condition can be caused by dermatitis (eczema) or environmental conditions, especially during winter (i.e., from hot dry air in the home and cold windy air outside). Keep in mind that generalized itching can also be a sign of systemic diseases, particularly liver and renal disorders. When itching is strong and unrelenting, suspect an underlying disease and encourage the patient to seek medical evaluation.

Slower healing and compromised tissue perfusion in the elderly makes them more susceptible to bacterial infection of wounds, appearing as cellutitis, impetigo, and, in the case of immunocompromised adults, staphylococcal scalded skin. The elderly also experience a higher incidence of fungal infections, partly because of decreases in the cutaneous immunological response. In addition, they suffer higher rates of **herpes zoster** (shingles), which peaks between ages 50 and 70. Although these skin disorders occur in the young, their duration and severity increases markedly with age.

In treating skin disorders, remember that many conditions may be drug-induced. Beta-blockers, for example, can worsen psoriasis, which occurs in about 3% of elderly patients. Question patients about their medications, keeping in mind that certain prescription drugs (e.g., penicillins and sulfonamides) and some over-the-counter drugs can cause skin eruptions. Also ask about topical home remedies, such as alcohol or soaps, which may cause or worsen the disorder. Find out if the patient is compliant with prescribed topical treatments. Finally, remember that some drugs and topical medications commonly used to treat skin disorders in the young can worsen or cause other problems for the elderly. Antihistamines and corticosteroids are two to three times more likely to provoke adverse reactions in the elderly than in younger adults.

Pressure Ulcers (Decubitus Ulcers)

Most pressure ulcers occur in people over age 70. As many as 20% of patients enter the hospital with a pressure ulcer or develop one while hospitalized. The highest incidence occurs in nursing homes where up to 25% of patients may develop this condition.

Pressure ulcers typically develop from the waist down, usually over bony prominences, in bedridden patients. However, they can occur anywhere on the body and with the patient in any position. Pressure ulcers usually result from tissue hypoxia and affect the skin, subcutaneous tissues, and muscle. Factors that can increase the risk of this condition include:

- External compression of tissues (i.e., pressure)
- Altered sensory perception
- **Maceration,** caused by excessive moisture
- Decreased activity
- Decreased mobility
- Poor nutrition
- Friction or shear

To reduce the development of pressure ulcers or to alleviate their condition, you may take these steps:

- Assist the patient in changing position frequently, especially during extended transport, to reduce the length of time pressure is placed on any one point.
- Use a pull sheet to move the patient, reducing the likelihood of friction.
- Reduce the possibility of shearing by padding areas of skin before movement.
- Unless a life-threatening condition is present, take time to clean and dry areas of excessive moisture, such as urinary or fecal incontinence and excessive perspiration.
- Clean ulcers with normal saline solution and cover with hydrocolloid or hydrogel dressings, if available. With severe ulcers, pack with loosely woven gauze moistened with normal saline.

MUSCULOSKELETAL DISORDERS

The skeleton, as you know, is a metabolically active organ. Its metabolic processes are influenced by a number of factors, including age, diet, exercise, and hormone levels. The musculoskeletal system is also subject to disease. In fact, musculoskeletal diseases are the leading cause of functional impairment in the elderly. Although usually not fatal, musculoskeletal disorders often produce chronic disability, which in turn creates a context for illness. Two of the most widespread musculoskeletal disorders include **osteoarthritis** and **osteoporosis**.

Osteoarthritis

Osteoarthritis is the leading cause of disability among people age 65 and older. Many experts think the condition may not be one disease but several with similar presentations. Although wear and tear as well as age-related changes such as loss of muscle mass predispose the elderly to osteoarthritis, other factors may play a role as well. Presumed contributing causes include:

- Obesity
- Primary disorders of the joint, such as inflammatory arthritis
- Trauma
- Congenital abnormalities, such as hip dysplasia

Osteoarthritis in the elderly presents initially as joint pain, worsened by exercise and improved by rest. As the disease progresses, pain may be accompanied by diminished mobility, joint deformity, and crepitus or grating sensations. Late signs include tenderness upon palpation or during passive motion.

The most effective treatment involves management before the disability develops or worsens. Prevention strategies include stretching exercises and activities that strengthen stress-absorbing ligaments (Figure 32-8). Immobilization, even for short periods, can accelerate the condition. Drug therapy is usually aimed at lessening pain and/or inflammation. Surgery, such as total joint replacement, is usually the last resort after more conservative methods have failed.

Osteoporosis

Osteoporosis affects an estimated 20 million people in the United States and is largely responsible for fractures of the hip, wrist, and vertebral bones following a fall or other injury. Risk factors include:

- *Age.* Peak bone mass for men and women occurs in their third and fourth decades of life and declines at varying rates thereafter. Decreased bone density generally becomes a treatment consideration at about age 50.
- *Gender.* The decline of estrogen production places women at a higher risk of developing osteoporosis than men. Women are more than twice as likely to

> **osteoarthritis** a degenerative joint disease, characterized by a loss of articular cartilage and hypertrophy of bone.

> **osteoporosis** softening of bone tissue due to the loss of essential minerals, principally calcium.

> *Wear and tear are the most common factors leading to osteoarthritis.*

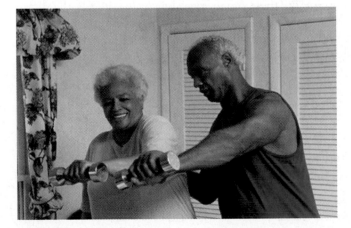

FIGURE 32–8 Regular stretching and weight-bearing exercises help prevent the development of osteoarthritis. *(The Stock Market Photo Agency)*

have brittle bone, especially if they experience early menopause (before age 45) and do not take estrogen replacement therapy.

- *Race.* Whites and Asians are more likely to develop osteoporosis than African Americans and Latinos, who have higher bone mass at skeletal peak.
- *Body weight.* Thin people, or people with low body weight, are at greater risk of osteoporosis than obese people. Increased skeletal weight is thought to promote bone density. However, weight-bearing exercise can have the same effect.
- *Family history.* Genetic factors (such as peak bone mass attainment) and a family history of fractures may predispose a person to osteoporosis.
- *Miscellaneous.* Late menarche, nulliparity, and use of caffeine, alcohol, and cigarettes are all thought to be important determinants of bone mass.

Unless a bone density test is conducted, persons with osteoporosis are usually asymptotic until a fracture occurs. The precipitating event can be as slight as turning over in bed, carrying a package, or even a forceful sneeze. Management includes prevention of fractures through exercise and drug therapy, such as the administration of calcium, vitamin D, estrogen, and other medications or minerals. Once the condition occurs, pain management also becomes a consideration.

RENAL DISORDERS

glomerulonephritis a form of nephritis, or inflammation of the kidneys; primarily involves the glomeruli, one of the capillary networks that are part of the renal corpuscles in the nephrons.

The most common renal diseases in the elderly include renal failure, **glomerulonephritis,** and renal blood clots. These problems may be traced to two age-related factors: (1) loss in kidney size and (2) changes in the walls of the renal arteries and in the arterioles serving the glomeruli. In general, the kidney loses approximately one-third of its weight between the ages of 30 and 80. Most of this loss occurs in the tissues that filter blood. When filtering tissue is gone, blood is shunted from the precapillary side directly to venules on the postcapillary side, thus bypassing any tissue still capable of filtering. The result is a reduction in kidney efficiency. This condition is complicated by changes in renal arteries, which promote the development of renal emboli and thrombi.

With renal changes, elderly patients are more likely to accumulate toxins and medications within the bloodstream. Occasionally, this will be obvious to the patient because he or she experiences a substantial decrease in urine output. More often, however, the elderly are prone to a type of renal failure in which urine output remains normal to high while the kidney remains ineffective in clearing wastes.

Processes that precipitate acute renal failure include hypotension, heart failure, major surgery, sepsis, angiographic procedures (the dye is nephrotoxic), and use of nephrotoxic antibiotics (i.e., gentamycin, tobramycin). Ongoing hypertension also figures in the development of chronic renal failure.

URINARY DISORDERS

urosepsis septicemia originating from the urinary tract.

Urinary tract infections (UTI) affect as much as 10% of the elderly population each year. Younger women generally suffer more UTIs than young men, but in the elderly the distribution is almost even. Most of these infections result from bacteria and easily lead to **urosepsis** due to reduced immune system function among the elderly.

A number of factors contribute to the high rate of UTIs among the elderly. They include:

- Bladder outlet obstruction from benign prostatic hyperplasia (in men)
- Atrophic vaginitis (in women)
- Stroke
- Immobilization
- Use of indwelling bladder catheters
- Diabetes
- Upper urinary tract stone
- Dementia, with resulting poor hygiene

Signs or symptoms of a UTI range from cloudy, foul smelling urine to the typical complaints of bladder pain and frequent urination. Urosepsis presents as an acute process, including fever, chills, abdominal discomfort, and other signs of septic shock. The septicemia generally begins within 24 to 72 hours after catheterization or cystoscopy.

Treatment of urosepsis commonly includes placement of a large-bore IV catheter for administration of fluids and parenteral antibiotics. Diagnosis of urosepsis is based on history and other physical findings. Prompt transport is critical. The prognosis for elderly patients with urosepsis is poor, with a mortality rate of approximately 30%. Maintenance of fluid balance as well as adequate blood pressure is essential.

Prompt transport is critical for elderly patients with suspected urosepsis.

ENVIRONMENTAL EMERGENCIES

As previously mentioned, environmental extremes represent a great health risk for the elderly. Nearly 50% of all **heatstroke** deaths in the United States occur among people over age 50. The elderly are just as susceptible to low temperatures, suffering about 750,000 winter deaths annually, primarily from hypothermia and "winter risks" such as pneumonia and influenza. As you may already know from your EMS experience, thermoregulatory emergencies represent some of the most common calls involving the elderly.

heatstroke life-threatening condition caused by a disturbance in temperature regulation; in the elderly, characterized by extreme fever and, in extreme cases, delirium or coma.

Hypothermia

A number of factors predispose the elderly to hypothermia. These include:

- Accidental exposure to cold
- CNS disorders, including head trauma, stroke, tumors, or subdural hematomas
- Endocrine disorders, including hypoglycemia and diabetes (Patients with diabetes are six times as likely to develop hypothermia as other patients.)
- Drugs that interfere with heat production, including alcohol, antidepressants, and tranquilizers
- Malnutrition or starvation
- Chronic illness
- Forced inactivity as a result of arthritis, dementia, falls, paralysis, or Parkinson's disease
- Low or fixed income, which discourages the use of home heating
- Inflammatory dermatitis
- A-V shunts, which increase heat loss

Signs and symptoms of hypothermia can be slow to develop. Many times, elderly patients with hypothermia lose their sensitivity to cold and fail to complain. As a result, hypothermia may be missed. Nonspecific complaints may suggest a metabolic disorder or stroke. Hypothermic patients may exhibit slow speech, confusion, and sleepiness. In the early stages, patients will exhibit hypertension and an increased heart rate. As hypothermia progresses, however, blood pressure drops and the heart rate slows, sometimes to a barely detectable level.

Remember that the elderly patient with hypothermia often does not shiver. Check the abdomen and back to see if the skin is cool to the touch. Expect subcutaneous tissues to be firm. If your unit has a low-temperature thermometer, check the patient's core temperature. (Regular thermometers often do not "shake down" far enough for an accurate reading.)

Remember that the elderly hypothermic patient often does not shiver.

As with other medical disorders, prevention is the preferred treatment. However, once elderly patients develop hypothermia, they become progressively impaired. Treat even mild cases of hypothermia, or suspected hypothermia, as a medical emergency. Focus on the rewarming techniques used with other patients and rapid transport. Maintain ongoing assessment to ensure that the hypothermia does not complicate existing medical problems or heretofore untreated disorders. Death most commonly results from cardiac arrest or ventricular fibrillation.

Treat even a mild case of hypothermia, or suspected hypothermia, as a medical emergency.

Hyperthermia (Heatstroke)

Heatstroke in the elderly is a serious medical emergency.

Age-related changes in sweat glands and increased incidence of heart disease place the elderly at risk of heat stress. They may develop heat cramps, heat exhaustion, or heatstroke. Although the first two disorders rarely result in death. Heatstroke, however, is a serious medical emergency. Risk factors for severe hyperthermia include:

- Altered sensory output, which would normally warn a person of overheating
- Inadequate liquid intake
- Decreased functioning of the thermoregulatory center
- Commonly prescribed medications that inhibit sweating such as antihistamines and tricyclic antidepressants
- Low or fixed income, which may result in a lack of air conditioning or adequate ventilation
- Alcoholism
- Concomitant medical disorders
- Use of diuretics, which increase fluid loss

As with hypothermia, early heatstroke may present with nonspecific signs and symptoms, such as nausea, light-headedness, dizziness, or headache. High temperature is the most reliable indicator, but consider even a slight temperature elevation as symptomatic if coupled with an absence of sweating and neurological impairment. Severe hypotension also exists in many critical patients.

Prevention strategies include adequate fluid intake, reduced activity, shelter in an air-conditioned environment, and use of light clothing. If hyperthermia develops, however, rapid treatment and transport are necessary.

TOXICOLOGICAL EMERGENCIES

As previously mentioned, aging alters pharmacokinetics and pharmacodynamics in the elderly. Functional changes in the kidneys, liver, and gastrointestinal system slow the absorption and elimination of many medications. In addition, the various compensatory mechanisms that help buffer against medication side effects are less effective in the elderly than these mechanisms are in younger patients.

Approximately 30% of all hospital admissions are related to drug-related illnesses. About 50% of all drug-related deaths occur in people over age 60. Accidental overdoses may occur more frequently in the aged due to confusion, vision impairment, self-selection of medications, forgetfulness, and concurrent drug use. Intentional drug overdose also occurs in attempts at self-destruction. Another complicating factor is the abuse of alcohol among the elderly.

It is essential for the EMT-I to be familiar with the range of side effects that can be caused by the polypharmacy (use of multiple medications) of medications taken by geriatric patients. In assessing the geriatric patient, always take these steps:

- Obtain a full list of medications currently taken by the patient, including prescribed medications, over-the-counter medications, and herbal and other dietary supplements.
- Elicit any medications that are newly prescribed. (Some side effects appear within a few days of taking a new medication.)
- Obtain a good past medical history. Find out if your patient has a history of renal or hepatic depression.
- Know your medications, their routes of elimination, and their potential side effects.
- If possible, always take all medications to the hospital along with the patient.

A knowledge of pharmacology is important in all patients. However, it is critical in recognizing potential toxicological emergencies in the geriatric patient. Some of the drugs or substances that have been identified as commonly causing toxicity in the elderly are described in the following sections. For additional information on pharmacology, pharmacokinetics, and pharmacodynamics, review Chapter 3, "Emergency Pharmacology."

Lidocaine

Lidocaine is used for the treatment of ventricular dysrhythmias. It is also a commonly used local anesthetic. The drug is primarily metabolized by the liver and excreted through the kidneys. In older patients, hepatic impairment can cause elevated lidocaine levels and possible toxicity. It is recommended that the lidocaine dose be reduced by 50% in patients greater than 70 years of age.

Beta Blockers

Beta blockers are used as antihypertensives, antidysrhythmics, and for glaucoma. In the elderly, beta blockers can cause depression, lethargy, and orthostatic hypotension. It is important to remember that patients taking beta blockers may not be able to increase their heart rate, which can mask the early findings of shock.

Antihypertensives/Diuretics

Diuretics can cause electrolyte abnormalities. In the elderly, decreased drug clearance can result in hypotension or dehydration. Other types of antihypertensives may affect the elderly differently. Because of this, it is sometimes necessary to reduce the dose or change to a less toxic agent.

Angiotensin-Converting Enzyme (ACE) Inhibitors

ACE inhibitors are popular antihypertensive agents because they have a good safety profile and are well tolerated by most patients. ACE inhibitors are also used to decrease afterload in CHF and pulmonary edema. In the elderly, ACE inhibitors can cause plasma volume reduction and hypotension. Also they have been associated with dizziness, lightheadedness, skin rashes, and cough.

Digitalis (Digoxin, Lanoxin)

Most patients who take digitalis on a regular basis are elderly. The drug is extremely effective at controlling the heart rate in tachydysrhythmias and at increasing cardiac output in congestive heart failure. Digitalis toxicity is the most common adverse drug effect that is seen in the elderly. It can cause visual disturbances, nausea, anorexia, abdominal discomfort, headache, and vomiting. Virtually any dysrhythmia can be seen in digitalis toxicity.

Antipsychotics/Antidepressants

Psychoactive medications affect mood, behavior, and other aspects of mental functioning. They are used in the elderly for depression and psychosis. The elderly are more vulnerable to the side effects of these medications and should be closely monitored. Be particularly alert for extrapyramidal system reactions with the antipsychotic medications.

Antiparkinsonian Agents

Drugs used in the treatment of Parkinson's disease can affect other body systems. Common complications include dyskinesia and psychological disturbances (such as hallucinations and nightmares).

Antiseizure Medications

Medications that prevent seizures can cause sedation in the elderly. They can also cause gastrointestinal distress, headache, lack of coordination, and skin rashes. The doses of these drugs often must be reduced in the elderly.

Analgesics and Anti-Inflammatory Agents

Pain medications, especially the narcotics, can cause sedation, mood changes, nausea, vomiting, and constipation. The anti-inflammatory agents can cause gastrointestinal distress, including gastritis and peptic ulcers. Elderly patients taking these classes of medications should be closely monitored.

Corticosteroids

Corticosteroids are necessary for the treatment of several diseases seen in the aged, including COPD, rheumatoid arthritis, and other inflammatory conditions. These drugs can cause ulcers, hypertension, glaucoma, and increased risk of infection. These side effects are more prevalent in the elderly.

SUBSTANCE ABUSE

substance abuse misuse of chemically active agents such as alcohol, psychoactive chemicals, and therapeutic agents; typically results in clinically significant impairment or distress.

Substance abuse is a widespread problem in the United States. It affects nearly all age groups, including the elderly. Up to 17% of people in the United States over age 60 are addicted to substances. That number is expected to rise as the baby boom generation increases the size of the elderly population.

In general, the factors that contribute to substance abuse among the elderly are different from those of younger people. They include:

- Age-related changes
- Loss of employment
- Loss of spouse or partner
- Multiple prescriptions
- Malnutrition
- Loneliness
- Moving from a long-loved house to an apartment

Like other age groups, the elderly may intentionally abuse substances, to escape pain or life itself. Other times, particularly in the case of prescription drugs, the abuse is accidental. Substance abuse in the elderly may involve drugs, alcohol, or both drugs and alcohol.

Drug Abuse

As previously mentioned, people age 65 and older have more illnesses, consume more drugs, and are more sensitive to adverse drug reactions than younger adults. The sheer number of medications taken by the elderly makes them vulnerable to drug abuse. Of the 1.5 billion prescriptions written each year in the United States, more than one-third goes to the elderly. People age 65 and older fill an average of thirteen prescriptions per year. The elderly also use a disproportionate percentage of over-the-counter drugs.

Polypharmacy, coupled with impaired vision and/or memory, increase the likelihood of complications. The elderly might experience drug-drug interactions, drug-disease interactions, and drug-food interactions.

The elderly who become physically and/or psychologically dependent on drugs (or alcohol) are more likely to hide their dependence and less likely to seek help than other age groups. Common signs and symptoms of drug abuse include:

- Memory changes
- Drowsiness
- Decreased vision/hearing
- Orthostatic hypotension
- Poor dexterity
- Mood changes
- Falling
- Restlessness
- Weight loss

In cases of suspected drug abuse, carefully document your findings. Collect medications for identification at the hospital, where the patient can be evaluated and, if necessary, referred for substance abuse treatment.

Alcohol Abuse

In a national survey, nearly 50% of the elderly reported abstinence from alcohol. However, the same survey found that 15% of the men and 12% of the women interviewed regularly drank in excess of the one-drink-a-day limit suggested by the National Institute on Alcohol Abuse and Alcoholism. Those percentages are expected to rise with the aging of the baby boom generation, which has generally used alcohol more frequently than their predecessors.

The use or abuse of alcohol places the elderly at high risk of toxicity. Physiological changes, such as organ dysfunction, make older adults more susceptible to the effects of alcohol. Consumption of even moderate amounts of alcohol can interfere with drug therapy, often leading to dangerous consequences. Severe stress and a history of heavy and/or regular drinking predispose a person to alcohol dependence or abuse in later life.

Unless a patient is openly intoxicated, discovery of alcohol abuse depends on a thorough history. Signs and symptoms of alcohol abuse in the elderly may be very subtle or confused with other conditions. Remember that even small amounts of alcohol can cause intoxication in an older person. If possible, question family, friends, or caregivers about the patient's drinking patterns. Pertinent findings include:

- Mood swings, denial, and hostility (especially when questioned about drinking)
- Confusion
- History of falls
- Anorexia
- Insomnia
- Visible anxiety
- Nausea

Treatment follows many of the same steps as for any other patient with a pattern of abusive drinking. DO NOT judge the patient. Evaluate the need for fluid therapy, and keep in mind the possibility of withdrawal. Transport the patient to the hospital for evaluation and referral for treatment. Ideally, these patients will seek support from community organizations such as Alcoholics Anonymous (AA). Many communities have AA groups specifically for senior citizens.

Unless an elderly patient is openly intoxicated, discovery of alcohol abuse often depends on a thorough history.

BEHAVIORAL/PSYCHOLOGICAL DISORDERS

When behavioral or psychological problems develop later in life, they are often dismissed as normal age-related changes. This attitude denies an elderly person the opportunity to correct a treatable condition and/or overlooks an underlying physical disorder. Studies have shown that the elderly retain their basic personalities and their adaptive cognitive abilities. In other words, intellectual decline and/or regressive behavior are not normal age-related changes. Unless an organic brain disorder is involved, alterations in behavior should be considered symptomatic of a possible psychological problem.

It is important to keep in mind the emotionally stressful situations facing many elderly people—isolation, loneliness, loss of self-dependence, loss of strength, fear of the future, and more. The elderly also face a higher incidence of secondary depression as a result of neuroleptic medications such as Haldol and Thorazine. Some of the common classifications of psychological disorders related to age include:

- Organic brain syndrome
- Affective disorders (depression)
- Personality disorders (dependent personality)
- Dissociative disorders (paranoid schizophrenia)

As with other people, the emotional well-being of the elderly impacts on their overall physical health. Therefore, it is important that you note evidence of altered behavior in any elderly patient who you assess and examine. Common signs and symptoms of a psychological disorder include lapses in memory, cognitive difficulty, changes in sleep patterns, fear of death, changes in sexual interest, thoughts of suicide, or withdrawal from society.

In general, management of psychological disorders in the elderly is the same as for other age groups. Two of the most common emotional disturbances that you may encounter in the elderly are depression and suicide.

Depression

Up to 15% of the non-institutionalized elderly experience depression. Within institutions, that figure rises to about 30%. The incidence of depression among the elderly is expected to rise in the early 2000s as the baby boomers, with their larger numbers and more prevalent depression at an earlier age, enter their 60s.

Some of the general signs and symptoms noted previously may indicate depression. Ask the patient about feelings of sadness or despair. Determine if he or she has suffered episodes of crying. Inquire about past psychological treatment and current stressful events, particularly the death of a loved one. Keep in mind that sensory changes, especially deafness and blindness, may make the patient vulnerable to depression. Serious acute diseases can have the same effect. If the patient recognizes the depression, ask about the duration and any prior bouts. Find out if the patient has been given any medications to treat the depression. If so, check compliance.

Some depressed patients may exhibit **hypochondriasis** (hypochondria). If this condition is a side effect of the depression, the patient will still show some degree of emotional pain and/or **dysphoria**. Although you may not be able to identify hypochondria in the field, remember that the condition is an illness and requires treatment by trained medical personnel.

In general, depressed patients should receive supportive care. Encourage them to talk, delicately raising questions about suicidal thoughts. The seriously depressed patient should be transported to the hospital. Treatment of depression usually entails psychotherapy and/or antidepressants.

Suicide

The highest suicide rates in the United States are among people over age 65, especially men. The elderly account for 20% of all suicides, but represent only 12% of the total population. Someone over age 65 completes suicide about every 90 minutes. Suicide is the third leading cause of death among the elderly, following falls and motor-vehicle collisions.

Depression is the leading cause for suicide among the elderly. As a group, the elderly are less likely to seek help than the young. They are also less likely to express their anger or sorrow, turning their feelings inward instead. Other stressors that put the elderly at risk of suicide include:

- Chronic illness
- Physical impairment
- Unrelieved pain
- Living in a youth-oriented society
- Family issues
- Financial problems
- Isolation and loneliness
- Substance abuse
- Low serotonin levels (Serotonin declines with age.)
- Bereavement
- Family history of suicide

Suicidal behavior is related to stress. As an EMT-I, you should try to evaluate the stress from an elderly patient's point of view, keeping the preceding factors in mind. In cases of a

hypochondriasis an abnormal concern with one's health, with the false belief of suffering from some disease, despite medical assurances to the contrary; commonly known as hypochondria.

dysphoria an exaggerated feeling of depression or unrest, characterized by a mood of general dissatisfaction, restlessness, discomfort, and unhappiness.

Remember that hypochondriasis is an illness, too.

seriously depressed patient, elicit behavior patterns from family, friends, or caregivers. Warning signs may include:

- Loss of interest in activities that were once enjoyable
- Curtailing social interaction, grooming, and self-care
- Breaking from medical or exercise regimens
- Grieving a personal loss ("I don't want to live without him/her.")
- Feeling useless ("Nobody would miss me.")
- Putting affairs in order, giving away things, finalizing a will
- Stockpiling medications or other lethal means of self-destruction, including firearms

Be particularly alert to suicide among the acutely ill. With more patients being returned home to care for themselves, there is a higher incidence of suicide among the terminally ill, especially cancer victims. A lack of post-acute hospital care can be interpreted as a lack of caring in general.

Prevention of suicide among the elderly involves intervention by all levels of society, from family to EMS to hospital workers. It is important to dispel the common myths about aging and age-related diseases. Recognition of warning signs and involvement of appropriate individuals and agencies is critical.

Your first priorities in the management of a suicidal elderly patient are to protect yourself and then to protect the patient from self-harm. To do this, you must gain access to the patient. This may require breaking into a house or room, particularly if the patient is unconscious or can be readily seen. Remember to summon law enforcement personnel as necessary. DO NOT RULE OUT FIREARMS AMONG THE ELDERLY.

If you reach the patient, emergency care has the highest priority secondary to crew safety. Conduct a brief interview with the patient, if possible, to determine the need for further action. DO NOT leave the suicidal patient alone. Administer medications with caution, keeping in mind polypharmacy and drug interactions in the elderly. (Consult with medical direction.) ALL SUICIDAL ELDERLY PATIENTS SHOULD BE TRANSPORTED TO THE HOSPITAL.

DO NOT rule out firearms among the elderly.

All suicidal elderly patients should be transported to the hospital.

TRAUMA IN THE ELDERLY PATIENT

Trauma is the leading cause of death among the elderly. Older patients who sustain moderate to severe injuries are more likely to die than their younger counterparts. Post-injury disability is also more common in the elderly than in the young.

CONTRIBUTING FACTORS

A number of factors contribute to the high incidence and severity of trauma among the elderly. Slower reflexes, arthritis, and diminished eyesight and hearing predispose the elderly to accidents, especially falls. The elderly, because of their physical state and vulnerability, are also at high risk from trauma caused by criminal assault. Purse snatching, armed robbery, and assault occur all too frequently in the elderly population, especially among those living in urban areas.

Age-related factors that place the elderly at risk of severe injury and complications include:

- Osteoporosis and muscle weakness—increased likelihood of fractures
- Reduced cardiac reserve—decreased ability to compensate for blood loss
- Decreased respiratory function—increased likelihood of **acute respiratory distress syndrome (ARDS)**
- Impaired renal function—decreased ability to adapt to fluid shifts
- Decreased elasticity in the peripheral blood vessels—greater susceptibility to tearing

acute respiratory distress syndrome (ARDS) respiratory insufficiency marked by progressive hypoxemia, due to severe inflammatory damage.

GENERAL ASSESSMENT

As with any other trauma patient, determine the mechanism of injury. Leading causes of trauma in the elderly include falls, motor vehicle crashes, burns, assault or abuse, and underlying medical problems such as syncope.

In assessing elderly trauma patients, remember that blood pressure readings may be deceptive. Older patients typically have a higher blood pressure than younger patients. Although a blood pressure of 110/70 may be normal for a 30-year-old person, it could represent a low blood pressure, and possibly shock, for an older patient. Elderly trauma patients also may not exhibit an elevated pulse, a common early sign of hypoperfusion. This may be because of a chronic heart disease or the use of medications to treat hypertension or myocardial infarction. Fractures may also be obscured or concealed because of a diminished sense of pain among the elderly. One of the best indicators of shock in the elderly is an altered mental status or changes in consciousness during assessment. Elderly trauma patients who exhibit confusion or agitation are candidates for rapid transport.

Observing for Abuse/Neglect

Make sure you observe the scene for signs of abuse and neglect. Abuse of the elderly is as big a problem in our society as child abuse and neglect. **Geriatric abuse** is defined as a syndrome in which an elderly person has received serious physical or psychological injury from family members or other caregivers. Abuse of the elderly knows no socioeconomic bounds. It often occurs when an older person is no longer able to be totally independent, and the family has difficulty upholding their commitment to care for the patient. It can also occur in nursing homes and other health-care facilities. The profile for the potential geriatric abuser may often show a great deal of life stress. In many cases, there is sleep deprivation, marital discord, financial problems, and work-related problems. As the abuser's life gets in further disarray, and as the patient further deteriorates, abuse may be the outcome.

Signs and symptoms of geriatric abuse and neglect are often obvious (Figure 32-9). Unexplained trauma is usually the primary presentation. The average abused patient is older than 80 and has multiple medical problems, such as cancer, congestive heart failure, heart disease, and incontinence. Senile dementia is often present. In these cases, it can be hard to determine whether the dementia is chronic or acute, especially if there is an increased likelihood of head trauma from abuse.

> *In assessing elderly trauma patients, remember that blood pressure and pulse readings can be deceptive indicators of hypoperfusion.*

geriatric abuse a syndrome in which an elderly person is physically or psychologically injured by another person.

FIGURE 32-9 When you encounter evidence of serious head injury, maintain a suspicion of geriatric abuse until proven otherwise.

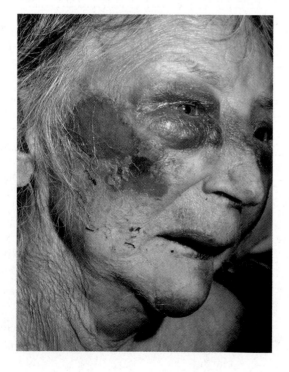

Whenever you suspect geriatric abuse, obtain a complete patient and family history. Pay particular attention to inconsistencies. DO NOT confront the family. Instead, report your suspicions to the emergency department and the appropriate governmental authority. Many states have very strong laws protecting the elderly from abuse or neglect. In fact, many states consider it a criminal offense not to report suspected geriatric abuse. These states also offer legal immunity to those who report geriatric abuse, as long as the report is made in good faith.

GENERAL MANAGEMENT

The priorities of care for the elderly trauma patient are similar to those for any trauma patient. However, you must keep in mind age-related systemic changes and the presence of chronic diseases. This is especially true of the cardiovascular, respiratory, and renal systems.

Cardiovascular Considerations

Recent or past myocardial infarction may contribute to the risk of dysrhythmia or congestive heart failure in the trauma patient. In addition, there may be a decreased response of the heart, in adjusting heart rate and stroke volume, to hypovolemia. An elderly trauma patient may require higher than usual arterial pressures for perfusion of vital organs, due to increased peripheral vascular resistance and hypertension. Care must be taken in IV fluid administration because of decreased myocardial reserves. Hypotension, hypovolemia, and hypervolemia are poorly tolerated in the elderly patient.

Respiratory Considerations

In managing the airway and ventilation in an elderly trauma patient, you must consider the physical changes that may affect treatment. Check for dentures and determine whether they should be removed. Keep in mind that age-related changes can decrease chest wall movement and vital capacity. Age also reduces the tolerance of all organs for anoxia. Remember, too, that COPD is widespread among the elderly.

Make necessary adjustments in treatment to provide adequate oxygenation and appropriate CO_2 removal. It is important to remember that use of 50% nitrous oxide (Nitronox) for elderly patients may result in more respiratory depression than would occur in younger patients. Positive pressure ventilation should also be used cautiously. There is an increased danger of resultant alkalosis and rupture of emphysematous bullae, making the elderly more vulnerable to pneumothorax.

Renal Considerations

The decreased ability of the kidneys to maintain normal acid/base balance, and to compensate for fluid changes, can further complicate the management of the elderly trauma patient. Any preexisting renal disease can decrease the kidney's ability to compensate. The decrease in renal function, along with a decreased cardiac reserve, places the elderly injured patient at risk for fluid overload and pulmonary edema. Remember, too, that renal changes allow toxins and medications to accumulate more readily in the elderly.

Transport Considerations

You may have to modify the positioning, immobilization, and packaging of the elderly trauma patient before transport. Be attentive to physical deformities such as arthritis, spinal abnormalities, or frozen limbs that may cause pain or special care (Figure 32-10). Recall the frailty of an elderly person's skin and avoid creating skin tears or pressure sores. Keep in mind that trauma places an elderly person at increased risk of hypothermia. Ensure that the patient is kept warm at all times.

SPECIFIC INJURIES

The elderly can be subject to a variety of injuries, just like any other age group. The three most common categories of injuries among the elderly include orthopedic injuries, burns, and injuries of the head and spine.

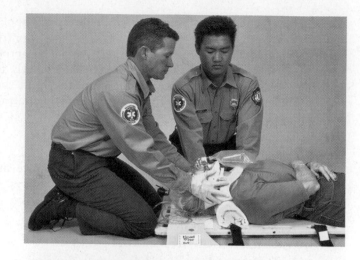

FIGURE 32-10A In an elderly patient with curvature of the spine, place padding behind the neck when immobilizing her to a long spine board.

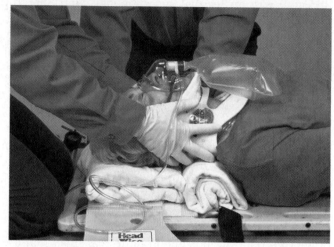

FIGURE 32-10B Additional padding, such as rolled blankets or towels behind the head, may be needed to keep the head in a neutral, in-line position.

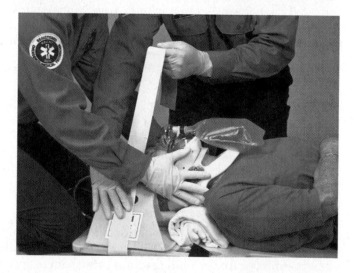

FIGURE 32-10C Secure the patient's head with a head immobilizer device. To prevent spinal damage, maintain manual stabilization until the head is secured.

Content Review

COMMON FRACTURES AMONG THE ELDERLY

- Hip or pelvis fractures
- Proximal humerus
- Distal radius
- Proximal tibia
- Thoracic and lumbar bodies

Orthopedic Injuries

As previously mentioned, the elderly suffer the greatest mortality and greatest incidence of disability from falls. Approximately 33% of falls in the elderly result in at least one fractured bone. The most common fall-related fracture is a fracture of the hip or pelvis (Figure 32-11). Osteoporosis and general frailty contribute to this. The older patient who has fallen should be assumed to have a hip fracture until proven otherwise. Signs and symptoms of a hip fracture include tenderness over the affected joint and shortening and external rotation of the leg. The patient is unable to bear weight on the affected leg. Those patients who live

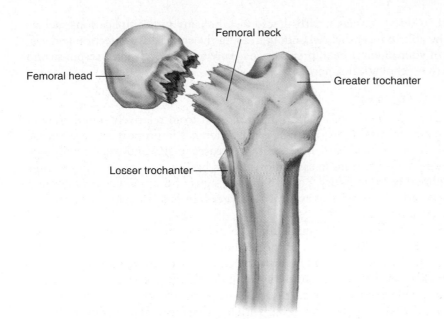

FIGURE 32-11 Subcapital femoral neck fracture. Patients with a displaced femoral neck fracture present with groin pain and a shortened externally rotated leg.

Femoral head

Femoral neck

Greater trochanter

Lesser trochanter

alone may not be able to get to a phone to summon help. Because of this, they may remain on the floor for a prolonged period of time. This can lead to hypothermia, hyperthermia, and/or dehydration.

Falls also result in a variety of other stress fractures in the elderly, including fractures of the proximal humerus, distal radius, proximal tibia, and thoracic and lumbar bodies. Falls may also lead to soft-tissue injuries and hot water burns, if the incident occurred in a tub or hot shower.

In treating orthopedic injuries, remember to ask questions aimed at detecting an underlying medical condition. Ask if the patient recalls "blacking out." Remain alert for evidence of potential cardiac emergencies. Package and transport the patient per the general guidelines mentioned earlier.

Burns

People age 60 and older are more likely to die from burns than any other age group except neonates and infants. Several factors help explain the high mortality rate among elderly burn victims. They include:

- Reaction time slows as people age, so the elderly often stay in contact with thermal sources longer than their younger counterparts.
- Pre-existing diseases place the elderly at risk of medical complications, particularly pulmonary and cardiac problems.
- Age-related skin changes (thinning) result in deeper burns and slower healing time.
- Immunological and metabolic changes increase the risk of infection.
- Reductions in physiological function and the reduced reserve of several organ systems make the elderly more vulnerable to major systemic stress.

Management of elderly burn patients follows the same general procedures as other patients. However, remember that the elderly are at increased risk of shock. Administration of fluids is important to prevent renal tubular damage. Assess hydration in the initial hours after a burn injury by blood pressure, pulse, and urine output (at least 1 to 2 mL/kg per hour).

In the case of the elderly, complications from a burn may manifest themselves in the days and weeks following the incident. For serious burns to heal, the body may use up to

20,000 calories a day. Elderly patients, with altered metabolisms and complications such as diabetes, may not be able to meet this demand, increasing the chances for infection and systemic failure. Part of your job may be to prepare the family for such a delayed response and to provide necessary psychological support.

Head and Spinal Injuries

As a group, the elderly experience more head injuries, even from relatively minor trauma than their younger counterparts. A major factor is the difference in proportion between the brain and the skull. As mentioned earlier, the brain decreases in size and weight with age. The skull, however, remains constant in size, allowing the brain more room to move, thus increasing the likelihood of brain injury. Because of this, signs of brain injury may develop more slowly in the elderly, sometimes over days and weeks. In fact, the patient may often have forgotten the offending injury.

The cervical spine is also more susceptible to injury due to osteoporosis and **spondylosis**. Spondylosis is a degeneration of the vertebral body. The elderly often have a significant degree of this disease. In addition, arthritic changes can gradually compress the nerve rootlets or spinal cord. Thus, injury to the spine in the elderly makes the patient much more susceptible to spinal cord injury. In fact, sudden neck movement, even without fracture, may cause spinal-cord injury. This can occur with less than normal pain, due to the absence of fracture. Therefore, it is important to provide older patients with suspected spinal injuries, especially those involved in motor vehicle accidents, with immediate manual cervical spinal stabilization at the time of initial assessment.

spondylosis a degeneration of the vertebral body.

S UMMARY

The practice of EMS in the twenty-first century means treating a growing elderly population. The "Graying of America" has resulted in a greater number of people age 65 and older, many of whom will be in home settings. When treating elderly patients, keep in mind the anatomical, physiological, and emotional changes that occur with age. However, never jump to conclusions based solely on age. Weigh normal age-related changes against abnormal changes, such as those resulting from a medical condition or trauma. Recall that elderly patients are much more susceptible to medication side effects and toxicity than younger patients. They also are more susceptible to trauma and environmental stressors. Abuse of the elderly occurs, and you should bear this in mind whenever injuries do not match the history. Any suspected abuse or neglect of an elderly patient should be reported to the emergency department and/or the appropriate governmental authorities.

O N THE WEB

For additional practice and review, go to the companion website at www.prenhall.com/bledsoe and click on *Intermediate Emergency Care: Principles & Practice.*

Chapter 33

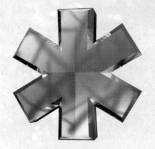

Assessment-Based Management

Objectives

After reading this chapter, you should be able to:

1. Explain how effective assessment is critical to clinical decision making. (pp.1310–1311)
2. Explain how the EMT-Intermediate's attitude and uncooperative patients affect assessment and decision making. (pp. 1311–1313)
3. Explain strategies to prevent labeling and tunnel vision and to decrease environmental distractions. (pp. 1310–1313)
4. Describe how personnel considerations and staffing configurations affect assessment and decision making. (pp. 1313–1314)
5. Synthesize and apply concepts of scene management and choreography to simulated emergency calls. (pp. 1313–1314)
6. Explain the roles of the team leader and the patient care person. (p. 1314)
7. List and explain the rationale for bringing the essential care items to the patient. (pp. 1314–1315)
8. When given a simulated call, list the appropriate equipment to be taken to the patient. (pp. 1314–1315)
9. Explain the general approach to the emergency patient. (pp. 1315–1319)
10. Explain the general approach, patient assessment differentials, and management priorities for patients with various types of emergencies that may be experienced in prehospital care. (pp. 1310–1319)
11. Describe how to effectively communicate patient information face to face, over the telephone, by radio, and in writing. (pp. 1319–1320)
12. Given various preprogrammed and moulaged patients, provide the appropriate scene size-up, initial assessment, focused assessment, and detailed assessment, then provide the appropriate care, ongoing assessments, and patient transport. (pp. 1310–1320)

Case Study

It's after midnight. In fact, a glance at the clock on the station wall tells me it's 3:05 on Sunday morning. I sigh with relief, thinking the worst is probably over for the weekend. Just then, the bell rings, signaling another call. Dispatch reports a single-vehicle crash on Moonglow Road, just outside of town. The caller has given no additional information.

I'm thinking: I wish the caller had provided more information. It's a single-vehicle crash, but I do not know how bad it is or how many patients there might be. The injuries could be minor or severe. Maybe the driver had a medical condition that caused the crash. My partner and I agree that we have to keep an open mind. No tunnel vision. We need to be prepared for anything. While my partner drives to the scene, I'm making a mental list of all the possible medical conditions and injuries that could be involved, and I'm mentally reviewing equipment that we'll need, including airway and ventilation devices, scissors to cut away clothing, dressings and bandages, immobilization equipment, and ECG monitor/defibrillator.

As we near the scene, I pull on gloves. Anticipating blood spatter, I have mask and eye protection ready, too. I look around carefully to determine scene safety. All the nearby telephone poles appear undamaged (so no electrical injuries, I'm thinking), and the police already have traffic under control. I spot the vehicle and surmise from the damage that it has rolled several times. Out in the field, about 50 yards from where the vehicle finally landed, I observe a crowd of people around someone lying on the ground. A police officer tells us this is the driver. There were no passengers and nobody else has been hurt, they say. However, the person who called in the crash seems to have left the scene, so no witnesses are present to interview.

I'm thinking: So only one patient, as far as we know. A roll-over and ejection, which make up a significant mechanism of injury. It'll be a big surprise if this person hasn't suffered multiple major injuries. So it's really important for us to be systematic about our assessment. We don't want to panic and miss something.

As we approach the patient, I notice that he is in a supine position with his right leg flexed under him at an unnatural angle. He appears unresponsive to the crowd and the glare of flashlights. Any blood would be soaking into the ground, so it's hard to estimate how much he's lost. But the only blood I see on his clothing is a spreading stain on the pants legs where one leg is bent under the other.

I'm thinking: There must have been multiple impacts when he struck the inside of the car and then the ground. Maybe the car even rolled over on him at some point. From the angle of that right leg and the blood on his pants, I'm anticipating an open fracture of the right tibia, but that may be the least of his problems. I may find more external bleeding when I do the rapid trauma assessment. And with all that blunt trauma, the patient will likely have internal injuries and internal bleeding, too. My general impression is that of a seriously injured male in his mid-twenties.

When we reach the patient, my partner immediately stabilizes his head and neck. I call out to the patient but get no response. I squeeze his shoulder and he makes a slight pushing-away gesture. I open the airway, using a jaw-thrust. The patient's breathing is shallow and only about eight times a minute. My partner has already grabbed a BVM out of the jump kit and is ready to assist the patient's ventilations with supplemental oxygen.

Checking pulses, I find that the patient has no radial pulses but does have a carotid pulse, indicating that his systolic blood pressure is probably somewhere between 60 and 80 mmHg. His skin is pale, cool, and clammy. As I noted earlier, a considerable amount of blood is coming from an injury to his right leg where it is bent under him. Two EMT-Basics have just arrived on the scene, and I assign one of them to quickly get the bleeding under control with direct pressure while I continue my assessment.

I'm thinking: Inadequate breathing, copious external bleeding, pale, cool, clammy skin, no peripheral pulses, and a low, possibly falling, blood pressure, all indicating shock. This is definitely a high priority patient. However, we mustn't get sidetracked by the apparent fracture and external bleeding. I'll complete the rapid trauma exam to be sure I've found all immediate life threats and so we can prioritize care and then prepare him for immediate transport.

I perform a head-to-toe rapid trauma assessment in less than 60 seconds, finding a reddened area over the right upper abdominal quadrant. When I palpate the area, the patient flinches. Reddening of the skin—the area hasn't had time to look bruised yet—and tenderness on palpation indicate internal injury and internal bleeding, making expedited transport an even more urgent priority.

As I expose and assess the extremities, I confirm an open right tibial fracture. I direct one of the EMT-Bs to assess vital signs while the other EMT-B and I apply gentle traction to straighten the right leg. I quickly place a pressure dressing over the open wound. Then, the EMT-Bs, my partner, and I log roll the patient and immobilize him to a long backboard.

I have found no medical ID medallion. The pulse is weak and rapid but steady. The patient has responded to painful stimulus with no indication of weakness or paralysis. The patient has a strong odor of alcohol on his breath, and one of the policemen says he found an open container of bourbon in the car.

I'm thinking: No medical ID that would tell me he's diabetic, for instance. No indication of a heart attack or stroke. Other than alcohol intoxication, there's no evidence of a medical condition as the cause of the crash. So far, this seems to be a straightforward case of alcohol leading to trauma, external and internal bleeding, and shock.

Further assessment and emergency care will have to be done en route to the emergency department. We have been on the scene for approximately 8 minutes.

One of the EMT-Bs offers to drive the ambulance to the hospital so my partner and I can both attend the patient. En route, I complete an ongoing assessment. The patient is stable, and I have time to perform a detailed physical exam but make no further findings. Meanwhile, my partner has started two IV lines of normal saline. I complete another ongoing assessment. By the time we arrive at the emergency department, the patient has begun to respond when we call to him.

INTRODUCTION

An EMT-I does more than just follow a standard sequence of assessment steps—scene size-up, initial assessment, focused history and physical exam, ongoing assessment, and detailed physical exam. While carrying out the assessment in a systematic way, an EMT-I is constantly thinking and reasoning.

The kind of reasoning an EMT-I needs to do has been described as an inverted pyramid, with the broad end at the top and the narrow point at the bottom (Figure 33-1). As soon as you receive the dispatch and the patient's chief complaint, you try to form a mental list of all the possible causes of the patient's problem. (Such a list is often called a "differential diagnosis.") You want to keep your mind wide open, avoiding tunnel vision.

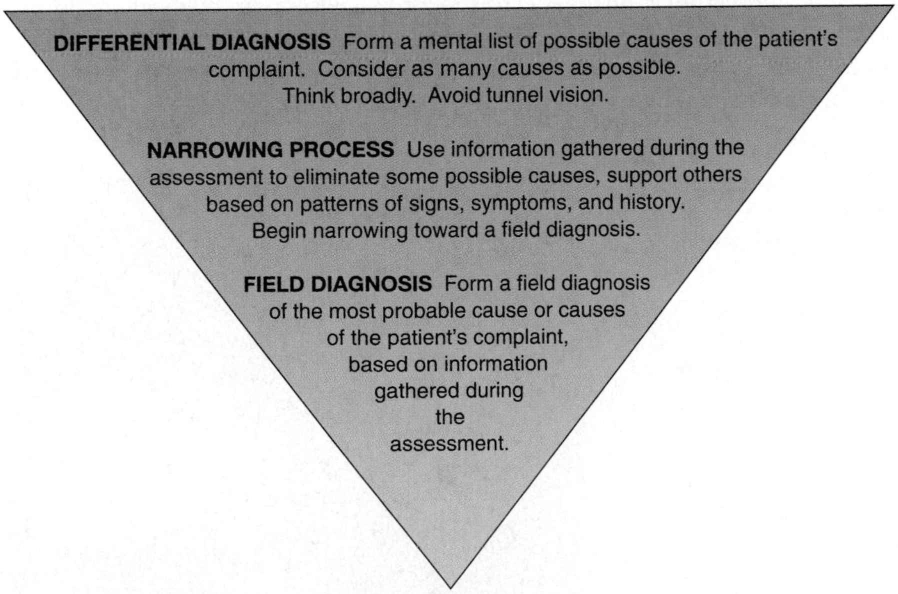

DIFFERENTIAL DIAGNOSIS Form a mental list of possible causes of the patient's complaint. Consider as many causes as possible. Think broadly. Avoid tunnel vision.

NARROWING PROCESS Use information gathered during the assessment to eliminate some possible causes, support others based on patterns of signs, symptoms, and history. Begin narrowing toward a field diagnosis.

FIELD DIAGNOSIS Form a field diagnosis of the most probable cause or causes of the patient's complaint, based on information gathered during the assessment.

FIGURE 33–1 Follow an inverted pyramid format to avoid tunnel vision while working toward a field diagnosis.

For example, the victim of an auto crash has an obvious open extremity fracture with associated external blood loss. Serious as it is, the EMT-I should resist being distracted by this injury. Suppose the patient had suffered a heart attack or cardiac arrest prior to or following the crash. Suppose the patient had other, more serious injuries, such as blunt abdominal trauma and internal bleeding. What if the EMT-I fails to consider these other possibilities, focuses on the obvious leg injury, and spends on-scene time splinting the fracture instead of completing the assessment and initiating rapid transport?

Far better if the EMT-I uses inverted-pyramid reasoning skills (which may also be called critical thinking, problem-solving, or clinical decision-making) to assess the patient and prioritize emergency care. The EMT-I begins by considering a wide variety of possible medical conditions and injuries. Then, while working through the standard sequence of assessment steps, the EMT-I uses the information gathered at each step of the assessment to eliminate some possibilities and support other possibilities. The EMT-I considers pertinent negatives (signs that are not present, such as paralysis or an erratic pulse) as well as findings that are present (such as reddening and tenderness in one abdominal quadrant) to narrow in on a field diagnosis.

EFFECTIVE ASSESSMENT

Assessment forms the foundation for patient care.

Assessment forms the foundation for patient care. You cannot treat or report a problem that is not found or identified. To find a problem, you must gather, evaluate, and synthesize information. Based on this process, you can then make decisions and take appropriate actions—formulate a management plan and determine the priorities for patient care.

An EMT-I is entrusted with a great deal of independent judgment and responsibility for performing the correct actions for each individual patient, including such advanced skills as ECG interpretation and medication administration. Additionally, the medical director and hospital staff must rely on your experience and expertise as you describe the patient's condition and your conclusions about it. Consequently, the ability to reason and to reach a field diagnosis is critical to EMT-I practice.

IMPORTANCE OF ACCURATE INFORMATION

The decisions you make as an EMT-I will only be as good as the information you collect.

The decisions that you make as an EMT-I will only be as good as the information that you collect. To make accurate decisions, you need to gather accurate information.

History

A patient's history is a crucial part of the medical record, especially in medical conditions (as contrasted to trauma, where the physical exam takes precedence over the history). Very often, doctors will base 80% of their diagnosis on the history. As a result, it is important for you to question the patient, family members, and bystanders (Figure 33-2). However, you

FIGURE 33-2 If the patient is unable to provide a history, gather information from family members or bystanders.

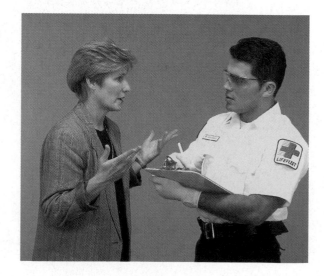

must not allow your knowledge of the disease—or your suspicion of the underlying problem—to affect the quality of the history you gather. Just because a patient has had a heart attack in the past does not mean that the person is having one now. Focus your questioning on the present complaint and associated problems.

Physical Exam

Never forget, or minimize, the importance of a thorough physical exam, especially when there is the possibility of trauma. Although the physical exam may be compromised by field conditions, it should never be done in a cursory manner. Even when you are dealing with angry family members or are in a bad physical environment, you must perform an effective examination. If field conditions make the exam difficult or nearly impossible, you may have to move the patient into the ambulance or some other controlled environment in order to perform the exam. If the patient is unresponsive or if there is a significant mechanism of injury, perform a complete head-to-toe assessment. If a patient is a responsive medical patient or has suffered minor trauma, focus your exam on the systems associated with the patient's chief complaint.

Pattern Recognition

In assessing a patient, remain alert to patterns. Compare the information that you gather with your knowledge base—what you have learned about the pathophysiology and presentation of various diseases and injuries. For example, a trauma patient with decreased mental status, unequal pupils, swelling or discoloration around the eyes, and bleeding from the ear is presenting a pattern typical of basilar skull fracture. A patient who complains of a cough, gradual onset of breathing difficulty, sharp chest pain, and shaking chills with an elevated temperature is displaying a pattern typical of pneumonia. There may be times when you do not recognize a pattern. Obviously, the greater your knowledge base, the greater the likelihood you will recognize patterns. The ability to recognize patterns also increases with experience, which is why new EMT-Is are generally assigned to work with experienced EMT-Is or paramedics for a time.

Assessment/Field Diagnosis

Sometimes your field diagnosis will be based on a combination of pattern recognition and intuition, which is also based on experience. Once you have determined the problem, your next step is to formulate a plan of action, based on the patient's condition and the environment.

BLS/ALS Protocols

All EMS systems have protocols devised by the medical director that guide both BLS and ALS patient care. However, protocols and standing orders do not replace the EMT-I's judgment. For example, you must exercise judgment, based on your assessment and field diagnosis, to know which protocol to use. You must exercise judgment to know when and how to follow a protocol—and you must also exercise judgment about when to deviate from a protocol. If a patient is allergic to a medication, for example, you do not administer it, even though a protocol calls for its use.

FACTORS AFFECTING ASSESSMENT AND DECISION MAKING

A number of factors—both internal (for example, your personal attitudes) and external (for example, the patient's attitude, distracting injuries, or environmental factors at the scene)—can affect your assessment of the patient and ultimately your decisions on how to manage treatment. By keeping these factors in mind, you can avoid the limitations that they impose on your collection and evaluation of patient information.

Personal Attitudes

Your attitude is one of the most critical factors in performing an effective assessment. You must be as nonjudgmental as possible to avoid "short circuiting" accurate data collection and pattern recognition by leaping to conclusions before completing a thorough assessment. Remember the popular computer mnemonic GIGO, garbage in/garbage out. You cannot reach valid conclusions about your patient based on a hasty or incomplete assessment. You

You must be as non-judgmental as possible to avoid "short circuiting" accurate data collection and the recognition of patterns.

will be unable to provide good medical management if, for example, you base decisions on the patient's social standing or likeability.

Seek to identify any preconceived notions that you may have about a group and then work to eliminate them. As mentioned in Chapter 32, for example, a number of signs and symptoms have been mistakenly ascribed to aging when in fact they may point to serious medical conditions. A preconception that decreased mental acuity in an elderly patient is "normal" may lead you to miss what is really wrong with this patient and cause you to provide inadequate care.

Uncooperative Patients

Admittedly, uncooperative patients make it difficult to perform good assessments. All too often these patients are perceived as being "high," either on alcohol or drugs. However, you must remember that there are many other possible causes for patient belligerence.

Whenever assessing an uncooperative or restless patient, consider medical causes—hypoxia, hypovolemia, hypoglycemia, or a head injury, such as a concussion or a subdural hematoma. Be careful not to jump to the conclusion that this patient is just another drunk or a "frequent flyer." The frequent flyer that you have transported for alcoholic behavior in the past may, this time, be suffering from trauma or a medical emergency.

If the person is in fact a substance abuser, keep in mind that abuse or addiction is an illness. No matter how difficult these patients are to manage, they still deserve the best care that you can provide (Figure 33-3). If you treat every patient in the manner in which you would want your loved ones treated, you will seldom go wrong.

Patient Compliance

Not all patients welcome the sight of an ALS team. Cultural and ethnic barriers, as well as prior negative experiences, may cause a patient to lack confidence in the rescuers. Such situations make it difficult for you to be effective at the scene, and the patients in fact may refuse to provide expressed consent for treatment or transport. It is your job to treat the patients in a way that will increase their confidence. If language is a barrier, try to speak through a friend, relative, or bystander who understands the patient's language, or in the case of deafness, signs. If you live in a community with a large ethnic population, try to become familiar with body language and customs of that culture. For example, some groups

If you treat every patient in the manner in which you would want your loved ones treated, you will never go wrong.

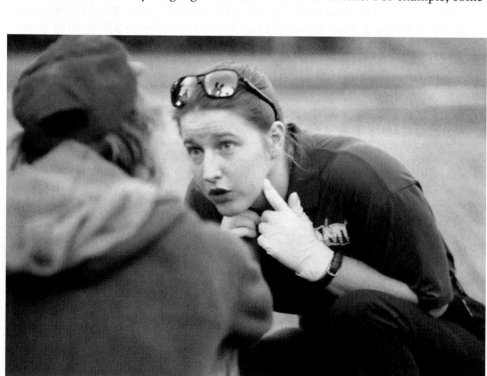

FIGURE 33-3 In treating substance abuse patients, maintain a nonjudgmental attitude.

consider it rude to make eye contact. Again, do not permit yourself to make snap judgments about the patient.

Distracting Injuries

Yet another factor that can affect your assessment and decisions involves obvious, but distracting injuries. A nasty-looking tibial fracture might cause the EMT-I to overlook the less obvious signs of internal bleeding. Scalp lacerations usually look worse than they really are and could divert your attention from more serious injuries, such as an open chest wound. You must resist the temptation to form a field diagnosis too early. While EMT-Is often have to rely on their "gut instinct," it may also lead them to make snap judgments. An open, bleeding fracture of the femur may be so distracting that an EMT-I rushes to treat it, missing the fact that the patient is also having difficulty breathing. Always take a systematic approach to patient assessment to avoid distractions and to find and prioritize care for all of the patient's injuries and conditions.

Environmental and Personnel Considerations

You have probably already experienced some of the environmental factors that can affect patient assessment and care. Among others, they include scene chaos, violent or dangerous situations, high noise levels, or crowds of bystanders. Even crowds of responders can be a problem, in some instances.

While having enough help is crucial, it is also important to use personnel wisely (Figure 33-4). A large number of rescuers moving around can be just as distracting as a large number of bystanders. In such situations, some of the rescuers might be staged nearby and brought to the scene when and if necessary. Some may also be assigned to control bystanders.

As a rule, assessment is best achieved by one rescuer. A single EMT-I can gather information and provide treatment sequentially. In the case of two EMT-Is, one EMT-I can assess the patient, while the other provides simultaneous treatment. With multiple responders, however, assessment and history may take place by committee, which often leads to disorganized management.

A large number of rescuers moving around can be just as distracting as a large number of bystanders.

ASSESSMENT/MANAGEMENT CHOREOGRAPHY

Although too many people, or multiple-tier responders, may make it hard to acquire a patient history and conduct a physical exam, it becomes even more difficult if the responders are all at the same professional level and have no clear direction. It is important to plan for these events so that personnel have predesignated roles. These roles may be rotated among team members so no one is left out, but there must be a plan to avoid "freelancing." If there is only one EMT-I, then that person must assume all ALS roles.

In the case of a two-EMT-I team, an effective plan involves the roles of team leader and patient care provider, assigned on an alternating basis. EMT-Is who work together regularly may develop their own plan, but a universally understood plan allows for other rescuers to participate in a rescue without interrupting the flow. While the dynamics of field situations may necessitate changes, a general game plan can go a long way toward preventing chaos.

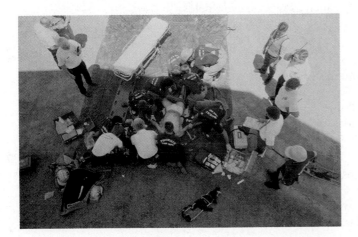

FIGURE 33-4 When multiple responders are on the scene, everyone should have a designated task.

If field dynamics dictate a change in planned roles, you are still working from a solid base. In setting up a two-person team, keep in mind the following descriptions of team leader and patient care provider roles.

Team Leader

The team leader is usually the person who will accompany the patient through to definitive care. The EMT-I charged with this role should establish contact and maintain dialogue with the patient. He or she obtains the history, performs the physical examination, and presents the patient, in both verbal and written reports. During multiple casualty situations, the team leader acts as the initial EMS commander.

The team leader must maintain overall patient perspective and provide leadership to the team by designating tasks and coordinating transportation. While the team leader must actively participate in critical interventions, it is important that this person not fall into the trap of trying to do everything alone. During ACLS calls, for example, the team leader's tasks might include the following: reading the ECG, talking on the radio and giving drug orders, controlling the drug box, and keeping notes on drug administrations and effects. Actual treatment, however, would be left to the designated patient care provider.

Patient Care Provider

The patient care provider should ensure scene cover (watching the team leader's back). This person should gather scene information, talk to relatives and bystanders, and obtain vital signs. The patient care provider performs any skills or interventions requested by the team leader, such as attaching monitoring leads, administering oxygen, obtaining venous access, administering medications, and securing transportation equipment. In multiple casualty situations, the patient care provider acts as the triage group leader. During ACLS calls, he or she administers drugs, monitors tube placement, and oversees BCLS.

THE RIGHT EQUIPMENT

Having the right equipment at the patient's side is essential. As an EMT-I, you must be prepared to manage many conditions and injuries or changes in the patient's condition. As already mentioned, assessment and management must usually be done simultaneously. If you do not have the right equipment readily available, then you have compromised patient care and, in fact, the patient may die.

Think of your equipment as items in a backpack. Just like backpacking, you must downsize your equipment to minimum weight and bulk to facilitate rapid movement. At the same time, you need certain essential equipment to ensure survival—in this case, patient survival. The following is a list of the essential equipment for EMT-I management of life-threatening conditions. You must bring these items to the side of every patient, regardless of what you initially think you may need:

- Infection control
  - Infection control supplies, such as gloves, eye shields
- Airway control
  - Oral airways
  - Nasal airways
  - Suction (electric or manual)
  - Rigid tonsil-tip and flexible suction catheters
  - Laryngoscope and blades
  - Endotracheal tubes, stylets, syringes, tape
- Breathing
  - Pocket mask
  - Manual ventilation BVM
  - Spare masks in various sizes
  - Oxygen tank and regulator
  - Oxygen masks, cannulas, and extension tubing

Content Review

ROLES OF TEAM LEADER

- Obtains history
- Performs physical exam
- Presents patient
- Handles documentation
- Acts as EMS commander

Content Review

ROLES OF PATIENT CARE PROVIDER

- Provides scene cover
- Gathers scene information
- Talks to relatives/bystanders
- Obtains vital signs
- Performs interventions
- Acts as triage group leader

If you do not have the right equipment readily available, you have compromised patient care.

- Occlusive dressings
- Large bore IV catheter for thoracic decompression
- Circulation
  - Dressings
  - Bandages and tape
  - Sphygmomanometer, stethoscope
  - Note pad and pen or pencil
- Disability
  - Rigid collars
  - Flashlight
- Dysrhythmia
  - Cardiac monitor/defibrillator
- Exposure and Protection
  - Scissors
  - Space blankets or something to cover the patient

You may also pack some optional "take in" equipment, such as drug therapy and venous access supplies. The method by which these supplies are carried may depend on how your system is designed (for example, EMT-I ambulances versus EMT-Is in non-transporting vehicles). It may also depend on local protocols, flexibility of standing orders, the number of EMT-I responders in your area, and the difficulty of accessing patients because of terrain or some other problem.

In most cases, venous access supplies should be carried with the drug box since venous access is required to administer most medications. The drug box should also contain any medications allowed in the formulary.

GENERAL APPROACH TO THE PATIENT

In addition to having the essential equipment, you need to have the essential demeanor to calm or reassure the patient. You must look and act the part of a professional, while exhibiting the compassion and understanding associated with an effective "bedside manner." Although patients may not have the ability to rate your medical performance, they can certainly rate your people skills and service. Be aware of your body language and the messages it sends, whether intentionally or unintentionally. Think carefully about what you say and how you say it—this includes your conversations with other members of the ALS team and anyone else at the scene.

Be aware of your body language and the messages it sends, whether intentionally or unintentionally.

Once again, it helps to preplan your general approach to the patient. This will prevent confusion and improve the accuracy of your assessment. One team member should engage in an active, concerned dialogue with the patient. This same person should also demonstrate the listening skills needed to collect information and to convey a caring attitude. Taking notes may prevent asking the same question repeatedly, as well as ensure that you acquire and pass on accurate data.

By approaching the patient with the right equipment and the right attitude, you minimize confusion and stand ready to provide effective emergency care.

The following sections briefly review the steps of the assessment that you will perform systematically on all patients. To review the assessment steps in detail, see Chapter 8.

SCENE SIZE-UP

The scene size-up has the following components:

- *Body substance isolation.* Be sure you are wearing disposable gloves and are wearing or have available other protective equipment that may be needed such as gown, mask, and eye protection.
- *Scene safety.* Observe the scene for any hazards to yourself, other rescuers, bystanders, and the patient. This is as important at a medical scene as at a trauma scene.

- *Locate all patients,* such as those who may have wandered away from a vehicle collision or additional patients in a household where the patient appears to be suffering from carbon monoxide or other toxic exposure.
- *Mechanism of injury or nature of the illness.* Determine this as well as possible at this stage of the call and remain observant for additional information as the call progresses.

If you determine that you may need additional equipment or support, now is the time to call for help.

INITIAL ASSESSMENT

After you size up the scene, you quickly begin the initial assessment for the purpose of detecting and treating immediate life threats. The components of the initial assessment are:

- Forming a general impression
- Mental status assessment (AVPU)
- Airway assessment
- Breathing assessment
- Circulation assessment
- Determining the patient's priority for further on-scene care or immediate transport

Depending on your findings during the initial assessment, you might determine that one of the following approaches is appropriate for the patient's priority status.

Resuscitative Approach

Take the resuscitation approach whenever you suspect a life-threatening problem, including:

- Cardiac or respiratory arrest
- Respiratory distress or failure
- Unstable dysrhythmias
- Status epilepticus (series of generalized motor seizures without an intervening return of consciousness)
- Coma or altered mental status
- Shock or hypotension
- Major trauma
- Possible C-spine injury

Patho Pearls

Providing competent, compassionate prehospital care is the goal of our profession. To be a competent field provider, you must first have a good knowledge of normal human anatomy and physiology. Then, you must learn about the problems that can develop. Understanding the pathophysiology of the various illnesses and injuries you encounter is essential to providing competent care.

You should also have excellent assessment skills. During the patient assessment you are actually serving as a detective. That is, you are looking for signs and symptoms that either point toward or away from a particular disease process or injury. Then, based on your assessment findings, you apply the skills you have learned. As you become more experienced, and as you are further away from your initial education, you must stay up to date with trends and practices of EMS.

Develop a habit of reading EMS research and staying abreast of changes in the profession through attendance at conferences, continuing education seminars, and symposia. Your education as an EMT-I does not end with graduation. That is where it begins.

In these cases, you must take immediate resuscitative action (such as CPR and defibrillation and ventilation) or other critical action (such as supplemental oxygen, control of major bleeding, or C-spine stabilization). Additional assessment and care can be performed after resuscitation and the rapid trauma assessment and/or en route to the hospital.

Contemplative Approach

Use the contemplative approach when immediate intervention is not necessary, such as with stable chest pain or a mild allergic reaction. In such situations, the focused history and physical exam, followed by any required interventions, will be performed at the scene, before transport to the hospital.

Immediate Evacuation

In some situations, you will need to immediately evacuate the patient to the ambulance (Figure 33-5). For example, a patient with severe internal bleeding requires life-saving interventions beyond an EMT-I's skills. You might also resort to immediate evacuation if the scene is too chaotic for rational assessment or if it is too unsafe or unstable.

FOCUSED HISTORY AND PHYSICAL EXAM

Following the initial assessment, you will perform the focused history and physical exam. Based on the patient's chief complaint and the information you have gathered during the initial assessment, you should consider your patient to belong to one of the following four categories:

- Trauma patient with a significant mechanism of injury or altered mental status
- Trauma patient with an isolated injury
- Medical patient who is responsive
- Medical patient who is unresponsive

For a trauma patient with a significant mechanism of injury or altered mental status or for an unresponsive medical patient, perform a complete head-to-toe physical examination (rapid trauma assessment for the trauma patient, rapid medical assessment for the medical patient). For the trauma patient with an isolated injury or for the responsive medical patient, perform a physical exam focused on body systems related to the chief complaint.

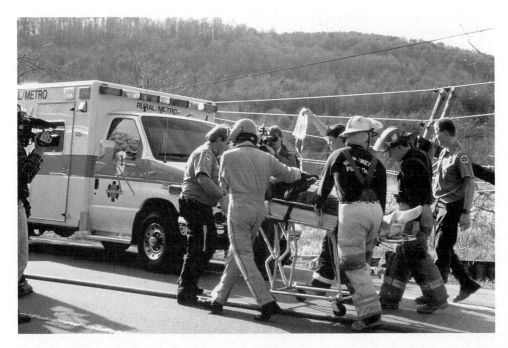

FIGURE 33–5 High-priority patients require immediate evacuation, with continued assessment and care done en route.

For a medical patient, gather the history before performing the physical exam, unless the patient is unable to provide one and there are no family members or bystanders present who can provide information. For a trauma patient, gather the history after you have performed the physical exam. (Of course, elements of the history and the physical exam are often obtained simultaneously if partners are working together or as you talk to the responsive patient while examining him.)

ONGOING ASSESSMENT AND THE DETAILED PHYSICAL EXAM

The ongoing assessment must be performed on all patients to monitor and to observe trends in the patient's condition—every 5 minutes if the patient is unstable, every 15 minutes if the patient is stable. Ongoing assessments must be performed until the patient is transferred to the care of hospital personnel. The ongoing assessment includes evaluation of the following:

- Mental status
- Airway, breathing, and circulation
- Transport priorities
- Vital signs
- Focused assessment of any problem areas or conditions
- Effectiveness of interventions
- Management plans

The detailed physical exam is similar to but more thorough than the rapid trauma assessment. It is generally performed only on trauma patients and only if time and the patient's condition permit. The purpose is to find any injuries or conditions that may have been missed during earlier assessments. In a critical patient, continuing ongoing assessments are more important than a detailed physical exam.

IDENTIFICATION OF LIFE-THREATENING PROBLEMS

At all stages of assessment, actively and continuously look for and manage any life-threatening problems.

At all stages of the assessment, from initial assessment through ongoing assessments, from the scene to the ambulance to arrival at the hospital, you must actively and continuously look for and manage any life-threatening problems.

You need to rapidly determine the chief complaint and to assess the distress in a systematic manner. Obtain baseline vital signs along with the focused physical exam, but if partners are working together, one may obtain the baseline vital signs earlier in the assessment. Focus on the relevant portions of the history and the physical findings. For example, a history of appendicitis would be relevant for a patient complaining of right lower quadrant pain, less relevant for a trauma patient with possible spinal injury.

If you have an educated suspicion of what you are looking for, then you will be able to ask more productive questions. However, you are less likely to find something if you do not suspect it. For this reason, throughout your assessment, keep in mind the mechanism of injury and the nature of the illness (as determined, starting with the initial assessment and the patient's chief complaint). Listen carefully to everything the patient says. With experience, you will develop the skill of multi-tasking—asking questions, listening to answers, and caring for the patient almost simultaneously. However, until you gain that experience, and unless you are actively managing a life-threatening condition, ask questions and just listen. Allow your partner to perform necessary tasks so that you do not miss any important clues.

The underlying principle of assessment-based management is to rapidly and accurately assess the patient and then treat for the worst-case scenario.

The ability of a patient to describe symptoms and an EMT-I's ability to listen greatly affect the quality and outcome of an assessment. The severity of pain does not always correlate well with the life-threatening potential of a condition. For example, a long splinter jammed under a fingernail will certainly cause pain, but few lives have been lost to such an injury. Conversely, some patients, especially the elderly, suffer myocardial infarctions with only vague symptoms that do not include chest pain. In addition, the location of pain and its source do not always correlate well, especially if it is visceral pain. For example, gallbladder attacks are often characterized by pain that is referred to the shoulder. As an EMT-I, you must listen with your ears and then use your knowledge base about various illnesses and diseases to interpret what the patient says.

Basically your role as EMT-I is to rapidly and accurately assess the patient and then to treat for the worst case scenario. This is the underlying principle of assessment-based management—your guide for providing effective emergency care.

PRESENTING THE PATIENT

The ability to communicate effectively is the key to transferring patient information, whether in an out-of-hospital setting or within the hospital itself. Although neither basic nor advanced life-support interventions may be required for every patient, a skill that will be used on every single patient is that of effective presentation, whether it is over the radio or telephone, in writing, or in face-to-face transfers at the receiving facility. Despite the frequency with which EMT-Is present patients, this is often the weakest link in patient care.

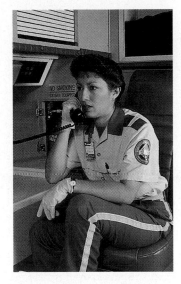

FIGURE 33-6 A clear, concise patient report will enable the hospital staff to prepare for the needs of the patient.

ESTABLISHING TRUST AND CREDIBILITY

Effective presentation and communication skills help establish an EMT-I's credibility (Figure 33-6). They also inspire the trust and confidence of patients and other medical personnel. If you present your assessment, your findings, and your treatment in a clear, concise manner, you give the impression of a job well done. A poor presentation, on the other hand, implies poor assessment and poor patient care.

Other health-care providers have little time or interest in listening to rambling, disjointed presentations that cover unimportant details while omitting vital information. Use the SOAP format or some variation of it. Not only does SOAP help you organize your presentation, most health-care providers have become accustomed to listening to it and know what to expect. (SOAP stands for *S*ubjective, *O*bjective, *A*ssessment, and *P*lan. For further description, see Chapter 11.)

The way in which you present the patient has direct implications for the person's care and recovery. Poor presentations compromise patient care. They lead to incomplete or even incorrect medical orders. If you do not communicate a patient's needs or status completely or accurately, a person may be denied some form of treatment based on the information that you have conveyed.

As an EMT-I, you will be an extension of the supervisory physician, working under his or her license. No doctor is going to issue orders for medications or other patient care based on guesswork. You are the doctor's eyes and ears at the emergency scene, and it is essential that you provide accurate information about both the patient and the emergency situation.

DEVELOPING EFFECTIVE PRESENTATION SKILLS

The most effective oral presentations usually meet these guidelines:

- Last less than 1 minute
- Are very concise and clear
- Avoid extensive use of medical jargon
- Follow a basic format, usually the SOAP format or some variation
- Include both pertinent findings and pertinent negatives (findings that might be expected, given the patient's complaint or condition, but are absent or denied by the patient)
- Conclude with specific actions, requests, or questions related to the plan

The best way to become proficient at presenting patients is to plan ahead and to practice. Start with an end in mind—know what particular areas of information will be asked for or expected so that you can be ready with that information. As you become more experienced, the flow of information will become second nature to you. Until that time, use a pre-printed form to help you organize your thoughts and information and to take notes during the patient work-up. Practice presenting both simulated and real patients, perhaps at company or unit drills. Listen to other EMT-Is as they present patients and learn from them. Adopt their good habits and avoid their bad ones.

An ideal presentation should include the following:

- Patient identification, age, sex, and degree of distress
- Chief complaint (why a patient called)
- Present illness/injury
  - Pertinent details about the present problem
  - Pertinent negatives
- Past medical history
  - Allergies
  - Medications
  - Pertinent medical history
- Physical signs
  - Vital signs
  - Pertinent positive findings
  - Pertinent negative findings
- Assessment
  - EMT-I impression
- Plan
  - What has been done
  - Orders requested

Remember, the key to developing presentation skills is repetition and an understanding of the format being used. Once you have mastered this, you can transfer the patient with the satisfaction and confidence of a job well done. (For more detail on this topic, review Chapters 10 and 11 on communications and documentation.)

REVIEW OF COMMON COMPLAINTS

In order to develop as an entry-level practitioner at the EMT-I level, it is important to participate in scenario-based reviews of commonly encountered complaints. As mentioned, you might take part in company or unit drills in which you will observe and work with experienced EMT-Is. You might also participate in laboratory-based simulations.

PRACTICE SESSIONS

The goal of practice sessions is to choreograph the roles and actions of the EMS response team. These sessions will give you the chance to practice assessment and decision making on cases that you are likely to encounter in out-of-hospital situations. They also give you the opportunity to provide intervention based on your assessment and to reinforce the modalities in local and/or regional treatment protocols. Finally, you can practice patient presentation, both verbally and in written form. At all phases, you get the benefit of feedback from the team members and crew with whom you will be working.

LABORATORY-BASED SIMULATIONS

Laboratory-based simulations require you to assess a pre-programmed patient or mannequin. You will make decisions relative to interventions and transportation. You will also provide interventions, package the patient (or mannequin), and transport. Ideally, you will work as part of a team and practice the various roles assigned to team members, including that of patient.

SELF-MOTIVATION

The chance to practice does not stop at the classroom or at your unit. While an EMT-I student or the new member of a team, take advantage of every opportunity to practice your new skills. Recruit family members or friends, or even a teddy bear, as volunteer patients. What is important is to practice, practice, practice until you feel comfortable with as many different situations as possible.

SUMMARY

Assessment forms the basis of patient care. In order to make correct decisions, you must gather information and then evaluate and synthesize it. A variety of factors may affect assessment and the decision-making process itself. Some of these factors include EMT-I attitude, uncooperative patients, obvious but distracting injuries, narrow or tunnel vision, the environment, patient compliance, and personnel considerations.

It is important to have the right equipment readily available to treat immediately life-threatening conditions. Effective communication and transfer of patient information—whether done face to face, over the telephone or radio, or in writing—is crucial to presenting the patient and assuring continuation of effective care.

Remember, the best way to develop good assessment skills is to practice until you become comfortable with a wide range of patient complaints.

ON THE WEB

For additional practice and review, go to the companion website at www.prenhall.com/bledsoe and click on *Intermediate Emergency Care: Principles & Practice.*

CHAPTER 34

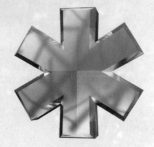

Responding to Terrorist Acts

Objectives *(Asterisks below indicate material supplemental to the U.S. DOT curriculum.)*

After reading this chapter, you should be able to:

*1. Identify the typical weapons of mass destruction likely to be used by terrorists. (pp. 1323–1324)

*2. Explain the mechanisms of injury associated with conventional and nuclear weapons of mass destruction. (pp. 1324, 1325, 1327, 1332)

*3. Identify and describe the major sub-classifications of chemical and biological weapons of mass destruction. (pp. 1327–1330, 1332–1333)

*4. List the scene evidence that might alert the EMS provider to a terrorist attack that involves a weapon of mass destruction. (p. 1334)

*5. Describe the special safety precautions and safety equipment appropriate for an incident involving nuclear, biological, or chemical weapons. (pp. 1326–1327, 1333, 1334; see also Chapters 8, 13, and 16)

*6. Identify the assessment and management concerns for victims of conventional, nuclear, biological, and chemical weapons. (pp. 1326–1327, 1330, 1331, 1333)

*7. Given a narrative description of a conventional, nuclear, biological, or chemical terrorist attack, identify the elements of scene size-up that suggest terrorism and identify the likely injuries and any special patient management considerations necessary. (pp. 1324–1334)

CASE STUDY

Late Monday morning during the first real cold spell of winter, Adam and Sean are called to transport a 54-year-old physician from a local OB/GYN clinic. He is found to have some "chest tightness" but no ECG abnormalities and the rest of his assessment is unremarkable. Shortly after delivering him to the emergency department, the pagers go off again, and Adam and Sean are requested to respond to the same address where several people are now complaining of fatigue, shortness of breath, and headache. Adam remembers that the clinic was the subject of a news report last week where abortion demonstrators became violent during a protest. As Adam and Sean call in service and en route, Adam requests that the fire department respond for a possible hazardous environment. Sean uses the cell phone (and a secure line) to contact the dispatch center to make their concerns known and suggests that dispatch call the clinic and request evacuation of the facility. Sean also requests that the center activate the county's WMD plan.

Adam and Sean are the first unit to arrive, so they establish incident command. They size up the scene and notice a dozen or so people in the parking lot and no signs of any smoke or gas clouds coming from the clinic. Adam notes the flag blowing gently from a northwesterly breeze. Sean parks the ambulance north and west of the building and, using the ambulance's public address system, requests the clinic employees approach his location. He also contacts dispatch with an approximate number of people at the scene and suggests the fire department approach the building from the northwest. Both EMT-Is don HEPA respirators and gloves. Sean speaks with some of the employees to ensure all personnel are out of the building and accounted for.

When the fire department arrives, Captain James approaches, receives a situation update from Adam, and then assumes incident command. He reports a team with SCBA gear is entering the building to investigate the problem. Adam and Sean establish a treatment sector and begin to assess the victims and administer high-flow, high-concentration oxygen to the patients with the worst complaints. Their initial evaluation reveals most patients are complaining of general fatigue, headache, some ringing in the ears, and mild dyspnea. Two other ambulances arrive and, at the direction of Adam, begin oxygen administration to the remaining patients. Captain James answers a radio call from the entry team and reports that carbon monoxide readings are very high in the building.

Adam and Sean remain at the scene but direct the other ambulances to begin transporting patients to the two local hospitals. Sean contacts medical direction and provides the number of patients, their signs and symptoms, and the likely cause of their problems. As Sean and Adam prepare the last of the patients for transport, Captain James reports that the furnace flue was intentionally redirected into the furnace room, generating the carbon monoxide. The police are informed and the area becomes a crime scene.

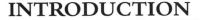

INTRODUCTION

The events of September 11, 2001, have greatly impacted our society and our sensitivity to the threat of terrorist acts. The extensive planning and coordination needed to bring down the World Trade Center and achieve such a great loss of life show just how intent some people are on causing public harm. This new awareness forces the EMS community to prepare itself to respond to acts of terrorism. These acts can come in many forms.

The weapon of choice used by terrorist groups worldwide is the conventional explosive. Conventional explosives have been used frequently in the Middle East and in the British Isles and were used by the Unibomber in the United States. We have also experienced major explosive events such as the destruction of the Physics Annex at the University of Wisconsin in the mid-1960s, the first attempt to destroy the World Trade Center (1993), and the bombing of the Oklahoma City Federal Building (1995). All these involved the use of vehicles filled with high nitrogen-content fertilizer soaked with diesel fuel and parked under or next to the facility.

It is clear that the twenty-first century will bring new terrorism threats using more unconventional means, such as commercial aircraft to bring down structures (Figure 34-1) and **weapons of mass destruction (WMD)** including nuclear, biological, and chemical (NBC) weapons. Harbingers of such acts include the attack on the Tokyo subway system with sarin gas (1996), and letters laced with anthrax spores sent through the mail in North America (2001). Both events underscore the real potential for massive and widespread injury and death caused by those intending to incite terror using WMDs. With the increasing likelihood of a **terrorist act,** EMS personnel become responsible for maintaining a higher index of suspicion for such an event. As an EMT, you also must prepare to protect yourself and your crew, your patients, and the public from the effects of such an attack.

Terrorists may be of foreign or domestic origin. They are likely to target locations that are symbolic of the government (a federal building such as the Pentagon) or that are influenced

The weapon of choice used by terrorist groups worldwide is the conventional explosive.

weapons of mass destruction (WMD) variety of chemical, biological, nuclear, or other devices use by terrorists to strike at government or high-profile targets, designed to create a maximum number of casualties.

terrorist act the use of violence to provoke fear and influence behavior for political, social, religious, or ethnic goals.

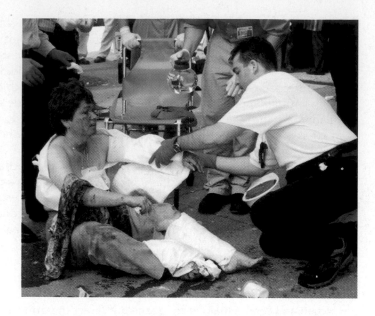

FIGURE 34-1 Providing treatment to a victim of the World Trade Center attack in New York City on September 11, 2001. *(Szenes Jason/Corbis Sygma.)*

Weapons of mass destruction include explosive and incendiary agents, nuclear detonation or contamination, and the release of biological or chemical agents.

by our country (such as an embassy). Domestic terrorists may further target corporations or their executives, who represent a threat to their cause. They may also target their own employer or the public through their employer's products (as in tainted food or pharmaceuticals). The objective of both the domestic and foreign terrorist is to incite terror (intense fear) in the public.

The likely mechanisms of mass destruction used by terrorists include explosive and incendiary agents, nuclear detonation or contamination, and the release of either biological or chemical agents.

EXPLOSIVE AGENTS

explosives chemical(s), when ignited, that instantly generate a great amount of heat resulting in a destructive shock wave and blast wind.

Explosives are the most likely method by which terrorists will strike. The bomb may range from a suicide bomber carrying a few sticks of dynamite to a large vehicle filled with highly explosive material. In an instant, the mechanism detonates and causes damage (Figure 34-2). The blast pressure wave may cause compression/decompression injury to the lungs, ears, and hollow, air-filled organs. Debris thrown by the blast may cause penetrating or blunt injuries, and similar additional injury may occur as the victim is thrown by the blast wind. Secondary combustion may induce burn injury, and structural collapse may cause blunt and crushing injuries. After the initial explosion, associated dangers include structural collapse, fire, electrical hazard, combustible or toxic gas hazards, and secondary explosions intended to disrupt rescue and injure emergency responders. Emergency responders are left to locate, extricate, and provide medical care for the victims. (See Chapter 13, "Blunt Trauma," for a detailed explanation of the blast process, the associated mechanisms of injury, and assessment and care of the blast victim.)

incendiary agents a special subset of explosives with less explosive power but greater heat and burn potential.

Incendiary agents are a special subset of explosives with less explosive power and greater heat and burn potential. Napalm, used extensively during the Vietnam War, is a military example, whereas the Molatov cocktail or gasoline bomb is more of a terrorist weapon. Some incendiary agents are of special concern. White phosphorus may spontaneously combust when exposed to air and may be a part of military munitions or a terrorist weapon. It can be very difficult to extinguish when it contacts the skin. Often, fire-resistant oil is used to exclude the air and extinguish any flame. Another example is magnesium, a metal that burns vigorously and at a high temperature (3,000°C). It also is difficult to extinguish. Incendiary agents are likely to cause severe and extensive burn injuries. (For more on burn injuries, see Chapter 16.)

Content Review

EXAMPLES OF INCENDIARY AGENTS

- Napalm
- Gasoline
- White phosphorus
- Magnesium

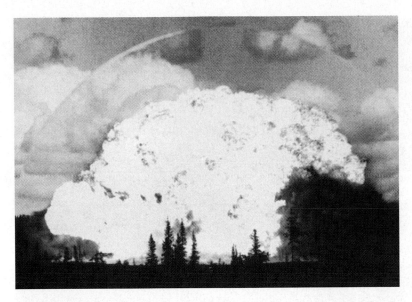

FIGURE 34-2   An explosion releases tremendous amounts of heat energy, generating a pressure wave, blast wind, and projection of debris.

NUCLEAR DETONATION

Nuclear detonation is the release of energy that is generated when heavy nuclei split (fission) or light nuclei combine (fusion) to form new elements. The unleashed energy is tremendous and creates an explosion of immense proportion. In addition to the extremes of the injury-producing mechanisms associated with conventional explosions, radiant heat is likely to incinerate everything in the immediate vicinity of the blast and induce burn injury to exposed skin even at great distances from the blast epicenter. Burn injuries are likely to be the most lethal and debilitating injuries associated with a nuclear detonation.

The damage associated with a typical nuclear detonation is extreme and results in concentric circles of total destruction and mortality, severe destruction and very high mortality, heavy destruction and moderate mortality, and light destruction and limited mortality (Figure 34-3). The explosive energy disrupts communications, power, water and waste service, travel, and the medical, emergency medical, and public safety infrastructures. It is an extreme disaster with great loss of life and injury and presents a great challenge to emergency responders.

The nuclear reaction also generates particles of debris and dust that give off nuclear radiation. Gases, heated by the explosion, draw these particles high into the atmosphere, where upper air currents carry the contamination until it falls to earth as fallout. This uplifting of irradiated debris leaves the scene almost radiation-free from moments after the blast until about one hour, post-ignition.

Nuclear radiation cannot be felt, seen, or otherwise detected by any of our senses. However, it damages the cells of the human body as it passes through them. Radiation passage changes the structure of molecules and essential elements of the cell. Damaged cells then go on to repair themselves, die, or to produce altered or damaged cells (cancer). As the intensity and duration of exposure increases, so do the degree and extent of cell damage and the risk to life. Nuclear radiation from the sun and other natural sources bombards us constantly. This exposure is very limited and the damage caused by it is minimal. However, the initial radiation produced by the nuclear chain reaction (the blast) and **fallout** can produce serious and life-threatening exposure. (See Chapter 16, "Burns," for the types of radiation, mechanisms of injury, and the assessment and care of the irradiated patient.)

A NUCLEAR INCIDENT RESPONSE

The first hour, post ignition, is generally spent moving the injured into structures that will protect them from fallout. Ideally, they are moved into the central areas of large, structurally

nuclear detonation the release of energy that is generated when heavy nuclei split (fission) or light nuclei combine (fusion) to form new elements. The unleashed energy is tremendous and creates an explosion of immense proportion.

Nuclear radiation cannot be felt, seen, or otherwise detected by any of our senses.

fallout radioactive dust and particles that may be life-threatening to people far from the epicenter of a nuclear detonation.

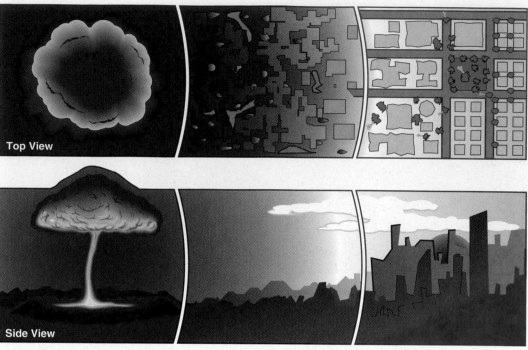

Top View

Side View

Total destruction and mortality   Severe destruction and mortality   Limited destruction and mortality

FIGURE 34-3 The concentric circles of destruction following detonation of a nuclear weapon.

sound buildings or at least to some cover from the falling contaminated dust. Simultaneously, the emergency responders organize, determine the direction of fallout movement, and begin to extricate the walking wounded and seriously injured from the perimeter of the explosion. During this time, evacuation of those in the anticipated path of fallout occurs. (They should remain outside the fallout pathway for at least 48 hours.) Entry into the scene is made from upwind and laterally to upper air movement in order to limit radioactive fallout exposure to rescuers.

As the response is organized, egress and evacuation routes are cleared, the injured are located and evacuated, and the response moves closer and closer to the blast epicenter. In general, some limited medical care is provided where the victims are found but most emergency medical care is provided at treatment sectors, remote from the seriously damaged areas and away from where fallout is expected. Patients are brought to a decontamination area, they are monitored for contamination, and decontaminated as needed, before care begins.

Care for victims of a nuclear detonation involves decontamination (as necessary), treatment associated with a conventional explosion (compression/decompression, blunt and penetrating injury care), and treatment for thermal burns. Burns are the most common and most immediate life-threatening injuries associated with a nuclear detonation and will likely be the focus of most care.

Before victims of a nuclear detonation arrive at an emergency medical treatment sector, someone must monitor them for radioactive contamination. This monitoring is accomplished using a device called a **Geiger counter.** The Geiger counter measures the passage of radioactive particles or rays through a receiving chamber and requires some training to use properly. (Usually, someone specially trained—and other than EMS—provides radioactive monitoring and decontamination.) If any significant radioactivity is noted, the patient's clothing is removed and he is washed with soap, water, and gentle scrubbing, and then rinsed. All contaminated clothing is bagged, and water is collected for proper disposal. A properly decontaminated patient does not pose a radiation threat either to himself or to you. During a response to a suspected nuclear incident, you will likely wear a **dosimeter**, a pen-like device used to record your total radiation exposure. This device is then monitored to determine when your exposure level is such that you should leave the scene for your own safety.

Burns are the most common and most immediate life-threatening injuries associated with a nuclear detonation and will likely be the focus of most care.

Geiger counter an instrument used to detect and measure the radiation given off by an object or area.

---

dosimeter an instrument that measures the cumulative amount of radiation absorbed.

If there is serious risk of fallout and continuing radiation exposure, EMTs may be asked to help distribute sodium iodine tablets. These tablets reduce the uptake of radioactive iodine (a common component of radioactive fallout) by the thyroid, which reduces the risk of thyroid injury or cancer. You may also be involved in the effort to evacuate the public from the expected fallout path.

Generally, patients with serious radiation exposure present with nausea, fatigue, and malaise (a general ill feeling). Treatment for these patients is limited to support, such as keeping them warm and well hydrated. The sooner these symptoms appear after the incident, the more serious the exposure. Generally, if symptoms occur earlier than six hours after the detonation, the exposure was very high. However, the effects of radiation exposure differ widely among individuals, so early diagnosis of the exposure extent and survivability from symptoms is unreliable. Due to the severity and nature of a nuclear detonation, disaster triage is necessary and many serious-to-critical burn patients will not survive, because of the inability of a medical system to care for the sheer number of victims.

> *The sooner symptoms appear after radiation exposure, the more serious the incident. If they appear sooner than 6 hours afterward, the exposure was very high.*

RADIOACTIVE CONTAMINATION

Radioactive contamination may also be spread using conventional explosives (the "**dirty bomb**"). This type of blast is of conventional origin and does not cause the great magnitude of destruction that a nuclear detonation would. However, the explosion distributes radioactive material over a large area and into the surrounding air. The result is an explosion site, with radioactive material contaminating the immediate vicinity. The greatest danger of this terrorist weapon is that the nature of the risk (the radiation) may not be recognized until well after the incident. Consequently, many more individuals and rescuers may be exposed or contaminated. Emergency care for victims of a recognized dirty bomb ignition includes decontamination and treatment (at a remote sector) for injuries that would be expected from a conventional bomb blast.

> **dirty bomb** a conventional explosive device that distributes radioactive material over a large area.

> *Emergency care for victims of a recognized "dirty bomb" includes decontamination and treatment for injuries that would be expected from a conventional bomb blast.*

CHEMICAL AGENTS

Another terrorist weapon of mass destruction is the release of chemical agents. These potential weapons range from simple hazardous materials common in our society, such as chlorine gas, to sophisticated chemicals, such as nerve agents specifically designed to do people harm. Since these chemical weapons are often gases or aerosols that disperse in the wind, the more common targets for their use are confined spaces such as subways or large buildings, which have central heating, air conditioning, or areas where people congregate such as arenas, shopping malls, and convention centers.

The concepts of volatility (vapor pressure) and specific gravity are important to understanding how the chemicals are distributed. **Volatility** is the ease by which a chemical changes from a liquid to a gas. Most chemical weapons are liquids that are moderately volatile. They are often deployed by an explosion or sprayed into the atmosphere creating an aerosol. A chemical that remains a liquid is said to be persistent and poses a contact or absorption threat, whereas vapors, gases, or aerosols present an inhalation danger. An example of a persistent chemical weapon is mustard agent.

Specific gravity refers to the density or weight of the vapor or gas as compared with air. A vapor or gas with a specific gravity less than air rises and quickly disperses into the atmosphere. This limits the effectiveness of the agent as a weapon. A gas with a specific gravity greater than air sinks beneath it, stays close to the ground, and accumulates in low places. Closed spaces, such as a basement, or low areas like a river valley resist dispersal of the vapor and maintain the danger. Common chemicals with high specific gravity include chlorine and phosgene.

Environmental conditions affect the dispersal of chemical weapons. In strong winds the gas or vapor mixes with large quantities of air and dilutes and disperses very quickly, limiting its concentration and effectiveness. Light wind moves the cloud downwind as a unit, increasing its effectiveness and the area involved. In windless conditions (which are infrequent) the cloud remains stationary, decreasing the area affected by it. Precipitation, especially rain, may deactivate or absorb some agents (such as chlorine). Early morning and

> **volatility** the ease by which a chemical changes from a liquid to a gas; the tendency of a chemical agent to evaporate.

> **specific gravity** refers to the density or weight of a vapor or gas as compared with air.

nerve agents chemicals that inhibit the degradation of a neurotransmitter (acetylcholine) and quickly facilitate a nervous system overload.

fasciculations involuntary contractions or twitchings of muscle fibers.

rhinorrhea watery discharge from the nose.

miosis abnormal contraction of the pupils; pinpoint pupils.

The actions of nerve agents can generally be reversed if the antidote is administered shortly after exposure.

Mark I kit a two-part auto-injector set the military uses as treatment for nerve-agent exposure; involves the administration of atropine and then pralidoxime chloride.

vesicants agents that damage exposed skin, frequently causing vesicles (blisters).

the time just before sunset are ideal for agent release because the winds are usually at their lowest velocity. The interior of a building with few open windows, especially when being heated or air-conditioned, is an especially controlled environment. A release of a chemical agent there can remain concentrated and deadly.

Chemical weapons are classified according to the way they cause damage to the human body. The chemicals include nerve agents, vesicants, pulmonary agents, biotoxins, and other hazardous chemicals.

NERVE AGENTS

Nerve agents (and some insecticides) damage nervous impulse conduction. These agents generally inhibit the degradation of a neurotransmitter (acetylcholine) and quickly cause a nervous system overload. This results in muscle spasms, convulsions, unconsciousness, and respiratory failure. Some common examples of nerve agents include GB (sarin), VX, GF, GD (soman), and GA (tabun). Although not designed as weapons, organophosphate and carbamate insecticides share a similar mechanism of action to nerve agents, but are much less potent.

Nerve agents, present as both vapor and liquid, are capable of being absorbed through the skin or inhaled and absorbed through the respiratory system. Exposure quickly leads to a series of signs and symptoms remembered as SLUDGE, or *S*alivation, *L*acrimation, *U*rination, *D*efecation, and *G*astric *E*mptying. In addition to these signs, the patient may experience dyspnea, **fasciculations** (these are prominent), **rhinorrhea**, blurry vision, **miosis**, nausea, and sweating. Ultimately, the patient may become unconscious, seize, stop breathing, and die.

The actions of nerve agents can generally be reversed if the antidote is administered shortly after exposure. However, many nerve agents permanently bind to the chemicals reabsorbing the neurotransmitters and their effects become more difficult to reverse. The prognosis for a patient exposed to a nerve agent is good if the antidote is administered quickly and artificial ventilation is provided.

Treatment for nerve-agent exposure includes the administration of atropine and then pralidoxime chloride. The military currently has these medications available in a two-part auto-injector set called a **Mark I kit.** As the threat of nerve agent release to the civilian population becomes greater, these kits may become more and more available to the EMS provider. The auto-injectors are designed for self-administration or buddy-administration (mainly for military personnel) or may be administered by rescue personnel. They are quick to use and may be necessary when confronted with numerous patients exposed to a nerve agent. The antidote combination is often followed by the administration of diazepam to reduce seizure activity. The auto-injector is a convenient way to administer this regimen of medications; however, the intravenous route is more rapid and preferred when available and as time permits.

The Mark I kit contains 2 mg of atropine and 600 mg of pradoxime chloride. It is administered for the first and mild symptoms of exposure (blurry vision, mild dyspnea, and rhinorrhea) and repeated in 10 minutes if symptoms do not improve. If serious signs and symptoms are present, three doses of both atropine and pralidoxime chloride may be administered. Intravenous administration should provide 2 mg of atropine every five minutes (until drying of secretions or 20 mg is administered) and 1 gm of pralidoxime chloride every hour (until spontaneous respirations return). A pediatric version of the Mark I kit is available overseas and may soon be available in the United States.

VESICANTS (BLISTERING AGENTS)

Vesicants are agents that damage exposed skin, frequently causing vesicles (blisters). They are capable of causing damage to the skin, eyes, respiratory tract and lungs, and are able to induce generalized illness as well. The mustard gas of World War I is an example of a vesicant. Other examples include sulfur mustard (HD), nitrogen mustard (HN), lewisite (L), and phosgene oxime (CX). With the exception of phosgene oxime, the vesicants are thick oily liquids that create a vapor threat in warm temperatures. The liquid form, however, is highly toxic to the touch. Lewisite and phosgene oxime induce immediate irritation on contact or inhalation, whereas the mustards produce only slight discomfort that becomes more severe with time. This is important because mustard-exposed patients may not realize it at the time.

Patients exposed to vesicants present with the signs and symptoms of injury to the skin, mucous membranes, and the lungs. Exposed skin exhibits the signs of a chemical burn including pain, **erythema,** and eventually blistering. The eyes and upper airway display a burning or stinging sensation with tearing and rhinorrhea. Respiratory tract exposure results in dyspnea, cough, wheezing, and pulmonary edema. Systemic signs and symptoms include nausea, vomiting, and fatigue. Signs and symptoms occur slowly with the mustard agents and may prolong exposure.

Emergency care for the patient exposed to a vesicant is immediate decontamination. Exposure of even a few minutes can result in permanent injury. The exposed areas should be irrigated immediately with water from a hose (using limited pressure if possible). Also, irrigate the eyes with a preference for saline over water, but do not delay irrigation awaiting the proper fluid. If blistering has occurred, treat the lesions as you would any chemical burn. Apply loose sterile dressings, patch any effected eyes and medicate the patient for any serious pain.

erythema general reddening of the skin due to dilation of the superficial capillaries.

Emergency care for the patient exposed to a vesicant is immediate decontamination.

PULMONARY AGENTS

Pulmonary agents are those that primarily cause chemical injury to the lungs. They are agents similar to phosgene and chlorine. Some of the by-products, created as synthetics such as plastic, combust. These agents attack the mucous membranes of the respiratory system from the oral pharynx and nasal pharynx to the smaller respiratory bronchioles and alveoli. They produce inflammation and pulmonary edema resulting in dyspnea and hypoxia. Early signs and symptoms of pulmonary-agent exposure are related to irritation of the upper airway. They include rhinorrhea, nasal and throat irritation, wheezing, and cough. The victim may also experience tearing and eye irritation. Pulmonary edema is generally a late sign of exposure.

Emergency care for the individual exposed to a pulmonary agent is removal from the environment; high-flow, high-concentration oxygen; and rest. Endotracheal intubation and ventilation may be required. In cases of moderate to severe respiratory distress, consider 0.5 mL of albuteral by nebulized inhalation.

pulmonary agents chemicals that primarily cause injury to the lungs; commonly referred to as choking agents.

Emergency care for pulmonary agent exposure is removal from the environment, high-flow, high-concentration oxygen, and rest.

BIOTOXINS

Another type of agent that is classified as a biological agent but behaves more like a chemical agent is the **biotoxin.** These toxins are produced by a living organism but are themselves not alive. Such agents include ricin, staphylococcal enterotoxin B (SEB), botulinum toxin, and trichothecene mycotoxins (T2). Ricin, a by-product of making castor oil, inhibits the body's ability to synthesize proteins. It may be either aerosolized and inhaled or ingested. Ricin causes pulmonary edema when inhaled and gastric symptoms when ingested. Poisoning by both routes may cause multiple organ failure and shock.

Staphylococcal enterotoxin (SEB) is produced by a bacterium, *Staphylococcus aureus,* and is the agent most commonly responsible for food poisoning. Contamination may occur either orally, causing nausea and vomiting, or by inhalation, causing dyspnea and fever. Though only a small amount of toxin may cause symptoms and 50% of those contaminated may be incapacitated, SEB is rarely fatal.

Botulinum, the most toxic agent known, is an infrequent result of improper canning technique. It is 15,000 times more potent that VX, the most lethal nerve agent. Like the nerve agents, botulinum attacks the nervous system. It interferes with impulse transmission and interrupts the central nervous system's control of the organs. The result is weakness, paralysis, and death by respiratory failure. Botulinum can be ingested or inhaled.

Trichothecene mycotoxins are a group of biotoxins produced by fungus molds. They prohibit protein and nucleic acid formulation and effect body cells that divide rapidly first. T2 acts very quickly, causing skin irritation (pain, burning, redness, and blistering), respiratory irritation (nasal and oral pain, rhinorrhea, epistaxis, wheezing, dyspnea, and hemoptysis), eye

biotoxin poisons that are produced by a living organism but are themselves not alive.

irritation (pain, redness pain, tearing, and blurry vision), and gastrointestinal symptoms (nausea, vomiting, abdominal cramping, and bloody diarrhea). Generalized signs and symptoms include central nervous system signs, hypotension, and death.

Management of a victim of a biotoxin is supportive; antitoxins are generally not available. A special concern is directed to careful decontamination as even a very small amount of biotoxin can endanger rescuers and others.

OTHER HAZARDOUS CHEMICALS

Any toxic chemical has a potential for use as a weapon of mass destruction. Industry produces countless hazardous materials with the potential to cause great harm if released into the air or water supply or ignited to release toxic gases. The only difference between an accidental release and one that is intended to incite terror is that the intentional release will likely be optimized to affect the greatest number of people. It may also be more difficult to identify the agent used by a terrorist because the container will likely not identify the agent. The Department of Transportation's *Emergency Response Guidebook* (Figure 34-4), which is carried on ambulances and fire apparatus, is a good guide to most common hazardous materials that might be used as a weapon. It can also be helpful in denoting isolation and evacuation distances and suggesting specific care management steps.

RECOGNITION OF A CHEMICAL AGENT RELEASE

A chemical-weapon release may be visible as a cloud of mist, vapor, dust, or as puddles, or it may be completely unrecognizable. There may be an associated smell such as that of newly mown grass (phosgene), the smell of rotten eggs (hydrogen sulfide), or other strange or unusual odors. However, never search out such an odor. You may also notice injured, inca-

FIGURE 34-4 Department of Transportation's *Emergency Response Guidebook. (Craig Jackson/In the Dark Photography)*

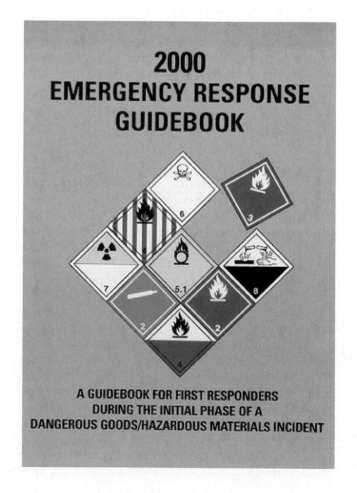

pacitated, or dead insects, birds, or animals. Given that the terrorist may be intent on optimizing the effect of the release, be especially wary of large public gatherings or large but confined spaces such as a public building, and low spaces that limit dissipation such as subway terminals. Terrorists may also target food or water supplies with either chemical or biological agents. This may result in very widespread effects.

A cardinal sign of a chemical release is the manifestation of common signs and symptoms occurring rapidly among a group of individuals. Common signs of a chemical release include inflamed mucosa (eye, nasal, oral, or throat irritation), exposed skin irritation, chest tightness, burning and/or dyspnea, gastrointestinal signs (nausea, abdominal cramping, vomiting, and diarrhea) and central nervous system disturbances (confusion, lethargy, nausea/vomiting, intoxication, headache, and unconsciousness).

MANAGEMENT OF A CHEMICAL AGENT RELEASE

Approach the scene from upwind and remain a good distance away from the site. Generally, evacuate the immediate area if the release is small and contained. However, if the release involves a great quantity of material, such as that in a tank car or large commercial storage container, evacuate the general population for a radius of 700 to 2,000 feet and 1½ miles downwind during the day. If the release occurs at night, then evacuate a 2,000-foot radius and as much as 6 to 7 miles downwind.

Once the public danger is reduced by scene isolation, make sure the injured are properly decontaminated before you begin care (Figure 34-5). The agency that provides spill containment and decontamination at the hazardous materials incident generally provides decontamination for both nuclear and chemical weapons of mass destruction. (This is most commonly the fire department.)

In addition to the emergency care steps noted earlier, most patients require oxygen administration and possibly respiratory support.

A cardinal sign of a chemical release is the manifestation of common signs and symptoms occurring rapidly among a group of individuals.

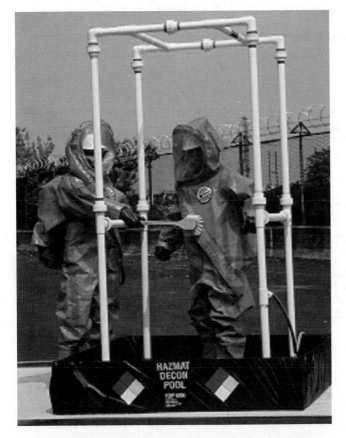

FIGURE 34-5 Rescuers in decontamination process.

BIOLOGICAL AGENTS

biological agents either living organisms or toxins produced by living organisms that are deliberately distributed to cause disease and death.

Biological agents are either living organisms or toxins produced by living organisms that are deliberately distributed to cause disease and death. Generally, these agents are grouped as non-contagious (anthrax and biotoxins) or as contagious and capable of spreading from human to human (smallpox, ebola, plague). Contagious agents are of greatest concern because the people originally infected can spread the disease, often before the medical community has recognized that a biological weapon attack has occurred. The EMS and other medical systems are especially vulnerable because they are called to treat those who first display the disease's signs and symptoms, possibly before the nature and significance of the disease is known. Non-contagious agents affect only those who received the initial dose, thus limiting the scope of the disease and making it somewhat easier to identify when and where the contact took place.

Recognition of biological agent release is difficult. Often there is no noticeable cloud of gas or any noticeable odor. Recognition is especially difficult because any signs and symptoms of the disease occur at the end of the incubation period, often days or weeks after the initial contact. Rapid identification is further complicated as many potential biological weapons present with signs and symptoms typical of influenza or many other general illnesses. (See Table 34-1.) Most commonly, the existence of a biological attack is recognized when numerous patients report to the emergency department or physician's office with similar signs and symptoms. Only then can the health department begin to work to identify the disease's nature and when and where the exposure most likely happened. By the time the disease outbreak is recognized as a bioterrorism event, secondary exposures from those affected by contagious agents may already be occurring. These secondary exposures may include family members, friends, workmates, and the medical system, including EMS, emergency department personnel, and other health-care providers.

Most commonly, the existence of a biological attack is recognized when numerous patients report to the emergency department with similar signs and symptoms.

Mother Nature may be the most sinister of all bioterrorists. Mutant strains of common diseases such as the more serious variations of influenza, multi-drug resistant strains of tuberculosis, or the recent cold-like virus called *severe acute respiratory syndrome (SARS)* may emerge and create epidemics of massive proportions. They even may be more likely than a terrorist's use of a biological weapon. Tracking the origin and combating these naturally occurring diseases is exactly like tracking and combating a biological weapon used by terrorists.

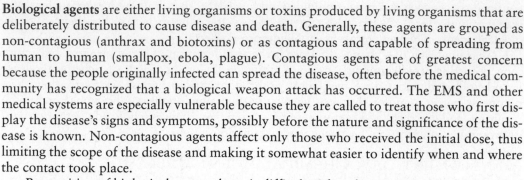

Disease	Incubation Period	Mortality	Signs and Symptoms				
			Fever	Chills	Cough	Malaise	Nausea/ Vomiting
Anthrax	1–6 days	90%	√		√	√	
Pneumonic plague*	1–6 days	57%–100%	√	√	√	√	
Tularemia	3–5 days	35%	√		√	√	
Q Fever	2–14 days	1%	√		√	√	
Smallpox*	12 days	30%	√			√	√
Venezuelan equine encephalitis	1–5 days	1%	√	√	√	√	√
Cholera	1–3 days	50%					√
Viral hemorrhagic fever	3–7 days	5%–20%	√			√	
Ebola*	3–7 days	80%–90%	√			√	

*Human-to-human contagious disease.

Currently the list of potential WMD diseases is extensive and contains pneumonia-like agents, encephalitis-like agents, and others.

PNEUMONIA-LIKE AGENTS

Pneumonia-like bioterror agents include anthrax, plague, tularemia, and Q fever, and are probably the most likely agents for a terrorist attack. They are sometimes called influenza-like agents because of common, non-specific symptoms. They all cause cough, dyspnea, fever, and malaise. Anthrax and plague are the most deadly, with 90% to 100% mortality. Anthrax is not contagious, thus limiting any human-to-human transmission. The strain of plague most likely used for bioterrorism is pneumonic, which carries not only a very high mortality (100% untreated and about 57% when treated), but also has minimum survival when left untreated for the first 18 hours after signs and symptoms appear. Q fever is more of an incapacitating disease with a very low death rate.

ENCEPHALITIS-LIKE AGENTS

Smallpox and Venezuelan equine encephalitis (VEE) are influenza-like diseases with a higher mortality, probably because they attack the central nervous system. They are very effective as biological weapons because small amounts of aerosolized agent can cause the disease. Smallpox is also very contagious. Human-to-human transmission does not occur with VEE. Smallpox is considered eradicated as a natural occurring disease, but it is thought to exist in the WMD programs of some countries.

OTHER AGENTS

Cholera is a common disease in underdeveloped countries and is frequently related to poor sanitation. It is most commonly transmitted through the fecal-oral route and primarily causes severe dehydration and shock because of profuse diarrhea. It is one of the few agents that is not transmitted by the inhalation route and may be delivered as a weapon by way of contamination of food or untreated water.

Viral hemorrhagic fever (VHF) is a class of disease that includes the deadly ebola virus. As the name suggests, hemorrhagic fever attacks the bloodstream and damages blood vessels, causing them to leak and bleed. The patient may bruise easily and display petechia (tiny red patches of dermal hemorrhage). Most diseases of this class can be spread through the inhalation route or through direct contact with infectious material.

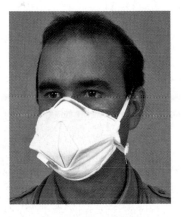

FIGURE 34-6 High efficiency particulate air (HEPA) respirator.

PROTECTION AGAINST BIOLOGICAL AGENT TRANSMISSION

Protection against the most common of biological agents used as weapons includes the prudent care steps used to prevent ordinary communicable disease transmission. If there is a heightened alert status for a WMD release or terrorist event, employ a more aggressive use of body substance isolation (BSI) precautions. Gloves are very effective in protecting against biological agent transmission from bodily fluids, as is rigorous and frequent hand-washing. Almost all biological agents are transmitted by the respiratory route, so be sure to take droplet inhalation precautions. A properly fitted HEPA respirator is very effective in preventing agent transmission (Figure 34-6). A sodium hypochlorite solution (0.5%) or other disinfectants are very effective in killing most biological agents. The ambulance interior and any equipment used or possibly contaminated should be vigorously cleaned with the solution.

Immunizations against many biological agents are not available. Those immunizations that are available usually carry a small risk of associated reaction. Hence, the prophylactic administration to a very large number of health-care workers may not be warranted unless or until a significant risk becomes apparent. Consult with your medical director for your system's recommendations and the method used to provide you with immunizations if the need arises.

Emergency care for most patients affected by biological weapons is limited to supportive care (maintain body temperature, administer oxygen and, in some cases, IV fluids). Once the exact organism is isolated (after prehospital care), then a regimen of antibiotic therapy may be prescribed.

Protection against biological agents used as weapons includes the prudent care steps used to prevent ordinary communicable disease transmission.

Emergency care for most patients affected by biological weapons is limited to supportive care.

If a biological attack is suspected, health officials will interview the victims carefully. They will try to determine when the patients first noticed symptoms and identify any close personal contacts since that time. These people may be infected if the agent is indeed contagious.

GENERAL CONSIDERATIONS REGARDING TERRORIST ATTACKS

SCENE SAFETY

One in every five victims of the World Trade Center collapse on September 11, 2001, was a member of an emergency response team. This great number of emergency personnel deaths underscores the need to recognize the dangers to EMS providers and ensure that safety is an active concern during the response to an act of terrorism.

Terrorists in other countries often set second explosive devices with the intent to disrupt any rescue attempt. A chemical release or radioactivity can linger and affect those who attempt unprotected rescue of patients. It is imperative that you carefully analyze a scene to determine the risk to you and other rescuers. Then ensure the scene is entered only by those trained and equipped to enter a hazardous or deadly environment.

Carefully analyze an emergency scene to determine the risk to you and other rescuers. Then make sure the scene is entered only by those trained and equipped to do so.

RECOGNIZING A TERRORIST ATTACK

It is relatively easy to recognize a nuclear or conventional explosion. However, remember that radioactive fallout travels with the upper wind current (not just those at ground level), so watch cloud movement. Stay upwind. Remember, too, that terrorists may use the conventional explosion to distribute radioactive material (the "dirty bomb"), and they may set secondary detonations through booby traps or secondary timers to target rescuers. Also be aware of structural collapse, because the explosion may weaken a building's structure. Do not enter the scene until you are sure it is safe from all hazards.

Recognition of a chemical release may not be as obvious. There may be no cloud of gas or aerosolized material. There may be no unusual odors either. However, groups of victims will be complaining of similar symptoms, though symptom development may take some time. Stay upwind of the site and request that victims and potential victims evacuate (or be evacuated) to you. Only personnel who are specially trained and equipped to deal with hazardous materials should enter the scene.

Identifying a biological agent at the time of release is probably impossible. There might be a cloud of dust or aerosolized material but there are no immediate signs and symptoms from those exposed. Such contamination also may be distributed by the mail (anthrax-laced letters, for instance) or other vehicles. The incident is likely to be recognized after the incubation period and only after several patients report to the emergency department with the disease. Then the local health department will try to find out what all victims have in common to identify where the biological agent release took place.

RESPONDING TO A TERRORIST ATTACK

Your first role in responding to a possible act of terrorism is to ensure your own safety and that of your patient, other rescuers, and the public. Once safety is ensured, make certain all patients are properly decontaminated (if need be), and then begin to provide the appropriate emergency medical care.

Your role as an emergency care provider for a terrorist attack is very similar to the other emergency responses you are more likely to encounter during your career. A nuclear incident is handled like a conventional explosion with a hazardous material (radiation) involved. The release of a chemical agent is a hazardous material incident. A biological weapon release is handled like an infectious disease outbreak. Although the location of the attack may optimize the number of people it affects, it is still a hazardous material incident (chemical or radiation agent), an infectious disease incident (biological event), a conventional explosion, or a combination of the above. Use your training and follow your system's protocols and disaster plans for each of these incidents.

SUMMARY

Many of the mechanisms of injury used by terrorists subtly induce their damage (toxic gases, radiation contamination, or biological agents) so that there is little scene evidence. Your responsibility is to maintain an enhanced lookout for any signs of NBC release or exposure and limit the contact you, the general population, and your patients have to such an agent. In general, it is not the role of EMS to deal with NBC agents. Your role as an EMT-I is likely to provide supportive care after patient decontamination.

ON THE WEB

For additional practice and review, go to the companion website at www.prenhall.com/bledsoe and click on *Intermediate Emergency Care: Principles & Practice*.

Glossary

2,3-diphosphoglycerate (2,3-DPG) chemical in the red blood cells that affects hemoglobin's affinity for oxygen.

abandonment termination of the EMT-I/patient relationship without assurance that an equal or greater level of care will continue.

ABCs airway, breathing, and circulation.

abduction movement of a body part away from the midline.

aberrant conduction conduction of the electrical impulse through the heart's conductive system in an abnormal fashion.

ABO blood group two antigens known as A and B. A person may have either (type A or type B), both (type AB), or neither (type O).

abortion termination of pregnancy before the twentieth week of gestation. The term "abortion" refers to both miscarriage and induced abortion.

abrasion scraping or abrading away of the superficial layers of the skin.

abruptio placentae a condition in which the placenta separates from the uterine wall.

absence seizure type of generalized seizure with sudden onset, characterized by a brief loss of awareness and rapid recovery.

absolute refractory period the period of the cardiac cycle when the myocardial cells have not completely repolarized and stimulation will not produce any depolarization whatever.

absorption *see* surface absorption.

acceleration the rate at which speed or velocity increases.

acclimatization the reversible changes in body structure and function by which the body becomes adjusted to a change in environment.

acetylcholinesterase (AChE) enzyme that stops the action of acetylocholine, a neurotransmitter.

acid a substance that liberates hydrogen ions (H+) when in solution.

acidosis a high concentration of hydrogen ions; a pH below 7.35.

ACLS advanced cardiac life support.

acquired immunity protection from infection or disease that is (a) developed by the body after exposure to an antigen (active acquired immunity) or (b) transferred to the person from an outside source such as from the mother through the placenta or as a serum (passive acquired immunity).

acquired immunodeficiency syndrome *see* AIDS.

acrocyanosis cyanosis of the extremities.

action potential the stimulation of myocardial cells, as evidenced by a change in the membrane electrical charge, that subsequently spreads across the myocardium.

activated charcoal a powder, usually pre-mixed with water, that will adsorb (bind) some poisons and help prevent them from being absorbed by the body.

active immunity acquired immunity that occurs following exposure to an antigen and results in the production of antibodies specific for the antigen; immunity developed after birth as a result of a direct exposure to an antigen or disease.

active listening the process of responding to your patient's statements with words or gestures that demonstrate your understanding.

active rescue zone area where special rescue teams operate; also known as the *hot zone* or *inner circle*.

active transport movement of a substance through a cell membrane against the osmotic gradient; that is, from an area of lesser concentration to an area of greater concentration, opposite to the normal direction of diffusion; requires the use of energy.

actual damages refers to compensable physical, psychological, or financial harm.

acuity the severity or acuteness of your patient's condition.

acute arterial occlusion the sudden occlusion of arterial blood flow.

acute effects signs and/or symptoms rapidly displayed upon exposure to a toxic substance.

acute gastroenteritis sudden onset of inflammation of the stomach and intestines.

acute myocardial infarction (AMI) *see* myocardial infarction.

acute pulmonary embolism blockage that occurs when a blood clot or other particle lodges in a pulmonary artery.

acute renal failure (ARF) the sudden-onset of severely decreased urine production.

acute respiratory distress syndrome (ARDS) respiratory insufficiency marked by progressive hypoxemia, due to severe inflammatory damage and fluid accumulation in the alveoli of the lungs. Also called *adult respiratory distress syndrome*.

acute retinal artery occlusion a non-traumatic occlusion of the retinal artery resulting in a sudden, painless loss of vision in one eye.

acute tubular necrosis a particular syndrome characterized by the sudden death of renal tubular cells.

addendum addition or supplement to an original report.

addiction compulsive and overwhelming dependence on a drug; may be physiological, psychological, or both.

Addison's disease endocrine disorder characterized by adrenocortical insufficiency. Symptoms may include weakness, fatigue, weight loss, and hyperpigmentation of skin and mucous membranes.

Addisonian crisis form of shock associated with adrenocortical insufficiency and characterized by profound hypotension and electrolyte imbalances.

adduction movement of a body part toward the midline.

adenosine triphosphate (ATP) a high-energy compound present in all cells, especially muscle cells; when split by enzyme action, it yields energy.

adhesion union of normally separate tissue surfaces by a fibrous band of new tissue.

adjunct medication agent that enhances the effects of other drugs.

administration tubing flexible, clear plastic tubing that connects the solution bag to the IV cannula.

administrative law law that is enacted by governmental agencies at either the federal or state level. Also called *regulatory law*.

adrenergic pertaining to the neurotransmitter norepinephrine.

adrenocorticotropic hormone hormone secreted by the anterior lobe of the pituitary gland that is essential to the function of the adrenal cortex, including production of glucocorticoids.

adult respiratory distress syndrome *see* acute respiratory distress syndrome.

advance directive a document created to ensure that certain treatment choices are honored when a patient is unable to express his choice of treatment.

advanced life support (ALS) advanced life-saving procedures such as intravenous therapy, drug therapy, intubation, and defibrillation.

aerobic with oxygen or requiring oxygen.

aerobic metabolism the stage of metabolism requiring the presence of oxygen, in which the breakdown of glucose (in a process called the Krebs or citric acid cycle) yields a high amount of energy.

aeromedical evacuations transport by helicopter.

affect visible indicators of mood.

afferent carrying impulses toward the central nervous system. Sensory nerves are afferent nerves.

affinity force of attraction between a drug and a receptor.

afterbirth the placenta and accompanying membranes that are expelled from the uterus after the birth of a child.

afterload the resistance a contraction of the heart must overcome in order to eject blood; in cardiac physiology, defined as the tension of cardiac muscle during systole (contraction).

against medical advice (AMA) when a patient refuses medical care after being advised that he needs it.

ageism discrimination against aged or elderly people.

aggregate to cluster or come together.

agonist drug that binds to a receptor and causes it to initiate the expected response.

agonist-antagonist drug that binds to a receptor and stimulates some of its effects but blocks others; also called *partial agonist*.

AIDS acquired immunodeficiency syndrome, a group of signs, symptoms, and disorders that often develop as a consequence of HIV infection.

air embolism air in the vein.

airbags inflatable high-pressure pillows that when inflated can lift up to 20 tons, depending upon the make.

airborne transmitted through the air by droplets or particles.

air-purifying respirator (APR) system of filtering a normal environment for a specific chemical substance using filter cartridges.

albumin a protein commonly present in plant and animal tissues. In the blood, albumin works to maintain blood volume and blood pressure and provides colloid osmotic pressure, which prevents plasma loss from the capillaries.

aldosterone hormone secreted by the adrenal cortex that increases sodium reabsorption by the kidneys; it plays a part in regulation of blood volume, blood pressure, and blood levels of potassium, chloride, and bicarbonate.

algorithm schematic flow chart that outlines appropriate care for specific signs and symptoms.

alkali a substance that liberates hydroxyl ions (OH^-) when in solution; a strong base.

alkalosis a low concentration of hydrogen ions; a pH above 7.45.

allergen a substance capable of inducing allergy of specific hypersensitivity.

allergic reaction an exaggerated response by the immune system to a foreign substance.

allergy exaggerated immune response to an environmental antigen.

allied health professions ancillary health-care professions, apart from physicians and nurses.

alloimmunity *see* isoimmunity.

alpha radiation low level form of nuclear radiation; a weak source of energy that is stopped by clothing or the first layers of skin.

ALS *see* advanced life support.

alveoli microscopic air sacs where most oxygen and carbon dioxide gas exchanges take place.

Alzheimer's disease a degenerative brain disorder; the most common cause of dementia in the elderly.

amniotic fluid clear, watery fluid that surrounds and protects the developing fetus.

amniotic sac the membranes that surround and protect the developing fetus throughout the period of intrauterine development.

ampere basic unit for measuring the strength of an electric current.

amphiarthrosis joint that permits a limited amount of independent motion.

ampule breakable glass vessel containing liquid medication.

amputation severance, removal, or detachment, either partial or complete, of a body part.

amyotrophic lateral sclerosis (ALS) progressive degeneration of specific nerve cells that control voluntary movement characterized by weakness, loss of motor control, difficulty speaking, and cramping. Also called *Lou Gehrig's disease*.

anabolism the constructive phase of metabolism in which cells convert nonliving substances into living cytoplasm.

anaerobic metabolism the stage of metabolism that does not require oxygen, in which the breakdown of glucose (in a process called glycolysis) produces pyruvic acid and yields very little energy.

anaerobic able to live without oxygen.

analgesia the absence of the sensation of pain.

analgesic medication that relieves the sensation of pain.

anaphylactic shock *see* anaphylaxis.

anaphylaxis a life-threatening allergic reaction; also called *anaphylactic shock*.

anastomosis communication between two or more blood vessels.

anatomy the structure of an organism; body structure.

anchor time set of hours when a night-shift worker can reliably expect to rest without interruption.

anemia a reduction in the hemoglobin content in the blood to a point below that required to meet the oxygen requirements of the body.

anesthesia the absence of all sensation.

anesthetic medication that induces a loss of sensation to touch or pain.

aneurysm a weakening or ballooning in the wall of a blood vessel.

anger hostility or rage to compensate for an underlying feeling of anxiety.

angina pectoris chest pain that results when blood supply's oxygen demands exceed the heart's.

angiocatheter *see* over-the-needle catheter.

angioneurotic edema marked edema of the skin that usually involves the head, neck, face, and upper airway; a common manifestation of severe allergic reactions and anaphylaxis.

anion an ion with a negative charge—so called because it will be attracted to an anode, or positive pole.

anithyperlipidemic drug used to treat high blood cholesterol.

anorexia nervosa psychological disorder characterized by voluntary refusal to eat.

anorexia absence of appetite.

anoxia the absence or near-absence of oxygen.

anoxic hypoxemia an oxygen deficiency due to disordered pulmonary mechanisms of oxygenation.

antacid alkalotic compound used to increase the gastric environment's pH.

antagonist drug that binds to a receptor but does not cause it to initiate the expected response.

antepartum before the onset of labor.

anterior toward the front of the body. *Opposite of* posterior.

anterior cord syndrome condition that is caused by bony fragments or pressure compressing the arteries of the anterior spinal cord and resulting in loss of motor function and sensation to pain, light touch, and temperature below the injury site.

anterior medial fissure deep crease along the ventral surface of the spinal cord that divides the cord into right and left halves.

anterograde amnesia inability to remember events that occurred after the trauma that caused the condition.

antibiotics substances that destroy or inhibit microorganisms; agents that kill or decrease the growth of bacteria.

antibody a substance produced by B lymphocytes in response to the presence of a foreign antigen that will combine with and control or destroy the antigen, thus preventing infection.

anticholinergic agent agent that blocks parasympathetic nerve impulses.

anticipatory thinking ahead.

anticoagulant drug that inhibits blood clotting.

antidiuresis formation and passage of a concentrated urine, preserving blood volume.

antidiuretic hormone (ADH) hormone released by the posterior pituitary that induces an increase in peripheral vascular resistance and causes the kidneys to retain water, decreasing urine output, and also causes splenic vascular constriction.

antidote a substance that will neutralize a specific toxin or counteract its effect on the body.

antidysrhythmic drug used to treat and prevent abnormal cardiac rhythms.

antiemetic medication used to prevent vomiting.

antigen protein on the surface of a donor's red blood cells that the patient's body recognizes as "self" or "not self."

antigen processing the recognition, ingestion, and breakdown of a foreign antigen, culminating in production of an antibody to the antigen or in a direct cytotoxic response to the antigen.

antigen-antibody complex the substance formed when an antibody combines with an antigen to deactivate or destroy it; also called *immune complex.*

antigen-presenting cells (APCs) cells, such as macrophages, that present (express onto their surfaces) portions of the antigens they have digested.

antihyperlipidemic drug used to treat high blood cholesterol.

antihypertensive drug used to treat hypertension.

antineoplastic agent drug used to treat cancer.

antiplatelet drug that decreases the formation of platelet plugs.

antiseptic cleansing agent that is not toxic to living tissue.

antitussive medication that suppresses the stimulus to cough in the central nervous system.

anuria no elimination of urine.

anxiety disorder condition characterized by dominating apprehension and fear.

anxiety state of uneasiness, discomfort, apprehension, and restlessness.

anxious avoidant attachment a type of bonding that occurs when an infant learns that his caregivers will not be responsive or helpful when needed.

anxious resistant attachment a type of bonding that occurs when an infant learns to be uncertain about whether or not his caregivers will be responsive or helpful when needed.

aortic dissection a degeneration of the wall of the aorta.

APGAR scoring a numerical system of rating the condition of a newborn. It evaluates the newborn's heart rate, respiratory rate, muscle tone, reflex irritability, and color.

aphasia absence or impairment of the ability to communicate through speaking, writing, or signing as a result of brain dysfunction; occurs when the individual suffers brain damage due to stroke or head injury.

apnea absence of breathing.

apneustic respiration breathing characterized by a prolonged inspiration unrelieved by expiration attempts, seen in patients with damage to the upper part of the pons.

apoptosis response in which an injured cell releases enzymes that engulf and destroy itself; one way the body rids itself of damaged and dead cells.

appendicitis inflammation of the vermiform appendix at the juncture of the large and small intestines.

appendicular skeleton bones of the extremities, shoulder girdle, and pelvis (excepting the sacrum).

aqueous humor clear fluid filling the anterior chamber of the eye.

arachnoid membrane middle layer of the meninges.

ARDS *see* acute respiratory distress syndrome.

arrhythmia the absence of cardiac electrical activity; often used interchangeably with dysrhythmia.

arterial gas embolism (AGE) an air bubble, or air embolism, that enters the circulatory system from a damaged lung.

arteries vessels that carry blood from the heart to the body tissues.

arteriole a small artery.

arteriosclerosis a thickening, loss of elasticity, and hardening of the walls of the arteries from calcium deposits.

arthritis inflammation of a joint.

articular surface surface of a bone that moves against another bone.

artifact deflection on the ECG produced by factors other than the heart's electrical activity.

ascending loop of Henle the part of the nephron tubule beyond the descending loop of Henle.

ascending reticular activating system a series of nervous tissues keeping the human system in a state of consciousness.

ascending tracts bundles of axons along the spinal cord that transmit signals from the body to the brain.

ascites bulges in the flanks and across the abdomen, indicating edema caused by congestive heart failure.

asepsis a condition free of pathogens.

asphyxia a decrease in the amount of oxygen and an increase in the amount of carbon dioxide as a result of some interference with respiration.

aspiration inhaling foreign material such as vomitus into the lungs.

assault an act that unlawfully places a person in apprehension of immediate bodily harm without his consent.

assay test that determines the amount and purity of a given chemical in a preparation in the laboratory.

asthma a condition marked by recurrent attacks of dyspnea with wheezing due to spasmodic constriction of the bronchi, often as a response to allergens, or by mucous plugs in the arterial walls.

ataxic respiration poor respirations due to CNS damage, causing ineffective thoracic muscular coordination.

atelectasis alveolar collapse; collapse of a lung or part of a lung.

atherosclerosis a progressive, degenerative disease of the medium-sized and large arteries.

atrophy a decrease in cell size resulting from a decreased workload.

atypical angina *see* Prinzmetal's angina.

augmented limb leads another term for unipolar limb leads, reflecting the fact that the ground lead is disconnected, which increases the amplitude of deflection on the ECG tracing.

auscultation listening with a stethoscope for sounds produced by the body.

authoritarian a parenting style that demands absolute obedience without regard to a child's individual freedom.

authoritative a parenting style that emphasizes a balance between a respect for authority and individual freedom.

autoimmune disease condition in which the body makes antibodies against its own tissues.

autoimmunity an immune response to self antigens, which the body normally tolerates.

automaticity pacemaker cells' capability of self-depolarization.

autonomic dysfunction an abnormality of the involuntary aspect of the nervous system.

autonomic ganglia groups of autonomic nerve cells located outside the central nervous system.

autonomic hyperreflexia syndrome condition associated with the body's adjustment to the effects of spinal shock; presentations include sudden hypertension, bradycardia, pounding headache, blurred vision, and sweating and flushing of the skin above the point of injury.

autonomic nervous system part of the nervous system controlling involuntary bodily functions. It is divided into the sympathetic and the parasympathetic systems.

autonomic neuropathy condition that damages the autonomic nervous system, which usually senses changes in core temperature and controls vasodilation and perspiration to dissipate heat.

autonomy a competent adult patient's right to determine what happens to his own body.

autoregulation process that controls blood flow to tissue by causing alterations in the tissue.

avulsion forceful tearing away or separation of body tissue; an avulsion may be partial or complete.

axial loading application of the forces of trauma along the axis of the spine; this often results in compression fractures of the spine.

axial skeleton bones of the head, thorax, and spine.

axis deviation *see* left axis deviation, right axis deviation.

axon extension of a neuron that serves as a pathway for transmission of signals to and from the brain; major component of white matter.

B lymphocytes white blood cells that, in response to the presence of an antigen, produce antibodies that attack the antigen, develop a memory for the antigen, and confer long-term immunity to the antigen.

Babinski response big toe dorsiflexes and the other toes fan out when sole is stimulated.

bacteria (singular *bacterium*) single-cell organisms with a cell membrane and cytoplasm but no organized nucleus.

bacterial tracheitis bacterial infection of the airway, subglottic region; in children, most likely to appear after episodes of croup.

bactericidal capable of killing bacteria.

bacteriostatic capable of inhibiting bacterial growth or reproduction.

bag-valve mask (BVM) ventilation device consisting of a self-inflating bag with two one-way valves and a transparent plastic face mask.

ballistics the study of projectile motion and its interactions with the gun, the air, and the object it contacts.

baroreceptor sensory nerve ending, found in the walls of the atria of the heart, vena cava, aortic arch, and carotid sinus, that is stimulated by changes in pressure.

barotrauma injury caused by pressure within an enclosed space; when occuring during a diving descent is commonly called *the squeeze*.

basal metabolic rate (BMR) rate at which the body consumes energy just to maintain stability; the basic metabolic rate (measured by the rate of oxygen consumption) of an awake, relaxed person 12 to 14 hours after eating and at a comfortable temperature.

basic life support (BLS) refers to basic life-saving procedures such as artificial ventilation and cardiopulmonary resuscitation (CPR).

basophil type of white blood cell that participates in allergic responses.

battery the unlawful touching of another individual without his consent.

Battle's sign black and blue discoloration over the mastoid process.

behavior a person's observable conduct and activity.

behavioral emergency situation in which a patient's behavior becomes so unusual that it alarms the patient or another person and requires intervention.

Bell's palsy one-sided facial paralysis with an unknown cause characterized by the inability to close the eye, pain, tearing of the eyes, drooling, hypersensitivity to sound, and impairment of taste.

bend fractures fractures characterized by angulation and deformity in the bone without an obvious break.

benign prostatic hypertrophy a noncancerous enlargement of the prostate associated with aging.

bereavement death of a loved one.

beta radiation medium-strength radiation that is stopped with light clothing or the uppermost layers of skin.

bilateral periorbital ecchymosis black-and-blue discoloration of the area surrounding the eyes. It is usually associated with basilar skull fracture. Also called *raccoon eyes*.

bioassay test to ascertain a drug's availability in a biological model.

bioavailability amount of a drug that is still active after it reaches its target tissue.

bioequivalence relative therapeutic effectiveness of chemically equivalent drugs.

bioethics the application of ethics to the life sciences.

biologic half-life time the body takes to clear one half of a drug.

biological/organic related to disease processes or structural changes.

biological agents either living organisms or toxins produced by living organisms that are deliberately distributed to cause disease and death.

biotoxin poison that is produced by a living organism but is itself not alive.

biotransformation changing a substance in the body from chemical to another; in the case of hazardous materials, the body tries to create less toxic materials.

BiPAP bilevel positive airway pressure.

bipolar disorder condition characterized by one or more manic episodes, with or without periods of depression.

bipolar limb leads electrocardiogram leads applied to the arms and legs that contain two electrodes of opposite (positive and negative) polarity; leads I, II, and III.

birth injury avoidable and unavoidable mechanical and anoxic trauma incurred by the newborn during labor and delivery.

blast wind the air movement caused as the heated and pressurized products of an explosion move outward.

blepharospasm twitching of the eyelids.

blood pressure force of blood against arteries' walls as the heart contracts and relaxes.

blood spatter evidence the pattern that blood forms when it is spattered or dropped at the scene of a crime.

blood tube glass container with color-coded, self-healing rubber top.

blood tubing IV administration tubing that contains a filter to prevent clots or other debris from entering the patient.

bloodborne transmitted by contact with blood or body fluids.

blood-brain barrier tight junctions of the capillary endothelial cells in the central nervous system vasculature through which only non-protein-bound, highly lipid-soluble drugs can pass.

BLS *see* basic life support.

blunt trauma injury caused by the collision of an object with the body in which the object does not enter the body.

body language *see* nonverbal communication.

body substance isolation (BSI) a strict form of infection control that is based on the assumption that all blood and body fluids are infectious.

body surface area (BSA) amount of a patient's body affected by a burn.

Bohr effect phenomenon in which a decrease in pCO_2/acidity causes an increase in the quantity of oxygen that binds with the hemoglobin and, conversely, an increase in pCO_2/acidity causes the hemoglobin to give up a greater quantity of oxygen.

bolus concentrated mass of medication.

bonding the formation of a close personal relationship (as between mother and child), especially through frequent or constant association.

borborygmi loud, prolonged, gurgling bowel sounds indicating hyperperistalsis.

bowel obstruction blockage of the hollow space within the intestines.

Bowman's capsule the hollow, cup-shaped first part of the nephron tubule.

bradycardia a slow heart rate; a heart rate less than 60 beats per minute.

bradypnea slow respiration.

brain abscess a collection of pus localized in an area of the brain.

brain ischemia injury to brain tissues caused by an inadequate supply of oxygen and nutrients.

brainstem part of the brain connecting the cerebral hemispheres with the spinal cord. It is comprised of the mesencephalon (midbrain), the pons, and the medulla oblongata.

branch functional level within the Incident Management System based upon primary roles and geographic locations. Also called *sector*.

breach of duty an action or inaction that violates the standard of care expected from an EMT-I.

bronchi tubes from the trachea into the lungs.

bronchiectasis chronic dilation of a bronchus or bronchi, with a secondary infection typically involving the lower portion of the lung.

bronchiolitis viral infection of the medium-sized airways, occurring most frequently during the first year of life.

Broselow tape a measuring tape for infants that provides important information regarding airway equipment and medication doses based on your patient's length.

Brown-Séquard's syndrome condition caused by partial cutting of one side of the spinal cord resulting in sensory and motor loss to that side of the body.

Brudzinkis's sign physical exam finding in which flexion of the neck causes flexion of the hips and knees.

bruit sound of turbulent blood flow around a partial obstruction.

bubble sheet scannable run sheet on which boxes or "bubbles" are filled in to record information.

buccal between the cheek and gums.

buckle fractures fractures characterized by a raised or bulging projection at the fracture site.

buffer a substance that tends to preserve or restore a normal acid-base balance by increasing or decreasing the concentration of hydrogen ions.

bulimia nervosa recurrent binge eating.

bundle branch block a kind of interventricular heart block in which conduction through either the right or left bundle branches is blocked or delayed.

bundle of Kent an accessory AV conduction pathway that is thought to be responsible for the ECG findings of pre-excitation syndrome.

burette chamber calibrated chamber of Berutrol IV administration tubing that enables precise measurement and delivery of fluids and medicated solutions.

burnout occurs when coping mechanisms no longer buffer job stressors, which can compromise personal health and well-being.

bursa sac containing synovial fluid that cushions adjacent structures.

bursitis acute or chronic inflammation of the small synovial sacs.

CAGE questionnaire a questionnaire designed to determine the presence of alcoholism.

calcaneus the largest bone of the foot; the heel.

caliber the diameter of a bullet expressed in hundredths of an inch. (0.22 caliber = 0.22 inches); the inside diameter of the barrel of a handgun, shotgun, or rifle.

callus thickened area that forms at the site of a fracture as part of the repair process.

CAMEO® Computer-Aided Management of Emergency Operations; website developed by the EPA and NOAA as a source of information, skills, and links related to hazardous substances.

cancellous having a lattice-work structure, as in the spongy tissue of a bone.

cannula hollow needle used to puncture a vein.

cannulation *see* intravenous access.

capillary one of the minute blood vessels that connect the ends of arterioles with the beginnings of venules; where oxygen is diffused to body tissue and products of metabolism enter the bloodstream.

capnography the measurement of exhaled carbon dioxide concentrations.

carbon dioxide waste product of the body's metabolism.

cardiac arrest the absence of ventricular contraction.

cardiac contractile force the strength of a contraction of the heart.

cardiac cycle the period of time from the end of one cardiac contraction to the end of the next.

cardiac depolarization a reversal of charges at a cell membrane so that the inside of the cell becomes positive in relation to the outside; the opposite of the cell's resting state in which the inside of the cell is negative in relation to the outside.

cardiac monitor machine that displays and records the electrical activity of the heart.

cardiac output the amount of blood pumped by the heart in one minute (computed as stroke volume × heart rate).

cardiac tamponade accumulation of excess fluid inside the pericardium.

cardioacceleratory center a sympathetic nervous system center in the medulla oblongata, controlling the release of epinephrine and norepinephrine.

cardiogenic shock shock caused by insufficient cardiac output; the inability of the heart to pump enough blood to perfuse all parts of the body.

cardioinhibitory center a parasympathetic center in the medulla oblongata, controlling the vagus nerve.

cardiovascular disease (CVD) disease affecting the heart, peripheral blood vessels, or both.

carina the point at which the trachea bifurcates into the right and left mainstem bronchi.

carpal bones bones of the wrist.

carrier mediated diffusion process in which carrier proteins transport large molecules across the cell membrane; also called *facilitated diffusion.*

cartilage connective tissue providing the articular surfaces of the skeletal system.

catabolism the destructive phase of metabolism in which cells break down complex substances into simpler substances with release of energy.

cataracts medical condition in which the lens of the eye loses its clearness.

catatonia condition characterized by immobility and stupor, often a sign of schizophrenia.

catecholamine a hormone, such as epinephrine or norepinephrine, that strongly affects the sympathetic nervous and cardiovascular systems, metabolic rate, temperature, and smooth muscle.

catheter a tube passed into or through the body.

catheter inserted through the needle Teflon catheter inserted through a large metal stylet; also called *intracatheter.*

cation an ion with a positive charge—so called because it will be attracted to a cathode, or negative pole.

cavitation the outward motion of tissue due to a projectile's passage, resulting in a temporary cavity and vacuum.

cell the basic structural unit of all plants and animals; a membrane enclosing a thick fluid and a nucleus. Cells are specialized to carry out all of the body's basic functions.

cell-mediated immunity the short-term immunity to an antigen provided by T lymphocytes, which directly attack the antigen but do not produce antibodies or memory for the antigen. Also called *cellular immunity.*

cell membrane also called *plasma membrane;* the outer covering of a cell.

cellular swelling swelling of a cell caused by injury to or change in permeability of the cell membrane with resulting inability to maintain stable intra- and extracellular fluid and electrolyte levels.

cellular telephone system telephone system divided into regions, or cells, that are served by radio base stations.

cellulitis inflammation of cellular or connective tissue.

central cord syndrome condition usually related to hyperflexion of the cervical spine that results in motor weakness, usually in the upper extremities and possible bladder dysfunction.

central IV line intravenous line placed into the superior vena cava for the administration of long-term fluid therapy.

central nervous system the brain and the spinal cord.

central neurogenic hyperventilation hyperventilation caused by a lesion in the central nervous system, often characterized by rapid, deep, noisy respirations.

central pain syndrome condition resulting from damage or injury to the brain, brainstem, or spinal cord characterized by intense, steady pain described as burning, aching, tingling, or a "pins and needles" sensation.

central venous access surgical puncture of the internal jugular, subclavian, or femoral vein.

cerebellum portion of the brain located dorsally to the pons and medulla oblongata. It plays an important role in the fine motor movement, posture, equilibrium, and muscle tone.

cerebral perfusion pressure (CPP) the pressure moving blood through the brain.

cerebrospinal fluid fluid surrounding and bathing the brain and spinal cord.

cerebrum largest part of the brain, consisting of two hemispheres. The cerebrum is the seat of consciousness and the center of the higher mental functions such as memory, learning, reasoning, judgement, intelligence, and the emotions.

certification the process by which an agency or association grants recognition to an individual who has met its qualifications.

cerumen ear wax.

C-FLOP mnemonic for the main functional areas within the IMS—command, finance/administration, logistics, operations, and planning.

chain of evidence legally retaining items of evidence and accounting for their whereabouts at all times to prevent loss or tampering.

chancroid highly contagious sexually transmitted ulcer.

chemoreceptor sense organ or sensory nerve ending located outside the central nervous system that is stimulated by and reacts to chemical stimuli.

chemotactic factors chemicals released by white blood cells that attract more white blood cells to an area of inflammation.

chemotaxis the movement of white blood cells in response to chemical signals.

CHEMTEL, Inc. Chemical Telephone, Incorporated; maintains a 24-hour, toll-free hotline at 800-255-3024; for collect calls and calls from other points of origin, dial 813-979-0626.

CHEMTREC Chemical Transportation Emergency Center; maintains a 24-hour, toll-free hotline at 800-424-9300; for collect calls and calls from other points of origin, dial 703-527-3887.

Cheyne-Stokes respiration a breathing pattern characterized by a period of apnea lasting 10-60 seconds, followed by gradually increasing depth and frequency of respirations; respiratory pattern of alternating periods of apnea and tachypnea.

chief complaint the pain, discomfort, or dysfunction that caused your patient to request help.

child abuse physical or emotional violence or neglect towards a person from infancy to eighteen years of age.

chlamydia group of intracellular parasites that cause sexually transmitted diseases.

choanal atresia congenital closure of the passage between the nose and pharynx by a bony or membranous structure.

cholinergic pertaining to the neurotransmitter acetylcholine.

chronic gastroenteritis non-acute inflammation of the gastric mucosa.

chronic obstructive pulmonary disease (COPD) a disease characterized by a decreased ability of the lungs to perform the function of ventilation.

chronic renal failure permanently inadequate renal function due to nephron loss.

chronotropy pertaining to heart rate.

chyme semifluid mixture of ingested food and digestive secretions found in the stomach and small intestine.

circadian rhythms physiological phenomena that occur at approximately 24-hour intervals.

circulation assessment evaluating the pulse and skin and controlling hemorrhage.

circulatory overload overload that occurs if too much medication is administered for the patient's condition.

circumcision the surgical removal of the foreskin of the penis.

circumduction movement at a synovial joint where the distal end of a bone describes a circle but the shaft does not rotate.

cirrhosis degenerative disease of the liver.

civil law division of the legal system that deals with noncriminal issues and conflicts between two or more parties.

claudication severe pain in the calf muscle due to inadequate blood supply. It typically occurs with exertion and subsides with rest.

clavicle bone that holds the scapula and shoulder joint at a fixed distance from the sternum.

cleaning washing an object with cleaners such as soap and water.

cleft lip congenital vertical fissure in the upper lip.

cleft palate congenital fissure in the roof of the mouth, forming a passageway between oral and nasal cavities.

clinical judgment the use of knowledge and experience to diagnose patients and plan their treatment.

clitoris highly innervated and vascular erectile tissue anterior to the labia minora.

clonal diversity the development, by B lymphocyte precursors in the bone marrow, of receptors for every possible type of antigen.

clonal selection the process by which a specific antigen reacts with the appropriate receptors on the surface of immature B lymphocytes, thereby activating them and prompting them to proliferate, differentiate, and produce antibodies to the activating antigen.

clonic phase phase of a seizure characterized by alternating contraction and relaxation of muscles.

closed fracture a broken bone in which the bone ends or the forces that caused it do not penetrate the skin.

closed incident an incident that is not likely to generate any further patients; also known as *contained incident* or *stable incident*.

closed pneumothorax *see* pneumothorax.

closed questions questions that ask for specific information and require only very short or yes-or-no answers. Also called *direct questions*.

closed stance a posture or body position that is tense and suggests negativity, discomfort, fear, disgust, or anger.

clotting the body's three-step response to stop the loss of blood.

coagulation necrosis the process in which an acid, while destroying tissue, forms an insoluble layer that limits further damage.

coagulation the third step in the clotting process, which involves the formation of a protein called fibrin that forms a network around a wound to stop bleeding, ward off infection, and lay a foundation for healing and repair of the wound.

cold zone location at a hazmat incident outside the warm zone; area where incident operations take place; also called *green zone* or *safe zone*.

colic acute pain associated with cramping or spasms in the abdominal organs.

collagen tough, strong protein that comprises most of the body's connective tissue.

collecting duct the larger structure beyond the distal nephron tubule into which urine drips.

colloid osmotic pressure *see* oncotic force.

colloids substances, such as proteins or starches, consisting of large molecules or molecule aggregates that disperse evenly within a liquid without forming a true solution; intravenous solutions containing large proteins that cannot pass through capillary membranes.

colostomy a surgical diversion of the large intestine through an opening in the skin where the fecal matter is collected in a pouch; may be temporary or permanent.

coma a state of unconsciousness from which the patient cannot be aroused.

command the individual or group responsible for coordinating all activities and who makes final decisions on the emergency scene; often referred to as the Incident Commander (IC) or Officer in Charge (OIC).

command post (CP) place where command officers from various agencies can meet with each other and select a management staff.

comminuted fracture fracture in which a bone is broken into several pieces.

common law law that is derived from society's acceptance of customs and norms over time. Also called *case law* or *judge-made law.*

communicable period time when a host can transmit an infectious agent to someone else.

communicable capable of being transmitted to another host.

communication the exchange of common symbols—written, spoken, or other kinds such as signing and body language; the process of exchanging information between individuals.

community-acquired infection an infection occurring in a nonhospitalized patient who is not undergoing regular medical procedures, including the use of instruments such as catheters.

comorbidity having more than one disease at a time.

compartment syndrome condition that occurs when circulation to a portion of the body is cut off; muscle ischemia that is caused by rising pressures within an anatomic fascial space.

compensated shock early stage of shock during which the body's compensatory mechanisms are able to maintain normal perfusion.

compensatory pause the pause following an ectopic beat where the SA node is unaffected and the cadence of the heart is uninterrupted.

competent able to make an informed decision about medical care.

competitive antagonism one drug binds to a receptor and causes the expected effect while also blocking another drug from triggering the same receptor.

complex partial seizure type of partial seizure usually originating in the temporal lobe characterized by an aura and focal findings such as alterations in mental status or mood.

compliance the stiffness or flexibility of the lung tissue.

concealment hiding the body behind objects that shield a person from view but that offer little or no protection against bullets or other ballistics.

concentration weight per volume.

concussion a transient period of unconsciousness. In most cases, the unconsciousness will be followed by a complete return of function.

conduction moving electrons, ions, heat, or sound waves through a conductor or conducting medium.

conductive deafness deafness caused when there is a blocking of the transmission of the sound waves through the external ear canal to the middle or inner ear.

conductivity ability of cells to propagate the electrical impulse from one cell to another.

confidentiality the principle of law that prohibits the release of medical or other personal information about a patient without the patient's consent.

confusion state of being unclear or unable to make a decision easily.

congenital present at birth.

congestive heart failure (CHF) condition in which the heart's reduced stroke volume causes an overload of fluid in the body's other tissues. *See also* heart failure.

congregate care living arrangement in which the elderly live in, but do not own, individual apartments or rooms and receive select services.

conjuctiva mucous membrane that lines the eyelids.

connective tissue the most abundant body tissue; it provides support, connection, and insulation. Examples: bone, cartilage, fat, blood.

consent the patient's granting of permission for treatment.

constitutional law law based on the U.S. Constitution.

contamination presence of an agent only on the surface of the host without penetrating it.

continuous quality improvement (CQI) a program designed to refine and improve an EMS system, emphasizing customer satisfaction.

CONTOMS Counter-Narcotics Tactical Operations; program that manages the training and certification of EMT-Tacticals and SWAT-Medics.

contractility ability of muscle cells to contract, or shorten.

contraction inward movement of wound edges during healing that eventually brings the wound edges together.

contrecoup injury occurring on the opposite side; an injury to the brain opposite the site of impact.

contusion closed wound in which the skin is unbroken, although damage has occurred to the tissue immediately beneath.

convection transfer of heat via currents in liquids or gases.

conventional reasoning the stage of moral development during which children desire approval from individuals and society.

convergent focusing on only the most important aspect of a critical situation.

cor pulmonale hypertrophy of the right ventricle resulting from disorders of the lung; congestive heart failure secondary to pulmonary hypertension.

core temperature the body temperature of the deep tissues, which usually does not vary more than a degree or so from its normal 37°C (98.6°F).

cornea thin, delicate layer covering the pupil and the iris.

coronary heart disease (CHD) a type of cardiovascular disease; the single largest killer of people in the U.S.

cortex the outer tissue of an organ such as the kidney.

cortisol a steroid hormone released by the adrenal cortex that regulates the metabolism of fats, carbohydrates, sodium, potassium, and proteins and also has an anti-inflammatory effect.

coup injury an injury to the brain occurring on the same side as the site of impact.

coupling interval distance between the preceding beat and a premature ventricular contraction (PVC).

cover hiding the body behind solid and impenetrable objects that protect a person from bullets.

CPAP continuous positive airway pressure.

crackles light crackling, popping, nonmusical sounds heard usually during inspiration.

cramping muscle pain resulting from overactivity, lack of oxygen, and accumulation of waste products.

cranial nerves twelve pairs of nerves that extend from the lower surface of the brain.

cranium vault-like portion of the skull encasing the brain.

creatinine a waste product caused by metabolism within muscle cells.

crepitation (or crepitus) crunching sounds of unlubricated parts in joints rubbing against each other.

cribbing wooden slates used to shore up heavy equipment.

cricothyroid membrane membrane between the cricoid and thyroid cartilages of the larynx.

cricothyrostomy the introduction of a needle or other tube into the cricothyroid membrane, usually to provide an emergency airway.

cricothyrotomy a surgical incision into the cricothyroid membrane, usually to provide an emergency airway.

criminal law division of the legal system that deals with wrongs committed against society or its members.

critical incident an event that has a powerful emotional impact on a rescuer that can cause an acute stress reaction.

critical incident stress debriefing (CISD) a process used to help rescuers work through their responses to a critical incident within 24 to 72 hours after the event.

critical incident stress management (CISM) a system of related interventions usually performed by regional, non-partisan, multi-disciplinary teams composed of EMS peers and specifically trained mental health workers.

critical thinking thought process used to analyze and evaluate.

Crohn's disease idiopathic inflammatory bowel disorder associated with the small intestine.

croup viral illness characterized by inspiratory and expiratory stridor and a seal-bark-like cough.

crowning the bulging of the fetal head past the opening of the vagina during a contraction. Crowning is an indication of impending delivery.

crumple zone the region of a vehicle designed to absorb the energy of impact.

crush injury mechanism of injury in which tissue is locally compressed by high-pressure forces.

crush syndrome systemic disorder of severe metabolic disturbances resulting from the crush of a limb or other body part.

crystalloids substances capable of crystallization. In solution, unlike colloids, they can diffuse through a membrane, such as a capillary wall; intravenous solutions that contain electrolytes but lack the larger proteins associated with colloids.

Cullen's sign discoloration around the umbilicus suggestive of intra-abdominal hemorrhage.

cultural imposition the imposition of one's beliefs, values, and patterns of behavior on people of another culture.

current the rate of flow of an electric charge.

Cushing's reflex a collective change in vital signs (increased blood pressure and temperature and decreased pulse and respirations) associated with increasing intracranial pressure.

Cushing's syndrome pathological condition resulting from excess adrenocortical hormones. Symptoms may include changed body habitus, hypertension, vulnerability to infection.

cyanosis bluish discoloration of the skin due to reduced hemoglobin in the blood.

cystic medial necrosis a death or degeneration of a part of the wall of an artery.

cystitis an infection and inflammation of the urinary bladder.

cytochrome oxidase enzyme complex, found in cellular mitochondria, that enables oxygen to create the adenosine triphosphate (ATP) required for all muscle energy.

cytokines proteins, produced by white blood cells, that regulate immune responses by binding with and affecting the function of the cells that produced them or of other, nearby cells.

cytoplasm the thick fluid, or *protoplasm*, that fills a cell.

cytotoxic toxic, or poisonous, to cells.

deafness the inability to hear.

debridement the cleaning up or removal of debris, dead cells, and scabs from a wound, principally through phagocytosis.

deceleration the rate at which speed or velocity decreases.

decerebrate posture sustained contraction of extensor muscles of the extremities resulting from a lesion in the brainstem. The patient presents with stiff and extended extremities and retracted head.

decode to interpret a message.

decompensated shock advanced stages of shock when the body's compensatory mechanisms are no longer able to maintain normal perfusion; also called *progressive shock*.

decompression illness development of nitrogen bubbles within the tissues due to a rapid reduction of air pressure when a diver returns to the surface; also called *the bends*.

decontaminate to destroy or remove pathogens.

decontamination the process of minimizing toxicity by reducing the amount of toxin absorbed into the body.

decorticate posture characteristic posture associated with a lesion at or above the upper brainstem. The patient presents with the arms flexed, fists clenched, and legs extended.

deep frostbite freezing involving epidermal and subcutaneous tissues resulting in a white appearance, hard (frozen) feeling on palpation, and loss of sensation.

deep venous thrombosis a blood clot in a vein.

defamation an intentional false communication that injures another person's reputation or good name.

defibrillation the process of passing an electrical current through a fibrillating heart to depolarize a "critical mass" of myocardial cells. This allows them to depolarize uniformly, resulting in an organized rhythm.

defusing a short, informal type of debriefing held within hours of a critical incident.

degenerative neurological disorders a collection of diseases that selectively affect one or more functional systems of the central nervous system.

degloving injury avulsion in which the mechanism of injury tears the skin off the underlying muscle, tissue, blood vessels, and bone.

degranulation the emptying of granules from the interior of a mast cell into the extracellular environment.

dehydration excessive loss of body fluid.

delayed effects signs, symptoms, and/or conditions developed hours, days, weeks, months, or even years after exposure to a toxic substance.

delayed hypersensitivity reaction a hypersensitivity reaction that takes place after the elapse of some time following reexposure to an antigen. Delayed hypersensitivity reactions are usually less severe than immediate reactions.

DeLee suction trap a suction device that contains a suction trap connected to a suction catheter. The negative pressure that powers it can come either from the mouth of the operator or, preferably, from an external vacuum source.

delirium tremens (DTs) disorder found in habitual and excessive users of alcoholic beverages after cessation of drinking for 48–72 hours. Patients experience visual, tactile, and auditory disturbances. Death may result in severe cases.

delirium condition characterized by relatively rapid onset of widespread disorganized thought.

delusions fixed, false beliefs not widely held within the individual's cultural or religious group.

demand valve device a ventilation device that is manually operated by a push button or lever.

dementia a deterioration of mental status that is usually associated with structural neurological disease.

demobilization establishment and staffing of a transition point with the object of providing crews time to regroup between a large-scale critical stress situation and going off duty or back to regular duty.

demobilized release of resources—personnel, vehicles, and equipment—for use outside the incident when they are no longer needed at the scene.

demographic pertaining to population makeup or changes.

demylenation destruction or removal of the myelin sheath of nerve tissue; found in Guillain–Barré syndrome.

denature alter the usual substance of something.

depersonalization feeling detached from oneself.

deployment strategy used by an EMS agency to maneuver its ambulances and crews in an effort to reduce response times.

depression a mood disorder characterized by hopelessness and malaise.

dermatome topographical region of the body surface innervated by one nerve root.

dermis true skin, also called *corium*. It is the layer of tissue producing the epidermis and housing the structures, blood vessels, and nerves normally associated with the skin.

descending loop of Henle the part of the nephron tubule beyond the proximal tubule.

descending tracts bundles of axons along the spinal cord that transmit signals from the brain to the body.

desired dose specific quantity of medication needed.

detailed physical exam careful, thorough process of eliciting the history and conducting a physical exam.

devascularization loss of blood vessels from a body part.

diabetes insipidus excessive urine production caused by inadequate production of antidiuretic hormone.

diabetes mellitus disorder of inadequate insulin activity, due either to inadequate production of insulin or to decreased responsiveness of body cells to insulin.

diabetic ketoacidosis complication of Type I diabetes due to decreased insulin intake. Marked by high blood glucose, metabolic acidosis, and, in advanced stages, coma. Ketoacidosis is often called diabetic coma.

diabetic retinopathy slow loss of vision as a result of damage done by diabetes.

dialysate the solution used in dialysis that is hypo-osmolar to many of the wastes and key electrolytes in blood.

dialysis a procedure that replaces some lost kidney functions.

diaphoresis sweatiness.

diaphragmatic hernia protrusion of abdominal contents into the thoracic cavity through an opening in the diaphragm.

diaphysis hollow shaft found in long bones.

diarthrosis a synovial joint.

diastole the period of time when the myocardium is relaxed and cardiac filling and coronary perfusion occur.

diastolic blood pressure force of blood against arteries when ventricles relax.

diencephalon portion of the brain lying beneath the cerebrum and above the brainstem. It contains the thalamus, the hypothalamus, and the limbic system.

differential field diagnosis the list of possible causes for your patient's symptoms.

difficult child an infant, who can be characterized by irregularity of bodily functions, intense reactions, and withdrawal from new situations.

diffuse axonal injury type of brain injury characterized by shearing, stretching, or tearing of nerve fibers with subsequent axonal damage.

diffusion the movement of molecules through a membrane from an area of greater concentration to an area of lesser concentration.

digestive tract internal passageway that begins at the mouth and ends at the anus.

digital communications data or sounds are translated into a digital code for transmission.

dilation enlargement. In reference to the heart, an abnormal enlargement resulting from pathology.

diplopia double vision.

direct pressure method of hemorrhage control that relies on the application of pressure to the actual site of the bleeding.

direct questions *see* closed-ended questions.

dirty bomb a conventional explosive device that distributes radioactive material over a large area.

disaster management management of incidents that generate large numbers of patients, often overwhelming resources and damaging parts of the infrastructure.

disease period the duration from the onset of signs and symptoms of disease until the resolution of symptoms or death.

disinfectant cleansing agent that is toxic to living tissue.

disinfecting cleaning with an agent that can kill some microorganisms on the surface of an object.

dislocation complete displacement of a bone end from its position in a joint capsule.

dissecting aortic aneurysm aneurysm caused when blood gets between and separates the layers of the arterial wall.

disseminated intravascular coagulation (DIC) a disorder of coagulation caused by systemic activation of the coagulation cascade.

dissociate separate; break down. For example, sodium bicarbonate, when placed in water, dissociates into a sodium cation and a bicarbonate anion.

dissociative disorder condition in which the individual avoids stress by separating from his core personality.

distal distant or far from the point of reference. *Opposite of* proximal.

distal tubule the part of the tubule beyond the ascending loop of Henle.

distributive shock shock that results from mechanisms that prevent the appropriate distribution of nutrients and removal of metabolic waste products; Examples include septic shock, neurogenic shock, and anaphylactic shock.

diuresis formation and passage of a dilute urine, decreasing blood volume; secretion of large amounts of urine.

diuretic an agent that increases urine secretion and elimination of body water; drug used to reduce circulating blood volume by increasing the amount of urine.

divergent taking into account all aspects of a complex situation.

diverticula small outpouchings in the mucosal lining of the intestinal tract.

diverticulitis inflammation of diverticula.

diverticulosis presence of diverticula, with or without associated bleeding.

Do Not Resuscitate (DNR) order legal document, usually signed by the patient and his physician, that indicates to medical personnel which, if any, life-sustaining measures should be taken when the patient's heart and respiratory functions have ceased.

domestic elder abuse physical or emotional violence or neglect when an elder is being cared for in a home-based setting.

dorsal toward the back or spine. *Opposite of* ventral.

dosage on hand the amount of drug available in a solution.

dose packaging medication packages that contain a single dose for a single patient.

dosimeter an instrument that measures the cumulative amount of radiation absorbed.

down time duration from the beginning of the cardiac arrest until effective CPR is established. *see also* total down time.

down-regulation binding of a drug or hormone to a target cell receptor that causes the number of receptors to decrease.

drag the forces acting on a projectile in motion to slow its progress.

drip chamber clear plastic chamber that allows visualization of the intravenous drip rate.

drip rate pace at which the fluid moves from the intravenous bag into the patient.

dromotropy pertaining to the speed of cardiac impulse transmission.

drop former device in a drip chamber that regulates the size of drops.

drowning asphyxiation resulting from submersion in liquid with death occurring within 24 hours of submersion.

drug overdose poisoning from a pharmacological substance in excess of that usually prescribed or that the body can tolerate.

drug chemical used to diagnose, treat, or prevent disease.

drug-response relationship correlation of different amounts of a drug to clinical response.

ductus arteriosus channel between the main pulmonary artery and the aorta of the fetus.

due regard legal terminology found in the motor vehicle laws of most states that sets up a higher standard for the operators of emergency vehicles.

duplex communication system that allows simultaneous two-way communications by using two frequencies for each channel.

dura mater tough layer of the meninges firmly attached to the interior of the skull and the spinal column.

duration of action length of time the amount of drug remains above its minimum effective concentration.

duty to act a formal contractual or informal legal obligation to provide care.

dynamic steady state homeostasis; the tendency of the body to maintain a net constant composition although the components of the body's internal environment are always changing.

dysmenorrhea painful menstruation.

dyspareunia painful sexual intercourse.

dysphagia inability to swallow or difficulty swallowing.

dysphoria an exaggerated feeling of depression or unrest, characterized by a mood of general dissatisfaction, restlessness, discomfort, and unhappiness.

dysplasia a change in cell size, shape, or appearance caused by an external stressor.

dyspnea an abnormality of breathing rate, pattern, or effort; the sensation of having difficulty in breathing.

dysrhythmia any deviation from the normal electrical rhythm of the heart.

dystonias a group of disorders characterized by muscle contractions that cause twisting and repetitive movements, abnormal postures, or freezing in the middle of an action.

dysuria painful urination often associated with cystitis.

easy child an infant, who can be characterized by regularity of bodily functions, low or moderate intensity of reactions, and acceptance of new situations.

ecchymosis blue-black discoloration of the skin due to leakage of blood into the tissues.

echo procedure immediately repeating each transmission received during radio communications.

ectopic beat cardiac depolarization resulting from depolarization of ectopic focus.

ectopic focus nonpacemaker heart cell that automatically depolarizes; *pl.* ectopic foci.

ectopic pregnancy the implantation of a developing fetus outside of the uterus, often in fallopian tubes.

eddies water that flows around especially large objects and, for a time, flows upstream around the downside of an obstruction; provides an opportunity to escape dangerous currents.

edema excess fluid in the interstitial space.

effacement the thinning of the cervix during labor.

efferent carrying impulses away from the brain or spinal cord to the periphery. Motor nerves are efferent nerves.

efficacy a drug's ability to cause the expected response.

egophony abnormal change in tone of patient's transmitted voice sounds.

Einthoven's triangle the triangle around the heart formed by the bipolar limb leads.

ejection fraction ratio of blood pumped from the ventricle to the amount remaining at end of diastole.

elder abuse *see* domestic elder abuse; institutional elder abuse.

elderly a person age 65 or older.

electrical alternans alternating amplitude of the P, QRS, and T waves on the ECG rhythm strip as the heart swings in a pendulum-like fashion within the pericardial sac during tamponade.

electrocardiogram (ECG) the graphic recording of the heart's electrical activity. It may be displayed either on paper or on an oscilloscope.

electrolyte a substance that, in water, separates into electrically charged particles.

emancipated minor a person under 18 years of age who is married, pregnant, a parent, a member of the armed forces, or financially independent and living away from home.

embolus undissolved solid, liquid, or gaseous matter in the bloodstream that may cause blockage of blood vessels; *pl.* emboli.

emergency doctrine *see* implied consent.

emergency medical dispatcher (EMD) EMS person responsible for assignment of emergency medical resources to a medical emergency.

emergency medical services (EMS) system a comprehensive network of personnel, equipment, and resources established for the purpose of delivering aid and emergency medical care to the community.

Emergency Medical Services for Children (EMSC) federally funded program aimed at improving the health of pediatric patients who suffer from life-threatening illnesses and injuries.

emergent phase first stage of the burn process that is characterized by a catecholamine release and pain-mediated reaction.

emesis vomitus.

empathy identification with and understanding of another's situation, feelings, and motives.

EMT-Tacticals (EMT-Ts) EMS personnel trained to serve with a tactical Emergency Medical Services or a law enforcement agency.

encephalitis acute infection of the brain, usually caused by a virus.

encode to create a message.

endocrine gland gland that secretes chemical substances directly into the blood; also called *ductless gland.*

endometriosis condition in which endometrial tissue grows outside of the uterus.

endometritis infection of the endometrium.

endometrium the inner layer of the uterine wall where the fertilized egg implants.

endotoxin toxic products released when bacteria die and decompose.

endotracheal intubation passing a tube into the trachea to protect and maintain the airway and to permit medication administration and deep suctioning.

end-stage renal failure an extreme failure of kidney function due to nephron loss.

enema a liquid bolus of medication that is injected into the rectum.

energy the capacity to do work in the strict physical sense.

enteral route delivery of a medication through the gastrointestinal tract.

enterotoxin an exotoxin that produces gastrointestinal symptoms and diseases such as food poisoning.

enucleation removal of the eyeball after trauma or illness.

environmental emergency a medical condition caused or exacerbated by the weather, terrain, atmospheric pressure, or other local factors.

epicardium serous membrane covering the outer surface of the heart; the visceral pericardium.

epidemiology the study of factors that influence the frequency, distribution, and causes of injury, disease, and other health-related events in a population.

epidermis outermost layer of the skin composed of dead or dying cells.

epididymis a saclike duct adjacent to a testis that stores sperm cells.

epidural hematoma accumulation of blood between the dura mater and the cranium.

epiglottitis infection and inflammation of the epiglottis.

epiphyseal fracture disruption in the epiphyseal plate of a child's bone.

epiphyseal plate area of the metaphysis where cartilage is generated during bone growth in childhood.

epiphysis end of a long bone, including the epiphyseal or growth plate, and supporting structures underlying the joint.

epistaxis nosebleed.

epithelial tissue the protective tissue that lines internal and external body tissues. Examples: skin, mucous membranes, the lining of the intestinal tract.

epithelialization early stage of wound healing in which epithelial cells migrate over the surface of the wound.

erythema general reddening of the skin due to dilation of the superficial capillaries.

erythrocyte red blood cell.

erythropoiesis the process of producing red blood cells.

erythropoietin a hormone produced by kidney cells that stimulates maturation of red blood cells in the bone marrow.

eschar hard, leathery product of a deep full-thickness burn; it consists of dead and denatured skin.

Esophageal Tracheal CombiTube (ETC) dual-lumen airway with a ventilation port for each lumen.

esophageal varices enlarged and tortuous esophageal veins.

essential equipment equipment/supplies required on every ambulance.

estimated date of confinement (EDC) the approximate day the infant will be born. This date is usually set at 40 weeks after the date of the mother's last menstrual period (LMP).

ethics the rules or standards that govern the conduct of members of a particular group or profession.

ETT endotracheal tube.

eustachian tube a tube that connects the ear with the nasal cavity.

evaporation change from liquid to a gaseous state.

evisceration a protrusion of organs from a wound.

excitability ability of cells to respond to an electrical stimulus.

exertional metabolic rate rate at which the body consumes energy during activity. It is faster than the basic metabolic rate.

exocrine gland gland that secretes chemical substances to nearby tissues through a duct; also called *ducted gland.*

exotoxin a soluble poisonous substance secreted during growth of a bacterium.

expectorant medication intended to increase the productivity of cough.

explosives chemical(s), that when ignited, instantly generate a great amount of heat resulting in a destructive shock wave and blast wind.

exposure any occurrence of blood or body fluids coming in contact with non-intact skin, mucous membranes, or parenteral contact (needle stick).

expressed consent verbal, nonverbal, or written communication by a patient that he wishes to receive medical care.

exsanguination the draining of blood to the point at which life cannot be sustained.

extension tubing IV tubing used to extend a macrodrip or microdrip setup.

extension bending motion that increases the angle between articulating elements.

external immune system *see* secretory immune system.

extracellular fluid (ECF) the fluid outside the body cells. Extracellular fluid is comprised of intravascular fluid and interstitial fluid.

extrauterine outside the uterus.

extravasation leakage of fluid or medication from the blood vessel that is commonly found with infiltration.

extravascular space the volume contained by all the cells (intracellular space) and the spaces between the cells (interstitial space).

extravascular outside the vein.

extrication use of force to free a patient from entrapment.

extubation removing a tube from a body opening.

facilitated diffusion diffusion of a substance such as glucose through a cell membrane that requires the assistance of a "helper," or carrier protein; *see also* carrier mediated diffusion.

facsimile machine device for electronically transmitting and receiving printed information.

factitious disorder condition in which the patient feigns illness in order to assume the sick role.

fallopian tubes thin tubes that extend laterally from the uterus and conduct eggs from the ovaries into the uterine cavity.

fallout radioactive dust and particles that may be life-threatening to people far from the epicenter of a nuclear detonation.

false imprisonment intentional and unjustifiable detention of a person without his consent or other legal authority.

fascia a fibrous membrane that covers, supports, and separates muscles and may also unite the skin with underlying tissue.

fasciculations involuntary contractions or twitchings of muscle fibers.

fasciculus small bundle of muscle fibers.

fatigue fracture break in a bone associated with prolonged or repeated stress.

fatigue condition in which a muscle's ability to respond to stimulation is lost or reduced through overactivity.

fatty change a result of cellular injury and swelling in which lipids (fat vesicles) invade the area of injury; occurs most commonly in the liver.

fear feeling of alarm and discontentment in the expectation of danger.

febrile seizures seizures that occur as a result of a sudden increase in temperature; occur most commonly between ages 6 months and 6 years.

fecal-oral route transmission of organisms picked up from the gastrointestinal tract (e.g., feces) into the mouth.

Federal Communications Commission (FCC) agency that controls all nongovernmental communications in the United States.

feedback a response to a message.

femur large bone of the proximal lower extremity.

fibrin protein fibers that trap red blood cells; the end product of the coagulation cascade that forms an intertwined "net" that traps blood elements and thickens blood.

fibrinolysis the process through which plasmin dismantles a blood clot.

fibroblasts cells that secrete collagen, a critical factor in wound healing.

fibrosis the formation of fiber-like connective tissue, also called *scar tissue* in an organ.

fibula the small bone of the lower leg.

field diagnosis prehospital evaluation of the patient's condition and its causes.

filtrate the fluid produced in Bowman's capsule by filtration of blood.

filtration movement of water out of the plasma across the capillary membrane into the interstitial space; movement of molecules across a membrane from an area of higher pressure to an area of lower pressure.

FiO_2 concentration of oxygen in inspired air.

first-pass effect the liver's partial or complete inactivation of a drug before it reaches the systemic circulation.

flail chest one or more ribs fractured in two or more places, creating an unattached rib segment. Breathing will cause paradoxical chest wall motion.

flanks the part of the back below the ribs and above the hip bones.

flat affect appearance of being disinterested, often lacking facial expression.

flechettes arrow-shaped projectiles found in some military ordnance.

flexion bending motion that reduces the angle between articulating elements.

fluid shift phase stage of the burn process in which there is a massive shift of fluid from the intravascular to the extravascular space.

focused history and physical exam problem-oriented assessment process based on initial assessment and chief complaint.

food poisoning nonspecific term often applied to gastroenteritis that occurs suddenly and that is caused by the ingestion of food containing preformed toxins.

foreign body airway obstruction (FBAO) blockage or obstruction of the airway by an object that impairs respiration.

Frank-Starling mechanism process by which an increase in cardiac output occurs in proportion to the diastolic stretch of the heart muscle fibers.

free drug availability proportion of a drug available in the body to cause either desired or undesired effects.

French unit of measurement approximately equal to one-third millimeter.

frostbite environmentally induced freezing of body tissues causing destruction of cells.

fugue state condition in which an amnesiac patient physically flees.

full-thickness burn burn that damages all layers of the skin; characterized by areas that are white and dry; also called *third-degree burn*.

functional impairment decreased ability to meet daily needs on an independent basis.

fungus plant-like microorganism.

gag reflex mechanism that stimulates retching, or striving to vomit, when the soft palate is touched.

galea aponeurotica connective tissue sheet covering the superior aspect of the cranium.

gamma radiation powerful electromagnetic radiation emitted by radioactive substances with powerful penetrating properties; it is stronger than alpha and beta radiation.

gangrene death of tissue or bone, usually from an insufficient blood supply; deep space infection usually caused by the anaerobic bacterium *Clostridium perfringens*.

gastric lavage removing an ingested poison by repeatedly filling and emptying the stomach with water or saline via a gastric tube; also known as *pumping the stomach*.

gastroenteritis nonacute inflammation of the gastrointestinal mucosa. Generalized disorder involving nausea, vomiting, gastrointestinal cramping or discomfort, and diarrhea. *See also* acute gastroenteritis.

gauge the size of a needle's or tube's diameter.

Geiger counter an instrument used to detect and measure the radiation given off by an object or area.

general adaptation syndrome (GAS) a sequence of stress response stages: stage I–alarm; stage II–resistance or adaptation; stage III–exhaustion.

general impression your initial, intuitive evaluation of your patient.

generalized seizures seizures that begin as an electrical discharge in a small area of the brain but spread to involve the entire cerebral cortex, causing widespread malfunction.

genitourinary system the male organ system that includes reproductive and urinary structures.

geriatric abuse a syndrome in which an elderly person is physically or psychologically injured by another person.

geriatrics the study and treatment of diseases of the aged.

German measles *see* rubella.

gerontology scientific study of the effects of aging and of age-related diseases on humans.

Glasgow Coma Scale scoring system for monitoring the neurological status of patients with head injuries.

glaucoma group of eye diseases that results in increased intraocular pressure on the optic nerve; if left untreated, can lead to blindness.

global aphasia a combination of motor and sensory aphasia.

glomerular filtration rate (GFR) the volume per day at which blood is filtered through capillaries of the glomerulus.

glomerular filtration the removal from blood of water and other elements, which enter the nephron tubule.

glomerulonephritis a form of nephritis, or inflammation of the kidneys; primarily involves the glomeruli, one of the capillary networks that are part of the renal corpuscles in the nephrons.

glomerulus a tuft of capillaries from which blood is filtered into a nephron.

glottic function opening and closing of the glottic space.

glottis lip-like opening between the vocal cords.

glucagon hormone that increases the blood glucose level by stimulating the liver to change stored glycogen to glucose.

glucocorticoids hormones released by the adrenal cortex that increase glucose production and reduce the body's inflammation response.

glucometer tool used to measure blood glucose level.

gluconeogenesis conversion of protein and fat to form glucose.

glucose intolerance the body cells' inability to take up glucose from the bloodstream.

glycogen a polysaccharide; one of the forms in which the body stores glucose.

glycogenolysis the breakdown of glycogen to glucose, primarily by liver cells.

glycolysis the first stage of the process in which the cell breaks apart an energy source, commonly glucose, and releases a small amount of energy.

glycosuria glucose in urine, which occurs when blood glucose levels exceed the kidney's ability to reabsorb glucose.

gold standard ultimate standard of excellence.

Golden Hour the 60-minute period after a severe injury; it is the maximum acceptable time between the injury and initiation of surgery for the seriously injured trauma patient.

gomphosis a joint that connects a tooth to the jaw.

gonorrhea sexually transmitted disease caused by a gram-negative bacterium.

Good Samaritan laws laws that provide immunity to certain people who assist at the scene of a medical emergency.

gout inflammation of joints and connective tissue due to build-up of uric acid crystals.

granulation filling of a wound by the inward growth of healthy tissues from the wound edges.

granulocytes white blood cells charged with the primary purpose of neutralizing foreign bacteria.

granuloma a tumor or growth that forms when foreign bodies that cannot be destroyed by macrophages are surrounded and walled off.

Graves' disease endocrine disorder characterized by excess thyroid hormones resulting in body changes associated with increased metabolism; primary cause of thyrotoxicosis.

gray matter areas in the central nervous system dominated by nerve cell bodies; central portion of the spinal cord.

Gray (Gy) a unit of absorbed radiation dose equal to 100 rads.

great vessels large arteries and veins located in the mediastinum that enter and exit the heart.

greenstick fracture partial fracture of a child's bone.

Grey-Turner's sign discoloration over the flanks suggesting intra-abdominal bleeding.

growth hormone hormone secreted by the anterior pituitary gland that promotes the uptake of glucose and amino acids in the muscle cells and stimulates protein synthesis.

growth plate the area just below the head of a long bone in which growth in bone length occurs in the epiphyseal plate.

gtts drops (Latin *guttae*, drops [*gutta*, drop]).

guarding protective tensing of the abdominal muscles by a patient suffering abdominal pain; may be a voluntary or involuntary response.

Guillain–Barré syndrome acute viral infection that triggers the production of autoantibodies, which damage the myelin sheath covering the peripheral nerves; causes rapid, progressive loss of motor function, ranging from muscle weakness to full-body paralysis.

gynecology the branch of medicine that deals with the health maintenance and the diseases of women, primarily of the reproductive organs.

hairline fracture small crack in a bone that does not disrupt its total structure.

half-life time required for half of the nuclei of a radioactive substance to lose activity by undergoing radioactive decay. In biology and pharmacology, the time required by the body to

metabolize and inactivate half the amount of a substance taken in.

hallucinations sensory perceptions with no basis in reality.

hantavirus family of viruses that are carried by the deer mouse and transmitted by ticks and other arthropods.

haptens molecules that do not trigger an immune response on their own but can become immunogenic when combined with larger molecules.

hate crimes crimes committed against a person solely on the basis of the individual's actual or perceived race, color, national origin, ethnicity, gender, disability, or sexual orientation.

haversian canals small perforations of the long bones through which the blood vessels and nerves travel into the bone itself.

hazardous material (hazmat) any substance that causes adverse health effects upon human exposure.

health-care professionals properly trained and licensed or certified providers of health care.

heart failure clinical syndrome in which the heart's mechanical performance is compromised so that cardiac output cannot meet the body's needs. *See also* congestive heart failure.

heat cramps acute painful spasms of the voluntary muscles following strenuous activity in a hot environment without adequate fluid or salt intake.

heat escape lessening position (HELP) developed by Dr. John Hayward. It is an in-water, head-up tuck or fetal position designed to reduce heat loss by as much as 60%.

heat exhaustion a mild heat illness; an acute reaction to heat exposure.

heat illness increased core body temperature due to inadequate thermolysis.

heatstroke acute, dangerous reaction to heat exposure, characterized by a body temperature usually above 105°F (40.6°C) and central nervous system disturbances. The body usually ceases to perspire.

HEENT head, eyes, ears, nose, and throat.

hematemesis vomiting blood.

hematochezia passage of stools containing red blood.

hematocrit the percentage of the blood consisting of the red blood cells, or erythrocytes.

hematology the study of blood and blood-forming organs.

hematoma collection of blood beneath the skin or trapped within a body compartment.

hematopoiesis the process through which pluripotent stem cells differentiate into various types of blood cells.

hematuria blood in the urine.

hemoconcentration elevated numbers of red and white blood cells.

hemocytoblasts *see* stem cells.

hemodialysis a dialysis procedure relying on vascular access to the blood and on an artificial membrane.

hemoglobin an iron-based compound found in red blood cells that binds with oxygen and transports it to body cells.

hemolysis destruction of red blood cells.

hemophilia a blood disorder in which one of the proteins necessary for blood clotting is missing or defective.

hemopneumothorax condition where air and blood are in the pleural space.

hemoptysis coughing up blood.

hemorrhage an abnormal internal or external discharge of blood.

hemorrhoid small mass of swollen veins in the anus or rectum.

hemostasis the body's natural ability to stop bleeding, the ability to clot blood.

hemothorax accumulation in the pleural cavity of blood or fluid containing blood.

HEPA high-efficiency particulate air.

heparin lock peripheral IV port that does not use a bag of fluid.

hepatic alteration change in a medication's chemical composition that occurs in the liver.

hepatitis inflammation of the liver characterized by diffuse or patchy tissue necrosis.

hepatomegaly enlarged liver.

hernia protrusion of an organ through its protective sheath.

herniation protrusion or projection of an organ or part of an organ through the wall of the cavity that normally contains it.

herpes simplex virus organism that causes infections characterized by fluid-filled vesicles, usually in the oral cavity or on the genitals.

herpes zoster an acute eruption caused by a reactivation of latent varicella virus (chicken pox) in the dorsal root ganglia; also known as *shingles*.

hiatal hernia protrusion of the stomach upward into the mediastinal cavity through the esophageal hiatus of the diaphragm.

high-pressure regulator regulator used to transfer oxygen at high pressures from tank to tank.

hilum the notched part of the kidney where the ureter and other structures join kidney tissue.

histamine substance released during the degranulation of mast cells and basophils that increases blood flow to the injury site due to vasodilation and increased permeability of capillary walls.

HIV human immunodeficiency virus, a virus that breaks down the immune defenses, making the body vulnerable to a variety of infections and disorders. *See also* AIDS.

HLA antigens antigens the body recognizes as self or non-self; present on all body cells except the red blood cells.

hollow-needle catheter stylet that does not have a Teflon tube but is itself inserted into the vein and secured there.

homeostasis the natural tendency of the body to maintain a steady and normal internal environment.

hookworm parasite that attaches to the host's intestinal lining.

hormone chemical substance released by a gland that controls or affects processes in other glands or body systems.

hospice program of palliative care and support services that addresses the physical, social, economic, and spiritual needs of terminally ill patients and their families.

hot zone location at a hazmat incident where the actual hazardous material and highest levels of contamination exist; also called *red zone* or *exclusionary zone*.

Huber needle needle that has an opening on the side of the shaft instead of the tip.

human immunodeficiency virus *see* HIV.

humerus the single bone of the proximal upper extremity.

humoral immunity the long-term immunity to an antigen provided by antibodies produced by B lymphocytes.

hydrolysis the breakage of a chemical bond by adding water, or by incorporating a hydroxyl (OH⁻)

group into one fragment and a hydrogen ion (H^+) into the other.

hydrostatic pressure blood pressure or force against vessel walls created by the heart beat. Hydrostatic pressure tends to force water out of the capillaries into the interstitial space.

Hymenoptera any of an order of insects such as bees and wasps.

hyperbaric oxygen chamber recompression chamber used to treat patients suffering from barotrauma.

hyperbilirubinemia an excessive amount of bilirubin—the orange-colored pigment associated with bile—in the blood. In newborns, the condition appears as jaundice. Precipitating factors include maternal Rh or ABO incompatibility, neonatal septis, anoxia, hypoglycemia, and congenital liver or gastrointestinal defects.

hypercarbia excessive pressure of carbon dioxide in the blood.

hyperglycemia excessive blood glucose.

hyperglycemic hyperosmolar nonketotic (HHNK) coma complication of type II diabetes due to inadequate insulin activity. Marked by high blood glucose, marked dehydration, and decreased mental function.

hypermetabolic phase stage of the burn process in which there is increased body metabolism in an attempt by the body to heal the burn.

hypernatremia excess of sodium in the blood.

hyperosmolar a solution that has a concentration of the substance greater than that of a second solution.

hyperplasia an increase in number of cells resulting from an increased workload.

hypersensitivity an exaggerated and harmful immune response; an umbrella term for allergy.

hypertension blood pressure higher than normal.

hypertensive emergency an acute elevation of blood pressure that requires the blood pressure to be lowered within one hour; characterized by end-organ changes such as hypertensive encephalopathy, renal failure, or blindness.

hypertensive encephalopathy a cerebral disorder of hypertension indicated by severe headache, nausea, vomiting, and altered mental status. Neurological symptoms may include blindness, muscle twitches, inability to speak, weakness, and paralysis.

hyperthermia unusually high core body temperature.

hyperthyroidism excessive secretion of thyroid hormones resulting in an increased metabolic rate.

hypertonic state in which a solution has a higher solute concentration on one side of a semi-permeable membrane than on the other side; one solution may be hypertonic to another.

hypertrophy an increase in cell size or organ size resulting from an increased workload.

hyphema blood in the anterior chamber of the eye, in front of the iris.

hypnosis instigation of sleep.

hypochondriasis an abnormal concern with one's health, with the false belief of suffering from some disease, despite medical assurances to the contrary; commonly known as *hypochondria*.

hypodermic needle hollow metal tube used with syringe to administer medications.

hypoglycemia deficiency of blood glucose. Sometimes called *insulin shock*.

hypoglycemic seizure seizure that occurs when brain cells aren't functioning normally due to low blood glucose.

hypo-osmolar a solution that has a concentration of the substance lower than that of a second solution.

hypoperfusion inadequate perfusion of the body tissues, resulting in an inadequate supply of oxygen and nutrients to the body tissues, also called *shock*.

hypotension lower than normal systolic and diastolic blood pressure.

hypothalamus portion of the brain important for controlling certain metabolic activities, including regulation of body temperature.

hypothermia decrease in body's core temperature.

hypothyroidism inadequate secretion of thyroid hormones resulting in a decreased metabolic rate.

hypotonic state in which a solution has a lower solute concentration on one side of a semi-permeable membrane than on the other side; one solution may be hypotonic to another.

hypoventilation reduction in breathing rate and depth.

hypovolemia reduced volume in the cardiovascular system.

hypovolemic shock shock caused by a loss of intravascular fluid volume.

hypoxemia decreased partial pressure of oxygen in the blood.

hypoxia state in which insufficient oxygen is available to meet the oxygen requirements of the cells.

hypoxic drive mechanism that increases respiratory stimulation when P_aO_2 falls and inhibits respiratory stimulation when P_aO_2 climbs.

iliac crest lateral bony ridge that is a landmark of the pelvis.

ilium large, flat innominate bone.

immediate hypersensitivity reaction a hypersensitivity reaction that occurs swiftly following reexposure to an antigen. Immediate hypersensitivity reactions are usually more severe than delayed reactions. The swiftest and most severe of such reactions is anaphylaxis.

immune complex *see* antigen-antibody complex.

immune response the body's reactions that inactivate or eliminate foreign antigens.

immune senescence diminished vigor of the immune response to the challenge and rechallenge by pathogens.

immune system the body system responsible for combating infection.

immunity exemption from legal liability. Also, long-term condition of protection from infection or disease; body's ability to respond to the presence of a pathogen.

immunogens antigens that are able to trigger an immune response.

immunoglobulins antibodies; proteins, produced in response to foreign antigens, that destroy or control the antigens.

impaled object foreign body embedded in a wound.

impetigo infection of the skin caused by staphylococci or streptococci.

implied consent consent for treatment that is presumed for a patient who is mentally, physically, or emotionally unable to grant consent. Also called *emergency doctrine*.

impulse control disorder condition characterized by the patient's failure to control recurrent impulses.

impulsive acting instinctively without stopping to think.

incendiary agent chemical(s) that combust easily or create combustion; a special subset of explosives with less explosive power but greater heat and burn potential.

Incident Management System (IMS) national system used for the management of multiple-casualty incidents, involving assumption of responsibility for command and designation and coordination of such elements as triage, treatment, transport, and staging; sometimes called the *Incident Command System*.

incision very smooth or surgical laceration, frequently caused by a knife, scalpel, razor blade, or piece of glass.

incontinence inability to retain urine or feces because of loss of sphincter control or cerebral or spinal lesions.

incubation period the time between contact with a disease organism and the appearance of the first symptoms.

index case the individual who first introduced an infectious agent to a population.

index of suspicion the anticipation of injury to a body region, organ, or structure based on analysis of the mechanism of injury.

induced active immunity immunity achieved through vaccination given to generate an immune response that results in the development of antibodies specific for the injected antigen; also called *artificially acquired immunity*.

inertia tendency of an object to remain at rest or remain in motion unless acted upon by an external force.

infarction area of dead tissue caused by lack of blood.

infection presence of an agent within the host, without necessarily causing disease.

infectious disease any disease caused by the growth of pathogenic microorganisms, which may be spread from person to person.

inferior beneath, lower, or toward the feet. *Opposite of* superior.

infestation presence of parasites that do not break the host's skin.

inflammation the body's response to cellular injury; also called *inflammatory response*. In contrast to the immune response, it develops swiftly, is nonspecific, and is temporary.

inflammatory process a nonspecific defense mechanism that wards off damage from microorganisms or trauma.

inflammatory response *see* inflammation.

influenza disease caused by a group of viruses.

informed consent consent for treatment that is given based on full disclosure of information.

infusion controller gravity-flow device that regulates fluid's passage through an electromechanical pump.

infusion pump device that delivers fluids and medications under positive pressure.

infusion rate speed at which a medication is delivered intravenously.

infusion liquid medication delivered through a vein.

ingestion entry of a substance into the body through the gastrointestinal tract.

inhalation entry of a substance into the body through the respiratory tract; drawing of medication into the lungs along with air during breathing.

initial assessment prehospital process designed to identify and correct life-threatening airway, breathing, and circulation problems.

injection entry of a substance into the body through a break in the skin; placement of medication in or under the skin with a needle and synringe.

injury intentional or unintentional damage to a person resulting from acute exposure to thermal, mechanical, electrical, or chemical energy or from the absence of such essentials as heat and oxygen.

injury current *see* current of injury.

injury risk a real or potentially hazardous situation that puts people in danger of sustaining injury.

injury-surveillance program the ongoing systematic collection, analysis, and interpretation of injury data essential to the planning, implementation, and evaluation of public health practice.

innominate one of the structures of the pelvis.

inotropy pertaining to cardiac contractile force.

insertion attachment of a muscle to a bone that moves when the muscle contracts.

inspection the process of informed observation.

institutional elder abuse physical or emotional violence or neglect when an elder is being cared for by a person paid to provide care.

insufflate to blow into.

insulin pancreatic hormone needed to transport simple sugars from the

interstitial spaces into the cells; substance that decreases blood glucose level.

integumentary system skin, consisting of the epidermis, dermis, and subcutaneous layers.

intercalated discs specialized bands of tissue inserted between myocardial cells that increase the rate in which the action potential is spread from cell to cell.

intermittent claudication intermittent calf pain while walking that subsides with rest.

intermittent mandatory ventilation (IMV) respirator setting where a patient-triggered breath does not result in assistance by the machine.

interpolated beat a premature ventricular contraction (PVC) that falls between two sinus beats without effectively interrupting this rhythm.

interstitial fluid the fluid in body tissues that is outside the cells and outside the vascular system.

interstitial nephritis an inflammation within the tissue surrounding the nephrons.

interstitial space space between cells.

intervener physician a licensed physician, professionally unrelated to patients on scene, who attempts to assist EMS providers with patient care.

intervertebral disk cartilaginous pad between vertebrae that serves as a shock absorber.

intracatheter *see* catheter inserted through the needle.

intracellular fluid (ICF) the fluid inside the body cells.

intracerebral hemorrhage bleeding directly into the tissue of the brain.

intracranial pressure (ICP) pressure exerted on the brain by the blood and cerebrospinal fluid.

intractable resistant to cure, relief, or control.

intradermal within the dermal layer of the skin.

intramuscular within the muscle.

intraosseous within the bone.

intrapartum occurring during childbirth.

intrarenal abscess a pocket of infection within kidney tissue.

intravascular fluid the fluid within the circulatory system; blood plasma.

intravascular space the volume contained by all the arteries, veins, capillaries, and other components of the circulatory system.

intravenous access surgical puncture of a vein to deliver medication or withdraw blood; also called *cannulation*.

intravenous fluid chemically prepared solution tailored to the body's specific needs.

intubation passing a tube into a body opening.

intussusception condition that occurs when part of an intestine slips into the part just distal to itself.

involuntary consent consent to treatment granted by the authority of a court order.

ion a charged particle; an atom or group of atoms whose electrical charge has changed from neutral to positive or negative by losing or gaining one or more electrons.

ionization the process of changing a substance into separate charged particles (ions).

ionize to become electrically charged or polar.

ionizing radiation electromagnetic radiation (e.g., x-ray) or particulate radiation (e.g., alpha particles, beta particles, and neutrons) that, by direct or secondary processes, ionizes materials that absorb the radiation. Ionizing radiation can penetrate the cells of living organisms, depositing an electrical charge within them. When sufficiently intense, this form of energy kills cells.

iris pigmented portion of the eye; the muscular area that constricts or dilates to change the size of the pupil.

irreversible antagonism a competitive antagonist permanently binds with a receptor site.

irreversible shock shock that has progressed so far that no medical intervention can reverse the condition and death is inevitable.

ischemia a blockage in the delivery of oxygenated blood to the cells.

ischial tuberosity one of the bony knobs of the posterior hip.

ischium irregular innominate bone.

isoimmunity an immune response to antigens from another member of the same species, for example Rh reactions between a mother and infant or transplant rejections; also called *alloimmunity*.

isolette also known as *incubator;* a clear plastic enclosed bassinet used to keep prematurely born infants warm.

isometric exercise active exercise performed against stable resistance, where muscles are exercised in a motionless manner.

isosthenuria the inability to concentrate or dilute urine relative to the osmolarity of blood.

isotonic exercise active exercise during which muscles are worked through their range of motion.

isotonic state in which solutions on opposite sides of a semi-permeable membrane are in equal concentration; solutions may be isotonic to each other.

J wave ECG deflection found at the junction of the QRS complex and the ST segment. It is associated with hypothermia and seen at core temperatures below 32°C, most commonly in leads II and V_6; also called *Osborn wave*.

Jackson's theory of thermal wounds explanation of the physical effects of thermal burns.

jargon language used by a particular group or profession.

joint capsule the ligaments that surround a joint; *synovial capsule*.

joint area where adjacent bones articulate.

Joule's law principle identifying that the rate of production of heat by a constant direct current is directly proportional to the resistance of the circuit and the square of the current.

justice the obligation to treat all patients fairly.

keloid a formation resulting from overproduction of scar tissue.

Kernig's sign inability to fully extend the knee with hips flexed.

ketone bodies compounds produced during the catabolism of fatty acids, including acetoacetic acid, b-hydroxybutyric acid, and acetone.

ketosis the presence of significant quantities of ketone bodies in the blood.

kidney transplantation implantation of a kidney into a person without functioning kidneys.

kinetic energy the energy an object has while it is in motion. It is related to the object's mass and velocity.

kinetics the branch of physics that deals with motion, taking into consideration mass and force.

Korotkoff sounds sounds of blood hitting arterial walls.

Korsakoff's psychosis psychosis characterized by disorientation, muttering delirium, insomnia, delusions, and hallucinations. Symptoms include painful extremities, bilateral wrist drop (rarely), bilateral foot drop (frequently), and pain on pressure over the long nerves.

Kreb's cycle process of aerobic metabolism that uses carbohydrates, proteins, and fats to release energy for the body; also known as *citric acid cycle*.

Kussmaul's respiration rapid, deep respirations caused by severe metabolic and CNS problems.

kyphosis exaggeration of the normal posterior curvature of the spine.

labia structures that protect the vagina and urethra, including the *labia majora* and the *labia minora*.

labor the time and processes that occur during childbirth; the physiologic and mechanical process in which the baby, placenta, and amniotic sac are expelled through the birth canal.

labrynthitis inner ear infection that causes vertigo, nausea, and an unsteady gait.

laceration an open wound, normally a tear with jagged borders.

lacrimal fluid liquid that lubricates the eye.

lactic acid compound produced from pyruvic acid during anerobic glycolysis.

laminae posterior bones of a vertebra that help make up the foramen, or opening, of the spinal canal.

laryngoscope instrument for lifting the tongue and epiglottis in order to see the vocal cords.

larynx the complex structure that joins the pharynx with the trachea.

latent period time when a host cannot transmit an infectious agent to someone else.

lateral toward the left or right of the midline.

laxative medication used to decrease stool's firmness and increase its water content.

Le Fort criteria classification system for fractures involving the maxilla.

leading questions questions framed to guide the direction of a patient's answers.

legislative law law created by law-making bodies such as Congress and state assemblies. Also called *statutory law.*

lesion any disruption in normal tissue.

leukemia a cancer of the hematopoietic cells.

leukocyte white blood cell.

leukocytosis too many white blood cells.

leukopenia too few white blood cells.

leukopoiesis the process through which stem cells differentiate into the white blood cells' immature forms.

leukotrienes also called *slow-reacting substances of anaphylaxis (SRS-A);* substances synthesized by mast cells during inflammatory response that cause vasoconstriction, vascular permeability, and chemotaxis; mediators released from mast cells upon contact with allergens.

leur lock adapter with a rubber-covered needle used to puncture a blood tube's self-healing top.

leur-sampling needle long, exposed needle that screws into the vacutainer and is inserted directly into the vein.

liability legal responsibility.

libel the act of injuring a person's character, name, or reputation by false statements made in writing or through the mass media with malicious intent or reckless disregard for the falsity of those statements.

lice parasitic infestation of the skin of the scalp, trunk, or pubic area.

licensure the process by which a governmental agency grants permission to engage in a given occupation to an applicant who has attained the degree of competency required to ensure the public's protection.

life expectancy based on the year of birth, the average number of additional years of life expected for a member of a population.

life-care community communities that provide apartments/homes for independent living and a range of services, including nursing care.

ligament connective tissue that connects bone to bone and holds joints together.

ligament of Treitz ligament that supports the duodenojejunal junction.

ligamentum arteriosum cord-like remnant of a fetal vessel connecting the pulmonary artery to the aorta at the aortic isthmus.

liquefaction necrosis the process in which an alkali dissolves and liquefies tissue.

living will a legal document that allows a person to specify the kinds of medical treatment he wishes to receive should the need arise.

local effects effects involving areas around the immediate site; should be evaluated based upon the burn model.

local limited to one area of the body.

lock-out/tag-out locking off of a machinery switch, then placing a tag on the switch stating why it is shut off; method of preventing equipment from being accidentally restarted.

lower gastrointestinal bleeding bleeding in the gastrointestinal tract distal to the ligament of Treitz.

lumen opening, or space, within a needle, artery, vein, or other hollow vessel.

Lyme disease recurrent inflammatory disorder caused by a tick-borne spirochete.

lymph overflow circulatory fluid in spaces between tissues.

lymphangitis inflammation of the lymph channels, usually as a result of a distal infection.

lymphatic system secondary circulatory system that collects overflow fluid from the tissue spaces and filters it before returning it to the circulatory system.

lymphocyte a type of leukocyte, or white blood cell, that attacks foreign substances as part of the body's immune response.

lymphokine a cytokine released by a lymphocyte.

lymphoma a cancer of the lymphatic system.

maceration process of softening a solid by soaking in a liquid.

macrodrip tubing administration tubing that delivers a relatively large amount of fluid.

macrophage immune system cell that has the ability to recognize and ingest foreign antibodies.

Magill forceps scissor-style clamps with circular tips.

major basic protein (MBP) a larvacidal peptide.

major histocompatibility complex (MHC) a group of genes on chromosome 6 that provide the genetic code for HLA antigens.

major trauma patient person who has suffered significant mechanism of injury.

malfeasance a breach of duty by performance of a wrongful or unlawful act.

malleolus the protuberance of the ankle.

Mallory-Weiss tear esophageal laceration, usually secondary to vomiting.

mammalian diving reflex a complex cardiovascular reflex, resulting from submersion of the face and nose in water, that constricts blood flow everywhere except to the brain.

mandible the jawbone.

manic characterized by excessive excitement or activity (mania).

manometer pressure gauge with a scale calibrated in millimeters of mercury (mmHg).

Marfan's Syndrome hereditary condition of connective tissue, bones, muscles, ligaments, and skeletal structures characterized by irregular and unsteady gait, tall lean body type with long extremities, flat feet, stooped shoulders. The aorta is usually dilated and may become weakened enough to allow an aneurysm to develop.

Mark I kit a two-part autoinjector set the military uses as treatment for nerve-agent exposure; involves the administration of atropine and pralidoxime chloride.

mask a device for protecting the face. *See also* respirator.

mass a measure of the matter that an object contains; the property of a physical body that gives the body inertia.

mast cell specialized cell of the immune system which contains chemicals that assist in the immune response.

material safety data sheets (MSDS) easily accessible sheets of detailed information about chemicals found at fixed facilities.

maxilla bone of the upper jaw.

maximum life span the theoretical, species-specific, longest duration of life, excluding premature or "unnatural" death.

McBurney's point common site of pain from appendicitis, one to two inches above the anterior iliac crest in a direct line with the umbilicus.

measured volume administration set IV setup that delivers specific volumes of fluid.

mechanism of injury the processes and forces that cause trauma.

meconium dark green material found in the intestine of the full-term newborn. It can be expelled from the intestine into the amniotic fluid during periods of fetal distress.

medial toward the midline or center of the body.

medical direction medical policies, procedures, and practices that are available to providers either on-line or off-line.

medical director a physician who is legally responsible for all of the clinical and patient-care aspects of an EMS system. Also referred to as *medical direction*.

medically clean careful handling to prevent contamination.

medicated solution parenteral medication packaged in an IV bag and administered as an IV infusion.

medication injection port in an intravenous administration set, a self-healing membrane into which a hypodermic needle is inserted for drug administration.

medications foreign substances placed into the human body. *See also* drug.

medulla oblongata lower portion of the brainstem, connecting the pons and the spinal cord. It contains major centers for control of respiratory, cardiac, and vasomotor activity.

medulla the inner tissue of an organ such as the kidney.

medullary canal cavity within a bone that contains the marrow.

melena dark, tarry, foul smelling stool resulting from gastrointestinal bleeding.

menarche the onset of menses, usually occurring between ages 10 and 14.

Meniere's disease a disease of the inner ear characterized by vertigo, nerve deafness, and buzzing in the ear.

meninges three membranes that surround and protect the brain and spinal cord: the dura mater, pia mater, and arachnoid membrane.

meningitis inflammation of the meninges, usually caused by an infection.

meningomyelocele hernia of the spinal cord and membranes through a defect in the spinal column.

menopause the cessation of menses and ovarian function due to decreased secretion of estrogen.

menorrhagia excessive menstrual flow.

menstruation sloughing of the uterine lining (endometrium) if a fertilized egg is not implanted. It is controlled by the cyclical release of hormones. Menstruation is also called a *period*.

mental status the state of the patient's cerebral functioning.

mental status examination (MSE) a structured exam designed to quickly evaluate a patient's level of mental functioning.

mesencephalon portion of the brain connecting the pons and cerebellum with the cerebral hemispheres; also called the *midbrain*. It controls motor coordination and eye movement.

mesenteric infarct death of tissue in the peritoneal fold (mesentery) that encircles the small intestine; a life-threatening condition.

mesentery double fold of peritoneum that supports the major portion of the small bowel, suspending it from the posterior abdominal wall.

metabolic acidosis acidity caused by an increase in acid, often because of increased production of acids during metabolism or from causes such as vomiting, diarrhea, diabetes, or medication.

metabolic alkalosis alkalinity caused by an increase in plasma bicarbonate resulting from causes including diuresis, vomiting, or ingestion of too much sodium bicarbonate.

metabolism the total changes that take place in an organism during physiological processes; the sum of cellular processes that produce the energy and molecules needed for growth and repair.

metacarpals bones of the palm.

metaphysis growth zone of a bone, active during the development stages of youth. It is located between the epiphysis and the diaphysis.

metaplasia replacement of one type of cell by another type of cell that is not normal for that tissue.

metatarsal one of the bones forming the arch of the foot.

metered dose inhaler handheld device that produces a medicated spray for inhalation.

microangiopathy a disease affecting the smallest blood vessels.

microcirculation blood flow in the arterioles, capillaries, and venules.

microdrip tubing administration tubing that delivers a relatively small amount of fluid.

midaxillary line an imaginary line from the middle of the armpit to the ankle; divides the body into anterior and posterior planes.

midbrain portion of the brain connecting the pons and cerebellum with the cerebral hemispheres.

midclavicular line an imaginary line from the center of either clavicle down the anterior thorax.

midline an imaginary line drawn vertically through the middle of the body, dividing it into right and left.

minimum effective concentration minimum level of drug needed to cause a given effect.

minimum standards lowest or least allowable standards.

minor depending on state law, this is usually a person under the age of 18.

minute volume amount of gas inhaled and exhaled in one minute.

miosis abnormal contraction of the pupils; pinpoint pupils.

miscarriage commonly used term to describe a pregnancy which ends before 20 weeks gestation; may also be called spontaneous abortion.

misfeasance a breach of duty by performance of a legal act in a manner that is harmful or injurious.

mitosis cell division with division of the nucleus; each daughter cell contains the same number of chromosomes as the mother cell.

mittelschmerz abdominal pain associated with ovulation.

Mix-o-Vial *see* nonconstituted drug vial.

mobile data terminal vehicle-mounted computer keyboard and display.

monoclonal antibody very pure and specific antibody to a single antigen.

monokine a cytokine released by a macrophage.

mononucleosis acute disease caused by the Epstein-Barr virus.

mons pubis fatty layer of tissue over the pubic symphysis.

mood disorder pervasive and sustained emotion that colors a person's perception of the world.

morals social, religious, or personal standards of right and wrong.

morgue area where deceased victims of an incident are collected.

Moro reflex occurring when a newborn is startled, arms are thrown wide, fingers spread, and a grabbing motion follows. Also called *startle reflex*.

motion the process of changing place; movement.

motor aphasia occurs when the patient cannot speak but can understand what is said.

mucolytic medication intended to make mucus more watery.

mucosal immune system *see* secretory immune system.

mucous membrane tissue lining of body cavities that handle air transport; usually contains small, mucus-secreting cells.

mucus slippery secretion that lubricates and protects airway surfaces.

multiple-casualty incident (MCI) incident that generates large numbers of patients and that often makes traditional EMS response ineffective because of special circumstances surrounding the event; also known as *mass-casualty incident*.

multiple myeloma a cancerous disorder of plasma cells.

multiple organ dysfunction syndrome (MODS) progressive impairment of two or more organ systems resulting from an uncontrolled inflammatory response to a severe illness or injury.

multiple personality disorder manifestation of two or more complete systems of personality.

multiple sclerosis disease that involves inflammation of certain nerve cells followed by demyelination, or the destruction of the myelin sheath, which is the fatty insulation surrounding nerve fibers.

multiplex duplex system that can transmit voice and data simultaneously.

mumps acute viral disease characterized by painful enlargement of the salivary glands.

Murphy's sign pain caused when an inflamed gallbladder is palpated by pressing under the right costal margin.

muscle tissue tissue that is capable of contraction when stimulated. There are three types of muscle tissue: *cardiac* (myocardium, or heart muscle), *smooth* (within intestines, surrounding blood vessels), and *skeletal*, or *striated* (allows skeletal movement). Skeletal muscle is mostly under voluntary, or conscious, control; smooth muscle is under involuntary, or unconscious, control; cardiac muscle is capable of spontaneous, or self-excited, contraction.

muscoviscidosis cystic fibrosis of the pancreas resulting in abnormally viscous mucoid secretion from the pancreas.

muscular dystrophy a group of genetic diseases characterized by progressive muscle weakness and degeneration of the skeletal or voluntary muscle fibers.

mutual aid agreements or plans for sharing departmental resources.

myesthania gravis disease characterized by episodic muscle weakness triggered by an autoimmune attack of the acetylcholine receptors.

myocardial infarction (MI) death and subsequent necrosis of the heart muscle caused by inadequate blood supply; also *acute myocardial infarction (AMI)*.

myocardium the cardiac muscle tissue of the heart.

myoclonus temporary, involuntary twitching or spasm of a muscle or group of muscles.

myometrium the thick middle layer of the uterine wall made up of smooth muscle fibers.

myotome muscle and tissue of the body innervated by spinal nerve roots.

myxedema coma life-threatening condition associated with advanced myxedema, with profound hypothermia, bradycardia, and electrolyte imbalance.

myxedema condition that reflects long-term exposure to inadequate levels of thyroid hormones with resultant changes in body structure and function.

nares the openings of the nostrils.

nasal cannula catheter placed at the nares.

nasal flaring excessive widening of the nares with respiration.

nasal medication drug administered through the mucous membranes of the nose.

nasal septum cartilage that separates the right and left nasal cavities.

nasogastric tube/orogastric tube a tube that runs through the nose or mouth and esophagus into the stomach; used for administering liquid nutrients or medications or for removing air or liquids from the stomach.

nasolacrimal duct narrow tube that carries into the nasal cavity the tears and debris that have drained from the eye.

nasopharyngeal airway uncuffed tube that follows the natural curvature of the nasopharynx, passing through the nose and extending from the nostril to the posterior pharynx.

nasotracheal route through the nose and into the trachea.

natural immunity inborn protection against infection or disease that is part of the person's or species' genetic makeup; genetically predetermined immunity that is present at birth; also called *innate immunity*.

naturally acquired immunity immunity that begins to develop after birth and is continually enhanced by exposure to new pathogens and antigens throughout life.

nature of illness a patient's general medical condition or complaint.

near-drowning an incident of potentially fatal submersion in liquid which did not result in death or in which death occurred more than 24 hours after submersion.

nebulizer inhalation aid that disperses liquid into aerosol spray or mist.

necrosis cell death; a pathological cell change; the sloughing off of dead tissue. Four types of necrotic cell change are *coagulative, liquefactive, caseous,* and *fatty. Gangrenous necrosis* refers to tissue death over a wide area.

needle adapter rigid plastic device specifically constructed to fit into the hub of an intravenous cannula.

needle cricothyrotomy surgical airway technique that inserts a 14-gauge needle into the trachea at the cricothyroid membrane.

negative feedback a mechanism of response that serves to maintain a state of internal constancy, or homeostasis. Changes in the internal environment trigger mechanisms that reverse or negate the change, hence the term "negative feedback."

negligence deviation from accepted standards of care recognized by law for the protection of others against the unreasonable risk of harm.

neonatal abstinence syndrome (NAS) a generalized disorder presenting a clinical picture of CNS hyperirritability, gastrointestinal dysfunction, respiratory distress, and vague autonomic symptoms. It may be due to intrauterine exposure to heroin, methadone, or other less potent opiates. Non-opiate central nervous system depressants may also cause NAS.

neonate an infant from the time of birth to one month of age.

nephrology the medical specialty dealing with the kidneys.

nephron a microscopic structure within kidney that produces urine.

nerve agents chemicals that inhibit the degradation of a neurotransmitter (acetylcholine) and quickly facilitate a nervous system overload.

nerve tissue tissue that transmits electrical impulses throughout the body.

net filtration the total loss of water from blood plasma across the capillary membrane into the interstitial space. Normally, hydrostatic pressure forcing water out of the capillary is balanced by oncotic force pulling water into the capillary for a net filtration of zero.

neuroeffector junction specialized synapse between a nerve cell and the organ or tissue it innervates.

neurogenic shock shock resulting from brain or spinal cord injury that causes an interruption of nerve impulses to the arteries with loss of arterial tone, dilation, and relative hypovolemia.

neuroleptanesthesia anesthesia that combines decreased sensation of pain with amnesia while the patient remains conscious.

neuroleptic antipsychotic (literally, *affecting the nerves*).

neuron nerve cell.

neurotransmitter chemical messenger that conducts a nervous impulse across a synapse. Examples include acetylcholine, norepinephrine, and dopamine.

neutron radiation powerful radiation with penetrating properties between that of beta and gamma radiation.

neutropenia a reduction in the number of neutrophils; a low neutrophil count.

neutrophil the most common phagocytic white blood cell.

newborn a baby in the first few hours of its life, also called *newly born infant*.

nitrogen narcosis a state of stupor that develops during deep dives due to nitrogen's effect on cerebral function; also called *raptures of the deep*.

nocturia excessive urination during the night.

noncardiogenic shock types of shock that result from causes other than inadequate cardiac output.

noncompensatory pause pause following an ectopic beat where the SA node is depolarized and the underlying cadence of the heart is interrupted.

noncompetitive antagonism the binding of an antagonist causes a deformity of the binding site that prevents an agonist from fitting and binding.

nonconstituted drug vial/Mix-o-Vial vial with two containers, one holding a powdered medication and the other holding a liquid mixing solution.

nonfeasance a breach of duty by failure to perform a required act or duty.

nonmaleficence the obligation not to harm the patient.

nonverbal communication gestures, mannerisms, and postures by which a person communicates with others; also called *body language*.

normal flora organisms that live inside our bodies without ordinarily causing disease.

normal sinus rhythm the normal heart rhythm.

nosocomial acquired while in the hospital.

nuclear detonation the release of energy that is generated when heavy nuclei split (fission) or light nuclei combine (fusion) to form new elements. The unleashed energy is tremendous and creates an explosion of immense proportion.

nucleus the organelle within a cell that contains the DNA, or genetic material; in the cells of higher organisms, the nucleus is surrounded by a membrane.

oblique having a slanted position or direction.

oblique fracture break in a bone running across it at an angle other than 90 degrees.

obstetrics the branch of medicine that deals with the care of women throughout pregnancy.

ocular medication drug administered through the mucous membranes of the eye.

off-line medical direction refers to medical policies, procedures, and practices that medical direction has set up in advance of a call.

ohm basic unit for measuring the strength of electrical resistance.

Ohm's law the physical law identifying that the current in amperes in an electrical circuit is directly proportional to the voltage and inversely proportional to the resistance.

old-old an elderly person age 80 or older.

oliguria decreased urine elimination to 400-500 mL or less per day.

omphalocele congenital hernia of the umbilicus.

oncotic force a form of osmotic pressure exerted by the large protein particles, or colloids, present in blood plasma. In the capillaries, the plasma colloids tend to pull water from the interstitial space across the capillary membrane into the capillary. Also called *colloid osmotic pressure*.

on-line medical direction occurs when a qualified physician gives direct orders to a prehospital care provider by either radio or telephone.

onset of action the time from administration until a medication reaches its minimum effective concentration.

open cricothyrotomy surgical airway technique that places an endotracheal or tracheostomy tube directly into the trachea through a surgical incision at the cricothyroid membrane.

open fracture a broken bone in which the bone ends or the forces that caused it penetrate the surrounding skin.

open incident an incident that has the potential to generate additional patients; also called *uncontained incident* or *unstable incident*.

open pneumothorax *see* pneumothorax.

open stance a posture or body position that is relaxed and suggests confidence, ease, warmth, and attentiveness.

open-ended questions questions that permit unguided, spontaneous answers.

ophthalmoscope handheld device used to examine interior of eye.

opportunistic pathogen ordinarily nonharmful bacterium that causes disease only under unusual circumstances.

opposition pairing of muscles that permits extension and flexion of limbs.

oral drug administration the delivery of any medication that is taken by mouth and swallowed into the lower gastrointestinal tract.

orbit the eye socket.

ordnance military weapons and munitions.

organ system a group of organs that work together. Examples: the cardiovascular system, formed of the heart, blood vessels, and blood; the gastrointestinal system, comprising the mouth, salivary glands, esophagus, stomach, intestines, liver, pancreas, gall bladder, rectum, and anus.

organ a group of tissues functioning together. Examples: heart, liver, brain, ovary, eye.

organelles structures that perform specific functions within a cell.

organic *see* biological.

organism the sum of all the cells, tissues, organs, and organ systems of a living being. Examples: the human organism, a bacterial organism.

organophosphates phosphorus-containing organic pesticides.

origin attachment of a muscle to a bone that does not move (or experiences the least movement) when the muscle contracts.

orogastric tube *see* nasogastric tube/orogastric tube.

oropharyngeal airway semicircular device that follows the palate's curvature.

orthopnea difficulty in breathing while lying supine.

orthostatic hypotension a decrease in blood pressure that occurs when a person moves from a supine or sitting to an upright position.

osmolality the concentration of solute per kilogram of water. *See also* osmolarity.

osmolarity the concentration of solute per liter of water (often used synonymously with *osmolality*).

osmosis the passage of a solvent such as water through a membrane; movement of solvent in a solution from an area of lower solute concentration to an area of higher solute concentration.

osmotic diuresis greatly increased urination and dehydration due to high levels of glucose that cannot be reabsorbed into the blood from the kidney tubules, causing a loss of water into the urine.

osmotic gradient the difference in concentration between solutions on opposite sides of a semipermeable membrane.

osmotic pressure the pressure exerted by the concentration of solutes on one side of a membrane that, if hypertonic, tends to "pull" water (cause osmosis) from the other side of the membrane.

osteoarthritis a degenerative joint disease, characterized by a loss of articular cartilage and hypertrophy of bone.

osteoblast cell that helps in the creation of new bone during growth and bone repair.

osteoclast bone cell that absorbs and removes excess bone.

osteocyte bone-forming cell found in the bone matrix that helps maintain the bone.

osteoporosis weakening of bone tissue due to loss of essential minerals, especially calcium.

otitis media middle ear infection.

otoscope handheld device used to examine interior of ears and nose.

ovaries the primary female sex glands, which secrete estrogen and progesterone and produce eggs for reproduction.

overdrive respiration positive pressure ventilation supplied to a breathing patient.

overhydration the presence or retention of an abnormally high amount of body fluid.

overpressure a rapid increase then decrease in atmospheric pressure created by an explosion.

over-the-needle catheter semi-flexible catheter enclosing a sharp metal stylet; also called *angiocatheter*.

ovulation the release of an egg from the ovary.

oxidation the loss of hydrogen atoms or the acceptance of an oxygen atom. This increases the positive charge (or lessens the negative charge) on the molecule.

oxidizer an agent that enhances combustion of a fuel.

oxygen gas necessary for energy production.

PA alveolar partial pressure.

Pa arterial partial pressure.

pack/year history a way to quantify your patient's smoking history by multiplying number of packs smoked per day by the number of years smoking.

pallor paleness.

palmar grasp a reflex in the newborn, which is elicited by placing a finger firmly in the infant's palm.

palpation using your sense of touch to gather information.

pancolitis ulcerative colitis spread throughout the entire colon.

panic attack extreme period of anxiety resulting in great emotional distress.

papilla the tip of a pyramid; it juts into the hollow space of the kidney.

paradoxical breathing assymetrical chest wall movement that lessens respiratory efficiency.

parasite organism that lives in or on another organism.

parasympathetic nervous system division of the autonomic nervous system that is responsible for controlling vegetative functions. Parasympathetic nervous system actions include decreased heart rate and constriction of the bronchioles and pupils. Its actions are mediated by the neurotransmitter acetylcholine.

parasympatholytic drug or other substance that blocks or inhibits the actions of the parasympathetic nervous system. Also called *anticholinergic*.

parasympathomimetic drug or other substance that causes effects like those of the parasympathetic nervous system. Also called *cholinergic*.

parenchyma principle or essential parts of an organ.

parent drug *see* prodrug.

parenteral route delivery of a medication outside of the gastrointestinal tract, typically using needles to inject medications into the circulatory system or tissues.

Parkinson's disease chronic and progressive motor system disorder characterized by tremor, rigidity, bradykinesia, and postural instability.

paroxysmal nocturnal dyspnea (PND) a sudden episode of difficult breathing that occurs after lying down; most commonly caused by left heart failure.

partial pressure the pressure exerted by each component of a gas mixture.

partial seizures seizures that remain confined to a limited portion of the brain, causing localized malfunction. Partial seizures may spread and become generalized.

partial-thickness burn burn in which the epidermis is burned through and the dermis is damaged; characterized by redness and blistering; also called a *second-degree burn*.

particulate evidence evidence such as hairs or fibers that cannot be readily seen with the human eye; also known as *microscopic evidence* or *trace evidence*.

partner abuse physical or emotional violence from a man or woman towards a domestic partner.

passive transport movement of a substance without the use of energy.

pathogens microorganisms capable of producing infection or disease, such as bacteria and viruses.

pathology the study of disease and its causes.

pathophysiology the study of how diseases alter normal physiology.

patient assessment problem-oriented evaluation of patient and establishment of priorities based on existing and potential threats to human life.

patient interview interaction with a patient for the purpose of obtaining in-depth information about the emergency and the patient's pertinent medical history.

peak load the highest volume of calls at a given time.

pedicles thick, bony struts that connect the vertebral bodies with the spinous and transverse processes and help make up the opening for the spinal canal.

PEEP *see* positive end-expiratory pressure.

peer review an evaluation of the quality of emergency care administered by an individual, which is conducted by that individual's peers (others of equal rank). Also, an evaluation of articles submitted for publication.

pelvic inflammatory disease (PID) an acute infection of the reproductive organs that can be caused by a bacteria, virus, or fungus.

pelvic space division of the abdominal cavity containing those organs located within the pelvis.

pelvis skeletal structure where the lower extremities attach to the body.

penetrating trauma injury caused by an object breaking the skin and entering the body.

penis the male organ of copulation.

peptic ulcer erosion caused by gastric acid.

percussion the production of sound waves by striking one object against another.

perforating canals structures through which blood vessels enter and exit the bone shaft.

perfusion the supplying of oxygen and nutrients to the body tissues as a result of the constant passage of blood through the capillaries.

pericardial tamponade filling of the pericardial sac with fluid, which in turn limits the filling and function of the heart.

pericardium fibrous sac that surrounds the heart.

perimetrium the serosal peritoneal membrane which forms the outermost layer of the uterine wall.

perinephric abscess a pocket of infection in the layer of fat surrounding the kidney.

perineum muscular tissue that separates the vagina and the anus.

periorbital ecchymosis black and blue discoloration surrounding the eye sockets.

periosteum the tough exterior covering of a bone.

peripheral arterial atherosclerotic disease a progressive degenerative disease of the medium-sized and large arteries.

peripheral nervous system part of the nervous system that extends throughout the body and is composed of the cranial nerves arising from the brain and the peripheral nerves arising from the spinal cord. Its subdivisions are the somatic and the autonomic nervous systems.

peripheral neuropathy any malfunction or damage of the peripheral nerves. Results may include muscle weakness, loss of sensation, impaired reflexes, and internal organ malfunctions.

peripheral vascular resistance the resistance of the vessels to the flow of blood: increased when the vessels constrict, decreased when the vessels relax.

peripheral venous access surgical puncture of a vein in the arm, leg, or neck.

peripherally inserted central catheter (PICC) line threaded into the central circulation via a peripheral site.

peristalsis wavelike muscular motion of the esophagus and bowel that moves food through the digestive system.

peritoneal dialysis a dialysis procedure relying on the peritoneal membrane as the semipermeable membrane.

peritoneal space division of the abdominal cavity containing those organs or portions of organs covered by the peritoneum.

peritoneum fine fibrous tissue surrounding the interior of most of the abdominal cavity and covering most of the small bowel and some of the abdominal organs.

peritonitis inflammation of the peritoneum caused by chemical or bacterial irritation.

permissive a parenting style that takes a tolerant, accepting view of a child's behavior.

persistent fetal circulation condition in which blood continues to bypass the fetal respiratory system, resulting in ongoing hypoxia.

personal protective equipment (PPE) equipment used by EMS personnel to protect against injury and the spread of infectious disease.

personal-care home living arrangement that includes room, board, and some supervision.

personality disorder condition that results in persistently maladaptive behavior.

pertussis disease characterized by severe, violent coughing.

pH abbreviation for *potential of hydrogen.* A measure of relative acidity or alkalinity. Since the pH scale is inverse to the concentration of acidic hydrogen ions, the lower the pH the greater the acidity and the higher the pH the greater the alkalinity. A normal pH range is 7.35 to 7.45.

phagocytes cells that have the ability to ingest other cells and substances, such as bacteria and cell debris.

phagocytosis process in which white blood cells engulf and destroy an invader.

phalanges bones of the fingers.

pharmacodynamics how a drug interacts with the body to cause its effects.

pharmacokinetics how a drug is absorbed, distributed, metabolized (biotransformed), and excreted; how drugs are transported into and out of the body.

pharmacology the study of drugs and their interactions with the body.

pharyngitis infection of the pharynx and tonsils.

pharyngo-tracheal lumen airway (PtL) a two-tube airway system.

pharynx a muscular tube that extends vertically from the back of the soft palate to the superior aspect of the esophagus.

phobia excessive fear that interferes with functioning.

phototherapy exposure to sunlight or artificial light for therapeutic purposes.

physiological stress a chemical or physical disturbance in the cells or tissue fluid produced by a change in the external environment or within the body.

physiology the functions of an organism; the physical and chemical processes of a living thing.

pia mater inner and most delicate layer of the meninges. It covers the convolutions of the brain and spinal cord.

Pierre Robin syndrome unusually small jaw, combined with a cleft palate, downward displacement of the tongue, and an absent gag reflex.

pill-rolling motion an involuntary tremor, usually in one hand or sometimes in both, in which fingers move as if they were rolling a pin back and forth.

pinna outer, visible portion of the ear.

pinworm parasite that is 3–10 mm long and lives in the distal colon.

pitting depression that results from pressure against skin when pitting edema is present.

placenta the organ that serves as a lifeline for the developing fetus. The placenta is attached to the wall of the uterus and the umbilical cord.

placental barrier biochemical barrier at the maternal/fetal interface that restricts certain molecules.

plasma membrane *see* cell membrane.

plasma thick, pale yellow fluid that makes up the liquid part of the blood.

plasma-level profile describes the lengths of onset, duration, and termination of action, as well as the drug's minimum effective concentration and toxic levels.

platelet phase a step in the clotting process in which platelets adhere to blood vessel walls and to each other.

platelet one of the fragments of cytoplasm that circulate in the blood and work with components of the coagulation system to promote blood clotting. Platelets also release serotonin, a vasoconstrictive substance.

pleura membranous connective tissue covering the lungs.

pleural friction rub the squeaking or grating sound of the pleural linings rubbing together.

pleuritic sharp or tearing, as a description of pain.

pluripotent stem cell a cell from which the various types of blood cells can form.

pneumatic anti-shock garment (PASG) garment designed to produce uniform pressure on the lower extremities and abdomen; used with shock and hemorrhage patients in some EMS systems.

pneumomediastinum the presence of air in the mediastinum.

pneumonia acute infection of the lung, including alveolar spaces and interstitial tissue.

pneumothorax a collection of air in the pleural space, causing a loss of the negative pressure that binds the lung to the chest wall. In an *open pneumothorax*, air enters the pleural space through an injury to the chest wall. In a *closed pneumothorax*, air enters the pleural space through an opening in the pleura that covers the lung. A *tension pneumothorax* develops when air in the pleural space cannot escape, causing a build-up of pressure and collapse of the lung. *See also* hemothorax, spontaneous pneumothorax.

Poiseuille's law a law of physiology stating that blood flow through a vessel is directly proportional to the radius of the vessel to the fourth power.

poliomyelitis (polio) infectious, inflammatory viral disease of the central nervous system that sometimes results in permanent paralysis.

polycythemia an excess of red blood cells.

polymorphonuclear cells *see* granulocytes.

polypharmacy multiple drug therapy in which there is a concurrent use of a number of drugs.

polyuria excessive urination.

pons process of tissue responsible for the communication interchange between the cerebellum, the cerebrum, midbrain, and the spinal cord.

portal system a venous subsystem that collects blood, fluids, and nutrients absorbed by the bowel and transports them to the liver.

positive end-expiratory pressure (PEEP) a method of holding the alveoli open by increasing expiratory pressure. Some bag-valve units used in EMS have PEEP attachments. Also EMS personnel sometimes transport patients who are on ventilators with PEEP attachments.

post partum depression the "let down" feeling experienced during the period following birth occurring in 70%–80% of mothers.

post-conventional reasoning the stage of moral development during which individuals make moral decisions according to an enlightened conscience.

posterior toward the back. *Opposite of* anterior.

posterior medial sulcus shallow longitudinal groove along the dorsal surface of the spinal cord.

post-ganglionic nerves nerve fibers that extend from the autonomic ganglia to the target tissues.

postrenal acute renal failure acute renal failure due to obstruction distal to the kidney.

posttraumatic stress syndrome reaction to an extreme stressor.

posture position, attitude, or bearing of the body.

PPD purified protein derivative, the substance used in a test for tuberculosis.

prearrival instructions dispatcher's instructions to caller for appropriate emergency measures.

pre-conventional reasoning the stage of moral development during which children respond mainly to cultural control to avoid punishment and attain satisfaction.

precordial (chest) leads electrocardiogram leads applied to the chest in a pattern that permits a view of the horizontal plane of the heart; leads V1, V2, V3, V4, V5, and V6.

precordium area of the chest wall overlying the heart.

prefilled syringe syringe packaged in a tamper-proof container with the medication already in the barrel; also called *preloaded syringe*.

pre-ganglionic nerves nerve fibers that extend from the central nervous system to the autonomic ganglia.

prehospital care report (PCR) the written record of an EMS response.

preload the pressure within the ventricles at the end of diastole; commonly called *end-diastolic volume*.

preloaded syringe *see* prefilled syringe.

premenstrual syndrome (PMS) a variety of signs and symptoms, such as weight gain, irritability, or specific food cravings associated with the changing hormonal levels that precede menstruation.

prerenal acute renal failure acute renal failure due to decreased blood perfusion of kidneys.

pressure ulcer ischemic damage and subsequent necrosis affecting the skin, subcutaneous tissue, and often the muscle; result of intense pressure over a short time or low pressure over a long time; also known as *pressure sore* or *bedsore*.

pressure wave area of overpressure that radiates outward from an explosion.

preventive strategy a management plan to minimize further damage to vital tissues.

primary area of responsibility (PAR) stationing of ambulances at specific high-volume locations.

primary care basic health care provided at the patient's first contact with the health-care system.

primary contamination direct exposure of a person or item to a hazardous substance.

primary immune response the initial development of antibodies in response to the first exposure to an antigen in which the immune system becomes "primed" to produce a faster, stronger response to any future exposures.

primary intention simple healing of a minor wound without granulation or pus formation.

primary prevention keeping an injury from ever occurring.

primary problem the underlying cause for your patient's symptoms.

primary triage triage that takes place early in the incident, usually upon first arrival.

Prinzmetal's angina variant of angina pectoris caused by vasospasm of the coronary arteries; not blockage per se. Also called *vasopastic angina* or *atypical angina*.

prions particles of protein, folded in such a way that protease enzymes cannot act upon them.

priority dispatching system using medically-approved questions and predetermined guidelines to determine the appropriate level of response.

proactive acting to prevent or deal with potential problems before they occur.

proctitis ulcerative colitis limited to the rectum.

prodrug medication that is not active when administered, but whose biotransformation converts it into active metabolites; also called *parent drug.*

profession refers to the existence of a specialized body of knowledge or skills.

professionalism refers to the conduct or qualities that characterize a practitioner in a particular field or occupation.

profile the size and shape of a projectile as it contacts a target; the energy exchange surface of the contact.

prognosis the anticipated outcome of a disease or injury.

prolonged QT interval QT interval greater than 0.44 seconds.

prompt care facilities hospital agencies that provide limited care and non-emergent medical treatment.

prostaglandins substances synthesized by mast cells during inflammatory response that cause vasoconstriction, vascular permeability, and chemotaxis and also cause pain. Prostaglandins also act to control inflammation by suppressing histamine release and releasing lysosomal enzymes.

prostate a gland that surrounds the male bladder neck and the first portion of urethra; it produces fluid that mixes with sperm to make semen.

prostatitis infection and inflammation of the prostate gland.

protocols the policies and procedures for all components of an EMS system; principles for managing certain patient conditions.

protozoan single-celled parasitic organism with flexible membranes and the ability to move.

proximal near the point of reference. *Opposite of* distal.

proximal tubule the part of the nephron tubule beyond Bowman's capsule.

proximate cause action or inaction of the EMT-I that immediately caused or worsened the damage suffered by the patient.

pruritus itching; often occurs as a symptom of some systemic change or illness.

PSAP public safety access point.

pseudo-instinctive learned actions that are practiced until they can be done without thinking.

psychogenic amnesia failure to recall, as opposed to inability to recall.

psychoneuroimmunological regulation the interactions of psychological, neurological/endocrine, and immunological factors that contribute to alteration of the immune system as an outcome of a stress response that is not quickly resolved.

psychosis extreme response to stress characterized by impaired ability to deal with reality.

psychosocial related to a patient's personality style, dynamics of unresolved conflict, or crisis management methods.

psychotherapeutic medication drug used to treat mental dysfunction.

pubis irregular innominate bone.

puerperium the time period surrounding the birth of the fetus.

pulmonary agents chemicals that primarily cause injury to the lungs; also called *choking agents.*

pulmonary embolism blood clot that travels to the pulmonary circulation and hinders oxygenation of the blood.

pulmonary hilum central medial region of the lung where the bronchi and pulmonary vasculature enter the lung.

pulmonary over-pressure expansion of air held in the lungs during ascent. If not exhaled, the expanded air may cause injury to the lungs and surrounding structures.

pulse oximeter noninvasive device that measures the oxygen saturation of blood.

pulse oximetry a measurement of hemoglobin oxygen saturation in the peripheral tissues.

pulse pressure difference between the systolic and diastolic blood pressures.

pulse quality strength, which can be weak, thready, strong, or bounding.

pulse rate number of pulses felt in one minute.

pulse rhythm pattern and equality of intervals between beats.

pulsus paradoxus drop in blood pressure of greater than 10 torr during inspiration.

puncture specific soft-tissue injury involving a deep, narrow wound to the skin and underlying organs that carries an increased danger of infection.

pupil dark opening in the center of the iris through which light enters the eye.

pyelonephritis an infection and inflammation of the kidney.

pyramids the visible tissue structures within the medulla of a kidney.

pyrexia fever, or above-normal body temperature.

pyrogen any substance causing a fever, such as viruses and bacteria or substances produced within the body in response to infection or inflammation.

QRS axis reduction of all the heart's electrical forces to a single vector represented by an arrow moving in a single plane. Also called *vector*.

QT interval period from the beginning of the QRS to the end of the T wave.

quality assurance (QA) a program designed to maintain continuous monitoring and measurement of the quality of clinical care delivered to patients.

quality improvement (QI) an evaluation program that emphasizes service and uses customer satisfaction as the ultimate indicator of system performance.

quality of respiration depth and pattern of breathing.

rabies viral disorder that affects the nervous system.

rad basic unit of absorbed radiation dose.

radiation transfer of energy through space or matter. *See also* ionizing radiation.

radio band a range of radio frequencies.

radio frequency the number of times per second a radio wave oscillates.

radius bone on the thumb side of the forearm.

rape Penile penetration of the genitalia or rectum without the consent of the victim.

rapid sequence intubation giving medications to sedate (induce) and temporarily paralyze a patient and then performing orotracheal intubation.

rapid trauma assessment quick check for signs of serious injury.

reabsorption the movement of a substance from a nephron tubule back into the blood.

reactive acting on problems after they occur.

reasonable force the minimal amount of force necessary to ensure that an unruly or violent person does not cause injury to himself or others.

rebound tenderness pain on release of the examiner's hands, allowing the abdominal wall to return to its normal position; associated with peritoneal irritation.

receptor specialized protein that combines with a drug resulting in a biochemical effect.

reciprocal in an ECG, a mirror image seen typically on the opposite wall of the injured area.

reciprocity the process by which an agency grants automatic certification or licensure to an individual who has comparable certification or licensure from another agency.

recirculating currents movement of currents over a uniform obstruction; also known as *drowning machine*.

recompression resubmission of a person to a greater pressure so that gradual decompression can be achieved; often used in the treatment of diving emergencies.

red bone marrow tissue within the internal cavity of a bone responsible for manufacture of erythrocytes and other blood cells.

reduced nephron mass the decrease in number of functional nephrons that causes chronic renal failure.

reduced renal mass the decrease in kidney size associated with chronic renal failure.

reduction returning of displaced bone ends to their proper anatomic orientation.

referred pain pain that is felt at a location away from its source.

reflective acting thoughtfully, deliberately, and analytically.

refractory period the period of time when myocardial cells have not yet completely repolarized and cannot be stimulated again. *See also* absolute refractory period, relative refractory period.

regeneration regrowth through cell proliferation.

registration the process of entering one's name and essential information within a particular record.

regulatory law *see* administrative law.

relative refractory period the period of the cardiac cycle when, although the myocardial cells have not completely repolarized, a sufficiently strong stimulus may produce depolarization.

remodeling stage in the wound healing process in which collagen is broken down and relaid in an orderly fashion.

renal acute renal failure ARF due to pathology within kidney tissue itself.

renal calculi kidney stones.

renal dialysis artificial replacement of some critical kidney functions.

renal pelvis the hollow space of the kidney at the junction with a ureter.

renal pertaining to the kidneys.

renin an enzyme produced by kidney cells that plays a key role in controlling arterial blood pressure.

repair healing of a wound with scar formation.

repolarization return of a muscle cell to its pre-excitation resting state.

reportable collisions collisions that involve over $1,000 in damage or a personal injury.

res ipsa loquitur a legal doctrine invoked by plaintiffs to support a claim of negligence, it is a Latin term that means "the thing speaks for itself."

reserve capacity the ability of an EMS agency to respond to calls beyond those handled by the on-duty crews.

reservoir any living creature or environment (water, soil, etc.) that can harbor an infectious agent.

resiliency the connective strength and elasticity of an object or fabric.

resistance a host's ability to fight off infection. Also, property of a conductor that opposes the passage of an electric current.

resolution the complete healing of a wound and return of tissues to their normal structure and function; the ending of inflammation with no scar formation.

respiration the exchange of gases between a living organism and its environment; exchange of oxygen and carbon dioxide during inhalation and exhalation in the lungs and at the cellular level.

respirator an apparatus worn that cleanses or qualifies the air.

respiratory acidosis acidity caused by abnormal retention of carbon dioxide resulting from impaired ventilation.

respiratory alkalosis alkalinity caused by excessive elimination of carbon dioxide resulting from increased respirations.

respiratory effort how hard patient works to breathe.

respiratory rate number of times a person breathes in one minute.

respiratory shock shock resulting from failure of the respiratory system to supply oxygen to the alveoli or remove CO_2 from them.

respiratory syncytial virus (RSV) common cause of pneumonia and bronchiolitis in children.

response time time elapsed from when a unit is alerted until it arrives on the scene.

resting potential the normal electrical state of cardiac cells.

restraint asphyxia death from positioning that prevents sufficient intake of oxygen.

resuscitation provision of efforts to return a spontaneous pulse and breathing.

reticular activating system (RAS) the system responsible for consciousness. A series of nervous tissues keeping the human system in a state of consciousness.

reticuloendothelial system (RES) the cells involved in the immune response.

retina light- and color-sensing tissue lining the posterior chamber of the eye.

retinal detachment condition that may be of traumatic origin and present with patient complaint of a dark curtain obstructing a portion of the field of view.

retinopathy any disorder of the retina.

retroauricular ecchymosis black-and-blue discoloration over the mastoid process (just behind the ear) that is characteristic of a basilar skull fracture. Also called *Battle's sign*.

retrograde amnesia inability to remember events that occurred before the trauma that caused the condition.

retroperitoneal space division of the abdominal cavity containing those organs posterior to the peritoneal lining.

return of spontaneous circulation resuscitation results in the patient's having a spontaneous pulse.

Rh blood group a group of antigens discovered on the red blood cells of rhesus monkeys that is also present to some extent in humans.

Rh factor an antigen in the Rh blood group that is also known as *antigen D*. About 85% of North Americans have the Rh factor (are Rh positive) while about 15% do not have the Rh factor (are Rh negative). Rh positive and Rh negative blood are incompatible.

rhabdomyolysis acute disease that involves the destruction of skeletal muscle.

rheumatoid arthritis chronic disease that causes deterioration of peripheral joint connective tissue.

rhinorrhea watery discharge from the nose.

rhonchi continuous sounds with a lower pitch and a snoring quality.

rhythm strip electrocardiogram printout.

rooting reflex occurring when an infant's cheek is touched by a hand or cloth, the hungry infant turns his head to the right or left.

rotation turning along the axis of a bone or joint.

rouleaux group of red blood cells that are stuck together.

rubella (German measles) systemic viral disease characterized by a fine pink rash that appears on the face, trunk, and extremities and fades quickly.

rule of nines method of estimating amount of body surface area burned by a division of the body into regions, each of which represents approximately 1% of total BSA (plus 1% for the genital region).

rule of palms method of estimating body surface area burned in comparison to the patient's palmar surface.

rules of evidence guidelines for permitting a new medication, process, or procedure to be used in EMS.

rust out an inability to keep abreast of new technologies and standards.

Ryan White Act federal law that outlines the rights and responsibilities of agencies and health care workers when an infectious disease exposure occurs.

SAMPLE history memory aid for gathering a complete patient history; letters stand for signs and symptoms, allergies, medications, pertinent past history, last oral intake, and events leading up to the emergency.

scabies skin disease caused by mite infestation and characterized by intense itching.

scene safety doing everything possible to ensure a safe environment.

scene-authority law legal state or local statute specifying who has ultimate authority at an MCI.

schizophrenia common disorder involving significant change in behavior often including hallucinations, delusions, and depression.

sclera the "white" of the eye.

scope of practice range of duties and skills EMT-Is are allowed and expected to perform.

scrambling climbing over rocks and/or downed trees on a steep trail without the aid of ropes. This can be especially dangerous when the surface is wet or icy.

scree loose pebbles or rock debris that can form on the slopes or bases of mountains; sometimes used to describe debris in sloping dry stream beds.

scrotum a muscular sac outside of the abdominal cavity that contains the testes, epididymis, and vas deferens.

scuba abbreviation for self-contained underwater breathing apparatus. Portable apparatus that contains compressed air which allows the diver to breathe underwater.

sebaceous glands glands within the dermis secreting sebum.

sebum fatty secretion of the sebaceous gland; it helps keep the skin pliable and waterproof.

second messenger chemical that participates in complex cascading reactions that eventually cause a drug's desired effect.

secondary contamination transfer of a hazardous substance to a non-contaminated person or item via contact with someone or something already contaminated by the substance.

secondary immune response the swift, strong response of the immune system to repeated exposures to an antigen.

secondary intention complex healing of a larger wound involving sealing of the wound through scab formation, granulation or filling of the wound, and constriction of the wound.

secondary prevention medical care after an injury or illness that helps to prevent further problems from occurring.

secondary triage triage that takes place after patients are moved to a treatment area to determine any change in status.

secretion the movement of a substance from the blood into a nephron tubule.

secretory immune system lymphoid tissues beneath the mucosal endothelium that secrete substances such as sweat, tears, saliva, mucus, and breast milk; also called *external immune system* or *mucosal immune system*.

sector *see* branch.

secure attachment a type of bonding that occurs when an infant learns that his caregivers will be responsive and helpful when needed.

sedative agent that exerts a soothing or tranquilizing effect.

seizure a temporary alteration in behavior due to the massive electrical discharge of one or more groups of neurons in the brain. Seizures can be clinically classified as generalized or partial.

Sellick's maneuver pressure applied in a posterior direction to the anterior cricoid cartilage, occludes the esophagus.

semantic related to the meaning of words.

semen male reproductive fluid.

semicircular canals the three rings of the inner ear. They sense the motion of the head and provide positional sense for the body.

semi-decontaminated patient another name for field-decontaminated patient.

semi-Fowler's position sitting up at 45°.

semipermeable able to allow some, but not all, substances to pass through. Cell membranes are semipermeable.

Sengstaken-Blakemore tube three-lumen tube used in treating esophageal bleeding.

senile dementia general term used to describe an abnormal decline in mental functioning seen in the elderly; also called *organic brain syndrome* or *multi-infarct dementia.*

sensitization initial exposure of a person to an antigen that results in an immune response.

sensorineural deafness deafness caused by the inability of nerve impulses to reach the auditory center of the brain because of nerve damage either to the inner ear or to the brain.

sensorium sensory apparatus of the body as a whole; also that portion of the brain that functions as a center of sensations.

sensory aphasia occurs when the patient cannot understand the spoken word.

septic shock shock that develops as the result of infection carried by the bloodstream, eventually causing dysfunction of multiple organ systems.

septicemia the systemic spread of toxins through the bloodstream. Also called *sepsis.*

septum cartilage that separates the right and left nasal cavities.

sequestration the trapping of red blood cells by an organ such as the spleen.

seroconversion creation of antibodies after exposure to a disease.

serotonin a substance released by platelets that, through constriction and dilation of blood vessels, affects blood flow to an injured or affected site.

serous fluid a cellular component of blood, similar to plasma.

serum solution containing whole antibodies for a specific pathogen.

sesamoid bone bone that forms in a tendon.

sexual assault Unwanted oral, genital, rectal, or manual sexual contact.

sexually transmitted disease (STD) illness most commonly transmitted through sexual contact.

sharps container rigid, puncture resistant container clearly marked as a biohazard.

shipping papers documents routinely carried aboard vehicles transporting hazardous materials; ideally should identify specific substances and quantities carried; also known as *bills of lading.*

shock a state of inadequate tissue perfusion. *See also* hypoperfusion.

short haul a helicopter extrication technique where a person is attached to a rope that is, in turn, attached to a helicopter. The aircraft lifts off with the person attached to it.

shunt surgical connection that runs from the brain to the abdomen for the purpose of draining excess CNS fluid and preventing increased intracranial pressure.

Shy-Drager syndrome chronic orthostatic hypotension caused by a primary autonomic nervous system deficiency.

sick sinus syndrome a group of disorders characterized by dysfunction of the sinoatrial node in the heart.

sickle cell anemia an inherited disorder of red blood cell production so named because the red blood cells become sickle-shaped when oxygen levels are low. Also called *sickle cell disease.*

side effect unintended response to a drug.

silent myocardial infarction a myocardial infarction that occurs without exhibiting obvious signs and symptoms.

simple diffusion the random motion of molecules from an area of high concentration to an area of lower concentration.

simple partial seizure type of partial seizure that involves local motor, sensory, or autonomic dysfunction of one area of the body. There is no loss of consciousness.

simplex communication system that transmits and receives on the same frequency.

singular command process where a single individual is responsible for coordinating an incident; most useful in single-jurisdictional incidents.

sinus air cavity that conducts fluids from the eustachian tubes and tear ducts to and from the nasopharynx.

sinusitis inflammation of the paranasal sinuses.

slander act of injuring a person's character, name, or reputation by false or malicious statements spoken with malicious intent or reckless disregard for the falsity of those statements.

slow-reacting substance of anaphylaxis (SRS-A) substance released from basophils and mast cells that causes spasm of the bronchiole smooth muscle, resulting in an asthma-like attack and occasionally asphyxia. *See also* leukotrienes.

sociocultural related to the patient's actions and interactions within society.

solvent a substance that dissolves other substances, forming a solution.

somatic nervous system part of the nervous system controlling voluntary bodily functions.

somatic pain sharp, localized pain that originates in walls of the body such as skeletal muscles.

somatoform disorder condition characterized by physical symptoms that have no apparent physiological cause and are attributable to psychological factors.

span of control number of people or tasks that a single individual can monitor.

spasm intermittent or continuous contraction of a muscle.

Special Weapons and Tactics (SWAT) Team a trained police unit equipped to handle hostage holders and other difficult law enforcement situations.

specific gravity refers to the density or weight of a vapor or gas as compared to air.

sperm cell male reproductive cell.

sphygmomanometer blood pressure measuring device comprising a bulb, a cuff, and a manometer.

spike sharp-pointed device inserted into the IV solution bag's administration set port.

spina bifida (SB) a neural defect that results from the failure of one or more of the fetal vertebrae to close properly during the first month of pregnancy.

spinal canal opening in the vertebrae that accomodates the spinal cord.

spinal cord central nervous system (CNS) pathway responsible for transmitting sensory input from the body to the brain and for conducting motor impulses from the brain to the muscles and organs.

spinal nerves 31 pairs of nerves that originate along the spinal cord from anterior and posterior nerve roots.

spinous process prominence at the posterior part of a vertebra.

spiral fracture a curving break in a bone as may be caused by rotational forces.

spondylosis a degeneration of the vertebral body.

spontaneous pneumothorax a pneumothorax (collection of air in the pleural space) that occurs spontaneously, in the absence of blunt or penetrating trauma.

spotter the person behind the left rear side of the ambulance who assists the operator in backing up the vehicle.

sprain tearing of a joint capsule's connective tissues.

staging location where ambulances, personnel, and equipment are kept in reserve for use at an incident.

standard of care the degree of care, skill, and judgment that would be expected under like or similar circumstances by a similarly trained, reasonable EMT-I in the same community.

standing orders preauthorized treatment procedures or protocol.

Starling's law of the heart law of physiology stating that the more the myocardium is stretched, up to a certain amount, the more forceful the subsequent contraction will be.

START acronym for *simple triage and rapid transport,* the most widely used disaster triage system.

startle reflex *see* Moro reflex.

status epilepticus prolonged seizure or multiple seizures with no regaining of consciousness between them.

statutory law *see* legislative law.

stem cells undifferentiated cells in the bone marrow from which all blood cells, including thrombocytes, erythrocytes, and various types of leukocytes, develop; stem cells are also called *hemocytoblasts.*

stenosis narrowing or constriction.

sterile free of all forms of life.

steroid agent that reduces the body's response to injury with effects that include reduction of swelling.

sterilizing use of a chemical or physical method such as pressurized steam to kill all microorganisms on an object.

stethoscope tool used to auscultate most sounds.

stock solution standard concentration of routinely used medications.

Stokes-Adams syndrome a series of symptoms resulting from heart block, most commonly syncope.

stoma opening in the anterior neck that connects the trachea with ambient air; a permanent surgical opening in the neck through which the patient breathes.

strain injury resulting from overstretching of muscle fibers.

strainers a partial obstruction that filters, or strains, the water such as downed trees or wire mesh; causes an unequal force on the two sides.

stress a hardship or strain; a state of physical or psychological arousal to stimulus.

stress response changes within the body initiated by a stressor.

stressor a stimulus that causes stress.

stridor predominantly inspiratory wheeze associated with laryngeal obstruction.

stroke volume the amount of blood ejected by the heart in one cardiac contraction.

stroke injury or death of brain tissue resulting from interruption of cerebral blood flow and oxygenation; also known as *cerebral vascular accident* or *brain attack.*

stylet plastic-covered metal wire used to bend the endotracheal tube into a J or hockey-stick shape.

subarachnoid hemorrhage bleeding that occurs between the arachoid and dura mater of the brain.

subcutaneous emphysema presence of air in the subcutaneous tissue; the resulting crackling sensation or sound.

subcutaneous tissue body layer beneath the dermis; the layer of loose connective tissue between the skin and muscle.

subdural hematoma collection of blood directly beneath the dura mater.

subendocardial infarction myocardial infarction that affects only the deeper levels of the myocardium; also called *non-Q-wave infarction* because it typically does not result in a significant Q wave in the affected lead.

subglottic referring to the lower airway.

sublingual beneath the tongue.

substance abuse use of a pharmacological substance for purposes other than medically defined reasons.

sucking reflex occurring when an infant's lips are stroked.

suction to remove with a vacuum-type device.

sudden death death within one hour after the onset of symptoms.

sudden infant death syndrome (SIDS) illness of unknown etiology that occurs during the first year of life, with the peak at ages 2–4 months.

sudoriferous glands glands within the dermis that secrete sweat.

superficial burn a burn that involves only the epidermis; characterized by reddening of the skin; also called *first-degree burn.*

superficial frostbite freezing involving only epidermal tissues resulting in redness followed by blanching and diminished sensation; also called *frostnip.*

superior above; toward the head. *Opposite of* inferior.

suppository medication packaged in a soft, pliable form, for insertion into the rectum.

supraglottic referring to the upper airway.

surface absorption entry of a substance into the body directly through the skin or mucous membrane.

surfactant substance that decreases surface tension.

survival when a patient is resuscitated and survives to be discharged from the hospital.

sutures pseudo-joints that join the various bones of the skull to form the cranium.

sympathetic nervous system division of the autonomic nervous system that prepares the body for stressful situations. Sympathetic nervous system actions include increased heart rate and dilation of the bronchioles and pupils. Its actions are mediated by the neurotransmitters epinephrine and norepinephrine.

sympatholytic drug or other substance that blocks the actions of the sympathetic nervous system. Also called *antiadrenergic.*

sympathomimetic drug or other substance that causes effects like those of the sympathetic nervous system. Also called *adrenergic.*

synapse space between nerve cells.

synarthrosis a joint that does not permit movement.

synchronized cardioversion the passage of an electric current through the heart during a specific part of the cardiac cycle to terminate certain kinds of dysrhythmias.

syncope transient loss of consciousness due to inadequate flow of blood to the brain with rapid recovery of consciousness upon becoming supine; fainting.

syncytium group of cardiac muscle cells that physiologically function as a unit.

synergism a standard pharmacological principle in which two substances or drugs work together to produce an effect that neither of them can produce on its own.

synovial fluid substance that lubricates synovial joints.

synovial joint type of joint that permits the greatest degree of independent motion.

syphilis blood-borne sexually transmitted disease caused by the spirochete *Treponema pallidum.*

syringe plastic tube with which liquid medications can be drawn up, stored, and injected.

system status management (SSM) a computerized personnel and ambulance deployment system

systemic effects effects that occur throughout the body after exposure to a toxic substance.

systemic throughout the body.

systole the period of the cardiac cycle when the myocardium is contracting.

systolic blood pressure force of blood against arteries when ventricles contract.

T cell receptor (TCR) a molecule on the surface of a helper T cell that responds to a specific antigen. There is a specific TCR for every antigen to which the human body may be exposed.

T lymphocytes white blood cells that do not produce antibodies but, instead, attacks antigens directly.

tachycardia pulse rate higher than 100.

tachycardia rapid heart rate; a heart rate greater than 100 beats per minute.

tachypnea rapid respiration.

tactile fremitus vibratory tremors felt through the chest by palpation.

teachable moments the time shortly after an injury when patients may be more receptive to teaching about how similar injury or illness could be prevented in the future.

ten-code radio communications system using codes that begin with the word ten.

tenderness pain that is elicited through palpation.

tendons long, thin, very strong collagen tissues that connect muscles to bones.

tension lines natural patterns in the surface of the skin revealing tensions within.

tension pneumothorax buildup of air under pressure within the thorax. The resulting compression of the lung severely reduces the effectiveness of respirations. *See* pneumothorax.

teratogenic drug medication that may deform or kill the fetus.

terminal-drop hypothesis a theory that death is preceded by a five-year period of decreasing cognitive functioning.

termination of action time from when the drug's level drops below its minimum effective concentration until it is eliminated from the body.

terrorist act the use of violence to provoke fear and influence behavior for political, social, religious, or ethnic goals.

tertiary prevention rehabilitation after an injury or illness that helps to prevent further problems from occurring.

testes primary male reproductive organs, which produce hormones responsible for sexual maturation and sperm; singular *testis.*

tetanus acute bacterial infection of the central nervous system.

thalamus switching station between the pons and the cerebrum in the brain.

therapeutic index the maximum tolerated dose divided by the minimum curative close of a drug; the range between curative and toxic dosages; also called *therapeutic window.*

therapy regulator pressure regulator used for delivering oxygen to patients.

thermal gradient the difference in temperature between the environment and the body.

thermogenesis the production of heat, especially within the body.

thermolysis loss of heat from the body.

thermoregulation the maintenance or regulation of a particular temperature of the body.

thoracoabdominal pump process by which respirations assist blood return to the heart.

thrill vibration or humming felt when palpating the pulse.

thrombocyte blood platelet.

thrombocytopenia an abnormal decrease in the number of platelets.

thrombocytosis an abnormal increase in the number of platelets.

thrombolytic drug that acts directly on thrombi by breaking them down.

thrombophlebitis inflammation of the vein.

thrombosis clot formation in coronary arteries or cerebral vasculature.

thrombus blood clot.

thyrotoxic crisis toxic condition characterized by hyperthermia, tachycardia, nervous symptoms, and rapid metabolism; also known as *thyroid storm.*

thyrotoxicosis condition that reflects prolonged exposure to excess thyroid hormones with resultant changes in body structure and function.

tibia the larger bone of the lower leg that articulates with the femur.

tidal volume average volume of gas inhaled or exhaled in one respiratory cycle.

tiered response system system that allows multiple vehicles to arrive at an EMS call at different times, often providing different levels of care or transport.

tilt test drop in the systolic blood pressure of 20 mmHg or an increase in the pulse rate of 20 beats per minute when a patient is moved from a supine to a sitting position; a finding suggestive of a relative hypovolemia.

tinnitus the sensation of ringing in the ears.

tissue a group of cells that perform a similar function.

tocolysis the process of stopping labor.

tolerance the need to progressively increase the dose of a drug to reproduce the effect originally achieved by smaller doses.

tone state of slight contraction of muscles that gives them firmness and keeps them ready to move.

tonic phase phase of a seizure characterized by tension or contraction of muscles.

tonic-clonic seizure type of generalized seizure characterized by rapid loss of consciousness and motor coordination, muscle spasms, and jerking motions.

tonicity solute concentration or osmotic pressure relative to the blood plasma or body cells.

topical anesthetic agent that produces partial or complete loss of sensation in the surface area to which it is applied.

topical medications material applied to and absorbed through the skin or mucous membranes.

tort a civil wrong committed by one individual against another.

total body water (TBW) the total amount of water in the body at a given time.

total down time duration from the beginning of the arrest until the patient's delivery to the emergency department.

total lung capacity maximum lung capacity.

touch pad computer on which you enter data by touching areas of the display screen.

tourniquet a constrictor used on an extremity to apply circumferential pressure on all arteries to control bleeding.

toxicology study of the detection, chemistry, pharmacological actions, and antidotes of toxic substances.

toxidrome a toxic syndrome; a group of typical signs and symptoms consistently associated with exposure to a particular type of toxin.

toxin any chemical (drug, poison, or other) that causes adverse effects on an organism that is exposed to it; any poisonous chemical secreted by bacteria or released following destruction of the bacteria.

trachea 10–12 cm long tube that connects the larynx to the mainstem bronchi.

tracheal deviation any position of the trachea other than midline.

tracheal tugging retraction of the tissues of the neck due to airway obstruction or dyspnea.

tracheobronchial tree the structures of the trachea and the bronchi.

tracheostomy a surgical incision that a surgeon makes from the anterior neck into the trachea; held open by a metal or plastic tube.

trajectory the path a projectile follows.

transdermal absorbed through the skin.

transection a cutting across a long axis; a cross-sectional cut.

transient ischemic attack (TIA) temporary interruption of blood supply to the brain; often seen as a precursor to a stroke.

transmural infarction myocardial infarction that affects the full thickness of the myocardium and almost always results in a pathological Q wave in the affected leads.

transverse fracture a break that runs across a bone perpendicular to the bone's orientation.

transverse process bony outgrowth of the vertebral pedicle that serves as a site for muscle attachment and articulation with the ribs.

trauma center medical facility that has the capability of caring for the acutely injured patient. Trauma centers must meet strict criteria to use this designation.

trauma registry a data retrieval system for trauma patient information, used to evaluate and improve the trauma system.

trauma triage criteria guidelines to aid prehospital personnel in determining which trauma patients require urgent transportation to a trauma center.

trauma a physical injury or wound caused by external force or violence.

trench foot a painful foot disorder resembling frostbite and resulting from exposure to cold and wet, which can eventually result in tissue sloughing or gangrene; also called *immersion foot.*

triage tag a tag containing vital information, affixed to a patient during a multi-patient incident.

triage a method of sorting patients by the severity of their injuries.

trichinosis disease resulting from an infestation of *Trichinella spriralis.*

trichomoniasis sexually transmitted disease caused by the protozoan *Trichomonas vaginalis.*

trocar a sharp, pointed instrument.

trunking communication system that pools all frequencies and routes transmissions to the next available frequency.

trust vs. mistrust refers to a stage of psychosocial development that lasts from birth to about 1½ years of age.

tuberculosis (TB) disease caused by a bacterium known as *Mycobacterium*

tuberculosis that primarily affects the respiratory system.

tunica adventitia outer fibrous layer of the blood vessels that maintains their maximum size.

tunica intima smooth interior layer of the blood vessels that provides for the free flow of blood.

tunica media the middle, muscular layer of the blood vessels that controls the vessels' lumen size.

turgor normal tension in a cell; the resistance of the skin to deformation.

turgor normal tension in the skin.

turnover the continual synthesis and breakdown of body substances that results in the dynamic steady state or homeostasis.

two-pillow orthopnea the number of pillows—in this case, two—needed to ease the difficulty of breathing while lying down; a significant factor in assessing the level of respiratory distress.

ulna bone on the little finger side of the forearm.

ultrahigh frequency radio frequency band from 300 to 3,000 megahertz.

umbilical cord structure containing two arteries and one vein that connects the placenta and the fetus.

UN number a four-digit identification number specific to a given chemical; some UN numbers are assigned to a group of related chemicals, but with different characteristics, such the UN 1203 designation for diesel fuel, gasohol, gasoline, motor fuels, motor spirits, and petrol. (The letters *UN* stand for "United Nations." Sometimes the letters *NA* for "North America" appear with or instead of the UN designation.)

unified command process in which managers from different jurisdictions—law enforcement, fire, EMS—coordinate their activities and share responsibility for command.

unipolar limb leads electrocardiogram leads applied to the arms and legs, consisting of one polarized (positive) electrode and a nonpolarized reference point that is created by the ECG machine combining two additional electrodes; also called *augmented limb leads*; leads aVR, aVL, and aVF.

unit predetermined amount of medication or fluid.

upper airway obstruction an interference with air movement through the upper airway.

upper gastrointestinal bleeding bleeding within the gastrointestinal tract proximal to the ligament of Treitz.

up-regulation a drug causes the formation of more receptors than normal.

urea waste derived from ammonia produced through protein metabolism.

uremia the syndrome of signs and symptoms associated with chronic renal failure.

ureter a duct that carries urine from kidney to urinary bladder.

urethra the duct that carries urine from the bladder out of the body; in men, it also carries reproductive fluid (semen) to the outside of the body.

urethritis an infection and inflammation of the urethra.

urinary bladder the muscular organ that stores urine before its elimination from the body.

urinary stasis a condition in which the bladder empties incompletely during urination.

urinary system the group of organs that produces urine, maintaining fluid and electrolyte balance for the body.

urinary tract infection (UTI) an infection, usually bacterial, at any site in the urinary tract.

urine the fluid made by the kidney and eliminated from the body.

urology the surgical specialty dealing with the urinary/genitourinary system.

urosepsis septicemia originating from the urinary tract.

urostomy surgical diversion of the urinary tract to a stoma, or hole, in the abdominal wall.

urticaria the raised areas, or wheals, that occur on the skin, associated with vasodilation due to histamine release; commonly called *hives*.

uterus hollow organ in the center of the abdomen that provides the site for fetal development.

vaccine solution containing a modified pathogen that does not actually cause disease but still stimulates the development of antibodies specific to it.

vacutainer device that holds blood tubes.

vagal response stimulation of the vagus nerve causing a parasympathetic response.

vagina canal that connects the external female genitalia to the uterus.

vagus nerve the tenth cranial nerve that monitors and controls the heart, respiration, and much of the abdominal viscera.

vallecula depression between the epiglottis and the base of the tongue.

valsalva maneuver forced exhalation against a closed glottis, such as with coughing. This maneuver stimulates the parasympathetic nervous system via the vagus nerve, which in turn slows the heart rate.

varicella viral disease characterized by a rash of fluid-filled vesicles that rupture, forming small ulcers that eventually scab.

varicose veins dilated superficial veins, usually in the lower extremity. Also called *varicosities*.

vas deferens the duct that carries sperm cells from epididymis to urethra.

vascular phase a step in the clotting process in which smooth blood vessel muscle contracts, reducing the vessel lumen and the flow of blood through it.

vasopresser agent causing contraction of the smooth muscle of the arteries and arterioles, thus increasing resistance to blood flow and elevating blood pressure.

vector a force that has both magnitude and direction. *See also* QRS axis.

vein a blood vessel that carries blood toward the heart.

velocity the rate of motion in a particular direction in relation to time.

venous access device surgically implanted port that permits repeated access to central venous circulation.

venous constricting band flat rubber band used to impede venous return and make veins easier to see.

ventilation the mechanical process of moving air in and out of the lungs.

ventral toward the front or toward the anterior part of the body. *Opposite of* dorsal.

Venturi mask high-flow face mask that uses a venturi system to deliver relatively precise oxygen concentrations.

vertebra one of 33 bones making up the vertebral column.

vertebral body short column of bone that forms the weight-bearing portion of a vertebra.

vertigo the sensation of faintness or dizziness; may cause a loss of balance.

very high frequency radio frequency band from 30 to 300 megahertz.

vesicants agents that damage exposed skin, frequently causing vesicles (blisters).

vial plastic or glass container with a self-healing rubber top.

virulence an organism's strength or ability to infect or overcome the body's defenses.

visceral pain dull, poorly localized pain that originates in the walls of hollow organs.

vital statistics height and weight.

vitreous humor clear watery fluid filling the posterior chamber of the eye. It is responsible for giving the eye its spherical shape.

volatility ease by which a chemical changes from liquid to gas; tendency of a chemical agent to evaporate.

voltage the difference of electric potential between two points with different concentrations of electrons.

volume on hand the available amount solution containing a medication.

volvulus twisting of the intestine on itself.

von Willebrand's disease condition in which the vWF component of factor VIII is deficient.

warm zone location at a hazmat incident adjacent to the hot zone; area where a decontamination corridor is established; also called *yellow zone* or *contamination reduction zone*.

warning placard diamond-shaped graphic placed on vehicles to indicated hazard classification.

washout release of accumulated lactic acid, carbon dioxide (carbonic acid), potassium, and rouleaux into the venous circulation.

weapons of mass destruction (WMD) variety of chemical, biological, or nuclear devices used by terrorists to strike at government or high-profile targets; designed to create a maximum number of casualties.

Wernicke's syndrome condition characterized by loss of memory and disorientation, associated with chronic alcohol intake and a diet deficient in thiamine.

wheezes continuous, high-pitched musical sounds similar to a whistle.

whispered pectoriloquy abnormal clarity of patient's transmitted whispers.

white matter material that surrounds gray matter in the spinal cord; made up largely of axons.

whole bowel irrigation administration of polyethylene glycol continuously at 1–2 L/hr through a nasogastric tube until the effluent is clear or objects are recovered.

window phase time between exposure to a disease and seroconversion.

withdrawal referring to alcohol or drug withdrawal in which the patient's body reacts severely when deprived of the abused substance.

wrap points mechanisms of injury in which an appendage gets caught and significantly twisted.

xiphisternal joint union between xiphoid process and body of the sternum.

yaw swing or wobble around the axis of a projectile's travel.

years of productive life a calculation made by subtracting the age at death from 65.

yellow bone marrow tissue that stores fat in semi-liquid form within the internal cavities of a bone.

Zollinger-Ellison syndrome condition that causes the stomach to secrete excessive amounts of hydrochloric acid and pepsin.

zone of coagulation area in a burn nearest the heat source that suffers the most damage and is characterized by clotted blood and thrombosed blood vessels.

zone of hyperemia area peripheral to a burn that is characterized by increased blood flow.

zone of stasis area in a burn surrounding the zone of coagulation and characterized by decreased blood flow.

zygoma the cheekbone.

Index